Diseases of the Kidney and Urinary Tract

Dedication

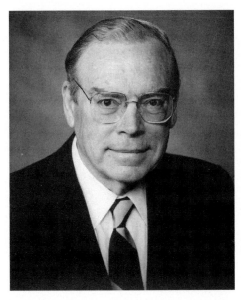

Carl William Gottschalk, MD, was a man for all seasons – brilliant scholar, committed mentor of students, dedicated citizen of the University of North Carolina and the broader academic community, and a gentleman in every sense of the word. Carl was a native Virginian whose southern manners and warm demeanor emanated a personal charm to his friends, colleagues, and students. He graduated Phi Beta Kappa from Roanoke College in 1942 and received an Honorary Doctor of Science from that institution in 1966. An Alpha Omega Alpha graduate from the University of Virginia School of Medicine, Carl Gottschalk then received his training in internal medicine at the Massachusetts General Hospital and his fellowship in Cardiology at the University of North Carolina. For the next forty years (1952–1992), his loyalty and many talents were an integral part of the University of North Carolina, which accounted for the respect and affection which he received from his many colleagues and friends. He was the Kenan Professor of Medicine and Physiology from 1969 until his untimely death on October 15, 1997, in Chapel Hill, North Carolina.

Carl Gottschalk's scientific contributions were recognized by his election to the National Academy of Science. He was President of the American Society of Nephrology from 1976–1977, and was a Councilor of the International Society of Nephrology (ISN). Carl founded the History of Medicine Commission of the ISN and the ISN Archives in Amsterdam, The Netherlands, which are appropriately named the Carl W. Gottschalk Archives of the ISN. Among many honors, awards, and distinguished named lectureships, Carl received the Homer W. Smith Award from the New York Heart Association and the David H. Hume Award from the National Kidney Foundation. The American Physiological Society has established the Carl W. Gottschalk Distinguished Lectureship in Renal Physiology and the University of North Carolina has inaugurated the Carl W. Gottschalk Lectureship in the Basic Sciences.

Scientist, medical historian, lepidopterist who has a butterfly (Strymon cecrops Gottshalki) named after him, recipient of many honors and awards, the written persona of Carl W. Gottschalk can only project a very modest picture of this Renaissance man. His kindness and consideration for others was unparalleled. It was my honor to have worked with him on three editions of Diseases of the Kidney and to dedicate this current edition to his memory.

Robert W. Schrier, MD

Contents

Section III. Hereditary Diseases

Section IV. Urological Diseases of the Genitourinary Tract

Section V. Neoplasms of the Genitourinary Tract

VOLUME II

Section VII. Acute Renal Failure

VOLUME III

Section X. Systemic Diseases of the Kidney

Section XIV. Nutrition, Drugs, and the Kidney

Color Figures for Volume I (Including Chapters 15, 16, and 28) Begin After Page 480.
Color Figures for Volume II (Including Chapters 60 and 65) Begin After Page 1582.
Color Figures for Volume III (Including Chapters 79, 88, 92, and 93) Begin After Page 2624.

Preface

The recent advances in all aspects of our knowledge of the kidney and its diseases mandate a new edition of *Diseases of the Kidney*. As in previous editions, a group of international experts was assembled to present this information in a comprehensive, authoritative, concise, and readily accessible fashion. The chapters have been extensively revised and updated.

Nephrology is a discipline that combines the basic and clinical sciences. Successful integration of this knowledge is the goal of this seventh edition. The fourteen sections of the three volume book are actually individual texts which can stand on their own. Moreover, because a unique feature of the book is a comprehensive inclusion of diseases of the urinary tract as well as the kidney, the seventh edition is named *Diseases of the Kidney and Urinary Tract*.

The first section presents an overall view of the structural, physiologic, and biochemical aspects of the kidney. This section incorporates the latest developments in cellular and molecular biology, emphasizing the most current information and concepts on cell signaling, receptors, and ion channels. For the last three editions the late Carl Gottschalk, MD, edited the nine chapters in the basic science section. I considered it a privilege to have worked with Dr. Gottschalk in editing this authoritative book, which has been totally reorganized from the first four editions. The goal was to publish the most comprehensive material for the practicing physician caring for patients with diseases of the kidney and urinary tract. The fourteen sections of the book covering 104 chapters are as follows:

I **Biochemical, Structural, and Functional Correlations in the Kidney** includes structural, hemodynamic, hormonal, ion transport and metabolic functions in nine chapters.

II **Clinical Evaluation** is covered in six chapters on urinalysis, laboratory evaluation, urography, tomography, angiography, and indications for renal biopsy.

III **Hereditary Diseases** in five chapters covers genetic mechanisms, medullary cystic and sponge disorders, polycystic kidney disease, Alport's syndrome, Fabry's disease, and nail-patella syndrome, as well as isolated renal tubular disorders.

IV **Urological Diseases of the Genitourinary Tract** are described in six chapters, including congenital abnormalities, urinary tract obstruction, renal calculi, reflux nephropathy, prostatic and micturition disorders.

V **Neoplasms of the Genitourinary Tract** are addressed in five chapters covering molecular mechanisms in malignancy, testicular carcinoma, prostate and bladder cancer, and primary neoplasms of the kidney and renal pelvis.

VI **Infections of the Urinary Tract and the Kidney** are contained in seven chapters, including host-defense mechanisms; urinary bacterial infections, including tuberculosis and fungal infections; renal abscesses, and cystitis.

VII **Acute Renal Failure** is described in twelve chapters, including the pathophysiology of cell ischemia and cell injury, acute tubular necrosis, acute interstitial nephritis, and nephrotoxic renal disease.

VIII **Hypertension** and its manifestations in the renal system are covered in seven chapters, which include pathophysiology, renal vascular and endocrine-related hypertension as well as hypertension in pregnancy and in diabetes.

IX **Glomerular, Interstitial, and Vascular Renal Diseases** are discussed in sixteen chapters, including collagen vascular diseases, chronic interstitial nephritis, primary glomerulonephritides and vasculitides.

X **Systemic Diseases of the Kidney** are covered in nine chapters, including diabetes, hepatorenal syndrome, sickle cell disease, gout, myeloma/amyloidosis, and tropical diseases.

XI **Disorders of Electrolyte, Water, and Acid—Base** are covered in eight chapters, including SIADH, central and nephrogenic diabetes insipidus, cardiac failure, cirrhosis and the nephrotic syndrome.

XII **Uremic Syndrome** section of six chapters covers pathophysiology, anemia, osteodystrophy, the nervous system, cardiovascular complications, and metabolic and endocrine dysfunctions.

XIII **Management of End-Stage Renal Disease** by transplantation, peritoneal dialysis and hemodialysis, including complications, outcomes, and ethical considerations is discussed in five chapters.

XIV **Nutrition, Drugs, and the Kidney** are covered in four chapters, including protein and caloric dietary issues as well as drug dosing recommendations in renal failure.

I would like to thank our authoritative and remarkably talented contributing authors, whose dedication to academic nephrology is unmatched.

Robert W. Schrier, MD

Contributing Authors

William T. Abraham, MD
Gill Professor
Department of Preventive Cardiology
Co-director
Gill Heart Institute
Chief
Department of Cardiovascular Medicine
University of Kentucky School of Medicine
Lexington, Kentucky

Gregory A. Achenbach, MD
Chairman
Department of Pathology
Rose Medical Center
Denver, Colorado

Horacio J. Adrogué, MD
Professor
Department of Medicine
Baylor College of Medicine
Chief
Renal Section
Houston Veterans Affairs Medical
    Center
Houston, Texas

Allen C. Alfrey, MD
Professor Emeritus
Department of Medicine
University of Colorado
Consultant
Veterans Administration Hospital
Denver, Colorado

Robert J. Alpern, MD
Dean
Southwestern Medical School
University of Texas Southwestern Medical Center
    at Dallas
Dallas, Texas

Robert J. Anderson, MD
Professor
Department of Medicine

Head
Division of General Internal Medicine
University of Colorado Health Sciences
    Center
Denver, Colorado

Sharon Anderson, MD
Professor of Medicine
Division of Nephrology
Oregon Health Sciences University
Chief
Nephrology Section
Portland Veterans Affairs Medical Center
Portland, Oregon

Thomas E. Andreoli, MD
Nolan Professor and Chairman
Department of Internal Medicine
University of Arkansas College of Medicine
Little Rock, Arkansas

Dennis L. Andress, MD
Professor
Department of Medicine
University of Washington
Staff Nephrologist
Veterans Affairs Puget Sound Health
    Care System
Seattle, Washington

Vincent T. Andriole, MD
Professor of Medicine
Department of Internal Medicine
Yale University School of Medicine
Attending Physician
Yale-New Haven Hospital
New Haven, Connecticut

William P. Arend, MD
Professor
Department of Medicine
University of Colorado Health
    Sciences Center
Denver, Colorado

William J. Arendshorst, MD, PhD
Professor and Interim Chair
Department of Cell and Molecular Physiology
University of North Carolina at Chapel Hill
*   School of Medicine*
Chapel Hill, North Carolina

Allen I. Arieff, MD
Professor
Department of Medicine
University of California School
*   of Medicine*
San Francisco, California

Anthony Atala, MD
Associate Professor
Department of Surgery
Harvard Medical School
Associate in Surgery
Department of Urology
Children's Hospital
Boston, Massachusetts

Curtis L. Atkin, PhD (deceased)
Research Associate Professor
Division of Rheumatology
Departments of Medicine and Biochemistry
University of Utah Medical Center
Salt Lake City, Utah

Robert C. Atkins, MSc, PhD, DSc, FRACP
Professor of Medicine
Department of Medicine
Monash University
Director of Nephrology
Department of Nephrology
Monash Medical Center
Clayton, Australia

Pierre Aucouturier, PhD
Associate
Department of Immunology
Faculty of Medicine, Necker
Poitiers, France

Kamal F. Badr, MD
Professor and Chair
Department of Medicine
American University
Beirut, Lebanon

David S. Baldwin, MD
Professor
Department of Medicine/Nephrology
New York University School of Medicine
Attending Physician
Department of Medicine/Nephrology
Tisch Hospital of New York University
New York, New York

Rashad S. Barsoum, MD, FRCP, FRCPE
Professor and Chairman
Department of Internal Medicine
Cairo University
Chairman
Cairo Kidney Center
Cairo, Egypt

Darren T. Beiko, MD, BSc
Chief Resident
Department of Urology
Kingston General Hospital
*   and Queen's University*
Kingston, ONT, Canada

William M. Bennett, MD
Professor of Medicine (Retired)
Director
Solid Organ and Cellular Transplantation
Transplant Services Department
Legacy Good Samaritan Hospital
Portland, Oregon

Tullio Bertani, MD
Associate Professor
Unit of Nephrology and Dialysis
Ospedali Riuniti di Bergamo
Azienda Ospedaliers
Bergamo, Italy

Anatole Besarab, MD
Professor of Medicine
Section of Nephrology
West Virginia University School of Medicine
Director
Renal Treatment Center
Department of Medicine
West Virginia University Hospital
Morgantown, West Virginia

Daniel G. Bichet, MD
Professor
Department of Medicine
Université de Montréal
Director
Clinical Research Unit
Hôpital du Sacré-Coeur de Montréal
Montreal, Quebec, Canada

Wayne A. Border, MD
Professor
Department of Medicine

University of Utah
Salt Lake City, Utah

George J. Bosl, MD
Professor
Department of Medicine
Weill Medical College
Cornell University
Chairman
Department of Medicine
Memorial Sloan-Kettering Cancer Center
New York, New York

Jean-Louis Bosmans, MD
Department of Nephrology
University Hospital Antwerp
Antwerp, Belgium

Mayer Brezis, MD
Professor
Department of Medicine
Hebrew University
Chief Physician
Department of Medicine
Hadasah University Hospital, Mount Scopus
Jerusalem, Israel

Verena A. Briner, MD
Professor
Department of Medicine
Basel University
Basel, Switzerland
Head
Department of Medicine
Kantonsspital
Lucerne, Switzerland

Keith E. Britton, MD, MSc, FRCR, FRCP
Professor and Consultant Physician
* in Charge*
Nuclear Medicine Department
Queen Mary College
University of London
St. Bartholomew's Hospital
London, United Kingdom

John M. Burkart, MD
Professor of Medicine
Head of Outpatient Dialysis
Department of Nephrology
Wake Forest University Medical Center
Winston-Salem, North Carolina

Melissa A. Cadnapaphornchai, MD
Assistant Professor
Departments of Pediatrics and Medicine

University of Colorado Health Sciences Center
Assistant Professor
Department of Pediatrics
The Kidney Center
The Children's Hospital
Denver, Colorado

John Stewart Cameron, MD, FRCP
Emeritus Professor
Department of Renal Medicine
Renal Unit
United Medical and Dental Schools of Guy's
* and St. Thomas's Hospitals*
London, United Kingdom

Andrés Cárdenas, MD
Liver Unit
Institute for Digestive Diseases
Hospital Clínic
University of Barcelona School of Medicine
Barcelona, Catalunya, Spain

Steven J. Chadban, MD, PhD
Senior Lecturer
Department of Medicine
Monash University
Senior Nephrologist
Department of Nephrology
Monash Medical Center
Clayton, Victoria, Australia

Laurence Chan, MD, PhD, FRCP, FACP
Professor of Medicine
Director, Transplant Nephrology
University of Colorado Health
* Sciences Center*
Denver, Colorado

Silvia D. Chang, MD, FRCPC
Clinical Instructor
Department of Radiology
University of British Columbia
Head
Abdominal MRI
Department of Radiology
Vancouver Hospital and Health
* Sciences Center*
Vancouver, British Columbia, Canada

Cyril Chantler, MD, FRCP
GKT Department of Pediatric Nephrology
Guy's Tower
Guy's Hospital
Vice Principal
King's College
London, United Kingdom

Devasmita Choudhury, MD
Assistant Professor
Department of Medicine
University of Texas Southwestern Medical
Center at Dallas
Director of Dialysis
Dallas Veterans Affairs Medical Center
Dallas, Texas

Godrey Clark, MD
GKT Department of Pediatric Nephrology
Guy's Tower
Guy's Hospital
London, United Kingdom

Anthony R. Clarkson, MD, FRACP, FRCP(Ed)
Associate Professor
Department of Medicine
University of Adelaide
Senior Consultant
Renal Unit
Royal Adelaide Hospital
Adelaide, South Australia, Australia

Carlos Cordon-Cardo, MD, PhD
Division of Molecular Pathology
Department of Pathology
Memorial Sloan-Kettering Cancer
Center
New York, New York

Howard L. Corwin, MD
Professor of Medicine and Anesthesiology
Dartmouth Medical School
Dartmouth-Hitchcock Medical Center
Lebanon, New Hampshire

E. David Crawford, MD
Professor of Surgery
Head
Section of Urologic Oncology
Department of Surgery and Radiation Oncology
University of Colorado Health Sciences Center
Denver, Colorado

Byron P. Croker, MD, PhD
Professor
Department of Pathology, Immunology,
and Laboratory Medicine
University of Florida
Chief
Department of Pathology and Laboratory
Medicine
North Florida/South Georgia Veterans
Health System
Gainesville, Florida

Robert E. Cronin, MD
Professor
Department of Internal Medicine
University of Texas Southwestern
Medical Center
Chief of Staff
Executive Office
Veterans Affairs North Texas Health
Care System
Dallas, Texas

Brian S. Cummings, MD
Postdoctoral Fellow
Department of Pharmacology
and Toxicology
University of Arkansas for Medical Sciences
Little Rock, Arizona

Nancy B. Cummings, MD
Clinical Professor of Medicine
Department of Nephrology
Georgetown University School of Medicine
Washington, D.C.
Senior Biomedical Advisor
National Institute of Diabetes & Digestive &
Kidney Diseases
National Institute of Health
Bethesda, Maryland

Giuseppe D'Amico, MD, FRCP
Professor
Department of Medicine
Postgraduate School of Nephrology
University of Milan
Director
Departments of Nephrology and Urology
San Carlo Hospital
Milan, Italy

Eugene Daphnis, MD
Attending Physician
Department of Nephrology
University of Crete School of Medicine
Attending Physician
Department of Nephrology
University Hospital of Heraklion
Crete, Greece

Scott F. Davies, MD
Professor
Department of Medicine
University of Minnesota
Division Chief
Pulmonary Division
Hennepin County Medical Center
Minneapolis, Minnesota

Marc E. De Broe, MD, PhD
Professor in Medicine
Department of Nephrology
University of Antwerp
Head
Department of Nephrology
University Hospital Antwerp
Antwerp, Belgium

Paul E. de Jong, MD, PhD
Professor and Head
Department of Internal Medicine
Division of Nephrology
University Hospital Groningen
Groningen, The Netherlands

Louise-Marie Dembry, MD
Associate Professor of Medicine and Epidemiology
Department of Internal Medicine/Infectious
*   Diseases*
Yale University School of Medicine
Hospital Epidemiologist
Department of Quality Improvement
*   Support Services*
Yale-New Haven Hospital
New Haven, Connecticut

Hugh E. de Wardener, MD, FRCP
Emeritus Professor of Medicine
Department of Clinical Chemistry
Imperial College School of Medicine
Charing Cross Campus
London, United Kingdom

Giovanni Barbiano di Belgiojoso, MD
Professor
Department of Kidney Diseases
University of Milan
Chief
Nephrology Unit
Luigi Sacco Hospital
Milan, Italy

Susan R. DiGiovanni, MD
Assistant Professor of Medicine
Department of Medicine
Division of Nephrology
Virginia Commonwealth University
Richmond, Virginia

Burl R. Don, MD
Associate Professor
Department of Medicine
Director
Department of Clinical Nephrology
Division of Nephrology
University of California Davis Medical Center
Sacramento, California

Michael S. Donnenberg, MD
Professor
Department of Medicine
University of Maryland, Baltimore
Head
Division of Infectious Diseases
Department of Medicine
University of Maryland Medical System
Baltimore, Maryland

Harry A. Drabkin, MD
Professor of Medicine
Department of Medicine/Medical Oncology
University of Colorado Health Sciences Center
Denver, Colorado

Michael J. Dunn, MD
Dean and Executive Vice President
Office of the Dean
Medical College of Wisconsin
Milwaukee, Wisconsin

Tevfik Ecder, MD
Associate Professor
Department of Medicine
University of Istanbul
Istanbul, Turkey

Charles L. Edelstein, MD, PhD
Associate Professor
Department of Renal Diseases
*   and Hypertension*
University of Colorado Health Sciences Center
University Hospital
Denver, Colorado

Garabed Eknoyan, MD
Professor
Department of Medicine
Baylor College of Medicine
Houston, Texas

David H. Ellison, MD
Chief
Division of Nephrology and Hypertension
Oregon Health and Science University
Portland, Oregon

Bryan T. Emmerson, AO, MD, PhD, FRACP
Professor Emeritus and Honorary Research
Consultant
Department of Medicine
University of Queensland

Princess Alexandra Hospital
Brisbane QLD, Australia

Raymond Estacio, MD
Associate Professor
Department of Medicine
University of Colorado Health Sciences Center
Denver, Colorado
General Internist
Department of Community Health
Denver Health Medical Center
Denver, Colorado

Ronald J. Falk, MD
Professor of Medicine
Department of Nephrology and Hypertension
University of North Carolina
Chapel Hill North Carolina

Randall J. Faull, MD
Senior Lecturer
Department of Medicine
Adelaide University
Consultant Nephrologist
Department of Renal Medicine
Royal Adelaide Hospital
Adelaide, South Australia

Franco Ferrario, MD
Head
Renal Immunopathology Center
Department of Nephro-Urology
Azienda Ospedaliera "Ospedale San Carlo"
Milan, Italy

Godela M. Fick-Brosnahan, MD
Assistant Professor
Department of Medicine
University of Colorado Health Sciences Center
Denver, Colorado

Paola Fioretto, MD
Assistant Professor of Endocrinology
Department of Internal Medicine
University of Padova
Padova, Italy

Cosmo L. Fraser, MD
Department of Medicine
University of California School of Medicine
San Francisco, California

Eli A. Friedman, MD
Distinguished Teaching Professor
Chief
Division of Renal Disease

Department of Medicine
SUNY, Health Science Center at Brooklyn
University Hospital of Brooklyn
Brooklyn, New York

Jørgen Frøkiaer, MD, PhD
Associate Professor
Institute of Experimental Clinical Research
University of Aarhus
Research Consultant
Department of Clinical Physiology
Aarhus University Hospital
Aarhus N, Denmark

Gloria R. Gallo, MD
Adjunct Professor
Department of Pathology
New York University School of Medicine
Department of Pathology
Tisch Hospital-New York University
 Medical Center
New York, New York

Robert M. Gemmill, PhD
Associate Professor
Department of Medicine/Medical Oncology
University of Colorado Health Sciences Center
Denver, Colorado

Christopher M. George, MD
Department of Medicine
Section of Hematology/Oncology
University of Chicago
Chicago, Illinois

Gregory G. Germino, MD
Associate Professor
Department of Internal Medicine
Division of Nephrology
Johns Hopkins University School of Medicine
Baltimore, Maryland

Pere Ginès, M.D.
Consultant in Hepatology
Associate Professor of Medicine
Liver Unit
Institute for Digestive Diseases
Hospital Clinic
University of Barcelona School of Medicine
Barcelona, Catalunya, Spain

Martin E. Gleave, MD, FACS, FRCSC
Professor
Department of Surgery
Division of Urology
University of British Columbia

Director
Department of Clinical Research
The Prostate Centre
Vancouver, British Columbia, Canada

L. Michael Glode, MD
Professor
Department of Medicine/Medical Oncology
University of Colorado Health Sciences Center
Denver, Colorado

Thomas A. Golper, MD
Professor
Department of Medicine
Division of Nephrology and Hypertension
Vanderbilt University Medical Center
Nashville, Tennessee

Martin C. Gregory, BM, BCh, DPhil
Adjunct Professor
Department of Medicine
University of Utah Health Sciences Center
Salt Lake City, Utah
Director of Nephrology
Department of Medicine
King Edward VII Memorial Hospital
Hamilton, Bermuda

Jean-Pierre Grünfeld, MD
Professor
Université Paris V-René Descartes
Chief
Department of Nephrology
Hospital Necker
Paris, France

Steven C. Hebert, MD
Professor and Chairman
Cellular and Molecular Biology
Professor of Medicine
Yale University School of Medicine
New Haven, Connecticut

William L. Henrich, MD
Professor
Department of Medicine
University of Maryland School of Medicine
Chairman
Department of Medicine
University of Maryland Medical Center
Baltimore, Maryland

Friedhelm Hildebrandt, MD
Professor
Department of Pediatrics
University Children's Hospital

Freiburg University
Freiburg, Germany

Thomas Heard Hostetter, MD
Department of Medicine Medical School
Division of Renal Diseases and Hypertension
University of Minnesota
Minneapolis, Minnesota

Luzma M. Houseal, MD
Department of Internal Medicine
Texas Tech University Health Sciences Center
Lubbock, Texas

Hedvig Hricak, MD, PhD
Professor and Chair
Department of Radiology
Memorial Sloan-Kettering Cancer Center
New York, New York

Keith A. Hruska, MD
Professor of Medicine and Associate Professor
    of Cell Biology
Department of Internal Medicine
Washington University School of Medicine
St. Louis, Missouri

Michael H. Humphreys, MD
Professor
Department of Medicine
University of California, San Francisco
    School of Medicine
Chief
Division of Nephrology
San Francisco General Hospital
San Francisco, California

Robert W. Janson, MD
Associate Professor
Department of Medicine
University of Colorado Heath Sciences Center
Chief
Rheumatology Section
Denver Veterans Affairs Medical Center
Denver, Colorado

J. Charles Jennette, MD
Brinkhous Distinguished Professor and Chair
Department of Pathology and Laboratory
Medicine
University of North Carolina
Chapel Hill, North Carolina

Paul Jungers, MD
Professor
Faculty of Medicine, Necker

University of René Descartes
Department of Nephrology
Hôpital Necker
Paris, France

George J. Kaloyanides, MD
Professor
Department of Medicine
Division of Nephrology and Hypertension
State University of New York at Stony Brook
School of Medicine
Health Sciences Center
Stony Brook, New York

Igal Kam, MD
Professor of Surgery
Chief, Transplant Surgery
University of Colorado School of Medicine
Denver, Colorado

Adrian I. Katz, MD
Professor
Department of Medicine
University of Chicago
Attending Physician
Department of Medicine
University of Chicago Medical Center
Chicago, Illinois

Peter G. Kerr, PhD, FRACP
Honorary Clinical Associate Professor
Department of Medicine
Monash University
Deputy Director
Department of Nephrology
Monash Medical Centre
Clayton, Victoria, Australia

Melanie S. Kim, MD
Associate Professor
Department of Pediatrics
Boston University School of Medicine
Associate Program Director
Department of Pediatrics
Boston Medical Center
Boston, Massachusetts

Paul L. Kimmel, MD
Professor
Department of Medicine
George Washington University Medical Center
Director, HIV Program
Division of Kidney, Urologic and
*   Hemtaologic Diseases*
National Institute of Diabetes, Digestive
*   and Kidney Diseases*

National Institutes of Health
Bethesda, Maryland
Attending Physician
Department of Medicine
George Washington University Hospital
Washington, DC

Saulo Klahr, MD
Simon Professor of Medicine
Department of Internal Medicine
Washington University School of Medicine
Director
Department of Research and Scientific Affairs
Barnes-Jewish Hospital
St. Louis, Missouri

Mark A. Knepper, MD, PhD
Chief
Renal Mechanisms Section
National Heart, Lung, Blood Institute
National Institutes of Health
Bethesda, Maryland

Sidney M. Kobrin, MD
Associate Professor
Department of Medicine
Director of Inpatient Dialysis
Renal Electrolyte Division
University of Pennsylvania
Philadelphia, Pennsylvania

Kenneth E. Kokko, MD
The Center for Cell and Molecular Signaling
*   and Renal Division*
Emory University School of Medicine
Departments of Physiology and Medicine
Veterans Affairs Medical Center
Atlanta, Georgia

Radko Komers, MD, PhD
Assistant Professor
Division of Nephrology and Hypertension
Oregon Health Science University
Portland, Oregon

Joel D. Kopple, MD
Professor
Departments of Medicine and Public Health
University of California Los Angeles
UCLA Schools of Medicine and Public Health
Los Angeles, California
Chief
Division of Nephrology and Hypertension
Department of Medicine
Harbor-UCLA Medical Center
Torrance, California

Brian L. Kotzin, MD
Professor
Departments of Medicine and Immunology
Co-Head
Division of Clinical Allergy and Immunology
University of Colorado Health Sciences Center
Denver, Colorado

Wilhelm Kriz, MD
Professor
Institute of Anatomy and Cell Biology
University of Heidelberg
Heidelberg, Germany

Tae-Hwan Kwon, MD
Assistant Professor
Department of Physiology
Dongauk University School of Medicine
Kyungju, South Korea

Richard A. Lafayette, MD
Assistant Professor
Department of Medicine
Associate Chief
Department of Nephrology
Stanford University Hospital
Stanford, California

Fadi G. Lakkis, MD
Assistant Professor
Department of Medicine
Emory University School of Medicine
Staff Physician
Renal Division
Emory University Hospital and Veterans Affairs
Medical Center
Atlanta, Georgia

Lucia R. Languino, PhD
Associate Professor
Department of Pathology
Yale University School of Medicine
New Haven, Connecticut

Andrew S. Levey, MD
Chief
Division of Nephrology
New England Medical Center
Professor
Department of Medicine
Tufts University
Boston, Massachusetts

Moshe Levi, MD
Professor
Department of Medicine
University of Texas Southwestern Medical Center
* at Dallas*
Chief
Nephrology Section
Dallas Veterans Administration Medical
* Center*
Dallas, Texas

Marshall D. Lindheimer, MD
Professor Emeritus
Departments of Obstetrics and Gynecology
University of Chicago Hospital
Chicago, Illinois

Francisco Llach, MD
Professor of Medicine
Department of Medicine
Georgetown University Medical Center
Director Clinical Nephrology
Department of Nephrology
Georgetown University Medical Center
Washington, DC

Graham A. MacGregor, FRCP
Professor of Cardiovascular Medicine
Blood Pressure Unit
St. George's Hospital Medical School
London, United Kingdom

Michael P. Madaio, MD
Professor
Department of Medicine
University of Pennsylvania
Philadelphia, Pennsylvania

Thomas M. J. Maling, MD, FRACR
Clinical Lecturer
Department of Radiology
Christchurch School of Medicine
Radiologist
Christchurch Hospital
Christchurch, New Zealand

Netar P. Mallick, MB, ChB, FRCP
Professor
Department of Renal Medicine
University of Manchester
Clinical Director and Consultant Physician
Department of Renal Medicine
Central M/CR Healthcare National Health
* Service Trust*
Manchester, United Kingdom

Shaul G. Massry, MD
Professor of Medicine
Department of Nephrology

University of Southern California
Los Angeles, California

Michael Mauer, MD
Professor
Department of Pediatrics
University of Minnesota
Minneapolis, Minnesota

Timothy W. Meyer, MD
Associate Professor
Department of Medicine
Stanford University School of Medicine
Stanford, California
Chief
Nephrology Section
Palo Alto VA Medical Center
Palo Alto, California

Dennis J. Mikolich, MD
Clinical Associate Professor
Department of Medicine
Brown University Medical School
Chief
Department of Infectious Diseases
Veterans Administration Medical Center
Providence, Rhode Island

Anne Marie Miles, MD
State University of New York Health Science
Center at Brooklyn
Division of Renal Disease
University Hospital of Brooklyn
Brooklyn, New York

William E. Mitch, MD
E. Garland Herndon Professor
Department of Medicine
Director
Renal Division
Emory University School of Medicine
Atlanta, Georgia

Harry L. T. Mobley, PhD
Professor
Department of Microbiology and Immunology
University of Maryland School
of Medicine
Baltimore, Maryland

Angel Montero, PhD
Assistant Professor
Department of Medicine
Emory University Renal Division and Veterans
Affairs Medical Center
Atlanta, Georgia

Jack Moore, Jr., MD
Associate Professor of Medicine
Department of Nephrology
Uniformed Services University of the
Health Sciences
Bethesda, Maryland
Director
Section of Nephrology
Department of Medicine
Washington Hospital Center
Washington, DC

Christopher S. Morris, MD
Assistant Professor
Department of Radiology
University of Vermont College
of Medicine
Attending Radiologist
Radiology Health Care Service
Fletcher Allen Health Care
Burlington, Vermont

Robert J. Motzer, MD
Associate Attending Physician
Department of Medicine
Joan and Sanford I Weill Medical College
Cornell University
New York, New York

Béatrice Mougenot, MD
Pathologist
Médecin des Hôpitaux
Department de Pathologie
Hôpital Tenon
Paris, France

Sean W. Murphy, MD, BSc, FRCP(C)
Assistant Professor
Department of Medicine
Memorial University of Newfoundland
Department of Medicine
Health Science Center
St. John's, Newfoundland, Canada

Patrick H. Nachman, MD
Assistant Professor
Department of Medicine
Division of Nephrology and Hypertension
University of North Carolina
Chapel Hill, North Carolina

L. Gabriel Navar, PhD
Professor and Chairman
Department of Physiology
Tulane University Health Sciences Center
New Orleans, Louisiana

Joel Neugarten, MD, JD
Professor
Department of Medicine
Albert Einstein College of Medicine
    of Yeshiva University
Site Director
Nephrology Division
Montefiore Medical Center
Renal Lab
Bronx, New York

J. Curtis Nickel, MD
Professor
Department of Urology
Queen's University
Kingston General Hospital
Kingston, Ontario, Canada

Lindsay E. Nicollé, MD, FRCPC
Professor and Head
Department of Internal Medicine
University of Manitoba
Head
Department of Medicine
Heath Science Centre and St. Boniface
    General Hospital
Winnipeg, Manitoba, Canada

Søren Nielsen, MD, PhD
Professor of Cell Biology
    and Pathophysiology
Department of Cell Biology
Institute of Anatomy
University of Aarhus
Aarhus C, Denmark

Nancy A. Noble, PhD
Research Professor
Department of Internal Medicine
University of Utah
Salt Lake City, Utah

Charles R. Nolan, MD
Associate Professor
Department of Medicine
Medical Director of Renal
    Transplantation
Department of Medicine/Surgery
University of Texas Health Sciences Center
    at San Antonio
San Antonio, Texas

Mark D. Okusa, MD
Associate Professor
Department of Nephrology
University of Virginia School of Medicine

Health Sciences Center
Charlottesville, Virginia

Biff F. Palmer, MD
Professor
Department of Internal Medicine
Clinical Director of Clinical Nephrology
Department of Internal Medicine
University of Texas Southwestern Medical Center
Dallas, Texas

Patrick S. Parfrey, MD
University Research Professor
Department of Medicine
Memorial University of Newfoundland
Department of Medicine
Health Sciences Center
St. John's, Newfoundland, Canada

Chirag Parikh, MD
Senior Fellow
Department of Renal Diseases and Hypertension
University of Colorado Heath Sciences Center
Denver, Colorado

Mark S. Pasternack, MD
Associate Professor
Department of Pediatrics
Harvard Medical School
Chief
Department of Pediatric Infectious Disease
Massachusetts General Hospital
Boston, Massachusetts

Mark A. Perazella, MD, FACP
Associate Professor
Department of Medicine
Yale University
Director
Acute Dialysis
Department of Nephrology
Yale-New Haven Hospital
New Haven, Connecticut

Ronald D. Perrone, MD
Professor
Department of Medicine
Tufts University
Associate Chief
Department of Nephorology
New England Medical Center
Boston, Massachusetts

Beth Piraino, MD
Professor
Department of Medicine

University of Pittsburgh School
of Medicine
Director
Peritoneal Dialysis Program
University of Pittsburgh Medical Center
Pittsburgh, Pennsylvania

Marc A. Pohl, MD
Ray W. Gifford Chair
Head, Section of Clinical Hypertension
and Nephrology
The Cleveland Clinic Foundation
Cleveland, Ohio

Patricia A. Preisig, PhD
Professor
Department of Internal Medicine
University of Texas Southwestern
Medical School
Dallas, Texas

Mahboob Rahman, MD, MS
Assistant Professor
Department of Medicine
Case Western Reserve University School
of Medicine
Department of Medicine
University Hospitals of Cleveland
Cleveland, Ohio

Asghar Rastegar, MD
Professor of Medicine
Associate Chair for Academic Affairs
Co-Chief
Nephrology Section
Department of Internal Medicine
Yale University School of Medicine
Departments of Internal Medicine
and Nephrology
Yale-New Haven Hospital
New Haven, Connecticut

W. Brian Reeves, MD
Professor
Department of Medicine
Penn State College of Medicine
Chief
Department of Nephrology
Hershey Medical Center
Hershey, Pennsylvania

Robert F. Reilly, Jr., MD
Associate Professor
Department of Medicine
Yale University Medical School
New Haven, Connecticut

Giuseppe Remuzzi, MD
Research Director
Negri Bergamo Laboratories
Head
Unit of Nephrology and Dialysis
Ospedali Riuniti di Bergamo
Azienda Ospedaliera
Bergamo, Italy

Claudio Rigatto, MD, FRCPC
Assistant Professor
Department of Medicine
University of Manitoba
Research Director
Department of Nephrology
St. Boniface General Hospital
Winnipeg, Manitoba, Canada

Jeffrey M. Rimmer, MD
Professor
Department of Medicine
University of Vermont College
of Medicine
Medical Director
Dialysis Department
Fletcher Allen Healthcare
Burlington, Vermont

Christophe Robino, MD
Service de Medecine Interne
Hôpital Broussais
Paris, France

Alan M. Robson, MD
Professor
Department of Pediatrics
Louisiana State University School of Medicine,
New Orleans
Tulane University School of Medicine
Medical Director
Children's Hospital of New Orleans
New Orleans, Louisiana

Françoise Roch-Ramel, MD
Professor
Institute of Pharmacology
and Toxicology
University of Lausanne
Lausanne, Switzerland

Rudolph A. Rodriguez, MD
Assistant Clinical Professor of Medicine
Medical Director
Renal Center
University of California, San Francisco
San Francisco, California

Allan R. Ronald, MD, FRCP
Professor
Departments of Internal Medicine and Medical
Microbiology
Section of Infectious Diseases
University of Manitoba Faculty of Medicine
Winnipeg, Manitoba, Canada

Pierre M. Ronco, MD, PhD
Professor of Renal Medicine
Medical Faculty Saint-Antoine
University Pierre et Marie Curie
Head
Department of Nephrology
Tenon Hôpital
Paris, France

Robert H. Rubin, MD
Gordon and Marjorie Osborne Professor of Health
*   Sciences and Technology*
Professor of Medicine
Harvard-MIT Division of Health Sciences
*   and Technology*
Harvard Medical School
Chief of Surgical and Transplant Infectious
*   Disease*
Department of Medicine
Massachusetts General Hospital
Boston, Massachusetts

Piero Ruggenenti, MD
Negri Bergamo Laboratories
Associate Professor
Unit of Nephrology and Dialysis
Ospedali Riuniti di Bergamo
Azienda Ospedaliera
Bergamo, Italy

Sandra Sabatini, PhD, MD, FACP
Professor
Departments of Internal Medicine
*   and Physiology*
The Combined Program in Nephrology and
*   Renal Physiology*
Texas Tech University School of Medicine
Attending Physician
Departments of Nephrology and
*   Internal Medicine*
University Medical Center
Lubbock, Texas

Robert L. Safirstein, MD
Professor and Vice Chair
Department of Medicine
University of Arkansas for Medical Sciences
Chief

Medical Services
Department of Medicine
Central Arkansas Veterans Healthcare System
Little Rock, Arkansas

George A. Sarosi, MD
Professor
Department of Medicine
Indiana University School of Medicine
Chief
Medical Service
Department of Medicine
Roudebush VA Medical Center
Indianapolis, Indiana

Howard I. Scher, MD
Chief
Genitourinary Oncology Service
Memorial Sloan-Kettering Cancer Center
New York, New York

Arrigo Schieppati, MD
Negri Bergamo Laboratories
Associate Professor
Unit of Nephrology and Dialysis
Ospedali Riuniti di Bergamo
Azienda Ospedaliera
Bergamo, Italy

Laurent Schild, MD
Professor
Institute of Pharmacology and Toxicology
Medical School, University of Lausanne
Lausanne, Switzerland

H. William Schnaper, MD
Professor
Department of Pediatrics
Northwestern University Medical School
Department of Pediatric Medicine
Children's Memorial Hospital
Chicago, Illinois

Rick G. Schnellmann, PhD
Professor
Department of Pharmacology and Toxicology
University of Arkansas for Medical Sciences
Little Rock, Arkansas

Anton C. Schoolwerth, MD, MSHA
Professor
Department of Internal Medicine
Virginia Commonwealth University
Chairman
Department of Internal Medicine
Division of Nephrology

Medical College of Virginia
Richmond, Virginia

Robert W. Schrier, MD
Professor and Chairman
Department of Medicine
University of Colorado Health Sciences Center
Denver, Colorado

Donald J. Sherrard, MD
Professor
Department of Medicine
University of Washington
Chief of Nephrology
Department of Medicine
VA Medical Center
Seattle, Washington

Colin D. Short, MD
Department of Renal Medicine
Manchester Royal Infirmary
Manchester, United Kingdom

Visith Sitprija, MD, PhD
Emeritus Professor
Department of Medicine
Chulalongkorn University
Director
Department of Medicine
Queen Saovabha Memorial Institute
Bangkok, Thailand

Eduardo Slatopolsky, MD
Professor of Medicine
Department of Medicine, Renal Division
Washington University School of Medicine
Physician
Department of Medicine
Renal Division
Barnes Hospital
St. Louis, Missouri

Michael C. Smith, MD
Professor
Department of Medicine
Case Western Reserve University School
  of Medicine
Physician
Department of Medicine
Division of Nephrology
University Hospitals of Cleveland
Cleveland, Ohio

Miroslaw J. Smogorzewski, MD, PhD
Associate Professor
Department of Medicine

Division of Nephrology
Keck School of Medicine
University of Southern California
Attending Physician
Department of Medicine
University of Southern California Hospital
Los Angeles, California

Walter M. Stadler, MD
Associate Professor
Department of Medicine
University of Chicago
Chicago, Illinois

Walter E. Stamm, MD
Professor
Department of Medicine
University of Washington School of Medicine
Head
Department of Allergy and Infectious Diseases
University Hospital Medical Center
Seattle, Washington

Lodewijk W. Statius van Eps, MD
Emeritus Professor of Geographic Pathology
Department of History of Medicine
Free University of Amersterdam
Consultant
Departments of Internal Medicine, Nephrology,
  and Tropical Diseases
Slotervaart Hospital
Amsterdam, The Netherlands

Gunnar Steineck, MD
Associate Professor
Department of Oncology and Pathology
Karolinska Institute
Radiumhemmet, Karolinska Hospital
Department of Clinical Cancer Epidemiology
Stockholm City Council
Stockholm, Sweden

Terry B. Strom, MD
Professor
Department of Medicine
Division of Nephrology
Harvard Medical School
Director
Departments of Immunology and Medicine
Beth Israel Hospital
Boston, Massachusetts

Manikkam Suthanthiran, MD
Stanton Griffs Distinguished Professor of Medicine
Department of Transplantation Medicine
  and Extracorporeal Therapy

Division of Nephrology
Weill Medical College
Cornell University
Chief
Departments of Nephrology and Transplantation
    Medicine
New York Presbyterian Hospital
New York, New York

Charles P. Swainson, MD, FRCP
Senior Lecturer
Department of Clinical and Surgical Sciences
University of Edinburgh
Consultant Nephrologist
Department of Renal Medicine
Royal Infirmary
Edinburgh, Scotland

Suzanne K. Swan, MD, FACP
Associate Professor
Department of Medicine
University of Minnesota
Department of Nephrology
Hennepin County Medical Center
Minneapolis, Minnesota

Isaac Teitelbaum, MD
Associate Professor
Department of Medicine
University of Colorado School of Medicine
Medical Director
Dialysis Services
University of Colorado Hospital
Denver, Colorado

C. Craig Tisher, MD
Professor
Departments of Medicine and Pathology
University of Florida College of Medicine
Department of Medicine
Division of Nephrology
Shands Hospital and Clinics, Inc
Gainesville, Florida

Vicente E. Torres, MD
Professor of Medicine
Departments of Nephrology and Internal
    Medicine
Mayo Clinic
Rochester, Minnesota

Heino E. Velázquez, PhD
Research Scientist
Department of Medicine
Yale University School of Medicine
New Haven, Connecticut

Joseph G. Verbalis, MD
Professor
Departments of Medicine and Physiology
Georgetown University School of Medicine
Georgetown University Medical Center
Washington, DC

Nicholas J. Vogelzang, MD
Fred C. Buffett Professor
Departments of Medicine and Surgery
University of Chicago
Director
University of Chicago Cancer Research Center
Chicago, Illinois

Wei Wang, MD
Assistant Professor of Medicine
University of Colorado Health Sciences
    Center
Denver, Colorado

John W. Warren, MD
Professor
Department of Medicine
University of Maryland School of Medicine
Baltimore, Maryland

Terry Watnick, MD
Department of Internal Medicine
Division of Nephrology
Johns Hopkins University School of Medicine
Baltimore, Maryland

Judith A. W. Webb, MD
Consultant Radiologist
Diagnostic Radiology Department
St. Bartholomew's Hospital
West Smithfield, London, United Kingdom

Richard P. Wedeen, MD
Professor
Departments of Medicine, Preventive Medicine,
    and Community Health
UMDNJ-New Jersey Medical School
Newark, New Jersey
Associate Chief of Staff for Research
    and Development
Department of Veterans Affairs
New Jersey Health Care System
East Orange, New Jersey

Myron H. Weinberger, MD
Professor
Department of Medicine
Indiana University School of Medicine
Indianapolis, Indiana

Sterling G. West, MD
Professor
Department of Medicine
University of Colorado Health Sciences
    Center
Denver, Colorado

Andrew J. Woodroffe, MD, FRACP
Director
Renal Unit
Fremantle Hospital
Fremantle, Western Australia

Yalem Woredekalz, MD
Assistant Professor
Department of Medicine
State University of New York
Health Science Center at Brooklyn
Brooklyn, New York

Fred S. Wright, MD
Professor
Cellular and Molecular Physiology
    and Physiology
Yale University
New Haven, Connecticut
Associate Chief of Staff
Department of Research

VA Connecticut Healthcare System
West Haven, Connecticut

Michael Yudd, MD
Assistant Professor of Medicine
University of Medicine and Dentistry
    of New Jersey
Newark, New Jersey
Medical Director Dialysis Unit
Nephrology Section
Department of Veterans Affairs New Jersey
    Health Care System
East Orange, New Jersey

Dirk-Henrik Zermann, MD
Department of Urology
University Hospital
Friedrich Schiller University
Jena, Germany

Stephen H. Zinner, MD
Charles S. Davidson Professor of Medicine
Department of Medicine
Harvard Medical School
Chair
Department of Medicine
Mount Auburn Hospital
Cambridge, Massachusetts

SECTION X

Systemic Diseases of the Kidney

CHAPTER 73

Diabetic Nephropathy

Michael Mauer, Paola Fioretto, Yalem Woredekal, and Eli A. Friedman

DEFINING THE EXTENT OF THE PROBLEM

After the widespread development of end-stage renal disease (ESRD) programs in the late 1960s, the number of diabetic patients accepted for ESRD treatment has been steadily increasing, especially since the early 1980s (1) (Fig. 73-1). Although a study from Sweden suggested a recent marked decline in the incidence of diabetic nephropathy in type 1 (insulin-dependent) diabetic patients (2), this is not the general experience (see later), and may have resulted from strategies of strict glycemic control among this unusual Swedish study cohort (2). There is now evidence to suggest that diabetic nephropathy is the most important single disorder leading to renal failure in adults. In the United States, more than 44% of patients entering renal support programs are diabetic (1) (Fig. 73-2), and the annual cost of caring for these patients exceeds $5 billion in the United States alone (1). This is not surprising because diabetic nephropathy will develop in approximately 25% to 35% of type 1 diabetic patients (3–6) and approximately 8% to 10% of type 2 diabetic patients (7). The prevalence of insulin-dependent diabetes in the Western countries differs: Approximately 0.5% of the population in the United States and central Europe have type 1 diabetes; the percentage is higher in the northern Scandinavian countries and lower in southern Europe as well as in Japan. The incidence of type 2 diabetes is rising rapidly throughout the Western world, and at least 80% of diabetic patients with ESRD have type 2 diabetes (8). Once long-term metabolic aberrations have resulted in overt nephropathy, prevailing therapeutic modalities are clearly insufficient. Thus, ESRD can be postponed, but not prevented, by effective antihypertensive treatment (9–11) and by careful attention to glycemic control (see later). Thus, during the last few years, much research has concentrated on early detection of minor changes in renal

M. Mauer: Department of Pediatrics, University of Minnesota, Minneapolis, Minnesota

P. Fioretto: Department of Medical and Surgical Sciences, University of Padova, Padova, Italy

Y. Woredekal and E. A. Friedman: Department of Medicine, State University of New York, Health Science Center at Brooklyn, Brooklyn, New York

function and structure that may be relevant to predicting further development of disease, to discerning pathophysiologic mechanisms, and to earlier institution of treatment (12–18).

It now is possible to predict the later development of overt diabetic nephropathy relatively early in the course of both type 1 and type 2 (non–insulin-dependent) diabetes, thus giving rise to the concept of patients at "high risk" for diabetic nephropathy, or "incipient nephropathy" (19). An early increase in urinary protein excretion, especially albumin (i.e., microalbuminuria), has emerged as an important clinical parameter. A general outline of changes in renal function and structure is shown in Fig. 73-3. Definitions of the stages of renal involvement are given in Table 73-1.

Only a small portion of patients who have escaped nephropathy despite having diabetes for 20 to 25 years seems to contract clinically important nephropathy later (4). The reason for this diversity of risk is not clear. Familial or genetic factors seem to be very important (20,21), but glycemic control (3,22–24) and blood pressure (BP) levels also may be critical variables (25,26).

DIAGNOSIS OF DIABETIC NEPHROPATHY

The diagnosis of diabetic nephropathy usually is based on clinical evidence. If a young patient with type 1 diabetes for more than a decade shows overt urinary protein loss exceeding 0.5 g/24 hours, the probability of diabetic nephropathy on renal biopsy is very high. In the typical course, the development of proteinuria is slow; at first it is intermittent, but thereafter it becomes permanent and increasing. The onset of overt proteinuria often is associated with hypertension and declining glomerular filtration rate (GFR). If diabetic retinopathy also is present and other causes of clinical proteinuria can be excluded, there may be no need for a renal biopsy because our studies indicate that approximately 95% of type 1 diabetic patients with these criteria have diabetic nephropathy. In fact, in proteinuric patients with type 1 diabetes of more than 10 years' duration, diabetic nephropathy is highly likely even in the absence of significant diabetic retinopathy.

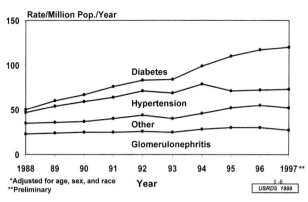

FIG. 73-1. End-stage renal disease (ESRD) incidence rates by primary diagnosis from 1997 to 1998, showing that diabetes is the major contributor to the increasing incidence of ESRD over the past decade. [From the United States Renal Data System (USRD) Report for 1999.]

Biopsy, however, clearly is indicated in an atypical course (e.g., if the protein loss and decline in renal function are rapidly progressive, if the onset of clinical renal disease is within the first 10 years of type 1 diabetes, or if the history or laboratory findings support a different disease process). However, in type 2 diabetes, especially in patients without retinopathy, the incidence of other renal diseases or atypical renal lesions may exceed 25% and renal biopsy may be a more important diagnostic tool (27). Renal biopsy, on the other hand, is an important research tool (13,28) and can be useful in the clinical evaluation of patients (29,30).

The development of overt (dipstick-positive) proteinuria, however, is a late event in the process, whereas changes in structure and more subtle changes in function occur much earlier in the course of diabetic kidney disease. In fact, abnormalities already are present at the time type 1 diabetes is diagnosed. Renal hypertrophy and glomerular hyperfiltration, and sometimes microalbuminuria, are characteristic early features (31). These early abnormalities appear related to the severity of the diabetic metabolic disturbances and improve with the establishment of good glycemic control, whereas with longer diabetes duration, reversal with good glycemic control is much more difficult to achieve.

RENAL DISEASE IN TYPE 2 DIABETES

Both type 1 and type 2 diabetic patients are at risk for development of nephropathy. However, ESRD is less common in type 2 diabetic patients (7,32,33), in part because type 2 diabetic patients with signs of renal dysfunction (e.g., microalbuminuria) have a very high cardiovascular mortality rate before ESRD can manifest (33–37). Nonetheless, because the prevalence of type 2 is much greater than that of type 1 diabetes, the total contribution of type 2 diabetes to ESRD far exceeds that of type 1 diabetes. The renal disease often is more dramatic and rapidly progressive in young patients with type 1 diabetes than in patients with type 2 diabetes. However, the clinical picture after the onset of overt diabetic nephropathy in the two types of patients probably is not very different (38). It can be speculated that severity of diabetes, age, and renal hemodynamic alterations may considerably modify the earlier course, resulting in higher risks and more rapid progression of the preclinical phase in the type 1 diabetic patient. Studies in Pima Indians, however, suggest that rapid progression also can be typical of patients with type 2 diabetes. Further, racial factors may play a role here. The incidence of ESRD is more than four times higher in black than in white type 2 diabetic patients (39). Although no significant excess incidence was seen among black type 2 diabetic patients in this study (39), other studies suggested that racial or ethnic background also may be an independent risk factor in type 1 diabetes (see later).

Differentiation between patients with type 1 and type 2 disease may be difficult (40,41). Problems may emerge in middle-aged and elderly patients who appear to need insulin treatment for proper metabolic control. Type 1 diabetes usually can be documented by the measurement of C-peptide at diagnosis, possibly after stimulation with glucagon, and by the presence of islet cell or glutamic acid decarboxylase antibodies (42). Some obese patients need insulin treatment for metabolic control, although they are not insulin dependent in the sense that they would not survive without insulin, and still have residual C-peptide production.

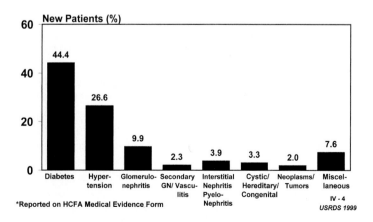

FIG. 73-2. Relative incidence of end-stage renal disease (ESRD) by primary diagnosis in 1997. [From the United States Renal Data System (USRDS) Report for 1999.]

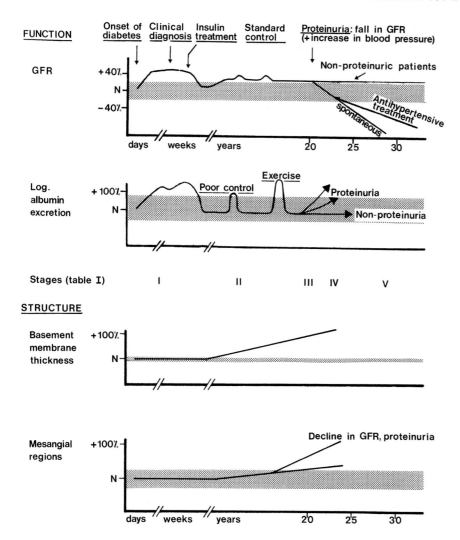

FIG. 73-3. Outline of renal function and structure in insulin-dependent diabetes mellitus (IDDM). Glomerular filtration rate (GFR), as measured by the exact clearance technique, is elevated at the time of clinical diagnosis but partially normalized during standard insulin treatment. However, during standard control, the GFR remains elevated in most patients. When clinical proteinuria is found, nephropathy is already advanced. Antihypertensive treatment postpones end-stage renal failure. The stages in diabetic nephropathy are defined in Table 73-1. Albumin excretion rate is the main parameter in this classification. Albumin excretion rate already may be increased at the time of clinical diagnosis, but can readily be normalized by standard treatment (stage I). In the following years, albumin excretion rate remains normal in many patients (stage II); it may increase during poor control or during exercise. When albumin excretion increases (stage III) and excretion rates remain high, the patients are at increased risk for the development of overt diabetic nephropathy. The two main early structural lesions are basement membrane thickening and mesangial expansion. Increased basement membrane thickness can be documented after a few years of diabetes, and mesangial lesions may be seen a few years later. Stage IV is overt diabetic nephropathy.

RENAL FUNCTION IN DIABETES

Careful and repeated measures of renal function in diabetic patients, discussed in detail later, are crucial to the effort to classify patients as to the risk for diabetic nephropathy and can stratify patients as to the risk for other diabetic complications. These renal functional measures are central to newer concepts regarding the development and institution of treatment strategies that may substantially influence the natural history of these complications that represent serious threats to quality of life and to survival.

This section describes the syndrome of microalbuminuria in patients with type 1 diabetes, compares this with the clinical significance of microalbuminuria in patients with type 2 diabetes, and details methodologies for appropriate measures of renal function in diabetes.

TABLE 73-1. *Definitions of stages of renal involvement in insulin-dependent diabetes mellitus[a]*

Stages	Designation	Time course
Stage I	Early hypertrophy–hyperfunction	Present at diagnosis
Stage II	Silent stage with normal albumin excretion, but glomerular lesions are present (e.g., basement membrane thickening, mesangial expansion)	Found after a few years of diabetes; may continue for decades
Stage III	Microalbuminuria characterized by persisting and increasing elevation of urinary albumin excretion but not clinical proteinuria	Typically found after >7 yr of diabetes
Stage IV	Overt diabetic nephropathy with clinical proteinuria	Typically found after 15–18 yr of diabetes
Stage V	End-stage renal failure	Typically found after approximately 25 yr of diabetes

[a]These definitions, based on renal function studies, are used throughout this chapter.

Microalbuminuria

Microalbuminuria is defined as the persistent excretion of albumin in the urine at rates that are above the normal range but below values detected by conventional methods, including ordinary urinary dipsticks. A 10-fold increase, or even more, in urinary albumin excretion (UAE) could occur without detection by standard clinical tests. Studies from three centers (14–16,43,44) agreed that microalbuminuria is a strong predictor of the subsequent development of overt diabetic nephropathy as manifested, typically, by overt proteinuria, hypertension, and ultimately declining GFR progressing toward ESRD (Table 73-1). These initial observations were confirmed by longer-term follow-up studies (44,45). However, the earlier studies, all retrospective in design, varied as to the lower limit of increased UAE that was predictive of the later development of overt nephropathy.

The normal values for UAE vary somewhat depending on the collection method, with a 30% to 50% lower excretion rate at night than during the day, but it is generally considered that the 95th upper percentile is less than 15 μg/minute (14,46) and certainly less than 20 μg/minute (47), and the definition of microalbuminuria as urinary albumin losses persistently between 20 and 200 μg/minute is now widely accepted (18) (Table 73-2). In fact, values of UAE between 12 and 20 μg/minute, although within the normal range, are uncommon in healthy people at rest, and type 1 diabetic patients whose UAE is in these upper ranges of normal are more likely to progress to persistent microalbuminuria (48).

Glomerular Filtration Rate and Microalbuminuria

Elevated GFR is a long-established phenomenon in patients with short-term type 1 diabetes (49–51). This increased GFR, which can be reduced but is difficult to normalize by glycemic control (49,52), has been suggested as a risk factor for diabetic nephropathy (see Pathogenetic Concepts). One study showed a 14% increase in GFR in 134 normoalbuminuric type 1 diabetic patients (mean, 135; range, 97 to 198 mL/minute) over control values (mean, 118; range, 93 to 143 mL/minute), with a further 5% increase in 50 microalbuminuric patients (mean, 142; range, 100 to 186 mL/minute) (53). Another study suggested that GFRs may be falling during the transition from microalbuminuria to overt nephropathy (54), and yet other studies indicated that reduced GFR can be seen in some normoalbuminuric and microalbuminuric patients with type 1 diabetes in association with more advanced glomerular lesions (55,56). From these studies it may be reasonable to conclude that among diabetic patients, microalbuminuria encompasses a quite wide range of renal structure and function (see also section on Structural–Functional Relationships in Diabetic Nephropathy).

The Predictive Value of Normoalbuminuria and Microalbuminuria for Diabetic Nephropathy

As suggested already, microalbuminuria derives its clinical utility as a strong predictor of the later development of overt nephropathy and, indeed, ESRD and death. Combining the initial longitudinal studies (14,15,17,43–45), microalbuminuria had a predictive value of approximately 75% to 80%. A recent review suggested that the predictive value of microalbuminuria may be somewhat less (56). In this review, the risk of progression of microalbuminuric patients to proteinuria over the subsequent decade was approximately 40% to 45% in patients with either type 1 or type 2 diabetes, with approximately 30% of microalbuminuric patients reverting to normoalbuminuria over 6 to 10 years of follow-up, whereas the remainder have persistent microalbuminuria. For example, in one study of patients with type 1 diabetes for at least 15 years, only 28% with microalbuminuria had overt nephropathy by 10-year follow-up, whereas 23% with normoalbuminuria at baseline subsequently had microalbuminuria (8%) or overt nephropathy (15%) (57).

Only a relatively small percentage ($\approx$10%) of patients who are normoalbuminuric despite 10 or more years of diabetes progress to microalbuminuria and overt proteinuria. Nonetheless, because at initial screening, most long-standing type 1 diabetic patients are normoalbuminuric, a sizable proportion ($\approx$40%) of the patients ultimately at risk for development of clinical diabetic nephropathy are normoalbuminuric

---

TABLE 73-2. *The Gentofte-Montecatini convention on persistent microalbuminuria*

Definitions of urinary albumin excretion in insulin-dependent patients. Consensus from a meeting at the Steno Memorial Hospital, Friday, January 11, 1985, and in Montecatini, April 1985.

Microalbuminuria is present when urinary albumin excretion rate is >20 μg/min and $\leq$200 μg/min. Urine should be collected in patients at rest or during 24 hr (e.g., as an outpatient procedure). Blood pressure should always be recorded.

Persistent microalbuminuria is suspected when values of 20–200 μg/min are found in two of three urine samples collected consecutively, preferably within 6 mo and no less than 1 mo. If more than three samples are available, mean values should correspond to the microalbuminuria level of 20–200 μg/min. Urine should be sterile in nonketotic patients, and other causes for increased urinary albumin excretion rate should be excluded. If duration of diabetes is <6 yr, other causes should be specifically excluded.

Best standard conventional diabetes control in the individual patients should be achieved.

Overt diabetic nephropathy is suspected when urinary albumin excretion rate is >200 μg/min in at least two of three consecutive urine samples, preferably collected within 6 mo. The urine sample should be sterile in nonketotic patients, and other causes of increased urinary albumin excretion rate should be excluded.

Dipsticks of urine for urinary protein should not be applied in the classification of renal disease in diabetes according to this proposal.

at baseline screening. Thus, microalbuminuria may be a less precise predictor of diabetic nephropathy risk than originally proposed and normoalbuminuria, despite long-term diabetes, is an imperfect predictor of safety. Nonetheless, given that microalbuminuria is associated with at least a 400% to 500% increase in risk of ultimate development of diabetic nephropathy, regular annual testing for this valuable marker should now be the standard of practice in the case of all type 1 diabetic patients with 5 or more years of duration and in all type 2 diabetic patients regardless of diabetes duration.

Systemic Hypertension and Microalbuminuria

Several studies found increased BP in microalbuminuric versus normoalbuminuric type 1 diabetic patients (14,43,58–60). In fact, before being detectable by standard BP measurement techniques, systemic BP may be increasing in type 1 diabetic patients whose UAE is rising. Thus, 24-hour ambulatory BP measurements are more closely correlated with UAE in the normal and microalbuminuric ranges than are standard office BPs (61,62). Nonetheless, even with standard methods there is a significant and direct relationship between BP and UAE (63–65).

Microalbuminuria and Diabetic Retinopathy

The complications of diabetes usually manifest in constellations; thus, there are strong associations in type 1 diabetes between UAE, diabetic retinopathy (66,67), and diabetic nephropathy lesions, but exceptions do exist (68,69). Thus, a few patients with advanced retinopathy (<15%) have normal or near-normal renal structure, whereas approximately 25% of patients with long-standing type 1 disease with overt nephropathy and advanced diabetic renal lesions have only mild retinopathy (68). These studies suggest that eye and kidney lesions of diabetes may have both common as well as organ-specific pathogeneses and susceptibilities. Microalbuminuric type 2 diabetic patients with proliferative retinopathy have typical lesions of diabetic nephropathy, whereas microalbuminuric type 2 patients with no or lesser retinopathy changes may have either little renal structural change or atypical patterns of renal injury (70). Given that type 1 diabetic patients with microalbuminuria are at increased risk for the later development of proliferative retinopathy (66,69) (Fig. 73-4), these patients should be advised to have close ophthalmologic monitoring. Conversely, patients in whom proliferative retinopathy is developing should be particularly closely watched for the emergence of signs of renal disease.

Microalbuminuria and Atherosclerosis

Diabetic patients with overt renal disease are at a markedly increased risk for cardiovascular mortality (4). Patients with microalbuminuria already manifest potentially atherogenic changes (71,72), including increased levels of low-density

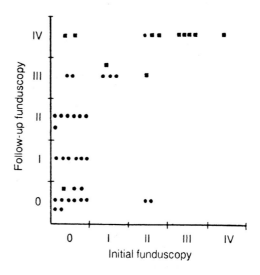

• Initial UAE < 15 µg/min or no progression in elevated albumin excretion (namely 2 patients with albumin excretion rate at 15.9 and 23.3 µg/min who did not have an increase in albumin excretion at follow-up)

■ Initial UAE ≥ 15 µg/min and increasing albumin excretion

FIG. 73-4. Follow-up funduscopy plotted against initial funduscopy in patients with insulin-dependent diabetes (10.4-year follow-up). IV, proliferative lesions; UAE, urinary albumin excretion. (From Miles DW, Mogensen CE, Gunderson HJG. Radioimmunoassay for urinary albumin: using a single antibody. *Scand J Clin Invest* 1970;26:5, with permission.)

lipoprotein cholesterol and fibrinogen and von Willebrand factor (73), the latter perhaps signaling widespread alterations in endothelial function. Although the nature of this interrelationship of diabetic nephropathy with macrovascular disease is not fully understood, common genetic risk pathways have been suggested (see Genetic Aspects of Diabetic Nephropathy). However, the abnormalities in these potentially atherogenic plasma factors that are associated with microalbuminuria are not secondary to urinary protein losses *per se,* which are far too small to account for the similar effects associated with nephrotic-range proteinuria.

Finally, microalbuminuria is associated with a generalized increased transcapillary escape rate for albumin in microalbuminuric versus normoalbuminuric type 1 diabetic patients (74), suggesting underlying abnormalities that may account for the strong tendency toward concordance of renal, eye, and macrovascular damage. However, as alluded to earlier regarding retinopathy, the exceptions, including uremic type 1 diabetic patients with negative coronary angiograms, suggest that a single unifying hypothesis will be inadequate (75).

Microalbuminuria in Type 2 Diabetes

Microalbuminuria predicts renal disease in diabetic Pima Indians (76), a group that tends to acquire type 2 diabetes at a relatively young age. However, in more elderly type 2 diabetic patients, the incidence of microalbuminuria and proteinuria (33,37,77–80) predicts an incidence of ESRD higher than the 8% to 10% of type 2 diabetic patients in whom uremia ultimately develops (7,32–34,37). This may have multiple explanations. First, microalbuminuria is a strong predictor of increased cardiovascular mortality in type 2 diabetes (33,35,36). Thus, many patients die before uremia supervenes. Second, because the nature of the underlying renal injury is more heterogeneous in type 2 diabetic patients (70) (see later), it is not surprising that the outcome is less predictable.

Measurement Techniques for Urinary Albumin

There are a number of possible urine sampling techniques, including:

Random urine samples. Random urine samples may be used for large-scale epidemiologic studies and clinical screening (81). Provided there is no extreme variation in urine output, a fair relationship with excretion rate is found (82). Simultaneous measurement of urine creatinine partly corrects for variations in urine output, and the urinary albumin–creatinine ratio in the first-voided, early-morning sample has the best correlation with measurements of timed overnight urine collections (83). A second, improved generation of dipstick tests has been developed (Micral-Test II) that has a good correlation with the immunochemically measured albumin concentration (84).

Twenty-four–hour urine samples. Many patients, when properly instructed, are able to provide complete collections (85,86), but often there are difficulties because of poor patient compliance. Further, measurements based on a 24-hour sample may show variability owing physical activity and metabolic control.

Overnight urine collection. Timed overnight urine collections are highly suitable for measurement of urinary albumin. Creatinine excretion can be used as a control, and multiple urine collections are advisable.

Variability in Urinary Albumin Excretion

Several studies have shown great variability in UAE, regardless of which urine collection method is used. In general, the variability is on the order of 40% to 50% when patients are studied during stable metabolic control (86,87), but patients studied repeatedly over a few months tend to remain within their categories (normoalbuminuria, microalbuminuria, or overt proteinuria). As mentioned earlier, however, approximately one-fourth to one-third of microalbuminuric patients may become normoalbuminuric when followed over 5 to 10 years. A number of factors, including physical exercise, poor metabolic control, and urinary infections, can influence these tests. Overnight collections reduce the exercise variability and avoid confusion with postural proteinuria.

Renal Function in Various Groups of Patients

Renal Function in Newly Diagnosed Diabetes

A marked increase in GFR of approximately 30% to 40% along with a concomitant increase in renal size has been documented in newly diagnosed type 1 diabetic patients without dehydration or acidosis at clinical presentation (49,52,88). Renal plasma flow also may be increased, but this is not consistent (52,88). These abnormalities are at least partially reversible within weeks by strict insulin treatment (89). UAE is almost always completely normalized within 1 to 2 weeks, but normalization of renal size seems to require months of precise glycemic control (52,88).

The GFR tends to be increased (hyperfiltration) but to a more limited extent in newly diagnosed type 2 diabetic patients (90). UAE may be increased at clinical presentation, but is quite variable (91,92). Compared with an appropriate control group, however, UAE is, on average, increased in these patients and a correlation of UAE to plasma glucose has been found (90). In one large study, GFR correlated best with glycated hemoglobin A (HbA$_{1c}$), BP, and microalbuminuria in newly diagnosed type 2 diabetic patients, and hyperfiltration was a fairly common finding (approximately 30%) (93).

Reversal of Renal Functional Changes

When patients with type 1 diabetes of some years' duration receive intensified insulin treatment (e.g., by insulin pump), a reduction in hyperfiltration is seen despite failure completely to normalize blood glucose (94,95). However, when diabetes has been present for some years (95), the enlarged kidney size does not normalize with improved control. UAE may be partially normalized by intensified insulin treatment (96). In type 2 diabetic patients, increased UAE at diagnosis may be reversed in some, but not all patients by normalizing the blood glucose (92).

Abnormalities in renal function early in type 1 diabetes are not strictly correlated with blood glucose levels (97). When diabetic patients are given oral glucose, GFR and renal plasma flow may increase slightly (2% to 3%), but only if these patients have normal or near-normal blood glucose levels before the glucose loads (98). When glucose is given to patients with already elevated plasma glucose levels (>10 mmol/L), a reduction in GFR may be seen. Correlations between daily glycemic excursions and GFR are more precise than that of GFR and HbA$_{1C}$ (99). Further, there is a good correlation between GFR and protein intake in type 1 diabetic patients and, corrected for protein intake, GFR in these patients is similar to that of control subjects (100). Whether the higher protein intake in many type 1 diabetic patients reflected hyperphagia resulting from poor glycemic control was not established in this study (100). Finally, ketone bodies, reflectors of poor glycemic control, can increase GFR in type 1 diabetic patients (101). Thus, hyperfiltration is not fully separable from poor glycemic control.

MECHANISMS RESPONSIBLE FOR DIABETIC NEPHROPATHY: GENERAL CONCEPTS

Although there might be important modulating factors, there is now overwhelming evidence indicating that diabetic nephropathy is secondary to the long-term metabolic aberrations found in diabetes. The two major early glomerular lesions, mesangial expansion and increased thickness of the glomerular basement membrane (GBM), are not found at diagnosis but develop thereafter and can be demonstrated after diabetes has been present for a few years (28,102). Moreover, in animal models, a number of changes in the kidney are prevented or reversed after normalization of metabolism (103–109). In human diabetes there is evidence that poor glycemic control is important for the development of lesions and clinical proteinuria (22,24,110). In identical twins discordant for type 1 diabetes, the kidneys of the nondiabetic member of these twin pairs were structurally normal, and in each instance GBM and mesangial measures were greater in the diabetic twin of the pair (111) (Fig. 73-5). In addition, normal kidneys from nondiabetic donors that are transplanted into diabetic patients develop all of the lesions of diabetic nephropathy (112–115). Further, mesangial matrix expansion does not develop in type 1 diabetic patients randomized to receive maximized glycemic control in the first 5 years after kidney transplantation, whereas this occurs in patients randomized to receive standard glycemic control (116). This study, along with the very large, multicenter Diabetes Control and Complications Trial (DCCT), which documented that patients with and those without baseline mild retinopathy randomized to strict control had less retinopathy progression and lower incidences of microalbuminuria and proteinuria after 7 to 8 years of follow-up (24), proves the role of glycemia as a risk factor for the specific eye and kidney abnormalities of type 1 diabetes. Similar trends were seen for the prevention of microalbuminuria and proteinuria in the large United Kingdom Prospective Diabetes Study (UKPDS) in type 2 diabetic patients (117). Perhaps most striking is the dramatic reversal of established diabetic nephropathy lesions in the native kidneys of type 1 diabetic patients with long-term (10 years) normoglycemia after successful pancreas transplantation (see later). On the other hand, it has been observed repeatedly that many patients show only a few, clinically insignificant vascular lesions even after decades of relatively poor control. It therefore is likely that important modulating factors exist, probably related to both genetic and environmental influences.

GENETIC ASPECTS OF DIABETIC NEPHROPATHY

Familial Clustering of Diabetic Nephropathy

Since 1989, evidence has mounted favoring a strong familial predisposition to the development of kidney disease associated with diabetes. Seaquist et al. (21) examined nephropathy risk in type 1 diabetes multiplex families with the proband (the first of the siblings to develop diabetes) having diabetes for at least 10 years, and the sibling for at least 7 years. Only 2 of the 12 type 1 siblings of probands free of diabetic nephropathy (17%) had UAE rates above 30 μg/minute. In contrast, 12 of the 29 siblings of probands with ESRD also had ESRD (41%), 12 had microalbuminuria or overt proteinuria, and only 5 (17%) were normal. Thus, the overall incidence of renal disease was 82% among the group of siblings whose probands had nephropathy. Studies of Borch-Johnsen et al. (118) and Quinn et al. (119) largely confirmed these findings in type 1 diabetes, and Freidman et al. (120) reported similar findings in type 2 diabetes. Also, in studies of two generations of Pima Indians with type 2 diabetes, proteinuria occurred among 14% of their offspring if neither parent had proteinuria, 23% if at least one parent had proteinuria, and 46% if both parents had diabetes and proteinuria (20).

Our studies indicate that the concordance of nephropathy among type 1 diabetic sibling pairs is based on concordance of renal lesions (121). Not only was the severity of individual glomerular lesions highly correlated, but the

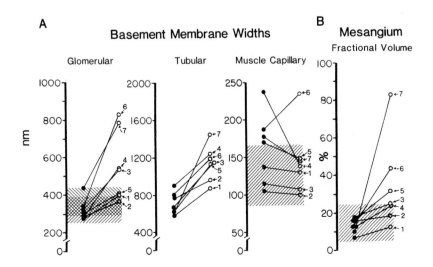

FIG. 73-5. Morphometric measurement of basement membrane width **(A)** and fractional volume of the mesangium (expressed as a percentage) **(B)** in kidney and skeletal muscle from identical twins discordant for type 1 diabetes mellitus. Values for nondiabetic twins *(closed circles)* are linked to values for their diabetic siblings *(open circles)*. The *hatched areas* indicate normal ranges. The normal range for glomerular basement membrane (GBM) width in men *(hatching* indicating higher normal values) overlaps the range in women *(hatching* indicating lower normal values). The diabetic twins differed significantly from their siblings in terms of GBM width (P = 0.002) and tubular basement membrane width (P = 0.0035), but not muscle capillary basement membrane width (P = 0.5).

patterns of lesions were similar among these sibling pairs. Thus, for example, if one sibling had relatively greater GBM width compared with the fractional volume of the glomerulus occupied by the mesangial matrix [Vv(mm/glom)], the other sibling was more likely to have the same pattern. The concordance of lesion severity was independent of measures of glycemia in these sib pairs. Moreover, the concordance in patterns of lesions indicated that there may be specific glomerular cellular responses to hyperglycemia that tend to be shared in siblings. These data and the studies indicating a concordance for sodium-hydrogen antiporter (Na/H) activity in cultured skin fibroblasts in these sibling pairs (122) support a strong genetic basis for diabetic nephropathy risk.

Ethnic Studies

Asian diabetic patients in the United Kingdom have greater prevalences of microalbuminuria, clinical nephropathy, and ESRD than do age-, sex-, and diabetes duration–matched European patients (123). African-American type 2 diabetic patients have a substantially increased risk of diabetic nephropathy compared with whites (39). There is an increased risk of diabetic nephropathy among Israeli Jews of non-Ashkenazi origin (124). In this study, both glycemic control and lower socioeconomic status also were significantly and independently correlated to albuminuria (124). These studies are consistent with genetic influences on diabetic nephropathy risk, although other variables may be involved.

Family Studies of Blood Pressure

Higher values of arterial pressure were found in parents of type 1 diabetic patients with microalbuminuria or proteinuria (125–127). More recently, it was shown that diabetic patients with advanced nephropathy had not only a greater prevalence of parental hypertension but higher mean arterial BPs during adolescence (128).

Familial Cardiovascular Disease and Diabetic Nephropathy

The prevalence of cardiovascular disease and cardiovascular death was found to be significantly greater in the parents of type 1 diabetic patients with nephropathy (129,130). Among the diabetic patients with nephropathy, a family history of cardiovascular disease was particularly more frequent in those diabetic patients who had had a cardiovascular event (129). These studies indicate that familial predisposition to cardiovascular disease increases the risk of nephropathy and the risk of cardiovascular disease in type 1 diabetic patients with nephropathy. Although this probably represents shared genetic risk factors, common environmental risk factors (e.g., diet, smoking) cannot yet be ruled out.

Sodium-Lithium Countertransport

Studies of intermediate phenotypes related to the risk of hypertension and cardiovascular disease such as red blood cell sodium-lithium countertransport activity (Na/Li CT) found increased activity of this membrane transport mechanism to be associated with essential hypertension and some of its renal and cardiovascular complications (131–133). Increased Na/Li CT rates were found in type 1 and type 2 diabetic patients with both microalbuminuria and clinical nephropathy (126,134,135), although not by all investigators (136).

In a confirmatory study, the prevalence of elevated Na/Li CT activity was found to be 21.5%, 42.8%, and 51.7% in normoalbuminuric, microalbuminuric, and clinically proteinuric patients, respectively (137), and, in multiple logistic regression analysis, Na/Li CT emerged as the factor most closely related to proteinuria, followed by duration of type 1 diabetes, mean BP, and glycated hemoglobin. In three studies, an interaction was observed between Na/Li CT and glycemia as predictors of proteinuria in that the highest frequency occurred in the patients with HbA_{1c} values above the median and Na/Li CT rates above the normal range (126,128,135). However, there is a significant correlation in Na/Li CT activity in identical twins discordant for diabetes (138). In a study of type 2 diabetic patients, albuminuria correlated with ambulatory BP but not with Na/Li CT activity (139).

Insulin Sensitivity

There is a greater resistance to peripheral insulin action in type 1 diabetic patients with high Na/Li CT activity (140). Reduced insulin sensitivity also is associated with increased serum triglycerides and apolipoprotein B, and with left ventricular hypertrophy (140), providing a possible link between nephropathy and cardiovascular risk. Reduced insulin sensitivity is associated with microalbuminuria in both type 1 and type 2 diabetic patients (141,142), itself a strong predictor of cardiovascular mortality (see earlier). Further, first-degree relatives of type 1 diabetic patients with microalbuminuria have greater abnormalities of carbohydrate and lipid metabolism than do first-degree relatives of normoalbuminuric type 1 diabetic patients (143). Insulin insensitivity also is a significant risk factor for cardiovascular disease in the general population. Finally, there may be an association between polymorphism of the insulin receptor gene and the development of overt proteinuria in type 1 diabetic patients (144).

Sodium-Hydrogen Antiport Activity

Sodium-lithium countertransport has parallels with the sodium-hydrogen (Na/H) antiporter exchange system that is involved in the regulation of intracellular pH, cell volume and growth, and proximal tubular sodium reabsorption (145). There is increased Na/H antiporter activity in leukocytes (146) and cultured skin fibroblasts (147) of type 1 diabetic patients with microalbuminuria and clinical proteinuria. The cultured skin fibroblasts of small groups of these patients also have increased proliferation rates (148–150) as well as increased expression of messenger RNA (mRNA) for $\alpha 3\beta 1$ integrin subunits (150) compared with normoalbuminuric patients and nondiabetic control subjects. Because integrins may regulate cell proliferation through the Na/H antiporter system (145), these abnormalities may be interrelated. Also, because cultured skin fibroblast Na/H antiporter activity is highly correlated among siblings concordant for type 1 diabetes and for nephropathy lesions (122), it is possible that these cultured skin fibroblast abnormalities are genetically regulated.

Diabetic Nephropathy Genes

As suggested previously, there are ongoing searches for genetic loci related to diabetic nephropathy susceptibility through genomic scanning and candidate gene approaches. Neither approach has yielded definitive results, but indications are that multiple genes may be involved (151,152). Several genes, in addition to those discussed already, have been proposed as plausible candidates based on the pathophysiology of diabetic nephropathy. Genetic polymorphism in genes related to the renin–angiotensin system (RAS) have been evaluated in many studies, yet it is still unclear that polymorphism of the angiotensin-converting enzyme (ACE) gene is important in the genesis of diabetic nephropathy (153–159). However, there is growing evidence that this polymorphism may be important in diabetic progression (160–162). In type 1 diabetic patients, the albumin excretion rate appears to increase faster in patients with the II genotype (162), and these patients appear to have the best response to ACE inhibitor therapy (161–163). Other studies, however, did not observe associations between polymorphisms of the ACE gene and diabetic nephropathy risk (163–165) or rate of decline in GFR (166) in type 1 or type 2 diabetic patients. One meta-analysis concluded that the D allele was significantly associated with diabetic nephropathy in both type 1 and type 2 diabetic patients (167), although one study found this association to be significant only in Japanese type 2 diabetic patients, but not in white type 1 or type 2 diabetic patients (168). A meta-analysis did not find associations between polymorphisms in the angiotensinogen gene and diabetic nephropathy risk (169). Further, two large studies did not find a role for angiotensin II type 1 receptor polymorphism in diabetic nephropathy (170,171), whereas another found that polymorphisms in the angiotensin II type 1 receptor contributed significantly to diabetic nephropathy risk only when accompanied by poor glycemic control (172).

Renin (173), endothelial nitric oxide synthetase (174), human inducible nitrogen oxide synthase (175,176), aldose reductase (177,178), PC-1 (179), atrial natriuretic peptide (180), apolipoprotein E (181–184), and heparan sulfate core protein (185) gene polymorphism also have been associated with diabetic nephropathy in some, but not all (186–189) studies.

Other genes studied (151) include type IV collagen (190), matrix metalloproteinase-9 (MMP-9) (191), endothelin and endothelin A receptor (192), transforming growth factor-β (TGF-β1) (193), plasminogen activator inhibitor-1 (165, 194), interleukin-1 (195,196), interleukin-1 receptor antagonist (197), G protein (198), β_3-adrenergic receptor (199), hepatocyte nuclear factor 1α (200), methylenetetrahydrofolate reductase (201,202), kallikrein (165,203), Werner's syndrome helicase (165), bradykinin B_2 receptor gene, paraoxonase gene, and insulin gene (204), but no clear consensus for a pathogenetic role of these genes in diabetic nephropathy risk has emerged.

Genomic scanning studies of Pima Indian families with type 2 diabetes suggested evidence for a nephropathy susceptibility locus on chromosome 18q[448]. Sibling pair linkage analysis in Pima Indians showed some evidence for linkage with diabetic nephropathy in four chromosomal regions (chromosome 3, 7, 9, and 20), with the strongest evidence in chromosome 7 (205). A study in white type 2 diabetic patients had previously shown linkage between diabetic nephropathy and chromosome 7 (206).

In summary, there is increasing evidence of familial and probably genetic predisposition to diabetic nephropathy. Preliminary data support linkages of diabetic nephropathy risk to factors regulating predisposition to hypertension and cardiovascular disease. It is reasonable to hypothesize that a single gene with a major effect or several genes with smaller effects interact with hyperglycemia to confer diabetic nephropathy risk. Further research in this area is likely to lead to important new information regarding risk factors, pathogenesis, and treatment of diabetic nephropathy.

PATHOGENETIC CONCEPTS

A complete discussion of all of the hypotheses that have been generated in an effort to explain the pathogenesis of diabetic nephropathy is beyond the scope of this chapter. Thus, this section is limited to concepts that have provided therapeutic directions that are currently being explored.

The Hemodynamic Hypothesis

Of potential general importance in all kidney disease, perhaps especially so in diabetes mellitus, is the concept proposed by Brenner, Hostetter, and coworkers (12,207,208) that glomerular hyperfiltration is causally related to progression of renal disease, regardless of the nature of the original initiating disease process. As emphasized already, glomerular hyperfiltration is a common abnormality of renal function among types 1 and 2 diabetic patients. In fact, marked hyperfiltration, like microalbuminuria, may predict an increased risk for development of clinical diabetic nephropathy (14,209), although this issue is not entirely settled (210). Berkman and Rifkin (211) described a diabetic patient with unilateral renal artery stenosis and marked diabetic lesions in the kidney exposed both to hypertension and diabetes, whereas the contralateral kidney in the same diabetic milieu that was protected from hypertension by the narrowed renal artery had only ischemic changes. A model of unilateral renal artery stenosis in diabetic rats seemed to confirm this single human observation (212). Insulin-treated diabetic rats have glomerular hyperfiltration explainable by increased single-nephron GFR, which is due to increased single-nephron blood flow and, in the Münich-Wistar rat strain, increased glomerular capillary pressure (213). Thus, there is reason to believe that alterations in intraglomerular hemodynamics could have important modulating influences on the rate at which lesions develop.

However, the genesis of diabetic nephropathy cannot be explained by hyperfiltration alone. Insulin-treated diabetic rats with hyperfiltration have slower development of diabetic renal lesions than do untreated diabetic rats with worse hypoglycemia and relative hypofiltration; these markedly hyperfiltrating, insulin-treated animals do not seem to acquire mesangial expansion disproportionate to the size of the glomerulus (214,215). Further, reduction in nephron mass in rats by uninephrectomy produces glomerular hemodynamic perturbations (216) that are similar to diabetes (214), but never produces the lesions (217,218) that are classic for diabetic nephropathy in animals (105–110), and reduced nephron mass has not been documented to produce diabetic nephropathy lesions in humans. The central lesion associated with hyperfiltration in rats, focal segmental sclerosis (219), is not an important lesion in human or animal diabetes (see Pathology of the Diabetic Kidney). ACE inhibitor treatment can lower glomerular capillary pressures in insulin-treated hyperfiltrating Münich-Wistar rats (220), but these drugs do not prevent GBM widening or an increase in Vv(mes/glom) in diabetic rats (221). The renal artery stenosis protection against diabetic nephropathy in rats and humans could be due to lower tissue glucose delivery because of impaired blood flow on the stenotic side and, thus, may have other than hemodynamic explanations. The rate of development of diabetic nephropathy in the single kidney (the human kidney transplant model) is virtually identical to that in two-kidney type 1 diabetic patients, arguing against the importance of glomerular hemodynamics and glomerular number in diabetic nephropathy pathogenesis.

Hemodynamic abnormalities may be more important in influencing the *progression* of established diabetic nephropathy lesions. Occlusion of glomerular capillaries or restriction of filtration surface in nonsclerosed glomeruli as a consequence of advanced diabetic renal lesions (see later) could cause compensatory enlargement of the remaining glomeruli associated with increased intraglomerular pressures and flows and permselectivity alterations (219). Such abnormal hemodynamic forces could accelerate disruption of the residual glomeruli, thus generating a destructive cycle that promotes progressive tissue injury and loss of renal function. It is our hypothesis that once advanced lesions of mesangial expansion and reduced capillary surface are established (see later), such destructive hemodynamic forces are set in motion. These forces manifest as microalbuminuria, progressing to proteinuria, and can propel the glomerulus to final destruction independent of the diabetic state. As suggested by Brenner (207,208) and Hostetter (219) and their respective colleagues, such a process may be common to a number of renal diseases. Moreover, proteinuria may lead to tubulointerstitial injury through complex mechanisms leading to further acceleration of loss of GFR (222). In fact, the magnitude of residual proteinuria after the institution of antihypertensive therapy, especially ACE inhibitors, in proteinuric diabetic patients is a strong predictor of the subsequent rate of decline of GFR.

Although we are arguing that a case has not been made that would allow the complete acceptance of the hypothesis that hemodynamic abnormalities are responsible for the *genesis* of the early lesions of diabetic nephropathy, it is nonetheless possible that manipulations that affect glomerular hemodynamics might also affect the genesis of diabetic renal lesions through influences other than hemodynamic ones. For example, the RAS could mediate renal growth responses and renal extracellular matrix (ECM) production and turnover. Angiotensin acts as an *in vitro* growth factor for mesangial (223) and smooth muscle (224) cells and can stimulate mesangial cell fibronectin synthesis (225). The increased *in vitro* fibronectin production of human mesangial cells grown in high glucose can be inhibited by the ACE inhibitor captopril (225). However, because various ACE inhibitors differ in their ability to block the glucose-induced increase in fibronectin (226), this effect may be independent of the RAS. Also, the glucose-stimulated increase in mesangial cell collagen production can be blocked by enalapril (227). Further, increased glomerular mRNA expression for ECM components, including $\alpha 1(I)$, $\alpha 1(III)$, and $\alpha 1(IV)$ collagen chains and laminin $\beta 1$, was attenuated by ACE inhibitor therapy in streptozotocin diabetic rats (228). Captopril inhibits the 72- and 92-kd MMPs, two distinct type IV collagenases (229), thus favoring ECM accumulation. However, lisinopril, a nonsulfhydryl ACE inhibitor, inhibited these metalloproteinases only at concentrations 1,000 times those of captopril. Further, zinc can reverse the inhibitory effect of captopril on metalloproteinases, arguing against a RAS-dependent effect (230). Thus, drugs affecting the RAS might also affect ECM dynamics and thereby renal structure in diabetes. However, the mechanisms of actions of these agents appear complex and are incompletely understood.

Transforming growth factor-β expression may be regulated in parallel with renin (231,232). Thus, increased juxtaglomerular apparatus prorenin production (see later) may be associated with other increased juxtaglomerular apparatus activities such as TGF-β production, and the latter has been linked to glomerular ECM abnormalities in diabetes (232).

Plasma Prorenin Levels and Diabetic Complications

Renin and its inactive precursor, prorenin, are secreted into the circulation from the kidney (233,234). Renin is derived almost entirely from the kidney (235,236), whereas prorenin, primarily of renal origin, also is produced in other sites (237–239). In long-standing diabetes with microvascular complications, plasma prorenin levels tend to be markedly elevated but renin levels tend to be normal or reduced (240–245). Proteinuria or retinopathy developed in only 1 of 20 young type 1 diabetic patients with consistently normal prorenin levels followed serially, whereas one or both developed in 8 of 14 patients with increased prorenin levels (241). Daneman et al. (243) studied 50 adolescents with type 1 diabetes for an average of 7 years, 25 with microalbuminuria. Prorenin was highest in the microalbuminuric patients versus the nonmicroalbuminuric patients, and the levels in all type 1 diabetic patients combined were higher than control values. Most interestingly, the nondiabetic siblings of the microalbuminuric patients in this study had higher prorenin values than did those of the nonmicroalbuminuric patients with type 1 diabetes (243). In another study, type 1 diabetic patients in whom microalbuminuria or proteinuria developed (progressors) had increased total renin content (which is predominantly prorenin) as early as 10 years before the onset of microalbuminuria (244). Increased plasma prorenin also antedates microalbuminuria in type 2 diabetic patients (245). Taken together, these studies suggest that elevated plasma prorenin may be a predictor of progressive diabetic nephropathy in type 1 and type 2 diabetes. The pathogenesis of increased plasma prorenin levels in diabetic patients with complications is incompletely understood, but is likely of renal origin (246).

BIOCHEMICAL PATHWAYS AND DIABETIC NEPHROPATHY: GENERAL CONCEPTS

The renal lesions of diabetic nephropathy are mainly due to accumulation of ECM components, such as collagens, tenascin, and fibronectin (247), as well as other, yet undescribed molecules. ECM accumulation occurs early on in the GBM (248) and tubular basement membrane (TBM) (249), is the principal cause of mesangial expansion, and also contributes to the later stages of interstitial expansion (250). This ECM accumulation is clearly secondary to an imbalance between synthesis and degradation of ECM components. However, not all renal ECM components change in parallel in diabetic nephropathy. Thus, $\alpha 3$ and $\alpha 4$ chains of type IV collagen persist or increase in density in the GBM of patients in whom diabetic renal lesions are developing, whereas $\alpha 1$ and $\alpha 2$ chains decrease in density in the peripheral capillary wall and mesangial matrix in patients with rapid development of diabetic nephropathy lesions, and remain unchanged in patients with slow development of diabetic nephropathy lesions despite long duration of type 1 diabetes (251,252). Thus, the ECM changes in diabetes are highly site specific, differing in direction in the GBM compared with the mesangial matrix and suggesting that variables related to cell type (e.g., glomerular epithelial cell for GBM, mesangial cell for mesangial matrix) are important determinants in the response

to the diabetic state. Moreover, these patterns of cell response may be genetically regulated. Type VI collagen, the other major glomerular collagen, is decreased in density of distribution in the endothelial aspect of the GBM and in the mesangial matrix in patients with both slow and fast development of diabetic nephropathy lesions, albeit with greater reduction in the latter (253). Thus, the exact ECM component responsible for mesangial matrix expansion in diabetic nephropathy remains to be described.

Mesangial cells cultured in high glucose concentration accumulate various matrix components (254–256), whereas MMPs have been implicated in the abnormal *in vitro* degradation of mesangial matrix by these cells (257,258). MMP activity is regulated at several levels, including gene expression, extracellular activation, and inhibition by specific tissue inhibitors of MMPs (TIMPs). MMPs and TIMPs can be modulated by PKC agonists, such as cytokines, hormones, and growth factors such as TGF-β (259–265).

The major hypotheses as to how hyperglycemia causes diabetic complications are (a) increased activity of a variety of growth factors, including TGF-β, growth hormone, insulin-like growth factor (IGF), vascular endothelial growth factor (VEGF), and epidermal growth factor (EGF); (b) activation of protein kinase C (PKC) isoforms; (c) activation of cytokines, including renin, angiotensin, endothelin, bradykinin; (d) formation of reactive oxygen species (ROS); (e) increased formation of advanced glycation end products; (f) increased activity of the aldose reductase pathway; and (g) altered glomerular proteoglycan metabolism. Polyol pathway–induced redox changes or hyperglycemia-induced formation of ROS could potentially account for most of the other biochemical abnormalities (266–268). These mechanisms, reviewed in the following sections, could be influenced by genetic determinants of susceptibility or resistance to hyperglycemic damage.

Growth Factors

This subject has recently been excellently reviewed in detail by Flyvberg (269) and, using this author's organizational scheme, is summarized here.

Transforming Growth Factor-β

Transforming growth factor-β isoforms (TGF-β1, TGF-β2, and TGF-β3) and receptors are present in all glomerular cells and in proximal tubular cells (270–274). Glomerular mesangial and epithelial cells exposed *in vitro* to TGF-β demonstrate increased ECM protein synthesis, decreased MMP synthesis, and increased TIMP production (275–279). Mitogen-activated protein kinases (MAPK) may play an important role in the glucose-induced TGF-β mediated increase in ECM production in mesangial cells (280,281). TGF-β1 gene overexpression has been described in rat (271,282) and human diabetic glomeruli. TGF-β1 stimulates glucose uptake by enhancing the expression of the glucose transporter

GLUT-1 in mesangial cells, perhaps aggravating the metabolic abnormalities of diabetes (283). Further, glomerular ECM accumulation was observed in nondiabetic transgenic mice overexpressing glomerular TGF-β1 (284), although the glomerular lesions resembled but did not fully mimic diabetic nephropathy lesions. Concentrations of TGF-β2 and TGF-β type II receptor proteins also are increased soon after induction of diabetes in rats (273). TGF-β–neutralizing antibodies reduce the in vitro increase in type IV collagen synthesis induced by high-glucose media (285). Further, neutralizing antibodies to TGF-β1, TGF-β2, and TGF-β3 limited the increases in renal TGF-β1, TGF-β type II receptor, collagen IV, and fibronectin mRNA expression and glomerular hypertrophy in diabetic mice (286). ACE inhibitor (enalapril) treatment decreases glomerular TGF-β type I, II, and III receptors, with no changes in TGF-β isoforms, completely prevents UAE increase and partially prevents renal hypertrophy in diabetic rats (287). ACE inhibitors may regulate the renal TGF-β system through decreases in TGF-β receptor (287). Specific PKCβ inhibitors also may have a role as antagonists of the TGF-β system (see below).

Growth Hormone and Insulin-Like Growth Factors

Diabetes leads to decreased hepatic production of IGF-I and the consequent decrease in serum IGF-I results in excess growth hormone secretion (288,289), which, in turn, stimulates local IGF-I pathways in other tissues, such as the kidney. IGF-I, in vitro, induces increased mesangial cell proliferation (290,291). Mesangial cells from nonobese diabetic mice secrete increased amounts of IGF-I (292), and the consequent reduction in MMP-2 activity (293) could lead to glomerular ECM accumulation. Increased kidney levels of IGF-I precede renal growth in diabetic rodents. This IGF-I renal accumulation and renal hypertrophy are influenced by glycemia (294–296). Renal accumulation of IGF-I is more likely caused by changes in renal IGF-I receptors and IGF-I binding proteins than by an increase in local kidney IGF-I production (297–299). Somatostatin analogs (300–304) and growth hormone receptor antagonists (305–307) prevent the rise in renal IGF binding protein-1 mRNA levels, renal IGF-I, and renal hypertrophy.

Vascular Endothelial Growth Factor

Vascular endothelial growth factor, a potent mitogen for vascular endothelial cells and a major regulator of angiogenesis, has been associated with proliferative retinopathy and neoangiogenesis in experimental and human diabetes. VEGF is normally expressed in glomerular and tubular epithelial cells (308–311), whereas the VEGF type 2 receptor is found in glomerular endothelial and cortical interstitial cells (310). Hypoxia is a powerful VEGF stimulator (312,313). Angiotensin II stimulates VEGF in mesangial cells (311,314,315). Glucose stimulates VEGF expression in smooth muscle cells (316,317). VEGF is increased in glomeruli in diabetic animals

(310). Mechanical stretch of human mesangial cells in vitro induces VEGF production, possibly linking glomerular hemodynamic abnormalities in diabetes to this system (315). VEGF mRNA glomerular expression was evaluated in microalbuminuric and proteinuric type 2 diabetic patients. No differences in VEGF mRNA levels were found between patients with or without typical diabetic glomerulopathy (318).

Epidermal Growth Factor

Epidermal growth factor is synthesized in the kidney, and mesangial, tubular, and interstitial cells have receptors for this peptide. EGF stimulates in vitro tubular cell proliferation (319,320) and thus may play a role in early diabetic renal hypertrophy (321,322). EGF strongly influences the synthesis and turnover of ECM proteins.

In summary, several growth factor pathways have the potential markedly to influence or control the role of development of diabetic nephropathy lesions, and some animal data are consistent with their significant role in the genesis of these lesions. Proof of these concepts in humans is lacking, but they are worthy of serious consideration.

Protein Kinase C

The PKC enzyme regulating Na^+/K^+-adenosine triphosphatase can be activated by diacylglycerol (323), and thus high glucose. High-glucose–induced PKC activation in glomerular cells in vitro raises TGF-β (324) and MAPK (325) activity. Although a link between PKC and TGF-β probably exists, TGF-β action is not directly mediated by PKC signaling. For example, the antioxidant α-tocopherol prevents the glucose-induced increase in PKC, TGF-β, and ECM production in mesangial cells without affecting the exogenous TGF-β–induced increase in ECM production (324). Treatment with a PKCβ isoform inhibitor blocks glomerular TGF-β1 mRNA and renal structural and functional changes in diabetic rats (326) and mice (327).

Cytokines

As discussed earlier (see section on The Hemodynamic Hypothesis), there are in vitro and animal model data linking the pathogenesis of diabetic nephropathy and the RAS. More than the other pathways described in this section, the RAS has been studied with regard to diabetic nephropathy in humans.

Angiotensin II

Angiotensin II also promotes mesangial cell proliferation through TGF-β activation (see also section on Plasma Prorenin Levels and Diabetic Complications, earlier) (328). Thus, angiotensin II can stimulate ECM synthesis through TGF-β activity. Mesangial cells exposed to angiotensin II in vitro showed increased TGF-β expression and ECM synthesis (328).

As already discussed, there are data supporting use of RAS blockade in the treatment of patients with established diabetic nephropathy. The question as to whether earlier intervention will prevent the genesis of the earlier lesions of diabetic nephropathy before renal functional abnormalities are detectable is unknown and under intensive study.

Glycosylation Products

Although the key points are summarized here, the reader is referred to the excellent review by Ziyadeh et al. (329) for greater detail on this subject.

One of the major metabolic effects of diabetes is the nonenzymatic reactions between reducing sugars, such as glucose, with free amino groups, lipids, or nucleic acids incorporation of glucose (330). This interaction, known as the *Maillard reaction* (331), is accelerated by hyperglycemia. Many proteins undergo nonenzymatic glycosylation in diabetes, such as hemoglobin (332), albumin (331), low-density lipoproteins (333), erythrocyte membrane proteins (334), and lens crystallines (335), leading to altered physicochemical properties of these molecules. This early glycation process proceeds through the formation of a labile Schiff base adducts, which then undergoes an intramolecular Amadori rearrangement to become a stable glucose-modified protein. Amadori products comprise the overwhelming majority of glucose-modified proteins in plasma, and receptors for some of those modified proteins have been defined (336). Further modifications of Maillard reaction products lead to intermolecular and intramolecular crosslinks and formation of advanced glycosylation end products (AGEs). These reactions are very complex and the reader is referred to excellent reviews for greater detail (337,338).

It has been suggested that the accumulation of Amadori and AGE products may be a major contributor to the development of diabetic complications (339). Increased AGEs can stimulate the synthesis of various growth factors, including IGF-I and TGF-β (340). A hallmark of the glomerular changes of diabetes is mesangial expansion, mainly due to increases in ECM (see later). Exposure to glycosylated ECM markedly increases the *in vitro* ECM production of mesangial cells (341). Further, intraperitoneal AGE-modified mouse albumin increases renal mRNA for TGF-β1 and ECM components (342). This effect is reduced by aminoguanidine (342), an AGE crosslink inhibitor (343). Glycosylated ECM has reduced turnover rates, favoring ECM accumulation. Thus, aminoguanidine was tested as a preventer of diabetic nephropathy lesions (344). Soulis-Liparota et al. (345) found that aminoguanidine diminished the increased collagen-related fluorescence in diabetic rat aorta, glomeruli, and renal tubules, as well as decreasing albuminuria. In this study, GBM width increased in both treated and untreated diabetic rats, but the Vv(mes/glom) increase was prevented by aminoguanidine. However, another study found that aminoguanidine ameliorated GBM thickening but not Vv(mes/glom) increase in diabetic rats (346). Moreover, in similar studies (M.W. Steffes, M. Mauer, unpublished data), aminoguanidine failed to have any effect on the GBM or mesangial expansion in severe, long-standing diabetes in rats. Thus, results from available studies of aminoguanidine on prevention of renal lesions in diabetic rats are inconsistent.

Amadori-Glycated Albumin and Diabetic Nephropathy

Renal cells grown in high glucose have upregulation of the TGF-β (347–350) and PKC (351–354) systems, and ECM overproduction (355,356). Amadori-glycated proteins, which are earlier consequences of the glycation process than AGEs, have similar effects even without high-glucose media (357). For example, glomerular epithelial cells exposed to glycated fetal bovine serum show increased levels of laminin and GBM antigens, unchanged type I collagen and fibronectin, and decreased collagenase activity (358). Glycated albumin and high-glucose media together cause an even greater *in vitro* increase in the TGF-β1 and type II TGF-β receptor mRNAs than either manipulation alone (359). Also, mouse mesangial cells incubated in normal glucose media containing glycated serum proteins have increased α1 type IV collagen and fibronectin mRNA, and these effects are intensified by high-glucose media (359,360). Moreover, antibody to glycated albumin prevented the increase in fibronectin and type IV collagen expression in glomerular cells (360–362), and reduced albuminuria in animals exposed to glycated albumin (362). For example, 8 weeks of antiglycated albumin antibody administration lowered plasma glycated albumin, reduced urinary albumin, and improved glomerular mesangial lesions in db/db diabetic mice (360,363,364). Type 1 diabetic patients showed higher plasma levels of glycated albumin than nondiabetic patients, and type 1 diabetic patients with diabetic nephropathy showed higher plasma levels of Amadori albumin than normoalbuminuric patients (365). However, studies examining the role of Amadori-glycated proteins in the progression of human diabetic renal disease have reached conflicting conclusions (366–371). Further studies of glycation's role in the pathogenesis of and treatment strategies for diabetic nephropathy are warranted. However, the fact that glycation is a nonenzymatic process dependent on the duration and magnitude of glycemia fails to explain why clinical diabetic nephropathy develops in only approximately half of patients with very poor glycemic control.

Increased Activity of Aldose Reductase

Insulin is required for entry of glucose into adipose and muscle cells, whereas the tissues that bear the brunt of injury in diabetes are freely permeable to glucose. Aldose reductase, the enzyme that catalyzes the reduction of glucose to sorbitol in the polyol pathway, has been extensively studied for its potential role in the development of diabetic nephropathy and other microvascular complications. Aldose reductase, not present in all mammalian cells, is present in all the target tissues of diabetic complications. These tissues include lens, retinal capillary wall pericytes, kidney, vascular endothelium, and peripheral nerve (Schwann cells).

Increased activity of aldose reductase leads to accumulation of sorbitol, which is further converted to fructose by the sorbitol dehydrogenase enzyme, which uses nicotinamide adenine dinucleotide (NAD^+) as substrate. The ratio NAD^+/NADH decreases and the conversion of glyceraldehyde-3-phosphate to 1,3-biphosphoglycerate is blocked, leaving more substrate (glyceraldehyde-3-phosphate) for the synthesis of α-glycerol phosphate, a diacylglycerol precursor. Diacylglycerol is a PKC activator that, as discussed, could regulate ECM synthesis and removal.

Hypertonicity stimulates aldose reductase gene expression, and kinases (p38-MAPK and mitogen-activated extracellular regulated kinase) are involved in the regulation of this response. PKC also has a role in controlling aldose reductase gene transcription. Raised glucose or H_2O_2 activates p38-MAPK, providing two potential mechanisms for glucose to contribute to increased aldose reductase expression that may or may not require concomitant hyperosmotic conditions. Moreover, ROS decrease the nitric oxide content, which activates aldose reductase.

Aldose reductase mRNA levels in circulating cells are increased in type 1 diabetic patients with diabetic nephropathy, but not in diabetic patients without nephropathy (372). However, in human studies, aldose reductase inhibitors have a partial (373,374) or no (375,376) effect in ameliorating renal microvascular complications. However, as already noted, the factors associated with progression of established damage to tissues may differ from the initial pathogenic mechanisms, and the latter has not yet been addressed by primary prevention trials.

The Steno Hypothesis

According to the "Steno hypothesis," albuminuria reflects widespread vascular damage (377). The abnormal charge permselectivity observed in rat (378) and human (379) studies suggests that loss of anionic proteoglycans may be responsible for the initial increase in the excretion of negatively charged albumin. Heparan sulfate, the main glycosaminoglycan component of basement membranes in human glomeruli (380,381), inhibits mesangial cell proliferation *in vitro* (382). Hyperglycemia can lead to partial depletion of heparan sulfate in the kidney as a result of both its decreased synthesis and a reduction in its sulfation level (383). Decreased heparan sulfate in the kidney can result in diminution of the physiologic electrostatic charge GBM barrier (384) and in mesangial expansion, a major pathogenic factor in diabetic nephropathy. The loss of this ionic barrier allows the escape of albumin (and later, other proteins) into the glomerular filtrate, causing albuminuria/proteinuria (380,385). Animal studies have shown that subcutaneous low-molecular-weight heparin administration, perhaps by inducing heparan sulfate synthesis, prevents an increase in UAE and GBM thickening in diabetic rats (386,387). Reduction in UAE also was reported in microalbuminuric type 1 diabetic patients treated with subcutaneous low-molecular-weight heparin (388). Ongoing studies suggest that oral glycosaminoglycan administration can reduce proteinuria in type 1 and type 2 proteinuric diabetic patients (389). Thus, this area of research may well expand in the next few years.

PATHOLOGY OF THE DIABETIC KIDNEY

In aggregate, the pathologic process of diabetic nephropathy in type 1 diabetic patients is unique to this disease (Table 73-3) and separable from all other renal disorders (13,105,405). This section describes renal structural changes in type 1 diabetes and is followed by a brief discussion of areas of overlap and difference with renal pathology in type 2 diabetes. The first of the changes that can be quantitated and documented is a thickening of the GBM (102). Although these findings are less carefully established, there also is thickening of the TBM (111,249) and Bowman's capsule. Within a few years after onset of diabetes or after transplantation of a normal kidney into a diabetic patient, afferent and efferent arteriolar hyalinosis can be noted (112). This hyalinosis

TABLE 73-3. *Pathology of established diabetic nephropathy in patients with insulin-dependent diabetes mellitus*

Always present[a]	Often or usually present	Sometimes present
Glomerular basement membrane thickening, especially lamina densa	Kimmelstiel-Wilson nodules[b] (nodular glomerulosclerosis)	Hyaline "exudative" lesions, subendothelial
Mesangial widening with increased matrix material predominating (diffuse glomerulosclerosis)	Afferent and efferent glomerular arteriolar hyalinosis[b]	Parietal Bowman's capsular surface "capsular drop"[b]
Intense glomerular basement membrane, tubular basement membrane, and Bowman's capsular immunofluorescent staining for albumin	Tubular basement membrane thickening, interstitial expansion, global glomerulosclerosis	

[a] In combination, diagnostic of diabetic nephropathy.
[b] Highly characteristic of diabetic nephropathy.
From Mauer SM, Steffes MW, Brown DM. The kidney in diabetes. *Am J Med* 1981;70:603.

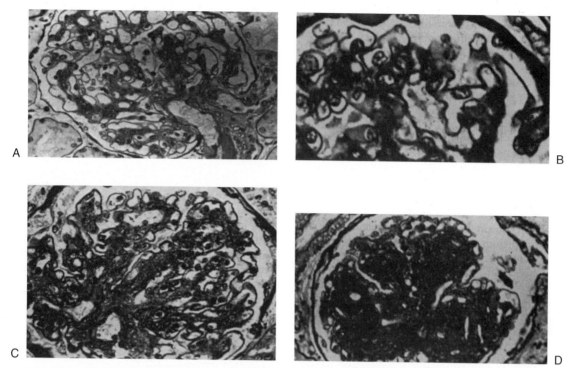

FIG. 73-6. Glomerulus from a patient with type 1 diabetes mellitus showing a mild, diffuse increase in mesangial area and replacement of smooth muscle cells in an efferent *(lower right)* arteriolar wall with "hyalin." [Periodic acid-Schiff (PAS), magnification ×325.] **B:** Glomerulus from a patient with type 1 diabetes mellitus showing a mild, diffuse increase in mesangial area, slight glomerular basement membrane (GBM) thickening, and capsular drops *(top left of center)* on the parietal surface of Bowman's capsule. (PAS, magnification ×630.) **C:** Glomerulus from a patient with type 1 diabetes mellitus showing moderate to severe mesangial expansion (diffuse diabetic glomerulosclerosis). (PAS, magnification ×300.) **D:** Glomerulus from a patient with type 1 diabetes mellitus showing severe nodular diabetic glomerulosclerosis (Kimmelstiel-Wilson lesions). (PAS, magnification ×400.)

ultimately can progress to the replacement of the smooth muscle cells of these small vessels by a waxy, homogeneous, translucent material (Fig. 73-6A). This and other "exudative" lesions of diabetes contain a variety of plasma proteins, especially immunoglobulins, complement, fibrinogen, and albumin (390,391). These exudative lesions may be related to inflammatory mediation cascades in that they are capable of fixing heterologous complement (392). Exudative lesions also may be seen in the glomerular capillary subendothelial space (hyaline caps) and along the parietal surface of Bowman's capsule (capsular drops; Fig. 73-6B). The latter most likely results from adhesion of capillary loops with hyaline caps to the parietal epithelium, deposition of the hyaline material, and retraction of the glomerular tuft (M. Mauer, personal communication).

Thickening of the GBM has been documented as early as 1.5 to 2.5 years after onset of type 1 diabetes, probably because minor changes in this parameter can be detected owing to the precision with which this dimension of GBM structure can be measured (104). Increases in the relative area of the mesangium appear to develop later (104), although this may be due to difficulty in measuring early changes, difficulties that are associated with variability in this structural measure among normal individuals (393). Nonetheless, it appears that increases in the volume of the cellular and matrix components of the mesangium can be detected in some patients as early as 5 to 7 years after the onset of diabetes (104,394,395) and within 2 to 5 years in the normal kidney transplanted into the diabetic patient (112–114).

These lesions appear to progress at rates that vary greatly between individuals and "spontaneous" improvement in lesions may sometimes be seen in renal biopsies spaced 5 years apart (M. Mauer and P. Fioretto, unpublished observations). However, the various renal structural changes do not necessarily develop at the same rate in the individual patients. Thus, changes in the GBM and mesangium are not highly correlated with one another (Fig. 73-7), with some patients having marked GBM thickening without much mesangial expansion and others uncommonly displaying the converse (13,394). Ultimately (13,394), marked renal extracellular basement membrane and mesangial expansion occurs in all type 1 diabetic patients who progress to renal insufficiency from diabetic nephropathy (see later).

The diffuse and generalized process of mesangial expansion has been termed *diffuse diabetic glomerulosclerosis* (Fig. 73-6C). *Nodular glomerulosclerosis* is diagnosed when there are areas of marked mesangial expansion forming large, round, fibrillar mesangial zones (seen with periodic

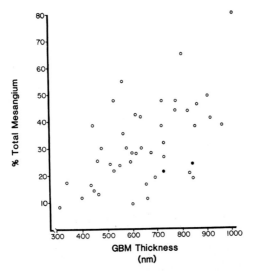

FIG. 73-7. Relationship of glomerular basement membrane (GBM) thickness and percent total mesangium (matrix + cells) in patients with type 1 diabetes. Percent total mesangium is equivalent to the mesangial fractional volume, or Vv(mes/glom).

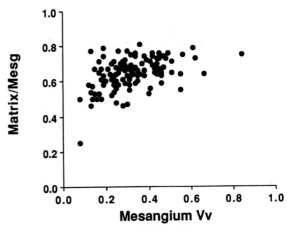

FIG. 73-8. The proportion of the mesangium that is matrix [matrix/mesangium (Matrix/Mesg)] in relation to mesangial fractional volume (mesangium Vv) in patients with long-standing type 1 diabetes. The normal value for Matrix/Mesg is 0.51 ± 0.08 (mean ± SD). Note that Matrix/Mesg is increased in most type 1 diabetic patients regardless of whether mesangium Vv is increased (>0.26).

acid-Schiff staining), with palisading of mesangial nuclei around the periphery of the nodule and extreme compression of the associated glomerular capillaries (Fig. 73-6D). This generally focal and segmental lesion has been hypothesized to be the consequence of dilatation of glomerular capillaries into microaneurysms (396). We have seen many examples of lesions that would clearly support this hypothesis. We have also noted examples of patients with occasional nodular lesions who have little or no diffuse glomerulosclerosis, thus supporting the contention that these two forms of diabetic mesangial expansion may, at least in part, have a different pathogenesis. In most instances, however, nodular glomerulosclerosis is seen in patients with advanced diffuse mesangial changes. Most important, nodular changes are not necessarily found in patients in whom overt diabetic nephropathy develops. In fact, approximately 50% of patients with clinical nephropathy have few or no nodular lesions.

The mesangial matrix fraction of the mesangial volume is increased in diabetic patients, often even in those in whom Vv(mes/glom) is still within the normal range (397) (Fig. 73-8). Thus, approximately two-thirds of the increase in mesangial volume in diabetes is due to ECM accumulation and one-third is due to mesangial cell expansion. Whether the latter is due to increased cell size, cell number, or both is unknown, but preliminary data are consistent with an increase in cell number (M. Steffes, personal communication).

These changes in mesangial and GBM ECM are characterized by expansion of all the intrinsic components of the mesangium, including types IV and VI collagen, laminin, and fibronectin (247), as well as additional intrinsic components of the normal renal ECM that have yet to be identified. These changes are consistent with increased production or decreased turnover, or both, of these intrinsic components. However, not all renal ECM components change in parallel

in diabetic nephropathy. Thus, α3 and α4 chains of type IV collagen persist or increase in the GBM of patients with developing diabetic renal lesions, whereas α1 and α2 chains are decreased in the peripheral capillary wall, even though initially persisting in the mesangium (251,252). Because the glomerular expression of "scar" collagen is very late in the evolution of diabetic glomerulopathy, the term *diabetic glomerulosclerosis* is, in fact, a misnomer. Accumulation of usual ECM components, not scar, represents most of the natural history of this disorder (247,251). Quantitative immunochemistry comparing type 1 diabetic patients on "slow" and "fast tracks" to nephropathy confirmed the aforementioned findings (252) and supported the view that the diabetic state has no uniform effect on ECM production and turnover, affecting different components in different locations variably. Nonetheless, the understanding of which ECM components are accumulating in the mesangium and GBM in diabetes is far from complete (252,253). Thus, quantitative electron microscopic immunohistochemical studies of mesangial types IV (252) and VI collagen (253), thought to be the dominant mesangial ECM molecules, have shown reduced densities in patients with rapid development of mesangial expansion, leaving the major ECM components responsible for this expansion yet to be described.

As the disease progresses and renal insufficiency ensues, more and more glomeruli either are totally sclerosed or, if incompletely scarred, have undergone closure of glomerular capillary lumina. We have noted that an increased fraction of glomeruli may be hyalinized in diabetic patients without the presence of advanced generalized diabetic glomerulosclerosis (398), and vice versa. Østerby and associates (399) showed that the distribution pattern of scarred glomeruli in diabetic patients with advanced renal disease is not random, but instead is oriented more often than expected by chance in the plane vertical to the capsule of the kidney. Perhaps this would be consonant with a pattern of glomerular scarring that results from obstruction of peripheral renal arteries (399). Our observations suggest that patients with increased numbers of sclerosed glomeruli tend to have more severe arteriolar hyalinosis lesions (398). Thus, both macrovascular and microvascular disease may contribute to renal injury in diabetic patients. Glomerular sclerosis and mesangial expansion are covariables (398), with these lesions tending to parallel one another in severity.

There is no precise relationship between duration of type 1 diabetes and the severity of the pathologic process described here (394). Although a statistically significant correlation between duration of diabetes and GBM and mesangial changes has been discerned, this was in selected groups of patients in three distinct clinical categories (i.e., patients early after onset, patients with microalbuminuria, and patients with established clinical diabetic nephropathy) (395). However, when patients with diabetes for at least 10 years with no other selection criteria are examined, no precise relationships between renal disease and duration of diabetes are found (394). This, in fact, is consonant with our knowledge of the natural history and marked variability in susceptibility to this disorder, such that some patients may be in renal failure after having diabetes for 15 years whereas others escape complications despite having type 1 diabetes for many decades. Thus, renal disease in a cross-section of patients with type 1 diabetes of long duration reflects the enormous variability in the ultimate clinical expression of diabetic renal involvement.

Structural–Functional Relationships in Diabetic Nephropathy

It is our view that the critical lesion of diabetic nephropathy that primarily leads to renal insufficiency in type 1 diabetic patients is expansion of the glomerular mesangium (394). A highly significant inverse correlation exists between GFR and mesangial expansion (394) (Fig. 73-9). However, when the absolute volume of mesangium per glomerulus is measured (i.e., mesangial fractional volume times glomerular

volume), this relationship, although statistically significant, is no longer very precise. Glomerular volume is an important variable that greatly clarifies these structural–functional interrelationships. Absolute mesangial volume per glomerulus and glomerular volume together predict peripheral glomerular capillary filtration surface per glomerulus with great accuracy, and filtration surface per glomerulus is directly and highly significantly correlated with GFR (400,401). More simply stated, moderate mesangial expansion occurring in a large glomerulus has relatively little effect in decreasing filtration surface, but the same degree of mesangial expansion in a small glomerulus is associated with a significant diminution of filtering surface and GFR. These and other data support the concept that expansion of the glomerular mesangium out of proportion to the size of the glomerulus is ultimately responsible for the decline in GFR associated with clinical diabetic nephropathy through effects on contiguous structures, specifically the glomerular capillary (compare Figs. 73-6A and 73-6D). As the mesangium expands, it ultimately restricts glomerular capillary luminal volume, distorts glomerular capillary diameter and length relationships, and diminishes the filtration surface (401) (Fig. 73-10). Although glomerular sclerosis (398) and capillary closure (402) also can influence this course of events, all the clinical manifestations of diabetic nephropathy in type 1 diabetes can occur in the context of minimal glomerular scarring (394).

Expressing the extent of mesangial expansion as a fraction of glomerular tuft area or volume fraction [Vv(mes/glom)] automatically factors for glomerular volume and is thus a good predictor of GFR. Fractional mesangial volume also is closely related to the presence or absence of overt proteinuria (Fig. 73-11) and hypertension (394,403). Thus, all of the major manifestations of clinical diabetic nephropathy are related to mesangial expansion and, necessarily, to distortions in glomerular capillary architecture. In contrast, the thickness of the GBM (394) is not closely related to GFR or to the presence or absence of hypertension. Although there is a direct relationship between UAE and GBM thickness (394) (Fig. 73-12), the finding that GBM width is more closely correlated with UAE among normal and microalbuminuric

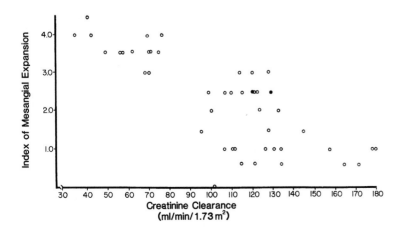

FIG. 73-9. Relationship of mesangial expansion and creatinine clearance in type 1 diabetes.

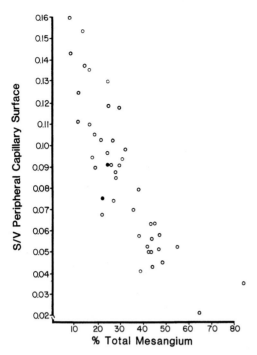

FIG. 73-10. Relationship of mesangial area and peripheral glomerular capillary filtration surface density (S/V) in type 1 diabetes.

patients (55,394), whereas Vv(mes/glom) is better correlated with UAE when all patient groups, including those with overt nephropathy, are included (394), suggests that different or additional mechanisms of injury to glomerular permselectivity may be operating in overtly nephropathic versus microalbuminuric patients. Total peripheral capillary filtration surface is highly correlated with GFR across the broad range from marked hyperfiltration to renal insufficiency (400,401,404).

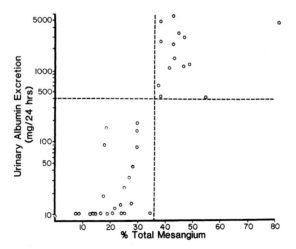

FIG. 73-11. Relationship of percent total mesangium and urinary albumin excretion in type 1 diabetes. Note that all patients with a total mesangium greater than 37% have clinical proteinuria (i.e., albumin excretion of 400 mg/24 hours), whereas the relationship between mesangial expansion and albuminuria at lower levels is not precise.

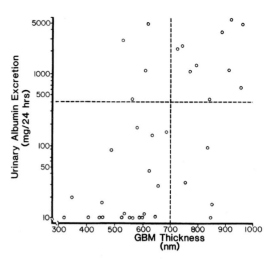

FIG. 73-12. Relationship of glomerular basement membrane (GBM) thickness and urinary albumin excretion in type 1 diabetes. Note the patients with marked GBM thickening and minimal or no increase in urinary albumin loss, and the patients with only modest GBM thickening and marked albuminuria.

Thus, hyperfiltration in type 1 diabetes is associated with increased filtration surface (400,401,404). Percentage global sclerosis (398) and interstitial expansion (405) also are correlated with the clinical manifestations of diabetic nephropathy and are, to some extent, variables independent of mesangial expansion in predicting the clinical manifestations of diabetic renal injury (i.e., proteinuria, hypertension, and declining GFR). In fact, some authors argue that it is the interstitial rather than the glomerular lesions that are more closely related to renal dysfunction in diabetes. However, this is seen only when interstitial measures are carefully taken and glomerular structure is subjectively estimated, and not when both are measured carefully. In fact, glomerular measures are stronger correlates of renal function in diabetes, especially at the earlier stages of the disease. Correlates of function with the interstitium are seen only when substantial numbers of late cases are included (405). Further, early interstitial expansion in type 1 diabetes is mainly due to expansion of the cellular component of this compartment, whereas increased interstitial fibrillar collagen is seen in patients whose GFR already is reduced (406). These and other findings suggest that interstitial and glomerular changes of diabetes have somewhat different pathogenetic mechanisms and that advancing interstitial fibrosis disease usually follows the glomerular processes. However, the exact contribution of these lesions to the renal dysfunction of diabetic nephropathy is very difficult to measure. Thus, progression from normal to microalbuminuria and from microalbuminuria to overt nephropathy is more closely related to progression of glomerular rather than interstitial disease (250).

Even more difficult and vexing has been the search for a clear structural basis for microalbuminuria. As emphasized already, persistent microalbuminuria in patients is a useful predictor for the development of clinical nephropathy, whereas the absence of microalbuminuria in patients with long-standing type 1 diabetes indicates a relatively low likelihood of overt nephropathy. Clinical nephropathy almost always is associated with advanced diabetic glomerular lesions in type 1 diabetic patients (394). One might reason that microalbuminuria is therefore predictive of the ultimate development of this pathologic process and, thus, would have a structural substrate. However, the relationship of renal structural changes to these low levels of UAE (i.e., normal or microalbuminuria) are complex and incompletely understood. Patients with long-standing type 1 diabetes (mean of 20 years) have, as a group, increased GBM width and Vv(mes/glom). These structural parameters in this group vary from within the normal range to rather advanced abnormalities (55). Patients with low-level microalbuminuria (≤ 30 μg/minute) are structurally similar to normoalbuminuric patients. Patients with microalbuminuric levels of UAE (>30 μg/minute) have even greater GBM and mesangial expansion, with essentially no values in the normal range, but overlap with normoalbuminuric patients (55) (Figs. 73-13 and 73-14). The incidence of hypertension and reduced creatinine clearance was greater in patients with microalbuminuria (>30 μg/minute) (55). Thus, higher-level microalbuminuria appears to be a marker of more advanced lesions as well as other functional disturbances (55). Nonetheless, patients with long-standing type 1 diabetes with normal UAE can have quite advanced diabetic renal lesions, although this is less common in normoalbuminuric patients with type 1 diabetes of shorter duration (406). Whether normoalbuminuric patients

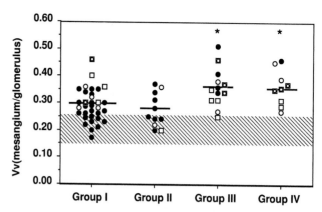

FIG. 73-14. Mesangial fractional volume [Vv(mesangium/glomerulus)] in the four groups of patients, as defined in Fig. 73-15. The *shaded area* represents the mean ±2 SD in a group of 52 age-matched normal control subjects. ● = Normal blood pressure and GFR; ○ = reduced GFR (<70 mL/minute/1.73 m²); □ = hypertension (≥140/85 mm Hg); ◙ = reduced GFR and hypertension. *P < 0.005 versus groups I and II. (From Fioretto P, Steffes MW, Mauer M. Glomerular structure and microalbuminuria in diabetes. *Diabetes* 1994;43:1362, with permission.)

with established lesions are more likely to progress to microalbuminuria and overt nephropathy than patients with less advanced lesions will require longitudinal study, but preliminary observations support this view (407,408).

Risk Factors for Nephropathy May Be Intrinsic to the Kidney

Nondiabetic members of identical twin pairs discordant for type 1 diabetes have GBM widths and Vv(mes/glom) values within the normal range (111). In each instance, the diabetic member of the identical twin pair had higher values for these measures than did the nondiabetic twin. This was true of TBM width as well. Several diabetic identical twins had values for GBM width and Vv(mes/glom) that were within the normal range, and could be discerned as having "lesions" only by comparison with their nondiabetic identical twin pair (111). However, some of the diabetic twins had severe lesions and overt nephropathy. Thus, the difference between individuals with type 1 diabetes appears to be the rate at which the diabetic lesions develop rather than their direction.

Some of the nondiabetic members of the identical twin pairs had increased muscle capillary basement membrane width (111) (Fig. 73-5), although there was no correlation between muscle capillary basement membrane width among the twin pairs. Further, this membrane width does not appear to be a useful predictor of the risk of kidney disease in patients with type 1 diabetes (409). Nonetheless, these data are compatible with the idea that there may be underlying cell or tissue characteristics in diabetic families that could confer susceptibility to or protection from important complications of diabetes, a highly controversial idea first proposed by Siperstein et al. (410,411) and by the renal biopsy studies in type 1 diabetic siblings discussed already. Supporting the

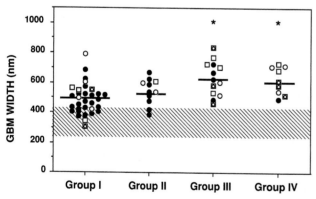

FIG. 73-13. Glomerular basement membrane (GBM) width in four groups of patients. Group I—normoalbuminuria [urinary albumin excretion (UAE) 22 mg/24 hours or approximately 45 μg/minute]; group II—low-level microalbuminuria (UAE = 23 to 45 mg/24 hours or approximately 15 to 30 μg/minute); group III—UAE = 46 to 100 mg/24 hours or approximately 31 to 70 μg/minute; group IV—UAE = 101 to 220 mg/24 hours or approximately 71 to 260 μg/minute. The *shaded area* represents the mean ± 2 SD in a group of 52 age-matched normal control subjects. ●, Normal blood pressure and GFR; ○ = reduced GFR (<70 mL/minute/1.73 m²); □ = hypertension ≤140/85 mm Hg; ◙ = reduced GFR and hypertension. *P < 0.005 versus groups I and II. (From Fioretto P, Steffes MW, Mauer M. Glomerular structure and microalbuminuria in diabetes. *Diabetes* 1994;43:1362, with permission.)

concept of risk factors intrinsic to the end organ are studies indicating a markedly variable rate of development of kidney lesions of diabetic nephropathy in transplanted kidneys, despite that each recipient had end-stage diabetic glomerulopathy in his or her own kidneys (113). This variability was only partially explained by differences in glycemia and was best explained by differences in susceptibility of the donor kidney to changes induced by the exposure to hyperglycemia (113). Preliminary data indicating that Na/H antiporter activity in the skin fibroblasts of kidney transplant donors is predictive of the rate of development of diabetic glomerular lesions in the type 1 diabetic recipient are consonant with this idea (J. Walker, L. Ng, G. Viberti, et al., unpublished data).

Mean glomerular volume and glomerular number have been proposed as structural determinants of nephropathy progression and risk. Filtration surface area per glomerulus is negatively correlated to mesangial expansion and positively correlated to mean glomerular volume (401). Mean glomerular volumes were significantly higher in a cohort of patients in whom nephropathy developed after type 1 diabetes of 25 years' duration compared with a group with nephropathy after only 15 years (412). Studies in normal humans showed that mean glomerular volume relates to body size, which is of course highly genetically determined. The number of glomeruli per kidney varies nearly threefold between normal individuals as well as in diabetic patients (413,414). This led to the hypothesis that fewer numbers of perhaps smaller glomeruli may influence nephropathy risk (415). However, although there appear to be fewer numbers of glomeruli in diabetic patients with advanced renal failure (414), this could be due to resorption of sclerotic glomeruli. In this same study (414), there was a small subgroup of type 1 diabetic patients with proteinuria whose glomerular number was not different from that of patients without proteinuria. If glomerular number were a determinant of nephropathy risk, fewer glomeruli in this subset would be predicted. Moreover, as already noted, rates of development of diabetic glomerulopathy in type 1 diabetic renal transplant recipients (one-kidney patients) are virtually identical to those seen in biopsies of native kidneys of type 1 diabetic patients (two-kidney patients) (416).

A Comparison of Nephropathy in Type 1 and Type 2 Diabetic Patients

Our knowledge of the natural history and of structural–functional relationships in nephropathy in type 2 diabetic patients lags behind that in type 1 diabetic patients, even though approximately 80% of diabetic patients with ESRD have type 2 diabetes. Renal structural–functional relationships in Japanese patients with type 2 diabetes (417) were initially reported to be similar to those described here for type 1 diabetes. Similarly, Danish proteinuric type 2 diabetic patients had structural changes similar to proteinuric type 1 diabetic patients, and the severity of these changes was strongly correlated with the subsequent rate of decline of GFR

(418). However, these authors found greater heterogeneity in glomerular structure in these type 2 than in type 1 patients with little or no diabetic glomerulopathy (418). Thus, the situation in patients with type 2 disease may be more complex than in type 1 diabetes, and a study of 52 northern Italian patients found that renal lesions in type 2 diabetes are quite heterogeneous (419). This study described three general groups of abnormalities. In the first group (19/52), patients had typical changes of diabetic nephropathy, including glomerular hypertrophy, diffuse and nodular mesangial expansion, and arteriolar hyalinosis. In the second group (16/52), there was a marked increase in the percentage of globally sclerosed glomeruli, whereas nonsclerosed glomeruli showed only mild diabetic changes. This was associated with severe tubulointerstitial lesions. In the third group (17/52), there were typical changes of diabetic glomerulosclerosis on which other nondiabetic lesions were superimposed, including proliferative glomerulopathy, membranous nephropathy, and others (419). In a Danish study (420), most type 2 diabetic patients (77%) with persistent proteinuria had diabetic renal disease, but 23% had a variety of nondiabetic glomerulopathies, including "minimal lesion nephropathy" (4/35), mesangial proliferative glomerulonephritis (2/35), mixed diabetic/mesangioproliferative glomerulonephritis (1/35), and chronic glomerulonephritis (1/35). All patients with proteinuria and diabetic retinopathy in this study had diabetic nephropathy. Although 40% of patients without retinopathy had diabetic nephropathy, 60% did not, suggesting that renal biopsies were more important in type 2 diabetic patients with overt proteinuria and no retinopathy. Similar results were obtained in a British study where, of 82 type 2 diabetic patients with renal impairment, 50 had typical diabetic nephropathy, 25 had other renal lesions, and 7 had mixed lesions (421). Again, retinopathy was a useful discriminator, but in this study as well, only approximately 40% of patients with diabetic nephropathy had retinopathy. In contrast, of 32 elderly Danish type 2 diabetic patients who underwent biopsy for clinical reasons, almost all had diabetic nephropathy lesions (422), and Ruggenenti et al. (423) reported typical diabetic lesions in microalbuminuric type 2 diabetic patients, but the latter were selected based on this criterion. Many proteinuric type 2 diabetic patients do not have retinopathy, however, and proliferative retinal lesions are less common in type 2 diabetes, suggesting a wider discrepancy in end-organ susceptibility than is seen in type 1 diabetes. Also, atypical patients tend to have renal biopsies for clinical indications, and this may explain some of the reported increase in incidence of nondiabetic renal disorders in type 2 diabetic patients.

Structural–Functional Relationships in Type 2 Diabetic Nephropathy

Østerby et al. found that type 2 diabetic patients tended to have less marked glomerular changes than type 1 diabetic patients with the same degree of proteinuria (424). However, in this comparison, the patients with type 1 disease had lower levels of GFR compared with type 2 diabetic patients with the same degree of proteinuria (424). One possible explanation of these findings is that the much larger glomerular volumes in the type 2 diabetic patients result in preservation of filtration surface. However, the explanation for the proteinuria in these type 2 diabetic patients, as alluded to earlier, was somewhat obscure. Nonetheless, these authors found a significant correlation between filtration surface per glomerulus and GFR, which ranged from 24 to 146 mL/minute/1.73 m^2 in these patients (424). In a study performed in type 2 diabetic Pima Indian patients, Vv(mes/glom) increased progressively from early diabetes to long-term diabetes with normoalbuminuria, to microalbuminuria, and finally to clinical nephropathy (425). There was no relationship between GFR and filtration surface per glomerulus in these various functional subgroups, but the range of GFRs in this patient population was not as great as in the Danish studies of Østerby et al. (424). Global glomerular sclerosis was considered an important correlative of reduced GFR in this study of Pima Indian type 2 diabetic patients (425). These authors also considered that glomerular podocyte loss was related to proteinuria in these patients, although this was not seen in microalbuminuric patients and thus is more likely to be a progression factor than one involved in the genesis of diabetic glomerulopathy. Moreover, further validation of the cell counting method used is needed.

The looser association between electron microscopic morphometric analysis of glomerular structure and renal function in type 2 diabetic patients compared with type 1 diabetic patients noted in the aforementioned studies may in part be explained by observations suggesting more complex patterns of renal injury in type 2 diabetic patients with microalbuminuria (426). Thirty-four white northern Italian type 2 diabetic patients with microalbuminuria underwent biopsy for research purposes. Three categories of renal structure were discerned by light microscopic analysis. In category I (CI; N = 10), renal structure by light microscopy was normal or near normal, showing only mild mesangial expansion, tubulointerstitial changes, or arteriolar hyalinosis, in any combination. In category II (CII; N = 10), patients had typical diabetic nephropathologic findings with balanced severity of glomerular, tubulointerstitial, and arteriolar changes, more typical of what is seen in type 1 diabetic patients. Category III (CIII; N =14) patients had atypical patterns of renal injury. These patients had absent or only mild glomerular diabetic changes with disproportionately severe renal structural lesions, including tubulointerstitial injury, advanced glomerular arteriolar hyalinosis, and global glomerular sclerosis exceeding 25%. That the lesions in CIII patients are of diabetic origin is suggested by the fact that HbA_{1c} was more elevated in this group and in CII than in CI patients. However, CIII patients differed from CII patients in having a higher body mass index and a lower incidence of proliferative retinopathy. Thus, the CII patients in this study may be similar to the type 2 diabetic patients with retinopathy in the Danish studies referred to previously (420,424). Findings in the CIII patients suggest that the kidney may react differently to hyperglycemia in different subpopulations with type 2 diabetes. This might reflect the heterogeneous nature of type 2 diabetes *per se* or different responses of the kidney to diabetes at different ages.

Recent unpublished observations suggest that these patterns also are seen in proteinuric type 2 diabetic patients; although a lower proportion of these patients are in CI compared with normoalbuminuric or microalbuminuric patients; approximately 15% of type 2 diabetic patients with proteinuria still had minimal renal lesions (P. Fioretto, unpublished data). A substantial proportion of proteinuric type 2 diabetic patients were in CIII, similar to the proportion for microalbuminuric patients. These categorizations have been confirmed by electron microscopic studies (P. Fioretto, unpublished data). Moreover, similar results have been found in Japanese type 2 diabetic patients studied by similar methods (T. Moriya, M. Mauer, unpublished data).

In summary, it appears that renal structural changes in type 2 diabetes are more complex than in type 1 disease. Approximately one-third of patients show atypical patterns of renal injury, and these are related to greater body mass index and a paucity of advanced retinopathy findings. Type 2 diabetic patients with microalbuminuria or proteinuria may have minimal lesions. Some subgroups of type 2 diabetic patients, such as Pima Indians, may more closely resemble type 1 diabetic patients, perhaps because of their young age of onset. Further cross-sectional and longitudinal studies in type 2 diabetic patients are required before the nature of these complexities can be better understood.

The heterogeneity of glomerular structure also appears to be related to the risk of progressive GFR loss in type 2 diabetic patients. Thus, Nosadini et al. showed that GFR decline over 4 years in microalbuminuric and proteinuric type 2 diabetic patients occurred among those patients with more advanced diabetic glomerulopathy as defined by electron microscopic morphometric analyses (427). Similarly, Christensen et al. found a more rapid GFR decline and rise in albuminuria in type 2 diabetic patients with typical diabetic glomerulopathy versus atypical cases (428).

It is particularly vexing that a combination of signs previously attributed to type 2 diabetes, including hypertension, coronary heart disease, increased plasma triglyceride levels, and decreased high-density lipoprotein cholesterol concentrations, accompany hyperglycemia in what Reaven termed *syndrome X* (429). Renal dysfunction in syndrome X, simulating nephropathy in type 2 diabetes, could be the consequence of hypertensive nephrosclerosis, hyperlipidemic renal artery atherosclerosis, renal hypoperfusion due to congestive heart failure, or the synergistic effects of two or more of these factors. Thus, population studies showed that an elevated UAE rate is associated with the features of this syndrome, namely, some degree of glucose intolerance, obesity, dyslipidemia, and elevated BP (E. Vestbo, unpublished results).

Other Renal Disorders in Diabetic Patients

Although it is suspected that other renal disorders such as nil lesion nephrotic syndrome (430) and membranous nephropathy (431) may occur with greater frequency in the type 1 diabetic patient population than among nondiabetic patients, in fact, less than 1% of type 1 diabetic patients with 10 or more years of diabetes and less than 4% of those with proteinuria and diabetes of long duration have conditions other than or in addition to diabetic nephropathy (personal observations). As already discussed, proteinuric type 2 diabetic patients with no retinopathy may have a high incidence of atypical renal biopsies or other diseases. Proteinuric type 1 diabetic patients with disease of less than 10 years' duration or type 2 diabetic patients without retinopathy should be thoroughly evaluated for other renal diseases, and renal biopsy for diagnosis and prognosis should be strongly considered.

DIABETIC NEPHROPATHY LESIONS ARE REVERSIBLE

Rats with long-term experimental diabetes show mesangial expansion that, by light microscopic studies, reverses within 2 months after the transplantation of their kidney into nondiabetic rats (104). Similarly, mesangial expansion reverses in long-standing diabetic rats by 2 months after successful islet transplantation (105). However, GBM width does not improve over this time (432), and in rats, unlike humans, mesangial expansion is due equally to matrix and cellular expansion, both of which improve with successful reversal of the diabetic state in these animals (433). It therefore was disappointing that no amelioration of established diabetic nephropathy lesions could be documented in long-standing type 1 diabetic patients (duration ≈20 years) at 5 years after the establishment of normoglycemia after successful pancreatic transplantation (434). However, after 10 years of pancreas transplant–induced normoglycemia, these patients had marked improvement in diabetic nephropathy lesions. Both GBM and TBM width were significantly improved compared with the baseline and 5-year values, with several measures falling into the normal range at the 10-year biopsy (435) (Fig. 73-15). Vv(mes/glom) also was improved at 10 years, mainly owing to a decrease in mesangial matrix fractional volume; again, in several instances, these parameters fell from the abnormal into the normal range (Fig. 73-15). Light microscopic observations confirmed these findings and showed remarkable glomerular architectural remodeling, including the disappearance of Kimmelstiel-Wilson nodular lesions (435). The reason for the long delay before the reversal process begins is a matter of speculation; however, it is clear that the mechanism for such architectural remodeling and healing exists. For this to be the case, the relevant renal cells must "know" that there is an abnormal ECM environment and must be able to respond to this with the expression of another form of ECM imbalance in which ECM removal exceeds production. This clearly is not the norm because

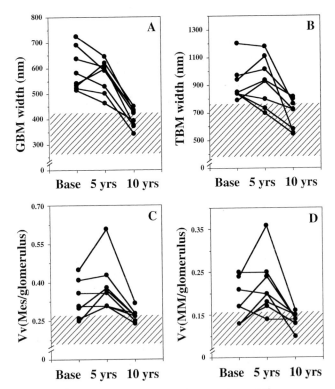

FIG. 73-15. Glomerular and tubular morphometric measures at baseline and 5 and 10 years after successful pancreas transplantation in nonuremic patients with long-standing type 1 diabetes. (From Fioretto P, Steffes MW, Sutherland DER, et al. Reversal of lesions of diabetic nephropathy after pancreas transplantation. *N Engl J Med* 1998;339:69, with permission.)

throughout adult life glomerular ECM production and removal remain in balance and GBM width and Vv(mes/glom) remain quite constant (393). Research into the control mechanisms for this healing process could lead to the prevention of these changes, even in the face of persistent hyperglycemia.

CLINICAL ASPECTS OF DIABETIC NEPHROPATHY

Diabetic nephropathy in both type 1 and type 2 diabetic patients characteristically follows a well-charted course, but coincident cardiac or hepatic disease may blur or mute its expression. Typically, the stages of diabetic nephropathy are as outlined previously. In this section, the stages at which renal functional changes are detectable and the management aspects of these stages are described.

Microalbuminuric Stage

The microalbuminuric stage is a clinically silent period, lasting 10 years or longer, before the first symptoms attributable to diabetic nephropathy appear (Fig. 73-16). Once microalbuminuria has progressed to proteinuria–a later marker of renal damage–leg swelling or generalized weight gain (reflecting fluid retention) signals substantive urinary protein loss, often

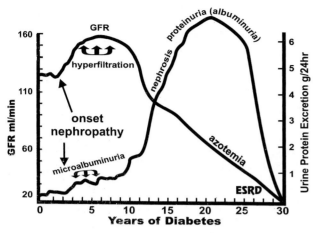

FIG. 73-16. The natural history of kidney disease in diabetes begins with the pathophysiologic perturbations of increased glomerular filtration rate (GFR), termed *hyperfiltration,* and the excretion of small amounts of albumin, termed *microalbuminuria.* Thereafter, proteinuria, nephrosis, azotemia, and end-stage renal disease follow in sequence. These stages are similar in type 1 and type 2 diabetes.

associated with hypoproteinemia. Microalbuminuria is an important sign and, as discussed earlier, is highly correlated with the subsequent development of clinical renal disease, proliferative diabetic retinopathy, and cardiovascular mortality (436–438).

In practice, the diagnosis of diabetic nephropathy almost always is based on clinical grounds, including a history of diabetes for a decade or longer, proteinuria preceding azotemia, and evidence of coincident extrarenal vasculopathy (retinopathy, peripheral vascular disease, coronary artery disease). However, as mentioned earlier, these are circumstances in which a complete nephrologic evaluation, perhaps including a renal biopsy, may be warranted. Also as noted earlier, although patients with syndrome X (in which type 2 diabetes is associated with hyperlipidemia, insulin resistance, hypertension, coronary artery disease, and low levels of high-density lipoproteins) may present with renal dysfunction simulating diabetic nephropathy; the etiology of their renal disease may be hypertensive nephrosclerosis, hyperlipidemic renal artery stenosis, poor renal perfusion due to congestive heart failure, or the synergistic effects of two or more of these factors. Kidney biopsy may be especially helpful in older patients in whom hypertension and degenerative vascular disease may simulate diabetic nephropathy. Illustrating this point is the impressive finding that in a clinicopathologic retrospective clinical kidney biopsy study of 334 patients 65 years of age or older, 33 had diabetes mellitus. Twenty-two of these 33 diabetic patients (66.7%) had pathologic findings not related to diabetes (439).

Nephrotic Stage

The nephrotic stage is defined as daily urinary protein excretion in excess of 3.5 g, associated with hypoalbuminemia,

hyperlipidemia, and varying degrees of extracellular fluid retention that may progress to anasarca. Diabetic proteinuric patients may retain fluid at higher levels of serum albumin than nondiabetic patients. The explanation for this observation is unclear. However, it is known that glycated albumin—a product of hyperglycemic protein denaturation—moves more freely than normal albumin across the GBM both *in vitro* (440) and in diabetic patients (441), and this could be true of other basement membranes in the body. There is little difficulty in ascribing nephrosis to diabetes in a young proteinuric person with type 1 diabetes, diabetic retinopathy, and no signs of heart disease. By contrast, however, the volume-overloaded older patient with type 2 diabetes often presents a perplexing mixture of heart and kidney disease. Relief from the burden of excess extracellular fluid by vigorous diuresis, using metolazone (5 to 20 mg once daily) plus furosemide (50 to 80 mg twice daily), either unmasks conjoint congestive heart failure by persistent effort intolerance and fatigue or, more commonly, answers the question of which organ system was responsible by inducing complete cardiac remission.

Azotemic Stage

The azotemic stage is an evolutionary transformation from the nephrotic stage of diabetic nephropathy as renal function declines (Fig. 73-16). Renal function appears to deteriorate at a slower rate in type 1 than in type 2 diabetes. This distinction may be illusory, however, because, according to the natural history of diabetic retinopathy, there often is a delay of 5 to 10 years in the diagnosis of type 2 diabetes in its incipient stages. Indicative of the relative rates of progression of the two types of diabetes is the study by Yokoyama et al., who reported that in a series of 1,578 Japanese patients with onset of diabetes before age 30 years, 39% (620 patients) had type 1 and 61% (958 patients) had type 2 diabetes (442). In these early-onset diabetic patients, the incidence of diabetic nephropathy was twice as high in those with type 2 compared with type 1 diabetes. Furthermore, these investigators noted a shorter interval from diagnosis of diabetes to development of nephropathy in the cohort with type 2 diabetes than in those with type 1 diabetes (442). Supporting the inference that the course of type 2 diabetic nephropathy may be more rapid in type 2 than in type 1 diabetes is a survey in Texas, where the interval between diagnosis of diabetes and development of ESRD in each of three ethnic/racial groups was 22 years for type 1 diabetes and 17 years for type 2 diabetes (443).

The DCCT and other studies in type 1 diabetic patients provide conclusive evidence that strict glycemic control in type 1 diabetes delays the onset of retinopathy and nephropathy (primary prevention) while also slowing progression of already established retinopathy (secondary prevention) (24,444–446). As noted earlier, confirmation of the value of careful metabolic control in type 2 diabetes was provided in the UKPDS, which included over 4,000 patients, with prolonged follow-up to 10 years. Participants in the UKPDS who achieved strict glycemic control effected a 25% reduction in the risk of microvascular complications (117), a direction similar to that of earlier studies (447–449). Shichiri et al. (450) also examined the effect of intensified glycemic control in a prospective study with an 8-year follow-up in 110 Japanese patients with type 2 diabetes, of whom 55 did not have retinopathy (primary prevention) and 55 had background retinopathy (secondary prevention). Rates of both retinopathy and nephropathy were significantly lower in those with superior glycemic control ($HbA_{1c} < 6.5\%$), and neurologic tests indicated improvement in this group compared with those assigned to conventional insulin injection therapy (450).

Reduction of systemic BP with antihypertensive therapy effectively slows progression of renal disease (451–453). Without question, the most seminal advance in efforts to delay the progression of diabetic nephropathy is application of increasingly effective BP reduction regimens using a variety of antihypertensive medications, including ACE inhibitors (454–457) and calcium channel blockers (458–460). Intensive antihypertensive therapy achieving a BP level below 130/80 mm Hg, with an optimal goal of 120/80, decreases the rate of progression of diabetic nephropathy, regardless of the pharmacologic means used.

The value of dietary protein restriction, once proposed as beneficial in retarding deterioration of renal function in diabetes, is based on studies with only short-term (<12 months) follow-up (461–468). Pijls et al. evaluated the effect of protein restriction on albuminuria in 121 type 2 diabetic patients with microalbuminuria or overt proteinuria (58 patients on protein restriction and 63 patients on a control diet). After completion of 6 and 12 months of dietary protein restriction, respectively, albuminuria was 28% (P < 0.001) and 18% (P = 0.08) lower in the experimental than in the control groups (461).

On the other hand, several trials of dietary protein restriction reported no benefit to progression of renal disease (469–472). Sampson et al., for example, discerned no relationship between mean dietary protein intake and GFR in a prospective study of 20 patients with type 1 diabetes and early nephropathy (470). A large, multicenter trial of protein restriction in nondiabetic patients conducted by Jameel et al. also was unable to retard the time to occurrence of ESRD and death (471). Consensus as to the renoprotective effect of protein restriction in diabetes still is incomplete because of contradictory reports. As a clinical compromise, many nephrologists advise avoidance of excess dietary protein in the belief that the rate of deterioration of renal function will be slowed.

COMORBID RISK FACTORS

To expedite management of the myriad microvascular and macrovascular complications that accompany ESRD in diabetic nephropathy, an inventory of comorbid risk factors should be made (Table 73-4). Subsequent selection of ESRD therapy for a diabetic patient whose kidneys are failing

TABLE 73-4. *Options in uremia therapy for diabetic patients with end-stage renal disease*

1. No specific uremia intervention = passive suicide
2. Peritoneal dialysis
   Intermittent peritoneal dialysis
   Continuous ambulatory peritoneal dialysis
   Continuous cyclic peritoneal dialysis
3. Hemodialysis
   Facility hemodialysis
   Home hemodialysis
4. Renal transplantation
   Cadaver donor kidney
   Living donor kidney
5. Pancreas plus kidney transplantation
   Type 1
   ?Type 2

requires a team approach, as well as appreciation of the patient's family, social, and economic circumstances. Home hemodialysis, for example, is unworkable for a blind diabetic patient who lives alone. Deciding on a kidney transplant requires knowledge of the patient's family structure, including willingness to participate by donating a kidney. Without a predetermined plan, the diabetic patient with ESRD is subjected to repetitive, inconclusive studies instead of implementation of urgently required treatment (e.g., panretinal photocoagulation or arterial bypass surgery).

A life plan may elect "no treatment" when life extension is unacceptable. Illustrating this point, a blind, hemiparetic diabetic patient experiencing daily angina and nocturnal diarrhea, who is scheduled for bilateral lower limb amputation, may chose death despite his family's plea that he start maintenance dialysis. Because azotemic diabetic patients typically are depressed, however, a rational decision to die must be distinguished from temporary despair over a current setback. Despondent diabetic patients, on occasion, respond to visits by rehabilitated dialysis patients or transplant recipients by reversing their decision to die. It is unwise, however, to coerce acceptance of dialysis or a kidney transplant when life has minimal (or even negative value) to the patient.

Management of diabetic patients with progressive renal insufficiency is a challenge because of comorbid conditions that accompany the nephropathy. For example, glucose control becomes more difficult as renal function deteriorates, requiring constant dose adjustment of insulin or oral hypoglycemic agents. Diabetic azotemic patients have a higher mortality rate than nondiabetic patients with equivalent renal insufficiency, usually because of cardiac disease, sepsis, cerebrovascular disease, and pulmonary disease (Fig. 73-17). Bisenbach and Zazgornik illustrated the role of specific extrarenal disease over time in diabetic patients during the pre-ESRD period (473). They studied 20 patients with type 2 diabetes who had a mean creatinine clearance of 81 mL/minute for a mean of 74 months (range, 40 to 119 months). Twelve deteriorated to the point where dialytic therapy was required to sustain life, whereas eight, whose residual renal function decreased to a mean creatinine clearance of 13 mL/minute,

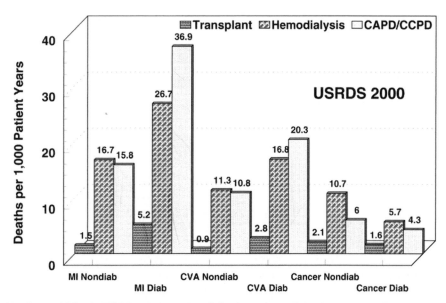

FIG. 73-17. Comorbidity in ESRD, 1996–1998, diabetic and nondiabetic patients by modality. Extracted from the United States Renal Data System 2000 Report, these data permit several inferences: (a) Renal transplant recipients, as a group, have markedly fewer deaths from myocardial infarction (MI), cerebrovascular disease (CVA), and cancer than do patients with end-stage renal disease (ESRD) undergoing either hemodialysis or continuous ambulatory peritoneal dialysis or continuous cyclic peritoneal dialysis (CAPD-CCPD); (b) whether treated with hemodialysis, CAPD-CCPD, or a kidney transplant, deaths from MI or CVA are greater in diabetic than in nondiabetic patients with ESRD; (c) in diabetic CAPD-CCPD–treated patients, the mortality rate is higher than in diabetic patients on hemodialysis; and (d) for undetermined reasons, cancer is a less common cause of death in diabetic compared with nondiabetic patients with ESRD. In all groupings, the effect of bias in assignment to treatment modality may override other factors determining outcome.

died owing to cardiac failure, sudden unexplained death, or stroke. Between the start of the study and initiation of dialysis or death, the prevalence of extrarenal disease rose sharply: retinopathy increased from 75% to 100%, cardiovascular disease increased from 45% to 90%, and cerebrovascular disease increased from 30% to 70%. Depression, often profound, results from the cumulative impact of vision loss, limb amputation(s), and cardiogenic limitation of routine daily activity. Withdrawal from dialytic therapy (tantamount to passive suicide) is observed more frequently in diabetic patients than nondiabetic patients (474). Listed in Table 73-5 are the most significant comorbid concerns in the management of diabetic patients with ESRD. Still to be ascertained as evidence-based conclusions are the contributions to diabetic morbidity from smoking, alcohol ingestion, and obesity, individually or in concert.

TABLE 73-5. *Diabetic complications that persist or progress during end-stage renal disease*

1. Retinopathy, glaucoma, cataracts
2. Coronary artery disease, cardiomyopathy
3. Cerebrovascular disease
4. Peripheral vascular disease: limb amputation
5. Motor neuropathy, sensory neuropathy
6. Autonomic dysfunction: diarrhea, dysfunction, hypotension
7. Myopathy
8. Depression

Diabetic Retinopathy

Retinopathy caused by diabetes is the leading cause of blindness in most developed countries. Of newly evaluated diabetic patients with ESRD, 97% have significant retinopathy (475), and 25% to 30% are blind or have severe vision loss (476,477). Many studies, including the DCCT and the UKPDS, have established that intense glycemic control can prevent or slow the progression of retinopathy in both type 1 and type 2 diabetic patients (24,117,478,479). In the ongoing, multicenter Wisconsin Epidemiologic Study of Diabetic Retinopathy in type 1 diabetic patients, the overall rate of progression of retinopathy was 86%, the rate of progression to proliferative retinopathy was 37%, and the incidence of macular edema was 26% over 14 years of observation. Regression of retinopathy was noted in 17% and was associated with lower HbA$_{1c}$ levels, whereas macular edema was associated with the presence of gross proteinuria (480). The ominous significance of retinopathy requiring laser photocoagulation in type 2 diabetes is evident from the study by Diglas et al. Of 157 patients followed for a mean of 5.1 years after laser treatment, greater than one-fourth (30.6%) of the study population died, 18.3% had a myocardial infarction, 14.7% had a limb amputation, and 8.3% developed uremia, but only 7.3% went blind (481). Laser treatment for diabetic retinopathy, in most cases, can prevent blindness, provided the diagnosis is made early enough. Advances in vitreoretinal surgery also have made possible the treatment of such late manifestations as vitreous hemorrhage and retinal detachment. Hayashi et al. assessed the outcome of vitrectomy performed on 76 eyes with proliferative diabetic retinopathy in 66 patients with ESRD. Visual acuity was improved in 60.5% of the eyes and remained unchanged in 31.5% (482). We advise that as a component of the initial evaluation of nephropathic diabetic patients, direct funduscopy, retinal photography, and fluorescein angiography be performed to provide a baseline facilitating interpretation of subsequent examinations.

Cardiovascular Disease

Cardiovascular disease is the comorbid condition that most frequently threatens life in diabetic patients with nephropathy. A number of studies have shown that microalbuminuria (the earliest stage of diabetic nephropathy) is an independent predictor for cardiovascular mortality in diabetic patients (483–486). Beilin et al. undertook a prospective longitudinal study of 666 type 2 diabetic patients, with a follow-up period from 1986 to 1993. When those with UAE of less than 30 mg/L were compared with those with urinary albumin levels of 30 to 300 mg/L, after adjustment for age, sex, and other cardiovascular risk factors, the hazard ratios were 1.77 (range, 1.22 to 2.57) for all causes, 2.34 (range, 1.38 to 3.99) for cardiovascular disease, and 1.78 (range, 97 to 3.26) for coronary artery disease (484).

Further to the point, Borch-Johnson and Kriener analyzed a study group comprising 2,890 type 1 diabetic patients diagnosed between 1933 and 1972. Those with proteinuria had a relative mortality risk from cardiovascular disease 37 times that of the general population, whereas in patients without proteinuria it was 4.2 times that of the general population (486). By the time diabetic patients reach ESRD, the relative mortality risk from cardiovascular disease is even higher. A study by Chantrel et al. consecutively evaluated 84 type 2 diabetic patients starting dialysis from 1995 and 1996. Cardiovascular disease was highly prevalent at the start of dialysis, with a history of myocardial infarction in 26%, angina in 36%, and acute left ventricular dysfunction in 67%; 32% (27 of 87 patients) died after a mean follow-up of 211 days, mostly from cardiovascular disease (487). Adding to the difficulty in management of diabetic nephropathy complicated by cardiac disease is the reality that extensive coronary artery disease often is asymptomatic in diabetes. Koch et al. evaluated cardiac integrity in 105 consecutive diabetic patients (77 type 1, 28 type 2), with a mean age of 43 years, during their first 6 months of dialysis treatment. Coronary angiography was performed in all regardless of clinical symptoms of coronary artery disease. Coronary artery disease was documented in 38 patients; 17 patients (36%) had single-vessel and 7 patients had two-vessel disease. In 11 of 38 patients, cardiac intervention was thought to be indicated, and 3 patients underwent coronary artery bypass grafting, whereas 8 patients had angioplasty (488). In this study, risk factors such as hypertension, smoking, and cholesterol and lipoprotein

(a) levels were not significantly different in patients with and without coronary artery disease. Manske et al. studied 151 type 1 diabetic patients with ESRD who were asymptomatic for coronary artery disease. Thirty-one had stenosis of greater than 75% in one or more coronary arteries, 26 of whom agreed to be randomly assigned to medical treatment (acetylsalicylic acid and calcium channel blockers) or revascularization (angioplasty or bypass surgery). Only 2 of 13 revascularized patients versus 10 of 13 medically treated patients reached a cardiovascular endpoint over a median of 8.4 months of follow-up (P < 0.01) (489).

In summary, coronary artery disease and congestive heart failure are the two most common causes of death in diabetic patients on renal replacement therapy, making a proactive approach necessary to reduce this risk. Investigation and intervention are warranted even in asymptomatic diabetic patients with ESRD and significant coronary artery disease. Whether prescription of aspirin, ACE inhibitors, and antilipid medication, as well as regular cardiac evaluations, will reduce mortality and morbidity caused by cardiovascular disease in diabetic patients with kidney disease is a subject under active investigation.

Limb Amputation

Almost half of all lower leg amputations are performed in patients with diabetes, and 5% to 25% of diabetic patients on hemodialysis undergo lower leg amputation each year (490). The threat of limb amputation persists in diabetic patients with a kidney or kidney–pancreas transplant (491,492). In over 70% of cases, amputation is preceded by trauma due to ill fitting shoes and precipitated by sensory and motor neuropathy with varying degrees of peripheral vascular disease.

Initiating a program to educate patients and family members about potential limb disease, with frequent examination of the feet, is a highly effective means of preventing limb loss (493). Van Gils et al. reported that in 124 high-risk patients (90/124 were diabetic), when simultaneous vascular surgery and podiatry triage and treatment were provided, only 18 of 124 required amputation after a mean follow-up of 55 months; 17 of these 18 patients had type 2 diabetes mellitus. Limb loss was avoided in 86.5% after 3 years, and in 83% after 5 years (494). Because failure of foot salvage in diabetic patients is due to problems of wound healing, early referral for revascularization before development of extensive tissue ischemia, gangrene, or infection is highly recommended. The appropriate treatment is prevention, consisting of daily washing, drying, and examination of the nails, soles, and interdigital creases of the feet, as well as wearing of comfortable, nonconstricting shoes with socks or stockings, and use of heel booties when confined to bed. Monthly visits to a podiatrist for nail and callus care complete the ideal program for the diabetic foot. Whether treatment with hyperbaric oxygen and application of genetically engineered skin grafts will reduce the rate of limb loss are subjects of current exploration.

Cerebrovascular Disease

The incidence of cerebrovascular disease increases as the severity of diabetic nephropathy progresses to ESRD (495). Once renal replacement therapy is initiated, death related to cerebrovascular disease is approximately twice as common in diabetic patients as in nondiabetic ones. Cerebrovascular disease also is regularly noted as a comorbid complication in diabetic recipients of a kidney or kidney–pancreas transplant. Nankivell et al. followed 82 type 1 diabetic patients who received kidney or kidney–pancreas transplants for as long as 10 years. Study subjects received carotid artery and lower limb vascular duplex scanning before transplantation, at 6 months posttransplantation, and then annually for up to 10 years. Carotid plaque was seen in 22% of patients at initial scanning, and this increased to 56.6% by 7 to 10 years (496).

Treatment options for stroke in diabetic patients with renal insufficiency require individualization and include risk factor modification—cessation of smoking, use of anticoagulation, adequate treatment of hypertension, and, in a selected group, carotid endarterectomy with or without arterial stent placement.

Autonomic Neuropathy

Autonomic neuropathy is a highly prevalent yet frequently overlooked disorder. Variably expressed in several organ systems, autonomic neuropathy impairs quality of life (gastroparesis, hypotension, and impotence) and may endanger the life of diabetic patients by inducing unawareness of hypoglycemia.

Diabetic cystopathy, although common, frequently is unrecognized and confused with worsening of diabetic nephropathy, and sometimes is mistaken for allograft rejection in kidney transplant recipients. Among 22 diabetic patients in whom renal failure developed (14 men, 8 women, with a mean age of 38 years), urodynamic study detected cystopathy in 8 (36%), manifested as detrusor paralysis in 1 patient, severe malfunction in 5 patients, and mild impairment in 1 patient (497).

Cardiac autonomic neuropathy is a common disorder seen in diabetic uremic patients. In one study, the prevalence of cardiac autonomic neuropathy was investigated in 117 patients, including 29 with diabetes (16 type 1 and 13 type 2) on dialysis, 40 patients on dialysis without diabetes, 32 diabetic patients without nephropathy, and 16 diabetic patients with a kidney transplant, as well as 25 healthy control subjects. Parasympathetic dysfunction was detected in 32% of the nondiabetic uremic subjects and 19% of those with diabetes without nephropathy. Cardiac autonomic neuropathy was evident in 88% of type 1 and 77% of type 2 diabetic patients on dialysis and in 75% of diabetic patients after kidney transplantation (498). Often manifested as loss of respiratory variation in heart rate and reduction in the physiologic nocturnal decrease in BP, it is clear that cardiac autonomic neuropathy affects most diabetic patients with advanced kidney disease (499). Silent myocardial infarction also is seen more often in diabetic patients with cardiac autonomic neuropathy (500).

Impaired gastric emptying (gastroparesis), a manifestation of autonomic neuropathy, affects approximately one-half of all diabetic patients (501,502) and is present in most azotemic diabetic groups when they are evaluated initially for renal disease (503). The diagnosis mostly a clinical one, but can be confirmed by a radionuclide gastric motility study that, if positive, prompts treatment with metoclopramide (preferably in liquid form) or erythromycin (504). Other manifestations of autonomic neuropathy of the gastrointestinal tract are obstipation and explosive nighttime diarrhea often coexisting with gastroparesis (505). Obstipation responds to a daily dose of cascara, whereas diarrhea is treated with psyllium seed dietary supplements one to three times daily plus loperamide (506) in repetitive 2-mg doses, to a total dose of 16 mg/day. Impairing quality of life and present in at least one-half of diabetic men with renal insufficiency is erectile dysfunction, which may improve with oral sildenafil, injected prostaglandins, or surgical insertion of a mechanical prosthesis (507).

Unawareness of hypoglycemia has been attributed to diabetic autonomic neuropathy, purportedly due to an inability to secrete counterregulatory hormones (glucagon and epinephrine) in response to hypoglycemia (508). In patients with diabetic autonomic neuropathy, decreased counterregulatory catecholamine responses may increase the risk for severe hypoglycemia (509). An important negative consequence of the struggle for tight metabolic control is the frightening increase in hypoglycemic episodes, some of which are detected late, at the point of loss of consciousness—a mean trade-off extracted as the price paid by patients who are dutifully compliant. Preliminary studies suggest that in uremic diabetic patients, autonomic neuropathy is, at least in part, reversible after pancreas–kidney transplantation (510,511).

These results are consistent with studies in nonuremic type 1 diabetic patients receiving pancreas transplant alone in whom diabetic neuropathy improved (512). Moreover, type 1 diabetic patients with autonomic cardiorespiratory reflex abnormalities had higher mortality rates that also were decreased by successful pancreas transplantation (513).

Motor Neuropathy

Sensory and motor neuropathy are common in long-standing diabetes. Uremic and diabetic neuropathy are indistinguishable by usual light microscopic techniques. Peripheral motor neuropathy progresses less frequently in diabetic patients with ESRD after successful renal transplantation.

Limited Joint Mobility

Along with an increased proclivity to proliferative retinopathy and diabetic nephropathy, diabetic patients manifest reduced range of motion for hand, finger, shoulder, and hip joints (514), a disorder compounded by the several arthropathies that affect the patient on long-term dialysis.

TABLE 73-6. *Variables in morbidity in diabetic kidney transplant recipients: the comorbidity index*

1. Persistent angina or myocardial infarction
2. Other cardiovascular problems, hypertension, congestive heart failure, cardiomyopathy
3. Respiratory disease
4. Autonomic neuropathy (gastroparesis, obstipation, diarrhea, cystopathy, orthostatic hypotension)
5. Neurologic problems, cerebrovascular accident, or stroke residual
6. Musculoskeletal disorders, including all varieties of renal bone disease
7. Infections including acquired immunodeficiency syndrome but excluding vascular access site or peritonitis
8. Hepatitis, hepatic insufficiency, enzymatic pancreatic insufficiency
9. Hematologic problems other than anemia
10. Spinal abnormalities, lower back problems, or arthritis
11. Vision impairment (minor to severe–decreased acuity to blindness)
12. Limb amputation (minor to severe–finger to lower extremity)
13. Mental or emotional illness (neurosis, depression, psychosis)

To obtain a numerical comorbidity index for an individual patient, rate each variable from 0 to 3 (0 = absent; 1 = mild— of minor import to patient's life; 2 = moderate; 3 = severe). By proportional hazard analysis, the relative significance of each variable isolated from the other 12 can be obtained.

Comorbidity Index for Diabetic Patients

To facilitate comparative grading within groups of patients, as well as to follow progress in individual patients during the course of ESRD treatment, we devised a rating system to inventory the type and severity of common comorbid problems. For each organ system, a numeric ranking score representing severity is assigned and the sum of all scores is taken as a comorbidity index (Table 73-6). Without some rating scheme, especially in very sick patients with multiple extrarenal disorders, it is difficult to gauge response to therapy, whereas deterioration may be overlooked. It is recognized that comparison between treatments [hemodialysis vs. continuous ambulatory peritoneal dialysis (CAPD) vs. renal transplantation vs. combined kidney and pancreas transplantation] demands more than simple scoring and that a more sophisticated tool for multivariate analysis, such as the Cox Proportional Hazard Model, is needed. For individual clinicians assessing their own patients repeatedly, however, the comorbidity index has proven helpful.

Comorbidity in diabetic patients on hemodialysis limits rehabilitation and results in an excess number of hospitalizations and longer hospital stays than in nondiabetic patients.

ENDING CONSERVATIVE MANAGEMENT

Although the development and progression of diabetic nephropathy may be retarded by normalizing BP, tightly controlling glucose, and adhering to a low-protein diet, many patients still progress to ESRD.

Continuing explanation to the patient of transpiring events and preparation for near-term developments builds confidence and minimizes panic, despair, and frantic behavior when the need for ESRD therapy becomes pressing. As the creatinine clearance falls to approximately 20 to 25 mL/minute, available options for ESRD therapy should be discussed and the patient's preference determined. Patient support groups, especially the American Association of Kidney Patients (AAKP), can play a vital role in guiding the patient with new ESRD in making appropriate choices regarding the type of therapy and location of facilities where treatment can be obtained. Membership in the AAKP should be encouraged as a key step in overcoming the shock, fear, bewilderment, and sometimes panic of first learning that one has ESRD. The AAKP's National Office telephone number is 1-800-749-2257.

Depending on the choice of treatment, there are specific preparatory steps that should be initiated. For example, for those opting for hemodialysis, construction of a vascular access—preferably an internal arteriovenous fistula—is of cardinal importance, thereby avoiding the pain and discomfort of percutaneous femoral or jugular venous cannulation until a suitable access is available. Predialysis management includes preserving forearm cutaneous veins by avoiding venous punctures and intravenous catheters. During the pre-ESRD interval, nutrition should be maintained and erythrocyte mass sustained above a hematocrit of 30%, as necessary, by administration of erythropoietin and supplemental iron. Metabolic bone disease due to secondary hyperparathyroidism may be minimized by use of intestinal phosphate binders along with synthetic vitamin D. Periodic (monthly) measurements of the serum calcium level to exclude hypercalcemia protect against vitamin D intoxication.

Resort to dialytic therapy or kidney transplantation should be effected before the patient loses muscle mass because of the catabolic state induced by uremia.

Although not proven by prospective alternative-case trials, consensus thinking suggests that renal replacement therapy should begin at a higher creatinine clearance (10 to 15 mL/minute) for diabetic than nondiabetic patients, because most diabetic patients become symptomatic at a higher creatinine clearance than do those with ESRD of other etiologies. Anorexia, nausea, vomiting, asterixis, and a reversed diurnal sleep pattern (insomnia coupled with daytime somnolence) are hallmark symptoms as uremia worsens. Indications for urgent dialysis include pericardial friction rub, unremitting gastric or colonic bleeding, seizures, and advancing uremic motor neuropathy (foot drop, paraplegia, quadriplegia, respiratory paralysis).

Preemptive kidney or kidney–pancreas transplantation is advocated at higher levels of residual renal function (creatinine clearance 15 to 20 mL/minute) in the belief that by avoiding the ravages of severe uremia, rehabilitation is more

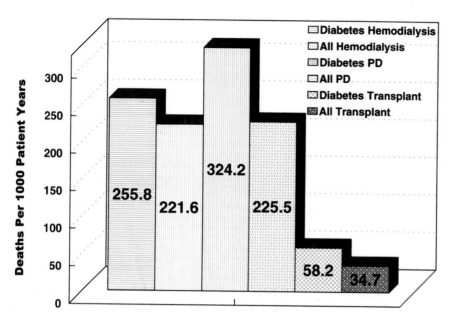

FIG. 73-18. ESRD death rates, 1998. These uncorrected death rates extracted from the United States Renal Data System 2000 Report demonstrate the adverse impact of diabetes on survival regardless of treatment modality, with transplant recipients evincing the best outcome. Although largely a product of selection bias in treatment assignment, treatment with peritoneal dialysis (PD), which combines continuous ambulatory peritoneal dialysis (CAPD) and continuous cyclic peritoneal dialysis (CCPD), had an inferior outcome in diabetes (higher death rate) than did treatment by hemodialysis.

likely to be successful. Even though evidence from a randomized, controlled trial showing a clear difference between early and late initiation of dialysis is sketchy and debated, an early start at a higher creatinine clearance level does ease management of BP and nutritional status, while probably retarding the progression of uremic motor neuropathy.

END-STAGE RENAL DISEASE

In the USRDS 2000 registry, as has been true for a decade, in the United States, Japan, and most of industrialized Europe, diabetes is the leading cause of treatment (incidence) of ESRD. The number of new diabetic patients accepted for renal replacement therapy has increased continuously during the 1990s, from 27% in 1988 to 40.5% in 1998 (1). Although the relative rates of ESRD treatment in Europe and Canada are approximately half that in the United States, a similar progressive increase in the proportion of incident patients with diabetes is reported (515).

Survival and medical rehabilitation of diabetic patients on renal replacement therapy is significantly inferior to that of other patients with ESRD (516,517) (Fig. 73-18). The highly prevalent comorbid conditions affecting diabetic patients when renal replacement therapy is initiated account for the greater risk of death and limited rehabilitation potential in these patients (515). With recognition and efforts to correct the impact of hypertension and dysmetabolism, survival of diabetic patients with ESRD has improved yearly since the mid 1980s (Fig. 73-19). A comprehensive team effort by both medical professionals and their patients, stressing the importance of preventive care to reduce hypertension, normalize blood glucose levels, and correct hyperlipidemia is rewarded by improved patient survival and rehabilitation.

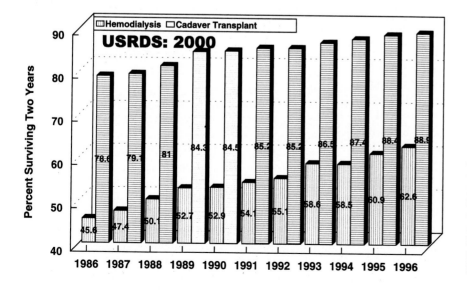

FIG. 73-19. Two-year survival rates of diabetic patients with end-stage renal disease (ESRD). Reflecting incremental improvements in management, especially better attention to blood pressure regulation and metabolic control, survival rates of patients with ESRD treated on hemodialysis or with a cadaver donor renal transplant have shown progressive improvement.

TABLE 73-7. *Comparison of end-stage renal disease options for diabetic patients*

Factor	Peritoneal dialysis[a]	Hemodialysis	Kidney transplantation
Extensive extrarenal disease	No limitation	No limitation except for hypotension	Excluded in cardiovascular insufficiency
Geriatric patients	No limitation	No limitation	Arbitrary exclusion as determined by program
Complete rehabilitation	Rare, if ever	Very few patients	Common as long as graft functions
Death rate	Much higher than for nondiabetic patients	Much higher than for nondiabetic patients	Approximately the same as nondiabetic patients
First-year survival	Approximately 75%	Approximately 75%	More than 90%
Survival to second decade	Almost never	Fewer than 5%	Approximately 1 in 5
Progression of complications	Usual and unremitting. Hyperglycemia and hyperlipidemia accentuated.	Usual and unremitting. May benefit from metabolic control.	Interdicted by functioning pancreas + kidney. Partially ameliorated by correction of azotemia.
Special advantage	Can be self-performed. Avoids swings in solute and intravascular volume level.	Can be self-performed. Efficient extraction of solute and water in hours.	Cures uremia. Freedom to travel.
Disadvantage	Peritonitis. Hyperinsulinemia, hyperglycemia, hyperlipidemia. Long hours of treatment. More days hospitalized than either hemodialysis or transplantation.	Blood access a hazard for clotting, hemorrhage, and infection. Cyclical hypotension, weakness. Aluminum toxicity, amyloidosis.	Cosmetic disfigurement, hypertension, personal expense for cytotoxic drugs. Induced malignancy. Human immunodeficiency virus transmission.
Patient acceptance	Variable, usual compliance with passive tolerance for regimen.	Variable, often noncompliant with dietary, metabolic, or antihypertensive component of regimen.	Enthusiastic during periods of good renal allograft function. Exalted when pancreas proffers euglycemia.
Bias in comparison	Delivered as first choice by enthusiasts though emerging evidence indicates substantially higher mortality than for hemodialysis.	Treatment by default. Often complicated by inattention to progressive cardiac and peripheral vascular disease.	All kidney transplant programs preselect those patients with fewest complications. Exclusion of those older than 45 yr for pancreas + kidney simultaneous grafting obviously favorably prejudices outcome.
Relative cost	Most expensive over long run	Less expensive than kidney transplant in first year, subsequent years more expensive.	Pancreas + kidney engraftment most expensive uremia therapy for diabetic. After first year, kidney transplant—alone—lowest-cost option.

[a]Continuous ambulatory peritoneal dialysis or continuous cyclic peritoneal dialysis.

Options in Uremia Therapy

End-stage renal disease in diabetic patients is treated similarly to that in nondiabetic patients, of all the options in therapy, a simultaneous pancreas and kidney transplant is restricted to diabetic recipients (Table 73-7). Although the choice of no treatment (passive suicide) is available to all patients with ESRD, this path is more likely to be elected by diabetic patients (518,519).

When advising a specific patient about the choice of treatment modality, medical, family, and personal factors must be taken into account. For example, a patient with severe cardiomyopathy may be restricted to CAPD because the stress of extracorporeal blood circulation would cause cardiac decompensation. By contrast, a young, motivated diabetic patient can choose from a menu of available treatments: hemodialysis at home or at a facility, peritoneal dialysis with CAPD or with a mechanical recycling device [continuous cyclic peritoneal dialysis (CCPD)], and kidney or kidney–pancreas transplantation.

Although the objective of uremic therapy is to provide different options to well-informed patients, in practice, most patients are assigned to the treatment preferred by the supervising nephrologist (520). This means that any subsequent comparison of outcome by modality is flawed by the nonrandom input. To illustrate, if healthier young patients are offered a renal transplant while near-moribund patients are relegated to peritoneal dialysis, it should not be surprising that rehabilitation and survival favor the transplant option.

No prospective, controlled trials of dialytic therapy of any type versus kidney transplantation have been reported. Therefore, what follows reflects an acknowledged bias in interpreting the bias of others. No distinction is made between ESRD treatment outcomes in type 1 and type 2 diabetes, mainly because key registries are flawed by counting all those treated with insulin as having type 1 diabetes. From several surveys of all treated patients on hemodialysis in Brooklyn, and a literature review, it is fair to estimate that more than 90% of newly treated diabetic patients with ESRD have type 2 diabetes. Therefore, even with partial correction of renal failure by dialytic therapy, the course of ESRD therapy in a diabetic patient is governed by the natural history of type 2 diabetes.

As a generalization, vasculopathic complications of diabetes are at least as severe in type 1 as in type 2 diabetes (521–523). Consequently, literature reports of the outcome of ESRD therapy by diabetes type are few and imprecise. We concur with Cantalano, who, when assessing the value of classifying diabetic patients with ESRD by type, remarked, "Classification does not appear to be useful when the individual patient is concerned, both in terms of management and outcome" (524).

Maintenance Hemodialysis

From the USRDS 2000 registry (Fig. 73-20), it is apparent that 74.3% of all diabetic patients with ESRD receive hemodialysis (center or home) as their renal replacement therapy, 7.3% are treated with CAPD or CCPD, and 17.1% receive a functioning kidney transplant (1). Given that effective hemodialysis is contingent on a continuous blood flow of up to 500 mL/minute, the need to establish a vascular access is an early concern. Peripheral vascular calcification in middle-sized arteries plus atherosclerosis of small vessels, as well as an increased risk of wound infection, may pose a

challenge for the vascular surgeon attempting to construct a vascular access in an azotemic diabetic patient. Although the preferable vascular access is an arteriovenous fistula, preexisting vascular disease limits its utility in diabetic patients, who have a primary failure rate of 30% to 40%. A less desirable, but necessary alternative vascular access can be constructed using a polytetrafluoroethylene graft with a half-life in excess of 1 year. Once it is established and functioning well enough to permit adequate hemodialysis, the mean 3-year survival rate of an arteriovenous fistula in diabetic patients is approximately 80%, whereas arteriovenous grafts remain viable in only 47% after 3 years (525). For many diabetic patients who survive beyond 1 year on hemodialysis, repetitive access revision, often requiring partial or total graft replacement, is the rule. The leading cause of hospitalization in diabetic patients with ESRD undergoing dialysis is complications of vascular access.

Hemodialysis treatment for diabetic patients is similar to that in nondiabetic patients, except for the interruption of dialysis because of intradialytic hypotension or painful, intractable muscle cramps. An ideal hemodialysis regimen consists of thrice-weekly dialyses, each lasting 4 to 5 hours, during which extracorporeal blood flow must be maintained at 300 to 500 mL/minute. Home hemodialysis can be performed by motivated patients wishing to maximize control over their bodies, a skill that is vital in managing diabetes. When dialysis sessions are timed precisely, it is noted that diabetic patients on hemodialysis actually receive a lower dialysis dose than nondiabetic patients because of the interruption of dialysis due to dialysis-induced hypotension or inadequate blood flow through the access (526). Intradialytic hypotension in diabetes is thought to be due to a depressed counterregulatory reflex in response to hypovolemia (527).

Glycemic control in a diabetic patient on a dialysis regimen is difficult. Insulin dosage is more complex in these patients because of unrecognized gastroparesis that disconnects absorption of ingested food from timed insulin administration, as well as reduced renal insulin catabolism that results in

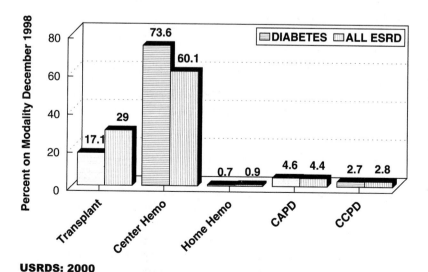

FIG. 73-20. ESRD treatment modality, diabetic versus total ESRD population. Compared with the entire group, as shown in these data extracted from the United States Renal Data System 2000 Report, diabetic patients with end-stage renal disease are more likely to be treated with maintenance hemodialysis even though their survival is best ensured by kidney transplantation.

prolonged action of exogenous insulin (528). This combination causes erratic glucose regulation complicated by frequent episodic hypoglycemia. Survival during the long-term management of ESRD in diabetes has been linked to the quality of glycemic control attained.

Defective bone matrix formation and mineralization without osteoid thickness characterize aplastic bone disease, a form of renal osteodystrophy affecting approximately one-third of uremic patients. Factors responsible for these mineralization defects have not been determined. Diabetic patients on dialysis are predisposed to adynamic bone disease, which is independent of exposure to aluminum (529). A prospective study of predialysis patients with a creatinine clearance of less than 10 mL/minute, none of whom had been treated with any form of vitamin D, showed that diabetic patients had low parathyroid hormone values and fewer bone lesions of advanced hyperparathyroidism (16% vs. 45%), whereas low bone turnover disease was noted in 56% of diabetic versus 41% of nondiabetic patients (530).

Maintenance hemodialysis does not restore vigor to diabetic patients, as documented first by Lowder et al. in 1986, who reported that of 232 diabetic patients on maintenance hemodialysis in Brooklyn, only 7 were employed, whereas 64.9% were unable to conduct routine daily activities without assistance (531). This finding was reaffirmed by an identical result in a survey conducted in 1999. Although in the United States the first-year death rate has decreased slightly in all patients with ESRD since the mid 1980s, diabetic patients on dialysis continue to evince the highest death rate of any large subset of U.S. patients with ESRD (1). Cardiac disease and infection are the first and second most prevalent causes of death in diabetic patients on hemodialysis.

Peritoneal Dialysis

Peritoneal dialysis is the ESRD treatment modality of choice for approximately 8% of diabetic patients in the United States. CAPD offers the advantages of freedom from a machine, performance at home, rapid training, slow and sustained ultrafiltration (less cardiovascular stress), and avoidance of heparin (532). As is true for hemodialysis, preparation of the patient for CAPD necessitates education, repetitive explanation, and facilitating surgery to insert an intraperitoneal permanent catheter. Motivated patients can learn the technique in approximately 1 week, although the usual training period ranges from 10 to 30 days. Volume exchanges of 2 to 3 L of sterile dialysate, containing insulin, antibiotics, and other drugs, three to five times daily are prescribed according to patient size, diet, and residual renal function. A satisfactory alternative to manual cycling of dialysate is the use of a mechanical cycling device in a regimen termed *CCPD,* which can be performed during sleep. During the course of both CAPD and CCPD, there is a constant risk of peritonitis as well as a gradual decrease in peritoneal surface area.

Diabetic patients with ESRD on CAPD experience twice as many hospitalization days as nondiabetic patients on CAPD; peritonitis accounts for 30% to 50% of these hospital days

(533). Surprisingly, despite the longer duration required for treatment of each episode, the overall risk of contracting peritonitis is no greater in diabetic than in nondiabetic patients with ESRD (534). Peritoneal dialysis is viewed by some nephrologists as the preferred choice of treatment for diabetic patients with ESRD (535), and there are specific indications for CAPD or CCPD when vascular access sites have been exhausted or in patients with severe hemodialysis-associated hypotension or angina related to atherosclerotic heart disease. An advantage of peritoneal dialysis for patients with poorly compensated congestive heart failure is its relatively slower ultrafiltration rate, coupled with less rapid removal of solutes resulting in smaller shifts in serum osmolality, which accounts for the absence of significant hypotension on CAPD. Hypotension may be provoked by repeated use of hypertonic (4.25%) dialysate exchanges. Another postulated advantage of peritoneal dialysis over hemodialysis is the avoidance of cytokine-mediated toxic responses provoked by contact of blood with biomaterials in the extracorporeal circuit and membranes used in hemodialysis (536).

To approach euglycemia when patients are continuously exposed to a dialysate glucose concentration of 1500 mg/dL, regular insulin (537) in large doses (60 to 130 U/day) is added to each bag of dialysate or injected through the connecting tubing (to avoid adsorption of insulin to polyvinyl chloride in the bag). Insulin requirements increase during peritonitis. A target 2-hour postprandial glucose level of between 150 to 200 mg/dL is advised.

Should insulin requirements exceed 100 U per exchange as gauged by widely fluctuating blood glucose levels, addition of subcutaneous injections of long-acting insulin usually is beneficial. Although intraperitoneal insulin administration minimizes the amplitude of glycemic excursion (538), high HbA_{1c} levels—even when glucose control appears satisfactory—may be noted. In all probability, what is being measured is carbamylated hemoglobin—a product of high ambient urea concentrations in uremia—which is indistinguishable from HbA_{1c} by usual chromatographic assays. An increased HbA_{1c} concentration also is found in nondiabetic patients with ESRD on CAPD; hence, HbA_{1c} as a measure of glucose control is rendered unreliable in this subset of uremic diabetic patients (539).

Malnutrition affects patients on both peritoneal dialysis and hemodialysis. CAPD-CCPD–treated diabetic patients become malnourished because of (a) reduced appetite caused by glucose infusion from dialysate, or early satiety due to increased intraabdominal pressure; and (b) large protein losses (8 to 10 g/day) in the dialysate fluid (540). With increasing duration of CAPD-CCPD, protein loss in the dialysate fluid rises in diabetic patients probably due to inflammation of peritoneum involving small peritoneal vessels (541). To maintain protein balance, patients on CAPD-CCPD should ingest at least 1.5 g/kg of protein per day, as well as between 130 and 150 g of carbohydrates per day. Although it is an impractical alternative because of high cost, malnourished patients on CAPD-CCPD reportedly extract nutritional benefit from dialysate containing essential amino acids (542). As is true for diabetic patients with ESRD treated by hemodialysis, the first and second leading causes of death during the course of CAPD-CCPD treatment are cardiovascular events and infections (other than peritonitis).

Switching of Dialysis Modalities

Patient acceptance of CAPD-CCPD may be less enthusiastic than for hemodialysis. An indication of patient preference is afforded by the decision, after 1 year of CAPD, by 49% of patients to transfer to a different ESRD treatment modality (543). Balancing the relative acceptance of the two major forms of dialytic therapy, only 37% of patients on hemodialysis opted to switch to peritoneal dialysis during the first year. Overall, more patients on CAPD-CCPD switch to hemodialysis (15.6%) than patients on hemodialysis switch to CAPD-CCPD (4.4%) (542). When technical failure prompts discontinuation of CAPD, peritonitis is the most common reason (544).

Kidney Transplantation

Diabetic nephropathy accounts for approximately 20% of kidney transplantations performed annually in the United States. One- and 5-year survival rates of diabetic patients with a kidney transplant, whether from a cadaver or live donor, have been improving consistently. In 1988, the 1- and 5-year survival rates of diabetic patients after kidney transplantation were 71.2% and 31.5%, respectively; survival rates improved by 1998 to 88.1% and 54.9%, respectively (1). Although improved survival of diabetic recipients of renal transplants is noted compared with survival on any form of dialysis (545–547), the comparison may be faulty because of a selection bias favoring healthier patients for transplantation.

Acknowledging this caveat, in the authors' view, the quality of life of a diabetic patient with ESRD with a functioning kidney transplant is substantially better than can be attained with either hemodialysis or CAPD-CCPD. More than half of all diabetic kidney transplant recipients, in most series, live for at least 3 years: many survivors return to occupational, school, or home responsibilities. Almost all diabetic patients with ESRD who have been treated by both dialysis (whether CAPD or hemodialysis) and a kidney transplant request a another transplant on loss of the allograft by rejection or other causes. In the patient's perspective, the vastly enhanced quality of life permitted by a functioning kidney transplant makes the choice between dialysis and solid organ replacement moot.

Kidney Plus Pancreas Transplant

Combined pancreas and kidney transplantation in type 1 diabetic patients is no longer an investigational procedure. Some centers have more than 10 years of experience with dual-organ grafting. The major benefit of a combined kidney–pancreas transplantation is the startling advancement in quality of life afforded by freedom from both insulin and dialysis; in this context, the improved patient survival rate is a bonus (548–551). Tyden et al. reported a 10-year follow-up on 14 type 1 diabetic patients subjected to combined pancreas–kidney transplantation, compared with 15 type 1 diabetic patients given a kidney transplant alone. After 10 years, recipients of a combined pancreas–kidney graft maintain normal glucose control, have improved nerve conduction and autonomic function, experienced better quality of life, and have a significantly lower mortality rate. Three of 14 recipients of a combined pancreas–kidney transplant died, contrasting starkly with the 12 of 15 kidney-alone recipients who died during follow-up (548).

Unique benefits of combined pancreas–kidney transplantation include normalization of both fasting glucose and HbA_{1c} levels, decreased plasma cholesterol, improved hypertension control, and a slowing of the rate of progression of both microvascular and macrovascular diabetic disease (552–555). As already mentioned, neuropathy can improve after combined pancreas and kidney transplantation (556–558). Further adding to the positive balance favoring dual-organ transplantation are studies indicating that diabetic retinopathy is stabilized in 75% to 90% of patients after a mean follow-up of 10 years (559,560). Kidney transplantation proffers better survival rates than any form of dialysis for diabetic patients, but combined pancreas–kidney transplantation may often even better survival rates and improved quality of life for type 1 diabetic patients. However, no randomized, controlled studies of dual transplantation versus kidney transplantation alone have been done, and selection bias could affect the studies published to date. Moreover, Manske et al. interjected a cautionary note in a study showing higher mortality rate among cadaver kidney–pancreas versus cadaver kidney-alone recipients (561), and urged careful selection of dual-transplant recipients (562). Finally, it may be reasonable to consider a well-matched living related donor kidney as a first step, with a cadaver pancreas transplant some time later. Whether patients with type 2 diabetes will gain biochemical or clinical improvement from either a pancreas or a pancreas plus kidney transplant is unclear. Preliminary reports from several clinical trials indicate that the dual-organ transplant may both normalize glycemic regulation and correct renal insufficiency to the same extent in selected type 2 diabetic recipients as has been observed in the type 1 recipient. Sasaki et al. described their unique experience providing 13 simultaneous pancreas–kidney transplants to type 2 diabetic recipients as documented by raised C-peptide levels. Unexpectedly, the graft survival rate in these type 2 diabetic recipients was 100% at a mean follow-up of 45.5 months (563). Although there are no prospective, randomized trials of available options in treating ESRD in the uremic diabetic patient, a compilation of advantages and concerns for the major treatment modalities is provided in Table 73-4.

SUMMARY

Diabetes is the disorder most often linked with development of ESRD in the United States, Europe, South America, Japan,

India, and Africa. Kidney disease is as likely to develop in long-standing type 2 diabetes as in type 1. Nephropathy in diabetes—if managed—follows a predictable course, starting with microalbuminuria, progressing through proteinuria and azotemia, and culminating in ESRD. The rate of renal functional decline in diabetic nephropathy is slowed by normalization of hypertension, establishment of euglycemia, and reduction of dietary protein intake. Compared with patients with ESRD of other causes, the diabetic patient sustains greater mortality and morbidity owing to concomitant (comorbid) systemic disorders, especially coronary artery and cerebrovascular disease. A functioning kidney transplant provides the uremic diabetic patient better survival with superior rehabilitation than does either CAPD-CCPD or maintenance hemodialysis. There are no reports, however, of prospective, controlled studies of dialysis versus kidney transplantation in diabetic patients whose therapy was assigned randomly. For the minority (<10%) of diabetic patients with ESRD, a combined pancreas and kidney transplant may cure diabetes and permit full rehabilitation. No matter which ESRD therapy has been elected, optimal rehabilitation in diabetic patients with ESRD requires that effort be devoted to recognition and management of comorbid conditions. Survival rates in diabetic patients with ESRD treated by dialytic therapy and renal transplantation are continuously improving.

REFERENCES

1. U.S. Renal Data System. *U.S. Renal Data System annual report.* Bethesda, MD: National Institutes of Health and National Institute of Diabetes and Digestive and Kidney Diseases, 2000.
2. Bojestig M, Arnqvist HJ, Hermansson G, et al. Declining incidence of nephropathy in insulin-dependent diabetes mellitus [published erratum appears in *N Engl J Med* 1994;330:584]. *N Engl J Med* 1994; 330:15.
3. Krolewski AS, et al. The changing natural history of nephropathy in type I diabetes. *Am J Med* 1985;78:785.
4. Andersen AR, et al. Diabetic nephropathy in nephropathic type I (insulin-dependent) diabetes: an epidemiological study. *Diabetologia* 1983;25:496.
5. Kofoed-Enevoldsen A, et al. Declining incidence of persistent proteinuria in type I (insulin-dependent) diabetic patients in Denmark. *Diabetes* 1987;36:205.
6. Rossing P, Rossing K, Jacobsen P, et al. Diabetic nephropathy: unchanged occurrence in patients with insulin-dependent diabetes mellitus. *Ugeskr Laeger* 1996;158:5940.
7. Caramori ML, Fioretto P, Mauer M. The need for early predictors of diabetic nephropathy risk: is albumin excretion rate sufficient? *Diabetes* 2000;49:1399.
8. Ritz E, Nowack R, Fliser D, et al. Type II diabetes: is the renal risk adequately appreciated? *Nephrol Dial Transplant* 1991;6:679.
9. Mogensen CE. Long-term antihypertensive treatment inhibiting progression of diabetic nephropathy. *BMJ* 1982;285:685.
10. Parving H-H, Andersen AR, Smidt UM. Early and aggressive antihypertensive treatment reduces the rate of decline in kidney function in diabetic nephropathy. *Lancet* 1983;1:1175.
11. Lewis EJ, et al. The effect of angiotensin-converting-enzyme inhibition on diabetic nephropathy. *N Engl J Med* 1993;329:1456.
12. Hostetter TH. Diabetic nephropathy. *N Engl J Med* 1985;312:642.
13. Mauer SM. Nephrology forum: structural-functional correlations of diabetic nephropathy. *Kidney Int* 1994;45:612.
14. Mogensen CE, Christensen CK. Predicting diabetes nephropathy in insulin dependent patients. *N Engl J Med* 1984;311:89.
15. Parving HH, Oxenbøll B, Svendsen PA. Early detection of patients at risk of developing diabetic nephropathy: a prospective study of urinary albumin excretion. *Acta Endocrinol (Copenh)* 1982;100:550.
16. Viberti GC, MacKintosh D, Keen H. Determinants of the penetration of proteins through the glomerular barrier in insulin-dependent diabetes mellitus. *Diabetes* 1983;32:92.
17. Viberti GC, Hill RD, Jarrett R.J. Microalbuminuria as a predictor of clinical nephropathy in insulin-dependent diabetes mellitus. *Lancet* 1982;1:1430.
18. Mogensen CE, Christensen CK, Christensen PD. The abnormal albuminuria syndrome in diabetes. In: Belfione F, et al, eds. *Curr Top Diabetes Res.* Basel:Karger, 1993;12.
19. Mogensen CE. Microalbuminuria and incipient diabetic nephropathy. *Diabet Nephropathy* 1984;3:75.
20. Pettitt DJ, Saad MF, Bennett PH. Familial predisposition to renal disease in two generations of Pima Indians with type II (non-insulin-dependent) diabetes mellitus. *Diabetologia* 1990;33:348.
21. Seaquist ER, Goetz FC, Rich S. Familial clustering of diabetic kidney disease. *N Engl J Med* 1989;320:1161.
22. Pirart J. Diabetes mellitus and its degenerative complications: a prospective study of 4,400 patients observed between 1947 and 1973. *Diabetes Care* 1978;1:168.
23. Hanssen KR, Dahl-Jørgensen K, Lauritzen, T. Diabetic control and microvascular complications. *Diabetologia* 1986;29:677.
24. Diabetes Complications and Control Trial Research Group. The effect of intensive treatment of diabetes on the development and progression of long-term complications of insulin dependent diabetes mellitus. *N Engl J Med* 1993;329:977.
25. Drury L. Diabetes and arterial hypertension. *Diabetologia* 1983;24:1.
26. Mogensen CE. Systemic blood pressure and glomerular leakage with particular reference to diabetes and hypertension. *J Intern Med* 1994;235:297.
27. Parving HH, Gall MA, Skott P. Prevalence and causes of albuminuria in non insulin-dependent diabetic patients. *Kidney Int* 1990;37: 243.
28. Østerby, R. Basement membrane morphology in diabetes mellitus. In: Ellenberg M, Rifkin H, eds. *Diabetes mellitus: theory and practice,* 3rd ed. New York: Medical Examination, 1983.
29. Østerby R. Lessons from kidney biopsies. *Diabetes Metab Rev* 1996; 12:51.
30. Mauer SM, Steffes MW, Ellis EN. Can the insulin-dependent diabetic patient be managed without kidney biopsy? In: Robinson RR, ed. *Proceedings of the IXth International Congress of Nephrology.* New York: Springer-Verlag, 1984.
31. Mogensen CE, Christensen CK. Blood pressure changes and renal function changes in incipient and overt diabetic nephropathy. *Hypertension* 1985;7:64.
32. Tung P, Levin SR. Nephropathy in non insulin-dependent diabetes mellitus. *Am J Med* 1988;85:131.
33. Schmitz A, Vaeth M. Microalbuminuria: a major risk factor in non insulin-dependent diabetes. A 10 year follow up study of 503 patients. *Diabet Med* 1988;5:126.
34. Moloney A, et al. Mortality from diabetic nephropathy in the United Kingdom. *Diabetologia* 1983;25:26.
35. Mogensen CE. Microalbuminuria predicts clinical proteinuria and early mortality in maturity-onset diabetes. *N Engl J Med* 1984;310:356.
36. Mattock M, et al. Microalbuminuria as a predictor of mortality in type 2 (non-insulin-dependent) diabetic patients: results from a 3-year prospective study. *Diabetologia* 1990;33:A49.
37. Fabre J, et al. The kidney in maturity onset diabetes mellitus: a clinical study of 510 patients. *Kidney Int* 1982;21:730.
38. Kunzelman CL, Knowler WC, Pettitt DJ. Incidence of proteinuria in type II diabetes in the Pima Indians. *Kidney Int* 1989;35:681.
39. Cowie CC, et al. Disparities in incidence of diabetic end-stage renal disease according to race and type of diabetes. *N Engl J Med* 1989; 321:1074.
40. Abourizk NN, Dunn JC. Types of diabetes according to National Diabetes Data Group Classification: limited applicability and need to revisit. *Diabetes Care* 1990;13:1120.
41. Sima EAH, Calles-Escandon J. Classification of diabetes: a fresh look for the 1990s? *Diabetes Care* 1990;13:1123.
42. Madsbad S, Krarup T, McNair P. Practical clinical value of the C-peptide response to glucagon stimulation in the choice of treatment in diabetes mellitus. *Acta Med Scand* 1981;210:153.

43. Mathiesen ER, et al. Incipient nephropathy in type I (insulin-dependent) diabetes. *Diabetologia* 1984;26:406.

44. Mau-Pedersen M, Christensen CK, Mogensen CE. Long term (18 year) prognosis for normo- and microalbuminuric type I (insulin-dependent) diabetic patients. *Diabetologia* 1992;35:A60.

45. Messent JWC, et al. Prognostic significance of microalbuminuria in insulin-dependent diabetes mellitus: a twenty-three year follow-up study. *Kidney Int* 1992;41:836.

46. Chavers BM, et al. Glomerular lesions and urinary albumin excretion in type I diabetic patients without overt proteinuria. *N Engl J Med* 1989;320:966.

47. Bangstad HJ, Dahl-Jørgensen K, Kjaersgaard P. Urinary albumin excretion rate and puberty in non-diabetic children and adolescents. *Acta Paediatr Scand* 1993;82:857.

48. Mathiesen ER, et al. Relationship between blood pressure and urinary albumin excretion in development of microalbuminuria. *Diabetes* 1990;39:245.

49. Mogensen CE. Kidney function and glomerular permeability in early juvenile diabetes. *Scand J Clin Lab Invest* 1971;28:79.

50. Mogensen CE. Glomerular filtration rate and renal plasma flow in short-term and long-term juvenile diabetes. *Scand J Clin Lab Invest* 1971;28:91.

51. Christiansen JS. On the pathogenesis of the increased glomerular filtration rate in short-term insulin-dependent diabetes. *Dan Med Bull* 1984;31:349.

52. Christiansen JS, et al. Kidney function and size in diabetics, before and during initial insulin treatment. *Kidney Int* 1982;21:683.

53. Hansen KW, et al. Normoalbuminuria ensures no reduction of renal function in type I (insulin-dependent) diabetic patients. *J Intern Med* 1992;232:161.

54. Mathiesen ER. Prevention of diabetic nephropathy: Microalbuminuria and perspectives for intervention in insulin dependent diabetes. *Dan Med Bull* 1993;40:273.

55. Fioretto P, Steffes MW, Mauer SM. Glomerular structure in non-proteinuric insulin-dependent diabetic patients with various levels of albuminuria. *Diabetes* 1994;43:1358.

56. Caramori ML, Fioretto P, Mauer M. The need for early predictors of diabetic nephropathy risk: is albumin excretion rate sufficient? *Diabetes* 2000;49:1399.

57. Forsblom CM, et al. Predictive value of microalbuminuria in patients with insulin-dependent diabetes of long duration. *BMJ* 1992;305:1051.

58. Wiseman MJ, et al. Glycaemia, arterial pressure and microalbuminuria in type I (insulin-dependent) diabetes mellitus. *Diabetologia* 1984;26:401.

59. Feldt-Rasmussen B, Borch-Johnsen K, Mathiesen ER. Hypertension in diabetes as related to nephropathy: early blood pressure changes. *Hypertension* 1985;7:18.

60. Mathiesen ER, et al. Prevalence of microalbuminuria in children with type I (insulin-dependent) diabetes mellitus. *Diabetologia* 1986;29:640.

61. Wiegman TB, et al. Comparison of albumin excretion rate obtained with different times of collection. *Diabetes Care* 1990;13:864.

62. Hansen KW, et al. Ambulatory blood pressure in microalbuminuric type I diabetic patients. *Kidney Int* 1992;41:847.

63. Christensen CK, Mogensen CE. The course of incipient diabetic nephropathy: Studies on albumin excretion and blood pressure. *Diabet Med* 1985;2:97.

64. Mogensen GE, et al. Blood pressure elevation versus abnormal albuminuria in the genesis and prediction of renal disease in diabetes. *Diabetes Care* 1992;15:1192.

65. Hansen KW. ACE inhibition and diabetic nephropathy. *BJM* 1991;303:1400.

66. Mogensen CE, Vigtrup J, Ehlers N. Microalbuminuria predicts proliferative diabetic retinopathy. *Lancet* 1985;1:1512.

67. Kostraba JN, et al. The Epidemiology of Diabetes Complications Study IV: correlates of diabetic background and proliferative retinopathy. *Am J Epidemiol* 1991;133:381.

68. Chavers BM, et al. Relationship between retinal and glomerular lesions in patients with type I diabetes mellitus. *Diabetes* 1994;43:441.

69. Cruicksh KJ, et al. A microalbuminuria as a predictor of the progression of retinopathy in younger-onset diabetic individuals. *Invest Ophthalmol Vis Sci* 1993;34:1182.

70. Brocco E, Fioretto P, Mauer M, et al. Renal structure and function in non-insulin dependent diabetic patients with microalbuminuria. *Kidney Int* 1997;63:S40.

71. Jensen T. Micro-albuminuria and large vessel disease in diabetes. *J Hypertens* 1992;10:S21.

72. Jensen T, Stender S, Deckert T. Abnormalities in plasmas concentrations of lipoproteins and fibrinogen in type I (insulin-dependent) diabetic patients with increased urinary albumin excretion. *Diabetologia* 1988;31:142.

73. Jones SL, et al. Plasma lipid and coagulation factor concentrations in insulin dependent diabetics with microalbuminuria. *BMJ* 1989;298:487.

74. Feldt-Rasmussen B. Increased transcapillary escape rate of albumin in type I (insulin-dependent) diabetic patients with microalbuminuria. *Diabetologia* 1986;29:282.

75. Manske CL, et al. Prevalence of, and risk factors for, angiographically determined coronary artery disease in type I-diabetic patients with nephropathy. *Arch Intern Med* 1992;152:2450.

76. Nelson S, et al. Assessment of risk of overt nephropathy in diabetic patients from albumin excretion in untimed urine specimens. *Arch Intern Med* 1991;151:1761.

77. Marshall SM, Alberti KG. Comparison of the prevalence and associated features of abnormal albumin excretion in insulin-dependent and non-insulin dependent diabetes. *QJM* 1989;70:61.

78. Gall AM, et al. Prevalence of micro- and macroalbuminuria, arterial hypertension, retinopathy and large vessel disease in European type 2 (non-insulin-dependent) diabetic patients. *Diabetologia* 1991;34:655.

79. Damsgaard EM. Prevalence and evidence of microalbuminuria in non-insulin dependent diabetes and relation to other vascular lesions. In: Mogensen CE, ed. *The kidney and hypertension in diabetes mellitus.* Boston: Martinus Nijhoff, 1988.

80. Ballard DJ, et al. Epidemiology of persistent proteinuria in type II diabetes mellitus: population-based study in Rochester, Minnesota. *Diabetes* 1988;37:405.

81. Mogensen CE. A complete screening of urinary albumin concentration in an unselected diabetic out-patient clinic population (1082 patients). *Diabet Nephropathy* 1983;2:11.

82. Ginsberg JM, et al. Use of single voided urine samples to estimate quantitative proteinuria. *N Engl J Med* 1983;309:1543.

83. Gatling W, Rowe DJF, Hill RD. Microalbumenuria: an appraisal of assay techniques and urine collection procedures for measuring urinary albumin at low concentrations. In: Mogensen CE, ed. *The kidney and hypertension in diabetes mellitus.* Boston: Martinus Nijhoff, 1988.

84. Poulsen P, Mogensen C. Evaluation of a new semiquantitative stix for microalbuminuria. *Diabetes Care* 1995;18:732.

85. Feldt-Rasmussen B, Mathiesen ER. Variability of urinary albumin excretion in incipient diabetic nephropathy. *Diabet Nephropathy* 1984;3:101.

86. Feldt-Rasmussen B, Mathiesen ER, Deckert T. Effect of two years of strict metabolic control on progression of incipient nephropathy in insulin-dependent diabetes. *Lancet* 1986;2:1300.

87. Mogensen CE. Urinary albumin excretion in early and long-term juvenile diabetes. *Scand J Clin Lab Invest* 1971;28:183.

88. Mogensen CE, Andersen MJF. Increased kidney size and glomerular filtration rate in untreated juvenile diabetes: normalization by insulin treatment. *Diabetologia* 1975;11:221.

89. Christensen CK. Rapidly reversible albumin and β2-microglobulin hyperexcretion in recent severe essential hypertension. *J Hypertens* 1983;1:45.

90. Schmitz A, Hansen H, Christensen T. Kidney function in newly diagnosed type II (non-insulin-dependent) diabetic patients, before and during treatment. *Diabetologia* 1989;32:434.

91. Damsgaard EM, Mogensen CE, Nielsen JR. Increased glomerular permeability to albumin in type 2 (non-insulin-dependent) diabetic patients before and after exercise. *Diabetologia* 1983;25:149.

92. Vasquez B, Flock E, Savage PJ. Sustained reduction of proteinuria in type 2 (non-insulin-dependent) diabetes following diet-induced reduction of hyperglycaemia. *Diabetologia* 1984;26:127.

93. Olivarius N de F, Andreasen AM, Keiding N, et al. Epidemiology of renal involvement in newly-diagnosed middle-aged and elderly diabetic patients: cross-sectional data from the population-based study "Diabetes Care in General Practice." *Diabetologia* 1993;36:1007.

94. Beck-Nielsen H, et al. Effect of insulin pump treatment for one year on renal function and renal morphology in patients with IDDM. *Diabetes Care* 1985;8:585.

95. Wiseman MJ, et al. Effect of blood glucose control on increased glomerular filtration rate and kidney size in insulin-dependent diabetes. *N Engl J Med* 1985;312:617.

96. Kroc Collaborative Study Group. Blood glucose control and the evolution of diabetic retinopathy and albuminuria: a preliminary multicenter trial. *N Engl J Med* 1984;311:365.

97. Mogensen CE, Christensen CK. Glomerular filtration rate, serum creatinine level and related parameters in incipient diabetic nephropathy. *Diabet Nephropathy* 1984;3:135.

98. Christiansen JS, Christensen, CK, Hermansen K. Enhancement of glomerular filtration rate and renal plasma flow by oral glucose load in well-controlled insulin-dependent diabetics. In: *Proceedings of the XII Congress I.D.F.* 1985.

99. Laborde K, Kevy-Marchal C, Kindermans C. Glomerular function and microalbuminuria in children with insulin-dependent diabetes. *Pediatr Nephrol* 1990;4:39.

100. Kupin WC, et al. Effect on renal function of changes from high to moderate protein intake in type I diabetic patients. *Diabetes* 1987;36:73.

101. Trevisan R, Nosadini R, Fioretto P. Ketone bodies increase glomerular filtration rate in normal man and in patients with type I diabetes mellitus. *Diabetologia* 1987;30:214.

102. Østerby R. Early phases in the development of diabetic glomerulopathy. *Acta Med Scand* 1975;475:1.

103. Brown DM, et al. Kidney complications. *Diabetes* 1982;31:71.

104. Lee CS, et al. Renal transplantation in diabetes mellitus in rats. *J Exp Med* 1974;139:793.

105. Mauer SM, Steffes MW, Brown DM. The kidney in diabetes. *Am J Med* 1981;70:603.

106. Mauer SM, Sutherland DER, Steffes MW. Pancreas islet transplantation: effects on the glomerular lesions of experimental diabetes in the rat. *Diabetes* 1974;23:748.

107. Rasch R. Prevention of diabetic glomerulopathy in streptozotocin diabetic rats by insulin treatment: kidney size and glomerular volume. *Diabetologia* 1979;16:125.

108. Rasch R. Prevention of diabetic glomerulopathy in streptozotocin diabetic rats by insulin treatment: glomerular basement membrane thickness. *Diabetologia* 1979;16:319.

109. Rasch R. Prevention of diabetic glomerulopathy in streptozotocin diabetic rats by insulin treatment: the mesangial regions. *Diabetologia* 1979;17:243.

110. Takazakura E, Nakamoto Y, Hayakawa H. Onset and progression of diabetic glomerulopathy. *Diabetes* 1975;24:1.

111. Steffes MW, Sutherland DER, Goetz FC. Studies of kidney and muscle biopsy specimens from identical twins discordant for type I diabetes mellitus. *N Engl J Med* 1985;312:1282.

112. Mauer SM, et al. Development of diabetic vascular lesions in normal kidneys transplanted into patients with diabetes mellitus. *N Engl J Med* 1976;295:916.

113. Mauer SM, et al. Long-term study of normal kidneys transplanted into patients with type I diabetes. *Diabetes* 1989;38:516.

114. Mauer SM, Steffes MW, Connett J. The development of lesions in the glomerular basement membrane and mesangium after transplantation of normal kidneys into diabetic patients. *Diabetes* 1983;32:948.

115. Mauer SM, Miller K, Goetz FC. Immunopathology of renal extracellular membranes in kidneys transplanted into patients with diabetes mellitus. *Diabetes* 1976;27:738.

116. Barbosa J, et al. The effect of glycemic control on early diabetic renal lesions. *JAMA* 1994;272:600.

117. UK Prospective Diabetes Study (UKPDS) Group. Intensive blood-glucose control with sulphonylureas or insulin compared with conventional treatment and risk of complications in patients with type 2 diabetes (UKPDS 33): UK Prospective Diabetes Study (UKPDS) Group. *Lancet* 1998;352:837.

118. Borch-Johnsen K, et al. Is diabetic nephropathy an inherited complication? *Kidney Int* 1992;41:719.

119. Quinn M, Angelico MC, Warram JH, et al. Familial factors determine the development of diabetic nephropathy in patients with IDDM. *Diabetologia* 1996;39:940.

120. Freedman BI, Tuttle AB, Spray BJ. Familial predisposition to nephropathy in African-Americans with non-insulin-dependent diabetes mellitus. *Am J Kidney Dis* 1995;25:710.

121. Fioretto P, et al. Glomerular structure in siblings with insulin dependent diabetes mellitus (IDDM). *J Am Soc Nephrol* 1991;2:289.

122. Trevisan R, Fioretto P, Barbosa J, et al. Insulin-dependent diabetic sibling pairs are concordant for sodium-hydrogen antiport activity. *Kidney Int* 1999;55:2383.

123. Allawi J, et al. Microalbuminuria in non-insulin-dependent diabetes: its prevalence in Indian compared with Europid patients. *BMJ* 1988;296:462.

124. Kalter-Leibovici O, VanDyk DJ, Leibovici L. Risk factors for development of diabetic nephropathy in Jewish IDDM patients. *Diabetes* 1991;40:204.

125. Viberti GC, Keen H, Wiseman MJ. Raised arterial pressure in parents of proteinuric insulin dependent diabetics. *BMJ* 1987;295:515.

126. Krolewski AS, Canessa M, Warram JH. Predisposition to hypertension and susceptibility to renal disease in insulin-dependent diabetes mellitus. *N Engl J Med* 1988;318:140.

127. Fagerudd JA, Tarnow L, Jacobsen P, et al. Predisposition to essential hypertension and development of diabetic nephropathy in IDDM patients. *Diabetes* 1998;47:439.

128. Barzilay J, et al. Predisposition to hypertension: risk factor for nephropathy and hypertension in IDDM. *Kidney Int* 1992;41:723.

129. Earle K, et al. Familial clustering of cardiovascular disease in patients with insulin-dependent diabetes and nephropathy. *N Engl J Med* 1992;326:673.

130. Tarnow L, Rossing P, Nielsen FS, et al. Cardiovascular morbidity and early mortality cluster in parents of type 1 diabetic patients with diabetic nephropathy. *Diabetes Care* 2000;23:30.

131. Canessa M, et al. Increased sodium-lithium countertransport in red cells of patients with essential hypertension. *N Engl J Med* 1980;302:772.

132. Carr SJ, Thomas TH, Wilkinson R. Erythrocyte sodium-lithium countertransport in primary and renal hypertension: relation to family history. *Eur J Clin Invest* 1989;19:101.

133. Nosadini R, et al. Sodium/lithium countertransport and cardiorenal abnormalities in essential hypertension. *Hypertension* 1991;18:191.

134. Mangili R, Bending JJ, Scott CR. Increased sodium-lithium countertransport activity in red cells of patients with insulin-dependent diabetes and nephropathy. *N Engl J Med* 1988;318:146.

135. Jones SL, et al. Sodium-lithium countertransport in microalbuminuric insulin-dependent diabetic patients. *Hypertension* 1990;15:570.

136. Gall M-A, et al. Red cell Na/Li countertransport in non-insulin-dependent diabetics with diabetic nephropathy. *Kidney Int* 1991;39:135.

137. Lopes de Faria JB, et al. Prevalence of raised sodium lithium countertransport activity in type I diabetic patients. *Kidney Int* 1992;41:877.

138. Hardman TC, et al. Erythrocyte sodium-lithium countertransport and blood pressure in identical twin pairs discordant for insulin-dependent diabetes. *BMJ* 1992;305:215.

139. Pinkney J, et al. The relationship of urinary albumin excretion rate to ambulatory blood pressure and erythrocyte sodium-lithium countertransport in NIDDM. *Diabetologia* 1995;38:356.

140. Lopes de Faria JB, et al. Sodium lithium countertransport activity in normoalbuminuric insulin dependent diabetic patients. *Diabetes* 1992;41:610.

141. Messent J, et al. Insulin sensitivity in microalbuminuric type I (insulin-dependent) diabetic patients. *Diabetologia* 1992;35:A95.

142. Groop L, et al. Insulin resistance, hypertension and microalbuminuria in patients with type II (non-insulin-dependent) diabetes mellitus. *Diabetologia* 1993;36:642.

143. Yip J, et al. Insulin resistance in family members of insulin-dependent diabetic patients with microalbuminuria. *Lancet* 1993;341:369.

144. Doria A, Warram JH, Krolewski AS. Insulin receptor gene polymorphism is associated with the development of overt proteinuria in IDDM. *J Am Soc Nephrol* 1992;3:757.

145. Mahnen Smith, R. L., and Aronson, P. S. The plasma membrane sodium hydrogen exchanger and its role in physiological and pathophysiological processes. *Circ Res* 1985;56:773.

146. Ng LL, et al. Leucocyte Na/H antiport activity in type I (insulin-dependent) diabetic patients with nephropathy. *Diabetologia* 1990;33:371.

147. Trevisan R, et al. Na/H antiport activity and cell growth in cultured skin fibroblasts of IDDM patients with nephropathy. *Diabetes* 1992;41:1239.

148. Morocutti A, et al. Early cell aging in diabetic nephropathy. *J Am Soc Nephrol* 1993;4:800.

149. Lurbe A, et al. Cell proliferation and Na/H exchange in cultured fibroblasts from patients with type I diabetes and nephropathy. *J Am Soc Nephrol* 1993;4:798.

150. Jin DK, et al. Skin fibroblast integrin expression in insulin dependent diabetic nephropathy (IDDM). *J Am Soc Nephrol* 1994;5:966.

151. Adler SG, Pahl M, Seldin MF. Deciphering diabetic nephropathy: progress using genetic strategies [Editorial]. *Curr Opin Nephrol Hypertens* 2000;9:99.

152. Krolewski AS. Genetics of diabetic nephropathy: evidence for major and minor gene effects [Clinical conference]. *Kidney Int* 1999;55:1582.

153. Marre M, Jeunemaitre X, Gallois Y, et al. Contribution of genetic polymorphism in the renin-angiotensin system to the development of renal complications in insulin-dependent diabetes: Genetique de la Nephropathie Diabetique (GENEDIAB) Study Group. *J Clin Invest* 1997;99:1585.

154. Hsieh M-C, Lin S-R, Hsieh T-J, et al. Increased frequency of angiotensin-converting enzyme DD genotype in patients with type 2 diabetes in Taiwan. *Nephrol Dial Transplant* 2000;15:1008.

155. Huang X-H, Rantalaiho V, Wirta O, et al. Angiotensin-converting enzyme gene polymorphism is associated with coronary heart disease in non-insulin-dependent diabetic patients evaluated for 9 years. *Metabolism* 1998;47:1258.

156. Doi Y, Yoshizumi H, Yoshinari M, et al. Association between a polymorphism in the angiotensin-converting enzyme gene and microvascular complications in Japanese patients with NIDDM. *Diabetologia* 1996;39:97.

157. Jeffers BW, Estacio RO, Raynolds MV, et al. Angiotensin-converting enzyme gene polymorphism in non-insulin dependent diabetes mellitus and its relationship with diabetic nephropathy. *Kidney Int* 1997;52:473.

158. Ohno T, Kawazu S, Tomono S. Association analyses of the polymorphisms of angiotensin-converting enzyme and angiotensinogen genes with diabetic nephropathy in Japanese non-insulin-dependent diabetics. *Metabolism* 1996;45:218.

159. Powrie JK, Watts GF, Ingham JN, et al. Role of glycaemic control in development of microalbuminuria in patients with insulin dependent diabetes.*BMJ* 1994;309:1608.

160. Oue T, Namba M, Nakajima H, et al. Risk factors for the progression of microalbuminuria in Japanese type 2 diabetic patients: a 10 year follow-up study. *Diabetes Res Clin Pract* 1999;46:47.

161. Parving H-H, Jacobsen P, Tarnow L, et al. Effect of deletion polymorphism of angiotensin converting enzyme gene on progression of diabetic nephropathy during inhibition of angiotensin converting enzyme: observational follow up. *BMJ* 1996;313:591.

162. Penno G, Chaturvedi N, Talmud PJ, et al. Effect of angiotensin-converting enzyme (ACE) gene polymorphism on progression of renal disease and the influence of ACE inhibition in IDDM patients: findings from the EUCLID Randomized Controlled Trial. EURODIAB Controlled Trial of Lisinopril in IDDM. *Diabetes* 1998;47:1507.

163. Schmidt S, Schone N, Ritz E. Association of ACE gene polymorphism and diabetic nephropathy? The Diabetic Nephropathy Study Group [published erratum appears in *Kidney Int* 1995;48:915]. *Kidney Int* 1995;47:1176.

164. Tarnow L, Cambien F, Rossing P, et al. Lack of relationship between an insertion/deletion polymorphism in the angiotensin I-converting enzyme gene and diabetic nephropathy and proliferative retinopathy in IDDM patients. *Diabetes* 1995;44:489.

165. De Cosmo S, Margaglione M, Tassi V, et al. ACE, PAI-1, decorin and Werner helicase genes are not associated with the development of renal disease in European patients with type 1 diabetes. *Diabetes Metab Res Rev* 1999;15:247.

166. Björck S, Blohme G, Sylven C, et al. Deletion insertion polymorphism of the angiotensin converting enzyme gene and progression of diabetic nephropathy. *Nephrol Dial Transplant* 1997;12:67.

167. Fujisawa T, Ikegami H, Kawaguchi Y, et al. Meta-analysis of association of insertion/deletion polymorphism of angiotensin I-converting enzyme gene with diabetic nephropathy and retinopathy. *Diabetologia* 1998;41:47.

168. Tarnow L, Gluud C, Parving H-H. Diabetic nephropathy and the insertion/deletion polymorphism of the angiotensin-converting enzyme gene. *Nephrol Dial Transplant* 1998;13:1125.

169. Staessen JA, Kuznetsova T, Wang JG, et al. M235T angiotensinogen gene polymorphism and cardiovascular renal risk. *J Hypertens* 1999;17:9.

170. Tarnow L, Cambien F, Rossing P, et al. Angiotensin-II type 1 receptor gene polymorphism and diabetic microangiopathy. *Nephrol Dial Transplant* 1996;11:1019.

171. Chowdhury TA, Dyer PH, Kumar S, et al. Lack of association of angiotensin II type 1 receptor gene polymorphism with diabetic nephropathy in insulin-dependent diabetes mellitus. *Diabet Med* 1997; 14:837.

172. Doria AT, Onuma T, Warram JH, et al. Synergistic effect of angiotensin II type 1 receptor genotype and poor glycaemic control on risk of nephropathy in IDDM. *Diabetologia* 1997;11:1293.

173. Deinum J, Tarnow L, van Gool JM, et al. Plasma renin and prorenin and renin gene variation in patients with insulin-dependent diabetes mellitus and nephropathy. *Nephrol Dial Transplant* 1999;14:1904.

174. Zanchi A, Moczulski DK, Hanna LS, et al. Risk of advanced diabetic nephropathy in type 1 diabetes is associated with endothelial nitric oxide synthase gene polymorphism. *Kidney Int* 2000;57:405.

175. Warpeha KM, Xu W, Liu L, et al. Genotyping and functional analysis of a polymorphic (CCTTT)(n) repeat of NOS2A in diabetic retinopathy. *FASEB J* 1999;13:1825.

176. Johannesen J, Tarnow L, Parving HH, et al. CCTTT-repeat polymorphism in the human NOS2-promoter confers low risk of diabetic nephropathy in type 1 diabetic patients [Letter] [In Process Citation]. *Diabetes Care* 2000;23:560.

177. Shah VO, Scavini M, Nikolic J, et al. Z-2 microsatellite allele is linked to increased expression of the aldose reductase gene in diabetic nephropathy. *J Clin Endocrinol Metab* 1998;83:2886.

178. Heesom AE, Hibberd ML, Millward A, et al. Polymorphism in the 5′-end of the aldose reductase gene is strongly associated with the development of diabetic nephropathy in type I diabetes. *Diabetes* 1997;46:287.

179. De Cosmo S, Argiolas A, Miscio G, et al. A PC-1 amino acid variant (K121Q) is associated with faster progression of renal disease in patients with type 1 diabetes and albuminuria. *Diabetes* 2000;49:521.

180. Schmidt S, Bluthner M, Giessel R, et al. A polymorphism in the gene for the atrial natriuretic peptide and diabetic nephropathy: Diabetic Nephropathy Study Group. *Nephrol Dial Transplant* 1998;13:1807.

181. Chowdhury TA, Dyer PH, Kumar S, et al. Association of apolipoprotein epsilon2 allele with diabetic nephropathy in Caucasian subjects with IDDM. *Diabetes* 1998;47:278.

182. Onuma T, Laffel LM, Angelico MC, et al. Apolipoprotein E genotypes and risk of diabetic nephropathy. *J Am Soc Nephrol* 1996;7:1075.

183. Kimura H, Suzuki Y, Gejyo F, et al. Apolipoprotein E4 reduces risk of diabetic nephropathy in patients with NIDDM. *Am J Kidney Dis* 1998;31:666.

184. Araki S-i, Moczulski DK, Zanchi A, et al. APOE ≥2 is causally related to the development of diabetic nephropathy. *J Am Soc Nephrol* 1998;9:113A.

185. Hansen PM, Chowdhury T, Deckert T, et al. Genetic variation of the heparan sulfate proteoglycan gene (perlecan gene): association with urinary albumin excretion in IDDM patients. *Diabetes* 1997;46:1658.

186. Fujita H, Narita T, Meguro H, et al. Lack of association between an ecNOS gene polymorphism and diabetic nephropathy in type 2 diabetic patients with proliferative diabetic retinopathy. *Horm Metab Res* 2000;32:80.

187. Maeda S, Haneda M, Yasuda H, et al. Diabetic nephropathy is not associated with the dinucleotide repeat polymorphism upstream of the aldose reductase (ALR2) gene but with erythrocyte aldose reductase content in Japanese subjects with type 2 diabetes. *Diabetes* 1999;48:420.

188. Dyer PH, Chowdhury TA, Dronsfield MJ, et al. The 5′-end polymorphism of the aldose reductase gene is not associated with diabetic nephropathy in Caucasian type I diabetic patients [Letter]. *Diabetologia* 1999;42:1030.

189. Moczulski DK, Scott L, Antonellis A, et al. Aldose reductase gene polymorphisms and susceptibility to diabetic nephropathy in type 1 diabetes mellitus. *Diabet Med* 2000;17:111.

190. Chen JW, Hansen PM, Tarnow L, et al. Genetic variation of a collagen IV alpha 1-chain gene polymorphism in Danish insulin-dependent diabetes mellitus (IDDM) patients: lack of association to nephropathy and proliferative retinopathy. *Diabet Med* 1997;14:143.

191. Maeda S, Haneda M, Hayashi K, et al. (A-C)n Dinucleotide repeat polymorphism at 5′ end of matrix metalloproteinase 9 gene is associated with nephropathy in Japanese subjects with type 2 diabetes. *J Am Soc Nephrol* 1998;9:118A.

192. Smyth JS, Savage DA, Maxwell AP. Lack of association between endothelin-1 and endothelin$_A$ receptor polymorphisms and diabetic nephropathy in IDDM. *J Am Soc Nephrol* 1998;9:123A.

193. Pociot F, Hansen PM, Karlsen AE, et al. TGF-beta1 gene mutations in insulin-dependent diabetes mellitus and diabetic nephropathy. *J Am Soc Nephrol* 1998;9:2302.

194. Wong TY, Poon P, Szeto CC, et al. Association of plasminogen activator inhibitor-1 4G/4G genotype and type 2 diabetic nephropathy in Chinese patients. *Kidney Int* 2000;57:632.

195. Loughrey BV, Maxwell AP, Fogarty DG, et al. An interleukin 1B allele, which correlates with a high secretor phenotype, is associated with diabetic nephropathy. *Cytokine* 1998;10:984.

196. Tarnow L, Pociot F, Hansen PM, et al. Polymorphisms in the interleukin-1 gene cluster do not contribute to the genetic susceptibility of diabetic nephropathy in Caucasian patients with IDDM. *Diabetes* 1997;46:1075.

197. Freedman BI, Yu H, Spray BJ, et al. Genetic linkage analysis of growth factor loci and end-stage renal disease in African Americans. *Kidney Int* 1997;51:819.

198. Fogarty DG, Zychma MJ, Scott LJ, et al. The C825T polymorphism in the human G-protein beta3 subunit gene is not associated with diabetic nephropathy in type I diabetes mellitus. *Diabetologia* 1998;41:1304.

199. Tarnow L, Urhammer SA, Mottlau B, et al. The Trp64Arg amino acid polymorphism of the beta3-adrenergic receptor gene does not contribute to the genetic susceptibility of diabetic microvascular complications in Caucasian type 1 diabetic patients. *Nephrol Dial Transplant* 1999;14:895.

200. Nishigori H, Yamada S, Kohama T, et al. Frameshift mutation, A263fsinsGG, in the hepatocyte nuclear factor-1beta gene associated with diabetes and renal dysfunction. *Diabetes* 1998;47:1354.

201. Odawara M, Yamashita K. A common mutation of the methylenetetrahydrofolate reductase gene as a risk factor for diabetic nephropathy [Letter]. *Diabetologia* 1999;42:631.

202. Neugebauer S, Baba T, Watanabe T. Methylenetetrahydrofolate reductase gene polymorphism as a risk factor for diabetic nephropathy in NIDDM patients [Letter]. *Lancet* 1998;352:454.

203. Yu H, Bowden DW, Spray BJ, et al. Identification of human plasma kallikrein gene polymorphisms and evaluation of their role in end-stage renal disease. *Hypertension* 1998;31:906.

204. Chowdhury TA, Dyer PH, Mijovic CH, et al. Human leucocyte antigen and insulin gene regions and nephropathy in type I diabetes. *Diabetologia* 1999;42:1017.

205. Imperatore G, Hanson RL, Pettitt DJ, et al. Sib-pair linkage analysis for susceptibility genes for microvascular complications among Pima Indians with type 2 diabetes: Pima Diabetes Genes Group. *Diabetes* 1998;47:821.

206. Patel A, Hibberd ML, Millward BA, et al. Chromosome 7q35 and susceptibility to diabetic microvascular complications [see comments]. *J Diabetes Complications* 1996;10:62.

207. Brenner BM, Meyer TW. Mechanisms of progression in renal disease. In Robinson RR, ed. *Proceedings of the IXth International Congress of Nephrology*, vol. 1. New York: Springer-Verlag, 1984.

208. Brenner BM. Hemodynamically mediated glomerular injury and the progressive nature of kidney disease. *Kidney Int* 1983;23:647.

209. Rudberg S, Persson B, Dahlquist G. Increased glomerular filtration rate as a predictor of diabetic nephropathy: an 8-year prospective study. *Kidney Int* 1992;41:822.

210. Jones SL, Wiseman MJ, Viberti GC. Glomerular hyperfiltration as a risk factor for diabetic nephropathy: five year report of a prospective study. *Diabetologia* 1991;34:59.

211. Berkman J, Rifkin H. Unilateral nodular diabetic glomerulosclerosis (Kimmelstiel-Wilson): report of a case. *Metab Clin Exp* 1973;22:715.

212. Mauer SM, et al. The effect of Goldblatt hypertension on the development of glomerular lesions of diabetes mellitus in the rat. *Diabetes* 1978;27:738.

213. Hostetter TH, Troy JL, Brenner BM. Glomerular dynamics in rats with diabetes mellitus. *Kidney Int* 1978;121:725.

214. Hagg E. Influence of insulin treatment on glomerular changes in rats with long-term alloxan diabetes. *Acta Pathol Microbiol Scand* 1974;82:228.

215. Rennke HG, et al. Pathogenesis of experimental diabetic microangiopathy: differential effects of hemodynamic and metabolic factors. *FASEB J* 1989;3:A444.

216. Azar S, et al. Single-nephron pressures, flaws and resistances in hypertensive kidneys with nephrosclerosis. *Kidney Int* 1977;62:28.

217. Steffes MW, Brown DM, Mauer SM. Diabetic glomerulopathy following unilateral nephrectomy in the rat. *Diabetes* 1978;27:35.

218. Steffes MW, et al. Diabetic glomerulopathy in the uninephrectomized rat resists amelioration following islet transplantation. *Diabetologia* 1982;23:347.

219. Hostetter TH, Olson JL, Rennke HG. Hyperfiltration in remnant nephrons: a potentially adverse response to renal ablation. *Am J Physiol* 1981;241:F85.

220. Zatz R, et al. Prevention of diabetic glomerulopathy by pharmacologic amelioration of glomerular capillary hypertension. *J Clin Invest* 1986;77:1925.

221. O'Brian RC, et al. The effect of perindopril and triple therapy in a normotensive model of diabetic nephropathy. *Diabetes* 1993;42:604.

222. Eddy AA. Molecular insights into interstitial fibrosis. *J Am Soc Nephrol* 1996;7:2495.

223. Ray PE, et al. Angiotensin II stimulates human fetal mesangial cell proliferation and fibronectin biosynthesis by binding to AT$_1$ receptors. *Kidney Int* 1994;45:177.

224. Campbell-Boswell M, Robertson AL Jr. Effects of angiotensin II and vasopressin on human smooth muscle cells in vitro. *Exp Mol Pathol* 1981;35:265.

225. Nahman NS Jr, Leonhart K, Cosio FG. Effect of captopril in fibronectin production by human mesangial cells cultured in high glucose. *J Am Soc Nephrol* 1990;1:552.

226. Nahman NS Jr, Leonhart K, Cosio FG. Variable effect of converting enzyme inhibitors on cell growth and fibronectin production by human mesangial cells grown in high glucose. *J Am Soc Nephrol* 1990;2:580.

227. Ihm CG, et al. Effect of angiotensin converting enzyme inhibition on collagen production by cultured mesangial cells. *Korean J Intern Med* 1994;9:9.

228. Nakamura T, et al. Enalapril attenuates increased gene expression of extracellular matrix components in diabetic rats. *J Am Soc Nephrol* 1995;5:1492.

229. Sorbi D, et al. Captopril inhibits the 72 kDa and 92 kDa matrix metalloproteinase. *Kidney Int* 1993;44:1266.

230. Hirokoshi S, et al. Water deprivation stimulates transforming growth factor β2 accumulation in the juxtaglomerular apparatus of mouse kidney. *J Clin Invest* 1991;88:2117.

231. Ray PE, et al. Renal vascular induction of TGFβ2 and renin by potassium depletion. *Kidney Int* 1993;44:1006.

232. Yamamoto T, et al. Expression of transforming growth factor β is elevated in human and experimental diabetic nephropathy. *Proc Natl Acad Sci USA* 1993;90:1814.

233. Sealey JE, et al. Plasma prorenin in normal, hypertensive, and anephric subjects and its effect on renin measurements. *Circ Res* 1977;40:1.

234. Derkx FHM, et al. Control of enzymatically inactive renin in man under various pathological conditions: implications for the interpretation of renin measurements in peripheral and renal plasma. *Clin Sci Mol Med* 1978;54:529.

235. Naruse K, Murakoshi M, Oasmura RY. Immunohistochemical evidence for renin in human endocrine tissues. *J Clin Endocrinol Metab* 1985;61:172.

236. Deschepper CF, et al. Analysis by immunohistochemistry and in situ hybridization of renin and its mRNA in kidney, testis, adrenal and pituitary of the rat. *Proc Natl Acad Sci USA* 1986;83:7552.

237. Ganten D, et al. The renin-angiotensin system in the brain. *Exp Brain Res* 1982;48:3.

238. Leutscher JA, et al. Increased plasma inactive renin in diabetes mellitus: a marker of microvascular complications. *N Engl J Med* 1985;312:1412.

239. Wilson DM, Luetscher JA. Plasma prorenin activity and complications in children with insulin-dependent diabetes mellitus. *N Engl J Med* 1990;23:1101.

240. Franken AAM, et al. Plasma prorenin as an early marker of microvascular disease in patients with diabetes mellitus. *Diabetes Metab* 1992;18:137.

241. Franken AAM, et al. Association of high plasma prorenin with diabetic retinopathy. *J Hypertens* 1988;6:S461.

242. Danser AHJ, et al. Renin, prorenin, and immunoreactive renin in vitreous fluid from eyes with and without diabetic retinopathy. *J Clin Endocrinol Metab* 1989;68:160.

243. Daneman D, et al. Plasma prorenin as an early marker in diabetic (IDDM) adolescents. *Kidney Int* 1994;46:1154.

244. Allen T, et al. Elevated plasma total renin precedes microalbuminuria and retinopathy in IDDM. In: *Proceedings of the International Diabetes Federation.* Kobe, Japan: 1994.

245. Anderson RW, et al. Plasma prorenin and diabetic nephropathy in NIDDM. *J Am Soc Nephrol* 1993;4:300.

246. Bryer-Ash M, Fraze EB, Luetscher JA. Plasma renin and prorenin (inactive renin) in diabetes mellitus: effects of intravenous furosemide. *J Clin Endocrinol Metab* 1988;66:454.

247. Falk RJ, Scheinman JI, Mauer SM, et al. Polyantigenic expansion of basement membrane constituents in diabetic nephropathy. *Diabetes* 1983;32[Suppl 2]:34.

248. Østerby R. Morphometric studies of the peripheral glomerular basement membrane in early juvenile diabetes: I. development of initial basement membrane thickening. *Diabetologia* 1972;8:84.

249. Brito PL, Fioretto P, Drummond K, et al. Proximal tubular basement membrane width in insulin-dependent diabetes mellitus. *Kidney Int* 1998;53:754.

250. Katz A, Kim Y, Sisson-Ross S, et al. An increase in the volume fraction of the cortical interstitium occupied by cells antedates interstitial fibrosis in type 1 diabetic patients. *J Am Soc Nephrol* 2000; 11:118A.

251. Kim Y, Kleppel MM, Butkowski R, et al. Differential expression of basement membrane collagen chains in diabetic nephropathy. *Am J Pathol* 1991;138:413.

252. Zhu D, Kim Y, Steffes MW, et al. Glomerular distribution of type IV collagen in diabetes by high resolution quantitative immunochemistry. *Kidney Int* 1994;45:425.

253. Moriya T, Groppoli TJ, Kim Y, et al. Quantitative immunoelectron microscopy of type VI collagen in glomeruli in type I diabetic patients. *Kidney Int* 2001;59:317.

254. Ayo SH, Radnik RA, Glass WFD, et al. Increased extracellular matrix synthesis and mRNA in mesangial cells grown in high-glucose medium. *Am J Physiol* 1991;260:F185.

255. Pugliese G, Pricci F, Pugliese F, et al. Mechanisms of glucose-enhanced extracellular matrix accumulation in rat glomerular mesangial cells. *Diabetes* 1994;43:478.

256. Sharma K, Ziyadeh FN. Hyperglycemia and diabetic kidney disease: the case for transforming growth factor-beta as a key mediator. *Diabetes* 1995;44:1139.

257. Baricos WH , Shah SV. Proteolytic enzymes as mediators of glomerular injury. *Kidney Int* 1991;40:161.

258. Davies M, Coles GA, Thomas GJ, et al. Proteinases and the glomerulus: their role in glomerular diseases. *Klin Wochenschr* 1990;68: 1145.

259. Birkedal-Hansen H, Moore WG, Bodden MK, et al. Matrix metalloproteinases: a review. *Crit Rev Oral Biol Med* 1993;4:197.

260. Kahari VM, Saarialho-Kere U. Matrix metalloproteinases and their inhibitors in tumour growth and invasion. *Ann Med* 1999;31:34.

261. Johansson N, Ahonen M, Kahari VM. Matrix metalloproteinases in tumor invasion. *Cell Mol Life Sci* 2000;57:5.

262. Murphy G. Matrix metalloproteinases and their inhibitors. *Acta Orthop Scand Suppl* 1995;266:55.

263. Matrisian LM. Metalloproteinases and their inhibitors in matrix remodeling. *Trends Genet* 1990;6:121.

264. Bruijn JA, Roos A, de Geus B, et al. Transforming growth factor-beta and the glomerular extracellular matrix in renal pathology. *J Lab Clin Med* 1994;123:34.

265. Lawrence DA. Transforming growth factor-beta: a general review. *Eur Cytokine Netw* 1996;7:363.

266. Brownlee M. Negative consequences of glycation. *Metabolism* 2000;49:9.

267. Nishikawa T, Edelstein D, Du XL, et al. Normalizing mitochondrial superoxide production blocks three pathways of hyperglycaemic damage. *Nature* 2000;404:787.

268. Nishikawa T, Edelstein D, Brownlee M. The missing link: a single unifying mechanism for diabetic complications. *Kidney Int* 2000;58[Suppl 77]:S26.

269. Flyvbjerg A. Putative pathophysiological role of growth factors and cytokines in experimental diabetic kidney disease. *Diabetologia* 2000;43:1205.

270. Wrana JL, Attisano L, Wieser R, et al. Mechanism of activation of the TGF-beta receptor. *Nature* 1994;370:341.

271. Nakamura T, Fukui M, Ebihara I, et al. mRNA expression of growth factors in glomeruli from diabetic rats. *Diabetes* 1993;42:450.

272. Choi ME, Kim EG, Huang Q, et al. Rat mesangial cell hypertrophy in response to transforming growth factor-beta 1. *Kidney Int* 1993; 44:948.

273. Hill C, Flyvbjerg A, Gronbaek H, et al. The renal expression of transforming growth factor-beta isoforms and their receptors in acute and chronic experimental diabetes in rats. *Endocrinology* 2000;141:1196.

274. Ziyadeh FN, Snipes ER, Watanabe M, et al. High glucose induces cell hypertrophy and stimulates collagen gene transcription in proximal tubule. *Am J Physiol* 1990;259:F704.

275. Nakamura T, Miller D, Ruoslahti E, et al. Production of extracellular matrix by glomerular epithelial cells is regulated by transforming growth factor-beta 1. *Kidney Int* 1992;41:1213.

276. Humes HD, Nakamura T, Cieslinski DA, et al. Role of proteoglycans and cytoskeleton in the effects of TGF-beta 1 on renal proximal tubule cells. *Kidney Int* 1993;43:575.

277. Roberts AB, McCune BK, Sporn MB. TGF-beta: regulation of extracellular matrix. *Kidney Int* 1992;41:557.

278. Davies M, Thomas GJ, Martin J, et al. The purification and characterization of a glomerular-basement-membrane-degrading neutral proteinase from rat mesangial cells. *Biochem J* 1988;251:419.

279. Marti HP, Lee L, Kashgarian M, et al. Transforming growth factor-beta 1 stimulates glomerular mesangial cell synthesis of the 72-kd type IV collagenase. *Am J Pathol* 1994;144:82.

280. Inoki K, Haneda M, Ishida T, et al. Role of nitrogen-activated protein kinases as demonstrated effectors of transforming growth factor-beta in mesangial cells. *Kidney Int* 2000;58:76.

281. Weigert C, Sauer U, Brodbeck K, et al. AP-1 proteins mediate hyperglycemia-induced activation of the human TGF-beta 1 promoter in mesangial cells. *J Am Soc Nephrol* 2000;11:2007.

282. Shankland SJ, Scholey JW, Ly H, et al. Expression of transforming growth factor-beta 1 during diabetic renal hypertrophy. *Kidney Int* 1994;46:430.

283. Inoki K, Haneda M, Maeda S, et al. TGF-beta 1 stimulates glucose uptake by enhancing GLUT1 expression in mesangial cells. *Kidney Int* 1999;55:1704.

284. Wogensen L, Nielsen CB, Hjorth P, et al. Under control of the Ren-1c promoter, locally produced transforming growth factor-beta1 induces accumulation of glomerular extracellular matrix in transgenic mice. *Diabetes* 1999;48:182.

285. Ziyadeh FN, Sharma K, Ericksen M, et al. Stimulation of collagen gene expression and protein synthesis in murine mesangial cells by high glucose is mediated by autocrine activation of transforming growth factor-beta. *J Clin Invest* 1994;93:536.

286. Sharma K, Jin Y, Guo J, et al. Neutralization of TGF-beta by anti-TGF-beta antibody attenuates kidney hypertrophy and the enhanced extracellular matrix gene expression in STZ-induced diabetic mice. Diabetes 1996;45:522.

287. Flyvbjerg A, Hill C, Grønbæek H, et al. Effect of ACE-inhibition on renal TGF-β type II receptor expression in experimental diabetes in rats. *J Am Soc Nephrol* 1999;10:679A.

288. Flyvbjerg A. Growth factors and diabetic complications. *Diabet Med* 1990;7:387.

289. Janssen JA , Lamberts SW. Circulating IGF-I and its protective role in the pathogenesis of diabetic angiopathy. *Clin Endocrinol (Oxf)* 2000;52:1.

290. Conti FG, Striker LJ, Lesniak MA, et al. Studies on binding and mitogenic effect of insulin and insulin-like growth factor I in glomerular mesangial cells. *Endocrinology* 1988;122:2788.

291. Doi T, Striker LJ, Elliot SJ, et al. Insulinlike growth factor-1 is a progression factor for human mesangial cells. *Am J Pathol* 1989;134:395.

292. Elliot SJ, Striker LJ, Hattori M, et al. Mesangial cells from diabetic NOD mice constitutively secrete increased amounts of insulin-like growth factor-I. *Endocrinology* 1993;133:1783.

293. Lupia E, Elliot SJ, Lenz O, et al. IGF-1 decreases collagen degradation in diabetic NOD mesangial cells: implications for diabetic nephropathy. *Diabetes* 1999;48:1638.

294. Flyvbjerg A , Orskov H. Kidney tissue insulin-like growth factor I and initial renal growth in diabetic rats: relation to severity of diabetes. *Acta Endocrinol (Copenh)* 1990;122:374.

295. Flyvbjerg A, Frystyk J, Osterby R, et al. Kidney IGF-I and renal hypertrophy in GH-deficient diabetic dwarf rats. *Am J Physiol* 1992; 262:E956.

296. Flyvbjerg A, Thorlacius-Ussing O, Naeraa R, et al. Kidney tissue somatomedin C and initial renal growth in diabetic and uninephrectomized rats. *Diabetologia* 1988;31:310.

297. Landau D, Chin E, Bondy C, et al. Expression of insulin-like growth factor binding proteins in the rat kidney: effects of long-term diabetes. *Endocrinology* 1995;136:1835.

298. Flyvbjerg A, Kessler U, Dorka B, et al. Transient increase in renal insulin-like growth factor binding proteins during initial kidney hypertrophy in experimental diabetes in rats. *Diabetologia* 1992;35:589.

299. Flyvbjerg A, Kessler U, Kiess W. Increased kidney and liver insulin-like growth factor II/mannose-6-phosphate receptor concentration in experimental diabetes in rats. *Growth Regul* 1994;4:188.

300. Flyvbjerg A, Frystyk J, Thorlacius-Ussing O, et al. Somatostatin analogue administration prevents increase in kidney somatomedin C and initial renal growth in diabetic and uninephrectomized rats. *Diabetologia* 1989;32:261.

301. Gronbaek H, Nielsen B, Frystyk J, et al. Effect of lanreotide on local kidney IGF-I and renal growth in experimental diabetes in the rat. *Exp Nephrol* 1996;4:295.

302. Steer KA, Sochor M, Kunjara S, et al. The effect of a somatostatin analogue (SMS 201-995, Sandostatin) on the concentration of phosphoribosyl pyrophosphate and the activity of the pentose phosphate pathway in the early renal hypertrophy of experimental diabetes in the rat. *Biochem Med Metab Biol* 1988;39:226.

303. Chen NY, Chen WY, Bellush L, et al. Effects of streptozotocin treatment in growth hormone (GH) and GH antagonist transgenic mice. *Endocrinology* 1995;136:660.

304. Chen NY, Chen WY, Kopchick JJ. A growth hormone antagonist protects mice against streptozotocin induced glomerulosclerosis even in the presence of elevated levels of glucose and glycated hemoglobin. *Endocrinology* 1996;137:5163.

305. Flyvbjerg A, Bennett WF, Rasch R, et al. Inhibitory effect of a growth hormone receptor antagonist (G120K-PEG) on renal enlargement, glomerular hypertrophy, and urinary albumin excretion in experimental diabetes in mice. *Diabetes* 1999;48:377.

306. Bellush LL, Doublier S, Holland AN, et al. Protection against diabetes-induced nephropathy in growth hormone receptor/binding protein gene-disrupted mice. *Endocrinology* 2000;141:163.

307. Segev Y, Landau D, Rasch R, et al. Growth hormone receptor antagonism prevents early renal changes in nonobese diabetic mice. *J Am Soc Nephrol* 1999;10:2374.

308. Simon M, Grone HJ, Johren O, et al. Expression of vascular endothelial growth factor and its receptors in human renal ontogenesis and in adult kidney. *Am J Physiol* 1995;268:F240.

309. Simon M, Rockl W, Hornig C, et al. Receptors of vascular endothelial growth factor/vascular permeability factor (VEGF/VPF) in fetal and adult human kidney: localization and [^{125}I]VEGF binding sites. *J Am Soc Nephrol* 1998;9:1032.

310. Cooper ME, Vranes D, Youssef S, et al. Increased renal expression of vascular endothelial growth factor (VEGF) and its receptor VEGFR-2 in experimental diabetes. *Diabetes* 1999;48:2229.

311. Williams B. A potential role for angiotensin II-induced vascular endothelial growth factor expression in the pathogenesis of diabetic nephropathy? *Miner Electrolyte Metab* 1998;24:400.

312. Shweiki D, Itin A, Soffer D, et al. Vascular endothelial growth factor induced by hypoxia may mediate hypoxia-initiated angiogenesis. *Nature* 1992;359:843.

313. Stavri GT, Hong Y, Zachary IC, et al. Hypoxia and platelet-derived growth factor-BB synergistically upregulate the expression of vascular endothelial growth factor in vascular smooth muscle cells. *FEBS Lett* 1995;358:311.

314. Pupilli C, Lasagni L, Romagnani P, et al. Angiotensin II stimulates the synthesis and secretion of vascular permeability factor/vascular endothelial growth factor in human mesangial cells. *J Am Soc Nephrol* 1999;10:245.

315. Gruden G, Thomas S, Burt D, et al. Interaction of angiotensin II and mechanical stretch on vascular endothelial growth factor production by human mesangial cells. *J Am Soc Nephrol* 1999;10:730.

316. Natarajan R, Bai W, Lanting L, et al. Effects of high glucose on vascular endothelial growth factor expression in vascular smooth muscle cells. *Am J Physiol* 1997;273:H2224.

317. Williams B, Gallacher B, Patel H, et al. Glucose-induced protein kinase C activation regulates vascular permeability factor mRNA expression and peptide production by human vascular smooth muscle cells in vitro. *Diabetes* 1997;46:1497.

318. Bortoloso E, Del Prete D, Anglani F, et al. Vascular endothelial growth factor expression in microdissected glomeruli of type 2 diabetic patients. *Diabetologia* 1999;42[Suppl 1]:A273.

319. Vehaskari VM, Hering-Smith KS, Moskowitz DW, et al. Effect of epidermal growth factor on sodium transport in the cortical collecting tubule. *Am J Physiol* 1989;256:F803.

320. Hamm LL, Hering-Smith KS, Vehaskari VM. Epidermal growth factor and the kidney. *Semin Nephrol* 1993;13:109.

321. Guh JY, Lai YH, Shin SJ, et al. Epidermal growth factor in renal hypertrophy in streptozotocin-diabetic rats. *Nephron* 1991;59:641.

322. Gilbert RE, Cox A, McNally PG, et al. Increased epidermal growth factor in experimental diabetes related kidney growth in rats. *Diabetologia* 1997;40:778.

323. Lee TS, Saltsman KA, Ohashi H, et al. Activation of protein kinase C by elevation of glucose concentration: proposal for a mechanism in the development of diabetic vascular complications. *Proc Natl Acad Sci U S A* 1989;86:5141.

324. Studer RK, Craven PA , DeRubertis FR. Antioxidant inhibition of protein kinase C-signaled increases in transforming growth factor-beta in mesangial cells. *Metabolism* 1997;46:918.

325. Haneda M, Kikkawa R, Sugimoto T, et al. Abnormalities in protein kinase C and MAP kinase cascade in mesangial cells cultured under high glucose conditions. *J Diabetes Complications* 1995;9:246.

326. Ishii H, Jirousek MR, Koya D, et al. Amelioration of vascular dysfunctions in diabetic rats by an oral PKC beta inhibitor. *Science* 1996;272:728.

327. Koya D, Haneda M, Nakagawa H, et al. Amelioration of accelerated diabetic mesangial expansion by treatment with a PKC beta inhibitor in diabetic db/db mice, a rodent model for type 2 diabetes. *FASEB J* 2000;14:439.

328. Kagami S, Border WA, Miller DE, et al. Angiotensin II stimulates extracellular matrix protein synthesis through induction of transforming growth factor-beta expression in rat glomerular mesangial cells. *J Clin Invest* 1994;93:2431.

329. Ziyadeh FN. Mediators of hyperglycemia and the pathogenesis of matrix accumulation in diabetic renal disease. *Miner Electrolyte Metab* 1995;21:292.

330. Day JF, Thorpe SR, Baynes JW. Nonenzymatically glucosylated albumin: in vitro preparation and isolation from normal human serum. *J Biol Chem* 1979;254:595.

331. Brownlee M, Vlassara H , Cerami A. Nonenzymatic glycosylation and the pathogenesis of diabetic complications. *Ann Intern Med* 1984;101:527.

332. Bunn HF, Shapiro R, McManus M, et al. Structural heterogeneity of human hemoglobin A due to nonenzymatic glycosylation. *J Biol Chem* 1979;254:3892.

333. Gonen B, Baenziger J, Schonfeld G, et al. Nonenzymatic glycosylation of low density lipoproteins in vitro. Effects on cell-interactive properties. *Diabetes* 1981;30:875.

334. Bailey AJ, Robins SP, Tanner MJ. Reducible components in the proteins of human erythrocyte membrane. *Biochim Biophys Acta* 1976;434:51.

335. Monnier VM, Stevens VJ, Cerami A. Nonenzymatic glycosylation, sulfhydryl oxidation, and aggregation of lens proteins in experimental sugar cataracts. *J Exp Med* 1979;150:1098.

336. Wu VY, Cohen MP. Evidence for a ligand receptor system mediating the biologic effects of glycated albumin in glomerular mesangial cells. *Biochem Biophys Res Commun* 1995;207:521.

337. Chen S, Cohen MP, et al. Amadori-glycated albumin in diabetic nephropathy: pathophysiologic connections. *Kidney Int* 2000;58[Suppl 77]:S40.

338. Raj DS, Choudhury D, et al. Advanced glycation end products: a nephrologist's perspective. *Am J Kidney Dis* 2000;35:365.

339. Monnier VM, Vishwanath V, Frank KE, et al. Relation between complications of type I diabetes mellitus and collagen-linked fluorescence. *N Engl J Med* 1986;314:403.

340. Brownlee M, Cerami A, Vlassara H. Advanced glycosylation end products in tissue and the biochemical basis of diabetic complications. *N Engl J Med* 1988;318:1315.

341. Anderson SS, Kim Y, Tsilibary EC. Effects of matrix glycation on mesangial cell adhesion, spreading and proliferation. *Kidney Int* 1994;46:1359.

342. Yang CW, Vlassara H, Peten EP, et al. Advanced glycation end products up-regulate gene expression found in diabetic glomerular disease. *Proc Natl Acad Sci USA* 1994;91:9436.

343. Brownlee M, Vlassara H, Kooney A, et al. Aminoguanidine prevents diabetes-induced arterial wall protein cross-linking. *Science* 1986;232:1629.

344. McLennan SV, Fisher EJ, Yue DK, et al. High glucose concentration causes a decrease in mesangium degradation: a factor in the pathogenesis of diabetic nephropathy. *Diabetes* 1994;43:1041.

345. Soulis-Liparota T, Cooper M, Papazoglou D, et al. Retardation by aminoguanidine of development of albuminuria, mesangial expansion, and tissue fluorescence in streptozocin-induced diabetic rat. *Diabetes* 1991;40:1328.

346. Ellis EN, Good BH. Prevention of glomerular basement membrane thickening by aminoguanidine in experimental diabetes mellitus. *Metabolism* 1991;40:1016.

347. Wolf G, Sharma K, Chen Y, et al. High glucose-induced proliferation in mesangial cells is reversed by autocrine TGF-beta. *Kidney Int* 1992;42:647.

348. Rocco MV, Chen Y, Goldfarb S, et al. Elevated glucose stimulates TGF-beta gene expression and bioactivity in proximal tubule. *Kidney Int* 1992;41:107.

349. Hoffman BB, Sharma K, Zhu Y, et al. Transcriptional activation of transforming growth factor-beta1 in mesangial cell culture by high glucose concentration. *Kidney Int* 1998;54:1107.

350. Han DC, Isono M, Hoffman BB, et al. High glucose stimulates proliferation and collagen type I synthesis in renal cortical fibroblasts: mediation by autocrine activation of TGF-beta. *J Am Soc Nephrol* 1999;10:1891.

351. Ayo SH, Radnik R, Garoni JA, et al. High glucose increases diacylglycerol mass and activates protein kinase C in mesangial cell cultures. *Am J Physiol* 1991;261:F571.

352. Fumo P, Kuncio GS, Ziyadeh FN. PKC and high glucose stimulate collagen alpha 1 (IV) transcriptional activity in a reporter mesangial cell line. *Am J Physiol* 1994;267:F632.

353. Hempel A, Maasch C, Heintze U, et al. High glucose concentrations increase endothelial cell permeability via activation of protein kinase C alpha. *Circ Res* 1997;81:363.

354. Kikkawa R, Haneda M, Uzu T, et al. Translocation of protein kinase C alpha and zeta in rat glomerular mesangial cells cultured under high glucose conditions. *Diabetologia* 1994;37:838.

355. Ziyadeh FN. The extracellular matrix in diabetic nephropathy. *Am J Kidney Dis* 1993;22:736.

356. Ziyadeh FN, Fumo P, Rodenberger CH, et al. Role of protein kinase C and cyclic AMP/protein kinase A in high glucose-stimulated transcriptional activation of collagen alpha 1 (IV) in glomerular mesangial cells. *J Diabetes Complications* 1995;9:255.

357. Cohen MP, Ziyadeh FN, Lautenslager GT, et al. Glycated albumin stimulation of PKC-beta activity is linked to increased collagen IV in mesangial cells. *Am J Physiol* 1999;276:F684.

358. Singh AK, Mo W, Dunea G, et al. Effect of glycated proteins on the matrix of glomerular epithelial cells. *J Am Soc Nephrol* 1998;9:802.

359. Ziyadeh FN, Han DC, Cohen JA, et al. Glycated albumin stimulates fibronectin gene expression in glomerular mesangial cells: involvement of the transforming growth factor-beta system. *Kidney Int* 1998;53:631.

360. Cohen MP, Ziyadeh FN. Amadori glucose adducts modulate mesangial cell growth and collagen gene expression. *Kidney Int* 1994;45:475.

361. Cohen MP, Wu VY, Cohen JA. Glycated albumin stimulates fibronectin and collagen IV production by glomerular endothelial cells under normoglycemic conditions. *Biochem Biophys Res Commun* 1997;239:91.

362. Chen S, Cohen MP, Ziyadeh FN. Amadori-glycated albumin in diabetic nephropathy: pathophysiologic connections. *Kidney Int* 2000;58[Suppl 77]:S40.

363. Cohen MP, Sharma K, Jin Y, et al. Prevention of diabetic nephropathy in db/db mice with glycated albumin antagonists: a novel treatment strategy. *J Clin Invest* 1995;95:2338.

364. Cohen MP, Hud E, Wu VY. Amelioration of diabetic nephropathy by treatment with monoclonal antibodies against glycated albumin. *Kidney Int* 1994;45:1673.

365. Schalkwijk CG, Ligtvoet N, Twaalfhoven H, et al. Amadori albumin in type 1 diabetic patients: correlation with markers of endothelial

function, association with diabetic nephropathy, and localization in retinal capillaries. *Diabetes* 1999;48:2446.

366. Cavallo-Perin P, Chiambretti A, Calefato V, et al. Urinary excretion of glycated albumin in insulin-dependent diabetic patients with micro- and macroalbuminuria. *Clin Nephrol* 1992;38:9.

367. Kverneland A, Feldt-Rasmussen B, Vidal P, et al. Evidence of changes in renal charge selectivity in patients with type 1 (insulin-dependent) diabetes mellitus. *Diabetologia* 1986;29:634.

368. Gragnoli G, Signorini AM, Tanganelli I. Non-enzymatic glycosylation of urinary proteins in type 1 (insulin-dependent) diabetes: correlation with metabolic control and the degree of proteinuria. *Diabetologia* 1984;26:411.

369. Donnelly SM. Accumulation of glycated albumin in end-stage renal failure: evidence for the principle of "physiological microalbuminuria." *Am J Kidney Dis* 1996;28:62.

370. Sakai H, Jinde K, Suzuki D, et al. Localization of glycated proteins in the glomeruli of patients with diabetic nephropathy. *Nephrol Dial Transplant* 1996;11:66.

371. Ghiggeri GM, Candiano G, Delfino G, et al. Glycosyl albumin and diabetic microalbuminuria: demonstration of an altered renal handling. *Kidney Int* 1984;25:565.

372. Shah VO, Dorin RI, Sun Y, et al. Aldose reductase gene expression is increased in diabetic nephropathy. *J Clin Endocrinol Metab* 1997;82:2294.

373. Passariello N, Sepe J, Marrazzo G, et al. Effect of aldose reductase inhibitor (tolrestat) on urinary albumin excretion rate and glomerular filtration rate in IDDM subjects with nephropathy. *Diabetes Care* 1993;16:789.

374. Pedersen MM, Christiansen JS, Mogensen CE. Reduction of glomerular hyperfiltration in normoalbuminuric IDDM patients by 6 mo of aldose reductase inhibition. *Diabetes* 1991;40:527.

375. Ranganathan S, Krempf M, Feraille E, et al. Short term effect of an aldose reductase inhibitor on urinary albumin excretion rate (UAER) and glomerular filtration rate (GFR) in type 1 diabetic patients with incipient nephropathy. *Diabetes Metab* 1993;19:257.

376. McAuliffe AV, Brooks BA, Fisher EJ, et al. Administration of ascorbic acid and an aldose reductase inhibitor (tolrestat) in diabetes: effect on urinary albumin excretion. *Nephron* 1998;80:277.

377. Deckert T, Feldt-Rasmussen B, Borch-Johnsen K, et al. Albuminuria reflects widespread vascular damage: the Steno hypothesis. *Diabetologia* 1989;32:219.

378. Cohen MP, Klepser H, Wu VY. Undersulfation of glomerular basement membrane heparan sulfate in experimental diabetes and lack of correction with aldose reductase inhibition. *Diabetes* 37:1324, 1988.

379. Deckert T, Feldt-Rasmussen B, Djurup, et al. Glomerular size and charge selectivity in insulin-dependent diabetes mellitus. *Kidney Int* 1988;33:100.

380. Vernier RL, Steffes MW, Sisson-Ross S, et al. Heparan sulfate proteoglycan in the glomerular basement membrane in type 1 diabetes mellitus. *Kidney Int* 1992;41:1070.

381. Tamsma JT, van den Born J, Bruijn JA, et al. Expression of glomerular extracellular matrix components in human diabetic nephropathy: decrease of heparan sulphate in the glomerular basement membrane. *Diabetologia* 1994;37:313.

382. Castellot JJ Jr, Hoover RL, Harper PA, et al. Heparin and glomerular epithelial cell-secreted heparin-like species inhibit mesangial-cell proliferation. *Am J Pathol* 1985;120:427.

383. Raats CJ, Van Den Born J, Berden JH. Glomerular heparan sulfate alterations: mechanisms and relevance for proteinuria. *Kidney Int* 2000;57:385.

384. Jensen T. Pathogenesis of diabetic vascular disease: evidence for the role of reduced heparan sulfate proteoglycan. *Diabetes* 1997;46[Suppl 2]:S98.

385. Yokoyama H, Hoyer PE, Hansen PM, et al. Immunohistochemical quantification of heparan sulfate proteoglycan and collagen IV in skeletal muscle capillary basement membranes of patients with diabetic nephropathy. *Diabetes* 1997;46:1875.

386. Gambaro G, Cavazzana AO, Luzi P, et al. Glycosaminoglycans prevent morphological renal alterations and albuminuria in diabetic rats. *Kidney Int* 1992;42:285.

387. Gambaro G, Venturini AP, Noonan DM, et al. treatment with a glycosaminoglycan formulation ameliorates experimental diabetic nephropathy. *Kidney Int* 1994;46:797.

388. Myrup B, Hansen PM, Jensen T, et al. Effect of low-dose heparin on urinary albumin excretion in insulin-dependent diabetes mellitus. *Lancet* 1995;345:421.

389. Gambaro G, Manitius J, Pont'uch P, et al. Long-lasting reduction of albuminuria by oral sulodexide in micro- and macro-albuminuric type 1 and type 2 diabetic patients: the Di.N.A.S. Trial. *J Am Soc Nephrol* 2000;11:114A.

390. Brown DM, Mauer SM. Diabetes mellitus. In: Holliday M, Barratt M, Vernier RL, eds. *Pediatric nephrology,* 2nd ed. Baltimore: Williams & Wilkins, 1987.

391. Miller K, Michael AF. Immunopathology of renal extracellular membranes in diabetes mellitus: specificity of tubular basement membrane immunofluorescence. *Diabetes* 1976;25:701.

392. Burkholder PM. Immunohistopathologic study of localized plasma proteins and fixation of guinea pig complement in renal lesions of diabetic glomerulosclerosis. *Diabetes* 1965;14:755.

393. Steffes MW, et al. Quantitative glomerular morphology of the normal human kidney. *Lab Invest* 1983;49:82.

394. Mauer SM, et al. Structural-functional relationships in diabetic nephropathy. *J Clin Invest* 1984;74:1143.

395. Østerby R, Andersen AR, Gundersen HJ. Quantitative studies of glomerular ultrastructure in type I diabetics with incipient nephropathy. *Diabet Nephropathy* 1984;3:95.

396. Saito Y, et al. Mesangiolysis in diabetic glomeruli: its role in the formation of nodular lesions. *Kidney Int* 1988;34:389.

397. Steffes MW, et al. Cell and matrix components of the glomerular mesangium in type I diabetes. *Diabetes* 1992;41:679.

398. Harris RD, et al. Global glomerular sclerosis and glomerular arteriolar hyalinosis in insulin-dependent diabetes. *Kidney Int* 1991;40:107.

399. Horlyc A, Gundersen HJG, Østerby R. The cortical distribution pattern of diabetic glomerulopathy. *Diabetologia* 1986;29:146.

400. Østerby R, et al. A strong positive correlation between glomerular filtration rate and filtration surface in diabetic nephropathy. *Diabetologia* 1988;31:265.

401. Ellis EN, et al. Glomerular filtration surface in type I diabetes mellitus. *Kidney Int* 1986;29:889.

402. Østerby R, et al. Advanced diabetic glomerulopathy: quantitative structural characteristics of nonoceluded glomeruli. *Diabetes* 1987;36:612.

403. Mauer SM, Sutherland DER, Steffes MW. Relationship of systemic blood pressure to nephropathy in insulin-dependent diabetes mellitus. *Kidney Int* 1992;41:736.

404. Hirose K, et al. A strong correlation between glomerular filtration rate and filtration surface in diabetic kidney hyperfunction. *Lab Invest* 1980;43:434.

405. Lane PH, et al. Renal interstitial expansion in insulin-dependent diabetes mellitus. *Kidney Int* 1993;43:661.

406. Fioretto P, Steffes M, Mauer M. Progression of glomerular vs. interstitial lesions over 5 years in longstanding type I diabetic (IDDM) patients (pts). *J Am Soc Nephrol* 1993;4:303.

407. Walker J, et al. Glomerular structure in type-I (insulin-dependent) diabetic patients with normo- and microalbuminuria. *Kidney Int* 1992;41:741.

408. Caramori ML, Fioretto P, Mauer M. Long-term follow-up of normoalbuminuric longstanding type 1 diabetic patients: progression is associated with worse baseline glomerular lesions and lower glomerular filtration rate. *J Am Soc Nephrol* 1999;10:126A.

409. Ellis EN, et al. Relationship of muscle capillary basement membrane and renal structure and function in diabetes mellitus. *Diabetes* 1986;35:421.

410. Siperstein MD, Unger RH, Madison LL. Studies of muscle capillary basement membranes in normal subjects, diabetic and prediabetic patients. *Clin Invest* 1968;47:1973.

411. Siperstein MD, Feingold KR, Bennett PH. Hyperglycemia and diabetic microangiopathy. *Diabetologia* 1978;15:365.

412. Bilous RW, et al. Mean glomerular volume and rate of development of diabetic nephropathy. *Diabetes* 1989;38:1142.

413. Nyengaard JR, Bendtsen TF. Glomerular number and size in relation to age, kidney weight and body surface in normal man. *Anat Rec* 1992;232:194.

414. Bendtsen TF, Nyengaard JR. The number of glomeruli in type I (insulin-dependent) and type II (non-insulin dependent) diabetic patients. *Diabetologia* 1992;35:844.

415. Brenner BM, Garcia DL, Anderson S. Glomeruli and blood pressure: less of one, more of the other? *Am J Hypertens* 1988;1:335.

416. Moriya T, Chow L, Moriya R, et al. Does glomerular number influence diabetic nephropathy risk in insulin dependent diabetes mellitus (IDDM) patients? *J Am Soc Nephrol* 1997;8:115A(abstr).

417. Hayashi H, et al. An electron microscopic study of glomeruli in Japanese patients with non-insulin dependent diabetes mellitus. *Kidney Int* 1992;41:749.

418. Østerby R, et al. Glomerular structure and function in proteinuric type II (non-insulin-dependent) diabetic patients. *Diabetologia* 1993;32:1064.

419. Gambara V, et al. Heterogenous nature of renal lesions in type II diabetes. *J Am Soc Nephrol* 1993;3:1458.

420. Parving H-H, et al. Prevalence and causes of albuminuria in non-insulin-dependent diabetic patients. *Kidney Int* 1992;41:758.

421. Lipkin GW, et al. More than one kind of type 2 diabetes with renal disease do not have diabetic nephropathy. *J Am Soc Nephrol* 1994;5:379.

422. Olsen S, Mogensen CE. How often is NIDDM complicated with non-diabetic renal disease? An analysis of renal biopsies and the literature. *Diabetologia* 1996;39:1638.

423. Ruggenenti P, et al. Long-term treatment with either enalapril or nifedipine stabilizes albuminuria and increases glomerular filtration rate in non-insulin-dependent diabetic patients. *Am J Kidney Dis* 1994;24:753.

424. Østerby R, Gall M-A, Schmitz A, et al. Glomerular structure and function in proteinuric type II (non-insulin-dependent) diabetic patients. *Diabetologia* 1993;1:1064.

425. Pagtalunan ME, Miller PL, Jumping-Eagle S, et al. Podocyte loss and progressive glomerular injury in type II diabetes. *J Clin Invest* 1997;99:342.

426. Fioretto P, Mauer M, Brocco E, et al. Patterns of renal injury in NIDDM patients with microalbuminuria. *Diabetologia* 1996;39:1569.

427. Nosadini R, Velussi M, Brocco E, et al. Course of renal function in type 2 diabetic patients with abnormalities of albumin excretion rate. *Diabetes* 2000;49:476.

428. Christensen PK, Gall MA, Parving H-H. Course of glomerular filtration rate in albuminuric type 2 diabetic patients with or without diabetic glomerulopathy. *Diabetes Care* 2000;23:B14.

429. Reaven GM. Syndrome X: 6 years later. *J Intern Med* 1994;236:13.

430. Urizar RE, et al. The nephrotic syndrome in children with diabetes mellitus of recent onset. *N Engl J Med* 1969;281:173.

431. Cavallo T, Pinto JA, Rajaramas S. Immune complex disease complicating diabetic glomerulosclerosis. *Am J Nephrol* 1984;4:347.

432. Steffes MW, Brown DM, Basgen JM, et al. Glomerular basement membrane thickness following islet transplantation in the diabetic rat. *Lab Invest* 1979;41:116.

433. Steffes MW, Brown DM, Basgen JM, et al. Amelioration of mesangial volume and surface alterations following islet transplantation in diabetic rats. *Diabetes* 1980;29:509.

434. Fioretto P, Mauer SM, Bilous RW, et al. Effects of pancreas transplantation on glomerular structure in insulin-dependent diabetic patients with their own kidneys. *Lancet* 1993;342:120.

435. Fioretto P, Steffes MW, Sutherland DER, et al. Reversal of lesions of diabetic nephropathy after pancreas transplantation. *N Engl J Med* 1998;339:69.

436. Valmadrid CT, Klein R, Moss SE, et al. The risk of cardiovascular disease mortality associated with microalbuminuria and gross proteinuria in persons with older-onset diabetes mellitus. *Arch Intern Med* 2000;160:1093.

437. Feldt-Rasmussen B. Microalbuminuria, endothelial dysfunction, and cardiovascular risk. *Diabetes Metab* 2000;26:464.

438. Nosadini R, Brocco E. Relationship among microalbuminuria, insulin resistance, and renal-cardiac complication in insulin dependent and non-insulin dependent diabetes. *Exp Clin Endocrinol Diabetes* 1997;105(2):1.

439. Preston RA, Stemmer CL, Materson BJ, et al. Renal biopsy in patients 65 years or older: an analysis of the results of 334 biopsies. *J Am Geriatr Soc* 1990;38:669.

440. Daniels BS, Hausen EB. Glycation of albumin, not glomerular basement membrane, alters permeability in an in vitro model. *Diabetes* 1992;41:1415.

441. Bundschuh I, Jackle-Meyer I, Luneberg E, et al. Glycation of serum albumin and its role in renal protein excretion and the development of diabetic nephropathy. *Eur J Clin Chem Clin Biochem* 1992;30:651.

442. Yokoyama H, Okudaira M, Otani T, et al. Higher incidence of diabetic nephropathy in type 2 than in type 1 diabetes in early onset diabetes in Japan. *Kidney Int* 2000;58:302.

443. Pugh JA, Medina R, Ramirez M. Comparison of the course to end stage renal disease of type1 (insulin-dependent) and type2 (non-insulin-dependent) diabetic nephropathy. *Diabetologia* 1993,328:1676.

444. Richard P, Nisson BY, Rosenquist V. The effect of long term intensified insulin treatment on the development of microvascular complications of diabetes mellitus. *N Engl J Med* 1993;329:304.

445. Nathan DM. Long-term complications of diabetes mellitus. *N Engl J Med* 1993;328:1676.

446. The Microalbuminuria Collaborative Study Group. Predictors of the development of microalbuminuria in patients with type1 diabetes mellitus: a seven year prospective study. *Diabet Med* 1999;16:918.

447. Vijan S, Hofer TP, Hayward RA. Estimated benefits of glycemic control in microvascular complication in type 2 diabetes mellitus. *Ann Intern Med* 1997;127:788.

448. Oue T, Namla M, Nakajima M, et al. Risk factor for the progression of microalbuminuria in Japanese type 2 diabetic patients: 10 years follow-up. *Diabetes Clin J Pract* 1999;46:47.

449. Ohkubo Y, Kishikawa H, Araki E. Intensive insulin therapy prevents the progression of diabetic microvascular complications in Japanese patients with non-insulin dependent diabetes mellitus: a randomized prospective 6 year study. *Diabetes Res Clin Pract* 1995;28:103.

450. Shichiri M, Kishikawa H, Ohkubo Y, et al. Long-term results of the Kumamoto Study on optimal diabetes control in type 2 diabetic patients. *Diabetes Care* 2000;23:B21.

451. Deedwania PC. Hypertension and diabetes: new therapeutic options. *Arch Intern Med* 2000;160:1585.

452. Christieb AR. Treatment selection consideration for the hypertensive diabetic patient. *Arch Intern Med* 1990;150:1167.

453. Chantrel F, Bouiller M, Kolb I, et al. Antihypertensive treatment in type 2 diabetes and diabetic nephropathy. *Nephrologie* 2000;21:47.

454. Ruggenenti P, Perna A, Gherardi G, et al. Chronic proteinuric nephropathies: outcomes and response to treatment in a prospective cohort of 352 patients with different patterns of renal injury. *Am J Kidney Dis* 2000;35:1155.

455. Viberti G, Mogensen CE, Groop LC, et al. Effect of captopril on progression to clinical proteinuria, in patients with IDDM and microproteinuria. *JAMA* 1994;271:275.

456. Keane WF, Shapiro BE. Renal protective effects of angiotensin-converting enzyme inhibition. *Am J Cardiol* 1990;65:491.

457. Chan JC, Ko GT, Leung DH, et al. Long-term effects of angiotensin-converting enzyme inhibition and metabolic control in hypertensive type 2 diabetic patients. *Kidney Int* 2000;57:590.

458. Bakris GI, Copley JB, Vicknair N, et al. Calcium channel blockers versus other antihypertensive therapies on progression of NIDDM associated nephropathy. *Kidney Int* 1996;50:1641.

459. Velussi M, Brocco E, Frigato F, et al. Effects of cilazapril and amlodipine on kidney function in hypertensive NIDDM patients. *Diabetes* 1996;45:216.

460. Rossing P, Tarnow I, Boelskifte S, et al. Difference between nisoldipine and lisinopril on glomerular filtration rates and albuminuria in hypertensive IDDM patients with diabetic nephropathy during the first year of treatment. *Diabetes* 1997;46:481.

461. Pijls LT, de Vries H, Donker AJ, et al. The effect of protein restriction on albuminuria in patients with type 2 diabetes mellitus: a randomized trial. *Nephrol Dial Transplant* 1999;14:1445.

462. Hansen HP, Christensen PK, Tauber-Lassen E, et al. Low protein diet and kidney function in insulin dependent diabetic patients with nephropathy. *Kidney Int* 1999;55:621.

463. Raal FJ, Kalk WJ, Lawson M, et al. Effects of moderate dietary protein restriction on the progression of overt diabetic nephropathy: a 6-month prospective study. *Am J Clin Nutr* 1994;60:579.

464. Evanoff G, Thompson C, Brown J, et al. Prolonged dietary protein restriction in diabetic nephropathy. *Arch Intern Med* 1989;149:1129.

465. Brouhard BH, LaGrone L. Effect of dietary protein restriction on functional renal reserve in diabetic nephropathy. *Am J Med* 1990;89:427.

466. Raal FJ, Kalk WJ, Lawson M, et al. Effects of moderate dietary protein restriction on the progression of overt diabetic nephropathy: a 6-month prospective study. *Am J Clin Nutr* 1994;60:579.

467. Dullaart RP, Beusekamp BJ, Meijer S, et al. Long-term effects of protein restricted diet on albuminuria and renal function in IDDM patients without clinical nephropathy and hypertension. *Diabetes Care* 1993;16:483.

468. Zeller K, Whittaker E, Sullivan L, et al. Effect of restricting dietary protein on the progression of renal failure in patients with insulin dependent diabetes mellitus. *N Engl J Med* 1990;324:78.

469. Kasiske BL, Lakatua JD, Ma JZ, et al. A meta-analysis of the effects of dietary protein restriction on the rate of decline in renal function. *Am J Kidney Dis* 1998;31:954.

470. Sampson MJ, Griffith VS, Drury PL. Blood pressure, diet and the progression of nephropathy in patients with type1 diabetes and hypertension. *Diabet Med* 1994;1:150.

471. Jameel N, Pugh JA, Mitchell BD, et al. Dietary protein intake is not correlated with clinical proteinuria in NIDDM. *Diabetes Care* 1992;15:178.

472. Klahr S, Levy AS, Beck GJ, et al. The effect of dietary protein restriction and blood pressure control on the progression of chronic renal disease: Modification of Diet in Renal Disease Study Group. *N Engl J Med* 1994;330:929.

473. Biesenbach G, Zazgornik J. High mortality and poor quality of life during predialysis period in type2 diabetic patients with diabetic nephropathy. *Ren Fail* 1994;16:263.

474. Roberts JC, Kjellstrand CM. Choosing death: withdrawal from chronic dialysis without medical reason. *Acta Med Scand* 1988;223:181.

475. Blagg CR. Visual and vascular problems in dialyzed diabetic patients. *Kidney Int* 1974;6:S27.

476. Goldstein DA, Massry SG. Diabetic nephropathy: clinical cause and effect on hemodialysis. *Nephron* 1978;20:286.

477. Jacobs C, Rottemburg J, Frantz P. Treatment of end-stage renal failure in the insulin dependent diabetic patient. *Adv Nephrol* 1979;8:101.

478. Gaede P, Vedel P, Parving HH, et al. Intensified multifactorial intervention in patients with type 2 diabetes mellitus and microalbuminuria: the Steno type 2 randomized study. *Lancet* 1999;353:617.

479. The Diabetes Control and Complications Trial/Epidemiology of Diabetes Interventions and Complications Research Group. Retinopathy and nephropathy in patients with type1 diabetes four years after a trial of intensive therapy. *N Engl J Med* 2000;342:381.

480. Klein R, Klein BE, Moss SE, et al. The Wisconsin Epidemiologic Study of Diabetic Retinopathy: XVII. The 14-year incidence and progression of diabetic retinopathy and associated risk factors in type1diabetes. *Ophthalmology* 1998;10:1801.

481. Diglas J, Willinger C, Neu C, et al. Morbidity and mortality in type 1 and type 2 diabetes mellitus after the diagnosis of diabetic retinopathy. *Dtsch Med Wochenschr* 1992;117:1703.

482. Hayashi H, Kurata Y, Imanaga Y, et al. Vitrectomy for diabetic retinopathy in patients undergoing hemodialysis for associated end-stage renal failure. *Retina* 1998;18:156.

483. Dinneen SF, Gerstein HC. The association of microalbuminuria and mortality in non-insulin dependent diabetes mellitus: a systematic overview of the literature. *Arch Intern Med* 1997;157:1413.

484. Beilin J, Stanton KG, McCann VJ, et al. Microalbuminuria in type 2 diabetes: an independent predictor for cardiovascular mortality. *Aust N Z J Med* 1996;26:519.

485. Agewall S, Wikstrand J, Ljungman S, et al. Usefulness of microalbuminuria in predicting cardiovascular mortality in treated hypertensive men with and without diabetes mellitus: Risk Factor Intervention Group. *Am J Cardiol* 1997;80:164.

486. Borch-Johnson K, Kreiner S. Proteinuria value as predictor of cardiovascular mortality in insulin dependent diabetes mellitus. *BMJ* 1987;294:1651.

487. Chantrel F, Enache I, Bouiller M, et al. Abysmal prognosis of patients with type 2 diabetes entering dialysis. *Nephrol Dial Transplant* 1999;14:129.

488. Koch M, Gradaus F, Schocbet FC, et al. Relevance of conventional cardiovascular risk factors for the prediction of coronary artery disease in diabetic patients on renal replacement therapy. *Nephrol Dial Transplant* 1997;12:1187.

489. Manske CL, Wang Y, Rector T, et al. Coronary revascularisation in insulin-dependent diabetic patients with chronic renal failure. *Lancet* 1992;340:998.

490. Legrain M, Rottemburg J, Bentchikou A, et al. Dialysis treatment of insulin-dependent diabetic patients: ten years experience. *Clin Nephrol* 1984;21:72.

491. Kalker AJ, Pirsch JD, Heisey D, et al. Foot problems in the diabetic transplant recipients. *Clin Transplant* 1996;10:503.

492. Bentley F, Sutherland D, Mauer S. The status of diabetic renal allograft recipients who survive for ten or more years after transplantation. *Transplant Proc* 1985;17:1573.

493. Caputo GM, Cavangh PR, Ulbrecht JS, et al. Assessment and management of foot disease in patients with diabetes. *N Engl J Med* 1994;331:854.

494. Van Gils CC, Wheeler LA, Mellstrom M, et al. Amputation prevention by vascular surgery and podiatry collaboration in high-risk diabetic and non-diabetic patients: The Operation Desert Foot experience. *Diabetes Care* 1994;22:678.

495. Schleiffer T, Holken H, Brass H. Morbidity in 565 type 2 diabetic patients according to the stage of nephropathy. *J Diabetes Complications* 1998;12:103.

496. Nankivell BJ, Lau SG, Chapman JR, et al. Progression of macrovascular disease after transplantation. *Transplantation* 2000;69:574.

497. Viswanathan V, Prasad D, Chamukuttan S, et al. The prevalence and early onset of cardiac autonomic neuropathy among south indian type 2 diabetic patients with nephropathy. *Diabetes Res Clin Pract* 2000;48:211.

498. Kastenbauer T, Auinger M, Irsigler K. Prevalence of cardiac autonomic neuropathies in uremia and diabetes mellitus. *Wien Klin Wochenschr* 1994;106:733.

499. Yoshioka K, Teerasake J. Relationship between diabetic autonomic neuropathy and peripheral neuropathy as assessed by power spectral analysis of heart rate variations and vibratory perception thresholds. *Diabetes Res Clin Pract* 1994;24:9.

500. Jalal S, Alai MS, Khan KA, et al. Silent myocardial ischemia and cardiac autonomic neuropathy in diabetics. *J Assoc Physicians India* 1999;47:767.

501. Horowitz DK, Fraser R. Disordered gastric motor function in diabetes mellitus. *Diabetologia* 1994;37:543.

502. Annese V, Bassotti G, Caruso N, et al. Gastrointestinal motor dysfunction, symptoms, and neuropathy in non-insulin dependent diabetes mellitus. *J Clin Gastroenterol* 1999;29:171.

503. Clark DW, Nowak TV. Diabetic gastroparesis: what to do when gastric emptying is delayed. *Postgrad Med* 1994;95:195.

504. Lux G. Disorders of gastrointestinal motility: diabetes mellitus. *Leber Magen Darm* 1989;19:84.

505. Drenth JP, Engels LG. Gastroparesis: a critical reappraisal of new treatment strategies. *Drugs* 1992;44:537.

506. Battle WM, Cohen JD, Snape WJ Jr. Disorders of colonic motility in patients with diabetes mellitus. *Yale J Biol Med* 1983;56:277.

507. Spollett GR. Assessment and management of erectile dysfunction in men with diabetes. *Diabetes Educ* 1999;25:65.

508. Amiel S. Glucose counter-regulation in health and disease: current concepts in hypoglycemia recognition and response. *QJM* 1991;80:707.

509. Meyer C, Grossmann R, Mitrakou A. Effects of autonomic neuropathy on counter-regulation and awareness of hypoglycemia in type 1 diabetic patients. *Diabetes Care* 1998;21:1960.

510. Hathaway DK, Abell T, Cardoso S, et al. Improvement in autonomic and gastric function following pancreas-kidney versus kidney alone transplantation and the correlation with quality of life. *Transplantation* 1994;57:816.

511. Nankivell BJ, al-Harbi IS, Morris J, et al. Recovery of diabetic neuropathy after pancreas transplantation. *Transplant Proc* 1997;29:658.

512. Navarro X, Sutherland DE, Kennedy WR. Long-term effects of pancreatic transplantation on diabetic neuropathy. *Ann Neurol* 1997;42:727.

513. Navarro X, Kennedy, WR, Aeppli D, et al. Neuropathy and mortality in diabetes: influence of pancreas transplantation. *Muscle Nerve* 1996;19:1009.

514. Arkkila PE, Kantola IM, Vikari JS. Limited joint mobility in type 1 diabetic patients: correlation to other diabetic complications. *Intern Med* 1994;236:215.

515. Maisonneuve P, Agodoa L, Gellert R, et al. Distribution of primary renal disease leading to end-stage renal failure in United States, Europe, Australia/New Zealand: results from an international comparative study. *Am J Kidney Dis* 2000;35:157.

516. Sesso R, Melargno CS, Luconi PS, et al. Survival of dialyzed diabetic patients. *Rev Assoc Med Bras* 1995;41:178.

517. Koch M, Thomas B, Tschope W, et al. Survival and predictor of death in dialyzed diabetic patients. *Diabetologia* 1993;36:1113.

518. Choh LM, Germain M. Dialysis discontinuation and palliative care. *Am J Kidney Disease* 2000;36:140.

519. Mailloux LU, Belluci AG, Napolitan B, et al. Death by withdrawal from dialysis: a 20 year clinical experience. *J Am Soc Nephrol* 1993;3:1631.

520. Friedman EA. Physician bias in uremic therapy. *Kidney Int* 1985;[Suppl A]:S38.

521. Mauer SM, Chavers RM. A comparison of kidney disease in type 1 and type 2 diabetes. *Adv Exp Med Biol* 1985;189:299.

522. Sims EAH, Calles-Escandon J. Classification of diabetes: a fresh look for the 1990s? *Diabetes Care* 1990;13:1123.

523. Abourizk NN, Dunn JC. Types of diabetes according to National Diabetes Data Group Classification: limited applicability and need to revisit. *Diabetes Care* 1990;13:1120.

524. Cantalano C. Diabetes mellitus classification in end-stage renal failure [Letter]. *Nephrol Dial Transplant* 1995;10:301.

525. Palder SB, Kirkman RL, Whittemore AD. Vascular access for hemodialysis: patency rates and results of revision. *Ann Surg* 1985;202:234.

526. Cheigh J, Raghavan J, Sullivan J, et al. Is insufficient dialysis a cause for high morbidity in diabetic patients? *J Am Soc Nephrol* 1990;317(abstr).

527. Hampl H, Berweck S, Ludat K, et al. How can hemodialysis associated hypotension and dialysis induced symptoms be explained and controlled—particularly in diabetic atherosclerotic patients? *Clin Nephrol* 2000;53[Suppl]:S69.

528. Tzamaloukas AH, Murata GH, Zager PG, et al. The relationship between glycemic control and morbidity and mortality for diabetics on dialysis. *ASAIO J* 1993;39:880.

529. Pei Y, Heres G, Segre G, et al. Renal osteodystrophy in diabetic patients. *Kidney Int* 1993;44:159.

530. Hernandez D, Concepcion MT, Lorenao B, et al. Adynamic bone disease with negative aluminium staining in predialysis patients: prevalence and evolution after maintenance dialysis. *Nephrol Dial Transplant* 1994;9:512.

531. Lowder GM, Perri NA, Friedman EA. Demographics, diabetes type, and degree of rehabilitation in diabetic patients on maintenance hemodialysis in Brooklyn. *J Diabetic Complications* 1988;2:218.

532. Lindblad AS, Nolph KD, Novak JW, et al. A survey of the NIH CAPD Registry population with end-stage renal disease attributed to diabetic nephropathy. *J Diabetic Complications* 1988;2:227.

533. Rottembourg J. Peritoneal dialysis in diabetics. In: Nolph KD, ed. *Peritoneal dialysis.* Boston: Martinus Nijhoff, 1985:363.

534. Maiorca R, Vonesh E, Cancarini GC. A six year comparison of patients and technique survival in CAPD and hemodialysis. *Kidney Int* 1988;34:518.

535. Legrain M, Rottembourg J, Bentchikou A, et al. Dialysis treatment of insulin dependent diabetic patients: ten years experience. *Clin Nephrol* 1984;21:72.

536. Nolph DK. Is residual renal function preserved better with CAPD than with hemodialysis? *AKF Nephrol Lett* 1990;7:1.

537. Flynn CT, Nanson JA. Intraperitoneal insulin with CAPD: an artificial pancreas. *Trans Am Soc Artif Int Organs* 1979;25:114.

538. Scarpioni LL, Ballocchi S, Castelli A, et al. Continuous ambulatory peritoneal dialysis in diabetic patients. *Contrib Nephrol* 1990;84:60.

539. Fluckiger R, Harmon W, Meier W, et al. Hemoglobin carbamylation in uremia. *N Engl J Med* 1981;304:823.

540. Blumenkrantz MJ, Gahl GM, Kopple JD, et al. Protein losses during peritoneal dialysis. *Kidney Int* 1981;19:593.

541. Krediet RT, Zuyderhoudt FMJ, Boeschoten EW, et al. Diagnosis of protein calorie malnutrition in diabetic patients on hemodialysis and peritoneal dialysis. *Nephron* 1986;42:133.

542. Held PJ, Port FK, Blagg CR, et al. The United States Renal Data System annual data report. *Am J Kidney Dis* 1990;16[Suppl 2]:34.

543. Yuan ZY, Balaskas E, Gupta A, et al. Is CAPD or hemodialysis better for diabetic patients? CAPD is more advantageous. *Semin Dial* 1992;5:181.

544. Port FK, Wolf RA, Mauger EA, et al. Comparison of survival probabilities for dialysis patients versus cadaveric renal transplant recipients. *JAMA* 1993;270:1339.

545. Khauli RB, Steinmuller DR, Novick AC, et al. A critical look at survival of diabetics with end-stage renal disease: transplantation versus dialysis. *Transplantation* 1986;41:598.

546. Grenfell A, Bewick M, Snowden S, et al. Renal replacement for diabetic patients: experience at King's College Hospital 1980–1989. *QJM* 1992;85:861.
547. Mazzuchi N, Gonzalez-Martinez F, Carbonell E, et al. Comparison of survival for hemodialysis patients vs renal transplant recipients treated in Uruguay. *Nephrol Dial Transplant* 1999;14:2849.
548. Tyden G, Bolinder J, Solders G, et al. A 10 year prospective study of IDDM patients subjected to combined pancreas and kidney transplantation or kidney transplantation alone. *Transplant Proc* 1998; 30:332.
549. Becker BN, Brazy PC, Becker YT, et al. Simultaneous pancreas-kidney transplantation reduces excess mortality in type 1 diabetic patients with end-stage renal disease. *Kidney Int* 2000;57:2129.
550. Secchi A, Martinenghi S, Castoldi R, et al. Effects of pancreas transplantation on quality of life in type1 diabetic patients undergoing kidney transplantation. *Transplant Proc* 1998;30:339.
551. Sudan D, Sudan R, Stratta R. Long-term outcome of simultaneous kidney-pancreas transplantation analysis of 61 patients with more than 5 years follow-up. *Transplantation* 2000;69:550.
552. Biesenbach G, Margreiter R, Konigstrainer A, et al. Comparisons of progression of macrovascular diseases after kidney-pancreas and kidney transplantation in diabetic patients with end-stage renal disease. *Diabetologia* 2000;45:231.
553. Cheung AT, Perez RV, Chen PC. Improvements of diabetic microangiopathy after successful simultaneous pancreas-kidney transplantation: a computer-assisted intravital microscopy study on the conjunctival microcirculation. *Transplantation* 1999;68:927.
554. Abendroth D, Schmand J, Landgraf R, et al. Diabetic microangiopathy in type1 (insulin dependent) diabetic patients after successful pancreatic and kidney or solitary kidney transplantation. *Diabetologia* 1991;34[Suppl 1]: S131.
555. La Rocca E, Gobbi C, Ciurlino D, et al. Improvement of glucose/insulin metabolism reduces hypertension in insulin-dependent diabetes mellitus recipients of kidney-pancreas transplantation. *Transplantation* 1999;65:390.
556. Allen RD, al-Harbi IS, Morris JG, et al. Diabetic neuropathy after pancreas transplantation determinants of recovery. *Transplantation* 1997;63:830.
557. Kennedy WR, Navararro X, Goetx FC, et al. Effects of pancreas transplantation on diabetic neuropathy. *N Engl J Med* 1990;320: 1031.
558. Gaver AO, Cardoso D, Pearson S, et al. Improvement in autonomic function following combined pancreas-kidney transplantation. *Transplant Proc* 1991;23:1660.
559. Pearce IA, Ilango B, Sells RA, et al. Stabilization of diabetic retinopathy following simultaneous pancreas and kidney transplant. *Br J Ophthalmol* 2000;84:736.
560. Chow VC, Pai RP, Chapman JR, et al. Diabetic retinopathy after combined kidney-pancreas transplantation. *Clin Transplant* 1999;13: 356.
561. Manske CL, Wang Y, Thomas W. Mortality of cadaveric kidney transplantation versus combined kidney-pancreas transplantation in diabetic patients. *Lancet* 1995;346:1658.
562. Manske CL. Risks and benefits of kidney and pancreas transplantation for diabetic patients. *Diabetes Care* 1999;22:B114.
563. Sasaki TM, Gray RS, Ratner RE, et al. Successful long-term kidney-pancreas transplants in diabetic patients with high C-peptide levels. *Transplantation* 1998;65:1510.

CHAPTER 74

The Normal and Diseased Kidney in Pregnancy

Marshall D. Lindheimer and Adrian I. Katz

Renal disease, regardless of severity, was once considered a major impediment to a successful pregnancy. Both maternal and fetal prognoses were considered quite poor, with special concern that conception frequently exacerbated the underlying disorder, thus hastening its progression to end-stage renal disease (1). Evidence accumulated since 1980, however, has led to a revision of these views, and we now know that there are many instances in which pregnancy in women with kidney disease carries little risk. This chapter, designed to aid physicians consulted when such patients contemplate conceiving or are already pregnant, focuses on the pathophysiology, risk assessment, and management of renal disease in pregnancy. Hypertension associated with pregnancy is dealt with elsewhere in this book (Chapter 53, Hypertension and Pregnancy). But first a review of the normal changes in the physiology and morphology of the urinary system during gestation is required if we are to detect abnormalities at an early stage.

PREGNANCY-INDUCED CHANGES IN ANATOMY AND FUNCTION

Anatomy

Kidney

Kidney weight, size, and volume increase in normal human gestation (2–6). Although autopsy data are obviously limited, there is a unique series in which the combined weight of "normal" kidneys of 97 women who expired during or shortly after pregnancy averaged 307 g, a value greater than published norms in nonpregnant women (4). Kidney length estimated by either pyelography or nephrotomography increases by about 1 cm, returning to nonpregnant values by the sixth postpartum month (5,6).

Increments in kidney weight also occur in rodent pregnancy, in which one group of investigators claimed that

M. D. Lindheimer: Department of Medicine and Department of Obstetrics and Gynecology, University of Chicago, Chicago, Illinois
A. I. Katz: Department of Medicine, University of Chicago; and University of Chicago Medical Center, Chicago, Illinois

proximal tubule length and renal dry weight increase, in a manner reminiscent of events during compensatory hypertrophy after uninephrectomy (7). Davison and Lindheimer (8), however, failed to detect biochemical evidence of new kidney growth in pregnant rats. They, as others (9), measured similar renal dry weights in gravid and nonpregnant rats and concluded that the increased total weight was entirely due to the increment in water content. In essence, the changes in kidney weight and length during either human or animal gestation are but a consequence of the increase in renal interstitial and intravascular volumes that accompany normal pregnancy (see later discussion).

There is very little information on the microscopic anatomy of kidneys from normal human or animal gestations. The light microscopic appearance in renal biopsies, usually obtained near term during cesarean delivery, has been described as similar to that in nonpregnant subjects. On the other hand, the glomerular diameter in 27 autopsy cases was substantially greater than that measured in nonpregnant subjects (4). Most autopsies described by Sheehan and Lynch (4) were performed within 2 hours of death, between 1935 and 1946, at the Glasgow Royal Maternity Hospital by the celebrated pathologist H. L. Sheehan. The monograph (4), which focuses on the histology of the kidneys, liver, and brains of women dying with preeclampsia or eclampsia, also contains approximately 1,700 references. The same authors also performed cell counts, concluding that increments in glomerular size were due to cellular hypertrophy, rather than hyperplasia.

Collecting System

The most prominent alterations in the urinary tract involve the collecting system. The calices, renal pelves, and ureters all dilate, accompanied by hypertrophy of ureteral smooth muscle and hyperplasia of its connective tissue (2,3,10–14) (Fig. 74-1). The dilatation, which tends to be more prominent on the right, may be observed in the initial trimester and is present in more than 90% of pregnant women at term (2,3,11,13). The "normal" limits of caliceal dilatation have

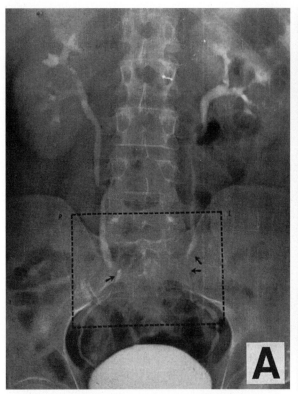

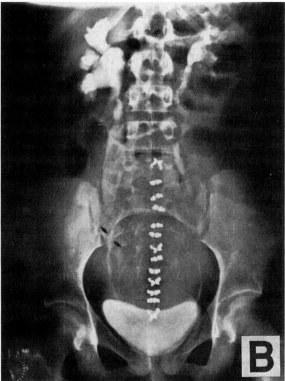

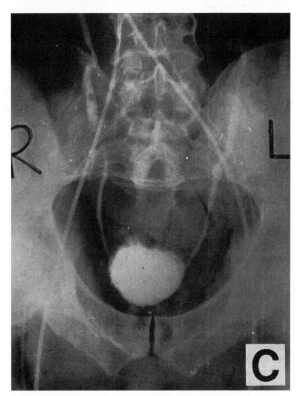

FIG. 74-1. The "physiologic" dilation of the urinary tract in pregnancy. **A:** Mild dilatation. The ureters are seen along their entire course. Note the sharp cutoff of the right ureter at the pelvic brim *(single arrow),* where it crosses the iliac artery ("iliac sign"). **B:** More severe dilatation, includes the renal pelvis and calices. Double arrow points to the pelvic brim. **C:** Postmortem injection study. Catheters in the iliac artery again demonstrate the iliac sign on the right. (From Dure-Smith P. Pregnancy dilation and the urinary tract. *Radiology* 1970;96:545, with permission.)

always been hard to define, but the reader may find recently published norms by Faúndes et al. (15) to be useful guidelines.

There are differing views about the cause of the urinary tract dilatation in pregnancy. Some believe the etiology to be hormonal in nature; others, obstructive in origin (2,3,14). The principal arguments favoring the former come from animal studies and evidence that in humans, the ureters may dilate before the uterus has enlarged sufficiently to become an obstructive factor, and from the failure of prolonged catheterization

TABLE 74-1. *Renal changes in normal pregnancy*

Alteration	Manifestation	Clinical relevance
Increased renal size	Renal length $\approx$1 cm greater on radiographs	Postpartum decreases in size should not be mistaken for parenchymal loss
Dilation of pelves, calices, and ureters	Resembles hydronephrosis on ultrasound or IVP (more marked on right)	Not to be mistaken for obstructive uropathy; retained urine leads to collection errors; upper urinary tract infections are more virulent; may be responsible for "over-distention syndrome"; elective pyelography should be deferred to $\geq$12 wk postpartum
Increased renal hemodynamics	Glomerular filtration rate and renal plasma flow increase 35–50%	Serum creatinine and urea nitrogen values decrease; >0.8 mg/dL (>72 μmol/L) creatinine already suspect; protein, amino acid, and glucose excretion all increase
Changes in acid–base metabolism	Renal bicarbonate threshold decreases; progesterone stimulates respiratory center	Serum bicarbonate and P_{CO_2} are 4–5 mmol/L and 10 mm Hg lower, respectively; a P_{CO_2} of 40 mm Hg already represents substantial CO_2 retention
Renal water handling	Osmoregulation altered (osmotic thresholds for AVP release and thirst decrease; hormonal disposal rates increase)	Serum osmolality decreases $\approx$10 mOsmol/L (serum Na $\approx$5 mEq/L); increased metabolism of AVP may cause transient diabetes insipidus in pregnancy

IVP, intravenous pyelography; AVP, vasporessin; P_{CO_2}, carbon dioxide tension.
Source: From Lindheimer MD, Grünfeld J-P, Davison JM. Renal disorders. In: Barron WM, Lindheimer MD, eds. *Medical disorders during pregnancy,* 3rd ed. St. Louis: Mosby–Year Book, 2000,39, with permission.

to reverse the dilatation (2,3). Support for the obstructive theory comes from studies in which intraureteral pressure was monitored in third-trimester gravidas subjected to several postural maneuvers (16). Pressure, which was greatest when the gravidas were supine or standing, decreased markedly when they assumed a lateral decubitus or knee-to-chest position or immediately after cesarian delivery of the fetus, observations that imply that the gravid uterus can obstruct the ureters. The increased pressure was only present above the pelvic brim, which is consistent with an elegant study performed by Dure-Smith (10). The latter, combining *in vivo* and postmortem observations, concluded that dilatation of the collecting system terminates at the level of the true bony pelvic brim. This is where the ureters and the iliac arteries cross (Fig. 74-1B) and where the weight of the enlarged uterus produces a pyelographic filling defect termed the "iliac sign" (Fig. 74-1A). One should note, however, that failure to observe dilatation below the pelvic brim is not conclusive evidence of obstruction. This is because Waldeyer's sheath, the connective tissue that envelops the ureters as they enter the true pelvis, hypertrophies during pregnancy, which could prevent hormonal dilatation below the pelvic brim.

Finally, there is another theory that ascribes obstruction of the ureters to dilatation of the ovarian and uterine veins (particularly on the right) during pregnancy, and in fact an "ovarian vein syndrome" characterized by ureteral colic due to the obstruction of the ureter by an enlarged ovarian vein has been described in patients ingesting oral contraceptives (2,17). In a sense, this postulate combines the hormonal and obstructive theories, but we find the concept of venous dilation as a cause of ureteral obstruction unconvincing.

Clinical Relevance

The anatomic changes during pregnancy described previously have considerable clinical significance (Table 74-1). Acceptable norms of kidney size should be increased by 1 cm, and therefore postpartum reductions in renal length from values estimated during pregnancy should not be attributed to pathologic decrements in renal mass. The dilated urinary tract often contains substantial volumes of urine, which may lead to errors in timed urine volumes, but these can be avoided if the patient is hydrated and assumes a lateral decubitus position 45 to 60 minutes before starting and again before completing the collection. These maneuvers minimize dead space errors by producing a diuresis and ensuring that any residual urine within the urinary tract or bladder is dilute and of recent origin.

Factors that may be responsible for these anatomic changes have also been linked to several pathologic problems that arise in pregnancy. There is an "overdistention" syndrome (Fig. 74-2) characterized by abdominal pain, marked hydronephrosis, variable increases in serum creatinine levels, and even hypertension (18–21). Symptoms may be ameliorated by assuming a knee-to-chest or lateral recumbent position. Some patients have responded to placement of ureteral stents with improvement of renal function and normalization of blood pressure; the stents were removed postpartum without recurrence of the syndrome. One should note that frank urinary obstruction may be difficult to diagnose during

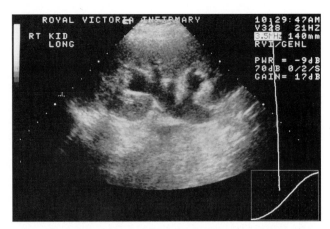

FIG. 74-2. Overdistention syndrome. This ultrasound demonstrates marked dilatation of the pelvic caliceal system. The patient complained of right-sided loin pain that worsened despite treatment of presumed pyelonephritis. The symptoms resolved immediately after stent placement and did not recur when the stent was removed 1 month after delivery. (From J. M. Davison, with permission.)

pregnancy, in which case the "iliac sign" may prove helpful. Finally, two rare but serious complications that occur in late pregnancy are acute urinary retention and nontraumatic rupture of the ureters (18,22). Whether they represent extreme instances of "physiologic" dilatation or reflect other underlying pathology is unclear.

Function

Renal Hemodynamics

Glomerular filtration rate (GFR) and renal plasma flow (RPF) increase markedly during gestation (Fig. 74-3). Detailed reviews of more than 50 reports can be found elsewhere (2,3,17, 23,24), including discussions of important methodological considerations that in the past led to discrepancies in the

literature. The best studies are those in which inulin clearance (C_{inulin}) and p-aminohippurate clearance (C_{PAH}) were measured serially and simultaneously, preferably with the subjects positioned in lateral recumbency during the test. The importance of the latter is that supine or upright posture may transiently decrease GFR and RPF, especially in late pregnancy, when assuming a supine position results in the enlarged uterus encroaching on the aorta and vena cava and obstructing their flow (2,23,24). These reviews and the more recent literature permit the following synthesis: An increase in GFR and RPF may already be present in the luteal phase of the menstrual cycle (24,25), and both are significantly increased by the sixth gestational week (26). The increments in GFR peak approximately 50% above nonpregnant values by the end of the second trimester, and these high levels are maintained through gestational week 36, after which a decrease of 15% to 20% may occur. There are disputes about whether this decrease actually occurs, but in some reports, 24-hour endogenous creatinine clearance does return to nonpregnant levels at term (17,24,27).

The increase in RPF during the first two trimesters (50% to 80%) surpasses that of GFR, so in many reports, filtration fraction falls slightly. Near term, however, C_{PAH} may decline about 25%, and filtration fraction returns to that observed in nonpregnant populations, even though RPF is still considerably elevated (17,24,27–29).

The mechanisms responsible for the changes in renal hemodynamics during human pregnancy are unclear. There are increases in cardiac output and extracellular volume that appear to parallel those of GFR and RPF (26), but vascular resistance and blood pressure fall at the same time. A number of endocrine changes—including increments in circulating levels of aldosterone, desoxycorticosterone, progesterone, prolactin, and chorionic gonadotropin—occur and could conceivably augment renal hemodynamics, but none of these hormones alone appears to have effects as large as those seen in pregnant women. Plasma albumin concentration and

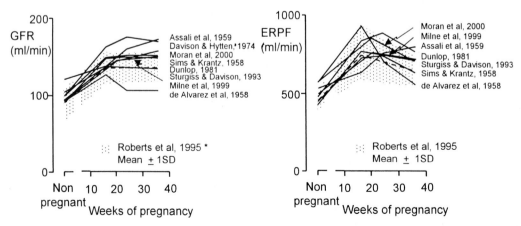

FIG. 74-3. Serial changes in glomerular filtration rate **(left)** and effective renal plasma flow **(right)** in pregnancy. Changes reported by several workers are superimposed on the mean *(dashed line)* ±1 standard deviation *(shaded area)* from the study by Roberts et al. (29). (From J. M. Davison, with permission.)

oncotic pressure decrease early in pregnancy, and if similar decrements are present within the glomerular capillary, they could explain a rise in GFR (17,24).

Renal hemodynamics also increase during pregnancy in several animal species (2,3,17,24,30). Results from micropuncture protocols designed to span the whole rat gestation suggest that increases in single nephron GFR are due exclusively to increments in glomerular plasma flow (30). Furthermore, the tubuloglomerular feedback mechanism appears to be operating normally in this species but is reset to "sense" the increased nephron filtration rate as normal (31). Gestational vasodilatation does not appear to alter the intrinsic renal autoregulatory ability in rats or rabbits (32,33). Renal vasodilatation during rat pregnancy involves an even reduction of the afferent and efferent arteriolar pressures so glomerular capillary pressure is kept constant (Fig. 74-4). In such a scenario, hyperfiltration should have no adverse effects on long-term renal morphology and function, a postulate elegantly shown to be true in rats after six repetitive pregnancies (34).

Direct micropuncture studies of the determinants of ultrafiltration are obviously proscribed in humans, but insight into these parameters can be obtained by measurements of the fractional clearance of neutral dextrans ($C_{dextran}/C_{inulin}$). Such data are subjected to mathematical modeling that explores the mechanism of solute transport across heteroporous membranes, and when combined with measured GFR, RPF, and plasma oncotic pressure predict the glomerular ultrafiltration coefficient (K_f) and glomerular membrane porosity. Permselectivity to neutral dextrans has been found to be altered in human pregnancy (Fig. 74-5), and theoretical analysis of these curves with either the "isoporous plus shunt" or lognormal models (29,35,36) suggests the following: Hyperfiltration during human gestation is primarily due to increases in RPF with a minor contribution due

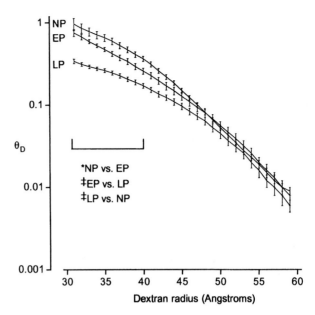

FIG. 74-5. Serial changes in fractional dextran clearance relative to water clearance (as C_{inulin}) (ΘD) in early pregnancy (*EP*, 16 weeks gestation), late pregnancy (*LP*, 36 weeks gestation), and nonpregnant (*NP*, 16 weeks postpartum) women (N = 11). (* $P < 0.02$; $P < 0.0001$.) (From Roberts M, Lindheimer MD, Davison JM. Altered glomerular permselectivity to neutral dextrans and heteroporous membrane modeling in human pregnancy. *Am J Physiol* 1996;270:F338, with permission.)

to decreased oncotic pressure. There is a small increment in K_f, and membrane porosity appears to be altered. There is no evidence of increased glomerular capillary pressure in pregnant women (Fig. 74-6), similar to findings in the pregnant rat. However, one must underscore the theoretical nature of this approach.

Studies in animal models before 1995, primarily involving rodent gestation and designed to gain insight into the factors responsible for the striking changes in renal hemodynamics are detailed and cited elsewhere (24,30,37). GFR increases in pseudopregnant rats, suggesting that the stimulus is maternal in origin. However, a host of studies designed to mimic the maternal hormonal milieu in pregnancy, including treatment with estrogens, progesterone, or prolactin, have been negative or contradictory. Similarly, neither acute nor chronic cyclooxygenase inhibition reversed the increased GFR in pregnant animals. More promising observations by Conrad et al. (38–43), appearing since 1995 and described later, are based on the following approach.. The preglomerular and postglomerular arterioles, as well as the contractile elements interposed between them (e.g., the mesangium), are sensitive to various vasoactive hormones and autocoids including angiotensin II, endothelins (ET), atrial natriuretic peptides, and endothelium-derived relaxing factors (EDRFs), as well as to the alterations in their receptors. These hormones, autocoids, or receptors are or may be altered during pregnancy.

First, Danielson and Conrad (38) measured GFR and RPF in awake, chronically instrumented rats at midpregnancy, the

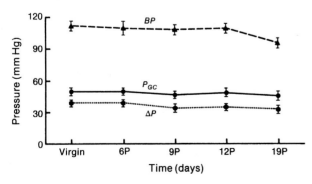

FIG. 74-4. Glomerular capillary pressure (P_{GC}), transglomerular hydrostatic pressure difference (ΔP), and arterial blood pressure (BP) measured in virgin, and 6-, 9-, 12-, and 19-day pregnant euvolemic Munich-Wistar rats. Data are mean ±1 standard error; only the BP on gestational day 19 is significantly lower than values in virgin animals. (From Baylis C. Glomerular filtration and volume regulation in gravid animal models. *Clin Obstet Gynaecol (Baillière)* 1994;8:235, with permission.)

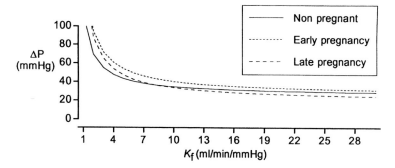

FIG. 74-6. The theoretical relationship between the ultrafiltration coefficient (K_f) and the transglomerular hydrostatic pressure difference (ΔP) in normal pregnancy. Note that over a large range of K_f chosen to include those we would expect in humans, there is little difference in the ΔP when results during early gestation, late pregnancy, and the nonpregnant state are compared with one another. (From Roberts M, Lindheimer MD, Davison JM. Altered glomerular permselectivity to neutral dextrans and hetero-porous membrane modeling in human pregnancy. *Am J Physiol* 1996;270:F338, with permission.)

period when gestational increments most resemble those observed in humans . Acute inhibition of nitric oxide synthases (NOSs) decreased GFR and RPF and increased renal vascular resistance to a greater extent in gravid than in virgin rats, eliminating the differences in renal hemodynamics among groups.

Consistent with these clearance results are *in vitro* data demonstrating that NOS inhibition restored the myogenic reactivity of resistance-sized renal arteries obtained from pregnant rats to that of virgin controls (40). However, their message became less clear in pregnant animal models undergoing chronic NOS inhibition (39). In these latter circumstances, the pregnant animals still manifested increases in GFR, suggesting that when the NO-EDRF system is suppressed, compensatory mechanisms take over. These appear to be mediated by vasodilatory prostaglandins, because now the gestational rise can be abolished with meclofenamate (although prostaglandin inhibitors alone have no influence on the increased renal hemodynamics of rat gestation). Conrad and colleagues (41) further suggested a role for ET and its receptors in the renal adaptation to pregnancy. ET is normally thought of as a potent vasoconstrictor, but using pharmacologic probes, the authors suggested that ET plays an important role in maintaining low vascular tone in pregnant rodents via stimulation of an ET$_B$ receptor subtype, tonic stimulation of NO-EDRF, feedback inhibition of ET production, or combinations of these actions. Finally, this same group has demonstrated that relaxin, a hormone that in women originates in the corpus luteum of the ovary and whose production is markedly stimulated by human chorionic gonadotropin (HCG), increases GFR and decreases plasma osmolality (P osm) in rats (42,43). These two observations led to an appealing hypothesis, for we now have in relaxin a hormone whose levels rise in the luteal phase of the menstrual cycle and even more markedly in gestation and whose actions can simultaneously explain both the enhanced renal hemodynamics and the changes in osmoregulation that occur in human gestation.

Because GFR and RPF are already markedly increased, the question has arisen whether renal vasodilatation is already maximal during pregnancy or whether gravidas possess a "functional reserve" akin to that demonstrated during protein loading or amino acid infusions in nonpregnant populations. Several investigators have demonstrated further increases in

renal hemodynamics during the infusion of amino acids into pregnant rats (44) and women (28,35,36). Effects of oral protein loading, however, have been equivocal (45–47). Furthermore, although some have suggested that GFR (measured as creatinine clearance, C_{cr}) correlates with protein intake during human gestation, others have observed similar renal hemodynamics when gravid women followed diets whose protein content was alternatively restricted or supplemented for 1 week before testing (48,49).

In summary, evidence from both pregnant rats and pregnant women suggests that hyperfiltration in pregnancy is primarily due to increased RPF, the latter being due to decreases in renal vascular resistance. There has been considerable progress toward understanding factors responsible for the increased renal hemodynamics during gestation, most made since the last edition of this text. This includes evidence implicating NO, ET or its receptor, and relaxin, but the results are still inconclusive. When finally identified, the putative mechanism must explain why the pregnancy-induced rise in GFR is so powerful (being far greater than that evoked by protein loading or amino acid infusions in nonpregnant individuals), and why it occurs in subjects with kidneys already hypertrophied after uninephrectomy as well as in transplant recipients (50,51). Finally, data from micropuncture in rats and modeling of fractional dextran clearances in pregnant humans suggest that despite hyperfiltration, glomerular capillary pressure is unaltered, indicating that the sustained gestational increments in GFR should not be harmful to the kidney.

Significance of the Increased GFR and RPF

Because there is, at most, a small increase in the production and excretion of creatinine during normal pregnancy (2,52), the large increments in C_{cr} lead to reduction in its plasma level. The concentration of serum urea also decreases, partly because of its augmented clearance, but also because there is enhanced protein synthesis. Therefore, levels of serum creatinine and urea nitrogen that average 0.7 mg/dL and 12 mg/dL (60 μmol/L and 4.3 mmol/L), respectively, in the nonpregnant state decrease to means of 0.5 mg/dL and 9 mg/dL (44 μmol/L and 3.2 mmol/L) during gestation (2,27). *Thus, values considered normal in nonpregnant women may reflect abnormal function in pregnancy.* For example, concentrations of serum creatinine and urea nitrogen exceeding 0.8 mg/dL and 13 mg/dL (80 μmol/L and 5 mmol/L), respectively, should alert the clinician to evaluate renal function further. Finally, the filtered loads of many solutes increase, explaining in part why glucosuria, aminoaciduria, and enhanced urinary excretion of water soluble vitamins often occur during normal pregnancy (2,27). These increments in urinary nutrients may enhance the susceptibility of gravidas to symptomatic urinary tract infections.

Tubular Function

Glucose and Amino Acids

Glucose excretion normally increases during pregnancy, exceeding the upper limits of normal in nonpregnant subjects (about 100 mg per 24 hours) 85% of the time and often reaching 1 g or more per day (2,27,37,53); urinary glucose then returns to nonpregnant levels during the first postpartum week (54). Gestational glucosuria is due mainly to increments in filtered load, but the tubular handling of glucose is also altered in pregnancy. Welsh and Sims (55) suggested in 1960 that women manifesting overt glucosuria in pregnancy had lower maximal tubular reabsorption capacities (T_m) than those who did not, and 15 years later, Davison et al. (56) demonstrated that both the T_m and fractional reabsorption of glucose (T/F glucose) decrease in all subjects during pregnancy. Of interest, those women most severely glucosuric during gestation had the lowest T/F glucose rates both when pregnant and postpartum. They were not, however, glucosuric when not pregnant, because filtered glucose had decreased substantially. Thus, even though the splay of the titration curve increases or the apparent T_m decreases, the striking increment in GFR remains the major cause of glucosuria in pregnancy.

Sturgiss et al. (27) have offered an interesting hypothesis. These authors propose that in some instances, marked gestational glucosuria reflects residual tubular damage from earlier untreated urinary tract infections, although the gravida is no longer bacteriuric. In such instances, subtle lesions may have been brought to the fore by pregnancy.

Glucosuria also occurs during pregnancy in the rat, where micropuncture studies reveal that proximal tubular reabsorption of glucose is enhanced commensurate with the increase in filtered load, and therefore the increment in urinary excretion reflects decreased distal reabsorption (57). It has also been suggested that this may reflect a change in epithelial permeability resulting from an increased backleak in the loop of Henle (57).

The excretion of many amino acids also increases in gestation and may reach 2 g per 24 hours (2,27,37,58). The few studies designed to determine its mechanism were inconclusive, but it appears that alterations in both GFR and tubular reabsorption would be needed to account for the magnitude of some of the amino acids' (e.g., glycine and histidine) excretion rates (2,27,37).

Uric Acid

Urate excretion (and presumably production) increases in pregnancy and its clearance, which is typically 6 to 12 mL per minute in nonpregnant populations, rises to 12 to 20 mL per minute during gestation (2,24,37,59,60). The absolute quantities of urate filtered and reabsorbed also increase, but there are conflicting data on whether the urate fractional clearance (C_{urate}/C_{inulin}) rises as well (23,24,37,60,61). Whatever the case might be, the net result is a fall in serum urate levels of at least 25%, so values range from 2.5 to 5.0 mg/dL (149 to 298 μmol/L), with 5.0 to 5.5 mg/dL (298 to 327 μmol/L) being the upper limit of normal at most centers (2,24,37,62). There may be racial variations of the normal range, as well as diurnal variations in urate levels during pregnancy, with the highest values noted in the morning and lowest in the evening (63–65). Circulating levels tend to be higher in the presence of multiple fetuses (65).

The changes in clearance and plasma levels are greatest in early pregnancy, whereas C_{urate} may decline and plasma levels rise near term (60–62,66,67). In some women, this may represent subclinical preeclampsia, because reductions in C_{urate}/C_{inulin} or increments in P_{urate} may precede overt manifestation of this disorder sometimes by many weeks (2,23,24,37,68,69), but nonrenal causes for the changes in urate levels near term have also been suggested (70).

Potassium Secretion

There is some uncertainty about the fate of body potassium stores during pregnancy. Some authors suggest that total body stores decrease early in gestation and then rise, and by gestational week 36 are about 100 mEq above prepregnancy levels (71). The more traditional view, however, is that cumulative potassium retention is approximately 350 mEq, most of which is stored in the fetal space and organs of reproduction (72). That potassium retention occurs is surprising, considering that gravidas have high circulating levels of aldosterone and other potent mineralocorticoids, although gravidas ingest and excrete normal quantities of sodium in their urine. Furthermore, gravidas tend to manifest bicarbonaturia at lower plasma levels than do nonpregnant women (see later discussion), which should also favor renal potassium loss. In contrast to nonpregnant subjects, gravidas have been shown to be quite resistant to the kaliuretic action of exogenous mineralocorticoids, especially when combined with a diet high in sodium content (73) (Fig. 74-7). This resistance to mineralocorticoids has been ascribed to the fact that gravidas also manifest high circulating levels of progesterone, a view supported by studies in both humans (37,73) and animals (37,74), but not accepted by all (75).

Resistance to the kaliuretic effects of mineralocorticoids may be advantageous and problematic during gestation. The hypokalemia due to excessive renal loss of potassium in both primary aldosteronism and Bartter's syndrome may remit during gestation (72,76). Such observations, however, are

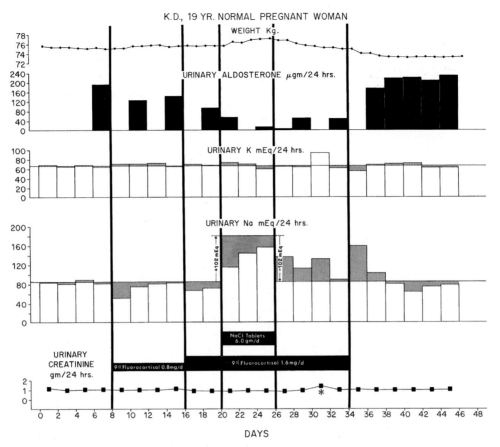

FIG. 74-7. Effect of a mineralocorticoid (Florinef acetate) in a normal pregnant woman. Ingestion of the potent mineralocorticoid led to sodium retention, but no kaliuresis was observed even when dietary sodium was substantially increased (days 20 to 26). The high baseline aldosterone excretion is normal for pregnancy. The different treatment periods *(heavy lines)* are shown, as are the arithmetic means of urinary sodium and potassium excretions *(horizontal lines)* during the pretreatment (control) days. A small kaliuresis was observed on day 31 only, but there was also increased creatinine excretion that day, suggesting a collection or measurement error. (From Ehrlich EN, Lindheimer MD. Effect of administered mineralocorticoids or ACTH in pregnant women. Attenuation of the kaliuretic influence of mineralocorticoids during pregnancy. *J Clin Invest* 1972;51:1301, with permission.)

variable, because instances of these diseases with substantial potassium depletion do occur in gravid women. On the other hand, patients with diseases that compromise potassium secretion (e.g., sickle cell anemia) or women receiving potassium-sparing diuretics may become hyperkalemic when GFR is seemingly normal or only modestly compromised (72). Finally, a very rare disorder, characterized by genetic alteration of the renal mineralocorticoid receptor in a manner in which hormones that normally antagonize the salt-retaining actions of aldosterone now act as agonists, has recently been described (77). When female heterozygotes from these families conceive, their 100-fold increase in progesterone results in marked salt retention, and hypertension in early gestation accompanied by renal potassium wasting, and hypokalemia, although plasma aldosterone levels remain undetectable.

Proton Excretion

There are alterations in acid–base metabolism in pregnancy that are both respiratory and renal in origin. Blood levels

of hydrogen ion decrease by 2 to 4 mmol/L early in gestation, a decrement sustained throughout pregnancy that results in an arterial (or arterialized capillary) blood pH level of 7.42 to 7.44, significantly higher than the 7.38 to 7.40 measured in nonpregnant subjects (17,78). Most of these changes appear to be due to the effects of increased progesterone on the respiratory center, which causes modest hyperventilation accompanied by a fall of PCO_2 from a mean of 39 mm Hg in the nonpregnant state to 30 mm Hg during gestation (17,78,79). These PCO_2 changes are accompanied by a decline in plasma bicarbonate of approximately 4 mmol/L, so normal values during pregnancy range from 18 to 22 mmol/L (17,78).

Studies of renal bicarbonate handling have revealed the following: Raising plasma bicarbonate levels to as high as 31 mmol/L results in concomitant increments in tubular reabsorption, and despite the presence of both hypocapnia and increased intravascular volume, there is no evidence of an increase in either the apparent tubular maximum or the "splay" of the titration curve depicting HCO_3 reabsorption as millimolar per liter of GFR (Fig. 74-8A) (78). On the other hand,

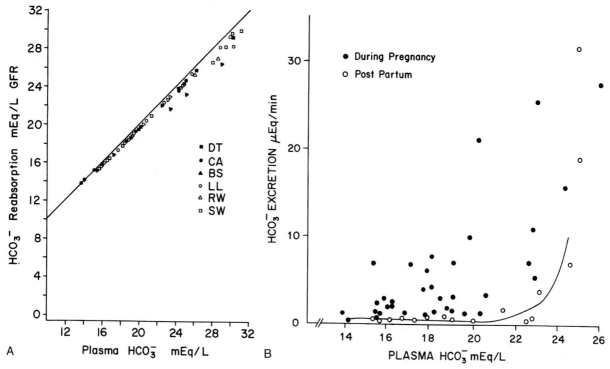

FIG. 74-8. Bicarbonate titration curves **(A)** measured in six third-trimester women during the slow infusion of a 5% NaHCO₃ solution. The infusion inadvertently ran faster for 30 minutes in subject *BS*, the only volunteer to display a wide splay. Bicarbonate excretion **(B)** as a function of plasma bicarbonate levels during pregnancy *(filled circles)* and in two of the subjects studied postpartum *(open circles)*. The bicarbonate threshold is lower in pregnant women (mean, 18 mmol/L), but even when surpassed during the infusion, the bicarbonaturia is still trivial. (From Lim VS, Katz AI, Lindheimer MD. Acid–base regulation in pregnancy. *Am J Physiol* 1976;231:1764, with permission.)

there is a small but persistent bicarbonate "leak" at lower plasma bicarbonate levels during pregnancy (even at levels of 15 to 16 mmol/L) compared with those of the same patient postpartum (Fig. 74-8B).

Urinary acidification has also been evaluated in pregnant women, and it appears that bicarbonate regeneration is comparable to or better than that in similarly tested nonpregnant women (17,78). During acute acidification induced by ammonium chloride ingestion, urinary pH level decreases and titratable acid and NH₄ excretion increase when blood pH, though reduced from 7.44 to 7.40, is still in the normal nonpregnant range. In essence, substantial bicarbonate regeneration occurs when blood pH would still be considered alkaline in nongravid women. Finally, distal proton secretory capacity appears unaltered in gestation (78), and the decrease of blood pH during exercise is similar in pregnant and nonpregnant women (80).

Renal Water Handling and Osmoregulation

Pregnant women experience a decline in body tonicity, as reflected in a decrement in P_{osm}. The decrease appears to start with the luteal phase of the missed menstrual cycle (25) and reaches a nadir about 10 mOsmol/kg below nonpregnant levels early in pregnancy, after which a new steady state is maintained until term (81–84). This decrement is a true decrease in effective P_{osm}, because most of it is due to a decline

in the concentration of sodium and its attendant anion, and data from both human and rodent gestation led to the following formulation of how these changes occur (82–89). First, the osmotic thresholds for thirst and antidiuretic hormone release decrease in parallel (Fig. 74-9). Lowering the threshold to drink stimulates increased water intake and dilution of body fluids. Because inhibition of arginine vasopressin (AVP) release also occurs at a lower level of body tonicity, the hormone continues to circulate and ingested water is retained. P_{osm} thus declines until it is below the osmotic thirst threshold and a new steady state with little change in water turnover is established.

Pregnancy also affects the disposal of AVP, its metabolic clearance rate (MCR) rising fourfold between early and midgestation (90). This increment seems to parallel both the increase in trophoblastic mass and the striking concomitant rise in the levels of circulating cystine aminopeptidase (vasopressinase). This has led to suggestions that vasopressinase is responsible for the rise in the MCR of vasopressin, which is also supported by studies demonstrating that the disposal rate of 1-desamino-8-D-arginine-vasopressin (dDAVP; desmopressin), an AVP analog resistant to inactivation by vasopressinase, is hardly altered by pregnancy (91) (Fig. 74-10).

Mechanisms responsible for the altered osmoregulation in pregnancy are obscure, although HCG (89,92), the constitutive NOS (93), and relaxin (42,94) have all been implicated

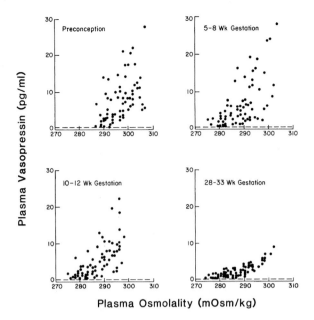

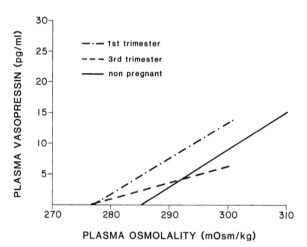

FIG. 74-9. Relationship of plasma arginine vasopressin (AVP) to plasma osmolality in eight healthy women who underwent hypertonic saline infusions starting before conception, then during gestation, and finally postpartum. Each point represents a value from a single blood sample; data from the postpartum test, similar to those taken preconception, are not shown. The cartoon **(lower panel)** depicts the highly significant regression lines from tests performed during pregnancy and in the nonpregnant state, which demonstrate a marked decrease in the abscissal intercept (the apparent threshold for AVP release) during gestation. Note the substantial decrease in the slope during the third trimester, which is discussed further in the text. (From Davison JM, et al. Serial evaluation of vasopressin release and thirst in human pregnancy: role for chorionic gonadotropin on the osmoregulatory changes of gestation. *J Clin Invest* 1988;81:798, with permission.)

in these changes. Relaxin, as noted previously (42,43), is a very interesting candidate because it will explain the effects of HCG on decreasing P_{osm} and osmotic thresholds in premenopausal women (89,92) but not men (89), the osmoregulatory changes in the menstrual cycle (25), and both the increases in renal hemodynamics and

alterations in osmoregulation during rodent and human gestation.

Some authors believe that despite measurable increments in absolute intravascular volume, gestation is a state of decreased "effective arterial volume," secondary to arterial vasodilation, and they have suggested that such nonosmotic influences are important effectors of the osmoregulatory changes in pregnancy (95–97). Studies describing serial hemodynamic and humoral alterations in pregnant baboons (98) and increased vascular sensitivity of gravidas to angiotensin-converting enzyme (ACE) inhibition (99) support the concept of a decreased "effective arterial volume" in pregnancy. Most interesting are studies by Ohara et al. (100), who suggest that borderline or undetectable elevations in plasma vasopressin concentrators (P_{AVP}) are present in gravid rats who also manifest upregulation of aquaporin-2 mRNA and its water channel protein in apical membranes of the collecting ducts. Others, based on both rodent and human studies, believe that the volume-sensing AVP-release mechanisms appear to adjust as pregnancy progresses so each new volume status is "sensed" as normal (30,37,82–84,92,101–103). We also find the observations of Ohara et al. (100) quite paradoxical, because any increments in AVP levels, even undetectable changes (presumably the result of decreased "effective arterial volume") causing increments in the density of apical water channels should blunt the animals' ability to excrete water loads, yet gravid rats excrete water loads more efficiently than virgin controls (85). The increased GFR and decreased aquaporin-2 trafficking to the apical membrane during vasopressin suppression could of course explain this capacity to excrete a water load.

Significance of the Altered Osmoregulation and AVP Metabolism

The osmoregulatory changes observed in humans do not occur in all species. For example, rats demonstrate decreases in P_{Na} and P_{osm} only at midgestation, whereas P_{osm} is unaltered in pregnant sheep (83,87). Also, the MCR of AVP remains unaltered in the latter species, whose placenta does not produce vasopressinase (83). Thus, the clinical relevance of these changes is still unclear. One answer may relate to the physiologic increase in extracellular volumes that accompanies normal gestation. In this respect, some believe that the increase in intravascular volume optimizes fetal development, and hypoosmolality would facilitate such expansion because the ingestion and retention of less solute is required per liter of extracellular water retained. In this case, the downward resetting of the osmotic threshold for AVP release would be advantageous, especially when sodium is scarce. More striking, however, are the clinical implications of the fourfold rise in the MCR of vasopressin, first with regard to the management of patients with vasopressin-deficient states and second as an explanation of a syndrome termed *transient diabetes insipidus (DI) of pregnancy.*

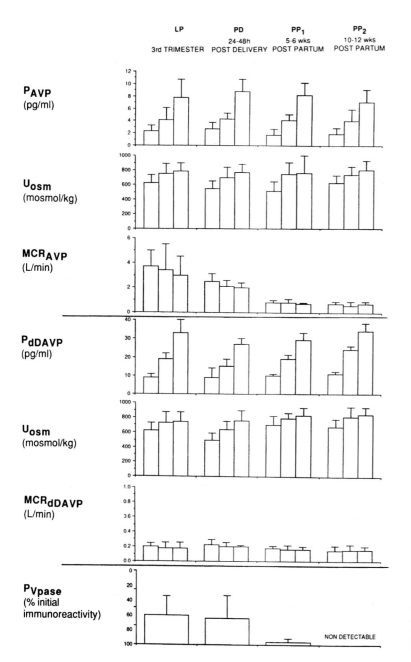

FIG. 74-10. Plasma levels and metabolic clearance rates (MCRs) of arginine vasopressin and l-desamino-8-D-arginine-vasopressin measured in the third trimester, 24 to 48 hours after delivery, as well as 5 to 6 and 10 to 12 weeks postpartum in six women. P_{vpase},-plasma vasopressinase. Above each bar is one standard deviation. (From Davison JM, et al. Metabolic clearance of vasopressin and an analogue resistant to vasopressinase in human pregnancy. *Am J Physiol* 1993;264:F348, with permission.)

Disorders of Water Metabolism in Pregnancy

Diabetes Insipidus in Pregnancy

The causes of DI antedating pregnancy are discussed elsewhere (104–107; Chapter 86, Nephrogenic and Central Diabetes Insipidus). Patients are rarely treated with AVP (e.g., pitressin) anymore, but if they are, the rise in hormonal disposal rates would obviously require an increase in dosage. Currently, however, virtually all women with known central DI are managed with desmopressin (dDAVP), the MCR of which, as mentioned, is not altered during pregnancy (91). Still, there are reports of increased dDAVP requirements in gestation, in which symptoms associated with the altered threshold for thirst seem to have been misinterpreted as

dDAVP "escape." In most instances, however, the preconception replacement dose has proved sufficient throughout gestation (82,83,104–107). Also, there is minimal, if any, transfer of dDAVP into breast milk (107).

Women who develop pituitary necrosis due to blood loss at delivery (Sheehan's syndrome) may manifest transient polyuria in the immediate puerperium. They also develop partial central DI, which is usually asymptomatic and detected only by special testing such as the P_{AVP} response during dehydration and/or hypertonic saline loading (107–110).

Nephrogenic DI in pregnancy is quite rare, although carriers of the X-linked variety may become polyuric in pregnancy (D. Bichet and G. Robertson, *personal communications*).

Diuretics, the mainstay of therapy in this disorder, work by depleting intravascular volume, which results in increased proximal reabsorption of sodium and the delivery of less fluid to the diluting site. The maintenance of hypovolemia may not be optimal for pregnancy, but when the polyuria is massive, such agents may have to be used.

Transient Diabetes Insipidus of Pregnancy

On occasion a gravida develops polyuria and polydipsia late in gestation, which disappear postpartum. This syndrome, described in the older literature, was characterized further in 1984, when Barron et al. (111) studied three women whose polyuria was resistant to the administration of synthetic vasopressin during the puerperium. Their disease, however, remitted soon afterward, and they regained the ability to concentrate their urine normally with overnight dehydration or after the administration of pitressin. Plasma AVP, measured in one of the women, was 7.3 pg/mL, a level that should have evoked maximum urine concentration. The authors, however, labeled the disorder "transient vasopressin-resistant DI of pregnancy," and avoided the term "nephrogenic," aware that the AVP measured in the patient's plasma might have been but fragments devoid of biological activity, but still recognized by radioimmunoassay; in other words, something was destroying the hormone. This led to the proposition that in certain women with transient DI of pregnancy, the disorder might reflect massive *in vivo* destruction of AVP by extremely elevated levels or exaggerated effects of vasopressinase. Figure 74-11 depicts the signal study by Dürr et al. (112) of a patient who became massively polyuric and hypernatremic and who failed to concentrate her urine after pharmacological doses of AVP, but whose U_{osmol} increased to 800 mOsmol/kg when dDAVP was administered. The authors used two methods to demonstrate that the P_{AVP} measured after the highest dose of AVP (surprisingly only 240 pg/mL) was not intact hormone but represented inactive fragments. In essence, the last dose of pitressin (25 μg) had been inactivated in less than 25 minutes. Both Barron and Dürr and their respective colleagues (111,112) also noted high levels of circulating vasopressinase in their patients, the latter group suggesting that this is the cause of the disorder; however, alterations in the enzyme's kinetics are another possibility.

Many other examples of this transient disorder have now been cited (82–84,105–107). Most of these gravidas also have preeclampsia or display coagulation and liver function abnormalities (113). The liver is a major site of vasopressinase inactivation.

There is a second form of transient DI of pregnancy in which some women with partial central DI, asymptomatic when nonpregnant, manifest polyuria after midpregnancy coincident with the normal fourfold increase in the MCR of AVP. This disorder also remits postpartum (114–117).

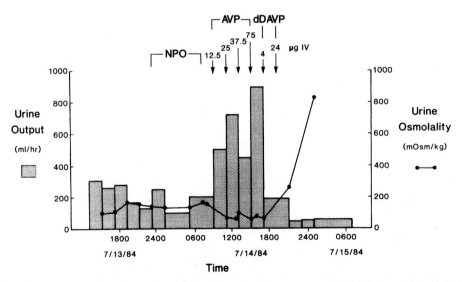

FIG. 74-11. Study during postpartum day 6 in a patient who developed diabetes insipidus late in gestation and remained polyuric in the puerperium. She was unable to concentrate her urine during fluid restriction (nothing per os), and plasma arginine vasopressin (AVP) was undetectable despite a P_{Na} level of 153 mEq/L. Her urine remained dilute despite the stepwise parenteral administration of large doses of AVP, but urinary osmolality increased to 800 mOsmol/kg after receiving l-desamino-8-D-arginine-vasopressin. Plasma AVP measured after the last dose of AVP was 240 ng/L (when values in the thousands were anticipated), but the material identified by radioimmunoassay was not bioactive and probably represented degraded fragments of AVP. Plasma vasopressinase measured on day 12 postpartum was tenfold higher than that in women at term. (From Dürr JA, et al. Diabetes insipidus in pregnancy associated with abnormally high circulating vasopressinase. *N Engl J Med* 1987;316:1070, with permission.)

Finally, at least one patient with transient DI postpartum resistant to both AVP and dDAVP has been described, the authors noting that both P_{AVP} and urinary prostaglandin E_2 were extremely elevated (118).

Transient Inappropriate Antidiuretic Hormone Secretion in Pregnancy

Gestational hyponatremia secondary to "inappropriate" secretion of AVP has been described. This disorder is extremely rare and may be associated with preeclampsia, both when the latter was characterized by marked proteinuria and hypoalbuminemia and when such evidence of marked intravascular volume depletion was less evident (119–121).

VOLUME REGULATION

There are alterations in volume homeostasis and in the control of blood pressure in pregnancy, both of which are incompletely understood. These topics, detailed in Chapter 53 (Hypertension and Pregnancy) and elsewhere (37,84,122,123), are summarized briefly here.

Weight Gain

Healthy women gain approximately 12.5 Kg in their first pregnancy, and 1 Kg less in subsequent gestations. However, these means have large standard deviations, and gravidas can gain twice such amounts or hardly any weight at all and still have normal pregnancies (37). Analysis of the distribution of this added weight reveals that not all the increase can be accounted for by the products of conception, by the tissues directly concerned with reproduction, or by the gain in total body water, but that 3 to 6 Kg of the increment is in maternal fat stores (37,71,84,124). Furthermore, these averages were compiled from subjects with no or only mild ankle edema during pregnancy, whereas about 15% of healthy gravidas develop generalized edema, characterized by swelling of the fingers and face as well. Weight gain in this latter group averages 14.5 Kg, of which about 5 Kg represents fluid accumulation within the extracellular space (37).

Fluid Volumes

Most of the weight added in pregnancy is in the form of fluid. The gain in total body water, measured by deuterium, by the stable isotope of oxygen (^{18}O) or by bioelectric impedance is between 6 and 9 L (2,17,37,71,124,125). Estimates of the gain in extracellular volume range from 4 to 7 L, suggesting that intracellular water also increases (0.5 to 1.0 L) during gestation (17,37,125). This area, however, requires further investigation, considering the wide variations reported by most authors and as the incomplete information on validation of their methods for use in pregnant women. Intravascular volume also increases in pregnancy, due to an estimated 40% increment in plasma volume and a small increase in red blood cell mass (37,84,122,123,126). Plasma volume increases most rapidly in the midtrimester, and the accumulation of interstitial volume is greatest in late pregnancy.

Renal Sodium Handling

There is a gradual cumulative retention of about 900 mEq of sodium during pregnancy, distributed between the products of conception and the increased maternal extracellular spaces described previously (17,37,122,123). However, late in pregnancy, when the accumulation is greatest, renal sodium retention is but a few milliequivalents per day and is difficult to detect in conventional balance studies. The reasons for these changes are obscure, with reports in the literature focusing on the hormonal changes in pregnancy that may affect renal salt handling or the effects of acute saline loading in pregnant women.

The concentration of several antinatriuretic hormones, mostly mineralocorticoids such as aldosterone and desoxycorticosterone, increases substantially during gestation (17, 37,127). The renin–angiotensin–aldosterone (RAA) system has been studied extensively in human pregnancy (17,122, 123,128). Figure 74-12 depicts the increments in renin substrate, plasma renin activity, and plasma and urinary aldosterone that accompany normal pregnancy (129). Note that urinary sodium excretion, and presumably intake, are similar or only slightly increased throughout gestation compared with values measured postpartum. Thus, inadequate sodium intake does not seem to account for these rises in the RAA system. Other studies have demonstrated that despite apparently high circulating levels, the renin–aldosterone system responds appropriately when gravidas undergo acute or chronic expansion with saline infusions or high salt diets or when they are sodium restricted or receive diuretics (2,17,37). Furthermore, inhibition of aldosterone biosynthesis results in an inappropriate diuresis and subtle signs of volume depletion (130). In essence, the activated renin–aldosterone system in pregnancy does not appear to function autonomously, as some have postulated, because the very high levels of aldosterone (which often exceed those in patients with primary aldosteronism) are appropriate and respond to homeostatic demands.

There are also increments in the concentration of several potentially natriuretic hormones during gestation (e.g., oxytocin, vasodilating prostaglandins, and melanocyte-stimulating hormone) (17,37,122,123). Progesterone, whose values increase many-fold over that measured during the luteal phase of the menstrual cycle, is the hormone studied most in this respect. Ironically, however, progesterone may contribute to antinatriuresis, because it is a major source of the increase in desoxycorticosterone production. The current view is that most of the maternal desoxycorticosterone arises by extraadrenal 21-hydroxylation of circulating progesterone (131,132). Activity of the enzyme responsible for this conversion may be enhanced when estrogen levels are increased, as they are in pregnancy, and renal steroid 21-hydroxylase

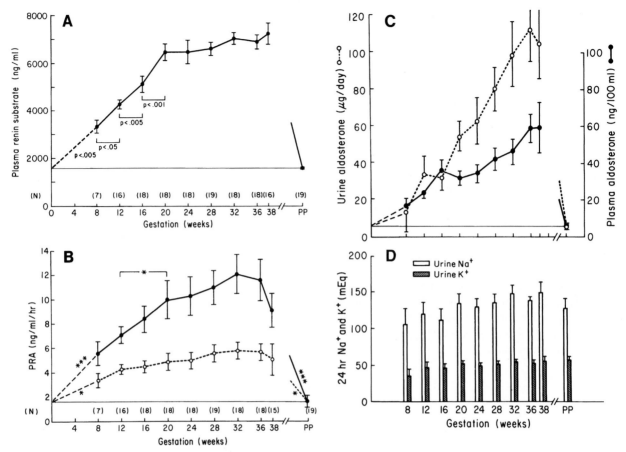

FIG. 74-12. Changes in plasma renin substrate **(A)**, its activity **(B)**, and plasma **(C)** and urinary **(D)** aldosterone, during normal gestation and their relationship to urinary sodium and potassium excretion **(right lower panel)**. Dashed line in **(B)** represents values normalized for postpartum substrate concentrations. (From Wilson M, et al. Blood pressure, the renin-angiotensin system, and sex steroids throughout normal pregnancy. *Am J Med* 1980;68:97, with permission.)

activity may be particularly high in pregnancy, so a considerable portion of maternal desoxycorticosterone may be produced near the renal mineralocorticoid receptor (133,134). Finally, and as noted in the section on renal potassium handling, a mutation of the mineralocorticoid receptor has been described (77) that recognizes traditional aldosterone antagonists as agonists. In these rare cases, therefore, the high progesterone levels paradoxically cause marked sodium retention and early pregnancy hypertension.

The role of natriuretic factors in pregnant women is poorly understood. The various circulating peptides and membrane pump inhibitors are usually described as elevated (17,122, 123,135), but these increases may be modest when related to the magnitude of the increase in intravascular and interstitial volumes that accompanies normal gestation.

Perhaps the major factor to consider when evaluating renal salt handling in pregnancy is the striking increase in GFR. Each day more than 10,000 mEq of sodium is filtered, which must be reabsorbed by the renal tubule, a quantity far greater than the expected salt-retaining effects of high circulating levels of aldosterone, desoxycorticosterone, or estrogens. Furthermore, filtration fraction is decreased throughout most of

gestation as is plasma albumin, additional factors that should enhance salt excretion.

Effects of Acute or Chronic Sodium Loads

Studies of the effect of acute saline infusions on urinary sodium excretion have produced conflicting results (17,23, 122,123) in that a decreased, increased, and unchanged ability to excrete the load have all been described. Of note are studies by Brown (122,123), Graves (52), and their respective colleagues in which salt intake before the infusion was controlled. The former found no differences in the sodium excretory capacity of normal gravidas compared with that of women in the nonpregnant state, whereas the latter suggested that both second- and third-trimester subjects respond with an enhanced natriuresis. Bay and Ferris (137) have reported that gravidas subjected to diets whose sodium content was as low as 10 mEq per day achieve urinary sodium balance as quickly as nonpregnant controls. The women studied by Bay and Ferris lost weight, and therefore, their data could be interpreted as suggesting that with extreme salt restriction, gravidas manifest subtle salt wasting (17,122,123). This is because sodium accumulation in late pregnancy should be in the range of 6 to 8 mEq per day, and restricting intake to 10 mEq should reveal differences between the pregnant and nonpregnant state.

Significance of the Volume Changes in Pregnancy

The reason maternal total body water—intravascular and interstitial volumes—increases during normal gestation is unclear, which is one reason interpretation of the meaning of these changes is disputed (17,84,123). Some authorities consider the physiologic hypervolemia of human gestation a suboptimal response to the general arterial vasodilation that accompanies pregnancy (the "underfill" theory), whereas others propose that it may be an epiphenomenon secondary to factors such as the marked increase in circulating mineralocorticoids (the "overfill" theory). Still others, including ourselves, postulate that the volume-sensing mechanisms are continually reset as gestation progresses so that the increments in absolute volume are "sensed" as normal ("normal fill"). These discordant hypotheses were mentioned briefly in the section on osmoregulation and AVP release and are clarified further here.

Views supporting "underfill" include activation of the renin–angiotensin system, manifested not only by an increase in all its circulating components (Fig. 74-11), but also by observations that gravidas manifest a greater increase in aldosterone release than nonpregnant subjects in response to small quantities of angiotensin II (138) and display exaggerated decreases in blood pressure when treated with ACE inhibitors (99). Those that rationalize the existence of increased absolute volume with "underfill" postulate further that marked peripheral vascular dilation precedes the rise in intravascular volume, the latter never completely compensating for this change (the "primary arterial vasodilatation" theory) (26,97,139). It is further suggested that this may be due to early upregulation of constitutive endothelial NOS in the vasculature (93). Studies of women and baboons in early pregnancy appear consistent with both the primary arterial vasodilatation and "underfill" hypotheses (26,98,139). As well, adrenalectomy or sodium restriction is tolerated more poorly by pregnant rats than by nonpregnant controls (140).

Support for the "overfill" theory includes absolute increments in extracellular volumes, high levels of circulating natriuretic factors or inhibitors of the membrane pump (17,123, 135), increases in renal hemodynamics, and observations by two groups of investigators (136,141) of increased sodium excretory capacity in response to saline infusions. Women with cardiac or renal disorders appear more susceptible to volume overload complications, whereas healthy gravidas seem to tolerate blood loss better than nonpregnant women. Finally, in most studies of gravid animals, the mean circulatory filling pressure appears slightly increased (84,142).

As noted, the "normal-fill" hypothesis is supported by animal experiments that probe relationships between intravascular volume depletion and AVP release (83,84,92, 101,102). In addition, studies in rats and humans suggest that sodium and water reabsorption in the proximal nephron (determined by indices such as fractional lithium or solute-free water clearances) is unaltered, and both species dilute their urine normally when water loaded during gestation (47,81, 84,102). These latter observations are important because failure to dilute the urine maximally and a blunted excretory response to water loading are major pathophysiologic features of the "underfill" status in hyponatremic patients with cirrhosis or cardiac failure, considered the prototypes of diseases in which absolute extracellular volumes are increased and "effective arterial volume" is low. Finally, the previously described data are in accord with studies demonstrating a similar sodium excretory response to saline infusions in the pregnant and nonpregnant states (17,23,122,123).

Controversies about the various "fill" hypotheses are yet to be settled. It may be that all are correct at some time during pregnancy. Hormone-induced vasodilation may create temporary "underfill" in early gestation, followed quickly by compensation to "normal-fill" as pregnancy progresses, whereas during the last trimester, antinatriuretic factors predominate, at least in some gravidas (26,84,92,139). The importance of settling this dispute, however, is not trivial, because a better understanding of how the gravida "senses" her volume changes will have an impact on our understanding and management of pregnant women with hypertensive complications and cardiac disorders. For the interested reader, we recommend discussions by Schrier et al. (96,97,143) and particularly Dürr and Lindheimer (84), who discuss these hypotheses and the latter includes a historical review in the form of an appendix entitled "On what is 'effective' in effective blood volume."

EVALUATION OF RENAL FUNCTION IN PREGNANCY

Examination of the Urine

Most, but not all (144), studies suggest that urinary protein excretion increases during normal gestation (17,50,84,145). Accepting the relative imprecision and variability of testing methods used by hospital laboratories, one should consider 300 mg per day (or twice the institution's cutoff for nonpregnant populations) the upper limit of normal protein excretion in pregnancy. It is unclear, however, whether urinary albumin excretion increases in normal pregnancy (84). We observed no difference in a small group of women studied serially when values obtained during gestation were compared with those measured 3 months postpartum (29), but follow-up collections made at 6 months or later suggest that nonpregnant levels may in fact have been slightly lower (Davison and Lindheimer, *unpublished observations*). In essence, if a difference can be demonstrated, it will be small, and thus, use of the upper limits of normal for nonpregnant populations is probably permissible. More research is needed here, because the detection of microabuminuria in pregnant women may have predictive value in relation to pregnancy outcome in women with diabetes and with regard to preeclampsia (17,84,146). Finally, there is sparse information (84) concerning the excretion of small-molecular-weight or tubule proteins, as well as enzymuria in both normal and abnormal gestation, and such tests have little current value in pregnancy.

There have been few attempts to quantitate the urine sediment of pregnant women. The excretion of red blood cells may rise (in pregnancy 1 to 2 red blood cells per high power field is acceptable), but whether increased leukocyturia occurs is unclear (2,5,147,148). One should be aware that microscopic and even gross hematuria may complicate otherwise uneventful gestations (149). The differential diagnosis includes all causes of hematuria in nongravid populations, but often no cause can be found and the bleeding subsides postpartum. Some of these episodes may be due to rupture of small veins around the dilated renal pelvis (149), and the hematuria may recur in subsequent pregnancies. Of importance, complete investigation of the hematuria can often be deferred until the postpartum period, and noninvasive techniques, including ultrasonography and magnetic resonance imaging, are helpful in arriving at such decisions.

Renal Function Tests

The endogenous creatinine clearance, the primary tool to assess GFR in nonpregnant subjects, is equally useful for evaluating function in gravidas (Table 74-1). The lower limit of normal for clearances measured during gestation should be about 30% above that of nongravid women, which in many institutions averages 90 to 110 mL per minute. As noted by some, the 24-hour endogenous creatinine clearance may fall toward nonpregnant values during the last gestational month (17,84), and therefore, a rise in serum creatinine 1 mg/dL per less (88 μmol/L) near term need not alarm the physician. Urinary creatinine results from tubular secretion and from glomerular filtration, but unfortunately, there is little information on whether the ratio of secreted to filtered creatinine is altered by gestation. However, it is fair to assume that when renal dysfunction is present (serum creatinine level, $\geq$1.5 mg/dL or 133 μmol/L), a substantial proportion of the clearance may be due to secretion, resulting in overestimation of the GFR. In such circumstances, the measurement of endogenous creatinine clearance can be performed during gestation during cimetidine (Food and Drug Administration [FDA] pregnancy class C) administration, and this might aid in assessing prognosis and managing the clinical course of the patient.

Urine concentration and dilution are similar in gravid and nonpregnant women. Supine posture can interfere with the ability of the gravida to produce a maximally dilute urine, whereas lateral recumbency interferes with optimal urine concentration (81). Such tests are therefore best performed with the patient seated quietly. Ammonium chloride loading to assess renal acidification (rarely indicated in gestation) gives results similar to those in nonpregnant women (78). Finally, when timed urine collections prove unreliable or are difficult to obtain, random urine protein : creatinine ratio and the Cockcroft-Gault formula (using preconception body weight) can be used to estimate protein excretion and creatinine clearances in pregnant women (150).

Renal Biopsy

Pregnancy was once considered a relative contraindication for the performance of renal biopsy because of earlier reports that stressed several complications, particularly excessive bleeding (2). This view may have stemmed from the fact that many of these biopsies were performed in hypertensive patients, at a time predating our current understanding of the coagulation abnormalities that may accompany preeclampsia. It is now evident that if the biopsy is performed in women with well-controlled blood pressure and normal clotting indices, its morbidity is similar to that in nonpregnant patients (151).

Although some authors (151) have recommended liberal use of renal biopsy during gestation, including for asymptomatic hematuria or proteinuria, we find few indications for this procedure in pregnancy and suggest the following guidelines (152). First, renal biopsy may be considered when there is sudden deterioration of renal function with no apparent cause, because certain forms of rapidly progressive glomerulonephritis when diagnosed early may respond to aggressive treatments such as high-dose steroid pulses or plasma exchange. Second, renal biopsy is helpful in symptomatic nephrotic syndrome (or when its biochemical abnormalities are marked), if present before the thirty-second gestational week. Although some may consider a therapeutic trial of steroids in such cases, we prefer to determine first whether the lesion is likely to respond to this regimen, thus avoiding the potential complications of corticoids, such as fetal anomalies, hyperglycemia, propensity to infection, and poor wound healing. Nephrotic range proteinuria alone in a normotensive woman with preserved renal function, who has neither severe hypoalbuminuria, marked hyperlipidemia, or intolerable edema, would lead us to examine the patient at frequent intervals and defer the renal biopsy to the postpartum period. This is because most investigators believe that prognosis is determined primarily by the level of renal function and the presence or absence of hypertension, rather than by the type of renal lesion (see later discussion). Similarly, as noted, decisions to perform a biopsy on the kidney are deferred to the postpartum period for pregnancies complicated by asymptomatic microscopic hematuria when there is no evidence of stone disease or tumor by ultrasonography. Finally, kidney biopsy should not be performed after the thirty-first gestational week. At this stage, the decision to terminate the gestation is usually made independently of biopsy results, and fetal survival is excellent, making even the minimal risk of an invasive procedure unnecessary.

THE CLINICAL SPECTRUM AND MANAGEMENT OF RENAL DISORDERS IN GESTATION

Acute Renal Failure

Acute renal failure (ARF) severe enough to require dialytic treatment is quite rare in pregnancy, its incidence being 1 : 20,000 or less of all gestations in industrialized nations (17,153,154). Such statistics are a considerable improvement over conditions that existed in the 1960s, when sudden and severe renal failure complicated 1 of every 8,000 gestations (2,17,153,154). This progress is due, most likely, to liberalization of abortion laws, as well as more aggressive antibiotic therapy and improved prenatal care (Fig. 74-13). Moreover, maternal mortality associated with ARF, once about 18%, is now unusual (153–156). Unfortunately, these reassuring statistics do not apply to developing nations, where pregnancy-related ARF may comprise up to 25% of referrals to dialysis centers and is associated with substantial maternal and fetal mortality (153,154,157,158).

Septic Abortion

Before the legalization of abortion in the United States, there were at least 200,000 (some estimate up to one million) illegal, usually nonsterile pregnancy terminations annually, and approximately 5% of these women became critically ill (154). A common presentation was septic shock with renal failure, and if the infecting organism was *Clostridium,* mortality was quite high (154). Because most of these events occurred during the initial trimester, ARF in pregnancy had a bimodal distribution, the first peak occurring early in pregnancy and comprising most of the cases of septic abortion, and a second peak between gestational week 35 and the immediate puerperium, due mainly to placental abruption, bleeding, or

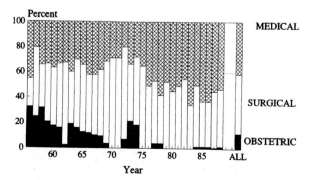

FIG. 74-13. The relative frequency of medical, surgical, and obstetric causes of acute renal failure at the General Infirmary at Leeds, England. Note the virtual disappearance of obstetric-related causes after 1980. (From Turney JH, Ellis CM, Parson FM. Obstetric acute renal failure. *Br J Obstet Gynaecol* 1989;96:679, with permission.)

preeclampsia (2,153,154). Fortunately, this initial peak has virtually disappeared because sterile terminations are readily available.

The clinical presentation of a gravida infected with clostridia is usually dramatic, the initial manifestations occurring several hours to 1 to 2 days after the attempted abortion. The patient is quite febrile and often manifests vomiting and diarrhea. Muscle pain, most intense in the upper limbs, thorax, and especially abdomen, may lead to erroneous diagnoses of an intraabdominal inflammatory process, particularly when a history of attempted abortion is denied or not sought. Also, there may be scant or no vaginal bleeding, and clostridia are difficult to culture or detect on the smear and are also normally present in the female genital tract. In essence, a high degree of suspicion is required, because once symptoms of clostridial infection develop, progression to shock and death is rapid.

Patients with clostridial sepsis are often jaundiced (because of hemolysis), which when combined with cutaneous vasodilatation and pallor produces a peculiar bronze skin coloration. Other features are marked anemia, a striking leukocytosis ($\geq 25,000/mm^3$), and thrombocytopenia associated with evidence of disseminated intravascular coagulation. Radiography may demonstrate air in the uterus and abdomen due to gas-forming organisms or perforation. Death occurs rapidly in some patients, but most respond rapidly to the antibiotic regimen (primarily high-dose penicillin) and volume resuscitation, and survival depends largely on the management of the renal failure. Review of the roles of hyperbaric oxygen, antitoxins, or exchange transfusions, and controversies concerning the conservative approach versus early surgical removal of the infected uterus, are beyond the scope of this chapter and are discussed in most obstetric texts (154).

Other Causes of Pregnancy-Associated Renal Failure

The etiology of ARF in pregnant women is often similar to that of nonpregnant populations, including volume depletion (with hyperemesis gravidarum) and bleeding (153,154). Antepartum uterine hemorrhage may be underestimated or difficult to diagnose when blood is trapped behind the placenta ("concealed hemorrhage"). In this respect, early blood replacement, even at the risk of slight overtransfusion, may forestall the development of acute tubular necrosis or cortical necrosis (see later discussion).

Sudden renal failure during pregnancy has been reported after drug ingestion, incompatible blood transfusions, various nephritides, collagen disorders, or rarely in sarcoidosis or lymphoma (153,154,159,160). There also seems to be a greater propensity for gravidas to develop ARF in association with acute infectious pyelonephritis (153,154,161). Of interest are a number of reports of ARF due to obstructive nephropathy, often in women with single kidneys (22,154, 162,163). Causes are again similar to those in nongravid women, including stone disease and tumors, as well as the "distention syndrome," which was described previously (18–22).

A number of renal failure syndromes are peculiar to pregnancy, which include those associated with preeclampsia, acute fatty liver, and idiopathic postpartum renal failure. Preeclampsia, characterized by generalized vasoconstriction, is the major cause of renal dysfunction in gestation, but fortunately function loss is mild to moderate at most (164) and renal replacement therapy is rarely required. However, when preeclampsia is superimposed on chronic renal disease or essential hypertension or is accompanied by marked coagulopathy (see "HELLP syndrome," Chapter 53, Hypertension and Pregnancy), preeclampsia may progress to acute tubular and even cortical necrosis (154,157,158,165–167)

The incidence of ARF in women with acute fatty liver of pregnancy was once estimated at 60%, but is considerably less today, perhaps due to earlier recognition of the disorder followed by rapid intervention to terminate the pregnancy (17,153,154). Both the etiology of the disease and its propensity to cause renal failure are obscure, though of interest are observations that some pregnant women developing either acute fatty liver of pregnancy or the microangiopathic *h*emolytic anemia, *e*levated *l*iver enzymes, and *l*ow *p*latelets (HELLP) syndrome harbor a long-chain 3-hydroxy acyl-CoA dehydrogenase deficiency or carry mutations of the enzyme's gene resulting in deficiencies in the fetus (168). Thus, ARF could be related to the coagulopathy that may accompany acute fatty liver of pregnancy or to hemodynamic factors akin to those observed in the "hepatorenal syndrome." Acute fatty liver of pregnancy was once associated with considerable maternal and fetal mortality, exceeding 70%, but maternal survival is now 90% or more (169). Such improved statistics may also be due to aggressive intervention but also reflect earlier recognition leading to the inclusion in reported series of patients with milder disease (154,169). However, irreversible cases still occur, and in these instances, orthotopic liver transplantation may be lifesaving (170).

Idiopathic postpartum renal failure is characterized by the onset of renal failure in the puerperium after an uneventful gestation. This disorder was first recognized in the 1960s (171–173), and fewer than 200 cases had been described by the year 2000 (under various names, including postpartum hemolytic-uremic syndrome, accelerated nephrosclerosis, postpartum malignant nephrosclerosis, and irreversible postpartum intravascular coagulation with ARF [153,154]).

Idiopathic postpartum renal failure may present 24 hours to several weeks after delivery, the patient manifesting oliguria, and at times anuria, rapidly progressive azotemia, and often evidence of microangiopathic hemolytic anemia or consumption coagulopathy. Blood pressure varies from normal or minimally elevated to severe hypertension. The cause of the syndrome is obscure, and suggestions have included an antecedent viral illness, retained placental fragments, and drugs, including oxytocic agents, ergotamine compounds, and oral contraceptives prescribed shortly after delivery (154). Hypocomplementemia noted in some cases has led

to speculation about immunologic causes. Deficiencies in prostaglandin production or antithrombin III levels similar to decreases observed in the hemolytic-uremic syndrome have also been ascribed to idiopathic postpartum renal failure (154). In the past, there were suggestions that preeclampsia and idiopathic postpartum renal failure had a common etiology (174). This concept has been extended with suggestions that those disorders, the "HELLP" syndrome, and acute fatty liver of pregnancy have a common pathogenesis, similar to that of thrombotic thrombocytopenic purpura and hemolytic-uremic syndrome (175). It has also been postulated that all these diseases are manifestations of a thrombotic microangiopathy induced by endothelial dysfunction, believed to be primarily due to a deficit in the NO-dependent endothelial relaxing factor. Although this hypothesis is intriguing, we note that there are many differences in both the manifestations and the prognosis of the various disorders listed previously.

The renal pathology findings in idiopathic postpartum renal failure are detailed elsewhere (154) and fall into two general categories. In one, changes in the glomerular capillaries resemble those seen in hemolytic-uremic syndrome, and in the other, there are arteriolar lesions reminiscent of malignant nephrosclerosis or scleroderma. It may be that the lesions resembling thrombotic microangiopathy are from biopsies obtained early in the course of the disease, whereas those suggesting accelerated nephrosclerosis represent a more chronic stage. There is also an increased incidence of bleeding associated with the performance of renal biopsy in these cases (153).

The prognosis of idiopathic postpartum renal failure is poor. Most of the patients succumb, require chronic dialysis, or survive with severely reduced function (153,154). Treatment is aimed at reduction of blood pressure and general supportive measures used in all patients with ARF (see later discussion). There are anecdotal claims that early anticoagulant therapy with heparin or fibrinolytic agents may reverse the renal failure, but the data are not convincing and these drugs are not harmless. Similarly, antiplatelet therapy, infusion of blood products such as antithrombin III concentrates, and plasma exchange remain unproven treatment modalities (although the latter may be useful in a variant of acute postpartum renal failure linked either to circulating lupus anticoagulant (176) or to circulating antiphospholipid antibodies (177,178). Because of the possible contributing role of retained placental fragments, dilation and curettage should be considered when the syndrome occurs very close to delivery.

Renal Cortical Necrosis

Cortical necrosis, the more ominous form of ARF, is fortunately rare, but in the past, it was more apt to be associated with pregnancy (4,153,154,179). The reason for this was obscure, but many of the women appeared to be older multiparas who perhaps had preexisting nephrosclerosis, suggesting that their kidneys were more vulnerable to inciting factors such as ischemia or coagulopathy. In this respect, cortical necrosis was most common late in gestation and occurred more frequently after placental abruption, especially when concealed hemorrhage was present (153,154). Another proposed reason was related to observations that the Sanarelli-Shwartzman reaction can be more easily produced in pregnant animals than in nongravid controls (2,154,180). Consistent with this possibility was a number of cases that followed prolonged retention of a dead fetus. The incidence of cortical necrosis related to gestation has now declined markedly in industrialized nations and is presently less than 1 of 80,000 births (179).

Although cortical necrosis may involve the entire renal cortex, resulting in irreversible renal failure, it is the incomplete ("patchy") variety that is most often associated with pregnancy (153,154,182). The latter condition is characterized by severe oliguria or even anuria, which lasts longer than uncomplicated acute tubular necrosis, followed by a variable return of renal function and a stable period of moderate renal insufficiency that in some patients progresses years later to end-stage renal disease.

Management of Acute Renal Failure in Pregnancy

Management of ARF during pregnancy is generally similar to that in nonpregnant subjects (Chapter 41, Acute Renal Failure), but several points pertinent to treatment of antepartum patients deserve emphasis. Both peritoneal dialysis and hemodialysis may be used (154,183,184). The former is theoretically preferable because it causes more gradual changes in fluid and solute levels and is thus less likely to be associated with precipitous hypotension or premature uterine contractions. If hemodialysis is the modality chosen, the problems listed previously can be minimized by daily treatments for shorter periods and avoidance of high-flux technology. Because urea, creatinine, and presumably many other metabolites (or toxins) that accumulate in the blood associated with uremia cross the placenta, dialysis should be undertaken early with the aim of maintaining blood urea nitrogen levels below 50 mg/dL (18 mmol/L), if possible, which may require substantial increments in the daily prescription in patients treated with peritoneal dialysis (185). Further details concerning the hemodialysis prescription are given in the section devoted to the management of women with end-stage renal disease treated with renal replacement therapy who conceive.

As noted, maternal prognosis has improved considerably compared with the dismal statistics published three decades ago. Survival for obstetric ARF is now markedly better than in patients whose disease is due to surgical or medical diseases. Prognosis for the fetus, however, appears worse than that for the mother, although here too the outlook is improving dramatically.

Finally, although this section stresses ARF requiring dialysis, we note that sudden renal dysfunction occurs more frequently, often in association with oliguria during labor or in the immediate puerperium (164,186). These events are transient, and the clinician should refrain from vigorous attempts at fluid resuscitation, because the latter is more apt to result in volume overload than to prevent any renal disaster.

Urinary Tract Infection

Infections of the urinary tract are the most frequent renal complications encountered during an otherwise normal pregnancy. In most instances, the problem is asymptomatic bacteriuria uncovered by routine screening. However, cystitis, overt pyelonephritis, and rarely perinephric abscess may also develop. The management of these conditions may be shared by obstetricians and nephrologists, especially in the latter two disorders, which may become life-threatening.

Asymptomatic Bacteriuria

The prevalence of covert urinary tract infection in gravidas is similar to that in nonpregnant women of reproductive age, ranging from 2% to 10%, with higher rates recorded in gravidas with sickle cell disease or diabetes (2,17,187–191). However, the natural history of asymptomatic bacteriuria is different during pregnancy than in the nonpregnant state. Outside of pregnancy, the situation is quite benign, but during gestation, covert bacteriuria progresses to acute pyelonephritis in 20% to 30% of patients. This may be particularly true in women with previous evidence of renal scarring, with or without reflux (192). In addition, there are claims that gravidas with asymptomatic bacteriuria have a higher incidence of anemia, hypertension, intrauterine growth retardation, or "preterm/low-birth-weight" infants (2,17,23,188,189), but data supporting these assertions are few and equivocal (23, 192–196). Most investigators currently recommend screening all gravidas and treating those with confirmed positive cultures (191). Screening is best performed during gestational week 16, because the onset of covert bacteriuria appears to be greatest between weeks 8 and 17 (197).

The practice of screening and treating asymptomatic bacteriuria is based on the as yet unproven assertion that such an approach prevents up to two-thirds of potential antepartum pyelonephritis (188,198). Even a more modest preventive effect would avoid substantial morbidity and result in significantly less hospitalization during pregnancy (190,191,199). Still, there are some who question the sensitivity and cost-effectiveness of routine screening (gravidas often generate contaminated and false-positive cultures, which require repeated testing and even catheterization) and suggest that testing be limited to those women with histories of recurrent infections, reflux, or nephrolithiasis (200–202). Until this issue is resolved, we continue to recommend universal screening. When considering screening, one should note that the dipstick method has a sensitivity of only about 70% compared with classic or semiquantitative culture techniques, but the former may still be more cost effective (191).

The incidence of bacteriuria increases immediately after delivery when it can be as high as 17% (203–205). This no doubt relates to the birth process and is not unexpected, because transient bacteriuria follows sexual intercourse and can be induced by massaging the urethra during gynecologic operations (37,206). Moreover, trauma occurring during labor impairs the resistance of the bladder to infection and facilitates colonization by pathogenic organisms. Still, in the absence of symptoms, "prophylactic" antibiotics are unwarranted, because in most instances the bacteriuria will clear spontaneously, falling to about 4% by the third postpartum day (203,205).

Symptomatic Infections

Cystitis or pyelonephritis complicates about 3% of all pregnancies (188,191). The incidence of acute cystitis (about 1% to 2%) does not seem to have been influenced by universal screening. Fortunately, however, the incidence of infectious pyelonephritis, the more ominous complication, has decreased from nearly 3% to 1% or less, a decline ascribed to aggressive screening for and treating of covert bacteriuria (188).

Cystitis

Acute cystitis in gestation is considered an entity unrelated to asymptomatic bacteriuria (188,191) for the following reasons: Cystitis occurs most frequently in the second trimester, in patients with previously negative screening cultures. The peak incidence of asymptomatic bacteriuria is much earlier, and its source is the upper urinary tract in about 50% of the women. Cystitis usually responds rapidly to treatment with a recurrence rate of about 17%, whereas that of asymptomatic bacteriuria may be as high as 35%. Finally, unlike covert bacteriuria, cystitis is not associated with a substantial risk of developing acute pyelonephritis (188)

Acute Pyelonephritis

Most (about 70%) patients who develop acute pyelonephritis during pregnancy have preexisting covert bacteriuria, and in a number of cases, the offending organism seems to have been newly acquired (187,188,191). Thus, although screening seems to have reduced the incidence of acute pyelonephritis by almost two-thirds, it has not and will not eradicate this disease (188,191). Ten percent of the cases occur in early pregnancy, and the rest present in equal proportions at midpregnancy and during the last trimester (207). Of interest is a report that women developing pyelonephritis antepartum manifest greater degrees of pelvicaliceal dilatation during gestation that may not regress after delivery, underscoring the need for postpartum investigation of this population (208).

The bacteriology of the various organisms that cause acute pyelonephritis are discussed in detail elsewhere (188,191). More than 90% of the uropathogens are aerobic Gram-negative rods, most of which are *Escherichia coli*. Pregnancy

seems to decrease tolerance to these infections, which may be related in part to observations that during gestation, there is immunosuppression of the cytokine and specific antibody responses to Gram-negative bacteria that invade the urinary tract (209). As a result, acute pyelonephritis in pregnancy can be often quite devastating to the health of both mother and fetus. This disorder was a cause of maternal mortality in the preantibiotic era, and currently about 20% of pregnant patients who present with pyelonephritis manifest bacteremia (188,191,207). Furthermore, there is substantial literature suggesting that upper urinary tract infections in gravidas are associated with the exaggerated effects of endotoxemia, including respiratory distress syndrome and various hematologic, hepatic, and renal functional abnormalities (2,37,188, 210). Concerning the latter, it is noteworthy that although upper urinary tract infections seem to have little effect on the renal hemodynamics of nonpregnant patients, acute pyelonephrixtis in pregnant women may result in transient and marked decrements in GFR (161). As for the fetus, acute pyelonephritis is associated with premature delivery, growth retardation, and intrauterine death (188,196,211). This disease should therefore be preferably treated in a hospital setting.

Perinephric or Cortical Abscess

These are very unusual events in pregnancy but should be considered in a setting of occult or resistant infections. This is especially true during the immediate puerperium, when physicians are apt to focus on uterine and abdominal sources of infection or on pelvic thrombophlebitis, and to overlook the renal problems noted previously.

Management of Urinary Tract Infections in Pregnancy

Table 74-2 lists the common antibiotics used to treat asymptomatic bacteriuria and cystitis during pregnancy (188,191).

TABLE 74-2. *Recommended therapy for asymptomatic bacteriuria and cystitis in pregnancy*

Agent[a]	Dosage
Standard courses of treatment (duration 7 d)	
Ampicillin	500 mg QID
Amoxicillin	250 mg TID
Nitrofurantoin[b]	50 mg QID or 100 mg BID
Cephalexin	250 mg QID or 500 mg BID
Amoxicillin/clavulanic acid	250/125 mg TID
Long-term prophylaxis	
Nitrofurantoin[b]	50 mg at night
Cephalexin	250 mg at night
Amoxicillin	250 mg at night

[a]All antibiotics in this table are in the Food and Drug pregnancy risk category B.
[b]Nitrofurantoin macrocrystals may reduce the incidence of gastrointestinal tract side effects.
Source: From Pedler SJ, Orr KE. Bacterial, fungal, and parasitic infections. In: Barrom WM, Lindheimer MD, eds. *Medical disorders during pregnancy,* 3d ed. St. Louis: Mosby, 2000, with permission.

In the past, given the tendency of asymptomatic bacteriuria to recur, many authorities suggested prolonged treatment, often for 6 or more weeks. Currently, however, most workers recommend a 7 day course, and even shorter periods are being evaluated (188,191,198). In this respect, there is a growing literature (191) describing success with single-dose therapy, which also has the theoretical advantages of being more cost effective, improving patient compliance, and minimizing drug toxicity. Some have suggested that failure of such treatment will identify patients at increased risk for recurrent asymptomatic bacteriuria who may benefit from suppressive regimens (191,212). Until these issues are resolved, we suggest the standard 7 day course (Table 74-2), which appears to treat successfully 90% of the women with cystitis and will eradicate bacteriuria for the remainder of pregnancy in more than 70% of the women with asymptomatic infections. Urine cultures should be repeated 1 or 2 weeks after completion of the initial antibiotic course, and then at 4- to 6-week intervals until delivery. Relapsing infections (reappearance of the same organism), which usually occur within the first 2 weeks and suggest a urinary tract abnormality (including nephrolithiasis) or renal involvement, should then be treated with a prolonged course (2 to 3 weeks), followed by suppressive therapy until delivery (Table 74-2). Reinfections (caused by a different strain or species) normally appear more than 3 weeks after treatment and are usually confined to the bladder. They may be treated with repeated short courses of antibiotics each time they occur or with long-term suppression. Alternatively, one may prescribe only post–coital prophylaxis (a single dose of either 250 mg of cephalexin or 50 mg of nitrofurantoin [213]). Trimethoprim-sulfamethoxazole combinations, frequently prescribed to nonpregnant women, are best avoided during gestation. Trimethoprim is teratogenic in animals and may also precipitate megaloblastic anemia during pregnancy, whereas sulfamethoxazole has been associated with kernicterus when prescribed near term (191).

Pregnant women with acute pyelonephritis are currently treated in a hospital setting, because they often require considerable supportive care and treatment with intravenous antibiotics (214). As of the year 2000, there were scattered reports (191) of successful management of gravidas with acute pyelonephritis in an outpatient setting, but we believe such data preliminary and await better-designed studies. A recent report that routine pretreatment urine and blood cultures are of limited use because only 6% of the patients require a change in therapy after the start of empiric treatment is of interest but should be confirmed (215). Because of an increase in the number of community-acquired pathogens resistant to ampicillin, many consultants recommend the addition of an aminoglycoside (usually gentamicin) and clindamycin initially, adjusting therapy when culture results become available. The "extended-spectrum" penicillins have also been used successfully in these women. The reader is referred elsewhere (188,191) for further discussion of individual antibiotics (the latter citation lists the current pregnancy risk classification according to definitions suggested by the FDA).

Most patients respond quickly, with the temperature returning to normal within 72 hours. Continued fever or evidence of sepsis should alert the physician to seek an obstructive cause using ultrasound or a plain abdominal x-ray film, because urinary calculi are the most common cause of obstruction in these patients, and about 90% of the stones are radiopaque. When clinical improvement is apparent, oral antibiotics may be substituted for parenteral medications, but there is little agreement concerning the treatment duration of uncomplicated infections. A minimum of 2 to 3 weeks seems appropriate, and many prescribe suppressive therapy through term thereafter, although urinary surveillance (see previous discussion of asymptomatic bacteriuria) has been claimed to be as effective as long-term suppression (216).

In summary, urinary tract infections are the most common renal complication of pregnancy, and most patients present with asymptomatic bacteriuria. Universal screening followed by treatment in culture-positive cases is debated but seems to have decreased the incidence of pyelonephritis, which in pregnant women can be a virulent disease. There is no consensus yet on the optimal treatment regimens of women with asymptomatic bacteriuria and those with acute pyelonephritis; at the start of the millennium, the effectiveness of single-dose antibiotic regimens for the former and outpatient management of the latter is still being debated. We screen all gravidas and treat those with covert bacteriuria for 7 to 10 days, initially hospitalize all patients with pyelonephritis, who then receive 2 to 3 weeks of the appropriate antibiotic, but underscore the need for further research in this area.

Preexisting Renal Disease

Perspectives

As noted, older views that underlying chronic renal disease of any severity precluded a successful pregnancy have been radically altered, because in many instances, prognosis for these patients is quite favorable (1). This more optimistic current approach is based on a series of studies dating from 1980, whose authors have reviewed the renal prognosis and gestational outcome in more than 1,000 patients, most with biopsy verification of their underlying kidney disorder (2,17, 217–227). Results of these largely retrospective studies permit the following guidelines, in which prognosis is mainly based on two functional parameters: the presence or absence of hypertension and the degree of renal insufficiency at conception. Women are arbitrarily classified in three categories: those with *mild, moderate,* or *severe* dysfunction.

Normotensive women with intact or only mildly decreased and stable renal function (serum creatinine, ≤ 1.4 mg/dL or 125 μmol/L) generally do well, experiencing more than 95% live births, about 75% of which are adequate for gestational age (217). These excellent fetal survival estimates are weighted to the more recent literature and reflect the marked advances in both perinatal and neonatal care. Gestation does not appear to alter the natural course of the renal disease (Fig. 74-14), but there is an increased incidence of superimposed preeclampsia or late pregnancy hypertension, as well as increased proteinuria that can exceed 3 g per day (17,217,223,225,227). Such increments rarely indicate functional deterioration; most patients with chronic renal disease and only mild dysfunction surprisingly experience a gestational-induced increase in GFR (217).

There are, however, exceptions to the optimistic outlook already described. Several nephropathies appear more sensitive to intercurrent pregnancy, including lupus nephropathy and perhaps membranoproliferative glomerulonephritis. In addition, women with scleroderma and periarteritis nodosa do poorly (especially when there is renal involvement and associated severe hypertension) and thus should be emphatically counseled to avoid pregnancy. Furthermore, authorities disagree on whether gestation influences adversely the natural history of IgA nephropathy, focal segmental glomerulosclerosis, and reflux nephropathy (17,218,223–225,228–236). Our view is that prognosis in the last three groups is similar to that of women with renal disease in general, being best when before pregnancy, function is preserved and high blood pressure absent. Although hypertension before conception increases the incidence of both maternal and fetal complications (218,237), the outlook of such patients has also improved dramatically, especially when the blood pressure is well controlled (238).

Prognosis is poorer when there are greater degrees of renal dysfunction. With moderate impairment (serum creatinine level, ≥1.5 to 3 mg/dL or 133 to 275 μmol/L), live births still approach 90%, but the incidence of fetal growth retardation or preterm deliveries exceeds 50% (17,239–242). In addition, one-third or more of such patients experience renal functional deterioration or the appearance of hypertension after midpregnancy. The latter may be severe and hard to control, and some women may experience an accelerated progression of their disease after delivery. Accordingly, pregnancy is not advisable in such patients. Note, however, that one group of investigators (227) suggests that maternal and fetal outcomes remain relatively favorable until serum creatinine levels approach 2 mg/L (or 177 μmol) and are more liberal in their recommendations.

When renal dysfunction before conception is severe (serum creatinine level, ≥3.0 mg/dL or ≥275 μmol/L, but some authorities consider the disease "severe" already at creatinine levels of 2.5 mg/dL or 210 μmol/L), the risk of maternal complications is far greater and the pregnancy success rate is rather poor (183,184,241,242). However, such patients are often infertile, especially when they have end-stage disease, but exceptions occur (184,243–245). For instance, women receiving renal replacement therapy occasionally conceive, and the incidence may be favorably influenced by erythropoietin therapy, which is associated with a return of ovulatory cycles and improvements in libido (245,246). However, fetal survival in women undergoing dialysis is barely more than 50%, (see later discussion), although there are serious maternal risks, including the occurrence of intraperitoneal hemorrhage and accelerated hypertension (183,184, 246). We therefore do not recommend planning or continuation of a pregnancy in women with preexisting severe renal dysfunction.

In summary, pregnancy in most women with renal dysfunction surveyed appears to have been successful. We must emphasize, however, that these views reflect literature that is primarily retrospective and that most of the patients described had but mild functional impairment. Published series dealing with greater degrees of dysfunction comprise less than 300 patients in aggregate. Thus, confirmation of our guidelines and a more definitive perspective require large prospective trials.

Specific Diseases

Table 74-3 lists specific diseases associated with pregnancy.

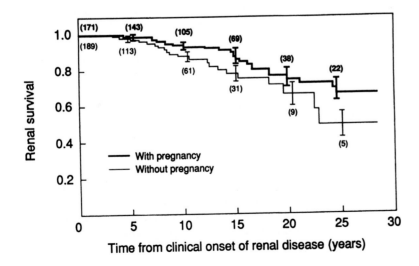

FIG. 74-14. Renal survival in women with preexisting renal disease who were pregnant at least once *(heavy line)* compared with those who never conceived. The long-term renal prognosis was similar in the two groups. (From Dr. P. Jungers, with permission.)

TABLE 74-3. *Preexisting renal disease and pregnancy*

Renal disease	Effects
Diabetic nephropathy	Most frequent nephropathy encountered. Pregnancy does not appear to accelerate functional loss; increased frequency of covert bacteriuria; high incidence of heavy proteinuria and hypertension after mid gestation.
Chronic glomerulonephritis and focal glomerular sclerosis (FGS)	There may be an increased incidence of high blood pressure late in gestation, but usually no adverse effect if renal function is preserved and hypertension absent before gestation; some disagree, believing that coagulation changes in pregnancy exacerbate these diseases, especially IgA nephropathy, FGS, and membranoproliferative glomerulonephritis.
Systemic lupus erythematosus	Expect more problems than in most glomerular diseases, but prognosis's more favorable if disease is in remission ≥6 mo before conception. Poorest maternal and fetal outcomes associated with antiphospholipid antibodies or with lupus anticoagulant.
Periarteritis nodosa and scleroderma	Fetal prognosis is poor; associated with maternal deaths; reactivation of quiescent scleroderma can occur during pregnancy or postpartum; therapeutic abortion should be considered.
Chronic pyelonephritis (infectious tubulointerstitial disease)	Bacteriuria in pregnancy may lead to acute exacerbations but otherwise is well tolerated. Frequent urine cultures are recommended and chronic suppressive antibiotic therapy may be necessary.
Reflux nephropathy	Some controversy but most now agree that these patients do well when function is preserved. They require frequent urine cultures.
Polycystic kidney disease	Patients with preserved function do well, but there is an increased tendency for late pregnancy hypertension and/or preeclampsia.
Urolithiasis	The "physiologic" ureteral dilation and stasis of pregnancy do not seem to affect natural history, but infections can be more frequent. Stents have been successfully placed during gestation.
Previous urologic surgery	Other urogenital tract malformations may be present; urinary infections increase, and functional decrements have been observed; cesarean section may be necessary to avoid disruption of the continence mechanism if artificial sphincters or neourethras are present.

Source: From Lindheimer MD, Grünfeld J-P, Davison JM. Renal disorders. In: Barron WM, Lindheimer MD, eds. *Medical disorders during pregnancy,* 3d ed. St. Louis: Mosby, 2000, with permission.

Diabetes

Diabetic nephropathy is the most common chronic renal disorder encountered during gestation. Most studies have focused on gravidas with overt disease (defined by the presence of abnormal proteinuria before conception or early in gestation), and there is very little information on the course of pregnancy in women with microalbuminuria only (227,247–261). The maternal long-term renal prognosis in patients with preserved function does not seem to be adversely affected by gestation, which is surprising because nephrotic range proteinuria and hypertension complicate two-thirds of these pregnancies. However, there are occasional observations of patients whose increased proteinuria does not remit or whose function deteriorates after delivery. Less surprising is limited evidence of rapid functional deterioration in diabetic women with moderate or greater renal dysfunction before pregnancy (247,256,257,260).

Fetal outcome, once considered poor is now quite good, with the success rates exceeding 95%. However, there is a high incidence of preterm deliveries as the rise in urinary protein excretion and blood pressure noted previously often occurs early in the third trimester, is difficult to differentiate from superimposed preeclampsia, and thus frequently leads to early termination of the pregnancy (247,249,252,256, 262,263). Of interest is a report of the appearance *de novo* of hypothyroidism during gestation in nephrotic diabetics (264).

Chronic Glomerulonephritis

Women with chronic glomerulonephritis, a general term that encompasses many morphologically and presumably pathogenetically distinct entities, seem to do well when renal function is preserved and hypertension absent (2,217–221,

224–227,235). There is evidence of transplacental transfer of nephritic factor(s) in association with membranoproliferative glomerulonephritis (265). This is also one of the entities in which pregnancy is said to have adverse effects on the course of the disease, such as an accelerated decline in renal function and an increased propensity to develop gestational hypertension or preeclampsia (the latter mainly ascribed to the type I renal lesion) (2,37,266). However, a review of the literature comprising 98 patients with membranoproliferative glomerulonephritis (225) suggests a maternal and fetal prognosis in this disease that is quite similar to that of gravidas with most other forms of chronic glomerulonephritis. Obviously more data are needed before firm conclusions can be reached.

IgA nephropathy is another disorder whose course in pregnancy is disputed. One group (228,231,232) persistently describes substantial declines in renal function that are only occasionally reversible, as well as the frequent appearance of *de novo* hypertension, which may fail to remit postpartum. In contrast, Jungers et al. (220,224,227) and Abe (223,233,235) reviewed more than 200 gestations in women with IgA nephropathy and also compared long-term renal function in 84 such patients who had experienced pregnancy with that of 80 who had never conceived. Both groups concluded that the natural history of this disorder and pregnancy outcome follow the generalization that the prognoses are excellent in normotensive women with minimal renal dysfunction. Lastly, we shall comment on acute poststreptococcal glomerulonephritis in this section, although it is obviously neither a preexisting nor a chronic renal disorder. Its occurrence in pregnant women is very unusual, perhaps due to the suppressed immune responsiveness characteristic of normal gestation (2,23,37,267–269). When it does occur, the recovery of renal function is usually complete and gestation is successful. Pregnancy in women with a remote history of acute glomerulonephritis is also uneventful (2,37).

Focal Segmental Glomerular Sclerosis

This is yet another disease whose course during gestation is disputed. Here, however, the reason may relate to the fact that focal segmental glomerular sclerosis (FSGS) has multiple causes. One group of Australian investigators (222,228,230)

noted hypertension, frequently severe, in 75% of their pregnant patients, functional deterioration in 45% of gestations, and a fetal loss of about 45%. The high blood pressure persisted postpartum in 20% of the women. Others (218,220, 227) dispute these data, again noting success when function before or in early pregnancy is preserved and hypertension absent. However, here too, the total published experience is sparse (100 or fewer patients described), and substantially more data are required to resolve this issue. Finally, there is an interesting report of women with FSGS experiencing two successful term deliveries, each followed by transient proteinuria in the neonate lasting several weeks (270). This is of interest because a circulating factor(s) that increases glomerular permeability to albumin has been described in some patients with FSGS by Savin and colleagues (271). This factor may therefore cross the placenta and affect the newborn.

Connective Tissue Disorders

The most common connective tissue disorder complicating pregnancy is, not surprisingly, systemic lupus erythematosus, a disease that primarily affects women during the childbearing years (272). The outlook for gravidas with lupus nephropathy and preserved kidney function is clearly more complex than that of a pregnant woman with the preexisting renal disorders discussed previously and is further complicated by the fact that the natural history of systemic lupus erythematosus is unpredictable regardless of gestation. However, reports appearing after 1980 have permitted a clearer understanding of the natural history and fetal outcome of gravidas with lupus nephropathy. Nine series that describe the gestational course of about 200 women with renal involvement are reviewed elsewhere (273). The best outcomes occur when the disease is in remission for 6 months before conception and when renal function is preserved (273). Prognosis is more guarded if the disease is active within 6 months of the pregnancy, when the lupus anticoagulant or an antiphospholipid antibody is present and, of course, if there is preexisting hypertension or greater degrees of renal insufficiency (176,272–274). Of note, lupus nephritis exacerbating or presenting *de novo* during late gestation may be difficult to differentiate from preeclampsia (2,272) (Table 74-4).

TABLE 74-4. *Comparison between preeclampsia and lupus nephritis*

Clinical measure	Preeclampsia	Lupus nephritis
C3, C4, CH$_{50}$	May be decreased but unusual	Commonly low
Urinalysis	Red blood cell (RBC) casts rare	RBC casts frequent
Onset of proteinuria	Commonly abrupt	Gradual or abrupt
Hepatic aminotransferases	May be increased	Rarely abnormal
Quantity of proteinuria	Will not differentiate	
Thrombocytopenia	Will not differentiate	
Hyperuricemia	Will not differentiate	
Hypertension	Will not differentiate	

Source: From Lockshin MD, Sammaratano LR. Rheumatic disease. In: Barron WM, Lindheimer MD, eds. *Medical disorders during pregnancy,* 3d ed. St. Louis: Mosby, 2000, with permission.

There is an increased incidence of first-trimester abortions, intrauterine growth retardation, and fetal death in women with systemic lupus erythematosus (272,275). These are also more apt to occur when circulating anticoagulants or antiphospholipid antibodies are present but may also be due to transplacental passage of the many other IgG autoantibodies that circulate in the blood of these patients. The latter are responsible for the occurrence of congenital heart block and the "neonatal lupus syndrome" including life-threatening thrombocytopenia, which are described further elsewhere (37,272). Still, it appears from most series that 85% to 90% of the fetuses survived (excluding first-trimester spontaneous abortions) (273). Management of lupus "flares" in the mother, including pulse steroids and chemotherapy, the treatment of the antiphospholipid syndrome, and the detection and management of congenital heart block are issues beyond the scope of this chapter and are detailed elsewhere (272,274).

In contrast to systemic lupus erythematosus, in which the disorder is usually sufficiently benign to allow conception in women who so desire, the outcome of pregnancy in patients with renal involvement with periarteritis nodosa or scleroderma is very poor, often because of the associated hypertension, which can be malignant in nature. In fact, many of the cases described in the older literature, albeit selective and anecdotal, were of maternal deaths, and fetal survival was dismal (2,37,272). The more recent literature, although still anecdotal, contains descriptions of successful pregnancies in women with scleroderma, but these were treated with ACE inhibitors, a drug category that should be avoided during gestation (272,276). We therefore continue to counsel against conception in women with these two entities and suggest pregnancy termination when the disease is present in the first trimester. Finally, there are reports that link pregnancy, via the passage to and persistence of fetal cells or DNA in the mother, to the pathogenesis of scleroderma, albeit years later (277,278).

Experience with other vasculitides, including Wegener's granulomatosis, is also sparse and anecdotal (272). Antenatal and postpartum exacerbations have been described, as well as successful pregnancies in women treated with azathioprine and cyclophosphamide. It should be noted, however, both are pregnancy risk class D agents (see *Physicians' Desk Reference*), although there is considerable experience with the former agent, primarily in gravid allograft recipients (see later discussion).

Miscellaneous Glomerular Disorders

The literature regarding minimal change nephropathy and pregnancy is quite favorable but is restricted to fewer than 200 gestations (217,220,227,223). Serum albumin levels usually decrease approximately 1 g in normal gestation, which should theoretically make gravidas more vulnerable to the complications attendant to massive urinary protein loss. Of interest, therefore, is a case description of a pregnant woman with steroid-responsive nephrotic syndrome who developed

in the first trimester renal insufficiency that responded rapidly to high-dose prednisone therapy (279). There is limited experience with membranous nephropathy as well in pregnancy, but for the most part, patients with preserved renal function do well (217,220,223,227). Their proteinuria may increase markedly, however, and at least one group has commented that severe nephrotic syndrome of any origin during the first trimester portends a poorer fetal prognosis (220,227).

Some Rarer Disorders

A retrospective report of 29 pregnancies in 17 women with renal amyloidosis secondary to familial Mediterranean fever is of concern; the authors suggested that gestation had an adverse effect on the natural history of the disease even when function was only minimally decreased (280). There is only anecdotal information on the course of Schönlein-Henoch disease and Goodpasture's syndrome in pregnancy (227,281,282). Concerning the latter are data from one report in which the authors postulated that the placenta ameliorated the disease during gestation by providing a large absorptive surface for the autoantibody (282). This would be consistent with an older report by Steblay (283) that sheep immunized to human placentas develop antibodies that react with both human placenta and glomerular basement membrane. He noted similar results when the sheep were immunized with glomeruli, suggesting that similar or identical antigens are present in the placenta and kidney.

Tubulointerstitial Disease and Reflux Nephropathy

There is sparse information on gestation in women with chronic interstitial nephritis and those with tuberculosis, but it would appear that here, too, outcome reflects functional status before conception (2,217). Of interest is the paucity of data relating to pregnancy in women with analgesic (primarily phenacetin) abuse, given the incidence of this disorder worldwide. One group of investigators (284) has suggested that women with interstitial nephritis were more prone to hypertension during pregnancy than those with glomerular disorders. This is contrary to our experience, in which pregnancy outcome was better than in those with primary glomerular diseases (217).

Reflux nephropathy is a disease that begins in childhood and affects a substantial number of women of reproductive age (285) (Chapter 24, Vesicoureteric Reflux and Reflux Nephropathy). Its presence may even remain undetected, and one should always consider this disorder in young women with frequent infections, especially if associated with unexplained hypertension. Some workers (228) have stressed that pregnancy affects adversely the course of this disease, but on careful review of their own data, these authors now note that gravidas who do poorly are mainly those who had hypertension and moderate renal dysfunction before conception (234). An analysis of 335 gestations in 135 women by Jungers' group (236) further revealed that when renal function was

TABLE 74-5. *Examples of inherited kidney diseases in which antenatal diagnosis may be technically possible*

	Mode of inheritance	Biochemical diagnosis	DNA study Linkage analysis	DNA study Gene defect[a]
ADPKD	AD		+	+
ARPKD	AR		+	
Alport's syndrome	XD		+	+
	AR		+	+
Primary hyperoxaluria type I	AR	+	+	+
Fabry's disease	XR	+	+	+
Finnish congenital nephrotic syndrome	AR	+ (raised amniotic fluid) alpha-fetoprotein concentration	+	+
Congenital diabetes insipidus	XR		+	+
	AR		+	+
Oculocerebrorenal syndrome of Lowe	XR		+	+
von Hippel-Lindau disease	AD		+	+

ADPKD, autosomal-dominant polycystic kidney disease; *ARPKD*, autosomal-recessive polycystic kidney disease; *AD*, autosomal dominant; *AR*, autosomal recessive; *XD*, X-linked dominant; *R*, X-linked recessive.
[a]In certain families in which the gene defect has been identified.
Source: From Lindheimer MD, Grünfeld J-P, Davison JM. Renal disorders. In: Barron WM, Lindheimer MD, eds. *Medical disorders during pregnancy,* 3d ed. St. Louis: Mosby, 2000, with permission.

preserved, 92% of the gestations succeeded, although 17% of the women delivered prematurely. Functional deterioration was only noted in patients with moderately or severely decreased GFR before conception or early in pregnancy.

Because of the nature of the disease, women with reflux nephropathy require frequent urine cultures and aggressive treatment when signs of urinary tract infection occur (285). Also, because the disease may be inherited, children who are born to parents with vesicoureteric reflux or reflux nephropathy or who have affected siblings should be screened in infancy (286). Finally, women who have undergone urinary tract reconstructive surgery, especially diversion, may develop reflux when pregnant (287). They also have a high incidence of asymptomatic bacteriuria. Still, and despite the risk of developing urinary tract obstruction as the uterus enlarges, their pregnancies are usually successful and fairly benign (287).

Inherited Renal Disorders

The most common genetic renal disorder is autosomal-dominant polycystic kidney disease (ADPKD), which affects 1 of 400 to 1,000 persons (288) (Chapter 18, Polycystic Kidney Disease). The other conditions encountered in women of childbearing age are renal amyloidosis associated with familial Mediterranean fever (an autosomal-recessive disorder clustering in Armenians and Sephardic Jews, discussed previously) and hereditary nephritis (289) (Chapter 19, Alport's Syndrome, Fabry's Disease, and Nail-Patella Syndrome). Most of the rarer disorders manifest during childhood and have usually progressed to end-stage renal disease before or by adolescence (e.g., nephronophthisis and

cystinosis). Still, such patients may conceive while receiving renal replacement therapy or after transplantation (290). Table 74-5 lists several inherited diseases that affect the kidney and for which antenatal diagnosis may be available (291). Women with these disorders should be referred for genetic counseling, preferably before they attempt conception or in early pregnancy.

Polycystic Kidney Disease. This disorder may remain undetected during gestation, but careful questioning for a family history of renal problems (10% or less of the cases are due to spontaneous mutations) and the judicious use of ultrasonography permit early detection. Women with ADPKD may have a greater propensity to develop late gestational hypertension or preeclampsia, but pregnancy outcomes are favorable when kidney function is preserved and hypertension absent (292). There is an increased risk for upper urinary tract infections that are at times severe and require treatment with lipophilic antibiotics such as ciprofloxacin or trimethoprim (both FDA pregnancy risk category class C) (288).

Although pregnancy does not appear to affect the natural history of the renal disorder, it may influence the effect of ADPKD on other organs. Liver cysts are more prevalent and larger in women, especially in those who have been pregnant, and enlargement of cysts (increasing the chance of rupture) may occur during gestation (Chapter 18, Polycystic Kidney Disease). One group of investigators (293,294) suggests that multiple pregnancies (defined as three or more) lead to an earlier onset of renal insufficiency. However, we believe that this may only reflect the effects of pregnancy once moderate dysfunction was present and that gestation does not influence the long-term renal prognosis of ADPKD. Finally, routine preconception screening of the intracerebral vasculature is not necessary and should be reserved for patients with a family history that reveals clustering of intracranial aneurysms or subarachnoid hemorrhage (295).

Hereditary Nephritis. Most patients with hereditary nephritis (85%) are men, having inherited the disease as an X-linked dominant disorder. In these families, most of carrier women manifest only mild or moderate degrees of urinary abnormalities (as dictated by the Lyon hypothesis) (289). The other 15% of patients with hereditary nephritis are examples of autosomal-dominant and autosomal-recessive inheritance. Thus, although hereditary nephritis is clinically silent in most women, there are exceptions, and the disease may manifest itself for the first time during a pregnancy. Because GFR is usually well preserved, most of these gestations succeed, but there is an interesting report describing two sisters with the disorder who developed rapidly progressive crescentic glomerulonephritis associated with pregnancy (296). Also, one should be aware of a variant of hereditary nephritis associated with macrothrombocytopenia and thrombocytopathy (2,289). Gestation in these women may be complicated by bleeding problems that appear to occur only at delivery or during surgical procedures.

Tuberous Sclerosis. This autosomal-dominant disorder is characterized by skin lesions, central nervous system involvement, and visceral lesions including renal angiomyolipomas (297). There may be renal aneurysms in these angiomyolipomas and in adjacent large branches of the renal arteries. One should attempt to detect and excise these aneurysms before a planned pregnancy, to prevent their rupture during gestation.

Von Hippel-Lindau Disease. This is also an autosomal-dominant disorder in which renal involvement includes cysts and bilateral multifocal renal carcinoma. Twenty-five percent of these patients also have pheochromocytoma, often bilateral, which may also cluster in families, and is sometimes the only manifestation of the disorder (298). Because pheochromocytomas are associated with fatal outcome and are especially prone to exacerbate during gestation, all patients with von Hippel-Lindau disease should be screened

for this disorder. The management of pheochromocytoma in pregnancy is discussed in Chapter 55 (Hypertension Associated with Endocrine Disorders). Details concerning genetic diagnosis and counseling are beyond the scope of this chapter and can be found elsewhere (299).

Urolithiasis

The incidence of stone disease in pregnant women varies by geographical location and is estimated to occur in 1 of every 1,500 pregnancies (300). The actual incidence, however, may be higher, because patients are often not identified until their disease is symptomatic and may even be overlooked if the symptoms are subtle (e.g., repeated urinary tract infections). There does not appear to be a marked increase in either the appearance or the recurrence rate of nephrolithiasis in pregnant women (301) (even in the face of marked calcium supplementation [302]). This is surprising because gravidas are normally hypercalciuric and their urinary supersaturation ratios for calcium oxalate and brushite are substantially increased (303) (Fig. 74-15). Urinary citrate and magnesium excretion also rise during pregnancy, but these increments are not enough to counter the marked increases in the supersaturation ratios (303). The answer, therefore, as to why there are no striking increases in stone disease during gestation may lie in the increased production and excretion of certain glycoproteins and of the Tamm-Horsfall protein, which decrease crystal aggregation and growth, thus inhibiting stone formation (300,304).

Presentation of the disease resembles that in nongravid subjects, the most common symptom being flank pain (about 89%), and more than 90% display either microscopic or macroscopic hematuria (305). Most stones passed during pregnancy contain calcium salts, others are infectious in origin ("struvite"), and very few are of the uric acid or cystine variety (37,300). The older literature anecdotally stressed the dramatic complications associated with obstruction or infection, whereas more recent reports describe more benign

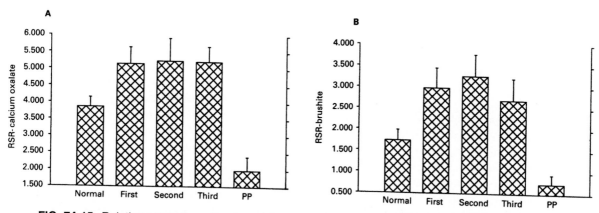

FIG. 74-15. Relative saturation ratios for calcium oxalate **(A)** and brushite **(B)** during each trimester of pregnancy and postpartum *(PP)*, as well as in a population of healthy women (normal). *P* < 0.01 for both comparisons. (From Maikrantz P, et al. Gestational hypercalciuria causes pathological urine calcium oxalate supersaturation. *Kidney Int* 1989;36:108, with permission.)

courses, except for increases in urinary tract infection and perhaps spontaneous abortion (37,300,301). Gestation does not appear to affect the course of urolithiasis, and there is even the impression that mobilized stones pass more easily because the ureters are dilated.

It should be stressed that the previous summary relates primarily to women with noninfectious calcium oxalate stones, whose course is also relatively benign in nonpregnant populations. Little is known, however, of the natural history of the more serious struvite stones during pregnancy. Experience with women who have cystinuria and conceive is also limited, although the results of one small series appear reassuring (306). In the latter disease, it is important to ensure hydration early in pregnancy when women are frequently nauseous, and thus far no adverse fetal effects have been ascribed to penicillamine (FDA pregnancy safety category D). There is virtually no information relating to urate stones, although acute renal dysfunction secondary to hyperuricemia has been described in pregnancy (307).

When stone disease is suspected, pregnancy should not be a deterrent to x-ray examination. A routine pyelogram involves about 0.4 rad, and exposure can be minimized further by restricting the number of films or using spiral computed tomography (308). If the stone obstructs the ureter, surgery may be necessary, and in this respect, about 30% of the patients described in the literature have undergone an operative procedure such as open lithotomy or percutaneous nephrostomy (37,300,309,310). Rigid ureteroscopy performed under general anesthesia has also been used in pregnancy (300,311). Currently, however, the placement of ureteral stents under ultrasonic guidance, a less invasive technique, has made it possible to manage gravidas through gestation and to defer more definitive surgical procedures until after delivery (37,300,312). Because there are very few data on lithotripsy during gestation, the procedure is best avoided. Finally, as noted previously, urinary tract infection in the presence of nephrolithiasis requires prolonged treatment (about 3 weeks), followed by suppressive therapy through the immediate puerperium, because the calculus represents a nidus of infection resistant to sterilization.

Guidelines on Managing Women with Preexisting Renal Disorders

Counseling

When counseling women on the advisability of conception or whether to continue a gestation already in progress, neither answers nor decisions come simply. These patients have high expectations, and the desire for motherhood is so strong as to tempt the sympathetic physician to take unwarranted risks. In addition, patients conceive against advise and refuse termination for religious, moral, or emotional reasons, in which case, both nephrologist and obstetrician (preferably a maternal-fetal-medicine subspecialist) must be ready to manage a difficult gestation and be prepared for serious complications.

We advise against attempting a pregnancy when serum creatinine levels exceed 1.4 mg/dL (124 μmol/L), but some permit gestation with preconception levels of up to 2 mg/dL (177 μmol/L), particularly in women with a single kidney, in those normotensive without treatment, and in those whose disorders are primarily interstitial in nature. As for blood pressure control, diastolic levels (Korotkoff V sound) should be 90 mm Hg or less.

In addition to the standard laboratory tests that permit the early detection of renal deterioration, the *database* should include serum uric acid and albumin levels, oxaloacetic and pyruvate transaminases, lactic acid dehydrogenase, and a platelet count, tests that will later aid in the differential diagnosis of an exacerbation of the renal disorder versus superimposed preeclampsia (Chapter 53, Hypertension and Pregnancy). We suggest biweekly visits, primarily to the obstetrician's clinic or office until gestational week 32, after which they are examined like all gravidas on a weekly basis. Renal parameters (primarily serum creatinine levels or its clearance) should be assessed every 4 to 6 weeks, unless more frequent evaluations become necessary. Fetal surveillance with electronic monitoring should be instituted after the thirty-second week, and even as early as the twenty-eighth to thirtieth week in frankly nephrotic patients.

Nephrotic gravidas are, in general, not prescribed diuretics because they may be oligemic and further intravascular volume depletion may compromise uteroplacental perfusion. Furthermore, both serum albumin concentrations and blood pressure normally decrease during gestation, in which case diuretics may be more prone to precipitate renal failure, circulatory collapse, or thromboembolic episodes. This is a relative recommendation, however, because there are nephrotic patients whose kidneys retain salt avidly and thus develop volume-induced hypertension. This is especially true in diabetic nephropathy, in which judicious use of diuretics may prevent or treat the presentation or aggravation of hypertension after midpregnancy and help avoid the early termination.

The treatment of hypertension in pregnancy is discussed elsewhere (313) (Chapter 53, Hypertension and Pregnancy). We use methyldopa, the preferred drug in the National High Blood Pressure Education Program's (NHBPEP) "consensus" report (313), because its safety during gestation is attested to by more than 20 years of postmarketing surveillance and several controlled trials; it also remains the only blood pressure medication for which there is a 7.5-year follow-up of the neonate. Currently, many hypertensive and diabetic patients who conceive are receiving either ACE inhibitors or angiotensin receptor antagonists. These drugs may cause fetopathies, neonatal oliguria anuria (which may be associated with irreversible renal failure), and possibly fetal anomalies or death (313, and an unpublished observation for the receptor antagonists). These medications are contraindicated during gestation and should be discontinued, and if necessary, another antihypertensive agent such as methyldopa should be substituted. Of note, although the NHBPEP report suggested that pregnant patients with chronic hypertension need not be treated until their diastolic levels reach 100 mm Hg or more (Korotkoff V sound), women with underlying renal disorders should receive therapy when these values are 90 mm Hg or more.

As of the year 2000, nephrologists have been treating many patients with renal disease, including nephrotic patients, with protein-restricted diets (Chapter 101, Protein Intake and Prevention of Chronic Renal Disease), but we caution against such a policy in pregnant patients, because little is known regarding fetal outcome in protein-restricted women. This is because of reports (whose citation and discussion is beyond the scope of this chapter) suggesting that protein restriction of gravid animals retards the development of the fetal kidney and is associated with hypertension in the offspring.

In the final analysis, GFR and blood pressure remain the two maternal parameters that determine the course of the gestation. Renal functional deterioration and the appearance or rapid acceleration of hypertension are best evaluated in a hospital setting, preferably one with an obstetrical tertiary care facility. It is important to remember that a decrement in creatinine clearance of 15% to 20% may occur normally near term, and increased proteinuria in the absence of hypertension need not cause alarm. In such circumstances, hospitalization is not necessary. When functional deterioration occurs earlier in pregnancy, there are no definite guidelines that permit prediction of postpartum reversibility, and the decision to terminate is always difficult. This is especially true when the gestation is approaching its twenty-fourth week, and 2 to 4 more weeks could improve substantially the chance for fetal survival. We usually recommend termination when serum creatinine levels have increased by 1 mg/dL, unless the values are still less than 2 mg/dL. Clearly this is an area in which more information is required.

Hemodialysis and Peritoneal Dialysis

Guidelines for the initiation and management of dialysis during pregnancy are detailed in several reviews (183,184,314). These patients are often rigidly protein restricted when not pregnant, but after conception, their protein intake should be liberalized (to at least 1.5 g/kg), especially in patients undergoing peritoneal dialysis (315,316). The concept of initiating early dialysis or increasing its frequency is based on the unproven but plausible hypothesis that fetal outcome is poorer in the face of marked azotemia even when uremic symptoms are not evident, and that fetal survival will improve in a less azotemic intrauterine environment. Thus, we recommend that renal replacement therapy be initiated when serum creatinine levels reach 5 to 6 mg/dL or if blood urea nitrogen levels are 60 mg/dL or more (183,184). Such a policy appears to facilitate volume and blood pressure control and permits a more liberal diet. Therapeutic goals include maintenance of predialysis blood urea nitrogen level at 50 mg/dL or less (17.9 mmol/L) while avoiding both hypotension and hypertension and rapid volume changes and maintaining pH and electrolyte levels near pregnancy norms (Table 74-1).

For example, dialysate bicarbonate levels may have to be reduced, and after midpregnancy, the average 0.5 kg per week weight gain should be taken into account when considering dry weight. These goals usually require daily dialysis.

Some of the problems encountered in these women include the following. Dialysis-induced uterine contractions, for which it is prudent to initiate uterine monitoring in association with dialysis when the patient has passed the twenty-fifth gestational week; the placenta produces Vitamin D and thus the calcitriol prescription may have to be reduced to avoid hypercalcemia; pregnancy is a hypercoagulable state, and intradialysis heparin requirements may be difficult to adjust; because pregnant women tolerate infection poorly, one should be extremely vigilant with patients receiving peritoneal dialysis. Some of the advantages of increasing the weekly dialysis prescription may be offset by increased loss of potassium, minerals, and water-soluble vitamins, often requiring nutritional supplementation and increases in dialysate potassium levels. Erythropoietin requirements increase markedly, and such needs may be the first indication that a patient on dialysis is pregnant (317). Although data are limited, erythropoietin seems to be well tolerated during gestation, and this drug has been used successfully even in women with moderate renal insufficiency and severe anemia who were not on dialysis (183,184).

Finally, as noted, pregnancy outcome in these women is poor and there are considerable maternal risks such as accelerated hypertension, cardiac decompensation, peritoneal bleeding (including venous erosion by the peritoneal catheter), and death (184,246,318). However, there are recent indications that prognosis may be improving, especially when the above-mentioned guidelines are adhered to (246,316,318–320). In this respect, a registry has been recently established at the Division of Nephrology, Loyola Stritch School of Medicine, Chicago, IL, directed by Dr. S. Hou, who can be contacted for up-to-date information.

Renal Transplantation

Transplantation reverses the abnormal reproduction associated with advanced renal disease. Ovulation and menses resume, and it has been estimated that as many as 1 of every 50 women of childbearing age with a functional kidney transplant become pregnant (321). Thus, it is not surprising that after a 1963 report of a successful pregnancy in a recipient of a renal allograft (322), thousands more followed. In many of these instances, the patient was unaware that she was fertile, suggesting a failure on the part of physicians to counsel these women properly.

In one extensive review of the literature through 1993, Davison (323) documented 3,382 gestations in 2,409 recipients of a renal allograft (it is our experience that many more are never reported). Most of these patients received azathioprine and prednisone, although experience with cyclosporine was then quite limited and newer immunosuppressive drugs (e.g., tacrolimus, mycophenolate mofetil) were yet to be used for the management of transplant recipients. About 35% of the pregnancies did not go beyond the first trimester, about 15% due to spontaneous miscarriages (an incidence similar to that of normal pregnant populations), and the remainder to selective inductions, often for nonmedical reasons. There was a 0.4% incidence of ectopic pregnancy. More encouraging, 93% of the gestations that continued beyond the first trimester succeeded, kidney prognosis and gestational outcome appearing to parallel those of pregnancy in women with preexisting renal disease in that the better the renal function before conception, the better the results. As expected, prognosis was best when the transplanted kidney came from a living related donor.

Many women with renal transplants experience increases in GFR during pregnancy, despite the presence of a single functioning kidney that often has undergone some degree of chronic rejection (50,51). The increments, however, are smaller than those observed in normal gestations. On the other hand, functional declines, usually in late gestation, are reported in about 15% of the patients, most frequently in the patients with the poorest prepregnancy creatinine levels. Fortunately, these are transient in most instances (37,323). Proteinuria also increases during these pregnancies, often to abnormal levels (50,323,324), but in most instances, these increments are functional in nature and unrelated to the health of the allograft.

This optimistic depiction must be tempered somewhat, because despite a high success rate, there are numerous maternal and fetal problems (17,323,325,326). These include steroid-induced hyperglycemia, leukopenia, serious infections including sepsis, uterine rupture, and even death in the mother. Hypertension complicates 30% of the gestations, and in such situations, plasma uric acid levels and protein excretion are not useful markers for diagnosing the presence of superimposed preeclampsia. This is because in allograft recipients, both indices could be above the norm at any stage of the gestation in otherwise uncomplicated pregnancies. There is also evidence that diabetic gravidas with renal allografts fare much worse than their nondiabetic counterparts, but the outlook may be better in patients who received combined pancreas and kidney transplants (323,328–330).

There are additional problems with the fetus and neonate as well (323,325,326). The incidence of prematurity, growth retardation, and low-birth-weight infants is increased, and congenital anomalies, serious infections, thrombocytopenia, hypoadrenalism, and hepatic insufficiency have been reported. Also, there are few, if any, long-term follow-up studies of the neonates, important as periodic reports of chromosomal damage, as well as subtle immunologic abnormalities (secondary to immunosuppression?) appear in the literature (323,331).

Finally, as mentioned, the surveys on which our summary is based primarily reflect results in patients managed with azathioprine and steroids alone, whereas virtually all allograft recipients now receive cyclosporine, tacrolimus, or mycophenolate, and newer agents are introduced all the time (for a review of immunosuppressive drugs in pregnancy, see reference 332). In this respect, regular reports have been generated by a National Transplantation Pregnancy Registry, established in late 1991 by Dr V. Armenti at the Thomas Jefferson University School of Medicine in the United States (325,329,333), and a similar registry has recently been activated in the United Kingdom (334). The initial reports from the former registry, which includes several hundred new patients, suggest outcomes similar to those in the review by Davison, although it appears that patients receiving cyclosporine tend to enter gestation with slightly higher creatinine levels and more hypertension, both adverse prognostic factors. These registries have also planned long-term surveillance of the newborns.

Effect of Pregnancy on Allograft Survival

There is a continuing controversy regarding the effect of pregnancy on the natural history of the renal allograft. Concerns that gestation might jeopardize the long-term health of the graft was revived in 1993 by a limited but well-designed case-control study by Salmela et al. (335). They described 29 posttransplant pregnancies in 22 women, each matched according to original disease, type of donor, immunosuppression, serum creatinine level at conception, and interval from transplant to pregnancy. Despite evidence of well-preserved renal function (serum creatinine averaging 1.1 mg/dL or 109 μmol/L before first gestation), the women who conceived had a lower 10-year graft survival rate (69% versus 100%; $P < 0.005$) compared with women who never did. This report rang alarm bells in transplant centers throughout the globe, even though we (336) noted in 1994 the atypical character of this study, in which the different results were primarily due to a highly unusual outcome in the controls, who in 10 years of follow-up had no graft failures! This is certainly contrary to the experience of most centers, in many of which statistics resemble (and may even be poorer than) those of the transplanted group who had conceived. Furthermore, the findings of Salmela et al. are at odds with results from the registry of the European Dialysis and Transplant Association (337) and three other recent reports (51,338,339). Most interesting among the latter is a survey by Sturgiss and Davison (338,339) of 18 women who had 34 pregnancies after transplantation, and which contained a considerable number of patients in the poorer prognostic category (e.g., moderate renal insufficiency, long-standing diabetes, and hypertension) (340). These women, too, were matched in case-control fashion to an equal number of women who had never conceived. There were no significant differences in GFR (measured by infusion techniques) or in the prevalence of hypertension between those who had conceived and those who had not, the posttransplant follow-up in each group averaging 12 years (Fig. 74-16). In summary, as of 2000, we believe there is no need to alter our generally optimistic counseling practices, although we do apprise the patients of the contrary findings of Salmela et al. (335). This is another area in which prospective data are needed.

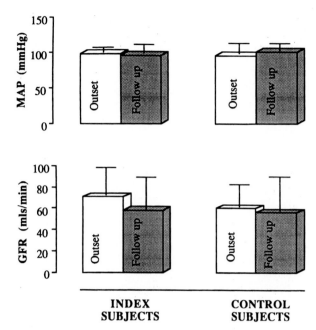

FIG. 74-16. Mean arterial pressure (MAP) **(upper panel)** and glomerular filtration rate (GFR) measured as the clearance of inulin **(lower panel)** in renal transplant recipients who underwent pregnancies **(left)**, compared with a control group who had never conceived. Open bars are at outset and closed bars are at follow-up studies. (From Dr. J. M. Davison, with permission.)

Management Guidelines

Pregnancy in allograft recipients has been reported since the 1960s, yet there have been no formal efforts by the many renal or transplantation societies to establish guidelines or criteria for preconception counseling. Ours are as follows:

1. Patients with transplants should wait 2 years before attempting conception (although we are aware that some authorities permit 1 year if graft is from a living related donor). This is because if renal function is stable and well preserved at 24 months, there is a high probability that it will remain so over the next several years. This strategy is supported by data emerging from the U.S. National Transplant Registry.
2. Serum creatinine levels should be no more than 2 mg/dL (177 μmol/L), and preferably less than 1.5 mg/dL (133 μmol/L), without evidence of rejection, pelvocaliceal dilatation, or infection. Proteinuria should be absent or minimal. The acceptance of higher initial serum creatinine levels by some is based on the assumption that in patients receiving cyclosporine, part of the functional loss is due to renal vasoconstriction.
3. Hypertension should be absent or easily managed.
4. Prednisone dosage should be less than or equal to 15 mg per day, and azathioprine 2 mg/kg per day or less. The azathioprine dose is based on limited data suggesting that fetal anomalies do not occur until more than 2.2 mg/kg per day is prescribed (341). A safe dosage for cyclosporine has

not been established because of the still-limited experience with this drug in pregnancy. We try to maintain a dosage of less than 5 mg/kg per day and to achieve circulating levels between 100 and 150 ng/mL.

These recommendations are relative and may require revision as more information on cyclosporine and other agents emerges.

Antenatal management is in general similar to that outlined for women with preexisting renal disease. Tests of liver function, calcium and phosphate levels, and red and white blood cell counts should be done at about 6-week intervals, because the liver of gravidas may be more sensitive to the hepatotoxic effect of azathioprine, and decreasing white cell counts may be predictive of neutropenia and thrombocytopenia in the newborn (both problems managed by decreasing the dose) (323). Monitoring calcium and phosphate levels is important because some women have had a subtotal parathyroidectomy, although others may manifest tertiary hyperparathyroidism. The hemogram is primarily monitored to detect marrow suppression secondary to the immunosuppressive therapy, but there are also data suggesting that the erythropoietin response to anemia may be suboptimal in these gestations (342). Because most patients receive steroids, they should also be screened for glucose intolerance during each trimester. Screening for toxoplasmosis and cytomegalovirus during each trimester, as well as for herpes simplex virus near term, is also advisable, although outcome studies to determine whether these policies are effective are sparse or lacking.

Gestations in transplant recipients are obviously "high risk" and require close prenatal and perinatal care. All pelvic examinations should be performed with strict aseptic techniques. The transplanted kidney is in the false pelvis and is not apt to obstruct the birth canal. Routine cesarean sections are therefore unnecessary, and the procedure is reserved for traditional indications. In this respect, many transplant patients have or have had pelvic osteodystrophy related to their previous renal failure or prolonged steroid therapy, which is of a severity that mandates an operative delivery (323). Regarding breast-feeding, steroids are secreted into breast milk but in the usual therapeutic doses are not sufficient to affect the infant. Metabolites of both azathioprine and cyclosporine also appear in breast milk (323). Their levels, too, are minimal, but in the absence of definitive data, we tend to discourage breast-feeding.

There are few guidelines concerning contraception in allograft recipients, a question frequently raised at counseling sessions or at the postpartum visit. The efficacy of intrauterine contraceptive devices (few are available in the United States) may be reduced because of the immunosuppressive and antiinflammatory agents these patients ingest (323). These devices may also aggravate menstrual problems and obscure signs and symptoms in early pregnancy, and their insertion and replacement is associated with transient bacteremia, which is an additional concern in immunosuppressed patients. Oral contraceptives may cause or aggravate hypertension or thromboembolism and may produce subtle changes in the immune system. Use of preparations with low estrogen content seems to have reduced these problems, but these drugs are yet to be systematically tested in transplant populations. Still, some prescribe them to allograft recipients, in preference to the less efficacious barrier method (323).

REFERENCES

1. Editorial. Pregnancy and renal disease. *Lancet* 1975;2:801.
2. Lindheimer MD, Katz AI. Philadelphia: *Renal function and disease in pregnancy.* Lea & Febiger, 1977.
3. Conrad KP. Renal changes in pregnancy. *Urol Annu* 1992;6:313.
4. Sheehan HL, Lynch JP. *Pathology of toxaemia of pregnancy.* Baltimore: Williams & Wilkins, 1973.
5. Bailey RR, Rolleston GL. Kidney length and ureteric dilatation in the puerperium. *J Obstet Gynaecol Br Commonw* 1971;78:55.
6. Cietak KA, Newton JR. Serial quantitative maternal nephrosonography in pregnancy. *Br J Radiol* 1985;58:405.
7. Garland HO, Green R, Moriarty RJ. Changes in body weight kidney weight and proximal tubular length during pregnancy. *Renal Physiol* 1978;1:42.
8. Davison JM, Lindheimer MD. Changes in renal haemodynamics and kidney weight during pregnancy in the unanaesthetized rat. *J Physiol (Lond)* 1980;301:129.
9. Baylis C. The mechanism of the increase in glomerular filtration in the twelve-day pregnant rat. *J Physiol (Lond)* 1980;305:405.
10. Dure-Smith P. Pregnancy dilatation of the urinary tract: the iliac sign and its significance. *Radiology* 1970;96:545.
11. Fried AM, Woodring JH, Thompson DS. Hydronephrosis of pregnancy. A prospective sequential study of the course of the dilatation. *J Ultrasound Med* 1983;2:255.
12. Cietak KA, Newton JR. Serial qualitative maternal nephrosonography in pregnancy. *Br J Radiol* 1985;58:399.
13. Rasmussen PE, Nielson FR. Hydronephrosis in pregnancy: a literature survey. *Eur J Obstet Gynecol Reprod Biol* 1988;27:249.
14. Croce JF, et al. Hydronephrosis in pregnancy. Ultrasonographic study [in Italian]. *Minerva Ginicologica* 1994;46:147.
15. Faúndes A, Bricola-Filho M, Pinto e Silva JL. Dilatation of the urinary tract during pregnancy: proposal of a curve of maximal caliceal diameter by gestational age. *Am J Obstet Gynecol* 1997;178:1083.
16. Rubi RA, Sala NL. Ureteral function in pregnant women III: effect of different positions and fetal delivery upon ureteral tonus. *Am J Obstet Gynecol* 1968;101:230.
17. Lindheimer MD, Katz AI. Renal physiology and disease in pregnancy. In: Seldin DW, Giebisch G, eds. *The kidney: physiology and pathophysiology,* 3d ed. Philadelphia: Lippincott Williams & Wilkins, 2000:2597.
18. Meyers SJ, Lee RV, Munschauer RW. Dilatation and nontraumatic rupture of the urinary tract during pregnancy. A review. *Obstet Gynecol* 1985;66:809.
19. Nielsen FR, Rasmussen PE. Hydronephrosis during pregnancy: four cases of hydronephrosis causing symptoms during pregnancy. *Eur J Obstet Gynecol Reprod Biol* 1988;27:245.
20. Eckford SD, Gingell JC. Ureteric obstruction in pregnancy: diagnosis and management. *Br J Obstet Gynaecol* 1991;98:1137.
21. Satin AJ, Seiken GL, Cunningham FG. Reversible hypertension in pregnancy caused by obstructive uropathy. *Obstet Gynecol* 1993;81:823.
22. Brandes JC, Fritsche C. Obstructive acute renal failure by a gravid uterus: a case report and review. *Am J Kidney Dis* 1991;18:398.
23. Chesley LC. *Hypertensive disorders of pregnancy.* New York: Appleton-Century-Crofts, 1978.
24. Conrad K, Lindheimer MD. Renal and cardiovascular alterations. In: Lindheimer MD, Roberts JR, Cunningham FG, eds. *Chesley's hypertensive disorders in pregnancy.* Stamford, CT: Appleton & Lange, 1999:263.
25. Chapman AB, et al. Systemic and renal hemodynamic changes in the luteal phase of the menstrual cycle mimic early pregnancy. *Am J Physiol* 1997;273:F777.
26. Chapman AB, et al. Temporal relationships between hormonal and hemodynamic changes in early pregnancy. *Kidney Int* 1998;54:2056.
27. Sturgiss SN, Dunlop W, Davison JM. Renal haemodynamics and tubular function in human pregnancy. *Clin Obstet Gynaecol (Baillière)* 1994;8:209.
28. Sturgiss SN, Wilkinson R, Davison JM. Renal reserve in human pregnancy. *Am J Physiol* 1996;271:F16.
29. Roberts M, Lindheimer MD, Davison JM. Altered glomerular permselectivity to neutral dextrans and heteroporous membrane modeling in human pregnancy. *Am J Physiol* 1996;270:F338.
30. Baylis C. Glomerular filtration and volume regulation in gravid animal models. *Clin Obstet Gynaecol (Baillière)* 1994;8:235.
31. Baylis C, Blantz RC. Tubuloglomerular feedback activity in virgin and 12-day pregnant rats. *Am J Physiol* 1985;249:F169.
32. Woods LL, Mizelle HL, Hall JE. Autoregulation of renal blood flow and glomerular filtration rate in the pregnant rabbit. *Am J Physiol* 1987;252:R69.
33. Recklehoff JR, Yokota F, Baylis C. Renal autoregulation in mid-term and late pregnant rats. *Am J Obstet Gynecol* 1992;166:1546.
34. Baylis C, Rennke HG. Renal hemodynamics and glomerular morphology in repetitively pregnant aging rats. *Kidney Int* 1985;28:140.
35. Milne JEC, Lindheimer MD, Davison JM. Glomerular heteroporous membrane modeling in the third trimester and postpartum before and during amino acid infusion. *(in review)*
36. Milne JEC, Lindheimer MD, Davison JM. Amino acid (AA) induced hyperfiltration in early pregnancy (EP), late pregnancy (LP),and postpartum: are different mechanisms involved? *Hypertens Pregnancy* 2000;19[Suppl 1]:111(abst).
37. Lindheimer MD, Katz AI. Renal physiology and disease in pregnancy. In: Seldin DW, Giebisch G, eds. *The kidney: physiology and pathophysiology,* 2nd ed. New York: Raven Press, 1992:3371.
38. Danielson LK, Conrad KP. Acute blockade of nitric oxide synthase inhibits renal vasodilation and ultrafiltration during pregnancy in chronically instrumented conscious rats. *J Clin Invest,* 1995;96:482.
39. Danielson LA, Conrad KP. Prostaglandins maintain renal vasodilation and hyperfiltration during chronic nitric oxide synthase blockade in conscious pregnant rats. *Circ Res* 1996;79:1161.
40. Gandley RE, Conrad KP, McLaughlin MK. Endothelin and nitric oxide mediate reduced myogenic reactivity of small renal arteries from pregnant rats. *Am J Physiol* 2001;280:R1.
41. Conrad KP, et al. Endothelin mediates renal vasodilation and hyperfiltration in pregnancy in chronically instrumented conscious rats. *Am J Physiol* 1999;276:F767.
42. Danielson LA, Sherwood OD, Conrad KP. Relaxin is a potent renal vasodilator in conscious rats. *J Clin Invest* 1999;103:525.
43. Danielson LA, Kerchner LJ, Conrad KP. Impact of gender and endothelin on renal vasodilation and hyperfiltration induced by relaxin in conscious rats. *Am J Physiol* 2000;279:R1298.
44. Baylis C. Effect of amino acid infusion as an index of renal vasodilatory capacity in pregnant rats. *Am J Physiol* 1988;254:F650.
45. Ronco C, et al. Renal functional reserve in pregnancy. *Nephrol Dial Transplant* 1988;2:157.
46. Woods LL, Davis LE. Renal hemodynamic response to protein intake in pregnant women. *Fed Am Soc Exp Biol J* 1994;8:A583.
47. Barron WM, Lindheimer MD. Effect of oral protein loading on renal hemodynamics in human pregnancy. *Am J Physiol* 1995;269:R888.
48. Schiffman RL, et al. Effect of dietary protein on glomerular filtration rate in pregnancy. *Obstet Gynecol* 1989;73:47.
49. Woods LL, Gaboury CL, Davis LE. Chronic protein feeding fails to increase renal hemodynamics in pregnant women. *J Am Soc Nephrol* 1994;5:616 (abst).
50. Davison JM. The effect of pregnancy on renal allograft recipients. *Kidney Int* 1985;27:74.
51. First MR, et al. Lack of effect of pregnancy on renal allograft survival or function. *Transplantation* 1995;59:472.
52. Graves SW, Cook SL, Seely EW. Fluid and electrolyte handling in normal pregnancy. *J Soc Gynecol Invest* 1995;2:291(abst).
53. Lind T, Hytten FE. The excretion of glucose during normal pregnancy. *J Obstet Gynaecol Br Commonw* 1972;79:961.
54. Davison JM, Lovedale C. The excretion of glucose during normal pregnancy and after delivery. *J Obstet Gynaecol Br Commonw* 1974;81:30.
55. Welsh GW, Sims EAH. The mechanism of renal glucosuria in pregnancy. *Diabetes* 1960;9:363.
56. Davison JM, Hytten FE. The effect of pregnancy on the renal handling of glucose. *J Obstet Gynaecol Br Commonw* 1975;82:374.

57. Atherton JC, Green R. Renal tubular function in the gravid rat. *Clin Obstet Gynaecol (Baillière)* 1994;8:265.
58. Hytten FE, Cheyne GA. The aminoaciduria of pregnancy. *J Obstet Gynaecol Br Commonw* 1972;79:424.
59. Boyle JA. Serum uric acid levels in normal pregnancy with observations on the renal excretion of urate in pregnancy. *J Clin Pathol* 1969;19:501.
60. Dunlop W, Davison JM. The effect of normal pregnancy on the renal handling of uric acid. *Br J Obstet Gynaecol* 1977;84:13.
61. Semple PF, Carswell W, Boyle JA. Serial studies of the renal clearance of urate and inulin during pregnancy and after the puerperium in normal women. *Clin Sci Mol Med* 1974;47:559.
62. Lockitch G. The effect of normal pregnancy on common biochemistry and hematology tests. In: Barron WM, Lindheimer MD, eds. *Medical disorders during pregnancy*, 3rd ed. St. Louis: Mosby, 2000:635.
63. Barry CL, Royle GA, Lake Y. Racial variation in serum uric acid concentration in pregnancy. A comparison between European, New Zealand Maori and Polynesian women. *Aust N Z J Obstet Gynaecol* 1992;32:17.
64. Hill LM, Furness C, Dunlop W. Diurnal variation in serum urate in pregnancy. *Br Med J* 1977;2:1520.
65. Fischer RL, et al. Maternal serum uric acid levels in twin gestations. *Obstet Gynecol* 1995;85:60.
66. Lind T, Godfrey KA, Philips PR. Changes in serum uric acid concentrations during normal pregnancy. *Br J Obstet Gynaecol* 1984;91:128.
67. Carter J, Child A. Serum uric acid levels in normal pregnancy. *Aust N Z J Obstet Gynaecol* 1989;24:13.
68. Dunlop W, et al. Clinical relevance of coagulation and renal changes in pre-eclampsia. *Lancet* 1978;ii:346.
69. Yoshimura A, et al. Significance of uric acid clearance in preeclampsia. *Am J Obstet Gynecol* 1990;162:1639.
70. Many A, Hubel CA, Roberts JM. Hyperuricemia and xanthine oxidase in preeclampsia revisited. *Am J Obstet Gynecol* 1996;174:288.
71. Forsum E, Sadurskis A, Wager J. Resting metabolic rate and body composition of healthy Swedish women during pregnancy. *Am J Clin Nutr* 1988;47:942.
72. Lindheimer MD, et al. Potassium homeostasis in pregnancy. *J Reprod Med* 1987;32:517.
73. Ehrlich EN, Lindheimer MD. Effect of administered mineralocorticoids or ACTH in pregnant women. Attenuation of the kaliuretic influence of mineralocorticoids during pregnancy. *J Clin Invest* 1972;51:1301.
74. Mujais SK, Nora NA, Chen Y. Regulation of the renal Na:K pump–role of progesterone. *J Am Soc Nephrol* 1993;3:1488.
75. Brown MA, et al. Potassium regulation and progesterone aldosterone relationships in human pregnancy. *Am J Obstet Gynecol* 1986;155:349.
76. August P, Lindheimer MD. Chronic hypertension in pregnancy. In: Lindheimer MD, Roberts JM, Cunningham FG, eds. *Chesley's hypertensive disorders in pregnancy*. Stamford, CT: Appleton & Lange, 1999:605.
77. Geller DS, et al. Activating mineralocorticoid receptor mutation in hypertension exacerbated by pregnancy. *Science* 2000;289:119.
78. Lim VS, Katz AI, Lindheimer MD. Acid–base regulation in pregnancy. *Am J Physiol* 1976;231:1764.
79. Takano M, Kaneda T. Renal contribution to acid–base during the menstrual cycle. *Am J Physiol* 1983;244:F320.
80. Heenan AP, Wolfe LA. Plasma acid–base regulation above and below the ventilatory thresholds. In late pregnancy. *J Appl Physiol* 2000;88:149.
81. Davison JM, Vallotton MB, Lindheimer MD. Plasma osmolality and urinary concentration and dilution during and after pregnancy: evidence that lateral recumbency inhibits maximal concentrating ability. *Br J Obstet Gynaecol* 1981;88:472.
82. Lindheimer MD, Barron WM. Water metabolism and vasopressin secretion during pregnancy. *Clin Obstet Gynaecol (Baillière)* 1994;8:311.
83. Lindheimer MD, Davison JM. Osmoregulation, the secretion of arginine vasopressin and its metabolism during pregnancy (minireview). *Eur J Endocrinol* 1995;132:133.
84. Dürr JA, Lindheimer MD. Control of volume and body tonicity. In: Lindheimer MD, Roberts JM, Cunningham FG, eds. *Chesley's hypertensive disorders in pregnancy,* 2nd ed. Stamford, CT: Appleton & Lange, 1999:103.
85. Dürr JA, Stamoutsos BA, Lindheimer MD. Osmoregulation during pregnancy in the rat. Evidence for resetting of the threshold for vasopressin secretion during pregnancy. *J Clin Invest* 1981;68:337.
86. Barron WM, et al. Osmoregulation and vasopressin secretion during pregnancy in Brattleboro rats. *Am J Physiol* 1985;248:R229.
87. Barron WM, Lindheimer MD. Osmoregulation in pseudopregnant and prolactin-treated rats: comparison with normal gestation. *Am J Physiol* 1988;254:R478.
88. Koehler EM, et al. Osmoregulation of the magnocellular system during pregnancy and lactation. *Am J Physiol* 1993;264:R555.
89. Davison JM, et al. Serial evaluation of vasopressin release and thirst in human pregnancy: role for chorionic gonadotropin on the osmoregulatory changes of gestation. *J Clin Invest* 1988;81:798.
90. Davison JM, et al. Changes in the metabolic clearance of vasopressin and plasma vasopressinase throughout human pregnancy. *J Clin Invest* 1989;83:1313.
91. Davison JM, et al. Metabolic clearance of vasopressin and an analogue resistant to vasopressinase in human pregnancy. *Am J Physiol* 1993;264:F348.
92. Davison JM, et al. Influence of humoral and volume factors on altered osmoregulation of pregnancy. *Am J Physiol* 1990;258:F900.
93. Xu DL, et al. Upregulation of endothelial and neuronal nitric oxide synthase in pregnant rats. *Am J Physiol* 1996;271:R1739.
94. Weisinger RS, et al. Relaxin alters plasma osmolality-arginine vasopressin relationship in the rat. *J Endocrinol* 1993;137:505.
95. Schrier RW, Dürr JA. Pregnancy: an overfill or underfill state? *Am J Kidney Dis* 1987;9:284.
96. Schrier RW. Pathogenesis of sodium and water retention in high output and low-output cardiac failure, nephrotic syndrome, cirrhosis, and pregnancy. *N Engl J Med* 1988;319:1065.
97. Schrier RW, Briner VA. Peripheral arterial vasodilation hypothesis and water retention in pregnancy: implications for the pathogenesis of preeclampsia-eclampsia. *Obstet Gynecol* 1991;77:632.
98. Phippard AF, et al. Circulatory adaptations to pregnancy-serial studies of haemodynamics, blood volume, and renin and aldosterone in the baboon (*Papio hamadryas*). *J Hypertens* 1986;4:773.
99. August P, et al. Role of renin–angiotensin system in blood pressure regulation in pregnancy. *Lancet* 1995;i:896.
100. Ohara M, et al. Upregulation of aquaporin 2 water channel in pregnant rats. *J Clin Invest* 1998;101:1076.
101. Barron WM, Stamoutsos BA, Lindheimer MD. Role of volume in the regulation of vasopressin secretion during pregnancy. *J Clin Invest* 1984;73:923.
102. Barron WM, et al. Role of hemodynamic factors in the osmoregulatory alterations of rat pregnancy. *Am J Physiol* 1989;257:R909.
103. Koehler EM, et al. Response of the magnocellular system in rats to hypovolemia and cholecystokinin during pregnancy and lactation. *Am J Physiol* 1994;266:R1327.
104. Amico JA. Diabetes insipidus and pregnancy. *Frontiers Horm Res* 1985;13:266.
105. Dürr JA. Diabetes insipidus syndrome in pregnancy. In: Cowley AJ Jr, Liard J-F, Aussiello DA, eds. *Vasopressin: cellular and integrative functions.* New York: Raven Press, 1988:257.
106. Dürr JA, Lindheimer MD. Diagnosis and management of diabetes insipidus during pregnancy. *Endocrinol Pract* 1996;2:353.
107. Molitch ME. Pituitary, thyroid, adrenal, and parathyroid disorders, In: Barron WM, Lindheimer MD, eds. *Medical disorders during pregnancy,* 3rd ed. St. Louis: Mosby, 2000:101.
108. Bakiri F, Benmiloud M, Vallotton MB. Arginine-vasopressin in post postpartum panhypopituitarism: urinary excretion and kidney response to an osmolar load. *J Clin Endocrinol Metab* 1984;58:511.
109. Iwasaki Y, et al. Neurohypophysial function in postpartum hypopituitarism: impaired plasma vasopressin response to osmotic stimuli. *J Clin Endocrinol Metab* 1989;68:560.
110. Arnaout MA, Ajlouni K. Plasma vasopressin responses in postpartum hypopituitarism. *Acta Endocrinol* 1992;127:494.
111. Barron WM, et al. Transient vasopressin-resistant diabetes insipidus of pregnancy. *N Engl J Med* 1984;310:442.
112. Dürr JA, et al. Diabetes insipidus in pregnancy associated with abnormally high circulating vasopressinase. *N Engl J Med* 1987;316:1070.
113. Kennedy S, et al. Transient diabetes insipidus and acute fatty liver of pregnancy. *Br J Obstet Gynaecol* 1994;101:387.

114. Baylis PH, et al. Recurrent pregnancy-induced polyuria and thirst due to hypothalamic diabetes insipidus: an investigation into possible mechanisms responsible for the polyuria. *Clin Endocrinol* 1986;24:459.

115. Hughes JM, Barron WM, Vance ML. Recurrent diabetes insipidus associated with pregnancy. pathophysiology and therapy. *Obstet Gynecol* 1989;73:462.

116. Iwasaki Y, et al. Aggravation of subclinical diabetes insipidus during pregnancy. *N Engl J Med* 1991;324:556.

117. William DJ, et al. Pathophysiology of transient cranial diabetes insipidus during pregnancy. *Clin Endocrinol* 1993;38:595.

118. Ford SM Jr, Lumpkin HL III. Transient vasopressin-resistant diabetes insipidus of pregnancy. *Obstet Gynecol* 1986;68:726.

119. Sutton RA, Schonholzer K, Kassen BD. Transient syndrome of inappropriate antidiuretic hormone secretion during pregnancy. *Am J Kidney Dis* 1993;21:444.

120. Hayslett JP, Katz DL, Knudson JM. Dilutional hyponatremia in preeclampsia. *Am J Obstet Gynecol* 1998;179:1312.

121. Magriples U, Laifer S, Hayslett JP. Dilutional hyponatremia in preeclampsia with and without nephrotic syndrome. *Am J Obstet Gynecol* 2001;184:231.

122. Brown MA, Gallery EDM. Volume homeostasis in normal pregnancy and pre-eclampsia: physiology and clinical implications. *Clin Obstet Gynaecol (Baillière)* 1994;8:287.

123. Gallery EDM, Lindheimer MD. Alterations in volume homeostasis. In: Lindheimer MD, Roberts JM, Cunningham FG, eds. *Chesley's hypertensive disorders in pregnancy,* 2nd ed. Stamford, CT: Appleton & Lange, 1999:327.

124. Catalano PM, et al. Estimating body composition in late gestation: a new hydration constant for body density and total body water. *Am J Physiol* 1995;268:F153.

125. Lukaski HC, et al. Total body water in pregnancy: assessment by using bioelectrical impedance. *Am J Clin Nutr* 1994;59:578.

126. Brown MA, Zammit VC, Mitar DM. Extracellular fluid volumes in pregnancy-induced hypertension. *J Hypertens* 1992;10:61.

127. August P, Lindheimer MD. Pathophysiology of preeclampsia. In: Laragh JH, Brenner BM, eds. *Hypertension: pathophysiology, diagnosis, and management,* 2nd ed. New York: Raven Press, 1995:2407.

128. Baylis C, et al. Recent insights into the roles of nitric oxide and renin-angiotensin in the pathophysiology of preeclamptic pregnancy. *Semin Nephrol* 1998;18:208.

129. Wilson M, et al. Blood pressure, the renin-angiotensin system, and sex steroids throughout normal pregnancy. *Am J Med* 1980;68:97.

130. Ehrlich EN. Heparinoid-induced inhibition of aldosterone secretion in pregnant women: the role of augmented aldosterone secretion in sodium conservation during normal pregnancy. *Am J Obstet Gynecol* 1971;109:963.

131. Winkel CA, et al. Conversion of plasma progesterone to deoxycorticosterone in men, nonpregnant and pregnant women, and adrenalectomized subjects: evidence for steroid 21-hydroxylase activity in nonadrenal tissues. *J Clin Invest* 1980;66:803.

132. Casey ML, MacDonald PC. Metabolism of deoxycorticosterone and deoxycorticosterone sulfate in men and women. *J Clin Invest* 1982;70:312.

133. Winkel CA, et al. Deoxycorticosterone biosynthesis in the human kidney: potential for the formation of a potent mineralocorticoid in its site of action. *Proc Natl Acad Sci USA* 1980;77:7069.

134. MacDonald PC, et al. Regulation of extraadrenal 21-hydroxylase activity: increased conversion of plasma progesterone to deoxycorticosterone during estrogen treatment of women pregnant with a dead fetus. *J Clin Invest* 1982;69:469.

135. Castro LC, Hobel CJ, Gornbein J. Plasma levels of atrial natriuretic peptide in normal and hypertensive pregnancies: a meta-analysis. *Am J Obstet Gynecol* 1994;171:1642.

136. Brown MA, et al. Sodium excretion in normal and hypertensive pregnancy: a prospective study. *Am J Obstet Gynecol* 1988;159:297.

137. Bay WH, Ferris TF. Factors controlling plasma renin and aldosterone in pregnancy. *Hypertension* 1979;1:410.

138. Brown MA, Broughton Pipkin F, Symonds EM. The effects of intravenous angiotensin II upon sodium and urate excretion in human pregnancy. *J Hypertens* 1988;6:457.

139. Duvekott JJ, et al. Early pregnancy changes in hemodynamics and volume homeostasis are consecutive adjustments triggered by a primary fall in systemic vascular tone. *Am J Obstet Gynecol* 1992;169:1382.

140. Barron WM, Nalbantian-Brandt C, Lindheimer MD. Role of adrenal mineralocorticoid in volume homeostasis and pregnancy performance in the rat. *Hypertens Pregnancy* 1993;12:59.

141. Weinberger MH, et al. The effect of posture and saline loading on plasma renin activity and aldosterone concentration in pregnant, non-pregnant, and estrogen treated women. *J Clin Endocrinol* 1977;44:69.

142. McLaughlin MK, Roberts JM. Hemodynamic changes. In: Lindheimer MD, Roberts JM, Cunningham FG, eds. *Chesley's hypertensive disorders in pregnancy,* 2nd ed. Stamford, CT: Appleton & Lange, 1999:69.

143. Schrier RW, et al. Pathophysiology of renal fluid retention. *Kidney Int* 1998;67:S127.

144. Kuo VS, Koumantakis G, Gallery EDM. Proteinuria and its assessment in normal and hypertensive pregnancy. *Am J Obstet Gynecol* 1992;167:723.

145. Higby K, et al. Normal values of urinary albumin and total protein excretion during pregnancy. *Am J Obstet Gynecol* 1994;171:984.

146. Barr J, et al. Microalbuminuria in early pregnancy in normal and high risk patients. *Early Pregnancy* 1996;2:197.

147. Gallery EDM, Györy AZ. Urinary concentration, white blood cell excretion, acid excretion, and acid base status in normal pregnancy: alterations in pregnancy-associated hypertension. *Am J Obstet Gynecol* 1979;135:27.

148. Gallery EDM, Ross M, Györy AZ. Urinary red blood cell and cast excretion in normal and hypertensive human pregnancy. *Am J Obstet Gynecol* 1993;168:67.

149. Danielli L, et al. Recurrent hematuria during multiple pregnancies. *Obstet Gynecol* 1987;69:446.

150. Quadri KHM, et al. Assessment of renal function during pregnancy using a random urine protein to creatinine ratio and Cockcroft-Gault formula. *Am J Kidney Dis* 1994;24:416.

151. Packham D, Fairley KF. Renal biopsy: Indications and complications in pregnancy. *Br J Obstet Gynaecol* 1987;94:935.

152. Lindheimer MD, Davison JM. Renal biopsy in pregnancy. "To b . . . or not to b . . . ? *Br J Obstet Gynaecol* 1987;94:932.

153. Pertuiset N, Grünfeld J-P. Acute renal failure in pregnancy. *Clin Obstet Gynaecol (Baillière)* 1994;8:333.

154. Lindheimer MD, et al. Acute renal failure in pregnancy. In: Brenner BM, Lazarus JM, eds. *Acute renal failure,* 3rd ed. New York: Churchill Livingstone, 1993:417.

155. Turney JH, Ellis CM, Parson FM. Obstetric acute renal failure. *Br J Obstet Gynaecol* 1989;96:679.

156. Stratta P, et al. Pregnancy-related acute renal failure. *Clin Nephrol* 1988;2:14.

157. Prakash J, et al. Pregnancy-related acute renal failure in Eastern India. *J Nephrol* 1995;8:214.

158. Randersee IGH, et al. Acute renal failure in pregnancy in South Africa. *Renal Fail* 1995;17:147.

159. Warren GV, Sprague SM, Corwin HC. Sarcoidosis presenting as acute renal failure during pregnancy. *Am J Kidney Dis* 1988;12:161.

160. Sheil O, Redman CWG, Pugh C. Renal failure in pregnancy due to primary lymphoma. Case report. *Br J Obstet Gynaecol* 1991;98:216.

161. Whalley PJ, Cunningham FG, Martin FG. Transient renal dysfunction associated with acute pyelonephritis of pregnancy. *Obstet Gynecol* 1975;46:174.

162. Jena M, Mitch WE. Rapidly reversible acute renal failure from ureteral obstruction in pregnancy. *Am J Kidney Dis* 1996;28:457.

163. Courban D, et al. Acute renal failure in the first trimester resulting from uterine lyomas. *Am J Obstet Gynecol* 1997;175:950.

164. Krane K, Cucuzzella A. Acute renal insufficiency in pregnancy: a review of 30 cases. *J Maternal-Fetal Med* 1995;4:12.

165. Chugh KS, et al. Spectrum of acute cortical necrosis in Indian patients. *Am J Med Sci* 1983;286:10.

166. Sibai BM, Villar M, Mabie BC. Acute renal failure in the hypertensive disorders of pregnancy. *Am J Obstet Gynecol* 1990;162:777.

167. Sibai BM, Ramadan M. Acute renal failure in pregnancies complicated by hemolysis, elevated enzymes and low platelets. *Am J Obstet Gynecol* 1993;168:1682.

168. Ibdah JA, et al. A fetal fatty-acid oxidation disorder as a cause of liver disease in pregnant women. *N Engl J Med* 1999;340:1723.

169. Baker AL. Liver and biliary tract diseases. In: Barron WM, Lindheimer MD, eds. *Medical disorders during pregnancy,* 3rd ed. St. Louis: Mosby, 2000:330.

170. Ockner SA, et al. Fulminant hepatic failure caused by acute fatty liver of pregnancy treated by orthotopic liver transplantation. *Hepatology* 1990;11:59.

171. Scheer RL, Jones DB. Malignant nephrosclerosis in women post partum: a note on microangiopathic hemolytic anemia. *JAMA* 1967;201:106.

172. Wagoner RD, Holley KE, Johnson WJ. Accelerated nephrosclerosis and post partum acute renal failure in normotensive women. *Ann Intern Med* 1968;69:237.

173. Robson JS, et al. Irreversible postpartum renal failure: a new syndrome. *Q J Med* 1968;37:423.

174. Kincaid-Smith P. The similarity of lesions and underlying mechanisms in preeclamptic toxemia and postpartum renal failure. In: Kincaid-Smith P, Mathew TH, Becker EL, eds. *Glomerulonephritis.* New York: John Wiley and Sons, 1973:1013.

175. Sibai BM, Kustermann L, Velasco J. Current understanding of severe preeclampsia, pregnancy-associated hemolytic uremic syndrome, thrombotic thrombocytopenic purpura, hemolysis, elevated liver enzymes, and low platelet syndrome, and postpartum acute renal failure: different clinical syndromes or just different names? *Curr Opinion Nephrol Hypertens* 1994;3:436.

176. Kincaid-Smith P, Fairley KF, Kloss M. Lupus anticoagulant associated with thrombotic microangiopathy and pregnancy related renal failure. *Q J Med* 1988;68:795.

177. Kniaz D, et al. Postpartum hemolytic-uremic syndrome associated with antiphospholipid antibodies. *Am J Nephrol* 1992;12:126.

178. Kupferminc MJ, et al. Severe postpartum pulmonary, cardiac, and renal syndrome associated with antiphospholipid antibodies. *Obstet Gynecol* 1994;83:806.

179. Madias NE, Donohoe JF, Harrington JT. Postischemic acute renal failure. In: Brenner BM, Lazarus JM, eds. *Acute renal failure,* 2nd ed. New York: Churchill Livingstone, 1988:251.

180. Conger JD, Falk S, Guggenheim SJ. Glomerular dynamics and morphologic changes in the generalized Shwartzman reaction in postpartum rats. *J Clin Invest* 1981;67:1334.

181. Raij L. Glomerular thrombosis in pregnancy: role of L-arginine-nitric oxide pathway. *Kidney Int* 1994;45:775.

182. Kleinknecht D, et al. Diagnostic procedures and long-term prognosis in bilateral renal cortical necrosis. *Kidney Int* 1973;4:390.

183. Hou S, Firanek C. Management of the pregnant dialysis patient. *Adv Renal Replacement Ther* 1998;5:24.

184. Hou S. Pregnancy in chronic renal insufficiency and end-stage renal disease. *Am J Kidney Dis* 1999;33:235.

185. Lew SQ, Watson JA. Urea and creatinine generation and removal in a pregnant patient on hemodialysis. *Adv Peritoneal Dial* 1992;8:131.

186. Nzerue CM, et al. Acute renal failure in pregnancy: a review of clinical outcomes at an inner city hospital from 1986–1996. *J Natl Med Assoc* 1998;90:486.

187. McFadyen IR, et al. Bacteriuria in pregnancy. *J Obstet Gynaecol Br Commonw* 1973;80:385.

188. Cunningham FG, Lucas MJ. Urinary tract infections complicating pregnancy. *Clin Obstet Gynaecol (Baillière)* 1994;8:353.

189. Millar LK, Cox SM. Urinary tract infections complicating pregnancy. *Infect Dis Clin North Am* 1997;11:13.

190. Bint AJ, Hill D. Bacteriuria of pregnancy: an update on significance, diagnosis and management. *J Antimicrob Chemother* 1994;33 [Suppl A]:93.

191. Pedler SJ, Orr KE. Bacterial, fungal, and parasitic infections. In: Barron WM, Lindheimer MD, eds. *Medical disorders during pregnancy,* 3rd ed. St. Louis: Mosby, 2000:411.

192. Schieve LA, et al. Urinary tract infection during pregnancy: its association with maternal morbidity and perinatal outcome. *Am J Public Health* 1994;84:405.

193. McGladdery SL, et al. Outcome of pregnancy in an Oxford-Cardiff cohort of women with previous bacteriuria. *Q J Med* 1992;303:533.

194. Romero R, et al. Meta-analysis of relationship between asymptomatic bacteriuria and preterm delivery/low birth weight babies. *Obstet Gynecol* 1989;72:576.

195. Meis PJ, et al. Factors associated with preterm birth in Cardiff, Wales. II. Indicated and spontaneous preterm birth. *Am J Obstet Gynecol* 1995;173:597.

196. Kaul AK, et al. Experimental gestational pyelonephritis induces preterm births and low birth weights in C3H/HeJ mice. *Infect Immun* 1999;67:5958.

197. Stenquist K, et al. Bacteriuria in pregnancy, frequency and acquisition. *Obstet Gynecol* 1989;72:576.

198. Harris RE. The significance of eradication of bacteriuria during pregnancy. *Obstet Gynecol* 1979;53:71.

199. Rouse DJ, et al. Screening and treatment of asymptomatic bacteriuria of pregnancy to prevent pyelonephritis: a cost-effective and cost-benefit analysis. *Obstet Gynecol* 1995;86:119.

200. Urinary tract infection during pregnancy [Editorial]. *Lancet* 1985;ii:190.

201. Campell-Brown M, et al. Is screening for bacteriuria in pregnancy worthwhile? *Br Med J* 1987;294:1579.

202. Dempsey C, et al. Characteristics of bacteriuria in a homogeneous maternity hospital population. *Eur J Obstet Gynaecol Reprod Biol* 1992;44:189.

203. Marraro RV, Harris RE. Incidence and resolution of spontaneous bacteriuria. *Am J Obstet Gynecol* 1977;128:722.

204. Eng J, Torkdsen EM, Christiansen A. Bacteriuria in the puerperium: an evaluation of methods for collecting urine. *Am J Obstet Gynecol* 1978;131:739.

205. Stray-Peterson B, Blakstad M, Eagan T. Bacteriuria in the puerperium. *Am J Obstet Gynecol* 1990;162:792.

206. Strom BL, et al. Sexual activity, contraceptive use, and other risk factors for symptomatic and asymptomatic bacteriuria. *Ann Intern Med* 1987;107:816.

207. Gilstrap LC, Cunningham FG, Whalley PJ. Acute pyelonephritis in pregnancy: an anterospective study. *Obstet Gynecol* 1981;57:409.

208. Twickler D, et al. Renal pelvicalyceal dilation in antepartum pyelonephritis: ultrasonographic findings. *Am J Obstet Gynecol* 1991;164:1115.

209. Petersson C, et al. Suppressed antibody and interleukin-6 response to acute pyelonephritis in pregnancy. *Kidney Int* 1994;45:571.

210. Twickler DM, et al. Ultrasonic evaluation of central and end-organ hemodynamics in antepartum pyelonephritis. *Am J Obstet Gynecol* 1994;170:814.

211. Graham JM, et al. Uterine contractions after antibiotic therapy for pyelonephritis in pregnancy. *Am J Obstet Gynecol* 1993;168:577.

212. Jakobi P, et al. Single dose antimicrobial therapy in the treatment of asymptomatic bacteriuria in pregnancy. *Am J Obstet Gynecol* 1987;156:1148.

213. Pfau A, Sacks TG. Effective prophylaxis for recurrent urinary tract infections during pregnancy. *Clin Infect Dis* 1992;14:810.

214. Wing DA, et al. A randomized trial of three antibiotic regimens for the treatment of pyelonephritis in pregnancy. *Obstet Gynecol* 1998;92:249.

215. Wing DA, et al. Limited clinical utility of blood and urine cultures in the treatment of acute pyelonephritis during pregnancy. *Am J Obstet Gynecol* 2000;182:1437.

216. Lenke RR, Van Dorsten JP, Schiffrin BS. Pyelonephritis in pregnancy: a prospective randomized trial to prevent recurrent disease evaluating suppressive therapy with nitrofurantoin and close surveillance. *Am J Obstet Gynecol* 1983;146:953.

217. Katz AI, et al. Pregnancy in women with renal disease. *Kidney Int* 1980;18:192.

218. Surian M, et al. Glomerular disease and pregnancy, a study of 123 pregnancies. *Nephron* 1984;36:101.

219. Abe S, et al. The influence of antecedent renal disease on pregnancy. *Am J Obstet Gynecol* 1985;153:508.

220. Jungers P, et al. Chronic kidney disease and pregnancy. *Adv Nephrol* 1986;15:103.

221. Barcelo P, Lopez-Lillo J, Del Rio G. Successful pregnancy in primary glomerular disease. *Kidney Int* 1986;30:914.

222. Packham DK, et al. Primary glomerulonephritis and pregnancy. *Q J Med* 1989;266:537.

223. Abe S. An overview of pregnancy in women with underlying renal disease. *Am J Kidney Dis* 1991;17:112.

224. Jungers P, et al. Specific controversies concerning the natural history of renal disease in pregnancy. *Am J Kidney Dis* 1991;17:116.

225. Imbasciati E, Ponticelli C. Pregnancy and renal disease: predictors of maternal outcome. *Am J Nephrol* 1991;11:353.

226. Jungers P, et al. Influence of pregnancy on the course of primary glomerulonephritis. *Lancet* 1995;346:1122.

227. Jungers P, Chauveau D. Pregnancy and renal disease. *Kidney Int* 1997;52:871.

228. Kincaid-Smith P, Fairley KF. Renal disease in pregnancy. Three controversial areas. Mesangial IgA nephropathy, focal glomerular sclerosis

(focal and segmental hyalinosis and sclerosis), and reflux nephropathy. *Am J Kidney Dis* 1987;9:328.

229. Jungers P, et al. Pregnancy in IgA nephropathy, reflux nephropathy, and focal glomerular sclerosis. *Am J Kidney Dis* 1987;9:334.

230. Packham DK, et al. Pregnancy in women with primary focal and segmental hyalinosis and sclerosis. *Clin Nephrol* 1988;29:185.

231. Packham DK, et al. IgA glomerulonephritis and pregnancy. *Clin Nephrol* 1988;30:15.

232. Packham DK, et al. Histological features of IgA glomerulonephritis as predictors of pregnancy outcome. *Clin Nephrol* 1988;30:22.

233. Abe S. Pregnancy and IgA nephropathy. *Kidney Int* 1991;40:1098.

234. El Khatib M, et al. Pregnancy related complications in women with reflux nephropathy. *Clin Nephrol* 1994;41:50.

235. Abe S. The influence of pregnancy on the long term renal prognosis in women with IgA nephropathy. *Clin Nephrol* 1994;41:61.

236. Jungers P, et al. Pregnancy in women with reflux nephropathy. *Kidney Int* 1996;50:593.

237. Sibai B, et al. Risk factors for preeclampsia, abruptio placenta, and adverse neonatal outcomes among women with chronic hypertension. *N Engl J Med* 1998;339:667.

238. Packham DK, et al. Comparison of pregnancy outcome between normotensive and hypertensive women with primary glomerulonephritis. *Clin Exp Hypertens Series B (Hypertens Pregnancy)* 1988;6:387.

239. Hou SH, Grossman SD, Madias N. Pregnancy in women with renal disease and moderate renal insufficiency. *Am J Med* 1985;78:185.

240. Imbasciati E, et al. Pregnancy in women with chronic renal failure. *Am J Nephrol* 1986;6:193.

241. Cunningham FG, et al. Chronic renal disease and pregnancy outcome. *Am J Obstet Gynecol* 1990;163:453.

242. Jones DC, Hayslett JP. Outcome of pregnancy in women with moderate and severe renal insufficiency. *N Engl J Med* 1996;335:226.

243. Schaefer RM, et al. Improved sexual function in hemodialysis patients on recombinant erythropoietin. A possible role for prolactin. *Clin Nephrol* 1989;31:1.

244. Lim VS. Reproductive endocrinology in uraemia. *Clin Obstet Gynaecol (Baillière)* 1994;8:460.

245. Schmidt RJ, Holley JL. Fertility and contraception in end-stage renal disease. *Adv Renal Replacement Ther* 1998;5:34.

246. Okundaye I, Abrinko P, Hou S. Registry for pregnancy in dialysis. *Am J Kidney Dis* 1998;31:776.

247. Star J, Carpenter MW. The effect of pregnancy on the natural history of diabetic retinopathy and nephropathy. *Clin Perinatol* 1998;25:887.

248. Sims EAH. Serial studies on renal function in pregnancy complicated by diabetes mellitus. *Diabetes* 1961;10:190.

249. Kitzmiller JL, et al. Diabetic nephropathy and perinatal outcome. *Am J Obstet Gynecol* 1961;141:741.

250. Jovanovic R, Jovanovic L. Obstetric management when normoglycemia is maintained in diabetic pregnant women with vascular compromise. *Am J Obstet Gynecol* 1984;149:617.

251. Grenfeld A, et al. Pregnancy in diabetic women who have proteinuria. *Q J Med* 1986;59:379.

252. Reece EA, et al. Diabetic nephropathy: pregnancy performance and feto-maternal outcome. *Am J Obstet Gynecol* 1988;159:56.

253. Mogensen CE, Klebe JG. Microalbuminuria and diabetic pregnancy. In: Mogensen CE, ed. *The kidney and hypertension in diabetes.* Norwell, MA: Kluwer Academic Publishers, 1988:223.

254. Bisenbach G, Zasgornick S. incidence of transient nephrotic syndrome in pregnancy in diabetic women with and without pre-existing nephropathy. *Br Med J* 1989;299:366.

255. Reece EA, et al. Does pregnancy alter the rate of progression of diabetic nephropathy. *Am J Perinatol* 1990;7:193.

256. Kimmerle R, et al. Pregnancies in women with diabetic nephropathy: long-term outcome for mother and child. *Diabetologia* 1995;38:227.

257. Miodovnik M, et al. Does pregnancy increase the risk of development for development and progression of diabetic nephropathy? *Am J Obstet Gynecol* 1996;74;1180.

258. Purdy LP, et al. Effect of pregnancy on renal function in patients with moderate to severe renal insufficiency. *Diabetes Care* 1996;9:1067.

259. Bar J, et al. Pregnancy outcome in patients with insulin dependent diabetes mellitus and diabetic nephropathy treated with ACE inhibitors before pregnancy. *J Pediatr Endocrinol Metab* 1999;12[Suppl 2]:659.

260. Bisenbach G, et al. How pregnancy influences renal function in nephropathic type 1 diabetic women depends on their pre-conceptual creatinine clearance. *J Nephrol* 1999;12:41.

261. Dunne FP, et al. Pregnancy outcome in women with insulin-dependent diabetes mellitus complicated by nephropathy. *Q J Med* 1999;92:451.

262. Combs CA, et al. Early pregnancy proteinuria in diabetes related to preeclampsia. *Obstet Gynecol* 1993;82:802.

263. Sibai BH, et al. Risk factors for preeclampsia and adverse neonatal outcomes in women with pregestational diabetes. *Am J Obstet Gynecol* 2000;182:364.

264. Jovanovic-Peterson L, Peterson CM. De novo clinical hypothyroidism in pregnancies complicated by type 1 diabetes, subclinical hypothyroidism, and proteinuria: a new syndrome. *Am J Obstet Gynecol* 1988;159:442.

265. Davis AE, et al. Transfer of C1 nephritic factor from mother to fetus. *N Engl J Med* 1977;297:144.

266. Morton MR, Bannister KM. Renal failure due to mesangiocapillary glomerulonephritis: use of plasma exchange therapy. *Clin Nephrol* 1993;40:74.

267. Singson E, Fisher KF, Lindheimer MD. Acute glomerulonephritis in pregnancy. *Am J Obstet Gynecol* 1980;137:857.

268. Shepherd J, Shepherd C. Poststreptococcal glomerulonephritis: a rare complication of pregnancy. *J Fam Pract* 1992;34:625.

269. Fervenza F, Green A, Layfyette RA. Acute renal failure due to postinfectious glomerulonephritis during pregnancy. *Am J Kidney Dis* 1997;29:273.

270. Lagrue G, et al. Pregnancy and glomerulonephritis. *Lancet* 1989;ii:1037.

271. Savin BJ, et al. Circulating factor associated with increased glomerular permeability to albumin in recurrent focal segmental glomerulosclerosis. *N Engl J Med* 1996;334:878.

272. Lockshin MD, Sammaritano LR. Rheumatic disease. In: Barron WM, Lindheimer MD, eds. *Medical disorders during pregnancy,* 3rd ed. St. Louis: Mosby, 2000:355.

273. Hayslett JP. the effect of systemic lupus erythematosus on pregnancy and pregnancy outcome. *Am J Reprod Immunol* 1992;28:199.

274. Arnout J, et al The antiphospholipid syndrome and pregnancy. *Hypertens Pregnancy* 1995;14:147.

275. Ogishima D, et al. Placental pathology in systemic lupus erythematosus with antiphospholipid antibodies. *Pathol Int* 2000;50:224.

276. Steen VD. Scleroderma and pregnancy. *Rheum Dis Clin North Am* 1997;23:133.

277. Nelson JL, et al. Michrochimerism and HLA compatible relationships in Ssc. *Lancet* 1998;351:559.

278. Artlett CM, Smth JB, Jiminez SA. Identification of fetal DNA and cells in skin lesions from women with systemic sclerosis. *N Engl J Med* 1998;338:1186.

279. Uribe LG, Vankur DK, Krane NK. Steroid-responsive nephrotic syndrome with renal insufficiency in the first trimester of pregnancy. *Am J Obstet Gynecol* 1991;164:568.

280. Livneh A, et al. Effect of pregnancy on renal function in amyloidosis of familial Mediterranean fever. *J Rheumatol* 1993;20:1519.

281. Yankowitz J, Kuller JA, Thomas RL. Pregnancy complicated by Goodpasture syndrome. *Obstet Gynecol* 1992;79:806.

282. Deubner H, Wagnild JP, Werner MH. Glomerulonephritis with anti-glomerular basement membrane antibody during pregnancy: possible role of the placenta in amelioration of the disease. *Am J Kidney Dis* 1995;25:330.

283. Steblay RW. Localization in human kidney of antibodies formed in sheep against human placenta. *J Immunol* 1962;88:434.

284. Klockars M, et al. Pregnancy in women with renal disease. *Acta Med Scand* 1980;207:207.

285. Bukowski TP, et al. Urinary tract infections and pregnancy in women who underwent antireflux surgery in childhood. *J Urol* 1998;159:1286.

286. Bailley RR. Familial and genetic aspects of primary vesicoureteric reflux. In: Morgan SH, Grünfeld J-P, eds. *Inherited disorders of the kidney.* Oxford: Oxford University Press, 1998:163.

287. Vordermark JS, Deshon GE, Agee RE. Management of pregnancy after major urinary reconstruction. *Obstet Gynecol* 1990;75:564.

288. Pirson Y, Chauveau D, Grünfeld J-P. Autosomal dominant polycystic kidney disease. In: Cameron JS, et al, eds. *Oxford textbook of clinical nephrology,* 2nd ed. Oxford: Oxford University Press, 1998:2393.

289. Grünfeld J-P, Knebelmann B. Alport's syndrome. In: Cameron JS, et al, eds. *Oxford textbook of clinical nephrology,* 2nd ed. Oxford: Oxford University Press, 1998:2427.

290. Reiss RE, et al. Successful pregnancy despite placental cystine crystals in a woman with nephropathic cystinosis. *N Engl J Med* 1988;319:233.

291. Knebelman B, et al. A molecular approach to inherited kidney disorders. *Kidney Int* 1993;44:1205.

292. Milutinovic J, et al. Fertility and pregnancy complications in women with autosomal dominant polycystic disease. *Obstet Gynecol* 1983;61:566.

293. Chapman AB, Johnson AM, Gabow PA. Pregnancy outcome and its relationship to progression of renal failure in autosomal dominant polycystic kidney disease. *J Am Soc Nephrol* 1994;5:1178.

294. Gabow PA, et al. Factors affecting progression of renal disease in autosomal polycystic renal disease. *Kidney Int* 1992;41:1311.

295. Wiebers DO, Torres VE. Screening for unrruptured intracranial aneurysms in autosomal dominant polycystic kidney disease. *N Engl J Med* 1992;327:953.

296. Harris JP, et al. Alport's syndrome presenting as crescentic glomerulonephritis: a report of two siblings. *Clin Nephrol* 1978;10:245.

297. Millner DS, Torres VE. Renal manifestations of neurofibromatosis and tuberous sclerosis. In: Morgan SH, Grünfeld J-P, eds. *Inherited disorders of the kidney.* Oxford: Oxford University Press, 1998:505.

298. Neumann HPH, et al. *Inherited disorders of the kidney.* Oxford: Oxford University Press, 1998:535.

299. Grünfeld J-P, Choukroun G, Knebelmann B. Genetic diagnosis and counseling in inherited renal diseases. In: Suki WN, Massry G, eds. *Therapy of renal diseases and related disorders,* 2nd ed. Boston, MA: Kluwer Academic Publishers, 1997:685.

300. Maikrantz P, Lindheimer MD, Coe FL. Nephrolithiasis and gestation. *Clin Obstet Gynaecol (Baillière)* 1994;8:375.

301. Coe FL, Parks JH, Lindheimer MD. Nephrolithiasis during pregnancy. *N Engl J Med* 1978;298:324.

302. Levine RJ, et al. Trial of calcium to prevent preeclampsia *N Engl J Med* 1997;337:69.

303. Maikrantz P, et al. Gestational hypercalciuria causes pathological urine calcium oxalate supersaturation. *Kidney Int* 1989;36:108.

304. Davison JM, et al. Increases in urinary inhibitor activity and the excretion of an inhibitor of crystalluria in pregnancy: a defense against the hypercalciuria of normal gestation. *Hypertens Pregnancy* 1993;12:25.

305. Stothers L, Lee LM. Renal colic in pregnancy. *J Urol* 1992;148:1383.

306. Gregory MC, Mansell MA. Pregnancy and cystinuria. *Lancet* 1983;ii:1958.

307. Alexopoulos E, et al. Acute uric acid nephropathy in pregnancy. *Obstet Gynecol* 1992;80:488.

308. Brent RL. The effect of embryonic and fetal exposure to X-rays and isotopes. In: Barron WM, Lindheimer MD, eds. *Medical disorders during pregnancy,* 3rd ed. St. Louis: Mosby, 2000:586.

309. Rodriguez PN, Klein AS. Management of urolithiasis during pregnancy. *Surg Gynecol Obstet* 1988;166:103.

310. van Sonnenberg E, et al. Symptomatic renal obstruction or urosepsis during pregnancy: treatment by sonographically guided percutaneous nephrostomy. *AJR: Am J Roentgenol* 1992;158:91.

311. Shokier AA, Mutagabani H. Rigid uteroscopy in pregnant women. *Br J Urol* 1998;81:678.

312. Loughlin KR, Bailey RB. Internal ureteral stents for conservative management of ureteral calculi during pregnancy. *N Engl J Med* 1986;315:1647.

313. Report of the National High Blood Pressure Education Program Working Group on high blood pressure during pregnancy. *Am J Obstet Gynecol* 2000;183:S1.

314. Hou SH. Pregnancy in end stage renal disease. *Adv Renal Replacement Ther* 1998;5:1.

315. Brookhyser J, Wiggens K. Medical nutrition therapy in pregnancy and kidney disease. *Adv Renal Replacement Ther* 1998;5:53.

316. Chan WS, Okun N, Kjellstrand CM. Pregnancy in chronic dialysis: a review and analysis of the literature. *Int J Artif Organs* 1998;21:259.

317. Maruyama H, et al. Requiring higher doses of erythropoietin suggests pregnancy in hemodialysis patients. *Nephron* 1998;79:413.

318. Toma H, et al. Pregnancy in women receiving renal dialysis or transplantation in Japan: a nationwide survey. *Nephrol Dial Transplant* 1999;14:1511.

319. Romao JE Jr, et al. Pregnancy in women on chronic dialysis. A single-center experience with 17 cases. *Nephron* 1998;78:416.

320. Nakabayashi M, et al. Perinatal and infant outcome of pregnant patients undergoing chronic hemodialysis. *Nephron* 1999;82:27.

321. Whitaker RH, Hamilton D. Effects of transplantation on non-renal effects of renal failure [Editorial]. *Br Med J* 1982;248:221.

322. Murray JE, et al. Successful pregnancies after transplantation. *N Engl J Med* 1963;269:3471.

323. Davison JM. Pregnancy in renal allograft recipients: problems, prognosis, and practicalities. *Clin Obstet Gynaecol (Baillière)* 1994;8:501.

324. Crowe AV, et al. Pregnancy does not adversely affect renal transplant function. *Q J Med* 1999;92:631.

325. Armenti VT, Moritz MJ, Davison JM. Medical management of the pregnant transplant recipient. *Adv Renal Replacement Ther* 1998;5:14.

326. Blowey DL, Warady BA. Neonatal outcome in pregnancies associated with renal replacement therapy. *Adv Renal Replacement Ther* 1998;5:45.

327. Ogborn PL, et al. Pregnancy following transplantation in class T diabetes mellitus. *JAMA* 1986;255:1911.

328. Tydén G, et al. Pregnancy after combined pancreas-kidney transplantation. *Diabetes* 1989;38[Suppl 1]:43.

329. Armenti VT, et al. The National Transplantation Pregnancy Registry: comparison between pregnancy outcomes in diabetic cyclosporine-treated female kidney recipients and Cy A-treated female pancreas-kidney recipients. *Transplantation Proc* 1997;29:669.

330. Barrou BM, et al. Pregnancy after pancreas transplantation in the cyclosporine era: report from the International Pancreas Transplant Registry. *Transplantation* 1997;65:524.

331. DiPaolo S, et al. Immunologic evaluation during the first year of life in infants born to cyclosporine-treated female transplant recipients: analysis of lymphocyte subpopulations and immunoglobulin serum levels. *Transplantation* 2000;69:2049.

332. Ghandour FZ, Knauss TC, Hricik DE. Immunosuppressive drugs in pregnancy. *Adv Renal Replacement Ther* 1998;5:31.

333. Armenti VT, et al. Pregnancy and transplantation [Review]. *Graft* 2000;3:59.

334. Davison JM, Redman CWG. Pregnancy post-transplant: the establishment of a UK registry. *Br J Obstet Gynaecol* 1997;104:1106.

335. Salmela KT, et al. Impaired renal function after pregnancy in renal transplant recipients. *Transplantation* 1993;56:1372.

336. Lindheimer MD, Katz AI. Pregnancy in women receiving renal replacement therapy [Editorial]. *Kidney* 1994;3:135.

337. Rizzoni G, et al. Successful pregnancies in women on renal replacement therapy. Report of the EDTA registry. *Nephrol Dial Transplant* 1992;7:279.

338. Sturgiss SN, Davison JM. Effect of pregnancy on long-term function of renal allografts. *Am J Kidney Dis* 1992;19:167.

339. Sturgiss SN, Davison JM. Effect of pregnancy on long-term function of renal allografts: an update. *Am J Kidney Dis* 1995;26:54.

340. Sturgiss SN, Davison JM. Perinatal outcome in allograft recipients: significance of hypertension and renal function before and during pregnancy. *Obstet Gynecol* 1991;78:573.

341. Registration Committee of the European Dialysis and Transplant Association. Successful pregnancies in women treated by dialysis and kidney transplantation. *Br J Obstet Gynaecol* 1980;87:839.

342. MaGee LA, et al. Erythropoiesis and renal transplant pregnancy. *Transplantation* 2000;14:127.

343. Lindheimer MD, Roberts JM, Cunningham FG, eds. *Chesley's hypertensive disorders in pregnancy,* 2nd ed. Stamford, CT: Appleton & Lang, 1999.

Space limitations dictate restriction of the reference list; we have therefore focused on citations during the past 25 years. More extensive literature surveys exceeding 2,000 citations can be found in texts and chapters by Chesley (23), Lindheimer and Katz (2,17), Lindheimer et al. (343), and Sheehan and Lynch (4).

CHAPTER 75

Liver Disease and the Kidney

Pere Ginès, Andrés Cárdenas, and Robert W. Schrier

The presence of abnormalities of kidney function in patients with liver diseases has been recognized for many years (1). More than a century ago, Frerichs in Europe and Flint in the United States reported the association between liver diseases and kidney dysfunction (2,3). These reports described the development of oliguria in patients with chronic liver disease in the setting of normal kidney histology and proposed the first pathophysiologic interpretation of kidney dysfunction in liver disease by linking the abnormalities in kidney function to the disturbances present in the systemic circulation. Since then, the relationship between the liver and kidney function has been the object of a considerable amount of research and substantial progress has been made in the last two decades with regard to the pathophysiology and management of kidney function abnormalities in liver diseases (Table 75-1).

Most abnormalities of kidney function in liver diseases occur in patients with cirrhosis and are pathophysiologically related to the presence of an expanded extracellular fluid volume which leads to the development of ascites and/or edema. Therefore, this chapter deals with the pathophysiology, clinical features, and treatment of ascites and renal function abnormalities in cirrhosis. The abnormalities in kidney function that may occur in other types of liver diseases are not discussed.

RENAL ABNORMALITIES IN CIRRHOSIS

Functional Renal Abnormalities

Most abnormalities of kidney function in cirrhosis are of functional origin (i.e., they occur in the absence of significant alterations in kidney histology) (4–8). These abnormalities are usually referred to as functional renal abnormalities, as opposed to nonfunctional or organic renal abnormalities, which may also develop in patients with cirrhosis (and are discussed later in this chapter).

P. Ginès and Andrés Cárdenas: Liver Unit, Institute for Digestive Diseases Hospital Clinic, University of Barcelona School of Medicine, Barcelona, Catalunya, Spain

R. W. Schrier: Department of Medicine, University of Colorado Health Sciences Center, Denver, Colorado

The most common functional renal abnormalities in cirrhotic patients are an impaired ability to excrete sodium and water and a reduction of renal blood flow (RBF) and glomerular filtration rate (GFR), the latter two being secondary to vasoconstriction of the renal circulation. Sodium retention is a key factor in the expansion of the extracellular fluid volume and ascites and edema formation, whereas water retention is responsible for the development of dilutional hyponatremia. Renal vasoconstriction, when severe, leads to hepatorenal syndrome (HRS). Chronologically, sodium retention is the earliest alteration of kidney function observed in patients with cirrhosis, whereas water retention leading to dilutional hyponatremia and HRS are late findings. In most patients, these abnormalities of kidney function usually worsen with time as the liver disease progresses. However, in some patients a spontaneous improvement or even normalization of sodium and, less often, in water excretion may occur during the course of their disease (9–11). This improvement in renal function may be seen after alcohol abstinence in patients with alcoholic cirrhosis but it may occur spontaneously in patients with nonalcoholic cirrhosis as well. The frequency and mechanism(s) of this improved renal function are not known. Improvement of renal function after the development of HRS is extremely unusual (12,13).

Sodium Retention and Ascites

Sodium retention is the most frequent abnormality of kidney function in patients with cirrhosis and ascites. The existence of sodium retention in cirrhosis was first documented more than 40 years ago when methods to measure electrolyte concentration in organic fluids became available (14–16). Since then, it has been well established that sodium retention plays a key role in the pathophysiology of ascites and edema formation in cirrhosis. The amount of sodium retained within the body is dependent on the balance between the sodium ingested in the diet and the sodium excreted in the urine. As long as the amount of sodium excreted is lower than that ingested, patients accumulate ascites and/or edema. The important role of sodium retention in the pathogenesis of ascites formation

TABLE 75-1. *Landmarks in ascites and renal dysfunction in liver disease*

1800s	First description of renal dysfunction in liver diseases
1940s	Demonstration of water retention in cirrhosis with ascites
1950s	Demonstration of sodium retention in cirrhosis with ascites and its relationship with increased mineralocorticoid activity
	Description of the hyperkinetic circulatory syndrome
	Clinical description of hepatorenal syndrome
1960s–1970s	Demonstration of renal vasoconstriction as the cause of hepatorenal syndrome
	Introduction of aldosterone antagonists in clinical practice
	Demonstration of increased activity of vasoconstrictor systems
	Demonstration of the role of prostaglandins in the maintenance of renal function
	Proposal of the overflow theory of ascites formation
1980s	Reintroduction of therapeutic paracentesis in clinical practice
	Proposal of the arterial vasodilation theory of ascites formation
1990s	Definition and diagnostic criteria of hepatorenal syndrome
	Description of functional renal failure after bacterial infections (i.e., ascites fluid infection) and its prevention by plasma volume expansion with albumin
	Use of splanchnic vasoconstrictors in hepatorenal syndrome

is supported by the fact that ascites can disappear just by reducing the dietary sodium content in some patients or by increasing the urinary sodium excretion with the administration of diuretics in others (16,17). Conversely, a high-sodium diet or diuretic withdrawal leads to the reaccumulation of ascites (15,16). The achievement of a negative sodium balance (i.e., excretion higher than intake) is the essence of pharmacologic therapy of ascites. Finally, studies in experimental animals have constantly shown that sodium retention precedes ascites formation, further emphasizing the important role of this abnormality of renal function in the pathogenesis of ascites in cirrhosis (18–22).

The severity of sodium retention in cirrhosis with ascites varies considerably from patient to patient. Some patients have relatively high urinary sodium excretion, whereas urine sodium concentrations are very low or even undetectable in others (Fig. 75-1). The proportion of patients with marked sodium retention depends on the population of cirrhotic patients considered. Most patients who require hospitalization because of severe ascites have marked sodium retention, as they excrete less than 10 mEq/day. Among patients who require hospitalization, sodium retention is particularly intense in patients with ascites refractory to diuretic treatment (23,24). By contrast, in a population of cirrhotic patients with mild or moderate ascites, the proportion of patients with marked sodium retention is low and most patients excrete more than 10 mEq/day spontaneously (without diuretic therapy). The response to diuretics is usually better in patients with moderate sodium retention than in those with marked sodium retention (17,25,26).

Nephron Sites of Sodium Retention

In most instances, sodium retention in cirrhosis is due to increased tubular reabsorption of sodium because it occurs

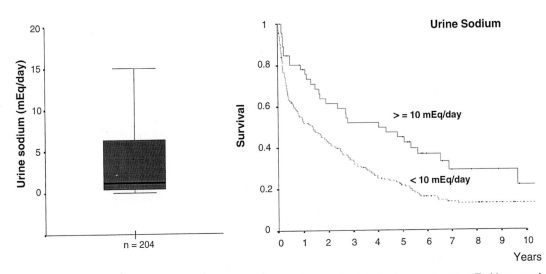

FIG. 75-1. Box plot of urinary sodium excretion (in conditions of a low-sodium diet—50 mEq/day—and without diuretics) **(left panel)** and long-term survival according to sodium excretion **(right panel)** in a series of 204 patients with cirrhosis admitted to the hospital for the treatment of ascites.

in the presence of normal or only moderately reduced GFR (17,27). The exact contribution of the different segments of the nephron to this increased sodium reabsorption is not completely known. Micropuncture studies in rats with cirrhosis and ascites have demonstrated an enhanced reabsorption of sodium in the proximal tubule (18,28). On the other hand, it has been shown that the development of a positive sodium balance and the formation of ascites in cirrhotic rats can be prevented by aldosterone antagonists, which suggests that the collecting ducts are important sites of the increased sodium reabsorption in experimental cirrhosis (21,29). Investigations in patients with cirrhosis have also provided discrepant findings. Results from earlier studies using sodium, water, or phosphate clearances to estimate the tubular handling of sodium suggest that the distal nephron is the main site of sodium retention (30–33). Studies using lithium clearance, which estimates sodium reabsorption in the proximal tubule, suggest that cirrhotic patients with ascites show a marked increase in proximal sodium reabsorption (34,35). Nevertheless, distal sodium reabsorption is also increased, especially in patients with more avid sodium retention (35). Clinical studies using spironolactone, to antagonize the mineralocorticoid receptor, indicate that this agent induces natriuresis in a large proportion of cirrhotic patients with ascites without renal failure, which supports a major role for an increased sodium reabsorption in distal sites of the nephron in these patients (26,36–39). Taken together, these results suggest that in patients with cirrhosis without renal failure, an enhanced reabsorption of sodium in both proximal and distal tubules contributes to sodium retention. Potential mediators of this increased sodium reabsorption include changes in the hydrostatic and colloidosmotic pressures in the peritubular capillaries and increased activity of the sympathetic nervous system and the renin–angiotensin–aldosterone system. Sodium retention is usually more marked in patients with renal failure than in those without renal failure due to both a reduction in filtered sodium load and a more marked activation of sodium-retaining systems.

Clinical Consequences

Because sodium is retained together with water isoosmotically in the kidney, sodium retention is associated with fluid retention, leading to expansion of extracellular fluid volume and increased amount of fluid in the interstitial tissue. In some patients with cirrhosis, the total extracellular fluid volume may increase up to 40 L or even more (compared to the average 14 L in a 70-kg healthy adult), which represents an approximate cumulative gain of 3,400 mEq of sodium (26 L of excess extracellular fluid volume times 130 mEq/L). In most patients with advanced cirrhosis, sodium retention is manifested by the development of ascites. The most common clinical symptom of ascites is discomfort due to abdominal swelling. In cases with marked accumulation of fluid, physical activity and respiratory function may be impaired. Other clinical consequences related to the presence of ascites are

the appearance of abdominal wall hernias and the spontaneous infection of ascitic fluid (also known as spontaneous bacterial peritonitis) (40). Both complications, especially infection, contribute markedly to the increased morbidity and mortality associated with the presence of ascites.

Accumulation of fluid in the subcutaneous tissue, as edema, is also common in patients with cirrhosis and sodium retention and in most cases occurs concomitantly with the existence of ascites. Edema is most commonly observed in the lower extremities, but generalized edema may occur as well. Mild or moderate edema may decrease or even disappear during bed rest and reappear during the daytime, reflecting an increased natriuresis in the supine position as compared with the upright position (41,42). Both hypoalbuminemia and increased venous pressure in the inferior vena cava due either to constriction of the vena cava within the liver or increased intraabdominal pressure caused by ascites may contribute to the high incidence of edema in cirrhotic patients with ascites. Leg edema is common in patients with cirrhosis treated with either surgical portacaval shunts or transjugular intrahepatic portosystemic shunts (TIPS), presumably because of the increased pressure in the inferior vena cava secondary to these procedures.

Other clinical manifestations of sodium retention in cirrhosis include pleural and/or pericardial effusions. Clinically significant pleural effusions occur in up to 10% of patients with cirrhosis (43,44). In most cases the effusion is mild or moderate, more frequent on the right side, and associated with the presence of ascites. Left-sided effusions are uncommon and usually occur in patients who have right-sided effusions as well. Occasionally, large right pleural effusions may exist in the absence of ascites and constitute the main manifestation of the disease (44,45). These cases usually recur after therapy and are due to the existence of anatomical defects in the diaphragm which cause a communication between the peritoneal and pleural cavities. The gradient between the positive intraabdominal pressure and the negative intrathoracic pressure explains the passage of all fluid formed in the peritoneal cavity to the pleural cavity. Although less commonly than ascitic fluid, pleural fluid may also become infected spontaneously, a condition known as spontaneous bacterial empyema (46). Finally, between one- and two-thirds of cirrhotic patients with ascites also have mild or moderate pericardial effusions as demonstrated by echocardiography (47). These disappear after the elimination of ascites and are not associated with clinical symptoms.

Assessment of Sodium Excretion in Clinical Practice

The assessment of the urinary excretion of sodium is very useful in the clinical management of patients with cirrhosis and ascites because it allows the precise quantification of sodium retention. Urine must be collected under conditions of fixed and controlled sodium intake (usually a low-sodium diet of 50 mEq/day during the previous 5 to 7 days), as sodium intake may influence sodium excretion. The amount of sodium ingested does not affect the excretion of sodium in patients with marked sodium retention who have very low urine sodium regardless of the amount of sodium taken with the diet, but may affect sodium excretion in patients with mild or moderate sodium retention. Diuretics should not be given during the 5- to 7-day period prior to urine collection to avoid a pharmacologic increase in sodium excretion. This period of time is particularly important in patients receiving spironolactone or other aldosterone antagonists that have a very prolonged half-life. Finally, although the measurement of sodium concentration in a spot of urine may provide a rough estimate of sodium excretion, the assessment of sodium excretion in a 24-hour period is preferable because it is more representative of sodium excretion throughout the day and takes into account the urine output.

In clinical practice, sodium excretion should be measured under the conditions stated above when patients with ascites are first seen or when there are signs suggestive of disease progression (e.g., marked increase in ascites or edema despite compliance with the sodium-restricted diet and diuretic therapy). On the other hand, the measurement of sodium excretion in patients under diuretic therapy is very useful to monitor the response to treatment.

Baseline sodium excretion is one of the best predictors of the response to diuretic treatment. Therefore, the measurement of urine sodium concentration and excretion is very helpful to establish the therapeutic schedule in cirrhotic patients with ascites. Patients with marked sodium retention in whom a positive sodium balance is anticipated despite a restriction in sodium intake should be started on moderately high doses of aldosterone antagonists (e.g., spironolactone 200 mg per day) alone or in association with loop diuretics (e.g., furosemide 40 mg per day). Conversely, patients with moderate sodium retention would likely respond to low doses of aldosterone antagonists (i.e., spironolactone 50 to 100 mg per day). Finally, the intensity of sodium retention also provides prognostic information in patients with ascites. Patients with baseline urine sodium lower than 10 mEq/day have a median survival time of only 1.5 years compared with 4.5 years in patients with urine sodium higher than 10 mEq/day (Fig. 75-1) (48–50).

Abnormalities of Renal Sodium Handling in Preascitic Cirrhosis

Patients with cirrhosis in the preascitic stage (without past or current history of ascites or edema) do not exhibit overt sodium retention but may have subtle abnormalities in renal sodium handling (Table 75-2) (41,51–66). The finding of increased blood volume in these patients strongly supports the existence of sodium retention sufficient enough to expand the intravascular volume but without causing ascites or edema (54–56). Preascitic cirrhotic patients come into sodium balance as long as their sodium intake is maintained within normal limits. However, some patients may be unable to handle a sodium load and develop ascites and/or edema in conditions of high-sodium intake (especially when they receive

TABLE 75-2. *Renal and circulatory abnormalities in patients with preascitic cirrhosis*

1. Increased cardiac output and blood volume
2. Portal hypertension and splanchnic arterial vasodilation
3. Inability to excrete an acute or chronic sodium load
4. Lack of escape from the sodium-retaining effect of mineralocorticoids
5. Reduced sodium excretion in upright posture and increased sodium excretion in recumbency
6. Increased atrial natriuretic peptide levels
7. Development of sodium retention and ascites and edema after treatment with vasodilators or nonsteroidal antiinflammatory drugs

intravenous saline solutions) or when treated with nonsteroidal antiinflammatory drugs or vasodilators (53,57,58, 67–70). This abnormal renal sodium handling of some preascitic patients is also evidenced by the lack of escape from the sodium-retaining effect of mineralocorticoids (51,52). Finally, it has been shown that patients in the preascitic stage under a normal sodium diet retain sodium while they are in upright posture, whereas they show an exaggerated natriuresis, as compared with healthy subjects, during bed rest (41,59). It has been suggested that this increased natriuresis during recumbency is responsible for the maintenance of sodium balance and may help prevent the formation of ascites or edema that would occur as a consequence of sodium retention that takes place during standing.

These subtle abnormalities in renal sodium handling present in compensated preascitic cirrhotic patients that are responsible for the increased blood volume are probably a homeostatic mechanism to compensate for the increased vascular capacitance of the splanchnic vascular bed in cirrhosis due to arterial vasodilation. This interpretation is supported by the observation that a pharmacologically induced vasodilation is followed by sodium retention and increased plasma volume and ascites and edema formation in most preascitic cirrhotic patients (68–71). It is also supported by the findings that patients who develop ascites or edema while on a high-sodium diet, or who fail to escape from the sodium-retaining effect of mineralocorticoids, are those with more marked abnormalities in systemic hemodynamics as indicated by higher cardiac output and lower total systemic vascular resistance (52). An alternative interpretation suggests that abnormal sodium handling in preascitic cirrhotic patients is related to the degree of liver dysfunction (58,61).

Water Retention and Dilutional Hyponatremia

Since the pioneer studies by Papper and Saxon and Shear and colleagues (72,73), it is well known that a derangement in the renal capacity to regulate water balance occurs commonly in advanced cirrhosis. Cirrhotic patients without ascites usually have normal or only slightly impaired renal water handling as compared with healthy subjects. Therefore, in these patients total body water, plasma osmolality, and serum sodium concentration are normal and hyponatremia does not develop, even in conditions of excessive water intake. By contrast,

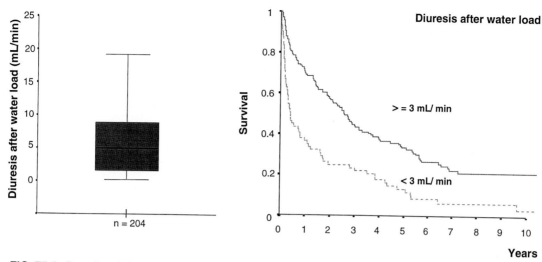

FIG. 75-2. Box plot of diuresis after a water load (20 mL/kg body weight of 5% dextrose IV) in conditions of a low-sodium diet—50 mEq/day—and without diuretics (**left panel**) and long-term survival according to diuresis after water load (**right panel**) in a series of 204 patients with cirrhosis admitted to the hospital for the treatment of ascites.

an impairment in the renal capacity to excrete solute-free water is very common in patients with ascites (72–76). In patients with ascites there is a direct correlation between urinary sodium excretion and water excretion as estimated by urine flow after a water load (73,76). However, no correlation exists between these two parameters when only patients with marked sodium retention are considered. Therefore, sodium retention is necessary but not sufficient for the development of water retention in cirrhotic patients.

As with sodium retention, the impairment of water excretion is not uniform in all patients with ascites; rather, it varies markedly from patient to patient (Fig. 75-2). In some patients, water retention is moderate and can only be detected by measuring solute-free water excretion after a water load. These patients are able to eliminate water normally and maintain a normal serum sodium concentration as long as their water intake is kept within normal limits, but they may develop hyponatremia when water intake is increased. In other patients, the severity of the disorder is such that they retain most of their water intake causing hyponatremia and hypoosmolality. Therefore, hyponatremia in cirrhosis with ascites is almost always dilutional in origin since it occurs in the setting of an increased total body water. Hyponatremia is also paradoxical in that it is associated with sodium retention and a marked increase in total body exchangeable sodium. The development of spontaneous dilutional hyponatremia requires a profound impairment in solute-free water excretion, since it usually occurs with a solute-free water clearance after a water load below 1 mL/minute (74). One-third of hospitalized cirrhotic patients with ascites have spontaneous dilutional hyponatremia (74). The existence of an impaired capacity to excrete solute-free water and/or dilutional hyponatremia is associated with a short survival in patients with cirrhosis and ascites (Fig. 75-2) (50,74,77–80).

Several factors may aggravate the impairment in water excretion in cirrhotic patients with ascites and/or precipitate the appearance of hyponatremia. These include the administration of hypotonic fluids in excess of the capacity to excrete solute-free water, treatment with diuretics or nonsteroidal antiinflammatory drugs (NSAIDs), large-volume paracentesis without plasma volume expansion, or administration of vasopressin analogs in patients with gastrointestinal bleeding (76,81–83).

Mechanisms of Impaired Renal Water Handling

The pathogenesis of water retention in cirrhosis is complex and probably involves several factors, including a reduced delivery of filtrate to the ascending limb of the loop of Henle, reduced renal synthesis of prostaglandins and nonosmotic hypersecretion of arginine vasopressin (AVP) (84–86). Although definitive data about the relative importance of these factors in the pathogenesis of water retention in patients with cirrhosis is lacking, it is likely that AVP hypersecretion plays a major role in water retention in patients without renal failure. This contention is supported by recent studies in animal cirrhosis as well as human cirrhosis showing that the administration of drugs that either reduce the secretion of AVP (κ-opioid agonists) or antagonize the tubular effects of AVP (V2 receptor antagonists) improve solute-free water excretion and increase serum sodium concentration (87–94). In patients with renal failure it is likely that besides AVP, a reduced distal delivery of filtrate due to decreased filtered load and increased proximal sodium and water reabsorption plays an important role in water retention.

Clinical Consequences

The clinical consequence of an impairment in solute-free water excretion is the development of dilutional hyponatremia. Dilutional hyponatremia is associated with sodium retention and increased total body sodium and should be distinguished from hyponatremia that, although less common, may develop in cirrhotic patients who are maintained on high doses of diuretics and sodium restriction after complete disappearance of ascites and edema. In some patients, dilutional hyponatremia is asymptomatic, but in others it is probably associated with clinical symptoms similar to those found in dilutional hyponatremia of other etiologies, including anorexia, headache, difficulty in mental concentration, sluggish thinking, lethargy, nausea, vomiting, and, occasionally, seizures. However, in many instances, it may be difficult to establish whether these symptoms are due to hyponatremia itself, the underlying liver disease, and/or associated conditions. Although hyponatremia and the subsequent hypoosmolality may increase the content of water in the brain cells and lead to cerebral edema and increased intracranial pressure, this situation is unlikely in cirrhotic patients because hyponatremia usually develops gradually, over days or weeks, and there is a progressive reduction in the number of osmotically active solutes in brain cells. This prevents the movement of excessive water into the brain cells and the subsequent development of brain edema. Nevertheless, no studies have been published investigating the existence of brain edema and its relationship with serum sodium concentration in hyponatremic cirrhotic patients as compared with other hyponatremic states.

Assessment of Water Excretion in Clinical Practice

As stated previously, the complete assessment of the renal capacity to excrete solute-free water in cirrhotic patients with ascites should include not only the determination of serum sodium concentration but also the evaluation of the acute response to the administration of water. The capacity to excrete solute-free water is a major prognostic factor of cirrhosis with ascites (77,80) and should be measured when a thorough evaluation of the disease is required, especially in patients who are considered for liver transplantation (discussed in more detail later). Moreover, the assessment of solute-free water excretion is of importance in the clinical management of patients, as it allows for the adjustment of fluid intake to the renal capacity to eliminate water, thus preventing the development of hyponatremia due to inappropriately high fluid intake.

Renal Vasoconstriction and Hepatorenal Syndrome

Investigations performed by Sherlock, Schroeder, and Epstein during the late 1960s and early 1970s provided conclusive evidence indicating that the renal failure of functional origin—the so-called hepatorenal syndrome (HRS)—was due to a marked vasoconstriction of the renal circulation (95–97). Later studies showed that, besides the striking renal vasoconstriction present in patients with HRS, mild or moderate degrees of vasoconstriction in the renal circulation are very common in patients with cirrhosis and ascites (98–101). When renal perfusion is estimated by sensitive clearance techniques, such as paraaminohippurate or inulin clearances, in a population of hospitalized patients with ascites, normal values are found in only one-fifth of cases. In another 15% to 20%, renal hypoperfusion is very intense and meets the criteria of HRS. In the remaining patients, mild or moderate reductions in renal perfusion exist (Fig. 75-3). These latter patients show slightly increased serum creatinine and/or blood urea nitrogen (BUN) levels in baseline conditions (in the absence of diuretic therapy). This moderate renal vasoconstriction is clinically relevant for several reasons: first, it is often associated with marked sodium and water retention

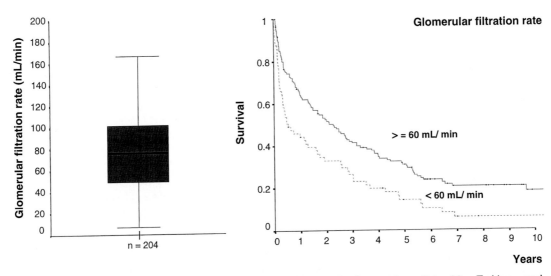

FIG. 75-3. Box plot of glomerular filtration rate (in conditions of a low-sodium diet—50 mEq/day—and without diuretics) (**left panel**) and long-term survival according to glomerular filtration rate (**right panel**) in a series of 204 patients with cirrhosis admitted to the hospital for the treatment of ascites.

and the presence of refractory ascites (102); second, it predisposes to the development of HRS (13,103); and third, it is associated with an impaired survival (50,80).

Definition of Hepatorenal Syndrome

The definition of HRS proposed by the International Ascites Club, which is the most widely accepted, is as follows: "Hepatorenal syndrome is a clinical condition that occurs in patients with advanced chronic liver disease, liver failure, and portal hypertension characterized by impaired renal function and marked abnormalities in the arterial circulation and activity of the endogenous vasoactive systems. In the kidney there is marked renal vasoconstriction that results in low GFR, whereas in the extrarenal circulation there is predominance of arterial vasodilation, which results in reduction of total systemic vascular resistance and arterial hypotension." (103) Although HRS occurs predominantly in advanced cirrhosis, it may also develop in other chronic liver diseases associated with severe liver failure and portal hypertension, such as alcoholic hepatitis, or in acute liver failure (104).

Pathogenic Mechanisms

The pathophysiologic hallmark of HRS is a vasoconstriction of the renal circulation (96,102,105,106). Studies of renal perfusion with renal arteriography, $_{133}$ Xe washout technique, paraaminohippuric acid excretion or, more recently, duplex Doppler ultrasonography, have demonstrated the existence of marked vasoconstriction in the kidneys of patients with HRS, with a characteristic reduction in renal cortical perfusion (96,106–112). The functional nature of HRS has been conclusively demonstrated by the lack of significant morphologic abnormalities in the kidney histology (5–8,113) and by the normalization of renal function after liver transplantation (114–118).

The mechanism of this vasoconstriction is incompletely understood and possibly multifactorial involving changes in systemic hemodynamics, increased pressure in the portal venous system, activation of vasoconstrictor factors, and suppression of vasodilator factors acting on the renal circulation (discussed later). Recent studies have shown that, contrary to the previous belief, other vascular beds besides the renal circulation are also vasoconstricted in patients with HRS, including the extremities and the cerebral circulation (119–121). This indicates the existence of a generalized arterial vasoconstriction in nonsplanchnic vascular beds of patients with HRS and suggests that the main vascular bed responsible for arterial vasodilation and reduced total peripheral vascular resistance in cirrhosis with HRS is the splanchnic circulation.

Clinical and Laboratory Findings

Hepatorenal syndrome is a common complication of patients with cirrhosis. In patients with ascites, the probability of

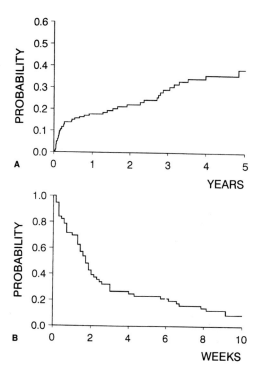

FIG. 75-4. A: Probability of developing hepatorenal syndrome in a series of 234 nonazotemic cirrhotic patients with ascites. **B:** Probability of survival after the development of hepatorenal syndrome in 56 cirrhotic patients with ascites. (From Ginès A, Escorsell A, Ginès P, et al. Incidence, predictive factors, and prognosis of the hepatorenal syndrome in cirrhosis with ascites. *Gastroenterology* 1993;105:229, with permission.) Reproduced with permission from (13).

developing HRS during the course of the disease is 18% at 1 year and increases up to 40% after 5 years of follow-up (13) (Fig. 75-4). The clinical manifestations include a combination of signs and symptoms related to renal, circulatory, and liver failure.

Renal failure may have a rapid or insidious onset and is usually associated with marked sodium and water retention which results in ascites and edema and dilutional hyponatremia, respectively (102,105). HRS may occur in two different clinical patterns, according to the intensity and form of onset of renal failure (Table 75-3) (102). Type 1 HRS is the classic type of HRS and represents the end of the spectrum of changes in renal perfusion in cirrhosis. The dominant clinical features of type 1 HRS are those of severe renal failure with oliguria or anuria and increased serum levels

TABLE 75-3. *Clinical types of hepatorenal syndrome*

Type 1	Rapid and progressive impairment of renal function as defined by a doubling of the initial serum creatinine to a level higher than 2.5 mg/dL or a 50% reduction of the initial 24-h creatinine clearance to a level lower than 20 mL/min in less than 2 weeks.
Type 2	Impairment in renal function (serum creatinine >1.5 mg/dL) that does not meet the criteria of type 1.

of urea and creatinine. Despite an important reduction of GFR in these patients, serum creatinine levels are commonly lower than values observed in patients with acute renal failure of similar intensity with respect to the reduction in GFR, but without liver disease (105,112,122,123). This is probably due to the lower endogenous production of creatinine secondary to reduced muscle mass in patients with cirrhosis compared with patients without liver disease. This type of HRS is often seen in patients with alcoholic cirrhosis, especially when associated with alcoholic hepatitis, but it occurs in nonalcoholic cirrhosis as well. Type 1 HRS is associated with a very low survival expectancy, the median survival time being only 2 weeks (Fig. 75-4) (13). Type 2 HRS is characterized by less severe and stable reduction of GFR that does not meet the criteria proposed for type 1. Patients are usually in a better clinical condition than those with type 1 HRS and their survival expectancy is longer. The dominant clinical feature of these patients is diuretic-resistant ascites due to the combination of intense sodium retention, reduced GFR, and marked stimulation of antinatriuretic systems (102). Severe spontaneous hyperkalemia is an uncommon feature of HRS. However, marked hyperkalemia may occur if patients are treated with aldosterone antagonists, especially patients with type 1 HRS. Severe metabolic acidosis and pulmonary edema, which are frequent complications of acute renal failure of patients without liver disease, are uncommon findings in patients with HRS. Because HRS is a form of functional renal failure, the characteristics of urine are those of prerenal azotemia, with oliguria, low urine sodium concentration, and increased urine osmolality and urine-to-plasma osmolality ratio (102,124). Nevertheless, there are nonoliguric forms of the syndrome and in some cases urine sodium concentration is not extremely reduced (124,125). As shown in Table 75-4, urinary indices are not currently considered essential for the diagnosis of HRS by the International Ascites Club.

Circulatory failure in patients with HRS is characterized by high cardiac output, arterial hypotension (most patients have a mean arterial pressure in the range of 60 to 80 mm Hg), and low total systemic vascular resistance, despite the existence of severe vasoconstriction in several vascular beds, as already discussed.

Finally, the third type of clinical manifestations of HRS is related to the existence of liver failure. Most patients show findings of advanced liver insufficiency, particularly jaundice, coagulopathy, poor nutritional status, and encephalopathy, although some patients with HRS may show only moderate liver failure. In general, patients with type 1 HRS have more severe liver failure compared with patients with type 2 HRS.

Precipitating Factors

In some patients, HRS develops without any identifiable precipitating factor, whereas in others it occurs in close chronologic relationship with bacterial infections, particularly

TABLE 75-4. *Diagnostic criteria of hepatorenal syndrome**

Major criteria

1. Low glomerular filtration rate, as indicated by serum creatinine greater than 1.5 mg/dL or 24-h creatinine clearance lower than 40 mL/min.
2. Absence of shock, ongoing bacterial infection, fluid losses, and current treatment with nephrotoxic drugs.
3. No sustained improvement in renal function (decrease in serum creatinine to 1.5 mg/dL or less or increase in creatinine clearance to 40 mL/min or more) following diuretic withdrawal and expansion of plasma volume with 1.5 L of a plasma expander.
4. Proteinuria lower than 500 mg/d and no ultrasonographic evidence of obstructive uropathy or parenchymal renal disease.

Additional criteria

1. Urine volume lower than 500 mL/day.
2. Urine sodium lower than 10 mEq/L.
3. Urine osmolality greater than plasma osmolality.
4. Urine red blood cells less than 50 per high power field.
5. Serum sodium concentration lower than 130 mEq/L.

*All major criteria must be present for the diagnosis of hepatorenal syndrome. Additional criteria are not necessary for the diagnosis, but provide supportive evidence.

spontaneous bacterial peritonitis (102,126,127). Approximately one-third of patients with spontaneous bacterial peritonitis develop an impairment of renal function during treatment with nonnephrotoxic antibiotics and in the absence of shock (126). This impairment in renal function is of functional origin and occurs in the setting of a further decrease in effective arterial blood volume of patients with ascites, as indicated by a marked activation of vasoconstrictor systems, and increased serum and ascitic fluid levels of cytokines (127,128). In approximately one-third of patients developing renal failure after spontaneous bacterial peritonitis, the impairment in renal function is reversible after resolution of infection. However, in the remaining patients the impairment in renal function is not reversible after the resolution of the infection and meets the criteria of HRS (type 1 in most cases). Patients who develop type 1 HRS after spontaneous bacterial peritonitis have a dismal outcome, with an in-hospital mortality close to 100% (126,128). Although uncommon, HRS has been reported after therapeutic paracentesis without plasma expansion (83). This is one of the reasons that supports the administration of intravenous albumin when large-volume paracentesis is performed (129). Gastrointestinal bleeding has been classically considered as a precipitating factor of HRS (124). However, the development of renal failure after this complication is uncommon in patients with cirrhosis (approximately 10%) and occurs mainly in patients with hypovolemic shock, in most cases associated with ischemic hepatitis, which suggests that renal failure in this setting is probably related to the development of acute tubular necrosis (ATN) and is not of functional origin (130). Diuretic treatment has also been classically described as a precipitating factor of HRS, but there is no clear evidence to support such a relationship.

Diagnosis

The diagnosis of HRS is currently based on several diagnostic criteria (Table 75-4) (102). The minimum level of serum creatinine required for the diagnosis of HRS is 1.5 mg/dL. Patients with cirrhosis with a serum creatinine above 1.5 mg/dL usually have a GFR below 30 mL/minute (105). In patients receiving diuretics, serum creatinine measurement should be repeated after diuretic withdrawal because in some patients serum creatinine may increase during diuretic therapy even in the absence of excessive diuresis causing volume depletion.

Because no specific laboratory tests are available for the diagnosis of HRS and patients with advanced cirrhosis may develop renal failure of other etiologies (prerenal failure due to volume depletion, ATN, drug-induced nephrotoxicity, and glomerulonephritis), the most important step in the diagnosis of HRS is to rule out renal failure secondary to volume depletion or organic renal causes (102). Gastrointestinal fluid losses, due to vomiting or diarrhea, or renal fluid losses, due to excessive diuresis, should be sought in all patients with cirrhosis presenting with renal failure. If renal failure is secondary to volume depletion, renal function improves rapidly after volume repletion and treatment of the precipitating factor. Shock is another common condition in patients with cirrhosis that may lead to renal failure due to ATN. While hypovolemic shock related with gastrointestinal bleeding is easily recognized, the presence of septic shock may be more difficult to diagnose because of the paucity of symptoms of bacterial infections in some patients with cirrhosis. Moreover, arterial hypotension due to the infection may be erroneously attributed to the underlying liver disease. In some patients with septic shock oliguria is the first sign of infection. These patients may be misdiagnosed as having HRS if signs of infection (cell blood count, examination of ascitic fluid) are not intentionally examined. On the other hand, as discussed before, patients with cirrhosis and spontaneous bacterial peritonitis may develop renal failure during the course of the infection, in the absence of septic shock (126,128). Renal failure in these patients may either improve with the antibiotic therapy or evolve into a true HRS, even after the resolution of the infection has been achieved. The administration of NSAIDs is another common cause of acute renal failure in patients with cirrhosis and ascites, which is clinically indistinguishable from a true HRS (81,131,132). Therefore, treatment with these drugs should always be ruled out before the diagnosis of HRS is made. Likewise, patients with cirrhosis are also at high risk of developing renal failure due to ATN when treated with aminoglycosides (131,133–136). Because of this high risk of nephrotoxicity and the existence of other effective antibiotics (e.g., third-generation cephalosporins) treatment with aminoglycosides should be avoided in patients with chronic liver disease. Finally, patients with cirrhosis may also develop renal failure due to glomerulonephritis (137). In these cases, proteinuria and/or hematuria are almost constant and provide a clue for the diagnosis, which may be confirmed by renal biopsy in selected cases.

Other Renal Abnormalities in Cirrhosis

Glomerular Abnormalities

The existence of glomerular abnormalities in patients with liver disease has been recognized for many years (138–141). Hepatitis C virus (HCV), hepatitis B virus (HBV), and cirrhosis have been implicated and their association with glomerular disease is well documented. The prevalence of these alterations varies depending on the condition. In the United States, HCV accounts for approximately 10% to 20% of all cases of glomerular disease, whereas in Japan it can account for approximately 60% of cases of glomerulopathy (142,143). In patients with HBV, the prevalence of associated glomerulonephritis has not been well documented because patterns of HBV also vary greatly depending on geographic location. Areas of low endemicity for HBV such as industrialized countries have a low prevalence of glomerular disease related to HBV, but areas of very high endemicity, such as Asia and Africa, have high rates of HBV-related glomerular disease (141). In regard to cirrhosis, the exact prevalence of glomerular disease is not well documented, however autopsy studies in cirrhotic patients indicate that glomerular alterations can occur in approximately 50% of cases (137). In fact, in a recent prospective study in unselected nonalcoholic cirrhotic patients in whom a renal biopsy was performed at the time of liver transplantation, glomerular abnormalities were found in all cases, although most patients had only minor changes (144).

In some cases renal glomerular abnormalities are clinically silent. However, when renal involvement is clinically present the manifestations commonly exist in the form of cryoglobulinemic and/or noncryoglobulinemic membranoproliferative glomerulonephritis (MPGN), membranous glomerulonephritis (MGN), and glomerular sclerosis. MPGN is the most common renal manifestation of HCV and HBV infection, whereas glomerular sclerosis occurs most commonly in patients with cirrhosis. The clinical presentation in all cases ranges from nonnephrotic proteinuria and microhematuria to overt nephrotic syndrome along with mild to moderate renal insufficiency (142,145).

Viral hepatitis is associated with the development of essential mixed cryoglobulinemia (EMC) (146,147). The prevalence of EMC is high (41%) in patients with chronic liver disease. When considering independent causes, HCV prevalence is higher (54%) than HBV (15%) or other causes of chronic liver disease (32%), however it is important to mention that these numbers vary according to geographic location

(148). EMC is a disorder in which mixed cryoglobulins (polyclonal IgG, and a monoclonal rheumatoid factor, IgM) precipitate at cool temperatures and cause a constellation of clinical findings characterized by arthritis, purpura, peripheral neuropathy, weakness, glomerulonephritis, and manifestations of vasculitis. There are two types: type II and type III, the strongest association with viral hepatitis is with type II (149). The development of renal disease, which occurs in half of the patients, carries a poor prognosis and the principal glomerular lesion is MPGN (146,147).

Renal involvement in patients with MPGN and HCV has been well documented (150–152). These patients often appear to have a primary glomerular disorder (50% to 60%). Although the majority have type II associated cryoglobulinemia, 30% to 40% do not have detectable circulating cryoglobulins at presentation (150). Approximately only 20% have physical signs of chronic liver disease, 75% have mild elevations of serum transaminase, and in most cases liver biopsy demonstrates chronic hepatitis with or without cirrhosis. Approximately 40% of patients will have signs consistent with extrarenal manifestations of cryoglobulinemia. The majority of patients present with nephrotic syndrome and mild renal insufficiency. Laboratory features include the presence of hypocomplementemia (low CH50, C4, and C3), presence of circulating rheumatoid factor, and elevated C1q binding (140,142,145,153). As mentioned previously, the most common glomerular lesion in patients with established alcoholic and nonalcoholic cirrhosis is glomerular sclerosis, which usually presents with mild proteinuria and hematuria.

The pathologic changes typically seen in glomerular nephropathy vary according to the underlying cause of liver disease. In HCV the renal biopsy of patients with MPGN shows an increased cellularity with accentuation of the lobular architecture of the glomerular tuft along with thickening of the capillary basement membrane (150,151). Mesangial proliferation, sclerosis, tubulointerstitial inflammation, and scarring may also be present. Immunofluorescence studies on renal biopsies reveal mesangial and capillary wall deposition of IgG, IgM, and C3 in most cases. Subendothelial deposits characteristic of MPGN can be demonstrated by electron microscopy, in addition other mesangial and subepithelial deposits can be observed. In some cases, these immune deposits have ultrastructural features of cryoglobulins such as granular, fibrillar, or immunotactoid structures. HCV- associated membranous nephropathy is indistinguishable from idiopathic membranous nephropathy (151). There is basement membrane thickening along with granular capillary wall deposits of IgG and C3 as seen by immunofluorescence. Subepithelial immune deposits with effacement of podocyte foot processes can be observed on electron microscopy.

Patients with HBV and MPGN have similar clinical and pathologic features compared with those with HCV-related MPGN. MGN is another common lesion found in patients with HBV (especially in children) and can present as a nephrotic syndrome (140,154). In adults, this type of glomerulopathy may sometimes progress to renal insufficiency in contrast to children who have a benign course. The characteristic pathologic finding in MGN is distinguished by the capillary wall deposition of hepatitis B e antigen (HBeAg), whereas HBV–MPGN is usually associated with mesangial and capillary wall deposits of hepatitis B s antigen (HbsAg) (155).

The pathologic findings in patients with glomerular sclerosis related to cirrhosis vary from patient to patient and are characterized by periglomerular fibrosis and hyaline thickening of the basement membrane, hypercellularity of epithelial and endothelial cells, and thickening of the mesangium by periodic acid-Schiff (PAS)-positive material (137,139,156). In some cases the glomerular lumen may become obliterated. Immunofluorescence studies have shown that these changes are associated with mesangial and subendothelial deposits of immunoglobulins, particularly IgA, although IgM, IgG, and complement can also be present (137,156,157). A classification of the glomerular lesions associated with cirrhosis has been proposed depending on the presence or absence of cellular proliferation (158). The most frequent type, without cell proliferation, is characterized by mesangial and subendothelial deposits of IgA often associated with IgG and IgM and, in some cases C1q. The less common type is associated with proliferative changes, marked basement membrane thickening and the immunoglobulin deposits are intramembranous and almost exclusively composed by IgA.

The pathogenesis of HCV- and HBV-related glomerulonephritis and cirrhotic glomerular sclerosis is associated with glomerular deposition of immune complexes containing antigens, antibodies, and rheumatoid factors. In HCV–MPGN circulating immune complexes deposit in the glomerular capillaries, where they localize in the subendothelium and mesangium and initiate a local cellular proliferation and leukocyte infiltration (141,151). This event can occur with or without the presence of cryoglobulins, which has led to the hypothesis that HCV can trigger autoantibody formation that reacts with local renal antigens or that the diseased liver contributes to the pathogenesis directly.

In HBV–MPGN, the exact mechanism of glomerular damage is not fully understood, however it most likely involves the deposition of circulating immune complexes containing HBV antigens (140,154). By contrast, in HBV–MGN it is believed that immune complexes develop in situ due to formation of autoantibodies in response to intrinsic glomerular antigens. The presence of immune complexes in patients with viral hepatitis without renal disease has also been documented, in fact autopsy studies of patients with acute or chronic HBV infection without clinical evidence of renal disease, revealed kidney lesions in approximately 15% to 20% (159).

Patients with cirrhosis, especially those with more severe glomerular alterations, often have hypocomplementemia, cryoglobulinemia, and increased serum levels of immunoglobulins. These findings may be due to the impaired activity of the reticuloendothelial system present in cirrhotic patients with portal hypertension (160). This would allow the passage of IgA and IgG complexes with bacterial, viral, or dietary antigens into the systemic circulation, which could then be deposited in the kidneys leading to glomerular lesions.

There are few studies that have focused specifically on the treatment of glomerular disease in the setting of chronic liver disease. In cryoglobulinemic or noncryoglobulinemic HCV–MPGN, patients receiving α-interferon therapy for 6 months or longer reduced proteinuria by 50%, but no significant change was observed in serum creatinine (161). Another controlled study of α-interferon reported an improvement in serum creatinine levels in 60% of treated patients and a better outcome was observed in those that cleared the virus, however renal disease returned upon discontinuation of therapy (162). In both studies clinical improvement occurred regardless of whether the viremia was suppressed or not; this might be explained by the previous duration of viremia, genotype of HCV, or variation of the host immune response. Other isolated reports have used a high-dose short course of α-interferon, with complete remission of nephrotic syndrome (163). Other treatments for HCV-associated renal disease, have focused on treating an underlying cause when present, such as EMC. Standard treatment of EMC includes corticosteroids, cytotoxic agents, and plasmapheresis, the goal is to control the formation and deposition of cryoglobulins. Corticosteroids, although beneficial in some cases, can elevate the levels of viremia and exacerbate hepatitis. However if EMC is present, pulse steroid therapy may rapidly improve renal function and vasculitis (164). Although the combination therapy of ribavirin and interferon for patients with HCV has been very successful, no reports are available regarding the efficacy of this combination on HCV-associated renal disease.

The treatment of HBV-associated renal disease is based on antiviral therapy with interferon. There are several reports that indicate that antiviral treatment can reverse renal disease (165–167). Two major studies have evaluated the effect of this treatment in patients with HBV-associated MGN and MPGN (168,169). The findings in both indicate that α-interferon therapy results in long-term remission in approximately 50% of patients treated and that this remission is accompanied by a significant improvement in renal function in the following months to years after interferon is stopped. The response to treatment is much better in children than in adults, due to the benign natural course in children.

Finally, in regard to the treatment of cirrhotic glomerular sclerosis, it has been reported that resolution of proteinuria and hematuria has occurred after liver transplantation (170). Unfortunately there is little information about the treatment of this renal manifestation in cirrhosis and more studies would be helpful in trying to define the response with liver transplantation or other treatments.

Renal Tubular Acidosis

Renal tubular acidosis (RTA) may occur in cirrhosis of different etiologies, particularly primary biliary cirrhosis, autoimmune hepatitis, and alcoholic cirrhosis (171–176). The most common type of RTA in cirrhosis is the incomplete distal RTA. This form is usually subclinical and can only be diagnosed by measuring urinary pH following acid loading. Forms of RTA associated with clinical symptoms are very unusual. It has been suggested that RTA may predispose to the development of hepatic encephalopathy (177), although there is no definitive proof for such association.

The pathogenesis of RTA associated with cirrhosis is unclear. In primary biliary cirrhosis and Wilson's disease, the impairment in renal acidification may be related to the deposition of copper in the tubules (174). In patients with other types of cirrhosis, a reduced delivery of sodium to the distal nephron has been suggested to be of pathogenic importance (178).

Drug-Induced Renal Dysfunction in Cirrhosis

Cirrhotic patients may develop sodium and water retention or renal failure when treated with a variety of drugs, especially NSAIDs, aminoglycosides, or vasodilators. NSAIDs are the paradigmatic drugs causing renal impairment in cirrhosis. The administration of NSAIDs is associated with a marked decrease in RBF and GFR in a significant proportion of patients with ascites (81,132,179–184). Patients with more avid sodium retention and marked activation of the renin–angiotensin—aldosterone system (RAAS) and sympathetic nervous system (SNS) have the highest risk of developing renal failure following NSAID administration because the maintenance of renal perfusion in these patients is dependent on an adequate renal prostaglandin synthesis (81,180,182, 184). In patients without ascites, NSAIDs may also cause mild reductions in RBF and GFR, which suggests that these drugs should be used with great caution even in cirrhotic patients without sodium retention (185). Renal failure has been reported to occur after treatment with a variety of NSAIDs, including indomethacin, aspirin (acetylsalicylic acid), ibuprofen, naproxen, and sulindac (67,81,132,180–184,186). In all these studies NSAIDs were given either in single doses or for short periods of time (usually 1 to 3 days) and GFR and RBF quickly returned to pretreatment values after cessation of the drug. However, it is not known whether renal failure may be reversible in patients treated for longer periods. NSAIDs may also impair water excretion and the natriuretic response to furosemide and spironolactone in patients with ascites (67,132,183,184,186). These effects may eventually lead to the development of dilutional hyponatremia and diuretic-resistant ascites. For all these reasons, the use of NSAIDs should be avoided in patients with cirrhosis, particularly in those with ascites and marked sodium retention. Some salicylates, like diflunisal or imidazole–salicylate, may be a safe alternative for cirrhotic patients requiring NSAIDs since they do not impair renal function or the renal response to furosemide in cirrhotic patients with ascites (187,188). However, since these drugs were only given for short periods of time in these studies, it is not known whether they may induce renal impairment when given for longer periods. A recent study in experimental cirrhosis showed that drugs that inhibit selectively cyclooxygenase-2 (COX-2) activity do not induce renal dysfunction (189). If these results are confirmed in human cirrhosis, selective inhibitors of COX-2 may be an alternative to classic NSAIDs in patients with cirrhosis and ascites.

The incidence of nephrotoxicity in cirrhotic patients treated with aminoglycosides is higher than in the general population, particularly when aminoglycosides are given in combination with cephalothin (32% compared to 14%) (190,191). Given this high rate of renal dysfunction and the availability of more effective and nonnephrotoxic antibiotics (e.g., the third-generation cephalosporins) (192), the use of aminoglycosides in cirrhotic patients does not seem to be justified except in very specific cases.

The use of diuretics in cirrhotic patients with ascites is often associated with abnormalities of renal function (193). The incidence of renal impairment during diuretic treatment ranges between 20% and 40% (194–196). This diuretic-induced renal failure is usually moderate and reversible after diuretic withdrawal (197) and is related to an imbalance between the fluid loss from the intravascular space caused by diuretic treatment and the passage of fluid from the peritoneal compartment to the general circulation. Ascites reabsorption is a rate-limited process that varies from patient to patient, ranging from as little as 200 mL to more than 1,000 mL/day (198). If diuretic therapy causes a loss of fluid above this limit, a contraction of circulating blood volume and a subsequent reduction of GFR occurs. Since fluid accumulated as edema in the interstitial space is more easily and rapidly reabsorbed than ascitic fluid, patients with peripheral edema may be treated with a more aggressive diuretic therapy because they have a low risk of diuretic-induced renal failure (197,199). Hyponatremia is another frequent complication of diuretic therapy in patients with cirrhosis and ascites. It may occur in up to 40% of patients (194–196). The most important pathogenic mechanism of diuretic-induced hyponatremia is an impairment of the renal ability to excrete solute-free water. This impairment is probably related to the inhibition of chloride and sodium reabsorption in the ascending limb of the loop of Henle caused by loop diuretics and to an increase in proximal sodium reabsorption and stimulation of AVP release secondary to intravascular volume depletion (200).

The use of vasodilators, has been recommended in the pharmacologic treatment of cirrhotic patients with portal hypertension because they reduce portal pressure by decreasing hepatic vascular resistance (201–203). However, their vasodilatory effect in the systemic circulation may induce deleterious effects on renal function. The acute administration of organic nitrates to cirrhotic patients causes renal vasoconstriction and sodium and water retention, these effects being particularly marked in patients with ascites (70,71, 204,205). Similarly, the oral long-term administration of prazosin, an α-adrenergic blocker, to compensated cirrhotic patients with portal hypertension causes vasodilation of the systemic circulation which leads to ascites and/or edema formation in a significant number of patients (68,206). Patients with lower baseline arterial pressure and systemic vascular resistance are those more predisposed to develop sodium retention following prazosin administration. Therefore, vasodilators should not be recommended as single therapy in patients with portal hypertension. The combination of vasodilators with β-adrenergic blockers has a more marked effect on portal pressure and does not seem to be associated with adverse effects on renal function (207,208).

FACTORS INVOLVED IN FUNCTIONAL RENAL ABNORMALITIES IN CIRRHOSIS

Circulatory Abnormalities

Hepatic and Splanchnic Circulation

The existence of cirrhosis causes marked structural abnormalities in the liver that result in severe disturbance of intrahepatic circulation causing increased resistance to portal flow and subsequent hypertension in the portal venous system (209). Progressive collagen deposition and formation of nodules alter the normal vascular architecture of the liver. Moreover, selective deposition of collagen in the space of Disse, the space between sinusoidal cells and hepatocytes, may constrict the sinusoids, resulting in further mechanical obstruction to flow (210,211). In addition to this passive resistance to portal flow there is an active component of intrahepatic resistance, which is due to the contraction of hepatic stellate cells (myofibroblastlike cells) present in sinusoids and terminal hepatic venules (212,213). The contraction of these cells is affected by endogenous vasoconstrictors and can be modulated by vasodilators and drugs that antagonize the vasoconstrictor factors (214–216). Moreover, there is a strong body of evidence indicating that despite the overproduction of the vasodilator nitric oxide (NO) in the systemic circulation in cirrhosis, there is a reduced production of NO in the intrahepatic circulation of cirrhotic livers that contributes further to the increased intrahepatic resistance characteristic of portal hypertension (217,218).

Portal hypertension induces profound changes in the splanchnic circulation (209,219). Classically, portal hypertension was considered to cause only changes in the venous side of the splanchnic circulation. However, studies in experimental animals indicate that portal hypertension also causes marked changes in the arterial side of the splanchnic vascular bed. In the venous side, the main changes consist of increased pressure and formation of portocollateral circulation, which causes the shunting of blood from the portal venous system to the systemic circulation. In the arterial side, there is marked arterial vasodilation which increases portal venous inflow (219,220). This high portal venous inflow plays an important role in the increased pressure in the portal circulation and may explain, at least in part, why portal pressure remains increased despite the development of collateral circulation. This arteriolar vasodilation is also responsible for marked changes in splanchnic microcirculation that may predispose to increased filtration of fluid. It has been shown that chronic portal hypertension causes a much greater increase in intestinal capillary pressure and lymph flow than does an acute increase in portal pressure of the same magnitude (221). This is probably due to a loss of the normal autoregulatory mechanism of the splanchnic microcirculation. The acute elevation of venous pressure in the intestine elicits a strong myogenic response, which leads to a reduction in blood flow. This phenomenon is thought to be a homeostatic response to protect the intestine against edema formation. This protective mechanism is not operative in chronic portal hypertension and arteriolar resistance is reduced and not increased (222). The resultant increases in capillary pressure and filtration may be important factors in the formation of ascites in cirrhosis. The mechanism(s) by which portal hypertension induces splanchnic arteriolar vasodilation is not completely understood although a number of vasoactive mediators have been proposed (and will be discussed subsequently).

Several lines of evidence indicate that portal hypertension is a major factor in the pathogenesis of ascites. First, patients with early cirrhosis without portal hypertension do not develop ascites or edema. Moreover, a certain level of portal hypertension is required for ascites formation. Ascites rarely develops in patients with portal pressure, as assessed by the difference between wedged and free hepatic venous pressure, below 12 mm Hg, (normal portal pressure: 5 mm Hg) (223–225). Second, cirrhotic patients treated with surgical portosystemic shunts for the management of bleeding gastroesophageal varices have a much lower risk of developing ascites than do patients treated with procedures that obliterate gastroesophageal varices but do not affect portal pressure (e.g., sclerotherapy, esophageal transection) (Fig. 75-5) (226). Finally, reduction of portal pressure with side-to-side or end-to-side portacaval anastomosis or TIPS (placement of a stent between a hepatic vein and the intrahepatic portion of the portal vein using a transjugular approach) is associated with an improvement of renal function and suppression of antinatriuretic systems (227–230). The mechanism(s) by which portal hypertension contributes to renal functional abnormalities and ascites and edema formation is not completely understood, yet three pathogenic mechanisms have been proposed: (a) alterations in the splanchnic and systemic circulation which would result in activation of vasoconstrictor and antinatriuretic systems and subsequent renal sodium and water retention; (b) hepatorenal reflex due to increased hepatic pressure which would cause sodium and water retention; and (c) putative antinatriuretic substances escaping from the splanchnic area through portosystemic collaterals that would have a sodium-retaining effect in the kidney (as discussed later in this chapter).

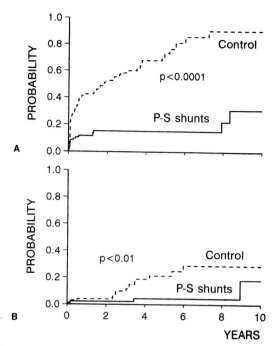

FIG. 75-5. Long-term probability of development of ascites (**A**) and hepatorenal syndrome (**B**) in a population of 204 cirrhotic patients with variceal bleeding treated with portosystemic shunts (P-S shunts), sclerotherapy, or esophageal transection (control) to prevent variceal rebleeding. (From Castells A, Saló J, Planas R, et al. Impact of shunt surgery for variceal bleeding in the natural history of ascites in cirrhosis: a retrospective study. *Hepatology* 1994;20:584, with permission.)

Systemic Circulation

The development of portal hypertension is associated with marked hemodynamic changes not only in the hepatic and splanchnic circulation but also in the systemic circulation. These changes, which have been well characterized in human and experimental cirrhosis, consist of reduced systemic vascular resistance and arterial pressure, increased cardiac index, increased plasma volume, and activation of systemic vasoconstrictor and antinatriuretic factors. These changes in systemic hemodynamics appear before the formation of ascites and are more marked as the disease progresses (29,231–237). The hemodynamic profile of patients with cirrhosis in different stages of the disease is summarized in Table 75-5. The factor that appears to trigger all these hemodynamic changes of cirrhosis is an arterial vasodilation located mainly in the splanchnic circulation (219,220,238,239). Whether or not arterial vasodilation occurs also in nonsplanchnic territories is still controversial (119,120,240). Whereas some studies using duplex Doppler have found arterial vasodilation and reduced vascular resistance in the upper and lower limbs, other studies have shown that blood flow in these arterial beds is normal or even reduced relative to the increased cardiac output. Whether exclusively or predominantly located in the splanchnic circulation, this arterial vasodilation causes an abnormal distribution of blood volume, which results in a reduction of

TABLE 75-5. *Hemodynamic profile of cirrhotic patients in different stages of disease*

	Preascitic cirrhosis	Cirrhosis with ascites	Hepatorenal syndrome
Cardiac output	Normal or increased	Increased	Increased
Arterial pressure	Normal	Normal or reduced	Reduced
Systemic vascular resistance	Normal or reduced	Reduced	Reduced
Plasma volume	Normal or increased	Increased	Increased
Portal pressure	Normal or increased	Increased	Increased
Vasoconstrictor systems activity	Normal	Increased*	Increased
Renal vascular resistance	Normal	Normal or increased	Increased
Brachial or femoral vascular resistance	Normal or reduced	Normal or increased	Increased
Cerebral vascular resistance	Normal	Increased	Increased

*May be normal in 20%–30% of patients

effective arterial blood volume (i.e., the blood volume in the central arterial tree that is sensed by baroreceptors) (237,241–244). This may explain why in most patients with cirrhosis and ascites systemic vasoconstrictor factors remain activated despite an increased plasma volume that in normal conditions would suppress the activation of these systems. The reduction in central blood volume correlates directly with systemic vascular resistance and inversely with portal pressure, indicating that the greater the vasodilation and the pressure in the portal system, the lower the central blood volume (237). The crucial role played by the reduced central blood volume in the activation of vasoconstrictor systems has been further corroborated by studies showing that improvement of central blood volume by the combination of expansion of plasma volume or head-out water immersion and administration of vasoconstrictor agents suppresses the activation of vasoconstrictor systems (245–248).

Despite extensive investigation, the mechanism(s) responsible for arterial vasodilation in cirrhosis is not completely understood. Several explanations have been proposed, including opening of arteriovenous fistulas, reduced sensitivity to vasoconstrictors, and increased circulating levels of vasodilator substances (235,249–251). This latter mechanism has been the most extensively studied. Increased plasma levels of glucagon, vasoactive intestinal peptide, prostaglandins, natriuretic peptides, platelet-activating factor, substance P, calcitonin gene-related peptide (CGRP), and adrenomedullin have been reported either in human and/or in experimental cirrhosis, but their role in the pathogenesis of vasodilation is unclear (249,252–256). At present, most available data, obtained mainly from experimental cirrhosis, indicate that NO is the main mediator of arterial vasodilation in cirrhosis (Table 75-6) (reviewed in reference 257). NO synthesis from cirrhotic arterial vessels is markedly increased compared to that of normal vascular tissue. This increased NO synthesis appears to be generalized, except for the intrahepatic circulation, but predominates in the splanchnic territory. Among the different isoforms of NO synthase, the constitutive form appears to be the one responsible for the increased NO synthesis. The normalization of NO synthesis in experimental cirrhosis by the administration of inhibitors of NO synthesis

is associated with a marked improvement of splanchnic and systemic hemodynamics, suppression of the increased activity of the RAAS and AVP concentration, increased sodium and water excretion, and reduction or disappearance of ascites (258).

Neurohumoral Systems

The functional renal abnormalities that occur in cirrhosis are probably the result of a complex interrelationship between different systems and factors with effects on renal function. The relative contribution of a particular system in the pathogenesis of these abnormalities in cirrhosis has, therefore, been difficult to assess. This section reviews the different systems

TABLE 75-6. *Evidences for a role of an increased vascular production of nitric oxide (NO) in the pathogenesis of arterial vasodilation and subsequent sodium and water retention in cirrhosis*

Experimental cirrhosis

1. Reversal of the impaired pressor response to vasoconstrictors of isolated aortic rings or splanchnic vascular preparations by NO synthase inhibition.
2. Enhanced vasodilator response to NO-dependent vasodilators.
3. Increased pressor effect of systemic NO synthase inhibition.
4. Increased NO synthesis in vascular tissue.
5. Normalization of the hyperdynamic circulation, activity of antinatriuretic systems, and sodium and water retention by chronic NO synthase inhibition.
6. Increased expression of NO synthase isoenzymes in vascular tissue.

Human cirrhosis

1. Correction of the arterial hyporesponsiveness to vasoconstrictors by NO synthase inhibition.
2. Enhanced vasodilatory response to NO-dependent vasodilators.
3. Increased plasma levels of NO and NO metabolites.
4. Increased NO in the exhaled air.
5. Increased NO synthase activity in polymorphonuclear cells and monocytes.

that may participate in renal dysfunction in cirrhosis. The evidence indicating their role in the pathogenesis of these abnormalities is discussed.

Renin–Angiotensin–Aldosterone System

Of all potential factors involved in the regulation of sodium excretion in cirrhosis, aldosterone has been the most extensively studied. Plasma aldosterone levels are increased in most cirrhotic patients with ascites and marked sodium retention (32,56,100,233,259–264). In ascitic patients with moderate sodium retention plasma aldosterone is either slightly elevated or normal. It should be pointed out, however, that these "normal" concentrations occur in the presence of an increase in total body sodium of a degree that generally suppresses aldosterone concentration in normal subjects. Three lines of evidence indicate that aldosterone plays an important role in the pathogenesis of sodium retention in cirrhosis: (a) there is an inverse correlation between urinary sodium excretion and plasma aldosterone levels (32,56,100,233,265); (b) studies in animals with experimental cirrhosis have shown the existence of a chronologic relationship between hyperaldosteronism and sodium retention (21); and (c) the administration of spironolactone, a specific aldosterone antagonist, is able to reverse sodium retention in the great majority of patients with ascites without renal failure (36,37,266–269). The observation that sodium retention may occur in cirrhotic patients in the absence of increased plasma aldosterone levels has raised the suggestion that other factors in addition to aldosterone may contribute to the increased sodium retention in cirrhosis (270). Nevertheless, it has also been suggested that cirrhotic patients may have an increased tubular sensitivity to aldosterone (32,56). This may explain the

natriuretic response to spironolactone observed in cirrhotic patients with ascites and normal plasma aldosterone concentration (37,268,269). Thus, the possibility exists that aldosterone may participate in renal sodium retention in cirrhosis even in the presence of normal plasma concentrations of the hormone. In addition to aldosterone, increased intrarenal levels of angiotensin II may also contribute to sodium retention in patients with cirrhosis by a direct effect on tubular sodium reabsorption. So far, however, no direct evidences exist to support this latter contention.

The increased plasma aldosterone concentration in cirrhotic patients with ascites are due to a stimulation of aldosterone secretion and not due to impaired degradation, as the hepatic clearance of aldosterone is normal or only slightly reduced in these patients (54,259,270). Among the different mechanisms that regulate aldosterone secretion an increased activity of RAAS is the most likely to be responsible for hyperaldosteronism in cirrhosis (Fig. 75-6). In fact, plasma renin activity (PRA), which estimates the activity of the RAAS, is increased in most patients with ascites and correlates closely with plasma aldosterone concentration (100, 233,260,261,271–273). Investigations using pharmacologic agents which interrupt RAAS have provided evidence suggesting that this system is activated as a result of a profound disturbance in systemic hemodynamics. The administration of angiotensin II receptor antagonists or converting-enzyme inhibitors to cirrhotic patients with ascites and increased PRA induces a marked reduction in arterial pressure and systemic vascular resistance, which suggests that the activation of RAAS is a homeostatic response to maintain arterial pressure in these patients (274–277).

The activation of RAAS is particularly intense in patients with HRS, suggesting a role for angiotensin II in the

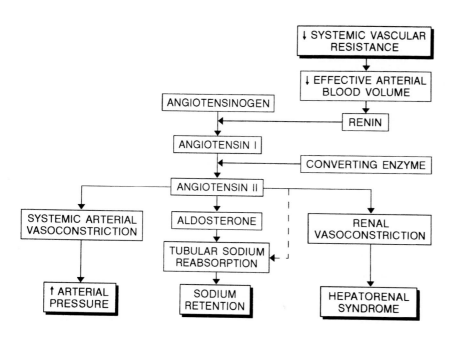

FIG. 75-6. Proposed mechanism of activation and renal and systemic effects of renin–angiotensin–aldosterone system in cirrhosis with ascites.

pathogenesis of renal vasoconstriction in HRS (179,180,278–281). This role is further supported by studies showing that the improvement of renal function in patients with HRS achieved by the administration of the vasopressin analogs ornipressin or terlipressin associated with albumin or the insertion of a TIPS is associated with a marked suppression of the activity of the RAAS (247,248,282). However, since the interruption of RAAS is associated with arterial hypotension in patients with high PRA, the effects of RAAS on renal function independent of those on systemic hemodynamics have been difficult to assess. At present, there are no inhibitors or antagonists of angiotensin II that are selective for the renal vasculature to examine this possibility.

Sympathetic Nervous System

Numerous studies have presented evidence indicating an increased activity of the SNS in cirrhosis. The plasma concentration of norepinephrine (NE) in the systemic circulation, an index of the activation of the SNS, is increased in most patients with ascites and normal or only slightly elevated in patients without ascites (180,283–288). This "normal" plasma NE concentration, however, is relatively increased in the presence of plasma volume expansion, which occurs in early cirrhosis. Investigations using titrated NE, to provide a more accurate assessment of the SNS activity, have confirmed that the high plasma NE levels are due to an increased activity of the SNS and not to an impaired elimination of NE, as the total spillover of NE to plasma is markedly increased in cirrhotic patients with ascites whereas the plasma clearance of NE is normal (289–293). Measurements of NE release and spillover in specific vascular beds have shown that the activity of the SNS is increased in many vascular territories, including kidneys, splanchnic organs, heart, and muscle and skin, supporting the concept of a generalized activation of the SNS (290–294). Direct evidence of the overactivity of the SNS in cirrhosis has been provided by measuring the sympathetic nerve discharge rates from a peripheral muscular nerve.

Muscular sympathetic nerve activity is markedly increased in patients with ascites and normal in patients without ascites and correlates directly with plasma NE concentration (295).

Because the SNS has profound effects on renal function (296), it is reasonable to presume that the increased renal sympathetic nervous activity in cirrhosis may play a role in the pathogenesis of functional renal abnormalities (Fig. 75-7). In fact, evidence suggests that the SNS is involved in sodium and water retention in cirrhosis. The activity of the SNS, either estimated by plasma NE or total NE spillover to plasma or measured from intraneural recordings, correlates inversely with sodium and water retention (284,290,295). In addition, bilateral renal denervation increases urine volume and sodium excretion in animals with experimental cirrhosis and ascites (297,298). Similarly, anesthetic blockade of the lumbar SNS, a maneuver that reduces the activity of the kidney SNS, improves sodium excretion in patients with cirrhosis and ascites (299). The acute inhibition of the renal sympathetic outflow with clonidine in patients with cirrhosis is associated with a reduction in renal vascular resistance and an increase in GFR and filtration fraction, suggesting that the activation of the SNS causes renal vasoconstriction by increasing arterial tone in the afferent arteriole (293). Finally, patients with HRS have significantly higher plasma levels of NE than do patients without renal failure, and arterial and renal venous NE correlate inversely with RBF, suggesting that the SNS may participate in the renal vasoconstriction observed in patients with HRS (180,264,300). Moreover, the circulating levels of neuropeptide Y, a neurotransmitter with a very potent vasoconstrictor action in the renal circulation released in the setting of a marked activation of the SNS, are increased in patients with HRS but not in those with ascites without renal failure (301).

The cause of the increased activity of the SNS in cirrhosis with ascites is not completely understood. Two major explanations have been proposed: either a baroreceptor-mediated response to a decrease in effective arterial blood volume due to arterial vasodilation (302) or a hepatorenal

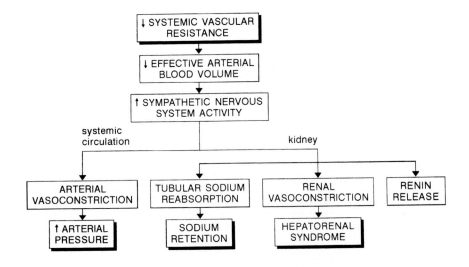

FIG. 75-7. Proposed mechanism of activation and renal and systemic effects of sympathetic nervous system in cirrhosis with ascites.

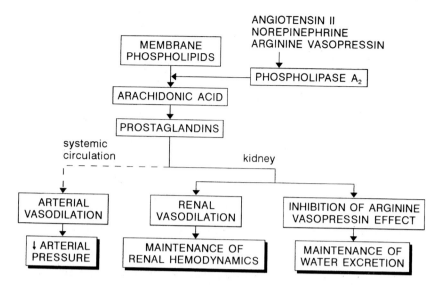

FIG. 75-8. Proposed mechanism of activation and renal and systemic effects of prostaglandins in cirrhosis with ascites.

reflex resulting from activation of hepatic baroreceptors due to sinusoidal hypertension (303–305). The first explanation seems more likely since the estimated central blood volume (i.e., the blood volume in the heart cavities, lungs, and central arterial tree) is reduced in cirrhotic patients and correlates inversely with SNS activity (241,242). The activity of the SNS can be suppressed by maneuvers that increase effective arterial blood volume, such as the administration of vasopressin analogs and albumin or the insertion of a peritoneovenous shunt (247,248,289,306).

Prostaglandins and Other Eicosanoids

Prostaglandins are known to have a protective effect on renal circulation in pathophysiologic situations associated with increased activity of renal vasoconstrictor systems (307). According to this formulation, prostaglandins appear to play a key role in the homeostasis of renal circulation and water excretion in cirrhotic patients with ascites (Fig. 75-8). The urinary excretion of prostaglandin E2 (PGE2) and 6-keto-prostaglandin F1α, which estimate the renal synthesis of PGE2 and PGI2, respectively, are increased in patients with cirrhosis and ascites without renal failure as compared to healthy subjects and patients without ascites (101,180, 181,308–312). Further evidence supporting a role for renal prostaglandins in the maintenance of RBF and GFR in cirrhosis with ascites derive from studies using NSAIDs to inhibit prostaglandin synthesis. The administration of NSAIDs, even in single doses, to cirrhotic patients with ascites causes a profound decrease in RBF and GFR in those who have a marked activation of vasoconstrictor systems but has little or no effect in patients without activation of these systems (81,132,180,183,184). An increased renal production of PGE2 also contributes to the maintenance of solute-free water excretion in nonazotemic cirrhotic patients with ascites as the inhibition of prostaglandin synthesis by NSAIDs in these patients impairs solute-free water excretion independently of changes in renal hemodynamics (186).

The relationship between the renal prostaglandin system and HRS is controversial. Several studies have reported that patients with HRS have lower urinary excretion of PGE2 and 6-keto-PGF1α than do patients with ascites without renal failure, which suggests that a reduced renal synthesis of vasodilator prostaglandins may play a role in the pathogenesis of HRS (101,180,309–311,313). The finding of low renal content of PGH2 synthase (medullary cyclooxygenase) in patients with HRS is consistent with this hypothesis (314). Other studies, however, did not find reduced urinary excretion of vasodilator prostaglandins in patients with HRS (315,316). Nevertheless, "normal" synthesis of prostaglandins may be low relative to the increased activity of vasoconstrictor systems in cirrhosis. Because patients with HRS have the greatest activation of renal vasoconstrictor systems, an imbalance between vasoconstrictor systems and the renal production of vasodilator prostaglandins has been proposed to explain the marked reduction of RBF and GFR that occurs in this condition (179). It has also been suggested that HRS could be the consequence of an imbalance between the renal synthesis of vasodilator and vasoconstrictor prostaglandins based on the observation of reduced urinary excretion of PGE2 and 6-keto-PGF1α and increased urinary excretion of TXB2 in patients with HRS (313,316). These findings, however, were not confirmed by subsequent investigations (101,310,311). Moreover, the administration of inhibitors of TXA2 synthesis does not improve renal function in these patients (317).

Prostaglandin synthesis in cirrhosis is also increased in extrarenal organs. Patients with cirrhosis have high urinary excretion of 2-3-dinor-6-keto-PGF1α, a metabolite of PGI2 considered to be an index of systemic PGI2 production (252, 315). As prostaglandins are potent vasodilators in the systemic circulation these observations raise the possibility that an increased prostaglandin synthesis may contribute to arterial vasodilation in cirrhosis. This suggestion is consistent with the observation that the NSAID indomethacin increases systemic vascular resistance and ameliorates the hyperdynamic circulation in cirrhotic patients (318).

Studies in rats with experimental cirrhosis and ascites have investigated the metabolic pathways leading to the increased synthesis of prostaglandins. Increased activity and expression of cytosolic phospholipase A2 (cPLA2) (the first enzyme of the metabolic cascade of eicosanoid synthesis) have been found in arterial and renal tissue of rats with cirrhosis and ascites compared with normal rats (319).

Little is known about the possible role of eicosanoids other than prostaglandins in the pathogenesis of functional renal abnormalities in cirrhosis. The urinary excretion of leukotriene E4 and N-acetyl-leukotriene E4, compounds with a vasoconstrictor effect in the renal circulation, is increased in cirrhotic patients with HRS as compared to healthy subjects and patients without ascites, suggesting that leukotrienes may participate in the pathogenesis of this syndrome (320,321).

Arginine Vasopressin

Studies in humans and experimental animals have provided several pieces of evidence indicating that AVP plays a key role in the pathogenesis of water retention in cirrhosis with ascites. These include: (a) plasma AVP levels are often increased in cirrhotic patients and correlate closely with the reduction in solute-free water excretion, patients with higher plasma AVP levels being those with the more severe impairment in water metabolism (76,186,322–326); (b) a chronologic relationship between AVP hypersecretion and impairment in water excretion can be found in rats with cirrhosis and ascites (327,328); (c) Brattleboro rats (rats with a congenital deficiency of AVP) with cirrhosis do not develop an impairment in water excretion (329); (d) kidneys from cirrhotic rats with ascites show increased gene expression of aquaporin, the AVP-regulated water channel (330); (e) the administration of specific antagonists of the tubular effect of AVP (V2 antagonists) restore the renal ability to excrete solute-free water in animal as well as in human cirrhosis (87–94).

The increased plasma AVP concentrations in cirrhosis are due to an increased hypothalamic synthesis and not to a reduced systemic clearance of the peptide (331–333). The increased synthesis of AVP is related to a nonosmotic hypersecretion of AVP, as most patients have a degree of hyponatremia and hypoosmolality that would suppress AVP release in normal subjects (186,322). The mechanism of this nonosmotic hypersecretion is probably hemodynamic, as plasma AVP levels correlate with PRA and plasma NE concentration (186,284) and are suppressed by maneuvers that increase effective arterial blood volume, such as head-out water immersion or peritoneovenous shunting in human cirrhosis (323,334) or inhibition of NO synthesis in experimental animal cirrhosis (258). This hemodynamic mechanism of AVP release in cirrhosis is also supported by the observation that the administration of a specific antagonist of the vascular effect of AVP (V1 antagonist) induces arterial hypotension in rats with experimental cirrhosis and ascites and water retention but not in control rats (335). This finding suggests that

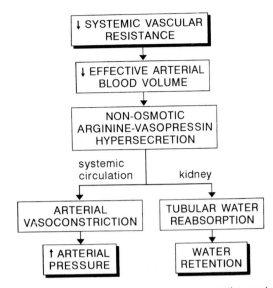

FIG. 75-9. Proposed mechanism of hypersecretion and renal and systemic effects of arginine vasopressin in cirrhosis with ascites.

AVP hypersecretion in cirrhosis contributes not only to water retention but also to the maintenance of arterial pressure (Fig. 75-9).

Natriuretic Peptides

Despite some controversial findings in early studies, most recent investigations showed that the plasma concentration of atrial natriuretic peptide (ANP) is increased in patients with ascites (336–344). In patients without ascites, plasma ANP levels may be either normal or increased. The high plasma levels of ANP in cirrhosis with ascites are due to increased cardiac secretion of the peptide and not reduced hepatic or systemic catabolism, as cardiac production of ANP is increased in cirrhotic patients with ascites but splanchnic and peripheral extraction are normal (336,345). Consistent with these observations is the finding of increased messenger RNA expression for ANP in ventricles from cirrhotic rats with ascites (346). In contrast to other diseases showing increased cardiac ANP secretion, in cirrhosis with ascites this increased secretion occurs in the presence of normal atrial pressure and reduced estimated central blood volume (241,336). The mechanism(s) responsible for this increased cardiac secretion of ANP is not known. The existence of increased plasma levels of ANP in cirrhosis with ascites sufficient to have a natriuretic effect in healthy subjects, together with the presence of renal sodium retention, indicates a renal resistance to the effects of ANP. This renal resistance has been confirmed in studies in human and experimental cirrhosis in which pharmacologic doses of natriuretic peptides (ANP or brain natriuretic peptide [BNP]) were administered (347–352). In these investigations patients with activation of antinatriuretic systems (RAAS and SNS) had a blunted or no natriuretic response after ANP infusion. This blunted response can be reversed by maneuvers that increase distal sodium delivery in human cirrhosis or by bilateral renal denervation in experimental cirrhosis, suggesting that the renal resistance to ANP in cirrhosis is related to the increased activity of antinatriuretic systems (298,353). Limited information exists on other peptides of the natriuretic peptide family. As with ANP, the plasma concentration of BNP is increased in cirrhotic patients with ascites as compared to healthy subjects (354). Finally, the urinary excretion of urodilatin, a member of the natriuretic peptide family exclusively synthesized in the kidney, which probably reflects the renal production of the peptide, is normal in patients with cirrhosis and ascites (355).

The role that the increased circulating levels of natriuretic peptides play in cirrhosis is not known. Because most of these peptides have vasodilator properties, a role in the pathogenesis of arterial vasodilation in cirrhosis has been proposed but not proved. By contrast, data from experimental studies suggest that they play an important role in the maintenance of renal perfusion and modulation of RAAS activity, as the selective blockade of the natriuretic peptide A and B receptors causes renal vasoconstriction and increased PRA and aldosterone levels in experimental cirrhosis (356).

Endothelins

Endothelins comprise three homologous peptides (ET-1, ET-2, and ET-3) with a very potent vasoconstrictor action (357). The intravenous infusion of ET-1, which was first described as a peptide synthesized by endothelial cells, causes a transient decrease in arterial pressure followed by a long-lasting increase in pressure. The effects of endothelins are mediated through two types of receptors, ET_A and ET_B, that exhibit distinct selectivity for endothelin isopeptides. The ET_A receptor binds ET-1 and ET-2 with a higher affinity than ET-3 while ET_B displays similar affinities for all three isopeptides. ET_A is responsible for the vasoconstrictor effect of ET-1, whereas the stimulation of ET_B mainly causes vasodilation (a vasoconstrictor effect has also been described) through the activation of NO and prostaglandins. Endothelin synthesized by endothelial cells is thought to participate in the regulation of vascular tone by acting as a paracrine substance on the underlying vascular smooth muscle cells. Because of its marked vasoconstrictor effect, ET-1 has been implicated in the pathogenesis of arterial hypertension as well as other disease states associated with increased vascular resistance and reduced perfusion in specific organs.

Increased plasma levels of ET-1 and ET-3 have been found in patients with cirrhosis and ascites and in patients without ascites, albeit to a lesser extent (358–365). The increased plasma levels of ET-1 found in cirrhosis derive either from an increased production in the splanchnic circulation and/or an increased intrahepatic production. Increased levels of ET-1 and its precursor Big-ET-1 have been found in plasma samples obtained from the portal and hepatic veins of patients with cirrhosis (366). Moreover, increased levels of ET-1 have

been demonstrated in hepatic tissue in human and experimental cirrhosis (367–370). In human cirrhosis, the increased hepatic ET-1 levels correlate with portal hypertension and the severity of ascites and liver failure (369,370). As opposed to other vasoconstrictor factors (e.g., angiotensin II or norepinephrine), the activity of which is increased in cirrhosis, it is unlikely that hyperendothelinemia in cirrhosis is a compensatory mechanism triggered by effective arterial hypovolemia. Endothelin levels are not suppressed by maneuvers that improve circulatory function, such as plasma volume expansion with or without concomitant administration of splanchnic vasoconstrictors (247,361,363). A role for endotoxemia in the increased endothelin levels in cirrhosis has also been proposed (358) but plasma endothelin concentration does not parallel endotoxin levels in cirrhotic patients (363).

The role that these increased circulating ET-1 levels play in the pathogenesis of abnormalities in renal, systemic, and hepatic circulation in cirrhosis is not known. A role for ET-1 in the pathogenesis of renal vasoconstriction in HRS has been proposed on the basis of markedly increased plasma endothelin levels in patients with HRS as compared with patients with ascites without HRS (360) and improvement of renal function after the administration of a selective antagonist of ET_A receptors in a small group of patients (371). However, the increased ET-1 levels in HRS have not been confirmed in other studies (361,372). A contribution of the increased endothelin levels to the maintenance of arterial pressure in cirrhosis is unlikely because most studies in experimental models of cirrhosis and portal hypertension have found no changes in arterial pressure after chronic endothelin receptor blockade (367,373–375). Because of the well-known vasoconstrictor effect of ET-1 in the intrahepatic circulation when infused through the portal vein, ET-1 has been postulated as a mediator of the increased intrahepatic resistance characteristic of diseases associated with portal hypertension. The results of these studies are conflicting and the role of endothelin in these abnormalities is unclear (376). Finally, recent studies suggest an important role for ET-1 in hepatic fibrogenesis by increasing collagen synthesis from hepatic stellate cells (368). In support of this hypothesis, a marked reduction in liver fibrosis has been demonstrated in bile duct-ligated rats chronically treated with an oral ET_A receptor antagonist (374).

Nitric Oxide

In addition to its effects in the regulation of systemic hemodynamics and arterial pressure, NO also participates in the regulation of renal function (377). Constitutive NO synthase has been found in several cell types in the kidney, including endothelial cells, mesangial cells, and some tubular epithelial cells. Inducible NO synthase has also been demonstrated in mesangial cells and epithelial cells. Under normal circumstances, NO participates in the regulation of glomerular microcirculation by modulating arteriolar tone and mesangial cell contractility. Moreover, NO facilitates natriuresis in response to changes in renal perfusion pressure, and regulates renin release (377).

Three lines of evidence indicate that the renal production of NO is increased in experimental cirrhosis. First, kidneys from cirrhotic rats show enhanced endothelium-dependent vasodilator response as compared to control animals (378). Second, infusion of L-arginine, the precursor of NO, causes a greater increase in renal perfusion in cirrhotic rats as compared to control rats (379). Finally, increased expression of NO synthase in kidney tissue from cirrhotic rats has been found in two studies (379,380). However, both studies showed discrepant findings with respect to the NO synthase isoform responsible for the increased NO synthesis.

The inhibition of NO synthesis in rats with cirrhosis and ascites does not result in renal hypoperfusion because of a marked rise in prostaglandin synthesis (381). However, the simultaneous inhibition of NO and prostaglandin synthesis in experimental cirrhosis results in a marked renal vasoconstriction suggesting that NO probably interacts with prostaglandins to maintain renal hemodynamics (382).

Renal Kallikrein–Kinin System

The kallikrein–kinin system is an enzyme system with important biological effects present in plasma as well as in many tissues. The kidney has all the components of the system, with the highest concentration being detected in the distal tubule (383). The system is activated by the enzyme kallikrein, a serine protease that acts on the substrate kininogen to release kinins, the effector substances of the system. The regulation of renal kallikrein production is poorly understood. The most important kinin formed within the kidney is kallidin, which is subsequently converted to bradykinin by an enzymatic process. The kinins are degraded to inactive peptides by kininase I and kininase II, which is the angiotensin-converting enzyme. This enzyme simultaneously converts angiotensin I to angiotensin II and hydrolyses kinins. The activity of the renal kallikrein–kinin system has been assessed by measuring the urinary kallikrein excretion, which estimates renal kallikrein production. The effects of kinins on renal function are characterized by renal vasodilation and increase in sodium and water excretion probably due to both increased RBF and direct inhibition of tubular sodium and water reabsorption. Despite these effects on renal function, the physiologic role of the renal kallikrein–kinin system has been difficult to estimate because of the complex interactions of this system with other renal systems, such as the RAAS and prostaglandins, and the lack of specific antagonists of the different components of the system (383).

For the same reasons, the role of the renal kallikrein–kinin system on renal function in cirrhosis has been difficult to assess. Some studies have reported that urinary kallikrein excretion is increased in patients with ascites without renal failure and reduced in patients with HRS and correlates directly with GFR, suggesting that the renal kallikrein–kinin system may contribute to the maintenance of renal hemody-

namics in cirrhosis (384,385). Other investigations, however, have found reduced urinary kallikrein excretion in patients with ascites (386,387). More specific methods to evaluate the activity of the kallikrein–kinin system are needed to define its role in the homeostasis of renal function in cirrhosis.

PATHOPHYSIOLOGY OF FUNCTIONAL RENAL ABNORMALITIES IN CIRRHOSIS

Ascites as Primary Edema: The Overflow Theory

The existence of a primary renal sodium retention in cirrhosis with ascites was proposed in an attempt to explain the paradox of coexistence of sodium retention and increased plasma volume in patients with ascites (388,389). According to this theory, the expansion of plasma volume would result in increased cardiac index and reduced systemic vascular resistance as adaptive circulatory mechanisms to the excess of intravascular volume. The existence of portal hypertension and circulating hypervolemia would lead to "overflow" of fluid within the peritoneal cavity. It has been proposed that the primary signal for sodium retention would arise from the liver, either as a consequence of intrahepatic portal hypertension, by means of hepatic low-pressure baroreceptors, or liver failure, by means of decreased hepatic clearance of a sodium-retaining factor or reduced hepatic synthesis of a natriuretic factor (58,303–305,390–392). However, the hemodynamic pattern of cirrhotic patients with ascites does not correspond with that predicted by the overflow theory because the arterial vascular compartment is not overfilled, as arterial pressure is low in most patients despite the increased plasma volume and cardiac index (Table 75-5). Moreover, there is marked overactivity of vasoconstrictor mechanisms, which would be suppressed if there were overfilling in the systemic circulation (237,244).

Because of the increasing evidence against the existence of vascular overfilling in cirrhosis with ascites, the overflow theory has been redefined recently to exclusively explain changes that occur in the preascitic stage of cirrhosis. Proponents of this theory suggest that in the preascitic stage of cirrhosis subtle sodium retention leading to plasma volume expansion would have two components: one related to the circulatory changes occurring in the splanchnic circulation aimed at maintaining the effective arterial blood volume (EABV) and one related to the existence of intrahepatic portal hypertension (393,394). Recent studies in patients with cirrhosis without ascites indicate that the existence of arterial vasodilation is of crucial importance in the development of sodium retention and ascites formation. In fact, preascitic cirrhotic patients with sinusoidal portal hypertension treated with mineralocorticoids do not show mineralocorticoid escape and develop ascites only when marked arterial vasodilation is present (52). Moreover, pharmacologically induced vasodilation in preascitic cirrhotic patients by means of the administration of prazosin, an α-adrenergic blocker, is associated with the development of ascites and/or edema in a significant proportion of patients (68). It is important to note that the development of sodium retention in these two studies was neither related to the degree of portal hypertension nor to the intensity of liver failure. In fact, in patients receiving prazosin, sodium retention occurred despite a marked reduction of portal pressure and improvement of liver perfusion.

Ascites as Secondary Edema: From the Traditional Theory to the Arterial Vasodilation Theory

The traditional concept of ascites formation in cirrhosis (395, 396) considers that the key event in ascites formation is a "backward" increase in hydrostatic pressure in the hepatic and splanchnic circulation due to the increased resistance to portal flow. This would cause a disruption of the Starling equilibrium and an increased filtration of fluid into the interstitial space. Initially, this capillary hyperfiltration is compensated by an increased lymphatic flow which returns the fluid to the systemic circulation via the thoracic duct. However, as portal hypertension increases, the lymphatic system is not able to drain the excess of interstitial fluid which then accumulates in the peritoneal cavity as ascites. Loss of fluid from the intravascular compartment results in true hypovolemia which is then sensed by cardiopulmonary and arterial receptors resulting in a compensatory renal sodium retention. The retained fluid cannot adequately fill the intravascular compartment and suppress the sodium-retaining signals to the kidney because fluid is continuously leaking in the peritoneal cavity, thus creating a vicious cycle. In cases with extreme hypovolemia, renal vasoconstriction develops, leading to HRS. This hypothesis is similar to the "backward" theory of edema

formation in heart failure, which suggests that sodium retention and formation of edema is secondary to the disruption of the Starling equilibrium in the microcirculation due to the backward increase in capillary hydrostatic pressure (397). The "classic underfilling" theory of ascites formation, however, does not correspond with the systemic hemodynamic abnormalities associated with cirrhosis (Table 75-5). If this theory were correct, changes in systemic circulation would consist of reduced plasma volume and cardiac index and increased systemic vascular resistance. However, findings in patients with cirrhosis and ascites are exactly the opposite, with increased plasma volume and cardiac index and reduced systemic vascular resistance (235,244).

These traditional backward theories of edema formation in cirrhosis and heart failure have been substituted by new theories that fit more precisely with the modern concepts of regulation of extracellular fluid volume, which consider that a reduction in EABV is the main determinant of sodium retention in major edematous states (398–400). Arterial vasodilation would be the triggering factor for sodium retention in cirrhosis, whereas a reduction in cardiac output would be the triggering factor in heart failure. The "arterial vasodilation" theory considers that the reduction in EABV in cirrhosis with ascites is not due to true hypovolemia, as proposed by the "traditional" theory, but rather to a disproportionate enlargement of the arterial tree secondary to arterial vasodilation (Fig. 75-10) (244,401,402). According to this theory, portal hypertension is the initial event with resultant splanchnic arteriolar vasodilation causing underfilling of the arterial circulation. The arterial receptors then sense the arterial underfilling and stimulate the SNS and the RAAS and cause nonosmotic hypersecretion of AVP. Renal sodium and water

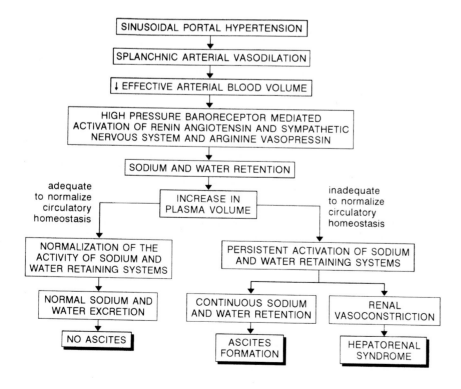

FIG. 75-10. Pathogenesis of functional renal abnormalities and ascites formation in cirrhosis according to the arterial vasodilation hypothesis.

retention are the final consequence of this compensatory response to a reduction in EABV. In early stages of cirrhosis, when splanchnic arteriolar vasodilation is moderate and the lymphatic system is able to return the increased lymph production to the systemic circulation, the EABV is preserved by transient periods of sodium retention. The fluid retained by the kidneys increases plasma volume and suppresses the signals stimulating the antinatriuretic systems and sodium retention terminates. Therefore, no ascites or edema is formed at this stage and the relationship between EABV and extracellular fluid volume is maintained. As liver disease progresses, splanchnic arterial vasodilation increases, thus resulting in a more intense arterial underfilling and more marked sodium and water retention. At this time, the EABV can no longer be maintained by the increased plasma volume, probably because the retained fluid leaks from the splanchnic circulation into the peritoneal cavity as ascites and/or from the systemic circulation to the interstitial tissue as edema. A persistent stimulation of vasoconstrictor systems occurs in an attempt to maintain EABV. The activation of these systems perpetuates renal sodium and water retention, which accumulates as ascites. The correlation between EABV and extracellular fluid volume is no longer maintained as EABV remains contracted despite progressive expansion of extracellular fluid volume. HRS probably represents the most extreme manifestation of the reduction in EABV. Studies in experimental models of portal hypertension aimed at carefully investigating the chronologic relationship between abnormalities in the systemic circulation and sodium retention indicate that arterial vasodilation with reduced systemic vascular resistance precedes sodium retention and subsequent plasma volume expansion (403,404).

The arterial vasodilation theory not only provides a reasonable explanation for the circulatory changes and activation of antinatriuretic systems observed in cirrhosis with ascites, but also for the preferential location of retained fluid in the peritoneal cavity. The existence of splanchnic arterial vasodilation causes a "forward" increase in splanchnic capillary pressure that enhances the effects of portal hypertension on the filtration coefficient in splanchnic capillaries, which facilitates the formation of ascites (219,221,222,405).

MANAGEMENT OF ASCITES AND FUNCTIONAL RENAL ABNORMALITIES IN CIRRHOSIS

In this section, the different methods used in the management of ascites and renal dysfunction in cirrhosis are discussed. A practical approach to the management of ascites in clinical practice is summarized in Tables 75-7 through 75-9.

Sodium Restriction

In all diseases associated with generalized edema (cirrhosis, heart failure, renal failure), the amount of exogenous fluid retained depends on the balance between sodium intake and the renal excretion of sodium. Because sodium is retained

TABLE 75-7. *Therapeutic approach to management of patients with cirrhosis and moderate ascites*

1. Start with low-sodium diet (50 mEq/d) and spironolactone (100–200 mg/d as single dose). Monitor body weight and urine sodium. Ideal weight loss should be 300–500 g/d in patients without peripheral edema and 800–1,000 g/d in patients with peripheral edema. Outpatients should be instructed to reduce the diuretic dosage in case of greater weight loss. Once ascites has decreased, maintain sodium restriction and reduce diuretic dosage approximately in half. If ascites or edema does not recur, increase sodium intake progressively and maintain a low dose of diuretics.
2. Low doses of loop diuretics (furosemide 20–40 mg/d) may be used initially in combination with spironolactone to increase the natriuretic effect. However, loop diuretics should be stopped when ascites and/or edema have decreased and patients should be monitored closely to prevent excessive diuresis.
3. If there is no response, check compliance with treatment and low-sodium diet. Increase the dose of diuretics stepwise every 7–10 d up to 400 mg/d of spironolactone and 160 mg/d of furosemide.

isoosmotically in the kidney, one liter of extracellular fluid is gained for every 130 to 140 mEq of sodium retained. If sodium excretion remains constant, the gain of extracellular fluid volume (and the consequent increase in weight) depends exclusively on sodium intake and increases proportionally to the amount of sodium taken with the diet. Nevertheless, because sodium excretion may be increased pharmacologically by the administration of diuretics, the sodium balance depends not only on sodium intake but also on the natriuretic response achieved by diuretics.

Based on this background, it seems reasonable that a reduction in sodium intake (low-salt diet) will favor a negative sodium balance and facilitate the disappearance of ascites and

TABLE 75-8. *Therapeutic approach to management of patients with cirrhosis and large ascites*

1. Total paracentesis plus intravenous albumin (8 g/L of ascites removed). As maintenance, low-sodium diet (50 mEq/d) associated with diuretic therapy.
2. If the patient was not on diuretics before the development of large ascites, start with spironolactone (200 mg/d as single dose) with or without loop diuretics (furosemide 40 mg/d) and then adjust the dose to maintain the patient with mild or no ascites or edema. Check body weight and urine sodium regularly. Monitor the patient closely during the first weeks of therapy.
3. If the patient was on diuretics before the development of large ascites, start with a dose slightly higher than the dose taken before paracentesis.
4. If ascites and/or edema increase, check compliance with treatment and low-sodium diet. Increase the dose of diuretics stepwise every 7–10 d up to 400 mg/d of spironolactone and 160 mg/d of furosemide. A reduction in physical activity may be beneficial.
5. If ascites or edema does not recur, a balance should be maintained between sodium intake and diuretic therapy.

TABLE 75-9. *Therapeutic approach to management of patients with cirrhosis and refractory ascites*

1. Total paracentesis plus intravenous albumin (8 g/L of ascites removed).
2. Maintain a low-sodium diet (50 mEq/d) constantly. A more severe sodium restriction is difficult to tolerate.
3. Check urine sodium under diuretic therapy (either spironolactone 400 mg/d and furosemide 160 mg/d or the maximum dose that does not induce complications). If urine sodium under diuretics is lower than 10 mEq/L, diuretic therapy should probably be stopped.
4. Total paracentesis plus intravenous albumin when necessary.

edema. This contention was demonstrated in earlier studies (14,16) and is supported by the common clinical observation that the management of ascites is more difficult in patients with no compliance to the low-sodium diet compared with compliant patients. Noncompliant patients usually require higher doses of diuretics to achieve resolution of ascites and are more often readmitted to the hospital for recurrence of ascites. Surprisingly, however, several randomized comparative studies have not demonstrated an advantage of low-sodium diet as compared with an unrestricted sodium diet in the management of ascites (26,406,407). Nevertheless, it should be pointed out that in these studies most patients had mild sodium retention (urine sodium in the absence of diuretic therapy was close to sodium intake) and showed an excellent response to diuretic therapy (only less than 5% of patients did not respond to diuretics).

Therefore, on the basis of available data, it can be concluded that in patients with mild sodium retention a restriction of dietary sodium is probably not necessary because the hypothetical benefit of low-salt diet in the achievement of a negative sodium balance is overridden by the marked natriuretic effect of diuretics. By contrast, in patients with marked sodium retention, who usually have a less intense natriuretic response to diuretics compared with patients with moderate sodium retention, dietary sodium restriction (40 to 60 mEq of sodium/day) may facilitate the elimination of ascites and delay the reaccumulation of fluid after ascites has been removed. A more severe restriction of sodium (less than 40 mEq/day) is not recommended because it is not well accepted by patients and may impair their nutritional status.

Diuretics

Diuretics eliminate the excess of extracellular fluid present as ascites and edema by increasing renal sodium excretion, thus achieving a negative sodium balance (408). Diuretics most often administered to patients with cirrhosis and ascites are aldosterone antagonists, mainly spironolactone and potassium canrenoate. These drugs selectively antagonize the sodium-retaining effects of aldosterone in the renal collecting tubules, and loop diuretics, especially furosemide, that

inhibit the Na^+–K^+–$2Cl^-$ cotransporter in the loop of Henle (39,408).

Despite the use of diuretics in clinical practice for more than 30 years, only a few randomized studies have been reported that compare the efficacy of different diuretic agents in the treatment of ascites (37,39,409). In patients without renal failure, aldosterone antagonists are more effective than loop diuretics (37). This higher efficacy of aldosterone antagonists has also been demonstrated in several prospective, yet not comparative, investigations (26,36,38,267). Based on these findings, aldosterone antagonists are considered the diuretics of choice in the management of cirrhotic ascites.

In clinical practice, aldosterone antagonists are often given in combination with loop diuretics. Theoretical advantages of this combination include greater natriuretic potency, earlier onset of diuresis, and less tendency to induce hyperkalemia. Two different schedules of combined administration have been proposed. First, the dose of aldosterone antagonists is increased progressively (usually up to 400 mg per day of spironolactone) and loop diuretics (furosemide up to 160 mg per day) are added only if no response is achieved with the highest dose of aldosterone antagonists. Second, both drugs are given in combination from the start of therapy. Whether one of these two combined schedules has advantages over the other has not been assessed.

Diuretic therapy is effective in the elimination of ascites in 80% to 90% of the whole population of patients with ascites, a percentage that may increase up to 95% when only patients without renal failure are considered (26,36,38,267,409–414). The remaining patients either do not respond to diuretic therapy or develop diuretic-induced complications that prevent the use of high doses of these drugs. This condition is known as refractory ascites (102). Diagnostic criteria of refractory ascites are shown in Table 75-10. Complications of diuretic therapy in patients with cirrhosis include hepatic encephalopathy, hyponatremia, renal impairment, potassium disturbances, gynecomastia, and muscle cramps (39,415). The incidence of renal and electrolyte disorders and encephalopathy varies depending on the population of patients studied, being higher in patients with marked sodium retention and renal failure (who require higher doses of diuretics) and lower in patients with moderate sodium retention and without renal failure. Although some of these complications may be unrelated to diuretic therapy and due to the existence of an advanced liver disease (416), diuretics no doubt play a major pathogenic role in these complications because their frequency is markedly lower if ascites is removed by therapeutic paracentesis (410–414).

Because therapeutic paracentesis has substituted diuretics as the treatment of choice for hospitalized cirrhotic patients with large ascites in most centers (417,418), current indications for use of diuretics in cirrhosis include: (a) treatment of patients with mild or moderate ascites or those with large ascites in whom paracentesis is not effective because of compartmentalization of ascitic fluid due to peritoneal adhesions; (b) treatment of patients with edema without

TABLE 75-10. *Definition and diagnostic criteria of refractory ascites*

Diuretic-resistant ascites	Ascites that cannot be mobilized or the early recurrence of which cannot be prevented due to a lack of response to sodium restriction (50 mEq/d sodium diet) and diuretic treatment (mean loss of weight less than 200 g/d during the last 4 days of intensive diuretic therapy–spironolactone 400 mg/d and furosemide 160 mg/d–and urinary sodium excretion less than 50 mEq/d).
Diuretic-intractable ascites	Ascites that cannot be mobilized or the early recurrence of which cannot be prevented due to the development of diuretic-induced complications (see below) that preclude the use of an effective diuretic dosage.
Diuretic-induced complications	Diuretic-induced hepatic encephalopathy: development of hepatic encephalopathy in the absence of other precipitating factors.
	Diuretic-induced renal failure: increase in serum creatinine by greater than 100% to a value above 2 mg/dL in patients with ascites responding to diuretic treatment.
	Diuretic-induced hyponatremia: decrease in serum sodium concentration by greater than 10 mEq/L to a level lower than 125 mEq/L.
	Diuretic induced hypokalemia or hyperkalemia: decrease of serum potassium concentration to less than 3 mEq/L or increase to more than 6.0 mEq/L despite appropriate measures to normalize potassium levels.

ascites; and (c) prevention of ascites recurrence after therapeutic paracentesis.

Therapeutic Paracentesis

During the last decade, therapeutic paracentesis has progressively replaced diuretics as the treatment of choice in the management of patients with cirrhosis and large ascites in many centers (417,418). This change in treatment strategy is based on the results of several randomized studies comparing paracentesis (either removal of all ascitic fluid in a single tap or repeated taps of 4 to 6 L/day) associated with plasma volume expansion versus diuretics (410–414). Because paracentesis does not modify renal sodium retention, patients should receive diuretics after paracentesis to avoid reformation of ascites (419).

Two aspects concerning the use of therapeutic paracentesis in patients with cirrhosis and ascites deserve specific discussion, (a) the population of patients with cirrhosis in whom therapeutic paracentesis should be used, and (b) the use of plasma expanders to prevent disturbances in circulatory function after paracentesis. While most physicians consider that therapeutic paracentesis is the treatment of choice for all patients with large ascites (417,418), others believe that therapeutic paracentesis should be used only in patients with refractory ascites (420). Results obtained in randomized, comparative studies indicate that therapeutic paracentesis is faster and associated with lower incidence of side effects compared with diuretics (410–414). Moreover, therapeutic paracentesis has a better cost-effectiveness profile compared with diuretic treatment, which requires prolonged hospital stays. Therefore, on the basis of available data, it

seems clear that the use of therapeutic paracentesis should not be restricted to patients failing to respond to diuretics and should be considered the treatment of choice for all patients with large ascites.

The removal of large volumes of ascitic fluid is associated with a circulatory dysfunction characterized by a reduction of effective blood volume (83,421–427). Four lines of evidence indicate that this circulatory dysfunction and/or the mechanisms activated to maintain circulatory homeostasis have detrimental effects in cirrhotic patients. First, circulatory dysfunction after therapeutic paracentesis is associated with rapid reaccumulation of ascites (427). Second, approximately 20% of these patients develop irreversible renal failure and/or water retention leading to dilutional hyponatremia (83). Third, portal pressure increases in patients developing circulatory dysfunction after paracentesis, probably owing to an increased intrahepatic resistance due to the action of vasoconstrictor systems on the hepatic vascular bed (425). Finally, the development of circulatory dysfunction is associated with a shortened survival (427).

At present, the only effective method to prevent circulatory dysfunction is the administration of plasma expanders. Albumin is more effective than other plasma expanders (dextran-70, polygeline) probably owing to its longer persistence in the intravascular compartment (427). When less than 5 L of ascites are removed, dextran-70 or polygeline show a similar efficacy compared with albumin. However, albumin is more effective than these two artificial plasma expanders when more than 5 L of ascites are removed (427). Despite this greater efficacy, randomized comparative studies have not shown differences in survival of patients treated with albumin compared with those treated with other plasma expanders (427–430). Larger trials would be required to demonstrate that the protective effect of albumin on circulatory function results in a survival benefit.

Taken together, the currently available data indicate that circulatory dysfunction after therapeutic paracentesis is potentially harmful to patients with cirrhosis and should be prevented. Albumin appears to be the plasma expander of choice when more than 5 L of ascites are removed.

Peritoneovenous Shunt

Peritoneovenous shunting causes the passage of ascitic fluid from the peritoneal cavity to the systemic circulation, which results in the improvement of effective arterial blood volume with subsequent reduction in the activity of vasoconstrictor and antinatriuretic systems (23). These favorable hemodynamic effects result in an increase in sodium excretion and, to a lesser extent RBF and GFR, which facilitate the management of ascites in most patients (431). Comparative studies of peritoneovenous shunting and therapeutic paracentesis plus intravenous albumin in patients with refractory ascites have shown no differences in survival, but the probability of readmission to the hospital for ascites as well as the number of readmissions for ascites recurrence are markedly lower in patients treated by peritoneovenous shunting compared with those treated by therapeutic paracentesis (24,432). Unfortunately, the use of the shunt is associated with a number of important complications, including coagulopathy, bacterial infections, peritoneal fibrosis, or shunt obstruction, which limit its clinical applicability (433,434). Obstruction is the most common complication and may be located either within the valve or due to thrombosis of the superior vena cava. Obstruction is associated with recurrence of ascites and requires surgical intervention with replacement of the clotted shunt (435). Although peritoneovenous shunting is an effective therapy for refractory ascites, the high incidence of side effects and the existence of an alternative therapy (e.g., therapeutic paracentesis) has resulted in a marked decline in its use in most centers.

In patients with type 1 HRS, peritoneovenous shunting prevents the progression of renal failure but does not prolong survival compared with supportive therapy (436). For this reason, peritoneovenous shunting is not regularly used in the management of patients with HRS.

Transjugular Intrahepatic Portosystemic Shunts

The reduction in portal pressure by surgical portosystemic shunts, especially side-to-side portacaval shunts, is associated with increased sodium excretion, suppression of antinatriuretic systems, and elimination of ascites in patients with cirrhosis and refractory ascites (227,228). Nevertheless, despite these favorable effects, surgical portosystemic shunts have not become a standard therapy of refractory ascites or HRS because of high operative mortality and an exceedingly high risk of chronic encephalopathy.

The usefulness of portosystemic shunting in the management of ascites is currently being reevaluated due to the introduction of transjugular intrahepatic portosystemic shunts (TIPS), a nonsurgical method of portal decompression that acts as a side-to-side portacaval shunt and has the advantage over surgical shunts of an extremely low operative mortality (437). The most frequent complication of TIPS are hepatic encephalopathy and obstruction of the stent. The available information regarding the use of TIPS in patients with ascites derives from several uncontrolled studies and two randomized comparative studies (229,230,438–442). As with surgical portosystemic shunts, TIPS are associated with favorable effects on renal function, including an increase in sodium excretion and reduction in the activity of antinatriuretic systems, which result in the elimination of ascites in some patients and the decrease of diuretic requirements in others. The only two published randomized studies comparing TIPS versus therapeutic paracentesis plus intravenous albumin showed a better control of ascites in patients treated with TIPS, but discrepant findings with respect to survival. In one study (447), TIPS were associated with a significantly impaired survival, whereas opposite findings were reported in the other study (442). Preliminary results of a third randomized study show no differences in survival between the two treatment options (442b). Further randomized comparative studies in large series of patients are needed before the role of TIPS in the management of refractory ascites in cirrhosis can be clearly defined (443).

Recent studies indicate that TIPS may also be of value in the management of HRS, yet the information available is still limited (282,444). TIPS improve renal perfusion and GFR and reduce the activity of vasoconstrictor systems (282). In patients with type 2 HRS, most of whom have refractory ascites, the improvement of renal perfusion is associated with an increase in urinary sodium excretion and improved renal response to diuretics. In patients with type 1 HRS, the use of TIPS is associated with a moderate increase in RBF and GFR and a reduction in serum creatinine levels in some, but not all, patients (282,444). It is not known whether the improvement in renal function is associated with an increased survival. Because the use of TIPS is often associated with significant side effects, particularly hepatic encephalopathy and impairment of liver function, its role in the management of HRS needs to be established by prospective controlled investigations.

Aquaretic Drugs

As discussed previously, cirrhotic patients with ascites often develop water retention and dilutional hyponatremia. At present, patients with dilutional hyponatremia are only managed with water restriction because no effective pharmacologic therapy exists for this complication. Recently, however, two types of drugs have been developed that selectively increase renal water excretion, nonpeptide antagonists of the V2 receptor of AVP and selective κ-opioid agonists. Both agents induce a dose-dependent increase in urine flow and solute-free water excretion in normal animals as well as in healthy human patients (445,446). Their renal effects are different than those of classic natriuretic agents because the increase in urine volume is associated with only mild or no increase in sodium excretion. The increased water excretion following the administration of κ-opioid agonists is accounted for both inhibition of AVP release from the neurohypophysis and direct intrarenal effect, while V2 receptor antagonists act by selectively inhibiting the water-retaining effect of AVP in the renal tubules. Investigations in experimental as well as human cirrhosis with ascites have shown that both types of drugs increase solute-free water excretion and improve serum sodium concentration (87–93). Although not yet available for use in clinical practice, these compounds will likely offer a novel therapeutic approach for the treatment of water retention and dilutional hyponatremia in cirrhotic patients with ascites in the near future.

Vasoconstrictor Drugs

The administration of vasoconstrictors represents the most promising pharmacologic approach to therapy of HRS. These drugs have been used in an attempt to improve renal perfusion by increasing systemic vascular resistance and suppressing the activity of endogenous vasoconstrictors. Because arterial vasodilation in HRS is exclusively located in the splanchnic circulation, the ideal vasoconstrictor for patients with HRS would be a drug with a selective action in the splanchnic arteries with no effect on the extrasplanchnic circulation. Although such a vasoconstrictor is not available at present, the family of drugs that are closer to these requirements are the agonists of the vasopressin V1 receptors (analogs of vasopressin with a predominant action on the V1 receptors and less effect on the V2 receptors). Alpha-adrenergic agonists (e.g., norepinephrine, metaraminol, or midodrine) and agonists of the angiotensin AT1 receptors have been used without significant clinical benefits (447). By contrast, the administration of V1 receptor agonists, such as ornipressin or terlipressin, is associated with suppression of the activity of endogenous vasoconstrictor systems and marked improvement of renal perfusion and GFR and normalization of serum creatinine levels in most patients (Fig. 75-11) (247,248,448). Although the information about the use of V1 agonists in patients with HRS is still very limited and based only on a few phase II studies conducted in small series of patients, several preliminary conclusions can be drawn while awaiting results of large randomized studies. These include: (a) V1 agonists should be given for prolonged periods, usually 7 to 15 days, because the improvement of renal function occurs slowly—in patients in whom normalization of serum creatinine has been achieved, recurrence of HRS after discontinuation of therapy is uncommon; (b) the effective doses of V1 agonists have not been defined precisely and may vary from patient to patient—ornipressin has been given in continuous IV infusion at doses ranging from 1 to 6 IU per hour while terlipressin has been given as IV boluses from 0.5 to 2 mg per 4 hours;

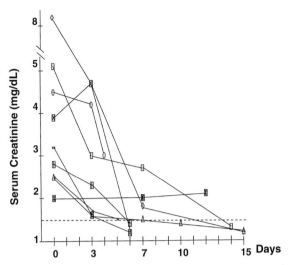

FIG. 75-11. Effects of administration of terlipressin (0.5 to 2 mg per 4 hours) IV and albumin (1 g per kg body weight at the initiation of treatment and 20 to 40 g per day thereafter) on serum creatinine in nine patients with cirrhosis and hepatorenal syndrome. From Uriz J, Ginès P, Cárdenas A, et al. Terlipressin plus albumin infusion: an effective and safe therapy of hepatorenal syndrome. *J Hepatol* 2000;33:43, with permission.)

(c) in some studies a concomitant administration of albumin has been used to further improve effective arterial blood volume; whether or not this maneuver increases the beneficial effects of these drugs on renal function is not known; (d) the incidence of important ischemic side effects requiring the withdrawal of the drug is high, especially with ornipressin; the ischemic complications appear to be less common in patients treated with terlipressin, which has a better safety profile than ornipressin; and the high frequency of ischemic complications should be weighed against the lack of alternative pharmacologic therapies for HRS; (e) the potential benefit of vasoconstrictor drugs on survival of patients with HRS has not been assessed and requires investigation in large placebo-controlled studies; and (f) because of limited information and relevant side effects, treatment with V1 agonists should probably be restricted at present to patients with type 1 HRS.

Liver Transplantation

Liver transplantation has become a frequent therapy for patients with cirrhosis and ascites. Although randomized studies comparing liver transplantation with conventional medical therapy in patients with ascites are obviously not available, the 70% to 80% 5-year probability of survival obtained in adult cirrhotic patients undergoing liver transplantation in most centers is markedly greater than the expected 20% survival probability for patients with cirrhosis and ascites who do not undergo transplantation (80,116–118).

Earlier recommendations suggested that ascites per se was not an indication for liver transplantation, and patients had to be considered for transplantation only when ascites was refractory to diuretic therapy or was associated with severe complications, such as spontaneous bacterial peritonitis or HRS. However, with these guidelines a large proportion of these patients die while on the waiting list for transplantation because of the short survival expectancy associated with these conditions (median survival time is less than 1 year for patients with refractory ascites and those recovering from spontaneous bacterial peritonitis and is even shorter for patients with HRS, particularly those with the progressive form of HRS type 1, who have a median survival time of less than 1 month) (13,24,432,449). With our growing knowledge on the natural history of ascites in cirrhosis, it is now understood that a number of factors can be used to predict survival accurately in these patients (50,80,450). The most useful predictive factors are related to abnormalities in renal function and systemic hemodynamics and include diuresis after a water load, arterial pressure, and serum creatinine and the intensity of liver failure, as assessed by the Child-Pugh score. By using these four variables, a prognostic model has been developed that allows us to estimate survival in individual patients (Table 75-11 and Fig. 75-12) (80). This prognostic model may be useful in the evaluation of patients for liver transplantation. The information provided may be of value in setting the priority for transplantation in countries in which this is decided by the severity of a patient's liver disease, or to propose a living donor liver transplantation in countries in which transplantation for patients with chronic liver disease is set by the time of entry on the waiting list and not by the severity of the disease.

Other Therapeutic Methods

Drugs with renal vasodilator activity have been used in patients with HRS in an attempt to counteract the effect of vasoconstrictor factors on the renal circulation. Dopamine was the first drug used owing to its renal vasodilatory effect when given in subpressor doses. Although there are isolated reports of reversal of HRS after dopamine administration, studies specifically assessing the effects of

TABLE 75-11. *The Barcelona prognostic model for predicting survival of cirrhosis with ascites. Survival time may be estimated from the prognostic index (Fig. 75-12)*

Variables[a]
Diuresis after water load (mL/min)[b]
Mean arterial pressure (mm Hg)
Child-Pugh class (B or C)[c]
Serum creatinine (mg/dL)

Prognostic index
$PI = -0.071 \times$ diuresis after water load[d] $-0.0178 \times$ mean arterial pressure[d] $+0.4738 \times$ Child-Pugh class (B=0; C=1) $+0.3433 \times$ serum creatinine[d]

[a]All variables should be obtained under low-sodium diet and without diuretic therapy.

[b]A water load of 20 mL/kg body weight of 5% dextrose IV is given for 45 min. Fifteen minutes later, urine is measured and then discarded. Immediately afterwards, urine is collected in three 30-min periods (in most cases without bladder catheter). The water load is kept constant throughout the whole study by infusing in each period an amount of 5% dextrose equal to the urine volume measured during the previous period. The final value given is the mean urine volume obtained in the three different periods. Normal values in healthy subjects are 14 ± 3 mL/min.

[c]The Child-Pugh class is calculated on the basis of the presence and degree of hepatic encephalopathy, the presence and degree of ascites, the serum bilirubin levels, the serum albumin level, and the prothrombin time.

[d]In mL/min.

dopamine on renal function in a series of patients with HRS have shown only minor effects—or no effects at all—on GFR (447). Despite its lack of efficacy, dopamine is still commonly used in clinical practice in patients with HRS. The second type of renal vasodilators used in patients with HRS are prostaglandins and prostaglandin analogs (447). The rationale for the use of prostaglandins was the belief that renal vasoconstriction in HRS could be due to reduced renal synthesis of prostaglandins. Unfortunately, however, no beneficial effects on renal function have been observed after the intravenous or intraarterial administration of PGE1 or PGE2 or the oral administration of the PGE1 analog misoprostol (447).

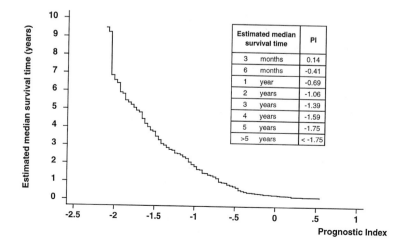

Estimated median survival time		PI
3	months	0.14
6	months	-0.41
1	year	-0.69
2	years	-1.06
3	years	-1.39
4	years	-1.59
5	years	-1.75
>5	years	< -1.75

FIG. 75-12. Assessment of prognosis of patients with cirrhosis and ascites. Estimated median survival time of patients with cirrhosis and ascites as a function of the prognostic index (PI) calculated using the following four prognostic parameters: diuresis after a water load, mean arterial pressure, intensity of liver failure (as assessed by the Child-Pugh score), and serum creatinine (Table 75-11). From Fernández-Esparrach G, Sánchez-Fueyo A, Ginès P, et al. A prognostic model for predicting survival in cirrhosis with ascites. *J Hepatol* 2001;34: 46, with permission.)

Plasma volume expansion with albumin or other plasma expanders has been used for many years in patients with ascites to improve renal function and facilitate elimination of ascites. However, the beneficial effects of plasma expansion are very modest, short-lived, and limited only to patients with slightly impaired renal function who respond to conventional therapy (421). Therefore, the available clinical evidence does not support its use for such indications. By contrast, a recent study showed that albumin infusion (1.5 g per kg body weight at the time of diagnosis of the infection and 1 g per kg 2 days later) is effective in preventing renal failure associated with spontaneous bacterial peritonitis, a condition known to cause an impairment of circulatory function in patients with cirrhosis and ascites (128). Moreover, albumin infusion improves survival in this setting.

Hemodialysis or peritoneal dialysis have been used in the management of patients with HRS, and sporadic cases of improvement of renal function have been reported (447). Unfortunately, there are no controlled studies evaluating the effectiveness of dialysis in HRS. Uncontrolled studies suggest that it is hardly effective because most patients die during treatment and there is a high incidence of severe side effects, including arterial hypotension, coagulopathy, and gastrointestinal bleeding. In some centers, hemodialysis is used to treat patients with HRS waiting for liver transplantation. The effectiveness of dialysis in this setting has not been appropriately studied. Continuous arteriovenous or venovenous hemofiltration have also been used but their efficacy also remains to be determined (447).

REFERENCES

1. Papper S. Liver–kidney interrelationships. A personal perspective. In: Epstein M, ed. *The kidney in liver disease*, 2nd ed. New York: Elsevier Biomedical, 1983:3.
2. Frerichs T. *Tratado práctico de las enfermedades del Hígado, de los vasos hepáticos y de las vías biliares*. Madrid: Librería Extranjera y Nacional, Científica y Literaria, 1877:362.
3. Flint A. Clinical report on hydro-peritoneum, based on an analysis of forty-six cases. *Am J Med Sci* 1863;45:306.
4. Papper S. The role of the kidney in Laënnec's cirrhosis of the liver. *Medicine (Baltimore)* 1958;37:299.
5. Papper S, Belsky JL, Bleifer KH. Renal failure in Laënnec's cirrhosis of the liver: I. Description of clinical and laboratory features. *Ann Intern Med* 1959;51:759.
6. Vesin P. Late functional renal failure in cirrhosis with ascites: pathophysiology, diagnosis and treatment. In: Martinin GA, Sherlock S, eds. *Aktuelle probleme der hepatologie*. Stuttgart: Georg Thieme Verlag, 1962;98.
7. Baldus WP, Feichter RN, Summerskill WHJ, et al. The kidney in cirrhosis. I. Clinical and biochemical features of azotemia in hepatic failure. *Ann Intern Med* 1964;60:353.
8. Shear L, Kleinerman J, Gabuzda GJ. Renal failure in patients with cirrhosis of the liver: I. Clinical and pathologic characteristics. *Am J Med* 1965;39:184.
9. Patek AJ Jr, Post J, Ratnoff OD, et al. Dietary treatment of cirrhosis of the liver. Results in one-hundred and twenty-four patients observed during a ten year period. *JAMA* 1948;138:543.
10. Post J, Sicam L. The clinical course of Laënnec's cirrhosis under modern medical management. *Med Clin North Am* 1960;44:639.
11. Pecikyan R, Kanzaki G, Berger EY. Electrolyte excretion during the spontaneous recovery from the ascitic phase of cirrhosis of the liver. *Am J Med* 1967;42:359.
12. Papper S. Hepatorenal syndrome. In: Epstein M, ed. *The kidney in liver disease*, 2nd ed. New York, Elsevier Biomedical, 1983;87.
13. Ginès A, Escorsell A, Ginès P, et al. Incidence, predictive factors, and prognosis of the hepatorenal syndrome in cirrhosis with ascites. *Gastroenterology* 1993;105:229.
14. Farnsworth EB, Krakusin JS. Electrolyte partition in patients with edema of various origins. *J Lab Clin Med* 1948;33:1545.
15. Falloon WW, Eckhardt RD, Cooper AM, et al. The effect of human serum albumin, mercurial diuretics, and a low sodium diet on sodium excretion in patients with cirrhosis of the liver. *J Clin Invest* 28:595–602, 1949.
16. Eisenmenger WJ, Blondheim SH, Bongiovanni AM, et al. Electrolyte studies on patients with cirrhosis of the liver. *J Clin Invest* 1950;29:1491.
17. Arroyo V, Rodés J. A rational approach to the treatment of ascites. *Postgrad Med J* 1975;51:558.
18. Levy M. Sodium retention in dogs with cirrhosis and ascites: efferent mechanisms. *Am J Physiol* 1977;233:F586.
19. Levy M, Allotey JB. Temporal relationships between urinary salt retention and altered systemic hemodynamics in dogs with experimental cirrhosis. *J Lab Clin Med* 1978;92:560.
20. López-Novoa JM, Rengel MA, Hernando L. Dynamics of ascites formation in rats with experimental cirrhosis. *Am J Physiol* 1980;238:F353.
21. Jiménez W, Martínez-Pardo A, Arroyo V, et al. Temporal relationship between hyperaldosteronism, sodium retention and ascites formation in rats with experimental cirrhosis. *Hepatology* 1985;5:245.
22. Gliedman ML, Carrol HJ, Popowitz L, et al. An experimental hepatorenal syndrome. *Surg Gynecol Obstet* 1970;131:34.
23. Blendis LM, Greig PD, Langer B, et al. The renal and hemodynamic effects of the peritoneovenous shunt for intractable hepatic ascites. *Gastroenterology* 1979;77:250.
24. Ginès P, Arroyo V, Vargas V, et al. Paracentesis with intravenous infusion of albumin as compared with peritoneovenous shunting in cirrhosis with refractory ascites. *N Engl J Med* 1991;325:829.
25. Ginès P, Arroyo V, Rodés J. Complications of cirrhosis: ascites, hyponatremia, hepatorenal syndrome and spontaneous bacterial peritonitis. In: Bacon D, DiBisceglie A, eds: *Liver disease: diagnosis and management*. Philadelphia: Churchill Livingstone, 2000;238.
26. Bernardi M, Laffi G, Salvagnini M, et al. Efficacy and safety of the stepped care medical treatment of ascites in liver cirrhosis: a randomized controlled clinical trial comparing two diets with different sodium content. *Liver* 1993;13:156.
27. Cardenas A, Bataller R, Arroyo V. Mechanisms of ascites formation. *Clin Liver Dis* 2000;4:447.
28. López-Novoa JM, Rengel MA, Rodicio JL, at al. A micropuncture study of salt and water retention in chronic experimental cirrhosis. *Am J Physiol* 1977;232:F315.
29. Clària J, Jiménez W. Renal dysfunction and ascites in carbon tetrachloride-induced cirrhosis in rats. In: Arroyo V, Ginès P, Rodés J, Schrier RW, eds. *Ascites and renal dysfunction in liver disease*. Malden, MA: Blackwell Science, 1999;379.
30. Chaimovitz C, Szylman P, Alroy G, et al. Mechanism of increased renal tubular sodium reabsorption in cirrhosis. *Am J Med* 1972;52:198.
31. Rochman J, Chaimovitz C, Szylman P, et al. Tubular handling of sodium and phosphate in cirrhosis with salt retention. *Nephron* 1978;20:95.
32. Wilkinson SP, Jowett TP, Slater JDH, et al. Renal sodium retention in cirrhosis: relation to aldosterone and nephron site. *Clin Sci* 1979;56:169.
33. Epstein M, Ramachandran M, DeNunzio AG. Interrelationship of renal sodium and phosphate handling in cirrhosis. *Miner Electrolyte Metab* 1982;7:305.
34. Angeli P, Gatta A, Caregaro L, et al. Tubular site of renal sodium retention in ascitic liver cirrhosis evaluated by lithium clearance. *Eur J Clin Invest* 1990;20:111.
35. Diez J, Simon MA, Anton F, et al. Tubular sodium handling in cirrhotic patients with ascites analysed by the renal lithium clearance method. *Eur J Clin Invest* 1990;20:266.
36. Eggert RC. Spironolactone diuresis in patients with cirrhosis and ascites. *Br Med J* 1970;4:401.
37. Pérez-Ayuso RM, Arroyo V, Planas R, et al. Randomized comparative study of efficacy of furosemide versus spironolactone in

nonazotemic cirrhosis with ascites. Relationship between the diuretic response and the activity of the renin-aldosterone system. *Gastroenterology* 1983;84:961.

38. Gatta A, Angeli P, Caregaro L, et al. A pathophysiological interpretation of unresponsiveness to spironolactone in a stepped-care approach to the diuretic treatment of ascites in nonazotemic cirrhotic patients. *Hepatology* 1991;14:231.

39. Angeli P, Gatta A. Medical treatment of ascites in cirrhosis. In: Arroyo V, Ginès P, Rodés J, Schrier RW, eds. *Ascites and renal dysfunction in liver disease*. Malden, MA: Blackwell Science, 1999:442.

40. Ginès P, Arroyo V, Rodés J. Pathophysiology, complications and treatment of ascites. *Clin Liver Dis* 1997;1:129.

41. Trevisani F, Bernardi M, Gasbarrini A, et al. Bed-rest-induced hypernatriuresis in cirrhotic patients without ascites: does it contribute to maintain "compensation"? *J Hepatol* 1992;116:190.

42. Ring-Larsen H, Henriksen JH, Wilken C, et al. Diuretic treatment in decompensated cirrhosis and congestive heart failure: effect of posture. *Br Med J* 1986;292:1351.

43. Lieberman FL, Hidemura R, Peters RL, et al. Pathogenesis and treatment of hydrothorax complicating cirrhosis with ascites. *Ann Intern Med* 1966;64:341.

44. Strauss RM, Boyer TD. Hepatic hydrothorax. *Semin Liver Dis* 1997;17:227.

45. Johnston RF, Loo RV. Hepatic hydrothorax. Studies to determine the source of the fluid and report of thirteen cases. *Ann Intern Med* 1964;611:385.

46. Xiol X, Castellví JM, Guardiola J, et al. Spontaneous bacterial empyema of cirrhotic patients: a prospective study. *Hepatology* 1996;23:719.

47. Shah A, Variyam E. Pericardial effusion and left ventricular dysfunction associated with ascites secondary to hepatic cirrhosis. *Arch Intern Med* 1991;151:186.

48. Arroyo V, Bosch J, Gaya J, et al. Plasma renin activity and urinary sodium excretion as prognostic indicators in nonazotemic cirrhosis with ascites. *Ann Intern Med* 1981;94:198.

49. Genoud E, Gonvers JJ, Schaller MD, et al. Valeur pronostique du système rénine-angiotensine dans la rèponse à la restriction sodée et le pronostic de l'ascite cirrhotique d'origine alcoolique. *Schweiz Med Wochenschr* 1986;116:463.

50. Llach J, Ginès P, Arroyo V, et al. Prognostic value of arterial pressure, endogenous vasoactive systems, and renal function in cirrhotic patients admitted to the hospital for the treatment of ascites. *Gastroenterology* 1988;94:482.

51. Denison EK, Lieberman FL, Reynolds TB. 9-fluorohydrocortisone induced ascites in alcoholic disease. *Gastroenterology* 1971;61:497.

52. La Villa G, Salmerón JM, Arroyo V, et al. Mineralocorticoid escape in patients with compensated cirrhosis and portal hypertension. *Gastroenterology* 1992;102:2114.

53. Papper S, Rosenbaum JD. Abnormalities in the excretion of water and sodium in "compensated" cirrhosis of the liver. *J Lab Clin Med* 1952;40:523.

54. Bosch J, Arroyo V, Rodès J. Hepatic and systemic hemodynamics and the renin–angiotensin–aldosterone system in cirrhosis. In: Epstein M, ed. *The kidney in liver disease*. New York, Elsevier Biomedical, 1983;286.

55. Lieberman FL, Reynolds TB. Plasma volume in cirrhosis of the liver: its relation to portal hypertension, ascites, and renal failure. *J Clin Invest* 1967;46:1297.

56. Bernardi M, Trevisani F, Santini C, et al. Aldosterone related blood volume expansion in cirrhosis before and after the early phase of ascites formation. *Gut* 1983;24:761.

57. Caregaro L, Lauro S, Angeli P, et al. Renal water and sodium handling in compensated liver cirrhosis: mechanism of the impaired natriuresis after saline loading. *Eur J Clin Invest* 1985;15:360.

58. Wood LJ, Massie D, McLean AJ, et al. Renal sodium retention in cirrhosis: tubular site and relation to hepatic dysfunction. *Hepatology* 1988;8:831.

59. Bernardi M, Di Marco C, Trevisani F, et al. Renal sodium retention during upright posture in preascitic cirrhosis. *Gastroenterology* 1993;105:188.

60. Bernardi M, Di Marco C, Trevisani F, et al. The hemodynamic status of preascitic cirrhosis: an evaluation under steady-state conditions and after postural change. *Hepatology* 1992;16:341.

61. Wong F, Massie D, Hsu P, et al. Renal response to a saline load in well-compensated alcoholic cirrhosis. *Hepatology* 1994;20:873.

62. Simon MA, Diez J, Prieto J. Abnormal sympathetic and renal response to sodium restriction in compensated cirrhosis. *Gastroenterology* 1991;101:1354.

63. Trevisani F, Colantoni A, Sica G, et al. High plasma levels of atrial natriuretic peptide in preascitic cirrhosis: indirect evidence of reduced natriuretic effectiveness of the peptide. *Hepatology* 1995;22:132.

64. Wong F, Liu P, Allidina Y, et al. Pattern of sodium handling and its consequences in patients with preascitic cirrhosis. *Gastroenterology* 1995;108:1820.

65. Naccarato R, Messa P, D'Angelo A, et al. Renal handling of sodium and water in early chronic liver disease. Evidence for a reduced natriuretic activity of the cirrhotic urinary extracts in rats. *Gastroenterology* 1981;81:205.

66. Warner LC, Campbell PJ, Morali G, et al. The response of atrial natriuretic factor (ANF) and sodium excretion to dietary sodium challenges in patients with chronic liver disease. *Hepatology* 1990;12:460.

67. Daskalopoulos G, Kronborg I, Katkov W, et al. Sulindac and indomethacin suppress the diuretic action of furosemide in patients with cirrhosis and ascites: evidence that sulindac affects renal prostaglandins. *Am J Kidney Dis* 1985;16:217.

68. Albillos A, Lledo JL, Rossi I, et al. Continuous prazosin administration in cirrhotic patients: effects on portal hemodynamics and liver and renal function. *Gastroenterology* 1995;109:1257.

69. Vorobioff J, Picabea E, Gamen M, et al. Propranolol compared with propranolol plus isosorbide dinitrate in portal-hypertensive patients: long-term hemodynamic and renal effects. *Hepatology* 1993;18:477.

70. Henriksen JH, Ring-Larsen H. Renal effects of drugs used in the treatment of portal hypertension. *Hepatology* 1993;18:688.

71. Salmerón JM, Ruiz del Arbol L, Ginès A, et al. Renal effects of acute isosorbide-5-mononitrate administration in cirrhosis. *Hepatology* 1993;17:800.

72. Papper S, Saxon L. The diuretic response to administered water in patients with liver disease. II. Laënnec's cirrhosis of the liver. *Arch Intern Med* 1959;103:750.

73. Shear L, Hall PW, Gabuzda GJ. Renal failure in patients with cirrhosis of the liver. II. Factors influencing maximal urinary flow rate. *Am J Med* 1966;39:199.

74. Arroyo V, Rodés J, Gutiérrez-Lizárraga MA, et al. Prognostic value of spontaneous hyponatremia in cirrhosis with ascites. *Am J Dig Dis* 1976;21:249.

75. McCullough AJ, Mullen KD, Kalhan SC. Measurements of total body and extracellular water in cirrhotic patients with and without ascites. *Hepatology* 1991;14:1103.

76. Vaamonde CA. Renal water handling in liver disease. In: Epstein M, ed. *The kidney in liver disease*, 4th ed. Philadelphia: Hanley & Belfus, 1996:33.

77. Cosby RL, Yee B, Schrier RW. New classification with prognostic value in cirrhotic patients. *Miner Electrolyte Metab* 1989;15:261.

78. Abad-Lacruz A, Cabré E, González-Huix F, et al. Routine tests of renal function, alcoholism, and nutrition improve the prognostic accuracy of Child-Pugh score in nonbleeding advanced cirrhosis. *Am J Gastroenterol* 1993;88:382.

79. Salerno F, Borroni G, Moser P, et al. Survival and prognostic factors of cirrhotic patients with ascites: a study of 134 outpatients. *Am J Gastroenterol* 1993;88:514.

80. Fernández-Esparrach G, Sánchez-Fueyo A, Ginès P, et al. A prognostic model for predicting survival in cirrhosis with ascites. *J Hepatol* 2001;34:46.

81. Boyer TD, Zia P, Reynolds TB. Effect of indomethacin and prostaglandin A1 on renal function and plasma renin activity in alcoholic liver disease. *Gastroenterology* 1979;215.

82. Ginès P, Jiménez W. Aquaretic agents: a new potential treatment of dilutional hyponatremia in cirrhosis. *J Hepatol* 1996;24:506.

83. Ginès P, Titó Ll, Arroyo V, et al. Randomized comparative study of therapeutic paracentesis with and without intravenous albumin in cirrhosis. *Gastroenterology* 1988;94:1493.

84. Ginès P, Abraham W, Schrier RW. Vasopressin in pathophysiological states. *Semin Nephrol* 1994;14:384.

85. Ginès P, Berl T, Bernardi M, et al. Hyponatremia in cirrhosis: from pathogenesis to treatment. *Hepatology* 1998;28:851.

86. Ishikawa SE, Schrier RW. Arginine Vasopressin in cirrhosis. In: Arroyo V, Ginès P, Rodés J, Schrier RW, eds. *Ascites and renal dysfunction in liver disease*. Malden, MA: Blackwell Science, 1999:220.

87. Tsuboi Y, Ishikawa SE, Fujisawa G, et al. Therapeutic efficacy of the non-peptide AVP antagonist OPC-31260 in cirrhotic rats. *Kidney Int* 1994;46:237.

88. Bosch- Marcé M, Poo JL, Jiménez W, et al. Comparison of two aquaretic drugs (niravoline and OPC-31260) in cirrhotic rats with ascites and water retention. *J Pharmacol Exp Ther* 1999;289:194.

89. Inoue T, Ohnishi A, Matsuo A, et al. Therapeutic and diagnostic potential of a vasopressin-2 antagonist for impaired water handling in cirrhosis. *Clin Pharmacol Ther* 1998;63:561.

90. Guyader MD, Ellis-Grosse EJ, Burke JT, et al. Dynamic effects of a novel, non-peptide ADH (V2) antagonist in cirrhotic patients with ascites. *Hepatology* 1998;28:1587A.

91. Bosch-Marcé M, Jiménez W, Angeli P, et al. Aquaretic effect of the k-opioid agonist RU 51599 in cirrhotic rats with ascites and water retention. *Gastroenterology* 1995;109:217.

92. Gadano A, Moreau R, Pessione F, et al. Aquaretic effects of niravoline, a kappa-opioid agonist, in patients with cirrhosis. *J Hepatol* 2000; 32:38.

93. Gerbes AL, Guelberg V, Decaux G, et al. VPA-985, an orally active vasopressin receptor antagonist improves hyponatremia in patients with cirrhosis. A double-blind placebo controlled multicenter trial. *Hepatology* 1999;30:1033A.

94. Jiménez W, Serradeil-Le Gal C, Ros J, et al. Long-term aquaretic efficacy of a selective non-peptide V2-vasopressin receptor antagonist in cirrhotic rats. *J Pharm Exp Ther* 2000;295:83.

95. Schroeder ET, Shear L, Sancetta SM, et al. Renal failure in patients with cirrhosis of the liver. Evaluation of intrarenal blood flow by para-aminohippurate extraction and response to angiotensin. *Am J Med* 1967;43:887.

96. Epstein M, Berck DP, Hollemberg NK, et al. Renal failure in the patient with cirrhosis. The role of active vasoconstriction. *Am J Med* 1970;49:175.

97. Hecker R, Sherlock S. Electrolyte and circulatory changes in terminal liver failure. *Lancet* 1956;2:1121.

98. Ginès P, Fernández-Esparrach G, Arroyo V, et al. Pathogenesis of ascites in cirrhosis. *Semin Liver Dis* 1997;17:175.

99. Ring-Larsen H. Renal blood flow in cirrhosis: relation to systemic and portal hemodynamics and liver function. *Scand J Clin Lab Invest* 1977;37:635.

100. Arroyo V, Bosch J, Mauri M, et al. Renin, aldosterone and renal hemodynamics in cirrhosis with ascites. *Eur J Clin Invest* 1979;9:69.

101. Rimola A, Ginès P, Arroyo V, et al. Urinary excretion of 6-keto-prostaglandin F1α, thromboxane B2 and prostaglandin E2 in cirrhosis with ascites. Relationship to functional renal failure (hepatorenal syndrome). *J Hepatol* 1986;3:111.

102. Arroyo V, Ginès P, Gerbes A, et al. Definition and diagnostic criteria of refractory ascites and hepatorenal syndrome in cirrhosis. *Hepatology* 1996;23:164.

103. Platt JF, Ellis JH, Rubin JM, et al. Renal duplex Doppler ultrasonography: a noninvasive predictor of kidney dysfunction and hepatorenal failure in liver disease. *Hepatology* 1994;20:362.

104. Wilkinson SP, Blendis LM, Williams R: Frequency and type of renal and electrolyte disorders in fulminant hepatic failure. *Br Med J* 1974;1:186.

105. Bataller R, Ginès P, Guevara M, Arroyo V. Hepatorenal syndrome. *Semin Liver Dis* 1997;17:233.

106. Ginès P, Rodés J. Clinical disorders of renal function in cirrhosis with ascites. In: Arroyo V, Ginès P, Rodés J, Schrier RW, eds. *Ascites and renal dysfunction in liver disease. Pathogenesis, diagnosis, and treatment*. Malden, MA: Blackwell Science, 1999:36.

107. Lancestremere RG, Davidson PL, Earley LE, et al. Renal failure in Laënnec's cirrhosis. II. Simultaneous determination of cardiac output and renal hemodynamics. *J Clin Invest* 1962;41:1922.

108. Epstein M. Renal sodium handling in liver disease. In: Epstein M, ed. *The kidney in liver disease*, 4th ed. Philadelphia: Hanley & Belfus, 1996:1.

109. Kew MC, Brunt PW, Varma RR, et al. Renal and intrarenal blood-flow in cirrhosis of the liver. *Lancet* 1971;2:504.

110. Sacerdoti D, Merlo A, Merkel C, et al. Redistribution of renal blood flow in patients with liver cirrhosis. The role of renal PGE2. *J Hepatol* 1986;2:253.

111. Platt JF, Marn CS, Baliga PK, et al. Renal dysfunction in hepatic disease: early identification with renal duplex Doppler US in patients who undergo liver transplantation. *Radiology* 1992;183:801.

112. Maroto A, Ginès A, Saló J, et al. Diagnosis of functional renal failure of cirrhosis by Doppler sonography. Prognostic value of resistive index. *Hepatology* 1994;20:839.

113. Lieberman FL. Functional renal failure in cirrhosis. *Gastroenterology* 1970;58:108.

114. Iwatsuki S, Popovtzer MM, Corman JL, et al. Recovery from "hepatorenal syndrome" after orthotopic liver transplantation. *N Engl J Med* 1973;289:1155.

115. Rimola A, Gavaler J, Schade RR, et al. Effects of renal impairment on liver transplantation. *Gastroenterology* 1987;93:148.

116. Gonwa TA, Morris CA, Goldstein RM, et al. Long-term survival and renal function following liver transplantation in patients with and without hepatorenal syndrome—experience in 300 patients. *Transplantation* 1991;51:428.

117. Gonwa TA, Wilkinson AH. Liver transplantation and renal function: results in patients with and without hepatorenal syndrome. In: Epstein M, ed. *The kidney in liver disease*, 4th ed. Philadelphia: Hanley & Belfus, 1996:529.

118. Rimola A, Navasa M, Grande L. Liver transplantation in cirrhotic patients with ascites. In: Arroyo V, Ginès P, Rodés J, Schrier RW, eds. *Ascites and renal dysfunction in liver disease. Pathogenesis, diagnosis, and treatment*. Malden, MA: Blackwell Science, 1999:522.

119. Fernández-Seara J, Prieto J, Quiroga J, et al. Systemic and regional hemodynamics in patients with liver cirrhosis and ascites with and without functional renal failure. *Gastroenterology* 1989;97:1304.

120. Maroto A, Ginès P, Arroyo V, et al. Brachial and femoral artery blood flow in cirrhosis: relationship to kidney dysfunction. *Hepatology* 1993;17:788.

121. Guevara M, Bru C, Ginès P, et al. Increased cerebral vascular resistance in cirrhotic patients with ascites. *Hepatology* 1998;28:39.

122. Papadakis MA, Arieff AI. Unpredictability of clinical evaluation of renal function in cirrhosis: a prospective study. *Am J Med* 1987;82:945.

123. Caregaro L, Menon F, Angeli P, et al. Limitations of serum creatinine level and creatinine clearance as filtration markers in cirrhosis. *Arch Intern Med* 1994;154:201.

124. Papper S. Hepatorenal syndrome. In: Epstein M, ed. *The kidney in liver disease*. New York: Elsevier Biomedical, 1978:91.

125. Dudley FJ, Kanel GC, Wood LJ, et al. Hepatorenal syndrome without sodium retention. *Hepatology* 1986;6:248.

126. Follo A, Llovet JM, Navasa M, et al. Renal impairment after spontaneous bacterial peritonitis in cirrhosis: incidence, clinical course, predictive factors and prognosis. *Hepatology* 1994;20;1495.

127. Navasa M, Follo A, Filella X, et al. Tumor necrosis factor and interleukin-6 in spontaneous bacterial peritonitis in cirrhosis: relationship with the development of renal impairment and mortality. *Hepatology* 1998;27:1227.

128. Sort P, Navasa M, Arroyo V, et al. Effect of intravenous albumin on renal impairment and mortality in patients with cirrhosis and spontaneous bacterial peritonitis. *N Engl J Med* 1999;5:403.

129. Ginès P, Arroyo V, Rodés J. Ascites, hepatorenal syndrome, and spontaneous bacterial peritonitis. In: McDonald J, Burroughs AK, Feagan B, eds. *Evidence based gastroenterology and hepatology*. London: BMJ Books, 1999:427.

130. Cardenas A, Ginès P, Uriz J, et al. Renal failure after gastrointestinal bleeding in cirrhosis: Incidence, characteristics, predictive factors and prognosis. *Hepatology* 2000;32:1463A.

131. Salerno F, Badalamenti S. Drug-induced renal failure in cirrhosis. In: Arroyo V, Ginès P, Rodés J, Schrier RW, eds. *Ascites and renal dysfunction in liver disease. Pathogenesis, diagnosis, and treatment*. Malden, MA: Blackwell Science, 1999:511.

132. Quintero E, Ginès P, Arroyo V, et al. Sulindac reduces the urinary excretion of prostaglandins and impairs renal function in cirrhosis with ascites. *Nephron* 1986;42:298.

133. Cabrera J, Arrroyo V, Ballesta AM, et al. Aminoglycoside nephrotoxicity in cirrhosis. Value of urinary beta-2 microglobulin to discriminate functional renal failure from acute tubular damage. *Gastroenterology* 1982;82:97.

134. Moore RD, Smith CR, Lietman PS. Increased risk of renal dysfunction due to interaction of liver disease and aminoglycosides. *Am J Med* 1986;80:1093.

135. Lietman PS. Liver disease, aminoglycoside antibiotics and renal dysfunction. *Hepatology* 1988;8:966.
136. McCormick PA, Greensdale L, Kibbler CC, et al. A prospective randomized trial of ceftazidime versus netilmicin plus mezlocillin in the empiric therapy of presumed sepsis in cirrhosis. *Hepatology* 1997;25:833.
137. Eknoyan G. Glomerular abnormalities in liver disease. In Epstein M, ed. *The kidney in liver disease*, 4th ed. Hanley & Belfus, 1996:123.
138. Raphael SS, Lynch MJG. Kimmelstiel-Wilson glomerulonephropathy: its occurrence in diseases other than diabetes mellitus. *Arch Pathol* 1958;65:420.
139. Bloodworth JMB, Sommers SC. "Cirrhotic glomerulosclerosis", a renal lesion associated with hepatic cirrhosis. *Lab Invest* 1959;8:962.
140. Willson RA. Extrahepatic manifestations of chronic viral hepatitis. *Am J Gastroenterol* 1997;92:4.
141. Levy M, Chen N. Worldwide perspective of hepatitis B-associated glomerulonephritis in the 80's. *Kidney Int* 1991;40[Suppl 35]:S24.
142. Stehman-Breen C, Johnson R. Hepatitis C virus-associated glomerulonephritis. *Adv Int Med* 1998;43:79.
143. Yamabe H, Johnson R, Gretch D, et al. Hepatitis C virus infection and membranoproliferative glomerulonephritis in Japan. *J Am Soc Nephrol* 1995;6:220.
144. Crawford DHG, Endre ZH, Axelsen RA, et al. Universal occurrence of glomerular abnormalities in patients receiving liver transplants. *Am J Kidney Dis* 1992;19:339.
145. Daghestani L, Pomeroy C. Renal manifestations of hepatitis C infection. *Am J Med* 1999;106:347.
146. D'Amico G. Renal involvement in hepatitis C infection: cryoglobulinemic glomerulonephritis. *Kidney Int* 1998;54:650.
147. Agnello V, Chung R, Kaplan L. A role for hepatitis C virus infection in type II cryoglobulinemia. *N Engl J Med* 1992;327:1490.
148. Lunel F, Musset L. Hepatitis C virus infection and cryoglobulinemia. *J Hepatol* 1998;29:848.
149. Agnello V. Hepatitis C virus infection and type II cryoglobulinemia: an immunological perspective. *Hepatology* 1997;26:1375.
150. Johnson RJ, Gretch DR, Yamabe H, et al. Membranoproliferative glomerulonephritis associated with hepatitis C virus infection. *N Engl J Med* 1993;328:465.
151. Johnson R, Willson R, Yamabe H, et al. Renal manifestations of hepatitis C virus infection. *Kidney Int* 1994;46:1255.
152. Harle D, Disder P, Dussol B, et al. Membranoproliferative glomerulonephritis and hepatitis C. *Lancet* 1993;341:904.
153. Itoh K, Tanaka K, Shiga J, et al. Hypocomplementemia associated with hepatitis C viremia in sera from voluntary donors. *Am J Gastroenterol* 1994;89:2019.
154. Johnson R, Couser WG. Hepatitis B infection and renal disease: clinical, immunopathogenic and therapeutic considerations. *Kidney Int* 1990;37:663.
155. Venkataseshan V, Lieberman K, Kim D, et al. Hepatitis B-associated glomerulonephritis: pathology, pathogenesis and clinical course. *Medicine* 1990;69:200.
156. Callard P, Feldman G, Prandi D, et al. Immune complex type glomerulonephritis in cirrhosis of the liver. *Am J Path* 1975;80:329.
157. Newell GC. Cirrhotic glomerulonephritis: incidence, morphology, clinical features and pathogenesis. *Am J Kidney Dis* 1987;9:183.
158. Berger J, Yaneva H, Nabarra B. Glomerular changes in patients with cirrhosis of the liver. *Adv Nephrol* 1978;7:3.
159. Morzycka M, Slosarczyk J. Kidney glomerular pathology in various forms of acute and chronic hepatitis. *Arch Pathol Lab Med* 1979;103:38.
160. Rimola A, Soto J, Bory F, et al. Reticuloendothelial system phagocytic activity in cirrhosis and its relation to bacterial infections and prognosis. *Hepatology* 1984;4:53.
161. Johnson R, Gretch D, Couser W, et al. Hepatitis C virus-associated glomerulonephritis. Effect of alpha-interferon therapy. *Kidney Int* 1994;46:1700.
162. Misiani R, Bellavita P, Domenico F, et al. Interferon alfa-2a therapy in cryoglobulinemia associated with hepatitis C virus. *N Engl J Med* 1994;330:751.
163. Yamabe H, Johnson R, Gretch D, et al. Membranoproliferative glomerulonephritis associated with hepatitis C virus infection responsive to interferon-alpha. *Am J Kidney Dis* 1995;25:67.
164. DeVecchi A, Montagnino G, Pozzi C, et al. Intravenous methylprednisolone pulse therapy in essential mixed cryoglobulinemia nephropathy. *Clin Nephrol* 1983;19:221.
165. Garcia G, Scullard G, Smith C, et al. Preliminary observation of hepatitis B-associated membranous glomerulonephritis treated with leucocyte interferon. *Hepatology* 1985;5:317.
166. Mizushima N, Kanai K, Matsuda H, et al. Improvement of proteinuria in a case of hepatitis B glomerulonephritis after treatment with interferon. *Gastroenterology* 1987;92:524.
167. De Man RA, Schalm SW, van der Heijden AJ, et al. Improvement of hepatitis B associated glomerulonephritis after antiviral combination therapy. *J Hepatol* 1989;8:367.
168. Lisker-Melman M, Webb D, Di Bisceglie AM, et al. Glomerulonephritis caused by chronic hepatitis B virus infection: treatment with recombinant human alpha-interferon. *Ann Intern Med* 1989;111:479.
169. Conjeevaran HS, Hoofnagle JH, Austin HA, et al. Long-term outcome of hepatitis B virus-related glomerulonephritis after therapy with interferon alpha. *Gastroenterology* 1995;109:540.
170. Ghabra M, Priano B, Greenberg A, et al. Resolution of cirrhotic glomerulonephritis following successful liver transplantation. *Clin Nephrol* 1991;35:6.
171. Oster JR, Hotchkiss JL, Carbon M, et al. Abnormal renal acidification in alcoholic liver disease. *J Lab Clin Med* 1975;85:987.
172. Golding PL. Renal tubular acidosis in chronic liver disease. *Postgrad Med J* 1975;51:550.
173. Charmes JP, Nicot G, Valette JP, et al. Acidose tubulaire renale latente du cirrhotique. *Nouv Presse Med* 1976;28:1731.
174. Parés A, Rimola A, Bruguera M, et al. Renal tubular acidosis in primary biliary cirrhosis. *Gastroenterology* 1981;80:681.
175. Puig JG, Anton FM, Gómez HE, et al. Complete proximal tubular acidosis (type 2, RTA) in chronic active hepatitis. *Clin Nephrol* 1980;13:287.
176. Caregaro L, Lauro S, Ricci B, et al. Distal renal tubular acidosis in hepatic cirrhosis: clinical and pathogenic study. *Clin Nephrol* 1981;15:143.
177. Shear L, Bonkowsky HL, Gabuzda GL. Renal tubular acidosis in cirrhosis. A determinant of susceptibility to recurrent hepatic precoma. *N Engl J Med* 1969;280:1.
178. Oster JR, Perez G. Acid-base homeostasis and pathophysiology in liver disease. In Epstein M, ed. *The kidney in liver disease*, 3rd ed. Baltimore: Williams & Wilkins, 1988:119.
179. Arroyo V, Ginès P, Rimola A, et al. Renal function abnormalities, prostaglandins, and effects of nonsteroidal anti-inflammatory drugs in cirrhosis with ascites. An overview with emphasis on pathogenesis. *Am J Med* 1986;81:104.
180. Arroyo V, Planas R, Gaya J, et al. Sympathetic nervous activity, renin–angiotensin system and renal excretion of prostaglandin E2 in cirrhosis. Relationship to functional renal failure and sodium and water excretion. *Eur J Clin Invest* 1983;13:271.
181. Zipser RD, Hoefs JC, Speckart PF, et al. Prostaglandins: modulators of renal function and pressor resistance in chronic liver disease. *J Clin Endocrinol Metab* 1979;48:895.
182. Laffi G, La Villa G, Pinzani M, et al. Lipid derived autacoids and renal function in liver cirrhosis. In: Epstein M, ed. *The kidney in liver disease*, 4th ed. Philadelphia: Hanley & Belfus, 1996:307.
183. Mirouze D, Zipser RD, Reynolds TB. Effect of inhibitors of prostaglandin synthesis on induced diuresis in cirrhosis. *Hepatology* 1983;3:50.
184. Planas R, Arroyo V, Rimola A, et al. Acetylsalicylic acid suppresses the renal hemodynamic effect and reduces the diuretic action of furosemide in cirrhosis with ascites. *Gastroenterology* 1983;84:247.
185. Wong F, Massie D, Hsu P, et al. Indomethacin-induced renal dysfunction in patients with well-compensated cirrhosis. *Gastroenterology* 1993;104:869.
186. Pérez-Ayuso RM, Arroyo V, Camps J, et al. Evidence that renal prostaglandins are involved in renal water metabolism in cirrhosis. *Kidney Int* 1986;26:72.
187. Antillon M, Cominelli F, Reynolds TB, et al. Comparative acute effects of diflunisal and indomethacin on renal function in patients with cirrhosis and ascites. *Am J Gastroenterol* 1989;84:153.
188. Salerno F, Lorenzano E, Maggi A, et al. Effects of imidazole-salicylate on renal function and the diuretic action of furosemide in cirrhotic patients with ascites. *J Hepatol* 1993;19:279.

189. Bosch-Marce M, Claria J, Titos E, et al. Selective inhibition of cyclooxygenase 2 spares renal function and prostaglandin synthesis in cirrhotic rats with ascites. *Gastroenterology* 1999;116:1167.

190. Moore RD, Smith CR, Petty BG, et al. Cephalotin plus an aminoglycoside is more nephrotoxic than methicillin plus an aminoglycoside. *Lancet* 1978;2:604.

191. Moore RD, Smith CR, Lipsky JJ, et al. Risk factors for nephrotoxicity in patients treated with aminoglycosides. *Ann Intern Med* 1984;100:352.

192. Felisart J, Rimola A, Arroyo V, et al. Cefotaxime is more effective than is ampicillin–tobramycin in cirrhotics with severe infections. *Hepatology* 1985;5:457.

193. Ginès P, Arroyo V, Rodés J. Pharmacotherapy of ascites associated with cirrhosis. *Drugs* 1992;43:316.

194. Ginès P, Arroyo V, Quintero E, et al. Comparison between paracentesis and diuretics in the treatment of cirrhotics with tense ascites. Results of a randomized study. *Gastroenterology* 1987;93:234.

195. Sherlock S, Senewiratne B, Scott A, et al. Complications of diuretic therapy in hepatic cirrhosis. *Lancet* 1966;1:1049.

196. Strauss E, De Sa MF, Lacet CM, et al. Standardization of a therapeutic approach for ascites due to chronic liver disease: a prospective study of 100 cases. *GED* 1985;4:79.

197. Rodés J, Bosch J, Arroyo V. Clinical types and drug therapy of renal impairment in cirrhosis. *Postgrad Med J* 1975;55:492.

198. Shear L, Ching S, Gabuzda GI. Compartmentalization of ascites and edema in patients with hepatic cirrhosis. *N Engl J Med* 1970;282:1391.

199. Pockros PJ, Reynolds TB. Rapid diuresis in patients with ascites from chronic liver disease: the importance of peripheral edema. *Gastroenterology* 1986;90:1827.

200. Forns X, Ginès A, Ginès P, et al. Management of ascites and renal failure in cirrhosis. *Semin Liver Dis* 1994;14:82.

201. Blei AT, Garcia-Tsao G, Groszmann RJ, et al. Hemodynamic evaluation of isosorbide dinitrate in alcoholic cirrhosis. Pharmacokinetic–hemodynamic interactions. *Gastroenterology* 1987;93:576.

202. Navasa M, Chesta J, Bosch J, et al. Reduction of portal pressure by isosorbide-5-mononitrate in patients with cirrhosis. Effects on splanchnic and systemic hemodynamics and liver function. *Gastroenterology* 1989;96:1110.

203. García-Pagán JC, Feu F, Navasa M, et al. Long-term haemodynamic effects of isosorbide 5-mononitrate in patients with cirrhosis and portal hypertension. *J Hepatol* 1990;11:189.

204. Bosch J, García-Pagán JC. Complications of cirrhosis. Portal hypertension. *J Hepatol* 2000;32[Suppl 1]:141.

205. Groszmann RJ. Beta-adrenergic blockers and nitrovasodilators for the treatment of portal hypertension: the good, the bad, the ugly. *Gastroenterology* 1997;113:1794.

206. García-Pagán JC, Escorsell A, Moitinho E, et al. Influence of pharmacological agents on portal hemodynamics: basis for its use in the treatment of portal hypertension. *Semin Liver Dis* 1999;19:427.

207. García-Pagán JC, Feu F, Bosch J, et al. Propranolol compared with propranolol plus isosorbide-5-mononitrate for portal hypertension in cirrhosis. A randomized controlled study. *Ann Intern Med* 1991;114:869.

208. Morillas RM, Planas R, Cabré E, et al. Propranolol plus isosorbide-5-mononitrate for portal hypertension in cirrhosis: long-term hemodynamic and renal effects. *Hepatology* 1994;20:1502.

209. García-Pagán JC, Bosch J. The splanchnic circulation in cirrhosis. In: Arroyo V, Ginès P, Rodés J, et al, eds. *Ascites and renal dysfunction in liver disease.* Malden, MA: Blackwell Science, 1999:330.

210. Scaffner F, Popper H. Capillarization of hepatic sinusoids in man. *Gastroenterology* 1963;44:239.

211. Orrego H, Medline A, Blendis LM, et al. Collagenisation of the Disse space in alcoholic liver disease. *Gut* 1979;20:673.

212. Bhathal PS, Grossman HJ. Reduction of the increased portal vascular resistance of the isolated perfused cirrhotic rat liver by vasodilators. *J Hepatol* 1985;1:325.

213. Rockey DC. New concepts in the pathogenesis of portal hypertension: hepatic wounding and stellate cell contractility. *Clin Liver Dis* 1997;1:13.

214. Bataller R, Nicolás JM, Ginès P, et al. Contraction of human hepatic stellate cells activated in culture: a role for voltage-operated calcium channels. *J Hepatol* 1998;29:398.

215. Bataller R, Ginès P, Nicolás JM, et al. Angiotensin II induces contraction and proliferation of human hepatic stellate cells *Gastroenterology* 2000;118:1149.

216. Görbig MN, Ginès P, Bataller R, et al. Atrial natriuretic peptide antagonizes endothelin-induced calcium increase and cell contraction in cultured human hepatic stellate cells. *Hepatology* 1999;30:501.

217. Gupta K, Toruner M, Chung MK, et al. Endothelial dysfunction and decreased production of nitric oxide in the intrahepatic microcirculation of cirrhotic rats. *Hepatology* 1998;28:926.

218. Wiest R, Groszmann RJ. Nitric oxide and portal hypertension: its role in the regulation of intrahepatic and splanchnic vascular resistance. *Semin Liver Dis* 1999;19:411.

219. Benoit JN, Granger DN. Splanchnic hemodynamics in chronic portal hypertension. *Semin Liver Dis* 1986;6:287.

220. Vorobioff J, Bredfeldt JE, Groszmann RJ. Increased blood flow through the portal system in cirrhotic rats. *Gastroenterology* 1984;87:1120.

221. Korthuis RJ, Kinden DA, Brimer GE, et al. Intestinal capillary filtration in acute and chronic portal hypertension. *Am J Physiol* 1988;254:G339.

222. Benoit JN, Granger DN. Intestinal microvascular adaptation to chronic portal hypertension in the rat. *Gastroenterology* 1988;94:471.

223. Rector WG. Portal hypertension: a permissive factor only in the development of ascites and variceal bleeding. *Liver* 1986;6:221.

224. Morali GA, Sniderman KW, Deitel KM, et al. Is sinusoidal portal hypertension a necessary factor for the development of hepatic ascites? *J Hepatol* 1992;16:249.

225. Casado M, Bosch J, Garcia-Pagan JC, et al. Clinical events after transjugular intrahepatic portosystemic shunt: correlation with hemodynamic findings. *Gastroenterology* 1998;114:1296.

226. Castells A, Saló J, Planas R, et al. Impact of shunt surgery for variceal bleeding in the natural history of ascites in cirrhosis: a retrospective study. *Hepatology* 1994;20:584.

227. Orloff MJ. Pathogenesis and surgical treatment of intractable ascites associated with alcoholic cirrhosis. *Ann NY Acad Sci* 1970;170:213.

228. Franco D, Vons C, Traynor, et al. Should portosystemic shunt be reconsidered in the treatment of intractable ascites in cirrhosis? *Arch Surg* 1988;123:987.

229. Quiroga J, Sangro B, Nuñez M, et al. Transjugular intrahepatic portosystemic shunt in the treatment of refractory ascites. Effect on clinical, renal, humoral and hemodynamic parameters. *Hepatology* 1995;21:986.

230. Ochs A, Rössle M, Haag K, et al. The transjugular intrahepatic portosystemic stent shunt procedure for refractory ascites. *N Engl J Med* 1995;332:1192.

231. Murray JF, Dawson AM, Sherlock S. Circulatory changes in chronic liver disease. *Am J Med* 1958;32:358.

232. Kontos HA, Shapiro A, Mauck HP, et al. General and regional circulatory alterations in cirrhosis of the liver. *Am J Med* 1964;57:526.

233. Bosch J, Arroyo V, Betriu A, et al. Hepatic hemodynamics and the renin–angiotensin–aldosterone system in cirrhosis. *Gastroenterology* 1980;78:92.

234. Abelmann WH. Hyperdynamic circulation in cirrhosis: a historical perspective. *Hepatology* 1994;20:1356.

235. Groszmann RJ. Hyperdynamic circulation of liver disease 40 years later: pathophysiology and clinical consequences. *Hepatology* 1994;20:1359.

236. Lee FY, Groszmann RJ. Experimental models in the investigation of portal hypertension. In: Arroyo V, Ginès P, Rodés J, et al, eds. *Ascites and renal dysfunction in liver disease.* Malden, MA: Blackwell Science, 1999:365.

237. Moller S, Henriksen JH. The systemic circulation in cirrhosis. In: Arroyo V, Ginès P, Rodés J, et al, eds. *Ascites and renal dysfunction in liver disease.* Malden, MA: Blackwell Science, 1999:307.

238. Kotelanski B, Groszmann R, Cohn JN. Circulation times in the splanchnic and hepatic beds in alcoholic liver disease. *Gastroenterology* 1972;63:102.

239. Sato S, Ohnishi K, Sugita S, et al. Splenic artery and superior mesenteric artery blood flow: nonsurgical Doppler US measurement in healthy subjects and patients with chronic liver disease. *Radiology* 1987;164:347.

240. Rodríguez-Pérez F, Isales CM, Groszmann RJ. Platelet cytosolic calcium, peripheral hemodynamics, and vasodilatory peptides in liver cirrhosis. *Gastroenterology* 1993;105;863.

241. Henriksen JH, Bendtsen F, Sorensen TIA, et al. Reduced central blood volume in cirrhosis. *Gastroenterology* 1989;97:1506.

242. Henriksen JH, Bendtsen F, Gerbes AL, et al. Estimated central blood volume in cirrhosis: relationship to sympathetic nervous activity, beta adrenergic blockade and atrial natriuretic factor. *Hepatology* 1992;16:1163.

243. Moller S, Sondergaard L, Mogelvang J, et al. Decreased right heart blood volume determined by magnetic resonance imaging: evidence of central underfilling in cirrhosis. *Hepatology* 1995;22:472.

244. Gines P, Schrier RW. The arterial vasodilation hypothesis of ascites formation in cirrhosis. In: Arroyo V, Gines P, Rodés J, et al, eds. *Ascites and renal dysfunction in liver disease.* Malden, MA: Blackwell Science, 1999:411.

245. Shapiro MD, Nichols KM, Groves BM, et al. Interrelationship between cardiac output and vascular resistance as determinants of "effective arterial blood volume" in patients with cirrhosis. *Kidney Int* 1985;28:206.

246. Nicholls KM, Shapiro MD, Kluge R, et al. Sodium excretion in advanced cirrhosis: effect of expansion of central volume and suppression of plasma aldosterone. *Hepatology* 1986;6:235.

247. Guevara M, Gines P, Fernández-Esparrach G, et al. Reversibility of hepatorenal syndrome by prolonged administration of orniplessin and plasma volume expansion. *Hepatology* 1998;27:35.

248. Uriz J, Gines P, Cárdenas A, et al. Terlipressin plus albumin infusion: an effective and safe therapy of hepatorenal syndrome. *J Hepatol* 2000;33:43.

249. Schrier RW, Caramelo C. Hemodynamics and hormonal alterations in hepatic cirrhosis. In: Epstein M, ed. *The kidney in liver disease.* Baltimore: Williams & Wilkins, 1988:265.

250. Norris SH, Buell JC, Kurtzman NA. The pathophysiology of cirrhotic edema: a reexamination of the "underfilling" and "overflow" hypotheses. *Semin Nephrol* 1987;7:77.

251. Fernández-Rodríguez F, Prieto J, et al. Arteriovenous shunting, hemodynamic changes, and renal sodium retention in liver cirrhosis. *Gastroenterology* 1993;104:1139.

252. Guarner F, Guarner C, Prieto J, et al. Increased synthesis of systemic prostacyclin in cirrhotic patients. *Gastroenterology* 1986;90: 687.

253. Bendtsen F, Schifter S, Henriksen JH. Increased calcitonin gene-related peptide (CGRP) in cirrhosis. *J Hepatol* 1991;12:118.

254. Gupta S, Morgan TR, Gordan GS. Calcitonin gene-related peptide in hepatorenal syndrome. *J Clin Gastroenterol* 1992;14:122.

255. Fernández-Rodríguez CM, Prieto J, et al. Plasma levels of substance P in liver cirrhosis: relationship to the activation of vasopressor systems and urinary sodium excretion. *Hepatology* 1995;21:35.

256. Guevara M, Gines P, Jiménez W, et al. Increased adrenomedullin levels in cirrhosis: relationship with hemodynamic abnormalities and vasoconstrictor systems. *Gastroenterology* 1998;114:336.

257. Martin PY, Gines P, Schrier RW. Nitric oxide as a mediator of hemodynamic abnormalities and sodium and water retention in cirrhosis. *N Engl J Med* 1998;339:533.

258. Martin PY, Ohara M, Gines P, et al. Nitric oxide synthase (NOS) inhibition for one week improves renal sodium and water excretion in cirrhotic rats with ascites. *J Clin Invest* 1998;101:235.

259. Rosoff L Jr, Zia P, Reynolds TB. Studies on renin and aldosterone in cirrhotic patients with ascites. *Gastroenterology* 1975;69:698.

260. Epstein M, Levinson R, Sancho J, et al. Characterization of the renin–aldosterone system in decompensated cirrhosis. *Circ Res* 1977;41: 818.

261. Chonko AM, Bay WH, Stein JH, et al. The role of renin and aldosterone in the salt retention of edema. *Am J Med* 1977;63:881.

262. Sellars L, Shore AC, Mott V, et al. The renin–angiotensin–aldosterone system in decompensated cirrhosis: its activity in relation to sodium balance. *Q J Med* 1985;56:485.

263. Bernardi M, De Palma R, Trevisani F, et al. Chronobiological study of factors affecting plasma aldosterone concentration in cirrhosis. *Gastroenterology* 1986;91:683.

264. Arroyo V, Gines P, Jiménez W, et al. Ascites, renal failure, and electrolyte disorders in cirrhosis. Pathogenesis, diagnosis, and treatment. In: McIntyre N, Benhamou JP, Bircher J, et al, eds. *Textbook of clinical hepatology.* Oxford: Oxford Medical Press, 1991:429.

265. Bernardi M, Santini C, Trevisani F, et al. Renal function impairment induced by change in posture in patients with cirrhosis and ascites. *Gut* 1985;26:629.

266. Epstein M. Aldosterone in liver disease. In: Epstein M, ed. *The kidney in liver disease,* 4th ed. Philadelphia: Hanley & Belfus, 1996:291.

267. Campra JL, Reynolds TB. Effectiveness of high-dose spironolactone therapy in patients with chronic liver disease and relatively refractory ascites. *Dig Dis Sci* 1978;23:1025.

268. Arroyo V, Jiménez W. Complications of cirrhosis. Renal and circulatory dysfunction. *J Hepatol* 2000;32[Suppl 1]: 157.

269. Bernardi M, Servadei D, Trevisani F, et al. Importance of plasma aldosterone concentration on the natriuretic effect of spironolactone in patients with liver cirrhosis and ascites. *Digestion* 1985;31:189.

270. Epstein M. Aldosterone in liver disease. In: Epstein M, ed. *The kidney in liver disease,* 3rd ed. Baltimore: Williams & Wilkins, 1988;356.

271. Mitch WE, Melton PK, Cooke CR, et al. Plasma levels and hepatic extraction of renin and aldosterone in alcoholic liver disease. *Am J Med* 1979;66:804.

272. Wernze H, Spech HJ, Muller G. Studies on the activity of the renin–angiotensin–aldosterone system (RAAS) in patients with cirrhosis of the liver. *Klin Wochenschr* 1978;56:389.

273. Wilkinson SP, Wheeler PG, Jowett TP, et al. Factors relating to aldosterone secretion rate, the excretions of aldosterone 18-glucuronide, and the plasma aldosterone concentration in cirrhosis. *Clin Endocrinol (Oxf)* 1981;14:355.

274. Schroeder ET, Anderson GH, Goldman SH, et al. Effect of blockade of angiotensin II on blood pressure, renin and aldosterone in cirrhosis. *Kidney Int* 1976;9:511.

275. Arroyo V, Bosch J, Mauri M, et al. Effect of angiotensin-II blockade on systemic and hepatic haemodynamics and on the renin–angiotensin–aldosterone system in cirrhosis with ascites. *Eur J Clin Invest* 1981;11:221.

276. Pariente EA, Bataille C, Bercoff E, et al. Acute effects of captopril on systemic and renal hemodynamics and on renal function in cirrhotic patients with ascites. *Gastroenterology* 1985;88:1255.

277. Lobden I, Shore A, Wilkinson R, et al. Captopril in the hepatorenal syndrome. *J Clin Gastroenterol* 1985;7:354.

278. Barnardo DE, Summerskill WH, Strong CG, et al. Renal function, renin activity and endogenous vasoactive substances in cirrhosis. *Am J Dig Dis* 1970;15:419.

279. Schroeder ET, Eich RH, Smulyan H, et al. Plasma renin level in hepatic cirrhosis. Relation to functional renal failure. *Am J Med* 1970;49:186.

280. Wong PY, Talamo RC, Williams GH. Kallikrein–kinin and renin–angiotensin systems in functional renal failure of cirrhosis of the liver. *Gastroenterology* 1977;73:1114.

281. Wilkinson SP, Smith IK, Williams R. Changes in plasma renin activity in cirrhosis: a reappraisal based on studies in 67 patients and "low-renin" cirrhosis. *Hypertension* 1979;1:125.

282. Guevara M, Gines P, Bandi JC, et al. Transjugular intrahepatic portosystemic shunt in hepatorenal syndrome: effects on renal function and vasoactive systems. *Hepatology* 1998;28:416.

283. Henriksen JH, Christensen NJ, Ring-Larsen H. Noradrenaline and adrenaline concentrations in various vascular beds in patients with cirrhosis. Relation to haemodynamics. *Clin Physiol* 1981;1:293.

284. Bichet DG, Van Putten VJ, Schrier RW. Potential role of increased sympathetic activity in impaired sodium and water excretion in cirrhosis. *N Engl J Med* 1982;307:1552.

285. Burghardt W, Wernze H, Schaffrath I. Changes of circulating noradrenaline and adrenaline in hepatic cirrhosis. Relation to stage of disease, liver and renal function. *Acta Endocrinol* 1982;99[Suppl 246]:100.

286. Bernardi M, Trevisani F, Santinin C, et al. Plasma norepinephrine, weak neurotransmitters and renin activity during active tilting in liver cirrhosis: relationship with cardiovascular hemostasis and renal function. *Hepatology* 1983;3:56.

287. Henriksen H, Ring-Larsen H, Christensen NJ. Sympathetic nervous activity in cirrhosis. A survey of plasma catecholamine studies. *J Hepatol* 1984;1:55.

288. Epstein M, Larios O, Johnson G. Effects of water immersion on plasma catecholamines in decompensated cirrhosis. Implications for deranged sodium and water homeostasis. *Miner Electrolyte Metab* 1985;11:25.

289. Nicholls KM, Shapiro MD, Van Putten VJ, et al. Elevated plasma norepinephrine concentrations in decompensated cirrhosis. Association with increased secretion rates, normal clearance rates, and suppressibility by central blood volume expansion. *Circ Res* 1985;56: 457.

290. Willett I, Esler M, Burke F, et al. Total and renal sympathetic nervous system activity in alcoholic cirrhosis. *J Hepatol* 1985;1:639.

291. Henriksen JH, Ring-Larsen H, Christensen NJ. Hepatic intestinal uptake and release of catecholamines in alcoholic cirrhosis. Evidence of enhanced hepatic intestinal sympathetic nervous activity. *Gut* 1987;28:1637.

292. MacGilchrist AJ, Howes LG, Hawksby C, et al. Plasma noradrenaline in cirrhosis: a study of kinetics and temporal relationship to ascites formation. *Eur J Clin Invest* 1991;21:238.

293. Esler M, Dudley F, Jennings G, et al. Increased sympathetic nervous activity and the effects of its inhibition with clonidine in alcoholic cirrhosis. *Ann Intern Med* 1992;116:446.

294. Henriksen JH, Ring-Larsen H, Kanstrup IL, et al. Splanchnic and renal elimination and release of catecholamines in cirrhosis. Evidence of enhanced sympathetic nervous activity in patients with decompensated cirrhosis. *Gut* 1984;25:1034.

295. Floras JS, Legault L, Morali GA, et al. Increased sympathetic outflow in cirrhosis and ascites: direct evidence from intraneural recordings. *Ann Intern Med* 1991;114:373.

296. DiBona GF. Neural control of the kidney: functionally specific renal sympathetic nerve fibers. *Am J Physiol* 2000;279:R1517.

297. Zambraski E. Effects of acute renal denervation on sodium excretion in miniature swine with cirrhosis and ascites. *Physiologist* 1985; 28:268.

298. Koepke J, Jones S, DiBona G. Renal nerves mediate blunted natriuresis to atrial natriuretic peptide in cirrhotic rats. *Am J Physiol* 1987;252:R1019.

299. Solís-Herruzo JA, Durán A, Favela V, et al. Effects of lumbar sympathetic block on kidney function in cirrhotic patients with hepatorenal syndrome. *J Hepatol* 1987;5:167.

300. Henriksen JH, Ring-Larsen H, Christensen NJ. Autonomic nervous function in liver disease. In Bomzon A, Blendis LM, eds. *Cardiovascular complications of liver disease*. Boca Raton, FL: CRC Press, 1990:63.

301. Uriz J, Ginès P, Jiménez W, et al. Increased circulating levels of neuropeptide Y in hepatorenal syndrome. A possible role in the pathogenesis of renal vasoconstriction. *J Hepatol* 2000;32:64A.

302. Better OS, Schrier RW. Disturbed volume homeostasis in patients with cirrhosis of the liver. *Kidney Int* 1983;23:303.

303. Kostreva DR, Castaner A, Kampine JP. Reflex effects of hepatic baroreceptors on renal and cardiac sympathetic nervous activity. *Am J Physiol* 1980;238:R390.

304. Levy M, Wexler MJ. Hepatic denervation alters first-phase urinary sodium excretion in dogs with cirrhosis. *Am J Physiol* 1987;253: F664.

305. Levy M, Wexler MJ. Sodium excretion in dogs with low grade caval constriction: role of hepatic nerves. *Am J Physiol* 1987;253:F672.

306. Blendis LM, Sole MJ, Campbell P, et al. The effect of peritoneovenous shunting on catecholamine metabolism in patients with hepatic ascites. *Hepatology* 1987;7:143.

307. Conrad KP, Dunn MJ. Renal prostaglandins and other eicosanoids. In: Windhager EE, ed. *Handbook of physiology*. "Renal physiology", section 8. New York: Oxford University Press, 1992:1707.

308. Epstein M, Lifschitz M, Ramachandran M, et al. Characterization of renal prostaglandin E responsiveness in decompensated cirrhosis: implications for renal sodium handling. *Clin Sci* 1982;63:555.

309. Guarner C, Colina I, Guarner F, et al. Renal prostaglandins in cirrhosis of the liver. *Clin Sci* 1986;70:477.

310. Laffi G, La Villa G, Pinzani M, et al. Altered renal and platelet arachidonic acid metabolism in cirrhosis. *Gastroenterology* 1986;90:274.

311. Uemura M, Tsujii T, Fukui H, et al. Urinary prostaglandins and renal function in chronic liver diseases. *Scand J Gastroenterol* 1986;21: 75.

312. Moore KP. Arachidonic acid metabolites and the kidney in cirrhosis. In: Arroyo V, Ginès P, Rodés J, et al, eds. *Ascites and renal dysfunction in liver disease*. Malden, MA: Blackwell Science, 1999:249.

313. Parelon G, Mirouze D, Michel F, et al. Prostaglandines urinaires dans le syndrome hépatorénal du cirrhotique: rôle du thromboxane A2 et d'un déséquilibre des acides gras polyinsaturés précurseurs. *Gastroenterol Clin Biol* 1985;9:290.

314. Govindarajan S, Nast CC, Smith WL, et al. Immunohistochemical distribution of renal prostaglandin endoperoxide synthase and prostacyclin synthase: diminished endoperoxide synthase in the hepatorenal syndrome. *Hepatology* 1987;7:654.

315. Moore K, Ward PS, Taylor GW, et al. Systemic and renal production of thromboxane A2 and prostacyclin in decompensated liver disease and hepatorenal syndrome. *Gastroenterology* 1991;100:1069.

316. Zipser RD, Radvan GH, Kronborg I, et al. Urinary thromboxane B2 and prostaglandin E2 in the hepatorenal syndrome; evidence for increased vasoconstrictor and decreased vasodilator factors. *Gastroenterology* 1983;84:697.

317. Zipser RD, Kronberg I, Rector W, et al. Therapeutic trial of thromboxane synthesis inhibition in the hepatorenal syndrome. *Gastroenterology* 1984;87:1228.

318. Bruix J, Bosch J, Kravetz D, et al. Effects of prostaglandin inhibition on systemic and hepatic hemodynamics in patients with cirrhosis of the liver. *Gastroenterology* 1985;88:430.

319. Niederberger M, Ginès P, Martin PY, et al. Increased renal and vascular cytosolic phospholipase A_2 activity in rats with cirrhosis and ascites. *Hepatology* 1998;27:42.

320. Huber M, Kastner S, Scholmerich J, et al. Analysis of cysteinyl leukotrienes in human urine: enhanced excretion in patients with liver cirrhosis and hepatorenal syndrome. *Eur J Clin Invest* 1989; 19:53.

321. Moore KP, Taylor GW, Maltby NH, et al. Increased production of leukotrienes in hepatorenal syndrome. *J Hepatol* 1990;11:263.

322. Bichet D, Szatalowicz V, Chaimovitz C, et al. Role of vasopressin in abnormal water excretion in cirrhotic patients. *Ann Intern Med* 1982;96:413.

323. Reznick RK, Langer B, Taylor BR, et al. Hyponatremia and arginine vasopressin secretion in patients with refractory hepatic ascites undergoing peritoneovenous shunting. *Gastroenterology* 1983;84:713.

324. Castellano G, Solís-Herruzo JA, Morillas JD, et al. Antidiuretic hormone and renal function after water loading in patients with cirrhosis of the liver. *Scand J Gastroenterol* 1991;26:49.

325. Arroyo V, Clària J, Saló J, et al. Antidiuretic hormone and the pathogenesis of water retention in cirrhosis with ascites. *Semin Liver Dis* 1994;14:44.

326. Ginès P, Abraham W, Schrier RW. Vasopressin in pathophysiological states. *Semin Nephrol* 1994;14:384.

327. Better OS, Aisenbrey GA, Berl T, et al. Role of antidiuretic hormone in impaired urinary dilution associated with chronic bile-duct ligation. *Clin Sci* 1980;58:493.

328. Camps J, Solá J, Arroyo V, et al. Temporal relationship between the impairment of free water excretion and antidiuretic hormone hypersecretion in rats with experimental cirrhosis. *Gastroenterology* 1987; 93:498.

329. Linas SL, Anderson RJ, Guggenheim SJ, et al. Role of vasopressin in impaired water excretion in conscious rats with experimental cirrhosis. *Kidney Int* 1981;20:173.

330. Asahina Y, Izumi N, Enomoto N, et al. Increased gene expression of water channel in cirrhotic rat kidneys. *Hepatology* 1995;21:169.

331. Kim JK, Summer SN, Howard RL, et al. Vasopressin gene expression in rats with experimental cirrhosis. *Hepatology* 1993;17:143.

332. Ardaillou R, Benmansour M, Rondeau E, et al. Metabolism and secretion of antidiuretic hormone in patients with renal failure, cardiac insufficiency and renal insufficiency. *Adv Nephrol* 1984;13:35.

333. Solís-Herruzo JA, González-Gamarra A, Castellano G, et al. Metabolic clearance rate of arginine vasopressin in patients with cirrhosis. *Hepatology* 1992;16:974.

334. Bichet DG, Groves BM, Schrier RW. Mechanisms of improvement of water and sodium excretion by immersion in decompensated cirrhotic patients. *Kidney Int* 1983;24:788.

335. Clària J, Jiménez W, Arroyo V, et al. Effect of V1-vasopressin receptor blockade on arterial pressure in conscious rats with cirrhosis and ascites. *Gastroenterology* 1991;100:494.

336. Ginès P, Jiménez W, Arroyo V, et al. Atrial natriuretic factor in cirrhosis with ascites: plasma levels, cardiac release and splanchnic extraction. *Hepatology* 1988;8:636.

337. Campbell PJ, Skorecki KL, Logan AG, et al. Acute effects of peritoneovenous shunting on plasma atrial natriuretic peptide in cirrhotic patients with massive refractory ascites. *Am J Med* 1988;84:112.

338. Klepetko W, Muller C, Hartter E, et al. Plasma atrial natriuretic factor in cirrhotic patients with ascites. Effect of peritoneovenous shunt implantation. *Gastroenterology* 1988;95:764.

339. Morgan TR, Imada T, Hollister AS, et al. Plasma human atrial natriuretic factor in cirrhosis and ascites with and without functional renal failure. *Gastroenterology* 1988;95:1641.

340. Skorecki KL, Leung WM, Campbell P, et al. Role of atrial natriuretic peptide in the natriuretic response to central volume expansion induced by head-out water immersion in sodium retaining cirrhotic subjects. *Am J Med* 1988;85:375.

341. Epstein M, Loutzenhiser R, Norsk P, et al. Relationship between plasma ANF responsiveness and renal sodium handling in cirrhotic humans. *Am J Nephrol* 1989;9:133.

342. Salerno F, Badalamenti S, Moser P, et al. Atrial natriuretic factor in cirrhotic patients with tense ascites. Effect of large-volume paracentesis. *Gastroenterology* 1990;98:1063.

343. Angeli P, Caregaro L, Menon F, et al. Variability of atrial natriuretic peptide plasma levels in ascitic cirrhotics: pathophysiological and clinical implications. *Hepatology* 1992;16:1389.

344. Warner L, Skorecki K, Blendis LM, et al. Atrial natriuretic factor and liver disease. *Hepatology* 1993;17:500.

345. Henriksen JH, Bendtsen F, Schutten HJ, et al. Hepatic-intestinal disposal of endogenous human alpha atrial natriuretic factor 99–126 in patients with cirrhosis. *Am J Gastroenterol* 1990;85:1155.

346. Poulos JE, Gower WR, Fontanet HL, et al. Cirrhosis with ascites: increased atrial natriuretic peptide messenger RNA expression in rat ventricle. *Gastroenterology* 1995;108:1496.

347. Salerno F, Badalamenti S, Incerti P, et al. Renal response to atrial natriuretic peptide in patients with advanced liver cirrhosis. *Hepatology* 1988;8:21.

348. López C, Jiménez W, Arroyo V, et al. Role of altered systemic hemodynamics in the blunted renal response to atrial natriuretic peptide in rats with cirrhosis and ascites. *J Hepatol* 1989;9:217.

349. Beutler JJ, Koomans HA, Rabelink TJ, et al. Blunted natriuretic response and low blood pressure after atrial natriuretic factor in early cirrhosis. *Hepatology* 1989;10:148.

350. Laffi G, Pinzani M, Meacci E, et al. Renal hemodynamic and natriuretic effects of human atrial natriuretic factor infusion in cirrhosis with ascites. *Gastroenterology* 1989;96:167.

351. Ginès P, Tító L, Arroyo V, et al. Renal insensitivity to atrial natriuretic peptide in patients with cirrhosis and ascites. Effect of increasing systemic arterial pressure. *Gastroenterology* 1992;102:280.

352. La Villa G, Riccardi D, Lazzeri C, et al. Blunted natriuretic response to low-dose brain natriuretic peptide infusion in nonazotemic cirrhotic patients with ascites and avid sodium retention. *Hepatology* 1995;22:1745.

353. Abraham WT, Lauwaars M, Kim J, et al. Reversal of atrial natriuretic peptide resistance by increasing distal tubular sodium delivery in patients with decompensated cirrhosis. *Hepatology* 1995;22:737.

354. La Villa G, Romanelli RG, Raggi VC, et al. Plasma levels of brain natriuretic peptide in patients with cirrhosis. *Hepatology* 1992;16:156.

355. Saló J, Jiménez W, Kuhn M, et al. Urinary excretion of urodilatin in patients with cirrhosis. *Hepatology* 1996;24:1428.

356. Angeli P, Jiménez W, Arroyo V, et al. Renal effects of natriuretic peptide receptor blockade in cirrhotic rats with ascites. *Hepatology* 1994;20:948.

357. Simonson MS. Endothelins: multifunctional renal peptides. *Physiol Rev* 1993;73:375.

358. Uchihara M, Izumi N, Sato C, et al. Clinical significance of elevated plasma endothelin concentration in patients with cirrhosis. *Hepatology* 1992;16:95.

359. Uemasu J, Matsumoto H, Kawasaki H. Increased plasma endothelin levels in patients with liver cirrhosis. *Nephron* 1992;60:380.

360. Moore K, Wendon J, Frazer M, et al. Plasma endothelin immunoreactivity in liver disease and the hepatorenal syndrome. *N Engl J Med* 1992;327:1774.

361. Asbert M, Ginès A, Ginès P, et al. Circulating levels of endothelin in cirrhosis. *Gastroenterology* 1993;104:1485.

362. Moller S, Emmeluth C, Henriksen JH. Elevated circulating plasma endothelin-1 concentrations in cirrhosis. *J Hepatol* 1993;19:285–290.

363. Saló J, Francitorra A, Follo A, et al. Increased plasma endothelin in cirrhosis. Relationship with systemic endotoxemia and response to changes in effective blood volume. *J Hepatol* 1995;22:389.

364. Trevisani F, Colantoni A, Gerbes A, et al. Daily profile of plasma endothelin-1 and -3 in pre-ascitic cirrhosis: relationships with the arterial pressure and renal function. *J Hepatol* 1997;26:808.

365. Bernardi M, Gulberg V, Colantoni A, et al. Plasma endothelin-1 and -3 in cirrhosis: relationship with systemic hemodynamics, renal function and neurohumoral systems. *J Hepatol* 1996;24:161.

366. Martinet JP, Legault L, Cernacek P, et al. Changes in plasma endothelin-1 and big endothelin-1 induced by transjugular intrahepatic portosystemic shunts in patients with cirrhosis and refractory ascites. *J Hepatol* 1996;25:700.

367. Leivas A, Jiménez W, Lamas S, et al. Endothelin-1 does not play a major role in the homeostasis of arterial pressure in cirrhotic rats with ascites. *Gastroenterology* 1995;108:1842.

368. Pinzani M, Milani S, DeFranco R, et al. Endothelin 1 is overexpressed in human cirrhotic liver and exerts multiple effects on activated hepatic stellate cells. *Gastroenterology* 1996;110:534.

369. Leivas A, Jiménez W, Bruix J, et al. Gene expression of endothelin-1 and ET(A) and ET(B) receptors in human cirrhosis: relationship with hepatic hemodynamics. *J Vasc Res* 1998;35:186.

370. Alam I, Bass NM, Bichetti P, et al. Hepatic tissue endothelin-1 levels in chronic liver disease correlate with disease severity and ascites. *Am J Gastroenterol* 2000;95:199.

371. Soper CP, Latif AB, Bending MR. Amelioration of hepatorenal syndrome with selective endothelin-A antagonist. *Lancet* 1996;347:1842.

372. Saló J, Fernández-Esparrach G, Ginès P, et al. Urinary endothelin-like immunoreactivity in patients with cirrhosis *J Hepatol* 1997;27:810.

373. Poo JL, Jiménez W, Maria Muñoz R, et al. Chronic blockade of endothelin receptors in cirrhotic rats: hepatic and hemodynamic effects. *Gastroenterology* 1999;116:161.

374. Cho JJ, Hocher B, Herbst H, et al. An oral endothelin-A receptor antagonist blocks collagen synthesis and deposition in advanced rat liver fibrosis. *Gastroenterology* 2000;118:1169.

375. Tièche S, DeGottardi A, Kappeler A, et al. Overexpression of endothelin-1 in bile duct ligated rats: correlation with activation of hepatic stellate cells and portal pressure. *J Hepatol* 2001;34:38.

376. Housset C. The dual play of endothelin receptors in hepatic vasoregulation. *Hepatology* 2000;31:1025.

377. Raij L. Nitric oxide and the kidney. *Circulation* 1993;87[Suppl V]:26.

378. Garcia-Estañ J, Atucha N, Mario J, et al. Increased endothelium-dependent renal vasodilation in cirrhotic rats. *Am J Physiol* 1994;267:R549.

379. Bosch-Marcé M, Morales-Ruiz M, Jiménez W, et al. Increased renal expression of nitric oxide synthase type III in cirrhotic rats with ascites. *Hepatology* 1998;27:1191.

380. Criado M, Flores O, Ortiz MC, et al. Elevated glomerular and blood mononuclear lymphocyte nitric oxide production in rats with chronic bile duct ligation: role of inducible nitric oxide synthase activation. *Hepatology* 1997;26:268.

381. Clària J, Jiménez W, Ros J, et al. Pathogenesis of arterial hypotension in cirrhotic rats with ascites: role of endogenous nitric oxide. *Hepatology* 1992;15:343.

382. Clària J, Ros J, Jiménez W, et al. Role of nitric oxide and prostacyclin in the control of renal perfusion in experimental cirrhosis. *Hepatology* 1995;22:915.

383. Knox FG, Granger JP. Control of sodium excretion: an integrative approach. In: Windhager EE, ed. *Handbook of physiology.* "Renal physiology", section 8. New York: Oxford University Press, 1992:927.

384. Greco AV, Porcelli G, Ghirlanda G, et al. L'escrezione di callicreina urinaria nella cirrosi epatica. *Min Med* 1975;66:1504.

385. Pérez-Ayuso RM, Arroyo V, Camps J, et al. Renal kallikrein excretion in cirrhotics with ascites: relationship to renal hemodynamics. *Hepatology* 1984;4:247.

386. Zipser RD, Kerlin P, Hoefs JC, et al. Renal kallikrein excretion in alcoholic cirrhosis. Relationship to other vasoactive systems. *Am J Gastroenterol* 1981;75:183.

387. Hattori K, Hasumura Y, Takeuchi J. Role of renal kallikrein in the derangement of sodium and water excretion in cirrhotic patients. *Scand J Gastroenterol* 1984;19:844.

388. Lieberman FL, Ito S, Reynolds. Effective plasma volume in cirrhosis with ascites. Evidence that a decreased value does not account for renal sodium retention, a spontaneous reduction in glomerular filtration rate (GFR), and a fall in GFR during drug-induced diuresis. *J Clin Invest* 1969;48:975.

389. Lieberman FL, Denison EK, Reynolds TB. The relationship of plasma volume, portal hypertension, ascites, and renal sodium retention in cirrhosis: the overflow theory of ascites formation. *Ann NY Acad Sci* 1970;170:202.

390. Wensing G, Sabra R, Branch RA. The onset of sodium retention in experimental cirrhosis in rats is related to a critical threshold of liver function. *Hepatology* 1990;11:779.

391. Rector WG Jr, Lewis F, Robertson AD, et al. Renal sodium retention complicating alcoholic liver disease: relation to portosystemic shunting and liver function. *Hepatology* 1990;12:455.

392. Ahloulay M, Dechaux M, Hassler C, et al. Cyclic AMP is a hepatorenal link influencing natriuresis and contributing to glucagon-induced hyperfiltration in rats. *J Clin Invest* 1996;98:2251.

393. Levy M. The genesis of urinary sodium retention in pre-ascitic cirrhosis: the overflow theory. *Gastroenterol Int* 1992;5:186.

394. Levy M. Pathogenesis of sodium retention in early cirrhosis of the liver: evidence for vascular overfilling. *Semin Liver Dis* 1994;14:4.

395. Witte MH, Witte CL, Dumont AE. Progress in liver disease: physiological factors involved in the causation of cirrhotic ascites. *Gastroenterology* 1971;61:742.

396. Witte CL, Witte MH, Dumont AE. Lymph imbalance in the genesis and perpetuation of the ascites syndrome in hepatic cirrhosis. *Gastroenterology* 1980;78:1059.

397. Braunwald E, Colucci WS, Grossman W. Clinical aspects of heart failure; high-output heart failure; pulmonary edema. In: Braunwald E, ed. *Heart disease. A textbook of cardiovascular medicine.* Philadelphia: WB Saunders, 1997:445.

398. Palmer BF, Alpern RJ, Seldin DW. Pathophysiology of edema formation. In: Seldin DW, Giebisch G, eds. *The kidney. Physiology and pathophysiology,* 2nd ed. New York: Raven Press, 1992:2099.

399. Schrier RW. Pathogenesis of sodium and water retention in high-output and low-output cardiac failure, nephrotic syndrome, cirrhosis and pregnancy. *N Engl J Med* 1988;319:1065.

400. Schrier RW. Body fluid volume regulation in health and disease: a unifying hypothesis. *Ann Intern Med* 1990;113:155.

401. Schrier RW, Arroyo V, Bernardi M, et al. Peripheral arterial vasodilation hypothesis: a proposal for the initiation of renal sodium and water retention in cirrhosis. *Hepatology* 1988;8:1151.

402. Schrier RW, Neiderbeger M, Weigert A, et al. Peripheral arterial vasodilation: determinant of functional spectrum of cirrhosis. *Semin Liver Dis* 1994;14:14.

403. Colombato LA, Albillos A, Groszmann RJ. Temporal relationship of peripheral vasodilatation, plasma volume expansion and the hyperdynamic circulatory state in portal-hypertensive rats. *Hepatology* 1991;15:323.

404. Albillos A, Colombato LA, Groszmann RJ. Vasodilatation and sodium retention in prehepatic portal hypertension. *Gastroenterology* 1992;102:931.

405. Harris NR, Granger N. Alterations of hepatic and splanchnic microvascular exchange in cirrhosis: local factors in the formation of ascites. In: Arroyo V, Ginès P, Rodés J, et al, eds. *Ascites and renal dysfunction in liver disease.* Malden, MA: Blackwell Science, 1999:351.

406. Reynolds TB, Lieberman FL, Goodman AR. Advantages of treatment of ascites without sodium restriction and without complete removal of excess fluid. *Gut* 1978;19:549.

407. Gauthier A, Levy VG, Quinton A, et al. Salt or no salt in the treatment of cirrhotic ascites: a randomised study. *Gut* 1986;27:705.

408. Bataller R, Ginès P, Arroyo V. Practical recommendations for the treatment of ascites and its complications. *Drugs* 1997;54:571.

409. Angeli P, Pria MD, De Bei E, et al. Randomized clinical study of the efficacy of amiloride and potassium canrenoate in nonazotemic cirrhotic patients with ascites. *Hepatology* 1994;19:72.

410. Ginès P, Arroyo V, Quintero E, et al. Comparison of paracentesis and diuretics in the treatment of cirrhotics with tense ascites. Results of a randomized study. *Gastroenterology* 1987;93:234.

411. Salerno F, Badalamenti S, Incerti P, et al. Repeated paracentesis and IV albumin infusion to treat "tense" ascites in cirrhotic patients: a safe alternative therapy. *J Hepatol* 1987;5:102.

412. Hagège H, Ink O, Ducreux M, et al. Traitement de l'ascite chez les malades atteints de cirrhose sans hyponatrémie ni insuffisance rénale. Résultats d'une étude randomisée comparant les diurétiques et les ponctions compensées par l'albumine. *Gastroenterol Clin Biol* 1992;16:751.

413. Acharya SK, Balwinder S, Padhee AK, et al. Large-volume paracentesis and intravenous dextran to treat tense ascites. *J Clin Gastroenterol* 1992;14:31.

414. Solá R, Vila MC, Andreu M, et al. Total paracentesis with dextran 40 vs diuretics in the treatment of ascites in cirrhosis: a randomized controlled study. *J Hepatol* 1994;20:282.

415. Angeli P, Albino G, Carraro P, et al. Cirrhosis and muscle cramps: evidence of a causal relationship. *Hepatology* 1996;23:264.

416. Gregory PB, Broekelschen PH, Hill MD, et al. Complications of diuresis in the alcoholic patient with ascites: a controlled trial. *Gastroenterology* 1977;73:534.

417. Ascione A, Burroughs AK. Paracentesis for ascites in cirrhotic patients. Gastroenterol Int 1990;3:120.

418. Arroyo V, Ginès A, Saló J. A European survey on the treatment of ascites in cirrhosis. *J Hepatol* 1994;21:667.

419. Fernández-Esparrach G, Guevara M, Sort P, et al. Diuretic requirements after therapeutic paracentesis in non-azotemic patients with cirrhosis. A randomized double-blind trial of spironolactone versus placebo. *J Hepatol* 1997;26:614.

420. Runyon BA. Treatment of patients with cirrhosis and ascites. *Semin Liver Dis* 1997;17:249.

421. Ginès P, Arroyo V. Is there still a need for albumin infusions to treat patients with liver disease? Gut 2000;46(5):588.

422. Pozzi M, Osculati G, Boari G, et al. Time course of circulatory and humoral effects of rapid total paracentesis in cirrhotic patients with tense, refractory ascites. *Gastroenterology* 1994;106:709.

423. Luca A, Garcia-Pagan JC, Bosch J, et al. Beneficial effects of intravenous albumin infusion on the hemodynamic and humoral changes after total paracentesis. *Hepatology* 1995;22:753.

424. Saló J, Ginès A, Ginès P, et al. Effect of therapeutic paracentesis on plasma volume and transvascular escape rate of albumin in patients with cirrhosis. *J Hepatol* 1997;27:645.

425. Ruiz del Arbol L, Monescillo A, Jiménez W, et al. Paracentesis-induced circulatory dysfunction: mechanism and effect on hepatic hemodynamics in cirrhosis. *Gastroenterology* 1997;113:579.

426. Vila MC, Solá R, Molina L, et al. Hemodynamic changes in patients developing effective hypovolemia after total paracentesis. *J Hepatol* 1998;28:639.

427. Ginès A, Fernández-Esparrach G, Monescillo A, et al. Randomized trial comparing albumin, dextran-70 and polygeline in cirrhotic patients with ascites treated by paracentesis. *Gastroenterology* 1996;111:1002.

428. Planas R, Ginès P, Arroyo V, et al. Dextran 70 vs albumin as plasma expanders in cirrhotic patients with tense ascites treated with total paracentesis. Results of a randomized study. *Gastroenterology* 1990;99:1736.

429. Salerno F, Badalamenti S, Lorenzano E, et al. Randomized comparative study of Hemaccel vs albumin infusion after total paracentesis in cirrhotic patients with refractory ascites. *Hepatology* 1991;13:707.

430. Fassio E, Terg R, Landeira G, et al. Paracentesis with dextran 70 vs paracentesis with albumin in cirrhosis with tense ascites: results of a randomized study. *J Hepatol* 1992;14:310.

431. Greig PD, Blendis LM, Langer B, et al. Renal and hemodynamic effect of the peritoneovenous shunt. II. Long-term effect. *Gastroenterology* 1981;1981;80:119.

432. Ginès A, Planas R, Angeli P, et al. Treatment of patients with cirrhosis and refractory ascites by LeVeen shunt with titanium tip. Comparison with therapeutic paracentesis. *Hepatology* 1995;22:124.

433. Epstein M. Peritoneovenous shunt in the management of ascites and hepatorenal syndrome. In: Epstein M, ed. *The kidney in liver disease,* 4th ed. Philadelphia: Hanley & Belfus, 1996:491.

434. Ring-Larsen H. Treatment of refractory ascites. In: Arroyo V, Ginès P, Rodés J, et al, eds. *Ascites and renal dysfunction in liver disease. Pathogenesis, diagnosis and treatment.* Malden, MA: Blackwell Science 1999:480.

435. LeVeen HH, Vujic I, D'Ovidio NJ, et al. Peritoneovenous shunt occlusion. Etiology, diagnosis, therapy. Ann Surg 1984;200:212.

436. Linas SL, Schaffer JW, Moore EE, et al. Peritoneovenous shunt in the management of the hepatorenal syndrome. Kidney Int 1986;30:736.

437. Shiffman ML, Jeffers L, Hoofnagle JH, et al. The role of transjugular intrahepatic portosystemic shunt for treatment of portal hypertension and its complications: a conference sponsored by the National Digestive Disease advisory board. *Hepatology* 1995;25:1591.

438. Ferral H, Bjarnason H, Wegryn SA, et al. Refractory ascites: early experience in treatment with transjugular intrahepatic portosystemic shunt. *Radiology* 1993;189:7905.

439. Somberg KA, Lake JR, Tomlanovich SJ, et al. Transjugular intrahepatic portosystemic shunt for refractory ascites: assessment of clinical and humoral response and renal function. *Hepatology* 1995;21:709.

440. Wong F, Sniderman K, Liu P, et al. Transjugular intrahepatic portosystemic stent shunt: effects on hemodynamics and sodium homeostasis in cirrhosis and refractory ascites. *Ann Intern Med* 1995;122: 816.

441. Lebrec D, Giuily N, Hadengue A, et al. Transjugular intrahepatic portosystemic shunts: comparison with paracentesis in patients with cirrhosis and refractory ascites: a randomized trial. *J Hepatol* 1996;25:135.

442. Rossle M, Ochs A, Gulberg V, et al. A comparison of paracentesis and transjugular intrahepatic portosystemic shunting in patients with ascites. *N Engl J Med* 2000;342:1701.

442b. Uriz J, Gines P. The International Study Group for Refractory Ascites. Randomized, multicenter, comparative study between TIPS and paracentesis with albumin in cirrhosis with refractory ascites. *J Hepatol* 2001;34:10.

443. Arroyo V, Ginès P. TIPS and refractory ascites. Lessons from recent history of ascites therapy. *J Hepatol* 1996;25:221.

444. Brensing KA, Textor J, Perz J, et al. Long-term outcome after transjugular intrahepatic portosystemic stent-shunt in non-transplant cirrhotics with hepatorenal syndrome: a phase II study. *Gut* 2000;47: 288.

445. Ohnishi A, Orita Y, Okahara R, et al. Potent aquaretic agent. A novel nonpeptide selective vasopressin 2 antagonist (OPC-31260) in men. *J Clin Invest* 1993;92:2653.

446. Hamon G, Fatin M, Le Matret O, et al. Pharmacological profile of niravoline, a new aquaretic compound. *J Am Soc Nephrol* 1994;5: 272A.

447. Arroyo V, Bataller R, Guevara M. Treatment of hepatorenal syndrome in cirrhosis. In: Arroyo V, Ginès P, Rodés J, et al, eds. *Ascites and renal dysfunction in liver disease. Pathogenesis, diagnosis and treatment.* Malden, MA: Blackwell Science, 1999:492.

448. Gulberg V, Bilzer M, Gerbes A. Long-term therapy and retreatment of hepatorenal syndrome type 1 with ornipressin and dopamine. *Hepatology* 1999;30:870.

449. Titó L, Rimola A, Ginès P et al. Recurrence of spontaneous bacterial peritonitis in cirrhosis. Frequency and predictive factors. *Hepatology* 1988;8:27.

450. Ginès P, Fernández-Esparrach G. Prognosis of cirrhosis with ascites. In: Arroyo V, Ginès P, Rodés J, et al, eds. *Ascites and renal dysfunction in liver disease. Pathogenesis, diagnosis and treatment.* Malden, MA: Blackwell Science, 1999:431.

CHAPTER 76

Monoclonal Gammopathies: Multiple Myeloma, Amyloidosis, and Related Disorders

Pierre M. Ronco, Pierre Aucouturier, Béatrice Mougenot

Monoclonal diseases of B-cell lineage, often referred to as plasma cell dyscrasias, are characterized by abnormal and uncontrolled proliferation of a single clone of B cells at different maturation stages, with a more or less marked differentiation to immunoglobulin (Ig)-secreting plasma cells. Thus, they are usually associated with the production and secretion in blood of a monoclonal Ig or a fragment thereof. A decreased production of normal polyclonal Ig may occur, thereby favoring infections. An ominous consequence of secretion of monoclonal Ig products is their deposition in tissues. These proteinaceous deposits can take the form of casts (in myeloma cast nephropathy [CN]), crystals (in myeloma-associated Fanconi's syndrome [FS]), fibrils (in light-chain [LC] and exceptional heavy-chain [HC] amyloidosis), or granular precipitates (in monoclonal Ig deposition disease [MIDD], (Table 76-1). They may disrupt organ structure and function, inducing life-threatening complications. In a large proportion of patients with crystals, fibrils, or granular deposits of Ig products, major clinical manifestations and mortality are related to visceral Ig deposition rather than to expansion of the B-cell clone. Indeed, except for myeloma CN that is generally associated with a large tumor mass malignancy, Ig precipitation or deposition diseases often occur in the course of a benign B-cell proliferation or of a smoldering or low-mass myeloma.

The presence of abnormal urine components in a patient with severe bone pain and edema was first recognized in the 1840s by Henry Bence Jones (1) and William MacIntyre (2) who described unusual thermal solubility properties of urinary proteins, far later attributed to Ig LCs (3). To perpetuate this discovery, monoclonal LC proteinuria is often referred to as *Bence Jones proteinuria*. This term is not appropriate because less than 50% of LCs show thermal solubility. Renal damage characterized by large protein casts surrounded by multinucleated giant cells within distal tubules was identified in the early 1900s, and termed *myeloma kidney*. This term must, however, be abandoned because CN with acute renal failure can occasionally occur in conditions other than myeloma and because other patterns of renal injury were subsequently found in patients with myeloma. The first of these was amyloidosis, where tissue deposits are characterized by Congo red binding and fibrillar ultrastructure. In 1971, Glenner and associates (4) showed that the amino acid sequence of amyloid fibrils extracted from tissue was identical to the variable region of a circulating Ig LC, thus providing the first demonstration that an Ig component could be responsible for tissue deposition. The spectrum of renal diseases due to monoclonal Ig deposition has expanded dramatically with the advent of routine staining of renal biopsy specimens with specific anti-κ and anti-λ LC antibodies, and of electron and immunoelectron microscopy (Table 76-1). These morphologic techniques associated with more sensitive and sophisticated analyses of blood and urine monoclonal components have led to the description of new entities, including nonamyloid monoclonal LC deposition disease (LCDD) (5,6), HC (or AH) amyloidosis (7), nonamyloid HC deposition disease (HCDD) (8,9), and chronic lymphocytic leukemia (CLL)-associated glomerulopathies with organized deposits (10,11). All these recently described pathologic entities principally involve the kidney, which appears as the main target for deposition of monoclonal Ig components. This is not only explained by the high levels of renal plasma flow and glomerular filtration rate (GFR), but also by the prominent role of the renal tubule in LC handling and catabolism (12–14).

Polymorphism of renal lesions may be due to specific properties of Ig components influencing their precipitation, their interaction with renal tissue, or their processing after deposition. Alternatively, the type of renal lesions may be driven by

P. M. Ronco: Medical Faculty Saint-Antoine, University Pierre et Marie Curie; and Department of Nephrology, Tenon Hospital, Paris, France

P. Aucouturier: Medical Faculty Necker, University René Descartes; and Department of Immunology, Necker Hospital, Paris, France

B. Mougenot: Department of Pathology, Tenon Hospital, Paris, France

TABLE 76-1. *Pathologic classification of diseases featuring tissue deposition or precipitation of monoclonal immunoglobulin-related material*

Organized			Nonorganized	
Crystals	Fibrillar	Microtubular	MIDD ("Randall type")	Other
Myeloma cast nephropathy[a]	Amyloidosis (AL, AH)	Cryoglobulinemia kidney	LCDD	Crescentic GN (IgA or IgM)
Fanconi's syndrome	Nonamyloid	GOMMID[b]	LHCDD	
Other (extrarenal)			HCDD	

AH, heavy-chain amyloidosis; *AL*, light-chain amyloidosis; *GN*, glomerulonephritis; *GOMMID*, glomerulonephritis with organized microtubular monoclonal immunoglobulin deposits; *HCDD, LCDD, LHCDD, MIDD*, heavy-chain, light-chain, light- and heavy-chain, monoclonal immunoglobulin deposition disease

[a]Crystals are predominantly localized within casts in the lumen of distal tubules and collecting ducts, but may also occasionally be found in the cytoplasm of proximal tubule epithelial cells.

[b]Nonamyloid microtubular monoclonal (or polyclonal) immunoglobulin deposits were reported under the term *immunotactoid glomerulopathy*.

(Adapted from Preud'homme JL, et al. Monoclonal immunoglobulin deposition disease (Randall type): relationship with structural abnormalities of immunoglobulin chains. *Kidney Int* 1994;46:965, with permission.)

the local response to Ig deposits, which may vary from one patient to another. That intrinsic properties of Ig components are responsible for the observed renal alterations was first suggested by *in vitro* biosynthesis of abnormal Ig by bone marrow cells from patients with lymphoplasmacytic disorders and visceral LC deposition (15) and by recurrence of nephropathy in renal grafts (16–18). A further demonstration of the specificity of Ig component pathogenicity was provided by Solomon and associates (19). They showed that the pattern of human renal lesions associated with the production of monoclonal LC, that is, myeloma CN, LCDD, and LC (or AL) amyloidosis could be reproduced in mice injected intraperitoneally with large amounts of LCs isolated from patients with multiple myeloma or AL amyloidosis. The good correlation between experimental findings and human lesions observed at biopsy or autopsy led to the conclusion that physicochemical or structural properties of LCs might be responsible for the specificity of renal lesions. This conclusion is also supported by the rare occurrence of pathologic associations such as CN and FS, or AL amyloidosis and LCDD.

A normal Ig is composed of two LCs and two HCs covalently assembled by disulfide bonds. LCs and HCs are themselves made up of so-called constant (C) and variable (V) globular domains. Whereas a limited number of genes encode the constant region, multiple gene segments are rearranged to produce a variable domain unique to each chain. Diversity is further amplified by mutations and variations of the linking peptide segment. While LCs (and HCs) have many structural similarities, they also possess a unique sequence that may be responsible for physicochemical peculiarities, hence their deposition in tissue or interaction with tissue constituents. A number of structural and physicochemical abnormalities of Ig have already been described (reviewed in references 20 and 21). They include deletions of C_H domains in HCDD (8,9) and HC amyloidosis (7), shortened or lengthened LCs and

abnormal LC glycosylation in LCDD (15,22), and resistance to proteolysis of the V_L fragment in FS (23,24). Moreover, overrepresentation of certain V_L gene subgroups was also reported in amyloidosis (26,27) and LCDD (28). The mechanisms generating Ig diversity may randomly create HCs or LCs with peculiar properties such as proneness to deposition, while mistakes in the rearrangement or hypermutation processes may result in altered genes encoding truncated Ig. It must be stressed, however, that some abnormal Ig chains produced in immunoproliferative disorders are not associated with any special clinical features. On the other hand, structural abnormalities of LCs are not a constant feature of diseases associated with LC deposition. These observations suggest the need to increase the number of nephritogenic Ig components to be analyzed at the complementary DNA (cDNA) and protein levels.

Myeloma- and AL amyloidosis-induced renal failure account for less than 2% of the patients admitted to a chronic dialysis program each year. This is due in part to the relative rarity of these immunoproliferative diseases, but also to deteriorated clinical condition of patients at the time of end-stage renal disease. A dramatic effort of prevention must therefore be carried out, relying on a better understanding of the structural and physicochemical properties of Ig components leading to deposition or precipitation in tissues. Any progress in this field may also enlighten the pathogenesis of immunologically mediated renal diseases, especially glomerulonephritides, because properties of monoclonal Ig components favoring their deposition may apply as well to polyclonal Ig involved in the formation of immune complexes. This is exemplified by type II mixed cryoglobulins that both contain a monoclonal Ig and form circulating immune complexes.

Because of the correlations already established between pathologic entities and physicochemical or binding properties of Ig components, and because of the lack of specificity of clinical manifestations such as acute renal failure or the nephrotic syndrome, we have classified the various forms of renal involvement in monoclonal gammopathies according to the lesions observed in renal biopsy specimens. We indeed consider that elucidation of the pathophysiologic mechanisms responsible for each type of lesion should result in the identification of patients at risk for this lesion and in the design of new therapeutic strategies.

MYELOMA-ASSOCIATED TUBULOPATHIES

The prevalence of tubular lesions or dysfunction in myeloma patients is difficult to assess because most patients do not undergo a renal biopsy, but it is most likely high. It can be approached histologically and functionally. In Kapadia's autopsy series (29), 46 (77%) of 60 consecutive myeloma patients had tubular atrophy and fibrosis, and 37 (62%) had tubular hyaline casts. A giant-cell reaction specific of myeloma CN was observed in 29 patients (48%). Only 3 patients (5%) had amyloidosis and 7 patients (12%) had apparently normal kidneys by light microscopic examination. In Ivanyi's more recent necropsy study including immunofluorescence (30), 18 of 57 patients (32%) had CN, while 6 (11%) had renal amyloidosis and 3 (5%) had κ-LCDD. Both series thus point out that tubular lesions are the major cause of renal disease in myeloma. The high prevalence of tubular alterations is also attested by increased urinary concentrations of the low–molecular-weight proteins normally reabsorbed by the proximal tubule (31), increased urinary elimination of the tubular lysosomal enzyme β-acetyl-D-glucosaminidase (31), and frequent abnormalities in renal tubular acidifying and concentrating ability (32) in patients with LC proteinuria. However, myeloma-associated FS remains exceptional; it was not detected in the 42 myeloma patients whose tubular function was systematically studied by Coward and associates (33).

CN is not only the most frequent lesion in myeloma patients, it is also the major cause of renal failure, as attested by its prevalence which is in the same range as that of renal insufficiency—about 45% in more recent series of myeloma patients (34,35). In nephrology departments that usually receive only myeloma patients with severe renal abnormalities, the prevalence of CN assessed histologically varies from 63% to 87% (37–40) among the myeloma patients with renal failure. It is most likely underestimated because patients with presumed CN do not systematically undergo a renal biopsy while those exhibiting significant albuminuria or a fortiori the nephrotic syndrome do, especially in the absence of amyloidotic deposits in nonrenal biopsy specimens. In myeloma patients with an albumin urinary output of less than 1 g/day, there is an almost perfect correlation between the diagnosis of CN and renal failure. Of note, CN may occur in other immunoproliferative disorders featuring urinary LC excretion. In a case of μ-HC disease, the urinary secretion of large amounts of free κ-chain was responsible for acute renal

failure with a typical histologic presentation of "myeloma kidney" (41).

Myeloma Cast Nephropathy

Clinical Presentation

Changing Presentation of Patients with Myeloma-Induced Renal Failure

When DeFronzo and associates reported the first series of 14 myeloma patients with acute renal failure in 1975 (42), it was established that renal failure occurred at some time during the illness in approximately half of the patients, but that the mode of presentation was usually chronic with a slow progression over a period of several months to years. Among the 187 patients collected by the DeFronzo group, 80 exhibited evidence of renal failure, but only 14 had acute renal failure occurring over a period of 2 to 10 days in the absence of previous renal impairment. Postmortem examination of 9 of the 14 patients showed specific myeloma casts in 6 and moderate to severe tubular atrophy in the remaining 3.

It seems that the mode of presentation of renal failure in myeloma has dramatically changed over the years. In their review of 141 patients treated in Nottingham between 1975 and 1988, Rayner and colleagues (35) showed that the absence of severe renal impairment at presentation predicted a low probability of subsequently developing renal failure. In only 5 of 34 patients in our own series (including 26 patients with typical CN, 2 with tubular necrosis, and 2 with nonspecific chronic interstitial nephritis) (37), the diagnosis of myeloma antedated the discovery of renal failure by more than 1 month. In 3 patients the presence of a monoclonal Ig was known for 10 to 18 years, but it only showed criteria of malignancy for less than 9 months. In 34 of the 53 cases (64%) collected in the Oxford series between 1989 to 1994 (43), renal failure was discovered within 1 month of the diagnosis of myeloma, and in more than half it antedated this diagnosis. Other recent series (38,39) also emphasize the simultaneous diagnoses of myeloma and renal failure. Such a change in epidemiology of renal failure may be interpreted in two ways. It is possible, although unlikely, that patients with established myeloma who subsequently develop renal failure are not referred for dialysis. Alternatively, more aggressive treatment of myeloma in the last decade resulting in better control of the tumor burden, decreased concentration of circulating monoclonal component, and reduced LC load in the tubules may have prevented LC precipitation within the tubule lumen, hence the development of CN (43).

Characteristics of Cast Nephropathy-Related Renal Failure

Table 76-2 summarizes the clinical and pathologic data in the four largest published series of myeloma patients with acute renal failure, in which a renal biopsy was performed in at

TABLE 76-2. *Clinical and pathologic characteristics of patients with myeloma-induced renal failure of presumed or established tubulointerstitial origin*

Series (ref. no.)	No. of patients	Age (yr)	Male–female ratio	Tumor mass		Serum creatinine (μmol/L)	Urinary light chain >2 g/day	Renal lesions in biopsy specimen
				IIB	IIIB			
Rota, et al., 1987 (37)	34	66 (33–90)	0.88	15%	73%	975 (164–2000)	53%	26 MCN 2 ATN 2 CIN
Pozzi, et al., 1987 (38)	50	63 (47–75)	1.38	12%	82%	798 (273–1518)	41%[a]	16 myeloma kidney[b] 8 other
Pasquali, et al., 1990 (39)	25	60 (48–74)	2.12	24%	72%	891 (455–1391)	72%	25 MCN
Winearls, 1995 (43)	42	66 (42–82)	2.0	Majority of patients		896 (302–2006)	NA	14 MCN 6 AIN[c]

AIN, acute interstitial nephritis; *ATN*, acute tubular necrosis; *CIN*, chronic interstitial nephritis; *MCN*, myeloma cast nephropathy; *NA*, not available; *IIB*, intermediate tumor mass; *IIIB*, high tumor mass.
[a]Total proteinuria, including light chains.
[b]Presumably myeloma cast nephropathy.
[c]"Compatible with myeloma."

least 40% of the patients. A diagnosis of myeloma CN was histologically established in 81 of 99 (82%) renal biopsies, and lesions compatible with this diagnosis were found in 10 further biopsy specimens (10%). In comparison with the Mayo Clinic series of 869 unselected myeloma cases (44) in which the mean age was 62 and the male–female ratio was 1.55, patients with acute renal failure did not show any particularity, except for a slight predominance of the female gender in the French series (37). As shown in Tables 76-2 to 76-4, myeloma patients with renal failure are characterized by high tumor mass, and virtually constant urinary LC loss, often of high output.

More than 72% of patients in the renal series have a high tumor burden (Table 76-2). This is confirmed by the Alexanian series, which collected 494 consecutive patients referred to an oncology center (36) (Table 76-3). Only 3% of patients with myeloma of low tumor mass had renal failure while 40% of those with high tumor burden had a serum creatinine concentration above 180 μmol/L. These data contrast with the hematologic characteristics of patients with other renal complications of dysproteinemia including FS, amyloidosis, and MIDD, in whom the monoclonal B

lymphocyte or plasma cell proliferation is either malignant but of low magnitude, or often benign from a hematologic point of view.

Another salient feature of myeloma associated with renal failure is the high prevalence of pure LC myelomas with no entire monoclonal Ig detectable in the serum by standard methods. While such LC myelomas represent only about 20% of all myelomas referred to hematology or cancer centers, they are found in between 37% and 64% of patients with renal failure of presumed or established tubulointerstitial origin. Development of CN in the two studies in which this diagnosis was established histologically (37,39) was associated with urinary excretion of LCs that exceeded 2 g/day in 53% and 72% of the patients, respectively (Table 76-2). This suggests that in myelomas producing complete Ig molecules, CN only occurs in those synthesizing an excess of LCs.

TABLE 76-3. *Relation between tumor mass and renal function*

Tumor mass	No. of patients*	% of patients with serum creatinine (μmol/L)		
		<180	180–270	>270
Low	151	97	1	2
Intermediate	183	89	5	6
High	160	60	17	23

*This series included 494 consecutive, previously untreated patients with multiple myeloma.
(From Alexanian R, et al. Renal failure in multiple myeloma: pathogenesis and prognostic implications. *Arch Intern Med* 1990;150:1693, with permission.)

TABLE 76-4. *Features associated with renal failure in myeloma*

	No. of patients[a]	% with renal failure	P
All patients	494	18	
Urinary LC (g/day)			0.00001
>2.0	123	39	
0.05–2.00	149	17	
<0.05	222	7	
Myeloma protein type			0.0003
Only LC protein	93	31	
Other	401	15	
Serum calcium (mmol/L)[b]			0.00001
>2.87	104	49	
≤2.87	390	10	

LC, light chain
[a]Same series of patients as in Table 76-3.
[b]Corrected calcium (mmol/L).
(From Alexanian R, et al. Renal failure in multiple myeloma: pathogenesis and prognostic implications. *Arch Intern Med* 1990;150:1693, with permission.)

TABLE 76-5. *Precipitants of acute renal failure in myeloma*

Series (ref. no.)	No. of patients	Dehydration	Infection	Hypercalcemia	Contrast medium	NSAIDs	None
Rota, et al., 1987 (37)	34[a]	65%	44%	44% (>2.60 mmol/L)	0%	24%	—
Pozzi, et al., 1987 (38)	50[a]	24%	10%	34% (≥2.75 mmol/L)	4%	0%	44%
Ganeval, et al., 1992 (40)	80[b]	10%	9%	30%	11%	—	35%
Winearls, 1995 (43)	42[a]	—	—	19%	—	10%	71%

NSAIDs, nonsteroidal antiinflammatory drugs
[a]Renal lesions are described in Table 76-2.
[b]Includes 29 patients with renal biopsies: 19 with myeloma cast nephropathy, 2 with amyloidosis, and 8 with light-chain deposition disease.
(Adapted from Rota S, et al. Multiple myeloma and severe renal failure: a clinicopathologic study of outcome and prognosis in 34 patients. *Medicine (Baltimore)* 1987;66:126; and Winearls CG. Nephrology forum: acute myeloma kidney. *Kidney Int* 1995;48:1347, with permission.)

Because of the increased proportion of pure LC myelomas in patients with renal failure, the percentages of IgG and IgA myelomas are reduced. IgD myeloma may be an exception because it is believed to have the greatest potential for causing renal disease (45,46). To give a balanced view on the prevalence of pure LC myeloma and on the output of urinary LCs in myeloma-associated renal failure, it is also necessary to analyze a nonrenal series (36). When specific disease features implicated in the pathogenesis of renal failure are examined, LC protein excretion emerges as a highly significant independent factor on multivariate analysis (Table 76-4). The risk of developing renal failure is twice as high in patients with pure LC myeloma, and five to six times greater in patients with a urinary LC protein loss greater than 2.0 g/day compared to those with a proteinuria less than 0.05 g/day. In contrast, the frequency of renal failure is identical in patients excreting κ- or λ-LCs, as it is in renal series except for the French one (37) that showed a predominance of the λ-isotype. In the Alexanian series (36), hypercalcemia also was a prominent independent pathogenetic factor on multivariate analysis, with a risk of renal failure five times greater in those patients with corrected calcium over 2.87 mmol/L.

The Clinical and Urinary Syndrome of Myeloma Cast Nephropathy

CN-induced renal failure is remarkably silent. Clinical accompanying signs, including weakness, weight loss, bone pain, and infection, are due to myeloma. Because of their nonspecificity and their frequency in older patients, they often do not lead patients to seek medical advice or physicians to prescribe serum and urinary electrophoreses—the key laboratory investigations for the diagnosis of myeloma including pure LC myeloma—when medical advice for such symptoms is sought. Peaks visible on serum or urine electrophoresis are typically identified by immunofixation.

The main urinary feature is the excretion of a monoclonal LC, which accounts for 70% or more of total proteinuria in 80% of patients (37). LC proteinuria is usually not detected by urinary dipsticks, but only by techniques measuring total proteinuria. Certain LCs fail to react or react weakly in some widely used precipitation assays such as the sulfosalicylic acid method, leading to false-negative or underestimated results. The remaining proteins are composed of albumin and low–molecular-weight globulins that have failed to be reabsorbed by proximal tubule cells. In the rare patients with albuminuria over 1 g/day, CN is usually associated with glomerular lesions due to amyloidosis or MIDD. There is no hematuria in pure CN.

Precipitants of Cast Nephropathy

Awareness of these precipitants is of paramount importance because it results in highly efficient preventive measures (Table 76-5). It is often difficult to indict a particular event as precipitating renal failure, for these patients have many of the complications of the disease at once. A common thread seems to be an effect on renal perfusion.

Hypercalcemia is an important precipitant found in 19% to 44% of the renal series (Table 76-5), and in 57% of the patients with renal failure in the nonrenal series by Alexanian and coworkers (36). In the latter series, hypercalcemia was identified as a major pathogenetic factor (Table 76-4). It acts presumably by inducing dehydration as a result of emesis and a nephrogenic diabetes insipidus. It may also enhance LC toxicity (47), and cause nephrocalcinosis. Calcium was shown to enhance the aggregation of LCs with Tamm-Horsfall protein (THP)(48).

Dehydration with or without hypercalcemia and infection are other major risk factors for acute renal failure. We carefully searched for infection foci in our own series (37), and found a high rate of urinary infections (10/34, 29%). In three cases these were associated with an increased proportion of polymorphonuclear leukocytes in the renal biopsy specimen, suggesting an etiologic link between infection and deterioration of renal function. Infection also causes dehydration and prompts the use of nephrotoxic antibiotics.

Contrast media have hitherto been considered an important precipitant of acute renal failure. It was hypothesized that the contrast medium bound to intratubular proteins, especially the LC and THP, causing them to precipitate and obstruct tubular flow (49). Contrast media are also vasoconstrictive agents, decreasing GFR and urinary output. McCarthy and

Becker (50) reviewed seven retrospective studies of myeloma patients receiving contrast media, involving 476 patients who had undergone a total of 568 examinations. The prevalence of acute renal failure (which was not defined) was 0.6% to 1.25% compared to 0.15% in the general population. This is a low risk that contradicts hypotheses that contrast media should not be used in myeloma patients. This change may reflect awareness of the risk and care taken to hydrate patients actively with alkaline solutes before and during the administration of contrast media. No clinical data currently support the preferential use of nonionic agents in myeloma patients to decrease the risk of acute renal failure.

A number of drugs are noxious in myeloma patients. They include antibiotics, particularly aminoglycosides, and nonsteroidal antiinflammatory drugs (NSAIDs). We first insisted on the harmful effects of NSAIDs that were given in 8 of the 34 patients (24%) of our series (37). We found that 6 of these 8 patients were oliguric and suggested that the chance of recovery was diminished if NSAIDs were a precipitating factor. Wu and colleagues (51) also report acute reversible renal failure in the absence of any other precipitant in two patients taking naproxen who were subsequently found to have myeloma. Shpilberg and associates (52) and Winearls (43) further describe two myeloma patients in whom the precipitating role of NSAIDs was clearly demonstrated. The mechanisms whereby NSAIDs precipitate renal failure in myeloma patients are most likely twofold (53). First, they reduce the production of vasodilatory prostaglandins that help to maintain an appropriate GFR in patients with renal hemodynamics compromised by dehydration. Second, inhibition of the diuretic effects of these prostaglandins presumably increases the tonicity of distal tubular fluid that would favor THP–LC coprecipitation and cast formation. Angiotensin-converting enzyme (ACE) inhibitors can also precipitate renal failure in myeloma patients because they reduce GFR dramatically in dehydrated patients (54). Their use as that of angiotensin type-1 receptor antagonists should be avoided in myeloma patients as long as a risk of decreased renal perfusion persists.

The lack of renal toxicity of recently introduced therapies including interferon α-2b, intravenous Igs, and thalidomide, remains to be established. Renal toxicity of interferon α was first demonstrated by our group (55) in mice injected at birth with interferon. They developed unusual lesions of glomerular basement membranes followed by immune complex deposition and in some cases, crescentic glomerulonephritis. Isolated cases of reversible or irreversible acute renal failure have also been reported in myeloma patients receiving interferon (43,56–58). Renal biopsy showed tubular lesions without casts, amyloid, or urate precipitation (56).

Renal Pathology and the Value of Renal Biopsy

A renal biopsy should not be systematically performed in patients with a presumed diagnosis of myeloma CN. It is, however, useful in three circumstances: (a) to establish the cause of renal failure in patients with clinically silent myeloma without evidence of serum monoclonal component on electrophoresis (59); (b) to analyze tubulointerstitial lesions and predict reversibility of renal failure in patients with presumed CN but multiple precipitating factors; and (c) to identify glomerular lesions in patients with urinary albumin loss of more than 1 g/day and no evidence of amyloid deposits in "peripheral" biopsies (e.g., accessory salivary glands, rectum, abdominal fat).

Myeloma Casts

Myeloma CN, also inappropriately referred to as *myeloma kidney*, is characterized by the presence of specific casts associated with severe alterations of the tubule epithelium. Myeloma casts were first described in 1920 by Thannhauser and Krauss (60). They are large and usually numerous. Their prevailing localization is the distal tubule and the collecting duct, but they may also be found in the proximal tubule (61) and even exceptionally in the glomerular urinary space. They often have a "hard" and "fractured" appearance, and show polychromatism upon staining with Masson's trichrome (Fig. 76-1). Casts may also have a stratified or laminated appearance. They may stain with Congo red, but only exceptionally show the typical yellow-green dichroism of amyloid under polarized light.

An important diagnostic feature of myeloma casts is the presence of crystals, which may be suspected by light microscopy (62). Such casts are often angular or heterogeneous because they contain multiple rhomboid or needle-shaped crystals surrounded by an amorphous material and cell debris.

Casts are often surrounded by mononuclear cells, exfoliated tubular cells, and more characteristically by multinucleated giant cells whose macrophagic origin has been established by specific antibodies (63). The diagnosis of myeloma casts by light microscopy can be definitely confirmed if multinucleated giant cells are present (Fig. 76-1). These cells are often seen engulfing the casts and at times actually

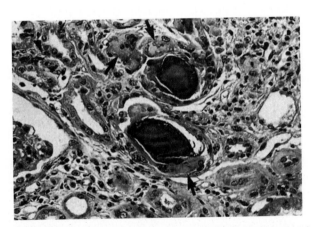

FIG. 76-1. Myeloma cast nephropathy. Typical myeloma casts with fractured appearance are surrounded by multinucleated macrophagic cells (*arrows*) in a patient with λ–light-chain myeloma. (Masson's trichrome ×312.)

phagocytizing fragments of the casts. In some cases, the cellular reaction is made of polymorphonuclear leukocytes in the absence of urinary tract infection.

In myeloma CN, there is a great variability in the respective percentage of typical myeloma casts and of nonspecific hyaline casts. In some instances, most casts have nonspecific characteristics by light microscopy, even if by immunofluorescence the vast majority consists predominantly of one of the two LC types. As emphasized by Pirani (63), the diagnosis of myeloma CN cannot be easily excluded, and the search for typical casts has to be conducted on all available sections if necessary. Typical "myeloma" casts with a giant, multinucleated cell reaction can be very occasionally detected in other hemopathies including μ-HC disease (41) and Waldenström's disease (E. Morelon, personal communication).

By immunofluorescence, myeloma casts are essentially composed of the monoclonal LCs excreted by the patient and the THP. In most cases, casts are stained exclusively or predominantly with either the anti-κ or the anti-λ antibody. In about 25% of myeloma biopsy specimens, however, casts stain for both antibodies because they contain polyclonal LCs, together with albumin and fibrinogen (62). Staining of angular casts is often irregular, and more intense at the periphery (Fig. 76-2). In heterogeneous casts, the crystals themselves fail to stain while the matrix of the cast and the surrounding cellular debris and amorphous material often stain positively for one of the LCs.

Cast ultrastructure has been studied by electron microscopy in 24 biopsy samples of myeloma CN by Pirani and associates (62). Crystals were detected in 14 biopsy specimens and suspected in another four. The authors have identified four major categories of casts depending on their content and ultrastructural appearance. One category characterized by large rectangular crystals, or fragments thereof, with a pentagonal or hexagonal cross-section, is found only in myeloma CN. It seems to be closely linked to the development of a giant-cell reaction around the cast. A second category also

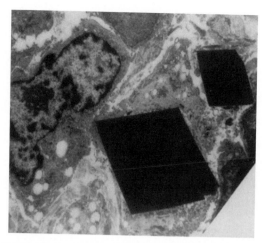

FIG. 76-3. Myeloma cast nephropathy. Rectangular crystals presumably composed of λ-light chains in tubular cells. (Electron micrograph, uranyl acetate and lead citrate $\times 7,000$.)

often contains crystals but they are small, electron-dense, and needle-shaped, and seemingly not associated with a cellular reaction. Similar large rectangular and small needle-shaped crystals can be found within plasma cells, suggesting that structural or physicochemical properties of LCs are directly responsible for crystal formation. Small and large crystals are also occasionally seen within the cytoplasm of either proximal or distal tubular cells (Fig. 76-3); they are surrounded by a single smooth membrane, indicating that they are located within lysosomes.

Tubules and Interstitium

Considerable tubular damage is almost always present in myeloma CN. Epithelial tubular lesions are seen not only in the distal tubules where casts are principally located, but also in proximal convoluted tubules whose epithelium undergoes atrophy and degenerative changes. Frank tubular necrosis may also be seen, with or without typical myeloma CN (37). By immunofluorescence, a variable number of tubule sections contain numerous "protein reabsorption droplets" staining for the monoclonal LC (64).

Interstitial lesions are often associated with the tubular damage. They may be mild and consist of inflammatory infiltrates and fibroedema, but fibrosis and its correlate, tubular atrophy, may also be fairly extensive. In severe cases with epithelial denudation and gaps in the continuity of the tubular basement membrane often in close contact with myeloma casts, granulomatouslike formations containing macrophages and histiocytes develop around the ruptured tubules (64) (Fig. 76-4).

Glomeruli and Vessels

The glomeruli are usually normal except for small clusters of globally sclerotic glomeruli and a mild thickening of the mesangial matrix. When mesangial thickening is more prominent, the possibility of an associated MIDD should be

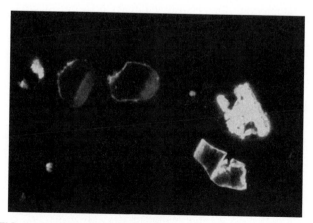

FIG. 76-2. Myeloma cast nephropathy. Several tubules contain large casts, one of which has an angular and fractured aspect. The stain with anti-κ antibody is more intense at the periphery of most casts. (Immunofluorescence $\times 312$.)

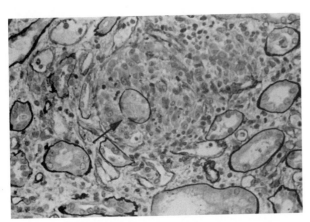

FIG. 76-4. Myeloma cast nephropathy. Interstitial granulomatouslike formations with macrophages surrounding disrupted tubular basement membrane (*arrow*) were numerous in this λ-chain cast nephropathy. (Silver stain ×312.)

considered. Amorphous deposits reminiscent of myeloma casts can exceptionally be seen in capillary loops or in the glomerular urinary space. In younger patients, severe chronic vascular lesions are sometimes observed, and may contribute to progression of sclerosis.

Pathophysiology of Myeloma Cast Nephropathy

CN occurs mainly in patients with myeloma with a high LC secretion rate (although there is no direct relation between this pathologic entity and the amount of urinary LCs). This suggests that LCs play a key pathogenetic role. That LCs are the main culprit is also supported by the following clinical, pathologic, and experimental data:

1. Renal lesions may recur on grafted kidneys (16).
2. Similar crystals may occasionally be seen within casts, proximal tubule cells, and plasma cells (63,65), suggesting that they are composed of the monoclonal LCs produced by the patient. Their usual lack of staining with anti-LC antibody is most likely due to degradation or masking of the relevant epitopes.

3. Mice injected with large amounts of LC purified from patients with CN developed extensive cast formation in the distal renal tubules (19,66). Electron microscopy showed that the casts contained elongated crystalloid structures (66) similar to those described later by Cohen and Border (64) and Pirani and associates (62) in patients with CN.

It is, however, surprising that a number of patients produce large amounts of LCs and yet fail to present significant signs of renal involvement throughout the course of the disease. This may be related to the absence of enhancing factors such as hypercalcemia, low urinary output and high urinary solute concentration, low urinary pH, and injection of contrast medium, but this also suggests that some LCs may be particularly prone to induce renal lesions, especially cast formation.

Because lesions observed in CN associate cast formation with proximal tubule cell lesions, it is usually believed that LCs are directly toxic to epithelial cells, resulting in decreased proximal reabsorption of the LCs and increased delivery to the distal tubule in which they coprecipitate with THP. Tubular obstruction by large and numerous casts may also contribute to the development of tubular lesions. For clarity, we will analyze separately the pathogenesis of proximal tubule lesions which result from renal metabolism of LCs, the mechanisms of cast formation, and the respective role of tubular obstruction and tubular lesions in the genesis of renal failure (Fig. 76-5). This mode of presentation is also warranted by the observation that certain LCs damage the proximal tubule while others precipitate in the distal tubule, obstructing the nephron, when perfused in rat nephrons *in vivo* (67).

Renal Metabolism of Light Chains and Pathogenesis of Proximal Tubule Lesions

An excess production of LCs over HCs appears to be required for efficient Ig synthesis, but it results in the release of free LCs, especially in myeloma. LCs are normally filtered by the glomerulus, then reabsorbed by the proximal tubule like

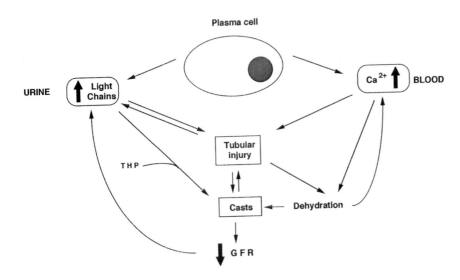

FIG. 76-5. Schematic representation of the pathogenesis of myeloma cast nephropathy. *GFR*, glomerular filtration rate; *THP*, Tamm-Horsfall protein; (Adapted from Winearls CG. Nephrology forum: acute myeloma kidney. *Kidney Int* 1995;48:1347.)

all filtered proteins. The λ-LCs and to a lesser extent κ-LCs circulate mainly as covalently linked dimers that have a mass-restricted glomerular filtration. In normal individuals, the small quantity of circulating free polyclonal LCs is filtered by glomeruli and approximately 90% of these are reabsorbed and catabolized by proximal tubular cells (14,68,69). LCs bind to a single class of low-affinity, high-capacity noncooperative binding sites described by Batuman and associates on both rat and human kidney brush-border membranes (70). These sites exhibit relative selectivity for LCs compared with albumin and β-lactoglobulin. They probably function as endocytotic receptors for LCs and possibly other low–molecular-weight proteins. It has recently been shown that LCs could bind to cubilin (71), a multiligand receptor belonging to the large family of low-density lipoprotein receptors and located in the intermicrovillar areas of the brush border. After binding to the luminal domain of proximal tubular epithelial cells, LCs are incorporated in endosomes that fuse with primary lysosomes where proteases, mainly cathepsin B, degrade the proteins into amino acids, which are returned to the circulation by the basolateral route. Decreased LC reabsorption can be induced by infusion of cationic amino acids that compete with the LC-binding sites (72), and by impairment of proximal tubule function.

When the concentration of filtered LCs is increased as in myeloma patients or experimental animals injected with LCs, profound functional and morphologic alterations of proximal tubule epithelial cells may occur. The functional disturbances include low–molecular-weight proteinuria (31,33), and inhibition of sodium-dependent uptake of amino acids and glucose by brush-border preparations (73). Morphologically, some of the LCs infused in mice (66) or rats (74) or perfused in rat nephron *in vivo* (67,75) accumulate in endosomes and lysosomes of the proximal convoluted tubule and sometimes of the distal convoluted tubule (66). Similar observations were made in a rat model of multiple myeloma in which spontaneously developing tumors that synthesized κ-LCs were transplanted to normal animals (76). Crystalloid formations were often seen within phagolysosomes in proximal tubule cells, and lysosomes often appeared markedly enlarged and distorted (76). Activation of the endosome/lysosome system was associated with mitochondrial alterations (74), prominent cytoplasmic vacuolation, focal loss of the microvillus border, and epithelial cell exfoliation (75).

These experiments thus establish that the proximal tubule epithelium is a main target of LC toxicity, but that not all LCs are toxic to this epithelium. These findings must, however, be interpreted with caution. In most cases, large amounts of LCs were injected or microperfused. Moreover, clinical characteristics and renal lesions of the patients from whom LCs were isolated were not defined or were poorly defined. Because of the heterogeneity of myeloma-associated tubulopathies, it might well be that some of the LCs, especially those prone to form crystals, were produced by patients with FS. On the other hand, these experimental models have served as an impetus for further experimental work, such as that carried out by Solomon and associates (19) who could establish

correlations between the type of LC deposits observed in the patient renal tubule (casts, crystals, or both) and the type of lesions induced 48 hours after intraperitoneal injection of the corresponding LC into mice. They also suggested that the proximal tubule endocytotic and lysosomal system might be overwhelmed when large quantities of LCs were filtered, thereby allowing LCs to proceed to the distal nephron. One may speculate that the more severe the LC-induced damage to the proximal tubule, the higher is the LC concentration is in the distal tubule.

Pathogenesis of Cast Formation

Because myeloma casts are composed principally of the monoclonal LC and THP, it has long been hypothesized that interaction of these two proteins was a key event in cast formation. THP is a highly glycosylated and acidic protein (isoelectric point (pI) = 3.2) synthesized exclusively by the cells of the ascending limb of Henle's loop (49). It is the major protein constituent of normal urine, and an almost universal component of casts whatever their nature and tubule location. This 80-kd protein is also remarkable for its ability to form reversibly high–molecular-size aggregates of about 7×10^6 daltons at high but physiologic concentrations of sodium and calcium, and at low urinary pH. The role of THP in cast formation has prompted a wealth of studies on its interactions with LCs. These studies were performed with the aim of defining a population of myeloma patients at risk of developing renal damage. The role of LC pI has long been suggested. As early as 1945, Oliver (61) proposed that the occurrence of casts in the distal tubules was the result of coagulation of globulins with a low pI in an acid urine. In 1979, Clyne and colleagues (77) suggested that LC with a high pI (greater than 5.6) and THP could bear opposite charges in the normal urine pH range, and undergo polar interaction between charged groups and precipitation. The Clyne group's hypothesis was supported by Coward and associates (78), who reported a significant negative correlation between pI and creatinine clearance. However, the nephritogenic potential of LCs with a high pI was not confirmed in further experimental and clinical studies (37,76,79,80). This does not rule out a role of LC interactions with THP based upon other physicochemical properties of the LC.

In an elegant series of works performed after the above reported studies, Sanders and coworkers implicated THP as a major pathogenetic factor. They first confirmed in a rat model that development of casts and injury to proximal tubule cells in renal tubules microperfused with human nephritogenic LC were not correlated with LC pI, molecular form, or isotype (67). Intranephronal obstruction was aggravated by decreasing extracellular fluid volume or adding furosemide. In perfused loop segments, cast-forming LCs reduced chloride absorption directly, thus increasing tubule fluid [Cl^-] and promoting their own aggregation with THP (81). Pretreatment of rats with colchicine completely prevented obstruction and cast formation in perfused nephrons (82).

THP from colchicine-treated rats did not contain sialic acid and did not aggregate with LCs *in vitro,* contrary to THP purified from control rats. More recent *in vitro* studies suggest that THP can undergo both self (homotypic) aggregation and heterotypic aggregation with LC (48). Homotypic aggregation is enhanced by calcium, furosemide, and low pH, and is dependent on THP sialic-acid content. Heterotypic aggregation requires previous binding of LC to the THP protein backbone (83). Studies on peptides identified by trypsin protection experiments allowed to identify a 9-residue sequence (amino acids 225 to 233) as the binding site on THP, including a histidine at position 226 that explains the pH dependence of LC–THP binding (84). The sugar moiety is also essential for coaggregation of LC and THP, perhaps by facilitating homotypic aggregation of THP.

These findings suggest that colchicine may be useful in the treatment of cast nephropathy and that new therapeutic strategies aimed at reducing LC–THP interactions can be envisioned. An increase in dietary salt and the loop diuretic, furosemide, may be harmful because they not only enhance THP homotypic aggregation, but they also increase THP expression in the rat (85). However, the mechanisms of cast nephropathy may not rely only on LC–THP interactions. First, we have found that five of 12 LCs purified from the urine of patients with CN failed to react with THP by enzyme-linked immunosorbent assay (ELISA) (24). Second, myeloma casts occasionally do not stain for THP in human biopsies (86), and casts induced in mice by LC injection do not seem to contain THP during the first 24 hours (66), indicating that some LCs may undergo aggregation or precipitation in the absence of THP. This hypothesis is supported by size-exclusion chromatography studies showing that the deposition of certain LCs *in vivo* may be related to their capability to aggregate *in vitro* (87). Other physicochemical properties of LCs may also play a pathogenetic role. We have found that 10 of the 12 LCs isolated from the urine of patients with CN showed significant resistance to trypsin or pepsin, or both; cathepsin B, a lysosomal enzyme, yielded small amounts of the variable domain of the LC in four cases (24). Resistance of LC to urinary and macrophage-released proteases may also contribute to cast formation and persistence since cells surrounding casts seem incapable of degrading cast proteins.

Role of Tubular Obstruction by Casts In the Genesis of Renal Failure

The role of casts as plugs obstructing the tubules has been clearly shown in micropuncture studies (88). In patients with myeloma the correlation between severity of renal insufficiency and the number of casts remains controversial. Hill and associates (89) find a good correlation between the extent of cast formation and degree of renal failure, whereas we (37) and others (32,90) fail to demonstrate this correlation. This may be explained partly by the prominent medullary

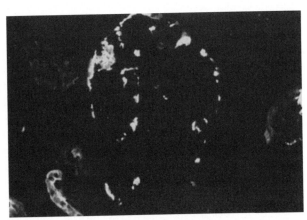

FIG. 76-6. Myeloma cast nephropathy. Immunofluorescence stain with anti–Tamm-Horsfall protein (THP) monoclonal antibody. Glomerular deposits in Bowman's space delineate the inner aspect of Bowman's capsule and penetrate between lobules of the capillary tuft. Identification of THP in the urinary spaces of glomeruli supports the obstructive role of casts with reflux of tubular urine. (Magnification ×312.)

localization of casts whose count is therefore underestimated in superficial kidney cortex biopsy specimens. The first indication that antibodies to THP could serve as probes of tubular obstruction was provided by Cohen and Border (64) who identified the protein in glomerular urinary spaces of two myeloma patients. This finding is indicative of intratubular urinary backflow (91). We detected THP in glomerular urinary spaces in 16 of 18 biopsies of patients with myeloma CN (92). Tamm-Horsfall deposits were often abundant, lining the inner aspect of Bowman's capsule and penetrating between lobules of the capillary tuft (Fig. 76-6). In other cases, they were segmental and localized between capillary loops. Fifty-five (46%) of the 119 glomeruli available for study stained for THP. Glomerular deposits of THP were also found in 10 of 13 mice grafted with a LC-secreting murine plasmacytoma, which developed severe renal lesions within 4 to 6 weeks (92). Although tubular obstruction is confirmed by this immunomorphologic study, the proportion of affected tubules is too small to account by itself for renal failure. As expected, renal failure induced by CN is multifactorial, implicating also tubular epithelial cell and interstitial lesions. From a clinical point of view, tubule obstruction by casts may explain the slow recovery of renal function noted in many patients (37).

Interstitial deposits of THP were also found in 8 (44%) of the 18 biopsies examined with specific antibodies (92). They probably result from a leakage of the protein through gaps in the tubular basement membrane favored by tubular obstruction. Clinical and experimental models have implicated the protein in the pathogenesis of tubulointerstitial nephritis. The role of THP has recently been partially elucidated by Thomas and associates (93,94). They identified a single class of sialic acid-specific cell surface receptors for THP on polymorphonuclear leukocytes, and further showed that *in vitro* activation of human mononuclear phagocytes by particulate

TABLE 76-6. *Histologic prognostic factors for recovery of renal function in patients with myeloma cast nephropathy[a]*

Group[b]	Tubular necrosis	Isolated	Myeloma cast nephropathy associated with			Chronic interstitial nephritis
			Tubular necrosis	Interstitial infiltrate	Fibrosis	
I (n = 7)	2	2	1	—	—	—
II (n = 9)	—	—	1	2	3	2
III (n = 18)	—	2	3[c]	1	11	—

[a]A renal biopsy was performed in 30 of 34 patients.
[b]I = complete; II = partial; III = no recovery of renal failure.
[c]Survival time less than 60 days.
(From Rota S, et al. Multiple myeloma and severe renal failure: a clinicopathologic study of outcome and prognosis in 34 patients. *Medicine (Baltimore)* 1987;66:126, with permission.)

THP led to the release of gelatinase and reactive oxygen metabolites, both probably contributing to tissue damage.

In conclusion, there is now considerable evidence that some LCs are intrinsically prone to induce tubular damage but the type of the predominant renal lesion (e.g., casts, crystals, or tubular epithelial cell alterations) varies from one LC to another. In addition, extrinsic factors including dehydration, hypercalcemia, low urine pH, and use of contrast medium or xenobiotics toxic to epithelial cells most likely enhance LC toxicity. Combined intrinsic and extrinsic factors account for the heterogeneity of renal lesions including typical and nonspecific (hyaline) casts, tubular epithelial atrophy and necrosis, and interstitial inflammatory infiltrates. Tubular obstruction plays an important but not exclusive role in the genesis of renal failure. Both tubular obstruction and acute tubular lesions are theoretically reversible.

Outcome and Prognosis of Myeloma Cast Nephropathy

Until the 1980s, myeloma-induced renal failure was associated with a very poor prognosis. In the first series reported by DeFronzo and colleagues (42), only 5 of 14 patients survived the early period of acutely impaired renal function, and 4 of these subsequently died within 2 months. A series of studies published between 1977 and 1984 (reviewed in reference 37) showed that although the overall prognosis was improving, the percentage of renal failure reversibility varied considerably from 0% to 60%. More recent studies have provided clear information on the renal and vital outcome.

Renal Outcome and Prognostic Factors

In 1987, we performed an exhaustive analysis of clinical and pathologic features in 34 patients with myeloma and severe renal failure in an attempt to reappraise the renal and vital outcome and to identify those factors predictive of complete or partial recovery of renal function (37). Sixteen of the 34 patients experienced completely or partially reversible renal failure, while 18 did not recover (9 of whom required dialysis). None of the clinical and biologic factors usually considered to be of prognostic value could predict a higher chance of recovering. Age, tumor mass, LC urinary output, oliguria, peak creatinine, hypercalcemia, infection, and LC pI were similar in both groups. The only difference was in the gender of patients: fewer females recovered than males. In contrast, main prognostic indicators were provided by renal histology, which was available in 88% of patients (Table 76-6). Return to normal renal function was seen only in patients with typical CN and/or tubular necrosis in the absence of interstitial damage. Global tubular atrophy and interstitial fibrosis were associated with partially or totally irreversible renal failure. The number of casts was not predictive.

We also found that recovery from renal failure after antitumor chemotherapy and symptomatic treatment might be delayed by several months. This observation is supported by the data from the Canadian Organ Replacement Register, which recorded that 7.2% of patients with myeloma on dialysis for more than 45 days recovered sufficient renal function to be independent of dialysis for more than 3 months (95). It is also in agreement with the patterns of evolution of serum creatinine described by Ganeval and associates (40). These authors noticed that patients with improved renal function showed a phase of rapid decrease in serum creatinine level within the first month, and then a second phase of much slower improvement. The first phase of improvement is mostly independent of chemotherapy since it takes place before the first signs of objective response and sometimes despite obviously uncontrolled growth of the tumor. The second phase is likely the result of both chemotherapy (in responders) and continuation of measures undertaken to suppress the toxic renal effect of remnant LCs.

Table 76-7 summarizes the renal outcome and prognostic factors identified in series subsequent to ours. The mean percentage of renal recovery was about 50%, with extremes of 17% and 83%. Such variations may be due to the way recovery is defined, the severity of renal failure, and the prevalence of precipitating factors. It must be pointed out that high serum creatinine level at presentation was quoted in two studies (38,40) as a marker of poor prognosis. This implies

TABLE 76-7. *Renal recovery, median survival, and prognostic indicators in 285 patients with severe renal failure and myeloma (1987–1995)*

Series (ref. no.)	No. of patients[a]	Renal recovery (%)	Median survival (mo.)	Renal predictors	Survival predictors
Rota, et al., 1987 (37)	34	47	19	Female gender (−)[b] Interstitial lesions, tubular atrophy	No renal recovery
Pozzi, et al., 1987 (38)	50	46	11	Serum creatinine Severity of renal lesions, number of casts	No renal recovery
Misiani, et al., 1987 (107)	23	83	9	NA	Response to chemotherapy
Pasquali, et al., 1990 (39)	37	43	17	NA	No renal recovery Hypercalcemia, early infection Interstitial fibrosis, tubular atrophy No plasma exchange
Johnson, et al., 1990 (111)	21	57	22	No. of casts Response to chemotherapy	NA
Ganeval, et al., 1992 (40)[c]	78	62	20	Serum creatinine at presentation	Response to chemotherapy Disease stage Renal function after 1 mo.
Winearls, 1995 (43) Mean (range)	42	17 51 (17–83)	20 17(9–22)	NA —	NA —

NA, not available.

[a]Includes early deaths.

[b](−) indicates pejorative prognostic factors.

[c]Includes 29 patients with renal biopsies: 19 with myeloma cast nephropathy, 2 with amyloidosis, and 8 with light-chain deposition disease.

that renal function impairment of any degree should be treated as a medical emergency (43).

The incidence of reversal of renal failure was about the same (51%) in Alexanian's series mixing renal and nonrenal patients (36). Reversibility of renal failure was more frequent only in patients with monoclonal IgG or IgA (63%) or with a serum creatinine level less than 270 μmol/L (67%); renal failure was reversible in only 24% of patients with pure LC myeloma. The median time for renal improvement was shorter (36 days) than in series including only patients with renal involvement (77 days in the series by Rota et al. [37]); the latter series, however, included patients with more severe renal failure.

Survival and Predictors

Median survival time in patients with myeloma and severe renal failure was 17 months (9 to 22 months) in the more recent series including mainly or exclusively patients with myeloma CN. However, careful scrutiny of our cases according to renal outcome showed that survival time was about 2 years in those patients whose serum creatinine returned to normal, compared to only 5 months in patients with irreversible renal failure (37). The effect of recovering renal function on survival was emphasized in three other series (38–40) (Table 76-7). Response to chemotherapy is another important predictor (Table 76-7). It is likely that the favorable effect of reversal of renal failure on survival is partly due to the reduction or disappearance of LCs observed in good responders.

In the Alexanian series of 494 consecutive myeloma patients (36), a large tumor mass was the only significant variable adversely affecting survival ($P < 0.001$) on multivariate analysis. For comparable patients with high tumor mass, the frequency of response was less and the remission and survival times were shorter with more severe renal failure, but the differences were not significant. Reversal of renal failure did not confer a survival advantage, contrary to response to chemotherapy. Myeloma remission was associated with an estimated 43% decrease in mortality rate.

In summary, contrary to a widely held belief, the presence or degree of renal failure *at diagnosis* is not a definite predictor of poor survival in myeloma patients. Tumor mass and response to chemotherapy are the two main predictors of survival. Reversibility of renal failure may also be a prognostic marker in patients with more severe deterioration of renal function (renal patient series). These conclusions suggest that myeloma patients with renal failure should be treated with the same chemotherapy as those without renal failure, and that any measure that could contribute to improve renal function (high fluid intake, urine alkalinization) should be taken on the day of diagnosis.

Treatment

The treatment of patients with CN-induced renal failure has two main objectives: (a) limiting further cast precipitation by reducing precipitability of the urinary LC and LC production rate, and (b) avoiding complications of uremia by dialysis and sometimes by transplantation. Even more importantly, preventive measures are essential to reduce the incidence of renal failure.

Decreasing Precipitability of the Urinary LC by Immediate Symptomatic Measures

Since coprecipitation in renal tubules of free LC and THP is the main nephritogenic event, measures to reduce concentration and precipitability of both partners are essential and urgent. They include rehydration, correction of hypercalcemia, stopping NSAIDs and ACE inhibitors, and treatment of infections with nonnephrotoxic antibiotics (40,96,97). Despite controversy about the role of LC pI in cast formation, alkalinization of urine remains recommended because solubility of THP is reduced at low pH and because an acidic environment increases LC binding to THP. Therefore a daily urine output greater than 3 L and a urine pH greater than 7.0 should be reached in all patients whose cardiac and renal function can tolerate a deliberate expansion of the extracellular fluid volume. These measures alone are sufficient to improve renal function in the majority of patients with renal impairment at presentation (36,96). However, they must be accompanied by therapeutic means aimed at decreasing the amount of urinary LCs filtered by glomeruli.

Reducing Production Rate (and Concentration) of the Monoclonal Light Chains

Most patients with myeloma reported to date in renal series were treated with conventional chemotherapy (i.e., alkylating agents and high-dose corticosteroids). No difference in survival time was observed between patients who received either continuous or discontinuous regimens (40). With these protocols, the response rate was 45% (40), similar to that found in series with few patients with renal failure (98). Many of the recent series described patients treated over a period when both chemotherapy and general management were evolving. It is therefore impossible to identify the best chemotherapy for patients with renal failure. The melphalan–prednisone combination remains the first-line conventional chemotherapy. Its drawbacks are slow antitumor action and necessity of reducing melphalan doses because the drug has renal elimination (99). Regimens including vincristine and doxorubicin ("VAD") induce earlier remission, which is an advantage in patients with hypercalcemia and renal failure, and are safer in patients with renal failure because the cytotoxic drugs are metabolized in the liver. Although a higher proportion of patients achieve remission with this regimen, its long-term efficacy in terms of median survival and

duration of remission is not better than that of melphalan–prednisone. The VAD protocol is efficient in the treatment of relapses (40% remission) (98) and of refractory myelomas (25% remission). Recombinant interferon α-2b might be beneficial in combination with chemotherapy or as a maintenance treatment. However, these therapeutic regimens have not radically changed the global prognosis of multiple myeloma.

In the past 10 years, the concept of high-dose chemotherapy regimens with hematopoietic stem cell support (to reduce the duration of the drug-induced myelosuppression with its high risks of morbidity and mortality) has modified the treatment of young patients with multiple myeloma (100). Transplantation from an allogeneic donor may have the advantage over autotransplantation of a potential "graft versus myeloma" effect, but the procedure still has a high level of related mortality. Many more patients are candidates for autologous transplantation that is now usually performed using peripheral blood stem cells. One can take advantage of $CD34^+$ cell selection to reduce the number of tumor cells in reinfused grafts. In 1996, a randomized controlled trial first demonstrated the benefits of high-dose therapy over conventional combination therapy in terms of complete remission rate, event-free survival, and overall survival in patients with normal renal function (101). High-dose therapy with autotransplantation may allow patients to obtain a median overall survival exceeding 5 years.

Until recently, however, high-dose therapy with stem cell transplantation had not been considered in patients with significant renal impairment. Small series are now appearing in the literature showing that this procedure is possible in these patients (102–104). It seems that transplant-related mortality is equivalent to that in similar patients with normal renal function.

The use of plasmapheresis was extensively discussed in a nephrology forum (43). It has been advocated by many to reduce LC concentration rapidly but its efficacy has not been convincingly established, except in patients with hyperviscosity syndrome (105–111). Two randomized controlled trials have been published thus far (109,111). Further randomized control trials enrolling more patients are required. However, it seems that those patients with more severe disease and acute renal failure may benefit from plasma exchanges. For this subpopulation of patients, it seems necessary to find new ways to remove more circulating monoclonal Ig more rapidly. In any case, plasma exchanges should not substitute for a vigorous treatment of precipitating factors of renal failure.

Supportive therapy in the form of blood transfusion, analgesia, and biphosphonates are important adjuncts to therapy. Berenson and coworkers demonstrated that pamidronate, a moderately potent biphosphonate, could reduce pain, hypercalcemia, radiotherapy episodes, and fractures in patients with Durie-Salmon stage III myeloma (112,113). Biphosphonates given intravenously may also be able to improve overall survival, perhaps by inducing apoptosis in myeloma cells (114). The total dose of pamidronate does not need to be reduced in renal impairment but regular review of renal function is recommended. Pamidronate has been used successfully in patients receiving hemodialysis (J. Berenson, personal communication). Infusion rate should not exceed 20 mg/hour in renal patients.

Dialysis and Renal Transplantation

Dialysis is clearly indicated for the treatment of acute renal failure and end-stage renal disease, except in patients with myeloma refractory to chemotherapy. It should be started early to avoid the added complications of uremia and to compensate for the hypercatabolic state induced by the use of high doses of corticosteroids. If peritoneal dialysis is chosen, early placement of a permanent indwelling dialysis catheter is recommended to avoid infectious peritonitis, the risk for which is increased by chemotherapy-induced leukopenia (43). Residual renal function must be carefully monitored because of possible improvement after several months of dialysis (95, 115). Two reports from Great Britain (116) and the United States (117) suggest that chronic dialysis is a worthwhile treatment in patients with myeloma and renal failure. Survival at 1 year was 45% in the British study (23 patients) and 54% in the American one (731 patients). At 30 months, survival rate declined to 25% compared with 66% in nondiabetic end-stage renal disease patients without myeloma (117). These data have been confirmed in more recent studies that showed a 1-year survival rate of 63% and a median survival of 12 to 20 months in patients with myeloma undergoing hemodialysis (review in reference 97). Hemodialysis and chronic ambulatory peritoneal dialysis (CAPD) appear to be equally effective treatments, but most authors emphasize the serious risk of infection in CAPD patients (116).

The experience with renal transplantation in myeloma is extremely limited (16,118,119). In one patient (16), lesions recurred early in the graft but normal renal function was sustained. Transplantation should be limited to carefully selected patients with an inactive hematologic disease.

Finally, if most cases of severe renal failure cannot be prevented because they occur simultaneously with the finding of myeloma, it is necessary to avoid or correct all precipitating factors of renal failure in patients with established myeloma. It is particularly important to reduce the use of NSAIDs as analgesic drugs to detect and control hypercalcemia as soon as possible and to correct dehydration.

Fanconi's Syndrome

Fanconi's syndrome (FS) is characterized by renal glycosuria, generalized aminoaciduria, hypophosphatemia, and often chronic acidosis, hypouricemia, and hypokalemia. It also often includes osteomalacia with pseudofractures. These manifestations result from functional impairment of the renal proximal tubule. The first association of FS with myeloma was reported by Sirota and Hamerman (120), although these authors considered FS and myeloma as two separate diseases. Engle and Wallis (121) first identified crystal-like inclusions in the tumor cells and in the renal tubule epithelial cells, and suggest that FS and myeloma could be related. Costanza and Smoller (122) describe cytoplasmic inclusions as round or rodlike electron–opaque structures with longitudinally oriented fibrils. Lee and associates (123) definitely establish myeloma as a cause of FS in the adult. Maldonado and associates (124) report the first review of 17 cases of FS with LC proteinuria and myeloma or amyloidosis, and a recent study including a review of 57 cases has been published (reviewed further in reference 25). Fewer than 70 documented cases have been reported to date. The rarity of FS in patients with myeloma contrasts with the high prevalence of tubule alterations in myeloma autopsy series (29) and after LC injection in animals. It suggests that unusual specific properties of LCs, mostly κ, are involved in the pathophysiology of FS.

Clinical Presentation

The clinical features of patients with plasma cell dyscrasia-associated FS are summarized in Table 76-8 (25). Most patients are over 50 years of age with a slight female predominance. Most common initial manifestations are bone pain and weakness, principally due to osteomalacia. The major cause of osteomalacia is hypophosphatemia, which results from increased urinary clearance of phosphate. Chronic acidosis and abnormal renal vitamin D metabolism further contribute to the development of bone lesions. Bone pain may also be the consequence of lytic lesions in patients with a high-mass myeloma. Other revealing signs are essentially due to the proximal tubule impairment or are related to hypokalemia. Renal failure occurs more frequently than one would expect in a disease of the proximal tubule.

Criteria for the diagnosis of FS (e.g., "orthoglycemic" glycosuria, increased phosphate and uric acid clearances, and generalized aminoaciduria) may not all be present, especially in patients with renal failure. Deterioration of renal function occurs in about half of the patients with plasma cell dyscrasia-associated FS, while it is rare in other causes of the syndrome. Generalized aminoaciduria is then a useful criterion in distinguishing FS from the nonspecific proximal tubular transport abnormalities found in chronic renal failure (123). The diagnosis of FS is often unrecognized for several years in patients presenting with proteinuria, bone pain, or renal failure. The mean time from onset to diagnosis of FS is about 3 years. Typically, the diagnosis of FS precedes that of the plasma cell dyscrasia, most often a κ–LC-excreting multiple myeloma, because the hematologic disease has a low tumor burden and a slow progression. In 21 out of 66 published cases, criteria for the diagnosis of myeloma are even lacking, and patients are momentarily classified as having a benign monoclonal gammopathy of undetermined significance (MGUS). In some patients, the diagnosis of the plasma cell dyscrasia remains undetermined between myeloma and MGUS because it may be difficult

TABLE 76-8. *Clinical characteristics of patients with plasma cell dyscrasia-associated Fanconi's syndrome*[a]

Total no. of patients	Age mean/ extremes	Gender	Initial manifestations	Bone lesions	Renal failure[c]	Plasma cell dyscrasia	Light chain isotype
68	57/22–81	30 males 38 females	Bone pain (25)[b] Weakness, fatigue (16) Weight loss (7) Polyuria–polydipsia (7) Hypokalemia-related signs (4) Proteinuria (18) Renal failure (16) Renal glycosuria (13)	Osteomalacia (25) High-mass myeloma (12) Plasmacytoma (1)	54	Myeloma (36)[d] MGUS (21)[e] MGUS/myeloma[f] (4) Lymphoma/CLL[g] (4) "Atypical" plasma cell dyscrasia (1)	49κ 7λ

[a]Figures in parentheses indicate number of patients.
[b]Related to osteomalacia.
[c]Serum creatinine >130 μmol/L, or creatinine clearance <80 mL/mn.
[d]Including 12 patients with a high-mass myeloma.
[e]Monoclonal gammopathy of undetermined significance (MGUS).
[f]Undetermined diagnosis, mostly due to cytoplasmic inclusions in plasma cells making interpretation of cytology difficult.
[g]Chronic lymphocytic leukemia (CLL).
(From Messiaen, et al. Adult Fanconi syndrome secondary to light chain gammopathy: clinicopathologic heterogeneity and unusual features in 11 patients. *Medicine* (Baltimore) 2000;19:135, with permission)

to recognize the cytologic characteristics of myeloma cells when the cytoplasm of plasma cells is stuffed with crystals.

Pathologic Data

FS is typically characterized by prominent crystals in enlarged proximal tubular cells and by degenerative changes of proximal tubules (25). In most cases, crystals are already visible by light microscopy. Proximal tubular cells are stuffed with microcrystals that stain red or green with Masson's trichrome and are periodic acid-Schiff negative. In the most severely affected tubules, crystal-containing exfoliated cells are seen in the tubule lumen while intracytoplasmic crystals are still present in atrophic tubules. In other cases, crystals can be only suspected by the presence of a finely granular material of glassy appearance in an enlarged proximal tubular epithelium (Fig. 76-7). Their presence is more easily demonstrated by toluidine-blue staining of semi-thin sections and by hematoxylin and eosin staining of cryostat sections. In all cases, crystals are present in the majority of proximal tubule cells. However, in the same tubule sections, all the cells are not equally affected: cells with a normal aspect coexist with crystal-stuffed cells. A common feature of all cases is the presence of severe lesions of the proximal tubule epithelium devoid of crystals. These lesions include vacuolization, loss of the luminal brush border, and focal cell sloughing, with cell fragments in the lumen of the tubules. Interstitial cellular infiltrate including plasma cells may contain analogous crystalline inclusion bodies. Patchy tubular atrophy and focal interstitial fibrosis together with a variable number of obsolescent glomeruli are often observed.

Immunologic confirmation of the nature of the crystalline deposits was first provided by Thorner and associates (126) in a case of λ–LC-FS, whereas in several cases, attempts to characterize the crystal proteins with anti-Ig conjugates

including anti-LC antibodies failed (127,128). When immunohistochemical studies are positive, crystals stain only (or predominantly) for the monoclonal LC, most often κ (Fig. 76-7). By electron microscopy, crystals of various size

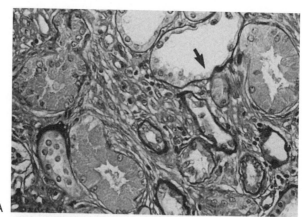

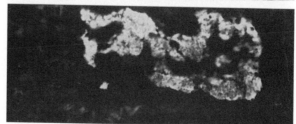

FIG. 76-7. Plasma cell dyscrasia-associated Fanconi's syndrome. **A:** Glassy appearance of the epithelium of several proximal convoluted tubules. Crystals were not evident by light microscopy, but were demonstrated by electron microscopy. Note also the severe lesions of the epithelial cells lining other tubules (*arrow*), interstitial fibrosis, and tubular atrophy. (Periodic acid-Schiff ×312.) **B:** Immunofluorescence stain of the same tubules with anti-κ monoclonal antibody. (Magnification ×312.)

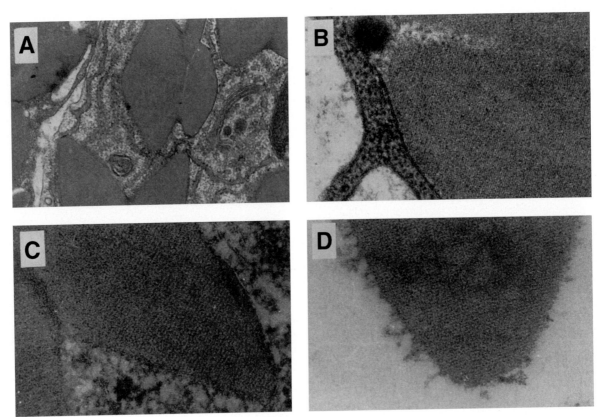

FIG. 76-8. Plasma cell dyscrasia-associated Fanconi's syndrome. Electron microscopic study of intracellular (*A, B,* and *C*) and *in vitro*-formed crystals in the same patient. **A:** Bone marrow plasma cell (and a macrophage on the left). (Magnification ×8,000.) **B:** Bone marrow macrophage. (Magnification ×50,000.) **C:** Proximal convoluted tubular epithelial cell. (Magnification ×50,000.) **D:** Crystal obtained *in vitro* from Sephadex G100 fraction C from the patient's urine. (From Aucouturier P, et al. Monoclonal Ig L chain and L chain V domain fragment crystallization in myeloma-associated Fanconi's syndrome. *J Immunol* 1993;150:3561, with permission.)

and shape (rectangular, rhomboid, round, or needle-shaped) are detected within the cytoplasm of proximal tubule cells (Fig. 76-8). Intracytoplasmic crystals are surrounded by a single smooth membrane, most likely of lysosomal origin (23,62,126). In rare cases, crystals are also seen in distal tubule cells (126,129). In other cases, crystals are not seen by light microscopy, but electron microscopy shows enlarged vesicular bodies containing dense tubular and rodlike structures (122–124,128,130,131) or fibrils and needle-shaped deposits very close to crystalline structures (129).

Crystal formation in plasma cell dyscrasia-associated FS is not limited to renal tubule epithelium but also occurs in bone marrow and tissue-infiltrating plasma cells, and in macrophages (23,121–124,130,132,133) (Fig. 76-8). The presence of crystals in macrophages close to the tumoral plasma cells might result from endocytosis of either freshly secreted LCs or lysed plasma cells. In plasma cells, the crystals are either unstained by anti-κ antibodies and clearly visible negatively on the strong diffuse cytoplasmic staining background, or stained more brightly than the rest of the cytoplasm, especially in their periphery (23). They are quasi-identical to those found in proximal tubule epithelial cells of the same patient (Fig. 76-8). They may be surrounded by smooth membranes, and therefore localized in lysosomes, but are also often found

inside the granular endoplasmic reticulum (134). These observations indicate that FS-LCs accumulate in lysosomes and in endoplasmic reticulum. LC degradation in plasma cells is well established (135–137) and may also occur in the endoplasmic reticulum (138). Crystal formation in these organelles therefore suggests incomplete proteolysis of LCs.

Although crystals are a salient feature of plasma cell dyscrasia-associated FS, they are neither specific nor absolutely constant. They can also be found in proximal tubule epithelial cells of patients with CN but in low amounts (24,62), and occasionally in myeloma patients with isolated tubular lesions, that is, in the absence of distal nephron myeloma casts (139,140). In addition, recent pathologic studies of 11 patients show that FS due to LC gammopathy is more heterogeneous than expected (25). A first group of seven patients presented with crystals in tubule cells, no myeloma casts, and a low-mass myeloma or a MGUS, thus corresponding to the typical form of FS described by Maldonado and colleagues (124). A second group of three patients showed myeloma casts in the setting of a high-mass myeloma. One patient of this group combined the typical histologic features of FS with those of myeloma CN. The two others did not show crystal inclusions in tubule cells even on electron microscopy examination. Only nine other patients with FS and high-mass myeloma have been reported, probably because the search for signs of FS is not routinely performed and crystal formation in proximal tubule cells is unusual in this setting. The last patient of our series had a MGUS and a full-blown FS but neither crystals nor casts.

These observations led to the following suggestions. First, the slow progression of myeloma disease in typical FS associated with crystal formation may be explained by the deleterious effects on cell growth of the accumulation of crystalline inclusions in the tumor plasma cells. Second, that FS may occur in the absence of overt crystal formation suggests that clogging of the endolysosomal system may be directly or indirectly responsible for the proximal tubule impairment. However, similar morphologic alterations including atypical lysosomes are also found in patients with LC deposits in the glomeruli and/or interstitium, but without FS (139). This leads to the conclusion that FS is not merely the consequence of lysosomal disturbances in proximal tubule epithelial cells, but that additional alterations are involved.

Pathophysiology of Plasma Cell Dyscrasia-Associated Fanconi's Syndrome

The rare occurrence of FS in multiple myeloma, the peculiar proneness of LCs to form crystals, and their unique ability to alter proximal tubular transports, indicate that LCs have unusual physicochemical properties. The peculiar propensity of certain LCs to form crystals *in vivo* is attested by experimental studies in mice (19) and rats (67,75,144). It is remarkable that the κ-LCs that induced crystallization *in vivo*, also significantly reduced the glucose, chloride, and volume fluxes (75,141). The clinical characteristics of the patients from whom the LCs were isolated, especially the presence of FS, were unfortunately not specified.

We have analyzed the crystal composition in a patient with myeloma-associated FS and hexagonal crystals in kidney proximal tubular cells, bone marrow plasma cells, and phagocytes (23). N-terminal sequencing and mass spectrometry studies showed that a 107-amino acid fragment corresponding to the variable domain of the κ-LC (Vκ) was the essential component of crystals forming spontaneously from the patient's urine (Fig. 76-9A). Vκ was also crystallized alone using the hanging drop technique (Fig. 76-9B). Crystals were hexagonal bipyramids and had the same 6.0-nm periodicity on electron micrographs as those found in the cells. The peculiar proneness of the V domain to resist proteolysis by trypsin, pepsin, and cathepsin B, to self-react, and to form crystals may explain its accumulation in phagolysosomes of plasma cells and proximal tubular cells. In further studies, we established that all four LC-V domains from patients with pure FS, but none of 12 LCs from patients with CN or four LCs from control patients, displayed resistance to cathepsin

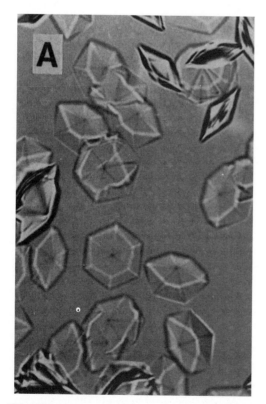
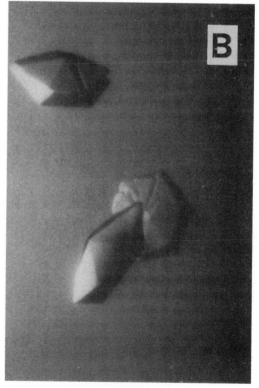

FIG. 76-9. Plasma cell dyscrasia-associated Fanconi's syndrome. Same patient as in Fig. 76-7. Crystals spontaneously obtained *in vitro* from a Sephadex G100 fraction of the patient's urinary proteins (**A**) and by the hanging drop technique from purified Vκ fragment (**B**). (**A**, magnification ×400; **B**, size of these crystals, 0.25 mm.) (From Aucouturier P, et al. Monoclonal Ig L chain and L chain V domain fragment crystallization in myeloma-associated Fanconi's syndrome. *J Immunol* 1993;150:3561, with permission.)

B (24). This property was not strictly associated with crystal formation, although crystals were shown to be made of V domain only. Furthermore, the Vκ domain was shown to be sensitive to proteolysis by cathepsin B in two patients with a high-mass myeloma from our more recent series (25), which suggests that the pathophysiology of tubule injury in FS might involve several distinct mechanisms. At variance with the observations made in patients with CN (24,83), LCs from patients with FS did not bind THP except in one case where both syndromes were associated.

The unusual physicochemical behavior of FS κ-chains was tentatively correlated with their structure in a number of cases (142). Sequence analyses showed that eight of nine (89%) LCs belonged to the VκI variability subgroup while this subgroup only accounts for 56% of all monoclonal κ-LCs. The VκI appeared to originate from only two germline genes, *LCO2/O12* in five cases and *LCO8/O18* in three. Analyses of the DNA sequence of germline, non-rearranged Vκ-gene segments in four patients revealed complete identity with the known *LCO2/O12* allele, which suggests that all structure peculiarities arose from somatic mutations in the proliferating clone (P. Aucouturier and Vidal, unpublished data). In the nine available sequences, residues had never or rarely been reported among VκI subgroup LCs. The unusual presence of nonpolar or hydrophobic residues in the CDR-L1 loop at position 30 was found in the five LCs derived from gene *LCO2/O12*. Nonpolar amino acids at position 30 can also be identified in LCs from AL-amyloidosis patients, however in such cases they have an aspartic acid at position 50, while all *LCO2/O12*-derived FS-LCs express a nonpolar (glycine or alanine) amino acid at this position (F.J. Stevens, personal communication). Moreover, besides sequence differences, FS and AL-amyloidosis display evident distinctive ultrastructural and biochemical features. FS-LCs appear to have low dimerization constants (F.J. Stevens, personal communication) while in AL-amyloidosis, V regions have a high propensity for forming dimers that might initiate their regular assembly into protofibrils (143). Monomeric LCs could expose hydrophobic surfaces that are buried in dimers. We recently showed the presence of unusually exposed hydrophobic residues on FS-LCs (142), while, on the other hand, amyloid fibril formation likely involves interactions between charged amino acids. Altogether, differences in polarity of the molecule surfaces may, at least partially, determine either the unidimensional pseudocrystallization of LC-V domains in amyloidogenesis (144), or the classic crystal formation observed in most cases of FS.

In summary, unusual properties of LCs in FS might explain crystal formation or LC accumulation in lysosomes. After endocytosis, LCs are processed in the endosomal and lysosomal compartment where "normal" LCs are degraded. In myeloma-associated FS, accumulation of the protease-resistant V domain fragment generated by lysosomal enzymes may induce crystal formation in this vesicular compartment. In two cases where crystals were not found in proximal tubule cells, similar protease resistance was observed (25), suggesting noncrystalline accumulation. Clogging of the endolysosomal system may subsequently alter apical membrane recycling and/or ATP production (hence, Na^+–K^+–ATPase functioning) as suggested by mitochondrial injury (123), and lead to progressive impairment of sodium-dependent apical transports. However, we do not know why FS does not occur in patients with apparently the same degree of distortion of the lysosomal compartment as can be seen in certain patients with myeloma with or without CN. The molecular mechanisms responsible for glycosuria, phosphaturia, generalized aminoaciduria, and uric acid loss remain poorly understood.

Treatment

There has been little information about the outcome and the response of FS to the treatment of the plasma cell dyscrasia (25,129,131,145). In patients with osteomalacia, considerable improvement can be obtained with α-hydroxy vitamin D, calcium, and phosphorus supplementation. The effect of chemotherapy on the proximal tubule impairment is much more debated. Uchida and associates (131) and Orfila and colleagues (129) reported that the treatment of myeloma could improve urinary signs and tubular transport abnormalities. On the other hand, it has been suggested (146) that the presence of crystals within plasma cells should be added to the list of criteria defined by Kyle and Greipp (147) against chemotherapy in myeloma. In our series of 11 cases, we have not observed a significant improvement of FS in the six patients who were treated with chemotherapy or α-interferon (25).

AMYLOIDOSIS

Amyloidosis has been known to be associated with or to cause renal disease for more than 100 years. Amyloid was originally identified as a waxy substance by Rokitansky in 1842 (148), but the term *amyloid* was coined by Virchow in 1854 (149) because the substance stained with iodine in a way that was similar to starch and cellulose. Although the protein content of amyloid was recognized subsequently, the term *amyloid* persisted. The diversity of amyloidotic disease was rapidly suspected on clinical grounds, but chemical studies in the late 1960s actually provided the basis of the present classification of amyloid (Table 76-9). In 1968, Pras and associates (150) isolated and purified amyloid fibrils, which opened the way to further chemical analyses. In 1971, Glenner and colleagues (4) found that the amyloid fibril proteins from two patients had an N-terminal sequence identical to Ig LCs, thus providing the first demonstration of a relation between amyloidosis and Ig. They also generated "amyloidlike" fibrils by proteolytic digestion of some human LCs, thus demonstrating their propensity of forming amyloid (151).

AL amyloidosis is certainly among the most severe complications of plasma cell proliferative disorders. From a practical point of view, it must be considered as such since the only efficient therapeutic tools to date are chemotherapeutic

TABLE 76-9. *Classification of amyloidoses*

Type	Precursor protein	Involved organs	Associated clinical syndrome
AL (AH)	Ig light chain (heavy chain)	Systemic (mostly kidneys, liver, heart, spleen, vessels, lungs, gastrointestinal tract, nerves, tongue)	Systemic amyloidosis (multiple organ involvement) Rarely, localized amyloidosis (orbital, for instance)
Aβ_2m	β_2-Microglobulin	Systemic (mostly musculoskeletal system, heart, synovium)	Hemodialysis-associated amyloidosis
AA	SAA apolipoprotein	Systemic (mostly spleen, liver, kidneys)	Systemic secondary amyloidosis Familial Mediterranean fever
AapoA1	Apolipoprotein A1	Nerves	Peripheral neuropathy
ATTR	Transthyretin	Nervous system, kidneys, thyroid, heart	Familial amyloid polyneuropathy Senile systemic amyloidosis
AGel	Gelsolin	Systemic (vessels)	Finnish hereditary systemic amyloidosis
Aβ	β-Amyloid precursor protein	Brain	Alzheimer's disease Down's syndrome
APrP	Prion protein	Brain	Creutzfeldt-Jakob disease and other spongiform encephalopathies
ACys	Cystatin C	Brain and other tissues	Iceland-type hereditary amyloid angiopathy
AIAPP	Islet amyloid polypeptide	Pancreas	Insulinoma, type II diabetes
ACal	Procalcitonin	Thyroid	Thyroid medullary carcinoma

(Adapted from Husby G, et al. The 1990 Guidelines for Nomenclature and Classification of Amyloid and Amyloidosis. In: Natvig JB, et al., eds. *Amyloid and amyloidosis.* Dordrecht: Kluwer Academic, 1991:7; Sipe JD. Amyloidosis. *Annu Rev Biochem* 1992;61:947.)

drugs against B-cell proliferations. However, ultrastructural as well as pathophysiologic considerations that may open new therapeutic avenues lead to include AL amyloidosis in the large entity of amyloidoses, covering conditions as different as familial polyneuropathies, Alzheimer's disease, type II diabetes, transmissible spongiform encephalopathies, hemodialysis-related amyloidosis, Iceland-type hereditary amyloidangiopathy, and secondary (AA) systemic amyloidosis, among others (Table 76-9). Amyloidogenesis seems to result from common mechanisms, which were highlighted by studies of Alzheimer's and the prion diseases (152,153).

General Characteristics of Amyloidosis

A Common Ultrastructural Molecular Organization Defining a Morphologic Entity

Amyloidosis is the general term for a morphologic entity, defined by visceral, extracellular deposition of protein material with unique tinctorial properties and ultrastructural characteristics. Amyloid deposits exhibit birefringence under polarized light, which indicates the presence of highly ordered structures. They have been extensively studied at the ultrastructural level by electron microscopy, infrared spectroscopy, and x-ray diffraction. In an important review published in 1980, Glenner (154) clustered all amyloidoses under the more convenient denomination of β-fibrilloses on the basis of the highly similar organization of the amyloid deposits. These are "typically composed of a felt-like array of 7.5- to 10-nm wide rigid, linear, non-branching, aggregated fibrils of

indefinite length." One amyloid fibril is made of two twisted 3–nm-wide filaments, each having a regular antiparallel β-pleated sheet configuration; the β-sheets are perpendicular to the filament axis. A regular packing of peptides or proteins with a β-sheet conformation results in the elongation of amyloid fibrils. The numerous hydrogen bonds between virtually all amide functions of the peptide backbones make such a structure highly stable. Other components, described below, are supposed to stabilize the fibrils.

Amyloid Protein Precursors and Classification of Amyloidoses

Amyloid protein precursors share the property of either a native β-pleated conformation or a high propensity to form β-sheets. All are globular structures, clearly distinct from fibrillar proteins such as collagen, which are proline-rich polymers with a longitudinal arrangement. The term *fibrils* is thus confusing, and one must keep in mind that in the case of amyloid, it actually refers to a quaternary arrangement of nonfibrillar proteins.

The International Committee for Amyloidosis recommended a nomenclature, essentially based on the nature of amyloid proteins (155); the abbreviated name of each amyloid protein is preceded by the letter A. The list provided in Table 76-9 is not exhaustive. More than 15 different amyloid protein precursors have been identified to date. This classification, favoring pathogenetic aspects, has the advantage of being less empirical than those based on clinical and pathologic presentations. However, it is worth noting that hereditary and secondary forms of a same disease exist and should

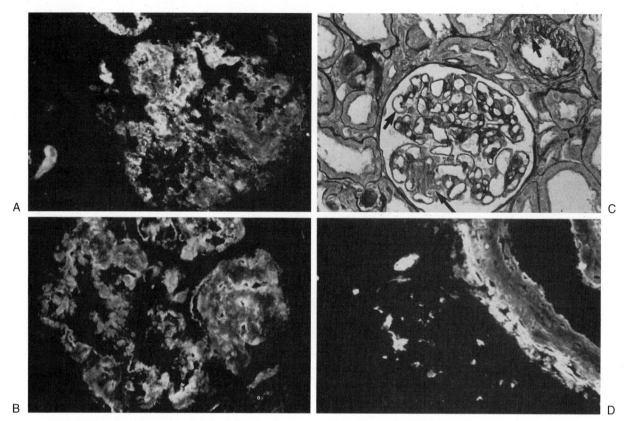

FIG. 76-10. Amyloidosis. **A:** Glomerular and vascular heavy amyloid deposits stained with anti-transthyretin antibody in a patient with Portuguese-type hereditary amyloidosis. (Immunofluorescence ×312.) **B:** Codeposition of amyloid P (AP) component in a glomerulus from the same patient as in (**A**). (Immunofluorescence stain with anti-AP component antibody ×312.) **C:** Glomerulus with early amyloid deposits in mesangium, capillary walls, and arteriolar wall (*arrows*) from a patient with AA amyloidosis. (Light microscopy, periodic acid-Schiff ×312.) **D:** Glomerulus from a patient with AL amyloidosis. Scanty glomerular deposits contrast with almost complete replacement of arterial walls by amyloid. (Immunofluorescence stain with anti-κ antibody ×312.)

be distinguished; for instance, systemic AA amyloidosis occurs in contexts of both chronic inflammatory or infectious diseases (secondary form), and familial Mediterranean fever. Normal transthyretin is responsible for senile systemic amyloidosis, while certain mutations are the cause of hereditary amyloid polyneuropathy (Fig. 76-10A). Thus, multiple different factors, either intrinsic (structural) or external (concentration of the precursor proteins, tissue factors, etc.), may influence the pathogenicity of a variety of potentially amyloidogenic proteins.

Other Constituents of Amyloid

In addition to the unique "pseudocrystalline" stacking of β-sheets just described, a few structural features are shared by all types of amyloid, and might help in understanding some aspects of the pathophysiology. Glycosaminoglycans (GAGs) have been found tightly associated to all isolated amyloid fibrils (156,157). GAGs are polysaccharide chains made of repeating uronic acid–hexosamine units of several types and normally linked to a protein core, thus constituting proteoglycans, which are important constituents of

extracellular matrices. The unvariable presence of GAGs in amyloid fibrils raises two suggestions:

1. Proteoglycans might interact with amyloidogenic precursors during the nucleation steps of amyloidogenesis (see below); indeed, most GAGs associated with fibrils are of the heparan sulfate type (158,159), and heparan sulfate proteoglycans are essential components of the basement membranes, which are preferential sites of amyloid deposition.
2. Sulfated GAGs might be important for inducing and stabilizing the β-pleated structure of the amyloid fibrils (160).

Another constituent of all amyloid deposits is a protein of the pentraxin family, the serum amyloid P component (SAP) (Fig. 76-10B). SAP is a decameric plasma glycoprotein made up of two noncovalently linked pentamers of identical subunits. The β-pleated structure of SAP (161) is strongly homologous to that of legume lectins such as concanavalin A. It shows no allelic polymorphism and displays striking interspecies homology. Furthermore, no occurrence of SAP deficiency has yet been described, which suggests that it has essential physiologic functions. SAP is a calcium-dependent lectin, with binding affinities toward DNA (162), C4-binding protein and the collagenlike region of C1q (163), and several constituents of extracellular matrices such as fibronectin and proteoglycans. SAP was shown to bind apoptotic cells and nuclear debris, and mice with targeted deletion of the SAP genes spontaneously develop anti-DNA antibody and a syndrome resembling human systemic lupus erythematosus (164). Two calcium sites are involved in carbohydrate binding. In the presence of calcium, SAP is remarkably resistant to proteolytic digestion, suggesting a physiologic role in maintaining extracellular matrix structures. Coating of amyloid fibrils with unaltered SAP is a constant feature that could result in their protection from catabolism. It is probable that SAP binding to amyloid deposits is mediated by GAGs through the formation of multicomponent complexes (165). The specific high affinity of SAP toward all types of amyloid was exploited for diagnosing, locating, and monitoring the extent of systemic amyloidosis using scintigraphy with ^{123}I-labeled SAP (166,167). SAP binding to all ligands is inhibited by specific sugars such as β-D-galactose cyclic pyruvate acetal. Moreover, the knowledge of SAP structure offers the opportunity of designing competitive inhibitors as potential drugs for the treatment of amyloidoses. However, the important physiologic role of SAP in protecting from autoimmunization (164) could make this approach hardly feasible.

Proteolysis and Nucleation

The process of amyloid formation involving amyloid precursors, GAGs, and SAP is starting to be understood, at least in certain amyloidoses. Proteolysis of a protein precursor proves to be a prerequisite for fibril formation in several types of amyloidosis. In systemic secondary (AA) amyloidosis, removing of the C-terminal part of an apolipoprotein acute-phase reactant, SAA, yields a 5- to 10-kd fibril-forming fragment; phagocytic cells, in particular macrophages, supposedly play a central role in this disease by providing the intralysosomal processing of the precursor (168). In Alzheimer's disease, the metabolism of an integral membrane protein, β-amyloid precursor protein (APP), generates a hydrophobic 39- to 43-amino acid fragment with amyloidogenic properties, the amyloid β-peptide (Aβ) (169). In other forms of amyloidosis, such as those involving transthyretin and Ig LCs, partial proteolysis has been demonstrated but may as well occur after fibrillogenesis. For instance in AA amyloidosis, cleavage of the precursor protein also occurs after fibril formation (170). The demonstration of small fragments from the LC constant domain in deposited fibrils also argues in favor of a postfibrillogenic proteolysis in AL amyloidosis (171).

Amyloidogenesis seems to be a nucleation-dependent polymerization process (144). Unlike other protein deposition diseases where amorphous aggregates are the consequence of insolubility of the pathogenic protein in the tissues, amyloid may result from a "one-dimensional crystallization."

In the latter process, formation of an ordered nucleus is the initial and limiting step, followed by a thermodynamically favorable addition of monomers leading to elongation of the fibrils. As shown in Alzheimer's and prion diseases, the nucleation step can be overrun by adding a preformed nucleus to a supersaturated solution of the amyloidogenic protein. A similar "seeding" phenomenon may explain the "amyloid-enhancing factor" activity of extracts from amyloid-containing tissues in AA amyloidosis animal models (172). The lag phase could also be shortened by injection of synthetic peptides corresponding to known amyloid fibril proteins (173).

Distribution of Amyloid: Localized Versus Systemic Amyloidosis

Tissue localization of the deposits is characteristic of many amyloidoses (Table 76-9). Single-organ involvement may reflect either local secretion or particular tropism of the amyloid precursor; for instance, pancreatic amyloidosis in patients with insulinoma or type II diabetes mellitus is related to cosecretion with insulin of islet amyloid polypeptide by β-cells (174). In some cases of Alzheimer's disease, molecules such as proteoglycans or lipids normally present in certain areas of the brain (amygdala, hippocampus, and neocortex) could behave as heterogeneous seeds for the polymerization of amyloid β-peptide (144). Systemic amyloidoses are derived from circulating precursors which either display unusual structural features or are present at abnormally high plasma levels, or both. Although most cases of LC amyloidosis are due to systemic organ deposition of LCs produced by bone marrow plasma cells, localized forms of LC amyloidosis have also been reported mostly in the orbit, the nasopharynx, and the genitourinary tract (reviewed in reference 175). A local infiltration of plasma cells is then usually found in proximity to the amyloid deposits, and may be responsible for the secretion of an amyloidogenic LC (176).

Pathologic Data with Special Emphasis on Renal Involvement

Despite the diversity of amyloidogenic proteins, they all deposit in tissue as fibrils constituted by the stacking of β-pleated sheets as identified by x-ray crystallography and diffraction studies (177). This unique protein conformation is responsible for the tinctorial and optical properties revealed by Congo red staining of tissue sections, and for the relative resistance of the fibrils to solution in physiologic solvents and to normal proteolytic digestion, which leads to their implacable accumulation in tissues (154).

By light microscopy, the deposits are extracellular, eosinophilic, and metachromatic. After Congo red staining, they appear faintly red and show the characteristic apple-green birefringence under polarized light. This light microscopic method is the most reliable to detect amyloid because it has virtually no false-positive findings. Sections thicker than those usually recommended for renal pathologic examination may be necessary to produce sufficient color density. Metachromasia is also observed with crystal violet, which stains the deposits in red. The use of other stains such as thioflavine T has been proposed, but the results lack specificity. The permanganate method of Wright and associates (178) may help to discriminate AA from AL fibrils if the sections are treated with permanganate before the Congo red procedure. AL amyloid is resistant, whereas AA amyloid is sensitive to permanganate digestion. There is usually good agreement between the sensitivity to permanganate and the staining of the deposits with a specific anti-AA antiserum (179). However in 8 of the 45 renal biopsy specimens of amyloid studied by Noel and associates (179), findings after permanganate treatment were either inconclusive because of the small size of the deposits, difficult to interpret because of only partial sensitivity, or conflicting with the immunostaining with anti-AA and anti-LC antibodies. It must be noted that sensitivity to permanganate treatment is not specific for AA amyloidosis but is shared by β_2-microglobulin amyloidosis.

In the kidney, the earliest lesions are located in the mesangium, along the glomerular basement membrane, and in the blood vessels (180) (Fig. 76-10C). Within the mesangium, deposits are primarily associated with the mesangial matrix, and subsequently irregularly increase by spreading from lobule to lobule and then invading the whole mesangial area. Amyloid deposits may also infiltrate the capillary basement membrane or be localized on both sides of it. When subepithelial deposits predominate, spikes recalling those seen in membranous glomerulopathy may be observed. Dikman and associates (181) showed that the severity of proteinuria correlated with the presence of spicules and podocyte destruction rather than with the amount of amyloid in the glomerulus. The spicules were associated with morphologic and clinical evidence of rapid amyloid deposition and a fulminant clinical course (181). Glomerular cell proliferation is infrequent. Advanced amyloid typically produces a nonproliferative, noninflammatory glomerulopathy, responsible for a marked enlargement of the kidney. The amyloid deposits replace normal glomerular architecture with loss of cellularity and usually without eliciting inflammation. When glomeruli become massively sclerotic, the deposits may be difficult to demonstrate by Congo red staining, and electron microscopy may then be helpful. The latter is required at very early stages, which may not be detected by light microscopy examination in patients presenting with the nephrotic syndrome (182,183). The media of the blood vessels is prominently involved at early stages. Vascular involvement may predominate, and occasionally may occur alone, particularly in AL amyloidosis (Fig. 76-10D). Deposits may also affect the tubules and the interstitium, leading to atrophy and disappearance of the tubular structures and to interstitial fibrosis.

Because of the heterogeneity of amyloidotic diseases, which results in specific diagnostic and therapeutic strategies adapted to the type of protein deposited within tissues,

immunofluorescence examination of snap-frozen biopsy specimens with specific antisera should be routinely performed (179,184,185). In the first series published by Gallo and associates (184), immunohistochemical classification of amyloid type was possible for 44 (88%) of 50 patients using anti-LC and anti-AA antisera. However, Noel and colleagues (179) point out that immunofluorescence with sera directed against HCs and LCs of Ig might be more difficult to interpret than with anti-AA antiserum. This is likely due to the frequent loss of LC constant domains in fibrils accounting for the absence of numerous epitopes normally recognized by antibodies. It is also possible that the pseudocrystalline structure of the fibrils makes these epitopes poorly accessible to conjugated antibodies. Two of eight renal biopsy specimens with presumed AL amyloidosis did not stain for any anti-Ig antibody whereas one showed coexistence of monotypic λ-LC and AA deposits of similar intensity (179), as previously noted by Gallo and associates (184). Both types of LCs may also be represented in AA deposits, probably as a consequence of increased protein permeability.

By electron microscopy, amyloid deposits are characterized by randomly oriented, nonbranching fibrils with an 8- to 10-nm diameter (Fig. 76-11). Early deposits can be found in close connection with mesangial cells that undergo important changes (186), and in the capillary walls distant from the mesangium on both sides of the basement membrane (187). As mentioned earlier, SAP has been found in all chemical

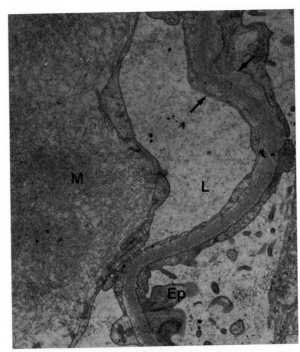

FIG. 76-11. Amyloidosis. Electron micrograph of glomerular deposits of amyloid. Randomly oriented fibrils invade the mesangium and are seen in the basement membrane on both sides of the lamina densa (*arrows*). *Ep*, epithelium; *L*, capillary lumen; *M*, mesangium. (Magnification ×12,000.) (Photo courtesy of Dr. L. H. Noël.)

types of amyloid thus far examined. In studies using double-label immunogold staining of AL and AA amyloid deposits, Yang and Gallo (188) show that SAP represented 1.5% and 6.5% of the total gold label in AL and AA, respectively. SAP occurred as widely separated single units while the major fibril protein was labeled in single rows, similar to beads on a string.

Histologic diagnosis may be achieved by rectal biopsy, provided that the biopsy specimen contains submucosal vessels in which early deposits are located; skin biopsy; biopsy of accessory salivary glands; bone marrow biopsy; or abdominal fat aspiration (189,190). A renal biopsy is usually performed when these diagnostic procedures have failed.

Epidemiology and Clinical Features of AL Amyloidosis

Epidemiology

Although less common than other forms, Ig LC-related (AL) amyloidosis was the first characterized at the biochemical level (191). This may be explained by the abundance of deposits, especially in certain organs (kidneys, liver, heart, spleen), and the often rapid fatal evolution of the disease, which prompted development of extraction methods from necropsy pieces (150). The incidence of primary AL amyloidosis in the United States per year is nine per million. Among systemic amyloidoses with predominant renal involvement, AL amyloidosis has become more common than AA amyloidosis since the widespread use of effective antimicrobial agents. Like myeloma patients, those with AL amyloidosis are more often males than females. The median age at diagnosis is 65 years (192) and 62 years in patients without an immunoproliferative disorder according to the series from the Mayo Clinic (193).

Amyloid deposits are found in approximately 10% of myeloma cases (30), and this incidence reaches 20% in patients with pure LC myeloma (194). The high frequency of amyloidosis associated with myeloma (56%) in Alexanian's series (195) was attributed to the referral of more myeloma patients for chemotherapy to the authors' institution. Conversely, a minority (probably less than one out of four) of patients with AL amyloidosis are considered to bear a patent immunoproliferative disease, which usually is a multiple myeloma, although other forms such as Waldenström's macroglobulinemia are not exceptional (196). In fact, the true incidence of myeloma depends on the criteria used for its diagnosis. AL amyloidosis without overt immunoproliferative disease is usually referred to as *primary amyloidosis*.

Clinical and Laboratory Features of AL Amyloidosis

The largest series published thus far on AL amyloidosis is that of the Mayo Clinic (197). It included 474 patients with biopsy-proved amyloidosis. Ninety-nine percent of the patients were 40 years of age or older; 69% were men and 31%

TABLE 76-10. *Clinical and laboratory features at presentation in 474 patients with proven AL amyloidosis*

Initial symptoms	
Fatigue	62%
Weight loss	52%
Pain	5%
Purpura	15%
Gross bleeding	3%

Physical findings[a]	
Palpable liver	24%
Palpable spleen	5%
Lymphadenopathy	3%
Macroglossia	9%

Laboratory findings	
Increased plasma cells (bone marrow ≥6%)	56%
Anemia (hemoglobin <10 g/dL)	11%
Elevated serum creatinine (≥1.3 mg/dL)	45%
Elevated alkaline phosphatase	26%
Hypercalcemia (>11 mg/dL)	2%
Proteinuria (≥1.0 g/24 h)	55%
Urine light chain	73%[b]
κ chain	23%
λ chain	50%

[a]A comparison of the prevalence of clinical syndromes according to the presence or the absence of myeloma is given in Table 76-11.
[b]Of 429 patients. All other figures refer to all 474 cases.
(Data from Kyle RA, Gertz MA. Primary systemic amyloidosis: clinical and laboratory features in 474 cases. *Semin Hematol* 1995;32:45.)

were women. Seventy-one patients (15%) had a myeloma according to the authors' criteria. Two hundred and nineteen (56%) of 391 patients had an increased number (≥6%) of plasma cells in the bone marrow.

The clinical and laboratory features at diagnosis are summarized in Tables 76-10 and 76-11 from the two latest series of the Mayo Clinic (192,197). The main clinical symptoms at presentation are weakness and weight loss. Except for bone pain, there is no difference in the incidence of initial symptoms in patients with and without myeloma. Nephrotic syndrome, orthostatic hypotension, and peripheral neuropathy were more common in patients with AL amyloidosis without myeloma than in those with associated myeloma

TABLE 76-11. *Syndromes at diagnosis in 229 patients with proven AL amyloidosis*

Syndromes	Without myeloma (182 patients)	With myeloma (47 patients)
Nephrotic syndrome	37%	13%
Carpal tunnel syndrome	21%	38%
Congestive heart failure	23%	23%
Peripheral neuropathy	20%	6%
Orthostatic hypotension	16%	4%

(Data from Kyle RA, Greipp PR. Amyloidosis (AL): clinical and laboratory features in 229 cases. *Mayo Clin Proc* 1983; 58:665.)

(Table 76-11). Renal insufficiency occurs usually in the presence of marked kidney enlargement and is usually not associated with hypertension. Proteinuria mainly composed of albumin is noted in 55% of the patients, indicating that glomerular involvement is a common feature of AL amyloidosis. Microscopic hematuria is, however, exceptional, and therefore should prompt the search of a bleeding lesion of the urinary tract.

Restrictive cardiomyopathy is found at presentation in up to one-third of patients and causes death in about half. Infiltration of the ventricular walls and the septum may be recognized by echocardiography. Amyloid may also induce arrhythmias and the sick sinus syndrome. Amyloid deposits in the coronary arteries may result in angina pectoris and myocardial infarction. Involvement of the gastrointestinal tract is also common and can cause motility disturbances, malabsorption, hemorrhage, or obstruction. Macroglossia occurs in about one-fifth of these patients. It may interfere with eating and obstruct airways. Hepatomegaly occurs initially in one-third of the patients, but abnormalities of hepatic function remain generally mild. Hyposplenism, usually associated with splenomegaly, is occasionally found. Peripheral neuropathy occurs in one-fifth of cases and is usually responsible for a painful sensory polyneuropathy followed later by motor deficits. Autonomic neuropathy causing orthostatic hypotension, lack of sweating, gastrointestinal disturbances, bladder dysfunction, and impotence may occur alone or together with peripheral neuropathy. Orthostatic hypotension is one of the major hampering complications of AL amyloidosis, causing some patients to be bedridden. Skin involvement may take the form of purpura characteristically around the eyes, ecchymoses, papules, nodules, and plaques usually on the face and upper trunk. AL amyloidosis may also infiltrate articular structures and mimic rheumatoid or an asymmetric seronegative synovitis. Infiltration of the shoulders may produce severe pain and swelling ("shoulder-pad" sign). A rare but potentially serious manifestation of AL amyloidosis is an acquired bleeding diathesis that may be associated with deficiency of factor X and sometimes also factor IX, or with increased fibrinolysis. It should be systematically looked for before any biopsy of a deep organ. It does not occur in AA amyloidosis, although widespread vascular deposits may also be responsible for bleeding. Actually, AL amyloidosis may infiltrate almost any organ other than the brain and thus be responsible for a wide variety of clinical manifestations.

On average, monoclonal LCs can be detected by immunoelectrophoresis in 73% of the urine samples, and the λ-isotype is twice as common as the κ-isotype, contrasting with the 1:2 λ-to-κ ratio observed in patients with multiple myeloma alone. With the use of more sensitive immunochemical techniques, a monoclonal Ig is found is nearly 90% of patients in the serum and/or the urine. It is, however, worth noting that, even under such conditions, there is no detectable monoclonal Ig in the serum and urine of some patients.

"Primary" Amyloidosis: A True Plasma Cell Dyscrasia

The broad similarities observed by Kyle and Greipp (192) between AL amyloidosis with and without myeloma, the high prevalence of urinary and circulating monoclonal Ig and/or LC in AL amyloidosis (197), and the finding of monotypic LC deposits in most patients with non-AA nonmyelomatous amyloidosis (179,184) supports the concept introduced by Osserman and coworkers (198) that "primary" amyloidosis (i.e., AL amyloidosis without myeloma) is probably a plasma cell dyscrasia. This concept is elegantly confirmed by immunofluorescence and biosynthetic studies of bone marrow cells. On the one hand, Preud'homme and associates (199) demonstrated, by immunofluorescence, monoclonal plasma cell populations in 12 of 14 patients with "primary" amyloidosis, even in those without detectable serum and urine monoclonal Ig and with a normal percentage of bone marrow plasma cells. This study also underscored the preponderance of patients with λ-LCs. The λ–κ ratio was 4:1, that is, higher than that previously noted in another series, which, however, had not analyzed bone marrow plasma cells (192,195,200). Moreover, the synthesis and excretion of large amounts of free monoclonal LCs were demonstrated in every patient studied by Buxbaum (201) and Preud'homme and associates (199), together with the presence of LC fragments in almost all patients. This contrasted with nonmyelomatous secondary amyloidosis, which was characterized by normal distribution of bone marrow plasma cells by immunofluorescence and by synthesis of normal-sized Ig, without free LC secretion and fragments (199).

AL amyloidosis thus illustrates the importance of a careful search of serum and urine monoclonal Ig for diagnostic, prognostic, and pathophysiologic purposes.

1. When sensitive methods including high-resolution agarose electrophoresis and immunofixation are used, a monoclonal LC can be detected in virtually all patients after sufficient concentration of the urine (202).
2. Detection of a urinary LC of the λ-isotype is significantly associated with a shorter survival compared with the κ-isotype (203).
3. Both the lack of a correlation between the amount of secreted LC with the disease progression and the overrepresentation of the λ-isotype point to the pathophysiologic importance of LC structure-related factors.

A definition of "primary" AL amyloidosis is certainly useful for inclusion of patients in prospective therapeutic trials. However, from a pathophysiologic point of view, myeloma-associated and "primary" AL amyloidoses represent two ends of a single entity. The intrinsic pathogenicity of the precursor free LC is probably highly variable from one patient to another, so that expression of the disease occurs in the context of very different tumor masses. Whatever the hematologic status, the amyloid disease is responsible for the predominant symptoms in most patients. AL amyloidosis is thus typical of these forms of plasma cell dyscrasias in which malignancy is conferred by the pathogenic LC rather than the underlying hematologic disease.

Outcome and Treatment of AL Amyloidosis

AL amyloidosis is among the most severe complications of plasma cell proliferative disorders. The median survival was 13 months in the series of 474 patients from the Mayo Clinic reported in 1995 (197). Despite the use of melphalan and prednisone, the median survival is still only 17 to 18 months (204). The records of all patients from the Mayo Clinic with a diagnosis of AL amyloidosis between January 1, 1966 and March 1, 1987 were recently reviewed (205). During the 21 years of the study, 841 patients with AL amyloidosis were seen. Actuarial survival was 51% at 1 year, 16% at 5 years, and 4.7% at 10 years. Unexpectedly, 30 patients survived for 10 years or more after the histologic diagnosis: all received alkylating-agent therapy. In these long-term survivors, the monoclonal protein disappeared from the serum or urine, and 4 of 10 patients with nephrotic syndrome showed an objective response. Congestive heart failure, older age, serum creatinine level of 2 mg/dL or more, bone marrow plasma cell value of 20% or more, platelet count of 500×10^9/L or less, and the presence of peripheral neuropathy were underrepresented in the 10-year survivors and are unfavorable prognostic features.

Because amyloid fibrils in AL amyloidosis consist of monoclonal immunoglobulin LCs produced by a clone of plasma cells, treatment with alkylating agents which are effective against plasma cell dyscrasias is warranted. However, the results of chemotherapy in amyloidosis are difficult to document because there is no easy way to measure the amount of amyloid in a patient. Investigators have long recognized that resolution of the nephrotic syndrome does not necessarily reflect that of amyloid deposits, and that the progressive deposition of amyloid can occur in the presence of improved clinical and laboratory findings. Scintigraphy after the injection of ^{123}I-labeled SAP component may be helpful for monitoring the extent of systemic amyloidosis (166,167), but this technique is not readily available. The definition of a response in amyloidosis should be hematologic and organ-based. Measurement of hematologic response includes disappearance of serum and urinary monoclonal protein or a decrease of more than 50%. Measurement of organ-based response includes improvement in renal involvement as demonstrated by a 50% decrease in the 24-hour urine albumin excretion in the absence of progressive renal insufficiency, and an increase of at least 1 g/dL in serum albumin (given an initial value of less than 3 g/dL) when the patient presents with nephrotic syndrome; a reduction in the size of the liver by at least 2 cm and a 50% decrease of serum alkaline phosphatase; improvement of the echocardiogram attested by a 2-mm reduction in the thickness of the interventricular septum or an increase of 20 percentage points in the ejection fraction (204). Unfortunately, it takes a long time to achieve an organ response in amyloidosis, probably because the body has a poor ability to mobilize preexistent amyloid deposits.

Chemotherapy without Stem Cell Support

All patients with amyloidosis deserve a trial of chemotherapy because of the improved survival of responders (206). The median survival time of 27 patients who fulfilled criteria for response was nearly 90 months, compared with 1 year for nonresponding patients.

Several studies were performed using alkylating agents. In the most important trial as yet performed, 220 patients with AL amyloidosis from the Mayo Clinic were randomly assigned to receive either colchicine alone (72 patients), melphalan and prednisone (77 patients), or melphalan plus prednisone and colchicine (71 patients) (204). Patients were stratified according to their major clinical manifestations, age, and sex. The median duration of survival was 8.5 months for the colchicine-treated group, 18 months for the melphalan and prednisone group, and 17 months for the melphalan, prednisone, and colchicine group ($P < 0.001$). Twenty-eight percent of patients receiving melphalan and prednisone showed a response compared with only 3% in the colchicine-treated group. Among patients who had a reduction in serum or urine monoclonal protein at 12 months, the overall length of survival was 50 months, whereas it was 36 months in nonresponders at 12 months ($P = 0.03$). Thirty-four patients (15%) survived for 5 years or longer. Another prospective randomized study including 100 patients has demonstrated a survival advantage for patients treated with melphalan and prednisone compared with colchicine (207).

In an effort to determine if more intensive therapy was beneficial, 101 patients were randomized to either melphalan and prednisone or a combination of drugs (vincristine, carmustine [BCNU], melphalan, cyclophosphamide, and prednisone) (208). Therapy with multiple alkylating agents did not result in a higher response rate or longer survival time when compared with standard melphalan and prednisone. High-dose dexamethasone produces some benefit in 15% to 20% of patients (209,210). Vitamin E and α2-interferon have not been beneficial.

Treatment, however, is not innocuous. As with all alkylating agents, the potential exists for late myelodysplasia or acute leukemia (211). In the Mayo Clinic's experience, approximately 6.5% of patients exposed to melphalan develop a myelodysplastic syndrome. Because of the age group of the patients, the development of myelodysplasia usually results in rapid death. Median survival from the onset of myelodysplasia is approximately 8 months.

High-Dose Chemotherapy with Stem Cell Support

Because most patients do not respond to conventional melphalan-based chemotherapy, alternatives need to be found. Based on the success of high-dose therapy followed by autologous stem cell transplantation (ASCT) in multiple myeloma, ASCT has been used to treat AL amyloidosis with the aim of eradicating the amyloidogenic plasma cell clone. An important report of about 25 consecutive autografted cases treated with 200 mg per m^2 IV melphalan was published in 1998 by Comenzo and associates (212), and this group has updated its results in abstract form for a series of 102 patients treated either with high-dose (200 mg per m^2) IV melphalan (high-dose melphalan [HDM]: 53 cases) or intermediate dose (100 or 140 mg per m^2) IV melphalan (intermediate-dose melphalan [IDM]: 49 cases) when patients had diminished cardiac or renal function or were of advanced age (213). Patients were classified according to their predominant organ involvement: renal, cardiac, or other. The 3-month treatment-related mortality was similar in both groups (15% to 17%). In both groups, the survival rate at 4 years was related to the predominant site of the disease: 83% with HDM and 75% with IDM in cases of renal disease, 33% with HDM and 37% with IDM for patients with cardiac amyloidosis. The rates of complete hematologic response and of objective clinical improvement were higher in the group of patients treated with HDM, 55% and 54%, respectively, compared with 38% and 29%, respectively, in the group of patients treated with IDM. Remarkably, some patients with neuropathy and cardiac symptoms experienced clinical improvement. These impressive results led the authors to conclude that high-dose therapy with ASCT could be considered a standard therapy for patients with AL amyloidosis who meet eligibility criteria for stem cell transplantation.

However, several retrospective reports recently reviewed by Moreau (214) highlight potential biases in the studies that were performed by Comenzo et al. in a selected population of patients with "adequate cardiac, pulmonary, hepatic, and renal function" (212). In the study by Moreau et al. (215), the transplant-related mortality was 40%, and the univariate analysis of prognostic factors showed that the only parameter predictive for both overall survival and event-free survival was the number of clinical manifestations. When patients had fewer than two clinical manifestations, the 4-year overall and event-free survivals were 92% and 46%, respectively, compared with 11% for both parameters when two or more major clinical manifestations were documented before treatment. That selection of patients for ASCT plays a significant role in survival was convincingly shown by the Mayo Clinic group in a review of 1,288 patients with AL amyloidosis (216). Two-hundred and thirty-four patients who met eligibility criteria for stem cell transplantation were treated with conventional alkylating agent therapy. The median survival was 45.6 months. The authors therefore concluded that eligibility for stem cell transplantation was an independent favorable prognostic factor for AL amyloidosis, and that a randomized clinical trial evaluating stem cell transplantation versus standard chemotherapy should be indicated in this group of patients.

Chemotherapy with 4′-Iodo-4′ Deoxydoxorubicin

The anthracycline drug, 4′-iodo-4′ deoxydoxorubicin (I-DOX), strongly binds to amyloid fibrils, and it has been suggested that it could inhibit fibril growth, increase the solubility of existing amyloid deposits, and facilitate their clearance (217). A preliminary evaluation in eight patients with AL amyloidosis shows some evidence of amyloid resorption (218). An update of the results observed in 12 additional patients treated with I-DOX at 10 to 30 mg per m^2 per week for 4 consecutive weeks has been recently published (219). Only a minor proportion of patients responded to I-DOX, and serious adverse effects were reported in three patients. According to the authors, this drug should only be used as an adjunct to more effective treatment for AL amyloidosis.

Therapy of Renal Failure

Most studies of the clinical course and outcome of patients on dialysis include both AL and AA amyloidoses. In 1976, Jones (220) summarized the first European experience in 29 patients, and pointed out that the patients' survival rate was about half that of patients without amyloidosis who were maintained on hemodialysis. The patients' survival rate is low, but it compares favorably with that of patients not requiring dialysis: From 66% to 72% at 1 year, it falls to 30% to 44% at 5 to 6 years (221–223). No difference in survival was observed at any time between the patients with AL and AA amyloidoses (222). The survival rate of patients treated with CAPD is similar to that of patients on hemodialysis.

Cardiac amyloid is the most important predictor of poor survival in patients with AL amyloidosis undergoing dialysis, and cardiac deaths represent the main cause of mortality in such patients (223). Congestive heart failure, atrioventricular or intraventricular conduction defects, and arrhythmias due to amyloid myocardial involvement often occur. The management of patients with AL amyloid on hemodialysis is also often complicated by permanent hypotension, gastrointestinal hemorrhage, chronic diarrhea, and difficulties in the creation and maintenance of vascular accesses. It has, therefore, been suggested that CAPD could have several advantages over hemodialysis in the management of end-stage renal amyloidosis, including avoiding vascular access and deleterious effect on blood pressure (224,225). However, it may induce protein loss in the dialysates and thus enhance malnutrition.

Renal transplantation is limited by the severity of heart involvement and the recurrence of deposits in the transplanted kidney.

Epidemiology and Specific Features of AA Amyloidosis

Although AA amyloidosis does not involve deposition of Ig fragments and thus should not be classified within the group of monoclonal gammopathies, it shares with AL amyloidosis pathogenetic pathways, high prevalence of renal involvement, and some therapeutic aspects that deserve

TABLE 76-12. *Changing spectrum of underlying diseases in secondary AA amyloidosis*[a]

	Mayo, 1949 (n = 30)	AFIP, 1971 (n = 100)	Bristol, 1985 (n = 75)	Mayo, 1991 (n = 64)
Rheumatic disease	2 (7)	15 (15)	55 (73)	42 (66)
Granulomatous infection (TB, fungus, leprosy)	9 (30)	28 (28)	8 (11)	0
Pyogenic infection	10 (33)	35 (35)	5 (7)	11 (17)
Inflammatory bowel disease	2 (7)	4 (4)	3 (4)	6 (9)
Malignancy	7 (23)	18 (18)	3 (4)	2 (3)
Other	—	—	2 (3)	3 (5)

AFIP, Armed Forces Institute of Pathology; *TB*, tuberculosis
[a]Data are number of patients (percentage).
(From Gertz MA, Kyle RA. Secondary systemic amyloidosis: response and survival in 64 patients. *Medicine (Baltimore)* 1991;70:246; Browning MJ, et al. Ten years' experience of an amyloid clinic—a clinicopathologic survey. *Q J Med* 1985;215:213, with permission.)

further consideration. An important epidemiologic aspect of AA amyloidosis is the changing spectrum of underlying diseases (Table 76-12). Pyogenic and granulomatous infections, especially tuberculosis, account for far fewer cases than in the older series. This is because of the efficacy of antibiotic treatments for bacteria, which shows that amyloidosis can be efficiently prevented when its cause is suppressed. In contrast, the prevalence (about 70%) of amyloid linked to autoimmune inflammatory diseases, such as rheumatoid arthritis, has increased dramatically. Amyloid-associated inflammatory bowel diseases remain stable at 5% to 10%. AA amyloidosis in patients with Hodgkin's disease has virtually disappeared with more efficient treatment of the hematologic disease.

There are a number of clinical manifestations of AA amyloidosis (226,227) (Table 76-13). The main target organ by far is the kidney. Gastrointestinal disturbances including diarrhea, constipation, and malabsorption are the most common after kidney manifestations. In contrast with AL amyloidosis, congestive heart failure, peripheral neuropathy, macroglossia, and carpal tunnel syndrome occur infrequently. The reason for the differential distribution of AA and AL tissue deposits is not understood, but should stimulate research because this clinical observation deals with the deposition process per se. The optimal method for diagnosing AA amyloidosis remains controversial. Although kidney biopsy is positive in 100% of symptomatic patients, less invasive biopsy procedures should be preferred first (Table 76-13).

Survival time of patients with AA amyloidosis is usually longer than in AL amyloidosis (Table 76-13). The percentage of survivors is about 40% at 3 years (226,227), whereas all patients with AL amyloidosis were dead at this time point in Browning's series (226). The median survival time is approximately 2 years, extending to 42 months for those who survive past this point (227). As in AL amyloidosis, an elevated serum creatinine and a low serum albumin are strong adverse prognostic indicators. Main causes of death are uremia and dialysis complications, but not cardiac complications.

Three large series of renal transplantation in patients with amyloidosis have been published (228–230). They all come from Scandinavia, and essentially include patients with rheumatic diseases. In the first series (228), the 3-year survival rate for 45 patients with amyloidosis who received a cadaver kidney transplant but no cyclosporine was statistically less (51%) than that of the control subjects (79%). However, the graft survival rate, was not different between groups (about 42% at 3 years). The second series included 32 new

TABLE 76-13. *Characteristics of patients with secondary AA amyloidosis*

Series	No. of patients	Age (yrs)	Male-female ratio	Presenting clinical syndrome—no. (%)	Source of tissue for diagnosis—no. (%)	Causes of death—no./totals (%)	Survival
Browning, et al., 1985 (226)	75	57 (18–81)	0.8	Proteinuria/renal failure—49 (65) Gastrointestinal disturbance—4 (5) Hepatosplenomegaly—3 (4)	Rectum—45 (60) Kidney—11 (15)	Renal failure—18/37 (49) Bronchopneumonia—7/37 (19) Cardiac—4/37 (11)	~40% at 3 yrs
Gertz and Kyle, 1991 (227)	64	56 (14–80)	1.5	Proteinuria/renal failure—58 (91) Gastrointestinal disturbance—14 (22) Goiter—6 (9) Neuropathy/carpal tunnel—2 (3)	Rectum—32 (50) Kidney—24 (38) Stomach/small bowel—15 (23) Marrow—12 (19)	Uremia/dialysis complications—32/47 (68) Sepsis—4/47 (9) Cardiac—4/47 (9)	~40% at 3 yrs Median = 24.5 mos. (Survivors = 42 mos.)

patients (31 with AA amyloidosis) from the same Finnish center who received cadaver transplants and cyclosporine (229). Patient and graft survival rates at 3 years in this series were 71% and 68%, respectively. In the third series of 62 renal transplantations including 29 grafts from related living donors (230), the 1-year actuarial patient survival rate was 79%, decreasing to 65% after 5 years. Amyloid deposits recur in about 10% of the grafts (228,230). There is a high risk of infection that is the main cause of early deaths. As with dialysis, cardiac involvement is a major threat for patients receiving renal transplants.

Familial Mediterranean Fever

Familial Mediterranean fever represents both a particular type of AA amyloidosis and is the most common cause of familial amyloidosis. Interestingly, colchicine has proved to be efficient both in the prevention and treatment of this type of amyloidosis (231,232). Familial Mediterranean fever is usually transmitted as an autosomal-recessive disorder and occurs most commonly in Sephardic Jews and Armenians (233,234). Mutations of the gene for proteins called pyrin or marenostrin have been demonstrated (235,236). Clinically, there are two independent phenotypes. In the first, brief, episodic, febrile attacks of peritonitis, pleuritis, or synovitis occur in childhood or adolescence and precede the renal manifestations. In the second, renal symptoms precede and may be the only manifestation of the disease for a long time. The attacks are accompanied by dramatic elevations of acute-phase reactants, including serum amyloid A protein. Amyloid deposits of the AA type are responsible for severe renal lesions with prominent glomerular involvement leading to end-stage renal disease at a young age, and early death. Zemer and associates (232) show that in a cohort of 1,070 patients with familial Mediterranean fever, colchicine, an agent effective in preventing attacks (237), could prevent the appearance of proteinuria and deterioration of renal function in patients with amyloidosis who had proteinuria but not the nephrotic syndrome or renal insufficiency. Life-table analysis showed that the cumulative rate of proteinuria was 1.7% after 11 years in the compliant patients and 48.9% after 9 years in the noncompliant patients ($P < 0.0001$). In 1992, the authors corrected their statement that colchicine did not improve amyloidotic kidney disease once it had reached the nephrotic stage, because colchicine reversed the nephrotic syndrome in three patients (238). They insisted on the importance of a dosage adapted to the clinical situation. The minimal daily dose of colchicine for prevention of amyloidosis is 1 mg even if attacks are suppressed by a smaller dose. Patients with clinical evidence of amyloidotic kidney disease and kidney transplant recipients should receive daily doses of between 1.5 and 2.0 mg. Most interestingly, the serum levels of amyloid A protein (SAA) during attacks in patients receiving colchicine were only slightly less elevated than those in untreated patients (239), suggesting that prevention of amyloidosis by colchicine might be due, at least in part, to a peripheral effect of the drug on fibril formation.

In summary, clinical experience of familial Mediterranean fever and infection-related AA amyloidosis demonstrates that it is possible to prevent and treat AA amyloidosis efficiently. Well-conducted trials of colchicine may be warranted in other causes of AA amyloidosis, especially rheumatoid arthritis. Rheumatic patients may also benefit from immunosuppressive therapy (227,240,241), the efficacy of which needs to be demonstrated in further prospective randomized studies.

Pathophysiologic Considerations of AL Amyloidosis

Studies on the mechanisms of AL amyloidogenesis are made particularly difficult by the unique degree of structural heterogeneity of the precursor: Each monoclonal LC is different from all others. An Ig LC typically includes two globular domains of 105 to 110 amino acids, strongly homologous to each other, that exhibit the classic conformation of all domains belonging to the "Ig superfamily" of proteins. The COOH-terminal domain (constant domain, C) is encoded by a single gene segment with very little allelic polymorphism in κ-chains and by no more than four different gene segments in λ-chains. The NH$_2$-terminal domain structure (variable domain, V), on the other hand, results from complex somatic rearrangement and mutation events occurring in the course of B-cell differentiation, and leads to a high degree of diversity. The antiparallel β-pleated ("β-barrel") structure of Ig domains seems particularly adapted to amyloid formation. It is worth noting that another protein of the Ig superfamily, β_2-microglobulin, may form amyloid fibrils.

The implication of Ig HC in amyloidosis is exceptional. In one case of "AH amyloidosis" almost entirely documented at the molecular level, the pathogenic IgG HC had an internal deletion of half the molecule so that the V domain was directly joined to the COOH-terminal C domain, thus strikingly resembling a LC (7).

Not all Light Chains are Amyloidogenic

Despite predisposing conformation, a majority of Ig chains are not amyloidogenic even at long-lasting high secretion rates. Several LC characteristics are considered amyloidogenic, particularly the LC isotype. First, the λ–κ ratio is between 2:1 and 4:1, depending on the series. Second, a homology family of LC V region, the $V_{\lambda VI}$ variability subgroup, was shown to be overrepresented in AL amyloidosis (26). In a more recent study, $V_{\lambda VI}$ was found to be expressed exclusively in amyloid-associated monoclonal Ig and to represent 41% (17/41) of amyloidogenic λ-chains (27). In contrast, no significant imbalance of the variability subgroups of κ-chains was found (242). That certain LC isotype and V region subgroups are more frequently implicated in amyloidosis suggests that important pathogenic factors are intrinsic to the LC precursors.

Empirical studies also show that amyloidogenicity is often associated with some physicochemical features such as the presence of low–molecular-mass LC fragments in the urine, and low pI; together with LC isotypy, these parameters allow the prediction of the amyloidogenic/nonamyloidogenic character of a monoclonal LC, with a correct allocation in 81% of tested cases (243).

The ability of two amyloidogenic LCs contrasting with the failure of one nonamyloidogenic LC to reproduce typical fibrillar deposits in mice definitely demonstrates that essential pathogenic factors are borne by the LC precursors (244). This experimental model required huge amounts (up to 5.3 g/mouse) of purified monoclonal LCs to be injected intraperitoneally. Nevertheless, several interesting findings were noted, such as the presence of mouse SAP in the deposits, confirming its crucial role in either the constitution or, more probably, the maintenance of fibrils in vivo. Water deprivation dramatically increased the amyloidogenic potential of the LCs.

Comparison of Structures of Amyloid Light-Chain Precursors and Deposited Light Chains: A Role for Proteolysis?

Considerable works have been devoted to the study of structures of circulating monoclonal LCs or extracted fibrils. After the demonstration by Glenner and colleagues (191) that a LC was the predominant constituent of amyloid fibrils, they showed that NH_2-terminal sequences (up to 36 residues) were identical in the deposited and urinary monoclonal LCs from three patients (4,245). However, the fact that a mutant form or a molecular variant of the soluble LC could be the amyloid precursor was not excluded, and only recently the complete sequence identity between a circulating and a deposited LC was established (246). Association of AL amyloidosis with other deposition diseases such as LCDD (247) will raise the same question of uncertain identity between LCs forming different kinds of deposits. Mutant subclones may be encountered in myeloma, especially after treatment with alkylating agents, and have also been described in AL amyloidosis (248).

Analyses of LC precursor primary structures were performed either at the protein (249–252) or at the cDNA levels (253). All cases had an overall normal structure including a normal C domain sequence.

The essential role of the V domain in fibrillogenesis was further supported by analyses of fibrils extracted using adaptations of the method of Pras and coworkers (150), which showed it to always be the main amyloid constituent. The C domain is often, but not always (245,246), partially or totally absent from the fibrils (191,248,254–268). In many cases, heterogeneity in the length of the COOH-terminal end was noted (255,256,262,263). In a few cases, intact LC was present together with fragments (262); in most others, such heterogeneity might have been present but unrecognized because the analyses were focused on a purified predominant

fragment. These results raise the hypothesis of a possible role of proteolysis, as already demonstrated in other forms of amyloidosis. Bellotti and coworkers (269) show the disappearance of a conformational LC idiotope in the course of fibril formation, and suggest that polymerization results from the loss of the dimer conformation, possibly due to proteolysis of the C domain.

The question of a role of LC proteolysis in the amyloidogenic process has been addressed in different ways, but has not yet received a fully satisfactory answer. Abnormally low–molecular-mass LCs were secreted in in vitro biosynthesis experiments on bone marrow cells from AL amyloidosis subjects but they might result from either abnormal synthesis or proteolytic processing, or both (199, 201). In vitro digestion experiments using pepsin, trypsin, and kidney lysosomes yielded fibrils resembling amyloid by electron microscopy and displaying typical Congo red binding and green polarization birefringence (270–272). However, most tested LCs were from patients without amyloidosis, and the in vitro fibrils generally contained smaller fragments than those found in vivo. Thus, instead of reproducing "normal" amyloidogenesis, these experiments merely showed the ability of peptides generated by cleavage of β-pleated structures to form amyloidlike fibrils. Another intriguing matter of all in vitro fibrillogenesis experiments is the absence of GAGs and SAP, which are invariable constituents in vivo. Although these studies contribute to the general understanding of the molecular mechanisms of fibril formation, we believe that their validity as models is questionable. In bone marrow cell culture from an AL amyloidosis patient, Durie and associates (273) found amyloidlike material immediately adjacent to macrophages, and conclude that a processing of the LCs by these cells, similar to that observed in AA amyloidosis, might lead to amyloid formation. On the other hand, several observations point to the amyloidogenic potential of intact LCs; specifically, experimental mouse amyloid fibrils are made essentially of the entire injected LC (244); in vitro fibrils with characteristic tinctorial and ultrastructural properties of amyloid can be generated after simple reduction of the interchain disulfide bond of an intact LC dimer (274). Considering the sensitivity of C domains to proteases (275), it is conceivable that they are digested after constitution of the fibrils and tissue deposition. The demonstration of C domain fragments as amyloid component argues in this sense (171).

Amyloidogenic Light Chains: Light Chains with Peculiar Structure or with Affinity for Extracellular (Matrix) Constituents?

The search for primary structure peculiarities of the LC V domains first led to disappointing conclusions. Several unusual features such as N-glycosylations (248,253,260–263), insertion of acidic residues (256,258), and changes of charged to hydrophobic residues (248,252) have been noted. Infrequent amino acids at certain positions have been believed to affect the secondary structure of the framework regions (258) or the LC dimerization (264). This led Stevens and colleagues (143) to determine amyloid-associated LC residues from the comparison of 52 pathogenic sequences with a bank of 128 other LCs. In a more recent report which collected 100 LCs of the VκI variability subgroup including 37 amyloidosis cases, Stevens defined a limited number of structural risk factors, based on three sites of amino-acid substitution and the occurrence of N-glycosylation (277).

A study with LC mutants bearing certain amino acids found in amyloidogenic precursors suggested that an unfolding step facilitated by these substitutions could be required for fibril formation (278); however, as stressed by the authors, the *in vitro* conditions were clearly nonphysiologic, and such models with single replacements in a structural context that is different from the original pathogenic LCs have an essentially theoretical interest.

One AL amyloidosis-associated LC, protein Mcg, has been extensively studied at the three-dimensional structure level by x-ray crystallography (279), although the fundamental results have rarely been discussed with respect to pathology. In spite of all speculations on possible abnormal conformation of amyloidogenic LC V domains, the dimer Mcg is strikingly "normal" and similar to other known mouse and human LCs and antigen-binding (Fab) fragments. An interesting observation is that the combination of hypervariable regions (complementarity-determining regions [CDRs]) from both monomers mimics a normal antigen-binding site with affinities toward haptenlike compounds such as dinitrophenyl (DNP)-lysine and opioid peptides (280,281). The number of contact residues and consequent binding affinity are decreased after reduction of the disulfide bond between COOH-terminal cysteinyls of the C domains (282). Because DNP-lysine can bind specifically amyloidogenic dimers (283), it is possible that covalent binding between LCs influences their pathogenicity. In other cases, specific antibodylike binding of isolated Ig LCs was shown to be dependent on the dimerization status (284,285). The hypothesis that specific recognition by amyloidogenic LCs plays a pathogenic role was recently enforced by the demonstration of their higher dimerization constants (286), and by the finding of high rates of somatic mutations clustered in the CDRs, suggesting antigen-driven selection (287).

Specific affinity of a LC toward an extracellular structure might create a nucleus that could lead to elongation of a fibril, in accordance with proposed mechanisms of other forms of amyloidogenesis. Indeed, four tested amyloidogenic LCs seemed to react more strongly than others with endothelial cell basement membranes *in vitro* (P. Aucouturier and D. Cines, unpublished results). This would also explain the specific tissue localization of amyloid and its close association with extracellular matrix components such as GAGs. Indeed, amylogenic LCs seem to display a special affinity to heparin and chondroitin sulfate B and C (288).

Therapeutic Prospects

Although the existence of amyloid has been known for about 150 years, therapeutic results have been modest so far, except in familial Mediterranean fever- and infection-related AA amyloidosis. This is partly due to the fact that the specific amyloid proteins have only recently been identified and the pathogenetic pathways remain obscure. New therapeutic strategies should be directed at the three steps of the amyloidogenic process: synthesis of the precursor, deposition of amyloid fibrils, and removal or dissolution of amyloid fibrils.

Prevention of Amyloid Precursor Synthesis

Curing the underlying disease has proved to be extremely effective, as shown in infectious causes of AA amyloid (289, 290). This objective must be envisioned, at least theoretically, in all forms of amyloidosis. In AL amyloidosis, high-dose chemotherapy with blood stem cell transplantation should be considered in the younger patients with less advanced disease (291). In AA amyloidosis, attempts to interfere with cytokines (such as interleukin-6) known to increase SAA synthesis are made possible by the finding of specific inhibitors of proinflammatory cytokines, including the soluble forms of their receptors. The possibility of immunotargeting against precursor synthesis is also worth exploring in both amyloid types.

Prevention of Amyloid Fibril Deposition

As previously discussed, the target of colchicine is debated. Because colchicine affects a number of cell functions including assembly of cytoskeleton fibers, the drug might alter fibril deposition or turnover. Its efficacy, however, remains controversial, except in familial Mediterranean fever. Enhancing the proteolysis of the amyloid precursor may be a rewarding approach, as serine proteases expressed on monocyte surfaces, in supernatants from monocyte cultures and in serum are capable of degrading SAA (292,293). Another promising therapeutic strategy is blockade of RAGE (receptor for advanced glycation end-products), a multiligand receptor of the immunoglobulin superfamily that also is a receptor for the amyloidogenic form of serum amyloid A (294). Antagonizing RAGE with a soluble form of the receptor or with blocking antibodies inhibits amyloid deposition in the spleen of mice injected with amyloid-enhancing factor and silver nitrate (294). Interestingly, interaction of RAGE with AA activates genes involved in cell stress. Whether these findings can apply to other types of amyloidosis remains to be determined.

On the other hand, rapidly growing data on the nucleation process might lead to the synthesis of nucleation inhibitors for all types of amyloid. For example, low–molecular-weight (135 to 1,000) anionic sulfate or sulfate compounds were recently shown to interfere with heparan sulfate-stimulated β-peptide fibril aggregation *in vitro* (295). When administered orally, these compounds substantially reduced murine splenic AA amyloid progression.

Removal or Dissolution of Amyloid Fibrils

The rare observations showing a regression of amyloid deposits under effective treatment of the underlying disease as well as the finding that amyloid deposits may undergo redistribution (296) suggest that amyloid fibrils can be catabolized and removed from tissues. This process is most likely restrained by proteinase inhibitors that have been detected in amyloid deposits of various types (297,298), and by fibril coating with the calcium-dependent lectin SAP (161). A potential approach, therefore, would be to block these inhibitors, to target proteolytic enzymes at the amyloid deposition site, or to dissociate SAP with competitive ligands. At present, most attempts to use dimethylsulfoxide (DMSO) as an amyloid solvent have been disappointing because of lack of efficacy and bad odor from the patient's breath. On the other hand, a novel anthracycline, I-DOX, was shown to favor resorption of AL-type amyloid deposits (217,218), but the more recent results are disappointing (219).

MONOCLONAL IMMUNOGLOBULIN DEPOSITION DISEASE

Historical Comments and Nomenclature

It has been known since the late 1950s that nonamyloidotic forms of glomerular disease can occur in multiple myeloma. Kobernick and Whiteside (299) and Sanchez and Domz (300) first described glomerular nodules "resembling the lesion of diabetic glomerulosclerosis," lacking the staining features and fibrillar organization of amyloid. The monoclonal LC content of these lesions was recognized in 1973 by Antonovych and colleagues (5) and confirmed by Randall and associates (6) who published the first description of LCDD in 1976.

Soon after this first description, monoclonal HCs were found together with LCs in the tissue deposits from certain patients (301), and the terms monoclonal Ig deposition disease (MIDD) (301,302) and LC- and HC-deposition disease (LHCDD) (303,304) were proposed. More recently, deposits containing monoclonal HCs in the absence of detectable LCs were observed in patients affected with otherwise typical Randall's disease (HC deposition disease [HCDD]) (8,9). Gallo and colleagues (303) and Buxbaum and associates (304) use the designation MIDD for LCDD, LHCDD, and amyloidosis. The distinction between AL amyloidosis and MIDD is justified by likely distinct pathophysiology of amyloid, which implicates one-dimensional elongation of a pseudocrystalline structure, and of MIDD, which apparently involves nonorganized amorphous precipitation of Ig chains.

Pathologic Features

In clinical and pathologic terms, LCDD, LHCDD, and HCDD are essentially similar and therefore are described together.

We do, however, emphasize some unexpected characteristics of patients with HCDD because they may shed new light on the pathophysiology of MIDD.

Light Microscopy

The morphologic features of these disorders are well established, and in retrospect, cases of undiagnosed "paraamyloid" or unidentified glomerulonephritis or even "diabetic" glomerulosclerosis in patients with normal glycemic control were presumably MIDD. MIDD should not be considered a pure glomerular disease. In fact, tubular lesions may be more conspicuous than the glomerular damage.

Tubular lesions are characterized by the deposition of a refractile, eosinophilic, periodic acid-Schiff (PAS)-positive, ribbonlike material along the outer part of the tubular basement membrane in virtually all patients with MIDD. The deposits predominate around the distal tubules, Henle's loops, and in some instances the collecting ducts in which the epithelium is flattened and atrophied. Typical myeloma casts are only occasionally seen. In advanced stages, a marked interstitial fibrosis including refractile deposits is often associated with tubular lesions.

Glomerular lesions are much more heterogeneous (182, 305,306). Nodular glomerulosclerosis is the most characteristic (182,307) (Fig. 76-12A), but it is found in only 60% of patients with MIDD. Nodules are composed of membranelike material with nuclei at the periphery. The glomerular basement membranes are refractile and moderately thickened. The capillary loops stretch at the periphery of florid nodules and may undergo aneurysmal dilation. The Bowman's capsule may contain a material identical to that present in the center of the nodules. These lesions resemble nodular diabetic glomerulosclerosis, but some characteristics are distinctive: The distribution of the nodules is fairly regular in a given glomerulus; the nodules are often poorly argyrophilic; and exudative lesions as "fibrin caps" and extensive hyalinosis of the efferent arterioles are not observed. On the other hand, in occasional cases with prominent endocapillary cellularity and mesangial interposition, the glomerular features mimic a lobular glomerulonephritis.

Milder forms simply show an increase in mesangial matrix and sometimes in mesangial cells, and a modest thickening of the basement membranes appearing abnormally bright and rigid. Glomerular lesions may not be detected by light microscopy, but require ultrastructural examination. These lesions may represent early stages of glomerular disease.

Arteries, arterioles, and peritubular capillaries all may contain LC deposits in close contact with their basement membranes.

Whatever their location, the refractile deposits seen with Masson's trichrome are stained by PAS and are argentaffin, except for glomerular nodules which are not argentaffin. They do not show the staining characteristics of amyloid.

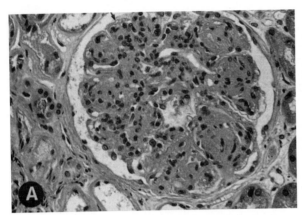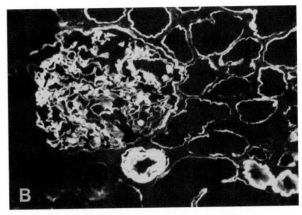

FIG. 76-12. Monoclonal immunoglobulin deposition disease. **A:** Typical nodular glomerulosclerosis. Note membranelike material in the center of the nodules and nuclei at the periphery. Some glomerular capillaries show double contours (*arrow*). Note also thickening of the basement membrane of atrophic tubules. (Light microscopy, Masson's trichrome ×312.) **B:** Bright staining of tubular and glomerular basement membranes, and of mesangium and arteriolar wall with anti-κ antibody in κ–light-chain deposition disease without nodular glomerular lesions. (Immunofluorescence ×312.)

Immunofluorescence

A key step in the diagnosis of the various forms of MIDD is immunofluorescence examination of the kidney. All biopsy specimens show evidence of monotypic LC and/or HC fixation along tubular basement membranes (Fig. 76-12B). This criterion is requested for the diagnosis of MIDD. In contrast with AL amyloidosis, the κ-isotype is markedly predominant.

The tubular deposits stain strongly and predominate along the loops of Henle and the distal tubules, but they are also often detected along the proximal tubules. In contrast, the pattern of glomerular immunofluorescence displays marked heterogeneity. In patients with nodular glomerulosclerosis, deposits of monotypic Ig chains are usually found along the peripheral glomerular basement membranes and to a lesser extent in the nodules themselves. The staining in glomeruli is typically weaker than that observed along the tubular basement membranes. This may not be a function of the actual amount of deposited material, since several cases have been reported in which glomerular immunofluorescence was negative despite the presence of large amounts of granular glomerular deposits by electron microscopy (62). Local modifications of deposited LCs might thus change their antigenicity (302). In patients without nodular lesions, glomerular staining occurs along the basement membrane, but it may involve the mesangium in some cases (Fig. 76-12B). Linear Ig-chain staining is usually present along Bowman's capsule basement membrane. Deposits of Ig chains are constantly found in vascular walls (Fig. 76-12B).

In the 19 patients with HCDD that have been studied so far, immunofluorescence with anti-LC polyclonal and monoclonal antibodies was negative despite typical nodular glomerulosclerosis (Table 76-14). Kidney deposits of γ-, α-, and μ-Ig classes have been identified. All γ-subclasses are represented. Analysis of the kidney biopsies with monoclonal antibodies directed to the various constant domains of the γ-HC showed that C_H1 domain determinants were undetectable in the six patients in whom this study was performed (Fig. 76-13). In addition, epitopes of the $\gamma1$ C_H2 domain were also missing in one patient. These findings are in agreement with immunochemical analyses of the patients' serum (Table 76-14).

Electron Microscopy

The most characteristic ultrastructural feature on electron microscopy is the presence of finely or coarsely granular electron-dense deposits that delineate the outer aspect of the tubular basement membranes (Fig. 76-14). They appear to be in contact with a well-preserved basal lamina. The deposits are usually quite large and may protrude into the adjacent part of the interstitium.

Ultrastructural glomerular lesions are characterized by the deposition of a nonfibrillar, electron-dense material in the mesangial nodules and along the glomerular basement membrane. The mesangial material is usually finely granular with a membranoid appearance (Fig. 76-15), but in some cases, it may contain strongly electron-dense granules identical to the peritubular deposits (306,307). The deposits along the glomerular basement membrane appear as a prominent but thin, continuous band delineating the endothelial aspect of the basement membrane. The limits between the deposits and the basement membrane may be difficult to distinguish. In rare cases the deposits invade the lamina densa. Glomerular endothelial cells are separated from this material by areas of electron-lucent fluffy material. Banded collagen fibrils have been reported in a few patients (319). Nonamyloid fibrils have also been noted in 2 patients with HCDD (313,318). Podocytes usually show extensive spreading. Mesangial proliferation predominates at the periphery of the nodules. Mesangial interposition with basement membrane

TABLE 76-14. *Characteristics of patients with heavy-chain deposition disease (HCDD)*

Reference (no.)	Sex, age (yr)	HTA	Hu (micro)	Pu (g/day)	Crea (μM)	Bone marrow	NGS	Serum			Kidney deposits		Serum complement
								Truncated Ig	Entire monoclonal Ig	Ig subclass	HC deletion	Complement	
(8)	F, 53	+	NS	4.4	133	8% pc (MM)	+	IgG1λ	IgG1λ	γ1	CH1, h, CH2	C3	NS
(9)	M, 58	+	+	1.0	130	16% pc (MM)	+	IgG1λ	none	γ1	CH1, (h?)	N	normal (C3,C4)
(9)	M, 71	++	++	nephrotic	280	5% pc	++	IgG1λ (minute amounts)	2 IgGκ	γ1	CH1	N	low C3, normal C4
(9)	M, 51	++	++	nephrotic	300	20% pc (MM)	++	free γ1 (minute amounts)	IgG1λ IgMκ free λ	γ1	CH1, (h?)	N	low (C3, C4, CH50)
(9,308)	F, 35	–	+	0.5	88	6% pc	+	free γ1 (minute amounts)	IgG1λ	γ1	NS	C1q, C3	low (C3, C4, CH50)
HARR[a] (309)	F, 58	NS	NS	NS	NS	NS	+	IgG1λ	free κ	γ1	CH1, (h?)	C1, C3	NS
(309)	F, 26	+	+	2.9	200	3% pc	+	NS	free κ	γ1	NS	C1q, C3	low C3, normal C4
(310)	F, 67	–	+	4.8	117	1% pc	+	NS	none	γ2	NS	C3 weak	normal
(311)	F, 79	++	+	3.9	125	4% pc	+	none	none	γ3	NS	C1q, C3 weak	low (C3,C4)
	F, 45	+	+	10	395	<5% pc	+	IgG3λ (minute amounts)	none	γ3	CH1, (h?)	C1q, C3	low (C3, C4, CH50)
(312)	F, 48	NS	NS	nephrotic	182	50% pc (MM)	NS	free γ	none	γ3	NS, but 1 domain missing	NS	NS
(313)	F, 73	+	+	3.0	204	14% pc	+	NS	IgG3λ IgG1λ	γ3	NS	C1q, C3, C4 weak	low (C3, C4)
(8)	F, 59	+	NS	18.0	140	normal	+	none	γ microscopic	γ4	CH1, (h?)	NS	NS
(314)	M, 50	+	+	+++	857	3% pc	+	NS	IgGλ	γ4	NS	NS	NS
(315)	M, 53	NS	NS	2.0	185	NS	+	NS	IgGκ	γ4	NS	C3 weak	NS
(316)	M, 74	NS	NS	nephrotic	NS	NS	+	NS	IgGκ	γ	NS	NS	NS
(317)	M, 62	+	+	3.0	288	<1% pc	+	ακ (48 kDa), α (26 kDa & 54 kDa)	none	α	NS	C3	normal
MOO[a]	M, 52	+	+	3.1	221	NS	+	NS	NS	α	NS	No	normal
(318)	F, 68	++	NS	6.0	NS	1% pc	+	NS	none	μ	NS	C3	normal

Crea, creatininemia; *h*, hinge; *HTA*, hypertension; *Hu*, hematuria; *micro*, microscopic; *MM*, multiple myeloma; *NGS*, nodular glomerulosclerosis; *NS*, not specified; *pc*, plasma cells; *Pu*, proteinuria
[a]Personal communication from V. D'Agati.

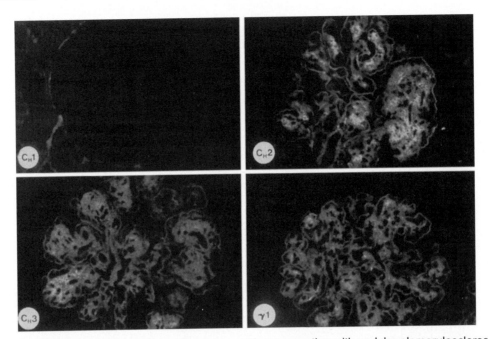

FIG. 76-13. Heavy-chain deposition disease in a patient presenting with nodular glomerulosclerosis in patient LOU (Table 76-15). Mesangial and parietal deposits stain with a monoclonal antibody specific for the γ1-isotype in the absence of detectable light chain (**bottom right**). Immunofluorescence with a panel of monoclonal antibodies directed to the various constant domains of the γ-heavy chain shows that the glomerular deposits are stained with anti-C_H2 and $-C_H$3, but not with anti-C_H1 antibodies. (Magnification $\times$312.) (From Moulin B, et al. Nodular glomerulosclerosis with deposition of monoclonal immunoglobulin heavy chains lacking C_H1. *J Am Soc Nephrol* 1999;10:519, with permission.)

duplication has been reported. Bowman's capsules may contain localized dense osmiophilic deposits.

The composition of glomerular matrix proteins has been examined comparatively in nodular glomerulosclerosis associated with LCDD and diabetes mellitus, using specific antibodies to basement membrane constituents (320). The glomeruli contained an excess of extracellular matrix molecules comparable to those found in many instances of progressive glomerular disease including diabetes. In a series of 36 patients with LC-related renal diseases including AL amyloidosis, CN, fibrillary glomerulopathy, and LCDD, transforming growth factor-β (TGF-β) was detected only

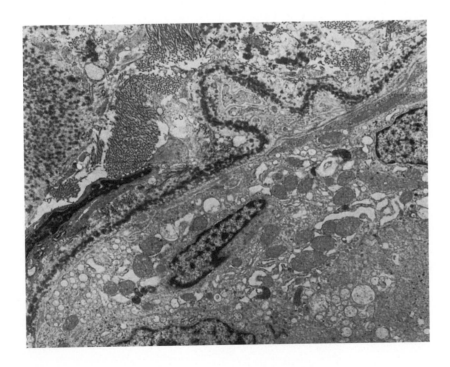

FIG. 76-14. Light-chain deposition disease. Coarsely granular dense deposits lining the outer aspect of the tubular basement membrane. (Electron microscopy, uranyl acetate and lead citrate $\times$6,000.) (From Ganeval D, et al. Visceral deposition of monoclonal light chains and immunoglobulins: a study of renal and immunopathologic abnormalities. *Adv Nephrol Necker Hosp* 1982;11:25, with permission.)

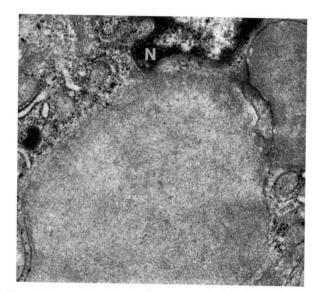

FIG. 76-15. Light-chain deposition disease. Detail of a mesangial nodule with finely granular, membranelike material. *N*, nucleus. (Electron microscopy, uranyl acetate and lead citrate ×15,000.) (Photo courtesy of Dr. L. H. Noël.)

in glomeruli of the three patients with LCDD and nodular glomerular lesions (321). In the control series, TGF-β was essentially found in nodular diabetic glomerulosclerosis, which may suggest that distinct initial insults to the glomerular mesangium may trigger similar fibrogenetic pathways. A similar accumulation of matrix proteins was found in the perisinusoidal space of the liver of patients with LCDD (322).

Clinical Presentation

Tables 76-15 and 76-16 summarize the main data from the four largest series published to date (304,305,323,324). They show an unexpectedly wide range of affected ages (31 to 77 years), but no clear gender preponderance.

Renal Features

Renal involvement is a constant feature of MIDD, and renal symptoms (primarily proteinuria and renal failure)

often dominate the clinical presentation (Table 76-15). In 23% to 67% of the patients, albuminuria is associated with the nephrotic syndrome. However, in 25% it is less than 1 g/day, and these patients mainly exhibit a tubulointerstitial syndrome. Albuminuria is not correlated with the existence of nodular glomerulosclerosis, at least initially, and may occur in the absence of significant glomerular lesions by light microscopy. Hematuria is more frequent than one would expect for a nephropathy in which cell proliferation is usually modest, with a few exceptions.

The high prevalence, early appearance, and severity of renal failure are other salient features of MIDD (6,325). In most cases, renal function declines rapidly, which is a primary reason for referral. It occurs with comparable frequency in patients with either low or heavy proteinuria (302), and thus presents in the form of a subacute tubulointerstitial nephritis or a rapidly progressive glomerulonephritis, respectively. The prevalence of hypertension is variable, but must be interpreted according to associated medical history.

Renal features of the 19 patients with HCDD were basically similar to those seen in LCDD and LHCDD (Table 76-14).

Extrarenal Manifestations

MIDD is a systemic disease (Table 76-16), but visceral LC deposits may be totally asymptomatic and found only at autopsy. Liver and cardiac deposits are most commonly found (305). Liver deposits were constant in patients whose liver was examined (326). They were either discrete, confined to sinusoids and basement membranes of biliary ductules without associated parenchymal lesions, or massive with marked dilation and multiple ruptures of sinusoids resembling peliosis. Hepatomegaly with mild alterations of liver function tests was the most usual symptom, but several patients developed hepatic insufficiency and portal hypertension. Three out of the 17 patients reported by Ganeval and associates (305) died of hepatic failure.

Cardiac involvement is also common. Of the 17 patients of the Necker and Tenon series (305), four developed cardiomegaly and two died of cardiac failure. As in the kidney

TABLE 76-15. *Renal manifestations at presentation in patients with light-chain deposition disease (LCDD) and light- and heavy-chain deposition disease (LHCDD)*

Series (ref. no.)	Age (yrs)	Male–female ratio	Proteinuria >1 g/d	Nephrotic syndrome	Hematuria	Renal failure	Hypertension
Necker/Tenon, 1982 (305) n = 17	57 (38–73)	1.8	13 (76%)	5 (29%)	5 (29%)	15 (88%)	3 (23%)[b]
Italy, 1988[a] (323) n = 15	53 (31–74)	0.7	11 (73%)	10 (67%)	NS	13 (87%)	12 (80%)
New York University, 1990 (304) n = 13	NS (35–71)	2.3	10 (77%)	3 (23%)	NS	12 (92%)	8 (61%)
Mayo Clinic, 1992 (324) n = 19	51 (37–77)	1.7	NS	10 (53%)	11 (58%)	17 (89%)	12 (63%)

NS, not specified
[a]Multicenter study.
[b]Plus 3 patients with past history of hypertension.

TABLE 76-16. *Hematologic features, extrarenal manifestations, and outcome of patients with light-chain deposition disease (LCDD) and light- and heavy-chain deposition disease (LHCDD)*

| Series (ref. no.) | Plasma cell dyscrasia | Bone marrow plasmacytosis >5% | Monoclonal component | | Extrarenal manifestations | Survival from onset of symptoms |
			Blood or urine	Tissue		
Necker/Tenon, 1982 (305) n = 17	Myeloma—9 Waldenström—1	10 (59%)	12/17 (71%) (8κ)	17	Liver—10 Heart—4 (+1)[b] Lung—2 Spleen—3 (+2)[b] Nervous system—4	1–46 mos 8/16 deceased
Italy, 1988[a] (323) n = 15	Myeloma—10	14 (93%)	11/14 (79%) (9κ)	15	Liver—7	5–54 mos 5/14 deceased
New York University, 1990 (304) n = 13	Myeloma—4	7 (54%)	10/12 (83%) (6κ)	11/11	Liver—3 Heart—6	1 mo–10 yrs 9/13 deceased
Mayo Clinic, 1992 (324) n = 19	Myeloma—6 Malignant LPD-1	10 (53%)[c]	16/19 (84%) (15κ)	19	Heart—4 Nervous system—2	89%: 1 yr 70%: 5 yrs

LPD, lymphoproliferative disease
[a]Multicenter study.
[b]Presence of light-chain deposits in otherwise asymptomatic patients.
[c]>10% plasma cells.

and liver, in all autopsy cases, immunofluorescence showed monotypic LC deposits in the vascular walls and perivascular areas of the heart (302).

Deposits may also occur along the nerve fibers and in the choroid plexus, as well as in the lymph nodes, bone marrow, spleen, pancreas, thyroid gland, submandibular glands, adrenal glands, gastrointestinal tract, abdominal vessels, lungs, and skin (see reference 302 for more detail).

Extrarenal deposits are less common in patients with HCDD. They have been reported in the heart (312), synovial tissue (312), skin (313), striated muscles (313), pancreas (8), around the thyroid follicles (8), and in Disse's spaces in the liver (8).

Hematologic Findings

The most common underlying disease in MIDD is myeloma (303) (Table 76-16). MIDD was found at postmortem examination in 5% of myeloma cases (30). It is often a presenting disease leading to the discovery of myeloma at an early stage. In some patients who first presented with common myeloma and with normal-sized monoclonal Ig without kidney disease, LCDD occurred when the disease relapsed after chemotherapy, together with Ig structural abnormalities (301,302). Since melphalan can induce Ig gene mutations (327), the disease in these patients might result from the emergence of a variant clone induced by the alkylating agent. Apart from myeloma, MIDD rarely complicates Waldenström's macroglobulinemia, including its apparently nonsecretory form (15). It often occurs in the absence of detectable malignant process (Tables 76-14 and 76-16), even after prolonged (more than 10 years) follow-up. In such "primary" forms, a monoclonal bone marrow plasma cell population is easily evidenced by immunofluorescence examination, whereas its detection requires a very careful analysis in primary amyloi-

dosis, in which clonal plasma cells usually account for less than 1% of bone marrow nucleated cells (199). This suggests that the plasma cell mass required for the clinical expression of the disease is larger in LCDD than in amyloidosis.

It is worth noting that in 15% to 30% of patients with LCDD, there is no detectable monoclonal Ig in the serum and urine (Table 76-16). Hence, some patients are affected with so-called nonsecretory myeloma or macroglobulinemia. Nonsecretory myeloma is inappropriately defined by the absence of detectable serum and urine monoclonal Ig. True nonsecretion is probably very rare (328). In most cases, there is a secretion of abnormal Ig molecules, which are either rapidly degraded postsynthetically or deposited in tissues (reviewed in reference 20).

In some patients also affected with HCDD, a monoclonal component may not be detected in serum and urine (8,310), (Table 76-14). In other patients, a monoclonal IgG1λ can actually be found in serum, but with a nondeleted HC component (9). Identification of the nephritogenic deleted HC, which circulates in low amounts, then requires serum fractionation followed by Western blotting (9).

Pathophysiology

The mechanisms leading to MIDD are more hypothetical than in AL amyloidosis for several reasons.

1. Similar pathologic conditions related to other protein precursors than monoclonal Ig are not known.
2. Circulating or urinary monoclonal Ig chain precursors are often absent or present at very low levels, making their purification and analysis particularly difficult.
3. Data on the precise nature of the visceral deposits remain speculative since they cannot be extracted like amyloid by suspension in distilled water.

Deposition does not Mean Pathogenicity

The finding by Solomon and colleagues (19) of unexpectedly frequent (14 out of 40) deposition of human monoclonal LCs along basement membranes in a mouse experimental model, raises the question of the relationship between tissue precipitation and pathogenic effects. While approximately 80% of MIDD cases are caused by κ-chains, human LCs which were found deposited along basement membranes in mice were predominantly of the λ type (9 out of 14) (19). In addition, LC deposition similar in type to LCDD by immunofluorescence but with only scanty granular electron-dense deposits in the tubular basement membrane may occur in the absence of glomerular lesions and tubular basement membrane thickening (329). Thus, the propensity of a given LC to form such deposits does not necessarily presume that it is pathogenic, and immunofluorescent staining should not be considered a sufficient criterion for pathologic diagnosis of MIDD. As shown by characteristic pathologic changes and experimental evidences, MIDD lesions are associated with local fibrosis, likely related to overproduction of extracellular matrix components.

MIDD is due to monoclonal κ-LC in most cases, with a probable overrepresentation of the rare $V_{\kappa IV}$ variability subgroup (28); however, $V_{\kappa IV}$ LCs may be encountered in myeloma without renal involvement (19).

Abnormal Glycosylation and Size of MIDD Light Chains

In vitro biosynthetic labeling experiments on short-term cultures showed that LCs absent from the urine were actually secreted by the bone marrow plasma cells (15,22,304). Undetectable circulating LCs were found to be N-glycosylated in all cases where they could be studied, either by *in vitro* inhibition of glycosylation with tunicamycin, analysis of the carbohydrate content of purified LCs (302), or by treatment with endoglycosidase-F (28). Another indirect evidence of glycosylation (i.e., the higher apparent molecular mass of the secreted LC compared with the cytoplasmic form) was found exclusively when the circulating LC was not detectable (21). Thus, glycosylation might increase the propensity of LC to precipitate in tissues and displace the equilibrium from soluble toward deposited forms so that these LCs are no longer detectable in the body fluids.

Structural abnormalities of Ig in MIDD have long been suggested by empirical studies of *in vitro* bone marrow cell biosynthesis products (301,302,305). In several cases with LC but no HC deposits, the bone marrow plasma cells contained both HCs and LCs. In such cases, normal-sized HCs were secreted together with LCs, both as assembled Ig molecules and free LC. In five cases, the deposits contained both HC and LC determinants; an Ig biosynthesis study performed in four of these showed truncated (short by about one domain) HCs (302,304). In a patient with HCDD (discussed below), normal-sized LCs and short HCs were noncovalently associated in a serum monoclonal IgG in the absence of detectable free HCs, and only the HCs were deposited (8). Hence, for both HCs and LCs there is a positive correlation between structural abnormalities, tissue deposition, and the absence of the corresponding chains in detectable amounts in serum and urine.

In a study of Ig biosynthesis by bone marrow plasma cells in eight consecutive patients (302), LCs were of normal size and secreted as monomers and dimers (as in common myeloma) in two cases, and grossly abnormal (short or apparently large) in the other six patients. These short or large LCs showed a striking ability to polymerize when secreted *in vitro*.

Sequence Analysis

Recent data collected in a patient (BLU) affected with nonsecretory κ-myeloma provided the first complete primary structure of a LC in LCDD (22). The 30-kd κ-chain found in the kidney was presumably identical to that secreted by the malignant plasma cells since they shared the same apparent molecular mass and 13 amino acid N-terminal sequence. It was encoded by a normal-sized κ-mRNA and N-glycosylation was proven by biosynthesis study with ^{14}C-glucose incorporation on a short-term bone marrow cell culture, and by endoglycosidase-F treatment. The C region was entirely normal and the V region belonged to the $V_{\kappa IV}$ subgroup. Comparison with germline sequence was made easy by the existence of a single germline $V_{\kappa IV}$ gene with no known allelic variant: Eight mutations were observed including replacement of Pro 95 (considered as essential for the conformation of the third hypervariable region). Replacement of Asp70 by Asn determined an N-glycosylation site. In another LC of the $V_{\kappa IV}$ subgroup from a patient with LCDD (330), 17 mutations were found, none of which was shared with the above κ chain. An extra cysteine was found at position 32; however, biosynthetic labeling experiments showed that the LC was secreted as monomer and dimer, as is usually seen for κ-LC.

The primary structures of a few further LCDD precursors were analyzed at the cDNA (330,331) and protein levels (332). As in AL amyloidosis, no common structural motif emerged from these studies. Most peculiarities are clustered in peptide loops corresponding to the complementary-determining regions (CDRs) (i.e., in parts of the molecules normally implicated in antigen binding), suggesting that a first step of the pathogenesis could be an LC tropism for extracellular components behaving as antigenlike structures. The most remarkable observations were unusual hydrophobic residues at positions where they could either be exposed to the solvent or strongly modify the conformation (331,332). In particular, molecular modeling experiments performed on $V_{\kappa IV}$ LCs underline the presence of hydrophobic residues (Leu, Ile, or Tyr) at position 27 or 31 or both in all known cases of LCDD. Other nonpolar groups may be exposed on CDRs, which suggests that hydrophobic interactions are important either in the amorphous precipitation of LCs or in the mechanisms leading to overproduction of extracellular matrix components (333).

Heavy-Chain Deposition Disease: A Disease Featured by Heavy-Chain Deletions

Nineteen cases of HCDD have been reported (see Table 76-14 for references). In all patients, an HC without LC was detected in the deposits. A deletion of the C_H1 domain was found in the deposited or circulating HC in the nine patients with γ-HCDD where it was searched for (Table 76-14). The C_H1 deletion was associated with a deletion of the C_H2 domain in one patient with γ-HCDD (8). It also occurred in a patient with α-HCDD (317). Thus, contrary to LCs, gross abnormalities seem to typify HC structures in MIDD. Complete primary structures, which were performed in two cases (8,334), showed precise deletions of entire domains, suggesting abnormal mRNA splicing. In the first patient in Table 76-14, an entire V domain of the V_{HIII} subgroup was directly joined to a normal third C domain, skipping the first C, hinge, and second C domains. This structure was strikingly similar to that reported in a case of AH amyloidosis (7), from which it differed by an unusual V domain: In particular, the invariant tryptophan at position 47 was replaced with a cysteine, and hydrophobic amino acids were found at positions exposed to the solvent in conserved framework regions. In the third patient in Table 76-14, the deposited γ-chain lacked the first C domain only, and was also remarkable by unusual substitutions in the V domain. Since a similar internal deletion of a γ-chain has been reported in a patient with HC disease without renal involvement or evidence of MIDD (335), it is probable that the V domain structures play a determining role in tissue precipitation. In two further cases termed pseudo-γ HCDD, predominant γ4-chain deposits were demonstrated with pathologic aspects similar to MIDD; the authors suggested that misfolding or denaturation of the LC was responsible for its nonreactivity with specific antibodies (336). It is worth noting that in most cases of HCDD, the circulating HC is associated with a λ-type LC. Whether the latter plays a role in deposition remains to be elucidated.

What is the Structure of Deposited Immunoglobulin Chains in Monoclonal Immunoglobulin Deposition Disease?

The precise structure of deposited Ig chains in MIDD remains speculative. Their strong immunoreactivity suggests that at least C domains are present in their native conformation. We are aware of two Western blot analyses of LCDD deposits. In one case, performed on myocardium after necropsy, the LC was predominantly deposited as an intact κ-chain with some fragments (337). In the second case the blot was done on an in vivo kidney biopsy and showed an intact κ-chain without detectable fragment (22).

Pathophysiology of Extracellular Matrix Accumulation

The strong periodic acid-Schiff reactivity of the deposits, even when the precursor LC is not glycosylated, suggests the invariable presence of carbohydrates. The latter might be responsible for the accumulation of extracellular matrix components, another striking feature in MIDD. The nature of these components, in particular the pattern of proteoglycans, is different in LCDD as compared with other conditions featuring renal fibrosis (338). Results of an in vitro study (339) suggest that deposited Ig chains may stimulate the mesangial cells through growth factors, in particular TFG-β, released either from blood-borne cells or produced by the local resident cells in an autocrine fashion. LC-induced overproduction of collagen IV, laminin, fibronectin, and tenascin is maximal at 72 hours of incubation with mesangial cells (340). Accumulation may be increased by a concomitant inhibition of collagenase IV, which is also mediated by TGF-β. None of these effects were found with amyloid LCs (340).

MIDD is a nice model to study the pathogenesis of glomerulosclerosis and interstitial fibrosis since the molecular culprit is a monoclonal Ig component of which the sequence is perfectly defined. Unfortunately, murine experimental models available to date do not reproduce the sclerotic phase of the disease (19,341).

Outcome and Treatment

The natural history of MIDD remains uncertain, mainly because extrarenal deposits of LCs observed in various organs can be totally asymptomatic or, on the contrary, cause severe organ damage leading to death. Survival from onset of symptoms varies from 1 month to 10 years (Table 76-16), whereas by comparison, the prognosis of a related disease, AL amyloidosis, is much more homogeneous. Heilman and associates (324) calculated that the 5-year actuarial rates for patient survival and survival free of end-stage renal disease under chemotherapy were 70% and 37%, respectively.

As in AL amyloidosis, the therapeutic strategy should be aimed at reducing Ig production by chemotherapy, hence improving or stabilizing renal failure and preventing extrarenal deposition of LCs. Chemotherapy is logical in patients with MIDD and myeloma. It is controversial in the absence of overt malignancy, given the uncertainties about the natural history of LCDD, the absence of reliable follow-up criteria, and the belief that MIDD is particularly resistant to chemotherapy.

At least two studies shed some light on the possible renal benefits of chemotherapy in MIDD (324,342). Both studies were retrospective and involved a small number of patients. In Ganeval's study that combined patients with myeloma and those without, only one of six patients treated with melphalan or cyclophosphamide associated with prednisone had reached end-stage renal failure at the end of follow-up (342). In contrast, renal death was observed in all eight patients who remained untreated or were treated late. However, it is noteworthy that treated patients initially had a lower serum creatinine concentration. In the Mayo Clinic's series (324), stabilization or improvement in renal function was essentially observed in patients with creatinine concentration less than 4.0 mg/dL.

It has been unclear, however, whether appropriate treatment can result in sustained remission in patients with LCDD. Barjon and colleagues (343) first provided the demonstration of relatively rapid clearance of deposits after syngeneic bone marrow transplantation to a patient with LCDD from his HLA-identical twin brother. Mariette and associates (344) also observed a striking recovery from multiorgan failure and clearing of LC deposits in the heart and liver of a patient with LCDD after intensive chemotherapy. Very recently, disappearance of nodular mesangial lesions and κ-LC deposits was reported in a patient with LCDD after long-term chemotherapy (345). These observations are of paramount importance. First, they demonstrate that fibrotic nodular glomerular lesions are reversible. Second, they argue for intensive chemotherapy in patients with severe visceral involvement.

Kidney transplantation has been performed in a few patients with MIDD. Recurrence of the disease is usually observed (17,18,346,347).

COMBINED GLOMERULAR AND TUBULAR LESIONS

Tubular Lesions Associated with Glomerular and Tubular Light-Chain Deposits

It is generally considered that CN and LC tissue deposition occur in mutually exclusive fashion. However, in CN, LC deposits are not exceptional along glomerular and tubular basement membranes (B. Mougenot and G. Touchard, personal communication) and small deposits of interstitial and vascular amyloid are occasionally seen. Conversely, in patients with glomerular lesions associated with LC, damage to proximal tubule epithelium often occurs and can become prominent in some patients (139,182), although typical myeloma casts are rare. In addition, the pattern of renal lesions may change with time under chemotherapy. In three patients with typical myeloma CN on initial biopsy, casts were replaced by massive tissue deposits of LC (κ-chains in two, amyloid in one) (89), suggesting chemotherapy-induced mutation of the LC, which might cause the LC to be deposited in tissues rather than giving rise to myeloma casts (301,327).

More exceptional is the association of FS with AL amyloidosis. In the three cases reported thus far (25,130,348), FS was not caused by amyloid infiltration of the kidney. Amyloid was diagnosed shortly before death or at autopsy. Nodular amyloid deposits were surrounded by atypical lymphoid cells containing numerous needle-shaped crystals, which suggested that "a product" from these cells "may have been involved with both crystal formation and amyloid production" (130). Since the nucleation process initiating amyloid and crystal formation may share similarities, it is tempting

to speculate that the responsible LCs bore unusual physicochemical properties, inducing both pathologic conditions (as previously discussed).

Combined AL Amyloidosis and Monoclonal Immunoglobulin Deposition Disease

Since the description of MIDD, it was expected that the two types of deposits might coexist at different sites in a single patient. The first observations were reported by Jacquot and associates in 1985 (247). A review by Gallo and colleagues (303) indicates that in approximately 7% of 135 patients with LCDD, amyloid was found in one or more organs. Because amyloid deposits were focal, the true incidence of the association may be markedly underestimated. In patients with both types of deposits, amyloid P component was found in the fibrillar, but not the nonfibrillar LC deposits by immunohistochemical methods (349). The pathophysiologic significance of this association remains controversial. On the one hand, some LCs may possess intrinsic properties that make them prone to form both fibrillar and nonfibrillar deposits, depending on the tissue microenvironment. On the other hand, in the absence of structural analysis of the deposited LCs, one cannot exclude that they are generated by different variant clones. In a patient with IgD myeloma, MIDD and amyloidosis were associated with CN (350).

OTHER DYSPROTEINEMIA-ASSOCIATED GLOMERULAR LESIONS

In this last section, we follow the same approach as in earlier sections, that is a description of pathologic entities based on immunomorphologic observations leading to pathophysiologic considerations is provided. We do not discuss cryoglobulinemia-associated glomerulonephritis, which is the subject of Chapter 69.

Glomerulonephritis with Intracapillary Thrombi of Immunoglobulin M

This glomerulonephritis is almost specific of Waldenström's macroglobulinemia (351). It is considered the most common renal lesion with amyloidosis in this condition, but like amyloidosis, it has become a rare entity probably because of the increased efficacy of chemotherapy. In the series of 16 autopsy and biopsy cases published by Morel-Maroger and associates (351), this lesion was found in six cases, and was associated with variable degrees of proteinuria and normal or slightly altered renal function. It was characterized by periodic acid-Schiff-positive, noncongophilic endomembranous deposits in a variable number of capillary loops. Deposits were sometimes so voluminous as to occlude the capillary lumens partially or completely, thus forming thrombi. By immunofluorescence, thrombi and deposits were stained with anti-IgM (three cases) and with anti-κ (one case) with antibodies. Two of the six patients had cryoglobulinemia and

TABLE 76-17. *Immunologic and clinical characteristics of fibrillary and immunotactoid glomerulopathies*

Characteristics	Amyloidosis (AL-type)	Fibrillary glomerulonephritis	Immunotactoid glomerulopathy (GOMMID)
Congo red staining	Yes	No	No
Composition	Fibrils	Fibrils	Microtubules
Fibril or microtubule size	8–15 nm	12–22 nm	>30 nm
Organization in tissues	Random (β-pleated sheet)	Random	Parallel arrays
Immunoglobulin deposition	Monoclonal LC (mostly λ)	Usually polyclonal (mostly IgG4), occasionally monoclonal (IgGκ)	Usually monoclonal (IgGκ or IgGλ)
Glomerular lesions	Deposits spreading from the mesanguim	MP, MPGN, CGN	Atypical MN, MPGN
Extrarenal manifestations (fibrillar deposits)	Systemic deposition disease	Pulmonary hemorrhage	Microtubular inclusions in leukemic lymphocytes
Association with LPD	Yes (myeloma)	Uncommon	Common (CLL, NHL) but debated
Renal presentation	Severe NS, absence of hypertension and hematuria	NS with hematuria, hypertension; RPGN	NS with microhematuria and hypertension
Treatment	Melphalan + prednisone; intensive therapy with blood stem cell autograft	Corticosteroids ± cyclophosphamide (crescentic GN)	Treatment of the associated LPD

CGN, crescentic glomerulonephritis; *CLL*, chronic lymphocytic leukemia; *GN*, glomerulonephritis; *GOMMID*, glomerulopathy with organized microtubular monoclonal immunoglobin deposits (see text); *LC*, light chain; *LPD*, lymphoproliferative disorder; *MN*, membranous nephropathy; *MP*, mesangial proliferation; *MPGN*, membranoproliferative glomerulonephritis; *NHL*, non-Hodgkin's lymphoma; *NS*, nephrotic syndrome; *RPGN*, rapidly progressive glomerulonephritis

slight glomerular cell proliferation. In the remaining four the amount of circulating IgM was higher than in the other patients of the series with amyloidosis or no detectable renal lesion, which suggested that hyperviscosity could favor IgM deposition in glomerular capillaries where ultrafiltration further increases the protein concentration. This pathophysiologic hypothesis is also supported by the study of Argani and Kipkie (352) in which formation of diffuse intracapillary thrombi was likely precipitated by severe dehydration.

Since renal biopsy may be hazardous in patients with Waldenström's macroglobulinemia with frequently increased bleeding time, it is wise to search for amyloid deposits first by a less invasive tissue biopsy. This is of utmost importance because amyloidosis is a major cause of morbidity associated with a much shorter survival time (196).

Glomerulonephritis with Nonamyloid Organized Monotypic Deposits

These entities are characterized by fibrillar or microtubular deposits in mesangium and glomerular capillary loops that are readily distinguishable from amyloid because fibrils are thicker and are not stained by Congo red. They have been termed fibrillary glomerulonephritis by Alpers and associates (353–355) and immunotactoid glomerulopathy by Korbet and colleagues (356–358). However, the two denominations may cover partly different morphologic entities as defined by the size and aspect of organized structures. For Alpers (354), the distinguishing morphologic features of immunotactoid

glomerulonephritis are the presence of organized deposits of large, thick-walled microtubules, usually greater than 30 nm in diameter, at times arranged in parallel arrays. On the other hand, fibrillary glomerulonephritis is characterized by more amyloidlike deposits with smaller fibrils (12 to 20 nm).

Although these criteria remain controversial (359), distinguishing immunotactoid from fibrillary glomerulonephritis may be of great clinical and pathophysiologic interest because the former seems to be more often associated with monotypic Ig deposits. However, it is difficult to assess precisely from the literature the respective prevalence in each entity of monotypic deposits and of circulating monoclonal Ig because studies of biopsies with anti-LC antibodies were often incomplete, urine and blood data uncertain, and even more, patients with dysproteinemias were excluded *a priori* from several series (356,360).

The characteristics of fibrillary and immunotactoid glomerulopathies are described in Table 76-17 by comparison with AL amyloid.

Pathology

In immunotactoid glomerulopathy, renal biopsy shows either membranous glomerulonephritis (often associated with segmental mesangial proliferation) or lobular membranoproliferative glomerulonephritis. By immunofluorescence, coarse granular deposits of IgG and C3 are observed along capillary basement membranes and in mesangial areas. Reviews of all published cases analyzed with anti-LC antibodies have

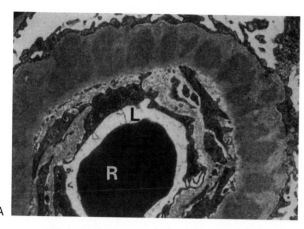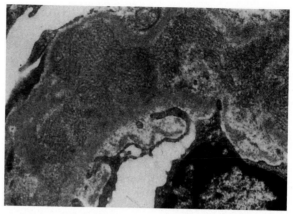

FIG. 76-16. Immunotactoid glomerulopathy. Atypical membranous glomerulonephritis showing exclusive staining of the deposits with anti-immunoglobulin G and anti-κ–light-chain antibodies, in chronic lymphocytic leukemia. **A:** Electron microscopy of a glomerular capillary showing subepithelial deposits with effacement of the foot-processes and mesangial interposition. *L*, capillary lumen; *R*, red blood cell. (Uranyl acetate and lead citrate ×4,400.) **B:** Higher magnification of the capillary wall showing microtubular structure of the deposits. (Magnification ×12,000.) (From Moulin B, et al. Glomerulonephritis in chronic lymphocytic leukemia and related B-cell lymphomas. *Kidney Int* 1992;42:127, with permission.)

concluded that monotypic deposits occur in 50% to 80% of patients with immunotactoid glomerulopathy, with both LC isotypes being represented (354–361). However, a circulating monoclonal Ig is detected only in a minority of patients, a finding reminiscent of MIDD. By electron microscopy, the distinguishing morphologic features of immunotactoid glomerulonephritis are the presence of organized deposits of large, thick-walled microtubules, usually greater than 30 nm in diameter, at times arranged in parallel arrays (Fig. 76-16). A particular form of immunotactoid glomerulopathy termed "glomerulonephritis with organized microtubular monoclonal immunoglobulin deposits" (GOMMID) has recently been described, often in the setting of chronic lymphocytic leukemia or related lymphoma (361). Inclusions showing the same microtubular organization and containing the same IgG subclass and LC type as the renal deposits are often detected in the cytoplasm of blood leukemic lymphocytes.

Mesangial proliferation and aspects of membranoproliferative glomerulonephritis are predominantly reported in series of fibrillary glomerulonephritis. Glomerular crescents are present in about 25% of the biopsies. Immunofluorescence studies mainly show IgG deposits (of the γ4-isotype in one series) with a predominant mesangial localization. Monotypic deposits containing mostly IgGκ, are detected in no more than 15% to 20% of patients. By electron microscopy, fibrils are randomly arranged and their diameter varies between 12 and 22 nm. Of note, the fibril size alone is not sufficient to distinguish nonamyloidotic fibrillary glomerulonephritis from amyloid.

Pathogenesis

The cause of fibrillary glomerulonephritis is not known. Fibril formation is thought to be mediated by the deposition of abnormal polyclonal or monoclonal proteins, or of immune complexes that are then able to form either random fibrillary structures or more organized microtubular deposits in the mesangium and along the capillary wall of the glomerulus. The exclusive or prevailing presence of IgG4 in the immune deposits of patients with fibrillary glomerulonephritis is of great interest. Although not monoclonal, this isotype-restricted homogeneous material made of highly anionic Ig may facilitate fibril formation. Amyloid P component has also been found in the fibrils. The recent description of fibrillar cryoprecipitates consisting of Ig-fibronectin complexes in the serum of patients with fibrillary glomerulonephritis without evidence of systemic disease indicates that serum precursors can lead to the formation of fibrillary deposits (362).

The mechanisms of Ig deposition in lymphocytes and kidney of patients with immunotactoid glomerulopathy or GOMMID are also poorly understood. Analysis of monoclonal Ig both at the protein and mRNA levels has not disclosed size abnormalities in two patients (361). Whether crystallization in lymphocytes and the glomerulus results from unusual intrinsic physicochemical properties of the monoclonal Ig, or from reactivity with a shared epitope remains to be established. These properties may also account for rapid disappearance of the Ig from the blood and its recurrence on renal graft noted in several patients.

Clinical Manifestations (353–361)

The incidence of glomerulopathies with nonamyloid deposition of fibrillary or microtubular material in a nontransplant adult biopsy population is estimated to be about 1% (equivalent to that of antiglomerular basement membrane [anti-GBM] disease). Despite a growing number of case reports, this is most likely underestimated because of the insufficient attention given to atypical reactions with

TABLE 76-18. *Renal lesions observed in B-cell proliferations*

Renal lesions	Multiple myeloma	Waldenström's macroglobulinemia	Chronic lymphocytic leukemia and related lymphomas
Tubular lesions			
Cast nephropathy	+++	−	−
(Proximal) tubule lesions[a]	+	−	−
Fanconi's syndrome	+ (smoldering)	−	−
Glomerular lesions[b]			
AL amyloidosis	++	+	+
MIDD (nodular, membranoproliferative, minimal change)	++	+	−
Nonamyloid organized deposits[c]	−	−	+
Type I and type II cryoglobulinemia	+	++	++
IgM capillary thrombi	−	+	−
Other (crescentic, minimal change, etc.)	+	+	+
Interstitial lesions			
B-cell infiltrate	+[d]	++	++
Nephrocalcinosis	+	−	−
Pyelonephritis (infections)	+	−	−

−, not or exceptionally observed; + to +++, semiquantitative rating of the prevalence of renal lesions;
MIDD, monoclonal immunoglobulin deposition disease
[a]Without detectable myeloma casts, sometimes acute tubular necrosis.
[b]Glomerular involvement is usually but not always preponderant.
[c]Usually atypical membranous (or membranoproliferative) glomerulonephritis.
[d]Exceptionally, plasmacytoma.

histochemical stains for amyloid and the lack of immunohistochemical and ultrastructure studies of most biopsy specimens.

The age range extends from 10 to 80 years with a peak incidence between 40 and 60 years. On average, patients with immunotactoid glomerulopathy are older than those with fibrillary glomerulonephritis. Nonamyloid fibrillary glomerulonephritis occurs with the same frequency in males and females while the male-to-female ratio is 2:1 in immunotactoid glomerulopathy.

Presenting renal manifestations include proteinuria, mostly in the nephrotic range, microhematuria, and hypertension. Renal insufficiency with rapid progression to end-stage renal disease occurs in approximately half of the patients followed for more than 2 years. Rapidly progressive glomerulonephritis is more often encountered in fibrillary glomerulonephritis, which seems more prone to superimposition of glomerular crescents.

Although fibril deposition is almost always confined to the kidney, similar fibrillary deposits have been reported in the alveolar capillary membrane in patients presenting with a pulmonary–renal syndrome and in the skin of a patient with a leukocytoclastic vasculitis. These observations suggest that the pathologic process may be systemic in nature. Recurrence of fibrillary or immunotactoid glomerulopathies has also been reported in patients receiving a renal allograft (363).

Associated Diseases

In addition to plasma cell dyscrasias, fibrillary and immunotactoid glomerulopathies have been reported in patients with hepatitis C infection (364), adenocarcinoma, Sjögren's syndrome, mixed connective tissue disease, and other conditions (reviewed in reference 365).

Treatment

Treatment with combined corticosteroids and intravenous cyclophosphamide has achieved variable results in patients presenting with crescentic fibrillary glomerulonephritis. In those with immunotactoid glomerulopathy, especially in the GOMMID subgroup, it is worth noting that corticosteroid therapy and/or chemotherapy are associated with partial or complete remission of the nephrotic syndrome, with a parallel improvement of the hematologic disease when present.

Renal transplantation has been performed in only a few patients, and recurrent disease occurred in several (363).

A better understanding of these unusual glomerulopathies, which most likely make up a new form of monoclonal Ig-related deposition disease with nonamyloid organization of the deposits will require: (a) detailed ultrastructural and immunomorphologic characterization of the renal deposits; (b) careful analysis of circulating Ig with sensitive techniques, including repeated search of cryoglobulins; (c) studies on bone marrow and circulating lymphocytes (ultrastructure, *in vitro* Ig biosynthesis); and (d) prolonged follow-up of patients to assess eventual occurrence of extrarenal manifestations and efficacy of treatment.

Glomerulonephritis with organized microtubular monoclonal immunoglobulin deposits must be added to the heterogeneous list of glomerulopathies caused by B-cell chronic lymphocytic leukemia and related lymphomas, including AL amyloidosis and the larger cohort of cryoglobulinemia-associated membranoproliferative glomerulonephritis (Table 76-18).

Other Types of Glomerulonephritis

Additional histologic forms of glomerulonephritis have occasionally been described in B-cell proliferations, and include crescentic and hypocomplementemic membranoproliferative glomerulonephritis apparently without cryoglobulinemia (reviewed in reference 366). However, most of these observations are old. Careful immunomorphologic, ultrastructural, and immunochemical studies should be performed before these histologic forms are recognized as distinct entities.

REFERENCES

1. Bence Jones H. On a new substance occurring in the urine of a patient with *mollities ossium. Philos Trans R Soc Lond* 1848;138:55.
2. MacIntyre W. Case of *mollities and fragilitas ossium*, accompanied with urine strongly charged with animal matter. *Med Chir Trans Lond* 1849;33:211.
3. Edelman GM, Gally JA. The nature of Bence Jones proteins: chemical similarities to polypeptide chains of myeloma globulins and normal γ-globulins. *J Exp Med* 1962;116:207.
4. Glenner GG, Terry W, Harada M, et al. Amyloid fibril proteins: proof of homology with immunoglobulin light chains by sequence analyses. *Science* 1971;172:1150.
5. Antonovych TT, Lin RC, Parrish E, et al. Light chain deposits in multiple myeloma. 7th Annual Meeting of the American Society of Nephrology, 1973. *Lab Invest* 1974;30:370A(abst 3).
6. Randall RE, Williamson WC Jr, Mullinax F, et al. Manifestations of systemic light chain deposition. *Am J Med* 1976;60:293.
7. Eulitz M, Weiss DT, Solomon A. Immunoglobulin heavy-chain-associated amyloidosis. *Proc Natl Acad Sci USA* 1990;87:6542.
8. Aucouturier P, et al. Brief report: heavy-chain deposition disease. *N Engl J Med* 1993;329:1389.
9. Moulin B, et al. Nodular glomerulosclerosis with deposition of monoclonal immunoglobulin heavy chains lacking C_H1. *J Am Soc Nephrol* 1999;10:519.
10. Moulin B, et al. Glomerulonephritis in chronic lymphocytic leukemia and related B-cell lymphomas. *Kidney Int* 1992;42:127.
11. Touchard G, et al. Nephrotic syndrome associated with chronic lymphocytic leukemia: an immunological and pathological study. *Clin Nephrol* 1989;31:107.
12. Wochner RD, Strober W, Waldmann TA. The role of the kidney in the catabolism of Bence Jones proteins and immunoglobulin fragments. *J Exp Med* 1967;126:207.
13. Mogielnicki RP, Waldmann TA, Strober W. Renal handling of low molecular weight proteins. I. L-chain metabolism in experimental renal disease. *J Clin Invest* 1971;50:901.
14. Maack T, Johnson V, Kau ST, et al. Renal filtration, transport and metabolism of low-molecular-weight proteins: a review. *Kidney Int* 1979;16:251.
15. Preud'homme JL, et al. Synthesis of abnormal immunoglobulins in lymphoplasmacytic disorders with visceral light chain deposition. *Am J Med* 1980;69:703.
16. De Lima JJ, Kourilsky O, Meyrier A, et al. Kidney transplant in multiple myeloma. Early recurrence in the graft with sustained normal renal function. *Transplantation* 1981;31:223.
17. Scully RE. Case records of the Massachusetts General Hospital (Case 1-1981). *N Engl J Med* 1981;304:33.
18. Gerlag PGG, Koene RAP, Berden JHM. Renal transplantation in light chain nephropathy: case report and review of the literature. *Clin Nephrol* 1986;25:101.
19. Solomon A, Weiss DT, Kattine AA. Nephrotoxic potential of Bence Jones proteins. *N Engl J Med* 1991;324:1845.
20. Cogné M, Silvain C, Khamlichi AA, et al. Structurally abnormal immunoglobulins in human immunoproliferative disorders. *Blood* 1992;79:2181.
21. Preud'homme JL, et al. Monoclonal immunoglobulin deposition disease (Randall type). Relationship with structural abnormalities of immunoglobulin chains. *Kidney Int* 1994;46:965.
22. Cogné M, Preud'homme JL, Bauwens M, et al. Structure of a monoclonal kappa chain of the $V_{κIV}$ subgroup in the kidney and

plasma cells in light chain deposition disease. *J Clin Invest* 1991;87:2186.
23. Aucouturier P, et al. Monoclonal Ig L chain and L chain V domain fragment crystallization in myeloma-associated Fanconi's syndrome. *J Immunol* 1993;150:3561.
24. Leboulleux M, et al. Protease resistance and binding of Ig light chains in myeloma-associated tubulopathies. *Kidney Int* 1995;48:72.
25. Messiaen T, et al. Adult Fanconi syndrome secondary to light chain gammopathy: clinicopathologic heterogeneity and unusual features in 11 patients. *Medicine* 2000;79:135.
26. Solomon A, Frangione B, Franklin EC. Bence Jones proteins and light chains of immunoglobulins: preferential association of the $V_{λVI}$ subgroup of human light chains with amyloidosis AL (λ). *J Clin Invest* 1982;70:453.
27. Ozaki S, Abe M, Wolfenbarger D, et al. Preferential expression of human λ-light chain variable region subgroups in multiple myeloma, AL amyloidosis, and Waldenström's macroglobulinemia. *Clin Immunol Immunopathol* 1994;71:183.
28. Denoroy L, Déret S, Aucouturier P. Overrepresentation of the $V_{κIV}$ subgroup in light chain deposition disease. *Immunol Lett* 1994;42:63.
29. Kapadia SB. Multiple myeloma: a clinicopathologic study of 62 consecutively autopsied cases. *Medicine* 1980;59:380.
30. Ivanyi B. Frequency of light chain deposition nephropathy relative to renal amyloidosis and Bence Jones cast nephropathy in a necropsy study of patients with myeloma. *Arch Pathol Lab Med* 1990;114:986.
31. Cooper EH, Forbes MA, Crockson RA, et al. Proximal renal tubular function in myelomatosis: observations in the fourth Medical Research Council trial. *J Clin Pathol* 1984;37:852.
32. DeFronzo RA, Cooke CR, Wright JR, et al. Renal function in patients with multiple myeloma. *Medicine (Baltimore)* 1978;57:151.
33. Coward RA, Mallick NP, Delamore IW. Tubular function in multiple myeloma. *Clin Nephrol* 1985;24:180.
34. MacLennan ICM, Drayson M, Dunn J. Multiple myeloma. *Br Med J* 1994;308:1033.
35. Rayner HC, Haynes AP, Thompson JR, et al. Perspectives in multiple myeloma: survival, prognostic factors and disease complications in a single centre between 1975 and 1988. *Q J Med* 1991;290:517.
36. Alexanian R, Barlogie B, Dixon D. Renal failure in multiple myeloma: pathogenesis and prognostic implications. *Arch Intern Med* 1990;150:1693.
37. Rota S, et al. Multiple myeloma and severe renal failure: a clinicopathologic study of outcome and prognosis in 34 patients. *Medicine (Baltimore)* 1987;66:126.
38. Pozzi C, et al. Prognostic factors and effectiveness of treatment in acute renal failure due to multiple myeloma: a review of 50 cases. Report of the Italian Renal Immunopathology Group. *Clin Nephrol* 1987;28:1.
39. Pasquali S, Casanova S, Zucchelli A, et al. Long-term survival patients with acute and severe renal failure due to multiple myeloma. *Clin Nephrol* 1990;34:247.
40. Ganeval D, et al. Treatment of multiple myeloma with renal involvement. *Adv Nephrol Necker Hosp* 1992;21:347.
41. Preud'homme JL, Bauwens M, Dumont G, et al. Cast nephropathy in μ heavy chain disease. *Clin Nephrol* 1997;48:118.
42. DeFronzo RA, Humphrey RL, Wright JR, et al. Acute renal failure in multiple myeloma. *Medicine (Baltimore)* 1975;54:209.
43. Winearls CG. Nephrology forum: acute myeloma kidney. *Kidney Int* 1995;48:1347.
44. Kyle RA. Multiple myeloma: review of 869 cases. *Mayo Clin Proc* 1975;50:29.
45. Fibbe WE, Jansen J. Prognostic factors in IgD myeloma: a study of 21 cases. *Scand J Haematol* 1984;33:471.
46. Blade J, Lust JA, Kyle RA. Immunoglobulin D multiple myeloma: presenting features, response to therapy and survival in a series of 53 cases. *J Clin Oncol* 1994;12:2398.
47. Smolens P, Barnes JL, Kreisberg R. Hypercalcemia can potentiate the nephrotoxicity of Bence Jones proteins. *J Lab Clin Med* 1987;110:460.
48. Huang ZQ, Sanders PW. Biochemical interaction between Tamm-Horsfall glycoprotein and Ig light chains in the pathogenesis of cast nephropathy. *Lab Invest* 1995;73:810.
49. Ronco P, et al. Pathophysiologic aspects of Tamm-Horsfall protein: a phylogenetically conserved marker of the thick ascending limb of Henle's loop. *Adv Nephrol Necker Hosp* 1987;16:231.
50. McCarthy CS, Becker JA. Multiple myeloma and contrast media. *Radiology* 1992;183:519.

51. Wu MJ, Kumar KS, Kulkarni G, et al. Multiple myeloma in naproxen-induced acute renal failure. *N Engl J Med* 1987;317:170.

52. Shpilberg O, Douer D, Ehrenfeld M, et al. Naproxen-associated fatal acute renal failure in multiple myeloma. *Nephron* 1990;55:448.

53. Dubose TD, Molony DB, Verani R, et al. Nephrotoxicity of non-steroidal anti-inflammatory drugs. *Lancet* 1994;344:515.

54. Rabb H, et al. Acute renal failure from multiple myeloma precipitated by ACE inhibitors. *Am J Kidney Dis* 1999;33:E5.

55. Gresser I, Maury C, Tovey M, et al. Progressive glomerulonephritis in mice treated with interferon preparations at birth. *Nature* 1976;263:420.

56. Fahal IH, Murry N, Chu P, et al. Acute renal failure during interferon treatment. *Br Med J* 1993;306:973.

57. Sawamura M, Matsushima T, Tamura J, et al. Renal toxicity in long-term alpha-interferon treatment in a patient with myeloma. *Am J Hematol* 1992;41:146.

58. Noel C, et al. Acute and definitive renal failure in progressive multiple myeloma treated with recombinant interferon alpha-2a: report of two patients. *Am J Hematol* 1992;41:298.

59. Border WA, Cohen AH. Renal biopsy diagnosis of clinically silent multiple myeloma. *Ann Intern Med* 1980;93:43.

60. Thannhauser SJ, Krauss E. Uber eine degenerative Erkrankung der Harnkanalchen (Nephrose) by Bence-Jones' scher Albuminurie mit Nirerenschwund (kleine, glatte, weisse Niere). *Dtsch Arch Klin. Med* 1920;133:183.

61. Oliver J. New directions in renal morphology: a method, its results and its future. *Harvey Lectures* 1945;40:102.

62. Pirani CL, Silva F, D'Agati V, et al. Renal lesions in plasma cell dyscrasias: Ultrastructural observations. *Am J Kidney Dis* 1987;10:208.

63. Pirani CL. Histological, histochemical and ultrastructural features of myeloma kidney. In: Minetti L, D'Amico G, Ponticelli C, eds. *The kidney in plasma cell dyscrasias.* Dordrecht: Kluwer Academic Publishers, 1988:153.

64. Cohen AH, Border WA. Myeloma kidney: an immunomorphogenetic study of renal biopsies. *Lab Invest* 1980;42:248.

65. Sikl H. A case of diffuse plasmocytosis with deposition of protein crystals in the kidneys. *J Path Bact* 1949;61:149.

66. Koss MN, Pirani CL, Osserman EF. Experimental Bence Jones cast nephropathy. *Lab Invest* 1976;34:579.

67. Sanders PW, et al. Differential nephrotoxicity of low molecular weight proteins including Bence Jones proteins in the perfused rat nephron in vivo. *J Clin Invest* 1988;82:2086.

68. Strober W, Waldmann TA. The role of the kidney in the metabolism of plasma proteins. *Nephron* 1974;13:35.

69. Sumpio BE, Maack T. Kinetics, competition and selectivity of tubular absorption of proteins. *Am J Physiol* 1982;243:F379.

70. Batuman V, Dreisbach AW, Cyran J. Light-chain binding sites on renal brush-border membranes. *Am J Physiol* 1990;258:F1259.

71. Batuman V, et al. Myeloma light chains are ligands for cubilin (gp280). *Am J Physiol* 1998;275:F246.

72. Mogensen CE, Solling K. Studies on renal tubular protein reabsorption: partial and near complete inhibition by certain amino acids. *Scand J Clin Lab Invest* 1977;37:477.

73. Batuman V, Sastrasinh M, Sastrasinh S. Light chain effects on alanine and glucose uptake by renal brush border membranes. *Kidney Int* 1986;30:662.

74. Smolens P, Barnes JL, Stein JH. Effect of chronic administration of different Bence Jones proteins on rat kidney. *Kidney Int* 1986;30:874.

75. Sanders PW, Herrera GA, Galla JH. Human Bence Jones protein toxicity in rat proximal tubule epithelium in vivo. *Kidney Int* 1987;32:851.

76. Smolens P, Venkatachalam M, Stein JH. Myeloma kidney cast nephropathy in a rat model of multiple myeloma. *Kidney Int* 1983;24:192.

77. Clyne DH, Pesce AJ, Thompson RE. Nephrotoxicity of Bence Jones proteins in the rat: importance of protein isoelectric point. *Kidney Int* 1979;16:345.

78. Coward RA, Delamore IW, Mallick NP, et al. The importance of urinary immunoglobulin light chain isoelectric point (pI) in nephrotoxicity in multiple myeloma. *Clin Sci* 1984;66:229.

79. Melcion C, et al. Renal failure in myeloma: relationship with isoelectric point of immunoglobulin light chains. *Clin Nephrol* 1984;22:138.

80. Johns EA, Turner R, Cooper EH, et al. Isoelectric points of urinary light chains in myelomatosis: analysis in relation to nephrotoxicity. *J Clin Pathol* 1986;39:833.

81. Sanders PW, Booker BB, Bishop JB, et al. Mechanisms of intranephronal proteinaceous cast formation by low molecular weight proteins. *J Clin Invest* 1990;85:570.

82. Sanders PW, Booker BB. Pathobiology of cast nephropathy from human Bence Jones proteins. *J Clin Invest* 1992;89:630.

83. Huang ZQ, Kirk KA, Connelly KG, et al. Bence Jones proteins bind to a common peptide segment of Tamm-Horsfall glycoprotein to promote heterotypic aggregation. *J Clin Invest* 1993;92:2975.

84. Huang ZQ, Sanders PW. Localization of a single binding site for immunoglobulin light chains on human Tamm-Horsfall glycoprotein. *J Clin Invest* 1997;99:732.

85. Ying WZ, Sanders PW. Dietary salt regulates expression of Tamm-Horsfall glycoprotein in rats. *Kidney Int* 1998;54:1150.

86. Verroust P, Morel-Maroger L, Preud'homme JL. Renal lesions in dysproteinemias. *Springer Semin Immunopathol* 1982;5:333.

87. Myatt EA, et al. Pathogenic potential of human monoclonal immunoglobulin light chains: relationship of in vitro aggregation to in vivo organ deposition. *Proc Natl Acad Sci USA* 1994;91:3034.

88. Weiss JH, et al. Pathophysiology of acute Bence Jones protein nephrotoxicity in the rat. *Kidney Int* 1981;20:198.

89. Hill GS, Morel-Maroger L, Mery JPh, et al. Renal lesions in multiple myeloma: their relationship to associated protein abnormalities. *Am J Kidney Dis* 1983;2:423.

90. Levi DF, Williams RC Jr, Lindstrom FD. Immunofluorescent studies of the myeloma kidney with special reference to light chain disease. *Am J Med* 1968;44:922.

91. McGiven AR, Hunt JS, Day WA, et al. Tamm-Horsfall protein in the glomerular capsular space. *J Clin Pathol* 1978;31:620.

92. Ronco P, et al. Pathophysiological aspects of myeloma cast nephropathy. In: Minetti L, D'Amico G, Ponticelli C, eds. *The kidney in plasma cell dyscrasias.* Dordrecht: Kluwer Academic Publishers, 1988: 93.

93. Thomas DBL, Davies M, Peters JR, et al. Tamm Horsfall protein binds to a single class of carbohydrate specific receptors on human neutrophils. *Kidney Int* 1993;44:423.

94. Thomas DBL, Davies M, Williams JD. Release of gelatinase and superoxide from human mononuclear phagocytes in response to particulate Tamm Horsfall protein. *Am J Pathol* 1993;142:249.

95. Pichette V, Quérin S, Desmeules M, et al. Renal function recovery in end-stage renal disease. Biochemical characterization. *Am J Kidney Dis* 1993;22:398.

96. MacLennan ICM, Cooper EH, Chapman CE, et al. Renal failure in myelomatosis. *Eur J Haematol* 1989;43[Suppl 51]:60.

97. Clark AD, Shetty A, Soutar, R. Renal failure and multiple myeloma: pathogenesis and treatment of renal failure and management of underlying myeloma. *Blood Rev* 1990;13:79.

98. Alexanian R, Dimopoulos M. The treatment of multiple myeloma. *N Engl J Med* 1994;330:484.

99. Osterborg A, Ehrsson H, Eksborg S, et al. Pharmacokinetics of oral melphalan in relation to renal function in multiple myeloma patients. *Eur J Cancer Clin Oncol* 1989;25:899.

100. Munshi NC, et al. Novel approaches in myeloma therapy. *Semin Oncol* 1999;26:28.

101. Attal M, et al. A prospective, randomised trial of autologous bone marrow transplantation and chemotherapy in multiple myeloma. *N Engl J Med* 1996;35:91.

102. Tricot G, et al. Safety of autotransplants with high dose melphalan in renal failure, a pharmacokinetic and toxicity study. *Clin Cancer Res* 1996;2:947.

103. Ballester AF, et al. High dose chemotherapy and autologous peripheral blood stem cell transplantation in patients with multiple myeloma and renal insufficiency. *Bone Marrow Transplant* 1997;20:653.

104. Parikh P, et al. Autografting in myeloma patients with renal impairment. *Ann Oncol* 1996;7[Suppl 5]:4100.

105. Misiani R, et al. Plasmapheresis in the treatment of acute renal failure in multiple myeloma. *Am J Med* 1979;66:684.

106. Pasquali S, Cagnoli L, Rovinetti C, et al. Plasma exchange therapy in rapidly progressive renal failure due to multiple myeloma. *Int J Artif Organs* 1984;8:27.

107. Misiani R, Tiraboschi G, Mingardi G, et al. Management of myeloma kidney: an anti-light-chain approach. *Am J Kidney Dis* 1987;10:28.

108. Wahlin A, Löfvenberg E, Holm J. Improved survival in multiple myeloma with renal failure. *Acta Med Scand* 1987;221:205.

109. Zucchelli P, Pasquali S, Cagnoli L, et al. Controlled plasma exchange trial in acute renal failure due to multiple myeloma. *Kidney Int* 1988;33:1175.

110. Kajtna-Koselj M, et al. Plasma exchange in myeloma renal failure. *Prog Clin Biol Res* 1990;337:271.

111. Johnson WJ, Kyle RA, Pineda AA, et al. Treatment of renal failure associated with multiple myeloma. *Arch Intern Med* 1990;150:863.

112. Berenson J, et al. Efficacy of pamidronate in reducing skeletal events in patients with advanced multiple myeloma. *N Engl J Med* 1996;334:488.

113. Berenson J, et al. Long-term pamidronate treatment of advanced multiple myeloma patients reduces skeletal events. *J Clin Oncol* 1998; 16:593.

114. Shipman CM, Rogers MJ, Apperley JF, et al. Biphosphonates induce apoptosis in human myeloma cell lines: a novel anti-tumour activity. *Br J Haematol* 1997;98:665.

115. Brown WW, et al. Reversal of chronic end-stage renal failure due to myeloma kidney. *Ann Intern Med* 1979;90:793.

116. Iggo N, et al. Chronic dialysis in patients with multiple myeloma and renal failure: a worthwhile treatment. *Q J Med* 1989;270:903.

117. Port FK, Nissenson AR. Outcome of end-stage renal disease in patients with rare causes of renal failure. II. Renal or systemic neoplasms. *Q J Med* 1989;272:1161.

118. Walker F, Bear RA. Renal transplantation in light-chain multiple myeloma. *Am J Nephrol* 1983;3:34.

119. Humphrey RL, Wright JR, Zachary JB, et al. Renal transplantation in multiple myeloma: a case report. *Ann Intern Med* 1975;83:651.

120. Sirota JH, Hamerman D. Renal function studies in an adult subject with the Fanconi syndrome. *Am J Med* 1954;16:138.

121. Engle RL, Wallis LA. Multiple myeloma and the adult Fanconi syndrome. *Am J Med* 1957;22:5.

122. Costanza DJ, Smoller M. Multiple myeloma with the Fanconi syndrome. Study of a case, with electron microscopy of the kidney. *Am J Med* 1963;34:125.

123. Lee DBN, Drinkard JP, Rosen VJ, et al. The adult Fanconi syndrome. Observations on etiology, morphology, renal function and mineral metabolism in three patients. *Medicine (Baltimore)* 1972;51:107.

124. Maldonado JE, et al. Fanconi syndrome in adults. A manifestation of a latent form of myeloma. *Am J Med* 1975;58:354.

125. Deleted in proofs.

126. Thorner PS, Bédard YC, Fernandes BJ. λ-Light chain nephropathy with Fanconi's syndrome. *Arch Pathol Lab Med* 1983;107:654.

127. Mullen B, Chalvardjian A. Crystalline tissue deposits in a case of multiple myeloma. *Arch Pathol Lab Med* 1981;105:94.

128. Chan KW, Ho FCS, Chan MK. Adult Fanconi syndrome in kappa light chain myeloma. *Arch Pathol Lab Med* 1987;111:139.

129. Orfila C, Lepert JC, Modesto A, et al. Fanconi's syndrome, kappa light-chain myeloma, non-amyloid fibrils and cytoplasmic crystals in renal tubular epithelium. *Am J Nephrol* 1991;11:345.

130. Finkel PN, Kronenberg K, Pesce AJ, et al. Adult Fanconi syndrome, amyloidosis and marked kappa light chain proteinuria. *Nephron* 1973;10:1.

131. Uchida S, et al. Adult Fanconi syndrome secondary to κ-light chain myeloma: improvement of tubular functions after treatment for myeloma. *Nephron* 1990;55:332.

132. Dedmon RE, West JH, Schwartz TB. The adult Fanconi syndrome: report of two cases, one with multiple myeloma. *Med Clin North Am* 1963;47:191.

133. Headley RN, King JS Jr, Cooper MR, et al. Multiple myeloma presenting as adult Fanconi syndrome. *Clin Chem* 1972;18:293.

134. Maldonado JE, Brown AL Jr, Bayrd ED, et al. Ultrastructure of the myeloma cell. *Cancer* 1966;19:1613.

135. Baumal R, Scharff MD. Immunoglobulin biosynthesis by the MOPC 173 mouse myeloma tumor and a variant spleen clone. *J Immunol* 1976;116:65.

136. Mosmann TR, Williamson AR. Structural mutations in a mouse immunoglobulin light chain resulting in failure to be secreted. *Cell* 1980;20:283.

137. Dul JL, Argon Y. A single amino acid substitution in the variable region of the light chain specifically blocks immunoglobulin secretion. *Proc Natl Acad Sci USA* 1990;87:8135.

138. Klausner RD, Sitia R. Protein degradation in the endoplasmic reticulum. *Cell* 1990;62:611.

139. Sanders PW, Herrera GA, Lott RL, et al. Morphologic alterations of the proximal tubules in light-chain related renal disease. *Kidney Int* 1988;33:881.

140. Pasquali S, et al. Renal histological lesions and clinical syndromes in multiple myeloma. *Clin Nephrol* 1987;27:222.

141. Clyne DH, et al. Renal effects of intraperitoneal kappa chain injection. Induction of crystals in renal tubular cells. *Lab Invest* 1974;31: 131.

142. Deret S, et al. Kappa light chain-associated Fanconi's syndrome: molecular analysis of monoclonal immunoglobulin light chains from patients with and without intracellular crystals. *Protein Eng* 1999;12:363.

143. Stevens FJ, et al. A molecular model for self-assembly of amyloid fibrils: immunoglobulin light chains. *Biochemistry* 1995;34:10697.

144. Jarrett JT, Lansbury PT Jr. Seeding "one-dimensional crystallization" of amyloid: a pathogenic mechanism in Alzheimer's disease and scrapie? *Cell* 1993;73:1055.

145. Gailani S, Seon BK, Henderson ES. κ-Light chain myeloma associated with adult Fanconi syndrome: response of the nephropathy to treatment of myeloma. *Med Pediatr Oncol* 1987;4:141.

146. Levine SB, Bernstein LD. Crystalline inclusions in multiple myeloma. *JAMA* 1985;254:1985.

147. Kyle RA, Greipp PR. Smoldering multiple myeloma. *N Engl J Med* 1980;302:1347.

148. Rokitansky KF. *Handbuch der pathologischen anatomie*. Berlin: Baumüller and Seidel, 1842.

149. Virchow R. Über eine im Gehirn und Rünckenmark des Menschen aufgefundene Substanz mit der Chemischen Reaction der Cellulose. *Virch Arch Path Anat* 1854;6:135.

150. Pras M, Schubert M, Zucker-Franklin D, et al. The characterization of soluble amyloid prepared in water. *J Clin Invest* 1968;47:924.

151. Glenner GG, et al. Creation of "amyloid" fibrils from Bence Jones proteins in vitro. *Science* 1971;174:712.

152. Come JH, Fraser PE, Lansbury PT Jr. A kinetic model for amyloid formation in the prion diseases: importance of seeding. *Proc Natl Acad Sci USA* 1993;90:5959.

153. Jarrett JT, Berger EP, Lansbury PT Jr. The carboxyterminus of the β amyloid protein is critical for the seeding of amyloid formation: implications for the pathogenesis of Alzheimer's disease. *Biochem* 1993;32:4693.

154. Glenner GG. Amyloid deposits and amyloidosis: the β-fibrilloses (first of two parts). *N Engl J Med* 1980;302:1283.

155. Husby G, et al. The 1990 guidelines for nomenclature and classification of amyloid and amyloidosis. In: Natvig JB, et al, eds. *Amyloid and amyloidosis*. Dordrecht: Kluwer Academic Publishers, 1991:7.

156. Snow AD, Willmer J, Kisilevsky R. Sulfated glycosaminoglycans: a common constituent of all amyloids? *Lab Invest* 1987;56:120.

157. Nelson SR, Lyon M, Gallagher JT, et al. Isolation and characterization of the integral glycosaminoglycan constituents of human amyloid A and monoclonal light-chain amyloid fibrils. *Biochem J* 1991;275:67.

158. Norling B, Westermark GT, Westermark P. Immunohistochemical identification of heparan sulphate proteoglycan in secondary systemic amyloidosis. *Clin Exp Immunol* 1988;73:333.

159. Magnus JH, Stenstad T, Husby G, et al. Isolation and partial characterization of heparan sulphate proteoglycans from human hepatic amyloid. *Biochem J* 1992;288:225.

160. Kisilevsky R. Proteoglycans, glycosaminoglycans, amyloid-enhancing factor, and amyloid deposition. *J Intern Med* 1992;232:515.

161. Emsley J, et al. Structure of pentameric human serum amyloid P component. *Nature* 1994;367:338.

162. Butler PJG, Tennent GA, Pepys MB. Pentraxin–chromatin interactions: serum amyloid P component specifically displaces H1-type histones and solubilizes native long chromatin. *J Exp Med* 1990;172:13.

163. Ying SC, Gewurz AT, Jiang H, et al. Human serum amyloid P component oligomers bind and activate the classical complement pathway via residues 14-26 and 76-92 of the A chain collagen-like region of C1q. *J Immunol* 1993;150:169.

164. Bickerstaff MCM, et al. Serum amyloid P component controls chromatin degradation and prevents antinuclear autoimmunity. *Nature Med* 1999;5:694.

165. Loveless RW, Floyd-O'Sullivan G, Raynes JG, et al. Human serum amyloid P is a multispecific adhesive protein whose ligands include 6-phosphorylated mannose and the 3-sulphated saccharides: galactose, N-acetylgalactosamine and glucuronic acid. *EMBO J* 1992;11:813.

166. Hawkins PN, Lavender JP, Pepys MB. Evaluation of systemic amyloidosis by scintigraphy with ^{123}I-labeled serum amyloid P component. *N Engl J Med* 1990;323:508.

167. Hawkins PN, Myers MJ, Lavender JP, et al. Diagnostic radionuclide imaging of amyloid: biological targeting by circulating human serum amyloid P component. *Lancet* 1988;1:1413.

168. Sipe JD. Amyloidosis. *Annu Rev Biochem* 1992;61:947.

169. Haass C, Selkoe DJ. Cellular processing of β-amyloid precursor protein and the genesis of amyloid β-peptide. *Cell* 1993;75:1039.

170. Kisilevsky R, Narindrasorasak S, Tape C, et al. During AA amyloidogenesis is proteolytic attack on serum amyloid A a pre- or postfibrillogenic event? *Int J Exp Invest* 1994;1:174.

171. Olsen KE, Sletten K, Westermark P. Fragments of the constant region of immunoglobulin light chains are constituents of AL-amyloid proteins. *Biochem Biophys Res Com* 1998;251:642.

172. Shirahama T, et al. Amyloid enhancing factor-loaded macrophages in amyloid fibril formation. *Lab Invest* 1990;62:61.

173. Ganowiak K, Hultman P, Engström U, et al. Fibrils from synthetic amyloid-related peptides enhance development of experimental AA-amyloidosis in mice. *Biochem Biophys Res Comm* 1994;199:306.

174. Johnson KH, O'Brien TD, Betsholtz C, et al. Islet amyloid, islet-amyloid polypeptide, and diabetes mellitus. *N Engl J Med* 1989;321:513.

175. Skinner M. Localized genitourinary amyloidosis: a new form of light chain disease. *Amyloid: Int J Exp Clin Invest* 1998;5:71.

176. Asl KH, Liepnieks JJ, Nakamura M, et al. Organ-specific (localized) synthesis of Ig light chain amyloid. *J Immunol* 1999;162:5556.

177. Eanes ED, Glenner GG. X-ray diffraction studies of amyloid filaments. *J Histochem Cytochem* 1968;16:673.

178. Wright JR, Calkins E, Humphrey RL. Potassium permanganate reaction in amyloidosis. A histologic method to assist in differentiating forms of this disease. *Lab Invest* 1977;36:274.

179. Noel LH, Droz D, Ganeval D. Immunohistochemical characterization of renal amyloidosis. *Am J Clin Pathol* 1987;87:756.

180. Suzuki Y, Churg J, Grishman E, et al. The mesangium of the renal glomerulus: electron microscopic studies of pathologic alterations. *Am J Pathol* 1963;43:555.

181. Dikman SH, Churg J, Kahn T. Morphologic and clinical correlates in renal amyloidosis. *Human Pathol* 1981;12:160.

182. Sanders PW, Herrera GA, Kirk KA, et al. Spectrum of glomerular and tubulointerstitial renal lesions associated with monotypical immunoglobulin light chain deposition. *Lab Invest* 1991;64:527.

183. Sanders PW, Herrera GA. Monoclonal immunoglobulin light chain related renal diseases. *Semin Nephrol* 1993;13:324.

184. Gallo GR, et al. Characterization of tissue amyloid by immunofluorescence microscopy. *Clin Immunol Immunopathol* 1986;39:479.

185. Shirahama T, et al. Histochemical and immunohistochemical characterization of amyloid associated with chronic hemodialysis as β2-microglobulin. *Lab Invest* 1985;53:705.

186. Shirahama T, Cohen AS. Fine structure of the glomerulus in human and experimental renal amyloidosis. *Am J Pathol* 1967;51:869.

187. Gise HV, Christ H, Bohle A. Early glomerular lesions in amyloidosis: electron microscopic findings. *Virchows Arch* 1981;390:259.

188. Yang GCH, Gallo GR. Protein A-gold immunoelectron microscopic study of amyloid fibrils, granular deposits, and fibrillar luminal aggregates in renal amyloidosis. *Am J Pathol* 1990;137:1223.

189. Duston MA, Skinner M, Shirahama T, et al. Diagnosis of amyloidosis by abdominal fat aspiration: analysis of four years' experience. *Am J Med* 1987;82:412.

190. Gertz MA, Li CY, Shirahama T, et al. Utility of subcutaneous fat aspiration for the diagnosis of systemic amyloidosis (immunoglobulin light chain). *Arch Intern Med* 1988;148:929.

191. Glenner GG, Harbaugh J, Ohms JI, et al. An amyloid protein: the amino-terminal variable fragment of an immunoglobulin light chain. *Biochem Biophys Res Comm* 1970;41:1287.

192. Kyle RA, Greipp PR. Amyloidosis (AL): clinical and laboratory features in 229 cases. *Mayo Clin Proc* 1983;58:665.

193. Kyle RA. Primary systemic amyloidosis. *J Intern Med* 1992;232:523.

194. Stone MJ, Frenkel EP. The clinical spectrum of light chain myeloma: a study of 35 patients with special reference to the occurrence of amyloidosis. *Am J Med* 1975;58:601.

195. Alexanian R, Fraschini G, Smith L. Amyloidosis in multiple myeloma or without apparent cause. *Arch Intern Med* 1984;144:2158.

196. Gertz MA, Kyle RA, Noel P. Primary systemic amyloidosis: a rare complication of immunoglobulin M monoclonal gammopathies and Waldenström's macroglobulinemia. *J Clin Oncol* 1993;11:914.

197. Kyle RA, Gertz MA. Primary systemic amyloidosis: clinical and laboratory features in 474 cases. *Semin Hematol* 1995;32:45.

198. Osserman EF, Takatsuki K, Talal N. Multiple myeloma. I. The pathogenesis of "amyloidosis." *Semin Hematol* 1964;1:3.

199. Preud'homme JL, Ganeval D, Grünfeld JP, et al. Immunoglobulin synthesis in primary and myeloma amyloidosis. *Clin Exp Immunol* 1988;73:389.

200. Isobe T, Osserman EF. Patterns of amyloidosis and their association with plasma-cell dyscrasia, monoclonal immunoglobulins and Bence Jones proteins. *N Engl J Med* 1974;290:473.

201. Buxbaum J. Aberrant immunoglobulin synthesis in light chain amyloidosis: free light chain and light chain fragment production by human bone marrow cells in short-term tissue culture. *J Clin Invest* 1986;78:798.

202. Pascali E. Bence Jones protein in primary systemic amyloidosis. *Blood* 1993;81:564.

203. Gertz MA, Kyle RA. Prognostic value of urinary protein in primary systemic amyloidosis (AL). *Am J Clin Pathol* 1990;94:313.

204. Kyle RA, et al. A trial of three regimens for primary amyloidosis: colchicine alone, melphalan and prednisone, and melphalan, prednisone, and colchicine. *N Engl J Med* 1997;336:1202.

205. Kyle RA, et al. Long-term survival (10 years or more) in 30 patients with primary amyloidosis. *Blood* 1999;93:1062.

206. Gertz MA, Kyle RA, Greipp PR. Response rates and survival in primary systemic amyloidosis. *Blood* 1991;77:257.

207. Skinner M, et al. Treatment of 100 patients with primary amyloidosis: a randomized trial of melphalan, prednisone, and colchicine versus colchicine only. *Am J Med* 1996;100:290.

208. Gertz MA, et al. Prospective randomized trial of melphalan and prednisone versus vincristine, carmustine, melphalan, cyclophosphamide, and prednisone in the treatment of primary systemic amyloidosis. *J Clin Oncol* 1999;17:262.

209. Gertz MA, et al. Phase II trial of high-dose dexamethasone for untreated patients with primary systemic amyloidosis. *Med Oncol* 1999;16:104.

210. Gertz MA, et al. Phase II trial of high-dose dexamethasone for previously treated immunoglobulin light-chain amyloidosis. *Am J Hematol* 1999;61:115.

211. Gertz MA, Kyle RA. Acute leukemia and cytogenetic abnormalities complicating melphalan treatment of primary systemic amyloidosis. *Arch Intern Med* 1990;150:629.

212. Comenzo RL, et al. Dose-intensive melphalan with blood stem-cell support for the treatment of AL (amyloid light-chain) amyloidosis: survival and responses in 25 patients. *Blood* 1998;91:3662.

213. Comenzo RL, et al. Treating AL amyloidosis with dose-intensive melphalan: outcome in 102 patients. *Blood* 1998;10 [Suppl 1]:324a.

214. Moreau P. Autologous stem cell transplantation for AL amyloidosis: a standard therapy? *Leukemia* 1999;13:1929.

215. Moreau P, et al. Prognostic factors for survival and response after high-dose therapy and autologous stem cell transplantation in systemic AL amyloidosis: a report on 21 patients. *Br J Haematol* 1998;101:766.

216. Dispenzieri A, et al. Eligibility for PBSCT for AL amyloidosis is a favorable independent prognostic factor for survival: survival of 234 patients with primary systemic amyloidosis (AL) functionally eligible for peripheral blood stem cell transplantation. *Proc Am Soc Clin Oncol* 1999;18:20a.

217. Merlini G, et al. Interaction of the anthracycline 4′-iodo-4′-deoxydoxorubicin with amyloid fibrils: inhibition of amyloidogenesis. *Proc Natl Acad Sci USA* 1995;92:2959.

218. Gianni L, Bellotti V, Gianni AM, et al. New drug therapy of amyloidoses: resorption of AL-type deposits with 4′-iodo-4′-deoxydoxorubicin. *Blood* 1995;86:855.

219. Merlini G, et al. Treatment of AL amyloidosis with 4′-iodo-4′-deoxydoxorubicin: an update. *Blood* 1999;93:1112.

220. Jones NF. Renal amyloidosis: pathogenesis and therapy. *Clin Nephrol* 1976;6:459.

221. Martinez-Vea A, Garcia C, Carreras M, et al. End-stage renal disease in systemic amyloidosis: clinical course and outcome on dialysis. *Am J Nephrol* 1990;10:283.

222. Moroni G, et al. Chronic dialysis in patients with systemic amyloidosis: the experience in Northern Italy. *Clin Nephrol* 1992;38:81.

223. Gertz MA, Kyle RA, O'Fallon WM. Dialysis support of patients with primary systemic amyloidosis. A study of 211 patients. *Arch Intern Med* 1992;152:2245.

224. Browning MJ, et al. Continuous ambulatory peritoneal dialysis in systemic amyloidosis and end-stage renal disease. *J Royal Soc Med* 1984;77:189.

225. Cantaluppi A. C.A.P.D. and systemic diseases. *Clin Nephrol* 1988; 30[Suppl 1]:S8.

226. Browning MJ, et al. Ten years' experience of an amyloid clinic—a clinicopathological survey. *Q J Med* 1985;215:213.

227. Gertz MA, Kyle RA. Secondary systemic amyloidosis: response and survival in 64 patients. *Medicine (Baltimore)* 1991;70:246.

228. Pasternack A, Ahonen J, Kuhlbäck B. Renal transplantation in 45 patients with amyloidosis. *Transplantation* 1986;42:598.

229. Isoniemi H, Eklund B, Höckerstedt K, et al. Renal transplantation in amyloidosis. *Transplant Proc* 1989;21:2039.

230. Hartmann A, et al. Fifteen years' experience with renal transplantation in systemic amyloidosis. *Transplant Int* 1992;5:15.

231. Goldfinger SE. Colchicine for familial Mediterranean fever. *N Engl J Med* 1972;287:1302.

232. Zemer D, et al. Colchicine in the prevention and treatment of the amyloidosis of familial Mediterranean fever. *N Engl J Med* 1986;314: 1001.

233. Sohar E, Gafni J, Pras M, et al. Familial Mediterranean fever: a survey of 470 cases and review of the literature. *Am J Med* 1967;43:227.

234. Schwabe AD, Peters RS. Familial Mediterranean fever in Armenians: analysis of 100 cases. *Medicine (Baltimore)* 1974;53:453.

235. The International FMF Consortium. Ancient missense mutations in a new member of the *Roret* gene family are likely to cause familial Mediterranean fever. *Cell* 1997;90:797.

236. The French FMF Consortium. A candidate gene for familial Mediterranean fever. *Nat Genet* 1997;17:25.

237. Zemer D, et al. A controlled trial of colchicine in preventing attacks of familial Mediterranean fever. *N Engl J Med* 1974;291:932.

238. Zemer D, Livneh A, Langevitz P. Reversal of the nephrotic syndrome by colchicine in amyloidosis of familial Mediterranean fever. *Ann Intern Med* 1992;116:426.

239. Knecht A, de Beer FC, Pras M. Serum amyloid A protein in familial Mediterranean fever. *Ann Intern Med* 1985;102:71.

240. Ahlmen M, Ahlmen J, Svalander C, et al. Cytotoxic drug treatment of reactive amyloidosis in rheumatoid arthritis with special reference to renal insufficiency. *Clin Rheumatol* 1987;6:27.

241. Berglund K, Keller C, Thyssel H. Alkylating cytostatic treatment in renal amyloidosis secondary to rheumatic disease. *Ann Rheum Dis* 1987;46:757.

242. Solomon A, Weiss DT. A perspective of plasma cell dyscrasias: clinical implications of monoclonal light chains in renal disease. In: Minetti L, D'Amico G, Ponticelli C, eds. *The kidney in plasma cell dyscrasias.* Dordrecht: Kluwer Academic Publishers, 1988:3.

243. Bellotti V, et al. Relevance of class, molecular weight and isoelectric point in predicting human light chain amyloidogenicity. *Br J Haematol* 1990;74:65.

244. Solomon A, Weiss DT, Pepys MB. Induction in mice of human light-chain-associated amyloidosis. *Am J Pathol* 1992;140:629.

245. Terry WD, et al. Structural identity of Bence Jones and amyloid fibril proteins in a patient with plasma cell dyscrasia and amyloidosis. *J Clin Invest* 1973;52:1276.

246. Klafki HW, et al. Complete amino acid sequence determinations demonstrate identity of the urinary Bence Jones protein (BJP-DIA) and the amyloid fibril protein (AL-DIA) in a case of AL-amyloidosis. *Biochemistry* 1992;31:3265.

247. Jacquot C, et al. Association of systemic light-chain deposition disease and amyloidosis: a report of three patients with renal involvement. *Clin Nephrol* 1985;24:93.

248. Dwulet FE, O'Connor TP, Benson MD. Polymorphism in a kappa I primary (AL) amyloid protein (BAN). *Mol Immunol* 1986;23:73.

249. Tonoike H, Kametani F, Hoshi A, et al. Amino acid sequence of an amyloidogenic Bence Jones protein in myeloma-associated systemic amyloidosis. *FEBS Lett* 1985;185:139.

250. Tonoike H, Kametani F, Hoshi A, et al. Primary structure of the variable region of an amyloidogenic Bence Jones protein NIG-77. *Biochem Biophys Res Comm* 1985;126:1228.

251. Eulitz M, Breuer M, Linke RP. Is the formation of AL-type amyloid promoted by structural peculiarities of immunoglobulin L-chains?

252. Ferri G, Stoppini M, Iadarola P, et al. Structural characterization of κ II Inc, a new amyloid immunoglobulin. *Biochim Biophys Acta* 1989;995:103.

253. Aucouturier P, et al. Complementary DNA sequence of human amyloidogenic immunoglobulin light-chain precursors. *Biochem J* 1992; 285:149.

254. Natvig JB, Westermark P, Sletten K, et al. Further structural and antigenic studies of light-chain amyloid proteins. *Scand J. Immunol* 1981;14:89.

255. Husby G, Sletten K, Blumenkrantz N, et al. Characterization of an amyloid fibril protein from localized amyloidosis of the skin as λ immunoglobulin light chains of variable subgroup I (AλI). *Clin Exp Immunol* 1981;45:90.

256. Sletten K, Natvig JB, Husby G, et al. The complete amino acid sequence of a prototype immunoglobulin-λ light-chain-type amyloid-fibril protein AR. *Biochem J* 1981;195:561.

257. Sletten K, Westermark P, Pitkänen P, et al. Amino acid sequences in amyloid proteins of κIII immunoglobulin light-chain origin. *Scand J Immunol* 1983;18:557.

258. Dwulet FE, Strako K, Benson MD. Amino acid sequence of a λ VI primary (AL) amyloid protein (WLT). *Scand J Immunol* 1985;22: 653.

259. Eulitz M, Linke R. Amyloid fibrils derived from V-region together with C-region fragments from a λII-immunoglobulin light chain (HAR). *Biol Chem Hoppe-Seyler* 1985;366:907.

260. Tveteraas T, Sletten K, Westermark P. The amino acid sequence of a carbohydrate-containing immunoglobulin-light-chain-type amyloid-fibril protein. *Biochem J* 1985;232:183.

261. Toft KG, Sletten K, Husby G. The amino-acid sequence of the variable region of a carbohydrate-containing amyloid fibril protein EPS (immunoglobulin light chain, type λ). *Biol Chem Hoppe-Seyler* 1985;366:617.

262. Holm E, Sletten K, Husby G. Structural studies of a carbohydrate-containing immunoglobulin-λ-light-chain amyloid-fibril protein (AL) of variable subgroup III. *Biochem J* 1986;239:545.

263. Fykse EM, Sletten K, Husby G, et al. The primary structure of the variable region of an immunoglobulin IV light-chain amyloid-fibril protein (AL GIL). *Biochem J* 1988;256:973.

264. Benson MD, Dwulet FE, Madura D, et al. Amyloidosis related to a λ IV immunoglobulin light chain protein. *Scand J Immunol* 1989;29:175.

265. Westermark P, Benson L, Juul J, et al. Use of subcutaneous abdominal fat biopsy specimen for detailed typing of amyloid fibril protein-AL by amino acid sequence analysis. *J Clin Pathol* 1989;42:817.

266. Kitajima Y, Hirata H, Kagawa Y, et al. Partial amino acid sequence of an amyloid fibril protein from nodular primary cutaneous amyloidosis showing homology to λ immunoglobulin light chain of variable subgroup III (A λ III). *J Invest Dermatol* 1990;95:301.

267. Liepnieks JJ, Dwulet FE, Benson MD. Amino acid sequence of a kappa I primary (AL) amyloid protein (AND). *Mol Immunol* 1990;27: 481.

268. Picken MM, Gallo GR, Pruzanski W, et al. Biochemical characterization of amyloid derived from the variable region of the κ light chain subgroup III. *Arthritis Rheum* 1990;33:880.

269. Bellotti V, et al. Use of an anti-idiotypic monoclonal antibody in studying amyloidogenic light chains in cells, urine and fibrils: pathophysiology and clinical implications. *Scand J Immunol* 1992;36:607.

270. Linke RP, Tischendorf RW, Zucker-Franklin D, et al. The formation of amyloid-like fibrils in vitro from Bence Jones proteins of the VλI subclass. *J Immunol* 1973;111:24.

271. Linke RP, Zucker-Franklin D, Franklin EC. Morphologic, chemical, and immunologic studies of amyloid-like fibrils formed from Bence Jones proteins by proteolysis. *J Immunol* 1973;111:10.

272. Epstein WV, Tan M, Wood IS. Formation of "amyloid" fibrils in vitro by action of human kidney lysosomal enzymes on Bence Jones proteins. *J Lab Clin Med* 1974;84:107.

273. Durie BGM, Persky B, Soehnlen BJ, et al. Amyloid production in human myeloma stem-cell culture, with morphologic evidence of amyloid secretion by associated macrophages. *N Engl J Med* 1982;307: 1689.

274. Klafki HW, et al. Reduction of disulfide bonds in an amyloidogenic Bence Jones protein leads to formation of "amyloid-like" fibrils in vitro. *Biol Chem Hoppe-Seyler* 1993;347:1117.

Primary structure of an amyloidogenic λ-L-chain (BJP-ZIM) *Biol Chem Hoppe-Seyler* 1987;368:863.

275. Solomon A, McLaughlin CL. Bence-Jones proteins and light chains of immunoglobulins. I. Formation and characterization of amino-terminal (variant) and carboxyl-terminal (constant) halves. *J Biol Chem* 1969;244:3393.

276. Deleted in proofs.

277. Stevens FJ. Four structural risk factors identify most fibril-forming kappa light chains. *Amyloid: Int J Exp Clin Invest* 2000.

278. Hurle MR, Helms LR, Li L, et al. A role for destabilizing amino acid replacements in light-chain amyloidosis. *Proc Natl Acad Sci USA* 1994;91:5446.

279. Schiffer M, Girling RL, Ely KR, et al. Structure of a λ-type Bence-Jones protein at 3.5-Å resolution. *Biochemistry* 1973;12:4620.

280. Edmundson AB, et al. Binding of 2,4-dinitrophenyl compounds and other small molecules to a crystalline λ-type Bence-Jones dimer. *Biochemistry* 1974;13:3816.

281. Edmundson AB, Ely KR, Herron JN, et al. The binding of opioid peptides to the Mcg light chain dimer: flexible keys and adjustable locks. *Mol Immunol* 1987;24:915.

282. Edmundson AB, Ely KR, He XM, et al. Cocrystallization of an immunoglobulin light chain dimer with bis(dinitrophenyl) lysine: tandem binding of two ligands, one with and one without accompanying conformational changes in the protein. *Mol Immunol* 1989;26:207.

283. Bertram J, Gualtieri RJ, Osserman EF. Amyloid-related Bence Jones proteins bind dinitrophenyl L-lysine (DNP). In: Glenner G, Costal P, Freitas F, eds. *Amyloid and amyloidosis*. Amsterdam: Excerpta Medica, 1980:351.

284. Masat L, Wabl M, Johnson JP. A simpler sort of antibody. *Proc Natl Acad Sci USA* 1994;91:893.

285. Sun M, Li L, Gao QS, et al. Antigen recognition by an antibody light chain. *J Biol Chem* 1994;269:734.

286. Wilkins-Stevens P, et al. Recombinant immunoglobulin variable domains generated from synthetic genes provide a system for in vitro characterization of light-chain amyloid proteins. *Protein Science* 1995;4:421.

287. Perfetti V, et al. Evidence that amyloidogenic light chains undergo antigen-driven selection. *Blood* 1998;91:2948.

288. Jiang X, Myatt E, Lykos P, et al. Interaction between glycosaminoglycans and immunoglobulin light chains. *Biochemistry* 1997;36:13187.

289. Lowenstein J, Gallo G. Remission of the nephrotic syndrome in renal amyloidosis. *N Engl J Med* 1970;282:128.

290. Dikman SH, Kahn T, Gribetz D, et al. Resolution of renal amyloidosis. *Am J Med* 1977;63:430.

291. Van Buren M, Hene RJ, Verdonck LF, et al. Clinical remission after syngeneic bone marrow transplantation in a patient with AL amyloidosis. *Ann Intern Med* 1995;122:508.

292. Lavie G, Zucker-Franklin D, Franklin EC. Degradation of serum amyloid A protein by surface-associated enzymes of human blood monocytes. *J Exp Med* 1978;148:1020.

293. Natvig JB, Skogen B, Amundsen E. Therapeutic prospects in amyloidosis. In: Minetti L, D'Amico G, Ponticelli C, eds. *The kidney in plasma cell dyscrasia*. Dordrecht: Kluwer Academic Publishers, 1988:271.

294. Yan SD, et al. Receptor-dependent cell stress and amyloid accumulation in systemic amyloidosis. *Nature Med* 2000;6:643.

295. Kisilevsky R, et al. Arresting amyloidosis in vivo using small-molecule anionic sulphonates or sulphates: implications for Alzheimer's disease. *Nature Med* 1995;1:143.

296. Shirahama T, Cohen AS. Redistribution of amyloid deposits. *Am J Pathol* 1980;99:539.

297. Abraham OR, Selkoe DJ, Potter H. Immunochemical identification of the serine protease inhibitor α_1-antichymotrypsin in the brain amyloid deposits of Alzheimer's disease. *Cell* 1988;52:487.

298. Campistol JM, et al. Demonstration of plasma proteinase inhibitors in β_2-microglobulin amyloid deposits. *Kidney Int* 1992;42:915.

299. Kobernick SD, Whiteside JH. Renal glomeruli in multiple myeloma. *Lab Invest* 1957;6:478.

300. Sanchez LM, Domz CA. Renal patterns in myeloma. *Ann Intern Med* 1960;52:44.

301. Preud'homme JL, et al. Synthesis of abnormal heavy and light chains in multiple myeloma with visceral deposition of monoclonal immunoglobulin. *Clin Exp Immunol* 1980;42:545.

302. Ganeval D, Noël LH, Preud'homme JL, et al. Light-chain deposition disease: its relation with AL-type amyloidosis. *Kidney Int* 1984;26:1.

303. Gallo G, Picken M, Buxbaum J, et al. The spectrum of monoclonal immunoglobulin deposition disease associated with immunocytic dyscrasias. *Semin Hematol* 1989;26:234.

304. Buxbaum JN, Chuba JV, Hellman GC, et al. Monoclonal immunoglobulin deposition disease: light chain and light and heavy chain deposition diseases and their relation to light chain amyloidosis. Clinical features, immunopathology, and molecular analysis. *Ann Intern Med* 1990;112:455.

305. Ganeval D, et al. Visceral deposition of monoclonal light chains and immunoglobulins: a study of renal and immunopathologic abnormalities. *Adv Nephrol Necker Hosp* 1982;11:25.

306. Noel LH, Droz D, Ganeval D, et al. Renal granular monoclonal light chain deposits: morphological aspects in 11 cases. *Clin Nephrol* 1984;21:263.

307. Gallo GR, et al. Nodular glomerulopathy associated with nonamyloidotic kappa light chain deposits and excess immunoglobulin light chain synthesis. *Am J Pathol* 1980;99:621.

308. Yasuda T, Fujita K, Imai H, et al. Gamma-heavy chain deposition disease showing nodular glomerulosclerosis. *Clin Nephrol* 1995;44:394.

309. Herzenberg AM, Kiaii M, Magil AB. Heavy chain deposition disease: recurrence in renal transplantation and report of IgG2 subtype. *Am J Kidney Dis* 2000;35:pE25.

310. Herzenberg AM, Lien J, Magil AB. Monoclonal heavy chain (immunoglobulin G3) deposition disease: report of a case. *Am J Kidney Dis* 1996;28:128.

311. Kambham N, Markowitz GS, Appel GB, et al. Heavy chain deposition disease: the disease spectrum. *Am J Kidney Dis* 1999;33:954.

312. Husby G, et al. Chronic arthritis and γ heavy chain disease: coincidence or pathogenic link? *Scand J Rheumatol* 1998;27:257.

313. Rott T, Vizjak A, Lindic J, et al. IgG heavy-chain deposition disease affecting kidney, skin, and skeletal muscle. *Nephrol Dial Transplant* 1998;13:1825.

314. Katz A, Zent R, Bargman JM. IgG heavy-chain deposition disease. *Mod Pathol* 1994;7:874.

315. Strom EH, Fogazzi GB, Banfi G, et al. Light chain deposition disease of the kidney: morphological aspects in 24 patients. *Virchows Arch* 1994;425:271.

316. Polski JM, Galvin N, Salinas-Madrigal L. Non-amyloid fibrils in heavy chain deposition disease. *Kidney Int* 1999;56:1601.

317. Cheng IK, Ho SK, Chan DT, et al. Crescentic nodular glomerulosclerosis secondary to truncated immunoglobulin alpha heavy chain deposition. *Am J Kidney Dis* 1996;28:283.

318. Liapis H, Papadakis I, Nakopoulou L. Nodular glomerulosclerosis secondary to μ heavy chain deposits. *Hum Pathol* 2000;31:122.

319. Schubert GE, Adam A. Glomerular nodules and long-spacing collagen in kidneys of patients with multiple myeloma. *J Clin Pathol* 1974;27:800.

320. Bruneval P, Foidart JM, Nochy D, et al. Glomerular matrix proteins in nodular glomerulosclerosis in association with light chain deposition disease and diabetes mellitus. *Hum Pathol* 1985;16:477.

321. Herrera GA, Shultz JJ, Soong SJ, et al. Growth factors in monoclonal light-chain-related renal diseases. *Hum Pathol* 1994;25:883.

322. Bedossa P, Fabre M, Paraf F, et al. Light chain deposition disease with liver dysfunction. *Hum Pathol* 1988;19:1008.

323. Confalonieri R, et al. Light chain nephropathy: histological and clinical aspects in 15 cases. *Nephrol Dial Transplant* 1988;2:150.

324. Heilman RL, Velosa JA, Holley KE, et al. Long-term follow-up and response to chemotherapy in patients with light-chain deposition disease. *Am J Kidney Dis* 1992;20:34.

325. Tubbs RR, et al. Light chain nephropathy. *Am J Med* 1981;71:263.

326. Droz D, et al. Liver involvement in nonamyloid light chain deposits disease. *Lab Invest* 1984;50:683.

327. Preud'homme JL, Buxbaum J, Scharff MD. Mutagenesis of mouse myeloma cells with melphalan. *Nature* 1973;245:320.

328. Cogné M, Guglielmi P. Exon skipping without splice site mutation accounting for abnormal immunoglobulin chains in nonsecretory human myeloma. *Eur J Immunol* 1993;23:1289.

329. Gallo G, Buxbaum J. Monoclonal immunoglobulin deposition disease: immunopathologic aspects of renal involvement. In: Minetti L, D'Amico G, Ponticelli C, eds. *The kidney in plasma cell dyscrasias*. Dordrecht: Kluwer Academic Publishers, 1988:171.

330. Khamlichi AA, et al. Primary structure of a monoclonal κ chain in myeloma with light chain deposition disease. *Clin Exp Immunol* 1992;87:122.

331. Rocca A, et al. Primary structure of a variable region of the $V_{\kappa}1$ subgroup (ISE) in light chain deposition disease. *Clin Exp Immunol* 1993;91:506.

332. Bellotti V, et al. Amino acid sequence of *k* Sci, the Bence Jones protein isolated from a patient with light chain deposition disease. *Biochim Biophys Acta* 1991;1097:177.

333. Deret S, et al. Molecular modeling of immunoglobulin light chains implicates hydrophobic residues in non-amyloid light chain deposition disease. *Protein Eng* 1997;10:1191.

334. Khamlichi AA, Aucouturier P, Preud'homme JL, et al. Structure of abnormal heavy chains in human heavy chain deposition disease. *Eur J Biochem* 1995;229:54.

335. Prelli F, Frangione B. Franklin's disease: Igγ 2H chain mutant BUR. *J Immunol* 1992;148:949.

336. Tubbs RR, et al. Pseudo-γ heavy chain (IgG$_4\lambda$) deposition disease. *Mod Pathol* 1992;5:185.

337. Picken MM, Frangione B, Barlogie B, et al. Light chain deposition disease derived from the κ_1 light chain subgroup. Biochemical characterization. *Am J Pathol* 1989;134:749.

338. Stokes MB, et al. Expression of decorin, biglycan, and collagen type I in human renal fibrosing disease. *Kidney Int* 2000;57:487.

339. Zhu L, et al. Pathogenesis of glomerulosclerosis in light chain deposition disease: role of transforming growth factor-β. *Am J Pathol* 1995;147:375.

340. Herrera GA, et al. Glomerulopathic light chain–mesangial cell interactions modulate in vitro extracellular matrix remodeling and reproduce mesangiopathic findings documented in vivo. *Ultrastruct Pathol* 1999;23:107.

341. Khamlichi AA, et al. Role of light chain variable region in myeloma with light chain deposition disease: evidence from an experimental model. *Blood* 1995;86:3655.

342. Ganeval D. Kidney involvement in light chain deposition disease. In: Minetti, D'Amico G, Ponticelli C, eds. *The kidney in plasma cell dyscrasias*. Dordrecht: Kluwer Academic Publishers, 1988:221.

343. Barjon P, et al. Traitement de la maladie par dépôts de chaînes légères par greffe de moelle. *Néphrologie* 1992;13:24.

344. Mariette X, Clauvel JP, Brouet JC. Intensive therapy in AL amyloidosis and light-chain deposition disease. *Ann Intern Med* 1995;123:553.

345. Komatsuda A, et al. Disappearance of nodular mesangial lesions in a patient with light chain nephropathy after long-term chemotherapy. *Am J Kidney Dis* 2000;35:E9.

346. Spence RK, et al. Renal transplantation for end-stage myeloma kidney. Report of a patient with long-term survival. *Arch Surg* 1979;114:950.

347. Briefel GR, et al. Renal transplantation in a patient with multiple myeloma and light chain nephropathy. *Surgery* 1983;93:579.

348. Short IA, Smith JP. Myelomatosis associated with glycosuria and aminoaciduria. *Scot Med J* 1959;4:89.

349. Gallo G, Picken M, Frangione B, et al. Nonamyloidotic monoclonal immunoglobulin deposits lack amyloid P component. *Mod Pathol* 1988;1:453.

350. Lam KY, Chan KW. Unusual findings in a myeloma kidney: a light- and electron-microscopic study. *Nephron* 1993;65:133.

351. Morel-Maroger L, Basch A, Danon F, et al. Pathology of the kidney in Waldenström's macroglobulinemia. Study of sixteen cases. *N Engl J Med* 1970;283:123.

352. Argani I, Kipkie GF. Macroglobulinemic nephropathy. Acute renal failure in macroglobulinemia of Waldenström. *Am J Med* 1964;36:151.

353. Alpers CE, Rennke HG, Hopper J, et al. Fibrillary glomerulonephritis. An entity with unusual immunofluorescence features. *Kidney Int* 1987;31:781.

354. Alpers CE. Immunotactoid (microtubular) glomerulopathy: an entity distinct from fibrillary glomerulonephritis? *Am J Kidney Dis* 1992;19:185.

355. Alpers CE. Fibrillary glomerulonephritis and immunotactoid glomerulopathy: two entities, not one. *Am J Kidney Dis* 1993;22:448.

356. Korbet SM, Schwartz MM, Rosenberg BF, et al. Immunotactoid glomerulopathy. *Medicine (Baltimore)* 1985;64:228.

357. Korbet SM, Schwartz MM, Lewis EJ. Immunotactoid glomerulopathy. *Am J Kidney Dis* 1991;17:247.

358. Korbet SM, Schwartz MM, Lewis EJ. Current concepts in renal pathology. The fibrillary glomerulopathies. *Am J Kidney Dis* 1994;23:751.

359. Fogo A, Qureshi N, Horn RG. Morphologic and clinical features of fibrillary glomerulonephritis versus immunotactoid glomerulopathy. *Am J Kidney Dis* 1993;22:367.

360. Mazzucco G, et al. Glomerulonephritis with organized deposits: a new clinicopathological entity? Light-, electron-microscopic and immunofluorescence study of 12 cases. *Am J Nephrol* 1990;1:21.

361. Touchard G, et al. Glomerulonephritis with organized microtubular monoclonal immunoglobulin deposits. *Adv Nephrol* 1994;23:149.

362. Rostagno A, et al. Fibrillary glomerulonephritis related to serum fibrillar immunoglobulin–fibronectin complexes. *Am J Kidney Dis* 1996;28:676.

363. Pronovost PH, Brady HR, Gunning ME, et al. Clinical features, predictors of disease progression and results of renal transplantation in fibrillary immunotactoid glomerulopathy. *Nephrol Dial Transplant* 1996;11:837.

364. Markowitz GS, Cheng JT, Colvin RB, et al. Hepatitis C viral infection is associated with fibrillary glomerulonephritis and immunotactoid glomerulopathy. *J Am Soc Nephrol* 1998;9:2244.

365. Brady HR. Nephrology forum: fibrillary glomerulopathy. *Kidney Int* 1998;53:1421.

366. Meyrier A, Simon P, Mignon F, et al. Rapidly progressive ("crescentic") glomerulonephritis and monoclonal gammopathies. *Nephron* 1984;38:156.

CHAPTER 77

Hyperuricemia, Gout, and the Kidney

Bryan T. Emmerson

Gout is now recognized as a clinical syndrome resulting from an inflammatory response to the deposition of monosodium urate monohydrate (MSUM or urate) crystals both within and around joints. While the clinical picture in most cases is sufficiently characteristic to be diagnosable from the history, significant hyperuricemia has usually been present for some years prior to the first acute attack. Such crystallization from hyperuricemic fluids implies that the concentration has exceeded the solubility of urate in these fluids. However, urate solubility varies in body fluids depending on electrolyte composition, protein content, pH, and the presence of substances such as proteoglycans that maintain urate in soluble form (1). Changes in the concentrations of these substances may initiate precipitation of urate.

Hyperuricemia implies an increase in urate concentration above normal. However, such a definition presents the problem of defining normality. Reference ranges for urate concentrations in plasma, reflecting 95% of a population, vary widely from one population to another and even in the same population over the years. A physicochemical definition is theoretically feasible but difficult to examine *in vitro* under conditions that reproduce those in body fluids *in vivo*. Pragmatically, one might define an upper limit of normal as the value above which complications of hyperuricemia, in particular urate crystal deposition, are likely to be seen. The point at which there is minimum overlap between the curves of distribution of the serum urate in a normal population and that in a gouty population would help to define a value that might be considered the upper limit of normal. This has generally been accepted as being 0.42 mmol/L (7 mg/dL) for males and 0.36 mmol/L (6 mg/dL) for females (2,3).

The serum urate concentration reflects the balance between urate production and elimination. Hyperuricemia can develop either when production of urate is greater than elimination or when elimination of a normal amount of produced urate is inadequate. Excessive production of urate does not result in

hyperuricemia if the ability of the body to eliminate urate can match the increased production (3). Similarly, a reduced excretory ability for urate may not lead to hyperuricemia if the urate load is reduced in proportion to the excretory capacity. However, excessive production of urate (commonly called overproduction) is often present in association with an impaired ability of the kidney to excrete urate (commonly referred to as underexcretion). Urate in the body is produced by degradation of either endogenous or dietary nucleoproteins. It is principally eliminated via the renal tract, but about one-third enters the alimentary tract in the *succus entericus*, apparently by passive processes, and is degraded by colonic bacteria.

The understanding of the pathogenesis of hyperuricemia (Table 77-1) is clarified by considering the causes of overproduction of urate separately from the causes of underexcretion. However, it is important to remember that, in many patients, both overproduction and underexcretion occur together, and several factors contributing to hyperuricemia can operate simultaneously. Genetic overproduction of urate occurs in the presence of mutations of two enzymes: hypoxanthine–guanine phosphoribosyltransferase (HGPRT) and phosphoribosyl pyrophosphate synthetase (PRPPS). All patients possessing mutations of these enzymes overproduce urate from birth (4). Acquired overproduction may result from excessive degradation of nucleoprotein that may occur in the myeloproliferative and lymphoproliferative disorders such as polycythemia vera and the leukemias. Dietary nucleoprotein also contributes, the extent depending on the amount of purine consumed. Urate production relates to body size and weight so that larger persons produce more urate than those who are smaller. However, the specific body constituent that causes this, whether muscle mass, fat, or merely total body size, has not been finally decided (5). Urate is also produced by excessive degradation of ATP, as occurs during the metabolism of fructose and ethanol, during exercise, and in the presence of tissue hypoxia (6).

Primary underexcretion of urate in the absence of renal disease is a common finding in patients with gout. Numerous studies over the years have shown diminished renal ability to

B. T. Emmerson: Department of Medicine, University of Queensland at the Princess Alexandra Hospital, Brisbane, Queensland, Australia

TABLE 77-1. *Pathogenesis of hyperuricemia*

I. Overproduction of urate
  A. Genetic
    1. HGPRT mutation
    2. PRPPS mutation
  B. Acquired
    1. Endogenous; myelo- and lymphoproliferative
       disorders
    2. Exogenous; dietary purines
    3. Increased body size
II. Underexcretion of urate
  A. Genetic: primary underexcretion gout
  B. Acquired permanent
    1. Acute–chronic renal failure
    2. Essential hypertension
  C. Acquired transient
    1. Drugs
      a. Thiazide diuretics
      b. Pyrazinamide
      c. Ethambutol
    2. Metabolites
      a. Lactate
      b. Ketone bodies
      c. Insulin
      d. Angiotensin
      e. Vasopressin
    3. Plasma volume contraction
    4. Suboptimal urine volume

HGPRT, hypoxanthine-guanine phosphoribosyltransferase;
PRPPS, phosphoribosylpyrophosphate synthetase

eliminate urate at a particular serum urate concentration in patients with gout who have normal urate production and normal renal function (7–9). This is most readily demonstrated in a patient by the finding of a reduced urate clearance at a time when the glomerular filtration rate (GFR) and all other discrete renal functions are completely normal. Relative to a particular serum urate, such kidneys exhibit a reduced excretory capacity for urate, and the raised serum urate facilitates urate elimination (10). Thus, a satisfactory excretory capacity for urate is achieved at the cost of hyperuricemia.

Hyperuricemia is also a frequent finding in the presence of either acute or chronic renal disease, although adaptive changes take place to minimize the severity of such hyperuricemia. A clear distinction must be drawn between this secondary underexcretion of urate due to renal disease and the primary underexcretion of urate by the healthy kidney, which contributes to the hyperuricemia in some patients with primary gout. Essential hypertension is also associated with hyperuricemia because of impaired tubular urate excretion (11), due to either a defect in proximal tubular sodium handling (12) or early renal vascular disease (13).

Urate transport across the luminal membrane of the tubular cell appears to be mediated by an anion exchanger with an affinity for urate, lactate, paraaminohippurate, and hydroxyl ions, whereas transport across the basolateral membrane is mediated by an anion exchanger with special affinity for urate and chloride (14–16). Transport of urate can also occur through both membranes by diffusion.

There are also many conditions that transiently reduce the ability of the kidney to eliminate urate, and these may contribute to hyperuricemia. Many drugs, especially the thiazide diuretics, will reduce renal excretion of urate. A number of drugs that are uricosuric in larger doses may reduce renal elimination of urate in small doses. This is most readily seen with low doses of aspirin. Any link with sodium reabsorption is probably indirect by alteration in the rate of solute flow in the proximal tubule (17), so that slowing of flow allows greater urate reabsorption. Increased lactate concentrations (18) or the presence of ketone bodies (19) will also reduce the renal excretion of urate. Both vasopressin and angiotensin (20) reduce the urate clearance. Contraction of the extracellular fluid volume will also reduce renal elimination of urate (21,22). In addition, a urine volume of less than 1 mL per minute is suboptimal for renal elimination of urate (23). The importance of hyperinsulinemia as a contributor to hyperuricemia has recently been established. It is mostly seen as part of a syndrome in which compensatory hyperinsulinemia develops because of insulin resistance within muscle and adipose tissue, while the kidney and the liver retain their insulin sensitivity. This leads on the one hand to excessive triglyceride production by the liver, while the kidney tubule responds to the hyperinsulinemia by the retention of both urate and sodium (24), leading to both hyperuricemia and hypertension. This provides a mechanism and an explanation for the commonly seen clinical syndrome of abdominal obesity, hyperuricemia and gout, dyslipidemia, hypertension, impaired glucose tolerance, and occasionally type 2 diabetes (25). The common clinical association is an increased waist–hip ratio. Thus, a wide variety of factors exist that can modify the serum urate by affecting either urate production or its renal excretion.

THE ROLE OF THE KIDNEY IN URATE HOMEOSTASIS

The Handling of Urate by the Normal Human Kidney

There is considerable direct information concerning the transport of urate in the different segments of the nephron in animals. However, details vary widely in different species and the applicability of the findings to humans is difficult to determine, particularly as so few other species lack uricase. Thus, there is no totally satisfactory animal model from which to draw conclusions concerning the normal renal excretory mechanism for urate in humans. Even the higher apes have significant differences.

Nonetheless, there is a body of knowledge concerning renal excretion of urate in humans that is well established:

1. The clearance of urate is normally about 10% of the GFR. Extensive studies have given a value of 8.7 ± 2.5 mL/ minute (26). The relatively wide standard deviation of the values reflects the wide range of normality. Twin studies

have shown that a major component of the urate clearance is under genetic control (27).

2. Urate is almost totally filterable at the glomerulus. Protein binding, if present, is of very low order (ranging from 0% to 4% at 37°C) and does not appear to be of physiologic significance (28).

3. A great proportion of the urate that is filtered (possibly 95% to 99%) is reabsorbed, probably in the proximal tubule.

4. Tubular secretion contributes considerably to the urate that is present in the urine (29).

5. A medullary urate gradient is present in humans, with a progressive increase in urate concentration from the cortex to the medulla, with the concentration greatest at the papilla. The mechanism appears to be analogous to the process that causes a sodium or urea gradient (30,31).

Thus, the handling of urate by the renal tubule in humans is complex, and the precise mechanisms and sites of tubular reabsorptive and secretory processes remain to be defined. However, there is now increasing evidence for the existence of active urate–anion exchangers in the brush-border membrane of human proximal tubular cells (32,33) (see Chapter 8 for more detail).

Pharmacologic studies of the effect of a variety of drugs on urinary urate excretion have provided indirect evidence concerning transport within the tubule. Current concepts concerning transport depend on the interpretation of particular actions by these drugs, and, while present knowledge supports these concepts, it should be remembered that they still depend on conclusions reached on indirect evidence and the belief that a particular drug blocks one mechanism specifically. Most of the uricosuric drugs such as probenecid, sulfinpyrazone, or aspirin in high dosage are thought to act by inhibiting the urate–anion exchange mechanism. Pyrazinamide, which greatly reduces urinary urate excretion, is considered to act by blocking tubular secretion of urate (29,34). However, it is uncertain how completely it blocks secretion and how accurately the change in urate excretion following the administration of pyrazinamide can provide a measure of the total tubular secretory flux (35). Similarly, the uricosuric response to benzbromarone is abolished by pretreatment with pyrazinamide, implying that benzbromarone acts principally by inhibiting reabsorption of urate that has been secreted, because its uricosuric response is not interfered with by agents transported by the organic acid pathway (36). It has been deduced that postsecretory reabsorption may be a distal nephron function.

Renal excretion of urate is therefore currently regarded as having four components (29,37). Urate is completely filterable at the glomerulus and 98% to 99% of filtered urate is reabsorbed in the proximal tubule. Further distally, active tubular secretion of urate appears to have a potentially considerable capacity. In addition, much of the urate secreted is then reabsorbed so that, ultimately, only one-tenth of the urate that was filtered appears in the urine. In many gouty patients who are underexcretors of urate, the urate clearance appears to be within the lower limit of the normal range. It has been shown that, in such patients with normal urate production, tubular secretion of urate is quantitatively less than that in overproducers of urate who overexcrete urate (36). While this evidence suggests that tubular secretion of urate is a dominant factor in determining urate excretion, it must be remembered that these conclusions are indirect and based on the interpretation of changes in urate excretion following the administration of pharmacologic agents (37).

Changes in the Renal Handling of Urate with Reduced Renal Function

In considering this aspect, it is important to remember that the kidney is normally responsible for only approximately two-thirds of urate elimination from the body. In addition, there is considerable variability in the renal excretory capacity of urate in the normal population, with a correspondingly large range in the urate clearance (26) and the serum urate concentration. Accordingly, it is not surprising that the pattern in renal insufficiency is not a uniform one, particularly because the nature of the renal disease and the portion of the nephron most affected will vary.

With the onset of chronic renal disease, there is an early reduction in the urate clearance with a corresponding tendency to an increase in the serum urate concentration. Whether this causes hyperuricemia will depend on the usual serum urate and the dietary purine load. As the GFR is reduced by the chronic renal disease, the tendency for reduction in urate clearance and hyperuricemia will increase (38). However, it is important to note that the elevation of the serum urate is never as great as that of the blood urea nitrogen. As the GFR falls, there is a steady increase in fractional urate excretion (clearance of urate–clearance of inulin ratio), indicating an increased urate excretion per nephron (39). Thus, in transplant nephrectomy donors, despite a 20% increase in the GFR in the remaining kidney, an increased urate excretion per nephron occurs due to an increase of secreted urate (40), which permits the maintenance of a normal serum urate concentration (41). If one accepts changes in urate excretion following the administration of pyrazinamide as reflecting tubular secretion of urate, it seems likely that the increased urate excretion per nephron in chronic renal failure is due to increased tubular secretion (39). When renal failure becomes severe (less than 10 mL/minute), reduced tubular reabsorption of urate may also contribute to the increased urate excretion per nephron (42). Hyperuricemia in this situation is the result of failure of the adaptive increase in urate excretion per nephron to compensate for the degree of nephron loss. However, despite this increase in urate excretion per nephron, the total excretion of urate in the urine in unit time is quantitatively less in chronic renal failure than in the presence of normal renal function, and a direct relationship exists between the 24-hour

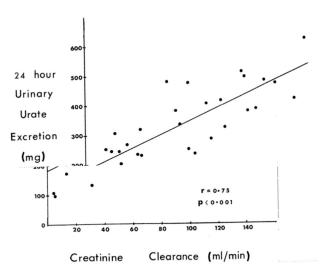

FIG. 77-1. The relationship between urinary urate excretion on a low-purine diet and creatinine clearance. (From Emmerson BT, Row PG. An evaluation of the pathogenesis of the gouty kidney. *Kidney Int* 1975;8:65. Reprinted by permission of Blackwell Science, Inc.)

urinary urate excretion on a low-purine diet and the creatinine clearance (Fig. 77-1). Increased urate excretion by extrarenal routes as well as reduced urate production also compensate for the reduced renal excretion (43).

TYPES OF INTERACTION BETWEEN HYPERURICEMIA, GOUT, AND THE KIDNEY

There are three principal ways in which hyperuricemia and gout can interact with the kidney resulting in three quite distinctive clinical syndromes. The first is an acute effect of urate overproduction on the kidney, resulting in a reversible deterioration of renal function with a characteristic pathology initiated by tubular obstruction due to uric acid crystals. As such, it is called a uric acid nephropathy. The second is a chronic interaction, usually referred to as a gout nephropathy, which may occur in sufferers from long-standing and severe gout, usually with tophi, in whom the gout was the primary problem and any renal damage occurred secondary to this. The continuing importance of this type of interaction in industrialized populations has been questioned (44) but a recent reappraisal has provided support for its continuing relevance (45). The third is one in which a patient with a chronic renal disease of definable nature (which often involves the renal interstitium) exhibits an unusual degree of hyperuricemia, which eventually leads to the development of a secondary gouty arthritis. In such a case, the renal disease would be primary and the gout a secondary development. In general, adverse effects attributable to hyperuricemia appear to be mediated by the formation of crystals either of urate (MSUM) or of uric acid and any adverse effects from this crystal formation would fit with one or other of the three types of interaction mentioned. Each of these syndromes will be considered in turn. However,

in any patient with both gout and renal disease, it is important to define the primary problem, and to distinguish this from secondary effects.

URATE AND URIC ACID CRYSTALS IN THE KIDNEY AND RESULTANT PATHOLOGY

When seeking a pathologic basis for disorders due to hyperuricemia and gout, one is drawn to the conclusion that most disease relating to hyperuricemia and gout is primarily the result of crystal formation. Other mechanisms, though postulated, have yet to be established. As far as such crystals are concerned, two different varieties may be formed; which type depends chiefly upon the pH at the site. At a lower pH, such as that of urine, a greater proportion of the molecules are present in the form of undissociated uric acid, in which form they are poorly soluble. Solubility increases greatly as pH rises from 5 to 7. When saturation occurs, the crystals formed usually consist of free uric acid. By contrast, the crystals formed at physiologic pH and ionic strength are the classic acicular (needle-shaped) crystals of MSUM (or urate) seen in tophi. Crystals will dissolve in a formalin fixative, whereas alcohol fixation leaves urate/uric acid crystals intact and in situ, they can be examined and identified by polarized light.

X-ray crystallography has demonstrated that tophaceous deposits consist of MSUM (46,47), whereas in renal calculi, the crystals are present as uric acid (48). Both types of crystal have been found within the kidney (49). In patients with gout, most of the crystals were in the form of urate, whereas in patients with acute leukemia, most of the crystals were in the form of uric acid. These latter crystals were found only within the lumina of the renal tubules and thus were in equilibrium with the components of tubular fluid (49). Because gout is a syndrome of varied etiologies in which some patients demonstrate urate overexcretion and others demonstrate urate underexcretion, the renal pathology might be expected to be diverse. Accordingly, it would be important to examine the types of renal lesion found in the presence of urate overexcretion and separately to study the effect of hyperuricemia without urate overexcretion on renal function and crystal deposition. Since urate overproduction can be of either genetic or acquired etiology, these are examined separately.

Genetic Urate Overproduction

In patients with mutations of the purine reutilization enzyme HGPRT, urate overproduction is present at least from the time of birth (4,50). Any renal lesion seen in such patients is most likely to have developed secondarily to this primary genetic urate overproduction. Thus, studies of the dynamics of renal function in a group of patients with HGPRT deficiency should provide clues to the mechanism whereby urate overproduction can cause renal disease. In addition, the extent of urate overproduction may cover a range in that hemizygotes for HGPRT deficiency are more severe overproducers of urate than the heterozygotes, which are only moderate overproducers (51). A follow-up of a large number of such patients (52) has allowed observations to be made about the possible sequence of events in such a situation. Study of the renal pathology in such patients revealed that acicular interstitial urate crystals could coexist in the one patient with intratubular deposits of uric acid. The pattern seen was consistent with the uric acid crystals having been deposited within the tubular lumen, whereas the acicular crystals were found chiefly within interstitial microtophi. It was also observed that, in some patients with primary urate overproduction, the serum urate concentration might still be within the normal range but that such patients would invariably have a very high urinary urate excretion. The normal serum urate concentration could persist as long as urate excretion remained in balance with urate production (53). Thus, overproduction of urate was accompanied by overexcretion of urate so long as renal excretory function for urate was maintained. In addition, in some patients with excessive urinary excretion of urate, episodes of acute renal failure were observed that were reversible by maneuvers that reduced the tendency to crystallization of uric acid within the urine, namely an alkaline diuresis. Such episodes might be precipitated by fluid restriction, but, if reversed, glomerular function could be completely restored to normal (54). Such rapid and complete reversibility of acute renal insufficiency would be consistent with intratubular uric acid deposition resulting from a high

uric acid concentration in tubular fluid and urine. Such acute renal failure should be considered as a *uric acid nephropathy* or a *hyperuricosuric nephropathy* rather than a hyperuricemic nephropathy. Observation of many patients with similar values for urinary uric acid excretion and presumably similar degrees of urate overproduction showed that the development of renal insufficiency was quite unpredictable in that some overproducers might develop renal insufficiency while others might maintain normal renal function for years. Although it was difficult to quantitate etiologic factors, it seemed that those who had experienced renal colic at any time or who tended to have a lower urine volume appeared to be the ones who were more likely to develop episodes of renal insufficiency.

These observations in primary overproducers of urate are consistent with much previous knowledge concerning the nature of urate deposits within the kidney and suggest a working hypothesis to explain the pathogenesis of renal disease in primary urate overexcretion (Fig. 77-2). Many overproducers of urate have a good renal excretory capacity for urate so that they remain normouricemic while urate excretion balances production. However, such a balance is associated with a high urinary uric acid excretion, usually exceeding 1 g or 6 mmol per 24 hours; thus, there is the potential for uric acid crystalluria to develop at times of concentrated or acid urine, either within the pelvis and ureter or within the renal

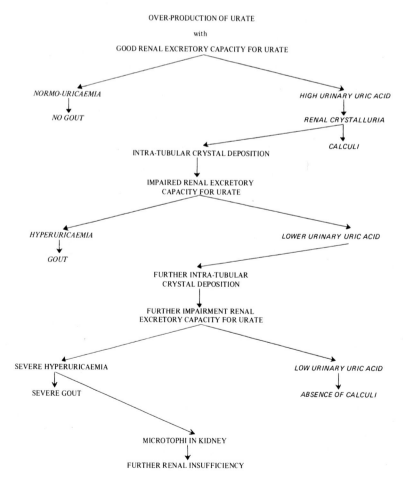

FIG. 77-2. Mechanisms whereby primary overproduction of urate may lead to the development of renal insufficiency. (From Emmerson BT, Row PG. An evaluation of the pathogenesis of the gouty kidney. *Kidney Int* 1975;8:65. Reprinted by permission of Blackwell Science, Inc.)

tubules. This may lead to the formation of uric acid calculi in some cases or to the intratubular formation of uric acid crystals or casts containing uric acid crystals in others. Such obstructive intratubular lesions, if uncorrected by an alkaline diuresis, can lead to loss of functioning nephrons and a fall in glomerular filtration. Any fall in glomerular function leads to a proportionate fall in renal excretion of urate (Fig. 77-1), and, in these overproducers, this will result in a lower level of urinary uric acid excretion (53). Such a fall in renal elimination of urate leads to a resetting of the balance between production and excretion and results in an elevation of the serum urate concentration and the potential to develop gout. Thus, repeated episodes of intratubular uric acid crystal deposition will progressively lead to a steady reduction in renal excretory capacity of urate, which, with the genetic overproduction of urate remaining unchanged, can lead not only to severe hyperuricemia but also to a fall in the urinary uric acid excretion to within the normal range. In such a situation, the risk of developing renal calculi or intratubular uric acid crystal deposits becomes greatly reduced. However, by this time, hyperuricemia may be severe and can lead to the formation of both gouty arthritis as well as the renal complications of an elevated serum urate in the form of interstitial microtophi. This could ultimately lead to increasing renal insufficiency because microtophi interfere with renal function.

Acute renal failure has been reported in several young children with HGPRT deficiency. Some of these have shown a crystal nephropathy on ultrasound, uric acid deposition on renal biopsy, and a high urinary uric acid concentration (55–57). Such reports suggest the need to determine the risks to renal function from the hyperuricosuria in these patients. The uric acid–creatinine ratio on a random urine specimen has been proposed as a screening test, but this ratio is normally very high and variable in infants. In the adult, a urate–creatinine ratio in urine that, if expressed in milligrams per deciliter, exceeds 1 (or if expressed in mmol/L, exceeds 0.66) indicates hyperuricosuria (58,59) and suggests uric acid crystalluria as a likely cause for the acute renal failure (60). Others have looked at uric acid excretion per deciliter of creatinine clearance and have found that this value is also useful in determining overexcretion in children (61). Values for these ratios vary with age in children, being greater in infancy, and the appropriate normal range needs to be sought for individual cases (62).

Acquired Overproduction of Urate Associated with Malignancy

Since most urate is normally produced by nucleoprotein degradation and the cellular turnover in bone marrow is greater than in any other tissue, there is a considerable increase in urate production in the presence of hemopoietic or lymphopoietic malignancy. In the presence of such an increased basal urate production, anticancer chemotherapy may cause such an acute increase in urate production that the renal complications of acute uric acid overexcretion may develop. It is well recognized that hydration and urinary alkalinization are valuable in preventing renal complications in patients with both a stable and moderate increase in urate production and in patients with the acute and severe increases that may occur during cellular damage caused either by chemotherapy or radiotherapy, often referred to as the tumor lysis syndrome. Wherever possible, such prophylaxis with an alkaline diuresis should be instituted before chemotherapy.

Chronic uric acid nephropathies may be found in association with a wide variety of malignancies, chiefly of hemopoietic origin. Sometimes it is present with disseminated neoplasms, including adenocarcinomas (63). The most common association, however, is with leukemias, lymphomas, and myeloproliferative disorders. During chemotherapy, an acute uric acid nephropathy may develop that can usually be reversed by treatment with measures aimed at reducing the concentration of uric acid in tubular fluid and increasing its solubility (i.e., an aggressive alkaline diuresis [64] and the administration of allopurinol [65]). Prevention is best achieved by the maintenance of a urine flow rate of at least 3 L/24 hours and the early use of allopurinol. The ready reversibility of the renal failure suggests a major obstructive component. Sometimes hemodialysis is needed, and this also promotes resolution (66–68). If the allopurinol can be administered before the chemotherapy, a high initial loading dose of up to 600 mg per day can be given, provided renal function is not impaired. This will maximally inhibit urate production. After chemotherapy, the dose of allopurinol needs to be related carefully to renal function (approximately 100 mg per day per 30 mL/minute GFR). However, allopurinol, though reducing production of urate, increases the production of its relatively insoluble precursor, xanthine, the concentration of which may readily exceed its solubility limit and cause crystal formation (69,70). Thus, the acute renal failure that develops after chemotherapy may not be due solely to uric acid deposition; other substances, particularly phosphate and xanthine, may also contribute.

Studies of the pathology of these kidneys are usually limited to the findings at autopsy when the tubules are blocked by extensive deposits of uric acid. With the recognition of the importance of prevention, such findings are less frequent. It is more difficult, however, to obtain information concerning the early changes within the kidney that accompany the very high rates of excretion of uric acid. In such a situation, no consistent glomerular changes have been found and the primary site of injury appears to be the renal tubules due to intratubular crystallization of urate–uric acid. Collecting ducts appear to be predominantly involved (Fig. 77-3) with a granulomatous reaction to the crystals. Some changes unrelated to crystal deposition have also been reported in the proximal tubules, but these were similar to those observed in hypoxia and ischemia. Electron microscopic examination of biopsy samples has shown phagocytosis of intraluminal crystals by lining epithelial cells of the distal tubules (Fig. 77-4). In some cases, the crystals appeared free within the cytoplasm

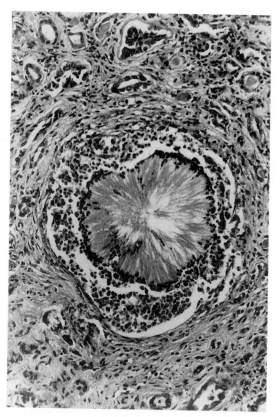

FIG. 77-3. From the kidney of a patient with urate overproduction of leukemia, this figure shows a central mass typical of acicular urate crystals, surrounded by an inflammatory cell infiltrate within a space suggesting the residuum of a dilated collecting duct. (Hematoxylin and eosin ×128.)

whereas other appearances suggested an initial association between the crystal and lysosomal structures. Sometimes urate crystals have been lodged between the wavy processes of histiocytes within the collecting tubules in close association with the tubular epithelial cells (Fig. 77-5). Such histiocytes could be involved in the formation of urate granulomas by passage from a luminal location to a more interstitial site via breaks in the tubular lining membranes (71).

Other Varieties of Urate Overproduction

Sickle cell anemia is regularly associated with hyperuricosuria (72). Usually this overproduction of urate is associated with an increase in urate clearance such that the serum urate remains normal for long periods. However, hyperuricemia is more often seen after the third decade (73). This seems to be associated with the development of renal damage and a reduced ability to eliminate urate. Whether this renal damage is due to sickling, to urate deposition, or to both is not known. The increased urate clearance in patients with sickle cell anemia is suppressible by pyrazinamide, which has caused it to be attributed to an increase in tubular secretion of urate (72). Hyperuricemia has also been reported in several other conditions where hemopoietic overactivity is present, such as cyanotic congenital heart disease.

Intense physical training in hot climates has been associated with hyperuricemia, an increase in urinary excretion of uric acid, and occasionally with acute renal failure (74,75). This increase in urate production was associated with features suggesting an associated muscle injury and, in hot weather, small

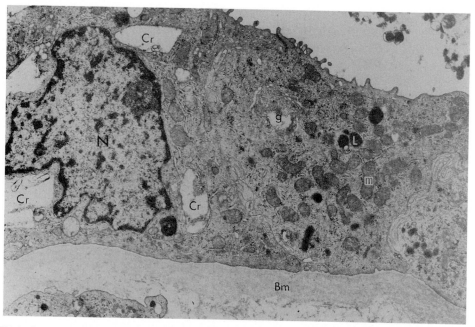

FIG. 77-4. Collecting tubule demonstrating various configurations of urate crystals (*Cr*). Golgi apparatus (*g*) is prominent. Lysosomal bodies (*L*) are increased. Nucleus (*N*) shows indentations and lobulations; (*m*) indicates mitochondria. Basement membrane (*Bm*) is intact. (Original magnification ×10,000.) (From Kanwar YS, Manaligod JR. Leukemic urate nephropathy. *Arch Pathol* 1975;99:467, © 1975, American Medical Association.)

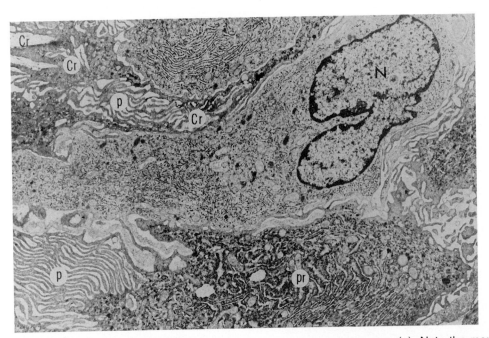

FIG. 77-5. Histiocyte with urate crystals (*Cr*) lodged between wavy processes (*p*). Note the marked increase in rough endoplasmic reticulum, ribosomes, and spiral-shaped polyribosomes (*pr*). Mitochondria are few and degenerated; nucleus (*N*) is lobulated. (Original magnification ×6,700.) (From Kanwar YS, Manaligod JR. Leukemic urate nephropathy. *Arch Pathol* 1975;99:467, © 1975, American Medical Association.)

urine volumes. Although myoglobinemia was not recorded in these cases, it has been found in marathon runners, and this has been correlated with the serum urate concentration. Thus, both the myoglobinuria and the increased urinary urate are potential factors that might contribute to the acute renal failure in this situation (76). A massive uricosuria may develop when a normal-calorie diet is resumed in subjects undergoing starvation for weight reduction, and renal damage may be found at these times (77). In addition, renal failure has been observed during the administration of uricosuric agents, chiefly the more potent ones such as sulfinpyrazone (78). Some of these episodes are reversible and appear during the first few days of therapy. They are particularly frequent when a high dose of sulfinpyrazone has been given initially, and especially when no precautions have been taken in the form of establishing an alkaline diuresis during the initial period of treatment (79). This is a particular problem when sulfinpyrazone is given in high dosage as an antiplatelet agent without special concern for the effect of the associated uricosuria on renal function (80). It seems much less common during the use of the less potent uricosuric agents such as probenecid or when sulfinpyrazone is used in more moderate doses.

Hyperuricosuria may occur without urate overproduction in patients with a reduced renal ability to reabsorb urate, resulting in a greatly elevated urate clearance together with marked hypouricemia (81). Such patients, though rare, may develop acute reversible renal failure by mechanisms similar to those seen with urate overproduction, either genetic or acquired by tumor lysis. This further supports the concept

that the high urate concentration in the urine is potentially damaging to renal function.

Studies of the Animal Kidney in Urate Overproduction

Most animals possess uricase, which makes it difficult to develop an animal model to study the effects of uric acid overproduction. However, the administration of the uricase inhibitor oxonate has enabled the alleviation of this problem and, with the addition of uric acid to the diet, has provided a reasonably satisfactory animal model of urate overproduction, albeit in an animal kidney that is not accustomed to handling urate. All degrees of urate overproduction can be induced by varying the dosages of oxonate and dietary uric acid; some regimens induce minimal hyperuricemia while others cause severe hyperuricemia. Similarly, the acuteness of the uric acid load on the kidney can be varied in this model from prolonged and low grade to acute and intense. Protection by a high tubular fluid flow has been established (82). In all cases, there was a considerable increase in the urine urate. Functionally, the pattern was that of an obstructive uropathy with a raised intraluminal pressure and a fall in the inulin clearance and single-nephron GFR. This could resolve in large part when the urate overproduction was terminated (83). Morphologically, multiple intraluminal deposits were seen within the tubule with dilation of collecting ducts, thinning of the lining epithelium, and urate deposits within and adjacent to the epithelium and the collecting ducts (84). Interstitial infiltrates were seen and there was a strong suggestion that neutrophil chemotaxis followed by degranulation and vacuolation was occurring with release of ingested crystals and possible precipitation of new crystals (85,86). The overall impression was that intraluminal obstruction by deposition of uric acid was playing a large part in the pathogenesis of the renal lesion. In the grossest lesions and the most acute studies, with the development of severe hyperuricemia as well as the presence of uric acid and urate within the tubular systems, crystalline material was also seen within the vasa recta between the corticomedullary junction and the papillary tip (87). The whole lesion was prevented by a high tubular fluid flow (82).

A similar pattern of a crystal nephropathy has been produced in the pig using an experiment that resulted in deposition of crystals of xanthine and oxypurinol in the ratio of 2:1. Intratubular deposit of these crystals was associated with erosion of the basement membrane and an interstitial nephritis. Tubular degeneration around an intratubular crystal mass appeared to transfer the crystals to the interstitium where, despite dissolution of the crystals, an interstitial nephritis persisted. Even short periods of intratubular obstruction by crystals in this model resulted in permanent changes with reduction in kidney size and impairment of renal function (88). These and other experimental studies emphasize the importance of intratubular crystal deposition, possibly of any sort, in the genesis of chronic renal disease and show that permanent changes in the interstitium may occur as secondary developments.

The Syndrome of Uric Acid Nephropathy

There is thus good evidence, both clinical and experimental, to support the concept of a uric acid nephropathy. The most important aspects of such a syndrome include:

1. The primary lesion is obstructive and relates to the deposition of uric acid within the distal tubules and the collecting ducts.
2. Secondary changes may develop in the tubular lining cells and in the interstitium, particularly within the medulla.
3. Although the syndrome may vary from acute and dramatic to chronic and low grade in its manifestations, the underlying pathogenesis remains similar.
4. The most important factor determining deposition is the concentration of uric acid within the tubular lumen and its varied solubility in relation to changes in pH.
5. The syndrome is potentially reversible although, unless treatment is rapidly instituted, permanent changes can result that may not be readily detected at an early stage by tests of renal or tubular function.
6. Despite very high rates of excretion of uric acid, the syndrome can be prevented by the maintenance of a high rate of flow of tubular fluid. Alkalinization of the urine, although helpful, is usually of secondary importance to a high flow rate.

Effect of the Serum Urate Concentration on Renal Function in Humans

The above considerations indicate that renal damage can develop in humans in the presence of excessive renal excretion of urate, irrespective of the presence or absence of an elevated serum urate concentration. Thus, in the presence of urate overexcretion, hyperuricemia is not necessary for the development of renal disease, and the presence of a high uric acid concentration in tubular fluid and urine is more important in the genesis of renal disease than elevation of the serum urate concentration.

Less information is available, however, concerning the risk of developing renal damage from an elevated serum urate concentration in the absence of urate overexcretion. In large part, this is due to the difficulty of excluding an associated overexcretion of urate or, in many subjects, even of knowing the status of their urate production or urate excretion. The position is further complicated by additional factors:

1. Because urate solubility varies with concentration, the risk of damage from an elevated urate concentration relates to the extent of its elevation. As the serum urate varies from day to day in any one individual, there is no single serum urate concentration that will be representative for that individual over a prolonged period in order to assess its potential in inducing renal disease.
2. The most important urate concentration in the genesis of urate-induced renal damage is that within the renal interstitium, and particularly the renal medulla and papilla (because of the medullary gradient of urate). It is almost impossible to obtain information about this *in vivo* or to know how it relates to the serum urate concentration at any time. Indeed the concentration of urate in the blood is probably the least important, although the most accessible, parameter.
3. Even in the presence of normal urate excretion, high concentrations of urate may appear in the urine at times of low urine flow rate. These may be associated with concentrations of urate similar to those that occur in urate overexcretion, which are known to be able to cause adverse effects on renal function. Accordingly, urine flow rate is a vital factor in assessing the effect of any urate parameter on renal function. Even in one individual, the urine flow rate can vary widely on different occasions. Thus, it is difficult to obtain good evidence concerning whether or not hyperuricemia of various degrees can induce renal damage in the absence of overt urate overexcretion.

Nonetheless, several longitudinal studies have examined renal glomerular function over many years in patients whose serum urate concentrations appear to have been reasonably stable. In general, such follow-up studies in patients with asymptomatic hyperuricemia have shown that levels of serum urate of less than 0.6 mmol/L (10 mg/dL) are rarely associated with the development of renal dysfunction. However, with serum urate concentrations greater than this, there is less confidence that renal dysfunction will not occur and values of up to 0.78 mmol/L (13 mg/dL) may well be significant in the genesis of renal insufficiency when present for prolonged periods (89). Follow-up of gouty patients with persisting hyperuricemia of between 0.6 and 0.7 mmol/L (10 to 12 mg/dL) has shown that renal dysfunction is not an invariable development. In view of the importance of the concentration of urate in tubular fluid and urine in the genesis of uric acid-induced renal disease, it would be better to avoid the term *hyperuricemic nephropathy*, implying as it does that the important urate concentration is in the blood.

RENAL DISEASE SECONDARY TO PRIMARY GOUT (GOUT NEPHROPATHY)

Historical Review and Tests of Renal Function

With the advent of effective treatment to restore a normal serum urate in gout, the complications from uric acid, particularly gout nephropathy, are seen less frequently. Inevitably, the question is asked whether such a condition ever really existed. Any answer to such a question requires examination of historic evidence, particularly that just prior to the availability of effective treatment to correct hyperuricemia.

The first mention of renal involvement in gout is attributed to Aretaeus the Cappadocian, in the second century A.D. (90). Little more is recorded until 1683, when Sydenham wrote that "gout breeds stones in the kidneys" (91). In 1823, Scudamore noted the frequent presence of proteinuria in patients with gout (92), and in 1843, Castelneau observed that uric acid deposits occurred in the kidneys as well as in the joints of gouty subjects (93). Todd (1857) referred to the "gouty kidney," which he regarded as being a "contracted state of the kidney peculiarly apt to be developed in the inveterate gouty diathesis" (94). He recorded "opaque streaks of lithate of soda, taking the direction of the tubules." Charcot and Cornil (1864) extended this observation by observing that urates were deposited between the tubules, as needle-shaped crystals chiefly in longitudinal directions, as well as within the tubules as amorphous urates that could cause obstruction (95). Garrod (1876) regarded the interstitial deposits of urate crystals as being specific for gout and observed contracted kidneys and urate crystal deposition "in all cases of chronic chalk gout where the opportunity of making the examination was afforded" (96). Lindsay (1913) emphasized the close relationship between gout and kidney disease and confirmed that the crystalline deposits scattered within the kidney consisted of interstitial urate identical to that found within the joints (97). Llewellyn (1920) claimed that "in early interstitial nephritis, the retention of uric acid preceded that of urea or creatinine," and that such hyperuricemia did not necessarily indicate or predispose to gouty arthritis (98). He commented that renal urate deposits might occur in nephritis in clinically occult form. He noted, however, that gouty subjects often have granular kidneys and distinguished this situation from that in which gout is a complication of primary renal disease.

He regarded the renal lesion in long-standing gout as an interstitial nephritis, similar to the ordinary "contracted kidney of the arteriosclerosis type" and that, the more severe the gout, the more likely it was that renal complications would develop. However, even though urate deposits might be present in the kidney of gouty subjects, Llewellyn was not persuaded that this established the gouty kidney as a distinct entity. He had difficulty in elucidating the relationship between gout and renal disease at a time when neither condition could be defined precisely.

Subsequent studies have eliminated the problem progressively in proportion to the ability to define the precise nature of the renal disease and the specific diagnosis of gout. In addition, objective assessment of renal function in gouty patients has become increasingly available. In their series of 55 cases in 1930, Schnitker and Richter (1936) found a "31% incidence of definite nephritis in true gout" with an 8% death rate due to uremia (99). Over 80% of those with nephritis had tophaceous gout and had suffered from gout for over 10 years. The evidence for nephritis consisted of proteinuria and impairment of tests of renal function. These authors found that vascular disease and hypertension were more frequent in patients with gout than in nongouty individuals of the same age, and, both clinically and pathologically, they regarded the underlying lesion in the kidney as being predominantly vascular. In 1940, Coombs and colleagues (100) also studied renal function in gouty subjects and found that most showed some evidence of renal damage. The earliest change was impairment of concentrating ability, whereas, with increasing renal impairment, the urate clearance was better maintained than the inulin clearance. They regarded the original deterioration as being due to the deposition of urate within the renal parenchyma. Hypertension was present in half the patients at a time when renal impairment was only of moderate degree. In 1941, Brøchner-Mortensen found evidence of renal disease in 25% of his 100 gouty patients (101).

In 1950, Brown and Mallory reported on the kidney pathology in five proven cases of gout "because of the frequency of renal dysfunction accompanying this disease" (102). They found urate deposits in the medulla, probably originating in the collecting tubules, together with nephrosclerosis. They reported a case with typical renal changes of a gout nephropathy but no clinical manifestations of joint disease, which they suggested might represent "primary renal gout." They also suggested that tubular blockage by urate predisposed to pyelonephritis, which might contribute to the renal damage. Fineberg (1958) emphasized the distinction between the primary nephropathy caused by crystal deposition or calculus formation and a secondary nephropathy caused by superimposed arteriosclerotic or pyelonephritis changes (103). He believed the specific lesion was caused by precipitation of urate within either the tubules or the interstitial tissue of the kidney. The most extensive study of the pathology of gout was reported by Talbott and Terplan in 1960 (104). They studied the kidneys of 191 patients and classified them as having mild or moderate clinical gout, severe tophaceous gout, or blood dyscrasias. They concluded that the only distinctive pathologic feature in the gouty kidney was the presence of urate crystals. They stressed that renal involvement was a frequent finding in patients with gout. Very few kidneys were normal; the most frequent abnormalities were microtophi, nephrosclerosis, and urinary tract infection. They regarded the presence of urate crystals with their surrounding giant-cell reaction as the distinctive pathologic feature of the gouty kidney. Renal insufficiency was "of critical degree" in 25% of patients.

At about this time, the modern era of nephrology with investigative techniques was developing. In addition, effective drug control of hyperuricemia was becoming feasible. The availability of such effective therapy greatly reduced the frequency of acute attacks and it was expected that such therapy would alter the frequency with which renal complications were found in gout. In 1961, renal biopsy techniques were directed toward the study of the kidney pathology in 10 gouty subjects, 8 of whom showed proteinuria and impaired renal function. From these biopsies, it was concluded that the renal lesion was consistent with the primary damage being tubular and the interstitial reaction secondary (105). By contrast, a biopsy study of 22 patients by Gonick and associates (1965) found widely varying features (106). They reported a distinctive glomerular lesion as well as vascular hypertrophy, tubular atrophy, and interstitial fibrosis and inflammation. Their evidence did not suggest that infection contributed and, although they found occasional microtophi in their biopsy specimens, they believed that this was rare. They regarded the glomerular lesion as a toxic effect from filtered urate. Similar glomerular changes have not been reported by others.

Renal disease in primary gout was again extensively studied in 1968 by Barlow and Beilin, who examined both renal function and renal histology in 80 biopsy specimens (107). Obesity, hypertension, and renal calculi were common in their patients, and renal insufficiency was present in 40%, even after allowing for the usual decline in renal function with age. Tubular function was impaired in proportion to glomerular function. The dominant lesion was a vascular nephrosclerosis, and bacterial infection was not a factor in the production of early lesions. They attributed the dilated tubules and focal interstitial lymphocytic infiltrate either to vascular ischemia or nephron obstruction. They focused on vascular nephrosclerosis as an important early feature in the pathogenesis of the renal lesion. Grahame and Scott (1970) found renal insufficiency in 25% of their gouty patients and hypertension in half (108). More recently, Gibson and coworkers (109) found that a relative impairment of GFR and concentrating ability in the gouty subjects was not fully explicable on the basis of aging and hypertension. As might be expected, when effective urate-lowering treatment had been available for over 20 years, renal dysfunction was found to be generally mild. These authors commented on the increased acidity of urine in their gouty subjects due to a defect in ammonium excretion and a relatively high excretion of titratable acid. However, interpretation of these data is difficult because urinary

acidification, even after loading, has been shown to be influenced in subjects with gout by the dietary intake of both purine and protein (110). Later, studies showed that the changes in renal function described by Gibson and coworkers could not be demonstrated over a 2-year period in patients treated with allopurinol (111).

Yu and associates have studied renal function in large groups of gouty patients over the years (112–114). Their earliest studies on 160 gouty patients reported that most subjects showed essentially normal renal function (24). However, they observed that in some patients the GFR declined progressively in association with deterioration of tubular function. They considered their clearance studies at that time to be compatible with the interpretation that the earliest manifestations of renal damage were principally tubular and attributable to the luminal and interstitial urate deposits, with associated infection and vascular changes as had been reported at autopsy. As the GFR declined, they believed that renal retention of urate would develop.

Studies of larger groups were reported some 20 years later (115). At the time, the presence of tophi was associated more with a low GFR and proteinuria. Yu and coworkers considered that the deterioration of renal function in gout was largely associated with aging, renal vascular disease, and renal calculi with pyelonephritis. Hyperuricemia alone, observed over a 12-year period, did not necessarily appear to have an adverse effect on renal function. They specifically emphasized the importance of coexisting vascular disease as part of any associated gout nephropathy. Except in rare cases, these authors considered that uncomplicated gout rarely led to renal function impairment and that the factors that had the greatest impact on renal function in gouty subjects were the coexistence of hypertension and vascular disease, the age of the patient, and the duration of the gout (113,114). This view was extended in a 1986 review (114a), which suggested not only that renal disease should no longer be a problem in gouty patients who are adequately treated, but that it had only been a problem in a minority of patients in whom the basic lesion was primary renal disease, often of the familial type.

These conclusions and the renal consequences of hyperuricemia and gout have recently been reexamined by Johnson and colleagues (45), and a strong association between hyperuricemia and chronic tubulointerstitial disease has been noted. These authors particularly questioned the interpretation of the data of Yu and coworkers (114) and concluded that the implication that gout was not directly injurious to the kidney was based on interpretations and assumptions that may not be valid. These included the question of whether hyperuricemia can lead to interstitial renal disease, which may then result in hypertension. The conclusion of the Johnson group was that renal disease may occur as a consequence of gout and that those patients with gout of longer duration or early onset were those most likely to develop the greatest degree of renal disease.

A recent clinical study from Taiwan by Tarng and associates (116) confirmed that gouty patients with tophi had significantly poorer renal function than those without such tophi. Moreover, 19 of the 21 patients in this study with tophaceous gout had echogenic regions scattered through the corticomedullary junction of both kidneys. The Tarng group's pathologic studies showed these to be characteristic micro-tophi in the medullary interstitium. The presence of hypertension caused an additional decline in renal function. The findings of Tarng and associates are reminiscent of those discovered in the United States at the time of the major study of Talbott and Terplan (104), carried out in the 1950s when effective treatment to correct hyperuricemia was not available and consequently gout more often became tophaceous. The Taiwanese study replicates the Talbott and Terplan experience, whereas the recently reduced frequency of renal disease as a sequel to gout in the United States (45) may reflect more frequent and more effective control of hyperuricemia in the U.S., with the result that tophi and microtophaceous renal disease occurs infrequently.

A recent autopsy study by Nickeleit and Mihatsch (117) showed that one-third of their group with gout demonstrated renal urate deposits. However, these authors also found such deposits in patients not known to have suffered from gout. They also reported a correlation between renal urate deposits and renal dysfunction, but the type of associated renal pathology was not always able to be defined clearly and included changes which could be attributable to hypertension, pyelonephritis, nephrolithiases, and chronic interstitial nephritis, as well as renal urate deposits. Thus, while there still remains the potential for urate or uric acid crystals to produce a nephropathy in gout, adequate therapeutic control of hyperuricemia would eliminate the contribution of these crystals and leave only other factors, such as hypertension, vascular disease, and nephrolithiases, to contribute to any nephropathy. In these days when effective treatment for hyperuricemia and gout is readily available, the classic gouty kidney as seen prior to the development of effective urate lowering therapy should be an uncommon finding.

Pathology and Pathogenesis

Since gout is a clinical syndrome resulting from multiple independent mechanisms, it is not to be expected that there will be a single or uniform abnormality found in the kidneys of all patients who have suffered from gout, even when the renal disease is secondary to primary gout. Thus, the pathologic findings in the gouty kidney are varied and consist of a number of different features that may occur either alone or in combination. Published descriptions of renal pathology in gout also often fail to distinguish between the renal disease that develops in some patients with gout and the gout that develops in some patients with renal disease. Such a failure also contributes to the somewhat confusing picture of the renal disease in patients who suffer from gout.

It is clear, particularly from the studies of Sokoloff (1957) (118) and Talbott and Terplan (1960) (104), that the essential and characteristic feature of the pathology of the gouty kidney

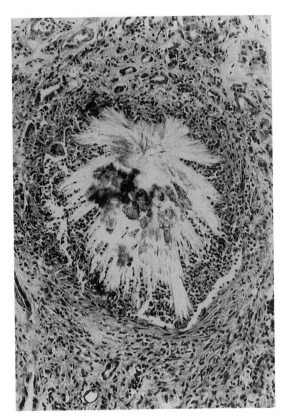

FIG. 77-6. A microtophus in the interstitium of the kidney with a central residuum of urate crystals, surrounded by spaces that once contained acicular crystals, together with an inflammatory infiltrate and giant-cell reaction. (Hematoxylin and eosin ×100.)

is the finding of acicular urate or uric acid crystals within the renal interstitium. These result in a cellular reaction that causes the formation of microtophi (Fig. 77-6) with resulting changes in the interstitial tissues and renal tubules.

The intratubular uric acid and urate deposits may result in tubular atrophy and eventually in nephron destruction. Likewise, the inflammatory response to the interstitial urate deposits may result in interstitial round-cell infiltration and peritubular fibrosis. Renal calculi, often consisting predominantly of uric acid, may be found in 10% to 20% of patients with gout. In addition, microcalculi formed within collecting ducts may cause their dilation. Such foreign material may predispose to secondary bacterial infection.

It is also clear that many subjects with gout suffer from prominent vascular nephrosclerosis, which in some subjects is aggravated by hypertension. Hypertension has been a frequent and early finding in patients with gout. Likewise, hyperlipidemia (chiefly hypertriglyceridemia) has been reported in over half the subjects with gout. Thus, changes within the blood vessels and renal changes attributed to ischemia and primary vascular disease have been prominent features of the kidney pathology in gouty subjects.

As discussed previously, two different types of crystal are formed within the kidney in gout. MSUM (or urate) is the characteristic long acicular crystal that indicates acute gout and tophus formation anywhere within the body. It tends to form at physiologic pH whenever urate saturation is exceeded and leads to a cellular response that varies with the site but most often results in a mononuclear and foreign body giant-cell reaction. On the other hand, uric acid forms only at an acid pH and therefore must precipitate initially within the lumen of a renal tubule (as in an acute uric acid nephropathy). The initial reaction to such a crystal occurs by tubular epithelial and histiocytic lining cells, which can sometimes ingest or digest it. However, larger amounts of crystals may cause tubular obstruction, which, if unrelieved, can cause loss of nephron function and its degeneration. These two varieties of crystal are not mutually exclusive and may occur together, but recognition of their differences helps clarify mechanisms. There is also evidence that intratubular uric acid crystals may disrupt tubular basement membranes and pass into the interstitium, where they may form a nidus on which further crystals may form and an interstitial microtophus may develop (88,119). Ultimately, a variable degree of chronic interstitial damage may develop, with loss of nephrons and dilation of tubules.

Superimposed on this primary crystal nephropathy are variable secondary manifestations, in the nature either of a bacterial infection or hypertensive and/or degenerative vascular disease (Fig. 77-7). The variety and relative frequency with which these features develop result in the variability seen in the renal pathology where the microscopic appearance of the kidney can vary from no detectable abnormality to irregularly scarred kidneys with granular surfaces containing white chalkish deposits within the parenchyma, particularly in the medulla.

The pathogenesis of the condition may be discussed by considering the various factors contributing to the pathologic changes, namely factors contributing to urate–uric acid crystal deposition, those contributing to vascular disease, and those promoting infection within the renal tract. The major factors determining the deposition of urate–uric acid in crystalline form are the local concentration at the site, the pH, and the presence or absence of solubilizing factors maintaining urate in solution. We know little about the concentrations of such substances in the renal interstitial fluid. However, one might expect that the concentration within the plasma might be an important determinant and, therefore, if there is a urate gradient increasing toward the medulla, the concentration of urate within the renal tubular lumen might also contribute. The risk of crystal deposition within the tubular fluid and urine will depend on the concentration of urate within the fluid, which will be dependent on both total urate excretion and the urine flow rate. Distal tubular fluid usually has a low pH as well; the factors predisposing to uric acid crystal formation within these tubules have already been discussed.

It is more difficult to determine the contribution of hypertensive and degenerative vascular disease to the nephropathy of gout, particularly as hypertension can be an early development in gout that may contribute to the nephropathy, and a nephropathy can be a cause of hypertension. Hyperuricemia has not been established as an independent risk factor for vascular disease, although it is a common association of many primary risk factors such as obesity, hypertension, and hyperlipidemia (89,120). Many of the exogenous factors that contribute to these risk factors also contribute to hyperuricemia. However, the hyperuricemia itself has no casual role in any associated vascular disease (120). Thus, exogenous risk factors for hypertension and vascular disease, if present, will contribute to any associated vascular disease in patients with gout and may thereby contribute to renal disease. Studies of platelet aggregation and adhesiveness in gout have not consistently shown any abnormality (121) and recent studies have not demonstrated any increased mortality from coronary or cerebrovascular disease in patients with gout or their families (120,122).

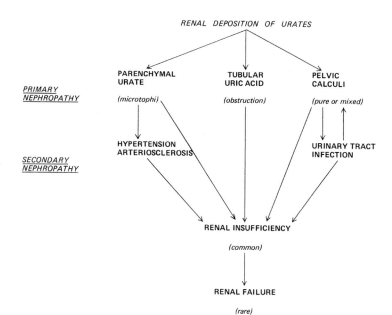

FIG. 77-7. Mechanisms whereby the different types of renal deposition of urate or uric acid can lead to the various pathologic findings in the kidneys of patients with gout. (From Emmerson BT. Gout, uric acid and renal disease. *Med J Aust* 1976;1:403. © 1976, The Medical Journal of Australia. Reproduced with permission.)

The presence of any foreign material within either the kidney or the urinary tract can predispose to the development and persistence of bacterial infection within a kidney. Thus, crystal formation at any site would increase the risk of superimposed infection. It does not seem to be a particular problem unless there is associated obstruction.

Clinical Features

As might be expected from the pathology and proposed pathogenesis, the clinical features of gouty renal disease are varied and somewhat unpredictable. Most patients with gout, especially if adequately treated with modern therapy, never develop renal disease attributable to the gout. Thus, renal disease is not a regular or necessary association of gouty arthritis. However, deterioration of renal function due to any associated vascular disease or aging may occur in any patient who has suffered from gout in the same way as it would had he or she never developed gout.

Nonetheless, in studies of large groups of patients with gout, some degree of renal disease is a fairly frequent finding in those with prolonged and untreated or inadequately treated gout. This is particularly so if the gout has been tophaceous and if the gouty arthritis has been prolonged and recurrent. In such patients, there is a rough correlation between the severity and duration of the gout and the severity of the renal disease. Yet, even in these patients, some of the renal disease is attributable to the associated hypertensive and vascular disease, particularly related to age changes. The risk factors for hypertensive and degenerative vascular disease are often ones that will promote hyperuricemia, and the risk of gout is proportional to the duration and severity of the hyperuricemia. When true gouty renal disease is present, however, the progression of the renal insufficiency may be quite intermittent, remaining nonprogressive for prolonged periods or showing only very slow deterioration.

In discussing gouty renal disease, one has to remember that gout is a dramatic clinical event that can usually be timed precisely, whereas the development of renal disease is usually asymptomatic in the early stages and difficult to date. Because of the great differences between patients, it is impossible to draw any conclusions concerning the risk of an individual patient with gout developing renal disease by any consideration of the frequency with which the various manifestations of renal disease can be seen in a group of patients with gout. An extensive review of many of the clinical features of gouty renal disease was undertaken by Barlow and Beilin in 1968 (107), who compared their 53 gouty patients with a review of 5,500 reported cases in the literature. It is noteworthy that they showed a 40% incidence of renal insufficiency in the 27 patients they investigated in detail, significantly higher than the 26% who had subcutaneous tophi. In 1970, Grahame and Scott (108) found hypertension in over half of their gouty patients and renal insufficiency with nitrogen retention in 25%. Of those with severe hypertension, half showed renal failure. Both hypertension and renal failure were more common in patients with a later age of onset of gout. They also identified another smaller group in whom renal failure and severe hypertension developed before the age of 20 years. In most patients, however, they found little, if any, deterioration in renal function with increasing duration of the gouty arthritis.

In view of the variability of the manifestations, only general comments can be made about the clinical features of gouty renal disease:

1. When gouty renal disease develops, patients have usually suffered from recurrent attacks of gout for a period of at least 10 years. Since the mean age of onset of gout is approximately 45 years, patients with gout nephropathy are usually about 55 years of age or more, a time when degenerative vascular disease may well be developing.
2. The development of proteinuria has been reported in between 20% and 50% of patients with gout and would usually signify renal damage. The presence of casts in the urine would support such a development.
3. A fall in the GFR beyond that which might be expected for age should alert the physician to the possible development of a gout nephropathy. Early studies suggested that the renal concentrating capacity was impaired prior to a reduction in glomerular function (100). However, more recent studies have not suggested any disproportionate impairment of concentrating capacity or evidence of other tubular dysfunction (112,113).
4. Hypertension is found twice as commonly in patients with gout as in matched normal controls (123). Such hypertension may be seen before any other evidence of renal impairment is apparent. However, precise measurements of renal glomerular function are rarely undertaken in the absence of nitrogen retention, and it is difficult to know whether the development of hypertension is an early sign of renal damage or whether it can occur prior to this and contribute to the renal insufficiency. It is not necessary to consider that hypertension, when present, is secondary to renal damage, although one might speculate concerning a possible contribution by renal microtophi.
5. Tophaceous deposits have been reported in 25% of the patients with gouty renal disease, a figure much higher than in the general group of patients with gout. Such a finding would be consistent with the hypothesis that the development of renal microtophi might also be determined by factors that confirm the formation of tophi elsewhere in the body and thereby explain the association of subcutaneous tophi with renal tophi and renal insufficiency.
6. Obesity, a common finding in many gouty patients, is reported to be present in at least half of those with gouty renal disease. It is not possible to indicate that the presence of obesity in a gouty subject increases the risk of developing renal disease, although it is associated with a higher incidence of hypertension and vascular disease.
7. The reported urolithiasis frequency of up to 15% of gouty subjects with renal disease would not be unexpected.
8. The coexistence of a vascular nephrosclerosis, a common biopsy finding in the renal disease of primary gout (107),

appears to be an important contributing factor to gout nephropathy. It is important therefore for the development of gout to be regarded as an indication that risk factors for vascular disease need to be examined and corrected when possible.

9. Although no definitive statement can be made concerning the degree of hyperuricemia associated with the development of renal disease, comparison with the risk of acute attacks of gout or tophus formation suggest that the risk is not significant at plasma urate concentrations below 0.6 mmol/L (10 mg/dL). The maintenance of a high urine flow rate may be more important in the prevention of gouty renal disease than any other therapy.

Management

The management of gouty renal disease is the same as that of all varieties of chronic renal disease with the added need to restore and maintain the serum urate within the normal range. Because patients with renal disease have a greater fall in the serum urate concentration with purine restriction than do patients without renal disease, moderate restriction of high-purine foods is desirable. A daily urine volume of at least 2 L should also be established. Maintenance of a normal serum urate can be achieved by either allopurinol or uricosuric drugs until significant renal insufficiency is present. Once significant renal failure is present (GFR less than 60 mL/minute), allopurinol is the drug of choice. The dose of allopurinol used should be the lowest that can maintain a normal serum urate concentration. The serum oxypurinol (the main metabolite of allopurinol) concentration for any dose level is proportional to the serum creatinine concentration, so that appropriate reductions below the usual dose level of 300 mg per day should be made in the presence of renal disease. The initial dose should be 50 mg per day, with 50-mg increments until the serum urate is controlled. As a rough guide, the dose should be 100 mg per day for every 30 mL/minute of glomerular filtration. Often a dose of 100 mg per day is sufficient. The chief risk from allopurinol is the development of an acute interstitial nephritis with rash, hepatitis, fever, and a lymphocytic and eosinophilic infiltration of the kidney with deteriorating renal function (124), which is potentially reversible. The risk of such an instance acute interstitial nephritis is increased by the use of the higher doses of allopurinol.

If hyperuricemia is not controlled with appropriate doses of allopurinol, correction of factors contributing to the hyperuricemia (such as a high-purine diet, alcohol consumption, the use of diuretics or other drugs tending to raise the serum urate, plasma volume contraction, or a suboptimal urine volume) should prevent further progression of renal insufficiency, provided hypertension can be adequately controlled and renal failure has not become advanced. If end-stage renal disease develops, hemodialysis will assist the allopurinol in controlling the hyperuricemia and other manifestations of renal failure (125). Renal transplantation is also effective, but any tendency to urate overproduction that might have contributed to the original development of the

renal failure should be controlled. The effect of azathioprine is greatly augmented by concurrent therapy with allopurinol, and the dose of azathioprine should be reduced to approximately 25% in such a situation.

Cyclosporine, the effect of which is not potentiated by allopurinol, might have been a useful alternative to azathioprine in transplant patients with gout. However, its use, either in transplant patients or in other conditions, is associated with a significant rise in the serum urate. This is attributable to an effect on proximal tubular transport of urate, together with some impairment of glomerular filtration (126–128). It usually remits promptly when the drug is withdrawn. The associated hyperuricemia may be sufficient to induce the development of secondary gout (129).

GOUT SECONDARY TO PRIMARY RENAL DISEASE

Most of the literature on this topic indicates that gout secondary to primary chronic renal disease is rare (130). Transplant registries record a diagnosis of gout in fewer than 1% of dialysis or transplant patients (131). However, a history of gout may not have been sought carefully and specifically in all of these patients. A recent study specifically directed at the frequency of gout in 200 patients with end-stage renal disease showed that 6% had suffered more than two attacks per year prior to maintenance dialysis (132) and that acute gout was rare in all dialysis patients. After transplantation, gout occurred principally in those receiving cyclosporine or diuretics (133), although a study from the Cleveland Clinic in 1999 reported a 23% frequency of gout in their long-term transplant patients (134). Gouty arthritis is not a frequent clinical problem in most patients with advanced renal failure, although the picture may well be different in the less severe and more chronic varieties of renal disease (135).

Gout may be simulated clinically by the acute inflammation caused by the deposition of crystals other than urate (MSUM). Thus, calcium pyrophosphate dihydrate (CPPD) deposition disease (often with chondrocalcinosis) which has been called "pseudo-gout" in its acute form, and hydroxyapatite ($Ca_{10}(PO4)_6OH$ or basic calcium phosphate, BCP) deposition disease may present with an acute calcific arthritis or periarthritis with calcific deposits radiologically. Thus, when an acute or chronic arthropathy occurs in a patient with renal insufficiency, it is important to define the nature of the crystals underlying the inflammation so that appropriate therapy can be targeted. This will usually require joint aspiration and examination of the synovial fluid. It is obviously of no value to correct hyperuricemia if the crystals causing the inflammation are CPPD or hydroxyapatite rather than urate (MSUM) (135a).

In considering this aspect, one needs to establish criteria to differentiate gout secondary to primary renal disease from renal disease that is secondary to primary gout. Two criteria should be helpful: (a) clear evidence of renal disease prior to the first attack of gouty arthritis, and (b) renal disease for which a specific diagnosis can be made with sufficient certainty to exclude gout nephropathy. This question was examined in 1965 by Richet and colleagues who reported 17 cases of gout secondary to chronic renal disease with renal insufficiency within the group of 1,600 patients in their nephrology service (136). Five of their cases had established renal failure, nine had compensated renal insufficiency with minimal nitrogen retention, and the remaining three cases had lead nephropathy. The Richet group then studied the clinical characteristics and nature of those nephropathies during the course of which gout had supervened. They noted that most of the nephropathies were very chronic and that hyperuricemia and nitrogen retention were of long duration. Additionally, they noted the frequent association with hypertension. All except the three patients with amyloidosis were hypertensive. These authors also postulated that renal amyloidosis was significantly associated with hyperuricemia and gout.

Twenty cases of gout considered to be secondary to chronic renal disease were also reported by Sorensen (137). Two demonstrated chronic glomerulonephritis and two had tubulointerstitial nephritis, but most of the other patients had a wide variety of renal diagnoses including arteriolar nephrosclerosis. In these patients, the author confirmed that urate production remained normal in the presence of progressive renal dysfunction despite a steady decrease in the percentage of urate excreted by the renal route. Urate balance was maintained by a proportionate increase in the nonrenal (alimentary) excretion of urate. An increasing proportion of filtered urate was excreted by each nephron as nephron numbers declined.

Another large study of 1,700 patients with gout revealed 253 with proteinuria or other evidence of renal disease (112). This group gives some indication of the pattern of renal disease currently seen in patients who present with both gout and renal disease. The serum urate concentration was significantly higher and the urinary urate excretion was significantly lower in the group with renal disease when compared to a group without renal disease. Of those with evidence of renal disease, hypertensive or arteriosclerotic vascular disease was the most common finding (45%), whereas 33% showed evidence of intrinsic chronic renal disease such as chronic glomerulonephritis, chronic pyelonephritis, or polycystic disease of the kidneys. The authors attributed to renal disease to long-standing tophaceous or fulminating gout in only 13% of the cases. In many of the patients the onset of the renal disease preceded that of gout by many years, and in these the recurrent acute gouty arthritis was infrequent and mild. In general, data from this report indicated that the great majority of patients with gout and renal insufficiency suffered from a nongouty intrinsic nephropathy, whereas relatively few cases of nephropathy were attributable to primary gout. Accordingly, the authors stressed the importance of considering the possibility, in patients with both gout and renal disease, of the renal disease being primary and the gout secondary.

A small group of gouty patients has recently been reported in whom primary renal disease was present at the time of, or before, their first attack of acute gout and in whom this renal disease was regarded as a major contributor to the development of gout (138). Patients with polycystic kidney disease or chronic lead nephropathy, or those who were receiving diuretics, were excluded from the study. In the remaining 12 patients, the degree of renal impairment was usually mild or moderate, the renal disease was of the tubulointerstitial rather than of the glomerular type, and the renal clearance of urate per unit of GFR (fractional excretion [FE] urate), rather than being increased as is usual in renal disease, was reduced, thus suggesting impairment of renal excretion of urate. Three-fourths of these patients were female and the common associations of gout, including regular alcohol consumption, obesity, and hypertension, were not prominent. The authors proposed that the intrinsic renal disease was a major contributor to their development of gout.

In determining whether renal disease may be the primary diagnosis with gout being a secondary development, three additional aspects need to be considered:

1. The effect of hypertension. It is clear that primary hypertension is not infrequently associated with hyperuricemia and is probably the cause thereof, possibly due to hypertensive renal vascular involvement (13). In addition, hypertension is a relatively common and early feature in many patients with gout; this hypertension is often recognized before significant nitrogen retention has developed. The mechanism whereby gouty patients develop hypertension is not well understood. In some it may be attributed to the associated development of vascular disease, whereas in others, an increase in renal renin production due to uric acid-induced renal damage has been neither established nor excluded.

2. The effect of diuretics. The ready availability and use of oral diuretic agents during the last 20 years has inevitably increased the incidence of hyperuricemia. This has happened both in patients with normal renal function and in patients with renal insufficiency. The degree of hyperuricemia resulting from these diuretics can vary considerably; in some cases the increase is only slight whereas in others the increase may be considerable. The frequent use of diuretics in patients with hypertension and renal disease would have contributed to an increased frequency of hyperuricemia in such patients, and this might have been expected to have increased the frequency with which gout would develop.

3. The presence of plasma volume depletion in patients with renal failure will promote renal tubular reabsorption of urate and the development of hyperuricemia. Thus, in any patient with chronic renal disease, the existence of volume depletion will increase tubular reabsorption of urate and result in an increase in the serum urate. In some, this state is a chronic one and such patients may be persistently hyperuricemic to a much greater extent than would be expected

from their glomerular function. Thus, the association between any particular type of chronic renal disease and gout may depend on its management and whether volume contraction is established or prevented (21,22,139).

Each of these aspects must therefore be considered in relation to any patient with gout secondary to primary renal disease because each will modify the degree and duration of hyperuricemia, which are probably the most important factors in determining whether or not gouty arthritis supervenes.

Specific Varieties of Renal Disease Associated with an Increased Incidence of Gouty Arthritis

Chronic Lead Nephropathy

For centuries lead poisoning has been thought to predispose to the development of gouty arthritis (140), and many of the old ideas of the association of alcohol with gout may have been due in part to its contamination with lead. Even Garrod in *A Treatise on Gout and Rheumatic Gout* (96), published in 1876, emphasized the high incidence of lead intoxication in gouty subjects. Since that time, there have been a number of reports of groups of persons with prolonged lead intoxication who suffered from gout. Thus, chronic lead nephropathy is now one of the best-documented varieties of chronic renal disease that is associated with the development of gout. In some series, 50% of patients with chronic lead nephropathy have a history of gouty arthritis. In this condition, the diagnosis of primary renal disease can be established unequivocally, and in many cases there is good evidence that the renal disease was present prior to the development of gout. Recent evidence has come from three countries: chronic lead nephropathy in Queensland, Australia, following childhood lead poisoning; "moonshine" drinkers in the southern United States; and studies of persons with industrial lead exposure in Paris and in the United States.

In the early years of the twentieth century, many children in Queensland developed lead poisoning due to the prolonged ingestion of flakes of lead paint. In some of these children, renal damage, which was not necessarily recognized, developed during this acute phase. After intervals of between 10 and 30 years, many presented with clinical features of chronic renal failure, by which time no overt signs of lead intoxication were present. This particular variety of nephropathy has a particularly slow rate of progression and unusual chronicity. The high frequency of gout was noted in many who had survived 10 to 20 years or more (141). In these subjects, the excessive storage of lead was confirmed by an increased renal excretion of lead following a standardized infusion of calcium ethylenediaminetetraacetic acid (calcium EDTA), although there were at that time no continuing signs of lead intoxication. The amount of lead excreted after the calcium EDTA increased with the degree of renal failure, and it appeared that the associated secondary hyperparathyroidism was an important contributing factor in this result by mobilizing lead stored in bone. Renal failure itself delayed the excretion of the lead

EDTA complex but did not increase the lead excretion in patients with renal failure not due to lead. An alternative index of bone lead can now be obtained *in vivo* and without invasion by measuring x-ray fluorescence of the phalanges.

An association between gout and the drinking of moonshine contaminated with lead was reported in the southern United States in the 1960s (142). In most of these patients, persisting signs of lead intoxication, in terms of alterations of hemoglobin and porphyrin metabolism, could still be detected, and a chronic nephropathy could be demonstrated.

The potential for industrial lead exposure and excessive absorption of lead to be associated with a nephropathy and gout was also emphasized about this time (136,143,144) in Paris in a group of lead workers with chronic renal disease, some of whom had also developed gout. More recently, the potential role of lead in the etiology of renal failure and gout has been studied in a variety of patients in whom past lead exposure was uncertain and acute signs of lead intoxication were lacking (145–147). Using the EDTA test to indicate excessive past lead absorption and storage, unrecognized excessive lead absorption was identified in patients with renal insufficiency who presented clinically with either hypertension or gout (148). These studies have suggested that many patients with both gout and renal disease, who might otherwise have been diagnosed as having gouty renal disease, may well be suffering from a primary renal disease in the form of chronic lead nephropathy with secondary gout (149).

However, more than an association between excessive lead absorption, renal disease, and gout is required for a diagnosis of chronic lead nephropathy. A lead worker who also reported a heavy consumption of alcohol and who developed chronic glomerulonephritis might well show evidence of excessive lead absorption, chronic renal disease, and gout, all of which would, in this case, be etiologically unrelated. A diagnosis of chronic lead nephropathy implies an etiologic relationship between the lead and the renal disease, and the feasibility of such a relationship ultimately requires epidemiologic studies if it is to be proved. In Queensland, this relationship has been established by the demonstration of an increased renal mortality in patients who suffered from lead poisoning in childhood, by the demonstration of an increased death rate from chronic renal failure some years after the lead poisoning, and by the demonstration of increased bone lead stores in patients dying with renal failure not due to any of the recognized varieties of chronic renal disease (150). The pathology and pathogenesis of this chronic lead nephropathy have been described (151). The clinical requirements for a diagnosis of chronic lead nephropathy in such patients include, in addition to definite evidence of excessive past lead absorption, the presence of bilaterally and equally contracted kidneys, chronic renal failure of long-standing and slow progression, and the exclusion as far as possible of any other variety of chronic renal disease. A search for an unrecognized lead etiology in patients receiving dialysis in Europe and the United States has suggested excessive lead stores in approximately 5% (152).

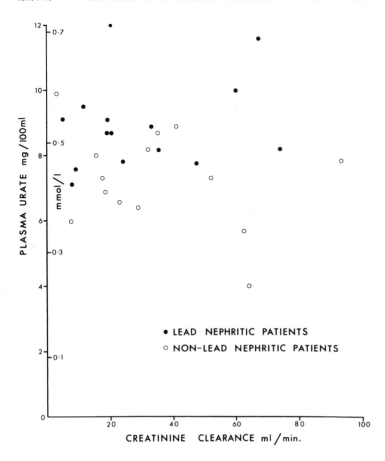

FIG. 77-8. Plasma urate concentrations after stabilization on a low-purine diet in relation to the creatinine clearance, showing the higher mean concentrations in patients with chronic lead nephropathy in comparison with a group with renal disease not due to lead.

Industrially, it has been more difficult to undertake the necessary epidemiologic studies to establish a relationship between lead exposure and impairment of renal function. In part, this has been because the risk is relatively low and the necessary duration of exposure (at levels currently seen in industrial processes) needs to be prolonged for up to 20 years. Extensive follow-up study of such lead workers has been reviewed by Ritz and associates (153) in several independent studies from countries as different as Romania, Spain, and the United States, all of which led to the conclusion that occupational lead exposure can cause impairment of renal function. However, such exposures appeared generally to exceed those currently existing in industry in developed countries. Only careful future studies will confirm this possibility, but it is interesting to consider the finding in a group of London civil servants without known industrial exposure that there was a slight rise in the serum creatinine concentration with each increment in blood lead concentration, suggesting that lead accumulation may slightly impair renal function (154). No influence on blood pressure was seen.

Even more controversial is any possible effect of low-level lead exposure on blood pressure. Evidence on this subject has been critically reviewed (153,155) and regarded as being consistent with an etiologic association. These studies suggest that it is mediated by a direct effect of lead on the arteriole, possibly secondary to intracellular alterations in calcium metabolism.

The mechanism to account for the high frequency of gout in chronic lead nephropathy has also been studied. In the Queensland cases, at all levels of renal function, the mean serum urate concentration in patients with chronic lead nephropathy was higher than that for patients whose renal disease was not caused by lead (Fig. 77-8). This has been the general experience in other studies as well. Urine uric acid values are particularly low in chronic lead nephropathy, and the disproportionate hyperuricemia is attributable to lower urate clearances in relation to corresponding creatinine clearances (156,157). In seeking the mechanism for this reduced urate clearance, studies using the pyrazinamide suppression test suggested that there was excessive tubular reabsorption of urate (158). Detailed study of urate kinetics in moonshine drinkers also demonstrated renal underexcretion of urate (156), and the French patients with chronic industrial lead intoxication also showed a selective impairment of renal excretion of urate (144). Thus, despite the various pathogenic mechanisms in the different varieties of chronic lead nephropathy, it appears that each variety exhibits a common specific impairment of urate excretion.

The Clinical Differentiation of Lead Gout from Primary Gout

The clinical findings in a group of patients with chronic lead nephropathy in Queensland were compared with those in another group of gouty patients in whom there had been no lead exposure (159). The lead gout group contained proportionately more women, half of whom were premenopausal. The lead gout group also showed a higher incidence of euphoria and mild mental impairment (possible sequelae of acute lead encephalopathy) together with renal disease and hypertension in the siblings (possibly unrecognized lead nephropathy). The number of attacks of gout and their severity was less in the lead gout group, whereas the primary gout group showed an increased frequency of regular alcohol consumption, obesity, and renal calculi. Tophi were present equally in both primary gout and lead gout, so that, although the gout was often less troublesome in lead nephropathy in many cases, urate retention and deposition were considerable. Evidence of renal disease prior to the first attack of gouty arthritis was present in half of these lead gout cases. These findings, together with the fact that significant renal disease was invariably present, should alert one to a possible underlying lead nephropathy in such patients. More recent studies in Italy have confirmed the value of seeking a lead etiology in patients with both gout and renal disease (160).

Polycystic Disease of the Kidneys

Gout has been reported in 25% to 35% of small groups of patients with adult polycystic kidneys (161–163). Because this implies an abnormality of renal handling of urate, urate homeostasis was studied in large groups of patients with adult polycystic kidney disease, especially at the stage before glomerular insufficiency developed (164). It was also compared with that in other family members without polycystic kidney disease. In this extensive study, no greater degree of hyperuricemia or impairment of urate excretion was demonstrated in the patients with polycystic kidney disease. However, the prevalence of gouty arthritis in these patients was not recorded, so that, while there is unequivocal evidence of normal renal handling of urate in this condition, the reason for the reported association with gout is not clear. Further study is needed of the specific prevalence of gouty arthritis in such patients with reduced filtration rates and of whether any gout from which they suffer is attributable to causes other than the kidney disease itself.

Amyloid Disease of the Kidney

This relatively uncommon variety of chronic renal disease was reported in 3 of 17 cases of primary renal disease with superimposed gout by Richet and associates in 1965 (136). They postulated defective renal elimination of urate as the cause. Their three subjects with amyloid nephropathy were the only ones in their series without hypertension, a fact that they attributed to concomitant involvement of the adrenal glands and the fact that hyperuricemia is common after adrenalectomy for arterial hypertension (perhaps the associated volume contraction would also contribute). They also noted that Talbott and Terplan (1960) (104) had included four cases of renal amyloidosis among the 190 gouty patients they studied at autopsy and questioned whether, in these cases, the gout was not more likely to be secondary to a primary amyloid nephropathy, rather than the renal amyloidosis being a sequel to primary gout.

Medullary Cystic Disease of the Kidneys

Three families with medullary cystic disease who presented with the early onset of hyperuricemia and gout have been described. In some of these cases, the hyperuricemia and gout antedated clinical evidence of renal failure by several years (165,166). However, the diagnosis of medullary cystic disease may be a difficult one while the patient is still living, and in the first family (166) typical gout had developed before the age of 20 years and had been present for many years before there was evidence of renal disease. At autopsy the kidneys were atrophic with granular surfaces, thin cortices, and multiple medullary cysts. Microscopically the characteristic hyaline sheathing of tubules and collecting ducts together with severe interstitial and glomerular scarring was found. There were no renal urate deposits. In one member, who developed acute podagra at the age of 20 years and who died in renal failure at the age of 38, a renal biopsy was undertaken at the age of 26 years. This showed patchy tubular atrophy, interstitial fibrosis, and scattered fibrotic glomeruli, and hyaline connective tissue sheathing of tubules was seen in some areas. Two children of an affected mother were hyperuricemic but showed no abnormality of glomerular or tubular function. The only abnormality detected in them was a reduced urate clearance (4% and 6% of creatinine clearance). Further follow-up of their renal function is needed.

In the second family, medullary cystic disease was diagnosed at ages that ranged between 4 and 32 years, with the age at death or commencement of dialysis ranging between 7 and 48 years (165). Burke and colleagues (165) believed that medullary cystic disease cannot be differentiated from juvenile nephrophthisis by the age of onset and the type of inheritance. These authors suggested that medullary cystic disease and juvenile nephrophthisis were essentially different manifestations of the same condition, which should best be classified as medullary cystic disease with either autosomal-dominant or autosomal-recessive inheritance. Three patients in this family presented with gout. Histologically, medullary cysts up to 5 mm in diameter were found with occasional similar cysts in the cortex. Most glomeruli were sclerosed and many showed periglomerular fibrosis that was present even in some in whom the glomerular tuft was normal. This report included details of the parent of a child with renal failure from medullary cystic disease who showed histologic evidence of medullary cystic disease at a time when renal function was normal. Such a key finding illustrates how easy it would be to wrongly attribute a renal lesion to hyperuricemia and gout because of the difficulty of establishing a firm alternative diagnosis. The diagnosis of medullary cystic disease is a difficult one in a living patient and even on renal biopsy, although computerized tomography of the kidney may prove useful in elucidating this problem. The third family, recently reported, was a large family from Cypriot. The members of this family presented with hyperuricemia and gout, hypertension, and medullary cysts, and progressed to end-stage renal failure in their early sixties. They did not show the same linkage markers as the other families studied (167).

These case reports need to be remembered when one reads reports of so-called familial urate nephropathy that show patients in whom the first symptom is gout and who later develop renal disease, the nature of which is not able to be diagnosed with certainty. For want of a better causative agent, the renal disease may be attributed to the associated hyperuricemia (168). There may well be many varieties of familial and primary nephropathy yet to be clearly defined, which, like medullary cystic disease, can predispose to the later development of gout.

Unusual Familial Nephropathies

There are many reports of unusual varieties of familial nephropathy associated with a high incidence of hyperuricemia and gout. The renal disease appears to involve tubular atrophy and interstitial fibrosis and has been classified as one of the hereditary degenerative renal diseases (169). The nature of this disease is difficult to determine with certainty, but a careful consideration of all aspects suggested that the renal disease was the primary phenomenon and the gout was secondary. A similar conclusion was drawn by Leumann and Wegmann (1983) concerning their familial nephropathy (170). They regarded the family they studied as having a primary tubulointerstitial nephropathy, inherited as a dominant character, with a defect in tubular excretion of urate resulting in hyperuricemia and gout.

The mechanism for the hyperuricemia and gout in some of these families has been established recently by the demonstration of a reduced urate clearance relative to the creatinine clearance (FE urate) (138,171). Although urinary urate excretion in absolute terms decreases with advancing renal failure, the amount excreted per nephron (reflected by the FE urate) actually rises. Accordingly, the demonstration of a low FE urate (less than 7%) in many of these patients can be taken to reflect a greater degree of impairment of renal excretion of urate, which could contribute to the hyperuricemia and gout. In some of these young patients, the low FE urate is detectable prior to the impairment of glomerular function and this has caused the condition to be referred to as *familial juvenile hyperuricemic nephropathy* (172). However, the renal disease as described is not due to urate or uric acid crystal deposits so that it is difficult to classify it as a gouty or hyperuricemic nephropathy. It fits best with the group of familial nephropathies with secondary hyperuricemia and gout.

Other Varieties of Renal Disease Predisposing to Gout

Hyperuricemia and gout have been described as complications of Bartter's syndrome and found to be due to a reduced renal clearance of urate (173). This reduced excretion of urate has been attributed to the coincident alkalosis, but the associated hypovolemia may provide a more ready explanation. The finding of gout in 24% of 30 patients with cystinuria also suggests an association between these conditions (174).

A high incidence of gout has been found in patients with analgesic nephropathy (175), and such a chronic nonprogressive type of renal disease may well be one that could be associated with prolonged hyperuricemia and the later development of gout. Bilateral hydronephrosis due to an obstructive uropathy is also associated with a reduced urate clearance and prolonged hyperuricemia and gout in some cases (176). Such suggestions support a concept that lesions that predominantly affect the renal tubules, or renal diseases that particularly affect the distal nephron, may be those that are more prone to be associated with undue hyperuricemia. Whether it is the duration of the hyperuricemia or the degree of hyperuricemia that is more important in the development of gout cannot be determined; most likely it is a combination of both. However, the concept of a distal nephron-type of disease as one commonly associated with gout needs to be explored further.

Serum urate concentrations exceeding 0.6 mmol/L (10 mg/dL) in patients with chronic renal failure are often referred to rather loosely as "disproportionate hyperuricemia." Such an observation might suggest that the underlying renal disease was one of those known to predispose to gout. However, in an individual patient, many factors other than the nature of the renal disease will determine the serum urate. These include the purine content of the diet, the urine flow rate, the blood pressure, drug treatment, and the presence or absence of plasma volume contraction. Each of these needs to be controlled if disproportionate hyperuricemia is to be claimed. A table in an article by Bulpitt (177) gives the theoretical upper limit of the average serum urate concentrations for hypertensive patients according to sex and the plasma urea concentration and whether or not the patient is receiving a thiazide diuretic. Nonetheless, a claim of disproportionate hyperuricemia is a difficult one to document if it is taken to imply the likelihood of a particular type of renal pathology.

Renal Medullary Microtophi

The finding of medullary microtophi at autopsy in the kidneys of patients who had never suffered from gout is also relevant to this consideration. Verger and coworkers (1967), who were responsible for highlighting this problem (178), described 17 patients (13 of whom had never suffered from articular gout) with medullary microtophi identical to those observed in primary gout. All of the patients had died of chronic renal failure, due to either interstitial nephritis, glomerulonephritis, vascular nephropathy, polycystic kidneys, or of undetermined nature. They also found medullary tophi in only half of those who had suffered from articular gout and who had died with renal failure. In most of these cases, the uric acid–urate appeared to have been deposited principally within the lumina of collecting ducts, but some of them were interstitial. There was invariably a tissue reaction to these deposits, which indicated that they were not a terminal development. All of the patients had been hyperuricemic in life and the authors queried whether these microtophi, although clearly not the cause, might have accelerated the patient's death. Similar findings were reported by Ostberg (179).

Subsequently, medullary microtophi were reported in 8% of 1,733 unselected autopsies in Brisbane, Australia (180). The larger microtophi were entirely interstitial, whereas some of the smaller urate deposits appeared to have become interstitial from a primary intratubular site. These authors compared the clinical features of these patients with medullary microtophi with those of a matched control group. Significant associations were demonstrated between the medullary microtophi and a history of gouty arthritis and the presence of preexisting, apparently primary, renal disease. However, it was noteworthy that the kidneys were otherwise completely normal in 25% of the cases in which medullary microtophi were found at autopsy, and no clear explanation for this was revealed. Moreover, some of the kidneys studied had come from previously healthy people who had died acutely and been subject to coroner's autopsies undertaken at the Institute of Forensic Pathology. Significantly greater nitrogen retention had been present in the group with medullary microtophi. However, the plasma urate concentration had not been significantly increased in this group over the control group.

These important findings bring up many unanswered questions, particularly about the causation of these medullary microtophi in otherwise normal subjects, as well as questions of whether they have any adverse effect on renal function, what their significance is, and if they indicate the need for therapy. In considering possible explanations for their development, one notes their association with gout and with primary renal disease, but also notices their lack of constant association with either gout or renal disease, which suggests that neither of these is an essential prerequisite. The problem has been discussed in detail by Linnane, Burry, and Emmerson (1981) (180), and the hypothesis was proposed that the dominant factors determining the formation of microtophi are the local intrarenal conditions at the site of the original crystal formation within the kidney. Gouty patients might, at times, have a high urate concentration within either the renal tubules or renal interstitium that might facilitate urate crystal formation. Patients with renal insufficiency have an increased urate excretion per nephron, so that high urate concentrations may again occur within tubular lumina. This explanation attributes the most important role in their development to the urine concentration of urate. The importance of urine flow rate was also supported by the finding of a negative association between the presence of microtophi and diabetes, in that this suggested that the polyuria of diabetes might be protective against the development of microtophi. A high tubular fluid flow rate has already been shown to be the most important protective mechanism against intratubular crystal formation both in patients with an acute uric acid nephropathy and experimentally in animals with severe overexcretion of urate. In this regard, it is worth emphasizing that the aforementioned studies of renal microtophi were done in patients living in a subtropical climate, and renal calculi have been shown to be more frequent in these areas than in colder climates (181).

Inevitably, these findings pose the question of whether allopurinol should be used more often in patients with hyperuricemia, gout, and renal disease. There is little doubt that allopurinol treatment of patients with gout and renal disease is justified. However, in patients with hyperuricemia alone, the use of allopurinol may cause additional problems that may counterbalance any benefit. First, its use in patients with renal disease is associated with an increased incidence of acute interstitial nephritis that may prove fatal. Second, while allopurinol reduces the concentration of urate, it increases the concentration of hypoxanthine and xanthine, and both of these, especially xanthine, may have their own solubility problems. Intratubular deposits containing both uric acid and hypoxanthine have been reported in newborn infants who suffered from anoxia; these have disappeared when adequate hydration was given (182). Accordingly, it seems likely that the best method of preventing the development of medullary microtophi is to constantly maintain a high tubular fluid flow.

It is difficult to further extend our understanding of the significance of these renal microtophi because their inaccessibility makes diagnosis during life extremely difficult. It would clearly be better to avoid their development, and yet their finding in apparently healthy subjects makes any drug prophylaxis impractical. A more widespread appreciation of the problem may facilitate a serendipitous solution.

Management

Patients with chronic renal disease who develop gouty arthritis should have their serum urate concentration restored to within the normal range and maintained there. This will involve maintenance of a high urine volume (preferably exceeding 2 L/24 hours), the correction of treatable causes for hyperuricemia, and, if significant hyperuricemia persists, the use of a drug to lower the serum urate. The potential complications from the use of allopurinol in the presence of renal disease have already been discussed (see "Management" in the "Renal Disease Secondary to Primary Gout (Gout Nephropathy)," earlier in this chapter), and similar considerations apply when the gout is secondary to the renal disease. The chief precaution is to keep the dose of allopurinol as low as possible, consistent with maintenance of a normal serum urate. If a dose of greater than 100 mg of allopurinol per day for every 30 mL per minute of GFR is not sufficient to normalize the serum urate, greater effort should be directed toward correcting any possible factor causing or contributing to the hyperuricemia (vide infra). If this does not normalize the serum urate, a potent uricosuric such as sulfinpyrazone may need to be added.

There is less uncertainty concerning the management of the asymptomatic hyperuricemia of chronic renal disease. A controlled trial has shown that the rate of progression of renal disease was no different in a group of patients with preexisting renal disease who were treated with allopurinol from an untreated control group (183). However, in that study, none of the subjects had been severely hyperuricemic and most serum urates were less than 0.6 mmol/L (10 mg/dL). Moreover, such a study could not have assessed the development of medullary microtophi in either group. Nonetheless, one would avoid drug treatment in hyperuricemic patients without gout in whom the usual serum urate is less than 0.6 mmol/L (10 mg/dL). However, that does not mean that the hyperuricemia should be ignored because, as already outlined, many of the causes of such renal hyperuricemia may be correctable. Such correctable factors include plasma volume contraction, an inadequate urine volume, the unnecessary use of drugs that promote hyperuricemia such as oral diuretics, inadequately treated hypertension, a high-purine diet, and regular alcohol consumption. Correction of these will usually lower the serum urate in patients with chronic renal insufficiency. However, it is easy to overlook the considerable benefit that may follow the restriction of high-purine foods and limitation of heavy alcohol consumption. Even severe hyperuricemia (greater than 0.6 mmol/L [10 mg/dL]) will usually respond to modest dietary modification and correction of the causes of hyperuricemia that have been mentioned previously. Should asymptomatic hyperuricemia greater than this become persistent and unresponsive to modification of causative features, low-dose allopurinol could be considered because of the potential risk of asymptomatic urate crystal deposition and the incompleteness of our understanding of its etiology. If correctable factors are first sought, however, such severe hyperuricemia will be persistent in very few patients.

THE CLINICAL DIFFERENTIATION OF PRIMARY GOUT FROM PRIMARY RENAL DISEASE IN PATIENTS WITH BOTH GOUT AND RENAL DISEASE

Because of the difficulty of determining whether patients with both renal disease and gout suffer from primary gout with secondary renal disease or primary renal disease with secondary gout, a group of patients with both renal disease and gout were studied (184). Patients with lead nephropathy were excluded and patients were then separated into two groups using the single criterion of whether the gout or the renal disease occurred first. The gout-first group consisted of patients in whom there was evidence that gout was present before any renal disease, and the renal disease-first group consisted of patients in whom there was clear evidence of renal disease being present prior to the first attack of gout. Because gout is dramatically symptomatic and renal disease is often asymptomatic, the finding that gout occurs first does not necessarily indicate the absence of renal disease at that time, especially knowing that the presence of minor degrees of renal disease may be difficult to establish without extensive investigation. Despite this limitation, it was thought that comparison of these groups might yield features that would be clinically useful in determining the primary process.

The gout-first group contained significantly more men, and the age of the patients at the time of the survey was significantly greater. The age of onset of the renal disease was also significantly different: 50 years in the gout-first group and 30 years in the renal disease-first group. The age of onset of the gout was approximately 40 years in each group. Thus, the renal disease-first group tended to develop renal disease at the age of 30 years and their gout some 10 years later, whereas the gout-first group first developed their gout at the age of 40 years, with renal disease supervening some 10 years later. Tophi were found only in the gout-first group. (It should be noted that the absence of tophi from this particular renal disease-first group was significantly different from the findings in patients with chronic lead nephropathy.)

The most dramatic difference, however, was in the number of attacks of gout suffered. The renal disease-first group had suffered on average only three attacks of gout, whereas the gout-first group had suffered an average of 50 attacks of gout; between 20 and 30 of these attacks occurred during the 10-year period before the renal disease was detected. By contrast, the renal disease-first group had been known to have renal disease for an average of 11 years (range 4 to 22 years) prior to the development of gout. Gout was more extensive and severe in the gout-first group and a moderately heavy alcohol consumption was more frequent. The factors contributing to the renal disease in the renal disease-first group included urinary tract infection, analgesic nephropathy, polycystic kidney disease, and essential hypertension. Of these, the dominant associated pathology in the gout-first group appeared to be essential hypertension.

In summary, two distinct symptom complexes emerge from this study. The patients in the gout-first group were older and suffered from more severe gout, as evidenced by the number of attacks, the more frequent tophi, and the more extensive joint involvement. Renal disease tended to be asymptomatic and to develop only after many attacks of gout over many years. By contrast, the renal disease-first group had usually suffered from renal disease for about 10 years before developing their first attack of gout, and the gout was less severe both in the number of attacks and in the joints involved. The relative mildness and infrequency of the gout in chronic renal disease and the fact that it needs to be sought specifically may be contributing to the relative infrequency with which gout has been recognized in patients with chronic renal disease.

Not all patients with gout and renal disease will be able to be classified by these procedures. However, if we are to advance our understanding of this problem, it is important that, when evidence is insufficient to decide unequivocally whether renal disease is caused by hyperuricemia and/or gout or whether they are secondary to the renal disease, the case or family is not reported as an example of renal disease due to hyperuricemia, urate, or gout (185,186). It is also important that we do not overlook a potentially treatable cause of renal dysfunction (187,188).

REFERENCES

1. Kippen I, et al. Factors affecting urate solubility in vitro. *Ann Rheum Dis* 1974;33:313.
2. Brøchner-Mortensen K, Cobb S, Rose BS. Report of Subcommittee on Criteria for the Diagnosis of Gout in Surveys. In: Kellgren JH, Jeffrey MR, Ball J, eds. *The epidemiology of chronic rheumatism.* Oxford: Blackwell, 1963:295.
3. Emmerson BT. *Hyperuricaemia and gout in clinical practice.* Sydney: ADIS Health Science Press, 1983.
4. Kelley WN, et al. A specific enzyme defect in gout associated with overproduction of uric acid. *Proc Natl Acad Sci USA* 1967;57:1735.
5. Talbott JH. Solid and liquid nourishment in gout. *Semin Arthritis Rheum* 1981;11:288.
6. Fox IH. Adenosine triphosphate degradation in specific disease. *J Lab Clin Med* 1985;106:101.
7. Nugent CA, Tyler FH. The renal excretion of uric acid in patients with gout and non-gouty subjects. *J Clin Invest* 1959;38:1890.
8. Rieselbach RE, et al. Diminished renal urate secretion per nephron as a basis for primary gout. *Ann Intern Med* 1970;73:359.
9. Seegmiller JE, et al. The renal excretion of uric acid in gout. *J Clin Invest* 1962;41:1094.
10. Lathem W, Rodnan GP. Impairment of uric acid excretion in gout. *J Clin Invest* 1962;41:1955.
11. Tykarski A. Evaluation of renal handling of uric acid in essential hypertension: hyperuricemia related to decreased urate secretion. *Nephron* 1991;59:364.
12. Cappuccio RP, Iacone R, Strazzullo P. Serum uric acid and proximal sodium excretion: an independent association in man (the Olivetti study). *J Hypertens* 1991;9[Suppl 6]:S280.
13. Messerli FH, et al. Serum uric acid in essential hypertension: an indicator of renal vascular involvement. *Ann Intern Med* 1980;93:817.
14. Knorr BA, Beck JC, Abramson RG. Classical and channel-like urate transporters in rabbit renal brush border membranes. *Kidney Int* 1994;45:727.
15. Knorr BA, et al. Isolation and immunolocalization of a rat renal cortical membrane urate transporter. *J Biol Chem* 1994;269:6759.
16. Polkowski CA, Grassl SM. Uric acid transport in rat renal basolateral membrane vesicles. *Biochim Biophys Acta* 1993;1146:145.
17. Kahn AM, Weinman EJ. Urate transport in the proximal tubule: in vivo and vesicle studies. *Am J Physiol* 1985;249:F789.
18. Yu TF, et al. Effect of sodium lactate infusion on urate clearance in man. *Proc Soc Exp Biol Med* 1957;96:809.
19. Scott JT, McCallum FM, Holloway VP. Starvation, ketosis and uric acid excretion. *Clin Sci* 1964;27:209.
20. Ferris TF, Gorden P. Effect of angiotensin and norepinephrine upon urate clearance in man. *Am J Med* 1968;44:359.
21. Steele TH. Evidence for altered renal urate reabsorption during changes in volume of the extra-cellular fluid. *J Lab Clin Med* 1969;74:288.
22. Weinman EJ, Eknoyan G, Suki WN. The influence of the extracellular fluid volume on the tubular reabsorption of uric acid. *J Clin Invest* 1975;55:283.
23. Brochner-Mortensen K. Uric acid in blood and urine. *Acta Med Scand* 1937;84[Suppl]:132.
24. Ter Maaten JC, Voorburg A, Heine RJ, et al. Renal handling of urate and sodium during acute physiological hyperinsulinaemia in healthy subjects. *Clin Sci* 1997;92:51.
25. Reaven GM. The kidney: an unwilling accomplice in syndrome X. *Am J Kidney Dis* 1997;30:928.
26. Gutman AB, Yu T-F. Renal function in gout. *Am J Med* 1957;23:600.
27. Emmerson BT, Nagel SL, Duffy DL, et al. Genetic control of the renal clearance of urate: a study of twins *Ann Rheum Dis* 1992;51:375.
28. Hardwell TR, et al. The binding of urate to plasma proteins determined by four different techniques. *Clin Chim Acta* 1983;133:75.
29. Steele TH. Urate secretion in man: the pyrazinamide suppression test. *Ann Intern Med* 1973;79:734.
30. Cannon PJ, Symchych PS, Demartini FE. The distribution of urate in human and primate kidney. *Proc Soc Exp Biol Med* 1968;129:278.
31. Epstein FH, Pigeon G. Experimental urate nephropathy: studies of the distribution of urate in renal tissue. *Nephron* 1964;1:144.
32. Roch-Ramel F, Werner D, Guisan B. Urate transport in brush-border membrane of human kidney. *Am J Physiol* 1994;266:F797.
33. Roch-Ramel F, Guisan B, Diezi J. Effects of uricosuric and antiuricosuric agents on urate transport in human brush-border membrane vesicles. *J Pharm Exp Therapeutics* 1997;280:839.
34. Steele TH, Rieselbach RE. The renal mechanism for urate homeostasis in normal man. *Ann J Med* 1967;43:868.
35. Holmes EW, Kelley WN, Wyngaarden JB. The kidney and uric acid excretion in man. *Kidney Int* 1972;2:115.
36. Levinson DJ, Decker DE, Sorensen LB. Renal handling of uric acid in man. *Ann Clin Lab Sci* 1982;12:73.
37. Diamond HS. Interpretation of pharmacologic manipulation of urate transport in man. *Nephron* 1989;51:1.
38. McPhaul JJ. Hyperuricemia and urate excretion in chronic renal disease. *Metabolism* 1968;17:430.
39. Steele TH, Rieselbach RE. The contribution of residual nephrons within the chronically diseased kidney to urate homeostasis in man. *Am J Med* 1967;43:876.
40. Magoula I, et al. Single kidney function: early and late changes in urate transport after nephrectomy. *Kidney Int* 1992;41:1349.
41. Rieselbach RE, Steele TH. Intrinsic renal disease leading to abnormal urate excretion. *Nephron* 1975;14:81.
42. Danovitch GM. Uric acid transport in renal failure. A review. *Nephron* 1972;9:291.
43. Vaziri ND, Freel RW, Hatch M. Effect of chronic experimental renal insufficiency on urate metabolism. *J Am Soc Nephrol* 1995;6:1313.
44. Reif MC, Constantiner A, Levitt MF. Chronic gouty nephropathy: a vanishing syndrome? *N Engl J Med* 1981;304:535.
45. Johnson RJ, Kivlighn SD, Kim YG, et al. Reappraisal of the pathogenesis and consequences of hyperuricemia in hypertension, cardiovascular disease, and renal disease. *Am J Kidney Dis* 1999;33:225.
46. Brandenberger E, DeQuervain F, Schinz HR. Zur frage der natur der ablagerungen in den gichtnoten. *Schweiz Med Wochenschr* 1947;77:642.
47. Howell RR, Eanes ED, Seegmiller JE. X-ray diffraction studies of the tophaceous deposits in gout. *Arthritis Rheum* 1963;6:97.
48. Prien EL, Frondel C. Studies in urolithiasis: I. The composition of urinary calculi. *J Urol* 1955;57:949.
49. Seegmiller JE, Frazier PD. Biochemical considerations of the renal damage of gout. *Ann Rheum Dis* 1966;25:668.
50. Seegmiller JE, Rosenbloom FM, Kelley WN. Enzyme defect associated with a sex-linked human neurological disorder and excessive purine synthesis. *Science* 1967;155:1682.
51. Emmerson BT, Wyngaarden JB. Purine metabolism in heterozygous carriers of hypoxanthine-guanine phosphoribosyltransferase deficiency. *Science* 1969;166:1533.
52. Emmerson BT, Gordon RB, Johnson LA. Urate kinetics in hypoxanthine-guanine phosphoribosyltransferase deficiency: their significance for the understanding of gout. *Q J Med* 1976;45:49.
53. Emmerson BT, Row PG. An evaluation of the pathogenesis of the gouty kidney. *Kidney Int* 1975;8:65.
54. Emmerson BT, Thompson L. The spectrum of hypoxanthine-guanine phosphoribosyl-transferase deficiency. *Q J Med* 1973;42:423.
55. Batch JA, et al. Renal failure in infancy due to urate over-production. *Aust NZ J Med* 1984;14:852.
56. Holland PC, et al. Hypoxanthine guanine phosphoribosyltransferase deficiency presenting with gout and renal failure in infancy. *Arch Dis Child* 1983;58:831.
57. Lorentz WB Jr, et al. Failure to thrive, hyperuricemia, and renal insufficiency in early infancy secondary to partial hypoxanthine-guanine phosphoribosyltransferase deficiency. *J Pediatr* 1984;104:94.
58. Kaufman JM, Greene ML, Seegmiller JE. Urine uric acid to creatinine ratio—a screening test for inherited disorders of purine metabolism. *J Pediatr* 1968;73:583.
59. Kelton J, Kelley WN, Holmes EW. A rapid method for the diagnosis of acute uric acid nephropathy. *Arch Intern Med* 1978;138:612.
60. Tungsanga K, et al. Urine uric acid and urine creatinine ratio in acute renal failure. *Arch Intern Med* 1984;144:934.
61. Stapleton FB, Nash DA. A screening test for hyperuricosuria. *J Pediatr* 1983;102:88.

62. Stapleton FB, et al. Uric acid excretion in normal children. *J Pediatr* 1978;92:911.
63. Crittenden DR, Ackermann GL. Hyperuricemic acute renal failure in disseminated carcinoma. *Arch Intern Med* 1977;137:97.
64. Lewis RW, et al. Molar lactate in the management of uric acid renal obstruction. *J Urol* 1981;125:87.
65. DeConti RC, Calabresi P. Use of allopurinol for prevention and control of hyperuricemia in patients with neoplastic disease. *N Engl J Med* 1966;274:481.
66. Barry KG, et al. Acute uric acid nephropathy. *Arch Intern Med* 1963; 111:452.
67. Kjellstrand CM, et al. Hyperuricemic acute renal failure. *Arch Intern Med* 1974;133:349.
68. Rieselbach RE, et al. Uric acid excretion and renal function in the acute hyperuricemia of leukemia. *Am J Med* 1964;37:872.
69. Jones DP, Mahmoud H, Chesney RW. Tumor lysis syndrome: pathogenesis and management. *Pediatr Nephrol* 1995;9:206.
70. Simmonds HA, et al. Allopurinol in renal failure and the tumour lysis syndrome. *Clin Chim Acta* 1986;160:189.
71. Kanwar YS, Manaligod JR. Leukemic urate nephropathy. *Arch Pathol* 1975;99:467.
72. Diamond HS, et al. Hyperuricosuria and increased tubular secretion of urate in sickle cell anemia. *Am J Med* 1975;59:796.
73. Reynolds MD. Gout and hyperuricemia associated with sickle-cell anemia. *Semin Arthritis Rheum* 1983;12:404.
74. Knochel JP, Dotin LN, Hamburger RJ. Heat stress, exercise and muscle injury: effects on urate metabolism and renal function. *Ann Intern Med* 1974;81:321.
75. Schrier RW, et al. Renal, metabolic and circulatory responses to heat and exercise. *Ann Intern Med* 1970;73:213.
76. Schiff HB, MacSearraigh ETM, Kallmeyer JC. Myoglobinuria, rhabdomyolysis and marathon running. *Q J Med* 1978;47:463.
77. Zuercher HU, et al. Acute renal failure complicating starvation for weight reduction. *Schweiz Med Wochenschr* 1977;107:1025.
78. Kovalchik MT III. Sulfinpyrazone induced uric acid urolithiasis with acute renal failure. *Conn Med* 1981;45:423.
79. Boelaert J, et al. Acute renal failure induced by sulfinpyrazone. *Kidney Int* 1981;20:305.
80. Wilcox RG, et al. Sulphinpyrazone in acute myocardial infarction: studies on cardiac rhythm and renal function. *Br Med J [Clin Res]* 1980;281:531.
81. Erley CMM, et al. Acute renal failure due to uric acid nephropathy in a patient with renal hypouricemia. *Klin Wochenschr* 1989;67:308.
82. Conger JD, Falk SA. Intrarenal dynamics in the pathogenesis and prevention of acute urate nephropathy. *J Clin Invest* 1977;59:786.
83. Brown EA, et al. Renal function in rats with acute medullary injury. *Nephron* 1980;26:64.
84. Spencer HW, Yarger WE, Robinson RR. Alterations of renal function during dietary induced hyperuricemia in the rat. *Kidney Int* 1976;9:489.
85. Waisman J, Bluestone R, Klinenberg JR. A preliminary report of nephropathy in hyperuricaemic rats. *Lab Invest* 1974;30:716.
86. Waisman J, et al. Acute hyperuricemic nephropathy in rats. An electron microscopic study. *Am J Pathol* 1975;81:367.
87. Conger JD, et al. A micropuncture study of the early phase of acute urate nephropathy. *J Clin Invest* 1976;58:681.
88. Farebrother DA, et al. Experimental crystal nephropathy (one year study in the pig). *Clin Nephrol* 1975;4:243.
89. Fessel WJ. Renal outcomes of gout and hyperuricemia. *Am J Med* 1979;67:74.
90. Aretaeus. *The extant works of Aretaeus, the Cappadocian.* London: New Sydenham Society, 1856.
91. Sydenham TA. Treatise of the gout. In: *The works of Thomas Sydenham*, vol II. London: Robinson, Otridge, Hayes and Newberry, 1788.
92. Scudamore C. *A treatise on the nature and cure of gout and gravel.* London: Joseph Mallett, 1823.
93. Castelneau NF. I. Gouty kidney. *Arch Gèn Mèd J Comp de Sci Med* 1843;3:285.
94. Todd RB. *Clinical lectures on certain diseases of the urinary organs, and on dropsies.* London: Churchill, 1857.
95. Charcot J, Cornil MV. Contributions à ètude des altérations anatomiques de la goutte et spècialement du rein chez les goutteux. *C R Soc Biol (Paris)* 1864;15:139.
96. Garrod AB. *A treatise on gout and rheumatic gout.* London: Longmans, Green, 1876.
97. Lindsay J. *Gout: its aetiology, pathology and treatment.* London: Hodder & Stoughton, 1913.
98. Llewellyn LJ. *Gout.* London: William Heinemann, Ltd., 1920.
99. Schnitker MA, Richter AB. Nephritis in gout. *Am J Med Sci* 1936; 192:241.
100. Coombs FS, et al. Renal function in patients with gout. *J Clin Invest* 1940;19:525.
101. Broøchner-Mortensen, K. One hundred gouty patients. *Acta Med Scand* 1941;106:81.
102. Brown JB, Mallory GK. Renal changes in gout. *N Engl J Med* 1950; 243:325.
103. Fineberg SK. Gout nephropathy. *J Am Geriatr Soc* 1958;6:10.
104. Talbott JH, Terplan KL. The kidney in gout. *Medicine (Baltimore)* 1960;39:405.
105. Greenbaum D, Ross JH, Steinberg VL. Renal biopsy in gout. *Br Med J [Clin Res]* 1961;1:1502.
106. Gonick HC, et al. The renal lesion in gout. *Ann Intern Med* 1965;62: 667.
107. Barlow KA, Beilin LJ. Renal disease in primary gout. *Q J Med* 1968; 37:79.
108. Grahame R, Scott JT. Clinical survey of 354 patients with gout. *Ann Rheum Dis* 1970;29:461.
109. Gibson T, et al. Renal impairment and gout. *Ann Rheum Dis* 1980;39: 417.
110. Plante GE, Durivage J, Lemieux G. Renal excretion of hydrogen in primary gout. *Metabolism* 1968;17:377.
111. Gibson T, et al. Allopurinol treatment and its effect on renal function in gout: a controlled study. *Ann Rheum Dis* 1982;41:59.
112. Yu T-F, Berger L. Renal disease in primary gout: a study of 253 gout patients with proteinuria. *Semin Arthritis Rheum* 1975;4:293.
113. Yu T-F, Berger L. Impaired renal function in gout. Its association with hypertensive vascular disease and intrinsic renal disease. *Am J Med* 1982;72:95.
114. Yu T-F, et al. Renal function in gout: V. Factors influencing the renal hemodynamics. *Am J Med* 1979;67:766.
114a. Beck LH. Requiem for gouty nephropathy. *Kidney Int* 1986;30:280.
115. Berger L, Yu T-F. Renal function in gout: IV. An analysis of 524 gouty subjects including long-term follow-up studies. *Am J Med* 1975; 59:605.
116. Tarng D, Lin H-Y, Shyong M-L, et al. Renal function in gout patients. *Am J Nephrol* 1995;15:31.
117. Nickeleit V, Mihatsch MJ. Uric acid nephropathy and end-stage renal disease—review of a non-disease. *Nephrol Dial Transplant* 1997;12:1832.
118. Sokoloff LB. The pathology of gout. *Metabolism* 1957;6:230.
119. Bluestone R, Waisman J, Klinenberg JR. The gouty kidney. *Semin Arthritis Rheum* 1977;7:97.
120. Culleton BF, Larson MG, Kannel WB, et al. Serum uric acid and risk for cardiovascular disease and death: the Framingham Heart Study. *Ann Intern Med* 1999;131:7.
121. MacFarlane DG, et al. A study of platelet aggregation and adhesion in gout. *Clin Exp Rheumatol* 1983;1:63.
122. Darlington LG, Slack J, Scott JT. Vascular mortality in patients with gout and in their families. *Ann Rheum Dis* 1983;42:270.
123. Hall AP. Hypertension and hyperuricaemia—discussion. *Proc R Soc Med* 1966;59:317.
124. Emmerson BT. Toxic nephropathy. In: Wyngaarden JB, Smith LH, eds. *Cecil's textbook of medicine*, 16th ed. Philadelphia: WB Saunders, 1982:551.
125. Johnson WJ, O'Duffy JD. Chronic gouty nephropathy treated by long-term hemodialysis and allopurinol. *Mayo Clin Proc* 1979;54:618.
126. Chapman JR, et al. Reversibility of cyclosporin nephrotoxicity after three months' treatment. *Lancet* 1985;1:128.
127. Palestine AG, Nussenblatt RB, Chan C-C. Side effects of systemic cyclosporine in patients not undergoing transplantation. *Am J Med* 1984;77:652.
128. Versluis DJ, et al. Cyclosporine A—related proximal tubular dysfunction: impaired handling of uric acid. *Transplant Proc* 1987;19:4029.
129. Hall BM, et al. Treatment of renal transplantation rejection. *Med J Aust* 1985;142:179.
130. Ross EJ. Chronic renal failure. In: Black DAK, ed. *Renal disease*, 3rd ed. Oxford: Blackwell, 1972:476.

131. Advisory Committee to the Renal Transplant Registry. The ninth report of the Human Renal Transplant Registry. *JAMA* 1972;220:253.

132. Ifudu O, et al. Gouty arthritis in end-stage renal disease: clinical course and rarity of new cases. *Am J Kidney Dis* 1994;23:347.

133. Noordzij TC, Leunissen KML, Van Hooff JP. Renal handling of urate and the incidence of gouty arthritis during cyclosporine and diuretic use. *Transplantation* 1991;52:64.

134. Braun WE, Richmond BJ, Protiva DA, et al. The incidence and management of osteoporosis, gout, and avascular necrosis in recipients of renal allografts functioning more than 20 years (level 5A) treated with prednisone and azathioprine. *Transplant Proc* 1999;31:1366.

135. Mertz DP, Schindera F. Secondary gout six years after acute renal failure. *Germ Med Mth* 1968;13:414.

135a. McCarthy GM. Crystal-related tissue damage. In: Smyth CJ, Holers VM, eds. *Gout, hyperuricemia and other crystal-associated arthropathies.* New York: Marcel Dekker Inc, 1999:39.

136. Richet G, Mignon F, Ardaillou R. Goutte secondaire des nephropathics chroniques. *Presse Med* 1965;73:633.

137. Sorensen LB. Gout secondary to chronic renal disease: studies on urate metabolism. *Ann Rheum Dis* 1980;39:424.

138. Vecchio PC, Emmerson BT. Gout due to renal disease. *Br J Rheum* 1992;31:63.

139. Feinstein EI, et al. Severe hyperuricemia in patients with volume depletion. *Am J Nephrol* 1984;4:77.

140. Wedeen RP. Punch cures the gout. *J Med Soc NJ* 1981;78:201.

141. Emmerson BT. Chronic lead nephropathy. The diagnostic use of calcium EDTA and the association with gout. *Aust Ann Med* 1963;12:310.

142. Morgan JM, Hartley MW, Miller RW. Nephropathy in chronic lead poisoning. *Arch Int Med* 1966;118:17.

143. Albahary C, et al. Le rein dans le saturnisme professionnel. *Arch Mal Profession* 1965;26:5.

144. Richet G, et al. Le rein du saturnisme chronique. *Rev Fr Etude Clin Biol* 1964;9:188.

145. Batuman V, et al. The role of lead in gout nephropathy. *N Engl J Med* 1981;304:520.

146. Wedeen RP. The role of lead in renal failure. *Clin Exp Dial Apheresis* 1982;6:113.

147. Wedeen R. Lead and the gouty kidney. *Am J Kidney Dis* 1983;11:559.

148. Batuman V, et al. Contribution of lead to hypertension with renal impairment. *N Engl J Med* 1983;309:17.

149. Batuman V. Lead nephropathy, gout, and hypertension. *Am J. Med Sci* 1993;305:241.

150. Henderson DA. The aetiology of chronic nephritis in Queensland. *Med J. Aust* 1958;1:377.

151. Inglis JA, Henderson DA, Emmerson BT. The pathology and pathogenesis of chronic lead nephropathy occurring in Queensland. *J Pathol* 1978;124:65.

152. Van de Vyver FL, et al. Bone lead in dialysis patients. *Kidney Int* 1988; 33:601.

153. Ritz E, Mann J, Stoeppler M. Lead and the kidney. *Adv Nephrol* 1988; 17:241.

154. Staessen J, et al. Blood lead concentration, renal function, and blood pressure in London civil servants. *Br J Ind Med* 1990;47:442.

155. Sharp DS, Becker CE, Smith AH. Chronic low-level lead exposure. Its role in the pathogenesis of hypertension. *Med Toxicol* 1987;2:210.

156. Ball GV, Sorensen LB. Pathogenesis of hyperuricemia in saturnine gout. *N Engl J Med* 1969;280:1199.

157. Emmerson BT. The renal excretion of urate in chronic lead nephropathy. *Aust Ann Med* 1965;14:295.

158. Emmerson BT, Mirosch W, Douglas JB. The relative contributions of tubular reabsorption and secretion to urate excretion in lead nephropathy. *Aust NZ J Med* 1971;1:353.

159. Emmerson BT. The clinical differentiation of lead gout and primary gout. *Arthritis Rheum* 1968;11:623.

160. Colleoni N, D'Amico G. Chronic lead accumulation as a possible cause of renal failure in gouty patients. *Nephron* 1986;44:32.

161. Martinez-Maldonado M. Polycystic kidney disease and hyperuricemia. *Ann Int Med* 1974;80:116.

162. Mejias E, et al. Hyperuricemia, gout and autosomal dominant polycystic kidney disease. *Am J Med Sci* 1989;297:145.

163. Newcombe DS. Gouty arthritis and polycystic kidney disease. *Ann Intern Med* 1973;79:605.

164. Kaehny WD, et al. Uric acid handling in autosomal dominant polycystic kidney disease with normal filtration rates. *Am J Med* 1990; 89:49.

165. Burke JR, et al. Juvenile nephrophthisis and medullary cystic disease—the same disease (report of a large family with medullary cystic disease associated with gout and epilepsy). *Clin Nephrol* 1982;18:1.

166. Thompson GR, et al. Familial occurrence of hyperuricemia, gout, and medullary cystic disease. *Arch Intern Med* 1978;138:1614.

167. Stavrou C, Pierides A, Zouvani I, et al. Medullary cystic kidney disease with hyperuricemia and gout in a large Cypriot family: no allelism with nephrophthisis type 1. *Am J Med Genet* 1998;77:149.

168. Duncan H, Dixon A St J. Gout, familial hyperuricaemia and renal disease. *Q J Med* 1960;29:127.

169. van Goor W, Kooiker CJ, Dorhout Mees EJ. An unusual form of renal disease associated with gout and hypertension. *J Clin Pathol* 1971; 24:354.

170. Leumann EP, Wegmann W. Familial nephropathy with hyperuricemia and gout. *Nephron* 1983;34:51.

171. Calabrese G, et al. Precocious familial gout with reduced fractional urate clearance and normal purine enzymes. *Q J Med* 1990;75:441.

172. McBride MB, Rigden S, Haycock GB, et al. Presymptomatic detection of familial juvenile hyperuricaemic nephropathy in children. *Pediatr Nephrol* 1998;12:357.

173. Meyer WJ III, Gill JR, Bartter FC. Gout as a complication of Bartter's syndrome. A possible role for alkalosis in the decreased clearance of uric acid. *Ann Intern Med* 1975;83:56.

174. Smith A, Wilcken B. Homozygous cystinuria in New South Wales. *Med J Aust* 1984;141:500.

175. Gulati PD, et al. Serum urate levels and uric acid clearance in obstructive and non-obstructive nephropathies. *J Assoc Physicians India* 1974;22:349.

176. Bastian P, Nanra RS. Analgesic nephropathy, uric acid and gout. *Aust NZ J Med* 1977;7:438(abst).

177. Bulpitt CJ. Serum uric acid in hypertensive patients. *Br Heart J* 1975; 37:1210.

178. Verger D, et al. Les tophus goutteux de la medullaire renale des uremiques chroniques. Etude de 17 cas decouverts au cours de 62 autopsies. *Nephron* 1967;4:356.

179. Ostberg Y. Renal urate deposits in chronic renal insufficiency. *Acta Med Scand* 1968;183:197.

180. Linnane JW, Burry AF, Emmerson BT. Urate deposits in the renal medulla. Prevalence and associations. *Nephron* 1981;29:216.

181. Burry AF. A profile of renal disease in Queensland. *Med J Aust* 1966; 1:826.

182. Manzke H, et al. Uric acid infarctions in the kidneys of newborn infants. A study on the changing incidence and on oxypurine ratios. *Eur J Pediatr* 1977;126:29.

183. Rosenfeld JB. Effect of long-term allopurinol administration on serial GFR in normotensive and hypertensive hyperuricaemic subjects. In: Sperling O, De Vries A, Wyngaarden JB, eds. *Purine metabolism in man. Adv Exp Med Biol* 1974;41B:581.

184. Emmerson BT, Stride PJ, Williams G. The clinical differentiation of primary gout from primary renal disease in patients with both gout and renal disease. *Adv Exp Med Biol* 1980;122A:9.

185. Klinenberg JR, Gonick HC, Dornfield L. Renal function abnormalities in patients with asymptomatic hyperuricemia. *Arthritis Rheum* 1975;18[Suppl 6]:725.

186. Nishida Y, et al. Tubular function impairment in patients with asymptomatic hyperuricemia. *J Urol* 1977;118:908.

187. Farebrother DA, et al. Uric acid crystal induced nephropathy: evidence for a specific renal lesion in a gouty family. *J Pathol* 1981;135:159.

188. Simmonds HA, et al. Familial gout and renal failure in young women. *Clin Nephrol* 1980;14:176.

CHAPTER 78

Sickle Cell Disease

Lodewijk W. Statius van Eps and Paul E. de Jong

In 1910, Herrick described the case of a young black student with severe anemia characterized by "peculiar elongated and sickle-shaped red blood corpuscles" (1). This was the first description of the condition later to be known as sickle cell anemia. He noted a slightly increased volume of urine of low specific gravity and thus observed the most frequent feature of sickle cell nephropathy: an inability of the kidney to concentrate urine normally. This "new disease," an inherited molecular disorder, was brought to the New World from West Africa, where it had probably been recognized for centuries, bearing many different tribal names (2).

The identification of this familial autosomal-codominant disorder as an abnormality of the hemoglobin molecule was made by Pauling and associates in 1949 (3). The exact nature of the defect, the substitution of valine for glutamic acid at the sixth residue of the beta chain, was established by Ingram (4), thus characterizing sickle cell anemia as a disease of molecular structure. The hemoglobin molecule is composed of two alpha and two beta chains. The beta chain has 146 amino acids and the alpha chain has 141 amino acids. The result of the point mutation in the beta chain is a slight change in the three-dimensional spatial configuration of the hemoglobin molecule. Glutamic acid is a charged amino acid and is therefore very soluble in water; valine is uncharged and poorly soluble in water. The loss of charge explains the slower migration of sickle cell hemoglobin with electrophoresis. Furthermore, the uncharged, poorly soluble valine residues create a "sticky spot," which causes the hemoglobin molecules to adhere to one another and to form elongated structures that distort the red cells into their characteristic sickle shape. Under conditions of hypoxia, acidosis, or hyperosmolality (the latter being present in the renal medulla), the physicochemical condition of sickle cell hemoglobin within the red blood cell changes and molecular aggregates are formed (5). These polymers form elongated

double-stranded fibers of hemoglobin molecules. The double-stranded fibers grow and elongate, finally resulting in 14 helical filaments grouped together to form the complete elongated large structure. The process of polymerization and the formation of these structures transform the erythrocyte into an elongated rigid shape (6) (Fig. 78-1).

The elongated structures stretch and rupture the protein skeleton and the bilipid membrane of the red blood cell (7,8). This morphologic change leads to leakiness of the red cell membrane, with eventual hemolysis. In addition, the conformational change causes an increase in blood viscosity and rheologic effects in the microcirculation that result in intravascular aggregates, ischemia, and infarction.

In the inner renal medulla and the renal papillae, where, especially during antidiuresis, osmolality is highly increased as a result of countercurrent multiplication and countercurrent exchange, shrinkage of red blood cells is observed (9). This results in an increase of intracellular hemoglobin concentration, which initiates the process of polymerization (10). This makes the renal medulla and papillae most vulnerable in sickle cell disease.

The homozygous form, sickle cell anemia (Hb-SS), is characterized by a severe hemolytic anemia (hemoglobin 5.9 to 9.6 g/dL). These patients suffer periodic attacks (crises) of severe pain in the joints, bones, muscles, and abdomen, associated with increased destruction of red blood cells. The hemoglobin of the homozygous patient is 80% or more Hb-S, the remainder being fetal hemoglobin (Hb-F). The patients are as a rule icteric and have a high percentage ($\pm 20\%$) of reticulocytes. Their mean red cell survival is 30 days ($N = 120$ days). In the heterozygous form, sickle cell trait (Hb-AS), only 30% to 45% of hemoglobin is Hb-S. Except under unusual circumstances this is a benign, asymptomatic condition, but renal abnormalities, such as disturbed urinary concentrating capacity, episodic hematuria, and sometimes even papillary necrosis with renal colic, may be observed. Blood hemoglobin content is normal or slightly decreased.

Hb-S can also occur in combination with another abnormal hemoglobin. These are called *double heterozygotes*. We

L. W. Statius van Eps: Department of History of Medicine, Free University of Amsterdam; and Department of Internal Medicine, Slotervaart Hospital, Amsterdam, The Netherlands

P. E. de Jong: Department of Internal Medicine, University Hospital Groningen, Groningen, The Netherlands

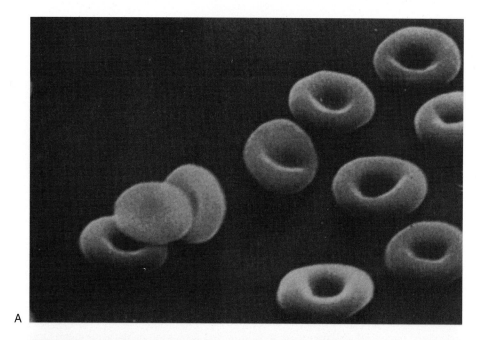

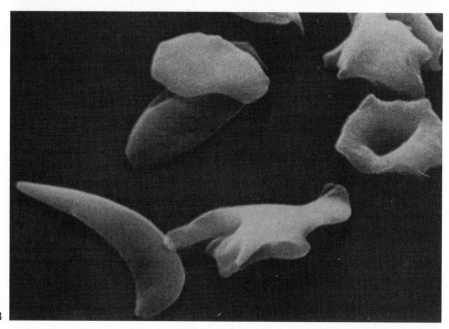

FIG. 78-1. A: Normal red blood cells from Hb-AA subject as seen by scanning electron microscope (SEM). (Magnification ×5,230.) **B:** Sickled red blood cells from Hb-SS subject viewed by SEM. The cells appear to be rigid and are deformed by the formation of intracellular elongated fibers formed as a result of polymerization of hemoglobin molecules. (From Barnhart MI, et al. *Sickle cell.* Kalamazoo, MI: Upjohn Co., 1974, with permission.)

describe some of these cell variants in order to stress the variability of these conditions. The many double heterozygotes have created a large group of hemoglobinopathies characterized by the phenomenon of sickling. In these patients, under conditions of hypoxemia, hyperosmolality, and acidosis, intracellular polymerization can occur, although in variable degrees. In sickle cell–hemoglobin C disease (Hb-SC), with about 50% Hb-S and the remainder Hb-C, the tendency to sickle is more pronounced than in Hb-AS. These Hb-SC patients can have severe clinical symptoms as do patients with other rare variants such as hemoglobin SD disease and sickle cell-beta thalassemia disease, clinically indistinguishable from Hb-SS. A renal concentration defect has been observed in patients with Hb-SC (11) and Hb-SD (12), as well as in Hb-S-beta thalassemia patients. The homozygote form of hemoglobin C disease has completely normal renal function

(13). Hemoglobin C$_{Harlem}$ has two substitutes on the beta chain, one of which is identical to the Hb-S abnormality, and has been found only in heterozygotes. Both sickling and hyposthenuria have been observed in these Hb-C$_{Harlem}$ patients (14). Hemoglobin C$_{Georgetown}$, another variant of hemoglobin C, also resembles Hb-S in its tendency to sickle. The same is the case with the recently described sickle cell–hemoglobin D$_{Iran}$, characterized by the substitution of glutamine for glutamic acid at position 22 in the beta chain. It has been identified in a Jamaican family of West African ancestry and is considered a benign sickle cell syndrome (15). Because patients with hemoglobin C$_{Georgetown}$ and those with sickle cell–hemoglobin D$_{Iran}$ have red blood cells that sickle, one can also expect concentration defects in their kidneys. However, this has not yet been investigated. Hemoglobin O$_{Arab}$ is a less common beta-chain variant, in which lysine is substituted for glutamic acid at position 121. Its origin is found in African people living in Arab territories. It has also been found in the African American population. Because the interaction of Hb-O$_{Arab}$ and Hb-S enhances gelling, the double heterozygote SO disease has all the clinical features of sickle cell anemia (16).

The incidence of sickle cell anemia varies in different parts of the world. It is estimated that 8% of African Americans have red cells that sickle, and that 1 in 40 persons with such cells is a homozygote (17). The frequency of HB-AC is estimated at 2% and that of Hb-SC at 0.04%. There are important geographic variations in the incidence of these important abnormal hemoglobins. One factor is the protection against infection with falciparum malaria by carriers of the sickle cell gene. This explains why the phenotypic frequencies for Hb-S vary from 10% to 40% in Africa and from 5% to 20% in Greece and Turkey. The phenotypic frequency for Hb-C is about 10% in West Africa (16).

This chapter is concerned with the renal manifestations of sickle cell disease, abnormalities that appear to result from the increased tendency of red blood cells to sickle while transversing the capillary circulation of the hyperosmotic renal medulla (9). Clinical impairment in concentrating function—and to a lesser degree in urinary acidification—is observed despite normal or even supernormal glomerular filtration rate (GFR) and renal plasma flow. Episodic hematuria, an increased tendency to pyelonephritis and papillary necrosis and, rarely, the nephrotic syndrome may be present.

PATHOLOGIC FEATURES

In 1923, Sydenstricker and colleagues first described macroscopic and microscopic postmortem studies of kidneys of patients with sickle cell disease (18). After a hiatus of 25 years and the development of electrophoretic techniques, which enable discrimination between the disease (Hb-SS), the trait (Hb-AS), and other sickling hemoglobinopathies, reports of functional and morphologic studies began to appear, making it possible to attempt to correlate function with structural changes.

Gross Anatomy

The kidneys of patients with sickle cell disease are usually of near-normal size and most do not show significant gross alterations (19). On cut surfaces, however, glomeruli often stand out very prominently as red "pinheads." Kidneys removed because of severe hematuria may demonstrate submucosal hemorrhages in the pelvis, medulla, and cortex (20). Calicectasis has been observed on pyelographic examination in 10 of 17 adult (Hb-SS) patients (21). Autopsy studies on three patients with calicectasis showed lesions consistent with acute and chronic pyelonephritis. However, these lesions could also have been caused by ischemia and necrosis as the result of the sickling process itself. Radiographic changes suggesting papillary necrosis—medullary cavitations, ring shadows, and calcifications in the pyramids—have also been observed (22–24). Occasionally, minimal papillary necrosis is apparent only on microscopic examination. Renal vein thrombosis is also an occasional finding in Hb-SS disease.

Whereas renal medullary pathology is often demonstrated, cortical infarctions are seldom reported. In a study on renal function in sickle cell anemia patients over 40 years of age, 20% of the patients exhibited irregularity of the renal outline on intravenous urography (25).

Morgan and associates (26) made a retrospective study of hospital necropsies of 21 patients with Hb-SS who died at the age of 40 or over. Renal failure had caused or contributed to death in 10 cases. All kidneys showed papillary damage. In 13 cases, moderate to severe cortical irregularity, including scarring, was seen. Hypertrophic glomeruli were observed with increased cellularity. Glomerulosclerosis was common, which the authors attributed to long-standing hyperfiltration. They considered glomerulosclerosis to be the major cause of renal failure in sickle cell anemia.

It is easy to envision that red blood cells sickle more readily in the relatively hypoxic and hyperosmotic renal medulla than in other capillary circulations. Consequently, increased viscosity of the medullary capillary blood slows the rate of flow, and intravascular aggregates may eventually develop into microthrombi, causing further impairment of the vasa recta circulation. Microradioangiographic studies have been performed on kidneys removed at autopsy from patients with normal hemoglobin, patients with Hb-SS disease, and patients with Hb-AS and Hb-SC disease (27) (Fig. 78-2). A significantly reduced number of vasa recta are seen in kidneys from Hb-SS patients. Even the vessels that are present are abnormal in that they are dilated, show spiral formation, and end bluntly. Patients with Hb-AS and Hb-SC disease show changes intermediate between those of the Hb-SS patients and normal subjects. In patients with Hb-AS, sparse bundles of vasa recta are surrounded by a chaotic pattern of dilated capillaries, with loss of the original bundle architecture. The

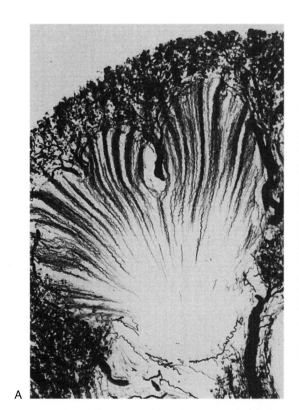
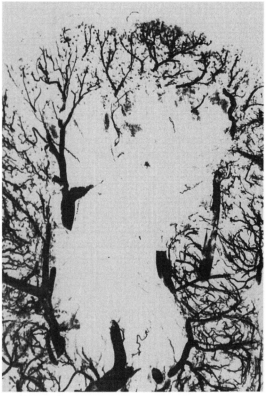
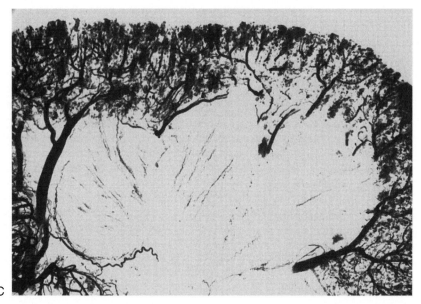

FIG. 78-2. Injection microradioangiographs of kidneys from a subject without hemoglobinopathy (**A**), a patient with sickle cell disease (**B**), and a patient with sickle cell–hemoglobin C disease (**C**). In the normal kidney (**A**), vasa recta are visible radiating into the renal papilla; in sickle cell anemia (**B**), vasa recta are virtually absent. Those vessels that are present are abnormal, are dilated, form spirals, and end bluntly, and many appear to be obliterated. The patient with Hb-SC (**C**) shows changes intermediately between the Hb-SS patients and the normal subjects. (From Statius van Eps, LW, et al. Nature of concentrating defect in sickle cell nephropathy, microradioangiographic studies. *Lancet* 1970;1:450, through courtesy of the editors.)

assumption is that these changes result from occlusion of vasa recta and represent the structural basis for the development of functional changes. The loss of the highly specialized structure of parallel running loops of Henle and vasa recta makes countercurrent multiplication and exchange impossible.

Microscopic Pathology

In the first description of structural changes in sickle cell kidneys, prominent glomeruli distended with blood and necrosis and pigmentation of tubular cells were observed (18). This description has been supplemented, but not altered substantially. An important point that has been stressed is that glomerular enlargement and congestion are more common in children beyond the age of 2 years and are most marked in juxtamedullary glomeruli (28,29). When the size of juxtamedullary glomeruli is systemically measured, there is a distinct difference between those of children with sickle cell disease and normal children. Both the afferent and efferent arterioles of the enlarged glomeruli may be dilated and engorged with sickled cells. In adult patients with Hb-SS and normal GFR, glomerular size as well as the total glomerular area per unit area of cortex have been found to be significantly greater than in patients with Hb-AS and normal control subjects. In older patients, this glomerular enlargement and congestion lead to progressive ischemia and fibrosis with obliteration of glomeruli (26,30). However, even in this older age group, the pathologic changes may be very mild if there is no clinical evidence of renal disease.

In the study by Falk and colleagues of 10 biopsied Hb-SS patients with proteinuria, glomerular enlargement was found along with peripheral focal segmental glomerulosclerosis (31). The mean ($\pm$SD) glomerular area of these patients was $28.7 \pm 4.1 \times 10^3$ μm^2 as compared with $15.8 \pm 4.3 \times 10^3$ μm^2 in control patients without renal disease.

Medullary lesions, however, are the most prominent; early changes consist of edema, focal scarring, and interstitial fibrosis. With progressive scarring there is tubular atrophy and infiltration of mononuclear cells. Most observers mention capillary stasis, ischemic infarction, and sporadic papillary necrosis. All these changes could be the result of the observed obliteration or attenuation of the medullary circulation (19).

Ultrastructural Pathology

Adults with Hb-SS disease (from 17 to 27 years) and limited ability to concentrate urine, but normal GFR and effective renal plasma flow (ERPF), show normal epithelial foot processes and glomerular basement membranes. Occasionally focal pedicle fusion and glomerular basement membrane thickening are observed (32). The cytoplasm of mesangial cells contains prominent electron-dense material with a homogeneous and sometimes granular or lamellated structure. The mesangial matrix may be increased in quantity with focal presence of fibrillar material. These findings cannot be considered specific for sickle cell disease, although the changes

mentioned previously increase with advancing clinical renal disease in the patient with Hb-SS. Moreover, these ultrastructural changes may be present without other signs of overt renal disease and may be the earliest effects of sickle cell disease on the kidney. Systematic follow-up studies will be necessary to establish this relationship. Interstitial cells of the outer medulla sometimes contain aggregates of granular electron-dense material. The normally close relationship of the interstitial cell processes and cytoplasmic fibrils to the interstitial capillaries appear to be at least partially interrupted by the interstitial collagen.

Pathologic Changes in the Nephrotic Syndrome

In studies of patients with sickle cell anemia who have nephrotic syndrome and marked renal insufficiency, much more striking electron-microscopic changes have been reported (33,34). There is effacement of foot processes, and sheets of epithelial cytoplasm cover the external surface of the basement membrane. Mesangial matrix is increased and basement membrane duplication is seen. Another feature is the appearance of electron-dense bodies, particularly in the mesangium and occasionally in the endothelial cytoplasm. Most of these ultrastructural changes are also observed in the nephrotic syndrome resulting from a variety of causes, and in the absence of concomitant sickle cell disease; therefore, they cannot be considered specific for the sickling disorders. Bakir and associates published a survey on 240 adults with sickle cell anemia over a period of 11 years (35). Twelve had the nephrotic syndrome. In nine, the glomerular lesion, which they proposed to call *sickle glomerulopathy,* consisted of mesangial expansion and basement membrane duplication. The prognosis of this complication of sickle cell nephropathy is very poor of 22 patients with sickle cell glomerulopathy, 9 from Bakir and colleagues' publication and 13 added from the literature, 11 died within 2 years, 10 from rapidly developing renal failure. Bakir and colleagues concluded, based on their very large group of sickle cell anemia patients, that the nephrotic syndrome, most often caused by sickle glomerulopathy, occurs in 4% of patients, leading to renal failure in two-thirds and death within 2 years in half of the patients. Hyperfiltration has been suggested to explain these findings (36).

Alternatively, the nephrotic syndrome in patients with both sickle cell anemia and sickle cell trait (37–39) has been interpreted as an autologous immune-complex nephritis. Immunologic studies in seven Hb-SS patients with clinical and laboratory evidence of glomerular disease revealed immunoglobulin and complement components and renal tubular epithelial antigens in a granular pattern along the glomerular basement membrane. Tubular epithelial antigens and cryoprecipitable renal tubular antigen-antibody complexes were detected in the circulation of some patients. It was suggested that an immune-deposit normocomplementemic nephritis develops in sickle cell anemia and that the involved antigen is released from tubules damaged by the vascular alterations characteristic of this disease.

Recently, more attention has been given to the occurrence of glomerulosclerosis in sickle cell anemia. Tejani and coworkers found glomerulosclerosis in 8 of 13 children in whom a renal biopsy was performed for persistent proteinuria or nephrotic syndrome, whereas mesangial proliferation was found in the other 5 children (40). Children with glomerulosclerosis were older at the onset of nephropathy and presented with nephrotic syndrome more often than did those with mesangial proliferation. In addition, several case reports mentioned the occurrence of the nephrotic syndrome with focal glomerulosclerosis in sickle cell anemia (10,29,33,34). All patients with mesangial proliferation and half of the patients with focal and segmental glomerulosclerosis had supernormal renal clearances at onset of nephropathy suggesting hyperfiltration (40). The latter, both in animals and humans, may be injurious to the integrity of glomeruli and lead to mesangial proliferation and focal segmental glomerulosclerosis. It has indeed been shown that hyperfiltration is a characteristic of the nephropathy in Hb-SS patients (13,19,41–43). This hyperfiltration may well be responsible for the glomerulosclerosis and the renal function decline in these patients (31,44). Bhathena and Sondheimer studied kidney biopsy specimens from six homozygous Hb-SS nephrotic patients (45). They observed a distinctive glomerulopathy of focal sclerosis developing in maximally hypertrophied glomeruli. The glomeruli were markedly enlarged, whether nephrotic (233.6 μm $\pm$ 25.3 [standard error, SE]) or not (control Hb-SS values 243.0 μm $\pm$ 12.5; normal control values 158.0 μm $\pm$ 12.7). As increased hyperfiltration and glomerular capillary hypertension are injurious to remnant glomeruli that undergo hypertrophy, the observed focal segmental glomerulosclerosis is the expected pathologic lesion. Hyperfiltration-related glomerular injury that supervenes in the form of progressive focal glomerulosclerosis causes renal insufficiency and increasing proteinuria, the nephrotic syndrome, and ultimately renal failure.

Although this form of sickle cell glomerulopathy is the most typical and specific lesion in sickle cell patients to cause the nephrotic syndrome and ultimately renal failure, other causes of nephrotic syndrome can occur with Hb-SS, such as poststreptococcal acute glomerulonephritis, membranoproliferative glomerulonephritis (46), and the autologous normocomplementemic membranoproliferative glomerulonephritis (38,39).

RENAL FUNCTION

Hemodynamics

Renal hemodynamics are, as a rule, either normal or supernormal in homozygous (Hb-SS) patients under 30 years of age (13,19,42,43). In Hb-SS infants, increased values have been observed for both GFR and effective renal blood flow (ERBF), as well as for the tubular transport maximum of para-aminohippurate (Tm$_{PAH}$). ERBF was found to be normal or elevated, although less elevated than effective renal plasma flow (ERPF) because of the very low hematocrit. The extraction ratio of para-aminohippurate (E$_{PAH}$) was decreased. Filtration fraction (GFR/ERPF) has been found to be decreased (mean 14% to 18%; normals 19% to 22%) (13,42,43,47). It has been suggested that selective damage of the juxtamedullary glomeruli might result in a lower filtration fraction because these nephrons appear to have the highest filtration fractions (48,49). Microradioangiographic studies lend support to this suggestion (27).

In sickle cell anemia, fractional creatinine excretion has been found to be increased (47); it is therefore advisable to employ inulin clearances when investigating GFR. In older patients (30 to 60 years of age) with Hb-SS, GFR and ERPF diminish with age to normal or even depressed levels. On the other hand, some patients with Hb-SS in their 40s or even older may have completely normal or even supernormal GFR and ERPF (19).

In sickle cell trait, sickle cell–hemoglobin C disease, homozygote–hemoglobin C disease, hemoglobin C trait (11), and sickle cell-beta thalassemia, GFR and ERPF were found to be within the range of normal. Conclusive data regarding renal function in different age groups in sickle cell trait patients are not available.

The mechanism responsible for the increase in renal hemodynamics in patients with sickle cell anemia is not certain. Multiple transfusions with Hb-A blood to patients with Hb-SS result in significant, although temporary, increases in hemoglobin concentration, with gradual and almost complete replacement of Hb-S by Hb-A. Because this procedure does not reduce the supernormal GFR and ERPF (13), the cause of the supernormal renal clearances in sickle cell nephropathy cannot be explained by the anemia per se or by the presence of the abnormal hemoglobin. Also GFR and ERPF may even be slightly reduced in chronic anemia from other causes, both in humans (50) and in dogs (51).

Alternatively, it is tempting to regard the increase in renal hemodynamics as an intrinsic characteristic of sickle cell nephropathy that is related to the medullary abnormalities. The ischemic damage to the medulla could be a stimulus for increased prostaglandin synthesis, leading to hyperfiltration (44,47,52). Indeed, during prostaglandin synthesis inhibition with indomethacin, a significant fall in GFR, ERPF, creatinine clearance, and urea clearance was observed in sickle cell anemia. In control subjects none of these variables changed after indomethacin. It is thus suggested that prostaglandins may play an important role in maintaining a normal GFR and ERPF in sickle cell anemia.

The increase in renal blood flow, whatever its cause, could secondarily cause both an increased GFR and a decreased E$_{PAH}$ (29), although a supernormal ERPF can be accompanied by normal GFR (52). There may also be a relationship between the supernormal GFR and ERPF of sickle cell nephropathy and the observed apparent increased reabsorption by the proximal renal tubule in these patients (see "Proximal Tubular Reabsorption") (53).

There is speculation on the possible mechanisms responsible for the decline in renal hemodynamics with age, sometimes ending in renal failure with, at necropsy, shrunken end-stage kidneys. It could well be that, over a number of years, continued loss of medullary circulation, interstitial fibrosis, and possibly superimposed pyelonephritis may lead to a progressive decline in GFR and advanced renal insufficiency in the patient with Hb-SS disease. Support for the idea of a reduction in medullary blood flow in sickle cell disease can be found in the microradioangiographic studies of Hb-SS kidneys (27) (Fig. 78-2). There was almost no perfusion of the vasa recta by the contrast medium in the kidneys obtained at autopsy. These findings suggest an almost complete absence of vasa recta in Hb-SS.

Another possible mechanism to explain the ultimate decrease of renal function in Hb-SS has been suggested (44). Histologic investigations of Hb-SS kidneys in children and young adults are consistent with the phenomenon of hyperfiltration. Microscopic studies have shown glomerular enlargement, most marked in juxtamedullary glomeruli, particularly in children (28). Also, in adult patients, glomerular size as well as total glomerular area per unit area of cortex have been found to be greater than in control subjects (31,34). As a relationship has been proposed between hyperfiltration, glomerulosclerosis, proteinuria, and even the nephrotic syndrome, these mechanisms may play a role in the natural history of sickle cell nephropathy. As mentioned previously, supernormal hemodynamics and hyperfiltration have been proposed as causative mechanisms of glomerulosclerosis (54). This pathogenetic pathway may explain the decrease in renal function in older Hb-SS patients. In Jamaica, 6 out of 25 Hb-SS patients over 40 years of age had a creatinine clearance lower than 80 mL/minute/1.73 M^2 (25).

Urinary Concentrating Capacity

An inability to achieve maximally concentrated urine has been the most consistent feature of sickle cell nephropathy. This inability has now been documented many times, in both the homozygous and the heterozygous states (11,13,55–59). The abnormality is unrelated to GFR and ERPF, since both as a rule are normal or even supernormal in sickle cell disease. There is, however, a definite relationship between concentrating capacity and age (Fig. 78-3). In Hb-SS patients older than 10 years, the maximal urinary concentration is reduced to about 400 mOsm/kg H$_2$O and does not decrease further with advancing age. In very young children with sickle cell anemia, a concentrating defect is present, but normal concentrating ability can be restored by multiple transfusions of Hb-A erythrocytes (13,57). This capacity for improvement is progressively lost with age, and in patients older than 15 years, impaired concentrating capacity is irreversible (Fig. 78-4). The renal concentrating capacity of the heterozygotes (Hb-AS) is affected too, but only later in life.

Maximally concentrated urine is produced by extraction of water from collecting duct fluid as it passes through the hy-

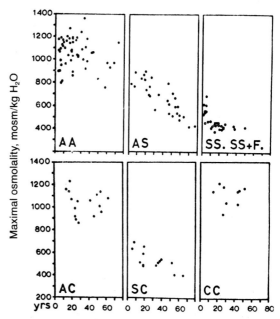

FIG. 78-3. Relationship between maximal urinary osmolality and age in normal subjects (*AA*), sickle cell trait (*AS*), sickle cell anemia (*SS, SS + F*), hemoglobin C trait (*AC*), sickle cell–hemoglobin C disease (*SC*), and hemoglobin C disease (*CC*). Normal subjects have a mean maximal urinary osmolality of 1,058 ± SD 128 mOsm/kg H$_2$O. The most marked impairment in concentrating capacity occurs in Hb-SS disease. Maximal urinary osmolality decreases significantly in the first decade of life to stabilize in patients older than 10 years at a mean of 434 ± SD 21 mOsm/kg H$_2$O. The latter has been designated the fixed maximum of sickle cell nephropathy. In Hb-AS and Hb-SC patients, a progressive decrease in maximal urinary osmolality with age can be observed. C Hemoglobin alone (AC or CC) does not impair concentrating ability. (From Statius van Eps, LW et al. The relation between age and renal concentrating capacity in sickle cell disease and hemoglobin C disease. *Clin Chim Acta* 1970;27:501, through courtesy of the editors.)

pertonic medullary interstitium in the presence of antidiuretic hormone (ADH). It does not increase further after exogenous ADH administration (58,60). In Fig. 78-5 it is demonstrated that sickle cell anemia patients are not able to increase urinary osmolality in spite of sufficiently stimulated vasopressin levels.

In the normal human kidney, approximately 85% of the nephrons have short loops of Henle restricted to the outer medullary zone. These nephrons may be largely responsible for achieving the interstitial osmolality of about 450 mOsm/kg H$_2$O that exists at the transition of the outer and inner medulla. The remaining 15% of human nephrons are juxtamedullary nephrons with long loops of Henle extending into the inner medullary zone and renal papillae. Together with the parallel hairpin vasa recta, these units are responsible for further increasing interstitial osmolality during antidiuresis in humans to about 1,200 mOsm/kg H$_2$O at the tip of the papillae. In experiments with rats (61), selectively removing the papillae destroys only nephrons originating in the

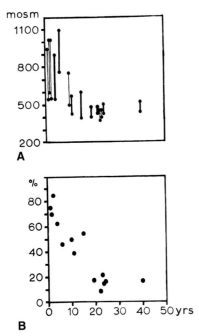

FIG. 78-4. Relationship between age and the ability to reverse the defect in urinary concentration in patients with sickle cell disease by blood transfusions. **A:** The maximal urinary osmolality achieved prior to transfusion (**lower point of each vertical line**) and after multiple transfusions with normal blood (**upper point of each vertical line**) in 14 patients with sickle cell disease ranging from 2 to 40 years of age (8 patients, *thick lines,* from Statius van Eps LW, et al. The influence of red blood cell transfusions on the hyposthenuria and renal hemodynamics of sickle cell anemia. *Clin Chim Acta* 1967;17:449; and 6 patients, *thin lines,* from Keitel HG, et al. Hyposthenuria in sickle cell anemia: a reversible renal defect. *J Clin Invest* 1956;35:998.). **B:** The percentage increase in maximal urinary osmolality resulting from transfusion. Maximal urinary osmolality prior to transfusion is depressed at all ages; significant improvement after transfusion occurs only in children and adolescents. (From Statius van Eps LW, et al. The influence of red blood cell transfusions on the hyposthenuria and renal hemodynamics of sickle cell anemia. *Clin Chim Acta* 1967;17:449, through courtesy of the editors.)

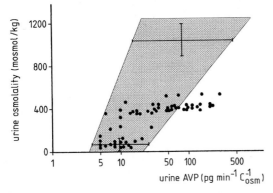

FIG. 78-5. The relation between urine osmolality and arginine vasopressin (AVP) excretion. The mean ± 2 standard deviations for AVP excretion and urine osmolality in control subjects, during water deprivation and water loading, is given. The individual values for Hb-SS patients are shown.

juxtamedullary cortex. In such animal preparations, a severe loss of concentrating capacity during fluid deprivation has been observed. Thus, juxtamedullary nephrons are necessary for achieving a maximal urine osmolality (29,62).

These pathophysiologic mechanisms help to clarify the abnormal findings in sickle cell nephropathy. On the basis of these mechanisms, the concentrating defect in sickle cell disease can be explained as a consequence of the sickling process per se and the resultant ischemic changes in the medullary microcirculation (27). It has been demonstrated that Hb-SS erythrocytes form sickle erythrocytes within seconds when placed in surroundings as hyperosmotic as the renal medulla during hydropenia (9).

Sickling of renal blood cells causes a significant increase in blood viscosity that could interfere with the normal circulation through the vasa recta, preventing both the active and passive accumulation of solute in the papillae necessary to achieve maximally concentrated urine. Increased viscosity of blood and intravascular aggregations of Hb-SS erythrocytes could also produce local hypoxia and eventually infarction of the renal papillae.

The vasa recta also provide the nutrient blood supply to the inner medulla and papillae, and it is at these sites that the most conspicuous lesions of established sickle cell nephropathy occur (e.g., focal scarring and patchy interstitial fibrosis). These lesions develop over many years, and it is probable that collateral capillary circulations are formed (Fig. 78-2). These collaterals probably lack the highly specialized spatial configuration—designated *zonation* (63)—of the normal vasa recta that run parallel to the long loops of Henle in the inner renal medulla. The loss of zonation and loss of countercurrent exchange function of the vasa recta, even with adequate nutrient blood flow through the medulla, could result in defective "trapping" of solute, so that the Hb-SS kidney would be unable to maintain a normally high papillary osmolality. The microradioangiographic studies thus offer the visible evidence for the mechanisms of the defect in renal concentrating capacity in sickle cell anemia (64).

Since it was demonstrated that fractional urea excretion fell markedly after indomethacin administration in sickle cell anemia patients and resulted in a rise in serum urea (53), the effect of indomethacin on renal concentrating capacity was also studied. Indeed, indomethacin normally promotes sodium reabsorption in the medulla with a consequent rise in papillary sodium and chloride concentration. Whereas indomethacin in normal patients improves renal concentrating capacity, it did not increase urinary osmolality in water-deprived Hb-SS patients (52,55) (Fig. 78-6A). This is therefore in favor of a defect in the capacity to trap solute in the medulla in sickle cell anemia. Also, the ability to concentrate urine was not increased in Hb-SS children placed on a high-protein diet (65), as observed in normal subjects. Both structurally and functionally, the sickle cell kidney has been compared to the beaver kidney because of a striking similarity of the vascular beds in the inner medulla—the lack of zonation (27). The beaver, which has only short loop nephrons and

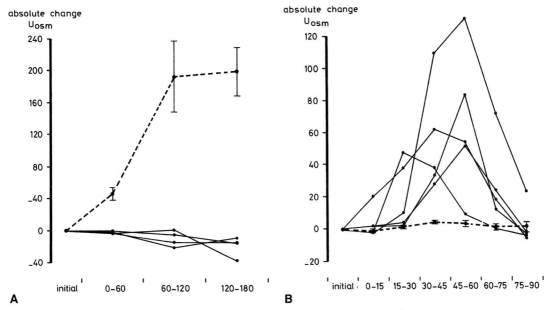

FIG. 78-6. The effect of indomethacin (75 mg as a suppository) in the water-depleted state (**A**) and the effect of indomethacin (0.25 mg/kg body weight IV) in the water-loaded state (**B**). The broken lines represent the means ± standard error of the mean in control subjects, and the continuous lines represent the individual data in patients with sickle cell anemia. (From De Jong PE, et al. The influence of indomethacin on renal concentrating and diluting capacity in sickle cell nephropathy. *Clin Sci* 1982;63:53, through courtesy of the editors.)

lacks an inner medullary zone, achieves a maximal urinary osmolality of only 500 mOsm/kg H_2O (66).

Loss of the ability to concentrate urine to more than 450 mOsm/kg H_2O is not of clinical importance under most circumstances because individuals usually drink more than the minimum amount of water necessary to excrete the average solute load of 600 to 800 mOsm/day. The obligatory urine volume to excrete this solute load in a patient with Hb-SS nephropathy amounts to about 2,000 mL/day, which is not an unusual urine volume for the normal person. Fluid deprivation or excessive fluid loss, however, will lead more rapidly to clinical dehydration in the patient with Hb-SS nephropathy than in the normal person. The clinician should be aware of this danger and should not limit the fluid intake of patients with sickle cell disease. Thus, in hot climates and in clinical syndromes attended by vomiting and diarrhea, the patient with sickle cell disease is vulnerable to more rapid dehydration than is the normal person.

Generation of Negative Solute-Free Water

The capacity to generate negative solute-free water (Tc_{H2O}) was studied in patients with sickle cell disease using different protocols. After mannitol loading, conflicting results have been obtained. Although Whitten and Younes find normal Tc_{H2O} levels in Hb-SS children (67), Levitt and colleagues describe two patients with a Tc_{H2O} of 3.2 mL/minute/100 mL glomerular filtrate (58). Hatch and associates find a mean Tc_{H2O} of 4.2 ± 0.9 SD mL/minute/100 mL glomerular filtrate in 11 Hb-SS patients compared to a mean Tc_{H2O}

of 5.7 ± 1.2 SD mL/minute/100 mL glomerular filtrate in 7 control subjects (56). These results suggest that Tc_{H2O} after mannitol loading is lower in sickle cell anemia.

After saline infusion, Hatch and associates (56) and Forrester and Alleyne (68) agree that Tc_{H2O} was impaired in Hb-SS patients. From these studies it was concluded that sickle cell anemia patients have a defect in the water-impermeable medullary loop of Henle that transports solute. The normal solute-free water clearance in Hb-SS patients argues against such an impairment in sodium chloride reabsorption from the ascending limb of Henle's loop. However, a normal solute-free water clearance only indicates a normal transport mechanism in the thick portion of the ascending limb in the outer medulla, whereas a normal Tc_{H2O} is depending on adequate function of the part of Henle's loop localized in the inner medulla. In agreement with this conclusion is the fact that the maximal concentrating capacity is generally not lower than 450 mOsm/kg H_2O. Thus, sickle cell anemia patients are able to increase urinary osmolality to the level that can be generated in the outer medulla. The pathology in the vasa recta, as shown in Fig. 78-2, is not contradictory to this conclusion of an adequate outer medullary transport. The capillary plexus surrounding short loops of Henle in the outer zone therefore does not necessarily penetrate into the inner zone.

A separation between the capillary plexus in the inner and outer zones has been suggested (69). One could thus propose that in sickle cell anemia the outer medullary circulation is adequate and the vascular pathology is confined primarily to the inner zone.

Urinary Diluting Capacity

Patients with sickle cell anemia are capable of diluting their urine normally (56,57,59). Under conditions of water diuresis, the fall in urinary osmolality has been found to be the same in control subjects and in patients with Hb-SS, and the percentage of filtered water excreted (C_{H2O}/GFR) was also identical in the two groups. Therefore, the capacity to reabsorb solute in the thick portion of the medullary ascending limb of Henle's loop apparently is intact in sickle cell anemia.

This combination of a defect in renal concentrating capacity with a normal diluting capacity is quite characteristic for sickle cell anemia. However, after indomethacin administration, the Hb-SS patient was not able to excrete water normally. There was a greater fall in C_{H2O}/GFR in sickle cell subjects compared to controls, and urinary osmolality rose from 42 to 125 mOsm/kg H_2O (19,55) (Fig. 78-6B). This result therefore suggests that renal prostaglandins are of importance in the normal diluting capacity in sickle cell anemia.

Urinary Acidification

Although systemic acidosis is generally not a feature of sickle cell disease in the absence of advanced renal failure, patients with Hb-SS or Hb-SC demonstrate an incomplete form of renal tubular acidosis (41,70–72). In response to a short-duration acid load (73), 79% of the patients with Hb-SS studied by Ho Ping Kong and Alleyne (70), 100% studied by Goossens and colleagues (71), and 29% of those studied by Oster and coworkers (72) were unable to decrease urine pH below 5.3, whereas normal subjects will achieve a urinary pH of 5.0 or lower. Titratable acid and total hydrogen ion excretion are lower in patients with Hb-SS or Hb-SC, but ammonia excretion is appropriate for the coexisting urine pH in most cases. The increased ammonia excretion induced by acid loading is reduced by indomethacin (41). This suggests that the assumed enhanced prostaglandin synthesis in sickle cell disease (74) may be important in maintaining a normal ammoniagenesis in sickle cell disease. When a maximal acidifying stimulus is employed, such as infusion of sodium sulfate, patients with Hb-SS may lower urine pH and increase net acid excretion to the same degree as normal subjects. Thus, the distal tubule of Hb-SS patients apparently requires a greater-than-normal stimulus to generate a normal urine-to-blood hydrogen ion gradient. In patients with sickle cell trait, renal acidification has been found to be normal (75).

The acidification defect has been classified as distal rather than proximal (71), because there is no associated wasting of bicarbonate and because it is characterized by failure to achieve a normal minimal urinary pH during acid loading. As none of the patients studied were acidemic or hyperchloremic before acid loading and no generalized proximal tubular reabsorptive defect was observed, the acidification defect was consistent with the incomplete syndrome of distal renal tubular acidosis (73,76). It has been suggested that the alterations in the microcirculation of the papillae may result in an inability of collecting ducts to maintain normally steep hydrogen ion gradients.

This very subtle defect in renal acidification generally does not cause systemic metabolic acidosis, which would increase sickling. For this reason, routine treatment with alkali is not indicated. Investigators in the West Indies (77), Nigeria (78), and the United States (72) find no evidence of metabolic acidosis in the absence of a sickle cell crisis, but find changes consistent with a mild chronic respiratory alkalosis. When metabolic acidosis occurs in a sickle cell patient, appropriate therapeutic measures should of course be taken as soon as possible.

Potassium Metabolism

In addition to the defect in hydrogen ion excretion, potassium excretion is also impaired in sickle cell patients (79–81). After administration of potassium chloride, sodium sulfate, or furosemide, potassium excretion was found to be subnormal in patients with sickle cell disease. Plasma renin activity and plasma aldosterone concentration in these patients were normal, both with normovolemia and after volume contraction. The defect could therefore not be explained by hypoaldosteronism. In spite of the impairment in renal potassium excretion, hyperkalemia did not develop during acute potassium chloride loading.

As with the defect in water and hydrogen ion excretion, the disturbance in potassium excretion could be due to an abnormality in the collecting duct secondary to the ischemic injury; potassium excretion is known to reflect primarily secretion in the distal nephron. The decreased potassium excretion, however, has not been well explored and other pathogenetic mechanisms could be involved. Potassium excretion in sickle cell trait is normal (82).

A hyperkalemic, hyperchloremic metabolic acidosis in sickle cell nephropathy has been observed (79). Three patients had Hb-SS, two had Hb-AS, and one had Hb-SC; all had impaired renal potassium excretion. Five of these six patients had a moderate to severe decrease of GFR and all patients had spontaneous metabolic acidosis. Selective aldosterone deficiency was recognized in three patients, two with normal and one with low plasma renin activity.

Other reports describe hyporeninemic hypoaldosteronism in patients with sickle cell disease (81,83). An impaired renin-secreting apparatus may result in impaired function of the adrenal glomerulosa cells, diminished aldosterone secretion, and an impaired ability to excrete potassium loads. In these cases, the hyperkalemia responded favorably to treatment with mineralocorticosteroids.

Proximal Tubular Secretion

Although severe disturbances in medullary transport occur in patients with sickle cell anemia, proximal tubular activity, both secretory and reabsorptive, appears to be supernormal. The tubular transport maximum of *para*-aminohippurate is elevated in sickle cell anemia, particularly in children (42). Other evidence of an increased proximal tubular secretory capacity has been obtained from studies regarding uric acid excretion. Notwithstanding the increased red cell turnover with consequent uric acid overproduction, most patients with sickle cell anemia are normouricemic. Urate clearance was found to be greater in these patients (84,85). This increased urate clearance was accounted for by increased pyrazinamide-suppressible urate clearance indicating an increased secretion of urate (84,86). Hyperuricemia in Hb-SS patients also can occur with decreased urate clearance, but these patients often have decreased *para*-aminohippurate clearance (85), proteinuria (87), or decreased inulin clearance (88). Urate clearance decreases with age in these patients and the incidence of hyperuricemia increases as renal function deteriorates (85). Attacks of gout can occur (88–91) and sometimes be clinically difficult to differentiate from an acute vasoocclusive crisis or from other bone and joint manifestations of sickle cell disease (i.e., sickle cell arthropathy) (92). Serum uric acid estimation may therefore be valuable in evaluating these patients.

As previously mentioned, the tubular secretion of creatinine has been found to be elevated with a 20% to 29% rise in fractional creatinine excretion in Hb-SS patients compared to control subjects (47,52). One should realize therefore that creatinine clearance in sickle cell anemia overestimates GFR considerably.

Proximal Tubular Reabsorption

Maximum tubular reabsorption of phosphate/L of glomerular filtrate (TmP/GFR) is also increased in sickle cell anemia. Consequent to this higher phosphate reabsorption, serum phosphate is elevated in these subjects (53,93). As is evident in Fig. 78-7, in both the fasting condition and after phosphate loading tubular reabsorption of phosphate is higher than expected for the corresponding serum phosphate level. It has been concluded that the high phosphate reabsorption reflects an increased reabsorptive activity of the proximal tubule (53). Because sodium reabsorption in the proximal tubule parallels phosphate reabsorption, this increased TmP/GFR suggests that increased sodium reabsorption may also occur in the proximal tubule. Indeed some studies reported an increased plasma volume in the noncrisis steady-state Hb-SS patients (94–96). On the other hand, this increased proximal tubular sodium reabsorption could be a secondary mechanism to correct for defects in salt reabsorption in a more distal part of the nephron. One might expect these patients to develop a volume-depleted state as a consequence of the defects in medullary water and sodium conservation. However, such distal compensatory mechanisms would not be expected to increase plasma volume.

An increased tubular uptake of beta-2-microglobulin has also been described in sickle cell anemia (97). A positive correlation between the reabsorption of phosphate and beta-2-microglobulin was reported. This positive correlation

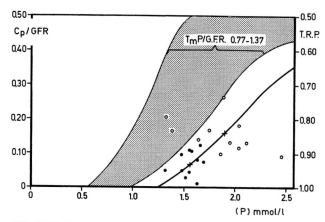

FIG. 78-7. Relation between C_p/glomerular filtration rate and serum phosphate (P). *Closed circles* represent values for the fasting patients; *open circles* are values obtained when U_pV was 0.032 mmol/minute. The *continuous line* shows the mean of the values in sickle cell anemia patients, and the *hatched area* indicates the range for normal persons. (From De Jong PE, et al. The tubular reabsorption of phosphate in sickle cell nephropathy. *Clin Sci* 1978;55:429, through courtesy of the editors.)

between phosphate and beta-2-microglobulin reabsorption is further evidence of an increased activity of the proximal tubule in sickle cell anemia. Zinc excretion has also been found to be abnormal in sickle cell anemia. Whereas the excretion of zinc in control subjects is lower than the filtered load of zinc, in Hb-SS patients zinc excretion exceeds the filtered load (98).

Thus, Hb-SS patients have a defect in renal medullary functions with a tendency to lose water and sodium, whereas ERPF, GFR, and proximal tubular activity are increased. In general, the ultimate result of this compensation will be normal homeostasis of fluid and electrolytes.

RENAL HORMONES

Erythropoietin

Data on plasma *erythropoietin* (EPO) levels in sickle cell anemia are conflicting. Increased values have been reported, both in asymptomatic patients and during infectious episodes (99). However, when comparing plasma EPO concentrations in sickle cell anemia with those in other causes of anemia, Hb-SS patients have similar (100) or decreased (101) values. EPO titers in patients with pure red cell aplasia, for instance, were 10-fold higher than those in patients with Hb-SS.

The observations of Sherwood and associates (102) that patients with sickle cell anemia produce less immunoreactive EPO at a given hemoglobin concentration than do patients with nonsickle cell anemias agree with previous results using biologic assay (103). Pediatric patients with sickle cell anemia have significantly higher EPO levels than do adults.

Morgan and Serjeant (25), in a study of patients older than 40 years, observed a fall in the Hb concentration among these individuals. They suggest that the lower Hb concentration is due to a reduced EPO production.

The potential mechanisms for the low EPO levels in sickle cell disease include interference with the renal synthesis of EPO, as a result of renal damage by the sickling process (microinfarctions), and the displacement to the right of the oxygen equilibrium curve. This displacement is caused by the lower affinity of the Hb-S polymer for oxygen in sickle cells and the increase in intracellular 2,3-diphosphoglyceric acid levels.

Renin–Angiotensin–Aldosterone System

Plasma renin activity and aldosterone concentration in general are found to be normal in patients with Hb-SS disease during steady-state conditions (47,80). After volume depletion, normal or increased values were found (104), and Hatch and associates (95) recently showed that both supine and upright plasma renin activities for different sodium intakes always were higher in Hb-SS patients than in control subjects. However, as mentioned earlier, some patients with hyporeninemic hypoaldosteronism and hyperkalemia have been described (81,83). Interestingly, high plasma renin activity has been described in a patient with intermittent hypertension occurring during a painful crisis. When the crisis had subsided, blood pressure normalized again (105). Possibly these episodes of hypertension were due to renal hypoperfusion at the time of the crisis. This is a unique finding in sickle cell anemia because hypertension seldom occurs in Hb-SS patients.

Renal Prostaglandins

Prostaglandin production has been documented in the interstitial medullary cells and collecting duct cells in the kidney (106), and production of renal prostaglandins is promoted by various vasoconstrictor stimuli (107). It might therefore be suspected that the ischemic insult to the inner medulla in sickle cell anemia induces synthesis of vasodilator prostaglandins. Indeed, the interstitial cells of the medulla in patients with sickle cell anemia contain aggregates of granular electron-dense material (32); this finding is compatible with increased prostaglandin synthesis in these cells. The role of renal prostaglandins in sickle cell anemia has been studied in two ways: first by indirect methods using indomethacin as a prostaglandin synthesis inhibitor, and second by direct measurement of urinary prostaglandin E_2 and $F_{2\alpha}$ (PGE_2 and $PGF_{2\alpha}$) excretion.

As already discussed, indomethacin administration does not change GFR and ERPF in control subjects, but a significant fall in these functions was found after indomethacin administration to Hb-SS patients (47,52). This suggests that prostaglandins are of importance in maintaining the supernormal or normal GFR and ERPF in sickle cell anemia. Prostaglandins may therefore be relevant with respect to the hyperfiltration observed in young patients with sickle cell

anemia. Prostaglandins induce a rise in renal blood flow, particularly in the juxtamedullary nephrons with a consequent rise in GFR. Such a prostaglandin-mediated hyperfiltration could cause glomerulosclerosis with ultimate loss of renal function and chronic renal failure in sickle cell anemia. The rise in renal blood flow and glomerular filtration could also explain the increased proximal tubular activity in these patients.

In normal subjects, indomethacin causes sodium and water retention and a rise in body weight. In Hb-SS patients, a similar sodium retention was observed after indomethacin administration. This sodium retention, however, was not accompanied by water retention or an increase in body weight. Rather, serum osmolality increased in these patients (44). In rats indomethacin promotes sodium reabsorption in the medulla with consequent rise in papillary sodium and chloride concentration (108); hence, the changes after indomethacin administration in Hb-SS patients point to a particular role for renal prostaglandins in volume homeostasis in these patients.

Indomethacin administration to water-deprived normal subjects caused a rise in urinary osmolality of 836 to 1,027 mOsm/kg H_2O, whereas the defect in urinary concentration in sickle cell anemia was not improved at all after indomethacin (55) (Fig. 78-6). This result supports a diminished solute gradient in the inner medulla of patients with Hb-SS, which is not modulated by prostaglandins.

During a water load, however, a rise in urinary osmolality occurred after indomethacin administration in patients with sickle cell disease, but not in control subjects. It is thus concluded that normal diluting capacity in patients with sickle cell anemia is dependent on adequate renal prostaglandin synthesis (52,55).

Both in the dehydrated and in the water-loaded state, PGE_2 excretion has been found to be normal in patients with sickle cell disease. $PGF_{2\alpha}$ excretion, however, is decreased, therefore, the $PGE_2/PGF_{2\alpha}$ ratio is higher than in normal persons (74). As PGE_2 and $PGF_{2\alpha}$ have different and sometimes opposite effects on renal hemodynamics, renin release, and sodium and water excretion (109,110), it is possible that an abnormal balance between these two prostaglandins may contribute to some of the characteristics of sickle cell nephropathy. For example, the relative excess of the vasodilating PGE_2 could explain the rise in renal blood flow and GFR, particularly in the juxtamedullary nephrons.

Hypertension and Sickle Cell Disease

The incidence of hypertension in the black population between the ages of 18 and 74 in the United States is 28.2%. This percentage sharply contrasts with that in sickle cell disease. Reports from both the Caribbean (111,112) and the United States (95,113) show that hypertension is present in only 2% to 6% of the Hb-SS patients (Fig. 78-8). These findings are difficult to interpret. Renal salt losing has been suggested (83), but these data are not convincing. Matustik and

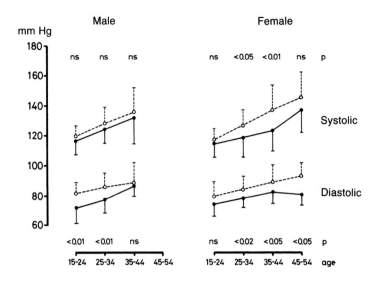

FIG. 78-8. Mean ± standard deviation of systolic and diastolic blood pressure in control subjects (*dotted lines*) and patients with sickle cell anemia (*closed lines*) who are age- and sex-matched. (Derived from De Jong PE, et al. Blood pressure in sickle cell disease. *Arch Intern Med* 1982;142:1239; and reproduced from De Jong PE, Statius van Eps LW. Sickle cell nephropathy. New insights into its pathophysiology. Editorial review. *Kidney Int* 1985;27:711, through courtesy of the editors.)

associates (104) and Hatch and coworkers (95) nicely show that Hb-SS patients are able to conserve sodium adequately on a severely restricted sodium diet. Moreover, the demonstration of an increased, instead of a lowered, plasma volume (94–96) does not support the hypothesis that the lower blood pressures in patients with sickle cell anemia are related to a volume loss. Another explanation has recently been forwarded. A decreased forearm vascular resistance that did not increase with cold-induced, sympathetic-mediated stimulation and an impaired pressor response to angiotensin II suggest that an altered vascular reactivity may protect these patients from hypertension (95).

Blood Coagulation and Vasa Recta Occlusion in Sickle Cell Disease

Statius van Eps and Leeksma (114) have suggested the occurrence of intravascular coagulation in sickle cell disease because of decreased platelet counts, increased platelet turnover, hyporeactive "exhausted" platelets, elevated fibrinopeptide A, and fragment D-dimer levels, all observed in patients suffering from a vasoocclusive crisis. The potential role of thrombotic occlusion in sickle cell disease was summarized by Francis (115). Activation of coagulation may contribute to the renal vasa recta occlusion and to a sickle cell crisis. Because this hypercoagulability has been observed associated with vasoocclusive crises in sickle cell disease (116), Wolters and colleagues studied the effect of low-dose acenocoumarol in sickle cell disease (117). The enhanced thrombin formation was corrected and normalized, and the increased plasma levels of prothrombin fragments 1 and 2, reflecting enhanced endogenous thrombin generation, became normal (117). Low-dose therapy with acenocoumarol to prevent sickle cell crisis is now under investigation.

Sickle erythrocytes and their spicules and vesicles have been shown to accelerate blood clotting *in vitro*. Their procoagulant activity has been explained by the presence of phosphatidylserine in the outer leaflet of their membrane (118). An increased adherence of sickle erythrocytes to monocytes and endothelial cells has been observed by many investigators (114). Hypertonicity as occurs in the vasa recta may facilitate adherence (119).

Diminished prostacyclin regenerating ability and increased prostacyclin inactivation in sickle cell anemia may explain the increased platelet aggregation in sickle cell disease. This agrees with our observations that intravenous prostacyclin can have a beneficial effect on a vasoocclusive crisis, provided therapy is started within 2 hours after the onset of symptoms (L. W. Statius van Eps, unpublished observations, 1992).

CLINICAL MANIFESTATIONS

Hematuria

In 1948, Abel and Brown were the first to discover a relationship between sickle cell disease and hematuria (120). They described a young black soldier who underwent nephrectomy because of severe and persistent unilateral hematuria. A renal neoplasm was suspected, but histopathologic examination of the excised kidney demonstrated only sickled red blood in the medullary vessels.

Hematuria is a very dramatic renal manifestation of sickle cell nephropathy. Gross hematuria occurs in patients who have heterozygous sickle hemoglobin (Hb-AS, Hb-SC) as well as in those who have the homozygous disease (Hb-SS) (120–126). The majority of cases have been reported in patients with Hb-AS and Hb-SC disease. The relative rarity of hematuria in cases of Hb-SS is more apparent than real, as sickle cell trait is approximately 40 times more common than the homozygous state. Gross hematuria in affected patients may occur at any age, including young children, and appears to be more common in males than in females. It has also been described in a white woman with sickle cell trait (127).

The pathologic abnormalities causing hematuria have not yet been elucidated. Kimmelstiel (128) describes the changes as temporary capillary stasis after spasm. The consequence is plugging of capillaries by sickle cells, resulting in vessel wall injury and, rarely, in true capillary thrombi with ischemia and necrosis. Mostofi and associates (20) studied 21 kidneys from patients with sickle cell disease that were removed because of massive blood loss and the possibility of renal neoplasm. The absence of significant gross alterations in most of these kidneys emphasizes the fact that the lesions are inconspicuous and may be easily missed. The most striking change consisted of severe stasis in peritubular capillaries of both the cortex and the medulla; the changes were most marked in the medulla. Extravasation of blood was observed, mainly into the collecting tubules.

These early observations are in accordance with our present insights into the pathophysiologic mechanisms in the inner medulla. Perillie and Epstein show that Hb-S erythrocytes transversing the hyperosmotic inner renal medulla undergo instant sickling as a result of an increase of intracellular hemoglobin concentration (9). Moreover, the renal medullary pH is quite acidic and oxygen tension is decreased; both factors promote sickling of red blood cells. Sickling in the vasa recta leads to increased blood viscosity, formation of microthrombi, ischemia, and necrosis, which could cause structural changes leading to hematuria.

The typical patient is a young black man with painless hematuria, often following mild or sometimes severe trauma to the renal area (126). Recurrences are frequent, and conservative therapeutic measures may not be immediately successful. In the majority of cases, however, bleeding eventually subsides spontaneously, although sometimes only after a period of weeks or even months. Interestingly, when hematuria is unilateral, which is generally the case (only about 10% of cases are bilateral), the left kidney appears to be involved four times more often than the right kidney.

Even in the absence of episodes of gross hematuria, most patients with sickle cell hemoglobin (Hb-SS) demonstrate microscopic hematuria. The finding of otherwise unexplained hematuria in a patient of African descent is a clear indication to perform appropriate tests for the presence of sickle cell disease or trait. The presence of gross hematuria in the patient with sickle cell disease can result in misleading findings on the intravenous urography. In almost one-half of all such patients with gross hematuria, blood clots produce filling defects in the renal pelvis that may be confused with neoplasm, calculus, or hemangioma. Such findings have led to unnecessary nephrectomy. Computed axial tomography (CT) can generally exclude the presence of a renal neoplasm.

Gross hematuria is thus a renal manifestation of sickle cell disease that can require major therapeutic decisions. Although hematuria can be massive and life-threatening, conservative measures are the treatment of choice. These include complete bed rest, urinary alkalinization, and the maintenance of a high rate of urine flow by infusion of mannitol or administration of diuretic agents and even infusion of distilled water (i.e., 500 mL over 15 minutes) (127). Repeated transfusions with normal Hb-A blood will both correct blood loss and increase the percentage of normal Hb-A. Also, hyperbaric oxygenation, which may decrease sickle cell formation, has been employed. Intravenous triglycyl vasopressin was successful in two sickle cell cases with persistent hematuria (128,129). Pelvic tamponade as a means of controlling hematuria has also been applied (130). Surgical intervention (i.e., nephrectomy) should be considered only in the presence of life-threatening hemorrhage that does not improve with conservative therapy or when multiple transfusions are not possible. If the bleeding can be localized in a distinct part of the kidney, one should consider the possibility of a renal autotransplantation after removal of that part of the kidney (131).

Until 1964 nephrectomy was necessary in about 50% of the sickle cell patients with severe, therapy-resistant hemorrhage. In that year, Immergut and Stevenson showed the favorable therapeutic effect of epsilon aminocaproic acid (EACA) in the control of hematuria associated with hemoglobinopathies (132).

Normal urine contains a fibrinolytic enzyme, urokinase, capable of destroying fibrin and thus dissolving clots in the urinary tract. EACA is a potent inhibitor of fibrinolysis and reaches a high urinary concentration after oral or parenteral ingestion.

Complete inhibition of fibrinolytic activity can normally be expected with 8 g of EACA daily. Urinary levels of EACA are 50 to 100 times those of plasma. With repeated oral dosage there is a gradual sustained renal excretion of the drug so that adequate urinary levels are maintained. Nilsson and associates, who treated 526 patients with hematuria of various origins with EACA, advocate the use of 3 to 4 g of EACA three to four times daily (115). The results of EACA in the treatment of hematuria of sickle cell nephropathy have been impressive, although the therapeutic regimens have varied (114,122,132–134).

Thrombotic complications have been reported to occur in patients receiving large doses of EACA, usually in excess of 12 g per day. Control of fibrinolytic hemorrhage often can be obtained, however, with doses as low as 2 or 3 g per day (135). Therefore, it is advisable to administer EACA on a short-term basis in the lowest dosage required to inhibit urinary fibrinolytic activity.

The therapy for hematuria in sickle cell patients must be individualized based on the severity and duration of each bleeding episode and should be reserved for those patients who have exhibited severe and prolonged or chronically recurrent hematuria (134). To conclude, a sickle cell patient with hematuria should first be treated with bed rest, blood transfusions in Hb-SS patients, urinary alkalinization (sodium bicarbonate, several grams q.i.d.), and diuresis with high volumes of fluid, preferably hypotonic solutions and furosemide (40 mg b.i.d.). If the hematuria continues, EACA should be added to this regimen. EACA should be given first in low doses, 1 g q.i.d., and gradually increased, when necessary, to 3 to 4 g q.i.d. (132). Intravenously, 5 g can be given followed by an infusion of 10 g per 12 hours.

The new antifibrinolytic drug, tranexamic acid, is a promising agent. It is 7 to 10 times more potent than EACA and merits a clinical trial in sickle cell hematuria. A suggested starting dose is 0.5 g q.i.d.

Gross hematuria has been observed in patients with combined sickle cell trait and von Willebrand's disease in the absence of extrarenal bleeding (136,137). These patients have been treated successfully with cryoprecipitate. It is therefore important to consider von Willebrand's disease and other hemorrhagic disorders in patients with sickle cell trait and hematuria.

Autosomal-dominant polycystic kidney disease (ADPKD) in blacks has been studied and its occurrence together with sickle cell hemoglobin analyzed (138). Sickle cell hemoglobin occurred more often than expected in ADPKD. The disease was more severe with earlier onset of end-stage renal disease in blacks compared with ADPKD whites and in blacks with sickle cell trait when compared with blacks without the trait. Both conditions can cause hematuria.

Urinary Tract Infections

The incidence of asymptomatic bacteriuria during pregnancy and the puerperium appears to be distinctively higher in women with sickle cell disease or sickle cell trait than in nonpregnant women or women without sickle cell disease or trait; a twofold increase has been observed in two surveys (139,140). This correlates with an increased incidence of "pyelonephritis" found at autopsy in Hb-AS patients (141). The pathologic changes due to Hb-SS nephropathy (medullary ischemia and fibrosis), however, may be easily confused with those of pyelonephritis.

Pyelonephritis or urosepsis may precipitate a crisis, as may other infections. For these reasons, all sickle cell patients in crisis should have a search performed for foci of infection, including one in the urinary tract.

Papillary Necrosis and Calicectasis

Renal papillary necrosis and calicectasis is a frequent occurrence in sickle cell disease, in both homozygotes and heterozygotes. Renal papillary necrosis as a complication of sickle cell nephropathy has an incidence ranging from 15% to 36% (23). Harrow and associates (24) were the first to stress the importance of this complication. As in sickle cell nephropathy, the distinctive abnormalities of the renal medulla and papillae are obliteration of vasa recta and medullary necrosis and fibrosis; papillary necrosis is a logical consequence of these processes.

In 45 patients, gross, painless hematuria (142) was the most common symptom reported. Renal colic caused by the passage of blood clots or ruptured particles of necrotic papillae is less frequent.

Intravenous pyelography is the method of choice to diagnose papillary necrosis (22,24).

Proteinuria and the Nephrotic Syndrome

Appreciable proteinuria is a frequent finding in sickle cell disease, occurring in about 30% of patients when observed over a prolonged period. Less common is proteinuria of nephrotic proportions (greater than 3 g/24 hour); however, severe proteinuria occurs often enough to suspect more than a fortuitous association between sickle cell disease and the nephrotic syndrome (143,144).

Tejani and associates (40) observed the frequent occurrence of focal segmental glomerulosclerosis in children with sickle cell disease. It can be assumed that the hyperfiltration in patients with sickle cell anemia makes them more prone to develop glomerulosclerosis (44).

Falk and colleagues investigated 381 patients with sickle cell disease for proteinuria and renal insufficiency (31). Twenty-six patients (7%) had serum creatinine concentrations above the normal range and 101 (26%) had proteinuria of at least 1+. Forty-four patients had a complete 24-hour urine collection. In these patients protein excretion ranged from 28 mg/24 hour to 10.8 g/24 hour, with a mean of 1.7 g/24 hour and SD of ±2.4 g. Twelve patients excreted more than 2.5 g of protein per 24 hours, associated with other features of the nephrotic syndrome. In the 10 biopsied patients with proteinuria, administration of an angiotensin-converting enzyme (ACE) inhibitor, enalapril, caused the 24-hour urinary protein excretion to decrease by 57% (range 23% to 79%) below the baseline value; it increased to 25% below baseline after discontinuation of enalapril. There was no significant change in GFR, ERPF, or filtration fraction nor was there a decrease in arterial pressure.

Sklar and coworkers reviewed the records of 386 patients with sickle cell anemia (145). Seventy-eight patients (20.4%) had proteinuria and 17 patients (4.6%) had renal insufficiency. Both renal insufficiency and proteinuria increased with age, reaching rates of 33% and 56%, respectively, in patients 40 years of age and older.

Falk and Jenette (146), compared the data regarding proteinuria in sickle cell disease found by Falk and associates (31), Bakir and coworkers (35), Powars and colleagues (147), and Sklar and others (145), and concluded that renal failure is virtually inevitable in sickle cell patients with the nephrotic syndrome.

All the findings of Falk and Jenette support the hypothesis that glomerular capillary hypertension is present in sickle cell nephropathy causing the major abnormalities observed: glomerular hypertrophy, focal segmental glomerulosclerosis, proteinuria, decrease in protein excretion with an ACE inhibitor, and the progressive decrease in renal function with age (146). As a possible cause of the glomerular hypertension and hypertrophy, investigators suggest the almost complete absence of vasa recta in the kidney of sickle cell patients (27) and that medullary ischemia results in increased renal production of prostaglandins (73). This leads in turn to vasodilation of afferent glomerular arterioles and to glomerular hypertension as proposed by de Jong and Statius van Eps (44).

Renal vein thrombosis has been diagnosed in some patients, and because Hb-SS predisposes to venous thrombosis, this complication should be considered in all patients with Hb-SS in whom massive proteinuria develops. However, the cause-and-effect relationship between renal vein thrombosis and the nephrotic syndrome is unclear.

Acute Renal Failure

Acute renal failure in association with sickle cell disease has rarely been described. Some reports describe a reversible acute oligoanuric renal failure in the setting of sickle cell crisis (148,149). In both of these studies rhabdomyolysis was suggested as the cause of this acute renal failure. In a study by Sklar and colleagues of 12 sickle cell anemia patients with acute renal failure, volume depletion in the setting of sickle cell crisis was the most common cause (150). Of the 12 patients, 10 survived and subsequently had recovery of renal function.

In a recent publication, Hassell and coworkers describe a syndrome of acute multiorgan failure in 14 sickle cell patients (10 Hb-SS, 4 Hb-SC) occurring during a painful event that was unusually severe for the patients (151). There was acute failure of at least two of three organs: lung, liver, or kidney. Acute renal insufficiency developed during 13 episodes, with a rapid, reversible elevation of serum creatinine concentration above 2.0 mg/dL during a period of 24 to 36 hours. Acute abnormalities of liver function and acute pulmonary infiltrates were observed. All but one patient recovered after treatment with multiple blood transfusions.

Chronic Renal Failure

Because renal function may deteriorate with age in Hb-SS patients, either as a result of the parenchymal damage due to sickling or because of primary glomerular disease, some patients with sickle cell disease will become candidates for chronic hemodialysis. Renal dysfunction is one of the most common causes of death in older patients with sickle cell anemia (152). Powars and coworkers performed a 25-year demographic and clinical cohort study to determine the incidence, clinical cause, and risk factors associated with the onset of chronic renal failure in 725 sickle cell anemia patients and 209 with sickle C disease (147). Of the sickle cell anemia group, 4.2% developed chronic renal failure compared with 2.4% of those with sickle C disease. The median ages at disease onset were 23.1 years for the sickle cell

anemia group and 49.9 years for the sickle C disease group. Survival time for sickle cell anemia patients after diagnosis of chronic renal failure, despite dialysis, was 4 years and the median age at the time of death, 27 years. Pathologic studies showed characteristic lesions of glomerular "dropout" and glomerulosclerosis. An interesting finding was that the risk for renal failure was increased in patients who had inherited the Central African Republic beta^{-s} gene cluster haplotype.

Sickle cell anemia patients are presenting with increasing frequency for renal replacement therapy. Both hemodialysis (153,154) and transplantation (155–157) can be performed successfully.

Nissenson and Port (154) report the course of 77 patients with sickle cell disease and end-stage renal failure. There is a marked male predominance, and renal failure appears most commonly in the third and fourth decades. The 2-year survival among those in this group receiving renal replacement therapy was approximately 60%.

Chatterjee shows that these patients do as well as others after transplantation with respect to patient survival and graft survival (155). Interestingly, hematocrit values after transplantation are found to be higher than in sickle cell anemia patients with normal renal function. A disturbance in renal concentrating capacity with a maximum urinary osmolality of 400 mOsm/kg H_2O was observed by us in one patient within 12 months after transplantation (L.W. Statius van Eps and P, de Jong, unpublished data). In one case report, the recurrence of sickle cell nephropathy was suggested in a transplanted kidney 3.5 years after transplantation (158).

Atrial Natriuretic Peptide

The renal effects of atrial natriuretic peptide (ANP) in sickle cell disease have been studied recently. In normal subjects, ANP exerts its natriuretic effects in several nephron segments dependent on prevailing ANP levels. Infusion of a low-dose ANP induced natriuresis in normal individuals but not in matched patients with sickle cell disease (159). This observation suggests that low-dose ANP inhibits sodium reabsorption in the long loops of Henle, possibly by increasing medullary blood flow and renal interstitial pressure. Natriuresis during supraphysiologic plasma levels of ANP appears to be multifactorial, by an increase in GFR and a decrease in both proximal and distal tubular sodium reabsorption. Infusion of high-dose ANP in patients with sickle cell disease and normal subjects induced a similar degree of natriuresis in both groups (159).

REFERENCES

1. Herrick JB. Peculiar elongated and sickle shaped red blood corpuscles in a case of severe anemia. *Arch Intern Med* 1910;6:517.
2. Konotey-Ahulu FID. Hereditary qualitative and quantitative erythrocyte defects in Ghana: a historical and geographical survey. *Ghana Med J* 1968;7:118.

3. Pauling L, et al. Sickle cell anemia, molecular disease. *Science* 1949; 110:543.

4. Ingram VM. Gene mutations in human hemoglobin. The chemical difference between normal and sickle cell hemoglobin. *Nature* 1959;180:326.

5. Murayama M. Molecular mechanisms of red cell "sickling." *Science* 1966;153:145.

6. Noguchi CT, Schechter AN. The intracellular polymerization of sickle hemoglobin and its relevance to sickle cell disease. *Blood* 1981; 58:1057.

7. Franck PFH, et al. Uncoupling of the membrane skeleton from the lipid bilayer. The cause of accelerated phospholipid flip-flop leading to an enhanced procoagulant activity of sickled cells. *J Clin Invest* 1985;75:183.

8. Lubin B, et al. Abnormalities in membrane phospholipid organization in sickled erythrocytes. *J Clin Invest* 1981;67:1643.

9. Perillie PE, Epstein FH. Sickling phenomenon produced by hypertonic solutions: a possible explanation for the hyposthenuria of sicklemia. *J Clin Invest* 1963;42:570.

10. Evans E, Mohandas N, Leung A. Static and dynamic rigidities of normal and sickle erythrocytes. Major influence of cell hemoglobin concentration. *J Clin Invest* 1983;73:477.

11. Statius van Eps LW, et al. The relation between age and renal concentrating capacity in sickle cell disease and hemoglobin C disease. *Clin Chim Acta* 1970;27:501.

12. Cawein MJ, et al. Hemoglobin S-D disease. *Ann Intern Med* 1966; 64:62.

13. Statius van Eps LW, et al. The influence of red blood cell transfusions on the hyposthenuria and renal hemodynamics of sickle cell anemia. *Clin Chim Acta* 1967;17:449.

14. Bookchin RM, Davis RP, Ranney HM. Clinical features of hemoglobin C_{Harlem}, a new sickling hemoglobin variant. *Ann Intern Med* 1968;68:8.

15. Serjeant B, et al. Sickle cell-hemoglobin D_{Iran}: a benign sickle cell syndrome. *Hemoglobin* 1982;6:57.

16. Serjeant GR. *Sickle cell disease,* 2nd ed. London: Oxford University Press, 1992:407.

17. Neel JV. The inheritance of sickle cell anemia. *Science* 1949;110:64.

18. Sydenstricker VP, Mulherin WA, Houseal RW. Sickle cell anemia, report of two cases in children with necropsy in one case. *Am J Dis Child* 1923;26:132.

19. Alleyne GAO, et al. The kidney in sickle cell anemia. *Kidney Int* 1975;7:371.

20. Mostofi FK, Vorder Brugge CF, Diggs LW. Lesions in kidneys removed for unilateral hematuria in sickle cell disease. *Arch Pathol* 1957;63:336.

21. Margulies SI, Minkin SK. Sickle cell disease: the roentgenologic manifestations of urinary tract abnormalities in adults. *Am J Roentgenol Radium Ther Nucl Med* 1969;108:702.

22. Akinkugbe OO. Renal papillary necrosis in sickle cell hemoglobinopathy. *Br Med J (Clin Res)* 1967;3:283.

23. Vaamonde CA. Renal papillary necrosis in sickle cell hemoglobinopathies. *Semin Nephrol* 1984;4:48.

24. Harrow BR, Sloane JA, Liebman NC. Röntgenologic demonstration of renal papillary necrosis in sickle cell trait. *N Engl J Med* 1963;268:969.

25. Morgan AG, Serjeant GR. Renal function in patients over 40 with homozygous sickle-cell disease. *Br Med J (Clin Res)* 1981;282:1181.

26. Morgan AG, Shah DJ, Williams W. Renal pathology in adults over 40 with sickle-cell disease. *West Indian Med J* 1987;36:241.

27. Statius van Eps LW, et al. Nature of concentrating defect in sickle cell nephropathy, microradioangiographic studies. *Lancet* 1970;1:450.

28. Bernstein J, Whitten CF. Histological appraisal of the kidney in sickle cell anemia. *Arch Pathol* 1960;70:407.

29. Buckalew VM, Someren A. Renal manifestations of sickle cell disease. *Arch Intern Med* 1974;133:660.

30. Walker BR, et al. Glomerular lesions in sickle cell nephropathy. *JAMA* 1971;215:437.

31. Falk RJ, et al. Prevalence and pathologic features of sickle cell nephropathy and response to inhibition of angiotensin-converting enzyme. *N Engl J Med* 1992;326:910.

32. Pitcock JA, et al. Early renal changes in sickle cell anemia. *Arch Pathol* 1970;90:403.

33. McCoy RC. Ultrastructural alterations in the kidney with sickle cell disease and the nephrotic syndrome. *Lab Invest* 1969;21:85.

34. Elfenbein IB, et al. Pathology of the glomerulus in sickle cell anemia with and without nephrotic syndrome. *Am J Pathol* 1974;77:357.

35. Bakir AA, et al. Prognosis of the nephrotic syndrome in sickle cell glomerulopathy. *Am J Nephrol* 1987;7:110.

36. Statius van Eps LW. Sickle cell nephropathy [Editorial]. *Kidney: Curr Survey World Lit* 1992;1:241.

37. Ozawa T, et al. Autologous immune complex nephritis associated with sickle cell trait: diagnosis of the hemoglobinopathy after renal structural and immunological studies. *Br Med J (Clin Res)* 1976;1:369.

38. Pardo V, et al. Nephropathy associated with sickle cell anemia: an autologous immune complex nephritis. II. Clinicopathologic study of seven patients. *Am J Med* 1975;59:650.

39. Strauss J, et al. Nephropathy associated with sickle cell anemia: an autologous immune complex nephritis. *Am J Med* 1975;58:382.

40. Tejani A, et al. Renal lesions in sickle cell nephropathy in children. *Nephron* 1985;39:352.

41. De Jong PE, et al. The influence of indomethacin on renal acidification in normal subjects and in patients with sickle cell anemia. *Clin Nephrol* 1983;19:259.

42. Etteldorf JN, Tuttle AH, Clayton GW. Renal function studies in pediatrics: I. Renal hemodynamics in children with sickle cell anemia. *Am J Dis Child* 1952;83:185.

43. Etteldorf JN, et al. Renal hemodynamic studies in adults with sickle cell anemia. *Am J Med* 1955;18:243.

44. De Jong PE, Statius van Eps LW. Sickle cell nephropathy. New insights into its pathophysiology [Editorial review]. *Kidney Int* 1985;27:711.

45. Bhathena DB, Sondheimer JH. The glomerulopathy of homozygous sickle hemoglobin (SS) disease: morphology and pathogenesis. *J Am Soc Nephrol* 1991;1:1241.

46. Freedman BI, Burkart JM, Iskander SS. Chronic mesangiolytic glomerulopathy in a patient with SC hemoglobinopathy. *Am J Kidney Dis* 1990;15:361.

47. De Jong PE, et al. The influence of indomethacin on renal haemodynamics in sickle cell anemia. *Clin Sci* 1980;59:245.

48. Hollenberg NK, Adams DF. Hypertension and intrarenal perfusion patterns in man. *Am J Med Sci* 1971;261:233.

49. Horster M, Thurau K. Micropuncture studies on the filtration rate of single superficial and juxtamedullary glomeruli in the rat kidney. *Pflugers Arch* 1968;301:162.

50. Bradley SE, Bradley GP. Renal function during chronic anemia in man. *Blood* 1947;2:192.

51. Aperia AC, Liebow AA, Roberts LE. Renal adaptation to anemia. *Circ Res* 1968;22:489.

52. Allon A, et al. Effects of nonsteroidal antiinflammatory drugs on renal function in sickle cell anemia. *Kidney Int* 1988;34:500.

53. De Jong PE, de Jong-van den Berg LTW, Statius van Eps LW. The tubular reabsorption of phosphate in sickle cell nephropathy. *Clin Sci* 1978;55:429.

54. Hostetter TH, et al. Hyperfiltration in remnant nephrons: a potentially adverse response to renal ablation. *Am J Physiol* 1981;241:F85.

55. De Jong PE, et al. The influence of indomethacin on renal concentrating and diluting capacity in sickle cell nephropathy. *Clin Sci* 1982;63:53.

56. Hatch FE, Culbertson JW, Diggs LW. Nature of the renal concentrating defect in sickle cell disease. *J Clin Invest* 1967;46:336.

57. Keitel HG, Thompson D, Itano HA. Hyposthenuria in sickle cell anemia: a reversible renal defect. *J Clin Invest* 1956;35:998.

58. Levitt MF, et al. The renal concentrating defect in sickle cell disease. *Am J Med* 1960;29:611.

59. Schlitt L, Keitel HG. Pathogenesis of hyposthenuria in persons with sickle cell anemia or the sickle cell trait. *Pediatrics* 1960;26:249.

60. McCrory WW, Goren N, Gornfeld D. Demonstration of impairment of urinary concentrating ability, or "Pitressin resistance" in children with sickle cell anemia. *Am J Dis Child* 1953;86:512.

61. Lief PD, Sullivan A, Goldberg M. Physiological contributions of thin and thick loops of Henle to the renal concentrating mechanism. *J Clin Invest* 1969;48:32a.

62. Jamison RL. Intrarenal heterogeneity. The case for two functionally dissimilar populations of nephrons in the mammalian kidney. *Am J Med* 1973;54:281.

63. Plakke RK, Pfeiffer EW. Blood vessels of the mammalian renal medulla. *Science* 1964;146:1683.

64. Visible proof [Editorial]. *Lancet* 1970;1:456.

65. Rubin MI. Effect of dietary protein on the renal concentrating process in sickle cell anemia. *Am J Dis Child* 1968;115:262.

66. Schmidt-Nielsen B, O'Dell R. Structure and concentrating mechanism in the mammalian kidney. *Am J Physiol* 1961;200:1119.

67. Whitten CF, Younes AA. A comparative study of renal concentrating ability in children with sickle cell anemia and in normal children. *J Lab Clin Med* 1960;55:400.

68. Forrester TE, Alleyne GAO. Excretion of salt and water by patients with sickle cell anemia: effect of a diuretic and solute diuresis. *Clin Sci* 1977;55:523.

69. Kriz W, Lever AF. Renal countercurrent mechanisms: structure and function. *Am Heart J* 1969;78:101.

70. Ho Ping Kong H, Alleyne GAO. Studies on acid excretion in adults with sickle cell anemia. *Clin Sci* 1971;41:505.

71. Goossens JR, et al. Incomplete renal tubular acidosis in sickle cell disease. *Clin Chim Acta* 1972;41:149.

72. Oster JR, et al. Renal acidification in sickle cell disease. *J Lab Clin Med* 1976;88:389.

73. Wrong O, Davies HEF. The excretion of acid in renal disease. *Q J Med* 1959;28:259.

74. De Jong PE, et al. Urinary prostaglandins in sickle cell nephropathy: a defect in 9-ketoreductase activity. *Clin Nephrol* 1984;22:212.

75. Oster JR, et al. Renal acidification in sickle cell trait. *Arch Intern Med* 1976;136:30.

76. Buckalew VM, et al. Incomplete renal tubular acidosis: physiologic studies in three patients with a defect in lowering urine pH. *Am J Med* 1968;45:32.

77. Ho Ping Kong H, Alleyne GAO. Acid-base status of adults with sickle-cell anemia. *Br Med J (Clin Res)* 1969;3:271.

78. Oduntan SA. Blood gas studies in some abnormal hemoglobin syndromes. *Br J Haematol* 1969;17:535.

79. Battle D, et al. Hyperkalemic hyperchloremic metabolic acidosis in sickle cell hemoglobinopathies. *Am J Med* 1982;72:188.

80. De Fronzo RA, et al. Impaired renal tubular potassium secretion in sickle cell disease. *Ann Intern Med* 1979;90:310.

81. De Fronzo RA. Hyperkalemia and hyporeninemic hypoaldosteronism. *Kidney Int* 1980;17:118.

82. Oster JR, Lanier DC, Vaamonde CA. Renal response to potassium loading in sickle cell trait. *Arch Intern Med* 1980;140:534.

83. Yoshino M, Amerian R, Brautbar N. Hyporeninemic hypoaldosteronism in sickle cell disease. *Nephron* 1982;31:242.

84. Diamond HS, et al. Hyperuricosuria and increased tubular secretion of urate in sickle cell anemia. *Am J Med* 1975;59:796.

85. Walker BR, Alexander F. Uric acid excretion in sickle cell anemia. *JAMA* 1971;215:255.

86. Diamond HS, Meisel AD, Holden D. The natural history of urate overproduction in sickle cell anemia. *Ann Intern Med* 1979;90:752.

87. De Ceulaer K, et al. Serum urate concentrations in homozygous sickle cell disease. *J Clin Pathol* 1981;34:965.

88. Ball GV, Sorensen LB. The pathogenesis of hyperuricemia and gout in sickle cell anemia. *Arthritis Rheum* 1970;13:846.

89. Gold MS, et al. Sickle cell anemia and hyperuricemia. *JAMA* 1968;206:1572.

90. Leff RD, Aldo-Benson MA, Fife RS. Tophaceous gout in a patient with sickle cell thalassemia: case report and review of the literature. *Arthritis Rheum* 1983;26:928.

91. Rotschild BM, et al. Sickle cell disease associated with uric acid deposition disease. *Ann Rheum Dis* 1980;39:392.

92. Espinoza LR, Spilberg I, Osterland CK. Joint manifestations of sickle cell disease. *Medicine* 1974;53:295.

93. Smith EC, et al. Serum phosphate abnormalities in sickle cell anemia. *Proc Soc Exp Biol Med* 1981;168:254.

94. Barreras L, Diggs LW, Lipscomb A. Plasma volume in sickle cell disease. *South Med J* 1966;59:456.

95. Hatch FE, et al. Altered vascular reactivity in sickle hemoglobinopathy. A possible protective factor from hypertension. *Am J Hypertens* 1989;2:2.

96. Wilson WA, Alleyne GA. O. Total body water, extracellular and plasma volume compartments in sickle cell anemia. *West Indian Med J* 1976;25:241.

97. De Jong PE, et al. Beta-2-microglobulin in sickle cell anemia—evidence of increased tubular reabsorption. *Nephron* 1981;29:138.

98. Yuzbasiyan-Gurkan VA, et al. Net tubular reabsorption of zinc in healthy man and impaired handling in sickle cell anemia. *Am J Haematol* 1989;31:87.

99. Haddy TB, et al. Erythropoiesis in sickle cell anaemia during acute infection and crisis. *Scand J Haematol* 1979;22:289.

100. Alexanian R. Erythropoietin excretion in bone marrow failure and hemolytic anemia. *J Lab Clin Med* 1973;82:438.

101. De Klerk G, et al. Serum erythropoietin (ESF) titers in anemia. *Blood* 1981;58:1164.

102. Sherwood JB, et al. Sickle cell anemia patients have low erythropoietin levels for their degree of anemia. *Blood* 1986;67:46.

103. Morgan AG, Gruber CA, Serjeant GR. Erythropoietin and renal function in sickle cell disease. *Br Med J* 1982;285:1686.

104. Matustik MC, et al. Hyperreninemia and hyperaldosteronism in sickle cell anemia. *J Pediatr* 1979;95:206.

105. Sellers BB. Intermittent hypertension during sickle cell crisis. *J Pediatr* 1978;92:941.

106. Nissen HM, Anderson H. On the localization of prostaglandin dehydrogenase activity in the kidney. *Histochemie* 1968;14:189.

107. Zins GR. Renal prostaglandins. *Am J Med* 1975;58:14.

108. Ganguli M, et al. Evidence that prostaglandin synthesis inhibitors increase the concentration of sodium and chloride in renal medulla. *Circ Res* 1977;40:135.

109. Levenson DJ, Simmons CJ, Brenner BM. Arachidonic acid metabolism, prostaglandins and the kidney. *Am J Med* 1982;72:345.

110. Tannenbaum J, et al. Enhanced renal prostaglandin production in the dog: I. Effect on renal function. *Circ Res* 1975;36:197.

111. De Jong PE, Landman H, Statius van Eps LW. Blood pressure in sickle cell disease. *Arch Intern Med* 1982;142:1239.

112. Grell GAC, Alleyne GAO, Serjeant GR. Blood pressure with homozygous sickle cell disease. *Lancet* 1981;2:1166.

113. Johnson CS, Giorgio AJ. Arterial blood pressure in adults with sickle cell disease. *Arch Intern Med* 1981;141:891.

114. Statius van Eps LW, Leeksma OC. Sickle cell nephropathy and haemostasis. In: Remuzzi G, Rossi EC, eds. *Haemostasis and the kidney*. London: Butterworth, 1989.

115. Francis RB Jr. Platelets, coagulation, and fibrinolysis in sickle cell disease: their possible role in vascular occlusion. *Blood Coagul Fibrinolysis* 1991;2:341.

116. Peters M, et al. Enhanced thrombin generation in children with sickle cell disease. *Thromb Haemost* 1994;71:169.

117. Wolters HJ, et al. Low intensity oral anticoagulation in sickle cell disease reverses the prethrombotic state: promises for treatment? *Br J Haematol* 1995;90:715.

118. Chiu D, Lubin B, Roelofsen B, et al. Sickled erythrocytes accelerate clotting in vitro: an effect of abnormal membrane lipid asymmetry. *Blood* 1981;58:398.

119. Hebbel RP, Moldow CF, Steinberg MH. Modulation of erythrocyte endothelial interactions and the vaso-occlusive severity of sickling disorders. *Blood* 1981;58:947.

120. Abel MS, Brown CR. Sickle cell disease with severe hematuria simulating renal neoplasm. *JAMA* 1948;136:624.

121. Allen TD. Sickle cell disease and hematuria: a report of 29 cases. *J Urol* 1964;91:177.

122. Bennet MA, Heslop RW, Meynell MJ. Massive haematuria associated with sickle-cell trait. *Br Med J (Clin Res)* 1967;1:677.

123. Chapman AZ, et al. Gross hematuria in sickle cell trait and sickle cell hemoglobin-C disease. *Am J Med* 1955;19:773.

124. Crone RI, et al. Gross hematuria in sickle cell trait. *Arch Intern Med* 1957;100:597.

125. Goodwin WE, Alston EF, Semans JH. Hematuria and sickle cell disease: unexplained gross unilateral renal hematuria in Negroes, coincident with the blood sickling trait. *J Urol* 1950;63:79.

126. Lucas WM, Bullock WH. Hematuria in sickle cell disease. *J Urol* 1960;83:733.

127. Marynick SP, Ramsey EJ, Knochel JP. The effect of bicarbonate and distilled water on sickle cell trait hematuria and in vitro studies on the interaction of osmolality and pH on erythrocyte sickling in sickle cell trait. *J Urol* 1977;118:793.

128. Kimmelstiel P. Vascular occlusion and ischemic infarction in sickle cell disease. *Am J Med Sci* 1948;216:11.

129. John EG, et al. Effectiveness of triglycyl vasopressin in persistent hematuria associated with sickle cell hemoglobin. *Arch Intern Med* 1980;140:1589.

130. Dees JE. Renal pelvic tamponade: a method for control of certain types of renal bleeding. *J Urol* 1965;93:136.

131. Quinibi WY. Renal autotransplantation for severe sickle cell haematuria. *Lancet* 1988;1:236.

132. Immergut MA, Stevenson T. The use of epsilon amino caproic acid in the control of hematuria associated with hemoglobinopathies. *J Urol* 1965;93:110.

133. Bilinsky RT, Kandel GL, Rabinez SF. Epsilon amino caproic acid therapy of hematuria due to heterozygous sickle cell diseases. *J Urol* 1969;102:93.

134. Black WD, Hatch FE, Acchiardo S. Amino caproic acid in prolonged hematuria of patients with sicklemia. *Arch Intern Med* 1976;136:678.

135. Gollub S, Deysine M, Cliffton EE. Mechanism of action of epsilon aminocaproic acid in the control of hemorrhage. *Ann NY Acad Sci* 1964;115:229.

136. Brody JI, Levison SP, Chung JJ. Sickle cell trait associated with von Willebrand syndromes. *Ann Intern Med* 1977;86:529.

137. Weinger RS, Benson GS, Villarreal S. Gross hematuria associated with sickle cell trait and von Willebrand's disease. *J Urol* 1979;122:136.

138. Yium J, et al. Autosomal dominant polycystic kidney disease in blacks: clinical course and effects of sickle-cell hemoglobin. *J Am Soc Nephrol* 1993;4:1670.

139. Pathak UN, et al. Bacteriuria of pregnancy: results of treatment. *J Infect Dis* 1969;120:91.

140. Whalley PJ, Martin FG, Pritchard JA. Sickle cell trait and urinary tract infection during pregnancy. *JAMA* 1964;189:903.

141. Amin UF, Ragbeer MMS. The prevalence of pyelonephritis among sicklers and nonsicklers in an autopsy population. *West Indian Med J* 1972;21:166.

142. Akinkugbe OO. Profuse haematuria in sickle cell trait. (With a note on renal papillary necrosis.) *W Afr J Med* 1966;15:151.

143. Berman LB, Tublin I. The nephropathies of sickle cell disease. *Arch Intern Med* 1959;103:602.

144. Sweeney MJ, Dobbins WT, Etteldorf JN. Renal disease with elements of the nephrotic syndrome associated with sickle cell anemia. *J Pediatr* 1962;60:42.

145. Sklar AH, et al. A population study of renal function in sickle cell anemia. *Int J Artif Organs* 1990;13:231.

146. Falk RJ, Jenette JC. Sickle cell nephropathy (review). *Adv Nephrol Necker Hosp* 1994;23:133.

147. Powars DR, et al. Chronic renal failure in sickle cell disease: risk factors, clinical course, and mortality. *Ann Intern Med* 1991;115:614.

148. Devereux S, Knowles SM. Rhabdomyolysis and acute renal failure in sickle cell anaemia. *Br Med J* 1985;290:1707.

149. Kelly CJ, Singer I. Acute renal failure in sickle-cell disease. *Am J Kidney Dis* 1986;8:146.

150. Sklar AH, Perez JC, Harp RJ, et al. Acute renal failure in sickle cell anemia. *Int J Artif Organs* 1990;13:347.

151. Hassell KL, Eckman JR, Lane PA. Acute multiorgan failure syndrome: a potentially catastrophic complication of severe sickle cell pain episodes. *Am J Med* 1994;96:155.

152. Thomas AN, Pattison C, Serjeant GR. Causes of death in sickle cell disease in Jamaica. *Br Med J (Clin Res)* 1982;285:633.

153. Friedman EA, et al. Uremia in sickle cell anemia treated by maintenance hemodialysis. *N Engl J Med* 1974;291:431.

154. Nissenson AR, Port FK. Outcome of end-stage renal disease in patients with rare causes of renal failure: I. Inherited and metabolic disorders. *Q J Med* 1989;271:1055.

155. Chatterjee SN. National study in natural history of renal allografts in sickle cell disease or trait: a second report. *Transplant Proc* 1987;21:33.

156. Gonzales-Carillo M, et al. Renal transplantation in sickle cell disease. *Clin Nephrol* 1982;18:209.

157. Spector D, et al. Painful crises following renal transplantation in sickle cell anemia. *Am J Med* 1978;64:835.

158. Miner DJ, et al. Recurrent sickle cell nephropathy in a transplanted kidney. *Am J Kidney Dis* 1987;10:306.

159. ter Maaten JC, Serne EH, van Eps WS, et al. Effects of insulin and atrial natriuretic peptide on renal tubular sodium handling in sickle cell disease. *Am J Physiol Renal Physiol* 2000;278(3):F499(abst).

CHAPTER 79

Tropical Nephrology

Rashad S. Barsoum and Visith Sitprija

The tropical zone is that region on earth lying between the tropics of Cancer (23.5 degrees North) and Capricorn (23.5 degrees South). The diversity of racial and ethnic backgrounds in this region considerably reflects on the population's susceptibility to diseases, modifies clinical patterns, and influences responses to treatment. A warm, humid atmosphere is the hallmark of tropical weather. However, the density of precipitation varies from one region to another, covering a whole spectrum from dryness in the Saharans of Africa and Arabia to the *tropical rain forest climate* of western and central Africa. These climatic features enrich the tropical ecology with many vectors of disease transmission. It also generates a large animal reservoir that ensures the development, persistence, and evolution of a dense microbial and parasitic environment.

The socioeconomic conditions and quality of governance vary widely in the tropical countries. Most acquired political independence within a few decades. Different political systems have developed and various cultures have interacted. Gross national products (GNPs) per capita vary from less than $250 U.S. dollars to more than $10,000 U.S. dollars (1) and partly explain the differences in standards of education, health care, and social services. These features have an immense impact on health care in this region.

Knowledge of tropical renal diseases is important. The general lack of effective disease prevention programs and delays in diagnosis and treatment have resulted in high morbidity and mortality rates associated with renal diseases. This has provided opportunities to observe the natural history of some diseases that cannot possibly be studied in developed countries. Tropical renal disease can serve as a model that may lead to better comprehension of nephrology in general. With rapid communication and globalization, renal diseases peculiar to the Tropics are no longer only of local concern.

In this chapter, diseases are discussed from the perspective of the Tropics. Many disorders are uniquely tropical and are not present in Western countries. Some are present in the West but have a different prevalence in the Tropics. However, emphasis is placed on the diseases that are common and unique in the Tropics, including tropical infections, poisonings from natural and chemical toxins, and some diseases related to the environment. Finally, the issue of end-stage renal disease (ESRD) and its management in different tropical regions is reviewed.

OVERVIEW

Epidemiology

Acute Renal Failure

Acute renal failure in the Tropics differs from that in Western countries with respect to etiology. Surgery and trauma account for more than 50% of cases in Western countries (2,3), whereas medical causes are the major etiologic factors in the Tropics (4–9). With socioeconomic development in the Tropics, the incidence of surgical causes is increasing, but the important causes are still medical, either tropical infections, drugs, or toxins (10,11). Obstetric acute renal failure, uncommon in Western countries (2,3), is still a problem in certain areas of the Tropics, with ominous outcome (10). There is a high incidence of bilateral cortical necrosis in India (5,12–14), probably related to late referral, as well as a high incidence of sepsis and massive blood loss. However, the incidence of obstetric causes is decreasing with better prenatal care and fewer criminal abortions. When community factors are excluded, the spectrum of hospital-acquired acute renal failure in northern India does not differ from that of developed countries (15).

Infections, toxins, and drugs or chemical agents are among the common medical causes of acute renal failure in the Tropics. Renal failure is often associated with fluid or electrolyte depletion, intravascular hemolysis, rhabdomyolysis, and jaundice. Falciparum malaria, leptospirosis, melioidosis, salmonellosis, and diarrheal diseases are representative of tropical infections frequently seen as causes of acute renal failure. Venoms of poisonous snakes and insects, raw

R. S. Barsoum: Department of Internal Medicine, Cairo University; and Cario Kidney Center, Cairo, Egypt

V. Sitprija: Department of Medicine, Chulalongkorn University; and Queen Saovabha Memorial Institute, Bangkok, Thailand

carp bile, and toxic plants represent natural toxins that cause nephrotoxicity (16).

Glomerular Diseases

The prevalence of glomerular diseases in the Tropics has been estimated to be 1 of 10,000, which is 2.5 times the rate in Western countries (17–21). The cause is not known but could be related to the environment. In Africa, glomerulonephritis has a high incidence in areas endemic for malaria and schistosomiasis. However, the incidence of glomerular diseases has decreased remarkably after malaria eradication programs (19,22), whereas the impact of schistosomiasis control remains to be elucidated (23). Nevertheless, postinfectious glomerulonephritis remains common in the Tropics.

Among the various forms of primary glomerular diseases, minimal change disease has a lower incidence (less than 10%) in the Blacks of South Africa (24) and Papua, New Guinea (25), than in Western countries (26). Focal segmental glomerulosclerosis is rare in India (27) and Pakistan (28). Mesangial proliferative glomerulonephritis is more frequent in the Tropics, especially in Southeast Asia, than in the West (29,30). The incidence of IgM nephropathy accounts for 50% of primary glomerular diseases in Thailand (29). IgA nephropathy also has a high prevalence in the Far East and Southeast Asia (31, 32) but is rare in Africa (33). Mesangiocapillary (membranoproliferative) glomerulonephritis is a common glomerular disease in South Africa (24) but is less common in Southeast Asia (29). Membranous glomerulonephritis is less common in Southeast Asia (29), South America (34), and the Caribbean (35) but is common in South Africa (36) and Pakistan (28,37–41).

Glomerulonephritis is the major cause of chronic renal failure in most countries in the Tropics. The incidence of diabetic nephropathy is increasing as the standard of living increases. Secondary glomerulonephritis resulting from infection has an impact on the development of chronic renal failure in Africa, but this is less so in Southeast Asia. Lupus nephritis has a high incidence in the Tropics, especially in Southeast Asia (29). The reason is not yet known.

Vascular Disease

Takayasu arteritis is a common vascular disease in the Oriental tropics and South Africa. Most reports have come from India (42), Sri Lanka (43), Singapore (44), Thailand (45), China (46), and Japan (47). It is the most common cause of renovascular hypertension, accounting for 61% of such patients in India (42).

Interstitial Nephritis

The incidence of interstitial nephritis in the Tropics perhaps does not differ from that of Western countries, although infection may play a larger role in the pathogenesis (16). The role of environmental pollution remains questionable. Chronic interstitial nephritis is emerging as an important cause of chronic renal failure in certain countries (48).

Clinical Presentation

Most acute tropical diseases, either infections or toxin poisonings, share common clinical renal manifestations.

Urinary Sediment Changes and Proteinuria

Mild urinary sediment changes are usually seen with tropical infection and toxin poisoning. Frequently, few erythrocytes and leukocytes in the urine are detected with infectious diseases. Mild urinary protein loss of less than 1 g per 24 hours may be observed (49). The urinary protein consists of albumin. These changes disappear quickly when infection is under control. Occasionally, proteinuria in the nephrotic range may be seen, but this resolves when infection subsides.

Persistent glomerulonephritis and proteinuria have been noted in diseases with a chronic course, such as quartan malaria, viral hepatitis, leprosy, schistosomiasis, and filariasis. Autoimmune mechanisms and associated infection may play a contributing role in these diseases. Glomerulonephritis usually does not resolve with treatment of the infection (40,50).

Hemoglobinuria

Intravascular hemolysis is frequently observed with tropical diseases. Bacterial hemolysin can induce hemolysis. The high incidence of glucose-6-phosphate dehydrogenase (G6PD) deficiency in the Tropics makes erythrocytes prone to hemolysis during infection and certain drug therapy. Intravascular hemolysis can be severe in patients with tropical infectious diseases. Malaria is a good example of intravascular hemolysis associated with G6PD deficiency. In the toxin model of viper venom, intravascular hemolysis can be produced through the activity of phospholipase A and the direct lytic factor (51). Certain chemical agents such as naphthalene and copper sulfate and plant toxins can also cause hemolysis. Hemoglobinuria contributes significantly to the development of acute renal failure in the Tropics.

Myoglobinuria

Infections and toxins are among the important causes of myoglobinuria in the Tropics. Rhabdomyolysis is often noted after sea snake bites and wasp, hornet, and bee stings (16). Certain infectious diseases affecting muscles such as trichinosis and leptospirosis can cause rhabdomyolysis. Because ischemia of the muscles can cause rhabdomyolysis, it is not surprising to see myoglobinuria in infectious diseases that compromise the microcirculation and result in muscular ischemia. Myoglobinuria has been observed in malaria, salmonellosis, and various viral diseases (49,52). Subclinical rhabdomyolysis has been observed in 70% of patients with acute renal failure living in tropical areas (53). The other causes of rhabdomyolysis such as hypokalemia, hypophosphatemia, and alcohol, heroin, and cocaine use are occasionally seen.

Electrolyte Changes

Hyponatremia is observed in 60% of the patients with febrile illness (54). The proposed causes are multiple and include increased antidiuretic hormone (ADH) release, resetting of osmoreceptors, cellular sodium influx, low sodium intake, and sodium loss by renal or extrarenal routes. Delayed response to a water load has been observed in malaria and has a clinical implication with respect to fluid administration. Fluid overload may lead to pulmonary edema. Hypernatremia caused by water deficit may be observed in the patient who has lost consciousness. Diabetes insipidus is rare and represents a bad prognostic sign.

Hypokalemia attributed to respiratory alkalosis is not uncommon in febrile illness. Interestingly, kaliuresis can be of a significant degree in leptospirosis (55) and in obstructive jaundice and could account for hypokalemia despite renal failure (56). Hypokalemia may also be observed in patients with severe diarrhea, especially with cholera. Hyperkalemia without renal failure is associated with intravascular hemolysis and rhabdomyolysis. It may be of an alarming degree and necessitate urgent treatment.

Hypocalcemia and hypophosphatemia have been observed in severe sepsis and malaria. The causes of hypocalcemia are multiple and include hypoalbuminemia, decreased activity of Ca-ATPase and Na-K-ATPase, parathyroid insufficiency, decreased 1α-hydroxylase activity, and the effect of interleukin-1 (IL-1) (57,58). Respiratory alkalosis is a frequent cause of hypophosphatemia.

Acute Renal Failure

Tropical acute renal failure is usually hypercatabolic, with rapid rises in blood urea nitrogen and serum creatinine levels (16). The blood urea nitrogen : serum creatinine ratio often exceeds 15 : 1, except in patients with rhabdomyolysis, in whom the ratio may be less than 10 : 1. Hyperuricemia and hyperphosphatemia may be noted. Jaundice may be present and is cholestatic, with only mild elevations of liver enzyme levels but with high serum alkaline phosphatase levels. With severe infections or certain toxin poisonings, intravascular coagulation and intravascular hemolysis may be present. The duration of renal failure averages 2 weeks but may last from a few days to several weeks. Nonoliguric renal failure is not uncommon. Renal failure is usually reversible, except in those patients with cortical necrosis.

General Management

Specific treatment of the basic tropical disease should be instituted. Proteinuria and abnormal urinary sediment usually resolve when the basic disease is controlled. Persistent glomerulonephritis is often problematic and usually does not respond to steroid and immunosuppressive treatment.

Treatment of acute renal failure in patients with tropical diseases does not differ from the standard treatment given for renal failure due to other causes. Because of hypercatabolism, dialysis, when indicated, should be performed frequently. Hemodialysis is preferred to peritoneal dialysis because with the latter, there is decreased solute exchange through the peritoneal membrane resulting from compromised microcirculation in severe infection. Fortunately, control of infection improves solute transport. Even so, in developing countries with poor socioeconomic standards, peritoneal dialysis is still used.

Exchange transfusion is useful in reducing the parasitic load in patients with falciparum malaria with heavy parasitemia (59) and in toxin poisoning. Severe jaundice with a total serum bilirubin concentration of more than 25 mg/dL can compromise renal function and should be treated by plasmapheresis (16). In acute renal failure associated with obstructive jaundice, decreasing jaundice by plasmapheresis can improve renal function.

Principal Pathophysiology

Most nephropathies associated with common tropical infections are attributed to three principal pathogenetic mechanisms: immune-mediated reactions, hemodynamic alterations, and direct invasion or direct nephrotoxicity (Fig. 79-1).

Immune-Mediated Reactions

The antigen load of an infective agent may provoke a complex host immune response (60) involving both humoral and cell-mediated systems, as, for example, in schistosomiasis (Fig. 79-2). This reaction often leads to renal parenchymal injury. Glomerulonephritis, usually immune complex mediated, is the classic expression, being reported with most of the viral, bacterial, and parasitic infections addressed in this chapter. Tubulointerstitial disease, on the other hand, may be encountered as the predominant immune-mediated injury in certain infections (e.g., leishmaniasis and toxoplasmosis). Secondary amyloidosis may result from the persistent antigenic load (e.g., leprosy, leishmaniasis, and schistosomiasis).

Hemodynamic Alterations

Various chemical mediators and cytokines are released during inflammation induced by infection or toxin (61–63). It is obvious that these substances have opposing effects: vasoconstriction and vasodilation. The net result is usually renal vasoconstriction and renal ischemia. Myocardial function can be depressed. Tumor necrosis factor (TNF), interleukins, platelet-activating factor (PAF), and myocardial depressant factors are known to be involved in the clinical picture of endotoxin shock (61,63). Oxygen radical generation in the

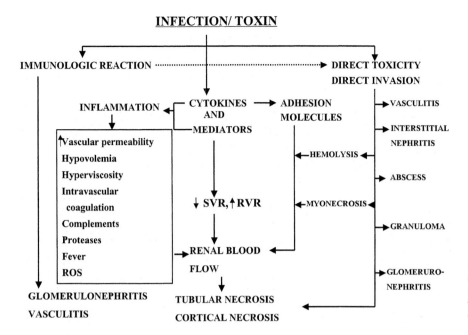

FIG. 79-1. Pathogenesis of infection and toxin-induced nephropathy. ROS, reactive oxygen species; SVR, systemic vascular resistance; RVR, renal vascular resistance.

inflammatory process and the reflow is an additional insult for the renal injury.

The role of hemorheologic change should be emphasized. In acute infections, acute-phase proteins are increased in the plasma (62). Plasma fibrinogen can rise significantly and accounts for an increase in plasma viscosity. Erythrocyte viscosity is also increased in intraerythrocytic parasitic infections such as malaria and babesiosis (59). The rise in blood viscosity and rouleaux formation can interfere with blood flow in the renal microcirculation (59). Cytoadherence of parasitized erythrocytes to the vascular endothelium in malaria can compromise the flow in the microcirculation. Cytoadherence between leukocytes and the vascular endothelium, which occurs in inflammation through the effects of cytokines, would further decrease the renal blood flow.

At the clinical level, several factors contribute to hemodynamic changes. These factors include volume depletion, pigmenturia, intravascular coagulation, and jaundice.

Volume Depletion

Volume depletion is common in severe tropical diseases. This can result from decreased fluid intake associated with increased fluid loss through the skin, urine, respiration, and gastrointestinal tract. After a viper bite, bleeding can result in significant hypovolemia. Increased vascular permeability due to mediators, free oxygen radicals, complement activation, and proteolytic enzymes from leukocytes, with fluid shift from the intravascular to the interstitial space, occurs frequently with severe infections (61,63). Hemorrhagic dengue, anthrax, falciparum malaria, and leptospirosis are among the diseases known to cause hypovolemia. Volume depletion due to diarrhea is a common cause of acute renal failure in India, Pakistan, and Bangladesh.

Pigmenturia

Intravascular hemolysis and rhabdomyolysis are seen in tropical disease; therefore, hemoglobinuria and myoglobinuria are risk factors and can contribute to acute renal failure by decreasing renal blood flow, direct tubular toxicity, and tubular obstruction (64,65).

Intravascular Coagulation

In most infectious diseases, intravascular coagulation is of a low grade and its role is therefore minimal. However, disseminated intravascular coagulation can be induced by sepsis and animal toxins (66). Disseminated intravascular coagulation can occur with Russell's viper venom, shigellosis, severe infection, and occasionally malaria and undoubtedly interferes with renal microcirculation (49).

Cardiac Dysfunction

Decreased cardiac function is observed in infectious diseases that involve the myocardium such as typhoid fever, leptospirosis, and diphtheria. Severe sepsis can also cause cardiac dysfunction through the effects of TNF, IL-2, PAF, and myocardial suppressant factor (61).

Jaundice

Severe jaundice is one of the risk factors for the development of acute renal failure, especially when the total serum bilirubin concentration exceeds 25 mg/dL. Hyperbilirubinemia at this level can inhibit tubular reabsorption of sodium and lead to sodium depletion and hypovolemia (67). It can also cause direct toxicity to the kidney. Cardiac dysfunction can be induced by severe jaundice (68).

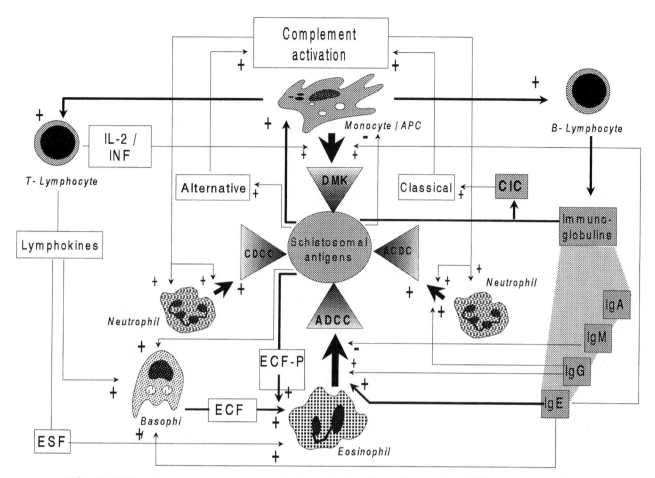

FIG. 79-2. The immune response to schistosomiasis. The principal four killing systems—direct macrophage killing (DMK), antibody-dependent cell-mediated cytotoxicity (ADCC), antibody and complement-dependent cytotoxicity (ACDC), and complement-dependent cytotoxicity (CDCC)—are shown. The close association of humoral and cell-mediated immunity in activating the parasite elimination mechanisms is displayed. Note the crucial role of the eosinophil and IgE. Also note the formation of pathogenic circulating immune complexes involving all major immunoglobulins. IL-2, interleukin-2; APC, antigen-presenting cell; INF, interferon; ESF, eosinophil-stimulating factor; ECF, eosinophil chemotactic factor; ECF-P, eosinophil chemotactic factor of parasitic origin; CIC, circulating immune complexes.

The role of a high body temperature in renal injury deserves comments. A temperature as high as 42°C can cause renal injury. Heat can induce tissue injury through complement activation and oxygen radical release (48). Although a fever of 42°C is unusual, it is possible that the combination of fever and other nonspecific factors contributes to renal injury. High temperature can decrease ATP and enhance ischemic renal injury (58).

These factors are nonspecific and can be shared by several inflammatory diseases. In most cases of renal injury, the causes are multiple. Therefore, severe infection of any etiology can cause acute renal failure.

Direct Invasion/Direct Nephrotoxicity

Viral, bacterial, and fungal agents and mature parasites may directly invade the renal parenchyma, lower urinary tract, or draining lymphatics. Pathogenicity is attributed to their physical or mechanical effects or to the local inflammatory reaction that they provoke. In the parasitic model, parasites migrate to the kidney and produce renal lesions through cellular reactions. These reactions consist of cellular proliferation, infiltration, and cystic and granulomatous changes around the parasites (69). This model has been shown in echinococcosis and filariasis.

Direct toxicity to the kidney has been demonstrated in several models. Of bacterial infections, leptospirosis is a good example (70). Leptospires penetrate the skin and enter the circulation to various organs. In the kidney, they produce mild glomerulonephritis within a few hours. Bacterial penetration through the peritubular capillaries to the interstitium causes interstitial nephritis. Tubular necrosis occurs when bacteria invade the renal tubules. Renal changes therefore consist of glomerulonephritis, interstitial nephritis, and tubular necrosis.

In the toxin model, viper venoms, particularly Russell's viper venom and green pit viper venom, are vasculotoxic and capable of causing vasculitis and glomerulonephritis (71,72).

Russell's viper venom also has tubular effects, as shown by an isolated renal perfusion experiment (73). A few plants are directly nephrotoxic. These include djenkol bean (*Pithecolobium lobatum*), Impila (*Callilepis laureola*), and toxic mushrooms (49).

TROPICAL INFECTIONS

Nephropathy in Bacterial Infections

Typhoid Fever and Salmonella Infections

Typhoid fever continues to be a common disease in tropical countries. Clinically significant renal disease with typhoid fever is uncommon, occurring in less than 6% of all patients (74–76). However, when careful and repeated urinalysis is performed, more than 50% of the patients are found to have definite findings of renal involvement (77). The spectrum of renal disease in typhoid fever includes mild to severe glomerular involvement (77–82) and acute tubular necrosis.

Hematuria and proteinuria are quite frequent during the febrile phase (77). The urinary protein loss is less than 1 g per 24 hours in most patients but can exceed this in few patients. The glomerular disease usually has a benign course, with complete recovery occurring in 1 to 2 weeks (77,82). Less commonly, fever, generalized edema, and hypertension mimicking acute poststreptococcal glomerulonephritis have been reported in South Africa (79). Recovery was complete with appropriate antimicrobial treatment. Renal histology, reported in several series (77,79,82), shows large glomeruli with mild to moderate mesangial proliferation. Immunofluorescent staining has shown variable amounts of C3, IgG, and IgM deposits (77,82). IgA deposition in the mesangial area has been described (83). The pathogenesis of typhoid glomerulonephritis is of an immunologic nature. Salmonella Vi antigen has been demonstrated in the glomerular capillary wall (82). The complement level is usually low during the acute phase in patients with renal involvement and normal in those without renal involvement (77,79,84). However, this has not been a consistent finding, particularly in experimental typhoid (85,86).

Acute renal failure has occurred with typhoid fever associated with intravascular hemolysis due to G6PD deficiency, disseminated intravascular coagulation, or severe jaundice (77,87–89). Rhabdomyolysis with renal failure associated with typhoid fever has been documented (90).

An interesting syndrome reported from Egypt is the nephrotic syndrome occurring in patients with chronic salmonellosis associated with schistosomiasis (91–94) (vide infra). It is amazing that although similar combinations of *Salmonella* and schistosomal infection occur in Brazil, the previously described pattern has not been reported (95).

Leptospirosis

Leptospirosis, an infectious disease caused by several serotypes of *Leptospira interrogans*, is worldwide in distribution. The disease is transmitted through contact of abraded skin or mucous membrane with blood, tissue, or urine of infected animals or through exposure to contaminated environments. It is an unusual cause of acute renal failure in Western countries (96,97); however, it plays an important role in certain tropical regions (98–100). In Southeast Asia and Sri Lanka, leptospirosis is one of the major causes of acute renal failure, accounting for 24% and 32% of all reported cases, respectively. The kidney is invariably involved in leptospirosis, and acute renal failure of variable severity occurs in most patients.

Clinically, patients present with sudden onset of chills, fever, generalized muscle pain, and variable degrees of jaundice. Urinary abnormality consists of mild proteinuria, a variable number of erythrocytes, occasional hemoglobinuria, granular casts, and bile-pigmented casts. Leptospiruria is demonstrated by dark-field illumination. Renal failure, occurring in 60% of the patients, may be mild and nonoliguric. Hypokalemia secondary to kaliuresis has been observed (55). Kaliuresis in leptospirosis is due to inhibition of potassium reabsorption in the medullary thick ascending limb of Henle (101) and increased sodium–potassium exchange in the principle cells of the collecting ducts secondary to decreased sodium reabsorption in the proximal tubules (102). Renal bicarbonate wasting similar to proximal renal tubular acidosis may be observed. In severe cases (Weil's disease), marked renal failure with a rapid rise in serum creatinine level and uric acid occurs in association with jaundice. Jaundice is usually cholestatic. Hepatocellular jaundice may be observed when associated with shock. In rare cases, hemolytic-uremic syndrome may be seen. In patients reported from Barbados (103) and French Polynesia (104), renal failure was associated with significant thrombocytopenia; however, full-blown disseminated intravascular coagulopathy is rare. Infection with different leptospiral serotypes does not seem to explain the marked variability in renal involvement.

Although leptospirosis involves every structure of the kidney, the primary lesion is interstitial, with local or diffuse mononuclear cell infiltration. Renal function can be normal. In acute renal failure, cellular degeneration of both proximal and distal tubules is seen. Glomerular changes are quite mild and limited to mild mesangial hypercellularity (105,106). On immunofluorescent staining, nonspecific C3 and IgM uptake is seen in the mesangial area and occasionally in the afferent arterioles (99,106). On electron microscopy, occasional dense deposits are seen in mesangial, paramesangial, and intramembranous locations (99). The organism itself is rarely seen in human biopsy studies. However, in hamster models, leptospires can be seen initially in the glomeruli and then in the interstitium and renal tubules a few hours after inoculation (106).

The pathogenesis of renal failure in leptospirosis is multifactorial.

1. Hemodynamic alterations. The renal blood flow is decreased through the effects of cytokines, mediators, and nonspecific inflammatory factors (Table 79-1) (107). Systemic vascular resistance is decreased along with

TABLE 79-1. *Hemodynamics in leptospirosis*

Severity	Anicteric	Icteric
Cardiac output	∼ or ↑	∼ or ↓
Blood volume	∼ or ↑	∼ or ↓
Systemic vascular resistance	↓	∼ or ↑
Renal vascular resistance	↑	↑↑
Renal blood flow	↓	↓↓
Glomerular filtration rate	↓	↓↓

increased cardiac output in anicteric leptospirosis but is increased in icteric leptospirosis with decreased cardiac output. The outer membrane of leptospires can cause a release of nitric oxide, TNFα, and monocyte chemoattractant protein from the medullary thick ascending limb of Henle (108). Peptidoglycans and lipopolysaccharide also induce monocytes to release proinflammatory cytokines and mediators.

2. Direct nephrotoxicity. Leptospire glycolipid can intercalate with the host cell membrane causing cellular injury (109). Membrane Na-K-ATPase is inhibited (110). Lipopolysaccharide, porin, and lipoprotein of the outer membrane have been shown to induce interstitial nephritis (111).

3. Immunologic mechanism. This mechanism plays a major role in canine leptospirosis. However, it probably does not play a significant role in human disease (106). Circulating immune complexes have only been demonstrated in one patient (99). An increased number of B lymphocytes has been observed in a patient with leptospirosis, along with a decrease in the number of CD3+ and CD4+ cells (112). In patients with severe jaundice (bilirubin level of more than 25 mg/dL), a causative role for bilirubin and bile salt has been postulated (67).

Management of renal failure in patients with leptospirosis should focus on treatment of the underlying abnormality. Penicillin is the drug of choice. Hemodialysis and peritoneal dialysis have been used successfully in patients with renal failure. Plasma exchange coupled with hemodialysis is advocated for patients with marked hyperbilirubinemia (113–115). In patients who recover from acute illness, renal function returns to normal. Prognosis is generally good. Bad prognostic indices include hyperbilirubinemia, hyperkalemia and pulmonary complications, and either pulmonary edema, adult respiratory distress syndrome, or hemorrhage. Continuous hemofiltration—either arteriovenous or venovenous—plasmapheresis, and blood exchange are useful in these clinical settings. In the rural area, blood exchange is preferred because of simplicity and the low cost.

Leprosy

Leprosy is a common infectious disease in tropical regions including Africa, Asia, and South America. It has been estimated that of 12 million cases of leprosy in the world, 3 million are in India. Renal involvement is frequent among patients with lepromatous leprosy, although it can also be seen in those with tuberculoid or borderline types (116,117). The prevalence of glomerulonephritis in leprosy varies from 6% to 50% in biopsy studies (118).

The clinical spectrum covers asymptomatic proteinuria and hematuria (119), nephrotic syndrome (120), nephritic syndrome, and even renal failure (121). Circulating immune complexes and cryoglobulinemia are detectable in most patients. Serum complement levels may be low (122). The cell-mediated immune response is depressed in the lepromatous type. Nephrotic syndrome is common in patients with amyloidosis but may be observed in patients with membranous and diffuse proliferative glomerulonephritis (123). Concentration and acidification defects have been described (116,118). Acute renal failure may occur (121,124) and chronic renal failure often results from complicated amyloidosis. Acute renal failure is mostly observed in lepromatous leprosy, with a prevalence of 63%, whereas only 2% of nonlepromatous patients have impaired renal function (124). Acute renal failure may also be a complication of multiple-drug treatment of leprosy (125). Treatment should concentrate on the leprosy; management of the renal involvement is only supportive.

Pathologically, diffuse proliferative glomerulonephritis and mesangial proliferative glomerulonephritis are common (78,116). Focal proliferative glomerulonephritis (116), membranous nephropathy (126), mesangiocapillary glomerulonephritis, crescentic glomerulonephritis (121), focal glomerulosclerosis (117), and interstitial nephritis (126) have been reported. Immunofluorescent study shows granular deposition of IgM, IgG, IgA, and C3 in the mesangial areas and along the glomerular capillary walls (127). Deposition of IgA alone has been occasionally demonstrated (120). There is electron-dense deposition in the mesangial, subendothelial, intramembranous, and subepithelial areas (116,128,129). The findings are compatible with that of immune complex glomerulonephritis. The nature of the antigen has not been identified. Glomerulonephritis may be only a nonspecific reaction. The possibilities exist among mycobacterial antigens, other microbial antigens, and autoantigen. Secondary amyloidosis is noted in 2.4% to 8.4% of patients, predominantly with lepromatous and borderline lepromatous leprosy, although it may be observed occasionally in tuberculoid leprosy (118).

Melioidosis

Melioidosis is an infectious disease caused by a Gram-negative bacillus, *Burkholderia pseudomallei*. The disease is prevalent in the Tropics, particularly in India, Thailand, Myanmar, Kampuchea (Cambodia), Laos, Vietnam, Malaysia, the Philippines, and Papua New Guinea. Melioidosis was an important health problem during the Vietnam War when many soldiers became the victims of this deadly disease. Significant serologic titers for the organism were detected in 29% of military personnel (130). Recently, antibodies to *B. pseudomallei* were detected in 39.5% of the people in northeastern Thailand. There are a few reports on melioidosis of the urinary tract (131,132). The data on renal involvement are scant, and according to a few reports, the rate of renal involvement varies from 2.4% to 35.0%. Yet, acute renal failure can occur in the septicemic form of the disease. In a series of 220 patients with melioidosis in northeastern Thailand, renal failure was noted in 35% (132). The underlying causes in 56% of the patients included diabetes mellitus, renal stone, cirrhosis, and glomerulonephritis. Hypoproteinemia was present in 60% of the patients. Hyponatremia was observed in 90% of the patients. The duration of renal failure varied from 1 week to 6 weeks, averaging 3 weeks. The mortality rate was close to 90%.

Renal pathologic changes include multiple renal abscesses, tubular necrosis, and interstitial nephritis (132). The bacteria are seen in the suppurative lesions (133). In the animal model, thrombi have been demonstrated in blood vessels and cortical necrosis has been observed (133). These have not been shown in human melioidosis. Renal changes are attributed to severe sepsis, which causes renal ischemia and inflammatory reactions to bacterial invasion.

Tetanus

Tetanus is capable of causing acute renal failure through stimulation of the sympathetic nervous system (134–136). The incidence of renal failure in tetanus is high in Brazil. In a report by Martinelli et al. (134), proteinuria was noted in 50% of the patients and impaired renal function was observed in 39% of patients in whom serum myoglobin levels were elevated. There is no correlation between the serum level of myoglobin or creatine phosphokinase and renal failure. Renal failure is usually nonoliguric and mild.

Scrub Typhus

Scrub typhus is widely distributed in the Tropics and can involve the kidney. As with the other infectious diseases, mild proteinuria with abnormal urine sediment is not uncommon. In most patients, renal function is normal. Renal failure can be observed with severe infection associated with either jaundice, intravascular coagulation, or hemolysis due to G6PD deficiency (137–139). The usual renal changes are those of mild mesangial proliferative glomerulonephritis. Deposition of IgM and C3 is seen in the mesangial area. In severe cases, platelet thrombi may be seen in the glomeruli, with focal thickening of the basement membrane. Tubular necrosis is observed in the presence of renal failure. Interstitial nephritis may be present (137,138,140). The infiltrate often occurs in the corticomedullary region and consists of mononuclear cells.

Perivascular infiltration and thrombophlebitis may be seen in the interlobular veins.

Diphtheria

Diphtheria can occasionally cause acute renal failure in children (141–143). In a review of 155 patients by Singh et al.

(143), renal failure was observed in only two. This could be attributed to decreased cardiac output due to myocarditis. Yet, diphtheria toxin may be nephrotoxic because it inhibits protein synthesis when it is added to the basolateral side of the renal tubular cells (144). Renal histologic changes in patients with acute renal failure are consistent with those of tubular necrosis (141). In a report of 70 patients by Kannerstein (142), tubular necrosis was observed in 16% and interstitial changes in 48%.

Cholera

Cholera is still endemic in Asian countries and renal failure attributed to fluid and electrolyte loss can occur. Acidosis in cholera is associated with an increased anion gap due to hyperproteinemia, hyperphosphatemia, and increased serum lactate levels (145). Hypokalemia can be striking. Interestingly, the ratio between blood urea nitrogen and serum creatinine may be lower than normal because of the larger loss of urea than creatinine through diarrhea and perhaps rhabdomyolysis due to hypokalemia. In addition to tubular necrosis, vacuolation of the proximal convoluted tubules due to hypokalemia may be present (146). Cortical necrosis has been described (147).

Shigellosis

Shigellosis can cause renal failure in the same fashion as cholera and other diarrheal diseases. In a series of 2,018 patients reported by Bennish et al. (119), renal failure occurred in 26%. By multivariate analysis, younger age, decreased serum protein level, altered consciousness, and thrombocytopenia were indices of a poor prognosis (119). Because shigella toxin causes endothelial injury, hemolytic-uremic syndrome may occur (148–150). In this setting, there may be cortical necrosis and diffuse fibrin deposition in the glomeruli. Srivastava et al. (151) reported an incidence of hemolytic-uremic syndrome of 34% in patients with acute renal failure mostly related to shigellosis. Renal histology showed cortical necrosis in 40% of the patients (151). The mortality rate was 60%.

Vibrio Vulnificus Infection

Vibrio vulnificus is a Gram-negative bacillus found in coastal and brackish waters. Infection by V. vulnificus usually occurs in immunocompromised host or chronic alcoholic hosts after consumption of contaminated seafood or injury to the skin in a marine environment. V. vulnificus infection in humans can be expressed as primary sepsis, wound infection, or gastrointestinal tract manifestation. The presenting symptoms include fever with chills, abdominal pain, vomiting, diarrhea, and lower extremity pain. Disseminated intravascular coagulation can occur. Acute renal failure is common with tubular necrosis as a significant pathologic change (152,153). Renal failure is ischemic in origin. Yet cellular injury can be induced by bacterial cytolysin, collagenase, protease, metalloproteinase, and phospholipases (154–157). The disease may be confused with leptospirosis, scrub typhus, malaria, and other forms of sepsis.

Nephropathy Due to Viral Infections

Many viral diseases can cause mild glomerular involvement. Rhabdomyolysis may be seen with viral infection and can be responsible for acute renal failure. It is, however, interesting that several viruses harbor in the kidney producing viruria without renal function changes.

Dengue

The disease is caused by dengue virus and is characterized by flu-like symptoms with headache, muscular pains, arthralgia, flushing of the face, conjunctival injection, and skin rashes. The disease is common in Southeast Asia (158,159) and is transmitted by the mosquito *Aedes aegypti. Aedes albopictus, Aedes scutellaris,* and *Aedes polynesiensis* may be important vectors in certain areas. Hypotension may occur during the second phase of the disease, a few days after the onset when fever declines. Complement activation, increased vascular permeability, and thrombocytopenia are the main pathophysiologic changes of the disease leading to hypovolemia and bleeding (160–163). Immune complexes play an important part in complement activation. Anaphylatoxins C3a and C5a, cytokines, and mediators are elevated and result in plasma leakage from the intravascular space. Usual renal manifestations in hemorrhagic dengue include mild urinary sediment changes, mild proteinuria, and hyponatremia. Renal failure in children is often mild and usually prerenal due to hypotension. In adults, renal failure can be severe and associated with cerebral symptoms and liver dysfunction. It is not clear why the disease is more severe in adults, but it could be related to virus virulence, associated infection, drugs used, and late hospitalization. Also, the disease may not be recognized earlier in adults. Jaundice is hepatocellular, with marked elevation of liver enzyme levels. The ratio between blood urea nitrogen and serum creatinine is lower than normal. Renal failure is oliguric with a prolonged clinical course.

Renal histologic changes include mesangial proliferation with IgM and C3 deposition, endothelial cell swelling, and perivascular infiltration by mononuclear cells (164). Tubules show degeneration along with interstitial edema (165). The diseases can be confused with Hantavirus infection, which can produce almost similar pathophysiology and symptoms.

Hantavirus Infection

Hantavirus is an RNA virus in the family Bunyaviridae. There are seven serotypes: Hantaan, Seoul, Puumala, Prospect Hill, Belgrade, Thottapalayam, and Sin Nombre. The disease is seen worldwide throughout Asia, Europe, North and South America, Australia, and Africa (166–169). It is considered a rare disease in tropical Asian countries. In Korea, Hantaan and Seoul serotypes are common. Hantaan virus causes severe disease with a renal syndrome. Seoul virus causes a disease of moderate severity, and Puumala virus produces the least severe disease. The epidemiologic significance of Prospect Hill serotype is not well understood. Belgrade virus is associated with severe disease in the Balkans. Sin Nombre serotype causes the most severe disease with a pulmonary syndrome in the United States. Thottapalayam virus is found in India. Rodents, especially rats, mice, and voles, are the important reservoirs. Infection is acquired mostly by inhalation of rodent excreta, although direct inoculation by abrasion or cuts of the skin is also possible. Increased vascular permeability is the main pathophysiology of the disease (168), because of the effects of various mediators, cytokines, complement activation, and vascular endothelial injury, which finally result in hypovolemia, decreased renal perfusion, and acute renal failure.

The symptoms of hantavirus infection with different serotypes vary greatly. Even in the same serotype, the symptoms can vary from mild to severe. The description of Hantaan virus infection with renal syndrome is classic.

Clinically, after the incubation period of 2 to 5 weeks, the disease is manifested by flu-like symptoms with fever, headache, flushed face, myalgia, abdominal pain, nausea, and vomiting. Periorbital edema, conjunctival hemorrhage, and palatal and axillary petechiae may be present. The clinical course can be divided into five phases: febrile, hypotensive, oliguric, diuretic, and convalescent (169). The febrile phase lasts for 3 to 7 days and is followed by the hypotensive phase due to hypovolemia, which develops with lysis of fever. The hypotensive phase lasts from 3 hours to 3 days and is followed by the oliguric phase, which may be prerenal or renal in origin. The duration of the oliguric phase, therefore, varies from a few days to several days. The diuretic and convalescent phases follow. In infection with other serotypes or in mild cases, these five phases may not be apparent. Hypotension and oliguria may not be present. The Sin Nombre serotype is associated with mild renal involvement but a severe pulmonary syndrome.

Renal involvement is common in Hantaan virus infection. Proteinuria, hematuria, and pyuria are usually observed. Renal failure is more common in Hantaan virus infection than in infections with the other serotypes and may be associated with pulmonary edema. Thrombocytopenia may occur in severe cases. Disseminated intravascular coagulation has been shown.

Renal pathologic changes are consistent with those of tubular necrosis. Medullary vessels are dilated and congested. Marked interstitial changes with edema and hemorrhage, with later infiltration by mononuclear cells, can be seen. The interstitial changes are pronounced in Puumala infection. Glomerular changes are not remarkable. Mild glomerular hypercellularity may be found. IgM, IgG, and C3 deposition in the glomeruli and interstitium may be observed.

Hepatitis B

Hepatitis B virus (HBV) infection is worldwide in distribution, with a low carrier rate in Western countries. The prevalence of the HBV surface antigen (HBsAg) carrier varies from 0.3% to 1.0% in North America to 1% in western Europe; 5% in South America, eastern Europe, Japan, and western Asia; 7% in Africa; and 10% to 20% in China, Taiwan, and Southeast Asia (170). The pathogenetic role of HBV in glomerulonephritis is a topic of great interest. The observations of a high incidence of HBsAg carriers among patients with various forms of glomerulonephritis, when compared with that of the general population, tend to support the role of HBV in the pathogenesis of glomerulonephritis. In Hong Kong, 22% of patients with glomerulonephritis are HBsAg-positive, which is higher than the carrier rate in the general population. In South Africa, 20% of the patients with glomerulonephritis are HBsAg-positive (171). In Zimbabwe, Japan, and Taiwan, HBs-antigenemia has been found in 80% to 100% of children with membranous glomerulonephritis (172–174). However, in Thailand and South Korea, the figure does not differ from that for the general population.

Clinical presentations vary from asymptomatic proteinuria and hematuria to nephrotic syndrome and impaired renal function with hypertension. Nephrotic syndrome is common with membranous and mesangiocapillary glomerulonephritis, whereas hematuria and asymptomatic proteinuria are present with mesangial proliferative glomerulonephritis. In about 33% of patients, the serum complement level is decreased. Patients with HBV may present with the clinical picture of essential cryoglobulinemia with purpura, arthralgia, and splenomegaly (175). Acute renal failure may occur with fulminant hepatitis (176) but may occasionally develop with uncomplicated HBV (177).

The natural history of HBV-associated glomerulonephropathy is not well understood (178). Spontaneous remission occurs in 50% of patients with membranous nephropathy. Seroconversion to positive anti–hepatitis B e antigen (anti-HBeAb) is associated with remission of proteinuria. In children, the disease may run a benign course and the pathology is mainly membranous. Among patients with IgA deposition, 19% had deterioration of renal function in 40 months. Clearance of HBsAg from blood has been associated with remission of polyarteritis. The use of steroids as treatment for glomerulonephritis should be discouraged. Corticosteroid therapy has been associated with active virus replication and hepatic dysfunction with an appearance of viruslike particles in the glomeruli (178,179). Interferon α (INFα) administration has been shown to suppress HBV expression with clearing of HBV e antigen (HBeAg) (178) and may be tried in HBV-associated glomerulonephritis with short duration of infection. The use of adenine arabinoside and thymic extract reduced proteinuria in 87% of patients with membranous nephropathy, with a reduction of HBV DNA in T cells, B cells, and macrophages along with seroconversion

from HBeAg-positive to anti-HBe-positive (180). The use of newer antiviral agents such as lamivudine requires further evaluation.

Renal pathologic changes include membranous glomerulonephritis, mesangial proliferative glomerulonephritis, mesangiocapillary glomerulonephritis, and polyarteritis nodosa (170). Among these, membranous nephropathy is usually associated with deposition of HBeAg in the immune complexes, whereas mesangial proliferative glomerulonephritis is associated with HBsAg complexes (181,182). HBV core antigen (HBcAg) has been found in patients with membranous nephropathy when polyclonal anti-HBcAg antiserum was used. Glomerular deposition of HBeAg and HBsAg is demonstrable in mesangiocapillary glomerulonephritis. The pathogenetic association between IgA nephropathy and HBV has attracted attention, because the geographic area with the highest endemicity of HBV infection also has the highest incidence of IgA nephropathy. Glomerular HBsAg deposition in a distribution similar to that of IgA immune staining is detected in 21% to 40% of patients (178,183). There is no HBeAg deposition.

Hepatitis C

The incidence of hepatitis C virus (HCV) carriers in the Tropics is less than 5%. Chronic HCV infection can be associated with mesangiocapillary glomerulonephritis (184–186), membranous glomerulonephritis (187), and diffuse proliferative glomerulonephritis (188). Mesangiocapillary lesion with mixed cryoglobulinemia is the common lesion. Glomerular immune complex deposition consists of HCV, anti-HCV IgG, and IgM rheumatoid factor. The cryoprecipitate containing HCV RNA and HCV antibody can be seen in the subendothelial glomerular deposits (189,190). Ohta et al. (191) demonstrated the core antigen in the glomeruli of patients with hepatitis C in the absence of circulating cryoglobulins. Electron microscopy of the renal tissue shows cryoglobulin-like structures. The patients have proteinuria, hematuria, decreased renal function and hypocomplementemia, rheumatoid factor, and circulating cryoglobulin. Nephrotic syndrome is a common presentation.

Treatment with INFα improves liver function and decreases urinary protein excretion with disappearance of HCV RNA (189). Exacerbation of glomerulonephritis with proteinuria and hematuria during interferon administration has been reported (192). It was suggested that renal damage was either a direct or an indirect effect of interferon on the glomerular endothelial and epithelial cells. The result of treatment by interferon therefore varies (192,193). The viral genotype and titer may be important determinants in response. In comparing with the other causes of secondary glomerulonephritis in the Tropics, HCV is a rather uncommon cause. However, it is an important cause of morbidity and mortality among recipients of renal transplantation and patients on chronic dialysis.

Hepatitis A

Fulminant hepatitis A can produce renal failure in a similar fashion to hepatorenal syndrome. Viral hepatitis associated with G6PD deficiency may present with massive intravascular hemolysis and acute renal failure (194). Recently, there have been several reports of acute renal failure developing in patients with hepatitis A in the nonfulminant form (195–197). The mechanism of renal failure is not well understood. In some patients, there are no apparent renal histologic changes, although in others, tubular necrosis is seen. Perhaps various nonspecific factors in inflammation that lead to renal ischemia superimposing on hepatic dysfunction produce the renal failure.

Mycotic Infections

Mycotic infections constitute an important part of tropical nephrology. Because no particular features distinguish such infections in the Tropics from those that occur in other parts of the world, this chapter does not include detailed accounts, which can be found elsewhere (Chapter 37, Fungal Urinary Tract Infections; Chapter 72, Chronic Tubulointerstitial Nephropathies; and Chapter 97, Outcomes and Complications of Renal Transplantation). For easy reference, however, the important mycotic infections of clinical significance in tropical countries are highlighted.

Mycotic Nephropathies in the Immunocompetent Individual

Coccidioidomycosis

The disease is widely distributed all over the globe, but endemic foci are identified in the tropical zone of the American continent, particularly Central America and Argentina. Infection is acquired through inhalation of dust containing the fungal hyphae, leading to predominantly pulmonary disease. The kidneys are involved in the rare disseminated form of the disease, particularly in non-Whites (198). The lesions are interstitial, either granulomatous or suppurative, usually multiple, and often associated with lung cavities (199).

Paracoccidioidomycosis

This is a chronic granulomatous disease, also endemic in Central and South America. It is characterized by mucocutaneous manifestations in addition to foci in different viscera including the kidneys (200).

Renal Disease Probably Caused by Fungal Toxins

Ochratoxins

These fungal products often contaminate stored cereals. They can induce a form of interstitial nephritis in pigs (201) that resembles and has been incriminated in the pathogenesis of Balkan nephropathy in humans (202). It is also a potent carcinogen that induces renal adenocarcinoma in small laboratory animals, but the relevance of this observation to humans is unknown.

Chronic interstitial nephritis associated with ochratoxin A has been reported from the tropical zone, including Egypt (203) and Northwest Africa (204).

Aflatoxins

Aflatoxins B_1 and B_2, produced by *Aspergillus flavus,* which contaminates many foods, particularly cereals, have been associated with hepatomas in humans and in experimental animals. They can also induce adenocarcinoma and pelvic neoplasms in rats (205).

Although aflatoxins are present all over the globe, they have recently attracted a lot of interest in the Tropics, where the cereal storage conditions are optimal for fungal growth. They have been incriminated in the remarkable increase in the incidence of hepatomas in most of Africa, particularly in association with persistent HBV-antigenemia (206). It is unknown whether aflatoxins are also responsible for a higher incidence of renal malignancy in the same continent.

Opportunistic Mycotic Infections in the Immunocompromised

Fungi are well-known opportunistic organisms worldwide. Fungal infections are even more prevalent in tropical countries, because of the uncontrolled use of antibiotics and immunosuppressive agents, poor general hygienic standards, and the high prevalence of acquired immunodeficiency syndrome (AIDS) in certain areas.

The principal opportunistic fungi encountered in the Tropics include the following:

1. Candidiasis is, by far, the most common. Urethritis, cystitis, and pyelonephritis are usually ascending infections (207). Disseminated candidiasis (208) is often a terminal event in patients with AIDS and overimmunosuppressed transplant recipients, intravascular catheters being a common source of infection (209).
2. *Pneumocystis carinii* infection is now regarded as a peculiar fungal infection on the basis of ribosomal RNA analysis. It causes serious pneumonia and occasional extrapulmonary manifestations in patients with AIDS and less often in those receiving immunosuppressive therapy including renal transplant recipients (210).
3. Disseminated histoplasmosis is an important risk to renal transplant recipients in Central and South America. Both primary infection and reactivation of dormant infection seem to occur. The disease is characterized by focal necrotic lesions in different viscera, bones, joints, meninges, endocardium, skin, and oral mucosa (211).
4. Invasive aspergillosis is a serious infection in renal transplant recipients, particularly after bacterial infection in

neutropenic patients (212). The disease is characterized by interstitial pneumonia or consolidation with or without cavitation, often accompanied by intracranial, gastrointestinal, hepatic, cardiac, and osseous lesions. Interstitial renal disease may also occur, presenting as proteinuria, pyuria, and hematuria, with rapid loss of function. Fungal "balls" have been observed in the urine of such patients (213).

5. The rhinocerebral, pulmonary, renal, and disseminated forms of mucormycosis are rare infections that may be encountered in patients with uncontrolled diabetes, particularly with ketoacidosis or renal failure (198,214). They often complicate desferrioxamine therapy in patients on dialysis and are occasionally seen in renal transplant recipients, being strongly associated with the use of azathioprine (215).

6. Cryptococcosis, which affects as many as 10% of patients with AIDS, is not a common opportunistic infection in patients on immunosuppressive treatment (216).

Parasitic Infections

Parasitic infestations influence the practice of clinical nephrology in the Tropics in three ways: (a) They are the causative agents of certain renal diseases, usually referred to as *parasitic nephropathies*; (b) they are among the important agents that may infect immunocompromised patients; and (c) they often modify the classic clinical picture, prognosis, and management of renal disorders at large.

Parasitic Nephropathies

Urinary tract disease that is due to parasitic infestation was known in pharaonic medicine. Several papyri, analogous to the medical textbooks of our time, accurately describe the clinical features of a disease called "aaa" attributed to a worm, acquired by exposure to Nile water (217). That this disease is indeed what we know today as *schistosomiasis* is suggested by the close similarity of the clinical features and by finding calcified schistosomal ova in the bladders of ancient Egyptian mummies (218). Schistosomiasis remains one of the most common parasitic nephropathies, exerting its effect mainly through the induction of lower urinary tract pathology. That the parasite may also lead to glomerular disease was suggested only a few decades ago (219,220), and subsequently confirmed by other investigators in Latin America (221,222), Africa (223–227), and Asia (228).

Malarial nephropathy was next on the list, being referred to in the Hippocrates collection, dating back to the fourth century BC, and suspected by Atkinson late in the nineteenth century (229). It remained for Giglioli (230) to present evidence for a potential cause-and-effect relationship between malaria and the nephrotic syndrome. Other investigators subsequently confirmed this suggestion on the basis of epidemiologic, experimental, and clinical grounds (20,231–236).

Schistosomiasis and malaria remain the most relevant parasitic nephropathies of epidemiologic concern. Renal lesions have been described with many other parasitic infections (Table 79-2), but these are generally either too mild to achieve clinical significance or geographically too restricted to be of epidemiologic importance. On the whole, the incidence of renal complications seems to be relatively low when depicted in relation to the global prevalence of parasitic diseases. However, there is a place for a lot of bias in this conclusion, because of the general unawareness of such complications, the lack of the necessary facilities to detect them in endemic areas, or the known difficulties in documentation and publication.

Parasitic Infections in the Immunocompromised

The renal patient may be immunocompromised as a feature of the primary disease, due to acquired infection with agents that impair the immune response such as human immunodeficiency virus (HIV), Epstein-Barr virus, and cytomegalovirus, or as a consequence of therapeutic immunosuppression. Such patients are susceptible to a number of well-defined infections (Chapter 97, Outcomes and Complications of Renal Transplantation). In the Tropics, the list of agents known to affect the immunocompromised host is even longer and involves a considerable number of parasites including *Toxoplasma, Cryptosporidium, Plasmodium, Schistosoma,* and *Strongyloides* species, which are discussed later in this chapter.

Some of these infections are acquired as a result of nonspecific impairment of the immune response against primary infection (e.g., cryptosporidiosis). Others represent activation of dormant infection, analogous to many bacterial and viral diseases (e.g., toxoplasmosis and strongyloidiasis). The occurrence of either pattern of parasitic infection in a compromised host usually indicates severe immunosuppression, hence, a grave prognosis. Other infestations may be caused by depression of the parasite-specific immune response, thereby disrupting the immunity against reinfection in endemic areas (e.g., schistosomiasis and malaria). Such infestations, although of considerable immunologic interest, are not particularly serious clinical problems.

Impact of Parasitic Infections on the Clinical Patterns and Management of Renal Disease

The clinical patterns of renal diseases in the Tropics may be modified in different ways by associated parasitic infestations. Many infestations cause or are associated with malnutrition, which, in addition to reflecting on the severity of the infestation per se (malaria, schistosomiasis, strongyloidiasis), augments nephrotic edema, increases anemia and bone disease in chronic renal failure, superimposes skin and peripheral nerve complications, and increases the risk of bacterial infection (237).

The associated chronic activation of the immune system is often blamed for increasing the incidence of secondary amyloidosis (238). The same was also attributed to impairment of

TABLE 79-2. *Reported clinical spectrum of parasitic nephropathies*

	Acute renal failure	Asymptomatic urinary abnormalities	Acute nephritic syndrome	Nephrotic syndrome	Chronic tubulointerstitial	Ureteral obstruction	Other features	Chronic renal failure	Infection in the immunocompromised
Caused by Protozoa									
Malaria									
Quartan		++		+++				+++	
Falciparum	+++	++	+	+					
Babesiosis	++[a]								
Visceral leishmaniasis		++		+[b]	+				
Trypanosomiasis									
African	++								
Toxoplasmosis									
Congenital		+		+					
Acquired									++
Caused by Cestoda									
Echinococcosis		+					+[c]		
Caused by Trematoda									
Schistosomiasis									
Hematobium		++	+	+[b]	+	+++		+++	+
Mansoni		+		+++		+		+++	
Opisthorchiasis	++	+					+[b,e]		++
Caused by Nematoda									
Filariasis									
Wuchereria bancrofti		+	+	++			+[d]		
Onchocerca volvulus		++		++				+	+
Loa loa		+							
Strongyloidiasis		+		+					++
Trichinosis		+							

Note: +, occasionally reported; ++, infrequently reported; +++, commonly reported.
[a]Usually with asplenia.
[b]Usually with amyloidosis.
[c]Mass effect of renal cysts.
[d]Chyluria.
[e]Jaundice.

macrophage function in kala azar (239). Immune activation may be expressed by hyperglobulinemia, which often poses diagnostic difficulties in the interpretation of false-positive results on serologic tests (225). What complicates the picture even further is the frequent association of autoimmunity with certain parasitic diseases such as schistosomiasis, malaria, and filariasis (240–242).

Most parasitic diseases are characterized by multisystem involvement, which compounds the clinical picture, prognosis, and management of the associated renal disorder. Common examples are the extensive microcirculatory disturbance in falciparum malaria associated with acute renal failure (243), the chronic hepatic and lower urinary tract pathology in schistosomiasis (244), and the chyluria of filariasis (245). Such elements in the scenario may have a considerable impact on treatment strategies, use of medications, and choice of acute (246) and chronic (247) dialysis modalities as well as on the safety and efficacy of dialysis (248). They often influence the donor selection, the recipient's immunosuppression, and the eventual outcome of renal transplantation (249).

Malaria

Malaria is a parasitic disease of great epidemiologic importance in the Tropics (Fig. 79-3), largely because of the warmth and humidity that favor the multiplication of mosquitoes, of which the anopheline species is the principal vector for malarial transmission. The incidence of malaria in the world is on the order of 300 to 500 million clinical cases each year with mortality averaging 2 million per year. The disease is caused by a protozoan, *Plasmodium,* of which four species

are pathogenic to humans, namely, *Plasmodium vivax, Plasmodium malariae, Plasmodium ovale,* and *Plasmodium falciparum* (250). The clinical pattern of the disease, the incidence of acute and chronic complications, and consequently the outcome are influenced by certain differences among the infective species. These include inherent features in their own life cycles as well as their selective adhesion to specific red cell and hepatocyte receptors (251). The age of infected erythrocytes is an important factor. Thus, whereas *P. vivax* and *P. ovale* infect only young red cells, and *P. malariae* infects only aging cells, *P. falciparum* infects erythrocytes at any age, explaining the heavy parasitemia associated with the latter (250). The expression of certain adhesion molecules on infected cells (252,253) determines the extent of their sequestration in the peripheral capillaries (254,255), which reflects on pathogenicity (256,257). The capacity of the infective strain to release cytokines (258), particularly TNFα and IL-6 (258–261), determines the severity of clinical disease. Enhanced synthesis of INFγ may influence the host resistance.

As with other parasitic infections, circulating malarial antigens (262) trigger a cascade of immune reactions including direct macrophage and complement activation (60,263) and a human leukocyte antigen–restricted specific immune response (250,264). The latter is largely modified by notorious interspecies, interstrain, and interstage antigenic variability. Although little is known about the cell-mediated response to the parasite (264), the humoral immune reaction is well documented. Most infected persons form antibodies against the sporozoite's surface-associated repetitive epitopes, as well as against most stages of the asexual cycle. Because of the heavy

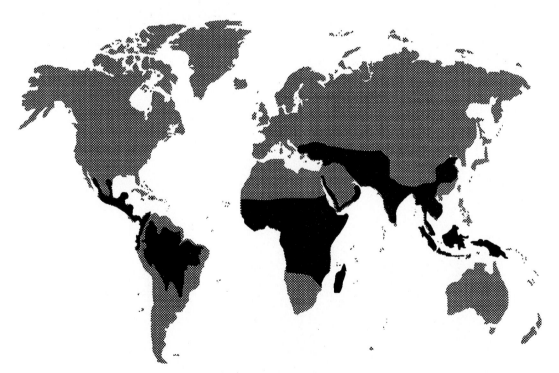

FIG. 79-3. Global distribution of malaria.

antigenic load, there is an abundance of circulating immune complexes in infected subjects.

Clinical Features. The disease is characterized by recurrent pyrexia with chills, the frequency of which varies according to the infective species (250). Constitutional features such as headache, malaise, and muscle and joint aches are usually encountered, more often with the first infection episode and in expatriates. Diarrhea, pulmonary edema, jaundice, coma, and circulatory failure may complicate falciparum infection, hence the term *malignant malaria.* The spleen is usually enlarged, particularly with relapsing disease. Anemia and neutrophil leukocytosis are prominent laboratory findings. The diagnosis is confirmed by direct visualization of the parasite in Giemsa-stained peripheral blood smears. Fluorescent staining with acridine orange enhances the diagnostic accuracy of peripheral blood examination. DNA probes have been recently introduced but are not widely applicable. Serology is of limited diagnostic value, particularly in endemic areas.

Renal Involvement in Malaria. Clinically significant renal disease may complicate infection with two malarial species, namely, *P. malariae* and *P. falciparum.* The former is associated with a chronic progressive syndrome, whereas infection with the latter is an acute complication, usually reversible by adequate management.

P. Malariae nephropathy. The causative link between *P. malariae* infection and glomerulonephritis is based on epidemiologic, experimental, and immunologic evidence (234,265–267). Thus, nephrotic syndrome and progressive glomerulonephritis are strikingly more prevalent in endemic areas; their prevalence was significantly reduced with eradication of malaria (20,231,268,269). Glomerular disease was experimentally induced by the closely related species *Plasmodium berghei* (234) and *P. brazilianum* (270), yielding ultrastructural changes identical to those seen in patients. Even more direct evidence was obtained by finding malarial antigen in the glomeruli (271), which also suggests that glomerular injury is indeed immune complex mediated (272).

Clinically significant renal involvement is relatively rare among patients with acute and chronic *P. malariae* infection,

which suggests the interaction of other factors in the pathogenesis of the renal lesion. Such other factors may include other bacterial and viral infections, of which Epstein-Barr virus infection has received particular attention (270) in view of its concomitantly high prevalence in endemic areas. It is presumed that a certain immunologic setting may be necessary for the malarial antigen to induce clinically significant glomerular disease (242). This may also be achieved by malnutrition (273), autoimmunity (272), or a genetic predisposition.

The glomerular lesion is dominated by subendothelial deposits. These are mainly seen by light microscopy (Fig. 79-4) as thickening of the capillary walls, giving a double contour appearance to the basement membrane (273). By immunofluorescence, the deposits usually exhibit a coarsely granular pattern along the capillary endothelium and contain IgG (most commonly IgG3), IgM, C3 (274), and in 25% to 33% of patients malarial antigens, particularly during early stages of disease (265,271). Less often, diffuse finely granular deposits containing IgG2 are encountered (274). Mixed patterns are not unusual. Electron microscopy shows subendothelial deposits of electron-dense or basement membrane–like material, associated with the formation of intramembranous lacunae (275).

In addition, a proliferative lesion, mainly involving the mesangium, is often encountered in adults. Crescents are rare in all age-groups. The extent of tubular involvement depends on the severity of glomerular lesions (265).

The pathology is initially focal and may indeed continue to be so, ending up with focal and segmental sclerosis. In most patients, however, the pathology is diffuse and progressive, leading to ESRD.

The clinical syndrome of quartan malarial nephropathy (265,269) is nonspecific, apart from its association with the features of the parasitic infection (vide supra). Most patients are children, with a mean age of 5 years. Proteinuria is encountered in a variable proportion of patients, up to 46% in the first published series (230). Microhematuria is occasionally noticed, particularly in the older age-groups. Overt nephrotic syndrome develops in a yet undefined fraction, and

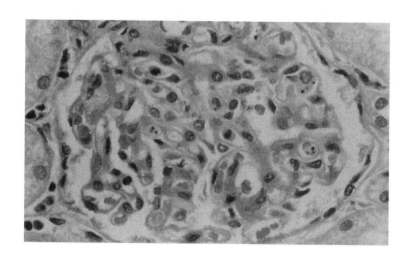

FIG. 79-4. Malarial nephropathy. Note the pigment-laden macrophages in glomerular capillary lumina. (hematoxylin and eosin stain, magnification ×200) (From Dr. V. Boonpucknavig, with permission.)

hypertension is a late encounter. Serum complement levels are normal, and blood cholesterol values are usually not elevated, owing to the associated nutritional deficiency. The disease progressively leads to chronic renal failure over 3 to 5 years (265,269). Response to antimalarial treatment is poor and limited to patients in early stages (231,265).

P. falciparum nephropathy. Renal complications encountered in falciparum malaria include acute renal failure, glomerulonephritis, and fluid and electrolyte changes. The former is, by far, the more important, being more frequent and more serious.

Acute renal failure usually occurs in those patients with heavy parasitemia (infected erythrocytes, more than 5%) or blackwater fever. The incidence of acute renal failure in patients with falciparum malaria is 1% to 4% (236), but it may reach up to 60% in those with severe malaria (246). In patients with sever malaria, the clinical and laboratory features of classic falciparum malaria are modified by profound disturbances of the microcirculation, closely similar to those encountered in septic shock (258,276). Disseminated intravascular coagulation may occur (277,278). Hyperbilirubinemia is almost invariable. The serum concentrations of both conjugated and unconjugated bilirubin are elevated (250), but the cholestatic element dominates. Left ventricular function may be compromised. With severe jaundice, hypoglycemia is a prominent feature that often contributes to coma. The hypoglycemia is attributed to excessive glucose consumption by millions of plasmodia, the effect of TNFα and hyperinsulinemia associated with quinine therapy (279). There is good correlation between the degree of parasitemia and the plasma level of TNFα.

Acute renal failure is usually oliguric and hypercatabolic, with the blood urea nitrogen : creatinine ratio being commonly more than 15. Hyperkalemia can be profound in patients with intravascular hemolysis. Hyperuricemia is

occasionally seen. Overproduction is suggested by a high urinary uric acid : creatinine ratio, particularly in jaundiced patients. The oliguric phase usually lasts for a few days to several weeks.

The prognosis depends on the severity of the condition, the response to antiparasitic treatment, the availability of dialysis, and the predominant pathogenetic factors involved; hence, there is great variability in outcome.

Therapy usually poses challenging problems, because of the complexity of the syndrome. Quinine remains the drug of choice. Artemisinin derivatives have been used with promising results in decreasing parasitemia, particularly in quinine-resistant patients. In mild renal failure, a combination of dopamine and furosemide can attenuate the progress of renal failure (280). Early in the development of renal failure, phenoxybenzamine increases the urine flow, glomerular filtration rate, and sodium excretion (281). Early dialysis is often needed to treat the hypercatabolic state. Although peritoneal dialysis is less effective because of the supervening circulatory disturbances, it becomes more effective as the flow in microcirculation is improved by treatment. It is often the only available dialysis modality in underdeveloped communities. In some cases, continuous peritoneal dialysis may be indicated. Exchange transfusion is helpful in patients with heavy parasitemia and those with severe jaundice (282). Prostacyclin may be useful in patients with severe intravascular hemolysis.

The pathogenesis is multifactorial, involving a complex interaction of mechanical, immunologic, and humoral components (243) (Fig. 79-5). The parasitized red cell and the parasite-activated monocyte are the cornerstones of all events. Characteristic of *P. falciparum* infection are particular red cell membrane abnormalities (283,284) with the formation of glycoprotein-rich knobs (254,255) (Fig. 79-6), expressing intercellular adhesion molecule 1 (ICAM-1), thrombospondin, and CD36 (256,257). Through these knobs, parasitized red

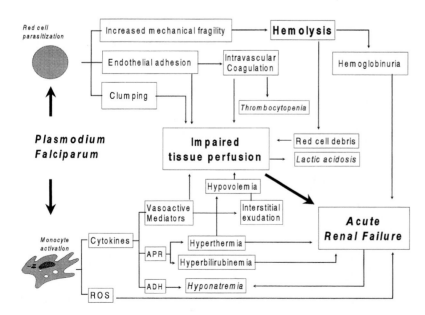

FIG. 79-5. The pathogenesis of acute renal failure in malaria. ADH, antidiuretic hormone; APR, acute-phase reactants; ROS, reactive oxygen species.

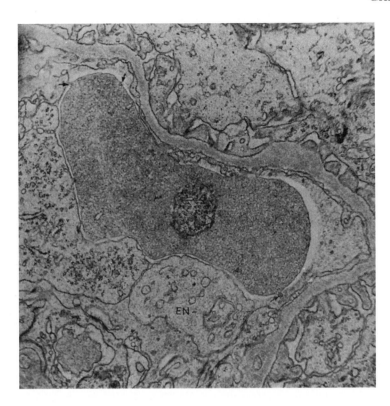

FIG. 79-6. Adherence knobs on the parasitized erythrocyte membrane *(arrows)* to the glomerular endothelium (EN). (From Sitprija V. Nephrology forum: nephropathy in falciparum malaria. *Kidney Int* 1988;34:866, with permission.)

cells are anchored together, forming large clumps, and stick to the endothelium of small capillaries (256).

The physiologic deformability of parasitized red cells is impaired (285) and their mechanical fragility increased (252), which leads to hemolysis. Although this is usually extravascular, intravascular hemolysis may also occur, particularly in patients with G6PD deficiency who are receiving quinidine or pyrimethamine therapy. In extreme forms, massive intravascular hemolysis leads to the frank hemoglobinuria characteristic of blackwater fever. Red cell debris and their free products exert their hemodynamic and toxic ill effects, which include vasoconstriction, renal tubular toxicity, and activation of intravascular coagulation. The latter has received considerable attention in malignant malaria (277,286). Activation of coagulation factors, thrombocytopenia, and increased plasma fibrin degradation products (263) has been well documented. However, glomerular capillary thrombosis is uncommon, and fibrin deposits have not been consistently seen by immunofluorescent study.

Massive monocyte activation is an integral component of the syndrome. In essence, it is almost identical to that encountered in response to endotoxin. Indeed, *bacterial* endotoxin, presumably of gut origin, has been detected in some patients with malignant malaria (276). Yet, this cannot be the whole explanation. No equivalent malarial endotoxin has ever been identified, but a direct effect of the plasmodium is suggested as a part of the innate immune response to infection (60). Monocyte activation by glycosylphosphatidylinositol moieties linked to the surface antigens of the malarial parasite leads to the release of several cytokines, of which TNFα,

IL-1, and IL-6 have been documented in malignant malaria (259,260,287).

A lot of humoral changes are seen in falciparum malaria. These include hypercatecholaminemia (288); increased levels of circulating plasma renin activity, kinins, and prostaglandins (236); ADH secretion (289–291); and hyperinsulinemia in quinine-treated patients (279). Most of these effects are nonspecific, being attributed to the severe acute infection. However, they seem to have a significant impact on the final target of all pathogenetic factors in malignant malaria, namely, the microcirculation.

The outcome of the whole scenario is hemodynamic and metabolic abnormalities. These include disturbed tissue eicosanoid balance (292,293), capillary dilatation and increased permeability (246), lactic acidosis (294), and the accumulation of reactive oxygen species (287). These may also be linked with the observed cell membrane abnormalities (251,284) associated with inhibition of magnesium-activated Na-K-ATPase (295,296), calmodulin depletion, and increased intracellular calcium influx (297,298).

Blood volume, initially increased in uncomplicated malaria (299,300), associated with increased cardiac output and decreased systemic vascular resistance, is reduced in severe malaria by both fluid transudation into the interstitial tissues and peripheral pooling (300,301). This leads to reduced cardiac output, increased systemic and renal vascular resistance, and decreased renal blood flow (Table 79-3). Acute renal failure in malaria is therefore ischemic in type. Tubular changes include cloudy swelling, hemosiderin granules, and cell necrosis of variable degrees. The tubular lumina often contain hemoglobin casts. The interstitium is edematous,

TABLE 79-3. *Hemodynamics in falciparum malaria*

Severity	Mild	Moderate	Severe
Infected erythrocytes	<1%	1–5%	>5%
Blood volume	~ or ↑	↑	~ or ↓
Cardiac output	~	↑	~ or ↓
Systemic vascular resistance	~	↓	↑
Renal vascular resistance	~	↑	↑↑
Renal blood flow	~	↓	↓↓
Glomerular filtration rate	~	↓	↓↓

with a moderate to dense mononuclear cellular infiltration, and the venules may show clumps of parasitized erythrocytes.

Glomerulonephritis may be associated with falciparum malaria at any age, although children remain the main population at risk (232,236,246). It is impossible to estimate the true incidence, because the disease is essentially mild, transient, and overshadowed by other complications. Glomerular lesions were detected in 18% of patients with falciparum malaria who underwent autopsy (302). Mild proteinuria, microhematuria, and casts are found in 20% to 50% of patients (246). Nephrotic (232) and acute nephritic (233,235) syndromes are occasionally seen, but hypertension is unusual. Serum C3 and C4 levels may be reduced during the acute phase. The disease is very rarely progressive. In contrast to quartan malarial nephropathy, falciparum glomerulopathy is reversible within 2 to 6 weeks after eradication of the infection.

The glomerular lesion is characterized by prominent mesangial proliferation with many transit cells. Mesangial matrix expansion is modest, and basement membrane changes are unusual. Deposition of an eosinophilic granular material has been noticed along the capillary walls, within the mesangium, and in Bowman's capsule (303). The glomerular capillaries are often empty, but they may contain a few parasitized red cells or giant nuclear masses in patients with intravascular coagulation (304). Immunofluorescent study shows finely granular IgM and C3 deposits along the capillary walls and in the mesangium. Malarial antigens are occasionally seen, analogous with an animal model (271), along the glomerular endothelium and the medullary capillaries (Fig. 79-7). ICAM-1 is expressed in the glomerular mesangium, vascular endothelium, and proximal tubular cells. The tubules and the vascular endothelium show expression of TNFα, IL-1, IL-6, and granulocyte–macrophage colony-stimulating factor (305). Electron microscopy shows subendothelial and mesangial electron-dense deposits along with granular, fibrillar, and amorphous material (334).

There is general agreement that the glomerular lesion in falciparum malaria, like that associated with quartan malaria, is immune complex mediated. The finding of specific circulating complexes and glomerular deposits supports this view. *P. falciparum* is a potent complement activator via the alternative pathway (263).

Fluid and electrolyte changes in malaria are of clinical and physiologic interest. Hyponatremia, usually asymptomatic, is observed in 67% of the patient (289). Hyponatremic patients have higher parasitemia than the patients with normal serum sodium levels (291). There are multiple courses including increased ADH, low sodium intake, sodium loss, cellular sodium influx, and a reset of osmoreceptor. Hypernatremia, usually associated with hypothalamic injury, is rare. Hypokalemia, attributed to respiratory alkalosis, is common. Hyperkalemia is seen in patients with intravascular hemolysis, rhabdomyolysis, or renal failure. As in sepsis, hypocalcemia and hypophosphatemia are seen in severe malaria (287,306). Hypocalcemia without renal failure is caused by decreased parathyroid hormone and the effect of IL-1. Phosphate shift into the cells induced by respiratory alkalosis accounts for hypophosphatemia (307). Both hypocalcemia and hypophosphatemia are transient and resolve with clinical improvement. Of clinical importance is the decreased response to water load, which can be observed in moderate and severe malaria. In this clinical setting, hemodynamic changes include hypervolemia, decreased peripheral vascular resistance, increased cardiac output, elevated plasma renin activity, and increased plasma norepinephrine levels, ADH, and renal vascular resistance (291). Hemodynamic alteration is therefore similar to that observed in cirrhosis of

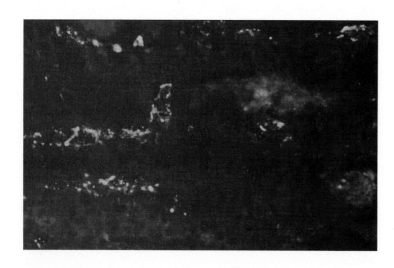

FIG. 79-7. Deposition of granular malarial antigen along the capillaries in the renal medulla. (anti–*Plasmodium falciparum*, magnification ×200) (From Dr. V. Boonpucknavig, with permission.)

the liver. Hyponatremia is an important clinical marker in these patients. A decreased response to water load occurs in 20% of hyponatremic patients. Fluid administration to the patient with moderate or severe malaria should be cautiously done to avoid fluid overload. Furosemide should be given when there is decreased response to fluid load.

Other malarial nephropathy. Mild mesangial proliferative glomerulonephritis with deposition of IgM and C3 can be observed in infection by *P. vivax* and *P. ovale*. Benign urinary sediment changes may be seen. Acute renal failure is rare.

Babesiosis

This rare febrile disease (308) is closely related to falciparum malaria. It is not strictly tropical, as most cases have been described in eastern Europe and the United States. However, it is often confused with falciparum malaria in patients returning from the Tropics. Either *Babesia microti* or *Babesia divergens* is responsible for infection. The disease manifests itself by fever, chills, and malaise associated with nausea and arthralgias. It is particularly severe in asplenic patients, who are more likely to develop acute renal failure as a result of hypotension, intravascular hemolysis, and disseminated intravascular coagulation. Mesangial proliferative glomerulonephritis with deposition of IgG and C3 is observed (309,310). Diagnosis is made by finding the intraerythrocytic parasite in a blood smear or by a serologic test. Therapy with quinine sulfate and clindamycin is usually effective in eradicating the parasite. Pentamidine is effective in resistant cases.

Visceral Leishmaniasis

This disease, also known as *kala azar* (or black sickness) (239), is one of three forms of human leishmaniasis with worldwide distribution, being highly prevalent in East and North Africa, northeastern China, Iran, the Mediterranean region, and Brazil. It is caused by *Leishmania donovani*, a protozoan that infects humans through a sandfly bite. The parasite lives and multiplies in the monocytes, being protected by a peculiar host–parasite interaction that involves depression of cell-mediated immunity.

Most patients remain asymptomatic, often with spontaneous cure. Overt disease ushers in with pyrexia, chills, sweating, asthenia, weight loss, and hepatosplenomegaly. Lymphadenopathy is often noticed but is seldom striking. Skin nodules containing the parasite may be seen, particularly at the inoculation site. If untreated, the disease may end fatally, usually due to intercurrent infections. Response to treatment with pentavalent antimony is slow and often incomplete. Primary resistance is encountered in 10% of patients.

In the kidney, the parasite induces a chronic inflammatory interstitial lesion (Fig. 79-8) that rarely progresses to any appreciable degree of fibrosis (311). The protozoan may be seen within the infiltrating monocytes, with little lymphocytic infiltration that reflects the characteristic depression of macrophage function (239). To the same mechanism is ascribed the frequent development of secondary amyloidosis (312). Immune complex–mediated glomerular lesions have also been described in kala azar (313–315), mesangioproliferative glomerulonephritis being the most common pattern (Fig. 79-9). IgM and C3 deposits are often found in the capillary walls and mesangium. Leishmania membrane antigen is detected (316).

Renal involvement in kala azar is usually subclinical. An occasional patient with secondary amyloidosis may present with gross proteinuria or even the nephrotic syndrome, but this is usually encountered as a terminal event in the patient's illness.

Trypanosomiasis

African trypanosomiasis (317), caused by *Trypanosoma brucei* and transmitted by the tsetse fly, is the cause of sleeping sickness. The Rhodesian version is an acute febrile illness with neurologic and cardiac manifestations, anemia, and disseminated intravascular coagulation that often ends fatally

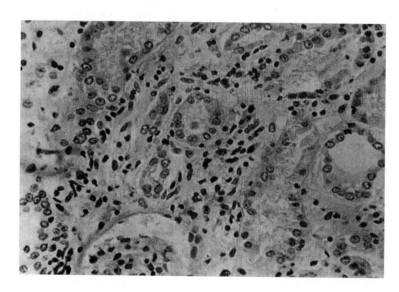

FIG. 79-8. Renal involvement in visceral leishmaniasis: interstitial edema, interstitial mononuclear infiltration, and degeneration of some tubular cells. (hematoxylin and eosin stain, magnification ×250)

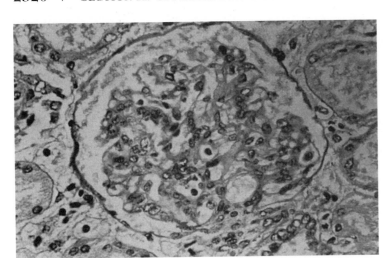

FIG. 79-9. Kidney involvement in visceral leishmaniasis: focal proliferative glomerulonephritis and mesangial expansion and presence of amorphous material in Bowman's space. (periodic acid-Schiff stain, magnification ×250)

within a few weeks. Acute renal failure may be encountered during the terminal phases as a component of multiorgan failure.

The Gambian type is more chronic, initially presenting with pyrexia, lymphadenopathy, and a skin eruption, followed several months or even years later by progressive meningoencephalitic manifestations.

Experimental infection in monkeys by *T. brucei* leads to proliferative glomerulonephritis, with IgM and C3 deposits in the mesangium and along the capillary walls. Serologic studies in this model showed high levels of circulating immune complexes and a reduction of serum C3 levels with normal C4 levels, suggestive of direct alternative complement activation by the parasitic antigens. Similar observations were made in a murine model, in which electron-dense deposits were also found in the mesangium and subendothelial space (318). Whether similar lesions also occur in humans is unknown. Clinically relevant renal complications have not been reported.

Toxoplasmosis

Toxoplasma gondii infection (319) is quite common worldwide, with a current estimate of 500 million infected humans. It is acquired through contact with cats and certain birds, by ingestion of cysts or oocysts. It can also occur through transplacental transmission (congenital toxoplasmosis). In most instances, the infection is dormant, with a few cysts lying in the lymph nodes, muscle, heart, or brain and little or no inflammatory response.

Overt clinical disease is rare in the immunocompetent individual. It usually manifests by cervical lymphadenopathy associated with pyrexia and malaise. The disease is self-limiting in most patients. Progressive chorioretinitis is the notorious expression of congenital toxoplasmosis in the immunocompetent individual.

In the immunocompromised, the disease is much more disseminated, presenting with pyrexia, hepatosplenomegaly, pneumonitis, maculopapular rash, myositis, myocarditis,

meningoencephalitis, or central nervous system mass lesions. The course is rapidly fatal.

Renal involvement in the immunocompetent and the immunocompromised host has been rarely described. The lesion is mainly glomerular, with a mesangioproliferative pattern. Mesangial IgM and Toxoplasma antigen deposits have been detected by immunofluorescent study. Renal infection is usually subclinical, although the nephrotic syndrome has been described in association with chorioretinitis in congenital toxoplasmosis (320).

Cryptosporidiosis

The causative protozoan, *Cryptosporidium*, belongs to the same family as *T. gondii*. The disease is also acquired through contact with infected domestic animals. It has recently emerged as an important opportunistic infection in immunocompromised patients in the Tropics and in the West, causing severe watery diarrhea, abdominal cramps, and occasional infection of the biliary system, leading to ascending cholangitis and rarely gangrene of the gallbladder. It is not surprising that renal involvement can occur through nonspecific inflammatory factors resulting in proteinuria and urinary sediment changes. There is currently no effective therapy for cryptosporidiosis (321).

Echinococcosis

Humans act as an intermediate host for *Echinococcus granulosus*, a parasite of worldwide distribution, mainly encountered among sheep-herding populations and those in close contact with dogs. Infection is acquired by ingestion of eggs contaminating the environment through the feces of infected dogs. The ova hatch in the gut; larvae migrate into the liver, lungs, brain, kidneys, muscles, and other tissues where they eventually yield cysts. The cysts contain and reproduce protoscoleces, which have the potential of completing the life cycle if ingested by a dog.

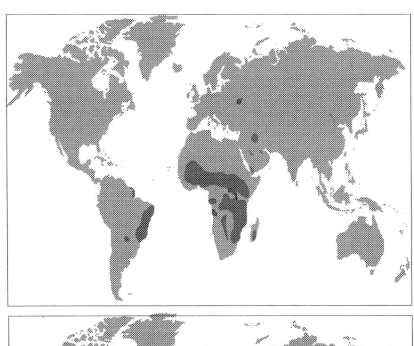

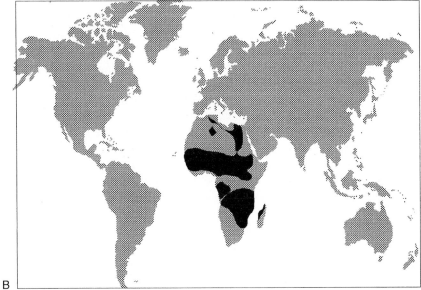

FIG. 79-10. Global distribution of schistosomiasis. **A:** *Schistosoma mansoni.* **B:** *Schistosoma haematobium.*

Echinococcosis (hydatid disease) in humans is characterized by multiorgan infection. Involvement of the kidneys may be silent, being discovered only during routine imaging. Hilar cysts have been described to cause caliceal back pressure and to stretch the arteries, leading to renovascular hypertension (322).

Immune-mediated glomerular injury has also been described. The disease is usually mild or subclinical. It affects young adults and presents with mild to moderate proteinuria and an increase in the urinary cellular elements. Renal biopsy results in several patients revealed a mesangioproliferative glomerulonephritis with IgM and C3 deposits (323). Parasitic antigens have not been searched for in the glomeruli, but they are readily detected in circulating immune complexes, particularly after mebendazole treatment or surgical intervention (322).

Schistosomiasis

Schistosomiasis is among the most widely spread of parasitic diseases, with an estimated 500 to 600 million people at risk (324) (Fig. 79-10). There are many strains of schistosomes, of which only five infect humans: *Schistosoma haematobium,* mainly in Africa; *Schistosoma mansoni* in Africa and South America; *Schistosoma japonicum* in China, Southeast Asia, and Japan; *Schistosoma intercalatum,* related to *S. mansoni* and found mainly in central Africa; and *Schistosoma mekongi,* related to *S. japonicum* and found in a few foci in Southeast Asia.

Infection is acquired through contact with fresh water harboring the specific snails, which act as the intermediate hosts and define the prevalence and density of infestation in different geographic areas. The infective agent is the *cercaria,* a fishlike organism with a bifid tail, 400 to 600 μm in length; the organism penetrates the skin or mucous membranes, loses its tail, and becomes a schistosomula. The latter gains access to the bloodstream through lymphatics and circulates in different capillary beds until it randomly reaches the portal or perivesical venous plexus. These sites contain trophic factors that promote the rapid growth of the schistosomula, which soon matures into an adult worm in the downstream veins. The adult worm is bisexual, the male being stronger and larger. The female stays in almost continuous copulation, with the male in a special groove called the *gynecophoral canal.* It only leaves to travel against the bloodstream to lay eggs in the submucosa of the urinary bladder (*S. haematobium*), colon, or rectum (*S. mansoni* and *S. japonicum*). During its active sexual life, the female *S. haematobium* or *S. mansoni* lays about 300 ova per day, whereas *S. japonicum* may lay up to 3,000 ova per day. Most ova find their way to the exterior by virtue of spines in their shells, aided by the muscle contractions of their habitat. Contact with fresh water leads to swelling and rupture of the shells, and release of *miracidia,* the infective stage to the snail, which completes the cycle (325).

Ova that fail to be exteriorized are the principal cause of pathogenicity. They cause a delayed hypersensitive reaction and granuloma formation that heals with fibrosis (326). The resulting functional consequences depend on the strategic anatomic sites of such fibrosis. Ova may be driven back along the bloodstream to deposit in different organs, where they also form granulomas. Most notorious are the hepatic granulomas, leading to periportal fibrosis and portal hypertension, and the pulmonary granulomas, which result in arteriolar occlusion and pulmonary hypertension. Other metastatic lesions include cerebral granulomas, often seen with *S. japonicum* infestations, subcutaneous nodules, and ocular granulomas, which are occasionally mistaken for other clinically similar conditions (327).

Renal Disorders Associated with Schistosomiasis

S. haematobium. The deposited ova form small tubercles that superficially resemble those of tuberculosis, hence, the name *pseudotubercles.* These coalesce to form nodules, which often get secondarily infected. With the evolution of the lesions, the underlying bladder wall gets fibrotic and the trapped ova become calcified. A thin mucosal layer may cover these lesions, which appear as pale granular areas called *sandy patches.* Other late lesions include mucosal cysts and fibrotic nodules, cystitis cystica and cystitis glandularis. Bladder malignancy often supervenes, a slowly growing squamous cell carcinoma being the predominant histopathologic pattern (328).

Functional consequences often complicate urinary schistosomiasis, depending on the site and extent of fibrosis. At the lower ends of the ureters, this leads to partial obstruction; at the bladder neck, it results in chronic outflow obstruction; and in the detrusor, it impairs contractility, resulting in an atonic viscus, which is often associated with vesicoureteric reflux. Upstream repercussions are attributed to ureteric obstruction, reflux, and chronic infection (244) (Chapter 24, Vesicoureteric Reflux and Reflux Neuropathy; and Chapter 25, Urinary Tract Obstruction).

The clinical features of schistosomiasis haematobium are encountered soon after the establishment of infection. Painful terminal hematuria is the time-honored presentation. It often affects children, more frequently men, reflecting the variance in exposure imposed by social constraints. The diagnosis is confirmed by finding the characteristic ova, with terminal spines, seen with routine urine microscopy. Pyuria and bacilluria are also detected in the presence of secondary infection. If untreated, hematuria persists for many years, although its intensity declines as the process of bladder fibrosis progresses. Eventually the patient is left with the symptoms of chronic cystitis, and upstream complications may develop.

Renal morbidity (Fig. 79-11) is reported in different endemic areas to vary from 2% to 52% of patients with lower urinary tract schistosomiasis haematobium, depending on the infective strain, intensity of infestation, availability of therapy, and probably genetic predisposition (329).

Because the pathology is usually localized in the submucosa of the lower ureteric sites, the proximal healthy part often undergoes significant hypertrophy, which allows adequate urodynamic compensation without any back-pressure sequelae. However, hydronephrosis develops in 9.7% to 48.0% of patients who fail to maintain this compensatory mechanism (244,329). Ascending infection is common, usually after instrumentation performed for various reasons. It is particularly common in patients with vesicoureteric reflux, again frequently induced by surgical or instrumental interventions. In addition to the regular features of acute and chronic pyelonephritis, infection often leads to the formation of stones. The proportion of patients with schistosomiasis haematobium who ultimately progress to end stage is unknown; a broad estimate in Egypt is 1 of 1,000 (330). With the high prevalence of infestation, even this small proportion amounts to 40 patients per million of the total population.

Early haematobium infestation is easy to cure. Several drugs have been used through the years, starting with the old-fashioned antimony preparations and ending up with the more modern, highly effective, and safe compounds niridazole and praziquantel (331). Surgical treatment is occasionally needed for the relief of obstruction or repair of reflux. ESRD management is classic, although often modified because of the problems imposed by active chronic pyelonephritis and bladder fibrosis (249).

S. mansoni. S. mansoni is principally an inhabitant of the portal venous tributaries, with colorectal disease and periportal hepatic fibrosis being the major consequences of infestation (319). Over the past three decades, experimental (332) and clinical (222,329) studies established that an immune-mediated glomerular injury may complicate this disease. Of the more than 100 antigens identified in the parasite, those of the adult worm's gut were incriminated in the pathogenesis of renal lesions. Particularly interesting are a proteoglycan and a glycoprotein, often referred to as *cathodal* and *anodal*

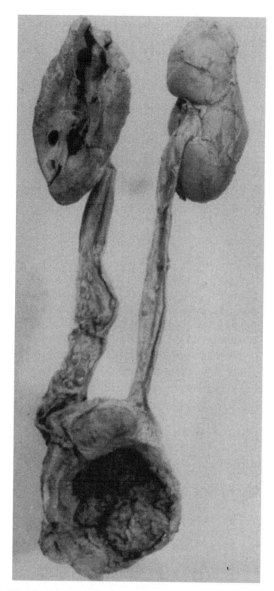

FIG. 79-11. Postmortem material showing the spectrum of urinary tract lesions in schistosomiasis haematobia. Note (a) the thickening of the bladder wall, dirty mucosa, and villous growth (squamous cell carcinoma); (b) the dilated ureters with cystic lesions (bilharzial cystitis cystica); (c) the dilated right pelvicaliceal system (due to obstruction/vesicoureteric reflux); and (d) the scarred left kidney of chronic pyelonephritis.

antigens, respectively, found by immunofluorescent study in the early glomerular lesions associated with schistosomiasis (333,334).

The initial glomerular response in humans (335) and in experimental animals (334,336,337) is essentially mesangial, with focal or diffuse axial cellular proliferation and no matrix expansion (Fig. 79-12). IgM and C3 deposits are detected by immunofluorescent study (336,338,339), often along with parasitic antigens (Fig. 79-13) (334,339). This lesion is not specific for *S. mansoni,* being also observed in humans with *S. haematobium* infection (224,340) and in experimental animals infected with *S. japonicum* (332). Apart from the nature of the antigen deposits (341), it is morphologically

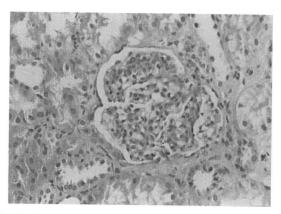

FIG. 79-12. Axial mesangial proliferation in early schistosomal glomerulopathy. (hematoxylin and eosin stain, magnification ×200) (From Barsoum RS. Schistosomal glomerulopathies. *Kidney Int* 1993;44:1, with permission.) (See Color Figure 79-12 following page 2624.)

similar to that seen with many other parasitic glomerulopathies.

Only mild clinical manifestations, usually limited to subnephrotic proteinuria and increased cellular excretion in urine, are associated with this lesion. There are considerable doubts about whether the lesion progresses in the absence of other factors (vide infra). The reported response to treatment with antiparasitic agents, steroids, and immunosuppressive agents has not been confirmed (342–346).

The initial glomerular lesions may subsequently progress into three distinct clinicopathologic syndromes.

1. Exudative glomerulonephritis (Fig. 79-14), which often complicates concomitant *Salmonella* infection, a frequent association in endemic areas (347,348), which leads to an acute, reversible nephrotic syndrome (222).

2. Progression into either mesangiocapillary glomerulonephritis (Fig. 79-15) or focal segmental sclerosis (Fig. 79-16), which seems to occur only in the presence of significant

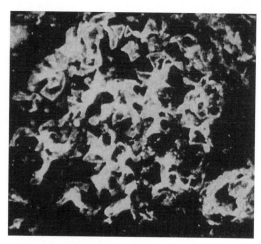

FIG. 79-13. Mesangial deposits of schistosomal Guy antigens in early schistosomal glomerulopathy. (See Color Figure 79-13 following page 2624.)

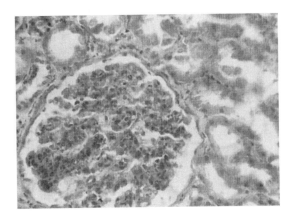

FIG. 79-14. Exudative glomerulonephritis in the nephrotic syndrome associated with combined *Schistosoma-Salmonella* infection. Note the abundance of neutrophils and monocytes in the glomerular capillaries and mesangium. (hematoxylin and eosin stain, magnification ×200) (From Barsoum RS. Schistosomal glomerulopathies. *Kidney Int* 1993;44:1, with permission.) (See Color Figure 79-14 following page 2624.)

hepatic disease. The crucial role of the liver has been well documented in experimental models (337,349) and clinical (350) and postmortem (351) studies. When associated with significant impairment of macrophage function (352), liver disease seems to permit a high worm antigen load to escape from the portal into the systemic circulation, thereby contributing to the formation of pathogenic immune complexes. Hepatic fibrosis has also been blamed for the defective clearance of IgA, originating in the gut in response to the parasite's antigenic products (353). Superimposed on the initial glomerular injury, IgA may be crucial in the progression of glomerular lesions into an overt nephropathy, and further on into ESRD. Autoimmunity may also have a potential role in disease progression (241).

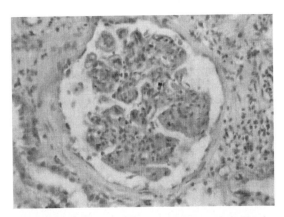

FIG. 79-15. Mesangiocapillary glomerulonephritis in advanced schistosomal glomerulopathy. Note the mesangial matrix expansion and the thickening of the glomerular basement membrane. (hematoxylin and eosin stain, magnification ×200) (From Barsoum RS. Schistosomal glomerulopathies. *Kidney Int* 1993;44:1, with permission.) (See Color Figure 79-15 following page 2624.)

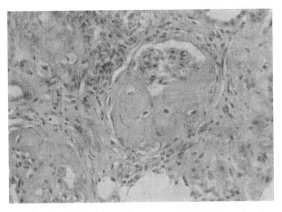

FIG. 79-16. Focal segmental glomerulosclerosis in advanced schistosomal glomerulopathy. (Masson trichrome stain, magnification ×200) (See Color Figure 79-16 following page 2624.)

The classic clinical presentation is the development of nephrotic edema and hypertension (50%) in a patient with typical hepatosplenic schistosomiasis. The diagnosis is supported by finding living schistosomal ova in the stools or rectal snips or by acquiring serologic evidence of active infestation. Liver biopsy results reveal the characteristic periportal fibrosis mostly sparing the hepatocytes and may also reveal deposited ova or worm pigments. This histopathologic pattern is reflected on conventional liver function tests, which are usually spared unless HBV or HCV infection is associated, which is fairly common. Endoscopic examination usually shows lower esophageal or fundal varices.

Examination of renal biopsy specimens usually reveals either of the two described patterns of glomerular injury, probably depending on genetic factors (354). Immunofluorescent study shows IgG and IgA deposits, and occasionally IgM and C3 deposits. Worm antigens are seldom seen at this stage. Variable degrees of nonspecific tubulointerstitial lesions have been observed, particularly with concomitant *S. haematobium* infection.

Both glomerular lesions are progressive (355,356). They do not respond to treatment. ESRD ultimately develops in those who survive the risks of ruptured esophageal varices or hepatocellular failure when the disease is compounded by viral hepatitis.

The epidemiologic importance of established schistosomal glomerulopathy as a cause of ESRD is not accurately quantitated; certain estimates suggest the figures of 10 per million of the general population (330) and 15% of those with schistosomal hepatic fibrosis (351).

3. Renal amyloidosis (Fig. 79-17) is the third potential outcome of schistosomal glomerulopathy, based on experimental findings in small laboratory animals (357, 358) and epidemiologic evidence in endemic areas (359,360).

It is suggested that the chronic parasitic antigen load of either *S. mansoni* or *S. haematobium* may lead to increased synthesis of AA protein and that local glomerular changes

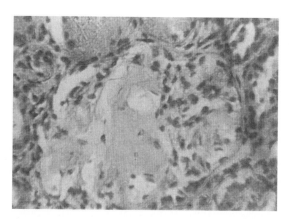

FIG. 79-17. Glomerular amyloid deposition in mixed *Schistosoma haematobium* and *Schistosoma mansoni* infection. (hematoxylin and eosin stain, magnification ×200) (From Barsoum RS, et al. Renal amyloidosis and schistosomiasis. *Trans R Soc Trop Med Hyg* 1979;73:367, with permission.) (See Color Figure 79-17 following page 2624.)

enhance deposition of this protein in the characteristic fibrillar structure (360). The clinical presentation of Schistosoma-associated amyloidosis resembles that of mesangiocapillary glomerulonephritis and focal segmental sclerosis, yet hepatosplenic disease may be less prominent and hypertension is less frequent. However, the disease more rapidly progresses to ESRD. Earlier reports of a favorable response to treatment (359) have not been substantiated.

S. japonicum. This infestation is similar to that with *S. mansoni* in causing hepatic fibrosis, portal hypertension, and splenomegaly. Metastatic lesions, particularly those in the central nervous system, are more common and more serious. Although most of the experimental background on schistosomal glomerulopathy is based on *S. japonicum* models (332), the clinical impact is extremely limited. Early mesangioproliferative lesions have been described, but overt disease is seldom reported and even denied (361). The reasons for this discrepancy are unclear; the nature of parasitic antigens, host genetic factors, limited hepatic involvement, and other factors may be incriminated. The high prevalence of IgA nephropathy in areas where *S. japonicum* infection is endemic (362) may mask the identity of *S. japonicum* glomerulopathy as a distinct disease.

Filariasis

Filariasis is highly prevalent in Africa, Asia, and South America (363) (Fig. 79-18). Of the eight filarial strains that infect humans, *Wuchereria bancrofti, Brugia malayi, Onchocerca volvulus,* and *Loa loa* are most frequently encountered in clinical practice. All species are transmitted by insect bites. The infective larvae migrate into the lymphatic vessels and slowly mature into adult worms over 3 to 18 months.

Adult *W. bancrofti* and *B. malayi* reside in the lymph nodes or afferent lymphatic vessels for decades. They mate and deliver the microfilariae, which either circulate in the bloodstream or migrate by way of the lymphatic channels to the dermis, awaiting their vector to complete the life cycle. *W. bancrofti* and *B. malayi* infections may be entirely dormant (*asymptomatic microfilaremia*), being usually identified by the accidental discovery of eosinophilia. Infected subjects with a pronounced immunologic response may present with

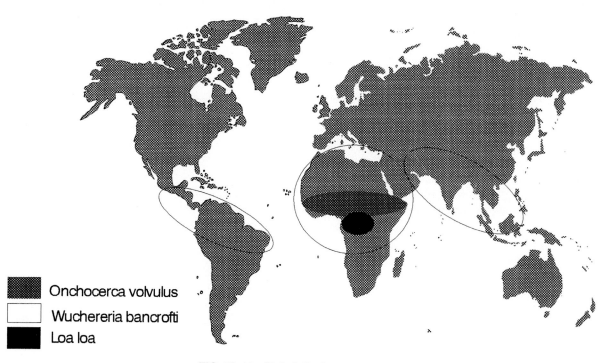

Onchocerca volvulus
Wuchereria bancrofti
Loa loa

FIG. 79-18. Global distribution of filariasis.

hypereosinophilia and pulmonary involvement. The classic presentation, however, is recurrent pyrexia with chills and lymphangitis caused by the local immune-mediated granulomatous response against the adult worms. In *B. malayi* infection, this reaction often leads to the formation of local abscesses that rupture and subsequently heal with characteristic scars. With *W. bancrofti,* the local reaction usually leads to lymphatic obstruction, gross upstream dilation, and distortion. Elephantiasis of the extremities and genitalia is the usual consequence. Rupture of the dilated lymphatic vessels may lead to chylous effusions, usually in the form of hydrocele or ascites. Rupture of the dilated retroperitoneal lymphatics into the renal pelvis leads to chyluria (Chapter 10, Urinalysis).

Adult *O. volvulus* coil up into spherical bundles in subcutaneous tissues and deep fascia, leading to characteristic nodules called *onchocercomas.* Regional lymph nodes may be enlarged. The worms deliver millions of microfilariae, which migrate into the skin and ocular tissues. In the latter tissues, they lead to keratitis, anterior uveitis, and less often chorioretinitis. Blindness (river blindness) supervenes in 1% to 4% of patients.

Adult *L. loa* worms live wandering in the subcutaneous and subconjunctival tissues. They may induce a peculiar hypersensitivity skin reaction, the *Calabar swellings,* which are localized erythematous and angioedematous lesions. Generalized angioedema may be encountered in expatriates and undernourished natives.

Renal Involvement in Filariasis. The best-documented renal lesion in filariasis is that associated with *O. volvulus.* In a large epidemiologic study in Cameroon, where this strain is hyperendemic, proteinuria was significantly more frequent among infected subjects (364). Minimal change, mesangioproliferative, mesangiocapillary, and chronic sclerosing glomerulonephritis lesions are most often encountered. Subendothelial and mesangial immune complexes containing IgM, IgG, C3 (245), and onchocercal antigens (364) were detected by immunofluorescence and mesangial electron-dense deposits (365), by electron microscopy. Onchocercal glomerulonephritis is known to recur in transplanted kidneys.

Similar lesions have also been described in bancroftiasis (366, 367) and loiasis (368), although specific antigens were not looked for. In addition, an exudative glomerulonephritis, referred to as *acute eosinophilic glomerulonephritis,* has been documented in patients with *W. bancrofti* infection (367), and membranous nephropathy in those with *L. loa* (364) infections. Microfilariae may be seen in the glomerular capillaries.

The clinical spectrum of filarial glomerulonephritis ranges from asymptomatic proteinuria to ESRD. Nephrotic syndrome is often ascribed to such infections in endemic areas. Acute nephritic syndrome in patients with bancroftiasis has been reported. Treatment with diethylcarbamazine may help to resolve early glomerular lesions, but it usually fails when the nephrotic syndrome is manifested (366). Proteinuria may even be aggravated by such treatment in some patients;

this is often attributed to further release of filarial antigens (369).

Trichinosis

Trichinosis is a nematodal infection of worldwide distribution, being particularly prevalent in communities where raw, smoked, or undercooked meat, especially pork, is eaten. It is fairly common in Southeast Asia and Latin America, but for obvious reasons, is rare in countries with large Muslim and Jewish populations.

Infection is acquired by ingestion of infective larvae encysted in striated muscles. Excystation occurs by acid-pepsin digestion in the stomach; parasites mature in the upper small intestine. The adult female produces larvae, which penetrate the blood and lymphatic vessels and migrate into different host organs. Those reaching the muscles become encysted and remain viable for many years.

Although trichinosis is often associated with nonspecific gastrointestinal symptoms, its main clinical impact is related to the eosinophilic granulomatous reaction that the encysted larvae provoke in different organs, including skeletal and cardiac muscles, lungs, and the central nervous system. Proptosis and periorbital edema associated with pyrexia and myalgia are the usual clinical clues to the diagnosis.

Renal involvement in trichinosis was vaguely reported as early as 1916 (370). It became more firmly established in recent years as more elaborate diagnostic criteria became established. The lesions are mainly glomerular, in the form of mesangial proliferation associated with immunoglobulin, C3, and occasionally fibrin deposits. Trichinella antigen has not been searched for in the glomeruli (371).

Renal involvement is usually subclinical, with mild proteinuria and microhematuria. Blood pressure is not elevated, and renal function is usually preserved or only mildly impaired (372). Hypoalbuminemia is occasionally noted, leading to contraction of the blood volume with a mild reduction of p-aminohippurate and creatinine clearances. Circulating immune complexes associated with a decrease in serum C3 level have been described. All clinical abnormalities are reversible by thiabendazole treatment (50 mg per kilogram of body weight per day for 2 days) (371).

Opisthorchiasis

The disease is caused by *Opisthorchis felineus* and *Opisthorchis viverrini* through the ingestion of raw or undercooked fish. *O. felineus* is common in the Philippines, Vietnam, and India, whereas *O. viverrini* is prevalent in Thailand, Laos, and Kampuchea. The liver is the target organ where the parasites lodge in the biliary tract. The incidence of cholangiocarcinoma is high in opisthorchiasis. Renal failure can occur in the patients with opisthorchiasis (373). Acute renal failure is seen in 49% of the patients with cholangiocarcinoma and severe jaundice (56). Hyponatremia and hypokalemia secondary to natriuresis and kaliuresis are frequently observed (67). The causes of renal failure are multiple and include hypovolemia, endotoxemia, cardiac dysfunction, effects of vasoactive mediators, hypotension, hyperbilirubinemia and hyperuricosuria.

Renal pathologic changes include tubular degeneration with bile staining and vacuolation of proximal tubules in the potassium-depleted patients. IgA deposition in the mesangium may be observed. In Syrian golden hamsters infected with *O. viverrini,* immune complex glomerulonephritis with deposition of IgG antibody specific to the integumental membrane of the adult worm has been shown (374). Renal amyloidosis with AA protein deposition in the glomeruli and interstitium can occur.

Strongyloidiasis

Infestation by *Strongyloides stercoralis* is endemic worldwide (375), particularly in the warm climates of the Tropics. Infection is acquired by skin contact with soil containing the free filariform larvae. The larvae migrate into the pulmonary capillaries where they break into the alveolar spaces, ascend through the airways to the pharynx, are then swallowed, and eventually mature in the duodenum into adult worms. In most infested subjects, only female worms are found in the small intestine. They reproduce by parthenogenesis, forming eggs that hatch in the gut and release rhabditiform larvae, which eventually transform into the infective filariform larvae in the soil. This transformation can also occur in the gut of an immunocompromised host.

Strongyloidiasis is a mild disease in the immunocompetent individual, being either asymptomatic or associated with vague abdominal symptoms. In the immunocompromised, however, reinfection with filariform larvae can occur through the intestinal walls or the perianal skin. As this process is repeated, hyperinfection occurs, leading to a potentially fatal disseminated disease. As the infective larvae migrate through the lungs, they can induce pulmonary hemorrhage and acute respiratory complications that mimic the adult respiratory distress syndrome. The larvae can also disseminate into various organs including the brain, eyes, pancreas, peritoneum, kidneys, and skin where they form creeping eruptions (376). Mesangial proliferative glomerulonephritis with nephrotic syndrome has been observed in association with strongyloidiasis. The nephrotic syndrome resolved after treatment of the disease (377). The response to thiabendazole treatment is remarkable, with parasitologic cure in more than 90% of patients.

Other Parasitic Diseases

Renal lesions rarely occur in visceral larva migrans caused by the migration of larval stages of *Toxocara canis* or *Toxocara cati* (378). Granulomatous changes consisting of eosinophils and histiocytes with giant cells may be observed.

Hematuria and eosinophiluria may be noted. Immune complex–mediated glomerulonephritis has been reported in amebiasis (379). However, ameba antigen was not demonstrated in the immune deposits.

TOXIC NEPHROPATHIES IN THE TROPICS

Nephropathy Due to Animal Toxins

Animal toxin poisoning is a common cause of acute renal failure and nephropathy in the Tropics.

Snakebites

Snakebites are a worldwide problem. It is estimated that 2,000 species of snakes exist, and 400 of them are poisonous (380). Snakebites are blamed for 40,000 deaths per year in the world; most occur in the tropical countries of Africa, South and Southeast Asia, and Latin America. In India alone, 15,000 patients die of snakebites per year, whereas in the United States, only 20 deaths per year are reported (381).

Renal involvement in snakebites has been reviewed extensively by Chugh (382). Renal failure complicates 5.5% to 26.0% of all snake poisonings (380,383,384). Most cases are due to the Viperidae family of snakes, which includes pit viper, rattlesnake, Russell's viper, saw scale viper, *Bothrops jararaca,* and puff adder (383,385). Other snakes such as the boomslang, mulga snake, dugite, gwardar, *Agkistrodon hypnale,* and *Cryptophis nigrescens* and sea snakes can also cause acute renal failure.

Clinical presentation is due to either local symptoms with pain, swelling, local bleeding, or infection at the site of bite, or systemic symptoms with generalized bleeding, hypotension, or oliguria. Oliguria usually occurs 24 to 72 hours after the bite. Patients can be hypotensive at presentation but often are normotensive. With viper bites, renal failure is usually associated with intravascular hemolysis and disseminated intravascular coagulation. Those patients with renal failure have higher urinary fibrin-degradation products levels than those with normal renal function, suggesting the role of intravascular coagulation in the pathogenesis of renal failure (386). With sea snake bites, renal failure is associated with rhabdomyolysis. Sepsis can be a complicating factor at presentation (380,383,387). Nephrotic syndrome has been reported in a rare patient after a snakebite (388). However, transient heavy proteinuria can occur in patients bitten by Russell's viper.

Renal histology has been studied by several groups (380, 389–394). Most patients show histologic findings compatible with acute tubular necrosis. Acute cortical necrosis is seen in significantly few patients (382). Electron microscopic study in Russell's viper poisoning complicated by acute renal failure has shown glomerular mesangial hypercellularity, vascular endothelial swelling, tubular epithelial necrosis, and interstitial infiltrates (395). Interstitial nephritis (396), proliferative glomerulonephritis (397–400), and arteritis of interlobular vessels (392) have been reported. Granular deposition of IgM and C3 in the mesangium is often observed.

There is evidence of deposition of immune complex *in situ* (72).

With sea snake poisoning (401,402), rhabdomyolysis is the primary event leading to myoglobinuric renal failure. Renal histology shows findings compatible with those of tubular necrosis (390,402). Muscle histology shows diffuse hyaline lesions involving muscle fiber (401).

Pathogenesis

Snake venom contains many proteolytic enzymes and phospholipases capable of triggering hemolysis, disseminated intravascular coagulopathy, fibrinolysis, complement activation, rhabdomyolysis, and tissue necrosis (385,387, 403–406). Hypotension can result from blood loss, anaphylaxis, myocardial depression, and generalized vasodilation due to bradykinin release. Systemic and renal hemodynamics in snake envenomation bear resemblance to that observed in infection and share the same cytokines and mediators (407–410). Given the protein nature of snake venom, acute renal failure is rarely caused by one factor but rather multiple factors. Chugh et al. (385) showed that a lethal dose of Russell's viper venom did not consistently cause renal failure, and histologically no renal lesion was observed. However, when a sublethal dose was used, renal failure occurred consistently, and histologically tubulointerstitial and glomerular fibrin deposition was seen. In an isolated perfused kidney, Russell's viper venom decreased the renal blood flow and glomerular filtration rate and increased the fractional excretion of sodium (411). The membrane potential of the proximal tubular cell is decreased in a dose-dependent fashion (73). Russell's viper venom decreases renal cortical mitochondrial oxygen consumption and increases the P/O ratio (410). Toxicity to glomeruli and tubular epithelial cells has been shown (412). Immune mechanism plays a role in the pathogenesis of glomerulonephritis. Therefore, there is evidence of hemodynamic changes, direct nephrotoxicity, and immunologic mechanism in snakebite nephropathy.

Treatment and Prognosis

Treatment of renal failure caused by snake poisoning is complicated by other systemic complications of the venom. Standard treatment includes local care, use of antivenom, generalized support, and if needed, dialysis (413). Dialysis in patients with a sea snake bite can improve muscular symptoms (402). Early administration of sodium bicarbonate to alkalinize urine prevents the development of acute renal failure (414,415). The prognosis for patients with renal failure is very good, and most recover with appropriate treatment (416). The prognosis in the few patients with cortical necrosis is poor (391,394,417,418).

Insect Stings

Proteinuria, nephrotic syndrome, and acute renal failure have been reported in association with bee, wasp, and hornet stings.

In a study by Elming and Solling of 20 healthy subjects stung by bees or wasps, pathologic albuminuria was found in three persons. The urine albumin excretion normalized in 2 months in two persons (419).

Nephrotic Syndrome

An association between bee stings and nephrotic syndrome has long been described (420). A relapse of nephrotic syndrome after a bee sting has been reported (421). From the pooled data including our experience, the onset of nephrotic syndrome varies from 2 to 14 days after the sting (421–426). Serum complement levels and renal function are usually normal. In most patients, the serum immunoglobulin profile is normal. One report described a decrease in serum IgA, IgM, and IgG levels (425). The response to steroid treatment is favorable in 50% of the patients.

Renal pathologic changes vary. Minimal change lesions, mesangial proliferative glomerulonephritis, membranous glomerulonephritis, and glomerulosclerosis are among the changes described (421,427). Deposition of C3, IgM, and IgG is demonstrable. However, no report has demonstrated the presence of bee venom antigens in the glomeruli. Although such a finding would indicate a role for an immunologic mechanism in the pathogenesis of glomerulonephritis, the cause-and-effect relationship between the bee venom and glomerulonephritis has not been substantiated. The association between the bee sting and nephrotic syndrome with minimal lesions, erythema of the skin, and eosinophilia described in one report (425) could be related to basophil sensitization (428).

The mechanism responsible for the development of glomerulonephritis is therefore not understood. The role of the bee venom (*Apis mellifera*) in inducing the alteration of T-cell function in mice, which might link with glomerulonephritis, deserves further study (429).

Renal Failure

Renal failure has occurred in patients stung by wasps (420, 430–433), hornets (427,430,434,435), and bees (426,436, 437). Stings are usually multiple. A single sting does not cause renal failure but can cause anaphylactic shock in the previously sensitized patient. Renal failure associated with rhabdomyolysis or intravascular hemolysis develops within 24 hours. Thrombocytopenia may be present with or without disseminated intravascular coagulation. Hepatocellular jaundice may be observed. Laboratory findings include hyperkalemia, hyperuricemia, hyperphosphatemia, hypocalcemia, hemoglobinuria, myoglobinuria, and elevation of muscle enzyme levels. Nonoliguric renal failure is not uncommon. Oligoanuria is often observed in older adults. The duration of renal failure varies from 1 week to several weeks. The course of renal failure is prolonged in older adults. Recovery of renal function is usual; however, residual renal damage can occur. Older adults and children are at high risk for a fatal outcome.

Renal pathologic changes include tubular necrosis and interstitial lesions with edema and mononuclear infiltration. The proximal, distal, and collecting tubules are affected. Renal failure is attributed to intravascular hemolysis, rhabdomyolysis, and hypotension.

Raw Carp Bile

Ingestion of raw carp bile, traditionally believed to improve visual acuity, stop coughing, decrease body temperature, and lower blood pressure, can result in renal failure. The problem is well known in Southeast Asia, Taiwan, China, and Korea. The raw bile of carp, belonging to the order of Cypriniformes, including *Ctenopharyngodon idellus, Cyprinus carpio, Hypophthalmichthys molitrix, Mylopharyngodon piceus,* and *Aristichthys nobilis,* is nephrotoxic (438). Clinical manifestations, which start from gastrointestinal symptoms, consist of abdominal pain, nausea, vomiting, and diarrhea occurring 10 minutes to 12 hours after the ingestion of raw bile (438,439). The amount of bile ingested varies from 15 to 30 mL. The gastrointestinal symptoms are followed by hepatitis and acute renal failure. The onset of oliguria varies from 2 to 48 hours after ingestion. Oliguria renal failure is noted in 54% of patients. Hematuria occurs in 77% and jaundice in 62%. The duration of renal failure varies from 2 to 3 weeks.

Renal pathologic changes are those of tubular necrosis. Glomeruli show no remarkable changes. The pathogenesis of renal failure is not well understood and perhaps is due to multiple factors. Nonspecific factors including diarrhea and jaundice leading to renal ischemia cannot be excluded. In rats, nephrotoxicity developed after the ingestion of carp raw bile but not hog raw bile. Therefore, mammalian bile is relatively nontoxic. Cyprinol, a bile alcohol, has been suggested to be nephrotoxic. Lin et al. (440) showed that the toxic compound exists in the ethanol-soluble fraction of bile, which has bile acids.

Jellyfish Stings

The tentacles of jellyfish (*Physalia physalis*) have the capsules or hematocytes that contain venom consisting of 5-hydroxytryptamine, histamine, and a glycoprotein with hemolytic properties (441). Severe poisoning can cause nausea, diarrhea, hypotension, intravascular hemolysis, and convulsions. Renal failure secondary to intravascular hemolysis has been reported (442).

Scorpion Stings

Scorpion venom can cause the release of acetylcholine, catecholamines, and various mediators, with toxic effects to the neuromuscular system. Among the clinical features after severe reaction to a scorpion sting are symptoms of autonomic nervous system stimulation, disseminated intravascular coagulation, myocarditis, cardiac failure, pancreatitis, pulmonary edema, convulsions, and hypotension (443,444).

Renal failure has been described in association with disseminated intravascular coagulation and massive hemorrhage in various organs (445).

Spider Bites

In most cases, the symptoms of spider bite are mild. Yet, severe reaction can occur from the bite of certain spiders. *Latrodectus* venom can cause severe pain at the site of the bite, nausea, vomiting, salivation, sweating, headache, muscular twitching, hypertension, and respiratory paralysis. *Sicarius* venom can cause disseminated intravascular coagulation with renal failure (446). Renal failure, intravascular hemolysis, and death presumably caused by the bite of the common brown spider (*Loxosceles reclusa*) have been reported (447).

Centipede Bites

A centipede bite usually causes local reactions. Severe systemic symptoms can occur after the bite of the giant desert centipede, *Scolopendra heros,* which is found in the southern part of the United States and Mexico. The venom contains phospholipase A_2, serotonin, and cardiotoxic protein (448). Nausea, vomiting, headache, rhabdomyolysis, and acute renal failure have been reported (449).

Lonomia Caterpillar Contact

The hemolymph and hair extract of caterpillar of moths in the genus *Lonomia* have strong fibrinolytic and enzymatic activities similar to tissue plasminogen activator, kallikrein, factor Xa, and urokinase causing both fibrinolysis and disseminated intravascular coagulation (450,451). Severe acute renal failure with a hemorrhagic syndrome resembling disseminated intravascular coagulation after contact with Lonomia caterpillars has been described (452,453).

Nephropathy Due to Plant Toxins

Several kinds of plants exert pharmacologic effects to the body. Certain effects are harmful and may directly or indirectly cause nephropathy. The subject has recently been reviewed (454).

Djenkol Bean

Djenkol beans (*Pithecolobium lobatum, Pithecolobium jiringa*) are consumed by people in Indonesia, Malaysia, and southern Thailand (455–460). The beans are eaten as food, either raw, fried, or roasted. Toxicity follows ingestion of the raw bean in large amounts (more than 5 beans), although there are different susceptibilities among individuals. Poisoning may be caused by a single bean in some individuals, whereas it may take 20 beans to cause toxicity in others (458). Ingestion of the boiled beans does not cause toxicity because the toxic substance, djenkolic acid, is removed from the bean. The amount of djenkolic acid may vary among beans from various sources. Poisoning is characterized by abdominal discomfort, loin pains, severe colic, nausea, vomiting, dysuria, gross hematuria, and oliguria occurring 2 to 6 hours after the beans are ingested. The patient may be anuric. Hypertension may be present. In a recent report of 22 patients with djenkol bean poisoning, dysuria was noted in 17 (77%), hematuria in 15 (68%), proteinuria in 10 (45%), hypertension in 8 (36%), and renal failure in 12 (55%) patients (457).

Urine analysis reveals erythrocytes, epithelial cells, protein, and the needlelike crystals of djenkolic acid. The symptoms are due to mechanical irritation of the renal tubules and urinary tract by the djenkolic acid crystals. Precipitation of djenkolic acid, causing tubular obstruction, occurs in acid and concentrated urine. Urolithiasis has been reported, with djenkolic acid as the nucleus (456). Most patients recover within a few days.

Diagnosis can easily be made by the history of bean ingestion and occasional sulfurous fetor in the breath. Treatment requires hydration to increase urine flow and alkalinization of urine by sodium bicarbonate. When the urine pH level is increased from 5.0 to 7.4, the solubility of djenkolic acid is increased by 43%, and at a pH level of 8.1, the solubility increases to 92% (455).

Callilepis Laureola

Callilepis laureola (Impila) is a perennial herb with a tuberous rootstock found widely in South Africa, Zambia, Zaire, Zimbabwe, and the neighboring countries. The plant is used in the form of infusion for coughs, constipation, intestinal worms, and many other illnesses. An alkaloid, atractyloside, found in the tuber of the plant, is believed to have nephrotoxic and hypoglycemic effects. It has an inhibitory effect on oxidative phosphorylation (461). After medication, toxic symptoms usually occur in less than 24 hours in 40% of the patients and within a few days in 72% (462–464). Clinically, the patient has abdominal pain, vomiting, and diarrhea. Hypoglycemia is observed in 81% of patients. Convulsions and coma are common. Hepatocellular jaundice is present. Renal failure ensues in most patients. Treatment is supportive. The mortality rate is more than 50%.

The kidney shows tubular necrosis involving the proximal tubules and the ascending loops of Henle. Interstitial edema and cellular infiltration are present.

Semecarpus Anacardium

Semecarpus anacardium is the name for the marking nut tree in India and tropical forests. The bark and the pericarp of the fruit have a black caustic juice that is irritating to the skin, causing eruptions and blisters. Prolonged exposure to the sap can cause abdominal pain, vomiting, fever, and renal failure (465). Cortical necrosis has been reported. Nephrotoxicity is attributed to the phenolic substance in the sap.

Mushrooms

The *Amanita* and *Galerina* species of mushrooms produce phallotoxins and are nephrotoxic. Toxic symptoms occur within 10 to 14 hours after ingestion and include abdominal pain, nausea, vomiting, and diarrhea, followed by jaundice, renal failure, convulsions, and coma (466). Renal failure is severe, with a mortality rate of more than 50%. In an animal model of poisoning with *Cortinarius orellanus* mushrooms, renal dysfunction occurred within 48 hours (467). The pattern of renal impairment included a decreased glomerular filtration rate, proteinuria, glycosuria, and a decreased tubular reabsorption of sodium, potassium, and water. Renal pathologic changes are those of tubular necrosis, with prominent necrosis of the proximal tubules with interstitial edema. There are no glomerular changes (468).

Cotton Seed Oil

The principal ingredient of the cotton seed oil is gossypol. Gossypol can cause kaliuresis and hypokalemia. The mechanism is not well understood. In central and southern China, where the dietary potassium intake is low, the incidence of gossypol-induced hypokalemia is between 4% and 5% (469). It has also been reported to cause distal renal tubular acidosis in Chinese people who consume cotton seed oil (470).

Several plants, including *Securidaca longipedunculata*, *Euphorbia matabelensis*, and *Crotalaria laburnifolia*, have been listed as being nephrotoxic (471,472), although there is no supporting scientific evidence. These plants are usually used as traditional medicine for the treatment of many illnesses and may cause renal failure through their side effects. For example, infusion of the leaves, bark, and root of *S. longipedunculata* can cause severe gastroenteritis with diarrhea and vomiting, which can result in acute renal failure through volume depletion without evidence of direct nephrotoxicity.

An association between the use of Chinese herbal medicine containing aristolochic acid and chronic renal disease has been described (473). Renal pathologic changes include tubular atrophy, interstitial fibrosis, glomerulosclerosis, and thickening of the wall of the interlobular artery and glomerular afferent arteriole. Urothelial malignancy has been observed. Multifocal atypia of the medullary collecting ducts, the pelvis and ureter with overexpression of p53 has been shown (474). On the positive side, traditional Chinese herbal medicine (Sairei-to) with the active principle saikosaponin-d has been shown to prevent glomerulosclerosis in uninephrectomized rats with anti-Thy-1 antibody injection (475).

Nephropathy Due to Other Chemicals

Accidental exposure to certain chemical toxins is well documented as a cause of acute renal failure in the Tropics, as it is in the West. This subject is addressed in Chapter 47 (Nephrotoxicity Secondary to Environmental Agents and Heavy Metals).

Chemical intoxication may also be associated with certain occupational hazards, involving exposure to industrial poisons such as lead, mercury, cadmium, uranium, and asbestos. This is highly prevalent in tropical countries, because of the inadequacy of environmental protection measures in industrial plants. The toxicologic aspects of such exposure are detailed in Chapter 47 (Nephrotoxicity Secondary to Environmental Agents and Heavy Metals).

Certain chemical hazards of particular importance in the Tropics deserve mentioning, namely, paraquat, copper sulfate, and diethylene glycol.

Paraquat Poisoning

This is mainly reported in Southeast Asia (476). Paraquat is a herbicide, widely used in agriculture, to which humans are exposed by ingestion (including suicidal intake), inhalation of sprays, or contact with skin abrasions (477). Pulmonary, hepatic, and renal manifestations occur with paraquat poisoning and are attributed to the massive generation of reactive oxygen radicals. Nephrotoxicity is expressed as acute tubular necrosis (478), which leads to accumulation of the poison and increases its systemic toxicity. Plasma paraquat levels of more than 2 mg/L at 24 hours and 1 mg/L at 48 hours are of grave prognostic significance (479).

As with many other chemical intoxications, the first line of treatment is to reduce absorption by gastric lavage and to the administer adsorbing substances such as fuller's earth. If renal function permits, forced diuresis should be attempted (480). Hemodialysis and charcoal hemoperfusion (481) are effective, whereas peritoneal dialysis is too inefficient. Attempts to reduce the oxygen radical load by suppressing leukocytic function with corticosteroids and even cyclophosphamide (482) are controversial.

Copper Sulfate Poisoning

This hazard is of considerable epidemiologic significance in India (483). Copper sulfate is used in the leather industry. Exposure occurs through accidental or intentional ingestion. Acute toxicity ushers in with prominent gastrointestinal manifestations, intravascular hemolysis, hepatic injury, and renal failure.

Renal injury is the result of massive intravascular hemolysis, induced by the action of the poison on intracellular enzyme systems including G6PD, glutathione reductase, and catalase (484,485). The associated hypovolemia, due to gastrointestinal fluid losses, further aggravates the renal insult. Acute tubular necrosis with rupture of the tubular basement membrane, copper deposits in the tubule cells, and hemoglobin casts in the tubule lumina are characteristic histopathologic features.

In addition to the conventional methods for reducing the absorption of the poison, fluid replacement and induction of diuresis, dimercaprol (100 to 150 mg intramuscularly every 4 hours) is effectively used for chelation in copper sulfate poisoning. Dialysis is often necessary during the critical hypercatabolic phase and also to assist in eliminating the toxin (486).

Diethylene Glycol Poisoning

Diethylene glycol is a known nephrotoxic agent. Poisoning with diethylene glycol in the Tropics has frequently been associated with contamination of ingestible pharmaceutical products. Outbreaks of acute renal failure by diethylene glycol contaminated acetaminophen have been reported in Nigeria (487) and Bangladesh (488). Recently there was a large outbreak of acute renal failure with deaths in children consuming diethylene glycol contaminated acetaminophen syrup in Haiti (489). Renal failure was severe and associated with hepatitis, pancreatitis, and central nervous system involvement with high mortality. It has been postulated that acetaminophen could provide an additive or potentiating effects for diethylene glycol toxicity. Hypovolemia caused by vomiting could be another contributing factor.

DIVERSE ENVIRONMENTAL PROBLEMS

In addition to the high prevalence of infections and intoxications, other features of tropical ecology may have a significant impact on the epidemiology of renal disease in certain geographic locations. These include the effects of climate, soil composition, and environmental pollution. Some of the available information on this issue is briefly reviewed.

Renal Stones

Renal stone disease is one of the common problems in tropical Asia. It accounts for 40% of renal problems in Pakistan, which is a country in the "stone belt" (490). The renal stones usually consist of mixed calcium, oxalate, and phosphate. The hot and dry climate and dietary factors play important roles. In the Arabian peninsula, the dietary ratio of oxalate to calcium and the dietary animal protein intake are higher than those in any other countries (491). In Israel, the high prevalence of renal stones is related to dehydration and solar hypervitaminosis D with absorptive hypercalciuria (492). In India and Pakistan, the cause of renal stones is not apparent but could be related to dehydration. The prevalence of upper urinary tract stones in the northeastern Thai population has been estimated to be 3.76 per 1,000 individuals, with a men : women ratio of 2 : 1 (493). The stones, like those in other Asian populations, are composed of calcium, oxalate, and phosphate. Urinary excretion rates for calcium, magnesium, oxalate, and urate are normal. Urinary phosphate excretion is slightly decreased. The low urinary citrate concentration could significantly contribute to stone formation (493,494).

Endemic Hypokalemia and Related Problems

Hypokalemia in northeastern Thailand is endemic and reflects the effects of the environment. Northeastern Thailand is a plateau in the arid area of the country, where the weather is dry and hot. Except for the areas close to the river basin, the land consists largely of sandstone. The soil, therefore, has low levels of potassium and is infertile. The people in the villages are of low socioeconomic status and consume the products of the land. Therefore, 38% of them have hypokalemia and are potassium depleted. The erythrocyte membranes of the villagers are found to have decreased Na-K-ATPase activity. The urine has a low citrate concentration. Both potassium depletion and decreased Na-K-ATPase activity lead to low urine citrate through intracellular acidosis, which enhances citrate reabsorption. Intracellular sodium concentration is increased, whereas intracellular potassium concentration is decreased. The basic abnormalities of these northeastern Thai villagers are, therefore, potassium depletion, decreased Na-K-ATPase activity, and low urinary citrate levels (494–496). These abnormalities resolved when they migrated to the capital city (495). Besides renal stones, sudden unexplained death and distal renal tubular acidosis are also important health problems of the region.

Sudden unexplained nocturnal death has recently received much attention. The incidence is 38 per 100,000 men between 20 and 49 years old (497). The victims are usually muscular young men of low socioeconomic class who die in their sleep without apparent organic lesion. Ventricular fibrillation has been observed and hypokalemia has been reported in some patients. They have decreased Na-K-ATPase activity of the erythrocyte membrane (498). It has been postulated that hypokalemia, the possible decrease in myocardial Na-K-ATPase, and sympathetic stimulation due to stress could lead to cardiac arrhythmias and death (499). The causes are likely multiple and could involve genetic variations. Recent evidence suggests that decreased activity of the sodium channel in the cardiac muscle could be incriminating.

The prevalence of distal renal tubular acidosis in northeastern Thailand is approximately 3.6%, with a female preponderance (500). The patients are usually admitted in the hospital during the mid summer because of muscular weakness or paralysis; nephrocalcinosis, renal stones, or both are noted in 27% of the patients. Interestingly, the patients have low urinary potassium levels, a finding different from Western reports. In addition, gastric acidity level is low (501), suggestive of decreased H-K-ATPase (HKα1) activity or decreased chloride bicarbonate exchange (AE2). Because of hypokalemia, aldosterone secretion is likely suppressed, and this would in turn decrease H-ATPase activity. Distal renal tubular acidosis is heterogeneous and requires further study on chloride bicarbonate exchange (AE), H-ATPase and HKα2 activities of the collecting ducts (502). In Southeast Asian, ovalocytosis with distal renal tubular acidosis *AE1* gene mutation has been reported (503).

Renal Disease and Environmental Pollution

A wide spectrum of chronic renal diseases is attributed to environmental pollution, which has been incriminated in the pathogenesis of glomerulonephritis (e.g., heavy metals, hydrocarbons), tubulointerstitial disease (e.g., lead), and renal and urothelial malignancies (cigarette smoking, cadmium, and aflatoxins). This subject is reviewed in Chapter 47 (Nephrotoxicity Secondary to Environmental Agents and Heavy Metals).

The epidemiologic significance of environmental pollution in the Tropics is unknown, but it may very well account for the high prevalence of renal disease in general, and particularly for the progressive increase in tubulointerstitial disease in the recently industrialized tropical countries (504,505). It is noteworthy that the item "unknown" accounts for 7.4% to 54.5% of ESRD on the tropical list of causes (504–508). Although this may be attributed to a lack of adequate diagnostic facilities (505,508) or to late patient presentation, it may also be accounted for by environmental pollution.

Experimental Background

Most of the available information in this field is derived from animal experiments. Nephrotoxicity can be induced by various chemicals in a number of animal models using rats, mice, hamsters, guinea pigs, chickens, ferrets, dogs, pigs, monkeys, and others. Three principal patterns are often encountered:

1. "Toxic" tubulointerstitial disease, in which the renal tubules, particularly the proximal ones, are the main target. Cell injury is mediated by various mechanisms including cell membrane disruption, disturbance of intracellular organelles, enzyme systems, and metabolic pathways. Cell necrosis and subsequent regenerative hyperplasia, luminal dilatation, interstitial edema, cellular infiltration, and ultimately fibrosis are the histopathologic hallmarks. Proteinuria, cylindruria, leukocyturia, and azotemia are the usual functional consequences. This pattern is attributed to a direct toxic effect on cell membranes or intracellular enzyme systems.

2. Acceleration of "spontaneous nephropathy" in adult male rats (509), with nephrotoxicity being expressed as a statistically significant increase in the incidence of nephropathy or the development of neoplastic lesions. The P$_2$ segment of the proximal tubule is the target. The lesions are ushered in by the appearance of intracellular hyaline droplets, which coalesce and eventually lead to cell necrosis. The resulting debris forms intraluminal granular casts that tend to block the tubules at the corticomedullary junction, leading to pressure necrosis of the surrounding cells and upstream tubular dilation. Spontaneously initiated clones expand, starting the process of regeneration. Adenomas and rarely adenocarcinomas may develop. Interstitial edema, cellular infiltration, and subsequent fibrosis and nephrocalcinosis cause progressive nephropathy in these animals.

The α_{2u}-globulin was recently brought into focus as an important sex-linked mediator of the renal lesions in this model (510). This protein is normally generated in the liver, filtered through the glomeruli, and taken up by the proximal tubule cells where it is metabolized in the lysosomes. Binding with certain chemicals slows its degradation, leading to its intracellular accumulation and subsequent crystallization in the form of hyaline droplets. The subsequent mechanisms of cellular injury in droplet nephropathy are unknown, but they may involve lysosomal disruption, release of reactive oxygen species, or others.

3. Carcinogenesis, in which expansion of particular cell clones leads to neoplastic growth. This may occur at the tubular level, leading to adenomas and adenocarcinomas, or at a urothelial cell level, leading to papillomas or transitional cell carcinomas of the pelvis, ureter, or bladder.

Recent emphasis has been on the levels of kidney lipid peroxidation after the administration of chemicals with carcinogenic potential. High levels were associated with more nephrotoxicity, the appearance of eosinophilic bodies in renal tubular cells, and the development of neoplasms. Cysteine or glutathione pretreatment was protective, whereas diethyl maleate resulted in exacerbation of the effects of lipid peroxidation (511).

Effects on Humans

It is difficult to substantiate the effect of environmental pollution on humans because of the complex interaction of a large number of factors, including the nature and magnitude of pollution, duration and continuity of exposure, individual susceptibilities, associated diseases, and drug intake. Inherent differences in body size, normal life span, metabolic pathways, defense mechanisms, and other factors make it impossible to extrapolate experimental observations to humans. Accordingly, the whole concept of renal disease due to environmental pollution remains disputable, although not necessarily unimportant, particularly in tropical countries where the international standards of air and water pollution and the acceptable qualities and quantities of food additives and contaminants are not stringently respected.

Specific Issues in Tropical Environmental Pollution

Exposure to Smoke, Dust, and Fumes

The relationship between tobacco smoking and bladder cancer is well established (512,513) (Chapter 29, Bladder Cancer). This problem is particularly relevant in tropical countries because of the lack of adequate control measures (514) and public education.

Compared with the rest of the world, the major cities in tropical countries have the highest levels of pollution from car, motorcycle, and other engine exhausts. There is unequivocal evidence that the combustion products of diesel fuel and unleaded gasoline (515), like other petroleum-derived jet fuels (516), are nephrotoxic to adult male rats, being mediated by α_{2u}-globulin. Other hydrocarbons such as paint, mineral

spirit, and aromatic solvents (517) have the same nephrotoxic potential.

It is uncertain whether human immunity, conferred by the low α_{2u}-globulin profile, against hydrocarbon-induced renal injury is absolute, even in the face of continuous exposure over many decades. It is noteworthy that lead nephropathy is an independent risk in most tropical countries where commonly used gasoline is not unleaded.

Exposure to lead is also carcinogenic, as suggested by a rat model (518) and by observations of an exposed human cohort (519).

Chronic exposure to cadmium (520) and asbestos (521), which in addition to industrial intoxication are often ingested with contaminated water or inhaled with dust, also carries a high risk for renal cell carcinoma.

Exposure to Food Additives

Many artificial flavors, colors, thickening substances, solvents, and even wrapping material to which humans are extensively exposed have documented nephrotoxic effects in experimental animals.

Toxic tubulointerstitial lesions have been associated with the administration of carotenes, used as artificial colors (522), and β-cyclodextrin, used as a flavor, color, and vitamin carrier and stabilizer and also in the decaffeination of coffee and tea and in reducing the cholesterol content of eggs (523,524). These lesions have also been reported with exposure to extraction solvents such as 1,2-dichloroethane (525), dichloromethane (526), α-methyl-benzyl alcohol (527), and diethylene glycol monoethyl ether (528).

Although no clinical nephrotoxicity has been attributed to most of these agents, acute renal failure was reported to complicate the accidental ingestion of large quantities of 1,2-dichloroethane (525), or inhalation of dichloromethane (529). Mild azotemia complicated acute intoxication with diethylene glycol monoethyl ether (530).

Protein droplet nephropathy has been associated with exposure of adult male rats to the flavoring agent limonene, used in beverages, chewing gum, candy, ice cream, gelatins, and puddings (531). Humans seem to be resistant to this type of nephrotoxicity because of the very small amounts of α_{2u}-globulin that they can produce (532).

Renal adenomas and *adenocarcinomas* have been induced in rats (533) and hamsters (534) by long-term ingestion of potassium bromide, which is often used as a flour-treatment agent. Accidental or suicidal administration in humans may be associated with acute renal failure, tubulointerstitial nephritis, interstitial fibrosis, and glomerulosclerosis (535).

Urothelial malignancy in the renal pelvis and urinary bladder has also been documented in experimental models. Of particular interest are the artificial sweeteners, most notoriously saccharin, which at high dietary concentrations of 5% or more induced bladder tumors in male rats (536). The relation between saccharin and bladder cancer in humans rests on soft evidence (537). Recent data, including a large postmortem study based on the examination of 6,503 sections obtained from 282 deceased patients (538) and a meta-analysis of 15 case-control studies (539), do not substantiate this relation in humans.

Exposure to Food Contaminants

Certain substances produced during food preparation or preservation have a nephrotoxic effect on experimental animals. Typical lesions were induced in rats by chloropropanols, which are produced during the preservation of vegetables (540–542). No human disease has been attributed to these contaminants.

Exogenous contaminants are more relevant to the question of human nephrotoxicity in the Tropics, where agriculture remains the predominant occupation. These include mycotoxins, pesticides, and veterinary drug residues.

Mycotoxins are discussed elsewhere in this and in other chapters, where reference is made to ochratoxin-associated interstitial renal disease and aflatoxin-associated neoplasias.

Pesticides are ingested with drinking water, plants, fish, poultry, and meat. Adequate control is beyond the capacity of most tropical countries, because of problems with analytical methodology, standardization, and so on. Large amounts, therefore, may be inevitably ingested by tropical inhabitants for lifelong periods.

Most pesticides are organophosphates; their main toxicity is on the red cells, thyroid gland, and nervous system. Weight loss, anemia, hepatic adenomas, esophageal and other gastrointestinal tract tumors, skin allergy, and teratogenicity are the principal toxic manifestations. There is some experimental evidence of toxicity to the liver and kidney (543), but no clinically significant renal disease has been ascribed to pesticides.

Veterinary drug residues constitute an important source of pollution in an agricultural environment where close contact between humans and animals is inevitable. These residues are ingested with vegetables, fruits, and meat. Some residues, including certain anthelmintics, antimicrobial agents, and production aids, are nephrotoxic to experimental animals.

The broad-spectrum anthelmintic tiabendazole induces tubular degeneration and hyperplasia in the short term in mice (544). However, nephrotoxicity was not observed in a 24-week study in humans (545).

Spiramycin, a macrolide antibiotic used for the treatment of bacterial and mycoplasmal infections in animals, causes "considerable kidney damage," particularly in the loops of Henle, and necrotic changes in several areas of the renal parenchyma in dogs (546). However, administration of this drug to human volunteers caused only mild gastrointestinal disturbances (547).

Ractopamine is a phenolethanolamine α-adrenergic agonist that increases weight, leanness, and feed efficiency in pigs. It causes a transient elevation of systolic blood pressure

in short-term studies in humans (548). Long-term follow-up studies are awaited.

END-STAGE RENAL DISEASE IN TROPICAL COUNTRIES

Prevalence

ESRD is highly prevalent in the Tropics, compared with Europe, although it matches with data on the United States (549), particularly among African and Native Americans (550,551). The reported figures range between 80 and 96 cases per million in Southeast Asia (362,552,553), 70 to 110 per million in Saudi Arabia (553,554), at least 120 per million in India (556), and 89 to 192 per million in Africa (508,557–560) and Latin America (561,562).

Glomerulonephritis remains the major cause of ESRD in the most economically underprivileged tropical countries such as Ethiopia (58.4%) (563), Bangladesh (47% to 54%) (506,564), and Sudan (36%) (507). Its impact is much less prominent in other tropical countries (505,508,554,565). Proliferative glomerulonephritis constitutes the major primary etiologic factor leading to ESRD. This is mainly attributed to bacterial, viral, and parasitic infections. The prevalence of certain types such as IgA and IgM nephropathies is strikingly different in various tropical regions, being quite rare in Africa (566,567) but is remarkably common in Australasia (565).

With increasing industrialization, chronic interstitial nephritis emerges as a prominent cause of ESRD in the Tropics (504,505). The role of environmental pollution in this trend remains questionable (206).

The reported contribution of diabetes is variable, usually ranging between 4.3% and 14.0% (505,563,568). However, the contribution of diabetic nephropathy is increasing in several tropical countries, reaching as high as 20% in Hong Kong (565), 24% in Bangladesh (506), and 26.8% in India (505).

The role of hypertensive nephrosclerosis is also variable, between 1.8% and 19.6%, probably depending on the definitions adopted. Polycystic disease is rare (1.9% to 4.5%). Other causes of chronic renal failure are even less frequent.

Clinical Patterns

The usual clinical syndrome of ESRD is modified in the Tropics by three factors: (a) associated manifestations of the primary disease, (b) manifestations of concomitant disorders, and (c) late diagnosis and poor management.

Associated Manifestations of the Primary Disease

As described earlier in this chapter, renal disease in the Tropics is often secondary to an endemic infection, is attributed to environmental pollution, or is caused by a drug or traditional medication. The associated features of the primary etiology frequently modify the clinical picture of ESRD.

Examples include the concomitant hepatic disease in schistosomal glomerulopathy; severe hypertension, arthropathy, and polyneuropathy with chronic exposure to lead; and persistent hyperkalemia with certain herbal intoxications.

Manifestations of Concomitant Disorders

Many patients have a concomitant illness, the features of which may overlap with or modify those of conventional ESRD. Such disorders reflect the general health status of the community, often dominated by endemic infections and infestations, malnutrition, and certain malignancies.

Endemic Infections and Infestations

Acute and chronic bacterial infections often complicate renal disease in the Tropics. In addition to those causing renal disease (vide supra) and those acquired during dialysis (vide infra), certain infectious agents may have an independent impact. One of the most outstanding infections is tuberculosis, which is encountered in 4.1% to 11.5% of the Saudi Arabian population on hemodialysis (569), Gulf countries (570), India (571,572), Bangladesh (506), and Indonesia (573). Tuberculous peritonitis has been reported in patients on chronic ambulatory peritoneal dialysis, in whom it poses notorious diagnostic difficulties (574). Evidence of previous *Salmonella* infection was detected in 42% of patients on regular hemodialysis in Egypt (575). Recent *Salmonella* infection–induced acute graft rejections in renal transplant recipients (576). The list includes many other infections, the most common being scabies, HBV, HCV, HIV infection (vide infra), and intestinal parasitic infections (206). In addition to imposing their specific symptomatology, these infections generally tend to induce a catabolic state that augments such uremic manifestations as asthenia, anemia, and bone disease.

Malnutrition

Protein-energy malnutrition is often a major problem in dealing with renal disease in the Tropics. This may be attributed to starvation, catabolic disorders, or physicians' instructions. It is unfortunate that general practitioners are still advising their patients to restrict protein intake to exceedingly low levels. Even nephrologists maintain this trend in patients on dialysis, as shown in a meta-analysis of recent European Dialysis and Transplant Association (EDTA) data (577), where 73.5% of uremic patients in developing countries were instructed to receive a daily protein intake of less than 0.6 g/kg, compared with 31.3% in western Europe.

Specific nutritional deficiencies of iron, calcium, Vitamin D, vitamins, and trace elements are also frequently encountered. The effects of these on anemia, bone, and peripheral nerve disease are obvious.

Malignancies

Infection-related malignancies are notoriously common in the Tropics. Examples include Burkitt's lymphoma and Kaposi's sarcoma (578). These often become a significant epidemiologic risk in immunocompromised patients.

Late Diagnosis and Poor Management

Owing to the prevailing standards of medical care, renal disease may not be suspected, may be neglected, or may be poorly managed for a long time before adequate nephrologic care is provided (568). Advanced uremic manifestations, of almost historic interest according to present-day Western standards, remain fairly common in the tropical glossary. It is not unusual to see a patient with extensive uremic frost on his or her cheeks or finger creases, or with multiple soft tissue swellings of metastatic calcification, or another crippled with bone deformities or motor polyneuropathy. Many patients are first seen in coma, in convulsions, or with a hematocrit level of 8% to 10%. The clinical picture is often further complicated by the use of medications without any dose adjustment in consideration of residual renal function.

Dialysis in the Tropics

Availability

Acute Dialysis

Hemodialysis is available for the management of acute renal failure in most of the major hospitals in the Tropics, even in those countries with the lowest GNPs (507,508,563,579–581). The efficiency of such units is widely variable, ultimately depending on socioeconomic development. For obvious reasons, acute peritoneal dialysis is more widely used. It is often implemented where limited or no specialized nephrologic care is available, at least as a first line of therapy. Unfortunately, the prevailing hygienic conditions in many tropical hospitals yield a high incidence of peritonitis.

Chronic Dialysis

The number of patients treated by chronic dialysis in the Tropics cannot be precisely defined, because of the scarcity of reliable registries. Data generated from sporadic publications (which are, unfortunately, mostly found in the nonindexed local literature), national registries (by personal communication with colleagues in charge), or supranational registries (African, Arabian, Latin American, and Asian Pacific registries) suggest that the chronic dialysis activity in the Tropics is fairly extensive. The chronic dialysis pools vary from less than 5 per million population in certain countries as Sudan (559), Tanzania (508), Ethiopia (563), Uganda (579), Nigeria (580), Ghana (581), and Bangladesh (582) to the 40 to 80 per million range in Thailand (553) and Algeria (560), 120 to 160 per million in Brazil (562), Argentina, Mexico (583),

Egypt (247), and Saudi Arabia (555), and to more than 300 per million in Singapore (584).

The Dialysis Environment

The Patient

Young adults in their 20s or early 30s constitute 70% to 80% of the dialysis population in the Tropics (556,557,584), which is attributed to the nature of the prevailing primary diseases. There is a male preponderance, partly explained by cultural factors and possibly the increased exposure to noxious environmental factors (vide supra). Most patients are poor and uneducated, which has a negative effect on the outcome of dialysis treatment because their health is poor to begin with (vide supra) and they do not adequately comply to the regularity of dialysis, diet, intake of medications, and rehabilitation. This inadequate compliance is often attributed to improper patient information, but the lack of motivation and financial shortcomings usually have a significant influence.

Medical Staff

Shortage of adequately trained medical and paramedical local staff is the rule in most tropical countries. In some of the better-off nations, the teams often include expatriates in key positions. When this is unaffordable, unqualified teams may take over. Several developing nations have their own training programs that generate nephrologists and dialysis specialists, technicians, and nurses. In-service training programs are already functional in a few countries, and successful regional conferences and postgraduate teaching courses have been conducted during the past decade.

Dialysis Units

The reported number of dialysis units varies, in different tropical countries, from less than 1 to 5 per million population (247,362,556,559,562). When detailed figures are compared with the respective numbers of patients actually receiving regular dialysis, it can be appreciated that the units are not kept sufficiently busy. The reasons for nonfunctional equipment are many and include lack of personnel, shortage of funds, poor maintenance, and inefficient organization.

Most units are located in hospitals, with a few satellite units in the better-developed countries. State-sponsored, insurance-sponsored, and private units are available in most countries, in proportions that differ according to the political systems and GNPs. Excellent state-sponsored units comprise most dialysis units in the economically better-off countries (544). However, the standard of service in state-sponsored units in most tropical countries with low GNPs is modest, which invites active participation of the private sector. Political system permitting, as in India, Egypt, Brazil, and most of Southeast Asia, private units tend to take the technical lead. Governments generally provide partial reimbursement for private dialysis in these countries. Insurance-sponsored units are also growing where health insurance systems are strong enough to support the cost.

Standard equipment is the rule, including nonvolumetric hemodialysis machines, acetate-based dialysate, cuprophane membrane hollow fibers, and so on. Peritoneal dialysis fluid is often locally manufactured, although at a very high cost (vide infra). A few units accept children and older adults, but almost none is specialized in pediatric or geriatric dialysis.

Chronic Dialysis Modalities

Hemodialysis is the predominant dialysis modality in most tropical countries, constituting 80% to 90% of the population on dialysis (562,585). In countries with the lowest GNPs, however, intermittent peritoneal dialysis (IPD) is the inevitable alternative (559,563,580). The implementation of continuous ambulatory peritoneal dialysis (CAPD) is widely variable, from sporadic experiences (586–588) to a national policy (Mexico, 90% [583]; Hong Kong, 70% [552]; Thailand, 40% [553]). Most other countries refrain from using CAPD because of the high cost (vide infra), high incidence of infection, and poor patient compliance. Accordingly, CAPD is offered only as a second choice to selected patients of the higher social classes.

IPD is still used for high-risk patients such as those with severe ischemic heart disease or complicated diabetes. On the whole, it accounts for at least 60% of all chronic peritoneal dialysis treatments in the developing world, compared with 2.7% in western Europe (577). Because adequate K_t/V can only be achieved by an impossible number of dialysis hours, IPD is associated with an extremely poor median survival time, 1 year, and modest quality of life (248,559,580). Although IPD is usually carried out in hospitals, the incidence of infection remains quite high.

The Cost of Regular Dialysis

Calculating dialysis costs is a difficult and complex procedure. Besides the direct costs including the prices of consumable items, overhead expenses, salaries, and fees, one must include the costs of interdialytic therapy, transfusions, hospital admissions, transportation, and so on. In even broader terms, one should also consider the days missed from work and the reduced productivity of some patients.

The items of typical annual direct dialysis cost per capita in a developing country (247) are essentially the same, with the differences being mainly influenced by the proportion of imported versus locally manufactured materials and by the prevailing standards of salaries and professional fees, which vary from 10% to 35% of the total cost (237,555).

Peritoneal dialysis is generally the most expensive modality of ESRD therapy in most tropical countries, even when locally manufactured solutions are used. This is attributed to the extremely high overhead expenses entailed in small-scale production lines. On the other hand, dialyzer reuse in many centers is often responsible for effectively reducing the comparative cost of hemodialysis.

Results and Limitations of Dialysis Treatment

The reported annual mortality rate after the first year for all dialysis modalities, for all ages, and irrespective of the primary renal disease in different tropical countries varies from 15% to 35%. The first-year mortality rate is about 25% to 45% higher. When considered separately, the mortality rate for IPD is much higher, whereas CAPD has yielded impressive results in certain series (588,589). There is a remarkable "center effect," in favor of economically privileged units that can afford recruiting better equipment and staff and that tend to a higher social class of patients (248).

Attention to the quality of life (248,566,590) is proportionate to individual nation's GNPs. In the poorer countries, which constitute the majority in the tropical zone, this issue is not even raised. Patients are often contented just being alive, even though they are disabled. The incidence of complications is quite high, mainly because of inadequate dialysis, poor water quality, undernutrition, dialysis-acquired infections, and deficient interdialytic care.

Dialysis-acquired infections are extremely common, mainly including the hepatitis viruses and cytomegalovirus. The prevalence of HIV infection is also high in endemic areas (591); further reports on its rate and epidemiologic and clinical sequelae in the dialysis population are awaited. HBV infection, with a prevalence approaching 90% among dialysis patients in certain countries a decade ago (592), has now considerably regressed to a rate of less than 40% in most tropical countries (591) and even to less than 7% in others (237,577). This decline is at least partly attributed to vaccination of the populations at risk. Unfortunately, HBV infection has been largely replaced by infection with HCV, antibodies to which have been reported in 24.3% to about 72% of populations from different tropical countries; the latter figure is the usual mode (593–598). Although the significance of HCV antibody detection remains unsettled, the available data from quite a few countries tend to support the presence of actual viremia, as shown by positive polymerase chain reactions, and concomitant hepatocellular injury, as shown by remittent elevation of the hepatic transaminases. Nevertheless, clinically significant chronic liver disease is apparently not alarming.

Cytomegalovirus infection is often overlooked in the population on dialysis, despite a prevalence amounting to 74% (575). This infection may lead to dialysis-associated rigors or pyrexia, yet its main importance lies in the potential risk that it imposes on the outcome of subsequent transplantation.

Similar implications seem to hold true for *Salmonella* infection, evidence of exposure to which has been detected in the pretransplantation assessment of as many as 42% of patients (575).

As a general rule, interdialytic medical care is extremely modest in tropical countries. Even such basic goals as blood pressure control, correction of anemia, and maintenance of the calcium and acid–base balance are often overlooked. Access to active Vitamin D and erythropoietin is a matter of affordability. In 1991, 7.9% of patients on hemodialysis and 2.9% of those on peritoneal dialysis in the seven developing countries (mostly tropical) reporting to the EDTA registry were treated with EPO, compared with 38.9% in western Europe. The subsequent need for multiple transfusions obviously facilitates the spread of dialysis-associated viral infections.

Renal Transplantation in the Tropics

Availability

Renal transplantation is widely available in many tropical countries. The precise data about different countries obtained from local, supranational, or different international registries are a bit controversial. The number of transplantations per million population ranges from less than 1 to more than 100 (553,585,599,600).

The Transplantation Environment

Renal transplantation activity in the Tropics follows two patterns: cadaver organ and living donor based. The major factor that determines this differentiation is cultural and depends on whether prevailing religions and heritage accept the concepts of brain death, removal of organs from the dead, and transplanting them into strangers.

Cadaver Organ–Based Programs

Such programs are currently running in South Africa, Southeast Asia, Latin America, and Saudi Arabia. Adequate legislation is established in those countries, even to the level of presumed consent in some (601). Despite earlier difficulties in harvesting and transporting donor kidneys, most of these programs are prosperous, expanding, and progressively limiting the growth of the dialysis pools. Recipients are generally selected according to standard rules and put on waiting lists with waiting times varying between 1 and 6 months.

Living Donor–Based Programs

In those countries where the law does not permit cadaver organ donation, transplantation of live donor organs is carried out instead. In almost all instances, such programs started with live-related donors, but soon unrelated donors were also accepted to a greater or lesser extent under different names and for different reasons. The social and moral reflections of this practice are discussed later in this chapter.

Recipients are those who can locate suitable donors. In some countries, they also have to get official permission to do so (575). Donors are either related or paid, the paid ones being usually men, in their third decade of life, educated to a medium level, unemployed or holding menial jobs, and depressed and in desperate need (602).

Transplantation Centers

Most transplantations are performed in general hospitals. There are virtually no independently standing specialized transplant centers. As with the dialysis activity and according to the same rules (vide supra), private transplantation teams share in providing the service in living donor–based programs.

The hygienic standards are variable. In some areas, they are far below average and are responsible for high postoperative morbidity and mortality rates, as well as for the transmission of infections such as AIDS, hepatitis, malaria, and others.

The Cost of Transplantation

The ultimate burden of renal transplantation on a national economy is less than that of dialysis. Despite the high initial expenses, and the cost of expensive medications such as cyclosporine and monoclonal antibodies, the ultimate analysis shows that transplantation is both cheaper and more cost effective. A local study in which cumulative survival rates were taken into consideration estimated that the annual steady-state budget for accepting 100 new patients for dialysis would be around $7.5 million U.S. dollars, compared with $6.2 million U.S. dollars for transplantation. The median survival times would be 2.0 and 7.1 years, respectively (603) (Fig. 79-19).

Results and Limitations of Renal Transplantation

Data obtained from national registries suggest that the outcome of renal transplantation in tropical countries is in accordance with international standards. However, it is presumable that most transplantations are not registered at all, because, for example, some countries do not have registries. It is therefore impossible to know the precise outcome of those thousands of grafts transplanted in patients in tropical countries.

However, the published sporadic data suggest that the recipient morbidity and mortality rates are relatively high, mainly due to postoperative wound and systemic infections. The latter include activation of dormant disease as well as *de novo* infections. Notorious for the Tropics are such infections as tuberculosis, salmonellosis, certain parasitic infections (vide supra), and others. As outlined earlier, the high incidence of certain malignancies such as Kaposi's sarcoma and Burkitt's lymphoma also accounts for the increased recipient mortality rate.

Socioeconomic Impact

ESRD is imposing a distinct socioeconomic strain on the economy, social integrity, and even morals of tropical communities at large. The financial burden in certain countries seems impossible to meet, whether by individuals or by the state. It is important to know that the cost of keeping one patient alive but partially rehabilitated on dialysis may literally exceed the average GNP generated by ten citizens (604). Yet, it is also important to realize the facts about the expenditures made by the same countries on such issues as political security, cigarette imports, and the purchase of weapons.

The meager social security services in most tropical countries usually leave the patients all by themselves, facing their physical disability, financial shortage, and a shaken position within family and community. In those countries in which the prevailing cultures do not permit using cadaver organs for transplantation even though the technical know-how is sufficiently developed, the practice of living unrelated donor transplantation became inevitable. In some places, selling kidneys subsequently emerged as an established trade, with all kinds of commercial dynamics including price negotiations, auctions, dealers, and commissions (605). Some countries have passed legislation against unrelated living donor kidney transplantation (576).

A few tropical countries (584,601) have established independent national kidney foundations that take care of the

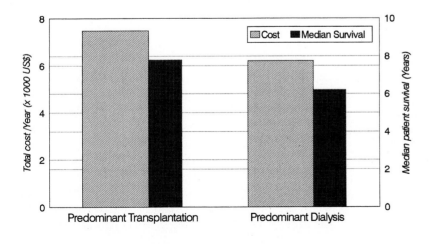

FIG. 79-19. Estimated average annual cost of treatment and respective median survival times in two hypothetical models of end-stage renal disease treatment strategies, predominant dialysis vs. predominant transplantation in a developing country. (See text for hypothesis and explanation.)

organization and funding of ESRD therapy, promote research and development, and support staff training. This positive trend has gained success in some tropical countries.

REFERENCES

1. *The World Bank Atlas.* International Bank for Reconstruction and Development/The World Bank. December 1993. ISBN 0 8213 1649 4. THE WORLD BANK ISBN 8213:1649 1993.
2. Hall JW, Johnson WJ, Maher FT, et al. Immediate and long-term prognosis in acute renal failure. *Ann Intern Med* 1970;73:515.
3. Kennedy AC, Burton JA, Luke RG, et al. Factors affecting the prognosis in acute renal failure. *Q J Med* 1973;42:73.
4. Adu D, Anim-Addo Y, Foli AK, et al. Acute renal failure in tropical Africa. *Br Med J* 1976;1:890.
5. Chugh KS, Singhal PC, Nath IV, et al. Spectrum of acute renal failure in North India. *J Assoc Physicians India* 1978;26:147.
6. El Reshaid K, Kapoor M, Johny KV, et al. Acute renal failure in Kuwait—a prospective study. *J Trop Med Hyg* 1993;96:323.
7. Ku G, Lim CH, Pwee HS, et al. Review of renal failure. *Ann Acad Med Singapore* 1975;4:115.
8. Sitprija V, Benyajati C. Tropical diseases and acute renal failure. *Ann Acad Med Singapore* 1975;4[Suppl]:112.
9. Seedat YK. Acute renal failure among Blacks and Indians in South Africa. *S Afr Med J* 1978;54:427.
10. Chugh KS, Sakhuja V, Malhotra HS, et al. Changing trends in acute renal failure in third world countries. Chandigarh Study. *Q J Med* 1989;73:1117.
11. Seedat YK, Nathoo BC. Acute renal failure in Blacks and Indians in South Africa. Comparison after 10 years. *Nephron* 1993;64:198.
12. Chugh KS, Singhal PC, Sharma BK, et al. Acute renal failure of obstetric origin. *Obstet Gynaecol* 1976;48:642.
13. Smith K, Browne JCM, Shackman R, et al. Renal failure of obstetric origin. *Lancet* 1965;2:351.
14. Kleinknect D, Grunfeld JP, Gomez PC, et al. Diagnostic procedure and long term prognosis in bilateral renal cortical necrosis. *Kidney Int* 1973;4:390.
15. Jha V, Malhotra HS, Sakhuja V, et al. Spectrum of hospital acquired acute renal failure in the developing countries. Chandigarh Study. *Q J Med* 1992;84:497.
16. Sitprija V. Acute renal failure in the Tropics. In: Husain I, ed. *Tropical urology.* London: Churchill Livingstone, 1987:48.
17. Cameron JS. The natural history of glomerulonephritis. In: Kincaid-Smith P, d'Apices AJF, Atkins RC, eds. *Progress in glomerulonephritis (perspectives in nephrology and hypertension series).* New York: Wiley, 1979:1.
18. The nephrotic syndrome in the Tropics [Editorial]. *Lancet* 1980; 2:461.
19. Kibukamusoke JW, Hutt MSR, Wilks NE. The nephrotic syndrome in Uganda and its association with quartan malaria. *Q J Med* 1967; 36:393.
20. Seedat YK. Nephrotic syndrome in the Africans and Indians of South Africa: a ten year study. *Trans R Soc Trop Med Hyg* 1978;72:506.
21. Powell KC, Meadows R. The nephrotic syndrome in New Guinea. A clinical and histological spectrum. *Aust N Z J Med* 1971;1:363.
22. Hendrickse RG. Epidemiology and prevention of kidney disease in Africa. *Trans R Soc Trop Med Hyg* 1980;74:8.
23. Barsoum RS. Schistosomal glomerulopathy, selection factors. *Nephrol Dial Transplant* 1987;2:488.
24. Seedat YK, Parag KB, Nathoo BC, et al. Glomerulonephritis in South Africa. *Proceedings of International Symposium on Geographical Nephrology.* Bangkok, 1990:99.
25. Powell KC, Meadows R, Anders R, et al. The nephrotic syndrome in Papua New Guinea: aetiological, pathological and immunological findings. *Aust NZJ Med* 1977;7:243.
26. Pesce AJ, First MR. Proteinuria: an Integrated Review. In: Cameron JS, Glassock RJ, eds. *Kidney disease series.* New York: Marcel Dekker Inc, 1979:131.
27. Sud A, Bhuyan UN, Tandon HD. Spectrum of morphological lesions in renal biopsies associated with primary nephrotic syndrome. *Ind J Med Res* 1978;68:811.
28. Sadiq S, Jafarey NA, Naqvi SAJ. An analysis of percutaneous renal biopsies in fifty cases of nephrotic syndrome. *J Pakistan Med Assoc* 1978;28:121.
29. Boonpucknavig V, Boonpucknavig S. Glomerulonephritis: pathogenesis, pathology and incidence in Thailand. *Ramathibodi Med J* 1982;5;5:16.
30. Sidabutar RP, Lumenta NA, Suharjono, et al. Glomerulonephritis in Indonesia. *Proc 3rd Asian Pacific Congress Nephrol.* Singapore, 1986:282.
31. Sinniah R. The pathology of IgA nephropathy. In: Clarkson AJ, ed. *IgA nephropathy.* Boston: Martinus Nijhoff, 1987:66.
32. Woo KT, Edmonson RPS, Wu AYT, et al. Clinical and prognostic indices in IgA nephritis. *Proceedings of the 3rd Asian Pacific Congress of Nephrology.* Singapore, 1986:119.
33. Seedat Y, Nathoo BC, Parag KB, et al. IgA nephropathy in Blacks and Indians of *Napal Nephron* 1988;50:137.
34. Queiroz FB, Brito E, Martinelli R. Influence of regional factors in the distribution of the histologic patterns of glomerulonephritis in the nephrotic syndrome. *Nephron* 1975;14:466.
35. Morgan AG, Shah DJ, Williams W, et al. Proteinuria and glomerular disease in Jamaica. *Clin Nephrol* 1984;21:205.
36. Seggie J, Davis PG, Ninin D, et al. Pattern of glomerulonephritis in Zimbabwe. Survey of disease characterized by nephrotic proteinuria. *Q J Med* 1984;53:104.
37. Coovadia HM, Adhikan MA, Morel Maroger L. Clinico pathological features of nephrotic syndrome in South African children. *Kidney Int* 1979;16:86.
38. Adu D, Anim-Addo Y, Foll AK, et al. The nephrotic syndrome in Ghana: clinical and pathological aspect. *Q J Med* 1981;50:297.
39. Kung'u A, Sitati SM. Glomerulonephropathies in Kenya. A histopathological study. *East Afr Med J* 1980;57:525.
40. Sitprija V, Boonpucknavig V. Tropical diseases and glomerulonephritis. *Proceedings of the 3rd Asian Pacific Congress of Nephrol.* Singapore, 1986:262.
41. Barnett HL. The natural and treatment history of glomerular diseases in children. What can we learn from international cooperative studies? *Proc 6th Int Congress Nephrol.* Florence, 1975:470.
42. Chugh KS, Jain S, Sakhuja V et al. Renovascular hypertension due to Takayasu's arteritis among Indian patients. *Q J Med* 1992;85:307.
43. Thenabadu PN, Rajasuriya K, Wickremasinghe HR. Nonspecific arteritis of the aorta and its main branches. *Br Heart J* 1979;32:181.
44. Teoh PC, Tan LK, Chia BL, et al. Nonspecific aortoarteritis in Singapore with specific reference to hypertension. *Am Heart J* 1978;95:683.
45. Vinijchaikul K. Primary arteritis of the aorta and its main branches. *Am J Med* 1967;43:15.
46. Dong Z, Li S, Lu X. Percutaneous transluminal angioplasty for renovascular hypertension in arteritis: experience in China. *Radiology* 1987;62:477.
47. Ishikawa KL. Natural history and classification of occlusive thromboaortopathy. *Circulation* 1978;57:27.
48. El-Reshaid K, Johny KV, Sugathan TN, et al. Epidemiological profile of end stage renal disease (ESRD) in Kuwait. *Saudi Kidney Dis Transplant Bull* 1993;4:82(abst).
49. Sitprija V. The kidney in acute tropical disease. In: Kibukamusoke JW, ed. *Tropical nephrology.* Canberra: Citforge Pty Ltd, 1984:48.
50. Chugh KS, Sakhuja V. Glomerular disease in the Tropics. *Am J Nephrol* 1990;10:437.
51. Condrea E. Hemolytic effects of snake venoms. In: Lee CY, ed. *Snake venoms.* Berlin: Springer, 1979:448.
52. Miller KD, White NJ, Lott JA, et al. Biochemical evidence of muscle injury in African children with severe malaria. *J Infect Dis* 1989;159:139.
53. Chusil S, Kasantikul V, Sitprija V. Subclinical rhabdomyolysis in tropical acute renal failure. *3rd Asian Pacific Congress Nephrol.* Singapore, 1986:60.
54. Choovichian P, Luvira U, Moolla-or P, et al. Renal function in acute febrile disease. *Int Med* 1988;4:105.
55. Seguro AC, Lomar AV, Rocha AS. Acute renal failure of leptospirosis: nonoliguric and hypokalemic form. *Nephron* 1990;55:146.
56. Mairiang P, Bhudhisawasdi V, Borirakchanyavat V, et al. Acute renal failure in obstructive jaundice in cholangiocarcinoma. *Arch Intern Med* 1990;150:2357.
57. Boyce BF, Yates AJ, Mundy GR. Bolus injection of recombinant human interleukin 1 causes transient hypocalcemic in normal mice. *Endocrinology* 1989;125:2780.

58. Zager RA. Temperature effects on ischemic and hypoxic renal proximal tubular injury. *Lab Invest* 1991;64:766.

59. Sitprija V. Nephrology forum: nephropathy in falciparum malaria. *Kidney Int* 1988;34:867.

60. Roitt I, Brostoff J, Male D. Immunity to protozoa and worms. In: Roitt IM, Brostoff J, Male DK, eds. *Immunology*. Edinburgh: Churchill Livingstone, 1985.

61. Bone RC. The pathogenesis of sepsis. *Ann Intern Med* 1991;115:4574.

62. Fauve RM. Inflammation and natural immunity. In: Fougereau M, Dausett J, eds. *Progress in immunology*. London: Academic Press, 1980:737.

63. Quezado ZMN, Natanson C. Systemic hemodynamic abnormalities and vasopressor therapy in sepsis and septic shock. *Am J Kidney Dis* 1992;20:214.

64. Sarrel PM, Lindsay DC, Poole-Wilson PA, et al. Hypothesis: inhibition of endothelium-derived relaxing factor by haemoglobin in the pathogenesis of pre-eclampsia. *Lancet* 1990;336:1030.

65. Zager RA. Myoglobin depletes renal adenine nucleotide pools in the presence and absence of shock. *Kidney Int* 1991;39:111.

66. Mahasandana S, Rungruxsirivon V, Chantarankul V. Clinical manifestations of bleeding following Russell's viper and green pit viper bites in adult. *S Asian J Trop Med Public Health* 1980;11:285.

67. Sitprija V, Kashemsant U, Sriratanaban A, et al. Renal function in obstructive jaundice in man: Cholangiocarcinoma model. *Kidney Int* 1990;38:948.

68. Lumlertgul D, Boonyaprapa S, Bunnachak D, et al. The jaundiced heart: evidence of blunted response to positive inotropic stimulation. *Renal Fail* 1991;13:15.

69. Sitprija V, Boonpucknavig V. Renal involvement in parasitic diseases. In: Tisher CC, Brenner BM, eds. *Renal pathology*. Philadelphia: Lippincott, 1989:575.

70. Sitprija V. Renal involvement in leptospirosis. In: Robinson RR, ed. *Tropical nephrology*. New York: Springer-Verlag New York, 1984:1041.

71. Chugh K. Nephrology forum: snake bite induced acute renal failure in India. *Kidney Int* 1989;35:891.

72. Sitprija V, Boonpucknavig V. Glomerular changes in tropical viper bite in man. *Toxicology* 1983;21:401.

73. Chaiyabutr N, Sitprija V, Sugino N, et al. Russell's viper venom–induced depolarization in the proximal tubule of triturus kidney. *ICMR Ann* 1985;5:181.

74. Gulati PD, Saxena SN, Gupta PS, et al. Changing patterns of typhoid fever. *Am J Med* 1968;45:544.

75. Nasrallah SM, Nassar VH. Enteric fever, a clinicopathologic study of 104 cases. *Am J Gastroenterol* 1978;69:63.

76. Samantray SK, Johnson SC, Chakrabarti AK. Enteric fever: an analysis of 500 cases. *Practitioner* 1977;2:400.

77. Khajehdehi P, Rastegar A, Kharazmi A. Immunological and clinical aspects of kidney disease in typhoid fever in Iran. *Q J Med* 1984;53:209.

78. Amerio A, Campese VM, Coratelli P, et al. Glomerulonephritis in typhoid fever. *Proc 5th Int Congress Nephrol*. 1972;316:62(abst).

79. Bouka I, Coovadia HM. Typhoid glomerulonephritis. *Br Med J (Clin Res)* 1970;2:710.

80. Choudhry VP, Srivastava RN, Vellodi A, et al. A study of acute renal failure. *Indian Pediatr* 1980;17:405.

81. Faierman D, Ross FA, Seckler SG. Typhoid fever complicated by hepatitis, nephritis and thrombocytopenia. *JAMA* 1972;221:60.

82. Sitprija V, Pipatanagul V, Boonpucknavig V, et al. Glomerulitis in typhoid fever. *Ann Intern Med* 1974;81:210.

83. Indraprasit S, Boonpucknavig V, Boonpucknavig S. IgA nephropathy associated with enteric fever. *Nephron* 1985;40:219.

84. Alarcon-Segovia D, Alcocer JC. Immunocomplex in typhoid fever. *Ann Intern Med* 1975;82:720.

85. Kontos HA, Wei EP, Povli shock JT, et al. Cerebral arteriolar damage by arachidonic acid and prostaglandin G$_2$. *Science* 1980;209:1242.

86. Shubart AF, Hornick RB, Ewald RW, et al. Changes of serum complement and properdin levels in experimental typhoid fever. *J Immunol* 93:387 1964;.

87. Baker NM, Mills AE, Rachman I, et al. Hemolytic-uremic syndrome in typhoid fever. *Br Med J (Clin Res)* 1974;2:84.

88. Glover SC, Smith CC, Porter IA. Fatal *Salmonella* septicaemia with disseminated intravascular coagulation and renal failure. *J Med Microbiol* 1982;15:117.

89. Lwanga D, Wing AJ. Renal complications associated with typhoid fever. *East Afr Med J* 1970;47:146.

90. Rheingold OJ, Greenwald RA, Hayas PJ, et al. Myoglobinuria and renal failure associated with typhoid fever. *JAMA* 1977;238:341.

91. Farid Z, Bassily S, Kent DC, et al. Chronic urinary Salmonella carriers with intermittent bacteremia. *J Trop Med Hyg* 1970;73:153.

92. Fari, Z, Higach, GI, Bassily S, et al. Chronic salmonellosis, urinary schistosomiasis and massive proteinuria. *Am J Trop Med Hyg* 1972;21:578.

93. Higashi GI, Farid Z, Bassily S, et al. Nephrotic syndrome in schistosomiasis mansoni complicated by chronic salmonellosis. *Am J Trop Med Hyg* 1975;24:713.

94. Bassily S, Farid Z, Barsoum RS, et al. Renal biopsy in Schistosoma/Salmonella associated nephrotic syndrome. *J Trop Med Hyg* 1976;79:256.

95. Rocha H, Kirk JW, Hearey CD. Prolonged Salmonella bacteremia in patients with schistosoma mansoni infection. *Arch Intern Med* 1971;128:254.

96. Kennedy ND, Pusey CD, Rainford DJ, et al. Leptospirosis and acute renal failure in clinical experience and a review of literature. *Postgrad Med* 1979;55:176.

97. O'Neill PG, Christie M, Cahill J, et al. Leptospirosis and renal failure: clinical experience over a one year period. *Ir J Med Sci* 1982;151:339.

98. Charoonruangrit S, Boonpucknavig S. Leptospirosis at Chulalongkorn Hospital: a report of 54 cases. *J Med Assoc Thai* 1964;47:653.

99. Lai KN, Aarons I, Woodroffe AJ, et al. Renal lesions in leptospirosis. *Aust N Z M Med* 1982;12:276.

100. Sitprija V. Renal involvement in human leptospirosis. *Br Med J (Clin Res)* 1968;2:656.

101. Yang CW, Pan MJ, Wu MS, et al. Leptospirosis: An ignored cause of acute renal failure in Taiwan. *Am J Kidney Dis* 1997;30:840.

102. Abdulkader RC, Seguro AC, Malheiro PS, et al. Peculiar electrolytic and hormonal abnormalities in acute renal failure due to leptospirosis. *Am J Trop Med Hyg* 1996;54:1.

103. Edwards CN, Nicholson GD, Everard CO. Thrombocytopenia in leptospirosis. *Am J Trop Med Hyg* 1982;31:827.

104. Raoult D, Jeandel PL, Mailloux M, et al. Thrombocytopenia and renal failure in leptospirosis. *Am J Trop Med Hyg* 1983;32:1464.

105. Sitprija V, Evans H. The kidney in human leptospirosis. *Am J Med* 1970;49:780.

106. Sitprija V, Pipatanagul V, Mertowidjojo K, et al. Pathogenesis of renal disease in leptospirosis. *Kidney Int* 1980;17:827.

107. Sitprija V. Leptospirosis. In: *Encyclopedia of life science, Macmillan Reference Limited*. London: Stockton Press *(in press)*.

108. Yang CW, Wu MS, Pan MJ. Leptospirosis renal failure in Taiwan. Abstracts. *8th Asian Pacific Congress Nephrol*. Taipei, 2000:161.

109. Vinh T, Adler B, Faine S. Glycolipoprotein cytotoxin from Leptospira interrogans serovar copenhageni. *J Genet Microbiol* 1986;132:111.

110. Younes-Ibrahim M, Burth P, Faris MV, et al. Inhibition of Na,K-ATPase by endotoxin extracted from Leptospira interrogans: a possible mechanism for the pathophysiology of leptospirosis. Comptes Rendu de l'Academie des Sciences. Serie III. *Science de la Vie* 1995;38:619.

111. Barnett JK, Barnett D, Bolin CA, et al. Expression and distribution of leptospiral outer membrane components during renal infection of hamsters. *Infect Immunol* 1999;67:853.

112. Yamashiro-Kanashiro EH, et al. Cellular immune response analysis of patients with leptospirosis. *Am J Trop Med Hyg* 1991;45:138.

113. Pecchini F, Borghi M, Bodini U, et al. Acute renal failure in leptospirosis: new trends in treatment. *Clin Nephrol* 1982;18:164.

114. Pochanugool C, Sitprija V. Hyperbilirubinemic renal failure in tropical disease: Treatment with exchange transfusion. *J Med Assoc Thai* 1978;61:75.

115. Sitprija V, Chusilp SK. Renal failure and hyperbilirubinemia in leptospirosis. Treatment with exchange transfusion. *Med J Aust* 1973;1:171.

116. Date A, Thomas A, Mathai R, et al. Glomerular pathology in leprosy. An electron inicroscopic study. *Am J Trop Med Hyg* 1977;26:266.

117. Johny KV, Karat ABA, Rao PS, et al. Glomerulonephritis in leprosy. A percutaneous renal biopsy study. *Lepr Rev* 1975;46:29.

118. Chugh KS, Damle PB, Kaur S. Renal lesions in leprosy amongst north Indian patients. *Postgrad Med J* 1983;59:707.

119. Bennish ML, Harris JR, Wojtyniak BJ, et al. Death in shigellosis: incidence and risk factors in hospitalized patients. *J Infect Dis* 1990;161:500.

120. Ramanujam K, Ramu G, Balakrishnam S. Nephrotic syndrome complicating lepromatous leprosy. *Indian J Med Res* 1973;61:548.
121. Singhal PC, Chugh KS, Kaur S, et al. Acute renal failure in leprosy. *Int J Lepr* 1977;45:171.
122. Shwe T. Serum complement (C3) in leprosy. *Lepr Rev* 1972;42:268.
123. Drutz DJ, Gutman RA. Renal manifestations of leprosy: glomerulonephritis, a complication of erythema nodosum leprosum. *Am J Trop Med Hyg* 1973;22:496.
124. Nigam P, Pant KC, Kapoor KK, et al. Histo-functional status of kidney in leprosy. *Indian J Lepr* 1986;58:567.
125. Peter KS, Vijayakumar T, Vasudevan DM, et al. Renal involvement in leprosy. *Lepr India* 1981;53:163.
126. Mittal MM, Maheshwari HB, Kumar S, et al. Renal lesions in leprosy. *Arch Pathol* 1972;93:8.
127. Shwe T. Immune complexes in the glomeruli of patients with leprosy. *Lepr Rev* 1972;42:282.
128. Bullock WE, Callerame ML, Panner BJ. Immunohistologic alterations of skin and ultrastructural changes of glomerular basement membranes in leprosy. *Am J Trop Med Hyg* 1974;23:81.
129. Cologlu AS. Immune complex glomerulonephritis in leprosy. *Lepr Rev* 1981;50:213.
130. Nigg C. Serological studies on subclinical melioidosis. *J Immunol* 1963;91:18.
131. Punyagupta S, Sirisanthana T, Stapatayavong B. *Melioidosis.* Bangkok: Medical Publisher, 1989.
132. Susaengrat W, Dhiensiri T, Sinavatana P, et al. Renal failure in melioidosis. *Nephron* 1987;46:167.
133. Piggott JA, Hochholzer L. Human melioidosis: a histopathologic study of acute and chronic melioidosis. *Arch Pathol* 1970;90:101.
134. Martinelli R, Matos CM, Rocha H. Tetanus as a cause of acute renal failure: possible role of rhabdomyolysis. *Revista da Sociedade Brasileira Medic Trop* 1993;26:1.
135. Seedat YK, Omar MA, Seedat MA, et al. Renal failure in tetanus. *Br Med J* 1981;282:360.
136. Daher EF, Abdulkader RC, Motti E, et al. Prospective study of tetanus-induced acute renal dysfunction: role of adrenergic over-activity. *Am J Trop Med Hyg* 1997;57:610.
137. Hsu GJ, Young T, Peng MY, et al. Acute renal failure associated with scrub typhus. Report of a case. *J Formosan Med Assoc* 1993;92:475.
138. Sitprija V. Interstitial nephritis in infection. *J Med Assoc Thai* 1974; 57:517.
139. Whelton A, Donadio JU Jr, Elisberg BL. Acute renal failure complicating rickettsial infection in G6PD deficient individuals. *Ann Intern Med* 1968;69:323.
140. Allen AC, Spitz S. A comparative study of the pathology of scrub typus (Tsutsugamushi disease) and other rickettsial diseases. *Am J Pathol* 1945;21:603.
141. Futrakul P, Sitprija V, Watana D, et al. Diphtheria with renal failure. *4th Colloquium in Nephrology.* Hong Kong, 1984:44(abst).
142. Kannerstein M. Histologic kidney changes in the common acute infectious diseases. *Am J Med Sci* 1942;203:65.
143. Singh M, Saidali A, Bakhtiar A, et al. Diphtheria in Afghanistan. Review of 155 cases. *J Trop Med Hyg* 1985;88:373.
144. Melby EI, Jacobsen J, Olsnes S, et al. Entry of protein toxins in polarized epithelial cells. *Can Res* 1993;53:1753.
145. Wang F, Butler T, Rabbani GH, et al. The acidosis of cholera. Contributions of hyperproteinemia, lactic acidemia and hyperphosphatemia to an increased serum anion gap. *N Engl J Med* 1986;315:1591.
146. Benyajati C, Keoplung M, Beisel WR, et al. Acute renal failure in Asiatic cholera: clinicopathologic correlations with acute tubular necrosis and hypokalemic correlations with acute tubular necrosis and hypokalemic nephropathy. *Am J Med* 1960;52:960.
147. De SN, Sengupta KP, Chanda NN. Renal changes including total cortical necrosis in cholera. *Arch Pathol* 1954;57:505.
148. Koster F, Levin J, Walker L, et al. Hemolytic-uremic syndrome after shigellosis. Relation to endotoxemia and circulating immune complexes. *N Engl J Med* 1978;298:927.
149. O'Riordan T, Kavanagh P, Mellotte G, et al. Haemolytic-uraemic syndrome in shigella. *Ir J Med* 1990;83:72.
150. Raghupathy P, Raghupathy P, Date A, et al. Haemolytic-uraemic syndrome complicating shigella dysentery in South Indian children. *Br Med J* 1978;2:1578.
151. Srivastava RN, Moudgil A, Bagga A, et al. Hemolytic-uremic syndrome in children in northern India. *Pediatr Nephrol* 1991;5:284.
152. Lerstloompleephunt N, Tantawichien T, Sitprija V. Renal failure in Vibrio vulnificus infection. *Renal Fail* 2000;22:337.
153. Kreger A, Lockwood D. Detection of extracellular toxin(s) produced by Vibrio vulnificus. *Infect Immunol* 1981;33:583.
154. Kothary MH, Kreger AS. Purification and characterization of an elastolytic protease of Vibrio vulnificus. *J Genet Microbiol* 1987; 133:1783.
155. Smith GC, Merkel JR. Collagenolytic activity of Vibrio vulnificus: potential contribution to its invasiveness. *Infect Immunol* 1982; 35:1155.
156. Miyoshi S, Hirata Y, Tomochika K, et al. Vibrio vulnificus may produce a metalloproteinase causing an edematous skin lesion in vivo. *FEMS Microbiol Lett* 1994;121:321.
157. Arnold M, Woo ML, French GL. Vibrio vulnificus septicemia presenting as spontaneous necrotizing cellulitis in a woman with hepatic cirrhosis. *Scand J Infect Dis* 1989;21:727.
158. Dengue fever cases and deaths in the Western Pacific Region 1991–1992 [Editorial]. *Dengue Newsletter* 1993;18:15.
159. Jatanasen S. DHF in the Southeast Asia Region. *Dengue Newsletter* 1992;17:1.
160. Futrakul P, Mitrakul C, Chumdermpadetsuk S, et al. Studies on the pathogenesis of dengue hemorrhagic fever: hemodynamic alteration and effect of alpha blocking agent. *J Med Assoc Thai* 1977; 60:610.
161. Futrakul P, Poshyachinda V, Mitrakul C, et al. Renal involvement and reticuloendothelial system clearance in dengue hemorrhagic fever. *J Med Assoc Thai* 1973;56:33.
162. Pongpanich B, Kumponpant S. Studies on dengue hemorrhagic fever. V. Hemodynamic studies of clinical shock associated with dengue hemorrhagic fever. *Pediatrics* 1973;83:1073.
163. Tuchinda P. Hemorrhagic fever in Thailand: physiologic derangement. *J Med Assoc Thai* 1973;56:1.
164. Boonpucknavig V, Bhamaraparavati N, Boonpucknavig S, et al. Glomerular changes in dengue hemorrhagic fever. *Arch Pathol Lab Med* 1976;100:206.
165. Bhamarapravati N, Tuchinda P, Boonpucknavig V. Pathology of Thailand hemorrhagic fever. A study of 100 autopsy cases. *Ann Trop Med Parasitol* 1967;61:500.
166. Gonzalez JP, Mc Cormick JG, Baudon D, et al. Serological evidence for Hantaan related virus in Africa. *Lancet* 1994;2:1036.
167. Tkachenko EA, Lee HW. Etiology and epidemiology of hemorrhagic fever with renal syndrome. *Kidney Int* 1991;40:54.
168. Cosgriff TM, Levis RM. Mechanisms of disease in hemorrhagic fever with renal syndrome. *Kidney Int* 1991;40:72.
169. Lee HW. Hantavirus infection in Asia. In: Davison AM, ed. *Nephrology.* London: Bailliere Tindall, 1988:816.
170. Outbreak of acute illness: Southwestern United States 1993 [Editorial]. *MMWR Morb Mortal Wkly Rep* 1993;42:421.
171. Vos GH, Grobbelaar G, Milnet LVA. Possible relationship between persistent hepatitis B antigenemia and renal disease in South African Bantus. *S Afr Med J* 1973;47:911.
172. Hsu HC, Lin GH, Chang MH, et al. Association of hepatitis B surface antigenemia and membranous nephropathy in children in Taiwan. *Clin Nephrol* 1983;20:121.
173. Seggie J, Nathoo K, Davies PG. Association of hepatitis B antigenemia and membranous glomerulonephritis in Zimbabwean children. *Nephron* 1984;38:115.
174. Takekoshi Y, Tanaka M, Shida N, et al. Strong association between membranous nephropathy and hepatitis B surface antigenemia in Japanese children. *Lancet* 1978;2:1065.
175. Levo Y, Gorevic PD, Hassab HJ, et al. Association between hepatitis B virus and essential mixed cryoglobulinemia. *N Engl J Med* 1977;296:1501.
176. Wilkinson SP, Blendis LM, Williams R. Frequency and type of renal and electrolyte disorders in fulminant hepatic failure. *Br Med J* 1974;1:186.
177. Wilkinson SP, Davies MH, Portmann B, et al. Renal failure in otherwise uncomplicated acute viral hepatitis. *Br Med J* 1978;2:338.
178. Lai KN, Lai FM. Clinical features and the natural course of hepatitis B virus related glomerulopathy in adults. *Kidney Int* 1991; 40:540.
179. Lai KN, Tam JS, Lin HJ, et al. The therapeutic dilemma of usage of corticosteroid in patients with membranous nephropathy and persistent hepatitis B virus surface antigenemia. *Nephron* 1990;54:12.

180. Lin CY, Lo S. Treatment of hepatitis B virus–associated membranous nephropathy with adenine arabinoside and thymic extract. *Kidney Int* 1991;39:301.

181. Ito H, Hattori S, Matsuda I, et al. Hepatitis B antigen mediated membranous glomerulonephritis. *Lab Invest* 1981;44:214.

182. Lai KN, Lai FM, Chan KW, et al. The clinicopathologic features of hepatitis B virus associated glomerulonephritis. *Q J Med* 1987;63:323.

183. Lai KN, Lai FM, Tam JS. IgA nephropathy associated with chronic hepatitis B virus infection in adults: the pathogenetic role of HBsAg. *J Pathol* 1989;157:321.

184. Burstein DM, Rodby RA. Membranoproliferative glomerulonephritis associated with hepatitis C virus infection. *J Am Soc Nephrol* 1993;4:1288.

185. Johnson RJ, Gretch DR, Yamabe H, et al. Membranoproliferative glomerulonephritis associated with hepatitis C virus infection. *N Engl J Med* 1993;328:465.

186. Pasquariello A, Ferri C, Moriconi L, et al. Cryoglobulinemic membranoproliferative glomerulonephritis associated with hepatitis C virus. *Am J Nephrol* 1993;13:330.

187. Davda R, Peterson J, Weiner R, et al. Membranous glomerulonephritis in association with hepatitis C virus infection. *Am J Kidney Dis* 1993;22:452.

188. Horikoshi S, Okada T, Shirato I, et al. Diffuse proliferative glomerulonephritis with hepatitis C virus–like particles in paramesangial dense deposits in a patient with chronic hepatitis C virus hepatitis. *Nephron* 1993;64:462.

189. Johnson RJ, Gretch DR, Couser WG, et al. Hepatitis C virus–associated glomerulonephritis. Effect of alpha-interferon therapy. *Kidney Int* 1994;46:1700.

190. Sansonno D, Gesualdo L, Manno C, et al. Hepatitis C virus–related proteins in the kidney tissue from hepatitis C virus–infected patients with cryoglobulinemic membranoproliferative glomerulonephritis. *Hepatology* 1997;26:1687.

191. Ohta S, Yokoyama H, Furuichi K, et al. Clinicopathological features of glomerular lesions associated with hepatitis C virus infection in Japan. *Clin Exp Nephrol* 1997;1:216.

192. Ohta S, Yokoyama H, Wada T, et al. Exacerbation of glomerulonephritis in subjects with chronic hepatitis C virus Infection after interferon therapy. *Am J Kidney Dis* 1999;33:1040.

193. Komatsuda A, Imai H, Wakui H, et al. Clinicopathological analysis and therapy in hepatitis C virus–associated nephropathy. *Intern Med* 1996;35:529.

194. Agarwal RK, Moudgil A, Kishore K, et al. Acute viral hepatitis, intravascular hemolysis, severe hyperbilirubinemia and renal failure in glucose-6-phosphate dehydrogenase deficient patients. *Postgrad Med J* 1985;61:971.

195. Eng C, Chopra S. Acute renal failure in nonfulminant hepatitis A. *J Clin Gastroenterol* 1990;12:717.

196. Mattoo TK, Mahmood MA, al Sowailem AM. Acute renal failure in nonfulminant hepatitis A infection. *Ann Trop Paediatr* 1991;11:213.

197. Faust RL, Pimstone N. Acute renal failure associated with nonfulminant hepatitis A viral infection. *Am J Gastroenterol* 1996;91:369.

198. Rippon JW. *Medical mycology,* 3rd ed. London: WB Saunders, 1988.

199. Petersen EA, Friedman BA, Crowder ED, et al. Coccidioiduria; clinical significance. *Ann Intern Med* 1976;85:35.

200. Cechella MS, Melo CR, Melo IS, et al. Male genital paracoccidioidomycosis. *Rev Inst Med Trop Sao Paulo* 1982;24:240.

201. Krogh P, Axelsen NH, Elling F, et al. Experimental porcine nephropathy. Changes of renal function and structure induced by ochratoxin A–contaminated feed. *Acta Pathol Microbiol Scand* 1974;246[Suppl]:1.

202. Krogh P. Environmental ochratoxin A and Balkan (endemic) nephropathy: evidence for support of a causal relationship. In: Strahinjic S, Stefanovic V, eds. *Endemic (Balkan) nephropathy. Proceedings of the 4th Symposium on Endemic (Balkan) Nephropathy.* Nis: University Press, 1979:35.

203. Saadi MG, Abdulla E, Fadel F, et al. Prevalence of ochratoxin A (OTA) among Egyptian children and adults with different renal diseases. *II Int Congress Geogr Nephrol, Hurghada, Egypt.* 1993:22(abst).

204. Achour A, et al. Chronic interstitial nephritis and ochratoxin A. *Int Congress Geogr Nephrol, Hurghada, Egypt.* 1993:52(abst).

205. Epstein SM, Bartus B, Farber E. Renal epithelial neoplasm-induced in male Wistar rats by oral aflatoxin B1. *Can Res* 1969;29:1045.

206. Barsoum R. Ecology and Egyptian nephrology. *Proc VIII Egypt Congress Nephrol, Fayoum, Egypt.* 1989:4.

207. Coltman KMD. Urinary tract infections. New thoughts on an old subject. *Practicioner* 1979;223:351.

208. Odds FC. *Candida and Candidiosis,* 2nd ed. London: Bailliere Tindall, 1988.

209. Hamory BH. Nosocomial bloodstream and intravascular device–related infections. In: Wenzel RP, ed. *Prevention and control of nosocomial infections.* Philadelphia: Williams & Wilkins, 1987:283.

210. Masur H, Lane HC, Kovacs JA, et al. Pneumocystis pneumonia: from bench to clinic. *Ann Intern Med* 1989;111:813.

211. Sarosi GA, Davies SF. Clinical manifestation and management of in the compromised patient. In: Warnock DW, Richardson MD, eds. *Fungal infection in the compromised patient.* Chichester: Wiley, 1982:187.

212. Howard RJ, Simmons RL, Najarian JS. Fungal infections in renal transplant recipients. *Ann Surg* 1978;88:598.

213. Torrington KG, Old CW, Urban ES, et al. Transurethral passage of Aspergillus fungus balls in acute myelocytic leukemia. *South Med J* 1979;72:281.

214. Scully RE, Mark EJ, McNeely WF, et al. Case 36. *N Engl J Med* 1988;319:629.

215. Morduchowicz G, Camuell D, Shapiro Z, et al. Rhinocerebral mucormycosis in renal transplant patients: report of three cases and review of the literature. *Rev Inf Dis* 1986;8:444.

216. Miller GP. The immunology of cryptococcal disease. *Semin Respir Infect* 1986;1:45.

217. Ghalioungui P. *Magic and medical science in Ancient Egypt.* London: Hodder and Stoughton, 1963.

218. Ruffer MA. Note on the presence of 'Bilharzia haematobia' in Egyptian mummies of the Twentieth Dynasty (1250–1000 BC). *Br Med J* 1910;1:1.

219. Gelfand GA. Possible relationship between the nephrotic syndrome and urinary schistosomiasis. *Trans R Soc Trop Med Hyg* 1963; 57:191.

220. Lopez M. *Aspectos renais da sindrome heaptoesplenica da esquistossomose mansonica.* Tese: Universidade de Minas Cerais, Escola de Medicina, Belo horizonte, Brasil, 1964.

221. Andrade ZA, Queiroz A. Lesoes renais na esquistossomose hepatoesplenica. *Rev Inst Med Trop Sao Paulo* 1968;10:36.

222. Andrade ZA, Rocha H. Schistosomal glomerulopathy. *Kidney Int* 1979;16:23.

223. Sabbour MS, El Said W, Abou Ganal IA. Clinical and pathological study of schistosomal nephritis. *Bull WHO* 1972;47:49.

224. Ezzat E, Osman R, Ahmed KY, et al. The association between Schistosoma haematobium infection and heavy proteinuria. *Trans R Soc Trop Med Hyg* 1974;68:315.

225. Barsoum RS, Bassily S, Baligh OK, et al. Renal disease in hepatosplenic schistosomiasis: a clinicopathological study. *Trans R Soc Trop Med Hyg* 1977;71:387.

226. Musa AM, Abu Asha H, Veress B. Nephrotic syndrome in Sudanese patients with schistosomiasis mansoni infection. *Ann Trop Med Parasitol* 1980;74:615.

227. Abdurrahman MB, Attah B, Narayana PT. Clinicopathological features of hepatosplenic schistosomiasis in children. *Ann Trop Paediatr* 1981;1:5.

228. Chandra-Shekkar K, Pathmanathan R. Schistosomiasis in Malaysia. *Rev Infect Dis* 1987;9:1026.

229. Atkinson LE. Bright's disease of Malarial origin. *Am J Med Sci* 1884;88:149.

230. Giglioli G. *Malarial nephritis: epidemiological and clinical notes on malaria, blackwater fever, albuminuria and nephritis in the interior of British Guiana, based on seven years' continual observation.* London: Churchill, 1930.

231. Gilles HM, Hendrichse RG. Nephrosis in Nigerian children. Role of malariae and effect of antimalarial treatment. *Br Med J (Clin Res)* 1963;2:27.

232. Berger M, Birch LM, Conte NF. The nephrotic syndrome secondary to acute glomerulonephritis during falciparum malaria. *Ann Intern Med* 1967;76:1163.

233. Hartenbower DL, Kantor GL, Rosen VJ. Renal failure due to acute glomerulonephritis during falciparum malaria: case report. *Milit Med* 1972;137:74.

234. Boonpucknaving V, Boonpucknaving S, Bhamarapravati N. Plasmodium berghei infection in mice: an ultrastructural study of immune complex nephritis. *Am J Pathol* 1973;70:89.

235. Futrakul P, Boonpucknavig V, Boonpucknavig S, et al. Acute glomerulonephritis complicating Plasmodium falciparum infection. *Clin Pediatr (Philadelphia)* 1974;13:281.

236. Sitprija V. Nephrology forum: nephropathy in falciparum malaria. *Kidney Int* 1988;34:866.

237. Barsoum R. Nephrology and African ecology. An overview. *Artif Organs* 1991;14:235.

238. Mandema E, Ruinen L, Sholten JH, et al, eds. *Amyloidosis*. Amsterdam: Excerpta Medica, 1968.

239. Manson Bahr PEC. Leishmaniasis. In: Manson Bahr PEC, Apted FIC, eds. *Tropical diseases*. London: Balliere Tindall, 1982:115.

240. Natali PG, Cioli D. Immune complex nephritis in mice infected with *S. mansoni*. *Fed Proc* 1974;33:757.

241. Thomas MA, Frampton G, Isenberg DA, et al. A common anti-DNA antibody idiotype and anti-phospholipid antibodies in sera from patients with schistosomiasis and filariasis with and without nephritis. *J Autoimmun* 1989;2:803.

242. Cohen S. Comments on immunopathology in malaria. *Adv Biosci* 1973;12:617.

243. Sitprija V, Vongsthongsri M, Poshyachinda V, et al. Renal failure in malaria: a pathophysiologic study. *Nephron* 1977;18:277.

244. Barsoum RS. Schistosomiasis. In: Cameron S, Davison AM, Grunfeld JP, et al, eds. *Oxford text book of clinical nephrology*. Oxford: Oxford University Press, 1993:1729.

245. Waugh DA, Alexander JH, Ibels LH. Filarial chyluria–associated glomerulonephritis and therapeutic consideration in the chyluric patient. *Aust N Z J Med* 1980;10:559.

246. Boonpucknaving V, Sitprija V. Renal disease in acute Plasmodium falciparum infection in man. *Kidney Int* 1979;16:44.

247. Barsoum RS. Dialysis in developing countries. In: Jacobs C, Winchester JF, Kjellstrand CM, et al, eds. *Replacement of renal function by dialysis, 4th ed.* Kluwer Academic Publishers, 1996.

248. Barsoum R, Shahrezad S, Abdel-Azim O, et al. Dialysis ward bio-ecology in a developing country. Effect on the results of treatment and impact of socio-economic factors. *VIII World Congress Int Soc Artif Organ.* 1991;15(abst).

249. Sobh MA, el-Agroudy AE, Moustafa FE, et al. Impact of schistosomiasis on patient and graft outcome after kidney transplantation. *Nephrol Dial Transplant* 1992;7:858.

250. Krogstad DJ. Malaria. In: Wyngaarden JB, Smith LH, Bennett JC, eds. *Cecil textbook of medicine,* 19th ed. Philadelphia: WB Saunders, 1992:1972.

251. Miller LH, Haynes D, McAuliffe FM, et al. Evidence for differences in erythrocyte surface receptors for malarial parasites Plasmodium falciparum and Plasmodium knowlesi. *J Exp Med* 1977;146:277.

252. Dvorak JA, Miller LH, Whitehourse WC, et al. Invasion of erythrocytes by malaria merozoites. *Science* 1975;187:748.

253. Aikawa M, Miller LH, Johnson J, et al. Erythrocyte entry by malarial parasites: a moving junction between erythrocyte and parasite. *J Cell Biol* 1978;77:72.

254. Kilejian A, Abati A, Trager W. Plasmodium falciparum and Plasmodium coatney: immunogenicity of knob-like protrusions on infected erythrocyte membrane. *Exp Parasitol* 1977;42:157.

255. Leech JH, Barnwell JW, Aikawa M, et al. Plasmodium falciparum malaria: association of knobs on the surface of infected erythrocytes with a histidine-rich protein and the erythrocyte skeleton. *J Cell Biol* 1984;98:1256.

256. Udeinya IJ, Schmidt JA, Aikawa M, et al. Falciparum malaria infected erythrocytes specifically bind to cultured human endothelial cells. *Science* 1981;213:555.

257. Roberts DD, Sherwood JA, Spitalnik SL, et al. Thrombospondin binds falciparum malaria parasitized erythrocytes and may mediate cytoadherence. *Nature* 1985;318:64.

258. Clark IA. Suggested importance of monokines in pathophysiology of endotoxin shock and malaria. *Klin Wochenschr* 1982;60:756.

259. Grau GE, Fajardo LF, Piguet PF, et al. Tumor necrosis factor (cachectin) as an essential mediator in murine cerebral malaria. *Science* 1987;237:1270.

260. Kern P, Hemmer CJ, Van Damme J, et al. Elevated tumor necrosis factor alpha and interleukin-6 serum levels as markers for complicated Plasmodium falciparum malaria. *Am J Med* 1989;87:139.

261. Grau GE, Taylor TE, Molyneux ME, et al. Tumor necrosis factor and disease severity in children with falciparum malaria. *N Engl J Med* 1989;320:1586.

262. McGregor IA, Turner MW, Williams K, et al. Soluble antigens in the blood of African patients with severe Plasmodium falciparum malaria. *Lancet* 1968;1:881.

263. Srichaikul T, Puwasatien P, Karnjanajetanee J, et al. Complement changes and disseminated intravascular coagulation in P. falciparum malaria. *Lancet* 1975;1:770.

264. Good M., Pombo D, Quakyi IA, et al. Human T cell recognition of the circumsporozoite protein of Plasmodium falciparum: immunodominant T cell domains map to the polymorphic regions of the molecule. *Proc Natl Acad Sci U S A* 1988;85:1199.

265. Hendrickse RG, Adeniyi A. Quartan malarial nephrotic syndrome in children. *Kidney Int* 1979;16:64.

266. Ehrich JHH, Horstmann RD. Origin of proteinuria in human malaria. *Trop Med Parasitol* 1985;36:39.

267. Davies DR, Wing AJ. Malaria, microscopy and marmoset. The saga of tropical medicine syndrome. *Q J Med* 1990;75:533.

268. Hendrickse RG, Gilles HM. The nephrotic syndrome and other renal diseases in children in Western Nigeria. *East Afr Med J* 1963;40:186.

269. Kibukamusoke JW. *Nephrotic syndrome of quartan malaria*. London: Edward Arnold, 1973.

270. Wedderburn N, Davies DR, Mitchell GH, et al. Glomerulonephritis in common marmosets infected with Plasmodium brasilianum and Epstein-Barr virus. *J Infect Dis* 1988;148:289.

271. Pakasa M, Van Damme B, Desmet VJ. Free intraglomerular malarial antigens. *Br J Exp Pathol* 1985;66:493.

272. Houba V. Immunologic aspects of renal lesions associated with malaria. *Kidney Int* 1979;16:3.

273. Hendrickse RG, Adeniyi A. Quartan malarial nephrotic syndrome in children. *Kidney Int* 1979;16:64.

274. Houba V, Lambert RG. Immunological studies on tropical nephropathies. *Adv Biosci* 1973;12:617.

275. Allison AC, Hendrickse RG, Edington GM, et al. Immune complexes in the nephrotic syndrome of African children. *Lancet* 1969;1:1232.

276. Clark IA. Does endotoxin cause both the disease and parasite death in acute malaria and babesiosis? *Lancet* 1978;2:75.

277. Borochovitz D, Crosley AL, Metz J. Disseminated intravascular coagulation with fatal haemorrhage in cerebral malaria. *Br Med J (Clin Res)* 1970;2:710.

278. Edwards IR. Malaria with disseminated intravascular coagulation and peripheral tissue necrosis successfully treated with streptokinase. *Br Med J (Clin Res)* 1980;280:1252.

279. White NJ, Warrell DA, Chanthavanich P, et al. Severe hypoglycemia and hyperinsulinemia in falciparum malaria. *N Engl J Med* 1983;309:61.

280. Lumlertgul D, Keoplung M, Sitprija V, et al. Furosemide and dopamine in malarial acute renal failure. *Nephron* 1989;52:40.

281. Sitprija V. Urinary excretion patterns in renal failure due to malaria: the effects of phenoxybenzamine in two cases. *Aust N Z J Med* 1971;1:44.

282. Nielson RL, Kohler RB, Chin W, et al. The use of exchange transfusions: a potentially useful adjunct in the treatment of fulminant falciparum malaria. *Am J Med Sci* 1979;277:325.

283. Yuthavong Y, Wilairat P, Panijpan B, et al. Alteration in membrane proteins of mouse erythrocytes infected with different species and strains of malarial parasite. *Comp Biochem Physiol* 1979;631:83.

284. Mikkelsen RB, Tanabe K, Wallack DFH. Membrane potential of Plasmodium infected erythrocytes. *J Cell Biol* 1982;93:685.

285. Cranston HA, Boylan CW, Carroll GL, et al. Plasmodium falciparum maturation abolishes physiologic red cell deformability. *Science* 1984;223:400.

286. Devakul K, Harinsuta T, Reid HA. ^{125}I labelled fibrinogen in cerebral malaria. *Lancet* 1966;2:886.

287. Eiam-Ong S, Sitprija V. Falciparum malaria and the kidney: a model of inflammation. *Am J Kidney Dis* 1998;32:316.

288. Skirrow MB, Chongsuphajaisiddhi T, Maegraith BG. The circulation in malaria: II. Portal angiography in monkeys (Macaca mulatta) infected with Plasmodium knowlesi and in shock following manipulation of the gut. *Ann Trop Med Parasitol* 1964;58:502.

289. Miller LH, Makaranond P, Sitprija V, et al. Hyponatremia in malaria. *Ann Trop Med Parasitol* 1967;61:265.

290. Fryatt RJ, Teng JD, Harries AD, et al. Plasma and urine electrolyte concentrations and vasopressin levels of patients admitted to hospital for falciparum malaria. *Trop Geogr Med* 1989;41:57.

291. Sitprija V, Napathorn S, Laorpatanaskul S, et al. Renal and systemic hemodynamics in falciparum malaria. *Am J Nephrol* 1996;16:513.

292. Clark IA. Thromboxane may be important in the organ damage and hypotension of malaria. *Med Hypotheses* 1981;7:625.

293. Weston M, Jackman N, Rudge C, et al. Prostacyclin in falciparum malaria. *Lancet* 1982;2:609.

294. White NJ, Warrell DA, Looareesuwan S, et al. Pathophysiological and prognostic significance of cerebrospinal fluid lactate in cerebral malaria. *Lancet* 1985;1:776.

295. Dunn MJ. Alteration of red cell sodium transport during malarial infection. *J Clin Invest* 1968;48:674.

296. Sarikabhuti B, Niyomkha P. Adenosine triphosphate levels in mouse erythrocytes infected with chloroquine-sensitive and choroquine-resistant Plasmodium berghei. *Ann Trop Med Parasitol* 1982;76:657.

297. Tanabe K, Mikkelsen RB, Wallach DFH. Calcium transport of Plasmodium chabaudi infected erythrocytes. *Cell Biol* 1982;93:680.

298. Krungkrai J, Yuthavong Y. Enhanced Ca uptake by mouse erythrocytes in malarial (Plasmodium berghei) infection. *Mol Biochem Parasitol* 1983;7:227.

299. Malloy JP, Brook MH, Barry KG. Pathophysiology of acute falciparum malaria: II. Fluid compartmentalization. *Am J Med* 1967;43:745.

300. Sitprija V, Suithichaiyakul T, Moollaor P. The kidney in malaria: renal and systemic hemodynamics. *Nephrology* 1996;2[Suppl l]:S94.

301. Chongsuphajaisiddhi T, Kasemsuth R, Tejavanija S, et al. Changes in blood volume in falciparum malaria. *Asian J Trop Med Public Health* 1971;2:344.

302. Spitz S. The pathology of acute falciparum malaria. *Milit Surgeon* 1946;99:555.

303. Bhamarapravati N, Boonpucknavig S, Boonpucknavig V, et al. Glomerular changes in acute Plasmodium falciparum infection: an immunologic study. *Arch Pathol* 1973;96:289.

304. Sinniah R, Churg J, Sobin LH. Protozoal infections. In: World Health Organization, ed. Renal disease. *Classification and atlas of infectious and tropical renal diseases.* Chicago: American Society of Clinical Pathology, 1988:13.

305. Rui-Mei L, Kara AU, Sinniah R. Dysregulation of cytokine expression in tubulointerstitial nephritis associated with murine malaria. *Kidney Int* 1998;53:845.

306. Petithory JC, Lebeau G, Galeazzi G, et al. Hypocalcemia in malaria. Study of correlations with other parameters. *Bull Soc Pathol Exot Filiales* 1983;76:455.

307. Mostellar ME, Tuttle EP Jr. The effects of alkalosis on plasma concentration and urinary excretion of inorganic phosphate in man. *J Clin Invest* 1964;43:138.

308. Ruebush TK, Juranek DD, Chisholm ES, et al. Human babesiosis on Nantucket Island. *Ann Intern Med* 1977;86:6.

309. Annable CR, Ward PA. Immunopathology of the renal complications of babesiosis. *J Immunol* 1974;112:1.

310. Itturri GM, Cox HW. Glomerulonephritis associated with acute haemosporidian infection. *Milit Med (Special Issue)* 1969;134:1119.

311. Duarte MIS, Silva MRR, Goto H, et al. Interstitial nephritis in human kala azar. *Trans R Soc Trop Med Hyg* 1983;77:531.

312. Weisinger JR, Pinto A, Velazquez GA, et al. Clinical and histological kidney involvement in human kala azar. *Am J Trop Med Hyg* 1978;27:357.

313. De Brito T, Hoshino-Shimizu S, Neto VA, et al. Glomerular involvement in human kala azar. A light, immunofluorescent, and electron microscopic study based on kidney biopsies. *Am J Trop Med Hyg* 1975;4:8.

314. Kager PA, Hack CE, Hannema AJ, et al. High C1q levels, low C13/C1q ratios, and high levels of circulating immune complexes in kala azar. *Clin Immunol Immunopathol* 1982;23:86.

315. Carvalho EM, Andrews BS, Martinelli R, et al. Circulating immune complexes and rheumatoid factor in schistosomiasis and visceral leishmaniasis. *Am J Trop Med Hyg* 1983;32:61.

316. Mancianti F, Poli A, Bionda A. Analysis of renal immune deposits in canine leishmaniasis: preliminary results. *Parasitologia* 1989;31:213.

317. Kirchhoff LV. Agents of African trypanosomiasis (sleeping sickness). In: Mandel GL, Douglas BJ, Bennet JE, eds. *Principles and practice of infectious disease,* 3rd ed. New York: Wiley, 1990:2085.

318. Nagle RB, Ward PA, Lindsley HB, et al. Experimental infections with African trypanosomiasis. *Am J Trop Med Hyg* 1974;23:15.

319. Mansor H. Toxoplasmosis. In: Wyngaarden JB, Smith LH, Bennett JC, eds. *Cecil textbook of medicine,* 19th ed. Philadelphia: WB Saunders, 1992:1987.

320. Ginsburg BE, Wasserman J, Huldt G, et al. Case of glomerulonephritis associated with acute toxoplasmosis. *Br Med J* 1974;3:664.

321. Crawford FG, Vermund SH. Human cryptosporidiosis. *CRC Crit Rev Microbiol* 1988;16:113.

322. Schantz PM, Okelo GBA. Echinococcosis (Hydatidosis). In: Warren KS, Mahmoud AAF, eds. *Tropical and geographical medicine,* 2nd ed. New York: McGraw Hill 1990:505.

323. Okelo GBA, Kyobe JA. Three-year review of human hydatid disease seen at Kenyata National Hospital. *East Afr Med J* 1981;58:695.

324. World Health Organization. The control of Schistosomiasis. Technical report series. *World Health Organ* 1985;1:113.

325. Manson-Bahr PEC, Bell DR. *Schistosomiasis Manson's tropical diseases.* London: Bailliere Tindall, 1987.

326. De Brito PA, Kazura IW, Mahmoud AF. Host granulomatous response in schistosomiasis mansoni. Antibody and cell mediated damage of parasite eggs in vitro. *J Clin Invest* 19854;74:1715.

327. Abdel Wahab MF. *Schistosomiasis in Egypt.* Florida: CRC Press, 1982.

328. Badr MM. Surgical management of urinary bilharziasis. In: Dudley H, Porres WJ, Carter DC, et al, eds. *Rob and Smith's operative surgery.* London: Butterworth, 1986.

329. Barsoum RS. Schistosomal glomerulopathies. *Kidney Int* 1993;44:1.

330. El-Said W, Barahat S, Khedr E, et al. Complications of schistosomiasis among Egyptian dialysis patients. *II Int Congress Geogr Nephrol, Hurghada, Egypt.* 1993:40.

331. Mahmoud AAF. Praziquantel for the treatment of helminthic infections. *Adv Intern Med* 1987;32:193.

332. Houba V. Experimental renal disease due to schistosomiasis. *Kidney Int* 1979;16:30.

333. Deelder AM, Kornelis D, Van Marck EAE. Schistosoma mansoni: characterization of two circulating polysaccharide antigens and the immunological response to these antigens in mouse: hamster and human infection. *Exp Parasitol* 1980;50:16.

334. De Water R, Van Marck EA, Fransen JA, et al. Schistosoma mansoni: ultrastructural localization of the circulating anodic antigen and the circulating cathodic antigen in the mouse kidney glomerulus. *Am J Trop Med Hyg* 1988;38:118.

335. Sobh M, Moustafa F, el-Arbagy A, et al. Nephropathy in asymptomatic patients with active Schistosoma mansoni infection. *Int Urol Nephrol* 1990;22:37.

336. Tada T, Kondo Y, Okumura K, et al. Schistosoma japonicum. Immunopathology of nephritis in Macaca fascicularis. *Exp Parasitol* 1975;38:291.

337. Natali PG, Cioli D. Immune complex nephritis in Schistosoma mansoni–infected mice. *Eur J Immunol* 1976;6:359.

338. Azevedo LS, de Paula FJ, Ianhez LE, et al. Renal transplantation and schistosomiasis mansoni. *Transplantation* 1987;44:795.

339. Sobh M, Moustafa FE, Sally SM, et al. Characterization of kidney lesions in early schistosomal-specific nephropathy. *Nephrol Dial Transplant* 1988;3:392.

340. Soliman M, Abdel-Salam E, Higashi GI, et al. Schistosomiasis haematobium glomerulopathy: a clinical or a pathological entity? *Xth International Congress of Nephrology.* Tokyo, Japan, 1987:362(abst).

341. Barsoum RS. Parasitic nephropathies. *Med For* 1990;35:19.

342. Falaco HA, Gould DB. Immune complex nephropathy in schistosomal mansoni. *Ann Intern Med* 1975;83:148.

343. Dutra M, de Carvalho Filho EM, Gusmao EA, et al. Tratamento da glomerulopatia da esquistossomose mansonica. Efeito de corticoesteroides, ciclofosfomida e esquistossomicidas. *Rev Inst Med Trop Sao Paulo* 1979;21:99.

344. Martinelli R, Pereira LJ, Rocha H. The influence of antiparasitic therapy on the course the glomerulopathy associated with schistosomiasis mansoni. *Clin Nephrol* 1987;27:229.

345. Sobh MA, Moustafa FE, Sally SM, et al. Effect of antischistosomal treatment on Schistosoma-specific nephropathy. *Nephrol Dial Transplant* 1988;3:744.

346. Martinelli R, Nobiat AC, Brito E, et al. *Schistosoma mansoni* induced mesangiocapillary glomerulonephritis: Influence of therapy. *Kidney Int* 1989;35:1227.

347. Hathout SE, El-Ghaffar YA, Awny AY. Chronic salmonellosis complicating schistosomiasis in Egypt. *Am J Trop Med Hyg* 1967;16:462.

348. Lambertrucci JR, Godoy P, Neves J, et al. Glomerulonephritis in Salmonella-Schistosoma mansoni association. *Am J Trop Med Hyg* 1988;38:97.

349. Van March E, Deelder AM, Gigase PLG. Effect of portal vein ligation on immune glomerular deposits in Schistosoma mansoni–infected mice. *Br J Exp Pathol* 1977;58:412.

350. Andrade ZA, Andrade SG, Sadigursky M. Renal changes in patients with hepatosplenic schistosomiasis. *Am J Trop Med Hyg* 1971;20:77.

351. Rocha H, Cruz T, Brito E, et al. Renal involvement in patients with hepatosplenic schistosomiasis mansoni. *Am J Trop Med Hyg* 1976;25:108.

352. Barsoum RS, Sersawy G, Haddad S, et al. Hepatic macrophage function in schistosomal glomerulopathy. *Nephrol Dial Transplant* 1988;3:612.

353. Barsoum RS, Nabil M, Saady G, et al. Immunoglobulin-A and the pathogenesis of schistosomal glomerulopathy. *Kidney Int* 1996;50:920.

354. Hassan AA. *Schistosomal nephropathy and HLA association* [Thesis]. Cairo: Cairo University; 1982.

355. De Brito T, Gunji J, Camargo ME, et al. Advanced kidney disease in patients with hepatosplenic Manson's schistosomiasis. *Rev Inst Med Trop Sao Paulo* 1970;12:225.

356. Sobh MA, Moustafa FE, el-Housseini F, et al. Schistosomal-specific nephropathy leading to end-stage renal failure. *Kidney Int* 1987;31:1006.

357. Robinson A, Lewert RM, Spargo BH. Immune complex glomerulonephritis and amyloidosis in Schistosoma japonicum infected rabbits. *Trans R Soc Trop Med Hyg* 1982;76:214.

358. Sobh M, Moustafa F, Ramzy R, et al. Schistosomal mansoni nephropathy in Syrian golden hamsters. Effect of dose and duration of infection. *Nephron* 1991;59:121.

359. Omer HO, Wahab SMA. Secondary amyloidosis due to schistosomiasis mansoni infection. *Br Med J* 1976;1:375.

360. Barsoum RS, Bassily S, Soliman MM, et al. Renal amyloidosis and schistosomiasis. *Trans R Soc Trop Med Hyg* 1979;73:367.

361. Watt G, Long GW, Calubaquib C, et al. Prevalence of renal involvement in Schistosoma japonicum infection. *Trans R Soc Trop Med Hyg* 1987;81:339.

362. Woo KT. Renal replacement therapy in Singapore. *Contrib Nephrol* 1990;82:30.

363. Ottesen EA, Filariasis. In: Wyngaarden JB, Smith LH, Bennett JC, eds. *Cecil textbook of medicine,* 19th ed. Philadelphia: WB Saunders, 1992.

364. Ngu JL, Chatelanat F, Leke R, et al. Nephropathy in Cameroon: evidence for filarial derived immune complex pathogenesis in some cases. *Clin Nephrol* 1985;24:128.

365. Ormerod AD, Petersen J, Hussey JK, et al. Immune complex glomerulonephritis and chronic anaerobic urinary tract infection; complication of filariasis. *Postgrad Med J* 1983;59:730.

366. Chugh KS, Singhal PC, Tewari SC. Acute glomerulonephritis associated with filariasis. *Am J Trop Med Hyg* 1978;27:630.

367. Date A, Gunasekaran V, Kirubakaran MG, et al. Acute eosinophilic glomerulonephritis with bancroftian filariasis. *Postgrad Med J* 1979; 55:905.

368. Pillay VKG, Kirch E, Kurtzman NA. Glomerulopathy associated with filarial loiasis. *JAMA* 1973;255:179.

369. Greene BM, Taylor HR, Humphrey RL. Proteinuria associated with diethylcarbamazine treatment of onchocerciasis. *Lancet* 1980;1:254.

370. Cummins WT, Carson GR. A study of 15 cases. *JAMA* 1916;67:806.

371. Sitprija V, Keoplung M, Boonpucknavig V, et al. Renal involvement in human trichinosis. *Arch Intern Med* 1980;140:544.

372. Guattery JM, Milne J, House RK. Observation on hepatic and renal dysfunction in trichinosis. *Am J Med* 1956;21:567.

373. Koompirochana C, Sonakul D, Chinda K, et al. Opisthorchiasis. A clinicopathologic study of 154 autopsy cases. *Southeast Asian J Trop Med Public Health* 1978;9:60.

374. Boonpucknavig S, Boonpucknavig V, Tanvanich S, et al. Opisthorchis viverrini: development of immune complex glomerulonephritis and amyloidosis in infected Syrian golden hamsters. *J Med Assoc Thai* 1992;75[Suppl]:7.

375. Genta RM. Global prevalence of strongyloidiasis. Critical review with epidemiologic insights into the prevention of disseminated disease. *Rev Infect Dis* 1989;11:755.

376. DeVault GA Jr, King JW, Rohr MS, et al. Opportunistic infection with Strongyloides stercoralis in renal transplantation. *Rev Infect Dis* 1990;12:653.

377. Churg J, Bernstein J, Glassock RJ. *Renal disease,* 2nd ed. Tokyo: Igaku-Shoin Medical Publishers, 1995:234.

378. Dent JH, Nichols RI, Beaver PC, et al. Visceral larval migrans. *Am J Pathol* 1956;32:777.

379. Westendorp RG, Doorenbos CJ, Thompson J, et al. Immune complex glomerulonephritis associated with an amebic liver abscess. *Trans R Soc Trop Med Hyg* 1990;84:385.

380. Chugh KS, Sakhuja V. Renal failure from snake bites. *Int J Artif Organs* 1980;3:319.

381. Minton SA, ed. *Snake venoms and envenomation.* New York: Marcel Dekker Inc, 1971.

382. Chugh KS. Snake bite induced renal failure in India. *Kidney Int* 1989;35:891.

383. Chugh KS, Aikat BK, Sharma BK, et al. Acute renal failure following snake bite. *Am J Trop Med Hyg* 1975;24:692.

384. Visuvaratnam M, Vinayagamoorthy C, Balakrishnam S. Venomous snake bites in North Ceylon. *J Trop Med Hyg* 1970;73:9.

385. Chugh KS, Pal Y, Chakravarty RN, et al. Pathogenesis of renal lesions in snake bites. *Proc 2nd Asian Pacific Congress Nephrol* 1983:183.

386. Han HE, Than T, Lwin M, et al. Urinary fibrin(ogen) degradation products in Russell's viper (Daboia russelli siamensis) bite victims. *Southeast Asian J Trop Med Public Health* 1993;24:198.

387. Warrell DA, Pope HM, Prentice CRM. Disseminated intravascular coagulation caused by the carpet viper (Echis carinatum) trial of heparin. *Br J Haematol* 1976;33:335.

388. Steinbeck VW. Nephrotic syndrome developing after snake bite. *Med J Aust* 1960;1:543.

389. Date A, Shastry JCM. Renal ultrastructure in cortical necrosis following Russell's viper envenomation. *J Trop Med Hyg* 1981;84:3.

390. Schmidt ME, Abdelbaki YZ, Tu AT. Nephrotoxic action of rattlesnake and sea snake venom. An electron-microscopic study. *J Pathol* 1976;118:75.

391. Shastry JC, Date A, Carman RH, et al. Renal failure following snake bite. A clinicopathological study of nineteen patients. *Am J Trop Med Hyg* 1977;26:1032.

392. Sitprija V, Benyajati C, Boonpucknavig V. Further observations of renal insufficiency in snake bite. *Nephron* 1974;13:396.

393. Sitprija V, Boonpucknavig V. The kidney in tropical snake bite. *Clin Nephrol* 1977;8:377.

394. Varagunam T, Panaboke RG. Bilateral cortical necrosis of the kidneys following snake bite. *Postgrad Med J* 1970;46:449.

395. Date A, Shastry JCM. Renal ultrastructure in acute tubular necrosis following Russell's viper envenomation. *J Pathol* 1982;137:225.

396. Sitprija V, Suvanpha R, Pochanugool C, et al. Acute interstitial nephritis in snake bite. *Am J Trop Med Hyg* 1982;31:408.

397. Acharya VN, Khanna UB, Almeida AF, et al. Acute renal failure due to viperine snake bite as seen in tropical western India. *Renal Fail* 1989;11:33.

398. Seedat YK, Reddy J, Edington DA. Acute renal failure due to proliferative nephritis from snake bite poisoning. *Nephron* 1974;13:455.

399. Sitprija V. Glomerular changes in tropical viper bite in man. *Toxicon* 1988;21:400.

400. Sitprija V, Boonpucknavig V. Extracapillary proliferative glomerulonephritis in Russell's viper bite. *Br Med J* 1980;280:1417.

401. Reid HA. Myoglobinuria and sea snake bite poisoning. *Br Med J (Clin Res)* 1961;1:1284.

402. Sitprija V, Sribhibhadh R, Benyajati C. Hemodialysis in poisoning by sea snake venom. *Br Med J (Clin Res)* 1971;3:218.

403. Chugh KS, Ganguly NK, Pal Y. Complement depletion following envenomation by Russell's viper and Echis carinatum venom in the Rhesus monkey. *Am J Trop Med Hyg* 1977;25:1039.

404. Chugh KS, Mohanthi D, Pal Y, et al. Coagulation abnormalities induced by Russell's viper venom in Rhesus monkey. *Am J Trop Med Hyg* 1979;28:763.

405. Nicholson JC, Ashby PA, Johnson ND, et al. Boomslang bite with haemorrhage and activation of complement by alternate pathway. *Clin Exp Immunol* 1976;16:295.

406. Warrell DA, Greenwood BM, Davidson NM, et al. Necrosis, hemorrhage and complement depletion following bites by spitting cobra. *Q J Med* 1976;45:1.

407. Tantawichien T, Khow O, Napathorn S, et al. Russell's viper venom induces cytokine secretion by human monocyte-derived macrophages. *5th Asia-Pacific Congress on Animal, Plant and Microbial Toxins; Pattaya, Thailand.* 1999:54(abst).

408. Thamaree S, Sitprija V, Leepipatpaiboon S, et al. Mediators and renal hemodynamics in Russell's viper envenomation. *J Nat Toxicol* 2000;9:43.

409. Sitprija V, Chaiyabutr N. Nephrotoxicity in snake envenomation. *J Nat Toxicol* 1999;8:271.

410. Chaiyabutr N, Sitprija V. Pathophysiological effects of Russell's viper venom on renal function. *J Nat Toxicol* 1999;8:351.

411. Ratcliff PJ, Pukrittayakamee S, Ledingham JGG, et al. Direct nephrotoxicity of Russell's viper venom demonstrated in the isolated perfused rat kidney. *Am J Trop Med Hyg* 1987;40:312.

412. Willingen CC, Thamaree S, Schramek H, et al. In vitro nephrotoxicity of Russell's viper venom. *Kidney Int* 1995;47:518.

413. Danzig LE, Abels GH. Hemodialysis for acute renal failure following rattle snake bite with recovery. *JAMA* 1961;175:136.

414. Ponraj D, Gopalakrishnakone P. Renal lesions in rhabdomyolysis caused by Pseudechis australis snake myotoxin. *Kidney Int* 1997;51:1956.

415. Sitprija V, Gopalakrishnakone P. Snake bite, rhabdomyolysis and renal failure. *Am. J Kidney Dis* 1998;31:1.

416. Mathai TP, Date A. Treatment and followup of cases of acute renal failure following snake bite. *9th Int Congress Nephrol.* Los Angeles, 1984(abst).

417. Da Silva OH, Lopez M, Godoy P. Bilateral cortical necrosis and calcification of the kidneys following snake bite: a case report. *Clin Nephrol* 1979;11:136.

418. Kaplinsky C, Frand M, Rubin Stein ZJ. Disseminated intravascular clotting and renal cortical necrosis complicating a snake bite. *Clin Pediatr (Philadelphia)* 1980;19:229.

419. Elming H, Solling K. Urine protein excretion after Hymenoptera sting. *Scand J Urol Nephrol* 1994;28:13.

420. Barss P. Renal failure and death after multiple stings in Papua New Guinea. Ecology, prevention and management of attacks by vespid wasps. *Med J Aust* 1989;151:659.

421. Cuoghi D, Venturi P, Cheli E. Bee sting and relapse of nephrotic syndrome. *Child Nephrol Urol* 1988;9:82.

422. Olivero JJ, Ayus JC, Eknoyan G. Nephrotic syndrome developing after bee stings. *South Med J* 1982;74:82.

423. Rytand DA. Onset of the nephrotic syndrome during a reaction to bee sting. *Standford Med Bull* 1955;13:224.

424. Sensirivatana R, Sukvichai P, Futrakul P. Nephrotic syndrome following a bee sting. *J Med Assoc Thai* 1984;67:525.

425. Tareyeva IE, Nikolaev AJ, Janushkevitch TN. Nephrotic syndrome induced by insect sting. *Lancet* 1982;2:825.

426. Tumwine JK, Nkrumah FK. Acute renal failure and dermal necrosis due to bee stings: report of case in a child. *Central Afr Med J* 1990;36:202.

427. Chugh KS, Sharma BK, Singhal PC. Acute renal failure following hornet stings. *J Trop Med Hyg* 1976;79:42.

428. Pirotsky E, Hieblot C, Benveniste J, et al. Basophil sensitization in idiopathic nephrotic syndrome. *Lancet* 1982;1:358.

429. Hyre HM, Smith RA. Immunological effects of honey bee (Apis mellifera) venom using BALB/c mice. *Toxicon* 1986;24:435.

430. Hoh TK, Soong CL, Cheng CT. Fatal haemolysis from wasp and hornet sting. *Singapore Med J* 1966;7:122.

431. Huang CC, Au C, Chen L, et al. Acute renal failure and hepatic injury following multiple wasp stings. Report of 2 cases. *J Formosan Med Assoc* 1983;82:623.

432. Laosombat V, Chub-uppakarn S. Acute renal failure following wasp sting. *J Med Assoc Thai* 1982;65:511.

433. Sitprija V, Boonpucknavig V. Renal failure and myonecrosis following wasp stings. *Lancet* 1972;1:749.

434. Korman SH, Jabbour S, Harari MD. Multiple hornet (Vespa orientalis) stings with fatal outcome in a child. *J Pediatr Child Health* 1994;26:283.

435. Sakhuja V, Bhalla A, Pereira BJ, et al. Acute renal failure following multiple hornet stings. *Nephron* 1988;49:319.

436. Humblet Y, Sonnet J, Van Ypersel de Strihou C. Bee stings and acute tubular necrosis. *Nephron* 1982;31:187.

437. Ramanathan M, Lam HS. Acute renal failure due to multiple bee stings: case reports. *Med J Malaysia* 1990;45:344.

438. Park SK, Kim DG, Kang SK, et al. Toxic acute renal failure and hepatitis after ingestion of raw carp bile. *Nephron* 1990;56:188.

439. Chen WY, Yen TS, Cheng JT, et al. Acute renal failure due to raw bile of grass carp (Ctenopharyngodon idellus). *J Med Assoc Thai* 1978;61:63.

440. Lin CT, Huang PC, Yen TS, et al. Partial purification and some characteristic nature of a toxic fraction of the grass carp bile. *Chin Biochem Soc* 1977;6:1.

441. Lim DC, Hessinger DA. Possible involvement of red cell membrane proteins in the haemolytic action of Portuguese Man of War toxin. *Biochem Biophys Res Com* 1979;91:761.

442. Spielman FJ, Bowe EA, Watson CB, et al. Acute renal failure as a result of Physalia physalis sting. *South Med J* 1982;75:1425.

443. Poon-King T. Myocarditis from scorpion stings. *Br Med J* 1963;1:374.

444. Waterman JA. Some notes on scorpion poisoning in Trinidad. *Trans R Soc Trop Med Hyg* 1993;32:607.

445. Reddy CRRM, Suvarnakumar G, Devi CS, et al. Pathology of scorpion venom poisoning. *J Trop Med Hyg* 1972;75:98.

446. Kibukamusoke JW, Chugh KS, Sakhuja V. Renal Effects of Envenomation. In: Kibukamusoke JW, ed. *Tropical nephrology.* Canberra, Australia: Citforge Ltd, 1984.

447. Taylor EH, Denny WF. Hemolysis, renal failure and death presumed secondary to bite of brown recluse spider. *S Afr Med J* 1966;59:1209.

448. Gomes A, Datta A, Sarangi B, et al. Isolation purification and pharmacodynamics of a toxin from the venom of the centipede Scolopendra subspinipes dehaani Brandt. *Indian J Exp Biol* 1983;21:203.

449. Logan JL, Ogden DA. Rhabdomyolysis and acute renal failure following the bite of the giant desert centipede, Scolopendra heros. *West. J. Med* 1985;142:549.

450. Arocha-Pinango CL, Layrisse M. Fibrinolysis produced by contact with a caterpillar. *Lancet* 1969;1:810.

451. Arocha-Pinango CL, de Bosch NB, Torres A, et al. Six new cases of a caterpillar- induced bleeding disorder. *Thromb Haemost* 1992;67:402.

452. Burdmann EA, Antunes I, Saldanha LB, et al. Severe acute renal failure induced by the venom of Lonomia caterpillars. *Clin Nephrol* 1996;40:337.

453. Duarte A, Walter G, Barros E, et al. Insuficiencia renal aguda por accidentes com lonomia obliqua. *Nephrol Latinoam* 1994;1:38.

454. Eiam-Ong S, Sitprija V. Tropical plant-associated nephropathy. *Nephrology* 1998;4:313.

455. Areekul S, Kirdudom P. Studies on the chemical components and toxic substances in Niang beans. *J Med Assoc Thai* 1977;60:3.

456. Areekul S, Muangman V, Bohkerd C. Djenkol bean as a cause of urolithiasis. *Southeast Asian J Trop Med Public Health* 1978;9:427.

457. Eiam-Ong S, Sitprija V, Saetang P, et al. Djenkol bean nephrotoxicity in Southern Thailand. *Proc First Asian Pacific Congress Animal, Plant and Microbial Toxins.* Singapore, 1987:628.

458. H'ng PK, Nayar SK, Lau WM, et al. Acute renal failure following jering ingestion. *Singapore Med J* 1991;32:148.

459. Reimann HA, Sukaton RV. Djenkol bean poisoning (djenkolism), a cause of hematuria and anuria. *Am J Med Sci* 1956;232:172.

460. West CE, Perrin DD, Shaw DC, et al. Djenkol bean poisoning (djenkolism): Proposal for treatment and prevention. *Southeast Asian J Trop Med Public Health* 1973;4:564.

461. Bye BN, Coetzer TH, Dutton MF. An enzyme immunoassay for atractyloside, the nephrotoxin of Callilepis laureola (Impila). *Toxicon* 1990;28:997.

462. Seedat YK, Hitchcock PJ. Acute renal failure from Callilepis laureola. *S Afr Med J* 1971;54:82.

463. Wainwright J, Schonland MM, Candy HA. Toxicity of Callilepis laureola. *S Afr Med J* 1977;52:313.

464. Watson AR, Coovadia HM, Bhoola KD. The clinical syndrome of Impila (Callilepis laurcola) poisoning in children. *S Afr Med J* 1979;55:190.

465. Matthai TP, Date A. Renal cortical necrosis following exposure to sap of the marking-nut tree (Semecarpus anacardium). *Am J Trop Med Hyg* 1979;28:773.

466. McClain JL, Hause DW, Clark MA. Amanita phalloides mushroom poisoning: a cluster of four fatalities. *J Forensic Sci* 1989;34:83.

467. Prast H, Pfaller W. Toxic properties of the mushroom Cortinarius orellanus (Fries) II. Impairment of renal function in rats. *Arch Toxicol* 1988;62:89.

468. Lahtipara S, Naukkarinen A, Collan Y. Mushroom poisoning due to Cortinarius speciosissimus: electron microscope study in rats. *Arch Toxicol* 1986;9[Suppl]:315.

469. Wang C, Yeung RTT. Gossypol and hypokalemia. *Contraception* 1985;32:237.

470. Gao H, Yang JT, Chang YT, et al. Gossypol in cotton seeds causes distal renal tubular acidosis: a preliminary observation in 177 patients. *Chin Med J* 1985;24:419.

471. Gold CH. Acute renal failure from herbal and patient remedies in Blacks. *Clin Nephrol* 1980;14:128.

472. Lowenthal MN, Jones IG, Mohelsky V. Acute renal failure in Zambia women using traditional herbal medicine. *J Trop Med Hyg* 1974;77:196.

473. Cosyns JP, Jadoul M, Squifflet JP, et al. Chinese herb nephropathy: a clue to Balkan endemic nephropathy? *Kidney Int* 1994;45:1860.

474. Cosyns JP, Jadoul M, Sqifflet JP, et al. Urothelial lesions in Chinese-herb nephropathy. *Am J Kidney Dis* 1999;33:1011.

475. Li P, Kawachi H, Suzuki Y, et al. The prevention of glomerulosclerosis in rats using traditional Chinese medicine, Sairei-to. *Nephrology* 2000;5:83.

476. Tungsanga K, Sitprija V, Suvanpha R, et al. Paraquat poisoning: experience in fourteen patients. *J Med Assoc Thai* 1981;64:215.

477. Newhouse M, McEvoy D, Rosenthalk D. Percutaneous paraquat absorption. An association with cutaneous lesions and respiratory failure. *Arch Dermatol* 1978;114:1516.

478. Oreopoulos DE, Soyannwo MA, Sinniah R, et al. Acute renal failure in case of paraquat poisoning. *Br Med J* 1968;1:740.

479. Proudfoot A, Stewart MS, Levitt T, et al. Paraquat poisoning: significance of plasma paraquat concentration. *Lancet* 1979;2:330.

480. Fisher HK, Humphries M, Balls R. Paraquat poisoning: recovery from renal and pulmonary damage. *Ann Intern Med* 1971;75:731.

481. Okonek S, Hofmann A, Henningsen B. Efficacy of gut lavage, haemodialysis, and haemoperfusion in the therapy of paraquat or diaquat intoxication. *Arch Toxicol* 1976;36:43.

482. Addo E, Poon-King T. Leukocyte suppression in treatment of 72 patients with paraquat poisoning. *Lancet* 1986;1:1117.

483. Chuttani HK, Gupta PS, Gulati S, et al. Acute copper sulfate poisoning. *Am J Med* 1965;39:849.

484. Metz EN. Mechanism of haemolysis by excess copper. *Clin Res* 1969;17:32(abst).

485. Fairbanks VF. Copper sulphate-induced haemolytic anemia. *Arch Intern Med* 1967;120:428.

486. Chugh KS, Singhal PC, Sharma BK. Methemoglobinemia in acute copper sulfate poisoning. *Ann Intern Med* 1975;82:226.

487. Okuonghae HO, Ighogboja IS, Lawson JO, et al. Diethylene glycol poisoning in Nigerian children. *Ann Trop Pediatr* 1992;12:235.

488. Hanif M, Mobarak MR, Ronan A, et al. Fatal renal failure caused by diethylene glycol in paracetamol elixir: the Bangladesh epidemic. *BMJ* 1995;311:88.

489. O'Brien KL, Selanikio JD, Hecdivert C, et al. Epidemic of pediatric deaths from acute renal failure caused by diethylene glycol poisoning. *JAMA* 1998;279:1175.

490. Naqvi SAJ. Regional problems in Pakistan-most prevalent kidney diseases and related problems. *Proceed 8th Colloquium in Nephrol.* Jakarta, 1989:283.

491. Robertson WG. The role of environment in the pathogeneses of renal stones. In: Mochizuki M, Sugino N, Sitprija V, eds. *Geographic nephrology.* Kobe: International Center for Medical Research, 1990.

492. Better OS, Shabtai M, Kedar S, et al. Increased incidence of nephrolithiasis in lifeguards in Israel. *Adv Exp Med Biol* 1980;128:487.

493. Sriboonlue P, Prasongwatana V, Chata K, et al. Prevalence of upper urinary tract stone disease in a rural community of Northeastern Thailand. *Br J Urol* 1992;69:240.

494. Tosukhowong P, Tungsanga K, Sriboonlue P, et al. Hypocitraturia and hypokaluria in renal stone farmers from northeastern Thailand: uncommon association with distal renal tubular acidosis. *J Nephrol* 1991;4:227.

495. Tosukhowong P, Tungsanga K, Kittinantavorakoon C, et al. Low erythrocyte Na/K pump activity and number in northeast Thailand adults: evidence suggesting an acquired disorder. *Metabolism* 1996; 45:804.

496. Tosukhowong P, Chotikasatit C, Tungsanga K, et al. Abnormal erythrocyte Na,K- ATPase activity in northeastern Thai population. *S Asian J Trop Med Public Health* 1992;23:526.

497. Tungsanga K, Sriboonlue P. Sudden unexplained death syndrome in northeast Thailand. *Int J Epidemiol* 1993;22:81.

498. Tosukhowong P, Chotigasatit C, Tungsanga K, et al. Hypokalemia, high erythrocyte Na and low erythrocyte Na,K-ATPase in relatives of patients dying from sudden unexplained death syndrome in

northeast Thailand and in survivors from near fatal attacks. *Am J Nephrol* 1996;16:369.

499. Sitprija V, Tungsanga K, Eiam-Ong S, et al. Metabolic syndrome caused by decreased activity of ATPases. *Semin Nephrol* 1991;11:249.

500. Nilwarangkur S, Nimmannit S, Chaovakul V, et al. Endemic primary distal renal tubular acidosis in Thailand. *Q J Med* 1990;74:289.

501. Sitprija V, Eiam-Ong S, Suvanapha R, et al. Gastric hypoacidity in distal renal tubular acidosis. *Nephron* 1988;50:395.

502. Tosukhowong P, Tungsanga K, Eiam-Ong S, et al. Environmental distal renal tubular acidosis in Thailand: an enigma. *Am J Kidney Dis* 1999;33:1180.

503. Vasuvattakul S, Yenchitsomanus PT, Vachuanichsanong P, et al. Autosomal recessive distal renal tubular acidosis associated with Southeast Asian ovalocytosis. *Kidney Int* 1999;56:1674.

504. Essamie MA, Soliman A, Fayad TM, et al. Serious renal disease in Egypt. *Int J Artif Organs* 1995;18:254.

505. Mani M. Chronic renal failure in India. *Nephrol Dial Transplant* 1993;8:684.

506. Rashid HU, Ahmed S, Rahman M, et al. Experience of hemodialysis in Bangaladesh. *The 1st Int Congress Dial Develop Countries.* Singapore, 1994:44.

507. Abboud O. Nephrology in the Sudan. *Proc ISN Afr Kid Electrolyte Conference.* Cairo: Cairo University Press, 1987:157.

508. Mtabaji JP, Kitinya J. Diseases of the kidney and urinary tract in Tanzania: a case for more comprehensive renal services. *Proc ISN African Kidney Electrolyte Conference.* Cairo: Cairo University Press, 1987:167.

509. Logothetopoulos J, Weinbren K. Naturally occurring protein droplets in the proximal tubule of the rat's kidney. *Br J Exp Pathol* 1955;36:402.

510. US Environmental Protection Agency. Alpha 2u globulin: association with chemically induced renal toxicity and neoplasia in the male rat. Washington, DC: U.S EPA/625/3-01/019F, 1991.

511. Kasai H, Nishimura S, Kurokawa Y, et al. Oral administration of the renal carcinogen, potassium bromate, specifically produces. β hydroxydeoxyguanosine in rat target organ DNA. *Carcinogenesis* 1987;8:1959.

512. Curvall M, Enzell C, Petersson B. An evaluation of the utility of four in vitro short- term tests for predicting the cytotoxicity of individual compounds derived from tobacco smoke. *Cell Biol Toxicol* 1984;1:173.

513. Florin I, Rutberg L, Curvall M, et al. Screening of tobacco smoke constituents for malignancy using the Ames test. *Toxicology* 1980;15:219.

514. Iscovich J, Castelletto R, Esteve J, et al. Tobacco smoking, occupational exposure and bladder cancer in Argentina. *Int J Cancer* 1987;40:734.

515. MacFarland HN. Toxicology of petroleum hydrocarbons. *Occup Med* 1988;3:445.

516. Bruner R. Pathologic findings in laboratory animals exposed to hydrocarbon fuels of military interest. In: Mehiman MA, ed. *Advances in modern environmental toxicology, renal effects of petroleum. Hydrocarbons.* Princeton: Princeton Scientific, 1984:133.

517. Philips RD, Cockrell BY. Effect of certain light hydrocarbons on kidney function and structure in male rats. In: Mehlman MA, ed. *Advances in Modern Environmental Toxicology, Renal Effects of Petroleum Hydrocarbons* Princeton: Princeton Scientific, 1984:89.

518. Van Esch GJ, Kroes R. The induction of renal tumors by feeding basic lead acetate to mice and hamsters. *Br J Cancer* 1969;23:765.

519. Paganini-Hill A, Glazer E, Henderson BE, et al. Case-specific mortality among newspaper web pressman. *J Occup Med* 1980;22:542.

520. Kolonel LW. Association of cadmium with renal cancer. *Cancer* 1976;37:1782.

521. Maclure M. Asbestos and renal adenocarcinoma. A case-control study. *Environ Res* 1987;42:353.

522. Furahashi T. Twenty-eight day oral subacute toxicity study on Dunaliella bardawil. Nihon Research Center, Inc, Hashima, Gifu, Japan. As submitted to WHO by Nikken Sohonsha Corporation, Hashima City, Japan 1989.

523. Perrin JH, Field FP, Hansen DA, et al. Beta-cyclodextrin as an aid to peritoneal dialysis. Renal toxicity of b cyclodextrin in the rat. *Chem Pathol Pharmacol* 1978;373:376.

524. Hiasa Y, Lin JC, Konishi N, et al. Histopathological and biochemical analyses of transplantable renal adenocarcinoma in rats induced by N-ethyl-N-hydroxyethylnitrosamine. *Cancer Res* 1984;44:1664.

525. WHO Environmental Health Criteria No. 62. 1,2-dichloroethane. Geneva: World Health Organization, 1987.

526. Condie LW, Smallwood CL, Laurie RD. Comparative renal and hepatotoxicity of halomethanes: bromodichloromethane, bromoform,

chloroform, dibromo-chloromethane and methylene chloride. *Drug Chem Toxicol* 1983;6:563.

527. Dieter MP. Toxicology and carcinogenesis studies of alpha methylbenzyl alcohol in F344/N rats and B6C3F1 mice (gavage studies). National Toxicology Program (NTP). Triangle Park, NC: Department of Health and Human Services Research; 1990; Technical report series no 369; NIH publication no 89-2824.

528. Smyth HF, Carpenter CP, Boyd Shaffer C. Summary of toxicological data: a 2-year study of diethylene glycol monoethyl ether in rats. *Fed Chem Toxicol* 1964;2:641.

529. Miller L, Pateras V, Friederici H, et al. Acute tubular necrosis after inhalation exposure to methylene chloride. Report of a case. *Arch Intern Med* 1985;145:145.

530. Brennaas O. Forgiftning med dietylenglykolmonoetyleter [a case of intoxication due to diethylene glycol monoethyl ether]. *Nord Med* 1960;64:1219.

531. Lehman-McKeeman LD, Caudill D, Takigiku R, et al. Comparative deposition of d limonene in rats and mice: relevance to male-rat–specific nephropathy. *Toxicol Lett* 1990;53:193.

532. Flamm WG, Lehman-Mackeeman L. The human relevance of the renal tumor- inducing potential of d limonene in male rats: implications for risk assessment. *Regul Toxicol Pharmacol* 1991;13:70.

533. Kurokawa Y, Matsushima Y, Takamura N, et al. Relationship between duration of treatment and the incidence of renal cell tumors in male F344 rats administered potassium bromate. *Jpn J Cancer Res (Gann)* 1987;78:358.

534. Takamura H, Yonemura Y, Hirono Y, et al. Long-term oral administration of potassium bromate in male Syrian golden Hamsters. *Sci Rep Res Inst Tokohu University Ser-C32:43* 1985.

535. Kurokawa Y, Maekawa A, Takahashi M, et al. Toxicity and carcinogenicity of potassium bromate. A new renal carcinogen. *Environ Health Perspect* 1990;87:309.

536. Vavasour E. Saccharin and its salts. *Toxicological evaluation of certain food additives and contaminants. 41st Meeting of the Joint FAO/WHO Expert Committee on Food Additives (JECFA). International Programme on Chemical Safety.* Geneva: World Health Organization, 1993;105.

537. Bravo MP, Del Rey-Calero J. Bladder cancer and the consumption of alcoholic beverages in Spain. *Eur J Epidemiol* 1987;3:365.

538. Auerbach O, Garfinkel L. Histologic changes in the urinary bladder in relation to cigarette smoking and use of artificial sweeteners. *Cancer* 1989;64:983.

539. Elcock M, Morgan RW. Update on artificial sweeteners and bladder cancer [Unpublished report]. 1992.

540. Wayss K, Bannasch P, Mattern J, et al. Vascular liver tumors induced in Mastomys (Praomys). Natalensis by single or two fold administration of dimethylnitrosamine. *J Natl Can Inst* 1979;62:1199.

541. Kluwe WM, Gupta BN, Lamb JC IV. The comparative effects of 1,2-dibromo-3-chloropropane (DBCP) and its metabolites, 3-chloro-1,2-propaneoxide (Epichlorohydrin), 3-chloro-1,2-propanediol (alphachlorohydrin) and oxalic acid on the urogenital system of male rats. *Toxicol Appl Pharmacol* 1983;70:67.

542. Jersy GC, Breslin WJ, Zielke GJ. Subchronic toxicity of 1,3-dichloro-2-propanol in the rat. *Toxicologist* 1991;11:353.

543. World Health Organization. *Pesticide residues in food 1993. Evaluations. Part II. Toxicology. International Programme on Chemical Safety.* Geneva: World Health Organization, 1993.

544. Tada Y, Yoneyama M, Kabashima J, et al. Effects of thiabendazole on the kidneys of ICR mice. *Fed Chem Toxicol* 1989;27:307.

545. Hennekeuser HH, Pabst K, Poeplau W, et al. Thiabendazole for the treatment of trichinosis in humans. *Texas Rep Biol Med* 1969;27:581.

546. Boyd, E. M. The acute oral toxicity of spiramycin. *Can J Biochem Physiol* 1958;36:103.

547. Descotes J, Vial T, Delattre D, et al. Spiramycin: safety in man. *J Antimicrob Chemother* 1988;22:207.

548. Ritter L. Ractopamine. *Toxicological evaluation of certain veterinary drug residues in food. 40th Meeting of the Joint WHO Expert Committee on Food Additives (JECFA). International Programme on Chemical Safety.* Geneva: World Health Organization, 1993.

549. United States Renal Data System. Incidence and causes of treated ESRD. Annual data report. *Am J Kidney Dis* 1991;18 2:30.

550. Gordon D. Racial differences in ESRD. *Dial Transplant* 1990;19:114.

551. Newman JM, Marfin AA, Eggers PW, et al. End stage renal disease among Native Americans 1983–86. *Am J Public Health* 1990;80:318.

552. Chan MK. Treatment of end stage renal failure in Hong Kong. In: Tanaka H, ed. *Dialysis therapy in the 1990s. Contributions to nephrology.* Basel: Krager, 1990:25.

553. Thailand renal replacement therapy registry report. Thailand: The Nephrology Society of Thailand, 1998.

554. Aswad S. Causes of chronic renal failure in Saudi Arabia. *NKF Bull* 1986;1:8.

555. Aldrees A. A cost evaluation of hemodialysis in Ministry of Health Hospitals, Saudi Arabia. An NKF Study. *Saudi Kidney Dis Transplant Bull* 1991;2:125.

556. Raj B, Jayaraman MA. Global perspective. *Dial Transplant* 1991; 20:470.

557. Barsoum RS, Rihan ZE, Ibrahim AS, et al. Long-term intermittent heamodialysis in Egypt. *Bull World Health Organ* 1974;51:647.

558. Abdullah MS. Development of renal services in Kenya. *East Afr Med J* 1981;58:309.

559. Abboud O. Special problems and challenges with dialysis. Sudan. *Saudi Kidney Dis Transplant Bull* 1993;4:35(abst).

560. Rayane T, Haddoum E. Chronic renal failure in Algeria. Renal replacement therapy strategies and progression. *Saudi Kidney Dis Transplant Bull* 1993;4[Suppl 1]:118(abst).

561. Friedman EA, Delano BG. Can the world afford uremia therapy? *Proc VIII Int Congress Nephrol.* Athens, 1981:57.

562. Rocha H. Nefrologia no Brasil: alguns aspectos de sua evoluccao historica. *J Bras Neprologia* 1993;15:107.

563. Habte B. Nephrology in Ethiopia. *Proc Int Soc Nephrol. African Kidney Electrolyte Conference.* Cairo: Cairo University Press, 1987:159.

564. Rahman M. Morbidity and mortality of patients on maintenance hemodialysis in Bangladesh. *1st Int Congress Dial Develop Countries.* Singapore, 1994:83.

565. Chan MK. Dialysis: a global perspective. *Dial Transplant* 1991;20:463.

566. Seedat YK, Macintosh C, Subban J. Quality of life for patients in an end-stage disease program. *S Afr Med J* 1987;71:500.

567. Philibos M, Francis M, Barsoum R. The histopathologic pattern of glomerulonephritis in a single specialized center experience. *XI Egypt Congress Nephrol.* Cairo, 1992:48(abst).

568. Huraib S. Causes of endstage renal disease in Saudi Arabia. *1st Int Congress Dial Develop Countries.* Singapore, 1994:80.

569. Shohaib SA, Scringeour EM, Shaerya F. Tuberculosis in active dialysis patients in Jeddah. *Am J Nephrol* 1999;19:34.

570. Pingle A, Shakuntala RV, Chowdhry Y, et al. Presentation, treatment and outcome of tuberculosis in an Oriental population with endstage renal disease. *1st Int Congress Dial Develop Countries.* Singapore, 1994:54(abst).

571. Malhotra KK, Parashar MK, Sharma RK, et al. Tuberculosis in maintenance hemodialysis patients. Study from an endemic area. *Postgrad Med J* 1981;57:492.

572. Pazianas M, Eastwood JB, MacRae KD, et al. Racial origin and primary renal diagnosis in 771 patients with end-stage renal disease. *Nephrol Dial Transplant* 1991;6:931.

573. Roesli RMA. Prevalence of tuberculosis in chronic hemodialysis patients. *1st Int Congress Dial Develop Countries.* Singapore, 1994:54(abst).

574. Thanaletchuml K, Lee GSL, Woo KT. TB peritonitis in patients on continuous ambulatory peritoneal dialysis (CAPD). Clinical features. *1st Int Congress Dial Develop Countries.* Singapore, 1994:59(abst).

575. Barsoum R. The Egyptian transplant experience. *Transplant Proc* 1992;24.

576. Saadi MG, Hassan AA, Asaad M, et al. Salmonella-associated rejection in renal transplant recipients. *XI Int Congress Nephrol.* Tokyo, Japan: 1990(abst).

577. Raine AE, Margreiter R, Brunner FP, et al. Report on the management of renal failure in Europe 1991. *Nephrol Dial Transplant* 1992;2:7.

578. Krown SE, Metroka C, Wernz J. Kaposi sarcoma in the acquired immune deficiency syndrome. A proposal for uniform evaluation response and staging criteria. *J Clin Oncol* 1989;7:1201.

579. Sezi CL. Nephrology in Uganda. *Proceedings ISN. African Kidney Electrolyte Conference.* Cairo: Cairo University Press, 1987:174.

580. Akinsola A, Adeiekun S. Renal replacement therapy in a Nigerian nephrological practice. *II Int Congress Geogr Nephrol.* Hurghada: Egypt, 1993:67(abst).

581. Ankrah T. Nephrology in Ghana. *Proceedings of the ISN. African Kidney Electrolyte Conference.* Cairo: Cairo University Press, 1987: 186.

582. Chugh K. Morbidity and mortality burden of infections and infestations in CMD patients in developing countries. *Proc 1st Int Congress Dial Develop Countries.* Singapore, 1994 *(in press).*

583. Trevino-Becerra A. Nefroeconomia en Mexico. *Nefrologia Mexicana* 1993;14:75.

584. Woods HF. A global perspective. *Dial Transplant* 1991;20:490.

585. Barsoum R. Renal transplantation in a developing country. The Egyptian 17-year experience. *Afr J Health Sci* 1994;1:30.

586. Parsoo I, Seedat YK, Naiker S, et al. Continuous ambulatory peritoneal dialysis in South Africa. A 4-year experience. *Periton Dial Bull* 1984;4:78.

587. Barsoum R, Ramzy M, Francis M, et al. Egyptian CAPD experience Budapest: EDTA/EDTNA. *Budapest* 1986:164(abst).

588. Abu-Aisha H, Huraib S, Al. Wakeel J, et al. Attitudes towards CAPD and hemodialysis of patients who had the choice or experienced both modalities of therapy modules. *Saudi Kidney Dis Transplant Bull* 1993;4:77(abst).

589. Lee, G. S. L. E, Thanaletchuml, K, Woo, K. CAPD in Singapore. Technical survival 1980–1993. *1st Int Congress Dial Develop Countries* Singapore, 1994:55(abst).

590. Bernal-Sundiang N, Chua AT. The quality of life of hemodialysis patients in the Philippines. *1st Int Congress Dial Develop Countries* Singapore, 1994:41(abst).

591. Barton EN, King SD, Douglas LL, et al. Antibodies to hepatitis virus (HBV, HCV, HDV) and retroviruses (HIV.I & T, HTLV.I) in Jamaican hemodialysis patients. *1st Int Congress Dial Develop Countries* Singapore, 1994:86(abst).

592. Barsoum R, Kamel M, Radwan N, et al. Concomitant association of hepatitis Bs antigen and anti HBs antibody in regular hemodialysis patients. *Proc IV Int Congress Mediter Countries Chemother* 1984:958.

593. Tohamy M, Abdul Naser M, Abdul Hafez A, et al. Hepatitis C infection in hemodialysis patients and staff in Assiut renal dialysis units. *Ain Shams Med J* 1992;43:625.

594. El-Banawy S, Zaki A, Heghazi T, et al. Hepatitis C virus antibodies in hemodialysis patients. *Proc 2nd Int Congress Geogr Nephrol.* Hurghada: Egypt, 1993(abst).

595. Al-Arrayed A, Chandra S, Al-Arrayed A. Prevalence of hepatitis C antibodies in patients on chronic hemodialysis. *Saudi Kidney Dis Transplant Bull* 1993;4:72(abst).

596. Huraib S, al-Rashed R, Aldrees A, et al. High prevalence of and risk factors for hepatitis C in haemodialysis patients in Saudi Arabia: a need for new dialysis strategies. *Nephrol Dial Transplant* 1995;10:470.

597. Adela RH, Roseli RMA, Widjojo J, et al. Prevalence of hepatitis C in hemodialysis patients in Bandung, Indonesia. *1st Int Congress Dial Develop Countries* Singapore, 1994:85(abst).

598. Sja'bani M, Hw S, Widians GR, et al. Risk factors for hepatitis C seroconversion in hemodialysis patients. A follow-up study. *1st Int Congress Dial Develop Countries* Singapore, 1994:96(abst).

599. Opelz G. Collaborative transplant study report. Heidelberg: Inst Immunol Heidelberg University, 1994.

600. Terasaki PI, Cecka JM. Clinical transplants 1993. The Regents of the University of California. 1994:601.

601. Aswad S, Paul T, Edrees A, et al. The role of the national kidney foundation in cadaveric renal transplantation in Saudi Arabia. *Saudi Kidney Dis Transplant Bull* 1990;1:145.

602. Farid MT, Torki AH, Barsoum RS. Psych-social profile in related and un-related live kidney donors. *Proc 2nd Int Congress Geogr Nephrol* Hurghada: Egypt, 1993:39(abst).

603. Barsoum RS. Dialysis in developing countries. In: Jacobs C, Kjellstrand CM, Winchester JF, eds. *Replacement of renal function by dialysis.* Dordrecht: 1996:1433.

604. Barsoum R. Ethical and moral dilemmas arising from uremia therapy in the Third World. A KAP review. *Prog Artif Organs* 1986;85:89.

605. Barsoum R. Ethical problems in dialysis and transplantation: Africa. In: Kjellstrands CM, Dossetor JB, eds. *Ethical problems in dialysis and transplantation.* Dordrecht: Kluwer Academic Publishers, 1991:169.

CHAPTER 80

Kidney Disease in Children

Godfrey Clark and Cyril Chantler

Renal disease or dysfunction in children commonly has different clinical features or therapies compared with that in adults. Although many pediatric renal conditions occur in common with adults, this chapter focuses on those kidney diseases whose clinical aspects differ in or pertain to children. Chapters dealing with renal conditions that affect both age groups also should be consulted for details.

KIDNEY DEVELOPMENT

Renal Embryogenesis

Normal kidney embryogenesis relies on specific gene function in a predefined spatial and temporal sequence; genes for tissue growth factors, cell adhesion proteins, and cell cycle control molecules have all been reported to play a role in the inductive interaction between epithelium and mesenchyme during renal differentiation. For example, differential expression of cadherins is important in renal tract development (1), and renal epithelium proliferation during differentiation depends on PAX2 (2). Altered levels of expression of PAX2 may produce renal hypoplasia, cystic dysplasia, or even renal tumors. Congenital renal anomalies may arise from genetic malfunction and, occasionally, they show strong familial inheritance.

The important role played by apoptosis during kidney development in balance with growth, division, and differentiation of renal epithelial and interstitial cells, particularly the controlling influence of the cell cycle gene bcl-2, has increased our understanding of normal renal morphogenesis as well as renal dysplasia (3). These events occur in the first trimester, before fetal urine production commences at 11 to 12 weeks of gestation.

The nephrons are fully formed by 36 weeks, but those in the superficial cortex are not functionally or morphologically mature at birth. The newborn kidney contains approximately 20% of its adult complement of cells [commensurate with its

G. Clark and C. Chantler: GKT Department of Paediatric Nephrology, King's College London, Guy's Hospital, London, United Kingdom

corrected glomerular filtration rate (GFR)], and cell division continues until 6 months of age (4). The glomerulus is lined by cuboidal epithelium at birth and is less permeable than in the older child. The high renal vascular resistance before birth is associated with a low renal blood flow, and renal function *in utero* is probably important only in relation to the volume and composition of the amniotic fluid (5), which determines proper lung development. Oligohydramnios is an important sign of an infant with renal agenesis or severely dysplastic kidneys, and such infants are born with compression deformities and an easily recognized facial appearance (Fig. 80-1). Neonatal mortality associated with these conditions often is due to lung hypoplasia.

Renal blood supply develops its interrelationship with nephron structures under the influence of angiotensin II. Angiopoeitin-1, angiopoeitin-2, and their tyrosine kinase receptor tie-1 control development of the main renal vessels and, together with vascular endothelial growth factor and its receptors, direct and maintain renal and glomerular vasculature. Cortical blood flow is restricted in the newborn kidney with a 1:1 ratio between cortical and juxtamedullary nephrons, and the high vascular resistance and low blood flow are associated with a high plasma angiotensin concentration (6). The rapid increase in renal blood flow after birth correlates with a decline in circulating angiotensin levels and an increase of GFR from approximately 20 to 60 mL/minute/ 1.73 m^2 by 6 months of age as glomerular blood flow increases.

The convoluted tubule is only approximately 10% of its adult length at birth, whereas glomerular diameter is approximately a third of its adult size; however, tubular glomerular balance is substantially intact (7), although tubular immaturity may lead to clinical features of Fanconi's syndrome. Tubular functions such as urinary concentrating capacity, glucose and phosphate reabsorption, and acidifying ability are normal if allowance is made for the low GFR. There is, however, greater nephron heterogeneity so that a wide splay is apparent in glucose and bicarbonate titration curves. There is some evidence that the low GFR may be controlled by the tubular function because the rise in GFR in extremely

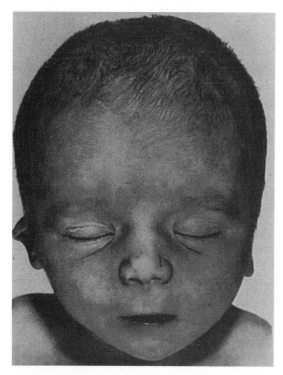

FIG. 80-1. Facial appearance of a child with renal agenesis (Potter's syndrome). (From Lieberman E. *Clinical pediatric nephrology.* Philadelphia: JB Lippincott, 1976:219, with permission.)

Functional limitations of the newborn kidney therefore are apparent mainly as a low GFR (Table 80-1) expressed in relation to kidney weight, body weight, surface area, or metabolic rate. The potential danger of a low renal capacity to maintain body composition in the face of a rapid turnover of fluid and electrolytes needs to be appreciated.

RENAL PHYSIOLOGY AND THE GROWING CHILD

The importance of the immaturity of the child and his or her kidneys and the relations between renal function, growth, nutritional requirements, and fluid and electrolyte balance are fundamental to pediatric nephrology. Normal kidney length is directly related to a child's height whether determined by ultrasound or scintigraphy (11,12); comparison with published normal ranges often is helpful when renal growth is being assessed clinically.

Infants and children have a higher metabolic rate in relation to body mass than do adults, and this is reflected by greater energy intakes and a higher turnover of fluid and electrolytes. Growth obviously contributes to this increased requirement for food and is most rapid in the first 2 years of life. The child grows 25 cm during the first year and trebles his birth weight; even during the prepubertal growth spurt the gain in height per year is only approximately a third of that achieved in the first year of life. Therefore, lack of growth in the first year of life is difficult to compensate for later in life. The main reason for this high metabolic rate is the larger proportion of body mass that consists of metabolically active organs, especially the brain (13). It is interesting that the higher energy turnover is reflected by a higher GFR in relation to body weight after the first year (Table 80-1), which obviously assists in the maintenance of body composition. This advantage is not present in the first few months because of the immature kidney, and disturbances of body composition can occur even in healthy infants fed inappropriate foods. Human milk or a modified cow's milk substitute is all that is required or should be given in the first 4 months of life in

premature infants begins only after sodium wasting ceases at a gestational age of approximately 32 weeks (8). The overall maintenance of total glomerular tubular balance obscures the differences in segmental tubular function in the neonatal kidney; specifically, the proportion of filtered sodium reabsorbed in the proximal tubule is reduced, whereas distal tubular sodium reabsorption is increased. The tubular glomerular balance, which is maintained by the low GFR and high plasma renin, angiotensin, and aldosterone levels, is precarious. Salt wasting may be apparent in the sick newborn and is common in infants whose distal tubular function is disturbed by cystic dysplasia or obstructive uropathy (9,10).

TABLE 80-1. *Glomerular filtration rate in children in relation to body size and kidney size*

Age	Kidney weight (g)	GFR mL/min	GFR/body weight (mL/min/kg)	GFR/SA (mL/min/1.73 m²) Mean	GFR/SA (mL/min/1.73 m²) Range ± 2 SD
Birth	27	2.5	0.7	20	
7 d	29	4.6	1.3	38	26–60
1 mo	32	6.4	1.6	48	28–68
6 mo	51	15.5	2.0	77	41–103
1 yr	71	28	2.9	115	49–157
2 yr	93	38	3.1	127	89–165
8 yr	149	70	2.7	127	89–165
Adult	290	131	2.1	131	88–174

GFR, glomerular filtration rate; SA, surface area.
From Oh W, Oh MA, Lind J. Renal function and blood volume in the newborn infant related to placental transfusion. *Acta Paediatr Scand* 1966;56:197; and Smith HW, et al. The application of saturation methods to the study of glomerular and tubular function in the human kidney. *J Mt Sinai Hosp* 1943;10:59.

normal infants, for it provides an adequate amount of energy, a large amount of fluid (required for an individual with high insensible losses and the inability to satisfy thirst), and an intake of other nutrients such as protein, sodium, potassium, and phosphate, which are sufficient for growth but do not provide a large excess that needs to be excreted by the kidneys.

The importance of these concepts in the management of renal failure is discussed later, but it is worth recognizing that disturbances in body composition such as uremia, acidosis, or alterations in electrolyte and volume status can occur rapidly if renal function is compromised. Even normal infants are at higher risk of renal dysfunction because the defense against infection is less well developed, so it is hardly surprising that gastroenteritis is a major cause of morbidity and mortality in infants throughout the world.

Water requirement is directly proportional to energy needs and, because metabolic rate correlates with body surface area (BSA), it is convenient to relate fluid requirements to surface area. Because 1 kilocalorie requires the consumption of 1 mL of water and basal metabolic activity requires 1,000 kcal/m^2 BSA, basal water requirement is 1 L/m^2 BSA. Normal activity increases energy needs by 50% so that the normal water requirement is 1,500 mL/m^2 BSA, of which 400 mL/m^2 BSA is for insensible losses in the nonpyrexial patient. The requirements should be increased by 12% for every degree celsius of body temperature above 37°C. BSA can be calculated from the formula BSA (m^2) = weight (kg)$^{0.5378}$ × height (cm)$^{0.3964}$ × 0.024265 (14) or can be obtained from nomograms.

An alternative method of calculating fluid requirements that avoids surface area calculations is to allow 100 mL/kg/day for the first 10 kg of body weight, 50 mL/kg/day for the next 10 kg, and 20 mL/kg/day for each kilogram over 20 kg. Insensible loss is one fourth of the total. Small or premature infants need even more fluid (Table 80-2).

It is apparent from these considerations that the fluid intake and urine output of small children is much higher in relation to body weight than for adults, and the importance of a low-solute intake in relation to energy and water intake should be appreciated. A large volume of dilute urine enables adequate conservation of water by urine concentration in response to extrarenal losses, whereas a solute intake of adult dimensions in relation to energy diminishes dilution and therefore the capacity for further urine concentration. This can easily lead to hypernatremia if excessive renal water losses occur. Sodium and potassium requirements are normally between 1 and 3 mmol/kg/day, though much of this is excreted in the urine, and intake in the oliguric child should be based on measured and estimated losses.

Relevance for Clinical Management

An infant's fluid and electrolyte status is important and the child with serious renal disease requires constant attention. The high-energy requirements are difficult to satisfy in the sick child and malnutrition can develop rapidly. Characteristically, infants and young children with chronic renal failure (CRF) are short and underweight and may never fulfill their growth potential during the three main phases of statural growth—infancy, childhood, and puberty. Nasogastric feeding or intravenous feeding with prolonged acute renal failure are used if necessary to supply an adequate energy intake. Dialysis is required earlier and more frequently to maintain body composition, and techniques such as continuous venovenous hemofiltration (15) to remove fluid and create space for energy and nutrient intake are invaluable in the catabolic child with acute renal failure in the intensive care setting. Fluid balance charts are difficult to maintain with any reliability, and by far the most useful parameter in clinical management is frequent weighing combined with a clinical assessment of the state of hydration and blood volume judged by the venous pressure, blood pressure, and toe temperature (see later).

In hyperosmolar dehydration, the normal signs of reduced skin turgor are absent because the water loss is largely intracellular; the child is irritable, the mucous membranes

TABLE 80-2. *Basal metabolic rate, body losses, and fluid requirements at different ages*

Age	Height (cm)	Weight (kg)	Surface area (m^2)	Basal energy (kcal)	Recommended energy intake (kcal)	Insensible fluid loss (mL/kg)	Normal water requirement (mL/kg)
1 wk	50	3.5	0.21	170	420	30	150
1 mo	54	4.0	0.23	210	476	30	
6 mo	66	7.7	0.35	430	850	30	150
1 yr	70	9.7	0.42	560	1,143	29	130
4 yr	101	16.4	0.68	760	1,592	23	110
12 yr	145	39	1.27	1,250	2,490	14	65
Adult	170	62	1.73	1,640	2,800	11	35

Note: 1 kcal = 4.18 kilojoules.
Data for basal energy from Talbot FB. Basal metabolism standards for children. *Am J Dis Child* 1938;55:455. Data for recommended daily allowance from Department of Health and Social Security. *Recommended intakes of nutrients for the United Kingdom*. Reports of Public Health and Medical Subjects, no. 120. London: HM Stationery Office, 1969; and Department of Health and Social Security. *Recommended daily amounts of food, energy, and nutrients for groups of people in the United Kingdom*. London: HM Stationery Office, 1979.

usually are parched, and the eyes are sunken. Extra fluid losses in vomitus and diarrhea may be considerable in proportion to body mass. Furthermore, infants lose heat extremely rapidly and constant attention to the thermal environment is imperative.

Two considerations are important in relation to drug therapy. The volume of distribution is determined by the body weight so that the loading dose can be calculated accordingly. The maintenance dose, however, is determined by the turnover or metabolic rate that correlates with the surface area rather than body weight and is therefore higher in relation to weight than for adults. If a constant blood level is required without large peaks, the drug must be administered more frequently than for an adult. Table 80-2 shows the surface area of children of different ages and body weight and, if the adult dose of the drug is known, it can be used to calculate the dose for a child if these considerations are kept in mind.

Because of the special metabolic requirements of this age group and the psychological vulnerability of the child and family, all operations and investigations should be planned with these considerations in mind. Precedence should be accorded to children when planning operating lists.

IDENTIFICATION AND INVESTIGATION OF RENAL DISEASE IN CHILDREN

Serious disease of the kidneys is rare in children and thus frequently is unsuspected until considerable damage has occurred. Congenital abnormalities of the urinary tract frequently are detected by prenatal fetal ultrasound (16), but routine abdominal palpation of all neonates should be performed and has led to an estimated incidence of abnormalities of 0.5% (17).

Imaging

The routine examination of pregnant women with views of the major organs of the fetus has led to the antenatal detection of congenital renal anomalies in 15 per 10,000 live births (Table 80-3); upper renal tract dilatation has been reported to occur in as many as 1 per 100 pregnancies. Fetal renal ultrasonography is accurate in detecting the number, size, and position of the kidneys, upper and lower tract dilatation, and liquor volume. It is reasonably good at revealing qualitative differences in renal echogenicity that may provide useful information about the presence of renal lesions, such as

TABLE 80-3. *Prevalence of congenital renal tract anomalies*

Anomaly	Rate per 10,000 births
Renal agenesis/dysplasia	4.7
Renal tract obstruction	8.0
Bladder or urethral obstruction	2.3
Exstrophy of bladder	0.3

From Schulman J, Edmonds LD, et al. Surveillance for and comparison of birth defects prevalences in two geographic areas—United States 1983–1988. *MMWR Mor Mortal Wkly Rep* 1993;42:1.

dysplasia and cysts (18). It provides little information about renal function so should not be relied on to give prognostic information to parents.

Detection of renal abnormalities antenatally allows the early proper investigation of the renal tract postnatally. In this way, obstructive uropathy can be relieved and antibiotic prophylaxis can be commenced immediately after the birth before serious urinary infection (19). It is hoped that early diagnosis will improve the long-term prognosis of these children, especially that of boys with congenital urethral valves. Drainage of the urinary tract can be accomplished *in utero* by inserting a suprapubic bladder catheter to drain the urine into the amniotic fluid. There is as yet no clear evidence that this modifies the outcome for renal function (20), and an accurate diagnosis is required if the fetus with a dilated but nonobstructed urinary tract is not to be placed at risk (16). Unfortunately, the hope that severe pulmonary hypoplasia, which so often is a fatal complication of severe urinary tract obstruction, could be prevented by early drainage *in utero* has not been sustained. This is not surprising because it is likely that the intervention would have to occur before the 16th week of gestation if pulmonary growth was to be enhanced (21).

Neonates and infants usually are investigated by renal tract ultrasound and micturating cystourography. The importance of detecting obstructive posterior urethral valves in boys and vesicoureteric reflux (VUR) in girls underlies the need for routine examination of the bladder for any infant with suspected renal tract anomalies (see Urinary Tract Infection, later).

Radiologic imaging in older children relies primarily on renal ultrasonography and radioisotope imaging. Intravenous urograms are used much less frequently today. Micturating cystourograms are still required to diagnose the grade of VUR, but indirect nuclide cystograms using ^{99m}Tc-mercaptotriacetylglycine (^{99m}Tc-MAG3) may be used in older children who can void at will to detect ongoing VUR. Computed tomography scanning and magnetic resonance imaging of the abdomen provide high-resolution imaging of the kidneys and renal tract in cases of pyelonephritis, tumors, or cysts (22), as well as defining spine and spinal cord anatomy, which is useful because obstructive uropathy and bladder dysfunction can coexist.

In addition to providing the information seen with antenatal ultrasound scanning, Doppler ultrasonography may demonstrate high-velocity arterial flow due to arterial narrowing from renal artery stenosis or middle aortic syndrome, renal venous blood flow in suspected cases of infantile renal venous thrombosis, and renal parenchymal perfusion abnormalities. Renal scarring may be identified by renal ultrasound scanning, particularly in the older child or when the scars are large or the kidney small and irregular, but it should not be used as the sole method to detect reflux nephropathy in infants because false-negative results occur in 11% (23). ^{99m}Tc-Dimercaptosuccinic acid (^{99m}Tc-DMSA) is more sensitive than renal ultrasound in detecting scars.

Scintigraphy with ^{99m}Tc-MAG3 provides dynamic and functional data in suspected obstructive uropathy and exposes the child to approximately one-third less radiation than ^{99m}Tc-diethylenetriaminepentaacetic acid (^{99m}Tc-DTPA) scanning; its use in children has superseded the latter.

Renal Function Tests

The measurement of renal function in children is difficult for two reasons. First, children hate blood tests, and the association of painful investigations with hospitals can dominate their reactions to doctors and nurses for years. Blood tests should be kept to a minimum. Never tell a child that it will not hurt because it always does. Instead, explain that the pain will be momentary and encourage one of the parents to be present; inducing anesthesia at the site of venipuncture by the use of local anesthetic creams or ethyl chloride spray may make procedure more acceptable. Always ask for help if the blood access is difficult because success is more likely when the child is not struggling and immobile; completing the procedure quickly also subjects the child to less physical and psychological trauma. Therefore, always ensure that the circumstances are propitious, that the child is comfortably warm and properly held, and that sufficient distractions are present to consume his or her interest.

Second, timed urine collections are difficult to obtain. They require constant supervision, although they can be obtained even in neonates. A plastic perineal bag properly applied can be kept empty by draining the urine as it is passed through a catheter placed in the plastic bag, which passes to a collecting vessel kept under constant low negative pressure (8). In practice, this is rarely required because most aspects of renal function can be measured without timed urine collection by factoring the measured substance by the urinary creatinine to account for differences in GFR.

Glomerular Filtration Rate

An assessment of GFR is the single most important test of renal function required in clinical practice. The 24-hour endogenous creatinine clearance is used most frequently in adults, but the urine collections usually are unreliable in infants and children. The 24-hour urine excretion of creatinine is a measure of creatinine production that is related to muscle mass and in turn correlates with the cube of height in boys and girls from the age of 6 months to maturity (24). Because GFR correlates with BSA or the square of height, it follows that GFR corrected for SA is related to height. Thus,

$$GFR = \frac{UcV}{Pc}$$

$$UcV \propto height^3$$

$$GFR \propto height^2$$

$$\frac{GFR}{BSA} \propto \frac{height}{Pc} \quad or \quad \frac{GFR}{BSA} = \frac{k(height)}{Pc}$$

where V is urine flow rate and Uc and Pc are the urine and plasma concentrations of creatinine, respectively. The value

for the constant k has been empirically derived (25–27). Thus,

$$GFR\,(mL/minute/1.73\ m^2) = 40 \times height\ (cm)/Pc\ (\mu mol/L)$$

or

$$GFR\,(mL/minute/1.73\ m^2) = 0.55 \times height\ (cm)/Pc\,(mg/dL)$$

when using automated methods for the measurement of plasma creatinine. The different relation of muscle mass to height in infants younger than 1 year and in adolescent boys results in k values of 0.45 and 0.7, respectively, when plasma creatinine is measured as milligrams per deciliter (27). Estimates of GFR from the height and plasma creatinine are more reliable than the 24-hour endogenous clearance in children and obviously are more convenient, and reliably detect a change in GFR of more than 19 mL/minute/1.73 m² (26). Obviously, the method is unreliable when body composition is severely disturbed and the normal relation between muscle mass and height is altered. Plasma creatinine concentration averages 0.88 mg/dL at birth, when the level is largely determined by the mother's plasma creatinine concentration. It falls to a nadir of 0.45 mg/dL at 2 years as GFR increases and then rises with the increase in muscle mass to 0.72 mg/dL at 12 years and 1.1 mg/dL in adult men. Therefore, it is apparent that the plasma creatinine can be used as a measure of GFR only if the normal values for children of different sizes are known or if the height correction to calculate GFR is applied.

The plasma creatinine provides a useful screening test for GFR, but like the 24-hour endogenous creatinine clearance, it does not provide an accurate measurement (28). More precision may be obtained by performing 3-hour creatinine clearance determinations under diuretic conditions or single-injection plasma clearance estimations using ^{51}Cr ethylenediaminetetraacetic acid, sodium iothalamate (29), or inulin (30). The single-injection method is particularly useful in children because the GFR is computed from the plasma decay curve and no urine collections are required (31).

Proteinuria

Quantitative assessment of albuminuria in children is affected by the unreliability of urine collections. However, its main purpose is to detect damage to the glomerular filter leading to increased permeability, and for this purpose the most sensitive parameter is the sieving coefficient (the relative concentration in glomerular filtrate and plasma water) of a molecule of a size that normally is just restrained by the glomerular filter. The albumin–creatinine clearance ratio or the fractional excretion of albumin provides a suitable approximation for use in clinical practice; being a ratio, it is independent of urine flow rate and can be estimated from a random urine and a coincident plasma sample. Thus,

$$Ca = \frac{UaV}{Pa}$$

$$Cc = \frac{UcV}{Pc}$$

$$\frac{Ca}{Cc} = \frac{Ua/Pa}{Uc/Pc}$$

where *Ua, Pa,* and *Ca* are urine concentration, plasma concentration, and clearance of albumin, respectively, and *Uc, Pc,* and *Cc* are urine concentration, plasma concentration, and clearance of creatinine, respectively; *V* is urine flow rate.

Most of the variation in Ca/Cc occurs in the urine concentration terms so that Ca/Cc may be predicted from the urine albumin–creatinine concentration ratio (mg/mg). A value of less than 0.1 is considered normal, 0.1 to 1.0 is mild, 1.0 to 10.0 is moderate, and over 10.0 is considered heavy proteinuria. The use of this ratio is preferred for children rather than the commonly performed 24-hour urine excretion when more than 300 mg per day usually is regarded as abnormal in children (32). The albumin excretion rate from a timed urine collection, or microalbuminuria in diabetic children, is an important predictive marker for diabetic nephropathy (33) or renal enlargement during puberty (34). Rarely, dipstick albuminuria due to predominantly tubular disease is encountered [e.g., Dent's disease (35)] (see later).

Proximal Tubular Function

The detection of proximal tubular dysfunction rather than its quantitation is all that is usually required, and for this purpose the presence of glycosuria, aminoaciduria, hyperchloremic acidosis with bicarbonate wasting, polyuria, polydipsia, rickets, or a combination of these features, which represent Fanconi's syndrome, usually are sought. Phosphaturia can be measured and is useful to detect both proximal tubular function and secondary hyperparathyroidism in children with CRF (see later). The fractional excretion of phosphate (FEPO$_4$) is the proportion of filtered phosphate that is excreted. Because this is calculated as a clearance ratio, a timed urine collection is not necessary.

$$\text{FEPO}_4 = \frac{\text{UPO}_4 \text{V}}{\text{PPO}_4} \times \frac{\text{Pc}}{\text{UcV}}$$

where *UPO$_4$* is the phosphate excretion and *PPO$_4$* × *UcV/Pc* is the filtered phosphate.

The fractional excretion of phosphate also can be used to calculate the theoretic phosphate threshold for renal tubular reabsorption (TmPO$_4$/GFR) (36). For children, the use of nomograms is unnecessary and the phosphate threshold can be calculated (37,38) using a random urine sample and simultaneous plasma sample from the following formula:

$$\text{TmPO}_4/\text{GFR} = \text{PPO}_4 - \frac{\text{UPO}_4 \times \text{Pc}}{\text{Uc}}$$

The phosphate threshold provides a useful index of parathyroid hormone (PTH) activity in children (39) and is relatively insensitive to changes in phosphate intake or GFR. FEPO$_4$ ranges between 2% and 12% in young children and rises to between 5% and 20% in adults: TmPO$_4$/GFR falls from an average of 6 mg/dL in children to 3.4 mg/dL in adults.

Tubular proteinuria can be measured by the clearance of retinol-binding protein, β_2-microglobulin, and α_1-microglobulin in urine relative to their ratio of urinary creatinine concentration. All are low-molecular-weight proteins (LMWP) that are present in plasma and filtered by glomerular filtration, after which 99.9% of the filtered LMWP is reabsorbed and catabolized by tubular cells. LMWP fractional excretion is high in infants, reflecting tubular immaturity, but falls from 1.68% to 0.5% between birth and 2 years of age (40). β_2-Microglobulin is unstable in acid urine and in clinical practice it is more convenient and accurate to use the excretion of retinol-binding protein as a measure of proximal tubular dysfunction. The normal range for the excretion of retinol-binding protein in a random sample is less than 1 to 24.5 mg per mole of creatinine (41). Tubular disease is associated with a marked increase in the excretion of LMWP (35,42), and this can be estimated again as a fractional excretion from a random urine and blood sample. The presence of excessive *N*-acetyl-glucosaminidase, an enzyme released from the proximal tubule cell brush border, in a child's urine is indicative of proximal tubular damage, being markedly raised in Fanconi's syndrome due to cystinosis.

Distal Tubular Function

Urine Acidification

Hydrogen ion is secreted by tubular cells and neutralizes filtered bicarbonate to form carbonic acid, which is then dehydrated using carbonic anhydrase, thus allowing carbon dioxide to diffuse into the tubular cells and then be reconstituted as bicarbonate (see Chapter 6). Distal tubular fluid is essentially free of bicarbonate, so that the appearance of bicarbonate in the urine (in effect, when the urine pH exceeds 6.1; at this pH, urine bicarbonate concentration is approximately 1 mmol/L) when the plasma bicarbonate is below the normal threshold for bicarbonate reabsorption implies a defect of proximal tubular bicarbonate handling. The threshold may need to be defined in a child with proximal renal tubular acidosis (RTA), and this can be achieved by raising the plasma bicarbonate concentration with an infusion of bicarbonate or by stopping the bicarbonate supplements and observing the urine pH as the plasma bicarbonate falls (43). The threshold for bicarbonate reabsorption is lower in infants than in older children and the splay on the bicarbonate reabsorption curve is wider so that the plasma bicarbonate concentrations are lower, ranging from 18 to 22 mmol/L for infants to 20 to 26 mmol/L for children. The range of normal in premature infants extends from 14.5 to 24.5 mmol/L (44).

The urine excretions of bicarbonate, titratable acid, and ammonium are essentially determined by the urine hydrogen ion concentration, so that much can be learned from measuring urine pH. Most children pass acid urine during the night and, if the plasma bicarbonate is normal, an early-morning urine pH of less than 5.3 excludes a defect of hydrogen ion excretion.

Renal tubular acidosis should be suspected in a child with a normal plasma anion gap [Na$^+$ − (Cl$^-$ + HCO$_3^-$) = 8 to

16 mmol/L] and a hyperchloremic acidosis; other possibilities are loss of HCO_3^- from the gastrointestinal tract or the administration of hydrochloric acid or its precursors. To differentiate between the RTA and the other conditions, the urine anion gap ($Na^+ + K^+ - Cl^-$) is measured because it estimates urine ammonium concentration; thus, a negative gap suggests gastrointestinal loss of HCO_3^-, whereas a positive gap ($Na^+ + K^+ > Cl^-$) indicates distal RTA (45).

The next step is to measure plasma K^+ concentration. If it is normal or decreased, the demonstration of an inability to lower urine pH below 5.3 either after ammonium chloride loading or after furosemide establishes the diagnosis of distal RTA (type 1) (45). In distal RTA, the defect is the inability of the distal tubule to generate or maintain a hydrogen ion gradient, so few hydrogen ions are excreted in the urine. Because carbon dioxide is generated in alkaline urine by the reaction of hydrogen ions with bicarbonate in tubular urine, the urine PCO_2 exceeds the blood PCO_2 by more than 30 mm Hg. This difference is not observed in children with distal RTA. Therefore, to test for distal RTA, it is kinder and safer to give a bicarbonate load to an acidotic child rather than exacerbate the acid load with ammonium chloride. The ingestion of oral sodium bicarbonate (3 mmol/kg) during antidiuresis should raise the urine pH above 7.4 and, when this has been achieved, the PCO_2 is measured on coincident urine and blood samples. Normal children have a urine–blood PCO_2 difference of 16 to 66 mm Hg, whereas the difference in children with distal renal acidosis ranges from -9 to $+8$ mm Hg (46). Alternatively, if it is necessary to perform this test to confirm distal renal acidosis, the dose of ammonium chloride for children is 150 mg (3 mmol)/kg (47), after which blood and urinary pH are documented when. Ammonium chloride should not be given to children with liver disease or defects of urea metabolism.

The urine calcium concentration (see later) always should be measured in children with suspected distal RTA because it usually is increased and its reduction to normal is a useful indication of adequate alkali replacement.

If the plasma K^+ is increased, then a urine pH of more than 5.3 after ammonium chloride identifies the rare type of distal RTA caused by a voltage-dependent defect. If the urine pH is less than 5.3, the diagnosis of hyperkalemic (type 4) RTA is established (45). (See Chapter 6 for the more complicated tests required to define the different types of distal RTA.)

Urine Concentrating Capacity

If the plasma osmolality is increased to more than 290 mOsm/kg and the urine is not concentrated, then a concentrating defect exists. Most children pass concentrated urine first thing in the morning, and if the osmolality exceeds 800 mOsm/kg, no further tests are required. If the child has frank polyuria and polydipsia, water deprivation tests should be carried out during the day with the child weighed at regular intervals and the test terminated when the weight loss exceeds 5%. A plasma osmolality can be obtained at this time to confirm

that an adequate stimulus for urine concentration has been achieved and desmopressin (DDAVP) given intranasally to check for nephrogenic diabetes insipidus. Normal children respond to a standard water deprivation test by producing a urine osmolality of $1,089 \pm 110$ mOsm/kg [standard deviation (SD)] (48). To perform this test, no fluid is allowed after 5:00 PM; the bladder is emptied at 8:00 PM, all the urine passed overnight is collected, and the osmolality is measured. An alternative is to administer vasopressin (DDAVP 20 μg intranasally; 10 μg for infants), but water intake should then be controlled to avoid water intoxication. The magnitude of the rise in urine osmolality with water deprivation depends partly on the urea excretion and the daily protein intake. Infants on low-protein milks or human milk concentrate urine less well, although the urine concentration of nonurea solutes and the ability to conserve water are similar to those of older children (49).

Plasma and Urine Electrolytes

Sodium

Hyponatremia does not necessarily imply a reduction in total body sodium because plasma sodium concentration measurement must be assessed in conjunction with extracellular fluid (ECF) volume. Careful clinical and laboratory appraisal is necessary to diagnose the cause. The renal conservation of sodium is limited in premature infants (see later) and hyponatremia is common if sodium supplements are not given; extrarenal losses of sodium from vomiting or diarrhea leading to hypovolemia also result in water retention from increased antidiuretic hormone (ADH) secretion. Hyponatremia is common in relapse of the nephrotic syndrome when the hypovolemia stimulates thirst and ADH secretion. Modern chemical analyzers do not produce "pseudohyponatremia" from the abnormal lipid content of plasma. In acute renal failure, the continued intake of water can lead to edema and dilutional hyponatremia, particularly in neonates with unsuspected renal failure. The syndrome of inappropriate secretion of ADH often is wrongly diagnosed in the sick newborn, particularly in those with a respiratory problem who are maintained on artificial ventilation. The diagnosis requires that the secretion of ADH should be inappropriate with regard both to the plasma osmolality and to the volume status of the plasma and ECF in the presence of normal thyroid function. The diagnosis of the cause of hyponatremia requires careful assessment of sodium and water intake, the clinical signs of ECF volume expansion or contraction, an estimation of renal function and GFR from the plasma creatinine and blood urea, and the analysis of urine sodium and urea content (50).

Hypernatremia is rare except in infants with diabetes insipidus, in whom lack of mobility and communication prevents them from being able to satisfy their thirst. Excessive sodium intake compared with water intake in infants with diarrhea or those fed unmodified cow's milk can cause hypernatremia; rarely, hypernatremia results from failure of normal thirst control (51) or from poisoning with salt (52). Hypernatremia due to inappropriate fluid prescription and abnormal thirst mechanism has been reported in the hospital setting (53).

The 24-hour urine sodium excretion is simply a measure of dietary intake and provides no other useful information in a normal person or in the patient in CRF with stable body composition. In acute renal failure, the measurement of urine sodium and urea concentration enables prerenal failure to be distinguished from established acute tubular necrosis. The fractional excretion of sodium (FENa%), again calculated as a clearance ratio on a random urine and plasma sample, provides the best discrimination; in established tubular necrosis it exceeds 2.5% (54):

$$FENa\% = \frac{UNa}{PNa} \times \frac{Pc}{Uc} \times 100$$

where *UNa, PNa, Uc,* and *Pc* are the urine and plasma concentrations of sodium and creatinine, respectively.

Calcium and Phosphate

Approximately 50% of total plasma calcium is protein bound and, in children who are dehydrated, this can cause an increase in total plasma calcium without an increase in the physiologically important ionized fraction. Total plasma calcium measurement should be corrected in children who have apparently high values but who are dehydrated because of polyuria or for other reasons by subtracting 0.09 mg/dL (0.0225 mmol/L) for every 1 g/L by which the plasma albumin exceeds 46 g/L. Values below 46 g/L can occur in children with nephrotic syndrome. Hypercalcemia can cause a renal concentrating defect, and cases of nephrogenic diabetes insipidus have been erroneously diagnosed because of failure to appreciate this potential error. Urine calcium excretion varies with diet, exposure to sunlight, and seasons, but the upper limit for normal is usually taken as 6 mg/kg/24 hours (0.15 mmol/kg/24 hours) or a calcium–creatinine ratio of 0.3 mg of calcium per milligram of creatinine (or 0.85 mmol/mmol). In British schoolchildren, these values rarely exceed 4 mg/kg/24 hours or 0.25 mg of calcium per milligram of creatinine (55).

Plasma inorganic phosphate concentration is higher in children, particularly during the first year of life, than in adults and thus is associated with a higher threshold for renal tubular phosphate reabsorption (see earlier). The normal range in infants is 3.7 to 8.6 mg/dL, falling to 3.4 to 5.9 mg/dL at 1 year, 3.6 to 5.0 mg/dL at 7 years, and 2.8 to 4.8 mg/dL after puberty (56). The upper limit for the solubility product for calcium × plasma phosphorus is 60.0 (mg/dL × mg/dL) or 4.8 (mmol/L × mmol/L), and it is important to monitor this parameter when managing children with CRF.

Miscellaneous

The upper limit for the urinary oxalate–creatinine ratio (mmol/mmol) falls from 0.26 before 1 year to 0.15 at 12 years and 0.083 after 12 years of age (28). The mean (SD) plasma oxalate–creatinine molar ratio is 0.033 (0.013) and is independent of age and renal function (57). Urinary vanillylmandelic acid excretion also is better expressed as the creatinine ratio, and the upper limit falls from 16.3 μmol vanillylmandelic acid per millimole creatinine at 6 months to 13.7 at 6 years and 7.6 in older children (58). Antenatal cord blood β_2-microglobulin concentrations have provided a measure of fetal renal function (59) in those fetuses that may have obstructive uropathy or renal anomaly.

GENETIC RENAL DISEASE

Genetic kidney disease more commonly presents in children than in adults, although there are notable exceptions (e.g., autosomal-dominant polycystic disease). Renal diseases due to genetic causes are recognized throughout childhood and have become an important area of clinical practice because increasingly more young children, even fetuses, are diagnosed with genetic disease by specialists in fetal medicine, geneticists, and pediatric nephrologists, with the latter being consulted about management for the postnatal kidney dysfunction. Neonates and infants may present with congenital nephrotic syndrome, chromosomal or syndromic abnormalities of the kidney (see later), and autosomal-recessive polycystic kidney disease. Toddlers may have severe renal failure from familial hemolytic-uremic syndrome (HUS) or renal dysplasia, whereas older children show clinical manifestations of juvenile nephronophthisis, Alport's syndrome, and occasionally autosomal-dominant polycystic disease.

Bartter's Syndrome and Related Disorders

Many genetic kidney conditions with "single-gene" inheritance patterns are now known to have several genetic loci producing superficially similar clinical phenotypes. Bartter's and Gitelman's syndromes are good examples because they often were confused in the early nephrology literature and genetic analysis has helped to differentiate them. Gitelman's syndrome with clinical features of hypokalemia–hypomagnesemia with hypocalciuria has been linked to a gene encoding a thiazide-sensitive Na/Cl-cotransporter on chromosome 16q13 (60,61), whereas families with Bartter's and hyperprostaglandin E syndrome did not show any linkage to this genomic region. Genetic analysis of patients with Bartter's syndrome has shown that the neonatal form, characterized by polyhydramnios, premature delivery, life-threatening episodes of fever and dehydration during the early weeks of life, growth retardation, hypercalciuria, and early-onset nephrocalcinosis, results from mutations in two genes. One encodes the bumetanide-sensitive Na/K/2Cl-cotransporter (NKCC2) and the other an adenosine triphosphate–sensitive, inwardly rectifying K channel (ROMK). This contrasts with older children presenting with classic Bartter's syndrome with symptoms of polyuria and failure to thrive but no nephrocalcinosis, who have either deletions or mutations at the gene encoding a renal chloride channel (ClC-Kb) (62).

Congenital Nephrotic Syndrome

The nephrotic syndrome is a common problem in children and has many causes (63) that relate to the age of presentation, but the diagnosis of congenital nephrotic syndrome may be confusing. Familial forms of nephrotic syndrome, such as Finnish-type congenital nephrotic syndrome and recessively inherited familial focal segmental glomerulosclerosis, are first diagnosed in infants when the patient either becomes nephrotic or manifests heavy proteinuria and renal impairment, as is frequently observed too in diffuse mesangial sclerosis–type congenital nephrotic syndrome. In practice, the age of presentation, if known, is more reliable than the histologic features and may determine the prognosis because those infants who present earliest (i.e., occurrence within the first 2 months of life) fare less well. Genetic analysis may offer an improved classification of these syndromes in the future. Although minimal change nephropathy, focal glomerulosclerosis, and diffuse mesangial proliferation as part of the idiopathic nephrotic syndrome of childhood may occur in the first 3 months of life, they usually present later, with 90% of these nephrotic children being toddlers or younger than 6 years of age.

Congenital nephrotic syndrome is extremely rare, difficult to treat, and often fatal. It usually is due to the two primary autosomal-recessive diseases mentioned previously (Finnish-type or diffuse mesangial sclerosis), so any child with nephrotic syndrome presenting in the first year should have the histologic lesion confirmed. Congenital nephrotic syndrome also may be secondary to intrauterine infections from syphilis, cytomegalovirus, toxoplasmosis, and measles, in which case treatment of the infection, where possible, may lead to resolution of the nephrotic syndrome (64). The gene for the more common Finnish-type congenital nephrotic syndrome, which occurs in all ethnic groups, has been identified on chromosome 19q13.1 and encodes a 1,242–amino acid transmembrane protein called *nephrin* that is expressed in podocytes. Clinically, the placental weight is increased to a third of the body weight in Finnish congenital nephrotic syndrome, and histologically there is mesangial hypercellularity and sclerosis, glomerular immaturity, and tubular cystic damage. An abnormal composition of the glomerular basement membrane with fewer sialic acid residues and a reduction in the anionic charge that normally opposes the filtration of plasma proteins (65) has been demonstrated (66), but these findings have not been confirmed (67). Antenatal diagnosis is possible from a raised amniotic α-fetoprotein level and genetic markers (68) .

Diffuse mesangial sclerosis, where glomerulosclerosis is not accompanied by mesangial hypercellularity, may occur in isolation or be associated with the Denys Drash syndrome of male pseudohermaphroditism (XY gonadal dysgenesis) (69) and the nephrotic syndrome presenting in infancy. Mutations in the tumor suppressor gene WT-1, which is known to have a role in podocyte embryogenesis, have been reported in both (63,70). Diffuse mesangial sclerosis progresses to end-stage renal failure (ESRF) more slowly than the Finnish type.

Maternal or amniotic α-fetoprotein concentrations are not raised in diffuse mesangial sclerosis, in contrast to Finnish congenital nephrotic syndrome.

The prognosis for congenital nephrotic syndrome is poor because no treatment is effective, and renal function slowly declines, although frequently the children die from septicemia provoked by the edema and malnutrition during the first year. An alternative clinical management is early bilateral nephrectomy and maintenance dialysis followed by transplantation (71). More recently, unilateral nephrectomy (72) together with indomethacin (up to 3 mg/kg/day), angiotensin-converting enzyme (ACE) inhibitors, and diuretics have greatly improved edema, hypovolemia, and patient well-being, reducing the time spent in hospital and the number of nephrotic complications. ESRF may not reached until 2 to 4 years of age, when dialysis and transplantation can be performed. Recurrence of the congenital nephrotic syndrome does not occur, but nephrotic syndrome related to viral infection posttransplantation has been reported (73). Minimal change nephropathy posttransplantation also has been observed (74).

Other Inherited Nephrotic Syndromes

New genes encoding for inherited nephrotic syndrome have been reported. NHPS2 on chromosome 1q25-31, which causes autosomal-recessive steroid-resistant nephrotic syndrome, has been mapped. Its relationship with other nephrotic syndromes, congenital or otherwise, is unknown, but NPHS2 is expressed in the podocytes of fetal and mature kidney glomeruli, and encodes a new integral membrane protein, podocin, belonging to the stomatin protein family (75). Autosomal-dominant focal segmental glomerulosclerosis has been linked to polymorphic markers on chromosome 13q19 (76), although others have not observed such a linkage (77). Clearly, the common clinical features of the nephrotic syndrome belie a heterogeneous group of disorders, many of which will have a genetic basis in children.

Cystinosis

Cystinosis is the most common cause of Fanconi's syndrome in children. It is an autosomal-recessive disease characterized by the abnormal accumulation of the amino acid cystine in lysosomes of all tissues due to a defective cystine transporter protein. The gene responsible for nephropathic cystinosis, CTNS on chromosome 17p, encodes for a 367–amino acid transmembrane protein called *cystinosin* (78). A common major deletion underlies most affected patients in Europe; other mutations have been reported (e.g., in Canadian patients of Irish ancestry and in intermediate cystinosis in adults; see Chapter 20).

Typically, cystinosis is a multisystem disease causing failure to thrive, dehydration, polyuria and polydipsia, vomiting, constipation, Fanconi's syndrome, and renal impairment in infancy. Indomethacin (3 mg/kg/day) may control the polyuria and improve the patient's biochemistry, but not growth (79). Further complications develop later in childhood: photophobia from corneal cystine crystal deposition and blindness from retinopathy, hypothyroidism (80), and diabetes mellitus from pancreatic involvement (81). Liver disease, portal hypertension, and hypersplenism usually occur in adolescents (82). The average age for renal replacement therapy is 9 years, with 95% of patients aged between 5 and 16 years.

Depletion of intralysosomal cystine is possible with cysteamine and related compounds that form mixed disulfides that are capable of being transported out of the lysosome. Improvement in the age to attain ESRF (83) and Fanconi's syndrome is possible, but growth has been disappointingly poor (84). This may relate to inadequate doses of cysteamine or its equivalents. Ultimately, approximately 35% of 25-year-old cystinotic adults, most of whom were untreated with cystine-depleting agents through most of their childhood years, manifested neurologic complications characterized by cerebral atrophy, pyramidal signs, difficulties with speech, cerebellar ataxia, and, finally, pseudobulbar palsy and death (82).

Mitochondrial Cytopathies

These rare but fascinating diseases commonly present in children and occasionally in adulthood (85). The genes encoding the 100 or so mitochondrial polypeptides of the respiratory chain reside in the nucleus and the mitochondrial genome. Because mitochondria are inherited from the ovum and the distribution of mitochondrial genomic mutations varies among the tissues of the fetus, the clinical presentation and severity of these disorders vary widely. One-third of children with respiratory chain protein mutations present in the first month of life. Muscle weakness and central nervous system disorders predominate, the latter universally so as the disease progresses (86), but gastrointestinal and cardiac symptoms occur. Renal manifestations include Fanconi's syndrome, reflecting the abnormal energy metabolism of the tubular cells or tubulointerstitial nephritis. Fanconi's syndrome predominantly occurs in girls with an autosomal-recessive inheritance. In older children, nephrotic syndrome with ocular muscle involvement may develop and may progress to chronic renal impairment (87).

RENAL DISEASE IN THE FETUS, NEONATE, AND INFANT

Neonatal Renal Problems

Over 90% of newborns pass urine within 24 hours, and failure to do so within 48 hours is abnormal (88). Proteinuria occurs in 20% of normal newborns and a few red cells occasionally are found in the urine (89). The main problems that occur are related to congenital abnormalities of the urinary tract (see later), including the renal vasculature, or to renal damage that occurs during birth (90). The development of routine ultrasonic scanning of the fetus for gross anatomic abnormalities

of organs during the first trimester has allowed infants with identified renal tract anomalies to be delivered in obstetric units with appropriate planned renal care, or has led to their early referral and investigation by pediatric renal units. Table 80-3 shows the relative prevalence of various congenital renal anomalies.

Many congenital renal tract anomalies are sporadic, but inherited or syndromic abnormalities are well described (91). Besides identifying those cases that form part of a syndrome, the pediatric nephrologist's role is to diagnose and relieve urinary tract obstruction, diagnose renal impairment, which also often is associated with renal tract infection, identify conditions that lead to progressive renal failure, promote normal growth of the infant, and prevent or treat urinary tract infection (UTI) and hypertension.

Structural Abnormalities

Antenatal ultrasonographic examination of the fetus is capable of detecting many structural renal anomalies, which occur in approximately 6 infants per 10,000 live births. Ultrasound may identify unilateral or bilateral renal agenesis, hypoplasia, dysplasia with or without cystic changes (the multicystic dysplastic kidney), hydronephrosis, hydroureter, and abnormal bladder, as well as abnormal renal shape (horseshoe kidney) and position (ectopic pelvic kidney). It cannot diagnose urinary tract obstruction, only dilatation. Over 300 congenital syndromes have been described that involve renal tract anomalies, and because many are inherited (e.g., Turner's syndrome), current hypotheses of renal tract maldevelopment involve genetic dysfunction in the embryo. Chromosomal abnormalities in children with renal dysplasia are very common. Although a genetic influence cannot be discounted, most cases are sporadic, so the etiology of renal structural anomalies must be multifactorial because many conditions occur only sporadically in families. The risk for more children being affected is low (92,93). Environmental factors are known to cause some anomalies (e.g., renal agenesis/hypoplasia in fetal alcohol syndrome).

Bilateral renal agenesis affects 1 in 7,000 fetuses. Estimates of unilateral renal agenesis vary from 1 in 400 to 1 in 1,600, and these children have a normal life expectancy if their single kidney is normal. Approximately 5% of first-degree relatives of patients with bilateral agenesis have unilateral agenesis, which suggests that the cause is either polygenic with a threshold-determining expression or multifactorial with genetic and environmental interactions.

Renal Dysplasia

Renal dysplasia is one of the most common congenital renal malformations (94) and on ultrasonography is characterized by loss of normal corticomedullary differentiation and usually bright echogenic appearances. The association between dysplasia and obstruction is important because the prognosis for renal function after surgical relief of the obstruction is

TABLE 80-4. *Causes of chronic/end-stage renal failure in children*

Diagnosis	BAPNRR[a] CRF + ESRF (age range, 0–18 yr)	(%)	NAPRTCS[b] CRF (age range, 0–20 yr)	(%)
Renal aplasia/hypoplasia/dysplasia	189	(27.4)	404	(23.5)
Obstructive uropathy	138	(20.0)	451	(26.3)
Glomerulonephritis	110	(16.0)	246	(14.3)
Reflux nephropathy	63	(9.1)	155	(9.0)
Interstitial disease	50	(7.3)	46	(2.7)
Renal vascular disease	31	(4.5)	48	(2.8)
Inherited disease				
Congenital nephrotic syndrome	47	(6.8)	11	(0.6)
Other inherited disease	46	(6.7)	123	(7.2)
Drug toxicity	4	(0.6)		(0.0)
Neoplasia	11	(1.6)	6	(0.3)
Other unclassified			228	(13.3)
Totals	689	(100.0)	1718	(100.0)

BAPNRR, British Association for Paediatric Nephrology Renal Registry, 1999; *NAPRTCS*, North American Pediatric Renal Transplant Cooperative Study, 1996; *CRF*, chronic renal failure; *ESRF*, end-stage renal failure.

[a]Adapted from Lewis M. Report of the Paediatric Renal Registry, 1999. In: *The UK Renal Registry: the second annual report.* London: The Renal Association, 2000:175–187.

[b]Adapted from Fivush BA, Jabs K, Neu AM, et al. Chronic renal insufficiency in children and adolescents: the 1996 annual report of NAPRTCS. *Pediatr Nephrol* 1998;12:328.

affected by the coexistent dysplasia. Dysplasia often arises from severe obstruction to urinary flow *in utero,* such as occurs with posterior urethral valve in boys, prune-belly syndrome (95), or severe VUR (96), or is syndromic [e.g., Ivermark's syndrome (97)]. It may be unilateral or bilateral, in which case it usually affects the kidneys asymmetrically and causes CRF early in childhood, often requiring renal replacement therapy (Table 80-4) (98,99). Renal histologic investigation shows developmental arrest, failure of differentiation, and the persistence of fetal mesonephric structures (100). Primitive ducts lined by columnar epithelium, nests of metaplastic cartilage, fetal glomeruli, and cysts may be found. The association of renal dysplasia and urinary obstruction and the abnormal tubular anatomy results in abnormal tubular physiology. Fractional reabsorption of sodium and bicarbonate in the proximal tubule is reduced. Distal reabsorption of sodium and hydrogen ion excretion may be impaired, causing the neonatal kidney to have an even higher fractional excretion of sodium. Chronic salt depletion compromises growth and cognitive function, and hypertension does not occur. Because urinary obstruction may damage the distal tubule and collecting ducts, urinary concentration is reduced, leading to variable but obligatory polyuria. These children require regular oral fluids, and drinks must be made readily available to them at all times. Dehydration and further renal impairment occur when these children are deprived of fluid, such as occurs for hospital investigations and anesthesia, or have increased extrarenal fluid and electrolyte losses (e.g., vomiting, gastroenteritis). Sodium wasting is treated by salt supplements, the dose being adjusted to maintain good growth, a normal plasma sodium, and normal blood pressure without clinical evidence of excessive ECF volume. The metabolic acidosis usually requires sodium bicarbonate supplements,

2 to 4 mmol/kg/day. If significant chronic renal impairment is present, attention to nutrition, which may require tube feeding to supply sufficient calories, and hyperparathyroidism is needed (see later). The physician should be aware that growth may be compromised in these children with renal dysplasia, which does not depend solely on their renal impairment.

If urinary obstruction is present then this must be relieved, such as when the upper moiety of a duplex kidney is drained by a dilated ureter whose distal end is obstructed by a ureterocele (101). A marked postoperative increase in urine production and salt loss may occur because of the reduced proximal tubular reabsorption of sodium and poor urinary concentrating ability of the dysplastic kidney. The consequent reduction in ECF further compromises renal perfusion and GFR, so careful postoperative fluid balance should be maintained and fluid prescription increased to anticipate the increased natriuresis and diuresis. Renal adaptation with reduction in polyuria may take days or even weeks to occur. Obstructed renal tracts are more prone to infection that will cause more kidney damage and thus compromise GFR further, so these infants should receive prophylactic antibiotics from birth at least until the obstruction is relieved, and they should have operative procedures covered with systemic broad-spectrum antibiotics.

Multicystic dysplasia is a form of renal dysplasia where the kidney has multiple cysts associated with an atretic ipsilateral ureter. Such kidneys undergo progressive atrophy during the first 2 years of life. Some are very large at birth and require surgical excision. They usually are not associated with a raised blood pressure, although malignant hypertension has been reported rarely. This small risk of hypertension, and an equally rare incidence of malignant change, has led to patients undergoing nephrectomy in many units. It is important to document by DMSA scan that the contralateral kidney is normal before nephrectomy of the multicystic dysplastic kidney because the contralateral ureter may reflux in approximately 30% of such infants. Although nephrectomy converts the child into a normal child with a single kidney who does not require medical observation, the anesthetic risk is comparable with the medical complication risk (102).

Congenital Hydronephrosis

Antenatal hydronephrosis has been identified by fetal ultrasonography in as much as 0.5% to 1% of pregnancies, but postnatally the prevalence is reduced. Several anatomic malformations cause hydronephrosis, such as pelviureteric junction narrowing (34%), minimal hydronephrosis (26%), ureterovesical junction stenosis or reflux (18%), neuropathic bladder with gross VUR, posterior urethral valves, duplex or cystic kidneys, ureteric duplications, or hydroureter (103,104). Protocols to investigate congenital hydronephrosis not only must identify the cause of the renal tract dilatation but identify the obstruction without being too invasive, expensive, or labor intensive, given the potential number of infants involved. A combined nephrology–urology team carries out the best clinical management. Approximately 1% or less of cases of hydronephrosis due to pelviureteric junction configuration are associated with significant obstruction to urinary flow (105). For unilateral hydronephrosis, we commence prophylactic antibiotics on postnatal day 1 and perform postnatal renal ultrasonography toward the end of the first week, thereby reducing the risk of missing a hydronephrotic kidney because of a reduced GFR during the first 3 days of life, which may cause the hydronephrosis to improve or disappear. This is followed by a micturating cystourethrogram and then, after 8 to 12 weeks, dynamic renal ^{99m}Tc-MAG3 scanning to identify impaired renal function from either obstruction or renal dysplasia. Some authors restrict micturating cystourograms to those infants with identifiable ureters on renal ultrasonography (106) but sometimes, moderate VUR is present without ureteric dilatation. There is no need for immediate surgery in children with pelviureteric junction configuration/obstruction because most will do well (107). Criteria for pyeloplasty for pelviureteric junction narrowing include differential GFR below 35%, severe hydronephrosis (>2.5 cm anteroposterior diameter), or deteriorating hydronephrosis or renal function of that kidney. Infants born with mild hydronephrosis (<1.5 cm anteroposterior diameter) are not likely to become obstructed. Equally, those having severe renal impairment on initial ^{99m}Tc-MAG3 scanning (<20% differential function) are unlikely to have significant recovery of function postpyeloplasty (105). All children should be followed for at least 3 months, with renal ultrasonography being repeated at this time because significant deterioration in the hydronephrosis occasionally may occur despite initial good prognostic features.

Bilateral hydronephrosis, particularly in male infants, should be more urgently investigated and treated. The presence of antenatal oligohydramnios and prematurity correlates with a poor postnatal renal outcome (108). However, antenatal renal ultrasonography is unreliable in predicting renal function postnatally (109,110). Besides prophylactic antibiotics on day 1, plasma creatinine should be measured daily for the first week to document the expected decrease in value or identify renal impairment if present. Renal ultrasonography with bladder views to measure bladder volume and wall thickness previoding and postvoiding, together with micturating cystourethrography should be obtained within the first week to diagnose posterior urethral valve or VUR. Urgent investigation is indicated if renal impairment is present. If a posterior urethral valve is the cause of obstruction, we recommend suprapubic catheter drainage of the bladder until a pediatric urologist carries out cystoscopic resection of the valve. Or, if VUR is not responsible for the bilateral hydronephrosis, early ^{99m}Tc-MAG3 scanning should be performed in an attempt to document differential GFR of each kidney and any degree of urinary obstruction. In children with spina bifida, early bladder videourodynamics should be performed rather than delayed to document the degree of bladder dysfunction, because significant renal damage may occur from high-pressure VUR and infection.

Acute Renal Failure

The newborn's kidneys are at risk for development of acute renal failure because of perinatal asphyxia, their low GFR, renal vasomotor constriction, and fluid/intravascular volume depletion. Consequently, acute tubular necrosis or infarction (acute cortical necrosis) may develop in up to 8% of neonates in intensive care (111). Although usually characterized by oliguria (<1 mL/hour/kg weight), polyuric acute renal failure commonly occurs, particularly with asphyxia, congenital abnormalities of the renal tract, and drug toxicity (aminoglycosides, antifungals); fractional excretion of sodium sometimes may be misleading in differentiating these two causes. Peripheral edema from fluid overload or hydrops may indicate renal failure occurring in the neonatal period. The large number of causes of hydrops and renal failure must be distinguished from hydrops due to hemolytic disease of the newborn, congenital heart disease, cardiac failure *in utero* secondary to cardiac arrhythmias, renal problems such as obstructive nephropathy or congenital nephrotic syndrome, pulmonary hypoplasia, intrauterine infections, chromosomal anomalies, and placental problems (112). Infants born with congenital heart disease also are more prone to development of acute renal failure caused either by heart failure or the effects of cardiac surgery (113). Maternal ACE inhibitor therapy causes acute renal failure in the newborn. Predicting which infants are at risk for development of neonatal renal failure from perinatal asphyxia in the intensive care unit may be assessed in a number of ways: by measuring plasma myoglobin, myoglobinuria, retinol-binding protein excretion (114), or asphyxia scores (115). Appropriate fluid restriction and salt balance can then be achieved before fluid overload and hyponatremia occur.

Rapid correction of prerenal causes of acute renal failure remains paramount for treating and avoiding prolonged renal dysfunction in neonates. Congenital obstruction and structural renal abnormalities such as dysplasia, hypoplasia, or agenesis should be excluded by ultrasonographic examination of the urinary tract, and a cystourethrogram usually is appropriate if hydronephrosis/hydroureter is demonstrated. Pulmonary edema should be prevented by positive-pressure ventilation, and acidosis should be corrected with intravenous sodium bicarbonate by initial half correction only of the metabolic acidosis to avoid precipitating intraventricular hemorrhage by use of excessive hyperosmolar solutions. Hyperkalemia should be treated with correction of any acidosis and nebulized, or intravenous salbutamol (4 μg/kg); intravenous 2% calcium gluconate; glucose and insulin; and rectal calcium–potassium exchange resin (in that order). These are only temporary measures while dialysis is being initiated. In an experienced unit, it is far safer to dialyze early with acute tubular necrosis, even though recovery often occurs quickly, because severe acidosis and hyperkalemia can recur very rapidly.

An adequate nutritional intake should be provided without causing water overload. Supportive therapy with provision of large numbers of calories by high-concentrate dextrose intravenous infusions and parenteral nutrition and antibiotics for infection is essential if control of the catabolic state and metabolic disturbance is to be achieved (116). Infants with heart problems and renal failure require inotropic support and early dialysis, particularly after surgery. Dialysis should be provided by continuous venovenous or arteriovenous diahemofiltration using small extracorporeal circuit volumes (117,118) and repeated flow across dialysis membranes before returning the blood to the patient, in preference to peritoneal dialysis. Although the latter technique may work well in the absence of expertise in diahemofiltration (119), accurate measurement of dialysate input and output, frequent weighing, temperature monitoring, and clinical examination of the child are required.

Other factors acting on renal blood flow such as angiotensin II, endothelin I, and nitric oxide appear important in maintaining GFR in the neonatal kidney (120–122), and therapeutic intervention in these areas may become possible in the future.

Renal Artery Thrombosis

Renovascular complications and abnormalities in renal blood flow commonly occur in neonates, particularly in the clinical setting of intensive care for premature infants. Umbilical artery catheters used for blood sampling may cause aortic intimal damage, mural clot formation and propagation, or embolism. If the tip of the catheter is placed above or around the orifices of the renal arteries, there is a significant risk of renal artery thrombosis or embolism. Depending on the degree of occlusion of the artery and on whether the main artery

or only interlobular arteries are involved, the resulting renal ischemia produces focal parenchymal scarring or complete infarction. Such infants usually present with hematuria, cardiovascular instability, collapse, shock or hypertension, renal impairment, anemia, and thrombocytopenia. A palpable renal mass may be present and if the aorta also is thrombosed, the femoral pulses become impalpable and leg circulation is poor, characterized by gray, mottled skin. Urgent Doppler ultrasonography of the aorta, inferior vena cava, and renal arteries and veins is required together with arteriography to confirm the diagnosis.

Intraaortic injection of a bolus of tissue plasminogen activator followed by a 24-hour infusion may dissolve the clot and salvage renal tissue and function (123,124). Although renal perfusion may recovery sufficiently to avoid long-term renal replacement therapy, ESRF usually results if bilateral involvement was present initially.

Renal Venous Thrombosis

This condition usually occurs within a few days of birth in infants with perinatal asphyxia and in infants of diabetic mothers, or later in infants with severe dehydration or nephrotic syndrome (125,126). Rarely, a predisposing coagulopathy may be present such as factor V (Leiden) mutation, protein S or C deficiency, or a maternal hypercoagulation state such as anticardiolipin syndrome (127). Such underlying diseases predisposing to thrombosis probably are more common than has been previously recognized, with new mutations in many coagulation factors being described that cause pathologic coagulation.

Renal venous thrombosis commences in the small venous tributaries of the renal cortex or medulla and propagates to the main renal vein; it may affect one or both kidneys and may produce inferior vena cava obstruction. The infant with renal venous thrombosis presents with hematuria, cardiovascular collapse, and a palpable mass in one or both renal areas. There is associated thrombocytopenia, anemia, hyperosmolality and acidosis, oliguria, and renal impairment (126). Clinical management entails resuscitation of the infant's circulation, correction of acidosis that persists once the cardiovascular volume has been restored, monitoring of coagulation parameters, fluid intake and output, and ultrasonography of the renal veins and inferior vena cava to document the extent of the thrombosis. Controlled trials of anticoagulation for unilateral or bilateral renal venous thrombosis, with or without inferior vena cava involvement, are lacking. Anticoagulation with heparin is required for bilateral disease and significant extension of clot into the lumen of the vena cava; surgical thrombectomy is not required unless inferior vena cava obstruction exists (128). This should be followed after 10 days with oral anticoagulation using coumarin derivatives. Full anticoagulation may be given (129) for at least 3 months for unilateral renal venous thrombosis, but the outcome usually is good. Bilateral renal involvement also requires anticoagulation. Dialysis usually is required for bilateral renal involvement to correct the acidosis and metabolic and electrolyte disturbances. Fibrinolytic therapy also has been used successfully (130). Long-term follow-up shows an increased incidence of hypertension and a decreased urinary concentrating ability, but good renal and cognitive function (131).

RENAL DISEASE IN CHILDREN

Urinary Tract Infection

Children of all ages may acquire UTI; UTI develops in 2.5% of boys and 8% of girls before the age of 7 years (132,133). The sex distribution with age has a large variation, with the M : F ratio being 0.6 between 1 month and 1 year and 0.09 in children aged 3 to 11 years. Few children or adults who have recurrent UTI progress to serious renal disease, but chronic pyelonephritis is an important cause of ESRF (Table 80-4). The epidemiology of chronic pyelonephritis is complicated by the virulence of the infecting organism and the specific susceptibility of the child. Investigation of children with UTI has shown that VUR is present in 25% to 33% and that the degree of VUR correlates well with the prevalence of renal scarring (134). P-fimbriated *Escherichia coli* are associated with the development of renal scars, and inappropriate antibiotic therapy may favor colonization with such organisms (135). Pyelonephritogenic *E. coli* bind specifically to epithelial cell receptors and have an affinity for receptors that exhibit the P1 blood group antigen. In the absence of reflux, these P-fimbriated *E. coli* may be associated with pyelonephritis in susceptible children (136). The understanding of UTI and its epidemiology with regard to congenital, genetic, and environmental aspects suggests that early diagnosis and treatment should lead to a reduction in morbidity and mortality rates.

The role of any pediatrician caring for children with UTI is to prevent recurrent UTI and new renal scar formation and consequently renal impairment, usually by identifying children with existing renal scars, underlying renal tract anomalies, or known complications of UTI or VUR. Indeed, without an underlying renal tract abnormality, progressive renal damage is rare in children with UTI. Population screening is not cost effective (132), but early diagnosis by primary health care workers, urgent treatment of acute pyelonephritis to minimize scar formation, and prevention of infection by long-term low-dose prophylactic antibiotics (137) or the surgical correction of reflux in selected children (138) can all contribute to an improved prognosis. Successful management of UTI in childhood by culturing urine from all febrile infants and toddlers in Sweden has reduced the prevalence of reflux nephropathy/chronic pyelonephritis causing ESRF in pediatric transplant recipients from 20% in the 1970s to less than 5% in 1990s in that country (139).

Reflux nephropathy or "scarring" in the presence of VUR may arise by two main independent mechanisms (140). Severe antenatal VUR causes segmental renal dysplasia or hypoplasia in the fetal kidney, whereas postnatal VUR with intrarenal reflux and urinary infection causes segmental renal pyelonephritic scars in both infants and older children (96). The presence of compound renal papillae, which allow the back-flow of infected urine from the calices into the collecting ducts (intrarenal reflux), is important in the generation of renal scars with VUR (141). The increased frequency of UTI in infants, the presence of congenital segmental renal dysplasia, the increased risk of true infective pyelonephritic scars developing in infants, and renal impairment at presentation all demonstrate that the target population in which to detect UTI and renal "scars" is children aged up to 18 months.

The clinical presentation of UTI varies with the age of the child. Fever above 38°C commonly occurs in all age groups with pyelonephritis (142). Infants often present with this symptom alone, but also may have failure to thrive, upper respiratory tract symptoms and signs, vomiting, diarrhea, seizures, and septicemic shock. Preschool-aged children often complain of abdominal pain with or without dysuria or frequency of micturition, and girls may have associated vulvovaginitis. Occasionally, acute urinary retention may occur due to anxiety of severe dysuria. Older children present mostly often with dysuria, frequency, abdominal pain, or hematuria. Occasionally, the presentation is acute with hypertensive encephalopathy or ESRF caused by renal scarring.

Unfortunately, making a definite diagnosis of UTI in these very young children often is difficult, but it should be undertaken because symptoms are variable and nonspecific, particularly in the target population (Table 80-5). Suprapubic aspiration, although providing definitive results in young infants, is difficult to perform in children older than 1 year of age and is becoming less popular. Bag urine specimens often are contaminated and need repeating at least twice for a definitive diagnosis. Preferably, a clean-catch urine specimen should be obtained, but both clean-catch urine and midstream urine specimens are difficult to acquire, particularly if parents are given the responsibility of obtaining them. A frequent mistake is to diagnose UTI from a significant growth of organisms after culture of a contaminated or improperly transported urine specimen. The specimen should be cultured within 2 hours or transported in a medium such as boric acid that prevents

TABLE 80-5. *Presenting symptoms in children with urinary tract infection*

Symptom	Age		
	0–2 yr (%)	2–5 yr (%)	5–12 yr (%)
Failure to thrive	33	3	
Irritability	5	2	
Cloudy, offensive urine	3	7	
Diarrhea, vomiting	32	8	2
Fever, convulsions	22	32	29
Hematuria	3	8	3
Urinary frequency, dysuria	2	16	22
Enuresis		13	15
Abdominal pain		11	29

From Smellie JM. Urinary tract infection in childhood. *Br J Hosp Med* 1974;12:485.

bacterial multiplication (143); alternatively, dip slide cultures inoculated at the bedside are reliable (144). Most truly infected urines contain an excess of pus cells and yield a pure growth of a single organism. Fresh urine without cells or visible organisms on microscopy is unlikely to be infected (145). Although more than 10^5 organisms per milliliter of urine is the standard criterion for UTI, in infants a moderate growth of 10,000 to 100,000 organisms per milliliter of urine may represent an infection, and further specimens should be obtained. Most mothers can collect a clean urine specimen from infants. Infants urinate frequently. A clean diaper should be applied after feeding and cleansing; if this diaper is dry 40 to 60 minutes later, the child probably has a full bladder and will urinate if woken and stimulated. Dipstick testing with leukocyte esterase and nitrite strips on fresh urine specimens may produce reliable predictive results (146,147), particularly if UTI is likely on clinical grounds (148). Negative results accurately predict absence of infection, but may be no more specific or sensitive than microscopy and, ultimately, urine dipsticks do not yield culture results (149).

A child with balanitis or sore vulva or terminal hematuria and infection but no other abnormalities on examination should have an ultrasonographic examination of the urinary tract, whereas a child with a fever greater than 38.5°C should be presumed to have acute pyelonephritis (150) and be studied more fully. A detailed history about fever accompanying the illness, the adequacy of the urinary stream in boys, and the presence of functional bladder problems, followed by careful palpation of the abdomen for renal masses and bladder enlargement, thorough examination of the genitalia, and assessment of perineal sensation and neurologic function in the lower limbs, should be carried out.

Appropriate investigations depend on the age of the child and the clinical assessment. Several medical committees have published guidelines on the appropriate protocol to investigate UTI in children (151–153). What is needed is appropriate investigation of all children with UTI if outcomes of children who present in middle or late childhood with ESRF due to reflux nephropathy are to be avoided (154). In general terms, in infants younger than 1 year of age, a micturating cystourethrogram is required together with renal ultrasonography and a functional study such as ^{99m}Tc-DMSA renal isotope scan to detect segmental renal dysplasia or scarring. In older children, the micturating cystourethrogram may be postponed until the infections are recurrent, unless the initial renal ultrasound or DMSA scan is abnormal. A straight abdominal radiograph, DMSA scan, and ultrasound examination or, alternatively, intravenous urography suffices in older children, although a cystogram should be ordered if further infections occur (155). An indirect DTPA scan is useful in older girls to exclude severe reflux and for following children with known reflux (156). Frequently repeated DMSA scanning is not necessary in children with known reflux nephropathy because ultrasonography detects medium or gross scarring. Failure to make the diagnosis (157), investigate thoroughly, and follow guidelines (158) remain the major obstacles

in identifying those children at risk of renal impairment or hypertension.

Management of Urinary Tract Infection

There is little evidence that older children with normal urinary tracts without renal scars who have recurrent UTI will sustain renal damage, and for such children, attention to hygiene, prevention of constipation, and an adequate fluid intake with regular bladder emptying are important. Mild or moderate reflux without upper tract dilatation in young children is likely to disappear in a reasonably short time so that, if the kidneys are not scarred, medical management seems appropriate, whereas severe reflux, especially with scarred kidneys, requires longer-term follow-up, and surgery may be advisable if the quality of the surgery can be guaranteed. However, the single most important action required to reduce the morbidity and mortality of chronic pyelonephritis is the diagnosis and treatment of UTI in infants with fever.

Management of UTI involves administration of appropriate antibiotics early to treat the infection and reduce the risk of renal scarring, attention to the voiding habits of children and avoidance of constipation, encouragement of good personal hygiene of the perineum and genitalia and fluid intake, and diagnosis of any underlying renal tract abnormality (159). Incontinence predisposes to infection, and the treatment of enuresis by bladder training is important. VUR associated with recurrent UTI may be treated medically with prophylactic antibiotics at night (160) or surgical reimplantation of the ureter (138,161,162). Recurrent infections, moderate or severe VUR, or anatomic abnormalities of the renal tract are indications for nightly prophylactic antibiotics because UTI causes considerable distress in children. The International Reflux Study has shown that medical management of VUR is equivalent to surgery in reducing the number of new renal scars (162,163). No advantage between medicine and surgery has been shown after 5 years of follow-up (164,165). Prophylactic antibiotics reduce the incidence of UTI, but doubt has been cast on whether regular prophylactic antibiotics or even surgery significantly alter the rate of new scar formation— most authors agree that making an early diagnosis of UTI is most important in this regard (157). In those children who continue to reflux with cessation of prophylactic antibiotics after 8 years of age, only 12% had another UTI (166). Antibiotic prophylaxis or surgery alone does not influence the number of children reaching ESRF—more effective and robust measures for diagnosis or therapy regimens are required (167).

Because most infections are caused by organisms from the bowel, at least in girls, successful antibiotic prophylaxis depends on the prevention of antibiotic resistance in the bowel flora. Suitable medicines are trimethoprim, 1 mg/kg; nitrofurantoin, 1 to 2 mg/kg; or nalidixic acid, 15 mg/kg, all given as a single dose at night. If infection occurs and the organism is still sensitive, the child or caregiver is likely to be noncompliant.

TABLE 80-6. *Clinical and pathologic correlations in children with glomerulonephritis*

Pathology	Acute nephritic syndrome	Nephrotic syndrome	Hematuria	Proteinuria	Hematuria and proteinuria
Minimal change	++	+++		+++	±
Proliferative disease					
Mesangial	++	++	++	++	++
Mesangiocapillary	++	++	−	−	++
Epithelial	++	++	−	−	+
Acute exudative	+++	+	−	−	++
Membranous	−	++	−	+	+
Focal proliferative	+	+	++	+	+
Focal sclerosis	−	++	−	++	+

+, present; −, not present.

The complications of UTI in children relate to those of renal scarring and renal calculi. *Proteus* infections more commonly cause renal calculi than any other infection because of the organism's ability to produce alkaline urine by degrading urea. In long-term follow-up studies over 10 to 41 years (168), hypertension was observed in young adults in approximately 10% of cases, with people in the higher percentile range for blood pressure being more at risk than others. Approximately 10% have significant renal impairment and may reach renal failure as young people (169). UTI, preeclampsia, fetal death, and low-birth-weight infants are more common in women with renal scarring (170,171).

Glomerulonephritis

The child with glomerulonephritis is likely to present in one of seven ways: acute nephritic syndrome (ANS), hematuria, nephrotic syndrome, proteinuria, hematuria and proteinuria, acute renal failure, or chronic renal insufficiency (Table 80-6). Like adults, the clinical syndrome does not always predict the pathologic process, and the long-term prognosis is related primarily to the pathologic process (see Chapter 71). However, the clinical and histologic features of mesangiocapillary nephritis (membranoproliferative nephritis) in children are similar to those in adults, but treatment with prolonged moderate-dose steroids produces a better outcome in children than adults (172,173); the prognosis of membranous nephropathy also is better in children than in adults. Renal biopsy is still undertaken primarily for prognostic purposes; it is not necessary in all children with glomerulonephritis, and the indications for it are important.

Acute Nephritic Syndrome

Acute nephritic syndrome can follow infection with a wide variety of different bacteria or viruses or be associated with primary glomerulonephritis of unknown origin (Table 80-6). It may be associated with multisystem diseases, such as Henoch-Schönlein purpura (HSP), systemic lupus erythematosus (SLE), Wegener's granulomatosis and other types of vasculitis, Goodpasture's syndrome, or bacterial endocarditis, or be due to an abnormal reaction to certain drugs, such as phenylbutazone or penicillin. Poststreptococcal nephritis is now uncommon in developed countries (174), yet is endemic in many developing countries. It is associated with skin sepsis, but ANS after other infections in children appears to have a good prognosis, as does poststreptococcal nephritis in children (see Chapter 58) (175). Renal biopsy is indicated in any child with postinfectious acute glomerulonephritis who does not follow the normal expected course to full recovery—specifically, in the child with ANS and acute renal failure, the child whose plasma creatinine does not fall to normal after the acute illness (176), or the child who continues to have a low C3 complement. Approximately 98% of children who present with ANS have uncomplicated disease (177) and a good prognosis (175), but the child with systemic disease (e.g., polyarteritis, SLE, or HSP), epithelial crescent formation, or Goodpasture's syndrome, in whom treatment may be urgent and effective, must not be missed (178).

Hematuria

Approximately 2.5% of children are identified as having hematuria by routine testing, defined as more than 10 red blood cells per high-power field on microscopic examination of urine (179), but only 0.05% still have hematuria when tested 3 months later. It occurs transiently during many acute systemic infections. Diseases causing hematuria in children are listed in Table 80-7, and care should be taken not to miss conditions that mimic it. A careful history and examination and simple investigations, such as a full blood count, plasma creatinine, GFR determination, urine microscopy and culture, urine protein estimation, urine calcium and uric acid–creatinine ratios (180), serum C3 and C4 complements, sickle cell preparation, antinuclear antibody factor, antineutrophil cytoplasmic antibodies, antistreptolysin titer concentration, abdominal radiograph for calculi, and ultrasonographic examination or intravenous urogram, are required. In marked contrast to adults, cystoscopy rarely is necessary unless the history suggests a bladder or urethral problem and urine examination reveals lower tract red blood cells (see Chapter 10). The family history is important and the urine of all first-degree relatives should be tested to exclude a familial cause such as autosomal-dominant thin membrane disease (181) or X-linked Alport's syndrome.

TABLE 80-7. *Causes of hematuria in children*

Infections, including tuberculosis
Trauma
Acute nephritic syndrome
Chronic nephritis
Recurrent hematuria syndrome
Familial nephritis
Tumors
Meatal ulcers
Renal calculi, hypercalciuria, hyperuricosuria
Henoch-Schönlein purpura
Hematologic disorders, including sickle cell disease and
    hemophilia
Systemic diseases (e.g., bacterial endocarditis and systemic
    lupus erythematosus)
Urologic malformations
Drugs

Most affected children do well, and extensive investigations, including renal biopsy, do not reveal serious disease and are not indicated (182). Prediction of long-term prognosis from screening of school children for hematuria is not possible and probably not worthwhile (183). Table 80-6 shows that conditions associated with isolated hematuria are those that usually have a good prognosis, whereas the combination of hematuria and proteinuria may be associated with serious disease; thus, such children should have a renal biopsy. Although studies have confirmed a good prognosis in children with intermittent microscopic or macroscopic hematuria, there is some suggestion that children with persistent hematuria do less well and may have more serious disease (181,184). A renal biopsy may be indicated in such children if the condition persists for more than a year even without proteinuria, and, in any case, a yearly follow-up for children with recurrent hematuria is advised. Immunoglobulin A (IgA) nephropathy has a good prognosis over 20 or more years in children without proteinuria, but overall, approximately 13% of children with IgA nephropathy reach ESRF in 10 years (185).

Henoch-Schönlein Nephritis

Henoch-Schönlein purpura was first described by Heberden; later, Schönlein described the typical rash and the joint pains, and Henoch then recognized the association of gastrointestinal involvement and nephritis. HSP affects 13.5/100,000 children per year (186) and can occur at any age (see Chapter 61), but is most common in children aged 2 to 8 years; boys are affected more frequently than girls. The diagnosis is made principally from the evolution and appearance of the rash, which in its typical form is not to be confused with any other condition. The generalized vasculitis affects skin (including nonpurpuric areas), the capsules of the joints, the gastrointestinal tract, and the glomerular capillaries. The pathognomonic feature on renal biopsy is mesangial deposition of IgA-containing immune complexes, although this is not invariable (187). The similarity of IgA nephropathy and HSP nephritis has been noted (see Chapter 61), and identical

twins have been described, one with IgA nephropathy and the other with HSP (188). Even hypertension in HSP without urinary abnormalities has been reported (189).

The cause of HSP is unknown (190), but many cases appear to follow infections, and for many years β-hemolytic streptococcal infections appeared to precipitate the disease, although this is now uncommon. Major histocompatibility antigen [human leukocyte antigen (HLA)] alleles DRB1*01 and DRB1*11 have been associated with the development of HSP, with or without nephritis, and DRB1*07 is protective (191). The C4 null genotype also is associated (192). Poststreptococcal nephritis with a rising antistreptolysin-O titer and a low C3 complement can occur with HSP, and the renal biopsy shows an acute exudative picture with mesangial IgA deposition. Electron microscopy reveals focal thinning of the glomerular basement membrane that resolves on remission. A case of poststreptococcal nephritis and all the clinical features of HSP without IgA deposition has been described in a child with selective IgA deficiency (193). Most children with HSP make a full recovery after 1 to 3 months, but during this period recurrent episodes of purpura may occur; one-third of patients have recurrences. Significant renal involvement is seen in 20% to 60% of cases. In some patients, attacks continue for months or years, and these patients cause particular anxiety because of the risk of serious renal involvement. However, only 1% to 2% reach ESRF (186).

Approximately one-third of children with HSP have abnormal urinary sediment for more than 1 month after the onset of the disease (194). The prognosis usually is good even for children with persistent urinary abnormalities, but children with combined nephritic and nephrotic syndrome, heavy proteinuria, crescentic glomerulonephritis involving more than 50% of glomeruli, or renal impairment at presentation are at greater risk for development of CRF (see Chapter 71) (186,195). Abnormal urine sediments may be found for some years before finally disappearing, and such children should be followed with 3-monthly determinations of blood pressure, plasma albumin, and serum creatinine because late deterioration may occur, which is difficult to predict on clinical features or biopsy findings for an individual.

Children with HSP who present with a combined nephrotic and nephritic syndrome tend to have more severe renal lesions on biopsy and fare less well. We obtain biopsies from children with HSP nephritis who have nephrotic-range proteinuria, sustained hypertension, or a raised plasma creatinine to detect those with extensive epithelial crescent formation. The presence of interstitial disease with tubular atrophy is a bad prognostic sign for long-term outcome, as is a mesangiocapillary-type appearance of the glomerulonephritis. There is some evidence that intensive immunosuppression with high-dose intravenous methylprednisolone (196) followed by prednisolone and azathioprine (197) [combined with plasmapheresis if necessary (198)] alters the poor prognosis in children with severe HSP crescentic nephritis (199). Methylprednisolone, cyclophosphamide, dipyridamole, and prednisolone for 3 months also is effective in severe HSP glomerulonephritis (200). The early use of prednisolone to prevent nephritis developing in children with HSP was supported by a controlled trial (201), although not confirmed in another study (202); it does not prevent recurrences of HSP.

Circulatory shock may occur during the acute phase of an attack of HSP with a massive transfer of plasma proteins into the extravascular fluid and intestines, as happens with intussusception; the plasma albumin concentration may fall below 2 g/dL without any significant proteinuria. Urgent resuscitation is required.

Symptomless Proteinuria

Mild, persistent proteinuria is prevalent in approximately 2% to 4% of children (179) and, in the absence of other evidence of renal disease, usually is benign (203). Orthostatic proteinuria has an excellent prognosis and affected children need not be kept under supervision. Its diagnosis should be made or excluded before planning more invasive investigations. Heavy proteinuria of more than $1 \text{ g}/1.73 \text{ m}^2/24$ hours, even in the absence of other evidence of renal disease, is an indication for renal biopsy because unexpected renal lesions may be discovered (Table 80-6; see Chapter 15). Hematuria in the presence of proteinuria is an indicator for renal biopsy because children with serious forms of idiopathic glomerulonephritis, such as epithelial crescentic nephritis, mesangiocapillary or membranoproliferative nephritis, and focal segmental sclerosis, may present in this way (Table 80-6).

Nephrotic Syndrome

Most children with nephrotic syndrome have minimal change disease, which responds to steroids with resolution of the proteinuria and has an excellent prognosis even if recurrent relapses occur into adult life (204). The main indication for renal biopsy, therefore, is if steroid resistance is present at the onset or develops later. A trial of prednisolone before biopsy at a dose of 60 mg/m^2 BSA for 4 weeks usually is advised except in children in whom suspicion of more serious disease is raised by factors such as age, sustained hypertension at onset, hematuria, or a low C3 complement (205). Although some children with focal glomerular sclerosis who respond to steroids are missed by this policy, this does not present a problem because the prognosis in such children is good (see Chapter 71). High-dose prednisolone therapy for more than 4 weeks, however, can cause side effects.

The subsequent clinical course of the nephrotic syndrome can be predicted from the initial response and the relapses in the first 6 months of the disease. Steroid resistance with the first course of prednisolone and heavy proteinuria in the first 6 months favor progression to ESRF in 21% to 35% of patients (206). Three relapses within the first 6 months after responding to the initial steroid therapy predicts that the child will continue to relapse frequently (207), as does the child's tissue type being HLA-DRB1*07 (208). The prevalence of frequently relapsing disease during 2 years of observation

in steroid-responsive children may be reduced from 50% to 27% by giving a weaning course of alternate-day steroids over a further 4 months after the initial 8-week therapy (209, 210).

Most steroid toxicity in children with steroid-sensitive nephrotic syndrome is caused by the frequency of relapses that require high-dose treatment. Once a child has been identified as a frequent relapser, several therapeutic options exist. A dose of alternate-day prednisolone may be given in the morning, which maintains remission without steroid toxicity (up to 0.5 mg/kg on alternate days), and the child maintained on treatment for a year before trying to discontinue the steroid therapy again by slowly weaning the dose (211). Levamisole 2.5 mg/kg on alternate days (212) or a course of an alkylating agent [cyclophosphamide (213), mustine, or chlorambucil (214)] are alternative therapies. Alkylating agents allow withdrawal of all medication with a risk of relapse of 45% at 2 years; however, approximately 15% are cured (215).

The main risk to a child with steroid-sensitive nephrotic syndrome is a complication of a relapse. Clinical signs of hypovolemia occur most commonly either with the first episode, or a relapse, and may be associated with septicemia due especially to pneumococcal bacterial infection, or vascular thrombosis. The physician should have a low threshold to perform paracentesis to diagnose primary peritonitis due to pneumococcal or Gram-negative organisms, particularly if the child is taking steroids. We maintain children on prophylactic penicillin during relapses. Trials of immunization with a pneumococcal vaccine show antibody responses are adequate (216) and persist for more than 5 years in more than 50% of immunized nephrotic children (217), but do not fully protect the child from *Streptococcus pneumoniae* infection (218). Hypovolemia should be considered in any child with a relapse, particularly if they are unwell, and especially with vomiting or abdominal pain. The most useful clinical sign is poor peripheral perfusion with cold feet and toes because the blood pressure may be raised from increased angiotensin production. The hematocrit rises and the urine output is low, with a low urinary sodium concentration. Acute renal failure requiring dialysis is rare, however. A raised blood urea nitrogen (BUN) with a normal plasma creatinine is common and is due to the reduced urea clearance associated with oliguria. Treatment consists of infusing salt-poor albumin at a concentration of 20 g/dL with careful monitoring to detect vascular overload (219).

Long-term cyclosporine at doses of 4 to 5 mg/kg/day effectively maintains remission for 2 to 4 years and is quite safe for 5 years providing regular monitoring of plasma creatinine, GFR, and cyclosporine trough levels is carried out. We give the patient or their parents the choice of having a renal biopsy every 2 years to detect histologic changes of cyclosporine toxicity or stopping the drug. After 5 years or more of cyclosporine treatment, less than 5% of patients have shown interstitial fibrosis or tubular atrophy attributed to drug toxicity, and usually this is accompanied by a decline in GFR. Seventy-five percent of steroid-responsive nephrotic children are able to discontinue steroids under cover of cyclosporine treatment.

Hemolytic-Uremic Syndromes

The HUS are broadly divided into the diarrhea-associated (D+) HUS, previously called *typical* or *epidemic form* (220), and non–diarrhea-associated (D−) HUS, previously called the *atypical* or *sporadic form* (221); familial forms exist and are usually, but not exclusively, D− HUS. Underlying C3 hypocomplementemia (222) associated with genetic mutations of complement factor H (223,224) predisposes to familial D− HUS. The diarrheal form is associated with infection by Shiga-like toxin–producing organisms, typically *E. coli* type 0157 [verotoxin-producing *E. coli* (VTEC)] in developed countries, *Shigella dysenteriae* type 1 in the Indian subcontinent and Africa, or occasionally *Shigella flexneri* infections. The severity after *Shigella* infection seems to be greater, but this may be related partly to malnutrition and socioeconomic factors (225). *S. pneumoniae* also may produce D− HUS because its neuraminidase toxin removes sialic acid residues from red blood cells, platelet membranes, and glomeruli to expose the Thomsen-Friedenreich antigen, which reacts with a circulating IgM (226). All forms of HUS, inherited or otherwise, have the ability to injure endothelial cells, and this seems to be a primary requisite for an agent to cause HUS (227), although circulating tissue factor levels are not increased (228). Neutrophils and complement may play important roles in this injury process, which results in thrombotic microangiopathy with hemolytic anemia (see Chapter 67). The pathogenesis of the acute renal failure seems to be related to damage to endothelial cells with platelet activation, a rise in nitric oxide, and intracapillary thrombi.

Diarrhea-associated HUS occurs in Europe and North America in the summer months after an episode of diarrhea, which often is bloody and usually is caused by VTEC. Sources of VTEC associated with HUS have been found in cows, pigs, contaminated cheese and dairy products, processed meats, and stagnant water such as wells and swimming lakes, in addition to other family members. D+ HUS is associated with a microangiopathic hemolytic anemia; thrombocytopenia is almost invariable and together with uremia, these results comprise the clinical features of HUS. Intravascular coagulation, clot fibrinolysis, and tissue-type plasminogen activator are increased, but not plasminogen activator inhibitor-1 (229). Prothrombin time and partial thromboplastin time usually are normal, and levels and activity of factors V and VIII are variable. Fibrin degradation products usually are elevated, but fibrinogen turnover is normal. Antithrombin III levels may be reduced, but protein C and S values usually are normal. Increased circulating concentrations of von Willebrand factor multimers have been described. Prostacyclin production by endothelial cells may be defective (230). It is not clear whether this failure is due to some toxic substance in the plasma of patients with HUS or the absence of a factor necessary for normal prostacyclin generation. Very high leukocyte counts are common in postdiarrheal HUS and this correlates with circulating interleukin-8 (IL-8) concentrations, whereas normal or low counts tend to be found in D− HUS. When present in D+ HUS cases, the higher the leukocyte count the worse the prognosis (231), probably signifying the greater involvement of endothelial tissue and therefore greater IL-8 release.

Hemolytic-uremic syndrome is the most common single cause of acute renal failure in infants and young children. The presentation is usually a child with an unremarkable episode of diarrhea (except for the fact that blood may be seen in the stools), who then becomes quiet, lethargic, and pale, and is noted to be oliguric. Extrarenal involvement in HUS, although common, rarely causes severe problems; however, catastrophic central nervous system complications can occur and are the usual cause of death (232). Treatment on admission to the hospital is directed toward dealing with the acute complications of renal insufficiency and, because these children often are extremely ill, urgent dialysis often is required. The prognosis in D+ HUS is good and full recovery of renal function after a period of a few days to a few weeks is expected, although renal functional reserve may be impaired (233,234). The most important component of management is the treatment of the acute renal failure with transfusions of packed red cells to alleviate the anemia after adequate dialysis has been established. The use of fresh frozen plasma is controversial. A controlled study in France demonstrated less hypertension and improved histologic appearances without acute cortical necrosis 1 year after D+ HUS in children treated with fresh frozen plasma compared with no fresh frozen plasma, but no difference in plasma creatinine (235). This result has not been confirmed in all studies (see Chapter 67). Because the prognosis in the postdiarrheal form is good, it is very difficult to perform adequate control trials to determine the efficacy of this treatment.

Hemolytic-uremic syndrome caused by neuraminidase from *S. pneumoniae,* which is rare, should be expected in any child who is toxic and has pneumonia and a positive Coombs' test. The diagnosis is important because blood transfusion may accelerate the agglutination. Such patients should be treated with penicillin to cure the infection and should not be given plasma until *S. pneumoniae* has been eliminated as the cause of the HUS (226).

The sporadic, familial, or D-forms of HUS are extremely uncommon. Familial autosomal-recessive forms of HUS have been described, and these need to be distinguished from the postdiarrheal form occurring in members of the same family at the same time. The sporadic familial form without diarrhea has a poor prognosis, and these children tend to progress to ESRF or die with complications such as cerebrovascular involvement in spite of treatment with fresh frozen plasma or plasmapheresis (236). HUS can recur after renal transplantation and it may be that such patients have the familial form of the disease. Autosomal-dominant inheritance of HUS has been described, but these patients are usually adult and have a very poor prognosis.

Hemolytic-uremic syndrome also can occur in other circumstances, such as in association with overwhelming sepsis, particularly in the newborn or young infant, and in association with some drugs such as cyclosporine.

HYPERTENSION

It is disappointing how frequently the measurement of blood pressure is neglected in pediatric practice. Population screening of children for UTI or urinary abnormalities is not cost effective (132), but this increases the responsibility of primary health care workers to identify the child with renal disease by measuring the blood pressure and testing the urine for blood and protein, and culturing where appropriate, at routine health checks. The sphygmomanometer cuff should be wide enough to cover the upper arm and long enough to encircle at least three-fourths of the arm circumference. The usual error is to use a cuff that is too small and results in a falsely high reading. The child, and in particular his or her arm, should be relaxed to avoid another source of error, especially with infants. Measurement is difficult in infants because auscultation of the Korotkoff sounds often is unsatisfactory. With Doppler devices, an accurate measurement of systolic pressure can be obtained. Values for normal blood pressure in children of different ages are given in Table 80-8.

Neonates and Infants

The upper limit for mean arterial blood pressure in infants weighing more than 2.5 kg rises from 68 mm Hg at birth to 87 mm Hg at 4 weeks (90). Systemic hypertension, not related to coarctation of the aorta, appears to be becoming more common in newborns, both because it is now easier to measure blood pressure using Doppler ultrasound and because of thromboembolic occlusions of the renal vasculature from umbilical arterial catheters (237). It is important to check that the tip of the catheter lies below the origin of the renal arteries. Rarer causes of hypertension include renal emboli from clots that originate in the ductus arteriosus, congenital renal artery stenosis, renal venous thrombosis, structural renal lesions, raised intracranial pressure, pheochromocytoma, and congenital adrenal hyperplasia. Affected infants often are ill with cardiac failure and neurologic problems. The most useful investigations are renal ultrasound and dynamic renal scintigraphy using ^{99m}Tc-labeled MAG3 scanning, which show a poorly functioning kidney with diminished blood flow. Additional information about the resolution of hypertension may be obtained using ACE scintigraphy (238). Control of the hypertension is vital; propranolol up to 3 mg/kg/day and the calcium channel blocking agent nifedipine up to 3 mg/kg/day with or without a diuretic are useful. The ACE inhibitor captopril or a longer-acting analog is useful but is contraindicated in renal artery stenosis [see Chandar et al. (238)]. More potent vasodilators such as minoxidil may be required. Acute control may be achieved with intravenous labetalol infusions at 1 to 3 mg/kg/hour, sodium nitroprusside 500 ng to 8 μg/kg/minute, or hydralazine in doses up to 3 mg/kg/day. In cases secondary to renal emboli, the prognosis often is good, with the hypertension resolving and the renal function improving with time if permanent renal ischemia is not present.

Causes and Investigation in Older Children

Severe hypertension, defined as a systolic or diastolic blood pressure at least 15 mm Hg above the 95th percentile for normal children of the same age, sex, and height (239), is rare, with a prevalence of approximately 1 in 500, and usually is secondary to a specific disease (Table 80-9). Although the possible causes are numerous, in practice approximately 67% of cases have parenchymal renal disease, 7% have renovascular problems, 22% have coarctation of the aorta, 1.5% have endocrine disease, and 2.5% have some other condition (240). Necessary investigations include the exclusion of coarctation of the thoracic or abdominal aorta on clinical examination; the examination of the urine for blood and protein; the measurement of plasma electrolytes, creatinine, and urea; renal imaging with ultrasound (including Doppler studies of aorta and renal arteries) and a DMSA scan; and the measurement of urinary catecholamine metabolite excretion (241). The rare cases of mineralocorticoid excess, real or apparent (242), can be distinguished by the presence of hypokalemic alkalosis in the clinical setting with salt and

TABLE 80-8. *Levels of blood pressure in children of different ages*

Age (yr)	Mean (mm Hg)		+2 Standard deviations (mm Hg)	
	Systolic	Diastolic	Systolic	Diastolic
0–3	95	60	110	70
4–7	100	65	115	75
8–10	105	70	125	80
11–15	120	75	135	85

TABLE 80-9. *Causes of hypertension in children*

Renovascular	Renal artery stenosis, neurofibromatosis, thrombosis, hemolytic-uremic syndrome
Parenchymal renal disease	Glomerulonephritis, nephrosis, pyelonephritis, trauma, Wilms' tumor, obstruction, dysplasia, Schönlein-Henoch disease, cortical necrosis
Cardiovascular disease	Coarctation of the aorta, anemia, polycythemia, Takayasu's arteritis, patent ductus arteriosus
Endocrine	Pheochromocytoma, neuroblastoma, hyperthyroidism, congenital adrenal hyperplasia, Conn's syndrome (primary hyperaldosteronism), Cushing's syndrome, Liddle's syndrome, hyperparathyroidism
Miscellaneous	Central nervous system lesions, traction, dehydration, drugs, licorice, vitamin D intoxication, hypernatremia

water excess rather than deficit, although the exact diagnosis requires analysis of plasma and urine steroids. Plasma renin and aldosterone concentrations should be measured on a venous blood sample taken after the patient has rested supine for 2 hours; the normal range is higher in children than in adults (243), and it is important to measure the plasma renin before starting treatment. Hypertension secondary to endocrine disease usually is associated with suppression of plasma renin, although a secondary rise can be found with a pheochromocytoma. Supine and upright plasma epinephrine and norepinephrine levels help to identify pheochromocytomas and give an indication whether they are adrenal or extraadrenal in origin (244). Computed tomography scans of thorax and abdomen are more sensitive than metaiodobenzylguanidine isotope scans in locating these tumors. Renal artery stenosis may be suspected from the raised plasma renin and from the clinical examination, but in the absence of a diagnosis, selective renal arteriography is indicated after the blood pressure has been controlled. The amount of contrast injected should be the minimum required and blood pressure should be monitored. Approximately 100 case reports of renal artery stenosis associated with pheochromocytoma exist, so the latter diagnosis should be excluded before selective renal arteriography. Evidence of renal ischemia is obtained from the differential renal vein renin determinations. A ratio of greater than 1.5:1.0 between the affected and nonaffected kidney is a useful predictor of renal ischemia and indicates that a favorable response to surgery is likely in children (245), although successful surgery has been reported in some cases when the ratio was less than 1.5:1.0 (246). A negative arteriogram with no significant difference between the renal vein renins and the systemic plasma renin excludes a renovascular cause for the hypertension.

Treatment

Children with hypertension should be admitted to the hospital for initial control of blood pressure; malignant hypertension is a medical emergency. Controlled lowering of the blood pressure by the use of intravenous labetalol or sodium nitroprusside infusions should be achieved slowly and steadily over a period of days if severe neurologic complications and blindness are to be avoided (247) (Table 80-10). The infusion rate of these drugs can be titrated to the blood pressure. If the child is having seizures, then an initial rapid reduction of systolic blood pressure by 20 to 40 mm Hg is necessary. Patients with malignant hypertension may be volume depleted, and the blood pressure may fall precipitously when a vasodilating agent such as nifedipine, hydralazine, or diazoxide is administered. In such cases, physiologic saline should be infused rapidly to correct the volume depletion and allow an even control of blood pressure. In fact, in salt-depleted hypertensive children, 0.9% saline may be necessary to gain control of the blood pressure. The calcium channel blocking agent nifedipine, administered orally, or β-adrenergic blocking drugs are useful to control less severe rises in blood pressure. ACE

TABLE 80-10. *Medications for use in hypertension*

Medication	Dosage
Oral	
Chlorothiazide	10 mg/kg/12 hr
Furosemide	0.5–7.5 mg/kg/d
Spironolactone	1 mg/kg/8 hr
Atenolol[a]	1–8 mg/kg/d
Propranolol	0.2–3.0 mg/kg/8 hr
Hydralazine	0.2–1.0 mg/kg/8 hr
Doxazosin[a]	1 mg, increasing gradually at fortnight intervals to 8 mg
Prazosin	Test dose 0.01 mg/kg; increase to 0.1 mg/kg/8 hr
Minoxidil	0.1–0.5 mg/kg/12 hr
Enalopril[a]	0.1–1.0 mg/kg/d
Captopril	0.3–5.0 mg/kg/d
Amlodipine[a]	2.5–10 mg per d
Nifedipine	0.25–1.0 mg/kg/8 h
Intravenous	
Labetalol	1–3 mg/kg/hr
Sodium nitroprusside	1–8 μg/kg/min
Hydralazine	0.15–0.50 mg/kg (IM or IV)
Diazoxide	1.5–5.0 mg/kg as rapid injection

[a]Once-daily dosing.

inhibitors should be avoided until renovascular disease or coarctation of aorta is excluded.

Oral regimens usually start with a long-acting calcium channel blocker such as amlodipine or a long-acting β-blocker, or both. A diuretic may be added if necessary with the aim to give smaller doses of synergistically acting drugs to reduce side effects, yet still keep the number of doses per day at a minimum to improve the child's compliance with therapy. Vasodilator drugs often lead to salt and water retention and escape from blood pressure control if a diuretic is not administered concomitantly. In children with renal insufficiency, the thiazide drugs are less effective and furosemide usually is advocated as the diuretic. The dose of furosemide must be increased to compensate for a low GFR because the drug action depends on its intraluminal concentration. A long-acting ACE inhibitor such as enalapril is used when renal ischemia or progressive CRF is the cause of the hypertension. This class of antihypertensive drug is especially valuable to control blood pressure in children with renin-dependent hypertension after HUS. When renal ischemia is caused by renal artery stenosis or coarctation of the aorta, captopril or related drugs may cause a precipitous fall in GFR because of efferent arteriolar dilatation; therefore, caution should be exercised. Concern exists over long-term metabolic effects (hypokalemia, hyperuricemia, and hyperglycemia) with prolonged thiazide therapy in growing children and the SLE syndrome associated with hydralazine treatment.

Essential Hypertension

It is usual to define essential hypertension in children as a blood pressure greater than the 95th percentile for age, taking into consideration the patient's height and sex; this inevitably defines 5% of the child population as hypertensive. However, screening studies have demonstrated that, on rechecking, only approximately 1% of a population of children has a persistently raised blood pressure. Ambulatory blood pressure monitoring discriminates between true and "white coat" hypertension. Although consistent measurement of blood pressure along percentile lines has been demonstrated in children between 1 and 5 years of age (248), the importance of identifying this group is not yet clear. One long-term follow-up study of young adults aged 21 to 30 years showed a threefold increased risk of hypertension in the children in the highest blood pressure quintile at 9 to 14 years of age (249); these data confirm the findings of others (250). The risk of hypertension in the offspring of hypertensive parents is increased (251). Certainly, there is no evidence that pharmacologic treatment should be instituted for mild hypertension in children, and the dangers probably outweigh the advantages. Although population screening may not be cost effective, blood pressure should be checked at office visits, on admission to the hospital, and in children with a family history of hypertension so that advice about weight reduction, exercise, smoking, and diet can be provided; because of familial predisposition to hypertension, this advice may well benefit other members of the family (252).

CHRONIC AND END-STAGE RENAL FAILURE IN CHILDREN

The overall prevalence of renal disease causing ESRF has remained constant since the late 1970s at 53.4 children per million population of children younger than 18 years of age (253). The annual rate in the United Kingdom of ESRF has been estimated at 5.2 to 7.5 per million children. However, some racial groups have higher rates than others. For example, Indian Asians have a threefold increase in demand for ESRF treatment in the United Kingdom, in part because of congenital renal tract anomalies (254). Whereas the overall prevalence of ESRF has not varied significantly since the late 1970s, its etiology and the age of reaching ESRF have changed as more young children with congenital or inherited renal disease are treated. Congenital renal tract abnormalities and inherited kidney conditions now account for 72% of the need for renal replacement therapy in children in the United Kingdom. In Sweden, reflux nephropathy has decreased from approximately 20% in the late 1970s to less than 5% of cases; this in not observed in all registries [Table 80-4; see Fivush et al. (255)]. The prevalence of CRF is unknown, but Leumann identified 28 children (or 18 per million population of children) in Switzerland with a plasma creatinine greater than 2 mg/dL (256).

Because CRF is rare in children compared with adults, it seems reasonable for a limited number of centers to specialize in providing treatment for children because treatment of an occasional child in adult treatment centers is likely to be unsatisfactory. A children's center should have the full range of general pediatric services, including intensive care facilities for children, a children's dialysis unit, pediatric nurses, social workers, dietitians, and the necessary educational and psychological staff to care for the needs of chronically handicapped children. The aim for most children with ESRF is a successful renal transplant, so it is advantageous if facilities for transplantation are available in the children's hospital. Obviously, such provision can be expensive, but is more economical if it is established in a hospital that already has well developed pediatric services and an active adult renal unit. A reasonable population base for a pediatric nephrology center would be 8 to 10 million people, providing an admission rate of approximately 15 children per year.

Pediatric nephrologists have the specter hanging over them of a short, malnourished child with bowed legs, due to renal rickets, presenting for treatment of ESRF. Today, this should not happen. Moreover, infants with end-stage disease and microcephaly and poor cognitive function from aluminum toxicity should not exist. Our knowledge of the factors that affect children in CRF is sufficient to ensure a better outcome, but our knowledge is far from complete. With proper diagnosis and investigation of the renal tract to ensure unobstructed urine flow, including bladder function, nutritional support, correction of electrolyte and acidosis imbalance, and control of secondary hyperparathyroidism, children with CRF should grow well and develop normally. It is these areas of the clinical care of pediatric CRF that differ greatly from the experience in adult nephrologic practice.

Management of the child with CRF/ESRF is time consuming, and careful clinical and biochemical assessment is required at regular intervals. This should include accurate measurement of height and weight, skinfold thickness, and upper arm circumference. The weight-for-height index is of particular value in detecting malnutrition. Pubertal status should be documented at intervals. Radiographs of the hand and wrist should be obtained annually for assessment of bone age and detection and supervision of renal osteodystrophy.

Growth Retardation in Children with Chronic Renal Failure

Nearly half of the children with CRF or ESRF were below the third percentile for height (257–259). The average height for young men and women treated by dialysis and transplantation during childhood is approximately 2 SD below the mean (260); this represents an average deficit of 15 cm in final height (261). This stunting of growth is a source of social embarrassment and psychological trauma. Children with congenital renal disease tend to be shorter than those with acquired disease because of a growth deficit during the first 2 years of life, when growth usually is so rapid. It reflects poor nutrition (262,263) and electrolyte, phosphate, and calcium imbalance (264). If dialysis is required, this mode of therapy provides suboptimal replacement of renal function and has many complications in infants (265,266). Moreover, children with syndromes, chromosomal anomalies, and some systemic conditions often have poor growth.

Improving dialysis improves growth (267). Although growth after transplantation may be normal (268), such accelerated growth to "catch up" is uncommon. Therefore, particular attention must be paid to maximize growth in the child with CRF before ESRF is reached, and this is especially important for the infant who is born with renal disease (269).

An integral part of the poor growth associated with uremia is the delay in skeletal and pubertal maturation. Although normal pubertal growth may occur in children with CRF on conservative medical management (270), growth hormone (GH) bursts from the pituitary gland are reduced in quantity, and in prepubertal and peripubertal boys, plasma insulin-like growth factor-1 (IGF-1) levels are reduced and IGF binding protein concentrations increased, leading to less growth-promoting activity of the pituitary-GH-IGF axis (271). In late puberty, GH burst frequency increases above normal but GH mass per burst remains low. Deranged (lower) overnight gonadotropin bursts from the pituitary also are observed in peripubertal children (272), which leads to an average delay in puberty onset in CRF of 2.5 years for both sexes (273). Children with ESRF do not fair so well, however, attaining only 48% to 58% of the normal pubertal height gain (273). The poor growth of CRF usually is associated with delayed skeletal maturation (274). During early puberty, height and skeletal development appear to advance in parallel, but later in puberty, skeletal maturation may advance more rapidly than the advance in chronologic age and growth, further limiting the final height. The mean age of onset for menarche in girls with ESRF is 15.1 years, compared with a mean age for normal girls of 13.4 years (275).

With transplantation, growth usually improves but is variable because of many complex factors, with only some patients showing "catch-up" growth (276). Certainly younger, prepubertal children, particularly those who are most stunted during CRF or who were dialyzed, grow better initially than older children or adolescents if they receive a good functioning renal transplant. Good posttransplantation renal function and alternate-day steroid therapy (277), or, better still, no long-term maintenance steroids, produce significantly better growth than daily maintenance doses without compromising allograft survival figures (278,279). However cystinotic children remain short despite restoration of good renal function posttransplantation (280).

Causes of Growth Failure

Determinants of growth at different ages are best described by growth velocity patterns, with final adult height being the outcome measure. Genetic, nutritional, hormonal, and metabolic determinants interact throughout each phase of growth. Potential for growth loss and recovery is greatest during infancy and early childhood. Growth retardation is particularly marked in children with generalized tubular dysfunction (Fanconi's syndrome), where sodium and bicarbonate wasting, polyuria and polydipsia, hypophosphatemia, and osteomalacia all contribute (281). Sodium wasting is particularly important both in these children and in infants with CRF caused by congenital obstruction or renal dysplasia/hypoplasia. Sodium is essential for growth (282), and salt supplements restore growth in children with isolated sodium wasting (283). Indomethacin reduces the increased fractional sodium excretion in cystinosis (79) and corrects the polyuria and polydipsia, and this may be associated with improvement in growth.

In children with CRF, renal osteodystrophy, osteomalacia, and osteitis fibrosa cystica due to secondary hyperparathyroidism are all potent inhibitors of growth. When the GFR is below 80 mL/minute/1.73 m^2, accumulation of phosphate and secondary hyperparathyroidism occur and can be prevented by using low-phosphate diets with or without phosphate-binding drugs. We routinely measure plasma PTH concentrations and adjust our therapy to keep the PTH levels within the normal physiologic range. The urinary fractional excretion of phosphate may be used instead of intact PTH, but direct PTH measurement is preferred. When the GFR reaches less than 25 mL/minute/1.73 m^2, high-dose phosphate binders together with extra vitamin D in the form of α-calcidol or 1,25-dihydroxycholecalciferol are used (284).

Chronic renal failure is associated with a complex derangement in the metabolism of protein (285) and energy (286) (see Chapter 103). These abnormalities tend to be worse in children because of their higher metabolic rate and energy and protein requirements. Peripheral uptake and metabolism of glucose under conditions of hyperglycemia are reduced by nearly 40% in uremic children (287), but this abnormality can be corrected either by suppression of the secondary hyperparathyroidism (288) or by reducing the nitrogen toxicity with low-protein diets (289).

The levels of the two most important growth hormones in humans, insulin and GH itself, are raised in CRF, with the balance of IGF-1 and its binding proteins in favor of there being less biologically active IGF-1 hormone (290–292). Daily injection of recombinant human GH (rhGH) improves the growth of children with CRF (293) and ESRF (294), as well as those posttransplantation (295), by normalizing IGF-1 bioactivity.

Body composition studies in uremic infants have demonstrated considerable reductions in cell mass in relation to height, with those children who have the most abnormal body composition being the smallest (269). Malnutrition due to these metabolic disturbances of uremia is common in adults, and in childhood it is equivalent to poor growth. Anorexia frequently accompanies CRF, and when the energy intake falls below 80% of the recommended dietary allowance, there is a correlation between the poor energy intake and poor growth (263,296). Energy intake can be increased by feeding and growth will improve, but, in many instances, will not become normal (266,297,298) . Feeding extra energy to children with adequate energy intakes does not improve growth. Although a poor spontaneous energy intake is an important cause of growth retardation, particularly in infants, and every attempt must be made to increase energy intake to normal levels (262), such measures do not guarantee good growth.

Nutritional Therapy

Prescribing a strict dietary regime for the anorectic child in CRF is futile because compliance is poor. We use a dietitian as an essential part of the clinical team to offer advice on diet. They prescribe an amount of low-phosphate food for infants, which contains supplements of glucose polymer or lipid to increase the daily calorie intake to a minimum of 120 but ideally 150 kcal/kg/day. Infants are fed high-protein milks and protein supplements up to a total of 2.5 g/kg/day. Older children with moderate or severe CRF initially fill out a prospective 3-day dietary assessment for the dietitian to analyze. Those with poor caloric intake and good urine output then are encouraged to drink cola, fizzy glucose drinks, and the like, which are high in calories, and if their weight gain is inadequate, glucose polymer supplements are added to these drinks. This strategy uses the obligate polyuria of CRF and thirst mechanisms. Eating commercially produced hamburgers and noncheese savory snacks also is encouraged, as is double cream. The only "dietary prescription" that is used is phosphate restriction by reducing dairy products to a minimum. Providing calories in this manner may account for a third of the daily total intake, usually produces good weight gains, and, by suppressing the spontaneous appetite, allows the clinician largely to ignore the remainder of the diet except if there is a particular problem such as hyperkalemia or hyperphosphatemia. If the weight gain is poor with the child's spontaneous food intake, early use of alimentary feeding with either a nasogastric feeding tube or gastrostomy is required (266). Care must be taken not to make the child obese with these measures.

Most important, this approach to food intake gets away from "prescribing" strict, controlled diets for older children in CRF and allows the child and family to choose a food according to their own preferences, thereby improving compliance and allowing the physician to concentrate on other aspects of the child's management.

The value of restricting protein in renal failure is scientifically based on recommended dietary allowances of foodstuffs and experimental animal and human evidence (289, 299,300). Although protein malnutrition is frequent in CRF, protein intake usually exceeds the minimum recommended intake (301) (Table 80-11), and the protein malnutrition is caused by either a poor energy intake or the severity of the uremic state. No great advantages were observed with dietary manipulation in three trials of protein restriction in CRF (302–304). Although the latter study did show improvement in growth, it required use of essential amino acid supplements and a high-calorie diet—both confounding factors in analyzing its efficacy. The Southwest Pediatric Nephrology Study Group controlled trial showed poorer growth in infants after 18 months of a low-protein diet. In clinical practice, the use of moderate or severe protein restriction in children with CRF is not required; excluding dairy products for phosphate restriction already reduces protein intake to some extent. Examination and adjustment of the average calorie intake, weight and height gain, BUN (which should be <60 mg/dL), and albumin is sufficient for a decision about dietary protein intake to be taken; restriction beyond dairy products rarely is required in our experience. When the BUN was maintained below 60 mg/dL, the peripheral consumption of glucose during sustained hyperglycemia was normalized, with normal insulin sensitivity for the peripheral uptake of glucose (289).

An adequate intake of vitamins such as pyridoxine and trace minerals should be ensured. The importance of an adequate sodium intake and the correction of a metabolic acidosis already has been emphasized.

Renal osteodystrophy is treated, and hopefully prevented, by giving supplements of active vitamin D when the GFR falls below 25 mL/minute/1.73 m^2 BSA. We usually prescribe α-calcidol (0.25 to 1.00 μg/day) or 1,25-dihydroxycholecalciferol (0.12 to 0.50 μg/day). Hyperphosphatemia should be controlled with dietary restriction of dairy products and

TABLE 80-11. *Recommended daily allowances of nutrients for children of different ages for use with chronic renal insufficiency*

Age	Height (cm)	Energy (kcal/kg)	Minimal protein	Calcium (g)	Phosphorus (g)
0–6 mo	60	120	2.2 g/kg	0.4	0.2
6–12 mo	72	100	1.8 g/kg	0.6	0.5
1–2 yr	81	1,100	18 g	0.7	0.7
2–4 yr	96	1,300	22 g	0.8	0.8
4–6 yr	110	1,600	25 g	0.8	0.8
6–8 yr	121	2,000	29 g	0.9	0.9
8–10 yr	131	2,200	31 g	1.0	1.0
10–12 yr	141	2,450	36 g	1.2	1.2
12–14 yr					
Male	151	2,700	40 g	1.4	1.4
Female	154	2,300	34 g	1.3	1.3
14–18 yr					
Male	170	3,000	45 g	1.4	1.4
Female	159	2,200	35 g	1.3	1.3

From Department of Health and Social Security. *Recommended intakes of nutrients for the United Kingdom.* Reports of Public Health and Medical Subjects, no. 120. London: HM Stationery Office, 1969.

phosphate-binding drugs such as calcium carbonate (10 to 200 mg/kg/day) (305) or cross-linked poly-(allylamine hydrochloride) (Renagel) (306). Monitoring therapy requires frequent measurement of serum PTH when the GFR falls below 25 mL/minute/1.73 m^2 BSA, reducing the phosphate content of the diet, and increasing the dose of phosphate binders as necessary (39). It also is important to monitor the plasma calcium frequently to prevent hypercalcemia, which usually occurs only when hyperparathyroidism has been controlled. The importance of suppressing secondary hyperparathyroidism must be emphasized, and we prefer PTH values to be normal. Adynamic bone disease has been described with low normal PTH values, but usually after high-dose intermittent intravenous active vitamin D metabolite treatment. There is concern about the use of aluminum hydroxide in infants (307), and we prefer calcium carbonate given with meals (308). If the child is hypercalcemic, it is best to lower the plasma phosphate by diet and Renagel and then substitute calcium carbonate when control has been established.

Concern exists among pediatric and adult nephrologists about the long-term metabolic consequences of a diet high in carbohydrate and fat and the cardiovascular disease risks they impose (309,310). Both hypertriglyceridemia and hypercholesterolemia are common in children with CRF and ESRF, although the observed derangement varies with the degree of uremia, mode of renal replacement therapy, and drug regimens (311–313). The abnormalities usually are proatherogenic (314), with some studies showing lipid metabolism being greatly deranged when the GFR is less than 40 mL/minute/1.73 m^2 (315), but not others (316). There are no large, controlled, long-term trials of therapy for hyperlipidemia in children with progressive renal disease. Short-term studies with fish oil, 5 to 8 g/day, show effectiveness in reducing hypertriglyceridemia but not hypercholesterolemia (317). Both triglyceride and cholesterol are reduced in nephrotic patients with 3-hydroxy-3-methylglutaryl coenzyme A (HMG-CoA) reductase inhibitors.

Growth Hormone Therapy

Growth hormone treatment is not a substitute for good management of the various abnormalities of body composition that occur in CRF (318) (see earlier). However, if these disturbances due to uremia are addressed and the child still fails to grow and is below the third percentile for height, recombinant human GH (rhGH) therapy at a dose of 30 U/m^2 BSA per week increases the height velocity SD score (SDS) in children with CRF (319,320), those undergoing dialysis (321), and those with transplants (322). It is more effective in prepubertal and younger children, when height velocity SDS may double or triple, compared with older, peripubertal children. "Catch-up" growth may occur in the first 2 or 3 years of therapy, but then height velocity reduces to more normal levels. If rhGH is stopped, "catch-down" growth is reported to occur in 75% of patients (323), whereas others report growth proceeding along the percentile lines (324). The therapy is

safe, with no common deleterious effects on GFR, long-term insulin insensitivity, or, in transplanted patients, allograft rejection (322,325). Although the parents' and patient's acceptance of the treatment is good (326), compliance still may be a problem in 60% of children and the issue should be raised, although there was little correlation with the response to therapy in one study (327). Although final heights are difficult to predict (328), early data show that many children with renal transplants are achieving heights close to the parental height predictions, provided the dosage of steroids is low, regardless of rhGH treatment (329).

Chronic Renal Failure

Because congenital abnormalities of the lower renal tract commonly cause progressive renal disease, a priority in caring for these children is to ensure that neither kidney is obstructed. This requires full investigation with renal tract ultrasonography, dynamic renal isotope scintillography (^{99m}Tc-MAG3), as well a micturating cystourethrogram or bladder videourodynamics. Treatment of urinary sepsis and its prevention by low-dose antibiotic prophylaxis is equally as important.

There are many types of electrolyte imbalance in the various causes of CRF, from salt wasting due to hydronephrosis or corrected lower tract obstruction to children with magnesium wasting in hypomagnesemic-hypercalciuric syndrome with nephrocalcinosis and CRF. Attention to detail with appropriate replacement is needed, and this is best performed in a clinic specifically allocated to children with low renal clearances. A raised plasma BUN above 60 mg/dL is more a reflection of inadequate calorie intake than excessive protein intake. Therefore, an important starting point is to ensure an adequate number of calories: at least 150 kcal/kg/day for infants, 120 to 150 kcal/kg/day for toddlers, and approximately 100 kcal/kg/day for young children, as detailed earlier. Children in CRF prefer savory foods to sweet food—"junk foods" are an excellent source of nourishment for these children.

Persistent acidosis is a common feature of CRF and disturbs tissue utilization of glucose, promotes protein catabolism (330), and increases insulin resistance and leaching of calcium from bones (331). It is essential to correct systemic acidosis in children with CRF if poor statural growth is to improve (332).

Secondary or tertiary hyperparathyroidism causes tissue insulin resistance and poor energy utilization, progression of renal disease, neurotoxicity, and decreased statural growth in children with renal failure. The essential goal in achieving adequate control of hyperparathyroidism in renal failure is to control the plasma phosphate in the lower half of the normal range and to keep the plasma calcium in the upper half of the normal range. Mak et al. showed that a dietary phosphate-binding agent, calcium carbonate, was more efficacious than aluminum hydroxide in lowering plasma phosphate and PTH (39). This was achieved with only very modest restriction of dietary phosphate by reducing milk, cheese, yogurt, and chocolate foods (39). Low or low-normal plasma calcium levels are increased by use of daily oral active vitamin D analogs like α-calcidol. Long-term control of hyperparathyroidism over a mean of 3 years using these techniques was reported to be successful, without serious side effects (308).

It must be realized that many children with CRF remain short because the diagnosis often is made late when the opportunity for growth is missed or their illness itself causes poor statural growth (e.g., cystinosis). Delayed pubertal development and growth spurt, particularly if it is delayed beyond 14 to 15 years, may lead to significant psychoemotional problems. It therefore is appropriate to initiate puberty with either intramuscular injections of testosterone (25, 50, or 100 mg monthly for 3 to 5 months) or oral oxandrolone (2.5 mg once daily) for 3 to 6 months in boys. Girls with CRF and pubertal delay may be prescribed estradiol 5 μg once daily to initiate pubertal changes.

Psychosocial Considerations

Chronic renal failure leads to severe psychological problems in some children, especially those on chronic hospital dialysis (333–337). The insecurity and painful procedures such as blood taking and fistula needling may elicit aggression toward parents and staff, and the insecurity this creates in both can lead to anxiety for all concerned. The aggression may be followed by withdrawal, or refusal to cooperate (which can at times make dialysis almost impossible), and can affect food intake and survival. The further stresses of retarded growth, retarded sexual and emotional maturation, loss of schooling, abnormal appearance, and dependence on hospital and machines inhibit the normal development of independence. The whole way of life for the child and family can be affected. Although the incidences of depression and anxiety do not differ from those in normal, healthy adolescents, personal and social adjustments often are poor. The coping strategies displayed by children on dialysis are better for those on home peritoneal dialysis than for those on hemodialysis (333). Children with functioning renal transplants fare much better (334).

In one survey of adults who had been treated in childhood for an average of 11 years, most were working full or part time in a variety of different jobs that were not dissimilar to those of their peers (260). Many, particularly the girls, were married and living normal sexual lives. However, 27% had additional disabilities in another long-term follow-up study (338). The mode of treatment is important in determining psychological morbidity, with transplanted children showing half the psychosocial problems of dialyzed children (339). Marriage occurred in approximately 50% of patients, with half of the couples having children of their own. Only 10% to 14% of pediatric patients with ESRF were unemployed (338,340). It was especially interesting that many families thought the experience had improved their family life rather than the reverse.

Stress in the care of the child with CRF/ESRF may be reduced if all the staff are aware of the problems and are willing to discuss them openly to alleviate anxiety, and take time to talk about the difficulties between themselves, with the families, and with the children. The environment where the children are treated is important: Schooling must be available, with a liaison between the hospital and the child's own school. Social service support to alleviate at least some of the family's difficulties, financial help for the unseen expenses, and an opportunity for relief by providing holidays for the children away from the family are important and aid in the development of independence. Access to skilled psychiatric assistance is important. Children need to grow emotionally and socially, and this is inhibited by overprotection; thus, families should be sympathetically discouraged from overindulgence. Children mature best with the love, discipline, and support of their families, and it is no surprise that dialysis at home, whether hemodialysis or automated peritoneal dialysis (APD), is associated with fewer problems (341). A multidisciplinary team is essential if the child and family are to overcome these problems and to provide holistic care for the patient (342,343).

Intellectual performance is reduced in adults with ESRF, and some studies in infants suggested a similar problem that may be compounded by the severe disturbances in body composition that occur in these younger children (344–347). With the advent of calcium carbonate and Renagel, aluminum neurotoxicity and bone disease should be not occur, but malnutrition strongly influences the development of microcephaly in infants with early, severe CRF from birth (348).

Dialysis

The management of anemia in children receiving hemodialysis has been revolutionized by the introduction of recombinant human erythropoietin. The dosage varies between 100 and 150 U/kg body weight given three times a week after dialysis (349). The dose should be adjusted to maintain the hemoglobin concentration in the lower half of the normal range for the child's age and sex. Erythropoietin treatment is associated with a fall in serum ferritin and, indeed, oral iron supplementation may be required (350). The amelioration of anemia is associated with increased well-being and exercise tolerance, and as long as the hemoglobin level is monitored carefully, hypertension does not appear to be a complication. Thrombosis of vascular access is, however, a risk. The avoidance of blood transfusions decreases the chance of sensitization to major histocompatibility complex (MHC) antigens and is associated with a fall in antibodies in previously sensitized children. We have not found it necessary routinely to use erythropoietin in children on conservative treatment for CRF or, indeed, in all children receiving continuous ambulatory peritoneal dialysis (CAPD) (351,352).

Children require more dialysis in relation to their body weight than adults do because their metabolic rates and therefore food intakes are higher. This means that they require larger dialyzers in relation to their body weight, but if too large a dialyzer is used with a volume exceeding more than 8% of the child's circulating blood volume (80 mL/kg body weight), there is a risk of hypotension on dialysis or hypertension after "wash-back" (353). Dialyzers should have low compliance and should be the largest that can be used while still maintaining an extracorporeal blood volume below 8% of the child's circulating blood volume. The dietary principles for the child on hemodialysis are similar to those discussed previously, and an adequate energy intake should be ensured and secondary hyperparathyroidism carefully controlled.

There are two types of peritoneal dialysis, APD and CAPD, as well as hemodialysis, which usually is hospital based, that are used long-term in children. Each has its advantages and disadvantages. In general, dialysis or preemptive transplantation is required in children when the GFR is 10 mL/minute/1.73 m^2 or lower, or if hyperkalemia, fluid overload, poor metabolic control, or poor growth (due to uremia) occur. Ideally, no child should be accepted onto a dialysis program unless renal transplantation is intended, because this offers the most successful therapy for ESRF in children (338).

Automated peritoneal dialysis may be used in infants as well as the older child or teenager. The nutritional problems of children are important, particularly in infants because of their need to achieve energy balance. They require greater dose of dialysis (354), and APD is most appropriate. Dialysis fill volumes are 0.8 to 1.2 L/m^2 or 35 mL/kg, and the amount of dialysis is set by the number of cycles per night. The large variation in body size of children of different ages means individual prescription volumes of peritoneal dialysate are required and should be reassessed at regular intervals (355,356). Peritoneal equilibration tests (PET) or formal timed clearances may be used to adjust dialysis prescriptions to gain better general health and growth (357). In general, children were thought to have higher solute transport than adults (358), but more recent evidence suggests the contrary when transport rates are corrected for BSA (359). By performing APD overnight, children may be left with their abdomen empty during the day, which adds to their daytime mobility and comfort. Using the "Y" system of connection, peritonitis rates of approximately one episode per 14 months per patient or better are easily achievable. CAPD may be used where dialysis machinery is not available, and like adult practice, requires four exchanges to be made per 24 hours (360); it is not as convenient for school-aged children or their parents. Both techniques can achieve creatinine clearances of approximately 70 L/week, giving the child a sense of well-being and permitting good school attendance.

The major problems with peritoneal dialysis are sepsis of the exit site or catheter tunnel, peritonitis, poor catheter position or malfunction, constipation interfering with dialysate drainage, and line breaks, in common with adult practice (see Chapter 98). Peritonitis caused by pets breaking the sterile circuit, usually by gnawing on the dialysis tubing, is well described in children on home dialysis. Attention to detail with regular cleaning and dressing of the exit site and a well

adherent catheter at the exit site protects against exit site and tunnel infections. Chronic colonization of the exit site often leads to peritonitis. Common pathogens that cause peritonitis in children are coagulase-negative staphylococci, *Staphylococcus aureus, Pseudomonas,* and occasionally *Candida.* The last two pathogens usually require the peritoneal catheter to be removed and hemodialysis commenced. Long-term peritoneal membrane failure may lead to high transporter status or ultrafiltration failure when assessed by PET. This may lead to an increased body mass index in the child because glucose is readily absorbed through the peritoneum. Sclerosing peritonitis does occur in children as well as adults, and is related to recurrent peritonitis and long-term use of peritoneal dialysis.

Criteria for adequacy of dialysis in children are not well researched. The hemodialysis prescription for children often is 4 hours three times per week, but recently kt/V or urea reduction ratio (>0.65) criteria have been calculated for children to assess the quality of dialysis (Chapters 98 and 99) (361–363). Hospital-based hemodialysis is becoming less popular, but it may have advantages in certain clinical settings. Nephrotic patients who have undergone recent bilateral nephrectomy are able to achieve better anabolism with hemodialysis than with peritoneal dialysis, when protein losses may further compromise a protein-malnourished child. Supervision by hospital staff also is possible in families who have difficulty coping with peritoneal dialysis, although hospital-based hemodialysis is more expensive. Long-term problems with hemodialysis arise from difficulty with vascular access. New double-lumen catheters with cuffs that are tunneled under the skin provide greatly improved access, particularly in small children and infants. Reliance on surgically performed arteriovenous fistulas or artificial arteriovenous grafts still occurs with older children and adolescents. Despite these advances, line sepsis, fistula stenosis or thrombosis, excessive interdialytic weight gains, and loss of schooling still pose significant problems to the child on hemodialysis.

Growth on dialysis remains suboptimal, as detailed previously. The mode of dialysis affects growth, with peritoneal dialysis having better growth rates than hemodialysis.

Renal Transplantation

Living related or cadaveric donor renal transplantation has been successfully performed routinely in children, from the age of 1 year, since the early 1970s. It remains the primary mode of therapy for renal failure in children and is most successful when carried out preemptively, because survival of children (and grafts) is no different from those who underwent dialysis initially (364,365). Successful transplantation gives the child with renal failure the best potential to achieve a normal life, growth, school performance, and psychosocial and emotional development. Adults who have been transplanted as children have a higher chance of being well rehabilitated, employed, and married than if they are undergoing dialysis (340).

Surgical and Perioperative Considerations of Very Young Children

Transplanting young children may present the surgeon with special problems—the discrepancy between the organ size and the recipient's abdomen may pose operative problems that the surgeon must address before surgery (366). Infants receiving kidneys from their parents commonly have the grafts placed in one renal bed, with native nephrectomy often being performed at the same operation. Renal vessels are anastomosed to the aorta and inferior vena cava, which may decrease the risk of postoperative graft thrombosis compared with anastomoses involving the common or internal iliac arteries. Age matching of donors and recipients does not improve graft survival for young children (367), although others have demonstrated in their units (368) that all recipients have less risk of graft loss if the donor age is 18 to 45 years. Graft function of adult and pediatric donors is similar within 2 years posttransplantation owing to adaptive changes dictated by the recipient's size (369). Vascular thrombosis of small allografts placed in young children is more common, as is renal artery stenosis (370). Young recipients often have renal tract anomalies or obstructed renal tracts as the cause of their ESRF, so a thorough preoperative assessment of urine drainage through the bladder and urethra is required (371), including videourodynamics in many cases, to enable the site of anastomosis of the transplant ureter to be planned. In those children with a urinary diversion, when graft function is optimal and good urine flow is present, bladder augmentation or urethral operations and anastomosis of the transplant ureter to the bladder can be carried out. Corrective bladder augmentation or other urologic operations often are unsuccessful unless good urine flow is ensured (372).

After surgery, the larger dissection associated with intraabdominal placement of the transplant kidney in very young children increases third-space fluid losses. The renal transplant's vascular capacity often greatly exceeds that of the child's native kidney, so extra care must be taken to maintain intravascular volume by adequate fluid replacement. Small discrepancies in fluid balance are critical to early graft function and even long-term outcome. Most important, postoperative tissue perfusion should be optimized by measurement of pulse, arterial blood pressure, central venous pressure, and the difference between central core temperature and peripheral skin temperature of the toe. The ideal postoperative cardiovascular status is to achieve an adequate central venous pressure, normal arterial blood pressure, a core–peripheral temperature gap of less than 2°C, and good urine output (>2 mL/kg/hour) (373). Ensuring good urine production optimizes graft function and leads to low primary nonfunction rates. Very young children with intraabdominal renal transplants often have postoperative ileus, temporary intolerance of feeds, and diarrhea, so the intravenous route for administration of fluid, immunosuppressive drugs, and, if gut malfunction is prolonged, parenteral feeding should be used.

Immunosuppression and Patient and Allograft Survival

The many successful immunosuppressive protocols used in children are similar to adult protocols, with adjustment of drug dosages based on BSA to reflect the discrepancy in body size and metabolic rate. Individual drugs require their pharmacokinetic parameters to be assessed in the pediatric transplant setting (374). Most commonly, the "triple regimen," comprising cyclosporine, azathioprine, and prednisolone (prednisone), is used. Variations on this basic protocol occur with the use of tacrolimus instead of cyclosporine and mycophenolate mofetil instead of azathioprine—approximately 55 variations are possible with the currently used drugs! The cyclosporine era has allowed a great reduction in the dose of steroid used posttransplantation, with improvement of graft survival, side effects, and growth. For example, our protocol reduces prednisolone doses from 60 mg/m^2 per day to 10 mg/m^2 on alternate days within 3 months. Long-term maintenance, alternate-day dosing of steroid has been shown greatly to improve pubertal growth, particularly in boys, compared with daily dosing at similar doses that were used in prednisolone and azathioprine protocols (277).

The North American Pediatric Renal Transplant Cooperative Study (NAPRTCS) has reported 1- and 6-year actuarial graft survival rates; living related donor graft survival rates are 90% and 74%, respectively, compared with cadaveric allograft survival rates of 80% and 58% (99). Approximately 22% to 33% of patients who are transplanted are younger than 5 years of age and their early graft survival is reduced (68% at 1 year), mainly for the technical reasons outlined previously (375). Graft thrombosis is overtaking acute rejection as the major cause of graft loss, despite the fact that rejection rates in the first 6 months of pediatric transplantation are approximately twice those of adult recipients in most centers. This should not deter parents or relatives from putting themselves forward as living related donors. Long-term survival rates in children who undergo renal transplantation before the age of 6 years are similar to those in older children and adults. Impressive patient and allograft survival rates with living related donors can be obtained in recipients younger than 2 years of age (376). This maximizes the potential for physical and neurologic development, with good catch-up growth and an increase in head circumference and developmental quotient being observed.

Loss of the renal transplant may occur from acute rejection, acute graft thrombosis, infection of the recipient that requires withdrawal of immunosuppression, or chronic allograft nephropathy, some of which is due to chronic rejection. Anti-HLA antibodies in children who have become sensitized are most troublesome when directed against MHC class II antigens and may complicate repeat transplantation. Because graft thrombosis is a common cause of graft loss in transplanted children, the pretransplantation workup of the recipient should include detailed screening for procoagulant conditions by functional and genetic testing, such as the presence of factor V (Leiden), homocystinuria, heterozygosity for factor C, S, prothrombin or antithrombin III deficiency, and others. For living related donor transplantation, these tests also should be performed on the donor.

Teenagers and Transplants

Delayed puberty and short stature are important potential problems of teenage life. Many transplanted teenagers have difficulty in meeting others socially, particularly in the case of boys meeting girls. Teenagers with renal transplants have anxiety about rejection (often reinforced by their doctors), which may lead to depression. When this is coupled with an abnormal body image and a chaotic lifestyle, noncompliance with medication may be very common (up to 60% of patients). Concerns over body image result from drug side effects, or a dialysis fistula may dominate a teenager's attitude to his or her treatment, leading to noncompliance. If this involves immunosuppression, the renal transplant is at risk. The severe, full-face acne and central obesity induced by steroids, the hypertrichosis of the trunk and limbs from cyclosporine, and the gum hypertrophy from cyclosporine and nifedipine are common concerns. Supportive counseling about their problems and a nonconfrontational approach to noncompliant teenagers is most constructive, as opposed to blaming them for their actions. The physician caring for such adolescents must show support and understanding for their concerns and adapt the drug regimen appropriately, and resist justifying the need for the drugs simply because the transplanted kidney is valuable to the patient. Such an approach is never helpful. Education about the importance and need for immunosuppressive drugs both before and after surgery reduces posttransplantation noncompliance.

Recurrent Disease and Long-Term Complications of Pediatric Renal Transplantation

Recurrent renal disease may occur after renal transplantation in approximately 11% of transplanted children. Steroid-resistant idiopathic nephrotic syndrome, usually due to focal segmental glomerulosclerosis, recurs in 30% to 50% of patients. The recurrence occurs very early in the transplant's clinical course, is slightly more common with living related kidneys, but is very common in second or subsequent grafts (70% to 80% of children) if it recurred in the first transplant. Heavy and prolonged immunosuppression has been successful in treating this posttransplantation complication, and recently both immunoadsorption of plasma and multiple plasmapheresis with standard triple therapy have been used successfully (377). In contrast to these clinical findings, mesangiocapillary glomerulonephritis commonly occurs later in the posttransplantation course, particularly if it is dense deposit disease.

Oxalosis recurs in 33% of newly transplanted kidneys and long-term graft survival rates at 3 years are only 17% to 23% (378). Successful transplantation is achieved by decreasing the oxalate load by extensive preoperative dialysis and postoperative diuresis. Alternatively, liver transplantation may be curative before severe CRF occurs.

Because of heavy immunosuppression with multiple drugs, their long-term administration with a successful allograft, and the relative lack of Epstein-Barr virus infection in young children, recipients transplanted at a young age are at increased risk for posttransplantation lymphoproliferative disorder (PTLD) and other neoplasms (see Chapter 97). Approximately 4% experience early PTLD. Our data in 530 renal allografts over 32 years give a prevalence of 1% to 2% for PTLD. Increased general use of more potent immunosuppression in the 1990s may increase this figure in future, a worrisome potential consequence of using potent immunosuppressive drugs in the effort to obtain better graft survival.

Transplanted children with chickenpox, which still is endemic in many countries, are at increased risk because the illness may be severe and even fatal in immunosuppressed hosts. We recommend all children who are placed on transplant waiting lists to be immunized against varicella. Immunizations usually are not contraindicated in children with renal transplants taking maintenance immunosuppression, although we recommend that live poliovirus vaccines not be used (379).

PEDIATRIC NEPHROLOGY CLINICAL SERVICES

The successful outcome of children with renal disease depends on many factors—early identification *in utero* for congenital renal malformations, early diagnosis of renal disease or infection in susceptible target populations of children, and appropriate clinical management of the patients' investigations and therapy. Because of the complex nature of most renal disease, which is due to the major role the kidneys play in homeostasis, it is clear that to attain the maximum potential well-being for a child with a serious renal condition, many skills are required. Moreover, for the child and his or her family, psychological and emotional, social, and financial support, together with education, usually are required.

There are no absolute contraindications to the treatment of a child with ESRF, but there are many relative ones. The purpose of treatment is to enable the child to survive and grow up to lead a full adult life. Most children can achieve this successfully only with the support of their families. Long-term dialysis and transplantation of newborns and infants with ESRF still are uncommon, but nearly every pediatric renal unit has had some experience with these children. Treatment of the child is not always the best or kindest option for the child or the family. The final decision, given that the resources are available, must rest with the family. Obviously, as the child grows older, these contraindications to treatment lessen, but the support that is required for the successful treatment of children in ESRF and their families must never be underestimated. Only a clinical team—nephrologists, other physicians and specialists, nurses, psychologists, social workers, teachers, play specialists, and parents—can provide all the necessary skills. Such clinical teamwork, coupled with research, holds the key to a successful future for children with renal disease.

REFERENCES

1. Cho EA, Patterson LT, Brookhiser WT, et al. Differential expression and function of cadherin-6 during renal epithelium development. *Development* 1998;125:803.
2. Ostrom L, Tang MJ, Gruss P, et al. Reduced Pax2 gene dosage increases apoptosis and slows the progression of renal cystic disease. *Dev Biol* 2000;219:250.
3. Winyard PJ, Nauta J, Lirenman DS, et al. Deregulation of cell survival in cystic and dysplastic renal development. *Kidney Int* 1996;49:135.
4. Widdowson EM, Crabb DE, Milner RD. Cellular development of some human organs before birth. *Arch Dis Child* 1972;47:652.
5. McCory WW. *Developmental physiology.* Cambridge, MA: Harvard University Press, 1972.
6. Kotchen JA, et al. A study of the renin-angiotensin system in newborn infants. *J Pediatr* 1972;80:938.
7. Nash MA, Edelmann CM, Jr. The developing kidney: Immature function is inappropriate standard. *Nephron* 1973;11:71.
8. Al-Dahhan J, Haycock GB, Chantler C, et al. Sodium homeostasis in term and preterm neonates: I. renal aspects. *Arch Dis Child* 1983;58:335.
9. Haycock GB, Aperia A. Salt and the newborn kidney. *Pediatr Nephrol* 1991;5:65.
10. Terzi F, Assael BM, Claris-Appiani A, et al. Increased sodium requirement following early postnatal surgical correction of congenital uropathies in infants. *Pediatr Nephrol* 1990;4:581.
11. Christophe C, Cantraine F, Bogaert C, et al. Ultrasound: a method for kidney size monitoring in children. *Eur J Pediatr* 1986;145:532.
12. Sisayan RM, Rossleigh MA, Mackey DW. Nomograms of renal length in children obtained from DMSA scintigraphy. *Clin Nucl Med* 1993;18:970.
13. Holliday MA. Metabolic rate and organ size during growth from infancy to maturity and during late gestation and early infancy. *Pediatrics* 1971;47:169.
14. Haycock G, Schwartz GJ, Wisotosky DH. Geometric method for measuring surface area: a height weight formula validated in infants, children and adults. *J Pediatr* 1978;93:62.
15. Yorgin PD, Krensky AM, Tune BM. Continuous venovenous hemofiltration. *Pediatr Nephrol* 1990;4:640.
16. Thomas DF. Urological diagnosis in utero. *Arch Dis Child* 1984;59:913.
17. Perlmann M, Williams J. Detection of renal anomalies by abdominal palpation. *BMJ* 1984;2:347.
18. Gray DL, Crane JP. Prenatal diagnosis of urinary tract malformation. *Pediatr Nephrol* 1988;2:326.
19. McLean RH, Gearhart JP, Jeffs R. Neonatal obstructive uropathy. *Pediatr Nephrol* 1988;2:48.
20. Freedman AL, Johnson MP, Smith CA, et al. Long-term outcome in children after antenatal intervention for obstructive uropathies. *Lancet* 1999;354:374.
21. Hislop A, Hey E, Reid L. The lungs in congenital bilateral renal agenesis and dysplasia. *Arch Dis Child* 1979;54:32.
22. Poustchi-Amin M, Leonidas JC, Palestro C, et al. Magnetic resonance imaging in acute pyelonephritis. *Pediatr Nephrol* 1998;12:579.
23. Christian MT, McColl JH, MacKenzie JR, et al. Risk assessment of renal cortical scarring with urinary tract infection by clinical features and ultrasonography. *Arch Dis Child* 2000;82:376.
24. Cheek DB, et al. Protein calorie malnutrition and the significance of cell mass relative to body weight. *Am J Clin Nutr* 1977;30:851.
25. Counahan R, Chantler C, Ghazali S, et al. Estimation of glomerular filtration rate from plasma creatinine concentration in children. *Arch Dis Child* 1976;51:875.
26. Morris MC, et al. Evaluation of a height/plasma creatinine formula in the measurement of glomerular filtration rate. *Arch Dis Child* 1982;57:611.
27. Schwartz GJ, Bryen LP, Spitzer A. The use of plasma creatinine concentration to estimate glomerular filtration rate in infancy, childhood and adolescence. *Pediatr Clin North Am* 1987;34:571.
28. Haycock GB. Creatinine, body size and renal function. *Pediatr Nephrol* 1989;3:22.
29. Mak RH, Al Dahhan J, Azzopardi D, et al. Measurement of glomerular filtration rate in children after renal transplantation. *Kidney Int* 1983;23:410.
30. Dalton RN, Turner C. A sensitive and specific method for the measurement of inulin. *Ann Clin Biochem* 1987;24:51.
31. Chantler C, Barratt TM. Estimation of glomerular filtration rate from plasma clearance of 51-chromium edetic acid. *Arch Dis Child* 1972;47:613.
32. Wagner MG, et al. Epidemiology of proteinuria. *J Pediatr* 1968;73:825.
33. Ellis EN, Warady BA, Wood EG, et al. Renal structural-functional relationships in early diabetes mellitus. *Pediatr Nephrol* 1997;11:584.
34. Lawson ML, Sochett EB, Chait PG, et al. Effect of puberty on markers of glomerular hypertrophy and hypertension in IDDM. *Diabetes* 1996;45:51.
35. Norden AG, Scheinman SJ, Deschodt-Lanckman MM, et al. Tubular proteinuria defined by a study of Dent's (CLCN5 mutation) and other tubular diseases. *Kidney Int* 2000;57:240.
36. Walton NG, Bijvoet OLM. Nomogram for the derivation of renal threshold phosphate concentration. *Lancet* 1975;2:183.
37. Brodehl J, Krause A, Hoyer PF. Assessment of maximal tubular phosphate reabsorption: comparison of direct measurement with the nomogram of Bijvoet. *Pediatr Nephrol* 1988;2:183.
38. Alon U, Hellerstein S. Assessment and interpretation of the tubular threshold for phosphate in infants and children. *Pediatr Nephrol* 1994;8:250.
39. Mak RHK, et al. Suppression of secondary hyperparathyroidsim in children with chronic renal failure by high dose phosphate binders $CaCO_3$ vs $Al(OH)_3$. *BMJ* 1985;291:623.
40. van Oort A, Monnens L, van Munster P. Beta 2 microglobulin clearance: an indicator of renal tubular maturation. *Int J Pediatr Nephrol* 1980;1:80.
41. Tomlinson PA. Low molecular weight proteins in children with renal disease. *Pediatr Nephrol* 1992;6:565.
42. Hall PW, Riccali ES. Renal handling of beta 2 microglobulin in renal disorders with special reference to the hepatorenal syndrome. *Nephron* 1981;27:62.
43. Rodriguez-Soriano J, Boichis H, Edelmann CM Jr. Bicarbonate reabsorption and hydrogen ion excretion in children with renal tubular acidosis. *J Pediatr* 1967;71:802.
44. Schwartz GJ, et al. Late metabolic acidosis: a reassessment of the definition. *J Pediatr* 1979;95:102.
45. Rodriguez-Soriano J, Vallo A. Renal tubular acidosis. *Pediatr Nephrol* 1990;4:268.
46. Donckerwolcke RA, et al. The diagnostic value of urine to blood carbon dioxide tension gradient for assessment of distal tubular hydrogen ion secretion in paediatric patients with renal tubular disorders. *Clin Nephrol* 1983;19:254.
47. Edelmann CM Jr. The renal response of children to acute ammonium chloride acidosis. *Pediatr Res* 1967;1:452.
48. Edelmann CM Jr, et al. A standardized test of renal concentrating capacity in children. *Am J Dis Child* 1967;114:639.
49. Edelmann CM Jr, Barnett HL, Stark H. Effect of urea on concentration of urinary non urea solute in premature infants. *J Appl Physiol* 1966;21:1021.
50. Judd BA, Haycock G, Dalton N, et al. Hyponatraemia in premature babies and following surgery in older children. *Acta Paediatr Scand* 1987;76:385.
51. Robertson GL, Aycinena P, Zerbe RL. Neurogenic disorders of osmoregulation. *Am J Med* 1982;72:339.
52. Rogers D, et al. Nonaccidental poisoning: an extended syndrome of child abuse. *BMJ* 1976;1:793.
53. Moritz ML, Ayus JC. The changing pattern of hypernatremia in hospitalized children. *Pediatrics* 1999;104:435.
54. Mathew OP, et al. Neonatal renal failure, usefulness of diagnostic indices. *Pediatrics* 1980;65:57.
55. Ghazali S, Barratt TM. Urinary excretion of calcium and magnesium in children. *Arch Dis Child* 1974;49:97.
56. Round JM. Plasma calcium, magnesium, phosphorus and alkaline phosphatase levels in normal British school children. *BMJ* 1973;3:137.
57. Barratt TM, Kasidas GP, Murdoch I, et al. Urinary oxalate and glycolate excretion and plasma oxalate concentration. *Arch Dis Child* 1991;66:501.

58. Niehaus CE, Ersser GP, Acherden SM. Routine laboratory investigation of urinary catecholamine metabolites in sick children. *Ann Clin Biochem* 1979;16:38.

59. Nolte S, Mueller B, Pringsheim W. Serum alpha 1-microglobulin and beta 2-microglobulin for the estimation of fetal glomerular renal function. *Pediatr Nephrol* 1991;5:573.

60. Pollak MR, Delaney VB, Graham RM, et al. Gitelman's syndrome (Bartter's variant) maps to the thiazide-sensitive cotransporter gene locus on chromosome 16q13 in a large kindred. *J Am Soc Nephrol* 1996;7:2244.

61. Karolyi L, Ziegler A, Pollak M, et al. Gitelman's syndrome is genetically distinct from other forms of Bartter's syndrome. *Pediatr Nephrol* 1996;10:551.

62. Rodriguez-Soriano J. Bartter and related syndromes: the puzzle is almost solved. *Pediatr Nephrol* 1998;12:315.

63. Salomon R, Gubler MC, Niaudet P. Genetics of the nephrotic syndrome. *Curr Opin Pediatr* 2000;12:129.

64. Wiggelinkhuizen J, Kaschula RO, Uys CJ, et al. Congenital syphilis and glomerulonephritis with evidence for immune pathogenesis. *Arch Dis Child* 1973;48:375.

65. Myers BD, Guasch A. Mechanisms of proteinuria in nephrotic humans. *Pediatr Nephrol* 1994;8:107.

66. Vernier RL, et al. Heparan sulphate rich anionic sites in the human glomerular basement membrane: decreased concentration in congenital nephrotic syndrome. *N Engl J Med* 1983;309:1001.

67. Van den Heuvel LP, Van den Born J, Jalanko H, et al. The glycosaminoglycan content of renal basement membranes in the congenital nephrotic syndrome of the Finnish type. *Pediatr Nephrol* 1992;6:10.

68. Mannikko M, Kestila M, Lenkkeri U, et al. Improved prenatal diagnosis of the congenital nephrotic syndrome of the Finnish type based on DNA analysis. *Kidney Int* 1997;51:868.

69. Habib R. Nephrotic syndrome in the 1st year of life. *Pediatr Nephrol* 1993;7:347.

70. Ito S, Ikeda M, Takata A, et al. Nephrotic syndrome and end-stage renal disease with WT1 mutation detected at 3 years. *Pediatr Nephrol* 1999;13:790.

71. Holmberg C, Antikainen M, Ronnholm K, et al. Management of congenital nephrotic syndrome of the Finnish type. *Pediatr Nephrol* 1995;9:87.

72. Coulthard MG. Management of Finnish congenital nephrotic syndrome by unilateral nephrectomy. *Pediatr Nephrol* 1989;3:451.

73. Laine J, Jalanko H, Holthofer H, et al. Post-transplantation nephrosis in congenital nephrotic syndrome of the Finnish type. *Kidney Int* 1993;44:867.

74. Lane PH, Schnaper HW, Vernier RL, et al. Steroid-dependent nephrotic syndrome following renal transplantation for congenital nephrotic syndrome. *Pediatr Nephrol* 1991;5:300.

75. Boute N, Gribouval O, Roselli S, et al. NPHS2, encoding the glomerular protein podocin, is mutated in autosomal recessive steroid-resistant nephrotic syndrome. *Nat Genet* 2000;24:349.

76. Vats A, Nayak A, Ellis D, et al. Familial nephrotic syndrome: clinical spectrum and linkage to chromosome 19q13. *Kidney Int* 2000;57:875.

77. Winn MP, Conlon PJ, Lynn KL, et al. Clinical and genetic heterogeneity in familial focal segmental glomerulosclerosis: International Collaborative Group for the Study of Familial Focal Segmental Glomerulosclerosis. *Kidney Int* 1999;55:1241.

78. Town M, Jean G, Cherqui S, et al. A novel gene encoding an integral membrane protein is mutated in nephropathic cystinosis. *Nat Genet* 1998;18:319.

79. Haycock GB, Al-Dahhan J, Mak RH, et al. Effect of indomethacin on clinical progress and renal function in cystinosis. *Arch Dis Child* 1982;57:934.

80. Burke JR, El-Bishti MM, Maisey MN, et al. Hypothyroidism in children with cystinosis. *Arch Dis Child* 1978;53:947.

81. Robert JJ, Tete MJ, Guest G, et al. Diabetes mellitus in patients with infantile cystinosis after renal transplantation. *Pediatr Nephrol* 1999;13:524.

82. Gagnadoux MF, Téte MJ, Guest G, et al. Hepatosplenic disorders in nephrotic cystinosis. Broyer M, ed. *Cystinosis*. Paris: Elsevier, 1999:70.

83. Manz F, Gretz N. Progression of chronic renal failure in a historical group of patients with nephropathic cystinosis: European Collaborative Study on Cystinosis. *Pediatr Nephrol* 1994;8:466.

84. van't Hoff WG, Gretz N. The treatment of cystinosis with cysteamine and phosphocysteamine in the United Kingdom and Eire. *Pediatr Nephrol* 1995;9:685.

85. Niaudet P, Rotig A. Renal involvement in mitochondrial cytopathies. *Pediatr Nephrol* 1996;10:368.

86. Munnich A, Rustin P, Rötig A, et al. Clinical aspects of mitochondrial disorders. *J Inherit Metab Dis* 1992;15:448.

87. Brun P, Ogier de Baulny H, Peuchmaur M, et al. Les Atteintes rénales des cytopathies mitochondriales. In: Arthuis M, et al., eds. *Journées Parisiennes des Pédiatrie*. Paris: Flammarion Médicine Sciences, 1994:227.

88. Kramer I, Sherry SN. The time of passage of the first stool and urine by the premature infant. *J Pediatr* 1957;51:373.

89. Rhodes PG, Hammel CL, Berman LB. Urinary constituents of the newborn infant. *J Pediatr* 1962;60:20.

90. Karlowicz MG, Adelman RJ. Acute renal failure in the neonate. *Clin Perinatol* 1992;19:139.

91. Woolf AS. A molecular and genetic view of human renal and urinary tract malformations. *Kidney Int* 2000;58:500.

92. Bernstein J. Is unilateral multicystic renal dysplasia sometimes heritable, and what is the risk of recurrence? *Pediatr Nephrol* 1990;4:662.

93. Al Saadi AA, Yoshimoto M, Bree R, et al. A family study of renal dysplasia. *Am J Med Genet* 1984;19:669.

94. Azimi F, Kodroff MB. Congenital renal dysplasia: Osathanondh-Potter type II polycystic kidneys. *Urology* 1976;7:550.

95. Hoagland MH, Hutchins GM. Obstructive lesions of the lower urinary tract in the prune belly syndrome. *Arch Pathol Lab Med* 1987;111:154.

96. Risdon RA, Yeung CK, Ransley PG. Reflux nephropathy in children submitted to unilateral nephrectomy: a clinicopathological study. *Clin Nephrol* 1993;40:308.

97. Larson RS, Rudloff MA, Liapis H, et al. The Ivemark syndrome: prenatal diagnosis of an uncommon cystic renal lesion with heterogeneous associations. *Pediatr Nephrol* 1995;9:594.

98. Ehrich JH, Rizzoni G, Brunner FP, et al. Renal replacement therapy for end-stage renal failure before 2 years of age. *Nephrol Dial Transplant* 1992;7:1171.

99. Benfield MR, McDonald R, Sullivan EK, et al. The 1997 Annual Renal Transplantation in Children Report of the North American Pediatric Renal Transplant Cooperative Study (NAPRTCS). *Pediatr Transplant* 1999;3:152.

100. Bernstein J. Developmental abnormalities of the renal parenchyma: renal hypoplasia and dysplasia. *Pathol Annu* 1968;3:213.

101. Gartell PC, MacIver AG, Atwell JD. Renal dysplasia and duplex kidneys. *Eur Urol* 1983;9:65.

102. Menster M, Mahan J, Koff S. Multicystic dysplastic kidney. *Pediatr Nephrol* 1994;8:113.

103. Tam JC, Hodson EM, Choong KK, et al. Postnatal diagnosis and outcome of urinary tract abnormalities detected by antenatal ultrasound. *Med J Aust* 1994;160:633.

104. Dudley JA, Haworth JM, McGraw ME, et al. Clinical relevance and implications of antenatal hydronephrosis. *Arch Dis Child Fetal Neonatal Ed* 1997;76:F31.

105. Nitzsche EU, Zimmerhackl LB, Hawkins RA, et al. Correlation of ultrasound and renal scintigraphy in children with unilateral hydronephrosis in primary workup. *Pediatr Nephrol* 1993;7:138.

106. Kitagawa H, Pringle KC, Stone P, et al. Postnatal follow-up of hydronephrosis detected by prenatal ultrasound: the natural history. *Fetal Diagn Ther* 1998;13:19.

107. Ransley PG, Dhillon HK, Gordon I, et al. The postnatal management of hydronephrosis diagnosed by prenatal ultrasound. *J Urol* 1990;144:584; discussion 593.

108. Oliveira EA, Diniz JS, Cabral AC, et al. Prognostic factors in fetal hydronephrosis: a multivariate analysis. *Pediatr Nephrol* 1999;13:859.

109. Blachar A, Blachar Y, Livne PM, et al. Clinical outcome and follow-up of prenatal hydronephrosis. *Pediatr Nephrol* 1994;8:30.

110. Thomas DF. Antenatal sonography revealed bilateral moderate hydronephrosis without dilatation of ureters or bladder in a fetus at 16 weeks' gestation. This was confirmed at 32 weeks. What advice should be given to the obstetrician regarding intra-uterine intervention, delivery, etc? *Pediatr Nephrol* 1991;5:292.

111. Stapleton FB, Jones DP, Green RS. Acute renal failure in neonates: incidence, etiology and outcome. *Pediatr Nephrol* 1987;1:314.

112. Etches PC, Lemons JA. Nonimmune hydrops fetalis: report of 2 cases including 3 siblings. *Pediatrics* 1979;64:326.

113. Rigden SP, Barratt TM, Dillon MJ, et al. Acute renal failure complicating cardiopulmonary bypass surgery. *Arch Dis Child* 1982;57:425.

114. Roberts DS, Haycock GB, Dalton RN, et al. Prediction of acute renal failure after birth asphyxia. *Arch Dis Child* 1990;65:1021.

115. Karlowicz MG, Adelman RD. Nonoliguric and oliguric acute renal failure in asphyxiated term neonates. *Pediatr Nephrol* 1995;9:718.

116. Shaw JC.L. Parenteral nutrition in the management of sick low birth weight infants. *Pediatr Clin North Am* 1973;20:333.

117. Bunchman TE, Donckerwolcke RA. Continuous arterial-venous diahemofiltration and continuous veno-venous diahemofiltration in infants and children. *Pediatr Nephrol* 1994;8:96.

118. Ellis EN, Pearson D, Robinson L, et al. Pump-assisted hemofiltration in infants with acute renal failure. *Pediatr Nephrol* 1993;7:434.

119. Matthews DE, et al. Peritoneal dialysis in the first 60 days of life. *J Pediatr Surg* 1990;25:110.

120. Proverbio MR, Di Pietro A, Coletta M, et al. Variations in renal hemodynamics during acute renal insufficiency in anoxic neonates. *Pediatr Med Chir* 1996;18:33.

121. Solhaug MJ, Ballevre LD, Guignard JP, et al. Nitric oxide in the developing kidney. *Pediatr Nephrol* 1996;10:529.

122. Toth-Heyn P, Drukker A, Guignard JP. The stressed neonatal kidney: from pathophysiology to clinical management of neonatal vasomotor nephropathy. *Pediatr Nephrol* 2000;14:227.

123. Takeda M, Katayama Y, Takahashi H, et al. Successful fibrinolytic therapy using tissue plasminogen activator in acute renal failure due to acute thrombosis of bilateral renal arteries. *Urol Int* 1993;51:177.

124. Rysava R, Zabka J, Peregrin JH, et al. Acute renal failure due to bilateral renal artery thrombosis associated with primary antiphospholipid syndrome. *Nephrol Dial Transplant* 1998;13:2645.

125. Arneil GC, MacDonald AM, Sweet EM. Renal venous thrombosis. *Clin Nephrol* 1973;1:119.

126. Arneil GC. Renal venous thrombosis. *Contrib Nephrol* 1979;15:21.

127. Bokenkamp A, von Kries R, Nowak-Gottl U, et al. Neonatal renal venous thrombosis in Germany between 1992 and 1994: epidemiology, treatment and outcome. *Eur J Pediatr* 2000;159:44.

128. Clark AG, Saunders A, Bewick M, et al. Neonatal inferior vena cava and renal venous thrombosis treated by thrombectomy and nephrectomy. *Arch Dis Child* 1985;60:1076.

129. McDonald MM, Hathaway WE. Neonatal hemorrhage and thrombosis. *Semin Perinatol* 1983;7:213.

130. Bromberg WD, Firlit CF. Fibrinolytic therapy for renal vein thrombosis in the child. *J Urol* 1990;143:86.

131. Mocan H, Beattie TJ, Murphy AV. Renal venous thrombosis in infancy: long-term follow-up. *Pediatr Nephrol* 1991;5:45.

132. Newcastle Covert Bacteriuria Research Group. Covert bacteriuria in schoolgirls in Newcastle upon Tyne: a 5-year follow-up. Newcastle Covert Bacteriuria Research Group. *Arch Dis Child* 1981;56:585.

133. Dickinson JA. Incidence and outcome of urinary tract infection in children. *BMJ* 1979;1:1330.

134. Panaretto K, Craig J, Knight J, et al. Risk factors for recurrent urinary tract infection in preschool children. *J Paediatr Child Health* 1999;35:454.

135. Herthelius M, Mollby R, Nord CE, et al. Amoxicillin promotes vaginal colonization with adhering *Escherichia coli* present in faeces. *Pediatr Nephrol* 1989;3:443.

136. Lomberg H, Hanson LA, Jacobsonn B. Correlation of P blood groups, vesicoureteric reflux and bacterial attachment in patients with recurrent pyelonephritis. *N Engl J Med* 1983;308:1189.

137. Smellie JM, Edwards D, Normand IC, et al. Effect of vesicoureteric reflux on renal growth in children with urinary tract infection. *Arch Dis Child* 1981;56:593.

138. Scott DJ, et al. Renal function following surgical correction of vesicoureteric reflux in childhood. *Br J Urol* 1986;58:119.

139. Esbjorner E, Aronson S, Berg U, et al. Children with chronic renal failure in Sweden 1978–1985. *Pediatr Nephrol* 1990;4:249; discussion 253.

140. Risdon RA. The small scarred kidney in childhood. *Pediatr Nephrol* 1993;7:361.

141. Ransley PG, Risdon RA. Renal papillary morphology and intrarenal reflux in the young pig and in infants and young children. *Urol Res* 1975;3:105.

142. Smellie JM. Urinary tract infection in childhood. *BMJ* 1974;12:485.

143. Porter IA, Brodie J. Boric acid preservative of urine samples. *BMJ* 1969;2:353.

144. Arneil GC, McAllister JA, Kay P. Detection of bacteriuria by dipslide culture. *Lancet* 1970;1:119.

145. Robins DJ, et al. Urine microscopy as an aid to detection of bacteriuria. *Lancet* 1975;1:476.

146. Lohr JA, Portilla MG, Geuder TG, et al. Making a presumptive diagnosis of urinary tract infection by using a urinalysis performed in an on-site laboratory. *J Pediatr* 1993;122:22.

147. Edwards A, van der Voort J, Newcombe R, et al. A urine analysis method suitable for children's nappies. *J Clin Pathol* 1997;50:569.

148. Lachs MS, Nachamkin I, Edelstein PH, et al. Spectrum bias in the evaluation of diagnostic tests: lessons from the rapid dipstick test for urinary tract infection. *Ann Intern Med* 1992;117:135.

149. Shaw KN, McGowan KL. Evaluation of a rapid screening filter test for urinary tract infection in children. *Pediatr Infect Dis J* 1997;16:283.

150. Schardijn GHC, et al. Comparison of reliability of tests to distinguish upper from lower urinary tract infections. *BMJ* 1984;289:284.

151. Elder JS, Peters CA, Arant BS Jr, et al. Pediatric Vesicoureteral Reflux Guidelines Panel summary report on the management of primary vesicoureteral reflux in children. *J Urol* 1997;157:1846.

152. American Academy of Pediatrics, Committee on Quality Improvement, Subcommittee on Urinary Tract Infection. Practice parameter: the diagnosis, treatment, and evaluation of the initial urinary tract infection in febrile infants and young children [published errata appear in *Pediatrics* 1999;103:1052, 1999;104:118 and 2000;105:141]. *Pediatrics* 1999;103:843.

153. Working Group of Research Unit, Royal College of Physicians. Guidelines for the management of acute urinary tract infection in childhood. *J R Coll Physicians* 1991;25:36.

154. Smellie JM, Rigden SP. Pitfalls in the investigation of children with urinary tract infection. *Arch Dis Child* 1995;72:251; discussion 255.

155. Haycock GB. A practical approach to evaluating urinary tract infection in children. *Pediatr Nephrol* 1991;5:401; discussion 403.

156. Merrick MV, Uttley W, Wild RA. A comparison of two techniques of detecting vesicoureteric reflux. *Br J Radiol* 1977;50:792.

157. Smellie JM, Poulton A, Prescod NP. Retrospective study of children with renal scarring associated with reflux and urinary infection. *BMJ* 1994;308:1193.

158. South Bedfordshire Practitioners' Group. Development of renal scars in children: missed opportunities in management. South Bedfordshire Practitioners' Group. *BMJ* 1990;301:1082.

159. Smellie JM. Reflections on 30 years of treating children with urinary tract infections. *J Urol* 1991;146:665.

160. Smellie JM, et al. Long term cotrimoxazole in the prophylaxis of childhood urinary infection: clinical aspects. *BMJ* 1976;111:203.

161. Group BRS. Prospective trial of operative versus nonoperative treatment of severe vesicoureteric reflux in children: five-year observation. *BMJ* 1987;295:237.

162. Olbing H, Claesson I, Ebel KD, et al. Renal scars and parenchymal thinning in children with vesicoureteral reflux: a 5-year report of the International Reflux Study in Children (European branch). *J Urol* 1992;148:1653.

163. Smellie JM, Tamminen-Mobius T, Olbing H, et al. Five-year study of medical or surgical treatment in children with severe reflux: radiological renal findings: the International Reflux Study in Children. *Pediatr Nephrol* 1992;6:223.

164. Piepsz A, Tamminen-Mobius T, Reiners C, et al. Five-year study of medical or surgical treatment in children with severe vesico-ureteral reflux dimercaptosuccinic acid findings: International Reflux Study Group in Europe. *Eur J Pediatr* 1998;157:753.

165. Jodal U, Hansson S, Hjalmas K. Medical or surgical management for children with vesico-ureteric reflux? *Acta Paediatr Suppl* 1999;88:53.

166. Cooper CS, Chung BI, Kirsch AJ, et al. The outcome of stopping prophylactic antibiotics in older children with vesicoureteral reflux. *J Urol* 2000;163:269; discussion 272.

167. Winberg J. Management of primary vesico-ureteric reflux in children: operation ineffective in preventing progressive renal damage. *Infection* 1994;22:S4.

168. Smellie JM, Prescod NP, Shaw PJ, et al. Childhood reflux and urinary infection: a follow-up of 10-41 years in 226 adults. *Pediatr Nephrol* 1998;12:727.

169. Jacobson SH, Eklof O, Lins LE, et al. Long-term prognosis of post-infectious renal scarring in relation to radiological findings in childhood—a 27-year follow-up. *Pediatr Nephrol* 1992;6:19.

170. Bukowski TP, Betrus GG, Aquilina JW, et al. Urinary tract infections and pregnancy in women who underwent antireflux surgery in childhood. *J Urol* 1998;159:1286.

171. Jungers P, Houillier P, Chauveau D, et al. Pregnancy in women with reflux nephropathy. *Kidney Int* 1996;50:593.

172. West CD. Childhood membranoproliferative glomerulonephritis: an approach to management. *Kidney Int* 1986;29:1077.

173. Braun MC, West CD, Strife CF. Differences between membranoproliferative glomerulonephritis types I and III in long-term response to an alternate-day prednisone regimen. *Am J Kidney Dis* 1999;34:1022.

174. Meadow SR. Post-streptococcal glomerular nephritis: a rare disease? *Arch Dis Child* 1975;50:379.

175. Clark G, White RH, Glasgow EF, et al. Poststreptococcal glomerulonephritis in children: clinicopathological correlations and long-term prognosis. *Pediatr Nephrol* 1988;2:381.

176. Gill D, et al. Progression of acute post-streptococcal nephritis to severe epithelial crescent formation. *Clin Nephrol* 1977;8:449.

177. Travis LB, et al. Acute glomerular nephritis in children: a review of the natural history with emphasis on prognosis. *Clin Nephrol* 1973;1:169.

178. Haycock GB. The treatment of glomerulonephritis in children. *Pediatr Nephrol* 1988;2:247.

179. Dodge WG, et al. Proteinuria and hematuria in school children: epidemiology and early natural history. *J Pediatr* 1976;88:327.

180. Stapleton FB. Hematuria associated with hypercalciuria and hyperuricosuria: a practical approach. *Pediatr Nephrol* 1994;8:756.

181. Piel CF, Biara CG, Goodman JR. Glomerular basement membrane attenuation in familial nephritis and benign hematuria. *J Pediatr* 1982;101:358.

182. Vehaskari VM. Asymptomatic hematuria: a cause for concern? *Pediatr Nephrol* 1989;3:240.

183. Benbassat J, Gergawi M, Offringa M, et al. Symptomless microhaematuria in schoolchildren: causes for variable management strategies. *QJM* 1996;89:845.

184. Miller PF, Speirs NI, Aparicio SR, et al. Long term prognosis of recurrent haematuria. *Arch Dis Child* 1985;60:420.

185. Wyatt RJ, Kritchevsky SB, Woodford SY, et al. IgA nephropathy: long-term prognosis for pediatric patients. *J Pediatr* 1995;127:913.

186. Stewart M, Savage JM, Bell B, et al. Long term renal prognosis of Henoch-Schonlein purpura in an unselected childhood population. *Eur J Pediatr* 1988;147:113.

187. West CD, McAdams AJ, Welch TR. Glomerulonephritis in Henoch-Schoenlein purpura without mesangial IgA deposition. *Pediatr Nephrol* 1994;8:677.

188. Meadow SR, Scott DG. Berger disease: Henoch-Schonlein syndrome without the rash. *J Pediatr* 1985;106:27.

189. Whyte DA, Van Why SK, Siegel NJ. Severe hypertension without urinary abnormalities in a patient with Henoch-Schonlein purpura. *Pediatr Nephrol* 1997;11:750.

190. Knight JF. The rheumatic poison: a survey of some published investigations of the immunopathogenesis of Henoch-Schonlein purpura. *Pediatr Nephrol* 1990;4:533.

191. Amoroso A, Berrino M, Canale L, et al. Immunogenetics of Henoch-Schoenlein disease. *Eur J Immunogenet* 1997;24:323.

192. Abe J, Kohsaka T, Tanaka M, et al. Genetic study on HLA class II and class III region in the disease associated with IgA nephropathy. *Nephron* 1993;65:17.

193. Martini A, Ravelli A, Notarangelo LD, et al. Henoch-Schonlein syndrome and selective IgA deficiency. *Arch Dis Child* 1985;60:160.

194. Koskimies O, et al. Henoch-Schonlein nephritis: long-term prognosis of unselected patients. *Arch Dis Child* 1981;56:482.

195. Counahan R, et al. The prognosis of Henoch-Schonlein nephritis. *BMJ* 1977;2:11.

196. Niaudet P, Habib R. Methylprednisolone pulse therapy in the treatment of severe forms of Schonlein-Henoch purpura nephritis. *Pediatr Nephrol* 1998;12:238.

197. Bergstein J, Leiser J, Andreoli SP. Response of crescentic Henoch-Schoenlein purpura nephritis to corticosteroid and azathioprine therapy. *Clin Nephrol* 1998;49:9.

198. Scharer K, Krmar R, Querfeld U, et al. Clinical outcome of Schonlein-Henoch purpura nephritis in children. *Pediatr Nephrol* 1999;13:816.

199. Saulsbury FT. Henoch-Schonlein purpura in children: report of 100 patients and review of the literature. *Medicine (Baltimore)* 1999;78:395.

200. Oner A, Tinaztepe K, Erdogan O. The effect of triple therapy on rapidly progressive type of Henoch-Schonlein nephritis. *Pediatr Nephrol* 1995;9:6.

201. Mollica F, Li Volti S, Garozzo R, et al. Effectiveness of early prednisone treatment in preventing the development of nephropathy in anaphylactoid purpura [see comments]. *Eur J Pediatr* 1992;151:140.

202. Saulsbury FT. Corticosteroid therapy does not prevent nephritis in Henoch-Schonlein purpura. *Pediatr Nephrol* 1993;7:69.

203. Antoine B, Stymvouldis A, Dardenne M. La stabilite evolutive des etats de proteinurie isolee. *Nephron* 1969;6:526.

204. Trompeter R, et al. Long-term outcome for children with minimal change nephrotic syndrome. *Lancet* 1985;1:368.

205. Mattoo TK. Kidney biopsy prior to cyclophosphamide therapy in primary nephrotic syndrome. *Pediatr Nephrol* 1991;5:617.

206. Tarshish P, Tobin JN, Bernstein J, et al. Prognostic significance of the early course of minimal change nephrotic syndrome: report of the International Study of Kidney Disease in Children. *J Am Soc Nephrol* 1997;8:769.

207. International Study of Kidney Disease in Children. Early identification of frequent relapsers among children with minimal change nephrotic syndrome: a report of the International Study of Kidney Disease in Children. *J Pediatr* 1982;101:514.

208. Konrad M, Mytilineos J, Ruder H, et al. HLA-DR7 predicts the response to alkylating agents in steroid-sensitive nephrotic syndrome. *Pediatr Nephrol* 1997;11:16.

209. Ueda N, Chihara M, Kawaguchi S, et al. Intermittent versus long-term tapering prednisolone for initial therapy in children with idiopathic nephrotic syndrome. *J Pediatr* 1988;112:122.

210. Ksiazek J, Wyszynska T. Short versus long initial prednisone treatment in steroid-sensitive nephrotic syndrome in children. *Acta Paediatr* 1995;84:889.

211. Srivastava RN, Vasudev AS, Bagga A, et al. Long-term, low-dose prednisolone therapy in frequently relapsing nephrotic syndrome. *Pediatr Nephrol* 1992;6:247.

212. Bagga A, Sharma A, Srivastava RN. Levamisole therapy in corticosteroid-dependent nephrotic syndrome. *Pediatr Nephrol* 1997;11:415.

213. International Study of Kidney Disease in Children. Prospective, controlled trial of cyclophosphamide therapy in children with nephrotic syndrome: report of the International Study of Kidney Disease in Children. *Lancet* 1974;2:423.

214. Niaudet P. Comparison of cyclosporin and chlorambucil in the treatment of steroid-dependent idiopathic nephrotic syndrome: a multicentre randomized controlled trial: the French Society of Paediatric Nephrology. *Pediatr Nephrol* 1992;6:1.

215. Arbeitsgemeinschaft für Pädiatrische Nephrologie. Cyclophosphamide treatment of steroid dependent nephrotic syndrome: comparison of eight week with 12 week course. Report of Arbeitsgemeinschaft für Pädiatrische Nephrologie. *Arch Dis Child* 1987;62:1102.

216. Fikrig SM, Schiffman G, Phillipp JC, et al. Antibody response to capsular polysaccharide vaccine of *Streptococcus pneumoniae* in patients with nephrotic syndrome. *J Infect Dis* 1978;137:818.

217. Tejani A, Fikrig S, Schiffman G, et al. Persistence of protective pneumococcal antibody following vaccination in patients with the nephrotic syndrome. *Am J Nephrol* 1984;4:32.

218. Primack WA, Rosel M, Thirumoorthi MC, et al. Failure of pneumococcal vaccine to prevent *Streptococcus pneumoniae* sepsis in nephrotic children. *Lancet* 1979;2:1192.

219. Reid CJ, Marsh MJ, Murdoch IM, et al. Nephrotic syndrome in childhood complicated by life threatening pulmonary oedema. *BMJ* 1996;312:36.

220. Trompeter RS, Schwartz R, Chantler C, et al. Haemolytic-uraemic syndrome: an analysis of prognostic features. *Arch Dis Child* 1983;58:101.

221. Taylor CM, Milford DV, White RH. A plea for standardized terminology within the haemolytic uraemic syndromes. *Pediatr Nephrol* 1991;5:97.

222. Noris M, Ruggenenti P, Perna A, et al. Hypocomplementemia discloses genetic predisposition to hemolytic uremic syndrome and thrombotic thrombocytopenic purpura: role of factor H abnormalities. Italian Registry of Familial and Recurrent Hemolytic Uremic Syndrome/Thrombotic Thrombocytopenic Purpura. *J Am Soc Nephrol* 1999;10:281.

223. Warwicker P, Donne RL, Goodship JA, et al. Familial relapsing haemolytic uraemic syndrome and complement factor H deficiency. *Nephrol Dial Transplant* 1999;14:1229.

224. Rougier N, Kazatchkine MD, Rougier JP, et al. Human complement factor H deficiency associated with hemolytic uremic syndrome. *J Am Soc Nephrol* 1998;9:2318.

225. Badami KJ, Srivastava RN, Kumar R, et al. Disseminated intravascular coagulation in post dysenteric haemolytic uraemic syndrome. *Acta Paediatr* 1987;76:919.

226. McGraw ME, Lendon M, Stevens RF, et al. Haemolytic uraemic syndrome and the Thomsen Friedenreich antigen. *Pediatr Nephrol* 1989;3:135.

227. Kaplan BS, Cleary TG, Obrig TG. Recent advances in understanding the pathogenesis of the hemolytic uremic syndromes. *Pediatr Nephrol* 1990;4:276.

228. Nevard CH, Blann AD, Jurd KM, et al. Markers of endothelial cell activation and injury in childhood haemolytic uraemic syndrome. *Pediatr Nephrol* 1999;13:487.

229. Van Geet C, Proesmans W, Arnout J, et al. Activation of both coagulation and fibrinolysis in childhood hemolytic uremic syndrome. *Kidney Int* 1998;54:1324.

230. Taylor CM, Lote CJ. Prostacyclin in diarrhoea-associated haemolytic uraemic syndrome. *Pediatr Nephrol* 1993;7:515.

231. Walters MD, Matthei IU, Kay R, et al. The polymorphonuclear leucocyte count in childhood haemolytic uraemic syndrome. *Pediatr Nephrol* 1989;3:130.

232. Gallo EG, Gianantonio CA. Extrarenal involvement in diarrhoea-associated haemolytic-uraemic syndrome. *Pediatr Nephrol* 1995; 9:117.

233. Georgaki H, Steed DM, Chantler C, et al. Renal function following acute renal failure in childhood: long-term follow-up study. *Kidney Int* 1989;35:84.

234. Tufro A, Arrizurieta EE, Repetto H. Renal functional reserve in children with a previous episode of haemolytic-uraemic syndrome. *Pediatr Nephrol* 1991;5:184.

235. Loirat C, Sonsino E, Hinglais N, et al. Treatment of the childhood haemolytic uraemic syndrome with plasma: a multicentre randomized controlled trial. The French Society of Paediatric Nephrology. *Pediatr Nephrol* 1988;2:279.

236. Mattoo T, Mahmood MA, al-Harlbi MS, et al. Familial recurrent haemolytic-uraemic syndrome. *J Pediatr* 1989;114:814.

237. Adelman RD. Long-term follow-up of neonatal renovascular hypertension. *Pediatr Nephrol* 1987;1:35.

238. Chandar JJ, Sfakianakis GN, Zilleruelo GE, et al. ACE inhibition scintigraphy in the management of hypertension in children. *Pediatr Nephrol* 1999;13:493.

239. National High Blood Pressure Education Program Working Group on Hypertension Control in Children and Adolescents. Update on the 1987 Task Force Report on High Blood Pressure in Children and Adolescents: a working group report from the National High Blood Pressure Education Program. National High Blood Pressure Education Program Working Group on Hypertension Control in Children and Adolescents. *Pediatrics* 1996;98:649.

240. Chantler C. Systemic hypertension. In: Anderson RH, et al., eds. *Paediatric cardiology.* London: Churchill Livingstone, 1986.

241. Dillon MJ. The diagnosis of renovascular disease. *Pediatr Nephrol* 1997;11:366.

242. Edwards CRW, et al. Localization of 11 hydroxysteroid dehydrogenase tissue specific protector of the mineralocorticoid receptor. *Lancet* 1988;11:986.

243. Dillon MJ, Ryness JM. Plasma renin activity and aldosterone concentration in children. *BMJ* 1975;4:316.

244. Eason JD, Evans N, Kenney I, et al. Clinical quiz. Left perirenal phaeochromocytoma and left upper pole renal artery stenosis: combined excision of tumor and left total nephroadrenalectomy, after full alpha- and beta-adrenergic blockade was achieved. *Pediatr Nephrol* 1996;10:804.

245. Dillon MJ, Shah V, Barratt TM. Renal vein renin measurements in children with hypertension. *BMJ* 1978;2:168.

246. Goddard C. Predictive value of renal vein renin measurements in children with various forms of renal hypertension. *Helv Paediatr Acta* 1977;32:49.

247. Hulse JA, Taylor DSI, Dillon MJ. Blindness and paraplegia in severe childhood hypertension. *Lancet* 1979;2:553.

248. de Swiet M, Fayers PM, Shinebourne EA. Value of repeated blood pressure measurements in children: the Brompton Study. *BMJ* 1980;1: 1567.

249. Bao W, Threefoot SA, Srinivasan SR, et al. Essential hypertension predicted by tracking of elevated blood pressure from childhood to adulthood: the Bogalusa Heart Study. *Am J Hypertens* 1995;8: 657.

250. Gillman MW, Cook NR, Rosner B, et al. Identifying children at high risk for the development of essential hypertension. *J Pediatr* 1993; 122:837.

251. Mongeau JG. Pathogenesis of the essential hypertensions. *Pediatr Nephrol* 1991;5:404.

252. Ellison RC. Should physicians intervene during childhood to prevent adult hypertension? *Schweiz Med Wochenschr* 1995;125:264.

253. Lewis M, for B.A.P.N. Report of the Paediatric Renal Registry 1999. In: Renal Association, *The UK Renal Registry: the second annual report.* London: 2000:175.

254. Roderick PJ, Raleigh VS, Hallam L, et al. The need and demand for renal replacement therapy in ethnic minorities in England. *J Epidemiol Community Health* 1996;50:334.

255. Fivush BA, Jabs K, Neu AM, et al. Chronic renal insufficiency in children and adolescents: the 1996 annual report of NAPRTCS. North American Pediatric Renal Transplant Cooperative Study. *Pediatr Nephrol* 1998;12:328.

256. Leumann EP. Chronic juvenile kidney insufficiency: results of a Swiss questionnaire. *Schweiz Med Wochenschr* 1976;106:244.

257. West CD, Smith WC. An attempt to elucidate the cause of growth retardation in renal disease. *J Dis Child* 1956;91:460.

258. Chantler C, Holliday M. Growth in children with renal disease and particular reference to the effects of calorie malnutrition: a review. *Clin Nephrol* 1973;1:230.

259. Betts PR, Magrath G, White RH. Proceedings: growth and dietary intake of children with chronic renal insufficiency. *Arch Dis Child* 1974;49:246.

260. Broyer M, Chantler C, Donckerwolcke R, et al. The paediatric registry of the European Dialysis and Transplant Association: 20 years' experience. *Pediatr Nephrol* 1993;7:758.

261. Hokken-Koelega AC, van Zaal MA, van Bergen W, et al. Final height and its predictive factors after renal transplantation in childhood. *Pediatr Res* 1994;36:323.

262. Abitbol CL, Zilleruelo G, Montane B, et al. Growth of uremic infants on forced feeding regimens. *Pediatr Nephrol* 1993;7:173.

263. Foreman JW, Abitbol CL, Trachtman H, et al. Nutritional intake in children with renal insufficiency: a report of the growth failure in children with renal diseases study. *J Am Coll Nutr* 1996;15:579.

264. Van Dyck M, Sidler S, Proesmans W. Chronic renal failure in infants: effect of strict conservative treatment on growth. *Eur J Pediatr* 1998;157:759.

265. Ellis EN, Pearson D, Champion B, et al. Outcome of infants on chronic peritoneal dialysis. *Adv Perit Dial* 1995;11:266.

266. Kari JA, Gonzalez C, Ledermann SE, et al. Outcome and growth of infants with severe chronic renal failure. *Kidney Int* 2000;57:1681.

267. Tom A, McCauley L, Bell L, et al. Growth during maintenance hemodialysis: impact of enhanced nutrition and clearance. *J Pediatr* 1999;134:464.

268. Bosque M, Munian A, Bewick M, et al. Growth after renal transplants. *Arch Dis Child* 1983;58:110.

269. Jones RW.A, et al. The effects of chronic renal failure in infancy on growth, nutritional status and body composition. *Pediatr Res* 1982;16:794.

270. Polito C, La Manna A, Iovene A, et al. Pubertal growth in children with chronic renal failure on conservative treatment. *Pediatr Nephrol* 1995;9:734.

271. Schaefer F, Veldhuis JD, Stanhope R, et al. Alterations in growth hormone secretion and clearance in peripubertal boys with chronic renal failure and after renal transplantation: Cooperative Study Group of Pubertal Development in Chronic Renal Failure. *J Clin Endocrinol Metab* 1994;78:1298.

272. Schaefer F, Veldhuis JD, Robertson WR, et al. Immunoreactive and bioactive luteinizing hormone in pubertal patients with chronic renal failure: Cooperative Study Group on Pubertal Development in Chronic Renal Failure. *Kidney Int* 1994;45:1465.

273. Schaefer F, Seidel C, Binding A, et al. Pubertal growth in chronic renal failure. *Pediatr Res* 1990;28:5.

274. Broyer M, et al. Maturation osseuse et development pubertaire chez l'enfant et l'adolescent en dialyse chronique. *Proc Eur Dial Transplant Assoc Eur Ren Assoc* 1972;9:181.

275. Broyer M, et al. Combined report on regular dialysis and transplantation of children in Europe, 1980. *Proc Eur Dial Transplant Assoc* 1981;18:60.

276. Kohaut EC. Chronic renal disease and growth in childhood. *Curr Opin Pediatr* 1995;7:171.

277. Broyer M, Guest G, Gagnadoux MF. Growth rate in children receiving alternate-day corticosteroid treatment after kidney transplantation. *J Pediatr* 1992;120:721.

278. Chao SM, Jones CL, Powell HR, et al. Triple immunosuppression with subsequent prednisolone withdrawal: 6 years' experience in paediatric renal allograft recipients. *Pediatr Nephrol* 1994;8:62.

279. Ellis D, Shapiro R, Jordan ML, et al. Comparison of FK-506 and cyclosporine regimens in pediatric renal transplantation. *Pediatr Nephrol* 1994;8:193.

280. Winkler L, Offner G, Krull F, et al. Growth and pubertal development in nephropathic cystinosis. *Eur J Pediatr* 1993;152:244.

281. Nash MA, et al. Renal tubular acidosis in infants and children. *J Pediatr* 1972;80:738.

282. Haycock GB. The influence of sodium on growth in infancy. *Pediatr Nephrol* 1993;7:871.

283. Rarvic JN, Roy JA. A salt-losing syndrome in infancy. *Arch Dis Child* 1962;37:548.

284. Turner C, Compston J, Mak RH, et al. Bone turnover and 1, 25-dihydroxycholecalciferol during treatment with phosphate binders. *Kidney Int* 1988;33:989.

285. Counahan R, El-Bishti M, Cox BD, et al. Plasma amino acids in children and adolescents on hemodialysis. *Kidney Int* 1976;10:471.

286. Mak RH. Carbohydrate metabolism in uremia. *Pediatr Nephrol* 1989;3:201.

287. Mak RH, Haycock GB, Chantler C. Glucose intolerance in children with chronic renal failure. *Kidney Int Suppl* 1983;15:S22.

288. Mak RH, et al. The role of secondary hyperparathyroidism in the glucose intolerance of chronic renal failure. *J Clin Endocrinol Metab* 1985;60:229.

289. Mak RH.K, et al. The effects of a low protein diet on glucose metabolism in uremia. *J Clin Endocrinol Metab* 1986;63:985.

290. Tonshoff B, Schaefer F, Mehls O. Disturbance of growth hormone—insulin-like growth factor axis in uraemia: implications for recombinant human growth hormone treatment. *Pediatr Nephrol* 1990;4:654.

291. Mak RH, Haycock GB, Chantler C. Insulin and growth in chronic renal failure. *Pediatr Nephrol* 1994;8:309.

292. Powell DR. Effects of renal failure on the growth hormone-insulin-like growth factor axis. *J Pediatr* 1997;131:S13.

293. Mehls O, Tonshoff B, Haffner D, et al. The use of recombinant human growth hormone in short children with chronic renal failure. *J Pediatr Endocrinol* 1994;7:107.

294. Fine RN, Koch VH, Boechat MI, et al. Recombinant human growth hormone (rhGH) treatment of children undergoing peritoneal dialysis. *Perit Dial Int* 1990;10:209.

295. Hokken-Koelega AC, de Jong RC, Donckerwolcke RA, et al. Use of recombinant human growth hormone (rhGH) in pubertal patients with CRI/dialysis/post-transplant: Dutch data. Dutch Study Group on Growth in Children with Chronic Renal Disease. *Br J Clin Pract Suppl* 1996;85:5.

296. Betts PR, Magrath G. Growth pattern and dietary intake of children with chronic renal insufficiency. *BMJ* 1974;2:189.

297. Arnold WC, Danford D, Holliday MA. Effects of caloric supplementation on growth in children with uremia. *Kidney Int* 1983;24:205.

298. Simmons JM, et al. Relations of caloric deficiency to growth failure in children on hemodialysis and the growth response to caloric supplementation. *N Engl J Med* 1971;285:653.

299. Hellerstein S, Holliday MA, Grupe WE, et al. Nutritional management of children with chronic renal failure: summary of the Task Force on Nutritional Management of Children with Chronic Renal Failure. *Pediatr Nephrol* 1987;1:195.

300. Salusky IB. The nutritional approach for pediatric patients undergoing CAPD/CCPD. *Adv Perit Dial* 1990;6:245.

301. Health and Social Security Department. *Recommended daily amounts of food, energy, and nutrients for groups of people in the UK.* London: Her Majesty's Stationery Office, 1979.

302. Uauy RD, Hogg RJ, Brewer ED, et al. Dietary protein and growth in infants with chronic renal insufficiency: a report from the Southwest Pediatric Nephrology Study Group and the University of California, San Francisco. *Pediatr Nephrol* 1994;8:45.

303. Sigstrom L, Attman PO, Jodal U, et al. Growth during treatment with low-protein diet in children with renal failure. *Clin Nephrol* 1984;21:152.

304. Kist-van Holthe tot Echten JE, Nauta J, Hop WC, et al. Protein restriction in chronic renal failure. *Arch Dis Child* 1993;68:371.

305. Clark AG, Oner A, Ward G, et al. Safety and efficacy of calcium carbonate in children with chronic renal failure. *Nephrol Dial Transplant* 1989;4:539.

306. Slatopolsky EA, Burke SK, Dillon MA. RenaGel, a nonabsorbed calcium- and aluminum-free phosphate binder, lowers serum phosphorus and parathyroid hormone: the RenaGel Study Group. *Kidney Int* 1999;55:299.

307. Randall ME. Aluminum toxicity in an infant not on dialysis. *Lancet* 1983;1:1327.

308. Tamanaha K, Mak RH, Rigden SP, et al. Long-term suppression of hyperparathyroidism by phosphate binders in uremic children. *Pediatr Nephrol* 1987;1:145.

309. Pennisi AJ, Heuser ET, Mickey MR, et al. Hyperlipidemia in pediatric hemodialysis and renal transplant patients: associated with coronary artery disease. *Am J Dis Child* 1976;130:957.

310. Querfeld U. Should hyperlipidemia in children with the nephrotic syndrome be treated? *Pediatr Nephrol* 1999;13:77.

311. El-Bishti M, Counahan R, Jarrett RJ, et al. Hyperlipidaemia in children on regular haemodialysis. *Arch Dis Child* 1977;52:932.

312. Papadopoulou ZL, Sandler P, Tina LU, et al. Hyperlipidemia in children with chronic renal insufficiency. *Pediatr Res* 1981;15:887.

313. Silverstein DM, Palmer J, Polinsky MS, et al. Risk factors for hyperlipidemia in long-term pediatric renal transplant recipients. *Pediatr Nephrol* 2000;14:105.

314. Ong CS, Pollock CA, Caterson RJ, et al. Hyperlipidemia in renal transplant recipients: natural history and response to treatment. *Medicine (Baltimore)* 1994;73:215.

315. Asayama K, Ito H, Nakahara C, et al. Lipid profiles and lipase activities in children and adolescents with chronic renal failure treated conservatively or with hemodialysis or transplantation. *Pediatr Res* 1984;18:783.

316. Corboy J, Sutherland WH, Walker RJ, et al. Cholesteryl ester transfer in patients with renal failure or renal transplants. *Kidney Int* 1994;46:1147.

317. Goren A, Stankiewicz H, Goldstein R, et al. Fish oil treatment of hyperlipidemia in children and adolescents receiving renal replacement therapy. *Pediatrics* 1991;88:265.

318. Jureidini KF, Hogg RJ, van Renen MJ, et al. Evaluation of long-term aggressive dietary management of chronic renal failure in children. *Pediatr Nephrol* 1990;4:1.

319. Hokken-Koelega AC, Stijnen T, de Muinck Keizer-Schrama SM, et al. Placebo-controlled, double-blind, cross-over trial of growth hormone treatment in prepubertal children with chronic renal failure. *Lancet* 1991;338:585.

320. Haffner D, Wuhl E, Schaefer F, et al. Factors predictive of the short- and long-term efficacy of growth hormone treatment in prepubertal children with chronic renal failure: the German Study Group for Growth Hormone Treatment in Chronic Renal Failure. *J Am Soc Nephrol* 1998;9:1899.

321. Berard E, Crosnier H, Six-Beneton A, et al. Recombinant human growth hormone treatment of children on hemodialysis: French Society of Pediatric Nephrology. *Pediatr Nephrol* 1998;12:304.

322. Maxwell H, Rees L. Randomised controlled trial of recombinant human growth hormone in prepubertal and pubertal renal transplant recipients: British Association for Pediatric Nephrology. *Arch Dis Child* 1998;79:481.

323. Schaefer F, Haffner D, Wuhl E, et al. Long-term experience with growth hormone treatment in children with chronic renal failure. *Perit Dial Int* 1999;19:S467.

324. Rees L, Ward G, Rigden SP. Growth over 10 years following a 1-year trial of growth hormone therapy. *Pediatr Nephrol* 2000;14:309.

325. Mentser M, Breen TJ, Sullivan EK, et al. Growth-hormone treatment of renal transplant recipients. The National Cooperative Growth Study experience: a report of the National Cooperative Growth Study and the North American Pediatric Renal Transplant Cooperative Study. *J Pediatr* 1997;131:S20.

326. Postlethwaite RJ, Eminson DM, Reynolds JM, et al. Growth in renal failure: a longitudinal study of emotional and behavioural changes during trials of growth hormone treatment. *Arch Dis Child* 1998;78:222.

327. Rees L. Compliance with growth hormone therapy in chronic renal failure and post transplant. *Pediatr Nephrol* 1997;11:752.

328. Gilli G, Mehls O, Wallstein B, et al. Prediction of adult height in children with chronic renal insufficiency. *Kidney Int Suppl* 1983;15:S48.

329. Aschendorff C, Offner G, Winkler L, et al. Adult height achieved in children after kidney transplantation. *Am J Dis Child* 1990;144:1138.

330. Boirie Y, Broyer M, Gagnadoux MF, et al. Alterations of protein metabolism by metabolic acidosis in children with chronic renal failure. *Kidney Int* 2000;58:236.

331. Grinspoon SK, Baum HB, Kim V, et al. Decreased bone formation and increased mineral dissolution during acute fasting in young women. *J Clin Endocrinol Metab* 1995;80:3628.

332. Kaiser BA, Polinsky MS, Stover J, et al. Growth of children following the initiation of dialysis: a comparison of three dialysis modalities. *Pediatr Nephrol* 1994;8:733.

333. Brem AS, Brem FS, McGrath M, et al. Psychosocial characteristics and coping skills in children maintained on chronic dialysis. *Pediatr Nephrol* 1988;2:460.

334. Reynolds JM, Garralda ME, Postlethwaite RJ, et al. Changes in psychosocial adjustment after renal transplantation. *Arch Dis Child* 1991;66:508.

335. Busschbach JJ, Rikken B, Grobbee DE, et al. Quality of life in short adults. *Horm Res* 1998;49:32.

336. Mongeau JG, Clermont MJ, Robitaille P, et al. Study of psychosocial parameters related to the survival rate of renal transplantation in children. *Pediatr Nephrol* 1997;11:542.

337. Foulkes LM, Boggs SR, Fennell RS, et al. Social support, family variables, and compliance in renal transplant children. *Pediatr Nephrol* 1993;7:185.

338. Offner G, Latta K, Hoyer PF, et al. Kidney transplanted children come of age. *Kidney Int* 1999;55:1509.

339. Roscoe JM, Smith LF, Williams EA, et al. Medical and social outcome in adolescents with end-stage renal failure. *Kidney Int* 1991;40:948.

340. Potter DE, Najarian J, Belzer F, et al. Long-term results of renal transplantation in children. *Kidney Int* 1991;40:752.

341. Wass VJ. Home dialysis in children. *Lancet* 1977;1:242.

342. Postlethwaite RJ, Garralda ME, Eminson DM, et al. Lessons from psychosocial studies of chronic renal failure. *Arch Dis Child* 1996;75:455.

343. Warady BA, Alexander SR, Watkins S, et al. Optimal care of the pediatric end-stage renal disease patient on dialysis. *Am J Kidney Dis* 1999;33:567.

344. Fennell RS, Fennell EB, Carter RL, et al. A longitudinal study of the cognitive function of children with renal failure. *Pediatr Nephrol* 1990;4:11.

345. Osberg JW, et al. Intellectual functioning in renal failure and chronic dialysis. *J Chronic Dis* 1982;35:445.

346. Rasbury WC, Fennell RS, Morris MK. Cognitive functioning of children with end stage renal disease before and after successful transplantation. *J Pediatr* 1983;102:589.

347. Rotundo A, Nevins TE, Lipton M, et al. Progressive encephalopathy in children with chronic renal insufficiency in infancy. *Kidney Int* 1982;21:486.

348. Elzouki A, Carroll J, Butinar D, et al. Improved neurological outcome in children with chronic renal disease from infancy. *Pediatr Nephrol* 1994;8:205.

349. Rigden SP, Montini G, Morris M, et al. Recombinant human erythropoietin therapy in children maintained by haemodialysis. *Pediatr Nephrol* 1990;4:618.

350. Morris KP, Watson S, Reid MM, et al. Assessing iron status in children with chronic renal failure on erythropoietin: which measurements should we use? *Pediatr Nephrol* 1994;8:51.

351. Offner G, Hoyer PF, Latta K, et al. One year's experience with recombinant erythropoietin in children undergoing continuous ambulatory or cycling peritoneal dialysis. *Pediatr Nephrol* 1990;4:498.

352. Braun A, Ding R, Seidel C, et al. Pharmacokinetics of recombinant human erythropoietin applied subcutaneously to children with chronic renal failure. *Pediatr Nephrol* 1993;7:61.

353. Gardiner AOP, et al. The assessment of dialysis requirement for children on regular haemodialysis. *Dial Transplant* 1982;11:754.

354. Warren S, Conley S. Nutritional considerations in infants on continuous peritoneal dialysis (CPD). *Dial Transplant* 1983;12:263.

355. Bunchman TE. Chronic dialysis in the infant less than 1 year of age. *Pediatr Nephrol* 1995;9:S18.

356. Fischbach M, Terzic J, Lahlou A, et al. Nutritional effects of KT/V in children on peritoneal dialysis: are there benefits from larger dialysis doses? *Adv Perit Dial* 1995;11:306.

357. Schaefer F, Klaus G, Mehls O. Peritoneal transport properties and dialysis dose affect growth and nutritional status in children on chronic peritoneal dialysis: Mid-European Pediatric Peritoneal Dialysis Study Group. *J Am Soc Nephrol* 1999;10:1786.

358. Sliman GA, Klee KM, Gall-Holden B, et al. Peritoneal equilibration test curves and adequacy of dialysis in children on automated peritoneal dialysis. *Am J Kidney Dis* 1994;24:813.

359. Bouts AH, Davin JC, Groothoff JW, et al. Standard peritoneal permeability analysis in children. *J Am Soc Nephrol* 2000;11:943.

360. Munoz-Arizpe R, Salazar-Gutierrez ML, Gordillo-Paniagua G. Adequacy of chronic peritoneal dialysis in low socioeconomic class uremic children. *Int J Pediatr Nephrol* 1986;7:81.

361. Evans JH, Smye SW, Brocklebank JT. Mathematical modelling of haemodialysis in children. *Pediatr Nephrol* 1992;6:349.

362. Buur T, Bradbury MG, Smye SW, et al. Reliability of haemodialysis urea kinetic modelling in children. *Pediatr Nephrol* 1994;8:574.

363. Verrina E, Brendolan A, Gusmano R, et al. Chronic renal replacement therapy in children: which index is best for adequacy? *Kidney Int* 1998;54:1690.

364. Offner G, Hoyer PF, Meyer B, et al. Pre-emptive renal transplantation in children and adolescents. *Transpl Int* 1993;6:125.

365. Vats AN, Donaldson L, Fine RN, et al. Pretransplant dialysis status and outcome of renal transplantation in North American children: a NAPRTCS Study. North American Pediatric Renal Transplant Cooperative Study. *Transplantation* 2000;69:1414.

366. Salvatierra O, Jr, Singh T, Shifrin R, et al. Successful transplantation of adult-sized kidneys into infants requires maintenance of high aortic blood flow. *Transplantation* 1998;66:819.

367. Arbus GS, Rochon J, Thompson D. Survival of cadaveric renal transplant grafts from young donors and in young recipients. *Pediatr Nephrol* 1991;5:152.

368. Gellert S, Devaux S, Schonberger B, et al. Donor age and graft function. *Pediatr Nephrol* 1996;10:716.

369. Dubourg L, Hadj-Aissa A, Parchoux B, et al. Role of the donor in post-transplant renal function. *Nephrol Dial Transplant* 1998;13:1494.

370. Henning PH, Bewick M, Reidy JF, et al. Increased incidence of renal transplant arterial stenosis in children. *Nephrol Dial Transplant* 1989;4:575.

371. Borzyskowski M, Mundy AR. The management of the neuropathic bladder in childhood. *Pediatr Nephrol* 1988;2:56.

372. Alfrey EJ, Salvatierra O Jr, Tanney DC, et al. Bladder augmentation can be problematic with renal failure and transplantation [see comments]. *Pediatr Nephrol* 1997;11:672.

373. Haycock G, ed. Intraoperative and immediate postoperative care in the management of the pediatric transplant recipient. In: Brodehl J, Ehrich J, eds. *Pediatric Nephrology: Proceedings of the Sixth International Symposium (Hanover, F.R.G.).* Berlin: Springer-Verlag, 1984: 146.

374. Kabasakul SC, Clarke M, Kane H, et al. Comparison of Neoral and Sandimmune cyclosporin A pharmacokinetic profiles in young renal transplant recipients. *Pediatr Nephrol* 1997;11:318.

375. Kari JA, Romagnoli J, Duffy P, et al. Renal transplantation in children under 5 years of age. *Pediatr Nephrol* 1999;13:730.

376. Najarian JS, Almond PS, Mauer M, et al. Renal transplantation in the first year of life: the treatment of choice for infants with end-stage renal disease. *J Am Soc Nephrol* 1992;2:S228.

377. Greenstein S, et al. Plasmapheresis treatment for recurrent focal sclerosis in pediatric renal allografts. *Pediatr Nephrol* 2000;14:1061.

378. Broyer M, Brunner FP, Brynger H, et al. Kidney transplantation in primary oxalosis: data from the EDTA Registry. *Nephrol Dial Transplant* 1990;5:332.

379. Furth SL, Neu AM, Sullivan EK, et al. Immunization practices in children with renal disease: a report of the North American Pediatric Renal Transplant Cooperative Study. *Pediatr Nephrol* 1997;11:443.

CHAPTER 81

Renal Function and Disease in the Aging Kidney

Devasmita Choudhury and Moshe Levi

Biologic senescence initiates a number of subtle structural and functional changes in the kidney. The aging kidney maintains homeostasis until renal reserve is overwhelmed by intercurrent insults such as infections, immunologic processes, drugs, toxins, or other organ system failure. The aged kidney, however, may be less tolerant of physiologic and pathophysiologic perturbations, predisposing the elderly to more significant renal compromise than expected. This can be seen with kidneys from donors older than 55 years of age, which are more likely to fail from chronic allograft nephropathy (1,2). The elderly are at least five times more prone to development of end-stage renal disease (ESRD) than young adults (3). Both European and U.S. registries highlight the growing incidence of elderly subjects initiating dialysis (3,4). The increasing prevalence of renal disease in a growing elderly population necessitates an understanding of the anatomic, physiologic, and pathologic mechanisms involved in the aging kidney. The ability to investigate the kidney using molecular probes has increased our understanding of the basic mechanisms that may be involved in hastening renal senescence. Accordingly, our current understanding of the interactions between aging, renal function, and renal disease is reviewed in this chapter.

CHANGES IN ANATOMY AND STUCTURE

Kidney mass progressively declines with advancing age. Intravenous urography and computed tomography scans of postmortem kidneys show a decrease in both renal size and volume (5,6). Glomerulosclerosis and tubulointerstitial fibrosis lead to a change in renal weight from 245 to 270 g during adulthood to 180 to 200 g by 90 years of age (7). These changes, however, may be age appropriate, as noted by a study evaluating 357 accidental death victims that excluded renal and other comorbid conditions (8). Little change

D. Choudhury and M. Levi: Department of Medicine, The University of Texas Southwestern Medical Center at Dallas, Dallas VA Medical Center, Dallas, Texas

in renal mass was found when renal weight was adjusted for the concurrent decrease in body surface area seen with aging (8).

A histologic predominance of ischemic cortical glomeruli is seen with a decrease in glomerular number by 30% to 50% by 70 years of age (9). Loss of glomerular tuft lobulation, an increase in mesangial volume by 8% to 12%, and progressive capillary collapse with obliteration of the lumen of the afferent arteriole characterize this histologic obsolescence (10). There is thickening and wrinkling of the basement membranes of both glomeruli and tubules, with eventual reduction and simplification of the vascular channels (11–13). The renal medulla appears relatively spared compared with the cortical glomeruli. At the molecular level, telomere shortening seems to occur in an age-dependent fashion in the renal cortex faster than in the medulla (14). Telomere length in human nephrectomy and autopsy kidneys of various ages investigated by Southern blotting of terminal restriction fragments and slot blotting using telomere-specific probes indicates a shortening in the telomere DNA of the renal cortex with age (14). Telomeres, DNA sequence repeats of (TTAGGG), protect ends of chromosomes and shorten with increasing age in somatic cells (14). Acting as a mitotic clock, telomeres reflect the replicative senescence of the cell (15,16). These findings raise the possibility that critical telomere shortening could become a limiting factor in some renal cell populations and contribute to some features seen in the senescent kidney (14). Juxtamedullary glomeruli see blood shunting from the afferent to the efferent arterioles, allowing redistribution of blood flow favoring the renal medulla (17) (Fig. 81-1). Blood flow is maintained to the medulla through the arteriolar recta vera, which do not decrease in number with age (18). Scarring with little cellular response occurs as hyaline is deposited in residual glomeruli and Bowman's space.

Tubule size and number decrease as tubules atrophy and develop diverticula of distal convoluted tubules. These outpouchings may represent the earliest formation of acquired cysts commonly seen in aged kidneys (19) (Fig. 81-2).

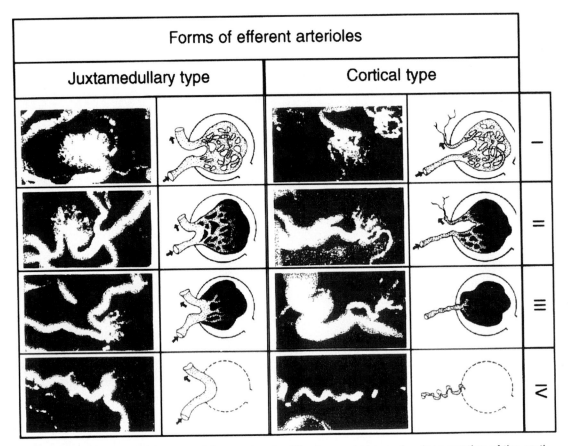

FIG. 81-1. Progressive (Stage I to IV) vascular simplification and glomerular degeneration of the cortical and juxtamedullary arteriole–glomerular units with corresponding microangiograms. (Reprinted with permission from Takazakura E, Sawabu N, Handa A, et al. Intrarenal vascular changes with age and disease. *Kidney Int* 1972;2:224.)

Bacteria and debris collect in these diverticula and may predispose to infection and pyelonephritis (20).

Tubulointerstitial fibrosis in aging may be an active process associated with interstitial inflammation, fibroblast activation, and accelerated apoptosis of cells in areas of fibrosis (21). Focal tubular cell proliferation, myofibroblast activation, macrophage infiltration, increased immunostaining for the adhesive proteins osteopontin and intracellular adhesion molecule-1, and collagen IV deposition are found in aged rats (21) (Fig. 81-3). Furthermore, age-related increases in types I and IV collagen and fibronectin messenger RNA (mRNA) expression were found in 24- and 30-month-old rats (21). Ischemia from peritubular capillary injury with altered endothelial nitric oxide synthase (eNOS) expression triggers this inflammation (21).

Changes in the aging intrarenal vasculature occur independent of hypertension or other renal disease. Walls of the larger renal vessels undergo variable sclerotic changes that are made worse by hypertension (11). Smaller vessels are spared, with less than 20% of senescent kidneys from nonhypertensive subjects displaying arteriolar changes (11). Pyelography and angiography on postmortem kidneys of normotensive subjects older than 50 years of age suggest that loss of renal

cortical tissue in the elderly may be related more to changes in the renal vasculature than to age alone (22).

RENAL BLOOD FLOW AND GLOMERULAR FILTRATION RATE

In addition to anatomic changes, functional changes occur in the aging renal vasculature and contribute to decreased renal blood flow. p-Aminohippurate (PAH) clearances of 600 mL/minute/1.73 m^2 at 20 to 29 years of age drop to 300 mL/minute/1.73 m^2 by 80 to 89 years, a change of approximately 10% per decade (23,24). Xenon washout scans in healthy kidney donors between 17 and 76 years of age demonstrate a preferential decrease in cortical blood flow and preservation of medullary flow with age, paralleling the selective loss of cortical vasculature seen histologically (25).

Whether this change in renal plasma flow (RPF) is affected by possible age-related changes in cardiac output is not clearly established because some studies have shown an age-related decrease in cardiac output, whereas other carefully designed studies have not shown such a change (26,27). There may be a small but definite decrease in the renal fraction of the cardiac output (28). This decrease in the proportion

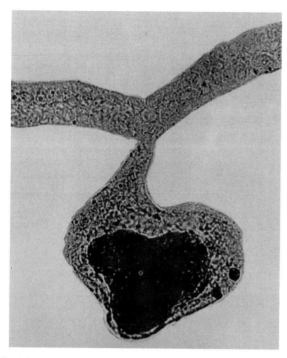

FIG. 81-2. Microdissection of collecting tubule and associated diverticulum showing continuity between tubular lumen and diverticulum. (Reprinted with permission from Baert L, Steg A. Is the diverticulum of the distal and collecting tubules a preliminary stage of the simple cyst in the adult? *J Urol* 1977;113:707.)

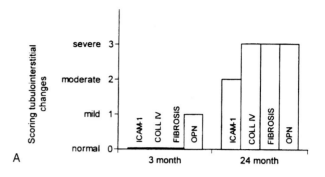

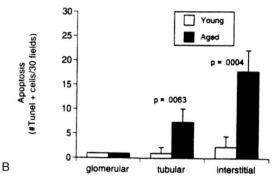

FIG. 81-3. A: Tubulointerstitial fibrosis as well as immunostaining for collagen IV (Coll IV), intracellular adhesion molecule-1 (ICAM-1), and osteopontin (OPN) are increased in aged rats compared with younger rats. **B:** Apoptosis in young and aged rats was quantified by the number of terminal deoxynucleotidyl transferase (Ttd)-mediated dUTP-biotin nick end labeling (TUNEL) cells in the glomeruli tubules and interstitium. Total number of TUNEL-positive cells/30 fields was 3.5 ± 2.5 in the 3-month-old versus 24.5 ± 5.3 in the 24-month-old rats (P = 0.0001). (Redrawn with permission from Thomas SE, Anderson S, Gordon KL, et al. Tubulointerstitial disease in aging: evidence for underlying peritubular capillary damage, a potential role for renal ischemia. *J Am Soc Nephrol* 1998;9:231.)

of renal blood flow relative to cardiac output may reflect the changes in anatomic and vascular responsiveness observed with renal aging.

An altered functional response of the renal vasculature in aged humans and animals may be an underlying factor in the decreased renal blood flow and increased filtration fraction noted in progressive renal aging. Although renal blood flow, as measured by PAH clearances, increases in elderly subjects with infusion of vasorelaxants, such as intravenous pyrogen (24) or atrial natriuretic peptide (ANP) (29), or intraarterial acetylcholine (25), the vasodilatory response is blunted compared with younger counterparts. Similarly, amino acid infusion results in an increase in glomerular filtration rate (GFR) and filtration fraction, whereas RPF remains unchanged (30) (Fig. 81-4). Impaired vasorelaxation may be the result of defective intracellular signaling (31). An exaggerated vasoconstrictive response is seen with stimulation of the renal sympathetic system, which may result from an inadequate response of cyclic adenosine monophosphate (cAMP) to β-adrenergic agonists or altered cyclic guanosine monophosphate (cGMP) response to ANP (32,33). Other mediators of vasorelaxation, including vasodilatory prostacyclin [prostaglandin (PG) I₂], also are decreased in aged human vascular cells and aged rat kidneys compared with the vasoconstrictive thromboxanes (34,35). Aging humans also are noted to excrete less vasodilatory natriuretic prostaglandin (PGE₂) (36). Inhibition

of angiotensin II, however, results in a preserved or exaggerated vasodilatory response in the elderly (37,38), suggesting a greater role for angiotensin II–mediated vasoconstriction of the aged renal vasculature. This is further demonstrated by significant increases in renal blood flow and GFR in aged rats treated with angiotensin-converting enzyme (ACE) inhibitors and angiotensin receptor blockers (39). The vasoconstrictive response to intraarterial angiotensin is identical in both young and older human subjects (25). A blunted vasodilatory capacity with appropriate vasoconstriction may indicate that the aged kidney is in a state of renal vasodilatation to compensate for underlying glomerular sclerotic damage. Intravenous glycine infusion in progressively aged groups of Sprague-Dawley rats mimics the change in RPF seen in humans and correlates histologically with progressive glomerulosclerosis (40). *N*-nitro-L-arginine-methyl-ester

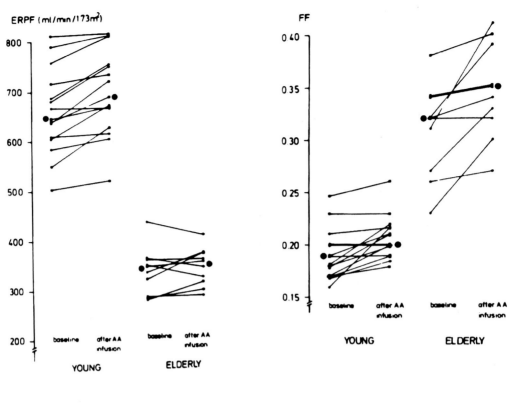

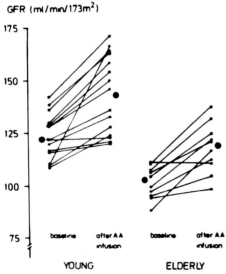

FIG. 81-4. Effective renal plasma flow (ERPF), glomerular filtration rate (GFR), and filtration fraction (FF) in young and elderly subjects at baseline and after amino acid (AA) infusion. ERPF remains unchanged, whereas GFR and FF increase. ■, Males; *females; ●, median. (Reprinted with permission from Fliser D, Zeier M, Nowack R, et al. Renal functional reserve in healthy elderly subjects. *J Am Soc Nephrol* 1993;3:1371.)

(L-NAME), an L-arginine analog that competitively inhibits the formation of endothelium-derived relaxing factor (EDRF), causes a marked increase in the vasoconstrictive response with a significant increase in renal vascular resistance (RVR) and a decrease in RPF in aged Sprague-Dawley rats compared with their younger counterparts (41). *In vivo* micropuncture of young and aged Sprague-Dawley rats also showed no age-related change in the magnitude of the pressor and vasoconstrictive response in angiotensin II infusion. Angiotensin II caused increased arteriolar resistances of both preglomerular and efferent vessels and decreased RPF and glomerular plasma flow. This was accompanied by a rise

in the glomerular hydraulic pressure gradient and increased filtration fraction in both young and older rats. However, the glomerular capillary ultrafiltration coefficient (K_f) decreased in the older rats, leading to a decrease in GFR and single-nephron GFR (SNGFR). In contrast, there was no change in K_f, GFR, or SNGFR in the younger rats. An angiotensin II–dependent decrease in K_f through contraction of glomerular mesangial cells, with a subsequent decrease in filtration surface area, is a possible explanation for the finding (42).

Despite a linear decrease in renal blood flow with age, the filtration fraction appears to increase. Because juxtamedullary nephrons have a higher filtration fraction than cortical nephrons, a combination of preserved medullary flow and decreased renal cortical plasma flow may explain this observation.

A decrease in nephron mass is expected with senescence of the kidney. However, the rate of decline in GFR in aging individuals can vary depending on methods of measurements, race, sex, genetic variance, and other underlying risk factors for renal dysfunction. Lewis and Alving noted a drop in urea clearance as early as 1938 (43), which others later confirmed by inulin, creatinine, and iothalamate clearances (44). Creatinine clearance drops linearly from 140 mL/minute/1.73 m^2 during the third and fourth decade to 97 mL/minute/1.73 m^2 by 80 years of age, a rate of decline of 0.8 mL/minute/1.73 m^2 per year (45). Iohexol clearance indicates a decrease of 1.0 mL/minute/1.73 m^2 per year (46). Inulin clearances, although slightly greater than 100 mL/minute/1.73 m^2 in healthy, normotensive elderly subjects without renal disease on a normal dietary protein intake of 1 g/kg/day, still were lower than in younger counterparts (47). Lew and Bosch also showed a drop in GFR with age. At the same time, however, they noted variability of creatinine clearance measurements in relation to protein intake (48). Despite variation in creatinine clearance measurements in relation to protein intake, GFR of aged subjects is lower than in younger subjects. Although a decrease in GFR is measured, a parallel increase in serum creatinine is not seen because muscle mass, from which creatinine is derived, concomitantly decreases with age. Clinically, this translates into an overestimation of GFR in the elderly. The importance of this lies in interpreting clearance values during medication dosing and in assessing risk to the aged kidney for ischemic, toxic, or metabolic events from the serum creatinine alone. Commonly used formulas either underestimate or overestimate GFR in the elderly (49–52) (Table 81-1). Although cumbersome, a more accurate formula derived from the Modification of Diet in Renal Disease study may be useful in assessing creatinine clearance

TABLE 81-1. *Commonly used formulas to estimate glomerular filtration rate*

1. Creatinine clearance (mL/min/1.73 m^2) = (1.33 − 0.64) × age^a

2. Creatinine clearance (mL/min) =
$$\frac{(140-\text{age}) \times \text{weight (kg)}}{72 \times \text{serum creatinine (mg/dL)}^a}$$

3. GFR = 170 × [P$_{cr}$]$^{-0.999}$ × [age]$^{-0.0176}$ × [0.762 if patient is female; 1.180 if patient is black] × [SUN]$^{-0.0170}$ × [alb]$^{+0.318}$

GFR, glomerular filtration rate; *SUN*, serum urea nitrogen; *alb*, albumin.

^{a}15% less in female patients.

*Formula 1 from Rowe JW, Andrew R, Tobin JD, et al. Age-adjusted standards for creatinine clearance. *Ann Intern Med* 1976;84:567. Formula 2 from Cockcroft DW, Gault MH. Prediction of creatinine clearance from serum creatinine. *Nephron* 1976;16:31. Formula 3 from Levey AS, Bosch J, Lewis JB, et al. A more accurate method to estimate glomerular filtration rate from serum creatinine: a new prediction equation. *Ann Intern Med* 1999;130:461.

in the elderly (52). Regardless of which formula is used to estimate GFR, when using drugs that are known to depend on the kidney for excretion or metabolism, appropriate dose adjustment followed by serial drug concentration monitoring is strongly recommended.

Some have recommended routine measurement of creatinine clearances. Again, variability in the collection may occur because of diet or other factors. Radionuclide clearance measurements with technetium-labeled diethylenetriaminepentaacetic acid (^{99m}Tc-DTPA) or ^{125}I-iothalamate, or radiocontrast clearance with single-injection iohexol fluorescence radiography analysis may be considered (44). Expense, exposure to radioactive substance, and test availability may be limiting factors.

Whether differences in sex have a significant effect on the rate of GFR decline in the aged is not clear. Some have suggested a more gradual decline in women than in men, although prospective cross-sectional human studies have not borne out this difference.

Racial and genetic differences, however, do seem to affect declining GFR in the elderly. African American subjects showed a more steeply declining slope in creatinine clearance with increasing age compared with whites, which in part may result from genetic variance (53). Increased nephrosclerosis also was noted in elderly subjects of Japanese origin versus elderly whites as a cause for worsening renal function (7).

A comparative analysis of GFR, RPF, and RVR between elderly normotensive, hypertensive, and heart failure subjects with the young was notable for worsening hemodynamics and increased RVR in all the elderly groups, but especially in those with heart failure (47). In this study, elderly hypertensive subjects did not show a significant decline in GFR compared with elderly normotensive subjects, although when elderly hypertensive subjects not receiving treatment were compared separately with those with a history of drug treatment for hypertension, the latter group had a lower GFR and higher RVR (47). Other studies also have noted age-related renal functional decline in hypertensive subjects (54,55). Intraglomerular hypertension hastening renal functional impairment in the elderly hypertensive person has been suggested as playing a possible role (56,57). Other risk factors leading to progressive renal dysfunction, including atherosclerosis of systemic and renal vasculature, diabetes mellitus, and abnormal lipid metabolism, also may play an important role in the functional decline of GFR in the elderly.

MEDIATORS OF GLOMERULOSCLEROSIS AND TUBULOINTERSTITIAL FIBROSIS: POTENTIAL STRATEGIES FOR MODULATION OF AGE-RELATED RENAL FUNCTIONAL DECLINE

Age-related glomerulosclerosis and tubulointerstitial fibrosis with loss of GFR may not necessarily be irreversible consequences of aging. Longitudinal follow-up of 254 healthy elderly subjects over 23 years with repeated creatinine clearances revealed that one-third of the subjects had no absolute

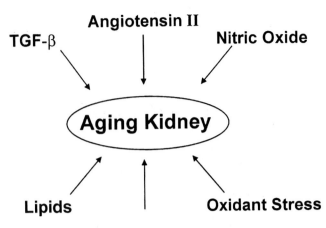

FIG. 81-5. Factors associated with the pathogenesis of age-related glomerulosclerosis and decline in renal function.

age-related decrease in creatinine clearance (58). Studies primarily conducted in animal models of aging have identified a number of factors that play a role in mediating glomerulosclerosis and tubulointerstitial fibrosis (Fig. 81-5). Whether alone or in combination, these pathophysiologic factors can incite age-related changes mimicking those occurring in diabetic nephropathy, with the process more accelerated in diabetes than in normal aging. The ability to modulate these factors can result in prevention of the progressive age-related decline in renal function.

Role of Angiotensin II

Known primarily for vasoactive effects on the renal vasculature and glomerular hemodynamics, angiotensin II mediates diverse biologic effects on the kidney, including proximal tubular transport of sodium and water (59,60), glomerular and tubular growth (61–65), decrease in nitric oxide synthesis (66), immunomodulation, growth factor induction, and accumulation of extracellular matrix proteins, all of which may modulate glomerulosclerosis and tubulointerstitial fibrosis. Intraglomerular hypertension mediated by angiotensin II–induced preferential efferent arteriolar vasoconstriction to maintain filtration pressure in aging nephrons has been implicated in age-dependent glomerular damage (67). Increased renal blood flow and GFR caused by ACE inhibitors, as noted previously, provides indirect evidence supporting this mechanism of glomerulosclerosis (39). Decreased RVR and intracapillary pressure decreased protein leak in aging rodents treated with ACE inhibitors (68). In addition, chronic ACE inhibitor administration decreases postprandial hyperfiltration, thereby decreasing the filtered load delivered to the kidney (69). ACE inhibitors also may play a role in modifying the size selectivity of the glomerular capillaries or changing the negative charge distribution in the glomerular barrier (68,70). Glomerular diameter, mesangial area, and total glomerulosclerosis were markedly decreased in ACE inhibitor–treated aged mice compared with age- and sex-matched untreated mice (68,71–74) (Fig. 81-6).

Beneficial effects of angiotensin antagonism are mediated by both hemodynamic and nonhemodynamic mechanisms. Angiotensin II induces growth-promoting, profibrotic cytokines. It stimulates collagen type IV transcription in medullary collecting tubule cells (75) through endogenous synthesis and autocrine action of transforming growth factor β (TGFβ) (76) as well as promote monocyte–macrophage influx stimulating mRNA and protein expression of the chemokine RANTES (regulated on activation, normal T-cell expressed and secreted) in endothelial cells (77). Angiotensin II inhibition of nitric oxide induces transcription of the proinflammatory chemokine, monocyte chemoattractant protein-1

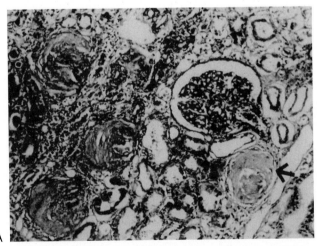

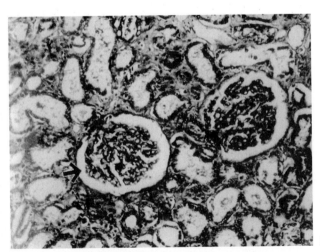

FIG. 81-6. Angiotensin-converting enzyme inhibitor (enalapril) decreases glomerulosclerosis in aged mice. A, Animals treated with placebo; B, animals treated with enalapril. (Reprinted with permission from Ferder L, Inserra F, Romano L, et al. Decreased glomerulosclerosis in aging by angiotensin-converting enzyme inhibitors. *J Am Soc Nephrol* 1994;5:1147.)

(MCP-1). With similar blood pressure control, enalapril-treated aged rats had significant reduction in tubulointerstitial fibrosis and alpha smooth muscle cell actin compared with nifedipine-treated aged rats or untreated aged rats (78). Furthermore, angiotensin II may promote matrix accumulation by stimulating plasminogen activator inhibitor-1 (PAI-1) secretion from the endothelium (79). Because PAI-1 inhibits tissue plasminogen activator and urokinase plasminogen activator, increased PAI-1 levels can lead to decreased proteolysis and fibrinolysis and increased matrix accumulation (80). Regression of age-related glomerular and vascular sclerosis and decreased collagen content were found in rats treated with angiotensin II antagonists (81). Taken together, these experimental data imply beneficial effects of angiotensin II antagonism in the elderly with age-related renal functional decline, although further conclusive data in humans are necessary.

Role of Transforming Growth Factor β

Ample evidence associates TGFβ with renal scarring, as is found with structural changes accompanying age-related renal decline. TGFβ, an active modulator of tissue repair, can be stimulated by a myriad of factors in the aging kidney, including increased angiotensin II activity, abnormal glucose metabolism, platelet-derived growth factor (PDGF), hypoxic or oxidative stress, mesangial stretch, and increased levels of advanced glycosylation end products (AGE). Renal fibrosis seen with aging may be the result of normal and or pathologic tissue repair. The response to injury is wound healing. In the face of persistent injury, this response can lead to tissue fibrosis. TGFβ stimulates gene transcription and production of collagen types III, IV, and I, as well as production of fibronectin, tenascin, osteonectin, osteopontin, thrombospondin, and matrix glycoaminoglycans (82). In addition, TGFβ inhibits collagenase and stimulates the synthesis of metalloproteinase inhibitors (83). The net result is the accumulation of extracellular matrix proteins with subsequent glomerulosclerosis and tubulointerstitial fibrosis (83–86). TGFβ mRNA abundance and TGFβ immunostaining are increased in the renal interstitium of aged rats (87,88) (Fig. 81-7.) Furthermore, the renal protective effects of long-term angiotensin II antagonism are associated with TGFβ downregulation, resulting in decreased interstitial fibrosis (87). Increased expression of TGFβ likely mediates in part age-related sclerosis, although specific proof still is lacking. Future use of TGFβ-neutralizing agents such as decorin, which antagonizes TGFβ action, or use of antiserum oligonucleotides, which specifically inhibit TGFβ expression in models of age-related renal sclerosis, may establish a more definite role for TGFβ in mediating age-related renal dysfunction.

Role of Nitric Oxide

Besides maintaining renal perfusion in the aging kidney (discussed elsewhere in this chapter), the role of nitric oxide as

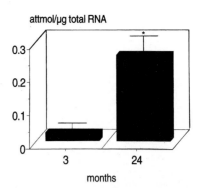

FIG. 81-7. Quantitative analysis of the amount of transforming growth factor-1 (TGF-1) mRNA in two groups of rats, 3 months and 24 months of age. Results expressed as mean ± SEM of ten animals, *P < 0.05 versus 3 month-old-rats; attmol/μg total RNA = attomolar TGF-1 cDNA concentration per milligram of total RNA. (Redrawn from Ruiz-Torres MP, Bosch R, O'Valle F, et al. Age-related increase in expression of TGF-β1 in the rat kidney: relationship to morphologic changes. *J Am Soc Nephrol* 1998;9:782.)

an interactive chemokine in ameliorating fibrosis is becoming more evident. Nitric oxide inhibits transcription factor family NFκB, which, in the presence of reactive oxygen intermediates, stimulates MCP-1 and promotes influx of monocyte–macrophages, causing inflammation injury (89,90). Therefore, nitric oxide acts in the negative feedback loop to decrease inflammation and subsequent fibrosis. Nitric oxide levels, however, are decreased in aged rats, as shown by decreased urinary excretion of stable nitric oxide oxidation products, nitrites and nitrates (91,92). In addition, there is decreased expression of eNOS in the peritubular capillaries of aged rats (21). Decreased eNOS expression and nitric oxide levels can lead to chronic tubulointerstitial ischemia and tubulointerstitial fibrosis seen with aging (21). Long-term dietary supplementation of aged rats with L-arginine results in significant increases in RPF and GFR and decreases in proteinuria and glomerulosclerosis (93) (Fig. 81-8). In addition, dietary L-arginine supplementation results in significant decreases in kidney collagen and N-ϵ-(carboxymethyl) lysine accumulation (CML) (94). The causes for the age-related decrease in eNOS are not known, but potential causes include increased angiotensin II activity, increased levels of AGE, hypoxia or oxidative stress, and perhaps dietary protein intake (92,95–98). Treatment of aged rats with angiotensin II antagonists or dietary protein restriction results in significant increases in and normalization of urinary nitric oxide excretion (92).

Role of Advanced Glycosylation End Products

Advanced glycosylation end products, crosslinks of glycoxidated proteins, lipids, and nucleic acids, slowly accumulate and produce tissue damage to the vascular and renal tissue with aging (99,100). In the presence of hyperglycemia, these end products accumulate more rapidly and accelerate tissue damage (101). These glycated proteins decrease

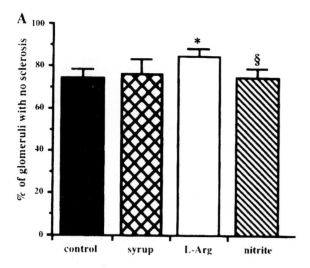

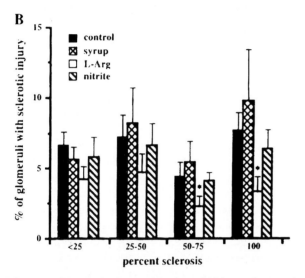

FIG. 81-8. Morphologic examination of kidneys from aging rats. **A:** Average percentage of glomeruli per kidney with no sclerosis. *$P < 0.05$ compared with untreated controls; §$P < 0.05$, nitrite-treated vs. L-arginine–treated groups. **B:** Average percentage of glomeruli per kidney with graded sclerotic injury. *$P < 0.05$, L-arginine–treated rats versus other groups. (Reprinted with permission from Reckelhoff JF, Kellum JA, Racusen LC, et al. Long-term dietary supplementation with L-arginine prevents age-related reduction in renal function. *Am J Physiol* 1997;272:R1768.)

vascular elasticity, induce endothelial cell permeability, and increase monocyte chemotactic activity through AGE receptor ligand binding, which stimulates macrophage activation and cytokine/growth factor secretion. AGE accumulation in the vascular endothelium and basement membrane results in defective nitric oxide vasodilation, possibly because of chemical inactivation of EDRF (102–106). Similar perturbations of the vascular endothelium are evident in diabetic patients and age-related vasculopathy. Both biochemical assay and immunohistochemistry have demonstrated increased levels of AGE and AGE receptors (RAGE) in aged kidneys of animals. In the kidney, there is increased mesangial matrix

with mesangial AGE deposition, increased basement thickening, increased vascular permeability, and induction of PDGF and TGFβ, resulting in glomerulosclerosis and tubulointerstitial fibrosis (102). Several factors contribute to accumulation of AGE and RAGE, including (a) a decline in GFR with age; (b) increased oxidative stress associated with age causing oxidative modification of glycated proteins and accumulation of CML; and (c) age-related insulin resistance, resulting in abnormal glucose metabolism and glycation of proteins. Studies also suggest that life-long consumption of AGE-enriched food substances and smoking also may result in increased AGE loads and increased AGE accumulation in tissues (107,108).

Further evidence for the significant role of AGE in age-related renal and cardiovascular disease comes from animal studies in aged rats and rabbits treated with aminoguanidine (109,110). Long-term aminoguanidine treatment in aged rats markedly diminished glomerulosclerosis, proteinuria (109) (Fig. 81-9), and age-related arterial stiffening and cardiac hypertrophy (111). Reversal of the AGE-associated increase in vascular permeability, prevention of defective vasodilatory response to acetylcholine and nitroglycerin, and prevention of mononuclear cell migratory activity were seen in the subendothelial and periarteriolar spaces in various tissues of rats and rabbits treated with aminoguanidine (110). Caloric restriction also may play a role in increasing the life span and ameliorating the renal lesions seen in aged animals. Caloric restriction imposed by 60% of the *ad libitum* diet in female brown Norway rats attenuated the burden of AGE and the other major oxidatively modified glycated proteins, CML and pentosidine (112,113). Similarly, 30-month-old lean WAG/Rij rats restricted to reduced caloric intake by 30% of the *ad libitum* diet (7 g/day) also showed a marked decrease in collagen AGE content in kidneys, glomeruli, and abdominal aorta compared with nonrestricted 30-month-old rats (114) (Fig. 81-10).

Cumulative evidence of AGE-associated acceleration of diabetic and age-associated vasculopathy and the possibility of treatment with aminoguanidine has led to clinical trials in humans. Results of these trials may change the progression of both diabetic and age-related changes in glomerulosclerosis. Cardiovascular side effects have precluded the completion of these early trials. Future studies may lead to further trials to change the progression of both diabetic and age-related glomerulosclerosis.

Role of Oxidative Stress

With aging, an increase in free radical production or an antioxidant enzyme deficiency can lead to lipid peroxidation and oxidative stress, resulting in tissue injury (115–118). Elevated levels of oxidized amino acids in urine indicate increased oxidized protein levels in the skeletal muscle of aged rats (119). As indicators of lipid oxidative damage, reactive oxygen species and thiobarbituric acid reactive substance levels are increased in the aged kidney (120), whereas

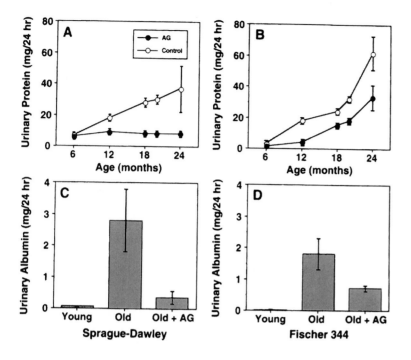

FIG. 81-9. Age-related urinary protein **(A and B)** and albumin loss **(C and D)** in the rat is suppressed by aminoguanidine (AG). Total urinary protein concentration was determined in 24-hour urine collected every 4 months over an 18-month period from S-D **(A)** or F344 **(B)** rats treated with AG (0.1% in drinking water) (●) or untreated, age-matched controls (○). Albuminuria was determined at baseline and at the end of the study in S-D **(C)** or F344 **(D)** rats. Data are expressed as means ± SEM. Comparisons (old vs. young; old vs. old + AG) of all experimental groups of both strains were significant at P < 0.05 (N = 5 to 7 rats per group). (Reprinted with permission from Li YM, Steffes M, Donnelly T, et al. Prevention of cardiovascular and renal pathology of aging by the advanced glycation inhibitor aminoguanidine. *Proc Natl Acad Sci USA* 1996;93:3902.)

antioxidant enzyme activities are decreased in aged rat kidneys (115). Other markers for oxidative stress and lipid peroxidation, including increased formation of isoprostanes, AGE, RAGE, and increase induction of heme oxygenase (121), also are elevated in aging rats. Furthermore, treatment of these rats with antioxidants, such as a high–vitamin-E diet, attenuated these changes with significant improvements noted in renal blood flow and GFR, and a decrease in glomerulosclerosis (121) (Fig. 81-11). Some studies have shown that

angiotensin II stimulates superoxide production by activating membrane-bound nicotinamide adenine dinucleotide phosphate (NADH)/NADPH oxidase, whereas ACE inhibitors can increase the activity of antioxidant enzymes (122,123). Ongoing studies also indicate that increased extracellular mesangial matrix synthesis resulting from TGFβ induction by reactive oxygen species in cultured mesangial cells and aged rats can be blocked with the antioxidant taurine or ACE inhibitor treatment (124).

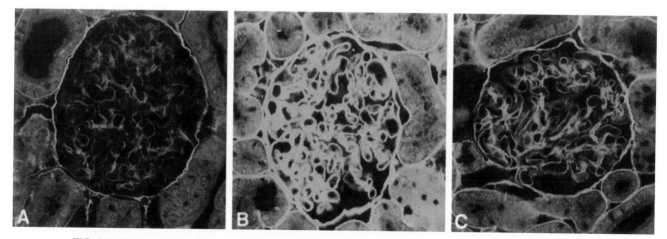

FIG. 81-10. Immunolocalization of advanced glycosylation end products (AGE) in the renal cortex of 10-month-old **(A)** and 30-month-old **(B)** female WAG/Rij rats fed *ad libitum,* and 30-month-old animals food-restricted by 30% **(C)**. AGE localized predominantly in extracellular matrix. Increased AGE accumulation was evident in tubular basement membranes, mesangial matrix, glomerular basement membranes, and Bowman's capsule between 10 to 30 months in rats fed *ad libitum.* Such accumulation was mostly prevented in food-restricted animals. (Magnification ×350.) (Reprinted with permission from Teillet L, Verbeke P, Gouraud S, et al. Food restriction prevents advanced glycation end products accumulation and retards kidney aging in lean rats. *J Am Soc Nephrol* 2000;11:1488.)

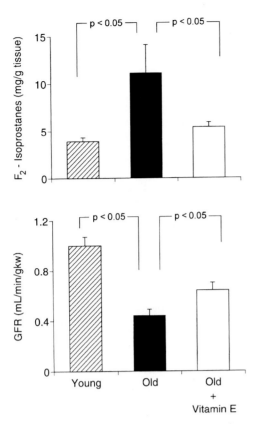

FIG. 81-11. Top: F_2 isoprostane levels in kidneys from young rats, aged 2 to 3 months, and old rats, aged 22 months, given either a control diet or a high–vitamin E diet. **Bottom:** Effect of a high–vitamin E diet on glomerular filtration rate (GFR) in old animals. (Redrawn with permission from Reckelhoff JF, Kanji V, Racusen LC, et al. Vitamin E ameliorates enhanced renal lipid peroxidation and accumulation of F2-isoprostanes in aging kidneys. *Am J Physiol* 1998;274:R767.)

Role of Lipids

Age-related accumulation of cholesterol occurs in several tissues, including the kidney (125–132), and may play an important in the progression of glomerulosclerosis and proteinuria in a number of disease states, including diabetes (132–136). Furthermore, in the presence of oxidative stress and AGE with aging, increased levels of modified low-density lipoprotein cholesterol and lipoprotein (a) may occur (137–139). These lipid products have been associated with increased oxygen radical formation, increased growth factor expression such as PDGF and TGFβ, inhibition of nitric oxide synthesis, migration and adherence of monocytes, and mesangial and vascular cell growth, effects that play an important pathogenic role in renal disease progression.

Lipoxidation stress induced by high-cholesterol feeding in type II diabetic rats has been shown to result in glomerulosclerosis and tubulointerstitial fibrosis (140). Streptozotocin-induced diabetic rats treated with HMG-CoA reductase inhibitors for 12 months had significant improvement in urinary albumin excretion and glomerular volume compared with untreated rats (141). Two other recent studies have shown a decrease in proteinuria and partial preservation of

GFR in type II diabetic patients treated long term with HMG-CoA reductase inhibitors (142,143). Similar trials may be important in aged patients.

RENAL TUBULAR FUNCTION

Anatomic, hemodynamic, and hormonal changes in the aged kidney affect crucial physiologic functions that maintain fluid–electrolyte, acid–base, and volume–water homeostasis. Under normal conditions, the aging kidney is able to maintain homeostasis. Under stress, however, the adaptive response of the kidney to maintain homeostasis is impaired.

Sodium Conservation

The aged kidney conserves sodium less efficiently under conditions of sodium deprivation. When sodium restriction is imposed on healthy elderly subjects, it takes nearly twice as long for the aged kidney to decrease urinary sodium excretion compared with younger control subjects; the half-time to decreased urinary sodium excretion with an abrupt decrease in sodium intake to 10 mmol/day was 30.9 hours in subjects older than 60 years compared with 17.6 hours in subjects younger than 30 years of age (144) (Fig. 81-12). Decreased

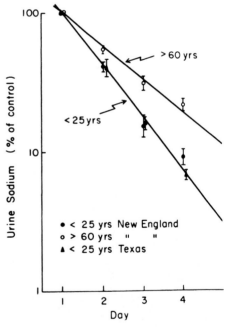

FIG. 81-12. Response of urinary sodium excretion to restriction of sodium intake in normal humans. The mean half-time ($t_{1/2}$) for eight subjects older than 60 years of age was −30.9 ± 2.8 hours, exceeding the mean half-time of −17.6 ± 0.7 hours for subjects younger than 25 years of age (P < 0.01). When the subjects younger than 25 years of age were separated according to geographic area, the mean half-time for the Texas group (>17.9 ± 0.7 hours) was similar to that of the New England group (>15.6 ±1.4 hours; P < 0.3). (Reprinted with permission from Epstein M, Hollenberg N. Age as a determinant of renal sodium conservation in normal man. *J Lab Clin Med* 1976;87:411.)

distal tubular reabsorption may be at fault, as demonstrated by clearance studies (145). Several factors may play a role in changing the age-related distal sodium conservation ability. It is possible that aging-induced renal interstitial scarring, decreased nephron number, and increased medullary flow may increase solute load per nephron, as found in patients with chronic renal failure.

Changes in levels of hormones regulating sodium excretion, such as renin, angiotensin, and aldosterone, as well as changes in the response to these hormones, also occur during the process of aging. Both circulating plasma renin and aldosterone concentrations have been found to decrease with aging in healthy elderly subjects. Basal plasma renin concentration or activity is decreased by 30% to 50% despite normal levels of renin substrate. Despite interventions to stimulate renin secretion, including assuming an upright position, a sodium intake of 10 mEq/day, furosemide administration, and air-jet stress, age-related differences in plasma renin activity become more pronounced (146–156) (Fig. 81-13). Studies in rats showed a decrease in juxtamedullary single-nephron renin content (152) and downregulation of renin mRNA abundance (Fig. 81-14) and renal ACE levels (157). One study also found a 56% decrease in type 1 angiotensin II receptor mRNA expression in aged rats (158).

Prehemorrhage and posthemorrhage plasma renin content was significantly decreased in older (15 months) versus younger (3 months) rats (157) (Fig. 81-14). Sodium-deprived aged rats showed a blunted rise in plasma renin activity with a delayed fall in urinary sodium excretion, despite a drop in mean arterial pressure (159). Measurements of plasma renin substrate concentrations in heathy, elderly subjects showed decreased conversion of inactive to active renin (155). Therefore, both decreased renin synthesis and impaired renin release may be responsible in part for reduced active renin content in the elderly. Similarly, plasma aldosterone decreases in parallel with aging. There is a 30% to 50% decrease in supine plasma aldosterone levels in elderly versus younger subjects. This becomes exaggerated with upright posture, sodium restriction, and furosemide administration (156,160–162) (Fig 81-13). This aldosterone deficiency is more likely related to a renin–angiotensin deficiency and not to an intrinsic adrenal defect because adrenocorticotropic hormone infusion in elderly subjects produces a normal aldosterone and cortisol response (156). The sluggish renal response to dietary sodium restriction seen in the elderly can be reproduced by ACE inhibitors and blockade of the renin–angiotensin–aldosterone system (163). Because aldosterone infusion results in marked improvement in sodium reabsorption in the elderly, tubular insensitivity seems less likely to be the cause of impaired sodium excretion, further supporting a deficiency in the renin–angiotensin–aldosterone mechanism (164). These data suggest that a renin–angiotensin or renin–aldosterone deficiency may be an important factor underlying the inability of the elderly to conserve sodium appropriately in the face of sodium deprivation.

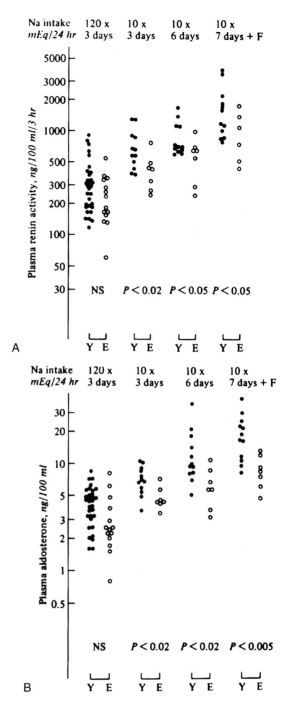

FIG. 81-13. Distribution of individual supine plasma renin **(A)** and aldosterone values **(B)** before and during progressive sodium depletion in young *(Y)* and elderly *(E)* healthy subjects. Values indicating statistical significance refer to differences between young and elderly subjects. Plasma renin activity values are those obtained at an incubation pH of 5.7. (Reprinted with permission from Weidmann P, De Chatel R, Schiffmann A, et al. Interrelations between age and plasma renin, aldosterone, and cortisol, urinary catecholamines, and the body sodium/volume state in normal man. *Klin Wochenschr* 1977;55:725.)

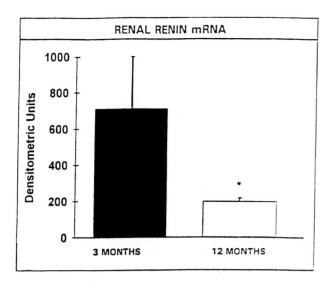

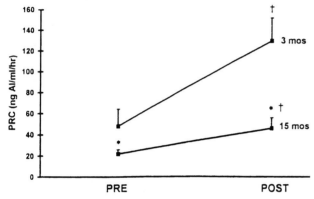

FIG. 81-14. Northern blot analysis of renin mRNA. Renal renin mRNA is significantly decreased in older (12 months) versus younger (3 months) rats. *P < 0.05. **Top:** Prehemorrhage *(Pre)* and posthemorrhage *(Post)* values for plasma renin content (PRC) revealed significantly lower levels in older rats, as well as a smaller increase after hemorrhage. *P < 0.05 versus young in same period; †P < 0.05 versus prehemorrhage. (Reprinted with permission from Jung FF, Kennefick TM, Ingelfinger JR, et al. Down-regulation of the intrarenal renin-angiotensin system in the aging rat. *J Am Soc Nephrol* 1995;5:1573.)

Sodium Excretion

The natriuretic ability of the aged kidney appears to be blunted in the face of Na loading or volume expansion (165–167). With a 2-L normal saline load, subjects older than 40 years of age excrete less Na compared with younger adults matched for size, sex, and race (53,168) (Fig. 81-15). Similarly, aged Sprague-Dawley rats with blood volume expansion excrete significantly less Na, especially when factored for body weight (167). Age also influences circadian variation in Na excretion in the elderly, with a greater percentage of the Na load being excreted at night (168). This may contribute to the nocturia observed in the elderly. Because Na excretion is affected by GFR, an age-associated decline in GFR may play a significant a role in limiting Na excretion.

Emerging studies, however, suggest that aging may affect changes in renal response to ANP, an important factor in the control of Na excretion. ANP is released from atrial myocytes in response to atrial stretch or volume loading. In the kidney, ANP acts through specific cell surface receptors on renal microvasculature and tubular epithelium to induce hyperfiltration, inhibit Na reabsorption, and suppress renin release. The ANP–cell surface receptor interaction results in activation of plasma membrane–associated guanylate cyclase to convert magnesium guanosine triphosphate to cGMP. cGMP then phosphorylates intracellular proteins, resulting in physiologic actions that include inhibition of luminal membrane Na channels. Stored as a 126–amino-acid prohormone (proANP), proteases in atrial tissue and serum are capable of cleaving proANP to the biologically active 28–amino-acid ANP [1-28]. ANP is rapidly degraded, but its serum half-life may be prolonged by selective blockade of degradative enzymes or clearance receptors (169). Elevated basal plasma ANP levels have been found in the healthy elderly to be three to five times those of the healthy young (166,170,171). With high salt intake, head-out body immersion in water, and saline loading, ANP secretion is stimulated to a greater extent in the elderly than in the young (166,170,172,173). With low salt intake, however, ANP levels are similar to those in the younger comparison group. Thus, ANP secretion in response to increased salt intake and volume loading appears to remain intact. Some have suggested that increased basal ANP levels may result from decreased metabolic clearance, increased half-life, and a larger volume of distribution in the elderly (174–177). It appears less likely that decreased GFR in the aged contributes significantly to high plasma ANP levels, given that patients with advanced chronic renal failure did not have significantly elevated ANP levels compared with normal (178). However, renal proximal tubule brush-border membrane, rich in degradative enzymes (endopeptidases), plays a major role in peptide degradation (169). Inhibitors of endopeptidases such as phosphoramidon, infused in rats with reduced renal mass, result in increased ANP levels that parallel increases in urinary cGMP (ANP second messenger) and urinary salt excretion (179). Renal neutral endopeptidase inhibition by candoxatril in 12 patients with New York Heart Association class II congestive heart failure significantly increased ANP and cGMP levels as well as urinary Na excretion without changing renal hemodynamics (180). Endopeptidase inhibition significantly decreases the metabolic clearance and prolongs the half-life of ANP in this population. The metabolic clearance of ANP in the elderly was decreased compared with the young at similar low ANP infusion rates (177,181). Perhaps with aging the number or quality of brush-border membrane degradative enzymes changes, resulting in decreased metabolic clearance. This possibility needs further investigation.

Several investigators have proposed that higher plasma ANP levels possibly represent a homeostatic adaptation to reduced sensitivity in the kidney (165,167,182). Although incremental increases in ANP infusion progressively increase

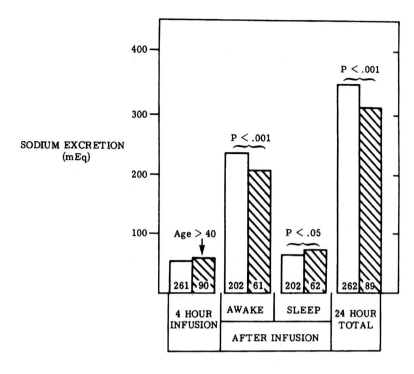

FIG. 81-15. Comparisons of urinary sodium excretion in younger *(clear bars)* and older *(hatched bars)* subjects after 2 L intravenous normal saline. Normal subjects older than 40 years of age excrete a sodium load slower than subjects younger than 40 years of age. Numbers at the base of the bars represent the number of subjects in each group. (Reprinted with permission from Luft FC, Grim CE, Fineberg NS, et al. Effects of volume expansion and contraction in normotensive whites, blacks, and subjects of different ages. *Circulation* 1979;59:643.)

urinary sodium excretion in the young, elderly subjects do not continue significantly to increase their sodium excretion beyond a physiologic ANP infusion of 2 ng/kg/minute (Fig. 81-16). Therefore, renal response to ANP appears to be blunted in the aged kidney. Other investigators have noted that baseline cGMP (ANP second messenger) levels show no change with age (166,173,177). However, with exogenous administration of low-dose ile[12]-ANP (101–126), cGMP increases significantly in plasma and urine of healthy elderly

subjects (177). Despite the increase in cGMP levels after ANP infusion, an increase in Na excretion is not seen (177). This suggests that the defect may be at the post-cGMP effector mechanism.

Because ANP can suppress the renin–angiotensin–aldosterone system and inhibit Na reabsorption, simultaneous measurements of plasma renin activity and aldosterone concentration during ANP infusion studies were done. These studies suggest that the natriuretic property of ANP differs

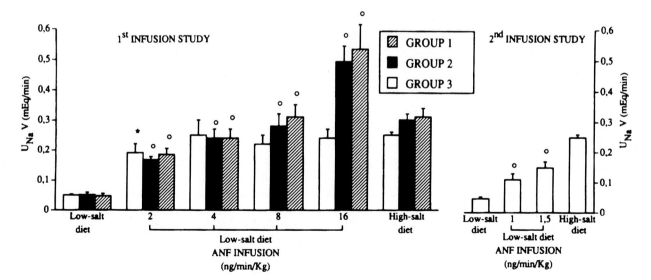

FIG. 81-16. Urinary sodium excretion for low-salt diet (during basal conditions and after atrial natriuretic factor infusion) and at high-salt diet conditions in young (group 1), middle-aged (group 2), and elderly subjects (group 3). The columns represent means and the bars standard errors of the mean. °P < 0.05 versus other steps and low-salt diet; *P < 0.01 versus low-salt diet. (Reprinted with permission from Leasco D, Ferrara N, Landino P, et al. Effects of age on the role of atrial natriuretic factor in renal adaptation to physiologic variations of dietary salt intake. *J Am Soc Nephrol* 1996;7:1045.)

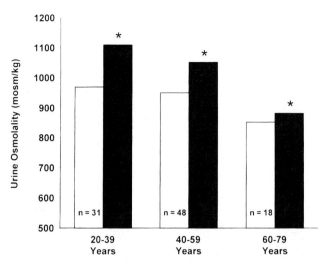

FIG. 81-17. The effect of age on urine osmolality in response to 12 hours of water deprivation. □, Pretreatment values; ■, posttreatment values. The number of subjects in each group is noted at the base of each bar. Urine osmolality decreases significantly with age after water deprivation (*P < 0.05). (Reprinted with permission from Rowe J, Shock N, DeFronzo R. The influence of age on the renal response to water deprivation in man. *Nephron* 1976;17:270.)

from its property of inhibiting Na reabsorption through suppression of the renin–angiotensin–aldosterone system. Each of these properties of ANP is influenced differently by age (165,166,177).

Renal Concentrating Capacity

Studies in the elderly have clearly demonstrated impaired renal concentrating ability compared with the young (43, 183–186) (Fig. 81-17). Appropriate maximal water conservation under hyperosmolar and water-deprived conditions depends on an intact osmoreceptor and volume receptor sensitivity for arginine vasopressin (AVP) release as well as an intact collecting tubule response to AVP in the face of maximal medullary tonicity. In the elderly, a combination of processes may be affected, leading to a defect in water conservation.

Arginine vasopressin release appears to be intact in the elderly in response to both osmotic stimulation and volume pressure stimulation, although the extent of the response depends on the type of stimulus. Osmoreceptor sensitivity to AVP release appears to be enhanced in the elderly. The hypothalamic–neurohypophyseal response to hypertonic saline in Long Evans rats indicates increased AVP release in response to osmotic stimuli (187,188). Similarly, osmoreceptor sensitivity is heightened in elderly subjects receiving a 3% saline infusion over 2 hours (189). Basal circulating AVP levels also are increased in the elderly (190–193) after 24 hours of water deprivation. Plasma AVP levels measured under conditions of water deprivation at 9 hours (194) and 14 hours (195) appear to be lower and only slightly higher,

respectively, than in the younger group. It may be that increased AVP response in the elderly depends on maximal osmoreceptor stimulation, as seen with prolonged water deprivation or hypertonic saline infusion. Some studies suggest that baroreceptor-mediated AVP release due to volume–pressure changes, such as an acute assumption of upright posture, decreases with age (196), as does the oropharyngeal inhibition of AVP release in response to drinking and cold liquids (192). However, plasma AVP levels increased significantly in 24 healthy elderly subjects 65 to 80 years of age who underwent a 60-degree head-up tilt stimulation compared with 24 younger subjects 20 to 34 years of age (197).

With AVP release reasonably intact, possibilities for an intrarenal defect in urinary concentrating ability have been investigated. Intrarenal resistance to AVP has been postulated as a possible cause for decreased urinary concentrating ability of the aged kidney. AVP infusion in healthy elderly subjects failed to correct the reduced concentrating capacity (198). Rowe and colleagues suggested a "washout" of medullary tonicity in the face of increased medullary blood flow in the aged kidney. In their study of 98 healthy, community-dwelling volunteers (20 to 79 years of age), a significant decrease in urine osmolality and an increase in solute excretion and osmolar clearance after 12 hours of overnight dehydration were found, independent of changes in creatinine clearance (187). This also may be explained by impaired solute transport in the ascending loop of Henle leading to inadequate medullary tonicity. In support of this possibility, water diuresis in elderly subjects indicates decreased sodium chloride transport in the ascending loop of Henle (145,199). However, data in aging rats are more suggestive of AVP resistance in the collecting tubules. Maximal urinary concentration despite 40 hours of dehydration and exogenous AVP was impaired in the aged rats. Although solute-free water formation was normal (CH_2O/GFR as a function of V/GFR), solute-free water reabsorption (TcH_2O/GFR as a function of Cosm/GFR) was impaired. Inner medullary solute content in both old and young rats was identical. Therefore, ascending limb solute transport appears to be intact, whereas collecting tubule water transport is diminished (200). An age-related decrease in cAMP generation in response to AVP also was found in inner medullary slices of both rats and mice (201,202). Maximum cAMP levels in older animals were lower compared with younger animals (201,202) (Fig. 81-18). In fact, older mice required a greater threshold dose of AVP to initiate a significant increase in cAMP (202). Downregulation of AVP receptors with a subsequent decreased cAMP response in the face of chronically elevated levels of AVP has been suggested (188); however, no change in receptor number or affinity for AVP was found (203). A postreceptor mechanism may play a role in this process. The abundance of stimulatory guanine nucleotide–binding protein (Gs) expression is decreased in aging kidneys (204). This may suggest a possible impairment in ATP-stimulated adenylate cyclase activity and cAMP levels. *In vitro* perfusion studies with cholera toxin and forskolin

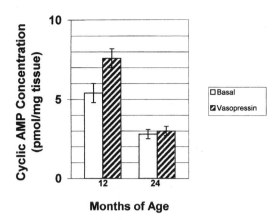

FIG. 81-18. Cyclic adenosine monophosphate (cAMP) concentration in renal papillary slices before and after stimulation by vasopressin (5 mU/mL). cAMP increased significantly postvasopressin in 12-month-old rats (N = 10; Δ2.81 ± 0.62 pmol/mg tissue) versus 24-month-old rats (N = 9; Δ + 0.25 ± 0.21 pmol/mg tissue); P < 0.05 in paired analysis. Each bar represents mean ± SEM. (Redrawn with permission from Beck N, Yu B. Effect of aging on urinary concentrating mechanisms and vasopressin-dependent cAMP in rats. *Am J Physiol* 1982;243:F121.)

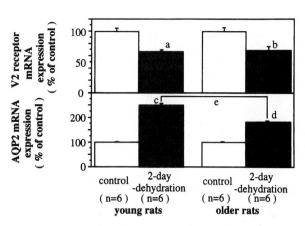

FIG. 81-19. Changes in expression of V2 receptor mRNA and aquaporin-2 (AQP-2) mRNA (Northern blot hybridization) after dehydration. The expression of mRNA after dehydration is presented as the mean percentage changes from control ± SE. [a]P < 0.005 versus young control group; [b]P < 0.05 versus older control group; [c]P < 0.01 versus young control group; [d]P < 0.001 versus older control group; [e]P < .01 between young and older rats after dehydration for 2 days. (Reprinted with permission from Terashima Y, Kondo K, Inaguki A, et al. Age associated decrease in response of rat aquaporin-2 gene expression to dehydration. *Life Sci* 1998;62:873.)

on freshly isolated cortical collecting tubules (CCT) of young (3 months), middle-aged (2 to 3 years), and old (4 to 5 years) rabbits showed that the ability of Gs to stimulate adenylate cyclase was severely compromised in collecting tubules from old animals. Infusion of cholera toxin, which induces adenosine diphosphate ribosylation of the Gs protein, thereby stimulating adenylate cyclase and generation of cAMP, resulted in only 32% stimulation in epithelia from old rabbit CCT compared with young control rabbits. Infusion of forskolin, a potent stimulator of adenylate cyclase at the level of the catalytic unit as well as of G protein interaction, yielded significantly lower adenylate cyclase stimulation (12% of young controls) in cultures from old rabbits. Gs proteins with the catalytic subunit of adenylate cyclase may be responsible for the age-associated decline in CCT response to AVP (205).

Arginine vasopressin regulates the collecting duct water channel aquaporin-2 (AQP-2), by downregulating V2 receptors on the basolateral membrane. Northern blot analysis of V2 receptor mRNA and AQP-2 mRNA in dehydrated young and old rats found similar degrees of downregulation of V2 receptor mRNA in both young and old rats. However, AQP-2 mRNA expression in old rats in response to dehydration was significantly less than in young rats (206) (Fig. 81-19). *In situ* hybridization of AQP-2 mRNA confirmed this finding (206). One study reported that there was decreased expression of AQP-2 and AQP-3 in the collecting ducts of 30-month-old female WAG/Rij rats compared with 10-month-old female counterparts, whereas papillary cAMP content measured by enzyme-linked immunosorbent assay in these normally hydrated animals was not significantly different between the two groups (207). Whether sex plays a role in these findings is not clear. Taken together, these results suggest that decreased expression of AQP-2 and AQP-3 in older rats is independent

of changes in circulating AVP and intracellular cAMP (207), and in part may explain the decrease in urine-concentrating ability seen with aging.

Renal Diluting Capacity

With aging, the ability to achieve minimal urinary dilution decreases (184,208–210). During water diuresis, subjects 77 to 88 years of age decreased their urine osmolality to 92 mosm/kg H_2O. This is significantly higher than the younger subjects (17 to 40 years of age), who were able to achieve a urine osmolality of 52 mosm/kg H_2O. Solute-free water clearance decreased from 16.2 to 5.9 mL/minute in old versus young subjects, respectively. Appropriate urinary dilution occurs if filtered fluid delivered distally undergoes appropriate solute extraction from the ascending loop of Henle with adequate AVP suppression in the face of water loading and hypoosmolality. GFR declines with age. Therefore, a decline in GFR with aging may be contributing to the decrease in the ability to excrete solute-free water. However, some investigators have found that despite correction for GFR, solute-free water clearance is decreased in older subjects (184,208). Whether adequate AVP suppression occurs with water loading or hypoosmolality or appropriate solute extraction occurs in the ascending Henle's loop remains to be investigated.

Acid–Base Balance

Although homeostatic maintenance of acid–base balance appears to be adequate in the elderly, acid loading demonstrates an impaired ability to excrete the acid load in the elderly. An age-related decline in renal mass and GFR has been

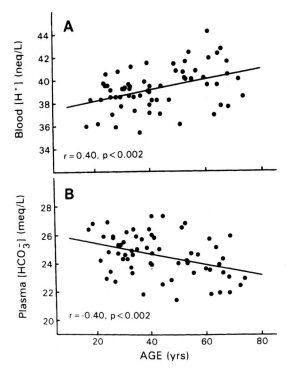

FIG. 81-20. Relation between $[H^+]_b$ and age **(A)** and between $[HCO_3^-]_p$ and age **(B)**, in normal adult humans (N = 64). Each data point represents the mean steady-state value in a subject eating a constant diet. Regression equations: $[H^+]_b = 0.045 \times$ age + 37.2; $[HCO_3^-]_p = -0.038 \times$ age + 26.0. (Reprinted with permission from Frassetto L, Morris RC Jr, Sebastian A. Effect of age on blood acid-base composition in adult humans: role of age-related renal functional decline. *Am J Physiol* 1996;271:F1112.)

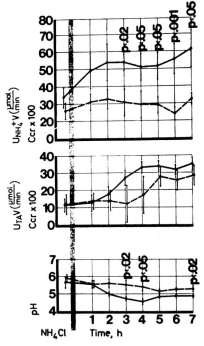

FIG. 81-21. Acid excretion over the entire study in young and elderly subjects. Ammonium ($U_{NH4}V$) and titratable acid ($U_{TA}V$) excretion corrected for GFR (Ccr × 100), and urinary pH were compared between young (group 1, *solid line*) and aged subjects (group 3, *dashed line*). Mean values (±SEM) along with P values of the differences between the two groups are shown. (Reprinted with permission from Agarwal BN, Cabebe FG. Renal acidification in elderly subjects. *Nephron* 1980;26:291.)

associated with this change (211). When endogenous acid production was held constant by a steady-state acid diet in a research setting with healthy subjects, a progressively worsening low-grade metabolic acidosis was observed with aging (212) (Fig. 81-20). The changes in GFR with age correlated significantly with decreases in blood pH and plasma HCO_3 (212). A decrease in plasma HCO_3 was accompanied by a reciprocal increase in plasma chloride concentration, similar to that found with early renal disease or renal tubular acidosis (212). Earlier studies by Adler et al. had shown decreased excretion of an oral ammonium load in elderly subjects between 72 and 93 years of age, with urinary ammonia accounting for less of the total acid excretion compared with younger subjects (211). When glutamine was given, the increases in ammonium excretion occurred as rapidly in old subjects as in young subjects, and with equal magnitude. Phosphate excretion increased and titratable acid accounted for a significantly greater percentage of total acid excretion. However, when acid excretion was factored for GFR, a decrease in renal tubular mass rather than a specific tubular defect was thought to be the etiology of decreased acid excretion. Agarwal and Cabebe, however, found that ammonium loading in older patients resulted in reduced ammonium excretion and ability to reach minimal pH even after correction for GFR, suggesting an intrinsic tubular defect (213) (Fig. 81-21). Whether this

defect is due to an anatomic or functional defect, such as impairment in the renin–angiotensin–aldosterone axis, which is frequently encountered in the aged, is not clear. Statistical significance was not reached for titratable acid. Studies in senescent rats fed equivalent amounts of NH_4Cl confirmed findings of a deficiency in the absolute amount of ammonium excreted after an acid load. This accounted for the more severe acidemia in the older rats (pH 7.40 to 7.09) compared with younger controls (pH 7.43 to 7.32) (214). Renal proximal tubular apical brush-border membrane vesicle transport studies revealed that sodium-hydrogen exchange activity (Na/H exchange), a major regulator of proximal tubular acidification, was similarly enhanced by the acid load in adult and aged rats (214). Phosphate transport was reduced to the same extent in both adult and aged rats. This suggests that impaired ammonium excretion also may mediate the age-related impairment in renal adaptation to metabolic acidosis even when compensating mechanisms appear to be intact (214).

Although a subtle degree of metabolic acidosis exists in the elderly (212), neither serum HCO_3 concentration nor pH values are found outside of the normal range. Bone demineralization and muscle wasting, complications of chronic metabolic acidosis, are common in the elderly. Underlying metabolic acidosis regulates mobilization of calcium and alkali from bone and inhibits renal calcium reabsorption, leading to calcium removal from the body. Increased protein intake increases endogenous acid production. Acidosis-induced enhanced muscle breakdown is mediated by activation of an ATP-dependent pathway involving ubiquitin and proteasome (215). Despite eubicarbonatemia, increased protein intake, often found in industrialized nations, in conjunction with aging and impaired acid excretion may be associated with a negative calcium balance, osteoporosis, and increased incidence of fractures as well as muscle wasting, as seen with aging (216). Studies in postmenopausal women have suggested improvement in nitrogen balance (217) and calcium balance (218) with potassium bicarbonate administration. Whether bicarbonate supplementation would be an important intervention in the elderly to prevent complications of chronic, subtle metabolic acidosis remains to be investigated.

MINERAL AND ELECTROLYTE BALANCE

Osmolar Disorders

Disorders of osmolality are common in the elderly (219–223). Subtle changes in both water and solute conservation and excretion in the elderly, added to underlying factors such as medications, infections, and emotional disability, can predispose the elderly to hyponatremia or hypernatremia.

Hyponatremia

Hyponatremia occurred in 11.3% of geriatric hospital inpatients over a 10-month period; the incidence has been found to be as high as 22.5% in a chronic disease facility (220,223). Enhanced osmotic AVP release along with impaired diluting ability predispose the elderly to a higher incidence of hyponatremia (224). Idiopathic syndrome of inappropriate antidiuretic hormone secretion has been reported in a subset of ambulatory geriatric clinic patients (225). Thiazide diuretics, implicated in 20% to 30% of hyponatremia cases in the elderly, further impair a preexisting renal diluting defect (220,221,223,226,227) (Fig. 81-22). A role for deficient prostaglandin synthesis in the elderly also has been suggested in the increased susceptibility to thiazide-induced hyponatremia, because water diuresis is impaired when prostaglandin synthesis is inhibited (226). Thiazide diuretics administered in combination with other medications, such as sulfonylurea compounds, chlorpropamide or tolbutamide, or

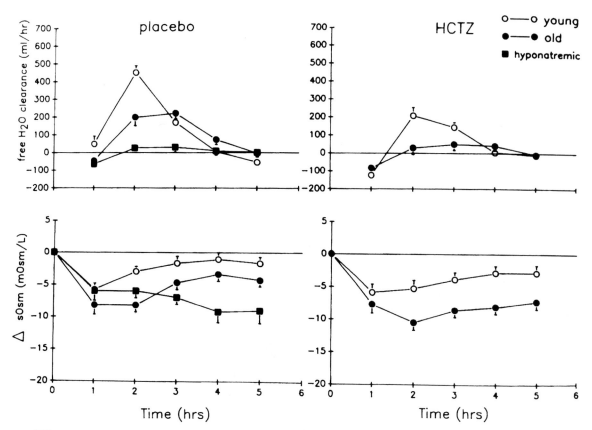

FIG. 81-22. Free water clearance (CH_2O) and change in serum osmolality ($\Delta sOsm$, mOsm/kg H_2O) after a water load with placebo versus hydrochlorothiazide (HCTZ) in young, old, and old with a prior history of thiazide-induced hyponatremia. CH_2O and decline in sOsm were significantly lower in the old than in the young [$P < 0.05$, analysis of variance (ANOVA)]. This difference was magnified after the use of HCTZ. Those with a history of hyponatremia had a lower CH_2O and decline in sOsm than did the healthy elderly ($P < 0.05$, ANOVA). (Reprinted with permission from Clark BA, Shannon RP, Rosa RM, et al. Increased susceptibility to thiazide-induced hyponatremia in the elderly. *J Am Soc Nephrol* 1994;5:1106.)

TABLE 81-2. *Mechanisms by which drugs can lead to impaired water metabolism*

Inhibit ADH release	Inhibit peripheral action of ADH	Potentiate ADH release	Potentiate peripheral action of ADH
Fluphenazine	Lithium	Nicotine	Tolbutamide
Haloperidol	Colchicine	Vincristine	Chlorpropamide
Promethazine	Vinblastine	Histamine	Nonsteroidal
Morphine (low doses)	Demeclocycline	Morphine (high doses)	antiinflammatory drugs
Alcohol	Glyburide	Epinephrine	
Carbamazepine	Methoxyflurane	Cyclophosphamide	
Norepinephrine	Acetohexamide	Angiotensin	
Cisplatinum	Propoxyphene	Bradykinin	
Clonidine	Loop diuretics		
Glucocorticoids			

ADH, antidiuretic hormone.

nonsteroidal antiinflammatory drugs (NSAIDs), which potentiate peripheral AVP action, can act in synergy to impair water excretion. Medications that stimulate the nonosmotic release of AVP or potentiate the renal tubular effects of AVP also act in synergy with an impaired diluting capacity and should be used with extreme caution in the elderly (Table 81-2).

An osmotic shift of water from the extracellular to intracellular space occurs with hyponatremia. This leads to a myriad of signs and symptoms, including apathy, disorientation, lethargy, muscle cramps, anorexia, nausea, agitation, depressed deep tendon reflexes, pseudobulbar palsy, and seizures (228). Recognition and appropriate institution of therapy are important to avoid severe neurologic sequelae, including central pontine myelinolysis.

Hypernatremia

Impaired renal concentrating and sodium conserving ability in the elderly also may increase their susceptibility to hypernatremia. Under normal physiologic conditions, thirst and fluid intake defend against hypernatremia and volume depletion. However, both of these defense mechanisms are impaired in the healthy elderly (192,229) (Fig. 81-23). Further impairment in fluid intake in geriatric patients with a depressed level of consciousness, immobility, or impaired ability to access free water can lead to lethal hypernatremic states with mortality rates ranging from 46% to 70% (219,222, 230,231). Acute increase of serum sodium above 160 mEq/L is associated with 75% mortality rate.

Because the elderly, with their impaired ability to conserve water or solute in combination with a decreased thirst and fluid intake, are prone to hypernatremia, use of medications that further inhibit the renal tubular action of AVP, such as lithium and demeclocycline, or medications that cloud the sensorium and decrease the thirst mechanism, such as sedatives and major tranquilizers, should be avoided. The use of osmotic diuretics, external feedings containing high levels of protein and glucose, and bowel cathartics should be monitored. Elderly patients with systemic illnesses, infections, dementia, fever, or neurologic disorders impairing AVP

release are at high risk for dehydration. Cellular dehydration can lead to severe neurologic sequelae, including obtundation, stupor, coma, seizures, and death. Therefore, cautious monitoring of elderly patients, especially debilitated elderly patients, receiving medications that affect tubular conservation of water or solute or affect the sensorium is warranted (Table 81-2).

Potassium Balance

With advancing age and loss of muscle mass, total body potassium (232) and total exchangeable potassium decrease. This is more pronounced in women than men. Plasma renin and aldosterone concentrations decrease with age (154,162). Because potassium excretion in the distal tubule is enhanced by the presence of aldosterone, relative hypoaldosteronism predisposes the elderly to hyperkalemia. Healthy elderly subjects, 65 to 85 years of age, had lower basal plasma aldosterone levels and a blunted aldosterone response to potassium infusion compared with younger subjects aged 20 to 35 years (233) (Fig. 81-24). Potassium loading studies in aging rats demonstrate a defect in both renal and extrarenal potassium adaptation. When an intravenous KCl infusion was administered to young and old rats on normal and high-potassium diets, the efficiency of potassium excretion was similar in both young and old rats on a normal diet (234). However, on the high-potassium diet, excretion of potassium was much less efficient in older rats than in the young rats (234). The rise in plasma potassium also was higher after KCl infusion in the aged rats on high-potassium intake compared with younger rats on high-potassium intake. KCl infusion after bilateral nephrectomy revealed that older rats on a high-potassium diet were unable to decrease the serum potassium to levels as low as compared with the younger rats (234). Na-K ATPase activity also was markedly reduced (by 38%) in the medulla of older rats compared with younger rats (234). These findings suggest that mechanisms protecting against acute hyperkalemia after potassium loading may not be affected by aging in rats, but renal and extrarenal potassium adaptation may be blunted (234). Whether these findings apply to human aging remains to be determined. No effect

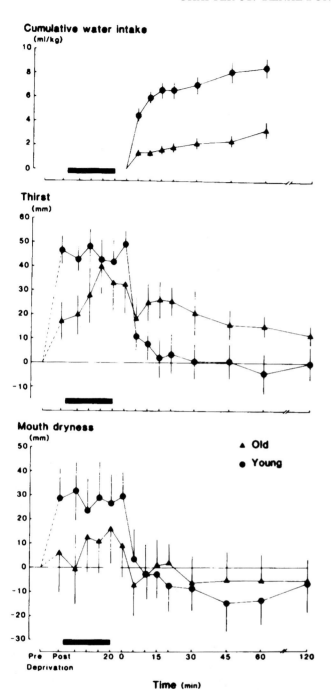

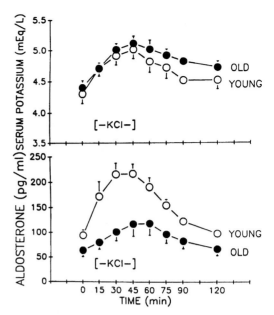

FIG. 81-24. Serum potassium and aldosterone levels before, during, and after infusion of potassium chloride (0.5 mEq/kg body weight over 45 minutes) in six healthy young and six healthy elderly men. Changes in serum potassium levels were similar, but elderly subjects had lower aldosterone responses (P < 0.005, analysis of variances). (Reprinted with permission from Mulkerrin E, Epstein FH, Clark BA. Aldosterone responses to hyperkalemia in healthy elderly humans. *J Am Soc Nephrol* 1995;6:1459.)

resulting in decreased activity of the Na-K-ATPase exchange pump in skeletal muscle (236).

A renal acidification defect in addition to decreased activity of the renin–angiotensin–aldosterone system may be an important cause of the increased incidence of type 4 renal tubular acidosis or the syndrome of hyporeninemic hypoaldosteronism in the elderly (237). In addition, given possible problems with chronic potassium adaptation with aging, medications that inhibit the renin–angiotensin–aldosterone system, such as ACE inhibitors, heparin, cyclosporine, tacrolimus, β-blockers, and NSAIDs, may increase the risk of hyperkalemia in the elderly. Similarly, sodium channel blocking agents such as trimethoprim and pentamidine and potassium-sparing diuretics such as amiloride, triamterene, and spironolactone can exacerbate underlying defects in potassium excretion in the elderly (238–240) (Fig. 81-25).

Calcium Balance

Renal tubular reabsorption of calcium appears to be unaffected with aging despite impaired calcium metabolism. Urinary calcium excretion and reabsorption remain appropriate under conditions of both increased and decreased dietary calcium in aged rats (241). In addition, there is no change in the absolute filtered load and proximal reabsorption of calcium per nephron between young and aged rats (242).

FIG. 81-23. Cumulative water intake and changes in thirst and mouth dryness in elderly (N = 7) and young (N = 7) groups. Symbols represent mean values, and bars SEM. Changes in thirst and mouth dryness were measured on a visual analog rating scale. The *hatched rectangle* represents the single-blind sham infusion. (Reprinted with permission from Phillips PA, Phil D, Rolls BJ, et al. Reduced thirst after water deprivation in healthy elderly men. *N Engl J Med* 1984;311:753.)

of aging was found for insulin-mediated potassium uptake in humans (235). However, a comparison of the exercise-induced elevation of plasma potassium in healthy young and elderly suggests that there may be an impaired response of the β-adrenergic–induced increase in adenylate cyclase activity,

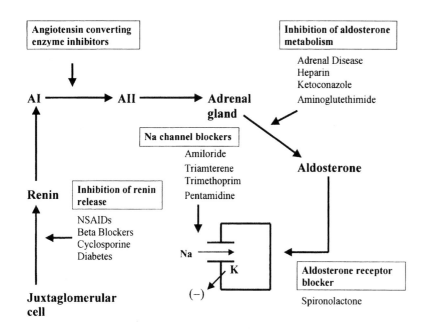

FIG. 81-25. Site of action of various pharmacologic agents and disease states that can further impair activity of the renin–angiotensin–aldosterone axis and exacerbate hyperkalemia in aged individuals with a progressive decline in renin and aldosterone levels. AI, angiotensin; AII, angiotensin II; NSAIDs, nonsteroidal anti-inflammatory drugs.

Aging is associated with decreased intestinal calcium reabsorption that seems to correlate with decreased 1-α-hydroxylase activity, decreased levels of 1,25-dihydroxycholecalciferol [1,25(OH)$_2$D$_3$], and increased basal parathyroid hormone (PTH) levels. The 1,25(OH)$_2$D$_3$-dependent calcium binding protein declines with age in parallel with the age-related decline in intestinal calcium absorption (241,243). Studies suggest that the rate of renal 1,25(OH)$_2$D$_3$ production with PTH infusion was initially lower in healthy elderly versus young; however, the final concentration of 1,25(OH)$_2$D$_3$ was not different in the two groups. Urinary cAMP and fractional phosphorus excretion also increased similarly in both groups, suggesting that the renal response to PTH infusion with aging is intact (244). These same investigators, however, found that calcium regulation of PTH release may be altered with aging when they studied the effect of calcium gluconate infusion and sodium ethylenediaminetetraacetic acid (NaEDTA) infusion in relation to PTH response. Their observations led them to conclude that the age-related increase in the serum concentration of PTH reflects an increase in both the set point for calcium and in the number of parathyroid cells. Whether the cell surface G-protein–coupled calcium sensing receptor, which may be responsible for the altered set point for PTH release seen in both primary and secondary hyperparathyroidism of uremia, plays a role in the increased set point for PTH release seen with aging awaits further investigation (245).

Phosphate Balance

Metabolic balance and clearance studies in humans and rats revealed an age-related decrement in renal tubular reabsorption of phosphate (246–254). This impairment in renal tubular phosphate occurs in addition to an age-related decrement in intestinal phosphate absorption (246). Furthermore, renal tubular adaptation to a low-phosphate diet also is impaired in aged rats (246,247,251,253). In spite of increased levels of serum PTH activity (255,256), the impairment in renal phosphate transport is independent of endogenous PTH activity because parathyroidectomy in aged rats results in a significant improvement, but not normalization of renal tubular reabsorption of phosphate (247,250–252).

A similar age-related impairment in phosphate transport also has been demonstrated in primary cultures of renal tubule cells from young and adult rats (257). In agreement with the *in vivo* studies (251), the decreases in phosphate transport are mediated by a decrease in the Vmax of sodium gradient–dependent phosphate transport (NaPi cotransport). Furthermore, adaptation to a low phosphate concentration in the culture medium also is significantly impaired in renal tubular cells cultured from old compared with young adult rats.

A study in aged rats indicates that the decrease in proximal tubular NaPi cotransport was associated with decreases in type II NaPi cotransporter (NaPi-2) protein and mRNA levels (258). In fact, immunohistochemistry revealed a marked decrease in the expression of NaPi-2 protein at the level of the apical brush-border membrane (258).

An additional factor that may play a role in the decrease in Na/Pi cotransport is the age-related increase in membrane cholesterol content (253,259–262). In fact, in brush-border membrane isolated from young adult rats, *in vitro* enrichment with cholesterol to levels similar to those measured in aged rats simulated the age-related impairment in the Vmax of NaPi cotransport (263). In opossum kidney cells with renal proximal tubular cell characteristics, direct alterations in cell cholesterol content per se were shown to modulate NaPi cotransport activity by causing alterations in the expression of the apical membrane NaPi-2 cotransport protein (264). This suggests that the age-related increase in membrane cholesterol also could play an important role in the age-related decrease in NaPi cotransport.

The role of impaired $1,25(OH)_2D_3$ metabolism in the age-related impairment in renal and intestinal phosphate transport also deserves to be determined because in vitamin D–deficient animals, administration of $1,25(OH)_2D_3$ results in significant improvements in renal (265–267) and intestinal (265) phosphate transport. The stimulatory effects of $1,25(OH)_2D_3$ on phosphate transport also are paralleled by significant alterations in brush-border membrane lipid composition and fluidity (268,269). It is therefore quite possible that similar lipid-modulating effects of $1,25(OH)_2D_3$ in the elderly also may result in significant improvements in renal and intestinal phosphate (and calcium) transport.

CLINICAL RENAL DISEASES IN THE ELDERLY

Acute Renal Failure

The elderly may be more susceptible to acute renal failure (ARF) because of the underlying compromise of renal function with aging. The incidence of ARF was found to be 3.5 times higher in patients older than 70 years than in those younger than 70 years of age in 437 prospective patients with ARF studied over a 9-year period in Spain (270). Increased prevalence of systemic diseases such as atherosclerosis, hypertension, diabetes, heart failure, and malignancy in a growing elderly population requiring various medical and surgical interventions can further exacerbate common causes of ARF including prerenal or volume depletion, sepsis, acute interstitial nephritis, nephrotoxin-induced glomerular and tubular dysfunction, and urinary tract obstruction. Specifically, cholesterol embolization, whether spontaneous or secondary to invasive procedures that manipulate the arterial vasculature, is more common in the elderly with generalized atherosclerosis. Less common but not to be overlooked, acute vasculitis or rapidly progressive glomerulonephritis (RPGN) may lead to significant morbidity and ESRD in the elderly.

Volume loss from vomiting, diarrhea, overzealous diuretic use, or bleeding, or decreased renal perfusion from drug- or sepsis-induced vasodilatation or low cardiac output frequently leads to prerenal azotemia in the elderly. In two prospective studies on the prevalence of renal failure, a prerenal etiology was found in over 50% of elderly patients (270,271). Underlying impaired ability to concentrate urine, regulate thirst, and conserve sodium in the aged may contribute to the high prevalence. In addition, age-related decreases in baseline renal blood flow and GFR and impairments in autoregulation of renal blood flow and renal functional reserve may render the kidney more susceptible to prerenal failure. Hemodynamic alterations with the use of prostaglandin inhibitors (NSAIDs) or ACE inhibitors, commonly used for the treatment of rheumatologic and cardiovascular disorders in the elderly, can further compromise renal vasoregulatory mechanisms. With appropriate intervention, including adequate and careful volume replacement and discontinuation of exacerbating medications, improvement of

cardiac output and renal recovery is expected. Sixty percent of prerenal elderly azotemic patients recovered renal function in one study (271).

Complications of major surgery account for approximately 30% of cases of ARF. Hypotension during or after surgery, postoperative fluid loss due to gastrointestinal fistulous drainage, arrhythmia, and myocardial infarction are common postoperative complications in the elderly that may result in ARF.

Vasodilation and hypotension from infection and sepsis with subsequent ARF often complicate the hospital course in the elderly. Infection, especially Gram-negative septicemia, accounts for 30% of cases of ARF in the elderly. Gram-negative infections frequently are associated with endotoxin-induced renovascular vasoconstriction, which in susceptible people can result in acute tubular necrosis. Frequently, these patients have multiorgan dysfunction or perioperative sepsis with an increased catabolic rate, which carries a poor prognosis in the elderly (272–274). Hemodynamic instability along with the need for complicated nephrotoxic antibiotic regimens such as aminoglycosides or amphotericin can prolong renal dysfunction. Antibiotic dosing needs to be carefully monitored in the elderly. GFR estimation by serum creatinine alone or by formulas using serum creatinine may be unreliable because bulk muscle mass decreases with aging. Further renal tubular and biochemical alterations with aging may enhance the toxic effects of antibiotics such as aminoglycosides on renal tubules. Age is a well known risk factor for aminoglycoside-induced nephrotoxicity (275).

Similarly, various common infections such as those caused by staphylococci, streptococci, legionellae, cytomegalovirus, and human immunodeficiency virus, as well as common antibiotics such as β-lactams and sulfonamides, and a myriad of other medications may cause interstitial inflammation and interstitial nephritis (276). Tubulointerstitial inflammation with activated macrophages releases degradative enzymes and may result in the loss of intact basement membranes, which hampers regeneration of the tubular segment. The fall in GFR may result from a loss of functioning nephrons and failure of the remaining nephrons to compensate with hyperfiltration (276).

Medications such as NSAIDs and ACE inhibitors not only compromise renal vasoregulating mechanisms that maintain GFR in the elderly but may cause interstitial inflammation and acute interstitial nephritis. With NSAIDs, presentation can be typical with pyuria and worsening ARF, or atypical with nephrotic-range proteinuria. Renal biopsy has shown both a minimal change lesion and membranous lesions with NSAIDs (277), especially propionic acid derivatives, and membranous lesions with the ACE inhibitor captopril.

Acute and prolonged vasoconstriction from radiocontrast infusion can significantly impair renal function in the elderly (278). With radiocontrast-induced renal failure, the initial increased osmotic load delivered to the macula densa also may trigger tubuloglomerular feedback, inducing renin release and reduction in GFR (279).

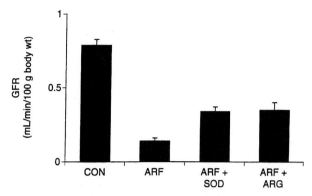

FIG. 81-26. The change in glomerular filtration rate (GFR) in aged (18-month-old) rats measured under basal conditions (CON), 1 day after acute renal failure (ARF), with superoxide dismutase infusion 1 day after ARF (ARF + SOD), and ARF aged rats pretreated with L-arginine (ARF + ARG). (Redrawn with permission from Sabbatini M, Sansone G, Uccello F, et al. Functional versus structural changes in the pathophysiology of acute ischemic renal failure in aging rats. *Kidney Int* 1994;45:1355.)

Experimental studies in aging rats indicate that the aging kidney has a greater propensity for ischemic and toxic ARF (280–284). Renal artery occlusion in young and aged rats produced a greater decline in the renal function in the older rats, which also had slower recovery (285,286). Glomerulosclerosis may not be the primary factor leading to ischemic renal failure in aging rats. In fact, when histologic variations between young and old rats were minimized by a low-protein diet, renal artery clamping still led to a significant decrease in GFR and RPF and an increase in RVR in older versus younger rats (285) (Fig. 81-26). Studies using blood oxygenation level–dependent magnetic resonance imaging in nine elderly female volunteers between 59 and 79 years of age showed a relative inability to improve medullary oxygenation with water diuresis compared with younger subjects, thus suggesting a possible predisposition to hypoxic renal injury in older patients (287). Oxygen free radicals can be generated during hemodynamically mediated ischemic ARF (288). When exogenous superoxide dismutase, a free radical scavenger, was infused into ischemic aged rats, renal hemodynamics significantly improved (285) (Fig. 81-26). Some have suggested that ischemic aged rats also may have impaired nitric oxide production or reduced intrarenal nitric oxide levels, which may predispose to renal failure (285). Nitric oxide is released tonically by vascular endothelium (289) to induce active vasodilatation and oppose vasoconstriction in order to maintain blood pressure (91). Basal tonically produced nitric oxide appears to play a pronounced role in maintenance of renal perfusion in aging (91,290). Nitric oxide production appears to be reduced with aging in isolated conduit arteries (291,292). Studies in aging rats have found a 40% decrease in serum levels of the NOS substrate L-arginine (293). Similar findings have been noted in aging humans (294). The maximum percent change in plasma cGMP, a marker for nitric oxide production, decreased with aging normotensive Japanese subjects given L-arginine

infusion (295). Older healthy subjects, despite a significant decrease in blood pressure while on a low-sodium diet, showed an age-related decline in urinary nitrate, nitrite, and cGMP, reflecting an age-dependent reduction in clearance (296). It may be that renal endothelial nitric oxide production is maximized in the normal elderly to maintain stable renal function. This appears to be consistent with a blunted vasodilatory response seen in the elderly (25). Measurements of nitric oxide production in the face of renal ischemia still need to be done in human subjects. When older rats were pretreated with L-arginine in their feed 7 days before renal artery occlusion, there was marked improvement in GFR (Fig. 81-26) and RPF, and a decrease in RVR. L-NAME, an NOS inhibitor, given to older L-arginine–fed rats abolished the renal hemodynamic response seen with L-arginine and superoxide dismutase (285). It is interesting to speculate whether a normal or high-protein diet would have altered these responses, given that rats fed a high-protein diet show an age-related decline in nitric oxide excretion as measured by urinary nitrite and nitrate excretion, whereas protein-restricted aged rats maintain urinary nitrite and nitrate excretion rates comparable with those of controls (92) (Fig. 81-27). L-Arginine supplementation in drinking water of aged animals appears to limit structural changes in the aging glomerular basement membrane (93,94). It remains to be seen whether nitric oxide plays a role in the beneficial effects of a low-protein diet on age-related glomerulosclerosis.

Alterations in metabolism and biochemistry of aging tubular cells also may play a role in mediating age-related enhancement of ischemic renal injury (284). When PAH and tetraethylammonium uptake was assessed in renal cortical slices after periods of *in vitro* anoxia, uptake was impaired to a greater extent in older compared with younger rats (284).

Atheroembolic renal disease may be a complication of intraarterial cannulation, especially in the elderly with

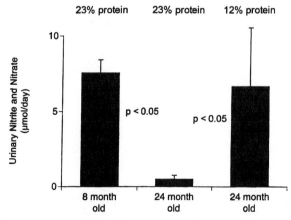

FIG. 81-27. Urinary excretion of nitrite and nitrate in control (8-month-old) rats, aged (24-month-old) rats fed a 23% protein diet, and aged rats fed a 12% protein diet. (Redrawn with permission from Sabbatini M, Sansone G, Uccello F, et al. Functional versus structural changes in the pathophysiology of acute ischemic renal failure in aging rats. *Kidney Int* 1994;45:1355.)

generalized atherosclerosis. Spontaneous cholesterol embolization also may occur (297), although it is seen more commonly after manipulation of the arterial vasculature for radiographic or surgical interventions such as carotid, coronary, renal, and abdominal angiography, aortic surgery, and percutaneous transluminal angioplasty (PTA) of coronary or renal arteries. Anticoagulants or fibrinolytic treatment in patients with diffuse atherosclerosis also can trigger cholesterol emboli (298). Renal failure can be irreversible and progressive, and may or may not be associated with other systemic findings of cholesterol embolization, such as purpura, livido reticularis of the abdominal and lumbar wall or lower extremities, Hollenhorst plaques with retinal ischemia, gastrointestinal bleeding, pancreatitis, myocardial infarction, cerebral infarction, and distal ischemic necrosis of the toes (299). Laboratory evidence for cholesterol embolization, including eosinophilia, eosinophiluria, and low complement levels, frequently is absent. Unfortunately, no specific therapy is available for reversal of this disease entity; instead, the clinician must carefully weigh the benefits and risks of angiographic procedures in elderly patients with widespread atherosclerotic disease and avoid excessive anticoagulation in these patients.

Symptomatic obstructive uropathy in the face of progressively rising blood urea nitrogen and creatinine can be a common presentation in elderly men with prostatic hypertrophy (300). Ureteric obstruction in women commonly arises from pelvic tumors of the uterus or cervix. Other retroperitoneal or pelvic neoplasm such as lymphoma, bladder carcinoma, and rectal tumors also can present as ARF in the geriatric population. However, typical symptoms of urinary tract obstruction, such as urinary frequency and difficulty with stopping and starting micturition, may not always be apparent in the elderly. Prolonged presence of obstruction may present with irreversible renal function. Careful review of medications such as anticholinergic agents and studies such as postvoid residual and renal ultrasonography may be necessary, followed by prompt urologic intervention. Infected residual urine may potentiate impairments in tubular function, blood flow, and GFR caused by obstruction.

Although the elderly may be at higher risk for development of ARF (270) and renal recovery may take longer (301), age per se is not an important determinant of survival in patients with ARF (271,302) and should not be used as a discriminating factor in therapeutic decisions concerning ARF (272,303). Most elderly patients respond well to treatment of ARF with dialysis. Therefore, prompt management with dialysis support as necessary to alleviate uremic symptoms and prevent uremic complications such as infection, congestive heart failure, myocardial infarction, and bleeding is recommended in elderly patients with ARF.

Renal Vascular Disorders

Atherosclerotic renovascular disease is an important cause of hypertension and is the cause of progressive ischemic renal failure and ESRD in up to 15% of patients with ESRD (304,305). Atheromatous involvement of the renal vasculature may present as (a) renal artery stenosis, (b) complex intrarenal lesions with multiple stenoses of intrarenal vasculature, and (c) cholesterol embolism. New onset of hypertension or progressive azotemia in the elderly, especially in the presence of other underlying risk factors for generalized atherosclerosis, indicates the need to consider atherosclerotic renal disease in this population (306,307). The natural history of atheromatous renal disease is progressive occlusion of the major renal arteries, especially when luminal narrowing is greater than 75% by angiography (308,309). Angiographic progression of renal artery stenosis was present in nearly 50% of 237 patients followed by Rimmer and colleagues (310). Mean GFR declined by 4 mL/minute in 51 patients with bilateral atherosclerotic renovascular disease followed for a median period of 52 months (311). Varying degrees of stenosis may be present in one or more renal arteries. Azotemic patients with a high-grade renal artery stenosis in a single kidney or unilateral renal artery occlusion and contralateral stenosis are at highest risk for progressive renal failure (309,312). Bilateral renal artery stenosis was associated with a crude mortality rate of 45% at 60 months in one study (311).

Smoking has emerged as an independent risk factor in the progression of macrovascular and microvascular renal disease in the elderly. Thirty smokers older than 55 years of age without other risk factors for vascular disease had significant decreases in RPF measured by radionuclide study and increased endothelin-1 (ET-1) concentrations compared with 24 age- and sex-matched nonsmokers (313). Smoking has been reported as a predictor of renal artery stenosis (314) as well as increasing the risk for development of ESRD (315). In a multivariate, best-fit model adjusted for sex, race, weight, age, and baseline serum creatinine of nondiabetic elderly patients older than 65 years of age in the Cardiovascular Health Study Cohort, the number of cigarettes smoked per day was independently associated with an increase in serum creatinine (316). Both norepinephrine and epinephrine are released as a result of smoking (317). In addition, smoking interferes with prostacyclin and thromboxane A_2 metabolism in the endothelium (318–321) with the vascular response to acetylcholine (322), nitric oxide, and ET-1 (323,324). ET-1 levels are increased in active smokers (325). A potent vasoconstrictor with mitogenic and atherogenic activity on vascular smooth muscle, ET-1 may be important in mediating the renal arteriolar thickening seen in pathologic studies (326–328).

Various methods have been used to help in the diagnosis of significant atherosclerotic renovascular disease. An increase in serum creatinine with the addition of an ACE inhibitor may provide a clinical clue to the presence of bilateral atherosclerotic renovascular disease or unilateral atherosclerotic stenoses in a single functional kidney (329). The decrease in GFR results from inhibition of the autoregulatory vasoconstrictive action of angiotensin II on the efferent arteriole, which maintains glomerular filtration in light of decreased glomerular perfusion (330). Renal scintigraphy using ^{99m}Tc-DTPA or ^{99m}Tc-mercaptoacetyltriglycine (^{99m}Tc-MAG3) before and after administration of an ACE inhibitor can be useful in solidifying clinical suspicion for a significant functional unilateral renal artery stenosis (331,332) Duplex ultrasound scanning of the renal arteries in some centers may provide noninvasive, highly sensitive and specific visualization of stenosis in the main renal arteries as well as blood flow velocity data to determine the significance of the stenosis (333). Alternatively, magnetic resonance angiography is used in some centers to visualize the renal arteries noninvasively. Carbon dioxide angiography also often is used in the presence of decreased GFR. Investigation with contrast renal angiography, however, remains the gold standard because the complete renal vasculature can be visualized, including the smaller intrarenal branches. Atheromatous narrowing of the distal branches of the renal arteries and microvasculature also may cause hypertension and ischemic renal failure (334).

Arterial cannulation and contrast injection of diffuse atherosclerotic vessels can lead to cholesterol embolization or contrast-induced nephropathy. An acute reversible rise in serum creatinine within 1 to 4 days after contrast administration can be attributed to the contrast dye. Irreversible and often progressive renal failure 1 to 4 weeks after arterial contrast injection, however, may be secondary to renal cholesterol embolization with or without systemic manifestations. Cholesterol crystals lodge in arteries with diameters of 100 to 200 μm or smaller, including glomerular tufts (335). Histologically, clear, biconvex clefts with surrounding inflammatory reaction can be seen because the lipid material is dissolved by tissue fixation (336). Blood pressure control, supportive management, and avoidance of further nephrotoxic insults are recommended in the face of cholesterol embolization or intrarenal atheromatous disease.

When technically possible, PTA or surgical revascularization should be considered to preserve renal function and improve blood pressure control in patients with significant atherosclerotic renal artery disease. Occasionally, the presence of collateral circulation may protect the renal parenchyma from ischemic injury despite progressive occlusive disease (337,338). Several cases have suggested reversibility of renal failure with angioplasty or surgical revascularization of renal artery stenosis (338–342). However, a serum creatinine of 3 mg/dL or more predicted poor outcome after technically successful PTA, with two-thirds of the patients in this group showing either no improvement in blood pressure, requiring dialysis within months of the procedure, or dying (343). These patients were noted to have a higher incidence of bilateral renal artery occlusion or high-grade stenosis of a solitary functioning kidney (343). Lesions amenable to angioplasty more commonly are unilateral, nonostial, and technically feasible to approach. Angioplasty may need to be repeated in at least 20% of cases with recurrence (307). Some investigators are considering intravascular stent placement (344). However, a serum creatinine of 2 mg/dL or more may be a poor prognostic indicator of poststent revascularization (345). Revascularization is recommended more commonly for ostial, bilateral, or totally occluding lesions (307).

Acute Glomerulonephritis

Acute glomerulonephritis in the elderly results most commonly from RPGN. Severe crescentic involvement, usually affecting over 50% of the glomeruli, is seen histologically. Clinically, a rapid decline in renal function associated with an active nephritic sediment (hematuria, pyuria, red blood cell casts, moderate to severe proteinuria) is seen. Pathogenesis is thought to be immune mediated, although clear-cut evidence for immunologic injury is absent in many cases. Immunohistologic presentations in the kidney are of three major types: type 1, presence of antiglomerular basement membrane antibody; type 2, with granular immune deposits; and type 3, with no immune deposits (346), although circulating antineutrophil cytoplasmic antibodies (ANCA) may be present. Typically, the type 2 and 3 histologic patterns are found more commonly in elderly with RPGN (347,348). Of 19 patients with crescentic glomerulonephritis in a biopsy series of 115 elderly patients, 9 patients had evidence for granular IgG deposition on immunofluorescence, whereas 6 patients had no immune deposits, and 3 patients had evidence for antiglomerular basement membrane disease (349). The pathologic findings were not described in one patient (349). Similarly, another study noted eight of ten elderly patients with RPGN had ANCA-positive sera, although no immune deposits were found (350). Pauciimmune crescentic glomerulonephritis was the diagnosis in 79 of 259 biopsies (31.2%) for ARF in adults aged 60 years or older (351).

In one series of 40 and another series of 60 patients with crescentic glomerulonephritis, the average or median age was older than 60 years (348,352). In general, the prognosis for elderly patients with RPGN is poor despite treatment successes in small, uncontrolled series (347,352,353). The risk–benefit ratio for treatment with pulse steroids, cyclophosphamide, or plasmapheresis for RPGN in the elderly must be individualized given the side effect profile of available treatment options.

Diffuse proliferative poststreptococcal acute glomerulonephritis in the elderly occurs in association with streptococcal infections of the throat and skin (354–357) and usually carries a favorable prognosis. In patients older than 55 years of age, an incidence of poststreptococcal glomerulonephritis as high as 22.6% (7 of 31 patients) has been reported (356,358).

Nephrotic Syndrome

The presentation of marked proteinuria, edema, and hypertension frequently leads to assessment by renal biopsy in the elderly. Thirty percent of patients in the Medical Research Council Glomerulonephritis Registry from 1978 to 1990 underwent biopsy for nephrotic syndrome (359). Membranous glomerulopathy (36.6%) was the most common histologic finding, followed by minimal change disease (11%) and renal

TABLE 81-3. *Histologic lesions in 489 elderly patients with primary nephrotic syndrome*

Authors	Minimal change	Membranous glomerulo-nephritis	Mesangial proliferative glomerulonephritis	Membrano-proliferative glomerulonephritis	Glomerulo-sclerosis	Chronic glomerulonephritis
Fawcett et al., 1971	6	5	—	4	16	5
Huriet et al., 1975	4	2	—	6	—	—
Moorthy and Zimmerman, 1980	9	15	7	2	1	—
Ishimuto et al., 1981	1	6	—	2	7	—
Lustig et al., 1982	2	16	—	2	3	—
Zech et al., 1982	19	31	2	4	—	3
Kingswood et al., 1984	2	16	11	3	—	—
Murphy et al., 1987	2	2	—	2	—	—
Sato et al., 1987	7	30	12	7	1	—
Johnston et al., 1992	35	116	18	—	5	—
Ozono et al., 1994	6	26	—	8	—	—
Total	93 (19%)	265 (54%)	50 (10%)	40 (8%)	33 (7%)	8 (2%)

amyloidosis (10.7%). Other reviews from the United States, France, Israel, England, and Japan corroborate these data (349,360–369). Cumulative data are shown in Table 81-3. Of 489 elderly patients with primary nephrotic syndrome, 54% were noted to have membranous glomerulonephritis, 19% with minimal change, 10% with mesangial proliferative, and 8% with membranoproliferative glomerulonephritis (347,357–367).

Glomerulosclerosis was evident in 7% of renal biopsies from the elderly. Glomerulosclerosis seen in the elderly resembles the focal segmental glomerulosclerosis seen more commonly in younger age groups. Juxtamedullary glomeruli frequently are affected and show positive immunofluorescence for IgM and C3. This lesion often is seen as an end result of other glomerulopathies and secondary advanced systemic diseases such as hypertension and diabetes (370), where hyperfiltration of functioning glomeruli may hasten the process of glomerulosclerosis (61,371). Juxtamedullary glomeruli may be more affected, given the significantly higher filtration fraction compared with superficial cortical nephrons. Glomerular ischemia from renovascular disease may lead to adaptive glomerular enlargement and segmental sclerosing lesions with nephrotic proteinuria in the elderly (372). Hyperlipidemia also may play an important role in glomerulosclerosis, as seen in both experimental animal models and patients.

Normal, healthy aging rats have shown a histologic appearance similar to that seen in human glomerulosclerosis, with IgM and C3 deposition and proteinuria (373–379). As a result, although the aging rat may represent an acceptable model for the study of various hemodynamic, metabolic, and immunologic factors mediating age-related glomerulosclerosis, studies using rats to evaluate the "normal aging" process should exclude animals with renal aging complicated by glomerulosclerosis.

The histopathologic pattern of nephrotic syndrome is unpredictable based only on clinical data. Given the greater number of aged patients being referred for renal replacement therapy, the number of renal biopsies performed in the elderly with proteinuria has been increased in the hope of early diagnosis and possible intervention. A retrospective review of idiopathic membranous nephropathy in the elderly revealed no evidence of improved outcome with prednisone therapy in 33 of 74 patients who received treatment. The rate of decline in renal function was not different compared with a younger group, although the incidence of chronic renal failure was much worse. This may have been secondary to a decreased renal functional reserve in the elderly (380). Others have reported partial or complete remission of nephrotic syndrome and protection from renal failure in patients with idiopathic membranous nephropathy treated with prednisone and cytotoxic agents (381). Therefore, the use of steroid and cytotoxic treatment needs to be considered cautiously and individualized in elderly patients with idiopathic membranous nephropathy. The outcome of treatment of proliferative glomerulonephritis was highly variable. However, because up to 19% of the elderly present with minimal change disease, which has a more favorable response and remission rate with corticosteroids, a complete workup, including renal biopsy, ought to be done in the elderly with nephrotic syndrome.

Nephrotic syndrome may coexist with or precede a malignancy (382). From 7% to 20% of patients with nephrotic syndrome may have an associated malignancy (369,383). The association between membranous lesions and malignancy is presumed to be mediated by immune complexes composed in part of tumor-associated antigens (383). Solid tumors of the lung, colon, rectum, kidney, breast, and stomach have been associated most commonly with membranous glomerulopathy. Therefore a thorough history, physical examination, and basic screening for an underlying malignancy should be done in elderly patients presenting with nephrotic syndrome.

Chronic Renal Failure

Progression of age-dependent medical diseases often leads to the chronic renal failure seen late in life. Long-standing diabetes, hypertension, chronic glomerulonephritis, ischemic atherosclerotic renovascular disease, and obstructive nephropathy are common diagnoses in chronic renal failure in the elderly. Clinical progression of chronic renal failure in the elderly frequently manifests as a decompensated preexisting medical illness such as congestive heart failure, gastrointestinal bleed, hypertension, or dementia rather than frank symptoms of uremia per se. Evidence for progression may not always be evident by laboratory testing because gradual loss of muscle mass in the elderly uremic patient may compensate for a lower creatinine clearance rate. Thus, actual renal reserve usually is lower than estimated by serum creatinine.

Advanced renal failure with no identifiable reversible causes, such as obstruction or renal artery stenosis, necessitates dialysis support before disabling symptoms of uremia and organ dysfunction become irreversible. Age itself should not be the sole criterion for exclusion from dialysis. In the absence of major extrarenal organ dysfunction, the elderly adjust fairly well to dialysis. Increasing numbers of elderly patients are being accepted for renal replacement therapy, with 55% of patients with ESRD older than 60 years of age (384–386). Longevity of older patients on dialysis is not markedly reduced, although not as favorable as in younger patients. Elderly patients with significant cardiovascular disease often do well with continuous ambulatory peritoneal dialysis (CAPD) (387–391). No major difference has been found in the incidence of peritonitis, type of infectious organism, or likelihood of technique failure between elderly and younger patients on CAPD (385,392). In fact, elderly patients may have less need for catheter replacement than younger patients on CAPD (385,392).

Neither mode of dialysis therapy, hemodialysis or peritoneal dialysis, is demonstrated to be clearly superior in the elderly (393–396). Variability in patient selection and underlying comorbid conditions such as diabetes, cardiovascular disease, malignancy, and peripheral vascular disease affect patient survival and contribute to conflicting study results (385). However, one study examining a historical prospective national sample from 1986 to 1987 of diabetic and nondiabetic Medicare patients with ESRD suggested that elderly diabetic patients may have a lower survival rate on CAPD versus hemodialysis (397). Controlled trials are lacking to assess actual mortality rates among diabetic patients on CAPD.

The mode of renal replacement therapy should be individualized in the elderly, taking into consideration underlying medical and psychosocial factors. For instance, CAPD may be the choice for those patients with widespread vascular disease and inability to maintain a patent vascular access, or those with significant hemodynamic instability during hemodialysis. Similarly, hemodialysis may be preferred for those patients with deconditioning or a home situation that prevents appropriate self-care dialysis. The socialization available at in-center hemodialysis units may be an important factor for many elderly patients who live alone or are depressed. Comorbid conditions such as vascular disease, infection, malnutrition, and malignancy as well as withdrawal from dialysis therapy have contributed to mortality in the elderly patient with ESRD.

Age alone does not preclude renal transplantation. Many elderly, medically eligible patients have undergone successful renal transplantation (398,399). In fact, patients older than 60 years of age with well matched demographics for comorbidities undergoing rigorous screening and with anticipated 5-year survival rates in excess of 80% had a substantial survival advantage over patients with ESRD on dialysis. Preoperative 1-, 3-, and 5-year survival rates were 98%, 95%, and 90% for elderly transplant recipients, versus 92%, 62%, and 27%, respectively, for those on dialysis (400). One-year posttransplantation patient and allograft survival rates are similar between young and elderly patients. A major cause of allograft loss in the elderly patient posttransplantation is death from cardiovascular disease or infection (399,401). A retrospective analysis of adult patients in the U.S. Renal Data System and United Network for Organ Sharing Renal Transplant Scientific Registry between 1988 and 1997 notes age as an independent factor increasing the relative risk of death from infection in the elderly transplant recipient (402). This analysis also confirmed previous data indicating a decrease in acute rejection in older transplant recipients (399). Therefore, underlying comorbid conditions such as significant cardiovascular disease and the ability of the elderly patient to tolerate immunosuppressive therapy in light of the patient's "biologic age" should be assessed carefully when considering renal transplantation in the elderly (403).

Urinary Tract Infection

Infection of the urinary tract is an important and significant problem in the aging population. Various factors contribute the increased prevalence of urinary tract infections in the elderly. These include altered bladder function and defenses, "immune senescence," changes in pelvic musculature and prostate size, and concomitant illnesses such as cerebrovascular accident or dementia that may lead to poor hygiene, impaired mobility, and neurogenic bladder dysfunction (404,405). Decreased prostate secretions in elderly men can predispose to lower tract infections, as can prostatic microcalculi, which can harbor bacteria and act as a nidus for prostate infections (406). Postmenopausal women have decreased estrogen levels that change the pH of vaginal secretions, allowing for vaginal colonization of bacteria and leading to subsequent cystitis (407). Intravaginal estrogen administration may prevent recurrent urinary tract infections in these women (408).

Asymptomatic bacteriuria has been found in 20% of healthy men older than 65 years of age with the prevalence increasing to 25% in both men and women who live in extended care facilities (409). Bacteriuria also has been noted in 30% to 50% of older hospitalized patients and over 35% of the aged admitted to nursing homes (410). Creatinine clearance is decreased in elderly with bacteriuria versus those without bacteriuria (210,411). Chronic pyelonephritis with glomerulosclerosis may contribute to this loss of renal function, although the association is not clear. Decreased survival rates with chronic bacteriuria may be related to underlying associated illnesses predisposing to bacteriuria (412). Treatment of asymptomatic bacteriuria has not resulted in improved survival rates (413,414). Treatment of asymptomatic bacteriuria in the absence of renal or other urologic abnormalities is not necessary because treatment failure and relapse rates are high (415). The benefits of chronic suppressive therapy need to be determined because long-term antibiotic therapy may lead to the emergence of resistant Gram-negative organisms (416,417).

Renal Cysts

There is an age-related increase in development of simple renal cysts. Incidental renal cysts are being recognized more commonly with increased use of sonography and computed tomography of the abdomen for various other diagnoses. Ectasia, diverticula, and microscopic cysts of the distal renal tubule are found more frequently by microdissection of adult kidneys older than 50 years of age compared with 20-year-old kidneys. Morphologically, these seem to progress to large cysts in the normal kidneys of adults (19). At least one renal cyst is found on postmortem examination in over half of patients older than 50 years of age (418). A sonographic study in 729 patients revealed a 22.1% prevalence of an acquired renal cyst in patients 70 years of age and older, whereas those in the age group from 15 to 29 years had a 0% prevalence (419). These acquired cysts frequently are simple, painless, and asymptomatic, although symptoms of abdominal or lumbar pain, hematuria, secondary infection, and renin-dependent hypertension have been associated. Simple acquired asymptomatic cysts, which have a thin, smooth wall and clear fluid-filled space with no internal echoes, usually require no treatment. Cysts filled with debris or internal echoes, thick walled cysts, or those in association with a possible renal mass are considered complicated. Complicated cysts need to be investigated by cyst puncture, angiography, or surgical exploration as indicated.

ACKNOWLEDGMENTS

The authors thank Patricia A. Wood for her expert secretarial assistance with this chapter and the Medical Media Department at Dallas Veterans Affairs Medical Center for their technical assistance with illustrations.

REFERENCES

1. Prommool S, Jhangri GS, Cockfield S, et al. Time dependency of factors affecting renal allograft survival. *J Am Soc Nephrol* 2000;11:565.
2. Terasaki PI, Gjertson DW, Cecka JM. Significance of the donor age effect on kidney transplants. *Clin Transplant* 1997;11:366.
3. United States Renal Data System. *1999 Annual data report.* Bethesda, MD: National Institutes of Health, 1999:31.
4. Gomez Campdera FJJ, Luno J, Garcia de Vinuesa S, et al. Renal vascular disease in the elderly [Review, 33 refs.]. *Kidney Int Suppl* 1998;68:S73.
5. Gourtsoyiannis N, Prassopoulous P, Cavouras D, et al. The thickness of the renal parenchyma decreases with age: a CT study of 360 patients. *Am J Radiol* 1990;155:541.
6. McLachlan M, Wasserman P. Changes in the distensibility of the aging kidney. *Br J Radiol* 1981;54:488.
7. Tauchi H, Tsuboi K, Okutomi J. Age changes in the human kidney of the different races. *Gerontologia* 1971;17:87.
8. Kasiske BL, Umen AJ. The influence of age, sex, race, and body habitus on kidney weight in humans. *Arch Pathol Lab Med* 1986;110:55.
9. Moore RA. The total number of glomeruli in the normal human kidney. *Anat Rec* 1958;48:153.
10. Sorensen FH. Quantitative studies of the renal corpuscles IV. *Acta Pathol Microbiol Scand* 1977;85:356.
11. Lindeman RD, Goldman R. Anatomic and physiologic age changes in the kidney. *Exp Gerontol* 1986;21:379.
12. MacCallum DB. The bearing of degenerating glomeruli on the problem of the vascular supply of the mammalian kidney. *Am J Anat* 1939;65:69.
13. McManus JFA, Lupton CH Jr. Ischemic obsolescence of renal glomeruli. *Lab Invest* 1960;9:413.
14. Melk A, Ramassar V, Helms L, et al. Telomere shortening in kidneys with age. *J Am Soc Nephrol* 2000;11:444.
15. Harley CB, Futcher AB, Greider CW. Telomeres shorten during ageing of human fibroblasts. *Nature* 1990;345:458.
16. Harley CB, Vaziri H, Counter CM, et al. The telomere hypothesis of cellular aging. *Exp Gerontol* 1992;27:375.
17. Takazakura E, Sawabu N, Handa A, et al. Intrarenal vascular changes with age and disease. *Kidney Int* 1972;2:224.
18. Ljungqvist A, Lagergren C. Normal intrarenal arterial pattern in adult and aging human kidney: a microangiographical and histological study. *J Anat* 1962;96:285.
19. Baert L, Steg A. Is the diverticulum of the distal and collecting tubules a preliminary stage of the simple cyst in the adult? *J Urol* 1977;113:707.
20. Darmady EM, Offer J, Woodhouse MA. The parameters of the aging kidney. *Pathology* 1973;109:195.
21. Thomas SE, Anderson S, Gordon KL, et al. Tubulointerstitial disease in aging: evidence for underlying peritubular capillary damage, a potential role for renal ischemia. *J Am Soc Nephrol* 1988;9:231.
22. Griffiths GJ, Robinson KB, Cartwright GO, et al. Loss of renal tissue in the elderly. *Br J Radiol* 1976;49:111.
23. Davies D, Shock N. Age changes in glomerular filtration rate, effective renal plasma flow, and tubular excretory capacity in adult males. *J Clin Invest* 1950;29:496.
24. McDonald R, Solomon D, Shock N. Aging as a factor in the renal hemodynamic changes induced by a standardized pyrogen. *J Clin Invest* 1951;30:457.
25. Hollenberg NK, Adams DF, Solomon HS, et al. Senescence and the renal vasculature in normal man. *Circ Res* 1972;34:309.
26. Danziger RS, Tobin JD, Becker LC, et al. The age associated decline in glomerular filtration in healthy normotensive volunteers: lack of relationship to cardiovascular performance. *J Am Geriatr Soc* 1990;38:1127.
27. Manyari DE, Patterson C, Johnson DE, et al. Left ventricular diastolic function in a population of healthy elderly subjects. An echocardiographic study. *J Am Ger Soc* 1985;33:758.
28. Lee TD Jr, Lindeman RD, Yiengst MJ, et al. Influence of age on the cardiovascular and renal responses to tilting. *J Appl Physiol* 1966;21:55.
29. Mulkerrin EC, Brain A, Hampton D, et al. Reduced renal hemodynamic response to atrial natriuretic peptide in elderly volunteers. *Am J Kidney Dis* 1993;22:538.
30. Clark B. Biology of renal aging in humans. *Adv Ren Replace Ther* 2000; 7:11.
31. Fliser D, Zeier M, Nowack R, et al. Renal functional reserve in healthy elderly subjects. *J Am Soc Nephrol* 1993;3:1371.
32. Lakatta EG. Cardiovascular regulatory mechanisms in advanced age. *Physiol Rev* 1993;73:413.
33. Moritoki H, Yoshikura T, Hisayama T, et al. Possible mechanism of age associated reduction of vascular relaxation caused by atrial natriuretic peptide. *Eur J Pharmacol* 1992;210:61.
34. Sato I, Kaji, K, Moreta I, et al. Augmentation of endothelial-1 prostacyclin and thromboxane A2 secretion associated with in vitro ageing in cultured human umbilical vein endothelial cells. *Mech Age Dev* 1993; 71:73.
35. Rathous M, Greenfeld AZ, Podjarny E, et al. Altered prostaglandin synthesis and impaired sodium conservation in the kidney of old rats. *Clin Sci* 1992;83:301.
36. Kuhlik A, Elahi D, Epstein FH, et al. Decline in urinary excretion of dopamine and PGE2 with age. *Geriatr Nephrol Urol* 1995;5:79.

37. Naeiji R, Fiasse A, Carlier E, et al. Systemic and renal hemodynamic effects of angiotensin converting enzyme inhibition by zabupril in young and old normal men. *Eur J Clin Pharmacol* 1993;44:35.

38. Hollenberg NK, Moore TJ. Age and the renal blood supply: renal vascular response to angiotensin converting enzyme inhibition in healthy humans. *J Am Geriatr Soc* 1994;42:805.

39. Baylis C. Renal responses to acute angiotensin II inhibition and administered angiotensin II in the aging, conscious, chronically catheterized rat. *Am J Kidney Dis* 1993;22:842.

40. Baylis C, Fredericks M, Wilson C, et al. Renal vasodilatory response to intravenous glycine in the aging rat kidney. *Am J Kidney Dis* 1990;15:244.

41. Tank JE, Vora JP, Houghton DC, et al. Altered renal vascular responses in the aging rat kidney. *Am J Physiol* 1994;266:F942.

42. Zhang XZ, Qiu C, Baylis C. Sensitivity of the segmental renal arterioles to angiotensin II in the aging rat. *Mech Ageing Dev* 1997;97:183.

43. Lewis WH, Alving AS. Changes with age in the renal function in adult men. *Am J Physiol* 1938;123:500.

44. Baracskay D, Jarjoura D, Cugino A, et al. Geriatric renal function: estimating glomerular filtration in an ambulatory elderly population. *Clin Nephrol* 1997;47:222.

45. Rowe JW, Andres R, Tobin JD, et al. The effect of age on creatinine clearance in men: a cross-sectional and longitudinal study. *J Gerontol* 1976;31:155.

46. Back SE, Ljungberg B, Nilsson-Ehle I, et al. Age dependence of renal function: clearance of iohexol and p-amino hippurate in healthy males. *Scand J Clin Lab Invest* 1989;49:641.

47. Fliser D, Franek E, Joest M, et al. Renal function in the elderly: impact of hypertension and cardiac function. *Kidney Int* 1997;51:1196.

48. Lew SQ, Bosch JP. Effect of creatinine clearance and excretion in young and elderly healthy subjects and in patients with renal disease. *J Am Soc Nephrol* 1991;2:856.

49. Goldberg TH, Finkelstein MS. Difficulties in estimating glomerular filtration rate in the elderly. *Arch Intern Med* 1987;147:1430.

50. Rowe JW, Andres R, Tobin JD, et al. Age-adjusted standards for creatinine clearance. *Ann Intern Med* 1976;84:567.

51. Cockcroft DW, Gault MD. Prediction of creatinine clearance from serum creatinine. *Nephron* 1976;16:31.

52. Levey A, Bosch J, Lewis J, et al. A more accurate method to estimate glomerular filtration rate from serum creatinine: a new prediction equation. *Ann Intern Med* 1999;130:461.

53. Luft FC, Fineberg NS, Miller JZ, et al. The effects of age, race, and heredity on glomerular filtration rate following volume expansion and contraction in normal man. *Am J Med Sci* 1980;279:15.

54. Lindeman RD, Tobin JD, Shock NW. Association between blood pressure and the rate of decline in renal function with age. *Kidney Int* 1984;26:861.

55. Wollom GL, Gifford RW Jr. The kidney as a target organ in hypertension [Review]. *Geriatrics* 1976;31:71.

56. Brenner BM. Nephron adaptation to renal injury or ablation. *Am J Physiol* 1985;249:F324.

57. Tolbert E, Weisstuch J, Feiner H. Onset of glomerular hypertension with aging precedes injury in the spontaneously hypertensive rat. *Am J Physiol* 2000;278:F839.

58. Lindeman RD, Tobin J, Shock NW. Longitudinal studies on the rate of decline in renal function with age. *J Am Geriatr Soc* 1985;33:278.

59. Schuster VL, Kokko JP, Jacobson HR. Angiotensin II directly stimulates sodium transport in rabbit proximal convoluted tubules. *J Clin Invest* 1984;73:507.

60. Cogan MG. Angiotensin II: a powerful controller of sodium transport in the early proximal tubule. *Hypertension* 1990;15:451.

61. Norman J, Badie-Dezfody B, Nord, EA, et al. EGF-induced mitogenesis in proximal tubular cells: potentiation by angiotensin II. *Am J Physiol* 1987;253:F299.

62. Norman JT. The role of angiotensin II in renal growth. *Ren Physiol Biochem* 1991;14:175.

63. Wolf G, Neilson EG. Angiotensin II induces cellular hypertrophy in cultured urine proximal tubular cells. *Am J Physiol* 1990;259:F768.

64. Maric C, Aldfred GP, Antoine AM, et al. Effects of angiotensin II on cultured rat renomedullary interstitial cells are mediated by AT_{1A} receptors. *Am J Physiol* 1996;271:F1020.

65. Wolf G, Ziyadeh FN, Zahner, G, et al. Angiotensin II is mitogenic for cultured rat glomerular endothelial cells. *Hypertension* 1996;27:897.

66. Wolf G, Ziyadeh FN, Schroeder R, et al. Angiotensin II inhibit inducible nitric oxide synthase in tubular MCT calls by a post-transcriptional mechanism. *J Am Soc Nephrol* 1997;8:551.

67. Anderson S, Brenner BM. Effects of aging on the renal glomerulus. *Am J Med* 1986;80:435.

68. Heudes D, Michel O, Chevalier J, et al. Effect of chronic ANG I-converting enzyme inhibition on ageing processes: I. kidney structure and function. *Am J Physiol* 1994;266:R1038.

69. Corman B, Chami-Khazraji S, Shaaeverbeke J, et al. Effect of feeding on glomerular filtration rate and proteinuria in conscious aging rats. *Am J Physiol* 1988;255:F250.

70. Remuzzi A, Puntorieri C, Battaglia T, et al. Angiotensin-converting enzyme inhibition ameliorates glomerular filtration of macromolecules and water and lessen glomerular injury in the rat. *J Clin Invest* 1990;85:541.

71. Zoha C, Remuzzi A, Corna D, et al. Renal protective effects of angiotensin-converting enzyme inhibition in aging rats. *Am J Med* 1992;92:603.

72. Anderson S, Rennke HG, Zatz R. Glomerular adaptations with normal aging and with long term converting enzyme inhibition in rats. *Am J Physiol* 1994;267:F35.

73. Michel JB, Heudes D, Michel O, et al. Effect of chronic ANG 1-converting enzyme inhibition on aging processes: II. large arteries. *Am J Physiol* 1994;267:R124.

74. Ferder L, Inserra F, Romano L, et al. Decreased glomerulosclerosis in aging by angiotensin-converting enzyme inhibitors. *J Am Soc Nephrol* 1994;5:1147.

75. Wolf G, Killen PD, Neilson EG. Intracellar signalling of transcription and secretion of type IV collagen after angiotensin II-induced cellular hypertrophy in cultured proximal tubular cells. *Mol Cell Biol* 1991;2:219.

76. Wolf G, Zahner G, Schoder R, et al. Transforming growth factor beta mediates the angiotensin II-induced stimulation of collagen type IV synthesis in cultured urine proximal tubular cells. *Nephrol Dial Transplant* 1996;11:263.

77. Wolf G, Ziyadeh FN, Thaiss F, et al. Angiotensin II stimulates expression of the chemokine RANTES in rat glomerular endothelial cells: role of angiotensin type receptor. *J Clin Invest* 100:1047,1997.

78. Inserra F, Romano LA, de Cavnaugh EMV. Renal interstitial sclerosis in aging: effects of enalapril and nifedipine. *J Am Soc Nephrol* 1996;7:676.

79. Vaughan DE, Lazos SA, Tong K. Angiotensin II the expression of plasminogen activator inhibitor-1 in culture endothelial cells. *J Clin Invest* 1995;95:995.

80. Fogo AB. The role of angiotensin II and plasminogen activator inhibitor-1 in progressive glomerulosclerosis. *Am J Kidney Dis* 2000;35:179.

81. Ma LJ, Nakamura S, Whitsett J, et al. Regression of glomerulosclerosis in aging by angiotensin II type I receptor antagonist (AIIRA) is linked to inhibition of plasminogen activator-1 (PAI-1). *J Am Soc Nephrol* 1999;10:576A(abstr).

82. Roberts AB, McCane BK, Sporn MB. TGF-beta: Regulation of extracellular matrix. *Kidney Int* 1992;41:557.

83. Wolf G. Link between angiotensin II and TGF-B in the kidney. *Miner Electrolyte Metab* 1998;24:174.

84. Noble NA, Border WA. Angiotensin II in renal fibrosis: should TGF-β rather than blood pressure be the therapeutic target? *Semin Nephrol* 1997;17:455.

85. Peters H, Noble NA, Border WA. Transforming growth factor-B1 in human glomerular injury. *Curr Opin Nephrol Hypertens* 1997;6:389.

86. Frishberg Y, Kelly CJ. TGF-β and regulation of interstitial nephritis. *Miner Electrolyte Metab* 1998;24:181.

87. Ruiz-Torres MP, Bosch R, O'Valle F, et al. Age-related increase in expression of TGF-β1 in the rat kidney: Relationship to morphologic changes. *J Am Soc Nephrol* 1998;9:782.

88. Ding G, Franki N, Singhal PC. Tubular cell senescence, expression of TGF-β1 and p21 WAFE/CIPL in interstitial fibrosis in aging rats. *J Am Soc Nephrol* 1998;9:493A(abstr).

89. Wolf G. Molecular mechanisms of angiotensin in the kidney: emerging role in the progression of renal disease beyond haemodynamics. *Nephrol Dial Transplant* 1998;13:1131.

90. Satriano JA, Shuldiner M, Hora K, et al. Oxygen radicals as second messengers for expression of the monocyte hemattractant protein, JE/MCP-1, and the monocyte colony-stimulating factor, CSF-1,

in response to tumor necrosis factor-alpha and immunoglobulin G: evidence for involvement of reduced nicotinamide adenine dinucleotide phosphate (NADPH)-dependent oxidase. *J Clin Invest* 1993;92:1564.

91. Hill C, Lateef AM, Engels K, et al. Basal and stimulated nitric oxide in control of kidney function in the aging rat. *Am J Physiol* 1997; 272:R1747.

92. Sonaka I, Futami Y, Maki T. L-arginine-nitric oxide pathway and chronic nephropathy in aged rats. *J Gerontol* 1994;49:B157.

93. Reckelhoff JF, Kellum JA Jr, Racusen LC, et al. Long-term dietary supplementation with L-arginine prevents age-related reduction in renal function. *Am J Physiol* 1997;272:R1768.

94. Radner W, Hoger H, Lubec B, et al. L-arginine reduces kidney collagen accumulation and N-ϵ-(carboxymethyl) lysine in the aging NMR-1 mouse. *J Gerontol* 1994;49:M44.

95. Nakayama I, Kawahara Y, Tsuda T, et al. Angiotensin II inhibits cytokine-stimulated inducible nitric oxide synthase expression in vascular smooth muscle cells. *J Biol Chem* 1994;269:11628.

96. Arima S, Ito S, Omata K, et al. High glucose augments angiotensin II action by inhibiting NO synthesis in in vitro microperfused rabbit afferent arterioles. *Kidney Int* 1995;48:683.

97. Hogan M, Cerami A, Bucala R. Advanced glycosylation end products block the antiproliferative effect of nitric oxide. *J Clin Invest* 1992;90:1110.

98. McQuillan LP, Leung GK, Marsden PA, et al. Hypoxia inhibits expression of eNOS via transcriptional and post-transcriptional mechanisms. *Am J Physiol* 1994;267:H1921.

99. Verbeke P, Perichon M, Borot-Laloi C, et al. Accumulation of advanced glycation endproducts in the rat nephron: link with circulating AGEs during aging. *J Histochem Cytochem* 1997;45:1059.

100. Schleicher ED, Wagner E, Nerlich A. Increased accumulation of the glycoxidation product N-(carboxymethyl) lysine in human tissues in diabetes and aging. *J Clin Invest* 1997;99:457.

101. Raj DSC, Choudhury D, Welbourne TC, et al. Advanced glycation end products: a nephrologists perspective. *Am J Kidney Dis* 2000;35: 365.

102. Vlassara H. Advanced glycosylation in nephropathy of diabetes and aging. *Adv Nephrol* 1996;25:303.

103. Bucala R, Tracey KJ, Cerami A. Advanced glycosylation products quench nitric oxide and mediate defective endothelium-dependent vasodilation in experimental diabetes. *J Clin Invest* 1991;87:432.

104. Saenz de Tejada I, Goldstein S, Azadzoi K, et al. Impaired neurogenic and endothelium-mediated relaxation of penile smooth muscle in diabetic men with impotence. *N Engl J Med* 1989;320:1025.

105. McVeigh GE, Brennan GM, Johnston GD, et al. Impaired endothelium dependent and independent vasodilation in patients with type 2 (non-insulin-dependent) diabetes mellitus. *Diabetolgia* 1992;35:771.

106. Gascho JA, Fanelli C, Zelis R. Aging reduces venous distensibility in normal subjects. *Am J Cardiol* 1989;63:1267.

107. He C, Sabol J, Mitsuhashi T, et al. Dietary glycotoxins: inhibition of reactive products by aminoguanidine facilitates renal clearance and reduces tissue sequestration. *Diabetes* 1999;48:1308.

108. Cerami C, Founds H, Nicholl I, et al. Tobacco smoke is a source of toxic reactive glycation products. *Proc Natl Acad Sci USA* 1997;94:13915.

109. Li YM, Steffes M, Donnelly T, et al. Prevention of cardiovascular and renal pathology of aging by the advanced glycation inhibitor aminoguanidine. *Proc Natl Acad Sci USA* 1996;93:3902.

110. Vlassara H, Fuh H, Makita Z, et al. Exogenous advanced glycosylation end-products induce complex vascular dysfunction in normal animals: a model for diabetic and aging complications. *Proc Natl Acad Sci USA* 1992;89:12043.

111. Corman B, Duriez M, Poitevin P, et al. Aminoguanidine prevents age-related arterial stiffening and cardiac hypertrophy. *Proc Natl Acad Sci USA* 1998;95:1301.

112. Cefalu WT, Bell-Farrow AD, Wang ZQ, et al. Caloric restriction decreases age-dependent accumulation of the glycoxidation products N^e-(carboxymethyl) lysine and pentosidine in rat skin collagen. *J Gerontol A Biol Sci Med Sci* 1995;50:B337.

113. Novelli M, Masiello P, Bombara M, et al. Protein glycation in the aging male Sprague-Dawley rat: effects of antiaging diet restrictions. *J Gerontol A Biol Sci Med Sci* 1998;53:B94.

114. Teillet L, Verbeke P, Gouraud S, et al. Food restriction prevents advanced glycation end products accumulation and retards kidney aging in lean rats. *J Am Soc Nephrol* 2000;11:1488.

115. Xia E, Rao G, Van Remmen H, et al. Activities of antioxidant enzymes in various tissues of male Fischer 344 rats are altered by food restriction. *J Nutr* 1995;125:195.

116. Oppenheim RW. Related mechanisms of action of growth factors and antioxidants in apoptosis: an overview. *Adv Neurol* 1997;72:69.

117. Papa S, Skulachev VP. Reactive oxygen species, mitochondria, apoptosis and aging. *Mol Cell Biochem* 1997;174:305.

118. Beckman KB, Ames BN. The free radical theory of aging matures. *Physiol Rev* 1998;78:547.

119. Leeuwenburgh C, Hansen PA, Holloszy JO, et al. Oxidized amino acids in the urine of aging rats: potential markers for assessing oxidative stress in vivo. *Am J Physiol* 1999;276:R128.

120. Ruiz-Torres P, Lucio J, Gonzalez-Rubio M, et al. Oxidant/antioxidant balance in isolated glomeruli and cultured mesangial cells. *Free Radic Biol Med* 1997;22:49.

121. Reckelhoff JF, Kanji V, Racusen LC, et al. Vitamin E ameliorates enhanced renal lipid peroxidation and accumulation of F2-isoprostanes in aging kidneys. *Am J Physiol* 1998;274:R767.

122. Ushio-Fukai M, Zafari AM, Fukui T, et al. p_{22}^{pho} is a critical component of the superoxide-generating NADH/NADPH oxidase system and regulates angiotensin II-induced hypertrophy in vascular smooth muscle cells. *J Biol Chem* 1996;38:23317.

123. de Cavanagh EM, Inserra F, Ferder L, et al. Superoxide dismutase and glutathione peroxidase activities are increased by enalapril and captopril in mouse liver. *FEBS Lett* 1995;361:22.

124. Cruz CL, Ruiz-Torres P, del Moral RG, et al. Age-related progressive renal fibrosis in rats and its prevention with ACE inhibitors and taurine. *Am J Physiol* 2000;278:F122.

125. Levi M, Jameson D, Van Der Meer BW. Role of BBM lipid composition and fluidity in impaired renal Pi transport in aged rats. *Am J Physiol* 1989;256:F85.

126. Cohen BM, Zubenko GS: Aging and the biophysical properties of cell membranes. *Life Sci* 1985;37:1403.

127. Eisenberg S, Stein Y, Stein O. Phospholipases in arterial tissue: IV. the role of phosphatide acyl hydrolase, lysophosphatide, acyl hydrolase, and sphingomyelin choline phosphohydrolase in the regulation of phospholipid composition in the normal human aorta with age. *J Clin Invest* 1969;48:2320.

128. Hegner D. Age dependence of molecular and functional changes in biological membranes properties. *Mech Ageing Dev* 1980;14:101.

129. Hegner D, Platt D, Heckers H, et al. Age-dependent physiochemical and biochemical studies of human red cell membranes. *Mech Ageing Dev* 1979;10:117.

130. Hubbard R, Garratt CJ. The composition and fluidity of adipocyte membranes prepared from young and adult rats. *Biochim Biophys Acta* 1980;600:701.

131. Rivnay B, Bergman S, Shinitzy M, et al. Correlations between membrane viscosity, serum cholesterol, lymphocyte activation and aging in man. *Mech Ageing Dev* 1980;12:119.

132. Yechiel EY. Relationship between membrane lipid composition and biological properties of rat myocytes: effects of aging and manipulation of lipid composition. *J Biol Chem* 1985;260:9123.

133. Ravid M, Rachmani R. Cholesterol as a predictor of progression in diabetic renal disease. *Contrib Nephrol* 1997;120:39.

134. Greco B, Breyer JA. Cholesterol as a predictor of progression in non-diabetic chronic renal disease. *Contrib Nephrol* 1997;120:48.

135. Neverov N, Kaysen G, Tareyeva I. Effects of lipid-lowering therapy on the progression of renal disease in nondiabetic nephrotic patients. *Contrib Nephrol* 1997;120:68.

136. Cheng IKP, Lau K, Janus E, et al. Treatment of hyperlipidemia in patients with non-insulin dependent diabetes mellitus with progressive nephropathy. *Contrib Nephrol* 1997;120:79.

137. Wanner C, Greiber S, Kramer-Guth A, et al. Lipids and progression of renal disease: role of modified low density lipoprotein and lipoprotein (a). *Kidney Int* 1997;52[Suppl 63]:S102.

138. Kamanna VS, Roh DD, Kirschenbaum MA. Hyperlipidemia and kidney disease: concepts derived from histopathology and cell biology of the glomerulus. *Histol Histopathol* 1998;13:169.

139. Wu ZL, Liang M-Y, Qui L-Q. Oxidized low density lipoprotein decreases the induced nitric oxide synthesis in rat mesangial cells. *Cell Biochem Funct* 1998;l16:153.

140. Dominguez JH, Tang N, Xu W, et al. Studies of renal injury: III. lipid-induced nephropathy in type II diabetes. *Kidney Int* 2000;57: 92.

141. Kim S, Han DC, Lee HB. Lovastatin inhibits transforming growth factor-β1 expression in diabetic rat glomeruli and cultured rat mesangial cells. *J Am Soc Nephrol* 2000;11:80.

142. Lam KSL, Cheng IKP, Janus ED, et al. Cholesterol-lowering therapy may retard the progression of diabetic nephropathy. *Diabetologia* 1995;38:604.

143. Tonolo G, Ciccarese M, Brizzi P, et al. Reduction of albumin excretion rate in normotensive microalbuminuric type 2 diabetic patients during long-term simvastatin treatment. *Diabetes Care* 1997;20:1891.

144. Epstein M, Hollenberg N. Age as a determinant of renal sodium conservation in normal man. *J Lab Clin Med* 1976;87:411.

145. Macias Nunez J, Garcia Iglesias C, Bonda Roman A, et al. Renal handling of sodium in old people: a functional study. *Age Ageing* 1978;7:178.

146. Anderson GH Jr, Springer J, Randall P, et al. Effect of age on diagnostic usefulness of stimulated plasma renin activity and saralasin test in detection of renovascular hypertension. *Lancet* 1980;2:821.

147. Bauer J. Age-related changes in the renin-aldosterone system. *Drugs Aging* 1993;3:238.

148. Baylis C, Engels K, Beierwaltes WH. β-Adrenoceptor-stimulated renin release is blunted in old rats. *J Am Soc Nephrol* 1998;9:1318.

149. Crane MG, Harris JJ. Effect of aging on renin activity and aldosterone excretion. *J Lab Clin Med* 1976;87:947.

150. Cugini P, Murano G, Lucia P, et al. The gerontological decline of the renin-aldosterone system: a chronobiological approach extended to essential hypertension. *J Gerontol* 1987;42:461.

151. Hall JE, Coleman TG, Guyton AC. The renin-angiotensin system normal physiology and changes in older hypertensives. *J Am Geriatr Soc* 1989;37:801.

152. Hayashi M, Samta T, Nakamura R, et al. Effect of aging on single nephron renin content in rats. *Ren Physiol* 1981;4:17.

153. Hayduk K, Krause DK, Kaufmann W, et al. Age-dependent changes of plasma renin concentration in humans. *Clin Sci* 1973;45:273S.

154. Noth RH, Lassman MN, Tan SY, et al. Age and the renin aldosterone system. *Arch Intern Med* 1977;137:1414.

155. Tsunoda K, Abe K, Goto T, et al. Effect of age on the renin-angiotensin-aldosterone system in normal subjects: simultaneous measurement of active and inactive renin, renin substrate, and aldosterone in plasma. *J Clin Endocrinol Metab* 1986;62:384.

156. Weidmann P, De Chatel R, Schiffmann A, et al. Interrelations between age and plasma renin, aldosterone, and cortisol, urinary catecholamines, and the body sodium/volume state in normal man. *Klin Wochenschr* 1977;55:725.

157. Jung FF, Kennefick TM, Ingelfinger JR, et al. Down-regulation of the intrarenal renin-angiotensin system in the aging rat. *J Am Soc Nephrol* 1995;5:1573.

158. Lu X, Li X, Li L, et al. Variation of intrarenal angiotensin II and angiotensin II receptors by acute renal ischemia in the aged rat. *Ren Fail* 1996;18:19.

159. Jover B, Dupont M, Geelen G, et al. Renal and systemic adaptation to sodium restriction in aging rats. *Am J Physiol* 1993;264:R833.

160. Flood C, Gherondache C, Pincus G, et al. The metabolism and secretion of aldosterone in elderly subjects. *J Clin Invest* 1967;46:961.

161. Hegstad R, Brown RD, Jiang NS, et al. Aging and aldosterone. *Am J Med* 1983;74:442.

162. Weidmann P, De Myttenaere-Bursztein S, Maxwell MH, et al. Effect of aging on plasma renin and aldosterone in normal man. *Kidney Int* 1975;8:325.

163. Mimran A, Ribstein J, Jover B. Aging and sodium homeostasis. *Kidney Int* 1992;41:S107.

164. Luft FC, Weinberger M, Grim CE. Sodium sensitivity and resistance in normotensive humans. *Am J Med* 1982;72:726.

165. Leasco D, Ferrara N, Landino P, et al. Effects of age on the role of atrial natriuretic factor in renal adaptation to physiologic variations of dietary salt intake. *J Am Soc Nephrol* 1996;7:1045.

166. Ohashi M, Fujio N, Nawata H, et al. High plasma concentrations of human atrial natriuretic polypeptide in aged men. *J Clin Endocrinol Metab* 1987;64:81.

167. Pollack JA, Skvorak P, Nazran SJ, et al. Alterations in atrial natriuretic peptide (ANP) secretion and renal effects in aging. *J Gerontol A Biol Sci Med Sci* 1997;52:B196.

168. Luft FC, Grim CE, Fineberg NS, et al. Effects of volume expansion and contraction in normotensive whites, blacks, and subjects of different ages. *Circulation* 1979;59:643.

169. Brenner BM, Ballermann BJ, Gunning ME, et al. Diverse biological actions of atrial natriuretic peptide. *Physiol Rev* 1990;70:665.

170. Haller B, Zust H, Shaw S, et al. Effects of posture and aging on circulating atrial natriuretic peptide levels in man. *J Hypertens* 1987;5:551.

171. McKnight JA, Roberts G, Sheridan B, et al. Aging and atrial natriuretic factor. *J Hum Hypertens* 1990;4:53.

172. Tajima F, Sagawa S, Iwamoto J, et al. Renal and endocrine responses in the elderly during head-out water immersion. *Am J Physiol* 1988;254:R977.

173. Tan AC, Hoefnagels WH, Swinkels LM, et al. The effect of volume expansion on atrial natriuretic peptide and cyclic guanosine monophosphate levels in young and aged subjects. *J Am Geriatr Soc* 1990;38:1215.

174. Clark BA, Elahi D, Shannon RM, et al. Influence of age and dose on the end-organ responses to atrial natriuretic peptide in humans. *Am J Hypertens* 1991;4:500.

175. Jansen TL, Tan AC, Smits P, et al. Hemodynamic effects of atrial natriuretic factor in young and elderly subjects. *Clin Pharmacol Ther* 1990;48:179.

176. Ohashi M, Fujio N, Nawata H, et al. Pharmacokinetics of synthetic alpha-human atrial natriuretic polypeptide in normal men: effect of aging. *Regul Pept* 1987;19:265.

177. Or K, Richards AM, Espiner EA, et al. Effect of low dose infusions of ile-atrial natriuretic peptide in healthy elderly males: evidence for a postreceptor defect. *J Clin Endocrinol Metab* 1993;76:1271.

178. Rascher W, Tulassay T, Lang RE. Atrial natriuretic peptide in plasma of volume overloaded children with chronic renal failure. *Lancet* 1985;2:303.

179. Lafferty HM, Gunning ME, Silva P, et al. Enkephalinase inhibition increases plasma atrial natriuretic peptide levels, glomerular filtration rate, and urinary sodium excretion in rats with reduced renal mass. *Circ Res* 1989;65:640.

180. Kimmelstiel CD, Perrone R, Kilcoyne L, et al. Effects of renal neutral endopeptidase inhibition on sodium excretion, renal hemodynamics and neurohormonal activation in patients with congestive heart failure. *Cardiology* 1996;87:46.

181. Gillies AH, Crozier IG, Nicholls MG, et al. Effect of posture on clearance of atrial natriuretic peptide from plasma. *J Clin Endocrinol Metab* 1987;65:1095.

182. Tonolo G, Soro A, Scardaccio V, et al. Correlates of atrial natriuretic factor in chronic renal failure. *J Hypertens* 1989;7:S238.

183. Lindeman RD, Lee TD Jr, Yiengst MJ. Influence of age, renal disease, hypertension, diuretics, and calcium on the antidiuretic responses to suboptimal infusions of vasopressin. *J Lab Clin Med* 1966;68:206.

184. Lindeman RD, Van Buren H, Maisz L. Osmolar renal concentrating ability in healthy young men and hospitalized patients without renal disease. *N Engl J Med* 1960;262:1306.

185. Meyer BR. Renal function in aging. *J Am Geriatr Soc* 1989;37:791.

186. Rowe J, Shock N, DeFronzo R. The influence of age on the renal response to water deprivation in man. *Nephron* 1976;17:270.

187. Handelmann GE, Sayson SC. Neonatal exposure to vasopressin decreases binding sites in the adult kidney. *Peptides* 1984;5:1217.

188. Miller M. Increased vasopressin secretion: an early manifestation of aging in the rat. *J Gerontol* 1987;42:3.

189. Helderman JH, Vestal RE, Rowe JW, et al. The response of arginine vasopressin to intravenous ethanol and hypertonic saline in man: the impact of aging. *J Gerontol* 1978;33:39.

190. Kirkland J, Lye M, Goddard C, et al. Plasma arginine vasopressin in dehydrated elderly patients. *Clin Endocrinol* 1984;20:451.

191. Phillips PA, Bretherton M, Risvanis J, et al. Effects of drinking on thirst and vasopressin in dehydrated elderly men. *Am J Physiol* 1993;264:R877.

192. Phillips PA, Phil D, Rolls BJ, et al. Reduced thirst after water deprivation in healthy elderly men. *N Engl J Med* 1984;311:753.

193. Rendeau E, de Lima J, Caillens H, et al. High plasma antidiuretic hormone in patients with cardiac failure: influence of age. *Miner Electrolyte Metab* 1982;8:267.

194. Faull C, Holmes C, Baylis P. Water balance in elderly people: is there a deficiency of vasopressin? *Age Ageing* 1993;22:114.

195. Li C, Hsieh S, Nagai I. The response of plasma arginine vasopressin to 14h water deprivation in the elderly. *Acta Endocrinol (Copenh)* 1984;105:314.

196. Rowe JW, Minaker KL, Sparrow D, et al. Age-related failure of volume-pressure-mediated vasopressin release. *J Clin Endocrinol Metab* 1982;54:661.
197. Ishikawa SE, Fujisawa N, Tsuboi Y, et al. Involvement of arginine vasopressin and renal sodium handling in pathogenesis of hyponatremia in elderly patients. *Endocr J* 1996;43:101.
198. Miller JH, Shock NW. Age differences in the renal tubular response to antidiuretic hormone. *J Gerontol* 1953;8:446.
199. Macias Nunez JF, Garcia Iglesias C, Tabernero Romo JM, et al. Renal management of sodium under indomethacin and aldosterone in the elderly. *Age Ageing* 1980;9:165.
200. Bengele H, Mathias R, Perkins J, et al. Urinary concentrating defect in the aged rat. *Am J Physiol* 1981;240:F147.
201. Beck N, Yu B. Effect of aging on urinary concentrating mechanisms and vasopressin-dependent cAMP in rats. *Am J Physiol* 1982;243:F121.
202. Goddard C, Davidson YS, Moser BB, et al. Effect of aging on cyclic AMP output by renal medullary cells in response to arginine vasopressin in vitro in C57 BL/Icrfa mice. *J Endocrinol* 1984;103:133.
203. Davidon YS, Davies I, Goddard C. Renal vasopressin receptors in ageing C57 BL/Icrfaᵗ mice. *J Endocrinol* 1987;115:379.
204. Liang CT, Barnes J, Hanai H, et al. Decrease in Gs protein expression may impair adenylate cyclase activity in old kidneys. *Am J Physiol* 1993;264:F770.
205. Wilson P, Dillingham MA. Age-associated decrease in vasopressin-induced renal water transport: a role for adenylate cyclase and G protein malfunction. *Gerontology* 1992;38:315.
206. Terashima Y, Kondo K, Inaguki, A, et al. Age associated decrease in response of rat aquaporin-2 gene expression to dehydration. *Life Sci* 1998;62:873.
207. Verbavatz JM, Preisser L, Berthonaud V, et al. Downregulation of AQP2 and AQP3 expression in aging rat kidney is independent of changes in circulating AVP and intracellular cAMP. *J Am Soc Nephrol* 1998;9:27A(abstr).
208. Crowe MJ, Forsling ML, Rolls BJ, et al. Altered water excretion in healthy elderly man. *Age Ageing* 1987;16:285.
209. Davis FB, VanSon A, Davis PJ. Urinary diluting capacity in elderly diabetic subjects. *Exp Gerontol* 1980;21:407.
210. Dontas AS, Marketos S, Papanayiotou PC. Mechanisms of renal tubular defects in old age. *Postgrad Med J* 1972;48:295.
211. Adler S, Lindeman RD, Yiengst MJ, et al. Effect of acute acid loading on urinary acid excretion by the aging human kidney. *J Lab Clin Med* 1968;72:278.
212. Frassetto L, Morris RC Jr, Sebastian A. Effect of age on blood acid-base composition in adult humans: role of age-related renal functional decline. *Am J Physiol* 1996;271:F1112.
213. Agarwal BN, Cabebe FG. Renal acidification in elderly subjects. *Nephron* 1980;26:291.
214. Rajendra P, Kinsella JL, Sacktor B. Renal adaptation to metabolic acidosis in senescent rats. *Am J Physiol* 1988;255:F1183.
215. Mitch WE, Medina R, Grieber S, et al. Metabolic acidosis stimulates muscle protein degradation by activating the adenosine triphosphate dependent pathway involving ubiquitin and proteasomes. *J Clin Invest* 1994;93:2127.
216. Alpern RJ, Sakhaee K. The clinical spectrum of chronic metabolic acidosis: homeostatic mechanisms produce significant morbidity. *Am J Kidney Dis* 1997;29:291.
217. Frassetto L, Morris RC Jr, Sebastian A. Potassium bicarbonate improves nitrogen balance in postmenopausal women. *J Am Soc Nephrol* 1995;6:308(abstr).
218. Sebastian A, Harris ST, Ottaway JH, et al. Improved mineral balance and skeletal metabolism in postmenopausal women treated with potassium bicarbonate. *N Engl J Med* 1994;330:1776.
219. Himmelstein DU, Jones AA, Woolhandler S. Hypernatremic dehydration in nursing home patients: an indicator of neglect. *J Am Geriatr Soc* 1983;31:466.
220. Kleinfeld M, Casimir M, Borra S. Hyponatremia as observed in a clinical disease facility. *J Am Geriatr Soc* 1979;27:156.
221. Shannon RP, Minaker KL, Rowe JW. Aging and water balance in humans. *Semin Nephrol* 1984;4:346.
222. Snyder NA, Fergal DW, Arieff AI. Hypernatremia in elderly patients. *Ann Intern Med* 1987;107:309.
223. Sunderam SG, Mankikar GD. Hyponatremia in the elderly. *Age Ageing* 1983;12:77.
224. Beck LH, Lavizzo-Morey R. Geriatric hyponatremia. *Ann Intern Med* 1987;107:768.
225. Miller M, Hecker M, Friedland D, et al. Apparent idiopathic hyponatremia in an ambulatory geriatric population. *J Am Geriatr Soc* 1996;44:404.
226. Clark BA, Shannon RP, Rosa RM, et al. Increased susceptibility to thiazide-induced hyponatremia in the elderly. *J Am Soc Nephrol* 1994;5:1106.
227. Hochman I, Cabili S, Peer G. Hyponatremia in internal medicine ward patients: causes, treatment, and prognosis. *Isr J Med Sci* 1989;25:73.
228. Arieff AI, Guisado R. Effects on central nervous system of hypernatremic and hyponatremic states. *Kidney Int* 1976;10:104.
229. Miller PD, Krebs RA, Neal BJH, et al. Hypodipsia in geriatric patients. *Am J Med* 1982;73:354.
230. Arieff AI, Guisado R, Lazarowitz VC. Pathophysiology of hyperosmolar states. In: Andreoli TE, Grantham JJ, Rector FC Jr, eds. *Disturbances in body fluid osmolality.* Bethesda, MD: American Physiological Society, 1977:227.
231. Mahowald JM, Himmelstein DU. Hypernatremia in the elderly: relation to infection and mortality. *J Am Geriatr Soc* 1981;29:177.
232. Allen TH, Anderson EC, Langham WH. Total body potassium and gross body composition in relation to age. *J Gerontol* 1960;15:348.
233. Mulkerrin E, Epstein FH, Clark BA. Aldosterone responses to hyperkalemia in healthy elderly humans. *J Am Soc Nephrol* 1995;6:1459.
234. Bengele H, Mathias R, Perkins J, et al. Impaired renal and extrarenal potassium adaptation in old rats. *Kidney Int* 1983;23:684.
235. Minaker KL, Rowe JW. Potassium homeostasis during hyperinsulinemia: effect of insulin level, β-blockade, and age. *Am J Physiol* 1982;242:E373.
236. Ford GA, Blaschke T, Wiswell R, et al. Effect of aging on changes in plasma potassium during exercise. *J Gerontol* 1993;48:M140.
237. Defronzo RA. Hyperkalemia and hyporeninemic hypoaldosteronism. *Kidney Int* 1980;17:118.
238. Meier DE, Myers WM, Swenson R, et al. Indomethacin-associated hyperkalemia in the elderly. *J Am Geriatr Soc* 1983;31:371.
239. Mor R, Pitilk S, Rosenfeld JB. Indomethacin- and Moduretic-induced hyperkalemia. *Isr J Med Sci* 1983;19:535.
240. Walmsley RN, White GH, Cain M, et al. Hyperkalemia in the elderly. *Clin Chem* 1984;30:1409.
241. Armbrecht HJ, Zenser TV, Gross CJ, et al. Adaptation to dietary calcium and phosphorus restriction changes with age in the rat. *Am J Physiol* 1980;239:E322.
242. Corman B, Rionel N. Single nephron filtration rate in proximal reabsorption in aging rats. *Am J Physiol* 1991;260:F75.
243. Armbrecht HJ, Zenser TV, Burns MEH, et al. Effect of age on intestinal calcium absorption and adaptation to dietary calcium. *Am J Physiol* 1979;236:E769.
244. Halloran BP, Lonergan ET, Portale AA. Aging and renal responsiveness to parathyroid hormone in healthy men. *J Clin Endocrinol Metab* 1996;81:2192.
245. Portale AA, Lonergan ET, Tanney DM, et al. Aging alters calcium regulation of serum concentration of parathyroid hormone in healthy men. *Am J Physiol* 1997;272:E139.
246. Armbrecht HJ, Gross CJ, Zenser TV. Effect of dietary calcium and phosphorus restriction on calcium and phosphorus balance in young and old rats. *Arch Biochem Biophys* 1981;210:179.
247. Caverzasio J, Murer H, Fleisch H, et al. Phosphate transport in brush border vesicles isolated from renal cortex of young growing and adult rats: comparison with whole kidney data. *Pflugers Arch* 1982;394:217.
248. Corman B, Michel J-B. Glomerular filtration, renal blood flow, and solute excretion in conscious aging rats. *Am J Physiol* 1987;253:R555.
249. Corman B, Pratz J, Poujeol P. Changes in anatomy, glomerular filtration, and solute excretion in aging rat kidney. *Am J Physiol* 1985;248:R282.
250. Haramati A, Mulroney S, Sacktor B. Age-related decrease in the tubular capacity for phosphate reabsorption in the rat. *Kidney Int* 1987;31:349(abstr).
251. Kiebzak GM, Sacktor B. Effect of age on renal conservation of phosphate in the rat. *Am J Physiol* 1986;251:F399.
252. Lee DBN, Yanagawa N, Jo O. Phosphaturia of aging: studies on mechanisms. *Adv Exp Med Biol* 1984;178:103.
253. Levi M, Jameson DM, Van Der Meer BW. Role of BBM lipid composition and fluidity in impaired renal Pi transport in aged rat. *Am J Physiol* 1989;256:F85.

254. Naafs MA, Fischer HR, Koorevaar G, et al. The effect of age on the renal response to PTH infusion. *Calcif Tissue Int* 1987;41:262.

255. Marcus R, Madvig P, Young G. Age-related changes in parathyroid hormone and parathyroid hormone action in normal humans. *J Clin Endocrinol Metab* 1984;58:223.

256. Wiske PS, Epstein S, Bell NH, et al. Increases in immunoreactive parathyroid hormone with age. *N Engl J Med* 1979;300:1419.

257. Chen ML, King RS, Armbrecht HJ. Sodium-dependent phosphate transport in primary cultures of renal tubule cells from young and adult rats. *J Cell Physiol* 1990;143:488.

258. Sorribas V, Lotscher M, Loffing J, et al. Cellular mechanisms of the age-related decrease in renal phosphate reabsorption. *Kidney Int* 1996;50:855.

259. Grinna LS. Age-related changes in the lipids of the microsomal and mitochondrial membranes of rat liver and kidney. *Mech Ageing Dev* 1977;6:197.

260. Grinna LS, Barber AA. Age-related changes in membrane lipid content and enzyme activities. *Biochim Biophys Acta* 1972;288:347.

261. Pratz J, Corman B. Age-related changes in enzyme activities, protein content, and lipid composition of rat kidney brush border membranes. *Biochim Biophys Acta* 1985;814:265.

262. Pratz J, Ripoche P, Corman B. Cholesterol content and water and solute permeabilities of kidney membranes from aging rats. *Am J Physiol* 1987;253:R8.

263. Levi M, Baird BM. Wilson PV. Cholesterol modulates rat renal brush border membrane phosphate transport. *J Clin Invest* 1990;85:231.

264. Zajicek H, Wang H, Widerkehr M, et al. Cholesterol modulates Na/Pi cotransport in OK cells. *J Am Soc Nephrol* 1997;8:570A(abstr).

265. Brandis M, Harmeyer J, Kaune R, et al. Phosphate transport in brush border membranes from control and rachitic pig kidney and small intestine. *J Physiol (Lond)* 1987;384:479.

266. Kurnik BR, Hruska KA. Effects of 1,25-dihydroxy-cholecalciferol on phosphate transport in vitamin D-deprived rats. *Am J Physiol* 1984;247:F177.

267. Liang CT, Barnes J, Cheng L, et al. Effects of 1,25-(OH)2D3 administered in vivo on phosphate uptake by isolated chick renal cells. *Am J Physiol* 1982;242:C312.

268. Brasitus TA, Dudeja PK, Eby B, et al. Correction by 1,25-dihydroxycholecalciferol of the abnormal fluidity and lipid composition of enterocyte brush border membranes in vitamin D-deprived rats. *J Biol Chem* 1986;261:16404.

269. Tsutsumi M, Alvarez V, Avioli LV, et al. Effect of 1,25-dihydroxyvitamin D3 on phospholipid composition of rat renal brush border membrane. *Am J Physiol* 1985;249:F117.

270. Pascual J, Orofino L, Uano F. Incidence and prognosis of acute renal failure in older patients. *J Am Geriatr Soc* 1990;38:25.

271. McInnes EG, Levy DW, Choudhuri MD, et al. Renal failure in the elderly. *QJM* 1987;64:583.

272. Gentric A, Cledes J. Immediate and long term prognosis in acute renal failure in the elderly. *Nephrol Dial Transplant* 1991;6:86.

273. Klouche K, Cristol JP, Kaaki M, et al. Prognosis of acute renal failure in the elderly. *Nephrol Dial Transplant* 1995;10:2240.

274. Santacruz F, Barreto S, Mayor MM, et al. Mortality in elderly patients with acute renal failure. *Ren Fail* 1996;18:601.

275. Moore RD, Smith CR, Lipsky JJ. Risk factor for nephrotoxicity in patients treated with aminoglycosides. *Ann Intern Med* 1984;100:352.

276. Michel DM, Kelly CJ. Acute interstitial nephritis. *J Am Soc Nephrol* 1998;9:506.

277. Kleinknecht D. Interstitial nephritis, the nephrotic syndrome, and clinic renal failure secondary to nonsteroidal anti-inflammatory drugs. *Semin Nephrol* 1995;15:228.

278. Rich MW. Incidence, risk factors, and clinical course of acute renal insufficiency after cardiac catheterization in patients 70 years of age or older: a prospective study. *Arch Intern Med* 1990;150:1237.

279. Porter GA. Radiocontrast-induced nephropathy. *Nephrol Dial Transplant* 1994;9:146.

280. Beierschmitt W, Keenan K, Weiner M. Age-related susceptibility of male Fischer-344 rats to acetaminophen nephrotoxicity. *Life Sci* 1986;39:2335.

281. Goldstein RS, Pasino DA, Hook JB. Cephaloridine nephrotoxicity in aging male Fischer-344 rats. *Toxicology* 1986;38:43.

282. Goldstein RS, Tarloff JB, Hook JB. Age-related nephropathy in laboratory rats. *FASEB J* 1988;2:2241.

283. Kyle ME, Kocsis JJ. The effect of age on salicylate-induced nephrotoxicity in male rats. *Toxicol Appl Pharmacol* 1985;81:337.

284. Miura K, Goldstein RS, Morgan DG, et al. Age-related differences in susceptibility to renal ischemia in rats. *Toxicol Appl Pharmacol* 1987;87:284.

285. Sabbatini M, Sansone G, Uccello F, et al. Functional versus structural changes in the pathophysiology of acute ischemic renal failure in aging rats. *Kidney Int* 1994;45:1355.

286. Zager RA, Alpers CE. Effects of aging on expression of ischemic acute renal failure in rats. *Lab Invest* 1989;61:290.

287. Prasad PV. Epstein FH. Changes in renal medullary pO2 during water diuresis as evaluated by blood oxygenation level-dependent magnetic resonance imaging: effects of aging and cyclooxygenase inhibition. *Kidney Int* 1999;55:294.

288. Paller MS, Moidal JR, Ferris TF. Oxygen-free radicals in ischemic acute renal failure in the rat. *J Clin Invest* 1984;74:1156.

289. Moncada S, Palmer RMJ, Higgs EA. Nitric oxide: physiology, pathophysiology, and pharmacology. *Pharmacol Rev* 1991;43:109.

290. Tan D, Cernad M, Aragoncillo P, et al. Role of nitric oxide-related mechanisms in renal function in ageing rats. *Nephrol Dial Transplant* 1998;13:594.

291. Kung CF, Luscher TF. Different mechanisms of endothelial dysfunction with aging and hypertension in rat aorta. *Hypertension* 1995;25:194.

292. Luscher TF, Bock HA. The endothelial L-arginine/nitric oxide pathway and the renal circulation. *Klin Wochenschr* 1991;69:603.

293. Reckelhoff JF, Kellum JA, Blanchard EJ, et al. Changes in nitric oxide precursor, L-arginine, and metabolites, nitrate and nitrite, with aging. *Life Sci* 1994;55:1895.

294. Sarwar GH, Botting HG, Collins M. A comparison of fasting serum amino acid profiles of young and elderly subjects. *J Am Coll Nutr* 1991;10:668.

295. Higashi Y, Oshima T, Ozono R, et al. Aging and severity of hypertension attenuate endothelium-dependent renal vascular relaxation in humans. *Hypertension* 1997;30:252.

296. Schmidt R, Sorkin M, Baylis C. Response of the nitric oxide (NO) system to variations in Na intake in aging man. *J Am Soc Nephrol* 1998;9:330A(abstr).

297. Cronin RE. Southwestern Internal Medicine conference: renal failure following radiologic procedures. *Am J Med Sci* 1989;298:342.

298. Gupta B, Spinowitz B, Charytan C, et al. Cholesterol crystal embolization-associated renal failure with recombinant tissue-type plasminogen activator. *Am J Kidney Dis* 1993;21:659.

299. Smith MC, Ghose MK, Henry AR. The clinical spectrum of renal cholesterol embolization. *Am J Med* 1981;71:174.

300. Feest T, Round A, Hamad S. Incidence of severe acute renal failure in adults: Results of a community based study. *BMJ* 1993;306:481.

301. Arora P, Kher V, Kohli HS, et al. Acute renal failure in the elderly: experience from a single centre in India. *Nephrol Dial Transplant* 1993;8:827.

302. Druml W, Lax F, Grimm G, et al. Acute renal failure in the elderly 1975. *Clin Nephrol* 1994;41:342.

303. Pascual J, Liano F, Ortuno J The elderly patient with acute renal failure. *J Am Soc Nephrol* 1995;6:144.

304. Scoble JE, Maher ER, Hamilton G, et al. Atherosclerotic renovascular disease causing renal impairment: a case for treatment. *Clin Nephrol* 1989;31:119.

305. Scoble JE, Sweny P, Stansby G, et al. Patients with atherosclerotic renovascular disease presenting to a renal unit: an audit of outcome. *Postgrad Med J* 1993;69:461.

306. Harding MB, Smith LR, Himmelstein SI, et al. Renal artery stenosis: prevalence and associated risk factors in patients undergoing routine cardiac catheterization. *J Am Soc Nephrol* 1992;2:1608.

307. Working Group on Renovascular Hypertension. Detection, evaluation, and treatment of renovascular hypertension: final report. *Arch Intern Med* 1987;147:820.

308. Jacobson HR. Ischemic renal disease: an overlooked entity. *Kidney Int* 1988;34:729.

309. Schreiber MJ, Pohl MA, Novick M. Natural history of atherosclerotic and fibrous renal artery disease. *Urol Clin North Am* 1984;11:383.

310. Rimmer JM, Gennari J. Atherosclerotic renovascular disease and progressive renal failure. *Ann Intern Med* 1993;118:712.

311. Baboolal K, Evans C, Moore RH. Incidence of end-stage renal disease in medically treated patients with severe bilateral atherosclerotic renovascular disease. *Am J Kidney Dis* 1998;31:971.

312. Connolly JO, Higgins RM, Walters HL, et al. Presentation, clinical features and outcome in different patterns of atherosclerotic renovascular disease. *QJM* 1994;87:413.

313. Gambara G, Budakovic A, Baggio B, et al. Cigarette smoking is associated with altered hemodynamics. *Nephrol Dial Transplant* 1996;11:A72.

314. Appel RG, Bleyer AJ, Reavis S, et al. Renovascular disease in older patients beginning renal replacement therapy. *Kidney Int* 1995;48:171.

315. Klag MJ, Whelton PK, Randall BL, et al. End-stage renal disease in African-American and white men: 16-year MRFIT findings. *JAMA* 1997;277:1293.

316. Bleyer AJ, Shemonski LR, Burke GL, et al. Tobacco, hypertension, and vascular disease: risk factors for renal functional decline in an older population. *Kidney Int* 2000;57:2072.

317. Cryer PE, Haymon MW, Santiago JV, et al. Norepinephrine and epinephrine release and adrenergic medication of smoking associated hemodynamic and metabolic events. *N Engl J Med* 1976;295:573.

318. Orth SR, Ritz E, Schrier RW. Renal risks of smoking. *Kidney Int* 1997;51:1669.

319. Nadler JD, Velasco JS, Horton R. Cigarette smoking inhibits prostacyclin formation. *Lancet* 1976;1:1248.

320. Welnnalm A, Bethin G, Grastrom EF, et al. Relation between tobacco use and urinary excretion of thromboxane A2 and prostacyclin metabolites in young men. *Circulation* 1991;83:1698.

321. Baggio B, Budakovic A, Gambaro G. Cardiovascular risk factors, smoking and kidney function. *Nephrol Dial Transplant* 1998;13[Suppl 17]:2.

322. Nitenberg A, Antony I, Foult JM. Acetylcholine-inducted coronary vasoconstriction in young, heavy smokers with normal coronary arteriographic findings. *Am J Med* 1993;95:71.

323. Celermajer D, Sorensen KE, Georgakapoulos D, et al. Cigarette smoking is associated with dose-related and potentially reversible impairment of endothelium-dependent dilatation in healthy young adults. *Circulation* 1993;88:2149.

324. Kiowski W, Linder L, Stoschitzky K, et al. Diminished vascular response to inhibition of endothelium-derived nitric oxide and enhanced vasoconstriction to exogenously administered endothelin-1 in clinically healthy smoker. *Circulation* 1994;90:27.

325. Haak T, Jungmann E, Raab C, et al. Elevated endorthelin-1 levels after cigarette smoking. *Metabolism* 1994;43:267.

326. Kohan DE. Endothelin in the kidney: physiology and pathophysiology. *Am J Kidney Dis* 1993;22:493.

327. Black HR, Zeevi GR, Silten RM, et al. Effect of heavy cigarette smoking on renal and myocardial arterioles. *Nephron* 1983;34:173.

328. Oberai B, Adams CW.M, High OB. Myocardial and renal arteriolar thickening in cigarette smoking. *Atherosclerosis* 1984;52:185.

329. Van de Ven PJ, Beutler JJ, Kaatee R, et al. Angiotensin converting enzyme inhibitor-induced renal dysfunction in atherosclerotic renovascular disease. *Kidney Int* 1998;53:986.

330. Anderson WP, Woods RL. Intrarenal effects of angiotensin II in renal artery stenosis. *Kidney Int* 1987;31[Suppl 20]:S157.

331. Erbslöh-Möller B, Dumas A, Roth D, et al. Furosemide 131I-hippuran renography after angiotensin-converting enzyme inhibition for the diagnosis of renovascular hypertension. *Am J Med* 1991;90:23.

332. Prigent A. The diagnosis of renovascular hypertension: the role of captopril renal scintigraphy and related issues. *Eur J Nucl Med* 1993;20:625.

333. Olin JW, Piedmonte MR, Young JR, et al. The utility of duplex ultrasound scanning of the renal arteries for diagnosing significant renal artery stenosis. *Ann Intern Med* 1995;122:833.

334. Bleyer AJ, Chen BS, D'Agostino RB, et al. Clinical correlates of hypertensive end-stage renal disease. *Am J Kidney Dis* 1998;31:28.

335. Meyrier A. Renal vascular lesions in the elderly: nephrosclerosis or atheromatous renal disease? *Nephrol Dial Transplant* 1996;11[Suppl 9]:45.

336. Kassirer JP. Atheroembolic renal disease. *N Engl J Med* 1969;280:812.

337. Morris GC Jr, Heider CF, Moyer JH. The protective effect of subfiltration arterial pressure on the kidney. *Surg Forum* 1995;6:623.

338. Schlanger LE, Haire HM, Zuckerman AM, et al. Reversible renal failure in an elderly woman with renal artery stenosis. *Am J Kidney Disease* 1994;23:123.

339. Beraud JJ, Calvet B, Durand A, et al. Reversal of acute renal failure following percutaneous transluminal recanalization of atherosclerotic renal artery occlusion. *J Hypertens* 1989;7:909.

340. Flye MW, Anderson RW, Fish JC, et al. Successful surgical treatment of anuria caused by renal artery occlusion. *Ann Surg* 1982;195:346.

341. O'Donohoe MK, Donohoe J, Corrigan TP. Acute renal failure of renovascular origin: cure by aortorenal reconstruction after 25 days of anuria. *Nephron* 1990;56:92.

342. Ramsey AG, D'Agati V, Dietz PA, et al. Renal functional recovery 47 days after renal artery occlusion. *Am J Nephrol* 1983;3:325.

343. Sandy DT, Vidt DG, Geisinger MA, et al. Serum creatinine prior to angioplasty (PTRA): a predictor of clinical success in atherosclerotic disease. *J Am Soc Nephrol* 1995;6:648.

344. Kuhn FP, Kutkuhn B, Toresello G, et al. Renal artery stenosis: preliminary results of treatment with the Strecker stint. *Radiology* 1991;180:367.

345. Dorros G, Jaff M, Dorros I, et al. Renal dysfunction is a poor prognosticator of patient survival after Palmaz stent revascularization for renal artery stenosis. *J Am Coll Cardiol* 1997;29:486A(abstr).

346. Couser WG. Idiopathic rapidly progressive glomerulonephritis. *Am J Nephrol* 1982;2:57.

347. Furci L, Medici G, Baraldi A, et al. Rapidly progressive glomerulonephritis in the elderly: long-term results. *Contrib Nephrol* 1993;105:98.

348. Jeffery RF, Gardiner DS, More IA, et al. Crescentic glomerulonephritis: experience of a single unit over a five year period. *Scot Med J* 1992;37:175.

349. Moorthy AV, Zimmerman SW. Renal disease in the elderly: clinicopathologic analysis of renal disease in 115 elderly patients. *Clin Nephrol* 1980;14:223.

350. Bergesio F, Bertoni E, Bandini S, et al. Changing pattern of glomerulonephritis in the elderly: a change of prevalence or a different approach? *Contrib Nephrol* 1993;105:75.

351. Haas M, Spargo BH, Wit E, et al. Etiologies and outcome of acute renal insufficiency in older adults: a renal biopsy study of 259 cases. *Am J Kidney Dis* 2000;35:433.

352. Bindi P, Mougenot B, Mentre F, et al. Necrotizing crescentic glomerulonephritis without significant immune deposits: a clinical and serological study [published erratum appears in *QJM* 1993;86: following 280] [see comments]. *QJM* 1993;86:55.

353. Donadio JV. Treatment and clinical outcome of glomerulonephritis in the elderly. *Contrib Nephrol* 1993;105:49.

354. Abrass CK. Glomerulonephritis in the elderly. *Am J Nephrol* 1985;5:409.

355. Arieff AI, Anderson RJ, Massry SG. Acute glomerulonephritis in the elderly. *Geriatrics* 1971;26:74.

356. Melby PC, Musick WD, Luger AM, et al. Poststreptococcal glomerulonephritis in the elderly. *Am J Nephrol* 1987;7:235.

357. Montoliu J, Darnell A, Torras A, et al. Acute and rapidly progressive forms of glomerulonephritis in the elderly. *J Am Geriatr Soc* 1981;29:108.

358. Washio M, Oh Y, Okuda S, et al. Clinicopathological study of poststreptococcal glomerulonephritis in the elderly. *Clin Nephrol* 1994;41:265.

359. Johnston PA, Brown JS, Davison AM. The nephrotic syndrome in the elderly: clinicopathologic correlations in 317 patients. *Geriatr Nephrol Urol* 1992;2:85.

360. Lustig S, Rosenfeld JB, BenBassat M, et al. Nephrotic syndrome in the elderly. *Isr J Med Sci* 1982;18:1010.

361. Fawcett IW, Hilton PJ, Jones NF, et al. Nephrotic syndrome in the elderly. *BMJ* 1971;2:387.

362. Huriet C, Rauber G, Kessler Cuny G, et al. Le syndrome nephrotique apres 60 ans, considerations etiologique d'apres une serie de 25 cas. *Ann Med Nancy* 1975;14:1021.

363. Ishimuto F, Shibasaki T, Nakano M, et al. Nephrotic syndrome in the elderly: a clinicopathological study. *Jpn J Nephrol* 1981;23:1251.

364. Kingswood JC, Banks RA, Tribe CR, et al. Renal biopsy in the elderly: clinicopathological correlations in 143 patients. *Clin Nephrol* 1984;22:183.

365. Lustig S, Rosenfeld J, Ben-Bassat M, et al. Nephrotic syndrome in the elderly. *Isr J Med Sci* 1982;18:1010.

366. Murphy PJ, Wright MG, Rai GS. Nephrotic syndrome in the elderly. *J Am Geriatr Soc* 1987;35:170.

367. Ozono Y, Harada T, Yamaguchi K, et al. Nephrotic syndrome in the elderly: clinicopathological study. *Jpn J Nephrol* 1994;36:44.
368. Sato H, Saito T, Furuyama T, et al. Histologic studies on the nephrotic syndrome in the elderly. *Tohoku J Exp Med* 1987;153:259.
369. Zech P, Colon S, Pointet P, et al. The nephrotic syndrome in adults aged over 60: etiology, evolution and treatment of 76 cases. *Clin Nephrol* 1982;17:232.
370. D'Agati V. The many masks of focal segmental glomerulosclerosis. *Kidney Int* 1994;46:1223.
371. Hostetter TH, Rennke HG, Brenner BM. The case for intrarenal hypertension in the initiation and progression of diabetic and other glomerulopathies. *Am J Med* 1985;72:375.
372. Thadhani R, Pascual M, Nickeleit V, et al. Preliminary description of focal segmental glomerulosclerosis in patients with renovascular disease. *Lancet* 1996;347:231.
373. Baylis C, Fredericks M, Leypoldt J, et al. The mechanisms of proteinuria in aging rats. *Mech Ageing Dev* 1988;45:111.
374. Bolton WK, Benton FR, Maclay JG, et al. Spontaneous glomerular sclerosis in aging Sprague-Dawley rats. *Am J Pathol* 1976;85:277.
375. Bolton WK, Sturgill BC. Spontaneous glomerular sclerosis in aging Sprague-Dawley rats. II. Ultrastructural studies. *Am J Pathol* 1980;98:339.
376. Couser WG, Stilmant MM. The immunopathology of the aging rat kidney. *J Gerontol* 1976;31:13.
377. Haley DP, Bulger RE. The aging male rat: structure and function of the kidney. *Am J Anat* 1983;167:1.
378. Meyer TW, Lawrence WE, Brenner BM. Dietary protein and the progression of renal disease. *Kidney Int* 1983;24:S243.
379. Yumura W, Sugino N, Nagasawa R, et al. Age-associated changes in renal glomeruli of mice. *Exp Gerontol* 1989;24:237.
380. Zent R, Nagai R, Cattran DC. Idiopathic membranous nephropathy in the elderly. *Am J Kidney Dis* 1997;29:200.
381. Ponticelli C, Attieri P, Scolari F, et al. A randomized study comparing methyl prednisolone plus chlorambucil versus methyl prednisolone plus cyclophosphamide in idiopathic membranous nephropathy. *J Am Soc Nephrol* 1998;9:444.
382. Eagen JW, Lewis EJ. Glomerulopathies of neoplasia. *Kidney Int* 1977;11:297.
383. Donadio JV. Treatment of glomerulonephritis in the elderly. *Am J Kidney Dis* 1990;16:307.
384. Agodoa L, Eggers P. Renal replacement therapy in the United States: data from the United States Renal Data System. *Am J Kidney Dis* 1995;25:119.
385. Nissenson A. Dialysis therapy in the elderly patient. *Kidney Int* 1993;43:S51.
386. Port F. Morbidity and mortality in dialysis patients. *Kidney Int* 1994;46:1728.
387. Gorban-Brennan N, Kliger A, Finkelstein F. CAPD therapy for patients over 80 years of age. *Perit Dial Int* 1993;13:140.
388. Ismail N, Hakim RM, Oreopoulos DG, et al. Renal replacement therapies in the elderly. Part 1: hemodialysis and chronic peritoneal dialysis. *Am J Kidney Dis* 1993;22:759.
389. Neves PL, Sousa A, Bernardo I, et al. Chronic haemodialysis for very old patients. *Age Ageing* 1994;23:356.
390. Vlachojannis J, Kurz P, Hoppe D. CAPD in elderly patients with cardiovascular risk factors. *Clin Nephrol* 1988;30:S13.
391. Williams AJ, Nicholl JP, El Nahas AM, et al. Continuous ambulatory peritoneal dialysis and hemodialysis in the elderly. *QJM* 1990;74:215.
392. Wolcott D, Nissenson A. Quality of life in chronic dialysis patients: a critical comparison of CAPD and hemodialysis. *Am J Kidney Dis* 1988;11:402.
393. Balaskas EV, Yuan ZY, Gupta A, et al. Long-term continuous ambulatory peritoneal dialysis in diabetics. *Clin Nephrol* 1994;42:54.
394. Lunde N, Port F, Wolfe R, et al. Comparison of mortality risk by choice of CAPD vs. hemodialysis in elderly patients. *Adv Perit Dial* 1991;7:68.
395. Maiorca R, Vonesh E, Cancarini GC, et al. A six year comparison of patient and technique survivals on CAPD and hemodialysis. *Kidney Int* 1988;34:518.
396. Maiorca R, Vonesh E, Cavalli P, et al. A multicenter, selection-adjusted comparison of patient and technique survivals on CAPD and hemodialysis [see comments]. *Perit Dial Int* 1991;11:118.
397. Held PJ, Port FK, Turenne MN, et al. Continuous ambulatory peritoneal dialysis and hemodialysis: comparison of patient mortality with adjustment for comorbid conditions. *Kidney Int* 1994;45:1163.
398. Cantarovich D, Baranger T, Tirouvanziam A, et al. One-hundred and five cadaveric kidney transplants with cyclosporine in recipients more than 60 years of age. *Transplant Proc* 1993;25:1323.
399. Ismail N, Hakim RM, Helderman JH. Renal replacement therapies in the elderly. Part 2: renal transplantation. *Am J Kidney Dis* 1994;23:1.
400. Johnson DW, Herzig K, Purdie D, et al. A comparison of the effects of dialysis and renal transplantation on the survival of older uremic patients. *Transplantation* 2000;69:794.
401. Nyberg G, Nilsson B, Hallste G, et al. Renal transplantation in elderly patients: survival and complications. *Transplant Proc* 1993;25:1062.
402. Meir-Kriesche HU, Ojo A, Hanson J, et al. Increased immunosuppressive vulnerability in elderly renal transplant recipients. *Transplantation* 2000;69:885.
403. Becker BN, Ismail N, Becker YT, et al. Renal transplantation in the older end stage renal disease patient. *Semin Nephrol* 1996;16:353.
404. Gardner ID. The effect of aging on susceptibility to infections. *Rev Infect Dis* 1980;2:801.
405. Sant GR. Urinary tract infection in the elderly. *Semin Urol* 1987;5:126.
406. Garibaldi RA, Nurse BA. Infections in the elderly. *Am J Med* 1986;81(1A):53.
407. Parson CL, Schmidt JD. Control of recurrent lower urinary tract infection in the post menopausal woman. *J Urol* 1982;128:1224.
408. Raz R, Stamm WA. A controlled trial of intravaginal estriol in postmenopausal women with recurrent urinary tract infections. *N Engl J Med* 1993;329:753.
409. Garibaldi RA, Brodine S, Matsumiya S. Infections among patients in nursing homes: policies, prevalence, problems. *N Engl J Med* 1981;305:731.
410. Kaye D. Urinary tract infections in the elderly. *Bull NY Acad Med* 1980;56:209.
411. Dontas AS, Kasviki-Charvati P, Papanayiotiu PC. Bacteriuria and survival in old age. *N Engl J Med* 1981;304:939.
412. Nordenstram GR, Brandberg CA, Odin AS, et al. Bacteriuria and mortality in an elderly population. *N Engl J Med* 1986;314:1152.
413. Abrutyn E, Mossey J, Berlin JA, et al. Does asymptomatic bacteriuria predict mortality and does treatment reduce mortality in elderly ambulatory women? *Ann Intern Med* 1994;120:827.
414. Nicolle LL, Bjornson J, Harding K. Bacteriuria in elderly institutionalized men. *N Engl J Med* 1983;309:1420.
415. Stamm W, Hooton T. Management of urinary tract infections in adults. *N Engl J Med* 1993;329:1328.
416. Abrutyn E, Boscia JA, Kaye D. The treatment of asymptomatic bacteriuria in the elderly. *J Am Geriatr Soc* 1988;36:473.
417. Boscia JA, Abrutyn E, Kaye D. Asymptomatic bacteriuria in elderly persons: treat or do not treat? *Ann Intern Med* 1987;106:764.
418. Kissane JM. The morphology of renal cystic disease. *Perspect Nephrol Hypertens* 1976;4:31.
419. Ravine D, Gibson RN, Donlan J, et al. An ultrasound renal cyst prevalence survey: specificity data for inherited renal cystic diseases. *Am J Kidney Dis* 1993;22:803.

Disorders of Electrolyte, Water, and Acid–Base

CHAPTER 82

Mechanisms of Diuretic Action

David H. Ellison, Mark D. Okusa, and Robert W. Schrier

The term diuretic derives from the Greek *diouretikos,* which means "to promote urine." Even though many substances promote urine flow, the term *diuretic* is usually taken to indicate a substance that can reduce the extracellular fluid volume by increasing urinary solute and water excretion. In 1553, Paracelsus recorded the first truly effective form of therapy for dropsy (edema), namely inorganic mercury (Calomel). Inorganic mercury remained the mainstay of diuretic treatment until the beginning of this century. In 1919, the ability of organic mercurial antisyphilitics to effect diuresis was discovered by Vogl, then a medical student (1). This observation led to the development of effective organic mercurial diuretics that continued to be used through the 1960s. In 1937, the antimicrobial, sulfanilamide, was found to cause metabolic acidosis. Carbonic anhydrase, which had been discovered in 1932, was inhibited by sulfanilamide. Pitts demonstrated that sulfanilamide inhibited Na bicarbonate reabsorption in dogs and Schwartz showed that sulfanilamide could induce diuresis when administered to patients with congestive heart failure. Soon, more potent sulfonamide-based carbonic anhydrase inhibitors were developed, but these drugs suffered from side effects and limited potency. Nevertheless, a group at Sharp & Dohme, Inc. was stimulated by these developments to explore the possibility that modification of sulfonamide-based drugs could lead to drugs that enhanced Na *chloride* rather than Na *bicarbonate* excretion. The result of this program was the synthesis of chlorothiazide and its marketing in 1957. This drug ushered in the modern era of diuretic therapy and revolutionized the clinical treatment of edema.

The search for more potent classes of diuretics led to the development of ethacrynic acid and furosemide in the United States and Germany, respectively (1). The safety and efficacy of these drugs led them to replace the organic mercu-

rials as drugs of first choice for severe and resistant edema. Spironolactone, marketed in 1961, was developed after the properties and structure of aldosterone had been discovered and steroidal analogs of aldosterone were found to have aldosterone-blocking activity. Triamterene was initially synthesized as a folic acid antagonist, but was found to have diuretic and K sparing activity.

The availability of safe, effective, and relatively inexpensive diuretic drugs has made it possible to treat edematous disorders and hypertension effectively. Driven by clinical need, the development of effective diuretic drugs led to the synthesis of ligands that interact specifically with Na and Cl transport proteins in the kidney. During the past 10 years, these ligands were used to identify and clone the Na and Cl transport proteins that mediate the bulk of renal Na and Cl reabsorption. The diuretic-sensitive transport proteins that have been cloned include the sodium hydrogen exchanger (NHE) family of proteins, the bumetanide-sensitive Na-K-2Cl cotransporters, the thiazide-sensitive Na-Cl cotransporter, and the epithelial Na channel. The information derived from molecular cloning has also permitted identification of inherited human diseases that are caused by mutations in transport proteins. The phenotypes of several of these disorders resemble the manifestations of chronic diuretic administration. Thus, the development of clinically useful diuretics permitted identification and later cloning of specific ion transport pathways. The molecular cloning is now helping to define mechanisms of diuretic action and diuretic side effects. The use of animals in which diuretic-sensitive transport pathways have been "knocked out" should permit a clearer understanding of which diuretic effects result directly or secondarily from actions of the drugs on specific ion transport pathways and which effects result from actions on other pathways or other organ systems.

D. H. Ellison: Division of Nephrology and Hypertension, Oregon Health and Science University, Portland, Oregon

M. D. Okusa: Division of Nephrology, University of Virginia School of Medicine, Charlottesville, Virginia

R. W. Schrier: Department of Medicine, University of Colorado Health Sciences Center, Denver, Colorado

NORMAL RENAL NACL HANDLING

The normal human kidneys filter approximately 23 moles of NaCl in 150 L of fluid each day. Approximately 10 g of salt (NaCl = 170 mmol = 4 g Na) are consumed each day by individuals on a typical Western diet. To maintain balance, renal NaCl excretion must be approximately 160 mmol/day (the difference owing to nonrenal losses). Under normal circumstances, approximately 99.2% of the filtered NaCl is reabsorbed by kidney tubules generating a normal fractional sodium excretion of less than 1%. Sodium, chloride, and water reabsorption by the nephron is driven by the metabolic energy provided by ATP. The ouabain-sensitive Na/K ATPase is expressed at the basolateral cell membrane of all Na transporting epithelial cells along the nephron. This pump maintains large ion gradients across the plasma membrane, with the intracellular Na concentration maintained low and the intracellular K concentration maintained high. Because the pump is electrogenic and because it associates with a K channel in the same membrane, renal epithelial cells have a voltage across the plasma membrane oriented with the inside negative relative to the outside.

The combination of the low intracellular Na concentration and the plasma membrane voltage generates a large electrochemical gradient favoring Na entry from lumen or interstitium. Specific diuretic-sensitive Na transport pathways are expressed at the apical (luminal) surface of cells along the nephron, permitting vectorial transport of Na from lumen to blood. Along the proximal tubule, where approximately 50% to 60% of filtered Na is reabsorbed, an isoform of the Na/H exchanger is expressed at the apical membrane (2). Along the thick ascending limb, where approximately 25% of filtered Na is reabsorbed, an isoform of the Na-K-2Cl cotransporter is expressed at the apical membrane (3,4). Along the distal convoluted tubule, where approximately 5% of filtered Na is reabsorbed, the thiazide-sensitive Na-Cl cotransporter is expressed (5,6). Along the connecting tubule and cortical collecting duct, where approximately 3% of filtered Na is reabsorbed, the amiloride-sensitive epithelial Na channel is expressed (7). These apical Na transport pathways form the targets for diuretic action.

This chapter discusses the molecular and physiologic bases for diuretic action in the kidney. Although some aspects of clinical diuretic usage are discussed, we have emphasized physiologic principles and mechanisms of action. Several recent texts provide detailed discussions of diuretic treatment of clinical conditions (8). Extensive discussions of diuretic pharmacokinetics are also available (9).

A rational classification of diuretic drugs (Table 82-1) is based on the primary nephron site of action. Such a scheme emphasizes, first, that more than one chemical class of drugs can affect the same ion transport mechanism. Second, although most diuretic drugs affect transport processes of several nephron segments, most owe their clinical effects primarily to their ability to inhibit Na transport by one particular nephron segment. An exception is the osmotic diuretics. Although these drugs initially were believed to inhibit solute and water flux primarily along the proximal tubule, subsequent studies have revealed effects in multiple segments. Other diuretics, however, will be classified according to their primary site of action.

OSMOTIC DIURETICS

Osmotic diuretics are substances that are freely filtered at the glomerulus, but are poorly reabsorbed (Fig. 82-1). The pharmacologic activity of drugs in this group depends entirely on the osmotic pressure exerted by the drug molecules in solution. It does not depend on interaction with specific transport proteins or enzymes. Mannitol is the prototypical osmotic diuretic (10). Because the relationship between the magnitude of diuretic effect and concentration of osmotic diuretic in solution is linear, all osmotic diuretics are small molecules. Other agents considered in this class include urea, sorbitol, and glycerol.

TABLE 82-1. *Effects of diuretics on electrolyte excretion*

	Na	Cl	K	Pi	Ca	Mg
Osmotic diuretics (14;15;229;4;36;437)	⇑ (10%–25%)	⇑ (15%–30%)	⇑ (6%)	⇑ (5%–10%)	⇑ (10%–20%)	⇑ (>20%)
Carbonic anhydrase inhibitors (55;144;229)	⇑ (6%)	⇑ (4%)	⇑ (60%)	⇑ (>20%)	⇑ or ⇔ (<5%)	⇑ (<5%)
Loop diuretics (141;142;144;207; 229;402)	⇑ (30%)	⇑ (40%)	⇑ (60%–100%)	⇑ (>20%)	⇑ (>20%)	⇑ (>20%)
DCT diuretics (142;207;229;230)	⇑ (6%–11%)	⇑ (10%)	⇑ (200%)	⇑ (>20%)	⇓	⇑ (5%–10%)
Na channel blockers (207;229;402)	⇑ (3%–5%)	⇑ (6%)	⇓ (8%)	⇔	⇔	⇓
Spironolactone (229)	⇑ (3%)	⇑ (6%)	⇓	⇔	⇔	⇓

Figures indicate approximate maximal fractional excretions of ions following acute diuretic administration in maximally effective doses. ⇑ indicates that the drug increases excretion; ⇓ indicates that the drug decreases excretion; ⇔ indicates that the drug has little of no direct effect on excretion. During chronic treatment, effects often wane (Na excretion), may increase (K excretion during DCT diuretic treatment), or may reverse as with uric acid (not shown).

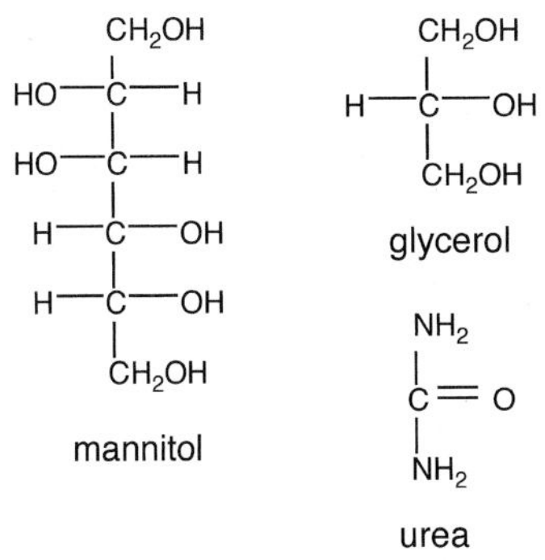

FIG. 82-1. Structures of osmotic diuretics.

Urinary Electrolyte Excretion

Ion transport is affected, although osmotic agents do not act directly on transport pathways. Following mannitol infusion, sodium, potassium, calcium, magnesium, bicarbonate, and chloride excretion rates increase (Table 82-1) (11–13). Rates of sodium and water fractional reabsorption are reduced by 27% and 12%, respectively, following the infusion of mannitol (14). Reabsorption of magnesium and calcium also is reduced in the proximal tubule and loop of Henle. In contrast, phosphate reabsorption is only inhibited slightly by mannitol in the presence of parathyroid hormone (11).

Mechanism of Action

The functional consequences that result from intravenous infusion of mannitol include an increase in cortical and medullary blood flow, a variable effect on glomerular filtration rate, an increase in sodium, water, calcium, magnesium, phosphorus, and bicarbonate excretion, and a decrease in medullary concentration gradient. The most pronounced effect observed with mannitol is a brisk diuresis and natriuresis. The mechanisms by which mannitol produces a diuresis include: (a) an increase in osmotic pressure in the lumens of the proximal tubule and loop of Henle, thereby retarding the passive reabsorption of water, and (b) an increase in renal blood flow and washout of medullary tonicity.

Mannitol is freely filtered at the glomerulus and its presence in tubule fluid minimizes passive water reabsorption. Normally, within the proximal tubule, sodium reabsorption creates an osmotic gradient for water reabsorption. When an osmotic diuretic is administered, however, the osmotic force of the nonreabsorbable solute in the lumen opposes the osmotic force produced by sodium reabsorption (15). Isosmolality of tubule fluid is preserved because molecules of mannitol replace sodium ions reabsorbed. However, sodium reabsorption eventually stops because the luminal sodium concentration is reduced to a point where a limiting gradient is reached and net transport of sodium and water ceases (11,14). This view was confirmed by stationary micropuncture studies (16). Quantitatively, mannitol has a greater effect on inhibiting Na and water reabsorption in the loop of Henle than in the proximal tubule. Free-flow micropuncture studies following mannitol infusion in dogs demonstrated a modest decrease in fractional reabsorption of sodium and water by the proximal tubule, but a much larger effect by the loop of Henle (11,14). Within the loop of Henle the site of action of mannitol appears to be restricted to the thin descending limb, resulting in a decrease in reabsorption of Na and water (17). In the thick ascending limb, reabsorption of Na continues in proportion to its delivery to this segment. The sum of net transport in the thin and thick limbs determines the net effect of mannitol in the loop of Henle. Further downstream in the collecting duct, mannitol reduces sodium and water reabsorption (18).

Renal Hemodynamics

During the administration of mannitol, its molecules diffuse from the bloodstream into the interstitial space. In the interstitial space, the increased osmotic pressure draws water from the cells to increase extracellular fluid volume. This effect increases total renal plasma flow (18). Cortical and medullary blood flow both increase following mannitol infusion (18,19). Single nephron glomerular filtration rate (GFR), on the other hand, increases in cortex and decreases in medulla (17,20); this action on the medulla washes out the medullary osmotic gradient by reducing papillary sodium and urea content (21–23). Experimental studies indicate that the osmotic effect of mannitol to increase water movement from intracellular to extracellular space leads to a decrease in hematocrit and blood viscosity. This fact contributes to a decrease in renal vascular resistance and increase in renal blood flow (22). In addition, secretion of vasodilatory substances is stimulated by mannitol infusion. Both prostacyclin (PGI2) (24) and atrial natriuretic peptide (25) could mediate the effect of mannitol on renal blood flow. The vasodilatory effect of mannitol is reduced when the recipient is pretreated with indomethacin or meclofenamate, suggesting that PGI2 is involved in the vasodilatory effect.

The effect of mannitol on GFR has been variable but most studies indicate that the overall effect is to increase GFR (10,14,26–28). Whereas mannitol was shown to increase both cortical and medullary blood flow, it increased cortical but decreased medullary single nephron GFR (17,20). The mechanisms by which mannitol reduces the GFR of deep nephrons are not known, but it has been postulated that mannitol reduces efferent arteriolar pressure. Micropuncture studies examining the determinants of GFR in superficial nephrons have demonstrated that the increase in single nephron GFR results from an increase in single nephron plasma flow and a decrease in oncotic pressure (28).

Alterations in renal hemodynamics contribute to the diuresis observed following administration of mannitol. An increase in medullary blood flow rate reduces medullary tonicity (23) primarily by decreasing papillary sodium and urea content (29) and increasing urine flow rate (22).

Pharmacokinetics

Mannitol is not readily absorbed from the intestine (10); therefore, it is routinely administered intravenously. Following infusion, mannitol distributes in extracellular fluid with a volume of distribution of approximately 16 L (30); its excretion is almost entirely by glomerular filtration (31). Of the filtered load, less than 10% is reabsorbed by the renal tubule, and a similar quantity is metabolized, probably in the liver. With normal glomerular filtration rate, plasma half-life is approximately 2.2 hours.

Clinical Use

Mannitol is used prophylactically or as treatment for established acute renal failure (10,32), although the basis for its use in established acute renal failure remains controversial (33,34). Mannitol improves renal hemodynamics in a variety of situations of impending or incipient acute renal failure. Mannitol (along with hydration and sodium bicarbonate) has been recommended for the early treatment in myoglobinuric acute renal failure (35) and in the prevention of posttransplant acute renal failure (36–38). Although some studies have shown a beneficial effect when used prophylactically to treat patients at risk for contrast nephropathy (39), other prospective controlled studies have not found mannitol beneficial in preventing acute renal failure (33,40).

Mannitol is used for short-term reduction of intraocular pressure (41). By increasing the osmotic pressure, mannitol reduces the volume of aqueous humor and the intraocular pressure by extracting water. Mannitol also decreases cerebral edema and the increase in intracranial pressure associated with trauma, tumors, and neurosurgical procedures (42). Mannitol is used perioperatively to treat patients undergoing cardiopulmonary bypass surgery. The beneficial effects may relate to its osmotic activity, thereby reducing intravenous fluid requirement (43) and its ability to act as a free radical antioxidant (44). Mannitol and other osmotic agents have been used to treat dialysis disequilibrium (45,46). This syndrome is characterized by acute symptoms during or immediately following hemodialysis. Most significant symptoms are attributable to disorders of the central nervous system such as: headache, nausea, blurred vision, confusion, seizure, coma, and death. Rapid removal of small solutes such as urea during dialysis of patients who are markedly azotemic is associated with the development of an osmotic gradient for water movement into brain cells producing cerebral edema and neurologic dysfunction. Dialysis disequilibrium syndrome can be minimized by slow solute removal and raising plasma osmolality with saline or mannitol.

Adverse Effects

Patients who have a reduced cardiac output may develop pulmonary edema when mannitol is infused. Intravenous mannitol administration increases cardiac output and pulmonary capillary wedge pressures (30). Acute and prolonged administration of mannitol leads to different electrolyte disturbances. Acute overzealous use or the accumulation of mannitol leads to dilutional metabolic acidosis and hyponatremia (47). Accumulation of mannitol also produces hyperkalemia (48,49) as a result of an increase in plasma osmolality. An increase in plasma osmolality increases potassium movement from intracellular to extracellular fluid from bulk solute flow and increase in the electrochemical gradient for potassium secretion. Prolonged administration of mannitol can lead to urinary losses of sodium and potassium leading to volume depletion, hypernatremia (as urinary loss of sodium is invariably less than water), and hypokalemia (50). Marked accumulation of mannitol in patients can lead to reversible acute renal failure that appears to be caused by vasoconstriction and tubular vacuolization (51–53). Mannitol-induced acute renal failure usually occurs when large cumulative doses of approximately 295 g are given to patients with previously compromised renal function (51).

PROXIMAL TUBULE DIURETICS (CARBONIC ANHYDRASE INHIBITORS)

Through the development of carbonic anhydrase inhibitors, important compounds were discovered that have utility as therapeutic agents and research tools. Carbonic anhydrase inhibitors have a limited therapeutic role as diuretic agents; however, because of that they are only weakly natriuretic. They are used primarily to reduce intraocular pressure in glaucoma and enhance bicarbonate excretion in metabolic alkalosis. Carbonic anhydrase inhibitors have been useful in developing other diuretic agents such as thiazide and loop diuretics and have been instrumental in elucidating transport mechanisms in proximal and distal nephron segments. Structures of carbonic anhydrase inhibitors are shown in Fig. 82-2.

Urinary Electrolyte Excretion

Through their effects on carbonic anhydrase in the proximal tubule, carbonic anhydrase inhibitors increase bicarbonate excretion by 25% to 30% (Table 82-1) (54–56). The increase in sodium and chloride excretion is minimal because these ions are reabsorbed by more distal segments

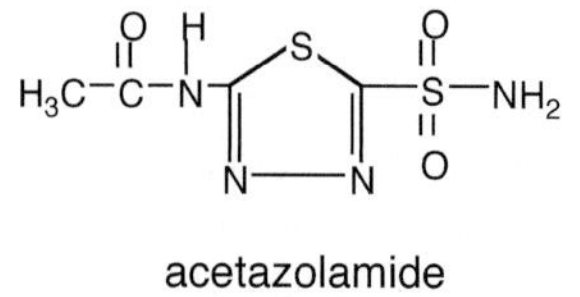

acetazolamide

FIG. 82-2. Structure of carbonic anhydrase inhibitor.

of the nephron (56). However, a residual small but variable amount of sodium is excreted along with bicarbonate. Rates of calcium and phosphate reabsorption are also blocked along the proximal tubule by carbonic anhydrase inhibitors. Because distal calcium reabsorption is stimulated, however, fractional calcium excretion does not increase (57). In contrast, phosphate appears to escape distal reabsorption following acetazolamide administration resulting, in an increase in fractional excretion of phosphate by approximately 3% (57,58). Although carbonic anhydrase inhibitors hinder proximal tubule magnesium transport, fractional excretion is either unchanged or increased as a result of variable distal reabsorption (58).

Carbonic anhydrase inhibitors increase potassium excretion (56,58–60). It is likely that several indirect effects of carbonic anhydrase inhibition contribute to the observed kaliuresis. Carbonic anhydrase inhibition could block proximal tubule potassium reabsorption and increase delivery to the distal tubule, but this has not been established clearly. Whereas carbonic anhydrase inhibitors decrease proximal tubule sodium, bicarbonate and water absorption during both free flow micropuncture and microperfusion, the effects of carbonic anhydrase inhibitors on proximal tubule potassium transport have been less consistent. In *free flow* micropuncture studies carbonic anhydrase inhibition did not affect proximal tubule potassium reabsorption (61), whereas carbonic anhydrase inhibition of *perfused* proximal tubules reduces net potassium transport (62). The effect of carbonic anhydrase inhibitors on the proximal tubule ion transport does, however, facilitate an increase in tubular fluid flow rate and sodium and bicarbonate but not chloride delivery to the distal nephron. This effect is thought to increase the concentration of nonreabsorbable anions in the distal tubule lumen, creating an increase in lumen-negative voltage (59) and increase in flow rate (63), factors known to increase potassium secretion by the distal tubule. Carbonic anhydrase inhibitors can also produce a luminal composition that is low in chloride and high in nonchloride anion. This luminal fluid composition has been demonstrated to stimulate potassium secretion by the distal nephron independent of a change in lumen-negative voltage (64).

Mechanism of Action

In the kidney, carbonic anhydrase inhibitors act primarily on proximal tubule cells to inhibit bicarbonate absorption. Carbonic anhydrase, a metalloenzyme containing one zinc atom per molecule, is important in sodium bicarbonate reabsorption and hydrogen ion secretion by renal epithelial cells. The biochemical, morphologic, and functional properties of carbonic anhydrase have been reviewed previously (65–67). Of the four major isozymes of carbonic anhydrase expressed in mammalian tissues, two appear relevant for luminal acidification in kidney. Type II carbonic anhydrase is distributed widely, comprising more than 95% of the overall activity in kidney and is sensitive to inhibition by sulfonamides (65,68).

Type II carbonic anhydrase is expressed in the cytoplasm and facilitates the secretion of H ions by catalyzing the formation of HCO_3 from OH and CO_2 (Eq. 3). Type IV carbonic anhydrase is bound to renal cortical membranes, comprising up to 5% of the overall activity in kidney, and is sensitive to sulfonamides (69,70). Type IV carbonic anhydrase, expressed on basolateral and luminal plasma membranes of proximal tubule cells (66,71,72) and luminal membrane of intercalated cells (73), catalyzes the dehydration of intraluminal carbonic acid generated from secreted protons (65,74). Evidence for the physiologic importance for carbonic anhydrase is apparent because a deficiency of Type II carbonic anhydrase leads to a renal acidification defect resulting in renal tubular acidosis (75). Furthermore, metabolic acidosis leads to an adaptive increase in both Type II and IV carbonic anhydrase mRNA expression in kidney (76), suggesting the importance of both carbonic anhydrase isoforms in this disorder.

Normally the proximal tubule reabsorbs 80% of the filtered load of sodium bicarbonate and 60% of the filtered load of sodium chloride. Early studies by Pitts and colleagues (77,78) and micropuncture studies indicated that hydrogen ion secretion was responsible for bicarbonate absorption and renal acidification (78–81). The cellular mechanism by which proximal tubules reabsorb bicarbonate is depicted in Fig. 82-3. The effect of carbonic anhydrase to accelerate bicarbonate is a result of the reactions that occur in both luminal fluid and in the cell. The mechanism of carbonic anhydrase action in luminal fluid (82), is shown in the following, where E represents the carbonic anhydrase enzyme:

Luminal Fluid

$$EH_2O + HCO_3^- \quad \Leftrightarrow \quad H_2O + CO_2 + EOH \qquad [1]$$

$$EOH + H^+ \quad \Leftrightarrow \quad EH_2O \qquad [2]$$

$$HCO_3^- + H^+ \quad \Leftrightarrow \quad CO_2 + H_2O \qquad [3]$$

Note that the addition of reactions 1 and 2 leads to the classic reaction 3. In this scheme, the enzyme is viewed as a superhydroxylator.

Luminal carbonic anhydrase prevents H from accumulating in tubule fluid, which would eventually stop all Na/H exchange (79). Once formed, carbon dioxide rapidly diffuses from the lumen into the cell across the apical membrane.

The mechanism by which intracellular carbonic anhydrase participates in net H^+ secretion is functionally the reverse of the reactions shown in the preceding.

Intracellular fluid

$$EH_2O \quad \Leftrightarrow \quad EOH + H^+ \qquad [2R]$$

$$EOH + H_2O + CO_2 \quad \Leftrightarrow \quad EH_2O + HCO_3^- \qquad [1R]$$

$$CO_2 + H_2O \quad \Leftrightarrow \quad HCO_3^- + H^+ \qquad [3R]$$

In this case, the enzyme splits water, thereby providing an hydroxyl ion to form bicarbonate. The bicarbonate ions then exit the basolateral membrane via $Na(HCO_3)_3$ cotransport (83–87). Thus in the early proximal tubule, the net effect

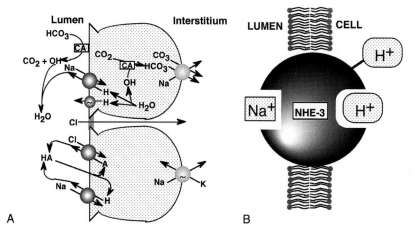

FIG. 82-3. Mechanisms of diuretic action in the proximal tubule. **A:** Functional models of cells along the early portion *(top cell)* and later portion *(bottom cell)* of the proximal tubule. Some transport proteins are omitted from each cell for clarity. Water splits into H and OH inside of proximal cells. Carbonic anhydrase (CA) catalyzes the formation of HCO_3 from OH and CO_2. Bicarbonate leaves the cell via the Na, HCO_3, CO_3 cotransporter (Based on information from Soleimani M, Grassl SM, Aronson PS. Stoichiometry of $Na + HCO_3^-$ cotransport in basolateral membrane vesicles isolated from rabbit renal cortex. *J Clin Invest* 1987;79:1276; Soleimani M, Aronson PS. Ionic mechanism of Na^+-HCO_3^- cotransport in rabbit renal basolateral membrane vesicles. *J Biol Chem* 1989;264:18302). A second pool of carbonic anhydrase is located in the brush border. This participates in disposing of filtered bicarbonate. Both pools of carbonic anhydrase are inhibited by acetazolamide and other carbonic anhydrase inhibitors (see text for details). Along the later portion of the proximal tubule, a component of Cl absorption is transcellular. **B:** A model of the Na/H exchanger, NHE-3.

of the process described results in the isosmotic reabsorption of $NaHCO_3$. The lumen chloride concentration increases because water continues to be reabsorbed, producing a lumen-positive potential (88). These axial changes provide an electrochemical gradient for transport of chloride via paracellular and transcellular pathways. The latter pathway for chloride likely involves a chloride/base exchanger operating in parallel with a Na/H proton exchanger (89,90). The dual operation of these parallel exchangers results in net NaCl absorption.

Carbonic anhydrase inhibitors act primarily on proximal tubule cells (91), where approximately 60% of the filtered load of sodium chloride is reabsorbed (92,93). The natriuretic potency of carbonic anhydrase inhibitors is relatively weak, however, despite the magnitude of sodium chloride reabsorption in the proximal tubule segment. Several factors explain this observation. First, proximal sodium reabsorption is generated by carbonic anhydrase-independent as well as carbonic anhydrase-dependent pathways. Second, these distal nephron segments largely reabsorb the increased sodium delivery to distal nephron segments (55–57). Third, carbonic anhydrase inhibitors generate a hyperchloremic metabolic acidosis further reducing the effects of subsequent doses of carbonic anhydrase inhibitor (94). Recent studies demonstrated that metabolic acidosis produces resistance of bicarbonate absorption to carbonic anhydrase inhibition (95). Following the induction of metabolic acidosis, the K_i for bicarbonate absorption by membrane impermeant carbonic anhydrase inhibitors was increased by a factor of 100 to 500, suggesting that metabolic acidosis is associated with changes in the physical properties of the carbonic anhydrase protein (95).

For these reasons, carbonic anhydrase inhibitors alone are rarely used as diuretic agents.

Following carbonic anhydrase inhibitor administration, proximal tubule bicarbonate reabsorption declines between 35% and 85% (54,81,96–100). Additional sites of action of carbonic anhydrase inhibitors include proximal straight tubule or loop of Henle (81,100,101), distal tubule (74), and the collecting and papillary collecting ducts (101–105). Yet, despite the effect of carbonic anhydrase inhibitors on proximal tubules as well as other nephron segments, compensatory reabsorption of bicarbonate at other downstream tubular sites limits net fractional excretion of bicarbonate to approximately 25% to 30%, even during acute administration (54,55).

The relative contributions of membrane-bound and intracellular components of cellular carbonic anhydrase have been examined. Both species contribute to bicarbonate absorption. Rector, Carter, and Seldin first suggested the role of membrane-bound carbonic anhydrase (80). The observation that carbonic anhydrase inhibitors produce an acid disequilibrium pH in the proximal tubule suggested that luminal fluid is normally in contact with carbonic anhydrase. Disequilibrium pH refers to the difference between the pH of tubule fluid *in situ* (pH_{is}) and the pH achieved after the tubule fluid is allowed to reach chemical equilibrium at known pCO_2. Thus in the presence of carbonic anhydrase, the pH measured in situ and at equilibrium should be similar. In the absence of carbonic anhydrase, the dehydration of H_2CO_3 to H_2O and CO_2 is slow, allowing H to accumulate in the lumen and reducing pH. The demonstration of an acid disequilibrium pH provided physiologic evidence in support of previous histochemical findings that a fraction of enzymatic activity was present in the tubule lumen. Although the cytoplasmic carbonic anhydrase constitutes the majority of enzyme activity in kidney, it is believed that the membrane-bound carbonic anhydrase plays a significant role in bicarbonate reabsorption by the proximal tubule. Studies addressing this question have employed carbonic anhydrase inhibitors that differ in their ability to penetrate proximal tubule cell membranes. Benzolamide is charged at normal pH and does not penetrate cell membranes well, whereas acetazolamide enters the cell relatively easily (106). Both intravenous (80,107) and intratubular administration of benzolamide (97) lead to an acid disequilibrium pH, indicating that luminal carbonic anhydrase inhibition contributes to bicarbonate absorption. Furthermore proximal tubular perfusion of benzolamide resulted in 90% inhibition of bicarbonate reabsorption. Despite near equal efficacy in inhibiting proximal tubule bicarbonate reabsorption, benzolamide lowered tubular fluid pH, whereas acetazolamide increased tubular fluid pH. These results suggest that the site of action of benzolamide is the brush border, whereas the site of action of acetazolamide is largely cellular. Inhibition of luminal carbonic anhydrase causes lumen pH to decrease because of the continued secretion of hydrogen ions and its accumulation in the tubular lumen. In contrast, acetazolamide does not produce an acid disequilibrium pH (97). The conclusion that tubular fluid is in direct contact with membrane carbonic anhydrase was substantiated by the use of dextran-bound carbonic anhydrase inhibitor (97,108). In proximal tubules perfused *in vivo,* Lucci and associates determined that dextran bound inhibitors, which inhibit only luminal carbonic anhydrase, decreased proximal tubule bicarbonate absorption by approximately 80% and reduced lumen pH.

Although these studies establish the importance of luminal carbonic anhydrase, they also support a role for intracellular or basolateral carbonic anhydrase. The observation that both acetazolamide and benzolamide inhibit proximal tubule bicarbonate reabsorption to a similar degree yet produce opposite effects on tubule fluid pH suggests that intracellular carbonic anhydrase contributes to proximal tubule luminal acidification.

The expression of carbonic anhydrase in the basolateral membrane of proximal tubule cells (71,72) suggests that this membrane-bound enzyme has an important role in basolateral bicarbonate transport (65,109). Carbonic anhydrase inhibitors, however, do not directly inhibit the basolateral bicarbonate exit transport system, $Na(HCO_3)$, but rather they inhibit intracellular generation of substrate for the transporter (110,111).

In the collecting duct, carbonic anhydrase facilitates acid secretion that is mediated by a vacuolar H adenosine triphosphatase (H-ATPase) (112) and a P-type gastric H-K-ATPase (113–115). Luminal administration of acetazolamide produced an acid disequilibrium pH in the outer medullary-collecting duct suggesting the contribution of luminal carbonic anhydrase (116). In recent studies, a membrane impermeant carbonic anhydrase inhibitor (F-3500; aminobenzolamide coupled to a nontoxic polymer polyoxyethylene) reduced bicarbonate absorption, thus confirming the presence of membrane bound carbonic anhydrase in the outer medullary-collecting duct (95). The K_i for inhibition of bicarbonate absorption was $5\mu M$, consistent with the inhibition of Type IV carbonic anhydrase.

Renal Hemodynamics

Inhibition of carbonic anhydrase decreases glomerular filtration rate (GFR) acutely by activating tubuloglomerular feedback (TGF) (62,117–119). Systemic acetazolamide infusion decreased GFR by 30%. Single nephron glomerular filtration rate (SNGFR) was 23% lower during acetazolamide infusion because increased solute delivery to the macula densa activates the TGF mechanism, which reduces GFR. Similar results were observed following infusion of benzolamide (118,119). Sar-ala[8]-angiotensin I, an angiotensin II antagonist, prevented the decrease in SGNFR, suggesting the involvement of local angiotensin II in response to benzolamide (118).

Pharmacokinetics

Acetazolamide is well absorbed from the gastrointestinal (GI) tract. More than 90% of the drug is plasma protein bound. The highest concentrations are found in tissues that contain large amounts of carbonic anhydrase (e.g., renal cortex, red blood cells). Renal effects are noticeable within 30 minutes and are usually maximal at 2 hours. Acetazolamide is not metabolized but is excreted rapidly by glomerular filtration and proximal tubular secretion. The half-life is approximately 5 hours and renal excretion is essentially complete in 24 hours (31). In comparison, methazolamide is absorbed more slowly from the GI tract, and its duration of action is long, with a half-life of approximately 14 hours.

Adverse Effects

Generally, carbonic anhydrase inhibitors are well tolerated with infrequent serious adverse effects. Side effects of carbonic anhydrase inhibitors may arise from the continued excretion of electrolytes. Significant hypokalemia and metabolic acidosis may develop (56). In elderly patients with glaucoma treated with acetazolamide (250 mg to 1,000 mg/day), metabolic acidosis was a frequent finding in comparison to a control group (120). Acetazolamide is also associated with nephrocalcinosis and nephrolithiasis owing to its effects on urine pH, facilitating stone formation (121). Premature infants treated with furosemide and acetazolamide are particularly susceptible to nephrocalcinosis, presumably because of the combined effect of an alkaline urine and hypercalciuria (122). Other adverse effects include drowsiness, fatigue, central nervous system depression, and paresthesias. Bone marrow suppression has been reported (123,124).

Clinical Use

The popularity of carbonic anhydrase inhibitors as diuretics has waned owing to the development of agents that are more effective with fewer toxic side effects. In general, tolerance develops rapidly and renders these drugs less effective. Daily use produces systemic acidemia from an increase in urinary excretion of bicarbonate. Nevertheless, acetazolamide can be administered for short-term therapy, usually in combination with other diuretics to patients who are resistant or do not respond adequately to other agents. The rationale for using a combination of diuretic agents is based on summation of their effect at different sites along the nephron. In addition to its use as a diuretic agent, carbonic anhydrase inhibitors are used in a number of other clinical situations.

The major indication for the use of acetazolamide as a diuretic agent is in the treatment of patients with metabolic alkalosis accompanied by edematous states (66,125) or chronic obstructive lung disease (126,127). In patients with cirrhosis, congestive heart failure, or nephrotic syndrome, aggressive diuresis with loop diuretics promotes intravascular volume depletion, secondary hyperaldosteronism and renal insufficiency, conditions that promote metabolic alkalosis. Administration of sodium chloride to correct the metabolic alkalosis may exacerbate edema. Acetazolamide can improve metabolic alkalosis by decreasing proximal tubule bicarbonate reabsorption, thereby increasing the fractional excretion of bicarbonate. An increase in urinary pH (>7.0) indicates enhanced bicarbonaturia. However, it should be noted that potassium depletion should be corrected prior to acetazolamide use because acetazolamide will increase potassium excretion. The time course of acetazolamide effect is rapid. In critically ill patients on ventilators, following the correction of fluid and electrolyte disturbances, intravenous acetazolamide produced an initial effect within 2 hours and a maximum effect in 15 hours (128).

Acetazolamide is used effectively to treat chronic open-angle glaucoma. The high bicarbonate concentration in aqueous humor is carbonic anhydrase dependent and oral carbonic anhydrase inhibition can be used to reduce aqueous humor formation. Newer topical formulations are currently in clinical trials (129,130) and could prove to be effective without the side effects of orally administered drugs.

Acute mountain sickness usually occurs in climbers within the 12 to 72 hours of ascending to high altitudes. A complex consisting of headache, nausea, dizziness, and breathlessness characterizes symptoms. Carbonic anhydrase inhibitors improve symptoms and arterial oxygenation (131,132).

The administration of acetazolamide has been used in the treatment of familial hypokalemic periodic paralysis (133,134), a disorder characterized by intermittent episodes of muscle weakness and flaccid paralysis. Its efficacy may be related to a decrease in influx of potassium as a result of a decrease in plasma insulin and glucose (135) or to metabolic acidosis. Carbonic anhydrase inhibitors can also be used as an adjunct treatment of epilepsy (136), pseudotumor cerebri (137), and central sleep apnea (138).

By increasing urinary pH, acetazolamide has been used effectively in certain clinical conditions. Acetazolamide is used to treat cystine and uric acid stones by increasing their solubility in urine. Acetazolamide in combination with sodium bicarbonate infusion is also used to treat salicylate toxicity. Salicylates are weak acids (pK_a 3.0); therefore, their ionic and nonionic forms exist in equilibrium. They are excreted primarily by the kidney through secretion via the organic anion transport pathway in the proximal tubule. Acetazolamide and sodium bicarbonate infusions increase urinary pH thereby favoring formation of a nondiffusible nonionic form of salicylate, thus increasing excretion of salicylates (139).

LOOP DIURETICS

The loop diuretics inhibit sodium and chloride transport along the loop of Henle. Although these drugs also impair ion transport by proximal and distal tubules under some conditions, these effects probably contribute little to their action clinically. The loop diuretics available in the United States include furosemide, bumetanide, torsemide, and ethacrynic acid (Fig. 82-4).

Urinary Electrolyte and Water Excretion

Loop diuretics increase the excretion of water, Na, K, Cl, phosphate, magnesium, and calcium (Table 82-1). The dose-response relationship between loop diuretic and urinary Na and Cl excretion is sigmoidal (Fig. 82-5). The steep dose response relation has led many to refer to loop diuretics as "threshold" drugs (9). Loop diuretics have the highest natriuretic and chloruretic potency of any class of diuretics; they can increase Na and Cl excretion up to 25% of the filtered load. If loop diuretics are administered during water loading, solute-free water clearance (C_{H2O}) decreases and osmolar clearance increases, although the urine always remains dilute (140–142). This effect contrasts with that of osmotic diuretics, which increase osmolar clearance and C_{H2O} (143). During hydropenia, loop diuretics impair the reabsorption of solute-free water (T^C_{H2O}) (140–142). During maximal loop diuretic action, the urinary Na concentration is usually 75 to 100 mM (144). Because urinary K concentrations during furosemide-induced natriuresis remain low, this means that the clearance of electrolyte free water (C_{H2Oe}) is increased when loop diuretics are administered during conditions of water diuresis or hydropenia (144). This effect of loop diuretics has been exploited to treat hyponatremia when combined with normal or hypertonic saline (145,146).

Mechanisms of Action

Na and Cl Transport

The predominant effect of loop diuretic drugs is to inhibit the electroneutral Na-K-2Cl cotransporter at the apical surface of thick ascending limb cells. The loop of Henle, defined as the

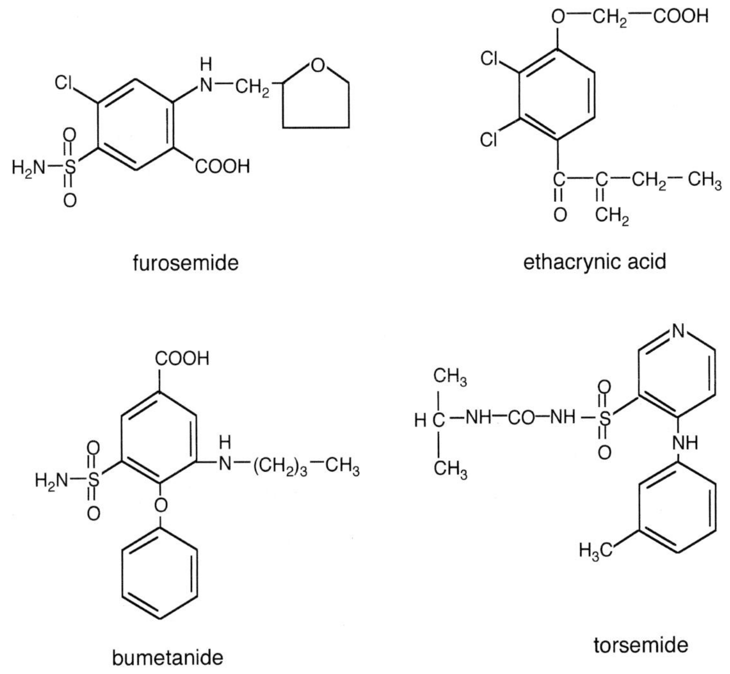

furosemide

ethacrynic acid

bumetanide

torsemide

FIG. 82-4. Structures of loop diuretics.

region between the last surface proximal segment and the first surface distal segment, reabsorbs 20% to 50% of the filtered Na and Cl load (147); thick ascending limb cells reabsorb approximately 10% to 20%. The model in Fig. 82-6 shows key components of Na, K, and Cl transport pathways in a thick ascending limb cell. As in other nephron segments, the Na/K ATPase at the basolateral cell membrane maintains the intracellular Na concentration low (approximately tenfold lower than interstitial) and the K concentration

high (approximately 20-fold higher than interstitial). Potassium channel(s) (148) in the basolateral cell membrane permits K to diffuse out of the cell, rendering the cell membrane voltage oriented with the intracellular surface negative, relative to extracellular fluid. A chloride channel in the basolateral cell membrane (149) permits Cl to exit the cell (148). Together with the apical K channel described in the following,

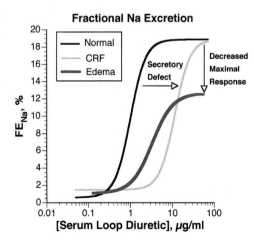

FIG. 82-5. Dose response curve for loop diuretics showing fractional Na excretion (FE_{Na}) as a function of serum loop diuretic concentration. Compared with normal patients, patients with chronic renal failure (CRF) show a rightward shift in the curve, owing to impaired diuretic secretion. The maximal response is preserved when expressed as FE_{Na} (although not when expressed as absolute Na excretion). Patients with edema demonstrate a rightward and downward shift, even when expressed as FE_{Na}.

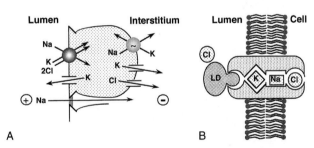

FIG. 82-6. Mechanisms of diuretic action along the loop of Henle. **A:** Models of thick ascending limb cells. Na and Cl are reabsorbed across the apical membrane via the loop diuretic-sensitive Na-K-2Cl cotransporter, NKCC2. Note that the transepithelial voltage along the thick ascending limb is oriented with the lumen-positive relative to blood. This transepithelial voltage drives a component of Na (and calcium and magnesium) reabsorption via the paracellular pathway. **B:** A model of NKCC interaction with ions. (Based on information from Lytle C, McManus TJ, Haas M. A model of Na-K-2Cl cotransport based on ordered ion binding and glide symmetry. *Am J Physiol* 1998;274:C299.) In this model, the transporter is first occupied by a Cl, then by a Na, then by a K, and finally by Cl. According to this model, loop diuretics (indicated as LD) interact with the Cl site and block Cl access. (Based on information from Haas M, McManus TJ. Bumetanide inhibits (Na + K + 2Cl) co-transport at a chloride site. *Am J Physiol* 1983;245:C235.)

this chloride channel generates a transepithelial voltage, oriented in the lumen-positive direction.

The transporter inhibited by loop diuretics is a member of the cation chloride cotransporter family (150,151). This protein, referred to as the bumetanide-sensitive cotransporter, first isoform (BSC-1) or as the Na-K-2Cl cotransporter, second isoform (NKCC2), is encoded by the gene SLC12A1 (152). It is believed to comprise 12 membrane-spanning domains and is expressed at the apical membrane of thick ascending limb (4) and macula densa (MD) cells (6,153). This transporter lies in parallel with a K channel (ROMK) permitting potassium to recycle from the cell to the lumen (154). Greger and Schlatter showed that the asymmetrical orientation of channels (apical versus basolateral) and the action of the Na/K ATPase and Na-K-2Cl cotransporter combine to create a transepithelial voltage that is oriented with the lumen positive, with respect to the interstitium (155). This lumen-positive potential drives absorption of Na, Ca, and Mg via the paracellular pathway. The paracellular component of Na reabsorption comprises 50% of the total transepithelial Na transport by thick ascending limb cells (156); it should be noted, however, that both the transcellular and the paracellular components of Na transport are inhibited by loop diuretics, the former directly and the latter indirectly. The thick ascending limb is virtually impermeable to water. The combination of solute absorption and water impermeability determines the role of the thick ascending limb as the primary diluting segment of the kidney.

Although direct inhibition of ion transport is the most important natriuretic action of loop diuretics, other actions may contribute. Thick ascending limb cells have been shown to produce prostaglandin E_2 following stimulation with furosemide (157), perhaps via inhibition of prostaglandin dehydrogenase (158,159). Blockade of cyclooxygenase reduces the effects of furosemide to inhibit loop segment chloride transport in rats (160); prostaglandin E_2 but not I_2 can restore this effect (161). Increases in renal prostaglandins may contribute to the hemodynamic effects of loop diuretics, described in the following.

Although high luminal concentrations of chloride might be suspected of inhibiting diuretic efficacy, based on the relation between luminal chloride concentration and diuretic binding to the transporter, there is no clinical information to suggest that that luminal chloride inhibits diuretic efficacy *in vivo*.

Ca and Mg Transport

Loop diuretics increase the excretion of the divalent cations, calcium, and magnesium. This effect to increase calcium excretion is used to advantage when furosemide is used together with saline to treat hypercalcemia (162). Although a component of magnesium and calcium absorption by thick ascending limbs may be active (especially when circulating parathyroid hormone levels are high) (163), a large component of their absorption is passive and paracellular, driven by the transepithelial voltage. As described, active NaCl transport

by thick ascending limb cells leads to a transepithelial voltage, oriented in the lumen-positive direction. The paracellular pathway in the thick ascending limb is believed to express a paracellular magnesium (and calcium) channel, parcellin (164). The positive voltage in the lumen, relative to interstitium, drives calcium and magnesium absorption through the paracellular pathway (165,166). Loop diuretics, by blocking the activity of the Na-K-2Cl cotransporter at the apical membrane of thick ascending limb cells, reduce the transepithelial voltage toward or to 0 mV (167–170). This stops passive paracellular calcium and magnesium absorption.

Renin Secretion

In addition to enhancing Na and Cl excretion, effects that result directly from inhibiting Na and Cl transport, loop diuretics also stimulate renin secretion. Although a component of this effect is frequently related to contraction of the extracellular fluid volume (see the following), loop diuretics also stimulate renin secretion by inhibiting Na-K-2Cl cotransport directly. Macula densa cells, which control renin secretion, sense the NaCl concentration in the lumen of the thick ascending limb (171). High luminal NaCl concentrations in the region of the macula densa lead to two distinct but related effects. First they activate the tubuloglomerular feedback (TGF) response, which suppresses glomerular filtration rate. Second, they inhibit renin secretion. The relation between these two effects is complex and has been reviewed (171), but both effects appear to result largely from NaCl movement across the apical membrane (172). Thick ascending limb cells express most of the ion transport pathways of macula densa cells. This includes the loop diuretic-sensitive Na-K-2Cl cotransporter (NKCC2 or BSC1) at the apical surface (6,153). Under normal conditions, an increase in luminal NaCl concentration in the thick ascending limb raises the NaCl concentration inside macula densa cells (172). Because the activity of the basolateral Na/K ATPase is lower in macula densa cells than in surrounding thick ascending limb cells (171), the cell NaCl concentration is much more dependent on luminal NaCl concentration in macula densa than thick ascending limb cells (173). When luminal and macula densa cell NaCl concentrations decline, production rates of nitric oxide and prostaglandin E2 are stimulated. Although the mechanisms by which Na and Cl transport regulate nitric oxide and prostaglandin production rates are not known, both mediators appear to participate importantly in effecting renin secretion.

The constitutive (neuronal) isoform of nitric oxide synthase (NOS I) is expressed by macula densa cells, but not by other cells in the kidney. Nitric oxide produced by macula densa cells has a paracrine effect to increase cellular concentrations of cAMP in adjacent juxtaglomerular cells. cAMP then stimulates renin secretion through protein kinase A. Recent data suggest that in juxtaglomerular cells, nitric oxide increases cellular concentrations of cGMP, which inhibit phosphodiesterase 3 (174). Inhibition of phosphodiesterase

3 permits cAMP accumulation. Several laboratories have reported that furosemide-induced stimulation of renin secretion is dependent on an intact nitric oxide system (175–177).

Prostaglandin production also participates in regulating renin secretion. Recently, the mRNA encoding an isoform of cyclooxygenase, COX-2, was identified in macula densa cells (178). This isoform is typically only found after induction by inflammatory cytokines. Blockade of prostaglandin synthesis either by nonspecific cyclooxygenase inhibitors (179) or by specific COX-2 blockers (178) reduces the renin secretory response to loop diuretics. Although the precise relation between nitric oxide and cyclooxygenase in stimulating renin secretion has not been defined, it has been suggested that prostaglandin synthesis is stimulated by nitric oxide (171).

Renal Hemodynamics

Unlike most other classes of diuretic drugs, glomerular filtration rate and renal blood flow tend to be preserved during loop diuretic administration (180), although GFR and RPF can decline if extracellular fluid volume contraction is severe. Loop diuretics reduce renal vascular resistance and increase renal blood flow under experimental conditions (181,182). This effect is believed related to the diuretic-induced production of vasodilatory prostaglandins.

Another factor that may contribute to the tendency of loop diuretics to maintain glomerular filtration rate and renal plasma flow despite volume contraction is their effect on the TGF system. The sensing mechanism that activates the TGF system involves NaCl transport across the apical membrane of macula densa cells by the loop diuretic sensitive Na-K-2Cl cotransporter. Under normal conditions, when the luminal concentration of NaCl reaching the macula densa rises, glomerular filtration rate decreases via TGF. To a large degree, the TGF-mediated decrease in GFR is believed to result from afferent arteriole constriction (171,183). Although the mechanisms by which ion transport across the apical membrane of macula densa cells translate to afferent arteriolar vasoconstriction are unclear, they may involve the production of adenosine (an afferent arteriolar vasoconstrictor) and the increase in mesangial and smooth muscle cell calcium concentrations (171). In a manner analogous to the effects on renin secretion, loop diuretic drugs block TGF by blocking the sensing step (184). In the absence of effects on the macula densa, loop diuretics would be expected to suppress GFR and RPF by increasing distal NaCl delivery and activating the TGF system (an effect that is observed during infusion of carbonic anhydrase inhibitors) (62); instead, blockade of the TGF permits GFR and RPF to be maintained.

Systemic Hemodynamics

Acute intravenous administration of loop diuretics increases venous capacitance (185). Some studies suggest that this effect results from stimulation of prostaglandin synthesis by the kidney (186,187). Other studies suggest that loop diuretics have effects in peripheral vascular beds as well (188). Pickers and coworkers examined the local effects of furosemide in the human forearm. Furosemide had no effect on arterial vessels, but did cause dilation of veins, an effect that was dependent on local prostaglandin production (189). Although venodilation and improvements in cardiac hemodynamics frequently result from intravenous therapy with loop diuretics, the hemodynamic response to intravenous loop diuretics may be more complex (190). Johnston and associates reported that low-dose furosemide increased venous capacitance, but that higher doses did not (191). It was suggested that furosemide-induced renin secretion leads to angiotensin II-induced vasoconstriction. This vasoconstrictor might overwhelm the prostaglandin-mediated vasodilatory effects in some patients. In two series, 1 to 1.5 mg/kg furosemide boluses, administered to patients with chronic congestive heart failure, resulted in transient *deteriorations* in hemodynamics (during the first hour), with declines in stroke volume index, increases in left ventricular filling pressure (192,193), and exacerbation of congestive heart failure symptoms. These changes may be related to activation of both the sympathetic nervous system and the renin–angiotensin system by the diuretic drug. Evidence for a role of the renin–angiotensin system in the furosemide-induced deterioration in systemic hemodynamics includes the temporal association between its activation and hemodynamic deterioration (192), and the ability of angiotensin I converting enzyme inhibitors to prevent much of the pressor effect (194). Many other studies have shown that acute loop diuretic administration frequently produces a transient decline in cardiac output; whether diuretic administration increases or decreases left atrial pressure acutely may depend primarily on the state of underlying sympathetic nervous system and renin–angiotensin axis activation.

Pharmacokinetics

The three loop diuretics that are used most commonly—furosemide, bumetanide, and torsemide—are absorbed quickly after oral administration, reaching peak concentrations within 0.5 to 2 hours. Furosemide absorption is slower than its elimination in normal subjects; thus the time to reach peak serum level is slower for furosemide than for bumetanide and torsemide. This phenomenon is called "absorption-limited kinetics" (9). The bioavailability of loop diuretics varies from 50% to 90%; when furosemide dosing is switched from intravenous to oral, the dose may need to be increased to compensate for its poor bioavailability (9). The half-lives of the loop diuretics available in the United States vary, but all are relatively short (ranging from approximately 1 hour for bumetanide to 3 to 4 hours for torsemide). The half-lives of muzolimine, xipamide, and ozolinone, none of which is available in the United States, are longer (6 to 15 hours).

Loop diuretics are organic anions that circulate tightly bound to albumin (>95%), thus their volume of distribution is small except during extreme hypoproteinemia (195).

Approximately 50% of an administered dose of furosemide is excreted unchanged into the urine. The remainder appears to be eliminated by glucuronidation, probably by the kidney. Torsemide and bumetanide are eliminated both by hepatic processes and renal excretion. The differences in metabolic fate mean that the half-life of furosemide is altered by renal failure, whereas this is not true for torsemide and bumetanide.

Clinical Use

Loop diuretics are used commonly to treat the edematous conditions, congestive heart failure, cirrhosis of the liver, and nephrotic syndrome. In addition, a variety of other electrolyte, fluid, and acid–base disorders can respond to loop diuretic therapy. Details of loop diuretic use for the treatment of edematous conditions are beyond the scope of this chapter.

Adverse Effects

There are at least three types of adverse effects of loop diuretics. The first and most common are those that result directly from the effects of these drugs on renal electrolyte and water excretion. The second are toxic effects of the drugs that are dose-related and predictable. The third are idiosyncratic allergic drug reactions.

Loop diuretics are frequently administered to treat edematous expansion of the extracellular fluid volume. Edema usually results from a decrease in the "effective" arterial blood volume. Overzealous diuretic usage or intercurrent complicating illnesses can lead to excessive contraction of the intravascular volume, leading to orthostatic hypotension, renal dysfunction, and sympathetic overactivity. Although patients suffering from congestive heart failure usually require diuretic therapy, the combination of diuretics and angiotensin converting enzyme (ACE) inhibitors is especially likely to cause renal dysfunction. High diuretic doses or extreme dietary NaCl restriction may predispose to renal dysfunction during therapy with diuretics and ACE inhibitors for congestive heart failure (196,197). In such cases, it is important to attempt to continue ACE inhibitors, in view of their effects on mortality. Functional renal failure in such patients often responds to a reduction in diuretic dose or liberalization in dietary NaCl intake, permitting continued administration of the ACE inhibitor.

Other populations at increased risk for relative contraction of the intravascular volume during loop diuretic therapy include elderly patients (198); those with preexisting renal insufficiency (199), right-sided heart failure, or pericardial disease; and patients taking nonsteroidal antiinflammatory drugs (NSAIDs).

Disorders of Na and K concentration are among the most frequent adverse effects of loop diuretics. Hyponatremia is less common with loop diuretics than with distal convoluted tubule diuretics but can occur (see the following). Its pathogenesis is usually multifactorial, but involves the effect of loop diuretics to impair the clearance of solute-free water.

Additional factors that may contribute include the nonosmotic release of arginine vasopressin (200), hypokalemia (201), and hypomagnesemia (202). Conversely, loop diuretics have been used to treat hyponatremia when combined with hypertonic saline, in the setting of the syndrome of inappropriate ADH secretion (146,203). The combination of loop diuretics and angiotensin I converting enzyme inhibitors has been reported to correct hyponatremia in the setting of congestive heart failure (204).

Hypokalemia occurs commonly during therapy with loop diuretics, although the magnitude is smaller than that induced by distal convoluted tubule diuretic (loop diuretics, 0.3 mM versus distal convoluted tubule diuretics, 0.5 to 0.9 mM) (205,206). Loop diuretics increase the delivery of potassium to the distal tubule because they block potassium reabsorption via the Na-K-2Cl cotransporter. In rats, under control conditions, approximately half the excreted potassium was delivered to the "early" distal tubule. During furosemide infusion, the delivery of potassium to the "early" distal tubule rose to 28% of the filtered load (207). Thus, it appears that a large component of the effect of loop diuretics to increase potassium excretion acutely reflects their ability to block potassium reabsorption by the thick ascending limb. Nevertheless, during chronic diuretic therapy, the degree of potassium wasting correlates best with volume contraction and serum aldosterone levels (208). These data suggest that, under chronic conditions, the predominant effect of loop diuretics to stimulate potassium excretion results from their tendency to increase mineralocorticoid hormones while increasing distal Na and water delivery.

Metabolic alkalosis is very common during chronic treatment with loop diuretics. Loop diuretics cause metabolic alkalosis via several mechanisms. First, they increase the excretion of urine that is bicarbonate free but that contains Na and Cl. This leads to contraction of the extracellular fluid around a fixed amount of bicarbonate buffer; a phenomenon known as contraction alkalosis. This probably contributes only slightly to the metabolic alkalosis that commonly accompanies chronic loop diuretic treatment. Loop diuretics directly inhibit transport of Na and Cl into thick ascending limb cells. In some species, these cells also express an isoform of the Na/H exchanger at the apical surface. When Na entry via the Na-K-2Cl cotransporter is blocked by a loop diuretic, the decline in intracellular Na activity will stimulate H secretion via the Na/H exchanger (209–211). Loop diuretics stimulate the renin–angiotensin–aldosterone pathway, both directly and indirectly, as discussed. Aldosterone directly stimulates H secretion by the medullary collecting tubule (212) and increases the magnitude of the transepithelial voltage in the cortical collecting duct. This effect stimulates H secretion via the electrogenic H ATPase present at the apical membrane of α intercalated cells. Hypokalemia itself also contributes to metabolic alkalosis by increasing ammonium production (213), stimulating bicarbonate reabsorption by proximal tubules (214,215), and increasing the activity of the H/K ATPase in the distal nephron (216). Finally, contraction of the extracellular fluid volume stimulates Na/H exchange in the proximal tubule and may reduce the filtered load of bicarbonate. All of these factors may contribute to the metabolic alkalosis observed during chronic loop diuretic treatment.

Ototoxicity is the most common nonrenal toxic effect of loop diuretics. Deafness, which is usually temporary, was reported shortly after the introduction of loop diuretics (217,218). It appears likely that all loop diuretics cause ototoxicity, because ototoxicity can occur during use of chemically dissimilar drugs such as furosemide and ethacrynic acid (217,218). The mechanism of ototoxicity remains unclear, although the stria vascularis, which is responsible for maintaining endolymphatic potential and ion balance (219) appears to be a primary target for toxicity (220). Loop diuretics reduce the striatal voltage from $+80$ mV to -10 to -20 mV within minutes of application (219). A characteristic finding in loop diuretic ototoxicity is strial edema. This suggests that toxicity involves inhibition of ion fluxes (220). Ikeda and Morizono detected functional evidence for the presence of a Na-K-2Cl cotransporter in the basolateral membrane of marginal cells in the inner ear (221). According to the model proposed by these investigators, marginal cells resemble secretory cells in other organ systems, with a Na-K-2Cl cotransporter and Na/K ATPase at the basolateral cell membrane and channels for K and Cl at the apical surface. According to this model, loop diuretic induced shrinkage of marginal cells results from inhibition of cell Na, K, and Cl uptake across the basolateral cell membrane. Recently, the secretory isoform of the Na-K-2Cl cotransporter, NKCC1, was localized in the lateral wall of the cochlea, using specific antibodies (222) and RT-PCR (223). Loop diuretics cause loss of outer hair cells in the basal turn of the cochlea, rupture of endothelial layers, cystic formation in the stria vascularis, and marginal cell edema in the stria vascularis (224).

Ototoxicity appears to be related to the peak serum concentration of loop diuretic and therefore tends to occur during rapid high-dose drug infusion. For this reason, it is most common in patients with uremia (225). It has been recommended that furosemide infusion be no more rapid than 4 mg/minute (226). In addition to renal failure, infants, patients with cirrhosis, and patients receiving aminoglycosides or *cis*-platinum may be at increased risk for ototoxicity (225).

DISTAL CONVOLUTED TUBULE DIURETICS

The first orally active drug that inhibited Na and Cl transport along the distal convoluted tubule (DCT) was chlorothiazide. Chlorothiazide was developed as sulfonamide-based carbonic anhydrase inhibitors were modified in pursuit of substances that increased Cl excretion rather than bicarbonate. The identification of a substance that increased Na and Cl excretion rates was immediately recognized as clinically significant, because extracellular fluid contains predominantly NaCl rather than $NaHCO_3$ (227,228), and because acidosis limits the effectiveness of carbonic anhydrase inhibitors. Subsequent development led to a wide variety of benzothiadiazide (thiazide) diuretics (Fig. 82-7); all are analogs of 1,2,4-benzothiadiazine-1,1-dioxide. Other structurally related diuretics include the quinazolinones (such as metolazone) and

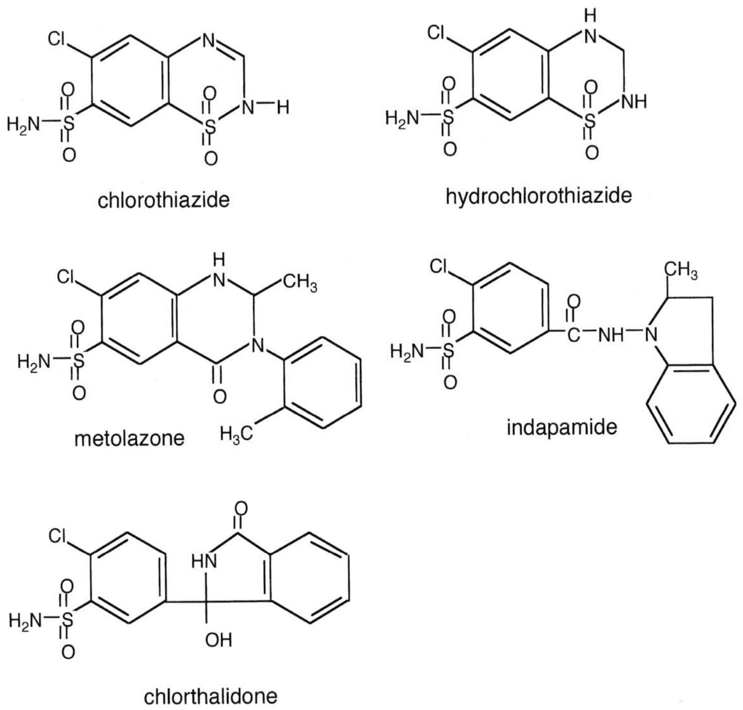

FIG. 82-7. Structures of distal convoluted tubule (DCT) diuretics.

substituted benzophenone sulfonamide (e.g., chlorthalidone). Although the primary site at which these drugs exert their action has been a source of confusion until recently, molecular identification of their target ion transporter has permitted precise delineation of their predominant site of action as the distal convoluted tubule. Although the term "thiazide diuretics" is frequently used to describe this class of drugs, a more accurate descriptor, one that is analogous to the descriptor "loop diuretics," is the term *distal convoluted tubule diuretics*.

Urinary Electrolyte and Water Excretion

Acute administration of these drugs increases the excretion of Na, K, Cl, HCO$_3$, phosphate, and urate (143,229,230), although the increases in HCO$_3$, phosphate, and urate excretion are probably related primarily to carbonic anhydrase inhibition (see the following). As such, the effects of DCT diuretics to increase HCO$_3$, phosphate, and urate excretion may vary, depending on the carbonic anhydrase inhibiting potency of a particular drug. Chronically, uric acid excretion declines and hyperuricemia can take place as contraction of the extracellular fluid volume occurs. Further, bicarbonate excretion ceases, and continuing losses of chloride without bicarbonate coupled with extracellular fluid volume contraction may lead to metabolic alkalosis. In contrast to loop and proximally acting diuretics, DCT diuretics tend to reduce urinary calcium excretion (231,232). Although the effects on urinary calcium excretion can be variable during acute administration (229,231,232), these drugs uniformly lead to calcium retention when administered chronically.

Distal convoluted tubule diuretics inhibit the clearance of solute free water (C_{H2O}) when administered during water diuresis. This effect is similar to that of loop diuretics and originally led to the mistaken inference that they act along the thick ascending limb. In contrast to loop diuretics, however, DCT diuretics do not limit T$^C_{H2O}$ during antidiuresis (142,233).

Mechanism of Action

Na and Water Transport in the Proximal Tubule

As discussed, DCT diuretics are related chemically to carbonic anhydrase inhibitors and most DCT diuretics retain carbonic anhydrase inhibiting activity (234). Carbonic anhydrase inhibitors interfere indirectly with the activity of the apical Na/H exchanger expressed at the luminal membrane of proximal tubule cells. Although this effect of DCT diuretics may be useful when these drugs are administered acutely (as during intravenous chlorothiazide administration), it probably contributes little to the overall natriuresis during chronic use (235,236). Yet this effect may play a role in the tendency for DCT diuretics to reduce the glomerular filtration rate and activate the TGF mechanism (62). The relative carbonic anhydrase inhibiting potency (shown in brackets) of

some commonly used DCT diuretics is chlorthalidone [67], benzthiazide [50], polythiazide [40], chlorothiazide [14], hydrochlorothiazide [1], and bendroflumethiazide [0.07] (237).

NaCl Absorption in the Distal Nephron

As the name indicates, the predominant site at which DCT diuretics inhibit ion transport is the DCT. Although clearance studies had identified one site of thiazide action as the cortical diluting segment (142) and a second site as the proximal tubule (238–240), micropuncture studies pinpointed the primary site of action as the superficial "distal tubule" (235). This region of the nephron, between the macula densa and the confluence with another nephron to form the cortical collecting duct, is cytologically heterogenous (241,242). It comprises a short stretch of post macula densa thick ascending limb, the DCT, the connecting tubule, and the initial portion of the cortical collecting duct. When this morphologic heterogeneity became evident, experiments were designed to determine the site of thiazide action more precisely. Microperfusion experiments in rats indicated that thiazide diuretics inhibit Na and Cl transport along the "early" portion of the distal tubule (243,244), a segment known to contain DCT cells predominantly (241,245).

Although microperfusion data from rats indicated that thiazide diuretics inhibit Na transport in the DCT, the transition between distal nephron segments in this species is gradual. For several years, therefore, it was impossible to attribute thiazide-sensitive Na-Cl transport to a specific cell type in the rat (246). In contrast rabbit distal nephron segments have abrupt transitions. Thus, it has been possible to perfuse DCTs, connecting tubules, and cortical collecting ducts separately *in vitro*. Imai and colleagues reported that thiazide-sensitive Na-Cl cotransport could be detected in connecting tubules, but not in distal convoluted tubules (247–249). In contrast, Velázquez and Greger reported evidence consistent with the presence of electroneutral Na transport in rabbit distal convoluted tubules (250,251), although thiazide-sensitive sodium or chloride transport was not measured directly. Pizzonia and colleagues immunodissected cells from mouse thick ascending limb and distal convoluted tubule (252). A clonal cell line was developed that expresses thiazide-sensitive sodium and chloride uptake, suggesting that thiazide-sensitive Na-Cl cotransport is expressed by distal convoluted tubule cells in the mouse (253,254). Definitive identification of cells that express the thiazide-sensitive Na-Cl cotransporter, however, required molecular identification of the protein.

Evidence for thiazide action in other nephron segments has also been obtained. *In vivo* catheterization experiments demonstrated a component of thiazide-sensitive Na transport in medullary collecting tubules of rats (255). Some (256,257) investigators have detected thiazide-sensitive Na-Cl transport in rat cortical collecting ducts perfused *in vitro*. In those experiments, pretreatment of animals with mineralocorticoid hormones was necessary to induce the thiazide-sensitive Na and Cl transport.

In 1984, Velázquez and colleagues reported the mutual dependence of Na and Cl transport in the superficial rat distal tubule (258). The same year, Stokes reported evidence that a directly coupled thiazide-sensitive Na-Cl cotransporter is expressed in the urinary bladder of the winter flounder (259). Gamba and coworkers expression cloned a thiazide-sensitive Na-Cl cotransporter from the flounder bladder (260) and detected a similar mRNA in rat and mouse kidney (260). Gamba and coworkers then cloned a rat form of the thiazide-sensitive Na-Cl cotransporter (261). Mouse, human, and rabbit forms were cloned shortly thereafter (262–264); the gene is SLC12A3. This transport protein has been variously termed the TSC (thiazide-sensitive cotransporter), NCCT (sodium chloride cotransporter), and NCC (sodium chloride cotransporter). In rat, human, and mouse, NCC message and protein are expressed by DCT cells (5,263,265–267). A model of NaCl transport by DCT cells is shown in Fig. 82-8. In human, rat, and mouse, expression of NCC extends into a transitional segment, referred to as the DCT2, which shares properties of DCT and connecting tubules (5,263). In the rabbit, the thiazide-sensitive Na-Cl cotransporter was also shown to be expressed *exclusively* by DCT cells (268); connecting tubule cells do not express the transporter (268). Thus, from a molecular standpoint, distal convoluted tubule cells in all mammalian species examined to date express the NCC.

Distal convoluted tubule diuretics are organic anions. Based on studies in which [^{3}H]metolazone binding to kidney cortical membranes was studied, DCT diuretics were believed to bind to the Na-Cl cotransporter at the anion site (269,270). This conclusion derives from the observation that chloride inhibits the binding of [^{3}H]metolazone in a competitive manner. Unlike loop diuretics binding to the Na-K-2Cl cotransporter, [^{3}H]metolazone binding to the Na-Cl cotransporter does not require the presence of Na, suggesting either that chloride binds first to the transporter or that binding of ions to the transporter is not "ordered" (269,270). Recently, studies using a heterologous expression system (271) found a Michaelis-Menten constant (K_m) for Na of 7.6 mM and for Cl of 6.3 mM. The Hill coefficients for Na and Cl were consistent with electroneutrality. The affinities of both Na and Cl were increased when the concentration of the counter ion was increased. The IC$_{50}$ values for thiazides were increased when either Na or Cl concentration was increased. These workers proposed a transport model featuring a random order of binding in which the binding of each ion facilitates the binding of the counter ion.

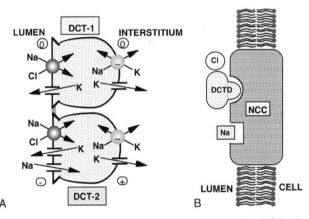

FIG. 82-8. Mechanisms of distal convoluted tubule (DCT) diuretics. **A:** Models of distal convoluted tubule cells. Two types of distal convoluted tubule cells have been identified in rat, mouse, and human, referred to here as DCT-1 and DCT-2. Na and Cl are reabsorbed across the apical membrane of DCT-1 cells only via the thiazide-sensitive Na-Cl cotransporter. This transport protein is also expressed by DCT-2 cells where Na can also cross through the epithelial Na channel, ENaC. (Based on information from Obermüller N, Bernstein PL, Velázquez H, et al. Expression of the thiazide-sensitive Na-Cl cotransporter in rat and human kidney. *Am J Physiol* 1995;269:F900; Bostanjoglo M, Reeves WB, Reilly RF, et al. 11β-hydroxysteroid dehydrogenase, mineralocorticoid receptor and thiazide-sensitive Na-Cl cotransporter expression by distal tubules. *J Am Soc Nephrol* 1998;9:1347; Schmitt R, Ellison DH, Farman N, et al. Developmental expression of sodium entry pathways in rat distal nephron. *Am J Physiol* 1999;276:F367.) Thus, the transepithelial voltage along the DCT-1 is near to 0 mV, whereas it is finite and lumen-negative along the DCT-2. **B:** A model of NCC interaction with ions and DCT diuretics. (Based on information from Tran JM, Farrell MA, Fanestil DD. Effect of ions on binding of the thiazide-type diuretic metolazone to kidney membrane. *Am J Physiol* 1990;258:F908, with permission.) In this model, DCT diuretics (indicated as DCTD) interact with the Cl site and block Cl access. (Based on information from Tran JM, Farrell MA, Fanestil DD. Effect of ions on binding of the thiazide-type diuretic metolazone to kidney membrane. *Am J Physiol* 1990;258:F908.)

Calcium and Magnesium Transport

Distal convoluted tubule diuretics reduce calcium excretion when administered chronically. This effect has been utilized clinically to treat calcium nephrolithiasis (see the following). Much progress in understanding mechanisms of the hypocalciuric effect of DCT diuretics has been made during the past 10 years. Acute administration of DCT diuretics has a variable effect on calcium excretion, sometimes leading to increases in calcium excretion (229,272). This probably reflects the carbonic anhydrase inhibiting capacity of these drugs, because carbonic anhydrase inhibitors increase urinary calcium excretion acutely. Ca reabsorption by proximal tubules is functionally coupled to sodium reabsorption; drugs that inhibit proximal Na reabsorption also inhibit proximal calcium reabsorption (273). During chronic treatment, however, the filtered calcium load decreases, owing to the hemodynamic effects discussed in the following, and the proximal calcium reabsorption increases, owing to extracellular fluid volume contraction.

The primary site where DCT diuretic increase renal calcium reabsorption is the same segment where they inhibit Na and Cl transport. Although rat distal nephrons reabsorb both Na and Ca, Constanzo and Windhager showed (274) that thiazide diuretics dissociate the two; Na reabsorption is inhibited, whereas calcium reabsorption is stimulated. Several

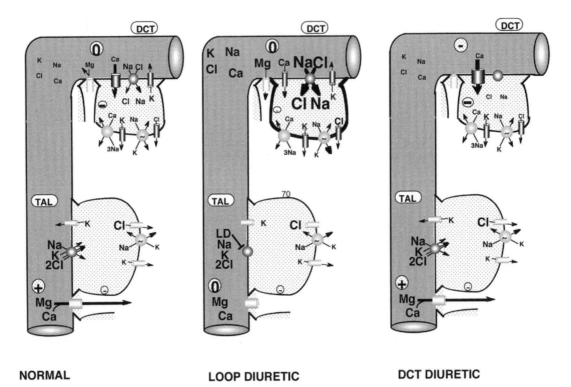

NORMAL **LOOP DIURETIC** **DCT DIURETIC**

FIG. 82-9. Summary of diuretic effects on calcium excretion. Compared with normal *(left panel)*, loop diuretics increase urinary calcium excretion. This effect occurs because loop diuretics (LD) *(middle panel)* block the 3 ion transporter and reduce the transepithelial voltage of the thick ascending limb. This reduces calcium (and magnesium) reabsorption across the paracellular pathway because the voltage drives such transport. In contrast, distal convoluted tubule (DCT) diuretics *(right panel)* block the Na-Cl cotransporter of the distal convoluted tubule (DCT). This increases the electrical negativity of DCT cells and opens apical calcium channels in the DCT. This leads to increased calcium reabsorption by DCT cells.

factors are now believed to contribute to the effect of DCT diuretics to stimulate calcium reabsorption (Fig. 82-9). As in most other cells, the intracellular calcium concentration of DCT cells is low, compared with extracellular fluid calcium (253). Calcium enters DCT cells passively, down its electrochemical gradient. Distal convoluted tubule diuretics increase the intracellular calcium activity, suggesting that a primary effect is to increase apical calcium entry (253). Brunette and colleagues (275,276) have proposed that two distinct pathways mediate apical calcium entry in DCT cells. One pathway has a high affinity for calcium and is stimulated by parathyroid hormone, whereas the other has a lower affinity for calcium and is stimulated by thiazide diuretics (275,276). Friedman and colleagues also have obtained evidence for distinct mechanisms of calcium entry. They have studied a calcium channel that is activated by hyperpolarization (163,253,277,278). When DCT cells were incubated with thiazide diuretics, the cells hyperpolarized, owing to the reduction in cellular chloride activity and the presence of a chloride channel at their basolateral membrane. The hyperpolarization was shown to activate calcium channels, leading to increased rates of calcium entry. These investigators provided evidence that the diuretic induced stimulation of calcium entry occurred via dihydropyridine-sensitive calcium

channel. Recently, a calcium channel has been cloned from a distal cell line that appears to have properties consistent with a role in distal calcium transport (279,280).

Distal convoluted tubule diuretics not only stimulate entry of calcium across the apical membrane, but also stimulate calcium transport across the basolateral cell membrane into the interstitium. Distal convoluted tubule cells, at least in rat, mouse, and human, express the Na/Ca exchanger (5,268, 281,282). The Na/Ca exchanger is believed to carry three Na ions in to the cell in exchange for one calcium ion; therefore, it is electrogenic. When DCT diuretics block the luminal entry pathway for Na and Cl, as noted, cells hyperpolarize and the intracellular Na activity declines. Both the hyperpolarization and the decline in cell Na concentration increase the electrochemical driving force favoring calcium movement from cell to interstitium. Although the data describing effects on apical and basolateral calcium transport were obtained in different model systems and from different species, taken together, they suggest that DCT diuretics stimulate both the apical entry pathway and the basolateral exit pathway that permit calcium reabsorption. The calcium reabsorptive pathway of the distal tubule is quite potent and the passive calcium permeability of this tubule segment is low; in stationary microperfusion experiments, the distal tubule was able to reduce the luminal calcium concentration below 0.1 mM (274).

Distal convoluted tubule diuretics increase urinary magnesium chronically and can cause hypomagnesemia (283–285), although the acute effects of DCT diuretics are more variable. The mechanisms of magnesium transport by DCT cells and their regulation by diuretics are not completely understood. Dai and colleagues proposed that magnesium is transported across the apical membrane of DCT cells by a hyperpolarization-activated magnesium channel (286). They found that DCT diuretics stimulated magnesium uptake into DCT cells by reducing the intracellular activity of chloride, hyperpolarizing the membrane voltage, and activating magnesium channels. The magnesium channels are sensitive to dihydropyridines but appear to be distinct from calcium channels (287). Amiloride was found to have similar effects on magnesium uptake (287). Quamme has proposed that magnesium wasting in Gitelman's syndrome, which results from mutations in the thiazide-sensitive Na-Cl cotransporter (262) and by analogy during DCT diuretic treatment, results from hypokalemia and from hyperaldosteronism (285). Yet a mouse with knockout of the thiazide-sensitive Na-Cl cotransporter demonstrates magnesium wasting in the absence of hypokalemia (288). Mechanisms of magnesium wasting in Gitelman's syndrome have been discussed recently (289).

Renal Hemodynamics

Distal convoluted tubule diuretics increase renal vascular resistance and decrease the glomerular filtration rate when given acutely (235,243,290–293). Okusa and coworkers (293) showed that intravenous chlorothiazide reduced the glomerular filtration rate by 16% when measured as whole kidney clearance or by micropuncture of a superficial distal tubule. In contrast, however, when flow to the macula densa was blocked and the single nephron glomerular filtration rate was measured by micropuncture of a proximal tubule, intravenous chlorothiazide had no effect on glomerular filtration rate. These data indicate that diuretic-induced stimulation of the TGF system mediates the effect of DCT diuretics on glomerular filtration rate; DCT diuretics are known to increase the concentration of Na in luminal fluid entering the superficial distal tubule. It is assumed that a change in the tubule fluid ion concentration mediates this effect.

Contraction of the extracellular fluid volume develops during chronic treatment with DCT diuretics, thereby increasing solute and water reabsorption by the proximal tubule. This effect reduces Na delivery to the macula densa below control levels. In view of the fact that the initial suppression of glomerular filtration rate resulted from TGF, initiated by distal NaCl delivery, the glomerular filtration rate usually returns close to control values during chronic treatment with DCT diuretics (236,294). Thus, when used chronically, DCT diuretics lead to a state of mild extracellular fluid volume contraction, increased fractional proximal reabsorption, and relatively preserved glomerular filtration (236,294).

The effect of DCT diuretics is variable when administered acutely (295). If urinary NaCl losses are replaced, these drugs tend to suppress renin secretion (296), probably by increasing NaCl delivery to the macula densa (293). In contrast, during chronic administration, renin secretion increases because solute delivery to the macula densa declines (236) and volume depletion activates the vascular mechanism for renin secretion.

Pharmacokinetics

Distal convoluted tubule diuretics are organic anions that circulate in a highly protein bound state. As with loop diuretics, the amount reaching the tubule fluid by filtration across the glomerular basement membrane is small. The predominant route of entry into tubule fluid is by secretion via the organic anion secretory pathway in the proximal tubule. Distal convoluted tubule diuretics are rapidly absorbed across the gut, reaching peak concentrations within 1.5 to 4 hours (9). The amount of administered drug that reaches the urine varies greatly (9) as does the half-life. Short-acting DCT diuretics include bendroflumethiazide, hydrochlorothiazide, tizolemide, and trichlormethiazide. Medium-acting DCT diuretics include chlorothiazide, hydroflumethiazide, indapamide, and mefruside. Long-acting DCT diuretics include chlorthalidone, metolazone, and polythiazide (9). The clinical effects of the differences in half-life are unclear, except in the incidence of hypokalemia, which is much more common in patients taking the longer acting drugs such as chlorthalidone (205,297).

Clinical Use

Distal convoluted tubule diuretics are used most commonly to treat essential hypertension. Despite a great deal of debate about the potential complications of DCT diuretics to treat essential hypertension, these drugs continue to be recommended as first line therapy for hypertension because they are clearly effective at reducing mortality (298). Distal convoluted tubule diuretics are also used commonly to treat edematous conditions, although they are frequently perceived as being less effective than loop diuretics. Although the maximal effect of loop diuretics to increase urinary Na, Cl and water excretion is greater than that of DCT diuretics, Leary and Reyes have shown that the cumulative effects of DCT diuretics on urinary Na and Cl excretion are greater than those of once-daily furosemide (299). Although these studies were conducted in normal volunteers, they may extend to patients with mild cases of edema. In addition, DCT diuretics have proved useful to treat edematous patients who have become resistant to loop diuretics. In this case, the addition of a DCT diuretic to a regimen that includes a loop diuretic frequently increases urinary Na and Cl excretion dramatically (see the following).

Distal convoluted tubule diuretics have become drugs of choice to prevent the recurrence of kidney stones in patients with idiopathic hypercalciuria. In several controlled and many uncontrolled studies, the recurrence rate for calcium stones has been reduced by up to 80% (300–302). Relatively high doses of DCT diuretics often are employed for the treatment of nephrolithiasis (303). Some studies suggest that the hypocalciuric effect of DCT diuretics wanes during chronic use in the setting of absorptive hypercalciuria (304). The observation that Gitelman's syndrome, an inherited disorder of the thiazide-sensitive Na-Cl cotransporter, may present during adulthood with hypocalciuria suggests that compensatory mechanisms may not exist for the effects of DCT diuretics on calcium transport (305). The ability of DCT diuretics to reduce urinary calcium excretion suggests that these drugs may prevent bone loss (306). Some (307,308), but not all (309,310), epidemiologic studies suggest that DCT diuretics reduce the risk of hip fracture and osteoporosis. Others have indicated that DCT diuretics can be effective in patients with primary hypoparathyroidism, when combined with a low-salt diet (311). A recent randomized controlled study confirmed that DCT diuretics reduce bone loss in women (312).

Distal convoluted tubule diuretics are also employed to treat nephrogenic diabetes insipidus, causing a paradoxic decrease in urinary volume flow rate. This action of DCT diuretics results from the combination of mild extracellular fluid volume contraction (owing to diuretic-induced natriuresis), suppression of glomerular filtration (owing largely to diuretic-induced activation of the TGF mechanism), and impaired solute reabsorption along the DCT. The DCT, like the thick ascending limb, is nearly impermeable to water (313). Solute reabsorption by the thiazide-sensitive Na-Cl cotransporter therefore contributes directly to urinary dilution. The central role of extracellular fluid volume contraction in the efficacy of DCT diuretics in diabetes insipidus was highlighted by the observation that dietary salt restriction is necessary to reduce urinary volume effectively (294). A recent report suggests that DCT diuretics may also increase the antidiuretic hormone-independent water permeability of the medullary collecting tubule (314).

Adverse Effects

Electrolyte disorders, such as hypokalemia, hyponatremia, and hypomagnesemia are common side effects of DCT diuretics. A measurable decline in serum K concentration is nearly universal in patients given DCT diuretics, but most patients do not become frankly hypokalemic (297). The clinical significance of diuretic-induced hypokalemia continues to be debated (315–321). Unlike the loop diuretics, DCT diuretics do not influence K transport directly (322,323). Instead, they increase K excretion indirectly. Distal convoluted tubule diuretics increase tubule fluid flow in the connecting tubule and collecting duct, the predominant sites of K secretion along the nephron. Increased flow stimulates K secretion (63). In addition, DCT diuretic-induced extracellular fluid volume contraction activates the renin–angiotensin–aldosterone system, further stimulating K secretion. Evidence for the central role

of aldosterone in diuretic-induced hypokalemia includes the observation that hypokalemia is much more common during treatment with long acting DCT diuretics, such as chlorthalidone, than with shorter-acting DCT diuretics, such as hydrochlorothiazide or with the very short-acting loop diuretics (205). Another reason that DCT diuretics may produce more potassium wasting than loop diuretics is the differences in effects on calcium transport. As discussed, loop diuretics inhibit calcium transport by the thick ascending limb, increasing distal calcium delivery. In contrast, DCT diuretics stimulate calcium transport, reducing calcium delivery to sites of potassium secretion. Okusa and colleagues (324) showed that high luminal concentrations of calcium inhibit the functional activity of ENaC in the distal nephron, thereby inhibiting potassium secretion. Distal convoluted tubule diuretics also increase urinary magnesium excretion and can lead to hypomagnesemia, as discussed. Hypomagnesemia may cause or contribute to the hypokalemia observed under these conditions (325,326). Some studies suggest that maintenance magnesium therapy can prevent or attenuate the development of hypokalemia (327), but this has not been supported universally.

Diuretics have been reported to contribute to more than one-half of all hospitalizations for serious hyponatremia. Hyponatremia is especially common during treatment with DCT diuretics, compared with other classes of diuretics, and the disorder is potentially life threatening (328). Several factors contribute to DCT diuretic-induced hyponatremia. First, as discussed, DCT diuretics inhibit solute transport in the terminal portion of the "diluting segment," the DCT. This impairs the ability to excrete solute-free water. Second, DCT diuretics can reduce the glomerular filtration rate, primarily by activating the TGF system. This limits solute delivery to the diluting segment and impairs solute-free water clearance. Third, DCT diuretics lead to volume contraction, which increases proximal tubule solute and water reabsorption, further restricting delivery to the "diluting segment." Fourth, hyponatremia has been correlated with the development of hypokalemia in patients receiving DCT diuretics (329). Finally, susceptible patients may be stimulated to consume water during therapy with DCT diuretics. Although the mechanisms are unclear, this may contribute importantly to the sudden appearance of hyponatremia that can occur during DCT diuretic therapy. Of note, one report suggests that patients who are predisposed to develop hyponatremia during treatment with DCT diuretics will demonstrate an acute decline in serum sodium concentration in response to a single dose of the drug (330).

Distal convoluted tubule diuretics frequently cause metabolic alkalosis. The mechanisms are similar to those described for loop diuretics, except that DCT diuretics do not stimulate Na/H exchange in the TAL.

Distal convoluted tubule diuretics cause several disturbances of endocrine glands. Glucose intolerance has been a recognized complication of DCT diuretic use since the 1950s. This complication appears to be dose related (331,332). The pathogenesis of DCT diuretic-induced glucose intolerance remains unclear, but several contributing factors have been suggested. First, diuretic-induced hypokalemia may decrease insulin secretion by the pancreas, via effects on the membrane voltage of pancreatic ß cells. When hypokalemia was prevented by oral potassium supplementation, the insulin response to hyperglycemia normalized, suggesting an important role for hypokalemia (333). Hypokalemia may also interfere with insulin mediated glucose uptake by muscle, but most patients demonstrate relatively normal insulin sensitivity (334). Other factors may contribute to glucose intolerance as well. Volume depletion may stimulate catecholamine secretion, but volume depletion during therapy with DCT diuretics is usually very mild. Recently, it has been suggested that DCT diuretics directly activate calcium-activated potassium channels that are expressed by pancreatic ß cells (335). Activation of these channels is known to inhibit insulin secretion.

Distal convoluted tubule diuretics increase levels of total cholesterol, total triglyceride, and LDL cholesterol, and reduce the HDL (334). Definitive information about the mechanisms by which DCT diuretics alter lipid metabolism is not available, but many of the mechanisms that affect glucose homeostasis have been suggested to contribute. Hyperlipidemia, like hyperglycemia, is a dose-related side effect, and one that wanes with chronic diuretic use. In several recent large clinical studies, the effect of *low-dose* DCT diuretic treatment on serum LDL was not significantly different from placebo (336). Further, hypertension treatment with DCT diuretics has now been shown clearly to reduce the risk of stroke, coronary heart disease, congestive heart failure, and cardiovascular mortality (337).

CORTICAL COLLECTING TUBULE DIURETICS

Diuretic drugs that act primarily in the cortical collecting tubule (potassium-sparing diuretics) comprise three pharmacologically distinct groups: aldosterone antagonists (spironolactone), pteridines (triamterene), and pyrazinoylguanidines (amiloride) (Fig. 82-10). The site of action for all diuretics of this class is the cortical collecting duct and the connecting tubule, where they interfere with sodium reabsorption and indirectly potassium secretion. Because of the ability to minimize the normal tendency of diuretic drugs to increase potassium excretion, amiloride (338), and triamterene (339,340) are considered potassium sparing. Diuretic activity is weak partly because fractional sodium reabsorption in the collecting tubule usually does not exceed 3% of the filtered load. Another reason, however, may relate to the tendency for these drugs to produce only partial blockade of Na channels. In support of this hypothesis, knockout or disruption of sodium channel (EnaC) function leads to profound renal salt wasting (341). Because potassium-sparing drugs are relatively weak natriuretic agents, they are most commonly used in combination with thiazides or loop diuretics, often in a single preparation, to restrict potassium losses and sometimes augment diuretic action. However, potassium-sparing diuretics

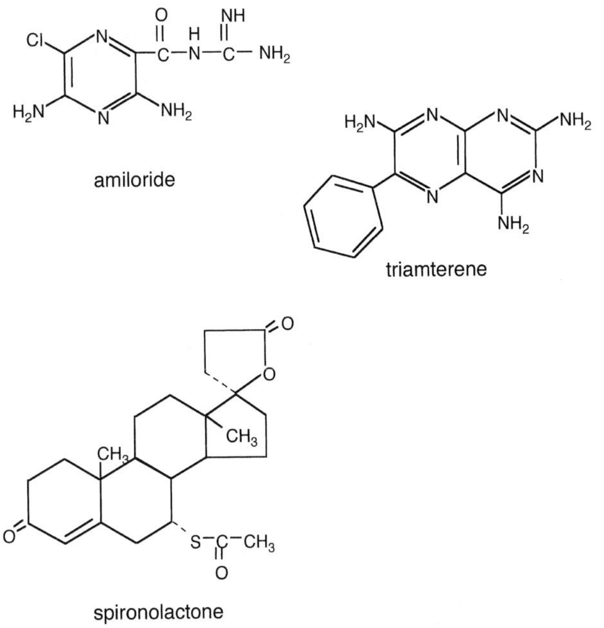

FIG. 82-10. Structure of collecting duct diuretics.

are used as first line agents in certain conditions. For example, spironolactone is used in the treatment of edema in patients with cirrhosis (342), and amiloride or triamterene is used as a first-line treatment of Liddle's syndrome (343) or Bartter's syndrome (344). Furthermore, spironolactone has been shown to improve mortality of patients with congestive heart failure (345).

Urinary Electrolyte Excretion

Amiloride, triamterene, and spironolactone are weak natriuretic agents when given acutely (Table 82-1), although some studies suggest that these drugs are as effective natriuretic agents as furosemide in some clinical settings (346). Additionally, these three diuretic agents decrease hydrogen ion excretion by the late distal tubule and collecting ducts. Evidence that spironolactone decreases hydrogen ion excretion comes from the finding of metabolic acidosis associated with mineralocorticoid deficiency (347,348), and the finding that spironolactone produces metabolic acidosis in patients with cirrhosis who have mineralocorticoid excess (349). In rats, the administration of amiloride and triamterene has been shown to inhibit urinary acidification (338,340). A common mechanism is likely to be involved in mediating the effects of all three diuretic agents on hydrogen ion secretion. These drugs reduce the lumen-negative potential and thus decrease the electrochemical gradient thereby favoring hydrogen ion secretion.

Clearance studies in rats have demonstrated that amiloride decreases calcium excretion (350). In these studies, amiloride produced both a decrease in the calcium clearance:Na clearance ratio ($C_{Ca} : C_{Na}$), as well as a decrease in the fractional excretion of calcium. The effect of triamterene on clearance of calcium was less clear, although it did decrease the $C_{Ca} : C_{Na}$ ratio. *In vivo* microperfusion of rat distal tubules demonstrated that the effect of chlorothiazide on calcium absorption was enhanced with amiloride, but that amiloride's action was along the "late" distal tubule (probably the connecting tubule) rather than in the true DCT (243). Furthermore, *in vitro* perfusion of connecting tubules has shown that amiloride stimulates calcium absorption (249). Amiloride is believed to stimulate calcium absorption through its ability to block sodium channels, thereby hyperpolarizing the apical membrane (351). Hyperpolarization of the apical membrane stimulates calcium entry through hyperpolarization-activated calcium channels, as discussed. Amiloride also has been reported to reduce magnesium excretion (283,352) and prevent the development of hypomagnesemia during therapy with a DCT diuretic (353).

Mechanism of Action

The sites of action of potassium-sparing diuretics are the distal tubule and collecting duct. In this discussion we define the distal tubule as that region of the nephron located between the macula densa and the junction with another distal tubule to form the collecting duct. This segment is a heterogeneous structure composed of at least four cell types: DCT cells, connecting tubule cells, intercalated cells, and principal cells. The collecting duct is the final site of sodium chloride reabsorption where approximately 3% of the filtered load is reabsorbed. In addition to actions on the cortical collecting duct, these diuretics inhibit Na and K transport by the connecting tubule, which is an important site of aldosterone stimulated Na absorption and K secretion (241,263,354). Recent molecular studies have indicated that sites of DCT diuretic action overlap considerably with sites of cortical collecting duct (CCD) diuretic action. Thus, in rat, mouse, and human, a transitional segment, with characteristics of both DCT and connecting tubule, is present along the distal tubule (263,268,313). This segment, which may comprise the bulk of the distal tubule in humans, expresses both the thiazide-sensitive Na-Cl cotransporter and the amiloride-sensitive epithelial Na channel.

Although the cortical collecting tubule reabsorbs only a small percentage of the filtered Na load, two characteristics render this segment important in the physiology of diuretic action. First, this nephron segment is the primary site of action of the mineralocorticoid aldosterone, a hormone that controls sodium reabsorption and potassium secretion. Second, virtually all of the potassium that is excreted is owing to the secretion of potassium by the connecting and collecting tubules. Thus, this segment contributes to the hypokalemia seen as a consequence of diuretic action.

The collecting tubule is composed of two cell types that have entirely separate functions. Principal cells (collecting duct cells) are responsible for the transport of sodium, potassium, and water, whereas intercalated cells are primarily responsible for the secretion of hydrogen or bicarbonate ions.

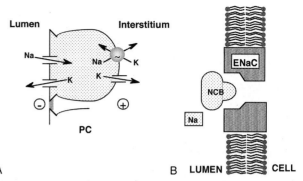

FIG. 82-11. Mechanism of collecting duct diuretics. **A:** Models of principal or connecting tubule cells. Na is reabsorbed via the epithelial Na channel (ENaC), which lies in parallel with a K channel. The transepithelial voltage is oriented with the lumen negative, relative to interstitium. **B:** shows a model of ENaC interaction with Na and with cortical collecting duct diuretics, such as amiloride and triamterene. (Based on information from Busch AE, Suessbrich H, Kunzelmann K, et al. Blockade of epithelial Na+ channels by triamterene-underlying mechanisms and molecular basis. *Pflugers Arch* 1996;432:760; Palmer LG. Epithelial Na channels: the nature of the conducting pore. *Renal Physiol Biochem* 1990;13:51.) In this model, Na channel blockers (indicated as CCDD) interact with the Na conducting pore, because of their positive charge and large size.

The apical membrane of principal cells express separate channels that permit selective conductive transport of sodium and potassium (Fig. 82-11). The mechanism by which sodium reabsorption occurs is through conductive sodium channels (355). The low intracellular sodium concentration as a result of the basolateral Na-K-ATPase generates a favorable electrochemical gradient for sodium entry through sodium channels. Because sodium channels are present only in the apical membrane of principal cells, sodium conductance depolarizes the apical membrane resulting in an asymmetric voltage profile across the cell. This effect produces a lumen-negative transepithelial potential difference. The lumen-negative potential difference together with a high intracellular to lumen potassium concentration gradient provides the driving force for potassium secretion.

Amiloride-sensitive sodium conductance is a function of the epithelial sodium channel (ENaC). The functional channel comprises at least three homologous subunits, α, ß, γ ENaC (356,357), comprising either four (2α, 1ß, 1γ) or nine subunits (358–360). Transcripts encoding the three subunits of ENaC have been identified in classic aldosterone-responsive tissues (361). A number of factors regulate this channel, including hormones (e.g., aldosterone, vasopressin, and oxytocin), intracellular signaling elements (e.g., G-proteins), and cAMP, protein kinase C, intracellular ions (e.g., sodium, hydrogen, and calcium) (361–368) and the cystic fibrosis transmembrane conductance regulator (369,370). Alterations in systemic acid–base balance (371) and sodium intake (372) also have been shown to regulate ENaC function. Studies using selective subunit antisera have demonstrated specific regulation of subunit abundance or pattern of expression. In mice adapted to a high-sodium diet, the α subunit was undetectable, and the ß and γ subunits were expressed in the cytoplasm (372). In contrast, mice on a low-sodium diet displayed subapical or apical expression of all three subunits (372). Administration of dDAVP to Brattleboro rats increased expression of all three subunits to varying degrees (364). Long-term acid loading decreases and base loading increases ß and γ subunits (371).

Nedd4 is a widely expressed ubiquitin-protein ligase that is believed to bind to the PY motif of the carboxy terminal tail of each ENaC subunit. Binding of Nedd4 to ENaC subunits leads to a decrease in Na channel activity (373,374) by decreasing surface expression through ubiquitination and degradation (373,374). It is thought that mutations in the PY motif of the carboxy terminal tail may prevent interaction of Nedd4 with ENaC, leading to Liddle's syndrome (374).

The amount of sodium and potassium present in the final urine is tightly controlled by aldosterone action on connecting and collecting duct cells. Extensive studies have demonstrated that in epithelia, aldosterone produces an early increase in sodium conductance (375,376) followed by a sustained increase in transepithelial sodium transport (375). As a result, transepithelial sodium transport is increased, an effect that depolarizes the apical membrane. An increase in the lumen-negative potential in turn enhances potassium secretion through conductive potassium channels located in the apical membrane. The cellular mechanisms that are responsible for these events have been extensively studied and reviewed (361,367,377). The hormone penetrates the basolateral membrane of principal cells and attaches to a cytosolic mineralocorticoid receptor, a heterotrimeric 8-9s complex of proteins. This receptor complex includes the steroid binding protein and heat shock proteins (HSP). Binding of aldosterone to this complex stimulates the release of HSPs leading to the translocation of the receptor–aldosterone complex to the nucleus (378). The function of HSPs is not clear; however, it is thought that they facilitate anchoring of unbound steroid receptors to the cytoskeleton, maintaining a high affinity conformation (379). Evidence also indicates that released HSP90 stimulates calcineurin, a protein phosphatase that regulates sodium transport, in a transcription-independent process (380). In the nucleus this complex induces the formation of specific messenger RNAs (mRNAs) encoding specific proteins called aldosterone-induced proteins (AIPs) (381). Newly formed mRNA leaves the nucleus to direct the production of AIPs. One such aldosterone-induced protein is the serum and glucocorticoid-induced kinase (sgk) (382–388) or represent ENaC or Na,K-ATPase subunits (381). Aldosterone has been shown to have heterogeneous effects on ENaC subunits. In mammals, aldosterone has been shown to increase the abundance of the α subunit of ENaC (367,389), to redistribute all three subunits to the apical region of principal cells (389) and to induce a shift in the molecular weight of the γ subunit from 85 to 70 kd (389). In contrast, however, a

mineralocorticoid knockout mouse demonstrated essentially normal expression of ENaC subunits in the kidney, suggesting aldosterone regulation ENaC function in a posttranscriptional manner (390).

Spironolactone

Spirolactones are compounds that have the principal effect of blocking aldosterone action (391,392). One of the spirolactones, spironolactone (Fig. 82-10), is an analog of aldosterone that is extensively metabolized (392,393). Spironolactone is converted by deacylation to 7α-thiospironolactone or diethioacetylation to canrenone (391). In the kidney, spironolactone and its metabolites enter target cells from the peritubular side, bind to cytosolic mineralocorticoid receptors, and act as competitive inhibitors of the endogenous hormone (378,394–396). In studies using radiolabeled spironolactone or aldosterone, [^{3}H]–spironolactone–receptor complexes were found to be excluded from the nucleus. In contrast, [^{3}H]–aldosterone–receptor complexes were detected in the nucleus (378). These results are consistent with the proposal that aldosterone antagonists block the translocation of mineralocorticoid receptors to the nucleus. The mechanism by which aldosterone antagonists block nuclear localization of antagonist–receptor complexes is not known; however, it has been suggested that they destabilize mineralocorticoid receptors, thereby facilitating proteolysis (397). As discussed, mineralocorticoid receptors like other steroid receptors contain a steroid-binding unit associated with other cellular components including HSP90, in its inactive state. Steroid binding produces dissociation of HSP90 from the steroid binding unit uncapping the DNA-binding sites. Spironolactone facilitates the release of HSP90 and could lead to degradation of the receptor in combination with rapid dissociation of ligand (397).

Spironolactone induces a mild increase in sodium excretion (1% to 2%) and a decrease in potassium and hydrogen ion excretion (394,398). Its effect depends on the presence of aldosterone. Spironolactone is ineffective in experimental adrenalectomized animals (399) and in patients with Addison's disease (400) or patients on a high-salt diet. In cortical collecting tubules perfused *in vitro*, spironolactone added to the bath solution reduced the aldosterone induced lumen-negative transepithelial voltage (339). By blocking sodium absorption in the collecting tubule, a decrease in lumen-negative potential reduces the driving force for passive sodium and hydrogen ion secretion (339).

Amiloride and Triamterene

Amiloride and triamterene (Fig. 82-10) are structurally different but are organic cations that use the same primary site of action (Fig. 82-11). Triamterene is an aminopteridine chemically related to folic acid and amiloride is a pyrazinoylguanidine. Systemically administered amiloride results in an increase in sodium excretion and decrease in potassium excretion (58,207,338,401). Their actions on sodium and potassium transport, unlike spironolactone, are independent of aldosterone (401). Systemically administered amiloride produces a small increase in sodium excretion and a much larger decrease in potassium excretion (207,402,403). Sampling of tubule fluid from the distal tubule demonstrated an inhibition of the normal rise in the tubule fluid to plasma potassium ratio. These results indicated that amiloride decreased distal tubule potassium secretion. Experiments employing *in vivo* microperfusion of distal tubules (323,404) and *in vitro* perfusion of isolated cortical collecting tubules (405,406) demonstrated that luminally administered amiloride reduced sodium absorption and potassium secretion. Similar results were obtained following *in vivo* microperfusion with benazamil (407), a more potent amiloride analog (408). Amiloride decreases potassium secretion by blocking sodium conductance in the apical membrane of distal tubule and collecting tubule cells (407,409,410), thereby decreasing the electrochemical gradient for potassium secretion.

In high concentrations ($>100~\mu$M), amiloride interacts with different transporters, enzymes, and receptors; however, at concentrations of 0.05 to 0.5 μM, amiloride interacts specifically with sodium channels (362,363). Furthermore, aromatic substitutions on the guanidinium moiety render the molecule even more potent (IC_{50} 10- to 20-fold lower than amiloride) (343,362). Only the parent compound, amiloride, however, is available for clinical use. The molecular mechanism by which amiloride blocks sodium channels has not yet been defined. It is likely, however, that the positive charge on the guanidinium moiety plays an important role in occluding the sodium channel (Fig. 82-11) (355,363). Amiloride has been demonstrated to bind to a 150-kd protein from the bovine renal papilla (411); however, the relationship between this protein and the putative Na channel components, α, ß, and γ rENaC, is not known (363). Other approaches using mutational analysis (412,413) and antiamiloride antibodies (414) have demonstrated contributions to amiloride binding by all three subunits in close proximity to the channel pore. A putative amiloride binding domain, WYRFHY, of the α subunit of ENaC has been identified (415).

Clearance and free-flow micropuncture studies using triamterene demonstrated results similar to studies with amiloride (207); however, the mechanism of action is not clearly defined. In earlier studies of rabbit cortical collecting tubules perfused *in vitro*, triamterene produced a gradual, reversible inhibition of the potential difference after a latent period of 10 minutes (339). Recent studies, however, suggest that triamterene binds to the epithelial sodium channel and thus has a mechanism of action similar to amiloride (416).

Pharmacokinetics

Spironolactone is poorly soluble in aqueous fluids. Bioavailability of an oral dose is approximately 90% in some but not all commercial preparations. The drug is rapidly metabolized in the liver into a number of metabolites. Until recently, canrenone was thought to be the major metabolite of spironolactone (392,393). This conclusion was based on fluorometric assays. Assays of spironolactone and its metabolites by the use of high performance liquid chromatography (HPLC), however, demonstrated that fluorometrically measured levels of canrenone overestimated true canrenone levels (417). Using HPLC, the predominant metabolite, 7α-methylspironolactone (418), is responsible for roughly 80% of the potassium-sparing effect. Spironolactone and its metabolites are extensively bound to plasma protein (98%). In normal volunteers, taking spironolactone (100 mg/day) for 15 days, the mean half-lives for spironolactone, canrenone, 7α-thiomethylspironolactone and 6ß-hydroxy-7α-thiomethyl-spironolactone were 1.4, 16.5, 13.8, and 15 hours, respectively. Thus, although unmetabolized spironolactone is present in serum, it has a rapid elimination time. The onset of action is extremely slow, with peak response sometimes occurring 48 hours or more after the first dose; effects gradually wane over a period of 48 to 72 hours. Spironolactone is used in cirrhotic patients to induce a natriuresis. In these patients, pharmacokinetic studies indicate that the half-lives of spironolactone and its metabolites are increased. The half-lives for spironolactone, canrenone, 7α-thiomethylspironolactone and 6ß-hydroxy-7α-thiomethyl-spironolactone are 9, 58, 24, and 126 hours, respectively (419).

Clinical Use

The most common side effect of loop and DCT diuretics is the depletion of body potassium with or without significant lowering of serum K concentration. Hypokalemia of sufficient magnitude may produce nonspecific weakness or may be life threatening. The more severe effects include impairment of neuromuscular function, cardiac dysrhythmia, intestinal disturbances, and partial loss of the ability to concentrate urine. Of particular concern is the potential for cardiac toxicity in patients with congestive heart failure who are maintained on cardiac glycosides. Given these potential problems, it is important to avoid potassium deficit through dietary intake of large amounts of potassium, avoidance of excessive NaCl intake, and monitoring of serum K concentrations. The most effective therapeutic measure is to add a potassium-sparing diuretic to the therapeutic regimen (420), but KCl supplements should be discontinued or plasma K monitored carefully if a K-sparing agent is used.

Spironolactone is most effective in patients with primary (adrenal adenoma or bilateral adrenal hyperplasia) (421) or secondary hyperaldosteronism (congestive heart failure, cirrhosis, nephrotic syndrome), and is ineffective in patients with a nonfunctional adrenal gland. Spironolactone is used for correction of hypokalemia. The drug is also administered alone, or with thiazides or a loop diuretic to reduce the ECF volume without causing potassium depletion or hypokalemia. The drug is especially appropriate for the treatment of cirrhosis with ascites, a condition invariably associated with secondary hyperaldosteronism. In comparison to loop or thiazide diuretics, spironolactone is equivalent or more effective (422). A combination of loop diuretic in addition to spironolactone can be used to boost natriuresis when the diuretic effect of spironolactone alone is inadequate. As noted, in low doses (25 mg/day) spironolactone has been shown recently to reduce morbidity and mortality in congestive heart failure when added to a regimen of ACE inhibitors and loop diuretics (345). This effect may be owing to blocking extrarenal effects of aldosterone (e.g., cardiac fibrosis or vascular compliance).

Spironolactone is the treatment of choice for hypertension resulting from adrenocortical hyperplasia (423).

Triamterene or amiloride is generally used in combination with potassium-wasting diuretics (thiazide or loop diuretics), especially when maintenance of normal serum potassium concentrations is clinically important. In addition, amiloride (or triamterene) has also been used as initial therapy in potassium wasting states such as primary hyperaldosteronism (424,425), Liddle's (426), Bartter's, or Gitelman's syndrome (344). Amiloride has been used in the treatment of lithium-induced nephrogenic diabetes insipidus (427). The efficacy of amiloride in this disorder relates to the ability of amiloride to block collecting duct sodium channels, a pathway by which lithium uses to gain entry into cells (428,429).

Adverse Effects

Hyperkalemia is the most serious adverse reaction encountered during therapy with spironolactone. Serum potassium should be monitored periodically even when the drug is administered with a potassium-wasting diuretic. Patients at highest risk are those with low glomerular filtration rates and those individuals who take potassium supplements concurrently. Hyperchloremic metabolic acidosis can develop independent of changes in renal function in patients with cirrhosis and ascites treated with spironolactone (349). Gynecomastia may occur in men, especially as the dose is increased (430); decreased libido and impotence also have been reported. Women may develop menstrual irregularities, hirsutism, or swelling and tenderness of the breasts. Spironolactone-induced agranulocytosis also has been reported (431).

Triamterene and amiloride may cause hyperkalemia. The risk of hyperkalemia is highest in patients with limited renal function (e.g., renal insufficiency, diabetes, and elderly patients). Additional complications included elevated serum blood urea nitrogen and uric acid, glucose intolerance, and gastrointestinal disturbances. Triamterene induces crystalluria or cylindruria (432), may contribute to or initiate formation of renal stones (433), and acute renal failure when combined with NSAIDs (434,435). The drugs are contraindicated in patients with hyperkalemia, individuals taking potassium supplements in any form, and patients with severe renal failure with progressive oliguria.

ACKNOWLEDGMENTS

The authors acknowledge with appreciation the contributions of Rainer Greger, an author of the previous version of this chapter.

REFERENCES

1. Eknoyan, G. A history of diuretics. In: Seldin DW, Giebisch G, eds. *Diuretic agents: clinical physiology and pharmacology.* San Diego: Academic Press, 1997:3.
2. Biemesderfer D, Pizzonia J, Abu-Alfa A, et al. NHE3: A Na+/H+ exchanger isoform of the brush border. *Am J Physiol* 1993;265:F736.
3. Ecelbarger CA, Wade JB, Terris J, et al. Localization and regulation of bumetanide-sensitive cotransporter protein in rat kidney. *J Am Soc Nephrol* 95;6:335.
4. Kaplan MR, Plotkin MD, Lee WS, et al. Apical localization of the Na-K-Cl cotransporter, *rBSC1*, on rat thick ascending limbs. *Kidney Int* 1996;49:40.
5. Obermüller N, Bernstein PL, Velázquez H, et al. Expression of the thiazide-sensitive Na-Cl cotransporter in rat and human kidney. *Am J Physiol* 1995;269:F900.
6. Obermüller N, Kuncharparty S, Ellison DH, et al. Expression of the Na-K-2Cl cotransporter by macula densa and thick ascending limb cells of rat and rabbit nephron. *J Clin Invest* 1996;98:635.
7. Duc C, Farman N, Canessa CM, et al. Cell-specific expression of epithelial sodium channel α, ß, and γ subunits in aldosterone-responsive epithelia from the rat: localization by in situ hybridization and immunocytochemistry. *J Cell Biol* 1994;127:1907.
8. Seldin DW, Giebisch G. *Diuretic agents: clinical physiology and pharmacology.* San Diego: Academic Press, 1997.
9. Brater DC. Diuretic pharmacokinetics and pharmacodynamics. In: Seldin DW, Giebisch G. *Diuretic agents: clinical physiology and pharmacology.* San Diego: Academic Press, 1997:189.
10. Better OS, Rubinstein I, Winaver JM, et al. Mannitol therapy revisited (1940–1997). *Kidney Int* 1997;51:886.
11. Wong NLM, Quamme GA, Sutton RAL, et al. Effects of mannitol on water and electrolyte transport in dog kidney. *J Lab Clin Med* 1979;94:683.
12. Duarte CG, Watson JF. Calcium reabsorption in proximal tubule of the dog nephron. *Am J Physiol* 1967;212:1355.
13. Stinebaugh BJ, Bartow SA, Eknoyan G, et al. Renal handling of bicarbonate: effect of mannitol diuresis. *Am J Physiol* 1971;220:1271.
14. Seely JF, Dirks JH. Micropuncture study of hypertonic mannitol diuresis in the proximal and distal tubule of the dog kidney. *J Clin Invest* 1969;48:2330.
15. Wesson LG Jr, Anslow WP. Excretion of sodium and water during osmotic diuresis in the dog. *Am J Physiol* 1948;153:465.
16. Winghager EE, Whittembury G, Oken DE, et al. Single proximal tubules of the Necturus kidney. III. Dependence of H_2O movement on NaCl concentration. *Am J Physiol* 1959;197:313.
17. Grennari RJ, Kassirer JP. Osmotic diuresis. *N Engl J Med* 1974; 291:714.
18. Buerkert J, Martin D, Prasad J, et al. Role of deep nephrons and the terminal collecting duct in a mannitol-induced diuresis. *Am J Physiol* 1981;240:F411.
19. Morris CR, Alexander EA, Bruns FJ, et al. Restoration and maintenance of glomerular filtration by mannitol during hypoperfusion of the kidney. *J Clin Invest* 1972;51:1555.
20. Thurau K. Renal hemodynamics. *Am J Med* 1964;36:698.
21. Nashat FS, Scholefield FR, Tappin JW, et al. The effect of acute changes in haematocrit in the anaesthetized dog on the volume and character of the urine. *J Physiol* 1969;205:305.
22. Nashat FS, Scholefield FR, Tappin JW, et al. The effects of changes in haematocrit on the intrarenal distribution of blood flow in the dog's kidney. *J Physiol* 1969;201:639.

23. Elpers MJ, Selkurt EE. Effects of albumin infusion on renal function in the dog. *Am J Physiol* 1920;153:161.

24. Johnston PA, Bernard DB, Perrin NS, et al. Prostaglandins mediate the vasodilatory effect of mannitol in the hypoperfused rat kidney. *J Clin Invest* 1981;68:127.

25. Yamasaki Y, Nishiuchi T, Kojima A, et al. Effects of an oral water load and intravenous administration of isotonic glucose, hypertonic saline, mannitol and furosemide on the release of atrial natriuretic peptide in men. *Acta Endocrinol (Copenhagen)* 1988;119:269.

26. Goldberg AH, Lilienfield LS. Effects of hypertonic mannitol on renal vascular resistance. *Proc Soc Exp Biol Med* 1965;119:635.

27. Lang F. Osmotic diuresis. *Renal Physiol* 1987;160:173.

28. Blantz RC. Effect of mannitol on glomerular ultrafiltration in the hydropenic rat. *J Clin Invest* 1974;54:1135.

29. Goldberg M, Ramirez MA. Effects of saline and mannitol diuresis on the renal concentrating mechanism in dogs: alterations in renal tissue solutes and water. *Clin Sci* 1967;32:475.

30. Anderson P, Boreus L, Gordon E, et al. Use of mannitol during neurosurgery: interpatient variability in the plasma and CSF levels. *Eur J Clin Pharmacol* 1988;35:643.

31. Weiner IM. Diuretics and other agents employed in the mobilization of edema fluid. In: Gilman AG, Rall TW, Nies AS, et al, eds. *The pharmacological basis of therapeutics*. New York: Pergamon Press, 1990:713.

32. Stevens MA, McCullough PA, Tobin KJ, et al. A prospective randomized trial of prevention measures in patients at high risk for contrast nephropathy: results of the P.R.I.N.C.E. study. Prevention of Radiocontrast Induced Nephropathy Clinical Evaluation. *J Am Coll Cardiol* 1999;33:403.

33. Conger JD. Interventions in clinical acute renal failure: what are the data? *Am J Kid Dis* 1995;26:565.

34. Thadhani R, Pascual M, Bonventre JV. Acute renal failure. *N Engl J Med* 1996;334:1448.

35. Better OS, Stein JH. Early management of shock and prophylaxis of acute renal failure in traumatic rhabdomyolysis. *N Engl J Med* 1990;322:825.

36. Van Valenberg PLJ, Hoitsma AJ, Tiggeler RGWL. Mannitol as an indispensable constituent of an intraoperative hydration protocol for the prevention of acute renal failure after renal cadaveric transplantation. *Transplantation* 1987;784:788.

37. Grino JM, Miravitlles R, Castelao AM. Flush solution with mannitol in the prevention of post-transplant renal failure. *Transplant Proc* 1987;19:4140.

38. Koning OH, Ploeg RJ, van Bockel JH, et al. Risk factors for delayed graft function in cadaveric kidney transplantation: a prospective study of renal function and graft survival after preservation with University of Wisconsin solution in multi-organ donors. European Multicenter Study Group. *Transplantation* 1963;63:1620.

39. Weisberg LS, Kurnick PB, Kurnik BR. Risk of radiocontrast in patients with and without diabetes mellitus. *Kidney Int* 1994;45:259.

40. Solomon R, Werner C, Mann D, et al. Effects of saline, mannitol, and furosemide on acute decreases in renal function induced by radiocontrast agents. *N Engl J Med* 1994;331:1416.

41. Quon DK, Worthen DM. Dose response of intravenous mannitol on the human eye. *Ann Opthalmol* 1981;13:1392.

42. McGraw CP, Howard G. Effect of mannitol on increased intracranial pressure. *Neurosurgery* 1983;13:269.

43. Jenkins IR, Curtis AP. The combination of mannitol and albumin in the priming solution reduces positive intraoperative fluid balance during cardiopulmonary bypass. *Perfusion* 1995;10:301.

44. England MD, Cavaroocchi NC, O'Brien JF, et al. Influence of antioxidants (mannitol and allopurinol) on oxygen free radical generation during and after cardiopulmonary bypass. *Circulation* 1986;74:134.

45. Gong G, Lindberg J, Abrams J, et al. Comparison of hypertonic saline solutions and dextran in dialysis-induced hypotension. *J Am Soc Nephrol* 1993;3:1808.

46. Arieff AI. Dialysis disequilibrium syndrome: current concepts on pathogenesis and prevention. *Kidney Int* 1994;45:629.

47. Aviram A, Pfau A, Czackes JW, et al. Hyperosmolality with hyponatremia caused by inappropriate administration of mannitol. *Am J Med* 1967;42:648.

48. Moreno M, Murphy C, Goldsmith C. Increase in serum potassium resulting from the administration of hypertonic mannitol and other solutions. *J Lab Clin Med* 1969;73:291.

49. Makoff DL, DaSilva JA, Rosenbaum BJ. On the mechanism of hyperkalemia due to hyperosmotic expansion with saline or mannitol. *Clin Sci* 1971;41:383.

50. Gipstein RM, Boyle JD. Hypernatremia complicating prolonged mannitol diuresis. *N Engl J Med* 1965;272:1116.

51. Dorman HR, Sondheimer JH, Cadnapaphornchai P. Mannitol-induced acute renal failure. *Medicine* 1990;69:153.

52. Visweswaran P, Massin EK, DuBose TD Jr. Mannitol-induced acute renal failure. *J Am Soc Nephrol* 1997;8:1028.

53. Temes SP, Lilien OM, Chamberlain W. A direct vasoconstrictor effect of mannitol on the renal artery. *Surg Gynecol Obstet* 1975;141:223.

54. DuBose TD, Lucci MS. Effect of carbonic anhydrase inhibition on superficial and deep nephron bicarbonate reabsorption in the rat. *J Clin Invest* 1983;71:55.

55. Cogan MG, Maddox DA, Warnock DG, et al. Effect of acetazolamide on bicarbonate reabsorption in the proximal tubule of the rat. *Am J Physiol* 1979;237:F447.

56. Buckalew VM Jr, Walker BR, Puschett JB, et al. Effects of increased sodium delivery on distal tubular sodium reabsorption with and without volume expansion in man. *J Clin Invest* 1970;49:2336.

57. Beck LH, Goldberg M. Effects of acetazolamide and parathyroidectomy on renal transport of sodium, calcium and phosphate. *Am J Physiol* 1973;224:1136.

58. Puschett JB, Winaver J. Efects of diuretics on renal function. In: Windhager EE, ed. *Handbook of physiology*. New York: Oxford University Press, 1992:2335.

59. Malnic G, Klose RM, Giebisch G. Micropuncture study of distal tubular potassium and sodium transport in rat nephron. *Am J Physiol* 1966;211:529.

60. Puschett JB, Rastegar A. Comparative study of the effects of metolazone and other diuetics on potassium excretion. *Clin Pharmacol Ther* 1973;15:397.

61. Beck LH, Senesky D, Goldberg M. Sodium-independent active potassium reabsorption in proximal tubule of the dog. *J Clin Invest* 1973; 52:2641.

62. Okusa MD, Persson AEG, Wright FS. Chlorothiazide effect on feedback mediated control of glomerular filtration rate. *Am J Physiol* 1989;257:F137.

63. Good DW, Wright FS. Luminal influences on potassium secretion: sodium concentration and fluid flow rate. *Am J Physiol* 1979;236:F192.

64. Velázquez H, Wright FS, and Good DW. Luminal influences on potassium secretion: chloride replacement with sulfate. *Am J Physiol* 1982; 242:F46.

65. Dobyan C, Bulger RE. Renal carbonic anhydrase. *Am J Physiol* 1982;243:F311.

66. Preisig PA, Toto RD, Alpern RJ. Carbonic anhydrase inhibitors. *Renal Physiol* 1987;10:136.

67. Maren TH. Carbonic anhydrase: chemistry, physiology, and inhibition. *Pharmacol Revs* 1967;47:597.

68. Wistrand PJ, Wahlstrand T. Rat renal and erythrocyte carbonic anhydrases: purification and properties. *Biochim Biophys Acta* 1977; 481:712.

69. Eveloff J, Swenson ER, Maren TH. Carbonic anhydrase activity of brush border and plasma membranes prepared from rat kidney cortex. *Biochem Pharmacol* 1979;28:1434.

70. Maren TH. Current status of membrane-bound carbonic anhydrase. *Ann NY Acad Sci* 1980;341:246.

71. Sanyal G, Pessah NI, Maren TH. Kinetics and inhibition of membrane-bound carbonic anhydrase from canine renal cortex. *Biochim Biophys Acta* 1965;1981:128.

72. Wistrand PJ, Kinne R. Carbonic anhydrase activity of isolated brush border and basal-lateral membranes of renal tubular cells. *Pflugers Arch* 1977;370:121.

73. Lonnerholm G, Wistrand PJ. Membrane-bound carbonic anhydrase CA IV in the human kidney. *Acta Physiol Scand* 1991;141:231.

74. Giebisch G, Malnic G, DeMello GB, et al. Kinetics of luminal acification in cortical tubules of the rat kidney. *J Physiol* 1977;267:571.

75. Sly WS, Whyte MP, Sundaram V, et al. Carbonic anhydrase II deficiency in 12 families with the autosomal recessive syndrome of osteopetrosis with renal tubular acidosis and cerebral calcification. *N Engl J Med* 1985;313:139.

76. Tsuruoka S, Kittelberger M, Schwartz J. Carbonic anhydrase II and IV mRNA in rabbit nephron segments: stimulation during metabolic acidosis. *Am J Physiol* 1998;274:F259.

77. Pitts RF, Alexander RS. The nature of renal tubular mechanism for acidifying the urine. *Am J Physiol* 1945;144:239.

78. DuBose TD Jr, Pucacco LR, Seldin DW, et al. Microelectrode determination of pH and PCO_2 in rat proximal tubule after benzolamide: evidence for hydrogen ion secretion. *Kidney Int* 1979;15:624.

79. DuBose TD Jr, Pucacco LR, Carter NW. Determination of disequilibrium pH in the rat kidney *in vivo*. Evidence for hydrogen ion secretion. *Am J Physiol* 1981;240:F138.

80. Rector FC Jr, Carter NW, Seldin DW. The mechanism of bicarbonate reabsorption in the proximal and distal tubules of the kidney. *J Clin Invest* 1965;44:278.

81. Vieira FL, Malnic G. Hydrogen ion secretion by rat renal cortical tubule as studied by an antimony microelectrode. *Am J Physiol* 1968;214:710.

82. Maren TH. Carbonic anhydrase. *N Engl J Med* 1985;313:179.

83. Akiba T, Alpern RJ, Eveloff J, et al. Electrogenic sodium/bicarbonate cotransport in rabbit renal cortical basolateral membrane vesicles. *J Clin Invest* 1986;78:1472.

84. Alpern, R. J. Mechanism of basolateral membrane $H^+/OH^-/HCO_3^-$ transport in the rat proximal convoluted tubule: a sodium-coupled electrogenic process. *J Gen Physiol* 1985;86:613.

85. Boron WF, Boulpaep EL. Intracellular pH regulation in the renal proximal tubule of the salamander. Basolateral HCO_3^- transport. *J Gen Physiol* 1983;81:53.

86. Grassl SM, Aronson PS. Na^+/HCO_3^- co-transport in basolateral membrane vesicles isolated from rabbit renal cortex. *J Biol Chem* 1986;261:8778.

87. Yoshitomi K, Burckhardt BC, Fromter E. Rheogenic sodium bicarbonate cotransport in the peritubular cell membrane of rat renal proximal tubule. *Pflugers Arch* 1985;405:360.

88. Lawrie GM, Morris GC, DeBakey ME. Long-term results of treatment of the totally occluded renal artery in forty patients with renovascular hypertension. *Surgery* 1980;88:753.

89. Schild L, Giebisch G, Karniski LP, et al. Effect of formate on volume reabsorption in the rabbit proximal tubule. *J Clin Invest* 1987;79:32.

90. Karniski LP, Aronson PS. Chloride/formate exchange with formic acid recycling: a mechanism of active chloride transport across epithelial membranes. *Proc Natl Acad Sci USA* 1985;82:6362.

91. Goldberg M. The renal physiology of diuretics. In: Orloff JJ, Berliner RW, eds. *Handbook of physiology*. Washington, DC: American Physiologic Society, 1973:1003.

92. Cortney MA, Mylle M, Lassiter WE, et al. Renal tubular transport of water, solute, and PAH in rats loaded with isotonic saline. *Am J Physiol* 1965;1199:1205.

93. Lassiter WE, Gottschalk CW, Mylle M. Micropuncture study of net transtubular movement of water and urea in nondiuretic mammalian kidney. *Am J Physiol* 1961;200:1139.

94. Maren TH. Carbonic anhydrase inhibition. IV. The effects of metabolic acidosis on the response to Diamox. *Bull Johns Hopkins Hosp* 1956;98:159.

95. Shuichi T, Schwartz GJ. HCO_3^- absorption in rabbit outer medullary collecting duct: role of luminal carbonic anhydrase. *Am J Physiol* 1998;274:F139.

96. Kunau RT Jr. The influence of carbonic anhydrase inhibitor, Benzolamide (CL-11,366), on the reabsorption of chloride, sodium, and bicarbonate in the proximal tubule of the rat. *J Clin Invest* 1972;51:294.

97. Lucci MS, Pucacco LR, DuBose TD Jr, et al. Direct evaluation of acidification by rat proximal tubule: role of carbonic anhydrase. *Am J Physiol* 1980;238:F372.

98. Lucci MS, Warnock DG, Rector FC Jr. Carbonic anhydrase-dependent reabsorption in the rat proximal tubule. *Am J Physiol* 1979;236:F58.

99. Burg M, Green N. Bicarbonate transport by isolated rabbit proximal convoluted tubules. *Am J Physiol* 1997;233:F307.

100. Malnic G, De Mello Aires M, Giebisch G. Micropuncture study of renal tubular hydrogen ion transport in the rat. *Am J Physiol* 1972;222:147.

101. McKinney TD, Burg M. Bicarbonate and fluid absorption by renal proximal straight tubule. *Kidney Int* 1977;12:1.

102. Koeppen BM, Helman SI. Acidification of luminal fluid by the rabbit cortical collecting tubule perfused in vitro. *Am J Physiol* 1982;242:F521.

103. Lombard WE, Kokko JP, Jacobson HR. Bicarbonate transport in cortical and outer medullary collecting tubules. *Am J Physiol* 1983;244:F289.

104. Ullrich KJ, Papavassiliou F. Bicarbonate reabsorption in the papillary collecting duct of rats. *Pflugers Arch* 1981;389:271.

105. Richardson RMA, Kunau RT Jr. Bicarbonate reabsorption in the papillary collecting duct: effect of acetazolamide. *Am J Physiol* 1982;243:F74.

106. Holder LB, Hayes SL. Diffusion of sulfonamides in aqueous buffers and into red cells. *Mol Pharmacol* 1965;1:266.

107. Lang F, Quehenberger P, Greger R, et al. Effect of benzolamide on luminal pH in proximal convoluted tubules of the rat kidney. *Pflugers Arch* 1978;375:39.

108. Tinker JP, Coulson R, Weiner IM. Dextran-bound inhibitors of carbonic anhydrase. *J Pharmacol Exp Ther* 1981;218:600.

109. Burckhardt BC, Sato K, Frömter E. Electrophysiological analysis of bicarbonate permeation across the peritubular cell membrane of rat kidney proximal tubule. I. Basic observations. *Pflugers Arch* 1874;401:34.

110. Sasaki S, Marumo F. Effects of carbonic anhydrase inhibitors on basolateral base transport of rabbit proximal straight tubule. *Am J Physiol* 1989;257:F947.

111. Soleimani M, Aronson PS. Effects of acetazolamide on Na^+-HCO_3^- cotransport in basolateral membrane vesicles isolated from rabbit renal cortex. *J Clin Invest* 1989;83:945.

112. Brown D, Hirsch S, Gluck S. An H^+-ATPase in opposite plasma membrane domains in kidney epithelial cell subpopulations. *Nature* 1988;331:622.

113. Wingo CS. Active proton secretion and potassium absorption in the rabbit outer medullary collecting duct: functional evidence for H-K-ATPase. *J Clin Invest* 1990;84:361.

114. Okusa MD, Unwin RJ, Velázquez H, et al. Active potassium absorption by the renal distal tubule. *Am J Physiol* 1992;262:F488.

115. Kone BC. Renal H,K-ATPase: structure, function and regulation. *Min Electrolyte Metab* 1996;22:349.

116. Star RA, Burg MB, Knepper MA. Luminal disequilibrium pH and ammonia transport in outer medullary collecting duct. *Am J Physiol* 1987;252:F1148.

117. Persson AE, Wright FS. Evidence for feedback mediated reduction of glomerular filtration rate during infusion of acetazolamide. *Acta Physiol Scand* 1982;114:1.

118. Tucker BJ, Blantz RC. Studies on the mechanism of reduction in glomerular filtration rate after benzolamide. *Pflugers Arch* 1980;388:211.

119. Tucker BJ, Steiner RW, Gushwa L, et al. Studies on the tubuloglomerular feedback system in the rat: the mechanism of reduction in filtration rate with benzolamide. *J Clin Invest* 1978;62:993.

120. Heller I, Halevy J, Cohen J, et al. Significant metabolic acidosis induced by acetazolamide. Not a rare complication. *Arch Intern Med* 1985;145:1815.

121. Parfitt AM. Acetazolamide and sodium bicarbonate induced nephrocalcinosis and nephrolithiasis: relationship to citrate and calcium excretion. *Arch Intern Med* 1969;124:736.

122. Stafstrom CE, Gilmore HE, Kurtin PS. Nephrocalcinosis complicating medical treatment of posthemorrhagic hydrocephalus. *Pediatr Neurol* 1992;8:179.

123. Johnson T, Kass MA. Hematologic reactions to carbonic anhydrase inhibitors. *Am J Opthalmol* 1986;101:410.

124. Werblin TP, Pollack IP, Liss RA. Blood dyscrasias in patients using methazolamide (Neptazane) for glaucoma. *Opthalmology* 1980;87:350.

125. Rose BD. *Clinical physiology of acid-base and electrolyte disorders.* New York: McGraw-Hill, 1994.

126. Bear R, Goldstein M, Phillipson M, et al. Effect of metabolic alkalosis on respiratory function in patients with chronic obstructive lung disease. *Can Med Assoc J* 1977;117:900.

127. Miller PD, Berns AS. Acute metabolic alkalosis perpetuating hypercarbia: a role for acetazolamide in chronic obstructive pulmonary disease. *JAMA* 1977;238:2400.

128. Marik PE, Kussman BD, Lipman J, et al. Acetazolamide in the treatment of metabolic alkalosis in critically ill patients. *Heart and Lung* 1991;20:455.

129. Strahlman E, Tipping R, Vogel R. A double-masked, randomized 1-year study comparing dorzolamide (Trusopt), timolol, and betaxolol. International Dorzolamide Study Group. *Arch Ophthamol* 1995;113:1009.

130. Serle JB. Pharmacological advances in the treatment of glaucoma. *Drugs and Aging* 1994;5:156.

131. Grissom CK, Roach RC, Sarnquist FH, et al. Acetazolamide in the treatment of acute mountain sickness: clinical efficacy and effect on gas. *Ann Intern Med* 1992;116:461.

132. Sutton JR, Houston CS, Mansell AL, et al. Effect of acetazolamide on hypoxemia during sleep at high altitude. *N Engl J Med* 1979;301:1329.

133. Griggs RC, Engel WK, Resnick JS. Acetazolamide treatment of hypokalemic periodic paralysis. Prevention of attacks and improvement of persistent weakness. *Ann Intern Med* 1970;73:39.

134. Resnick JS, Engle WK, Griggs RC, et al. Acetazolamide prophylaxis in hypokalemic periodic paralysis. *N Engl J Med* 1968;278:582.

135. Johnsen T. Effect upon serum insulin, glucose and potassium concentrations of acetazolamide during attacks of familial periodic hypokalemic paralysis. *Acta Neurol Scand* 1977;56:533.

136. Reiss WG, Oles KS. Acetazolamide in the treatment of seizures. *Ann Pharmacother* 1996;30:514.

137. Shoeman JF. Childhood pseudotumor cerebri: clinical and intracranial pressure response to acetazolamide and furosemide treatment in a case series. *J Child Neurol* 1994;9:130.

138. Shore ET, Millman EP. Central sleep apnea and acetazolamide therapy. *Arch Intern Med* 1983;143:1278.

139. Prescott LF, Balali-Mood M, Critchley JA, et al. Diuresis or urinary alkalinization for salicylate poisoning? *Br Med J* 1982;285:1383.

140. Goldberg M, McCurdy DK, Foltz E, et al. Effects of ethacrynic acid (a new saluretic agent) on renal diluting and concentrating mechanisms: evidence for site of action in the loop of Henle. *J Clin Invest* 1964;43:201.

141. Earley LE, Friedler RM. Renal tubular effects of ethacrynic acid. *J Clin Invest* 1964;43:1495.

142. Suki W, Rector FC Jr, Seldin DW. The site of action of furosemide and other sulfonamide diuretics in the dog. *J Clin Invest* 1965;44:1458.

143. Suki WN, Eknoyan G. Physiology of diuretic action. In: Seldin DW, Giebisch G, eds. *The kidney: physiology and pathophysiology.* New York: Raven Press, 1992:3629.

144. Puschett JB, Goldberg M. The acute effects of furosemide on acid and electrolyte excretion in man. *J Lab Clin Med* 1968;71:666.

145. Decaux G, Waterlot Y, Genette F, et al. Treatment of the syndrome of inappropriate antidiuretic hormone with furosemide. *N Engl J Med* 1981;304:329.

146. Hantman D, Rossier B, Zohlman R, et al. Rapid correction of hyponatremia in the syndrome of inappropriate secretion of antidiuretic hormone: an alternative treatment to hypertonic saline. *Ann Intern Med* 1973;78:870.

147. Khuri RN, Wiederholt M, Strieder N, et al. Effects of graded solute diuresis on renal tubular sodium transport in the rat. *Am J Physiol* 1975;228:1262.

148. di Stefano A, Greger R, Desfleurs E, et al. A Ba(2+)-insensitive K+ conductance in the basolateral cell membrane of rabbit cortical thick ascending limb cells. *Cell Physiol Biochem* 1998;8:89.

149. Vandewalle A, Cluzeaud F, Bens M, et al. Localization and induction by dehydration of ClC-K chloride channels in the rat kidney. *Am J Physiol* 1997;272:F678.

150. Hebert SC, Gamba G, Kaplan M. The electroneutral Na^+-(K^+)-Cl^- cotransport family. *Kidney Int* 1996;49:1638.

151. Delpire E, Kaplan MR, Plotkin MD, et al. The Na-(K)-Cl cotransporter family in the mammalian kidney: molecular identification and function(s). *Nephrol Dial Transplant* 1996;11:1967.

152. Quaggin SE, Payne JA, Forbush BI, et al. Localization of the renal Na-K-Cl cotransporter gene (Slc12a1) on mouse chromosome 2. *Mammalian Genome* 1995;6:557.

153. Ecelbarger CA, Terris J, Hoyer JR, et al. Localization and regulation of the rat renal Na^+-K^+-$2Cl^-$ cotransporter, BSC-1. *Am J Physiol Renal Fluid Electrolyte Physiol* 1996;271:F619.

154. Xu JZ, Hall AE, Peterson LN, et al. Localization of the ROMK protein on the apical membranes of rat kidney nephron segments. *Am J Physiol* 1997;273:F739.

155. Greger R, Schlatter E. Cellular mechanism of the action of loop diuretics on the thick ascending limb of Henle's loop. *Klin Wochenschrift* 1983;61:1019.

156. Hebert SC, Reeves WB, Molony DA, et al. The medullary thick limb: function and modulation of the single-effect multiplier. *Kidney Int* 1987;31:580.

157. Miyanoshita A, Terada M, Endou H. Furosemide directly stimulates prostaglandin E_2 production in the thick ascending limb of Henle's loop. *J Pharmacol Exp Ther* 1989;251:1155.

158. Abe K, Yasuima M, Cheiba L, et al. Effect of furosemide on urinary excretion of prostaglandin E in normal volunteers and patients with essential hypertension. *Prostaglandins* 1977;14:513.

159. Wright JT, Corder CN, Taylor R. Studies on rat kidney 15-hydroxyprostaglandin dehydrogenase. *Biochem Pharmacol* 1976;25:1669.

160. Kirchner KA. Prostaglandin inhibitors alter loop segment chloride uptake during furosemide diuresis. *Am J Physiol* 1985;248:F698.

161. Kirchner KA, Martin CJ, Bower JD. Prostaglandin E2 but not I2 restores furosemide response in indomethacin-treated rats. *Am J Physiol* 1986;250:F980.

162. Bilezikian JP. Management of hypercalcemia. *J Clin Endocrinol Metab* 1993;77:1445.

163. Friedman PA. Codependence of renal calcium and sodium transport. *Annu Rev Physiol* 1998;60:179.

164. Simon DB, Lu Y, Choate KA, et al. Paracellin-1, a renal tight junction protein required for paracellular Mg2+ resorption [see comments]. *Science* 1999;285:103.

165. Friedman PA. Basal and hormone-activated calcium absorption in mouse renal thick ascending limbs. *Am J Physiol* 1988;254:F62.

166. Bourdeau JE, Hellstrom-Stein RJ. Voltage-dependent calcium movement across the cortical collecting duct. *Am J Physiol* 1982;242:F285.

167. Burg MB. Tubular chloride transport and the mode of action of some diuretics. *Kidney Int* 1976;9:189.

168. Burg MB, Isaacson L, Grantham JJ, et al. Electrical properties of isolated perfused rabbit renal tubules. *Am J Physiol* 1968;215:788.

169. Burg MB, Green N. Effect of ethacrynic acid on the thick ascending limb of Henle's loop. *Kidney Int* 1973;4:301.

170. Burg MB, Stoner L, Cardinal J, et al. Furosemide effect on isolated perfused tubules. *Am J Physiol* 1973;225:119.

171. Schnermann J. Juxtaglomerular cell complex in the regulation of renal salt excretion. *Am J Physiol* 1998;274:R263.

172. Schlatter E, Salomonsson M, Persson AEG, et al. Macula densa cells sense luminal NaCl concentration via furosemide sensitive $Na^+2Cl^-K^+$ cotransport. *Pflugers Arch* 1989;414:286.

173. Lapointe J-Y, Laamarti A, Hurst AM, et al. Activation of Na:2Cl:K cotransport by luminal chloride in macula densa cells. *Kidney Int* 1995;47:752.

174. Kurtz A, Gotz KH, Hamann M, et al. Stimulation of renin secretion by nitric oxide is mediated by phosphodiesterase 3. *Proc Natl Acad Sci USA* 1998;95:4743.

175. Reid IA, Chou L. Effect of blockade of nitric oxide synthesis on the renin secretory response to frusemide in conscious rabbits. *Clin Sci* 1995;88:657.

176. Tharaux PL, Dussaule JC, Pauti MD, et al. Activation of renin synthesis is dependent on intact nitric oxide production. *Kidney Int* 1997;51:1780.

177. Schricker K, Hamann M, Kurtz A. Nitric oxide and prostaglandins are involved in the macula densa control of renin system. *Am J Physiol* 1995;269:F825.

178. Harding P, Sigmon DH, Alfie ME, et al. Cyclooxygenase-2 mediates increased renal renin content induced by low-sodium diet. *Hypertension* 1997;29:297.

179. Frölich JC, Hollifield JW, Dormois JC, et al. Suppression of plasma renin activity by indomethacin in man. *Circ Res* 1976;39:447.

180. Hook JB, Blatt AH, Brody MJ, et al. Effects of several saluretic-diuretic agents on renal hemodynamics. *J Pharmacol Exp Ther* 1966;154:667.

181. Dluhy RG, Wolf GL, Lauler DP. Vasodilator properties of ethacrynic acid in the perfused dog kidney. *Clin Sci* 1970;38:347.

182. Ludens JH, Hook JB, Brody MJ, et al. Enhancement of renal blood flow by furosemide. *J Pharmacol Exp Ther* 1968;163:456.

183. Jamison RL, Lacy FB, Pennel JP, et al. Potassium secretion by the descending limb or pars recta of the juxtamedullary nephron in vivo. *Kidney Int* 1976;9:323.

184. Wright FS, Schnermann J. Interference with feedback control of glomerular filtration rate by furosemide, triflocin, and cyanide. *J Clin Invest* 1974;53:1695.

185. Dikshit K, Vyden JK, Forrester JS, et al. Renal and extrarenal hemodynamic effects of furosemide in congestive heart failure after acute myocardial infarction. *N Engl J Med* 1973;288:1087.

186. Bourland WA, Day DK, Williamson HE. The role of the kidney in the early nondiuretic action of furosemide to reduce elevated left atrial pressure in the hypervolemic dog. *J Pharmacol Exp Ther* 1977;202:221.

187. Mukherjee SK, Katz MA, Michael UF, et al. Mechanisms of hemodynamic actions of furosemide: differentiation of vascular and renal effects on blood pressure in functionally anephric hypertensive patients. *Am Heart J* 1981;101:313.

188. Schmieder RE, Messerli FH, deCarvalho JGR, et al. Immediate hemodynamic response to furosemide in patients undergoing chronic hemodialysis. *Am J Kidney Dis* 1987;9:55.

189. Pickkers P, Dormans TP, Russel FG, et al. Direct vascular effects of furosemide in humans. *Circulation* 1997;96:1847.

190. Ellison DH. Intensive diuretic therapy: high doses, combinations, and constant infusions. In: Seldin DW, Giebisch G. *Diuretic agents: clinical physiology and pharmacology.* San Diego: Academic Press, 1997:281.

191. Johnston GD, Nicholls DP, Leahey WJ. The dose-response characteristics of the acute non-diuretic peripheral vascular effects of frusemide in normal subjects. *Br J Clin Pharmacol* 1984;18:75.

192. Francis GS, Siegel RM, Goldsmith SR, et al. Acute vasoconstrictor response to intravenous furosemide in patients with chronic congestive heart failure. *Ann Intern Med* 1985;103:1.

193. Curran KA, Hebert MJ, Cain BD, et al. Evidence for the presence of a K-dependent acidifying adenosine triphosphatase in the rabbit renal medulla. *Kidney Int* 1992;42:1093.

194. Goldsmith SR, Francis G, Cohn JN. Attenuation of the pressor response to intravenous furosemide by angiotensin converting enzyme inhibition in congestive heart failure. *Am J Cardiol* 1989;64:1382.

195. Inoue M, Okajima K, Itoh K, et al. Mechanism of furosemide resistance in analbuminemic rats and hypoalbuminemic patients. *Kidney Int* 1987;32:198.

196. Packer M. Identification of risk factors predisposing to the development of functional renal insufficiency during treatment with converting-enzyme inhibitors in chronic heart failure. *Cardiology* 1989;76:50.

197. Packer M, Lee WH, Medina N, et al. Functional renal insufficiency during long-term therapy with captopril and enalapril in severe congestive heart failure. *Ann Intern Med* 1987;106:346.

198. Smith WE, Steele TH. Avoiding diuretic related complications in older patients. *Geriatrics* 1983;38:117.

199. Kaufman AM, Levitt MF. The effect of diuretics on systemic and renal hemodynamics in patients with renal insufficiency. *Am J Kidney Dis* 1985;5:A71.

200. Bichet DG, Van Putten VJ, Schrier RW. Potential role of increased sympathetic activity in impaired sodium and water excretion in cirrhosis. *N Engl J Med* 1982;307:1552.

201. Tichman MP, Vorherr H, Kleeman CR, et al. Diuretic-induced hyponatremia. *Ann Intern Med* 1971;75:853.

202. Dyckner T, Webster PO. Magnesium treatment of diuretic-induced hyponatremia with a preliminary report on a new aldosterone antagonist. *J Am Coll Nutr* 1982;1:149.

203. Schrier RW. New treatments for hyponatremia. *N Engl J Med* 1978;298:214.

204. Dzau VJ, Hollenberg NK. Renal response to captopril in severe heart failure: role of furosemide in natriuresis and reversal of hyponatremia. *Ann Intern Med* 1984;100:777.

205. Ram CVS, Garrett BN, Kaplan NM. Moderate sodium restriction and various diuretics in the treatment of hypertension: effects of potassium wastage and blood pressure control. *Arch Intern Med* 1981;141:1015.

206. Palmer BF. *Potassium disturbances associated with the use of diuretics.* San Diego: Academic Press, 1997:571.

207. Hropot M, Fowler NB, Karlmark B, et al. Tubular action of diuretics: distal effects on electrolyte transport and acidification. *Kidney Int* 1985;28:477.

208. Wilcox CS, Mitch WE, Kelly RA, et al. Factors affecting potassium balance during frusemide administration. *Clin Sci* 1984;67:195.

209. Good DW. Sodium-dependent bicarbonate absorption by cortical thick ascending limb of rat kidney. *Am J Physiol* 1985;248:F821.

210. Good DW, Knepper MA, Burg MB. Ammonia and bicarbonate transport by thick ascending limb of rat kidney. *Am J Physiol* 1984;247:F35.

211. Oberleithner H, Lang F, Messner G, et al. Mechanism of hydrogen ion transport in the diluting segment of frog kidney. *Pflugers Arch* 1984;402:272.

212. Stone DK, Seldin DW, Kokko JP, et al. Mineralocorticoid modulation of rabbit medullary-collecting duct acidification. *J Clin Invest* 1983;72:77.

213. Tannen RL. The effect of uncomplicated potassium depletion on urine acidification. *J Clin Invest* 1970;49:813.

214. Soleimani M, Grassl SM, Aronson PS. Stoichiometry of Na+HCO$_3^-$ cotransport in basolateral membrane vesicles isolated from rabbit renal cortex. *J Clin Invest* 1987;79:1276.

215. Soleimani M, Aronson PS. Ionic mechanism of Na$^+$-HCO$_3^-$ cotransport in rabbit renal basolateral membrane vesicles. *J Biol Chem* 1989;264:18302.

216. Wingo CS, Straub SG. Active proton secretion and potassium absorption in the rabbit outer medullary collecting duct. Functional evidence for proton-potassium-activated adenosine triphosphatase. *J Clin Invest* 1989;84:361.

217. Maher JF, Schreiner GF. Studies on ethacrynic acid in patients with refractory edema. *Ann Intern Med* 1965;62:15.

218. Nochy D, Callard P, Bellon B, et al. Association of overt glomerulonephritis and liver disease: a study of 34 patients. *Clin Nephrol* 1976;6:422.

219. Bosher SK. The nature of ototoxicity actions of ethacrynic acid upon the mammalian endolymph system. I. Functional aspects. *Acta Otolaryngol* 1980;89:407.

220. Ikeda K, Oshima T, Hidaka H, et al. Molecular and clinical implications of loop diuretic ototoxicity. *Hear Res* 1997;107:1.

221. Ikeda K, Morizono T. Electrochemical profiles for monovalent ions in the stria vascularis: cellular model of ion transport mechanisms. *Hear Res* 1989;39:279.

222. Mizuta T. *Hear Res* 1997;106:154.

223. Hidaka H, Oshima T, Ikeda K, et al. The Na-K-Cl cotransporters in the rat cochlea: RT-PCR and partial sequence analysis. *Biochem Biophys Res Commun* 1996;220:425.

224. Ryback LP. Ototoxicity of loop diuretics. *Otolaryngol Clin N Am* 1993;26:829.

225. Star RA. *Ototoxicity.* San Diego: Academic Press, 1997.

226. Wigand ME, Heidland A. Ototoxic side effects of high doses of furosemide in patients with uremia. *Postgrad Med J* 1971;47:54.

227. Beyer KH Jr. The mechanism of action of chlorothiazide. *Ann NY Acad Sci* 1958;71:363.

228. Beyer KH Jr. Lessons from the discovery of modern diuretic therapy. *Perspect Biol Med* 1976;19:500.

229. Eknoyan G, Suki WN, Martinez-Maldonado M. Effect of diuretics on urinary excretion of phosphate, calcium, and magnesium in thyroparathyroidectomized dogs. *J Lab Clin Med* 1970;76:257.

230. Demartini FE, Wheaton EA, Healy LA, et al. Effect of chlorothiazide on the renal excretion of uric acid. *Am J Med* 1962;32:572.

231. Duarte CG, Bland JH. Calcium, phosphorous and uric acid clearances after intravenous administration of chlorothiazide. *Metabolism* 1965;14:211.

232. Costanzo LS, Weiner IM. On the hypocalciuric action of chlorothiazide. *J Clin Invest* 1974;54:628.

233. Earley LE, Kahn M, Orloff J. The effects of infusions of chlorothiazide on urinary dilution and concentration in the dog. *J Clin Invest* 1961;40:857.

234. Maren TH. Relations between structure and biological activity of sulfonamides. *Annu Rev Pharmacol Toxicol* 1976;16:309.

235. Kunau RT Jr, Weller DR, Webb HL. Clarification of the site of action of chlorothiazide in the rat nephron. *J Clin Invest* 1975;56:401.

236. Walter SJ, Shirley DG. The effect of chronic hydrochlorothiazide administration on renal function in the rat. *Clin Sci* 1986;70:379.

237. Friedman PA, Hebert SC. *Site and mechanism of diuretic action.* San Diego: Academic Press, 1997:75.

238. Fernandez PC, Puschett JB. Proximal tubular actions of metolazone and chlorothiazide. *Am J Physiol* 1973;225:954.

239. Edwards BR, Baer PG, Sutton RAL, et al. Micropuncture study of diuretic effects on sodium and calcium reabsorption in the dog nephron. *J Clin Invest* 1973;52:2418.

240. Burke TJ, Marshall WH, Clapp JR, et al. Renal hemodynamic determinants of chlorothiazide effectiveness. *Clin Res* 1972;20:88.

241. Reilly RF, Ellison DH. Mammalian distal tubule: physiology, pathophysiology, and molecular anatomy. *Physiol Rev* 2000;80:277.

242. Kriz W, Kaissling B. Structural organization of the mammalian kidney. In: Seldin DW, Giebisch G, eds. *The kidney: physiology and pathophysiology.* New York: Raven Press, 1992:779.

243. Costanzo LS. Localization of diuretic action in microperfused rat distal tubules: Ca and Na transport. *Am J Physiol* 1985;248:F527.

244. Ellison DH, Velázquez H, Wright FS. Thiazide sensitive sodium chloride cotransport in the early distal tubule. *Am J Physiol* 1987;253:F546.

245. Dørup J. Ultrastructure of three-dimensionally localized distal nephron segments in superficial cortex of the rat kidney. *J Ultrastruct Res* 1988;99:169.

246. Berry CA, Rector FC Jr. Renal transport of glucose, amino acids, sodium, chloride, and water. In: Brenner BM, Rector FC Jr, eds. *The kidney.* Philadelphia: WB Saunders, 1991:245.

247. Shimizu T, Yoshitomi K, Nakamura M, et al. Site and mechanism of action of trichlormethiazide in rabbit distal nephron segments perfused in vitro. *J Clin Invest* 1988;82:721.

248. Yoshitomi K, Shimizu T, Taniguchi J, et al. Electrophysiological characterization of rabbit distal convoluted tubule cell. *Pflugers Arch* 1989;414:457.

249. Shimizu T, Nakamura M, Yoshitomi K, et al. Interaction of trichlormethiazide or amiloride with PTH in stimulating Ca2+ absorption in rabbit CNT. *Am J Physiol* 1991;261:F36.

250. Greger R, Velázquez H. Role of the cortical thick ascending limb of the loop of Henle and of the early distal convoluted tubule in the urinary concentrating mechanism. *Kidney Int* 1987;31:590.

251. Velázquez, H. and R. Greger. K and Cl permeabilities in cells of the rabbit early distal convoluted tubule. *Kidney Int* 27:322, 1985.

252. Pizzonia JH, Gesek FA, Kennedy SM, et al. Immunomagnetic separation, primary culture, and characterization of cortical thick ascending limb plus distal convoluted tubule cells from mouse kidney. *In Vitro Cell Dev Biol* 1991;27A:409.

253. Gesek FA, Friedman PA. Mechanism of calcium transport stimulated by chlorothiazide in mouse distal convoluted tubule cells. *J Clin Invest* 1992;90:429.

254. Gesek FA, Friedman PA. On the mechanism of parathyroid hormone stimulation of calcium uptake by mouse distal convoluted tubule cells. *J Clin Invest* 1992;90:749.

255. Wilson DR, Honrath U, Sonnenberg H. Thiazide diuretic effect on medullary-collecting duct function in the rat. *Kidney Int* 1983;23:711.

256. Terada Y, Knepper MA. Thiazide-sensitive NaCl absorption in rat cortical collecting duct. *Am J Physiol Renal Fluid Electrolyte Physiol* 1990;259:F519.

257. Rouch AJ, Chen L, Troutman SL, et al. Na+ transport in isolated rat CCD: effects of bradykinin, ANP, clonidine, and hydrochlorothiazide. *Am J Physiol Renal Fluid Electrolyte Physiol* 1991;260:F86.

258. Velázquez H, Good DW, Wright FS. Mutual dependence of sodium and chloride absorption by renal distal tubule. *Am J Physiol* 1984;247:F904.

259. Stokes JB. Sodium chloride absorption by the urinary bladder of the winter flounder: a thiazide-sensitive electrically neutral transport system. *J Clin Invest* 1984;74:7.

260. Gamba G, Saltzberg SN, Lombardi M, et al. Primary structure and functional expression of a cDNA encoding the thiazide-sensitive, electroneutral sodium-chloride cotransporter. *Proc Natl Acad Sci USA* 1993;90:2749.

261. Gamba G, Miyanoshita A, Lombardi M, et al. Molecular cloning, primary structure, and characterization of two members of the mammalian electroneutral sodium-(potassium)-chloride cotransporter family expressed in kidney. *J Biol Chem* 1994;269:17713.

262. Simon DB, Nelson-Williams C, Bia MJ, et al. Gitelman's variant of Bartter's syndrome, inherited hypokalemic alkalosis, is caused by mutations in the thiazide-sensitive Na-Cl cotransporter. *Nat Genet* 1996;12:24.

263. Bostanjoglo M, Reeves WB, Reilly RF, et al. 11ß-hydroxysteroid dehydrogenase, mineralocorticoid receptor and thiazide-sensitive Na-Cl cotransporter expression by distal tubules. *J Am Soc Nephrol* 1998;9:1347.

264. Velázquez H, Náray-Fejes-Tóth A, Silva T, et al. The distal convoluted tubule of the rabbit coexpresses NaCl cotransporter and 11ß-hydroxysteroid dehydrogenase. *Kidney Int* 1998;54:464.

265. Plotkin MD, Kaplan MR, Verlander JW, et al. Localization of the thiazide sensitive Na-Cl cotransporter, rTSCl, in the rat kidney. *Kidney Int* 1996;50:174.

266. Yang TX, Huang YNG, Singh I, et al. Localization of bumetanide- and thiazide-sensitive Na-K-Cl cotransporters along the rat nephron. *Am J Physiol Renal Fluid Electrolyte Physiol* 1996;271:F931.

267. Loffing J, Valderrabano V, Froesch P, et al. Segmentation of the mouse distal nephron: morphology and distribution of transport proteins. *J Am Soc Nephrol* 1998;9:39A.

268. Bachmann S, Velázquez H, Obermüller N, et al. Expression of the thiazide-sensitive Na-Cl cotransporter by rabbit distal convoluted tubule cells. *J Clin Invest* 1995;96:2510.

269. Tran JM, Farrell MA, Fanestil DD. Effect of ions on binding of the thiazide-type diuretic metolazone to kidney membrane. *Am J Physiol* 1990;258:F908.

270. Ellison DH, Morrisey J, Desir GV. Solubilization and partial purification of the thiazide diuretic receptor from rabbit renal cortex. *Biochim Biophys Acta* 1991;1069:241.

271. Monroy A, Plata C, Hebert SC, et al. Characterization of the thiazide-sensitive Na(+)-Cl(−) cotransporter: a new model for ions and diuretics interaction. *Am J Physiol Renal Physiol* 2000;279:F161.

272. Popovtzer MM, Subryan VL, Alfrey AC, et al. The acute effect of chlorothiazide on serum-ionized calcium. Evidence for a parathyroid hormone-dependent mechanism. *J Clin Invest* 1975;55:1295.

273. Bomsztyk K, George JP, Wright FS. Effects of luminal fluid anions on calcium transport by proximal tubule. *Am J Physiol* 1984;246:F600.

274. Costanzo LS, Windhager EE. Calcium and sodium transport by the distal convoluted tubule of the rat. *Am J Physiol* 1978;235:F492.

275. Lajeunesse D, Brunette MG. The hypocalciuric effect of thiazides: subcellular localization of the action. *Pflugers Arch* 1991;417:454.

276. Lajeunesse D, Bouhtiauy I, Brunette MG. Parathyroid hormone and hydrochlorothiazide increase calcium transport by the luminal membrane of rabbit distal nephron segments through different pathways. *Endocrinology* 1994;134:35.

277. Bacskai BJ, Friedman PA. Activation of latent Ca2+ channels in renal epithelial cells by parathyroid hormone. *Nature* 1990;347:388.

278. Matsunaga H, Stanton BA, Gesek FA, et al. Epithelial Ca2+ channels sensitive to dihydropyridines and activated by hyperpolarizing voltages. *Am J Physiol Cell Physiol* 1994;267:C157.

279. Hoenderop JG, van der Kemp AW, Hartog A, et al. The epithelial calcium channel, ECaC, is activated by hyperpolarization and regulated by cytosolic calcium. *Biochem Biophys Res Commun* 1999;261:488.

280. Hoenderop JG, van der Kemp AW, Hartog A, et al. Molecular identification of the apical Ca2+ channel in 1,25-dihydroxyvitamin D3-responsive epithelia. *J Biol Chem* 1999;274:8375.

281. Reilly RF, Shugrue CA, Lattanzi D, et al. Immunolocalization of the Na+/Ca2+ exchanger in rabbit kidney. *Am J Physiol* 1993;265:F327.

282. White KE, Gesek FA, Friedman PA. Structural and functional analysis of Na+/Ca2+ exchange in distal convoluted tubule cells. *Am J Physiol Renal Fluid Electrolyte Physiol* 1996;271:F560.

283. Douban S, Brodsky MA, Whang DD. Significance of magnesium in congestive heart failure. *Am Heart J* 1996;132:664.

284. Hollifield JW. Thiazide treatment of systemic hypertension: effects on serum magnesium and ventricular ectopy. *Am J Cardiol* 1989;63:22G.

285. Quamme GA. Renal magnesium handling: new insights in understanding old problems. *Kidney Int* 1997;52:1180.

286. Dai LJ, Friedman PA, Quamme GA. Cellular mechanisms of chlorothiazide and potassium depletion on Mg2+ uptake in mouse distal convoluted tubule cells. *Kidney Int* 1997;51:1008.

287. Dai LJ, Friedman PA, Quamme GA. Mechanisms of amiloride stimulation of Mg2+ uptake in immortalized mouse distal convoluted tubule cells. *Am J Physiol* 1997;F249:F256.

288. Schultheis PJ, Lorenz JN, Meneton P, et al. Phenotype resembling Gitelman's syndrome in mice lacking the apical Na+-Cl− cotransporter of the distal convoluted tubule. *J Biol Chem* 1998;273:29150.

289. Ellison DH. Divalent cation transport by the distal nephron: insights from Bartter's and Gitelman's syndromes. *Am J Physiol Renal Physiol* 2000;F616.

290. Cassin S, Vogh B. Effect of hydrochlorothiazide on renal blood flow and clearance of para-aminohippurate and creatinine. *Proc Soc Exp Biol Med* 1966;122:970.

291. Aperia AC. Tubular sodium reabsorption and the regulation of renal hemodynamics. The effect of chlorothiazide on renal vascular resistance. *Acta Physiol Scand* 1969;75:360.

292. Pitts RF, Krück F, Lozano R, et al. Studies on the mechanism of diuretic action of chlorothiazide. *J Pharmacol Exp Ther* 1958;123:89.

293. Okusa MD, Erik A, Persson G, et al. Chlorothiazide effect on feedback-mediated control of glomerular filtration rate. *Am J Physiol* 1989;257:F137.

294. Earley LE, Orloff J. The mechanism of antidiuresis associated with the administration of hydrochlorothiazide to patients with vasopressin-resistant diabetes insipidus. *J Clin Invest* 1962;41:1988.

295. McGuffin WL Jr, Gunnells JC. Intravenously administered chlorothiazide in diagnostic evaluation of hypertensive disease. *Arch Intern Med* 1969;123:124.

296. Brown TC, Davis JO, Johnston CI. Acute response in plasma renin and aldosterone secretion to diuretics. *Am J Physiol* 1966;211:437.

297. Siegel D, Hulley SB, Black DM, et al. Diuretics, serum and intracellular electrolyte levels, and ventricular arrhythmias in hypertensive men. *JAMA* 1992;267:1083.

298. The sixth report of the Joint National Committee on Prevention, Detection, Evaluation and Treatment of High Blood Pressure. *Arch Intern Med* 1997;157:2413.

299. Leary WP, Reyes AJ. Renal excretory actions of diuretics in man: correction of various current errors and redefinition of basic concepts. In: Reyes AJ, Leary WP, eds. *Clinical pharmacology and therapeutic uses of diuretics.* Stuttgart: Gustav Fischer Verlag, 1988: 153.

300. Ettinger B, Citron JT, Livermore B, et al. Chlorthalidone reduces calcium oxalate calculous recurrence but magnesium hydroxide does not. *J Urol* 1988;139:679.

301. Laerum E, Larson S. Thiazide prophylaxis of urolithiasis: a double-blind study in general practice. *Acta Med Scand* 1984;215:383.

302. Yendt ER, Cohanim M. Prevention of calcium stones with thiazides. *Kidney Int* 1978;13:397.

303. Breslau NA. Use of diuretics in disorders of calcium metabolism. In: Seldin DW, Giebisch G. *Diuretic agents: clinical physiology and pharmacology.* San Diego: Academic Press, 1997:495.

304. Preminger GM, Pak CYC. Eventual attenuation of hypocalciuric response to hydrochlorothiazide in absorptive hypercalciuria. *J Urol* 1987;137:1104.

305. Simon DB, Karet FE, Rudin A, et al. The molecular basis of inherited hypokalemic alkalosis: Bartter's and Gitelman's syndromes. *J Am Soc Nephrol* 1996;7:1623.

306. Wasnich R, Davis J, Ross P, et al. Effect of thiazide on rates of bone mineral loss: a longitudinal study. *Br Med J* 1990;301:1303.

307. Felson DT, Sloutskis D, Anderson JJ, et al. Thiazide diuretics and the risk of hip fracture. Results from the Framingham study. *JAMA* 1991;265:370.

308. Ray WA, Griffin MR, Downey W, et al. Long-term use of thiazide diuretics and risk of hip fracture. *Lancet* 1989;1:687.

309. Cauley JA, Cummings SR, Seeley DG, et al. Effects of thiazide diuretic therapy on bone mass, fractures, and falls. *Ann Intern Med* 1993;118:666.

310. Heidrich FE, Stergachis A, Gross KM. Diuretic drug use and the risk for hip fracture. *Ann Intern Med* 1991;115:1.

311. Porter RH, Cox BG, Heaney D, et al. Treatment of hypoparathyroid patients with chlorthalidone. *N Engl J Med* 1978;298:577.

312. Reid IR, Ames RW, Orr-Walker BJ, et al. Hydrochlorothiazide reduces loss of cortical bone in normal postmenopausal women: a randomized controlled trial. *Am J Med* 2000;109:362.

313. Coleman RA, Knepper MA, Wade JB. Rat renal connecting cells express AQP2. *J Am Soc Nephrol* 1997;8:16A.

314. Cesar KR, Magaldi AJ. Thiazide induces water absorption in the inner medullary-collecting duct of normal and Brattleboro rats. *Am J Physiol* 1999;277:F756.

315. Kassirer JP, Harrinton JT. Diuretics and potassium metabolism: a reassessment of the need, effectiveness and safety of potassium therapy. *Kidney Int* 1977;11:505.

316. Flaker G, Villarreal D, Chapman D. Is hypokalemia a cause of ventricular arrhythmias. *J Crit Ill* 1986;66:74.

317. Harrington JT, Isner JM, Kassirer JP. Our national obsession with potassium. *Am J Med* 1982;73:155.

318. Kaplan NM. Our appropriate concern about hypokalemia. *Am J Med* 1984;77:1.

319. Freis ED. Critique of the clinical importance of diuretic-induced hypokalemia and elevated cholesterol level. *Arch Intern Med* 1989; 149:2640.

320. Kaplan NM. How bad are diuretic-induced hypokalemia and hypercholesterolemia? *Arch Intern Med* 1989;149:2649.

321. Myers MG. Diuretic therapy and ventricular arrhythmias in persons 65 years of age and older. *Am J Cardiol* 1990;65:599.

322. Velázquez H, Wright FS. Control by drugs of renal potassium handling. *Ann Rev Pharmacol Toxicol* 1986;26:293.

323. Velázquez H, Wright FS. Effects of diuretic drugs on Na, Cl, and K transport by rat renal distal tubule. *Am J Physiol* 1986;250:F1013.

324. Okusa MD, Velázquez H, Ellison DH, et al. Luminal calcium regulates potassium transport by the renal distal tubule. *Am J Physiol* 1990;258:F423.

325. Rude RK. Physiology of magnesium metabolism and the important role of magnesium in potassium deficiency. *Am J Cardiol* 1989;63:31G.

326. Dorup I. Magnesium and potassium deficiency. Its diagnosis, occurrence and treatment in diuretic therapy and its consequences for growth, protein synthesis and growth factors. *Acta Physiol Scand* 1994;150:7.

327. Dorup I, Skjaaa K, Thybo NK. Oral magnesium supplementation restores the concentrations of magnesium, potassium and sodium-potassium pumps in skeletal muscle of patients receiving diuretic treatment. *J Intern Med* 1993;233:117.

328. Ashraf N, Locksley R, Arieff A. Thiazide-induced hyponatremia associated with death or neurologic damage in outpatients. *Am J Med* 1981;70:1163.

329. Fichman MP, Vorherr H, Kleeman CR, et al. Diuretic-induced hyponatremia. *Ann Intern Med* 1971;75:853.

330. Friedman E, Shadel M, Halkin H, et al. Thiazide-induced hyponatremia: reproducibility by single dose rechallenge and an analysis of pathogenesis. *Ann Intern Med* 1989;110:24.

331. Carlsen JE, Kober L, Torp-Pedersen C, et al. Relation between dose of bendrofluazide, antihypertensive effect, and adverse biochemical effects. *Br Med J* 1990;300:975.

332. Harper R, Ennis CN, Heaney AP, et al. A comparison of the effects of low- and conventional-dose thiazide diuretic on insulin action in hypertensive patients with NIDDM. *Diabetologia* 1995;38:853.

333. Helderman JH, Elahi D, Andersen DK, et al. Prevention of the glucose intolerance of thiazide diuretics by maintenance of body potassium. *Diabetes* 1983;32:106.

334. Toto RA. Metabolic derangements associated with diuretic use: insulin resistance, dyslipidemia, hyperuricemia, and anti-adrenergic effects. In: Seldin DW, Giebisch G. *Diuretic agents: clinical physiology and pharmacology.* San Diego: Academic Press, 1997:621.

335. Pickkers P, Schachter M, Hughes AD, et al. Thiazide-induced hyperglycaemia: a role for calcium-activated potassium channels? *Diabetologia* 1996;39:861.

336. Grimm RH Jr, Flack JM, Granditis GA. Treatment of Mild Hypertension Study (TOMHS) Research Group. Long-term effects on plasma lipids of diet and drugs to treat hypertension. *JAMA* 1996;275: 1549.

337. Psaty BM, Smith NL, Siscovick DS, et al. Health outcomes associated with antihypertensive therapies used as first-line agents. *JAMA* 1997;277:739.

338. Baer JE, Jones CB, Spitzer SA, et al. The potassium sparing and natriuretic activity of amidino-3,4-diamino-6-chloropyrazinecarboxamide hydrochloride dihydrate (amiloride hydrochloride). *J Pharmacol Exp Ther* 1967;157:472.

339. Gross JB, Kokko JP. Effects of aldosterone and potassium-sparing diuretics on electrical potential differences across the distal nephron. *J Clin Invest* 1977;59:82.

340. Guignard JP, Peters G. Effects of triamterene and amiloride on urinary acidification and potassium excretion in the rat. *Eur J Pharmacol* 1970;10:255.

341. McDonald FJ, Yang B, Hrstka RF, et al. Disruption of the beta subunit of the epithelial Na+ channel in mice: hyperkalemia and neonatal death associated with a pseudohypoaldosteronism phenotype. *Proc Natl Acad Sci USA* 1999;96:1727.

342. Perez-Ayuso RM, Arroyo V, Planas R, et al. Randomized comparative study of efficacy of furosemide versus spironolactone in nonazotemic cirrhosis with ascites. *Gastroenterology* 1983;84:961.

343. Casavola V, Guerra L, Reshkin SJ, et al. Effect of adenosine on Na$^+$ and Cl$^-$ currents in A$_6$ monolayers. Receptor localization and messenger involvement. *J Membr Biol* 1996;151:237.

344. Okusa MD, Bia MJ. Bartter's syndrome. In: Foa PP, Cohen MP, eds. *Endocrinology and metabolism.* New York: Springer-Verlag, 1987: 231.

345. Pitt B, Zannad F, Remme WJ, et al. The effect of spironolactone on morbidity and mortality in patients with severe heart failure. *N Engl J Med* 1999;341:709.

346. Perez-Ayuso RM, Arroyo V, Planas R, et al. Randomized comparative study of efficacy of furosemide versus spironolactone in nonazotemic cirrhosis with ascites. Relationship between the diuretic response and the activity of the renin-aldosterone system. *Gastroenterology* 1983;84:961.

347. Hulter HN, Ilnicki LP, Harbottle JA, et al. Impaired renal H$^+$ secretion and NH$_3$ production in mineralocorticoid-deficient glucocorticoid replete dogs. *Am J Physiol* 1977;232:F136.

348. Kurtzman NA, White MG, Rogers PW. Aldosterone deficiency and renal bicarbonate reabsorption. *J Lab Clin Med* 1971;77:931.

349. Gabow PA, Moore S, Schrier RW. Spironolactone-induced hyperchloremic acidosis in cirrhosis. *Ann Intern Med* 1979;90:338.

350. Costanzo LS, Weiner IM. Relationship between clearances of Ca and Na: effect of distal diuretics and PTH. *Am J Physiol* 1976;230:67.

351. Friedman PA, Gesek FA. Stimulation of calcium transport by amiloride in mouse distal convoluted tubule cells. *Kidney Int* 1995;48:1427.

352. Bundy JT, Connito D, Mahoney MD, et al. Treatment of idiopathic renal magnesium wasting with amiloride. *Am J Nephrol* 1995;15:75.

353. Dyckner T, Wester P-O, Widman L. Amiloride prevents thiazide-induced intracellular potassium and magnesium losses. *Acta Med Scand* 1988;224:25.

354. Ellison DH, Reilly RF, Obermüller N, et al. Molecular localization of Na and Ca transport pathways along the renal distal tubule. *J Am Soc Nephrol* 1995;6:947.

355. Garty H, Palmer LG. Epithelial sodium channels: function, structure, and regulation. *Physiol Rev* 1997;77:359.

356. Canessa CM, Horisberger J-D, Rossier BC. Epithelial sodium channel related to proteins involved in neurodegeneration. *Nature* 1993;361:467.

357. Canessa CM, Schild L, Buell G, et al. Amiloride-sensitive epithelial Na$^+$ channel is made of three homologous subunits. *Nature* 1994;367:463.

358. Eskandari S, Snyder PM, Kreman M, et al. Number of subunits comprising the epithelial sodium channel. *J Biol Chem* 1999;274:27281.

359. Kosari F, Sheng S, Li J, et al. Subunit stoichiometry of the epithelial sodium channel. *J Biol Chem* 1998;273:13469.

360. Firsov D, Gautschi I, Merillat AM, et al. The heterotetrameric architecture of the epithelial sodium channel (ENaC). *EMBO J* 1998;17:344.

361. Gründer S, Rossier BC. A reappraisal of aldosterone effects on kidney: new insights provided by epithelial sodium channel cloning. *Curr Opin Nephrol Hypertens* 1997;6:35.

362. Garty H, Benos DJ. Characteristics and regulatory mechanism of the amiloride-blockable Na+ channel. *Physiol Rev* 1988;68:309.

363. Garty H. Molecular properties of epithelial, amiloride-blockable Na$^+$ channels. *FASEB J* 1994;8:522.

364. Ecelbarger CA, Kim G-H, Terris J, et al. Vasopressin-mediated regulation of epithelial sodium channel abundance in rat kidney. *Am J Physiol Renal Physiol* 2000;279:F46.

365. Chalfant ML, Denton JS, Berdiev BK, et al. Intracellular H$^+$ regulates the alpha-subunit of ENaC, the epithelial Na+ channel. *Am J Physiol* 1999;276:C477.

366. Masilamani S, Kim GH, Mitchell C, et al. Aldosterone-mediated regulation of ENaC alpha, beta, and gamma subunit proteins in rat kidney [see comments]. *J Clin Invest* 1999;104:R19.

367. Verrey F. Early aldosterone action: toward filling the gap between transcription and transport. *Am J Physiol* 1999;277:F319.

368. Stockand JD, Bao H-F, Schenck J, et al. Differential effects of protein kinase C on the levels of epithelial Na+ channel subunit proteins. *J Biol Chem* 2000;275:25760.

369. Ismailov II, Awayda MS, Jovov B, et al. Regulation of epithelial sodium channels by the cystic fibrosis transmembrane conductance regulator. *J Biol Chem* 1996;271:4725.

370. Jiang Q, Li J, Dubroff R, et al. Epithelial sodium channels regulate cystic fibrosis transmembrane conductance regulator chloride channels in xenopus oocytes. *J Biol Chem* 2000;275:13266.

371. Kim G-H, Martin SW, Fernandez-Llama P, et al. Long-term regulation of renal Na-dependent cotransporters and ENaC: response to altered acid-base intake. *Am J Physiol Renal Physiol* 2000;279:F459.

372. Loffing J, Pietri L, Aregger F, et al. Differential subcellular localization of ENaC subunits in mouse kidney in response to high- and low-sodium diets. *Am J Physiol Renal Physiol* 2000;279:F252.

373. Harvey KF, Dinudom A, Komwatana P, et al. All three WW domains of murine Nedd4 are involved in the regulation of epithelial sodium channels by intracellular Na+. *J Biol Chem* 1999;274:12525.

374. Goulet CC, Volk KA, Adams CM, et al. Inhibition of the epithelial Na+ channel by interactions of Nedd4 with a PY motif deleted in Liddle's syndrome. *J Biol Chem* 1998;273:30012.

375. Sansom SC, O'Neil RG. Mineralocorticoid regulation of apical cell membrane Na+ and K+ transport of the cortical collecting duct. *Am J Physiol* 1985;248:F858.

376. Garty H. Mechanisms of aldosterone action in tight epithelia. *J Membr Biol* 1986;90:193.

377. Garty H. Regulation of epithelial Na+ channel by aldosterone: open questions and emerging answers. *Kidney Int* 2000;57:1270.

378. Marver D, Stewart J, Funder JW, et al. Renal aldosterone receptors: studies with [^{3}H]aldosterone and the antimineralocorticoid [^{3}H]spirolactone (SC26304). *Proc Natl Acad Sci USA* 1974;71:1431.

379. Miyata Y, Yahara I. Cytoplasmic 8S glucocorticoid receptors binds to actin filaments through the 90-kDa heat shock protein moiety. *J Biol Chem* 1991;266:8779.

380. Tumlin JA, Lea JP, Swanson CE, et al. Aldosterone and dexamethasone stimulate calcineurin activity through a transcription-independent mechanism involving steroid receptor-associated heat shock proteins. *J Clin Invest* 1997;99:1217.

381. Verrey F. Transcriptional control of sodium transport in tight epithelia by adrenal steroids. *J Membr Biol* 1995;144:93.

382. Alvarez de la Rosa D, Zhang P, Naray-Fejes-Toth A, et al. The serum and glucocorticoid kinase sgk increases the abundance of epithelial sodium channels in the plasma membrane of Xenopus oocytes. *J Biol Chem* 1999;274:37834.

383. Brennan FE, Fuller PJ. Rapid upregulation of serum and glucocorticoid-regulated kinase (sgk) gene expression by corticosteroids in vivo. *Mol Cell Endocrinol* 2000;166:129.

384. Chen SY, Bhargava A, Mastroberardino L, et al. Epithelial sodium channel regulated by aldosterone-induced protein sgk. *Proc Natl Acad Sci USA* 1999;96:2514.

385. Naray-Fejes-Toth A, Canessa C, Cleaveland ES, et al. sgk is an aldosterone-induced kinase in the renal collecting duct. Effects on epithelial na+ channels. *J Biol Chem* 1999;274:16973.

386. Naray-Fejes-Toth A, Fejes-Toth G. The sgk, an aldosterone-induced gene in mineralocorticoid target cells, regulates the epithelial sodium channel. *Kidney Int* 2000;57:1290.

387. Pearce D, Verrey F, Chen SY, et al. Role of SGK in mineralocorticoid-regulated sodium transport. *Kidney Int* 2000;57:1283.

388. Shigaev A, Asher C, Latter H, et al. Regulation of sgk by aldosterone and its effects on the epithelial Na(+) channel. *Am J Physiol Renal Physiol* 2000;278:F613.

389. Masilamani S, Kim G-H, Mitchell C, et al. Aldosterone-mediated regulation of ENaCα,ß and γ subunits. *J Clin Invest* 1999;104:R19.

390. Berger S, Bleich M, Schmid W, et al. Mineralocorticoid receptor knockout mice: pathophysiology of Na+ metabolism. *Proc Natl Acad Sci USA* 1998;95:9424.

391. Fanestil DD. Mechanism of action of aldosterone blockers. *Semin Nephrol* 1988;8:249.

392. Shackleton CR, Wong NLM, Sutton RA. Distal (potassium-sparing) diuretics. In: Dirks JH, Sutton RAL, eds. *Diuretics: physiology, pharmacology and clinical use.* Philadelphia: WB Saunders, 1986;117.

393. Karim A. Spironolactone: disposition, metabolism, pharmacodynamics and bioavailability. *Drug Metab Rev* 1978;8:151.

394. Liddle GW. Aldosterone antagonists and triamterene. *Ann NY Acad Sci* 1966;134:466.

395. Corvol P, Claire M, Oblin ME, et al. Mechanism of the antimineralocorticoid effects of spironolactones. *Kidney Int* 1981;20:1.

396. Rossier BC, Wilce PA, Edelman SI. Spironolactone antagonism of aldosterone action on Na+ transport and RNA metabolism in toad bladder epithelium. *J Membrane Biol* 1977;32:177.

397. Couette B, Lombes M, Baulieu E-E, et al. Aldosterone antagonists destabilize the mineralocorticoid receptor. *Biochem J* 1992;282:697.

398. Kagawa CM. Blocking the renal electrolyte effects of mineralocorticoids with an orally active steroidal spirolactone. *Endocrinology* 1960;65:125.

399. Liddle GW. Specific and nonspecific inhibition of mineralocorticoid activity. *Metabolism* 1961;10:1021.

400. Coppage WS, Liddle GW. Mode of action and clinical usefulness of aldosterone antagonists. *Ann NY Acad Sci* 1960;88:815.

401. Bull MB, Laragh JH. Amiloride. A potassium-sparing natriuretic agent. *Circulation* 1968;37:45.

402. Duarte CG, Chomety G, Giebisch G. Effect of amiloride, ouabain, and furosemide on distal tubular function in the rat. *Am J Physiol* 1971;221:632.

403. Giebisch G. Amiloride effects on distal nephron function. In: Straub RW, Bolis L, eds. *Cell membrane receptors for drugs and hormones: a multidisciplinary approach.* New York: Raven Press, 1978:337.

404. Costanzo LS. Comparison of calcium and sodium transport in early and late rat distal tubules: effect of amiloride. *Am J Physiol* 1984;246:F937.

405. Stoner LC, Burg MB, Orloff J. Ion transport in cortical collecting tubule: effect of amiloride. *Am J Physiol* 1974;227:453.

406. Stokes JB. Ion transport by the cortical and outer medullary collecting tubule. *Kidney Int* 1982;22:473.

407. Okusa MD, Velázquez H, Wright FS. Effect of Na-channel blockers and lumen Ca on K secretion by rat renal distal tubule. *Am J Physiol* 1991;260:F459.

408. Li JHY, Cragoe EJ, Lindemann B. Structure-activity relationship of amiloride analogs as blockers of epithelial Na channels. II. side-chain modifications. *J Membr Biol* 1987;95:171.

409. O'Neil RG, Sansom SC. Characterization of apical cell membrane Na+ and K+ conductances of cortical collecting duct using microelectrode techniques. *Am J Physiol* 1984;247:F14.

410. Koeppen BM, Biagi BA, Giebisch G. Intracellular microelectrode characterization of the rabbit cortical collecting duct. *Am J Physiol* 1983;244:F35.

411. Benos DJ, Saccomani G, Sariban-Sohraby S. The epithelial sodium channel. Subunit number and location of the amiloride binding site. *J Biol Chem* 1987;262:10613.

412. Schild L, Schneeberger E, Gautschi I, et al. Identification of amino acid residues in the α, ß and γ subunits of the epithelial sodium channel (ENaC) involved in amiloride block and ion permeation. *J Gen Physiol* 1997;109:15.

413. Waldmann R, Champigny G, Lazdunski M. Functional degenerin-containing chimeras identify residues essential for amiloride-sensitive Na+ channel function. *J Biol Chem* 1995;270:11735.

414. Ishmailov II, Kieber-Emmons T, Lin C, et al. Identification of an amiloride binding domain within the α-subunit of the epithelial Na+ channel. *J Biol Chem* 1997;272:21075.

415. Kieber-Emmons T, Lin C, Foster MH, et al. Antiidiotypic antibody recognizes an amiloride binding domain within the a subunit of the epithelial Na+ channel. *J Biol Chem* 1999;274:9648.

416. Busch AE, Suessbrich H, Kunzelmann K, et al. Blockade of epithelial Na+ channels by triamterene-underlying mechanisms and molecular basis. *Pflugers Arch* 1996;432:760.

417. Merkus FWHM, Overdiek JWPM, Cilissen J, et al. Pharmacokinetics of spironolactone after a single dose: evaluation of the true canrenone serum concentrations during 24 hours. *Clin Exp Hypertens* 1983;[A]5:249.

418. Gardiner P, Schrode K, Quinlan D, et al. Spironolactone metabolism: steady-state serum levels of the sulfur-containing metabolites. *J Clin Pharmacol* 1989;29:342.

419. Sungaila I, Bartle WR, Walker SE, et al. Spironolactone pharmacokinetics and pharmacodynamics in patients with cirrhotic ascites. *Gastroenterology* 1992;102:1680.

420. Widmer P, Maibach R, Künzi UP, et al. Diuretic-related hypokalaemia: the role of diuretics, potassium supplements, glucocorticoids and ß2-adrenoceptor agonists. Results from the comprehensive hospital drug monitoring programme, Berne (CHDM). *Eur J Clin Pharmacol* 1995;49:31.

421. Brown JJ, Davies DL, Ferriss JB, et al. Comparison of surgery and prolonged spironolactone therapy in patients with hypertension, aldosterone excess, and low plasma renin. *Br Med J* 1972;2:729.

422. Laffi G, La Villa G, Carloni V, et al. Loop diuretic therapy in liver cirrhosis with ascites. *J Cardiovasc Pharmacol* 1993;22:S51.

423. Ganguly A. Primary aldosteronism. *N Engl J Med* 1998;339:1828.

424. Ganguly A, Weinberger MH. Triamterene-thiazide combination: alternative therapy for primary aldosteronism. *Clin Pharmacol Ther* 1981;30:246.

425. Griffing GT, Cole AG, Aurecchia SA, et al. Amiloride for primary hyperaldosteronism. *Clin Pharmacol Ther* 1982;31:56.

426. Botero-Velez M, Curtis JJ, Warnock DG. Brief report: Liddle's syndrome revisited—a disorder of sodium reabsorption in the distal tubule. *N Engl J Med* 1994;174:178.

427. Batlle DC, von Riotte AB, Gaviria M, et al. Amelioration of polyuria by amiloride in patients receiving long-term lithium therapy. *N Engl J Med* 1985;312:408.

428. Mehta PK, Sodhi B, Arruda JAL, et al. Interaction of amiloride and lithium on distal urinary acidification. *J Lab Clin Med* 1979;93:983.

429. Leblanc G. The mechanism of lithium accumulation in the isolated frog skin epithelium. *Pflugers Arch* 1972;337:1.

430. Rose LI, Underwood RH, Newmark SR, et al. Pathophysiology of spironolactone-induced gynecomastia. *Ann Intern Med* 1977;87:398.

431. Whitling AM, Pergola PE, Sang JL, et al. Spironolactone-induced agranulocytosis. *Ann Pharmacother* 1997;31:582.

432. Fairley KF, Woo KT, Birch DF, et al. Triamterene-induced crystalluria and cylindruria: clinical and experimental studies. *Clin Nephrol* 1986;26:169.

433. Carr MC, Prien EL Jr, Babayan RK. Triamterene nephrolithiasis: renewed attention is warranted. *J Urol* 1990;144:1339.

434. Weinberg MS, Quigg RJ, Salant DJ, et al. Anuric renal failure precipitated by indomethacin and triamterene. *Nephron* 1985;40:216.

435. Favre L, Glasson P, Vallotton MB. Reversible acute renal failure from combined triamterene and indomethacin: a study in healthy subjects. *Ann Intern Med* 1982;96:317.

436. Wesson LG. Magnesium, calcium and phosphate excretion during osmotic diuresis in the dog. *J Lab Clin Med* 1967;60:422.

437. Benabe JE, Martinez-Maldonado M. Effects on divalent ion excretion. In: Eknoyan G, Martinez-Maldonado M, eds. *The physiological basis of diuretic therapy in clinical medicine.* Orlando: Grune & Stratton, 1986:109.

438. Biemesderfer D, DeGray B, Aronson PS. Membrane topology of NHE3. Epitopes within the carboxyl-terminal hydrophilic domain are exoplasmic. *J Biol Chem* 1998;273:12391.

439. Lytle C, McManus TJ, Haas M. A model of Na-K-2Cl cotransport based on ordered ion binding and glide symmetry. *Am J Physiol* 1998;274:C299.

440. Haas M, McManus TJ. Bumetanide inhibits (Na + K + 2Cl) cotransport at a chloride site. *Am J Physiol* 1983;245:C235.

441. Isenring P, Jacoby SC, Forbush BI. The role of transmembrane domain 2 in cation transport by the Na-K-Cl cotransporter. *Proc Natl Acad Sci USA* 1998;95:7179.

442. Isenring P, Forbush BI. Ion and bumetanide binding by the Na-K-Cl cotransporter. Importance of transmembrane domains. *J Biol Chem* 1997;272:24556.

443. Schmitt R, Ellison DH, Farman N, et al. Developmental expression of sodium entry pathways in rat distal nephron. *Am J Physiol* 1999;276:F367.

444. Palmer LG. Epithelial Na channels: the nature of the conducting pore. *Renal Physiol Biochem* 1990;13:51.

445. Fuller CM, Berdiev BK, Shlyonsky VG, et al. Point mutations in alpha bENaC regulate channel gating, ion selectivity, and sensitivity to amiloride. *Biophys J* 1997;72:1622.

446. Li XJ, Xu RH, Guggino WB, et al. Alternatively spliced forms of the alpha subunit of the epithelial sodium channel: distinct sites for amiloride binding and channel pore. *Mol Pharmacol* 1995;47:1133.

CHAPTER 83

Idiopathic Edema

Graham A. MacGregor and Hugh E. de Wardener

Idiopathic edema is an ill-defined syndrome characterized by intermittent edema secondary to sodium and water retention. It occurs almost exclusively in women and is much worse with prolonged standing. Typically, patients gain excessive amounts of weight during the day compared with normal women. Although pitting edema, particularly in the ankles and legs, may be a prominent symptom, the clinical findings are not always as impressive as the patient's symptoms may suggest. A concern about weight amounting to an obsession is common in some patients with a defect in body image. Abdominal bloating often occurs. Many patients spend their lives alternately dieting and bingeing.

Many claims have been made about the etiology of this syndrome, and practically all the known mechanisms that control sodium and water excretion have been suggested at one time as possible causes of idiopathic edema. The idea that idiopathic edema may result from a defect in capillary permeability has been proposed, although there is little evidence to support this hypothesis (1). All investigations in these women are difficult because they often continue to take diuretics while telling investigators that they have stopped. In the majority of women with idiopathic edema, symptoms are made worse by diuretics, and initially may have been caused either by diuretics or the intermittent fasting and bingeing to which many of these women subject themselves (2).

Thorn pointed out many years ago that many patients with idiopathic edema are emotionally labile, depression being a particularly common feature (3). Some patients find that intermittent vomiting or laxative abuse has the same effect as diuretics in that it causes a transient loss of weight and an improved sense of well being, which is then followed, as with diuretics, by a worsening of the edema.

CLINICAL FEATURES

The typical features of idiopathic edema are intermittent swelling of the legs, hands, and rarely, the face, with abdominal bloating. In particular, there is no pattern to the weight gain, which can occur at any time and is unrelated to the menstrual cycle. Thorn arbitrarily applied a criterion of a weight gain >1.4 kg/day as essential for a diagnosis of idiopathic edema, stating that normal women gain <1 kg/day (3). Unfortunately, it is not clear from what studies Thorn chose these arbitrary figures and, in particular, whether the patients were taking diuretics at the time. Nevertheless, this criterion often has been used for diagnostic purposes (1). In our experience and others (4), it is not very helpful because some normal women can gain >1.5 kg/day without any symptoms, whereas other women gain only small amounts of weight but have a large number of symptoms directly attributable to sodium and water retention. Indeed, one recent study showed that one in six women attending a gynecologic outpatient clinic would be classified as having idiopathic edema (4).

In symptomatic subjects the weight gain, particularly the edema in the legs, is made worse by standing during the day and is also aggravated by warm weather. In other patients the most prominent symptom may be abdominal bloating (5). Many patients who do not have clinical evidence of edema may often complain of fullness and tightness of the face, ankles, and hands, particularly the fingers on which there are rings. At the time the physician sees the patient, in spite of what may seem to the patient almost disabling symptoms, there is usually no clinically detectable swelling or edema.

In addition, there may be substantial psychological and emotional disturbances, which Thorn regarded as one of the criteria for diagnosis of idiopathic edema (3). Typically, the patient is emotionally labile with depressive features. Nearly all patients have an excessive concern about their weight, and invariably they are trying to lose weight. They may have a defect in the image they have of their body size, a feeling that they are overweight and appear bloated when in fact they may seem to others to be underweight. Attempts to lose weight often consist of alternately fasting for as long as possible, followed by a short period of excessive food consumption. Such a binge is accompanied by severe sodium and water retention, perhaps by edema, and certainly by all the usual symptoms (6). At this time diuretics may temporarily relieve the sodium and water retention, or, if the patient has not yet

G. A. MacGregor: Blood Pressure Unit, St. George's Hospital Medical School, London, United Kingdom

H. E. de Wardener: Department of Clinical Chemistry, Imperial College School of Medicine, London, United Kingdom

discovered diuretics, temporary relief may be obtained by the use of laxatives or surreptitious vomiting.

DIAGNOSIS

Usually the syndrome is straightforward diagnostically, but other causes of sodium and water retention must be excluded. By far the most frequent cause of intermittent water and sodium retention that must be distinguished from idiopathic edema is the menstrual cycle. In patients with idiopathic edema, the "edema" has no relation to the menstrual cycle. It is useful for diagnostic purposes to ask patients to record for a period of time their morning and evening weight and the days on which they menstruate.

A typical feature of idiopathic edema is that true gain in weight is not nearly as impressive as that claimed by the patient. There is no doubt that many patients exaggerate their symptoms, often as a result of the indifference they have encountered from doctors who have dismissed their symptoms as trivial. The patient then feels that the only way to get attention is by claiming daily weight gains that are physiologically impossible. For instance, it is not unusual for patients to claim that they gain from 6 to 8 kg in a single day. If this were owing to sodium and water retention, there would have to be a minimum fluid intake of at least 6 to 8 liters, yet most patients deny drinking this amount of fluid in a single day.

In patients in whom the diagnosis is not clear-cut, Streeten and colleagues suggested that a water-loading test in the supine and upright positions might be useful (7). In this test, patients are instructed to drink 20 mL of water per kilogram of ideal body weight over 30 minutes; urine output is then followed for 4 hours. According to Streeten and colleagues, normal subjects excrete 70% of the water load within 4 hours, in both the supine and the upright positions, whereas patients with idiopathic edema excrete only 70% of the water load in the supine position and much less when upright. Such a test is positive in any subject who is volume depleted for any reason; therefore, if patients are furtively taking diuretics or are covertly sodium-depleting themselves in other ways, a positive test will not be diagnostic of some primary abnormality (8). There is also the risk with this test that hyponatremia may occur.

Idiopathic edema must be distinguished from other well-known causes of sodium and water retention such as heart failure and cirrhosis. Although this is not difficult in most patients, there have been occasional case reports of cardiomyopathy being diagnosed mistakenly as idiopathic edema (9). Renal disease, particularly the nephrotic syndrome, can cause edema but is relatively simple to exclude. Allergic causes of localized edema such as angioneurotic edema can usually be excluded by the history.

Prediabetic patients, who often experience intermittent edema before or at the time of developing diabetes, are more difficult (10). Patients with myxedema also may suffer intermittent swelling that disappears with correction of their thyroid deficiency (11). All patients who are seen for edema should have a fasting blood sugar measured, if not a glucose tolerance test and tests of thyroid function.

Many drugs can cause sodium and water retention, in particular, all the nonsteroidal antiinflammatory drugs. Estrogen therapy may cause sodium and water retention, and steroids with mineralocorticoid action (e.g., fludrocortisone and drugs that inhibit 11-beta hydroxy steroid dehydrogenase), so that drugs such as carbenoxolone and liquorice also may cause edema. Chlorpromazine and similar psychotropic drugs can cause fluid retention and mimic some of the symptoms of idiopathic edema (12). Many blood pressure-lowering drugs may cause edema, particularly the postadrenergic blocking drugs (e.g., guanethidine) and the direct arteriolar vasodilators (e.g., hydralazine). Minoxidil is almost invariably associated with severe sodium and water retention with edema unless diuretics are given concomitantly. The calcium entry antagonists, which are natriuretic and cause a long-term reduction in sodium balance (13), may paradoxically cause edema of the ankles and legs, particularly the dihydropyridine derivatives (e.g., nifedipine). This edema is thought to result from local arteriolar vasodilatation with an imbalance in capillary filtration.

Edema of the legs also may be caused by venous or lymphatic obstruction, and the differentiation from idiopathic edema may be difficult in some patients. This entity may occur particularly with the familial lymphatic syndromes, which may initially present with intermittent pitting edema. There may also be difficulties in some patients with severe varicose veins with thromboses who develop severe dilatation of the veins. They may then develop intermittent edema on standing upright, secondary to pooling of blood in the legs (a form of blood volume translocation that diminishes the "effective" blood volume). Many patients may conceal that they are taking diuretics or laxatives. It is very common for patients to alternately binge and fast. This in itself causes exaggerated swings in sodium and water balance.

ETIOLOGY

It is not surprising to find considerable controversy about the potential mechanisms whereby some women develop intermittent edema because the normal mechanisms controlling sodium and water balance in humans are not fully understood. Sodium balance plays an important role in regulating the volume of extracellular fluid in mammals. During evolution, as mammals moved away from the sea, they had difficulty in obtaining enough sodium and developed powerful mechanisms to conserve sodium in urine and sweat as well as an instinctual appetite for sodium. During evolution the average sodium intake of humans has been estimated to be around 5 to 10 mmol/day. However, the more recent ability of humans to obtain salt either from mines or evaporation of sea water and the finding that salt is a good preservative of food have meant that sodium intake has now increased to around 100 to 400 mmol/day. There is no doubt that such a marked increase in salt intake has been associated with an increase in extracellular fluid volume.

Surprisingly, idiopathic edema was not described until 1955 after the introduction of oral diuretics (14); however, Streeten claimed that he saw patients with idiopathic edema as early as 1952, that is, just before the introduction of oral diuretics (15). In the earlier literature, a case report in 1922 is often cited as the first case of idiopathic edema (16); however, this case report is that of a 28-year-old man with sodium and water retention who had clinical and radiologic evidence of a pituitary tumor that had already caused visual field defects. It hardly fits the description of idiopathic edema, although it may represent the first case report of a defect in the secretion of a natriuretic hormone.

Nearly all the potential mechanisms that may influence sodium excretion have at one time been claimed to be the underlying cause of idiopathic edema; however, the cause of the syndrome (assuming it exists) has proved elusive. In our view, most of the abnormal findings in these women are owing to the prior use of diuretics that have been stopped a few days before, the continued use of diuretics either knowingly or covertly during the test, excessive amounts of laxatives or surreptitious vomiting, or recurrent fasting followed by bingeing. A recurring problem in the literature of idiopathic edema is that it is often not clear whether patients were studied while taking diuretics, and if they were not, when the diuretics were stopped and what steps were taken to detect patients who continued to consume diuretics surreptitiously, take laxatives, or vomit.

Potential Etiologic Factors

Upright Posture

Whatever the cause of idiopathic edema, all investigators agree that the edema itself is made worse by prolonged periods of standing; indeed, in most patients the symptoms largely disappear if the patient lies flat during the day (1,3,7). Even in normal subjects, it is well established that adoption of the upright posture causes a reduction in sodium and water excretion. In careful studies, Streeten and coworkers showed that there is excessive sodium and water retention on tilting in patients with idiopathic edema compared with normal subjects (7). Indeed, they were able to classify patients with idiopathic edema into those who had what they termed "orthostatic water retention," others who had "orthostatic sodium retention," and a few in whom the edema apparently was unrelated to the upright position. This division of patients into those who retain water and/or sodium on standing upright has been criticized and seems to relate more to the severity of the patient's symptoms than to a different underlying mechanism (1). As with many other studies of patients with idiopathic edema, patients stopped the diuretic only a short time before the studies were performed, and Streeten and coworkers admit that some of the balance data on potassium excretion had to be discarded because of the previous

effects of the diuretics (7). It is therefore impossible to exclude the possibility, and in our view the probability that, compared with control subjects who had never had diuretics, the long-term use of diuretics would have caused increased sodium and water retention on tilting, even though the diuretics had been stopped a few weeks before (8). One possible mechanism for this excessive sodium and water retention on standing upright even when the diuretic has been discontinued is juxtaglomerular hyperplasia secondary to prolonged use of diuretics, which would give an exaggerated response of renin and aldosterone to the upright posture, even though the diuretic had been stopped some time previously.

Increased Renin or Aldosterone Level

Early reports of idiopathic edema claimed that patients had increased renin and aldosterone levels or an exaggerated renin and aldosterone response to standing (17–19). Most investigators now agree that these findings are likely to result from previous diuretic therapy. Our own experience and that of others is that if plasma renin activity or plasma aldosterone is raised, it is very suggestive that the patient either was taking a diuretic or was in some other way depleting herself of sodium. Assessment of the level of plasma renin activity or plasma aldosterone must be done in conjunction with a 24-hour urinary sodium excretion test, because subjects who are restricting salt intake also have raised plasma renin activity and increased aldosterone secondary to salt restriction rather than to the use of diuretics, laxatives, or vomiting.

With the realization that plasma aldosterone concentrations are normal in patients with idiopathic edema who were not taking diuretics, it was then suggested that in spite of normal levels, a possible mechanism might be a failure to escape from these normal levels of aldosterone. However, studies in which large amounts of fludrocortisone were given to patients with idiopathic edema have shown that they were able to escape from the sodium-retaining effect of the steroid, albeit at a slightly slower rate than normal subjects, and that they did not develop edema, making it extremely unlikely that the "idiopathic" edema could result from a failure to escape from a normal level of aldosterone (1).

Antidiuretic Hormone

The claimed abnormal response to sodium and water excretion in the upright posture in "idiopathic edema" has prompted some authors to suggest that there may be abnormalities of antidiuretic hormone (ADH) secretion. Thibonnier and colleagues, measuring urinary ADH, found that patients with idiopathic edema failed to show the normal suppression of ADH after a water load but only when they were in the upright posture, suggesting perhaps a posturally related defect in the feedback mechanisms controlling ADH (8). However, even if it is accepted that these results are not related to previous diuretic therapy, it is not clear how an increase in ADH secretion in the upright posture could cause edema. Excess secretion of ADH is well known to be associated with a fall in plasma sodium but not to cause sodium and water retention. It would seem, therefore, very unlikely that increased ADH secretion could have any direct role in the pathogenesis of idiopathic edema (5).

Hypothalamic Disorders

A report by Young and colleagues claimed that there is a greater release of prolactin, luteinizing hormone, and follicle-stimulating hormone following administration of luteinizing-releasing hormone and thyrotropin-releasing hormone in some patients with idiopathic edema (20). However, three of the 14 patients were studied while taking diuretics, and eight had stopped the diuretics 3 months previously. Furthermore, it is not clear from the paper whether any subjects were surreptitiously taking diuretics during the study. No comment is made as to whether the three who were known to be taking diuretics during the study had the most abnormal results. This study concluded that there might be some hypothalamic abnormality that would be compatible with the well-known psychological problems that occur in many patients with idiopathic edema. Some case reports of idiopathic edema associated with raised plasma prolactin concentration and a subsequent favorable response to bromocriptine support a hypothalamic disturbance (21). However, the study by Young and colleagues showed no significant difference between prolactin levels in the 14 patients compared with controls (20).

Estrogen and Progesterone

The fact that idiopathic edema occurs predominantly in women has led to the suggestion that the edema might be related to an imbalance among estrogen, progesterone, or other sex hormones. However, there is little evidence of a quantitative alteration in sex hormone secretion in these patients compared with normal controls (5). Although Lagrue and colleagues found some evidence for reduced progesterone levels and normal estrogen levels, progesterone administration did little to relieve the symptoms (22). The reason why the condition is primarily confined to women remains elusive, although there is little doubt that women are much more conscious of their weight and appearance than are men. It is extremely unusual to see men who are addicted to diuretics or laxatives or who vomit surreptitiously to adjust their weight and appearance.

Natriuretic Hormone

Several authors have suggested that there might be an abnormality of secretion of natriuretic factors in idiopathic edema. Mach and Favre have shown that of six patients on a restricted salt diet, three had urinary natriuretic factor levels that were above the normal range and in the same range as normal controls taking 9α-fludrocortisone, suggesting therefore that in idiopathic edema there is some abnormality in the way the kidney responds to natriuretic factors (23). However,

Anderson and Streeten have shown no difference in plasma atrial natriuretic peptide levels in patients with and without idiopathic edema (24).

Hypothyroidism

Many patients with hypothyroidism, and even some with subclinical hypothyroidism, may go through a phase of retaining sodium and water, developing symptoms suggesting idiopathic edema (11). It is therefore very important that thyroxine and triiodothyronine levels and, if available, thyroid-stimulating hormone levels are measured in all patients. If the results are in the low range of normal, it may be worthwhile doing a thyrotropin hormone-releasing test to exclude latent myxedema. The edema associated with thyroid deficiency responds well to treatment with thyroxine. Nevertheless, the majority of patients with idiopathic edema have completely normal thyroid function.

Diabetes

There is evidence that patients with diabetes or latent diabetes may go through a phase of retention of sodium and water mimicking the symptoms of idiopathic edema (10). At the very least, all patients should have a test of fasting blood glucose levels. If there is any suspicion of an abnormality, a full glucose tolerance test should be performed. Insulin can cause sodium and water retention and a change in insulin sensitivity could possibly play a role. The majority of patients with idiopathic edema have normal glucose metabolism. However, importantly, the condition may be aggravated or even initiated by sudden changes in carbohydrate and sodium intake.

Defective Venous Tone

If there is a severe defect of venous tone in the legs, then there will be pronounced pooling of blood on standing, which causes excessive sodium and water retention by the kidney owing to a reduction in renal blood flow (5). This pooling of blood is usually associated with severe varicose veins or previous thrombotic disorders of the veins of the legs. For instance, we have seen one patient who had long-standing venous problems in her legs. When she stood up, she developed severe orthostatic hypotension owing to the pooling of a considerable portion of the blood volume in her legs, and she then retained sodium and water. Eventually she developed edema if she was unable to lie down. This is a relatively rare cause of sodium and water retention and is not found in the majority of patients with idiopathic edema.

Abnormal Capillary Permeability

The idea that there may be an abnormality of capillary permeability in patients with idiopathic edema is attractive and has been accepted by some authorities without, in our view, critical appraisal of the evidence (1,15). There is, in fact, no definitive evidence to support an abnormality of capillary permeability in patients with idiopathic edema. The early case reports that have been cited seem to be describing patients that almost certainly had vasculitis associated with connective tissue disorders (25). More recently, Edwards and Bayliss have claimed that when they gave radiolabeled albumin intravenously, there was an increased disappearance of radioactive albumin from the plasma in patients with idiopathic edema compared with control subjects (1). This paper has been widely cited as evidence of abnormal capillary permeability; however, for ethical reasons, no measurements of the disappearance of radiolabeled albumin were made in control subjects. The authors therefore were in no position to decide whether the rate of loss of isotopically labeled albumin in their patients was abnormal (26,27).

The only groups that have attempted to measure directly the permeability of capillaries to albumin in patients with idiopathic edema and normal subjects are Lagrue and associates (28) and Behar and associates (29). Isotopically labeled albumin was injected intravenously, and the forearm was then monitored for radioactivity before, during, and after venous occlusion. Radioactivity rises and falls rapidly in such a maneuver, and failure of radioactivity to return to baseline levels is considered an indication of increased permeability to albumin. The results in patients with edema are difficult to interpret. The most pronounced abnormalities were found in patients with cirrhosis who were grossly edematous and in patients with edema associated with the menstrual cycle, but the abnormality was only present when the patients were edematous. Thus, it is not clear whether the prolonged retention of albumin in the extravascular compartment of the forearm was a consequence of the edema or its cause. In other words, the possibility that an increased volume of interstitial fluid can delay the removal of radioactive albumin from the interstitial space has not been eliminated (26).

Gill and colleagues found that some patients with idiopathic edema had a low plasma albumin level and also claimed that there may be a low circulating albumin pool in women with idiopathic edema (31). However, this has not been confirmed. Even if such a mechanism existed in Gill and coworkers' patients, it is unlikely that it would be relevant to other patients with idiopathic edema, because plasma albumin was in the normal range in all other reports.

If there is a defect in the capillaries, it is more likely that it relates to an attenuation of the reflex postural vasoconstriction of the precapillary sphincter on standing, as occurs in some diabetics and with treatment with nifedipine (30). This could well explain the few patients with idiopathic edema who are not in some way intermittently depleting and repleting themselves with sodium. Further studies of such patients would be very valuable.

Diuretics

Many patients find that when their symptoms are severe, the use of diuretics may temporarily alleviate both the edema and their symptoms. However, diuretics stimulate compensatory

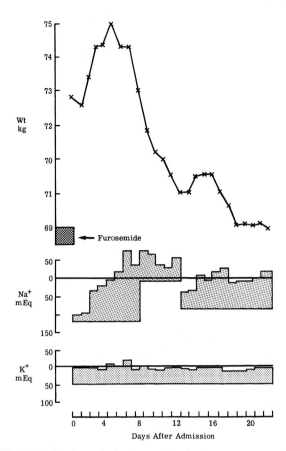

FIG. 83-1. Changes in body weight, sodium balance, and potassium balance in a 22-year-old nurse with idiopathic edema. She was edematous while on furosemide, which was then stopped. She noted an initial 3-kg weight gain with stopping of furosemide, followed by a 6- to 7-kg weight loss. (From: MacGregor GA, Tasker PRW, de Wardener HE. Diuretic induced oedema. *Lancet* 1975;1:489, with permission.)

mechanisms to retain sodium and water, and these compensatory mechanisms are longer acting than the natriuretic effect of the diuretic. Therefore, whenever diuretics are stopped, there is pronounced retention of sodium and water (2,6). Many patients who regularly consume diuretics may be able to keep themselves edema free. However, one of the first patients that we studied came to us with edema while taking furosemide, 160 mg/day, which she had been taking for over a year and a half (6). On admission to the metabolic ward, she had marked edema, and she remained edematous until the diuretic was stopped. When the furosemide was stopped, she gained 3 kg over 5 days, following which she began to lose weight. Figure 83-1 illustrates how her weight continued to fall until it leveled out at about 4 kg less than her weight when she was taking diuretics.

These remarkable findings led us to study 10 other patients with idiopathic edema who were taking diuretics (2). All patients were admitted to the metabolic ward and placed on a fixed sodium and potassium intake. Control observations were made while they continued to take diuretics, and the diuretics were then stopped. When the diuretics were stopped,

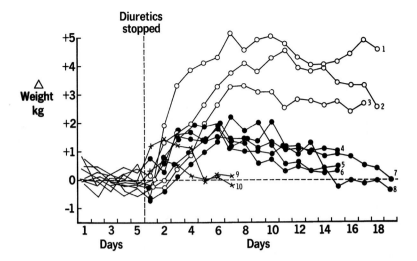

FIG. 83-2. Changes in weight in 10 patients while taking diuretics and after stopping them. Note that weight returned to the level present while taking diuretics within 3 weeks of stopping them in patients 4 to 10, whereas weight remained elevated 3 weeks after stopping the diuretics in patients 1, 2, and 3. (From: MacGregor GA, et al. Is "idiopathic" oedema idiopathic? *Lancet* 1979;1:397, with permission.)

all 10 patients retained sodium and water, as judged by a reduction in urinary sodium excretion and an increase in weight (Fig. 83-2). This retention of sodium and water and gain in weight appeared to be directly related to the degree of stimulation of the renin–angiotensin–aldosterone system by the diuretics. During the next 5 to 6 days after stopping diuretics, plasma renin activity (Fig. 83-3) and urinary aldosterone excretion (Fig. 83-4) gradually returned toward normal, urinary sodium excretion increased, and most patients then lost weight and their edema subsided. In seven patients no further treatment was necessary, and they remained well on follow-up without further attacks of edema. However, in

three patients who had been taking the largest amounts of diuretics and who had the greatest stimulation of the renin–angiotensin–aldosterone system before stopping the diuretics, weight remained elevated and edema recurred subsequently during the next few months in spite of the absence of diuretics. In view of the recurring edema, they were placed on a moderately restricted sodium diet of approximately 50 mmol/day. In two patients the edema then disappeared, and within a year they were able to increase their sodium intake to normal without developing edema. The third patient was not able to control her sodium or her calorie intake, and she continued to take diuretics and to have intermittent edema.

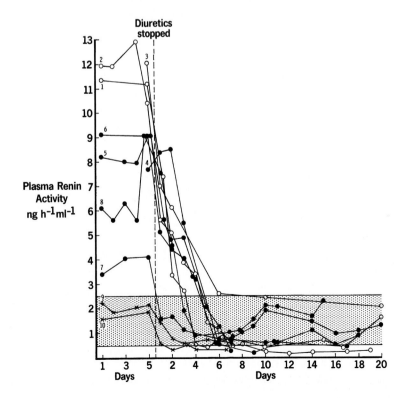

FIG. 83-3. Changes in plasma renin activity in 10 patients before and after stopping diuretics. (From: MacGregor GA, et al. Is "idiopathic" oedema idiopathic? *Lancet* 1979;1:397, with permission.)

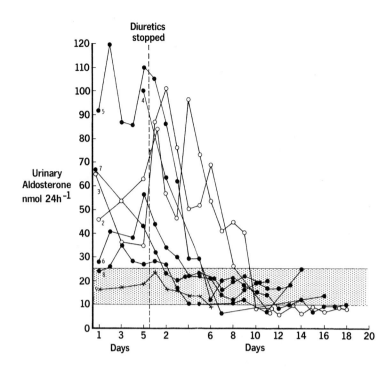

FIG. 83-4. Changes in urinary aldosterone levels in 10 patients taking diuretics and after stopping them. (From: MacGregor GA, et al. Is "idiopathic" oedema idiopathic? *Lancet* 1979;1:397, with permission.)

Claims have been made that some patients who have never taken diuretics present with idiopathic edema (15). In our own practice, the reason for starting diuretics was often trivial. These patients are almost always obsessed about their weight and appearance. Many patients confess that in attempting to control their weight, they vary the amount of food they consume, both before and after they started taking diuretics. In an attempt to lose weight they may starve themselves for several days and then lose control and eat several substantial meals. Sudden changes in carbohydrate intake can cause sodium and water retention with edema (32,33). In addition, prolonged low sodium intake also stimulates the renin–angiotensin–aldosterone system, and, as with diuretics, the effect of this stimulation persists for some time after sodium intake is suddenly raised. Therefore, a sudden increase in sodium intake causes sodium retention; this is compounded by the effect of a sudden increase in carbohydrate intake, which also causes retention of sodium and water, perhaps because of an increase in sympathetic tone (34).

To study the effect of sudden changes in carbohydrate and salt intake in young women, we studied four normal women aged 20 to 26 years, who were first placed on a low-sodium (10 mmol/day), low-carbohydrate (80 g/day) diet and then suddenly changed to a high-sodium (350 mmol/day), high-carbohydrate (350 g/day) diet (2). This sudden, simultaneous change in sodium and carbohydrate intake caused marked retention of sodium and water with a weight gain that varied from 3 to 4 kg over 24 to 36 hours (Fig. 83-5). With this retention of sodium and water and weight gain all of these normal women complained of the typical features of idiopathic edema—that is, tightness of the ankles, hands, and face, with detectable edema in two subjects and abdominal bloating. In subsequent studies we looked at the effect of

alteration of carbohydrate intake alone on sodium excretion and showed that when normal women change from a similar low- to a high-carbohydrate diet, there is a small degree of

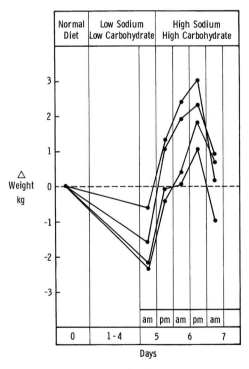

FIG. 83-5. Changes in weight in four normal young women after changing from their normal diet to a low-sodium, low-carbohydrate diet, and then to a high-sodium, high-carbohydrate diet. (From: MacGregor GA, et al. Is "idiopathic" oedema idiopathic? *Lancet* 1979;1:397, with permission.)

sodium retention and weight gain. These same women were then studied a second time when they were kept on a constant carbohydrate intake and changed from a low- (10 mmol/day) to a high-sodium (350 mmol/day) diet. This caused greater retention of sodium and weight gain, but the weight gain was less than when carbohydrate and sodium intakes were both suddenly increased. It would seem likely, therefore, that it is the combination of the change in both carbohydrate and sodium intake that causes severe sodium and water retention.

These observations in normal women suggest that the initial complaints in some patients with idiopathic edema might be owing to fluctuations in sodium and carbohydrate intake caused by the patients' concern for their weight and appearance. Sudden gains in weight with their attendant discomforts cause these women to seek medical advice. The absence of any obvious cause for the edema and the patient's persistence eventually overcome the doctor's reluctance to prescribe diuretics. Once on diuretics, the renin–angiotensin–aldosterone system is persistently stimulated both by the diuretics themselves and continued fluctuations in sodium and carbohydrate intake. Severe edema occurs if the diuretics are stopped, and both the patient and her doctor believe that the edema can be prevented only by the continuous use of diuretics.

Many of the previous findings in patients with idiopathic edema, such as reduced blood volume (1), raised plasma renin activity, and increased aldosterone level (17,18), could be directly owing to the previous use of diuretics. Associated findings, including a tendency toward sodium and water retention, especially when the patient receives a large sodium or water load, particularly on standing (7), could also be related to the prior administration of diuretics. There is no doubt that many patients with idiopathic edema show all the characteristics of chronic volume depletion (35). It is likely that the prolonged administration of diuretics causes persistent stimulation of the renin–angiotensin system and juxtaglomerular hypertrophy and may well cause other long- standing changes in mechanisms regulating sodium and water balance, so that even when diuretics have been stopped for some time there may be abnormal responses in these patients. Pelosi and colleagues claimed that idiopathic edema was a psychosomatic disease that was unrelated to diuretics. However, of the 25 patients they studied, 23 admitted to having taken diuretics (36)!

Patients who have not had diuretics often find that the fasting they subject themselves to leads to constipation. To seek relief from constipation, they start using laxatives and then find that when used to excess, laxatives are helpful in relieving them of the large volume of sodium and water they retain when they eat excessively. The incidence of laxative abuse in these patients is probably greatly underestimated, and all patients should have routine tests to make sure they are not abusing laxatives. Clearly, laxatives can induce exactly the same syndrome as diuretics (37).

Indeed, a study in which chronic laxative abusers had the laxatives withdrawn showed rebound retention of sodium and

water followed by resolution in seven of the nine patients studied (38). Other patients find that after bingeing, surreptitious vomiting stops their abdominal bloating and sodium and water retention (39). In our experience, surreptitious vomiting can be very difficult to exclude because most patients are ashamed of their habit and are very adept at hiding their vomiting from both their physicians and families.

In our view, therefore, idiopathic edema is related to the patient's habit of bingeing and fasting and then using some method of obtaining relief from the excess sodium and water retained. This usually involves the use of diuretics, laxatives, or surreptitious vomiting. All of these cause long-term stimulation of the renin–angiotensin–aldosterone system and subsequent worsening of sodium and water retention, which is compounded by continued fluctuations in sodium and carbohydrate intake.

MANAGEMENT

The management of idiopathic edema is not satisfactory. It is necessary first to obtain a full history of exactly what has precipitated the edema—diuretics, laxatives, surreptitious vomiting, or persistent fasting and bingeing. Sympathetic understanding and handling of the patient can help in elucidating a full history. Many patients feel rejected by their doctors, and this rejection compounds their feelings of resentment and leads to exaggeration of symptoms to try to get the doctor to take notice of them. Clearly, other causes of sodium and water retention need to be excluded, but this is usually not difficult. All patients should have the investigations detailed in Table 83-1, and further investigations should be done as appropriate and when indicated. Management largely depends on whether the patient is using diuretics or not.

Patients on Diuretics

All patients taking diuretics should stop taking them; however, patients develop edema if diuretics are stopped suddenly. Therefore, it is better to withdraw diuretics gradually and, at the same time, advise patients to restrict salt intake. Our experience indicates that most patients do not experience any severe rebound retention of sodium and water and therefore do not become edematous if they are able to restrict salt intake to approximately 50 mmol/day (40). It is helpful

TABLE 83-1. *Investigations for idiopathic edema*

Blood	Full blood count, urea, electrolytes, creatinine, liver function tests, total plasma albumin, fasting blood sugar, thyroid-stimulating hormone, renin activity
Urine tests	Urinary protein, 24-hr urinary sodium excretion, test for phenolphthalein
Other tests	Chest x-ray, electrocardiogram, glucose tolerance test. In selected cases only; venography, lymphangiogram

if patients continue to restrict salt intake; this usually controls edema satisfactorily if they maintain moderate sodium restriction without excessive fluctuations in salt intake. Some patients soon find that they can return to a normal salt intake without developing edema, particularly if they had been taking small doses of diuretics previously. Others find they are unable to maintain a constant moderate sodium restriction, and consequently their sodium and carbohydrate intake continues to fluctuate. In these patients, sympathetic understanding and careful work by a dietitian may be helpful in an attempt to regulate sodium and carbohydrate intake to regular amounts compatible with the patient's usually overwhelming desire to lose weight.

Patients Not on Diuretics

In this group of patients it is very important to exclude laxative abuse, covert use of diuretics, or surreptitious vomiting. Measurement of plasma renin activity and/or aldosterone while on a normal sodium intake is a good indicator of whether patients are depleting themselves of sodium. In patients who are not depleting themselves of sodium and are definitely not taking diuretics, who still have edema, we have found that moderate restriction of sodium intake to around 50 mmol/day usually relieves the symptoms, provided there is no fluctuation in food intake. Some studies have claimed that ß-blockers or a converting enzyme inhibitor such as captopril (41) may be helpful in treating unusual patients with persistent edema in spite of moderate sodium restriction, but there are no proper randomized control trials. Many patients find that lying flat during the day for a period may be helpful, particularly during a bad attack of edema, but this is not practical for most active women. Ephedrine has been reported to reduce edema formation in patients with diabetes and possibly may be helpful in some patients with idiopathic edema; however, there are no well-controlled studies. Even amphetamines such as dexamphetamine have been used, but the dangers of addiction of these controlled drugs are far too great to contemplate their use without a well-designed randomized double-blind control trial.

Occasional patients are encountered in whom edema persists. The use of a long-acting diuretic at the lowest effective dose may be justified, often combined with distally acting drugs. Loop diuretics should be avoided because they cause large fluctuations in sodium balance. It is interesting that there are very few women over the age of 60 who complain of the symptoms of idiopathic edema; apparently, the syndrome eventually resolves with increasing age.

Subjects who continue to fast and binge intermittently, surreptitiously take diuretics, vomit, or abuse laxatives are much more difficult to deal with and usually have the most severe associated psychological disorders, often merging into the same type of psychological disorder found in anorexia nervosa. Such patients can be extremely difficult to help and usually drift on a tide of discontent from one doctor to another.

REFERENCES

1. Edwards OM, Bayliss RIS. Idiopathic oedema of women. *Q J Med* 1976;45:125.
2. MacGregor GA, et al. Is "idiopathic" oedema idiopathic? *Lancet* 1979;1:397.
3. Thorn GW. Approach to the patient with "idiopathic oedema" or "periodic swelling." *JAMA* 1968;206:333.
4. Denning DW, et al. The relationship between 'normal' fluid retention in women and idiopathic oedema. *Postgrad Med J* 1990;66:363.
5. Feldman HA, Jayakumar S, Puschett JB. Idiopathic oedema: a review of aetiological concepts and management. *Cardiovasc Med* 1978;3:475.
6. MacGregor GA, Tasker PRW, de Wardener HE. Diuretic induced oedema. *Lancet* 1975;1:489.
7. Streeten DHP, et al. Studies of pathogenesis of idiopathic oedema: the roles of postural changes in plasma volume, plasma renin activity, aldosterone secretion rate and glomerular filtration rate in the retention of sodium and water. *Clin Sci Mol Med* 1973;45:347.
8. Thibonnier MJ, Marchetti JP, Corvol P. Influence of previous diuretic intake on the humoral and hormonal profile of idiopathic oedema. *Eur J Clin Invest* 1981;11:19.
9. Obeid AL, et al. Cardiac function in idiopathic oedema. *Arch Intern Med* 1974;134:253.
10. Dunnigan MG, Lawrence JR. Idiopathic oedema. *Lancet* 1979;1:776.
11. Al-Khader AA, Aber GM. The relationship between the 'idiopathic oedema syndrome' and subclinical hypothyroidism. *Clin Endocrinol* 1979;10:271.
12. Witz L, Shapiro MS, Shenkman L. Chlorpromazine induced fluid retention masquerading as idiopathic oedema. *Br Med J* 1987;294:807.
13. Cappuccio FP, et al. Acute and sustained changes in sodium balance during nifedipine treatment in essential hypertension. *Am J Med* 1991;91:233.
14. Mach RS, et al. Oedemes par retention de chlorure de sodium avec hyperaldosteronurie. *Schweiz Med Wochenschr* 1955;85:1229.
15. Streeten DHP. Idiopathic oedema. *Lancet* 1979;1:775.
16. Jungmann P. Uber eine isolierte Storung des Salztoff-Wechsels. *Klin Wochenschr* 1933;1:1546.
17. Luetscher JA, Lieberman AH. Idiopathic edema with increased aldosterone excretion. In: Baulieu EE, Robel P, eds. *Aldosterone.* Oxford: Blackwell Scientific, 1964.
18. Streeten DHP, Louis LH, Conn JW. Secondary aldosteronism in "idiopathic edema." *Trans Assoc Am Phys* 1960;73:227.
19. Veyrat R, Robert M, Mach RS. Etude de la renine dans les oedemes idiopathiques avec hyperaldosteronisme secondaire. *Schweiz Med Wochenschr* 1968;98:1499.
20. Young JB, et al. Evidence for a hypothalamic disturbance in cyclical oedema. *Br Med J* 1983;286:1691.
21. Edwards CRW, Besser GM, Thorner MO. Bromocriptine-responsive form of idiopathic oedema. *Lancet* 1979;1:94.
22. Lagrue G, Behar A, Morville R. Etude de la fonction ovarienne au cours des oedemes idiopathiques orthostatiques. *Presse Med* 1983;12:2859.
23. Mach RS, Favre H. Idiopathic oedema. *Lancet* 1979;1:826.
24. Anderson GH Jr, Streeten DHP. Effect of posture on plasma atrial natriuretic hormone and renal function during salt loading in patients with and without postural (idiopathic) edema. *J Clin Endocrinol Metab* 1990;1:243.
25. Emmerson K, Armstrong SH. High protein edema due to diffuse abnormality of capillary permeability. *Trans Am Clin Climatol Assoc* 1955;67:59.
26. MacGregor GA, de Wardener HE. Idiopathic oedema. *Lancet* 1979;1:670.
27. MacGregor GA, de Wardener HE. Idiopathic oedema. *Lancet* 1979;2:355.
28. Lagrue G, et al. Le syndrome d'oedemes cycliques idiopathiques. *J Urol Nephrol* 1976;12:929.
29. Behar A, et al. Untersuchungen zur bestimmung der kapillaren durchlassigkeit mit markiertem menschlichem albumin. *Nucklearmedizin* 1976;15:214.
30. Williams SA, Rayman G, Tooke JE. Dependent oedema and attenuation of postural vasoconstriction associated with nifedipine therapy for hypertension in diabetic patients. *Eur J Clin Pharmacol* 1989;37:333.
31. Gill JR, Waldmann TA, Bartter FC. Idiopathic edema: the occurrence of hypoalbuminemia and abnormal albumin metabolism in women with unexplained edema. *Am J Med* 1972;52:444.

32. Bloom WL. Inhibition of salt excretion by carbohydrate. *Arch Intern Med* 1962;109:26.
33. Garnett ES, Nahmias C. The effect of glucose on the urinary excretion of sodium and hydrogen ion in man. *Clin Sci Mol Med* 1974;47:589.
34. Landsberg L, Young JB. Fasting, feeding and regulation of the sympathetic nervous system. *N Engl J Med* 1978;298:1295.
35. Ferris TF, et al. Studies of the mechanism of sodium retention in idiopathic edema. *Trans Assoc Am Phys* 1973;86:310.
36. Pelosi AJ, et al. A psychiatric study of idiopathic oedema. *Lancet* 1986;ii:999.
37. Gross DJ, et al. Edema associated with laxative abuse and excessive diuretic therapy. *Isr J Med Sci* 1980;16:789.
38. Meyers AM, et al. Chronic laxative abusers with pseudo-idiopathic oedema and autonomous pseudo-Bartters' syndrome. *South Afr Med J* 1990;78:631.
39. Pelosi AJ, Lough M. Cyclical oedema. *Br Med J* 1983;287:2101.
40. Missouris CG, Cappuccio FP, Markandu ND, et al. Diuretics and oedema: how to avoid rebound sodium retention. *Lancet* 1992;339:1546.
41. Docci D, Turci F, Salvi G. Therapeutic response of idiopathic edema to captopril. *Nephron* 1983;34:198.
42. Edmonds M, Arocher A, Warkins P. Ephedrine: a new treatment for diabetic neuropathic oedema. *Lancet* 1983;1:548.
43. Streeten D. Idiopathic edema: pathogenesis, clinical features and treatment. *Endocrinol Metabol Clin North Am* 1995;25:531.

CHAPTER 84

Cardiac Failure, Liver Disease, and the Nephrotic Syndrome

William T. Abraham, Melissa A. Cadnapaphornchai, and Robert W. Schrier

The kidney plays a central role in the sodium and water retention and edema formation associated with cardiac failure, liver disease, and the nephrotic syndrome. In these edematous disorders, renal sodium and water retention is observed despite an excess of total body sodium and water. This finding is in contrast to the renal response of normal persons to extracellular fluid (ECF) volume expansion, where the administration of isotonic saline results in the urinary excretion of the excess amount of sodium and water with restoration of the normal ECF volume. This clinical paradox of continued renal sodium and water retention despite total body sodium and water excess defines the edematous disorders and has been under intense investigation for many years.

In the circumstances of acute or chronic intrinsic renal failure discussed elsewhere in this text, it is apparent why diseased kidneys with diminished filtration rates of sodium and water may retain sodium and water to the point of pulmonary or peripheral edema. However, in patients with cardiac failure or liver cirrhosis and in some nephrotic syndrome patients, the integrity of the kidney as the definitive effector organ of body fluid volume regulation is clearly intact. For example, transplantation of the kidney from cirrhotic patients with ascites and edema into subjects with normal hepatic function completely reverses the renal sodium and water retention (1). Conversely, transplantation of a normal liver into an edematous cirrhotic patient also abolishes the renal sodium and water retention (2). These observations demonstrate the reversible or functional nature of the abnormalities

in renal function and excretory capacity seen in these edematous states.

Although the kidney can be isolated from its extrarenal environment and yet be demonstrated to excrete a salt load added to its renal arterial perfusion circuit (3), it is now clear that extrarenal factors play a major role in the renal sodium and water retention of cardiac failure, liver disease, and the nephrotic syndrome. Thus, a strictly nephrocentric view of the pathogenesis of sodium and water retention in these edematous disorders is no longer tenable. Both systemic circulatory alterations and activation of various neurohormonal mechanisms contribute to the observed sodium and water retention. This chapter reviews the mechanisms of edema formation and sodium and water retention associated with cardiac failure, liver disease, and the nephrotic syndrome.

MECHANISM OF EDEMA FORMATION

Edema is a clinical sign that indicates an increase in the volume of sodium and water in the interstitial space. This increase in interstitial space volume is caused by an alteration of the Starling forces that govern the transfer of fluid from the vascular compartment into the surrounding tissue spaces (4). Edema may result from local factors such as obstruction of lymphatic or venous flow. However, the types of edema considered in this chapter reflect a generalized disturbance of sodium and water balance and are associated with a net increase in ECF volume, a situation that is usually not present when edema results from a local disruption of normal capillary mechanisms. Generalized edema results when altered Starling forces affect all capillary beds. The development of generalized edema thus indicates a widespread disturbance in the normal balance between tissue capillary and interstitial hydrostatic and colloid osmotic pressures, which control the distribution of ECF between the vascular and extravascular (interstitial) compartments. In cardiac failure, liver disease, and the nephrotic syndrome, sodium and water retention by

W. T. Abraham: Department of Medicine; and GIH Heart Institute, University of Kentucky College of Medicine, Lexington, Kentucky

M. A. Cadnapaphornchai: Department of Pediatrics and Medicine, University of Colorado Health Sciences Center; and Department of Pediatrics, The Kidney Center, The Children's Hospital, Denver, Colorado

R. W. Schrier: Department of Medicine, University of Colorado Health Sciences Center, Denver, Colorado

the kidney leads to the progressive expansion of the ECF volume and alteration of the Starling forces that subsequently result in edema formation.

Transcapillary solute and fluid transport consists of two types of flow, convective and diffusive. Bulk water movement occurs via convective transport induced by the imbalance between transcapillary hydraulic pressure and colloid osmotic pressure (4). Transcapillary hydraulic pressure is influenced by a number of factors, including systemic arterial and venous blood pressures, regional blood flow, and the resistances imposed by the precapillary and postcapillary sphincters. Systemic arterial blood pressure, in turn, is determined by cardiac output, intravascular volume, and systemic vascular resistance. Systemic venous pressure is determined by right atrial pressure, intravascular volume, and venous capacitance. These latter hemodynamic parameters are largely determined by sodium and water balance and by various neurohormonal factors. For example, right atrial pressure or right ventricular preload is modulated both by changes in the intravascular volume, which are largely determined by the kidney, and alterations in venous capacitance, which are governed in part by neuroendocrine mechanisms such as the sympathetic nervous system, renin–angiotensin system, nonosmotic release of arginine vasopressin (AVP), and the natriuretic peptides. As discussed in this chapter, activation of these two mechanisms (i.e., renal sodium and water retention and neurohormonal activation), which may influence transcapillary hydraulic and oncotic pressures, is observed with cardiac failure, liver disease, and the nephrotic syndrome.

Several mechanisms are capable of minimizing edema formation or diminishing the transudation of solute and water across the capillary bed. In several vascular beds, the local transcapillary hydraulic pressure gradient exceeds the opposing colloid osmotic pressure gradient throughout the length of the capillary bed so that filtration occurs across its entire length (5). Filtered fluid consequently must return to the circulation via lymphatics. Increased lymphatic drainage and the ability of lymphatic flow to increase may thus be seen as one protective mechanism that minimizes edema formation. Other protective mechanisms that reduce interstitial fluid accumulation include precapillary vasoconstriction, increased net filtration with a resultant rise in intracapillary plasma protein concentration, and increased interstitial fluid volume with a resultant augmentation of tissue hydraulic pressure. For example, increased net filtration itself, such as that associated with hypoalbuminemia and the resultant decreased plasma oncotic pressure, leads to a dissipation of capillary hydraulic pressure, a dilution of interstitial fluid protein concentration, and a corresponding rise in intracapillary protein concentration, all of which alter the balance of Starling forces to mitigate against further interstitial fluid accumulation.

These buffering factors directed against interstitial fluid accumulation may explain why, in patients with congenital analbuminemia, positive sodium and water balance and edema formation do not occur and sodium loads are excreted (6). Because the continued loss of intravascular fluid volume

TABLE 84-1. *Disturbances in microcirculatory hemodynamics associated with edema and expansion of extracellular fluid volume*

Increased venous pressure transmitted to the capillary
Adjustments in precapillary and postcapillary resistances to favor interstitial fluid accumulation
Inadequate lymphatic flow of drainage
Altered capillary permeability (K_f)

to the interstitial space without renal sodium and water retention may result in cessation of interstitial fluid formation, the presence of generalized edema therefore implies concomitant renal sodium and water retention. This is unquestionably the case in cardiac failure, liver disease, and the nephrotic syndrome. The disturbances in microcirculatory hemodynamics associated with edema and expansion of the ECF volume are described in Table 84-1.

CARDIAC FAILURE

Cardiac failure may be defined as the inability of the heart to deliver enough blood to peripheral tissues to meet metabolic demands. In the case of low-output cardiac failure, a decrease in cardiac output initiates a complex set of compensatory mechanisms in an attempt to maintain circulatory integrity. The adjustments that serve to stabilize cardiac performance and arterial perfusion in such patients include increases in plasma volume, atrial and ventricular filling pressures, peripheral vasoconstriction, and cardiac contractility and heart rate. The retention of sodium and water is a major renal compensation for a failing myocardium but it also accounts to a great extent for the familiar clinical syndrome of heart failure, which consists of pulmonary or peripheral edema, or both, and exercise intolerance. In fact, the ability to excrete a sodium load has been used as an index of the presence of heart failure (7), and a defect in water excretion is regularly encountered in such patients (8).

Classically, two theories have tried to explain how the kidney becomes involved in the renal sodium and water retention of heart failure. According to the "backward failure" hypothesis advanced by Hope (9) and Starling (4), central venous pressure and then peripheral venous pressure rise as the cardiac pump fails. With this increase in peripheral venous pressure, the hydraulic pressure in the capillaries exceeds opposing forces and causes the transudation of fluid from the intravascular compartment to the interstitial space, and thus the development of edema. This loss of intravascular fluid volume then signals the kidney to retain sodium and water in an attempt to restore the circulating volume to normal. The "forward failure" theory states that as the heart fails, there is inadequate perfusion of the kidney, resulting in decreased sodium and water excretion (10). As will become apparent from the following discussion, both an increase in central venous pressure or "backward failure" and a decrease in cardiac output or "forward failure" may contribute to the sodium and water retention of low-output cardiac failure via systemic and renal hemodynamic effects and through activation of various vasoconstrictor and antinatriuretic neuroendocrine systems. According to our recently described unifying hypothesis of body fluid volume regulation (11–17), neurohormonal activation plays a central role in the efferent limb of the sodium and water retention in cardiac failure, liver disease, and the nephrotic syndrome, whereas the afferent limb of this volume regulatory system is initiated by altered systemic hemodynamics. The following discussion addresses this unifying hypothesis of body fluid volume regulation and the afferent and efferent mechanisms for sodium and water retention in these edematous disorders.

Afferent Mechanisms for Renal Sodium and Water Retention in Heart Failure

The kidney alters the amount of dietary sodium excreted in response to signals from volume receptors and chemoreceptors in the circulation. These receptors may affect kidney function by altering renal sympathetic nerve activity and changing levels of circulating hormones with vasoactive and nonvasoactive (e.g., direct sodium-retaining) effects on the kidney. Important "effector" hormones include angiotensin II (ANG II), aldosterone, AVP, endothelin, nitric oxide, prostaglandins, and atrial and brain natriuretic peptides (ANP and BNP, respectively). Both high-and low-pressure baroreceptors as well as cardiac and hepatic chemoreceptors have been implicated in the activation of these neurohormonal systems.

High-Pressure Baroreceptors

In humans, evidence for the presence of volume-sensitive receptors in the arterial circulation originated from observations in patients with traumatic arterial-venous (AV) fistulae (18). Closure of AV fistulae is associated with a decreased rate of emptying of the arterial blood into the venous circulation, as demonstrated by closure-induced increases in diastolic arterial pressure and decreases in cardiac output. This results in an immediate increase in renal sodium and water excretion without changes in either glomerular filtration rate (GFR) or renal blood flow (18). This observation implicates the "fullness" of the arterial vascular tree as a "sensor" in modulating renal sodium and water excretion. In fact, the fullness of the arterial vascular compartment or the so-called effective arterial blood volume (EABV) (19) has been proposed as a major determinant of renal sodium and water handling, according to the unifying hypothesis of body fluid volume regulation (11–17).

The EABV is a measure of the adequacy of arterial blood volume to "fill" the capacity of the arterial circulation. Normal EABV exists when the ratio of cardiac output to peripheral vascular resistance maintains venous return and cardiac output at normal levels. Arterial or high-pressure volume receptors therefore may be stimulated when either cardiac output falls or peripheral vascular resistance diminishes to such

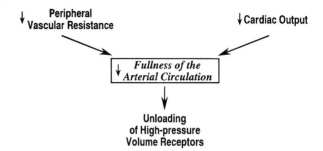

FIG. 84-1. Peripheral vascular resistance and cardiac output as the determinants of arterial filling or the "effective arterial blood volume." Here, either a decrease in vascular resistance or diminished cardiac output results in decreased fullness of the arterial circulation with unloading of high-pressure volume receptors and activation of various neurohormonal responses (see text).

an extent that the arterial circulation is no longer effectively "full" (Fig. 84-1). Thus, in the case of low-output cardiac failure, it is the diminution of cardiac output that is perceived by the arterial circulation as inadequate to maintain EABV. In high-output cardiac failure, decreased peripheral vascular resistance may serve as the signal for arterial underfilling (11–17). The concept of arterial underfilling in low- and high-output cardiac failure is discussed in the following.

Studies using one model of low-output cardiac failure—constriction of the vena cava in the dog—support the notion that a fall in cardiac output may be a primary stimulus for sodium and water retention by the kidney. Using this model, Schrier and associates (20–22) showed that constriction of the thoracic inferior vena cava (TIVC) is associated with a decrease in cardiac output, arterial pressure, and urinary sodium excretion even when renal perfusion pressure and renal venous pressure were held constant. Of note, renal denervation and adrenalectomy did not abolish this antinatriuresis. Furthermore, sodium retention did not correlate with changes in GFR or renal vascular resistance. Constriction of the superior vena cava to cause a decrease in cardiac output similar to that observed in the TIVC studies resulted in a similar fall in urinary sodium excretion despite the absence of concomitant hepatic, renal, and abdominal venous congestion. These findings support the hypothesis that the kidney decreases sodium excretion in response to a decrease in cardiac output and the associated arterial underfilling.

The preceding proposal was questioned by Migdal and colleagues (23), who compared the renal response in three different models of experimental heart failure. Specifically, they compared models of TIVC constriction, pulmonary artery occlusion (which is similar to caval constriction except that right-sided heart pressures are increased rather than decreased), and acute left ventricular infarction, another model of low-output heart failure but with increased left-sided heart pressures. This investigation demonstrated that with comparable decrements in cardiac output in all three models, only the TIVC constriction animals exhibited an antinatriuresis. The authors concluded that low cardiac output per se is not the afferent signal for sodium retention in low-output heart failure. These authors and others (24) suggested that in some way, decreased right-sided heart pressure mediates the antinatriuresis.

An alternative interpretation of the findings of Migdal and coworkers (23) is that a decrease in cardiac output is a stimulus for renal sodium and water retention, but an acute rise in atrial or ventricular end-diastolic pressures, in animals with acute pulmonary hypertension or acute left ventricular infarction, with the release of the natriuretic peptides ANP and BNP, initially obscures this effect. Support for this interpretation may be found in a report from Lee and colleagues (25), who examined sodium excretion in two models of low-output heart failure in the dog, acute heart failure produced by rapid ventricular pacing, and a TIVC constriction model. Similar to Migdal's animals, the dogs with TIVC constriction demonstrated diminished cardiac outputs and arterial pressures without an increase in atrial pressures or plasma ANP level but with avid renal sodium retention. Of note, plasma renin activity (PRA) and plasma aldosterone concentrations were substantially elevated in these TIVC constriction animals. In the case of pacing-induced heart failure, cardiac output and arterial pressure were similarly decreased, whereas atrial pressures and the plasma ANP concentration were significantly increased. In the animals with elevated rather than normal circulating ANP concentrations, urinary sodium excretion was maintained and PRA and plasma aldosterone concentration were not increased. Finally, dogs with TIVC constriction were given exogenous ANP to achieve circulating concentrations comparable to that seen in the pacing-induced heart failure animals. Exogenous administration of ANP to such levels prevented sodium retention, renal vasoconstriction, and activation of the renin–angiotensin–aldosterone system. These observations support the notion that decreased cardiac output is a stimulus for renal sodium retention in heart failure and suggest an important role for the natriuretic peptides in acutely attenuating this renal response. A further discussion of the role of ANP and BNP in heart failure is presented elsewhere in this chapter.

Other experimental evidence supports a role for diminished cardiac output as a determinant of the sodium and water retention of heart failure. Rats with small to moderate myocardial infarctions and decreased cardiac outputs exhibit decreased fractional sodium excretion despite normal right and left ventricular end-diastolic pressures (26). Using the model of TIVC constriction, Priebe and associates (27) demonstrated that the renal retention of sodium and water was reduced markedly when cardiac output was restored to normal by autologous blood transfusions. Moreover, reduction of pressure or stretch at the carotid sinus, like that produced by decreased cardiac output or arterial hypotension, activates the sympathetic nervous system and promotes renal sodium and water retention (28,29). Pharmacologic or surgical interruption of sympathetic afferent neural pathways emanating from high-pressure baroreceptor sites also inhibits the natriuretic response to volume expansion (21,22,30–34). High-pressure

baroreceptors also appear to be important factors in regulating the nonosmotic release of AVP, thus affecting renal water excretion (35,36). Finally, the juxtaglomerular apparatus, an arterial baroreceptor located in the afferent arterioles within the kidney, has been implicated in the modulation of renal renin release (28,37,38) and thus may stimulate increases in circulating ANG II and aldosterone, both of which promote sodium retention by the kidney.

Low cardiac output cannot be the only cause of sodium and water retention in heart failure, because diminished renal sodium and water excretion is also observed in states of high-output cardiac failure. In heart failure secondary to beriberi, anemia, thyrotoxicosis, or AV fistulae, cardiac output is increased as a consequence of a decrease in peripheral vascular resistance. This decrease in vascular resistance diminishes EABV (i.e., causes arterial underfilling) and serves as the stimulus for neurohormonal activation and renal sodium and water retention in these instances of high-output heart failure (11–17). As noted already in humans (18) and dogs (39), closure of an AV fistula causes increased sodium excretion, whereas opening of an AV fistula decreases urinary sodium excretion. These changes in renal sodium excretion correlate with changes in arterial pressure and peripheral vascular resistance rather than GFR or renal blood flow, supporting the importance of arterial circulatory "fullness" as a determinant of the renal response to heart failure.

These observations of decreased sodium and water excretion in both low- and high-output cardiac failure support the theory that arterial underfilling initiates reflex stimuli for the kidneys to retain sodium and water. In this regard, high-pressure baroreceptors in the carotid sinus, aortic arch, left ventricle, or the juxtaglomerular apparatus may comprise an important part of this reflex loop. Although these data support a role for arterial underfilling as the primary stimulus of the renal sodium and water retention of heart failure, low-pressure baroreceptors also may play an important role.

Low-Pressure Baroreceptors

In addition to the high-pressure arterial baroreceptors, the venous side of the circulation seems to be a logical place for receptors sensitive to changes in blood volume to be found. In fact, 85% of blood volume may be found in the venous circulation, whereas just 15% of circulatory volume resides in the arterial circulation (40). Although the smaller arterial blood volume may result in a higher sensitivity to detect blood volume changes, the larger amount of venous blood volume also may constitute an important component of the body fluid volume regulatory system.

The atria of the heart are highly distensible and densely populated with nerve endings sensitive to small changes in passive distention (41). Similar afferent low-pressure volume receptors may also be found in the pulmonary vasculature (42). Increased filling of the thoracic vascular and cardiac atria would be expected to signal the kidney to increase urinary sodium excretion in order to return the blood volume to normal. As expected, maneuvers that increase this thoracic or "central" blood volume such as weightlessness, negative pressure breathing, head-out water immersion, recumbency, and exposure to cold all produce a natriuresis (43–48). Similarly, measures that decrease intrathoracic blood volume, including positive pressure breathing, upright posture, and application of tourniquets to the lower extremities result in renal sodium retention (45,49,50). Thus, effective "central" blood volume, in addition to EABV, may serve as the afferent stimulus for regulation of renal sodium and water excretion.

Considerable evidence implicates the left atrium as an important site of low-pressure receptors (51–53). It is believed that changes in pressure or distention within the left atrium modulate electrical activity of the atrial receptors, which in turn may regulate renal sympathetic nerve activity. Left atrial nerves therefore can alter blood volume through changes in sodium excretion (53–55) as well as solute-free water excretion by influencing AVP release (56–58). Acutely increasing left atrial volume by inflation of a balloon within the left atrium results in increased urinary volume excretion (52), whereas hypotensive hemorrhage (59,60) and atrial tamponade (61) cause decreased atrial volume and diminish urine volume. However, in the setting of chronic heart failure, renal sodium and water retention occur despite left atrial distention and, frequently, loading of the other central baroreceptors (pulmonary veins, right atrium). Thus, in chronic heart failure, diminished cardiac output with arterial underfilling may exert the predominant effect via unloading of high-pressure arterial baroreceptors. Chronic studies in animals employing either experimental tricuspid insufficiency (62) or right atrial distention with an inflatable balloon (63) support this hypothesis. In these animal models, the increase in right atrial pressure was associated with avid renal sodium retention rather than the expected natriuresis. However, a concomitant fall in cardiac output could explain the sodium retention. Alternatively, alterations in cardiopulmonary baroreceptor function may occur in chronic but not acute heart failure.

Zucker and colleagues (64) demonstrated that the inhibition of renal sympathetic nerve activity seen during acute left atrial distention is lost during chronic heart failure in the dog. Moreover, a decrease in cardiac preload fails to produce the expected parasympathetic withdrawal and sympathetic activation in humans with heart failure (65–67). Nishian and colleagues (67) described paradoxical forearm vasodilation and hemodynamic improvement during acute unloading of cardiopulmonary baroreceptors in patients with severe chronic heart failure. This paradoxical response to lower body negative pressure was associated with static plasma norepinephrine levels (67), rather than the expected increase in plasma norepinephrine concentrations, further demonstrating this altered response to low-pressure baroreceptor unloading in heart failure. These observations confirm those made in heart failure patients during other forms of orthostatic stress (65,66). These findings are also consistent with the observation of a strong positive correlation between left atrial pressure and coronary sinus norepinephrine, a marker

of cardiac adrenergic activity, in patients with chronic heart failure (68). Taken together, these findings suggest that the normal inhibitory control of sympathetic activation accompanying increased atrial pressures is lost in heart failure patients and somehow may be converted to a stimulatory signal.

Cardiac and Pulmonary Chemoreceptors

In the heart and lungs, both vagal and sympathetic afferent nerve endings respond to a variety of exogenous and endogenous chemical substances, including capsaicin, phenyldiguanidine, bradykinin, substance P, and prostaglandins (PGs). Baker and associates (69) demonstrated stimulation of sympathetic afferent nerve endings by bradykinin in the heart of the cat. In conscious dogs, the administration of PGE_2 and arachidonate inhibited the cardiac baroreflex (70). Moreover, Zucker and associates (71) showed that PGI_2 attenuates the baroreflex control of renal nerve activity via an afferent vagal mechanism. Because substances such as bradykinin and PGs may circulate at increased concentrations in subjects with heart failure (72), it is possible that altered central nervous system input from chemically sensitive cardiac or pulmonary afferents contributes to the neurohormonal activation and sodium retention of chronic heart failure. This possibility may have important implications for the treatment of heart failure, because commonly prescribed medications such as angiotensin converting enzyme (ACE) inhibitors may alter circulating bradykinin and PG levels. At the present time, however, the exact roles of these hormones and cardiac and pulmonary chemoreceptors in heart failure are incompletely understood.

Hepatic Receptors

Theoretically, the liver should be in an ideal position to monitor dietary sodium intake and thus adjust urinary sodium excretion. Indeed, when compared with peripheral venous administration, infusion of saline solution into the portal circulation was reported to result in greater natriuresis (73,74). Similarly, the increment in urinary sodium excretion has been claimed to be greater when the sodium load is given orally than when given intravenously (75–77). In addition, the pathophysiologic retention of sodium in patients with severe liver disease is also consistent with an important role for the liver in the control of sodium excretion. However, some investigators (78,79) were unable to demonstrate a difference in sodium excretion between animals infused with 5% sodium chloride systemically and animals receiving the same solution via the portal vein. Moreover, Obika and colleagues (80) found similar sodium excretions after sodium loads given intravenously or by gastric lavage. Thus, the experimental evidence in favor of sodium or volume hepatic receptors remains controversial.

In summary, the afferent mechanisms for sodium and water retention in chronic heart failure may be preferentially localized on the arterial or high-pressure side of the circulation where EABV may serve as the primary determinant of the renal response. However, reflexes from the low-pressure cardiopulmonary receptor system also may be altered so as to influence renal sodium and water handling in heart failure. In this regard, increases in atrial and ventricular end-diastolic pressures also stimulate the release of the natriuretic peptides and inhibit AVP release, which may be important attenuating factors in renal sodium and water retention.

Efferent Mechanisms for Renal Sodium and Water Retention in Heart Failure

The Neurohormonal Response to Cardiac Failure

As mentioned, activation of various neurohormonal vasoconstrictor and antinatriuretic systems mediates to a large extent the renal sodium and water retention associated with the edematous disorders. Arterial underfilling secondary to a diminished cardiac output or peripheral vasodilation, perhaps in association with an alteration in low-pressure baroreceptor function, elicits these "compensatory" neuroendocrine responses in order to maintain the integrity of the arterial circulation by promoting peripheral vasoconstriction and expansion of the ECF volume through renal sodium and water retention (Fig. 84-2). The three major neurohormonal vasoconstrictor systems activated in response to arterial underfilling are the sympathetic nervous system, the renin–angiotensin–aldosterone system, and the nonosmotic release of AVP. Baroreceptor activation of the sympathetic nervous system appears to be the primary integrator of the hormonal vasoconstrictor systems involved in renal sodium and water retention. The nonosmotic release of AVP involves sympathetic stimulation of the supraoptic and paraventricular nuclei in the hypothalamus (81), whereas activation of the renin–angiotensin–aldosterone system involves renal ß-adrenergic stimulation (82). However, this latter system may provide positive feedback stimulation of the sympathetic nervous

system and nonosmotic AVP release. Various counterregulatory, vasodilatory, and natriuretic hormones, including the natriuretic peptides and prostaglandins, are also activated in heart failure and the other edematous disorders, and may attenuate the renal effects of vasoconstrictor hormone activation. The effects of these neurohormonal systems, as well as the effects of alterations in systemic hemodynamics, on renal hemodynamics and tubular sodium and water reabsorption in heart failure are discussed in the following.

Glomerular Filtration Rate

The GFR is usually normal in mild heart failure and is reduced only as cardiac performance becomes more severely impaired. Until 1961, it was generally accepted that the rate of glomerular filtration was a major determinant of renal sodium excretion. In 1961, de Wardener and colleagues (83) published their classic paper indicating that acute expansion of ECF volume by saline loading was accompanied by a brisk natriuresis even when GFR was reduced. Moreover, in sodium-retaining heart failure patients, GFR is often normal and may even be elevated in states of high-output cardiac failure. These observations argue against an important role for diminished GFR in the sodium retention of heart failure. However, it should be emphasized that the contribution of GFR to sodium balance is difficult to evaluate because very minute changes in GFR are difficult to measure and may account for important changes in sodium excretion. For example, under normal conditions, with a GFR of 100 mL/minute, the filtered load of sodium amounts to approximately 20,000 mEq/day. This amount of filtered sodium is enormous compared to the normal urinary sodium excretion of approximately 200 mEq/day. In view of this considerable difference, it is apparent that very small changes in GFR can result in major alterations in sodium excretion if tubular reabsorption remains unaltered. In any event, although GFR

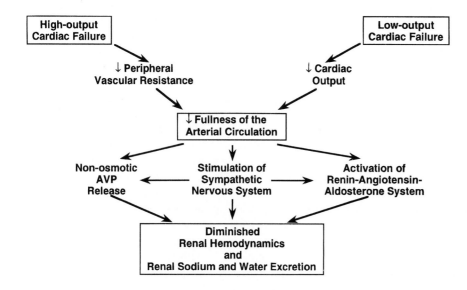

FIG. 84-2. Mechanism explaining the defect in renal sodium and water excretion in both high- and low-output heart failure. *AVP,* arginine vasopressin.

may be diminished in patients with advanced heart failure, a reduction in GFR alone is probably not an important cause of fluid retention in these patients because sodium retention can be observed in heart failure patients who have GFRs comparable to normal subjects who are capable of maintaining sodium balance.

Renal Blood Flow

Heart failure is commonly associated with an increase in renal vascular resistance and a decrease in renal blood flow (84). In general, renal blood flow decreases in proportion to the decrease in cardiac output. Some investigators also showed a redistribution of renal blood flow from the outer cortical nephron to juxtaglomerular nephrons during experimental heart failure (85,86). It was proposed that deeper nephrons with longer loops of Henle reabsorb sodium more avidly. Thus, the redistribution of blood flow to these nephrons in patients with heart failure might account for or substantially contribute to the renal sodium retention observed. However, other investigators were not able to demonstrate such a redistribution of blood flow in other models of cardiac failure (87,88). At the present time, the role of redistribution of renal blood flow in the sodium retention of cardiac failure therefore remains uncertain.

The increased renal vascular resistance in heart failure could be owing to enhanced renal sympathetic activity or increased circulating concentrations of ANG II, norepinephrine, vasopressin, or other vasoconstricting substances. Alternatively or in addition, decreased synthesis of or the development of tachyphylaxis to known vasodilating substances such as the natriuretic peptides and PGE_2 and PGI_2 may contribute to the increased renal vascular resistance. Studies performed in rats demonstrated the ability of the adrenergic neurotransmitter norepinephrine and ANG II to promote efferent arteriolar constriction (89,90). In a rat model of low-output heart failure caused by myocardial infarction, the marked elevation in efferent arteriolar resistance was abolished after infusion of an ACE inhibitor (90), thus implicating the renal vasoconstrictor properties of ANG II in heart failure. Clinical results from our laboratory also favor ANG II as a major renal vasoconstrictive substance in patients with heart failure (91). In patients with advanced heart failure, GFR was improved after 1 month of treatment with the ACE inhibitor captopril. However, similar patients receiving another vasodilating agent, prazosin, with identical improvement in cardiac output and left ventricular end-diastolic pressure but without any effect on the renin–angiotensin system had no improvement in GFR (91). Moreover, a published review of the literature on renal function alterations induced by ACE inhibition during heart failure concluded that the net effect of ACE inhibitors in patients with heart failure is to augment renal blood flow to a greater extent than cardiac output (92). This observation also supports an important role for ANG II in the renal hemodynamic alterations of heart failure. However, the renal response to ACE inhibition in patients with heart failure is variable;

as a result it is acknowledged that volume status and the degree of neurohormonal activation may influence this response (see the following).

In heart failure, the interaction between norepinephrine or ANG II and prostaglandins may also provide a means of preserving near-constancy of renal blood flow in response to arterial underfilling. Although inhibition of prostaglandin synthesis does not generally impair GFR in normovolemic animals (93,94) or humans (95), in states of high plasma concentrations of endogenous ANG II induced by volume depletion, blockade of prostaglandin synthesis may be associated with substantial declines in renal blood flow and GFR (93,94). Recent clinical results have underlined the importance of prostaglandins in the maintenance of renal function in patients with heart failure (72,96). In patients with heart failure, prostaglandin activity is increased and correlates with the severity of disease as assessed by the degree of hyponatremia (72). In these 15 patients, plasma levels of the metabolites of vasodilator PGI_2 and PGE_2 were found to be elevated three to 10 times above those seen in normal subjects. Of note, plasma levels of both metabolites also correlated positively with PRA and plasma ANG II concentrations. Administration of the prostaglandin synthesis inhibitor indomethacin in three of the hyponatremic heart failure patients resulted in a marked increase in peripheral vascular resistance and a fall in cardiac output. Riegger and associates (96) recently evaluated the renal effects of another prostaglandin synthesis inhibitor, acetylsalicylic acid, in patients with moderate heart failure consuming a normal sodium diet. In these patients, acetylsalicylic acid in doses that decreased the synthesis of renal PGE_2 resulted in a significant reduction in urinary sodium excretion. Moreover, the administration of a cyclooxygenase inhibitor in heart failure patients occasionally may result in acute reversible renal failure, an effect proposed to be owing in part to the inhibition of vasodilating renal prostaglandins and the resultant renal vasoconstriction (97). It should be noted, however, that the extent to which the effects on renal function and sodium and water handling result from renal hemodynamic or the tubular actions of the prostaglandins remains unclear.

As mentioned, norepinephrine may also contribute to the increased renal afferent arteriolar resistance in heart failure patients. In this regard, Oliver and associates (98) demonstrated that the venous to arterial norepinephrine concentration gradient across the kidney, a crude measure of renal nerve traffic, is increased in response to acute reduction of cardiac output. Moreover, Hasking and associates (99) showed that during a steady-state tritiated norepinephrine infusion, the spillover of norepinephrine to plasma from the kidney is significantly elevated in patients with heart failure. In these patients, the increased renal norepinephrine spillover substantially contributed to the increase in whole-body norepinephrine spillover. These findings demonstrate that renal adrenergic activity is increased in patients with heart failure, and thus contribute to the renal vasoconstriction. In support of this latter hypothesis, the administration of α-adrenergic receptor antagonists increased renal blood flow in edematous patients with heart failure (100).

Filtration Fraction, Proximal Tubular Sodium and Water Reabsorption, and Factors Acting Beyond the Proximal Tubule

Because renal blood flow falls as cardiac output decreases and GFR is usually preserved, filtration fraction often is increased in early heart failure. An increase in filtration fraction results in increased protein concentration and oncotic pressure in the efferent arterioles and peritubular capillaries that surround the proximal tubule (90). Such an increase in peritubular oncotic pressure has been proposed to increase sodium and water reabsorption in the proximal tubule (101–105). Direct evidence for increased single-nephron filtration fraction was provided by micropuncture studies in rats with myocardial infarction induced by coronary ligation (90). In rats with large myocardial infarctions involving approximately 40% of the left ventricular circumference, the single-nephron filtration fraction was markedly elevated (0.38 ± 0.02 versus 0.25 ± 0.02, $P < 0.005$) when compared with that in sham-operated control rats. The measurement of preglomerular, glomerular, and postglomerular pressures and flows revealed that these reductions in glomerular plasma flow rate and elevations in filtration fraction were associated with a profound constriction of the efferent arterioles. The effect of the latter was to sustain glomerular capillary hydraulic pressure, thereby preventing a marked fall in GFR. Significantly, fractional proximal fluid reabsorption was elevated in this model. Of interest, in these animals with myocardial infarction, the intravenous infusion of the ACE inhibitor teprotide led to the return of glomerular plasma flow rate, single-nephron filtration fraction, single-nephron GFR, efferent arteriolar resistance, and fractional proximal fluid reabsorption to, or toward, the levels found in the control rats (90). Consistent with these experiments, micropuncture studies performed in other models of heart failure such as acute TIVC constriction (106) and acute cardiac tamponade (107) in dogs showed that the proximal tubule was at least one major nephron site responsible for renal sodium retention or a blunted response to saline infusion.

Despite the convincing nature of many studies, not all investigators have been able to detect an effect of peritubular oncotic pressure on proximal tubular sodium and water reabsorption. Rumrich and Ullrich (108), Lowitz and associates (109), Bank and coworkers (110), and Holzgreve and Schrier (111) were unable to find changes in proximal reabsorption in spite of marked changes in peritubular oncotic pressures. Moreover, Conger and associates (112) directly perfused peritubular capillaries with either a protein-free or -rich solution and found that neither perfusate influences the rate of proximal reabsorption. Trying to reconcile these observations, Ott and associates (113) found that proximal reabsorption was different after changes in peritubular oncotic pressure in volume-expanded dogs compared with hydropenic animals. These authors suggested that expansion of ECF volume resulted in an increased passive backleak that could be reversed by raising the peritubular oncotic pressure. During hydropenia, however, when passive backleak was relatively less, raising the peritubular capillary oncotic pressure did not influence proximal reabsorption.

The effects of increased filtration fraction might be expected to be exerted primarily on proximal tubular sodium reabsorption. Nevertheless, although clearance and micropuncture studies in animals with heart failure have demonstrated increased sodium reabsorption in the proximal tubule, distal sodium reabsorption also seems to be involved. In this regard, clearance and micropuncture studies performed in dogs with AV fistulae (114), chronic pericarditis (107), and chronic partial thoracic vena caval obstruction (115) documented enhanced distal nephron sodium reabsorption. Levy (115) also showed that the inability of dogs with chronic vena caval obstruction to excrete a sodium load is a consequence of enhanced reabsorption of sodium at the loop of Henle. This nephron segment was similarly implicated in rats with AV fistulae (88). Physical factors also could be involved in the augmented reabsorption of sodium chloride by the loop of Henle in dogs with constriction of the vena cava (115).

Intrarenal mechanisms, specifically decreased delivery of tubular fluid to the distal diluting segment of the nephron, may also contribute to the impaired water excretion observed in heart failure. Evidence supporting this intrarenal mechanism of water retention in heart failure has been provided by studies involving the administration of mannitol (116) or the loop diuretic furosemide (117) to patients with heart failure and hyponatremia. Administration of either of these agents converted the cardiac patient's hypertonic urine to a dilute urine (116,117). Both mannitol and furosemide may diminish the tubular reabsorption of sodium and water in the more proximal portions of the nephron, thus increasing fluid delivery to the more distal nephron sites of urinary dilution. Other factors may, however, be implicated to explain these results: (a) the infusion of mannitol may produce volume expansion, thus suppressing the baroreceptor-mediated release of AVP, and (b) the furosemide-induced hypotonic urine was found not to be responsive to the administration of exogenous AVP, thus suggesting antagonism of AVP by furosemide (117). In support of this latter hypothesis, Szatalowicz and colleagues (118) provided further evidence that furosemide interferes with the renal action of AVP in humans.

In summary, the exact contribution of proximal versus distal nephron sites in the augmented sodium and water reabsorption seen in heart failure may depend on the severity of the heart failure and the concomitant degree of arterial underfilling. The fact that changes in filtration fraction have been observed in patients with heart failure before changes in sodium balance occur may question the dominance of peritubular factors and proximal reabsorption in the sodium retention characteristic of heart failure (119). This observation suggests that other factors, such as the direct tubular effects of neurohormonal activation, may play a significant role in the renal sodium and water retention of heart failure. The renal effects of these various neurohormonal systems are discussed in detail in the following, starting with activation of the vasoconstrictor mechanisms.

Vasoconstrictor Systems

Activation of the Sympathetic Nervous System in Heart Failure

The sympathetic nervous system is activated early in patients with heart failure. Numerous studies have documented elevated peripheral venous plasma norepinephrine concentrations in heart failure patients (99,120–123). In advanced heart failure, using tritiated norepinephrine to determine norepinephrine kinetics, Hasking and colleagues (99) and Davis and coworkers (122) demonstrated that both increased norepinephrine spillover and decreased norepinephrine clearance contribute to the elevated venous plasma norepinephrine levels seen in these patients, suggesting that increased sympathetic nerve activity is at least partially responsible for the high circulating norepinephrine levels. Our laboratory (123) has demonstrated that in earlier stages of heart failure, the rise in plasma norepinephrine in patients with heart failure was owing solely to increased norepinephrine secretion (Fig. 84-3), supporting the notion that sympathetic nervous system activity is increased early in the course of heart failure. Significantly, in our heart failure patients with mild to moderate symptoms, plasma epinephrine, a marker of adrenal activation, was not substantially elevated, confirming the neuronal source of the increased norepinephrine.

The Studies of Left Ventricular Dysfunction (SOLVD) investigators (124) reported the presence of adrenergic activation in patients with asymptomatic left ventricular dysfunction. In this substudy of the SOLVD trials, neurohormonal activation was assessed in 56 control subjects, 151 patients with left ventricular dysfunction (ejection fractions ≤35%) but no overt heart failure, and 81 patients with overt heart failure, prior to randomization to receive placebo versus an ACE inhibitor. The plasma norepinephrine concentration was significantly increased by 35% in subjects with asymptomatic left ventricular dysfunction compared to healthy control subjects, and by 65% above control values in the overt heart failure patients. These data also demonstrate that adrenergic activation occurs early in the course of heart failure or left ventricular dysfunction and are consistent with the observation that plasma norepinephrine concentrations or the degree of adrenergic activation are directly correlated with the degree of left ventricular dysfunction in heart failure patients (120,121,125,126). Finally, studies employing peroneal nerve microneurography to directly assess sympathetic nerve activity to muscle (MSNA) confirmed increased adrenergic nerve traffic in patients with heart failure (127).

As mentioned, studies in human heart failure demonstrated the presence of renal adrenergic activation (99). In this study of whole-body and organ-specific norepinephrine kinetics in heart failure patients, cardiac and renal norepinephrine spillovers were increased 504% and 206%, respectively, whereas norepinephrine spillover from the lungs was normal. These findings demonstrate the presence of selective cardiorenal adrenergic activation in heart failure. A discussion of the cardiac effects of this adrenergic activation is beyond the scope of this chapter. However, numerous adverse effects of increased cardiac adrenergic activity have been documented in humans (128), and recent positive experience with the use of ß-adrenergic receptor antagonists in heart failure patients (128–130) supports the hypothesis that norepinephrine is harmful to the myocardium. In this regard, it should be noted that a single resting venous plasma norepinephrine level provides a better guide to prognosis than do other commonly measured indices of cardiac performance, where high plasma norepinephrine levels are associated with a poor prognosis in patients with heart failure (131).

Renal Tubular Effects of Adrenergic Activation in Heart Failure

Renal nerves exert a direct influence on sodium reabsorption in the proximal tubule. Bello-Reuss and colleagues (54) demonstrated this direct effect of renal nerve activation to enhance proximal tubular sodium reabsorption in whole-kidney and nephron studies in the rat. In these animals, renal nerve stimulation produced an increase in the tubular fluid:plasma inulin concentration ratio in the late proximal tubule, a result of increased fractional sodium and water reabsorption in this segment of the nephron. Based on results of an elegant series of studies, DiBona and colleagues (132) implicated activation of the renal nerves in the sodium and water retention observed in the various edematous disorders. Experiments were conducted in conscious, chronically instrumented rats with either heart failure (myocardial infarction), cirrhosis (common bile duct ligation), or the nephrotic syndrome

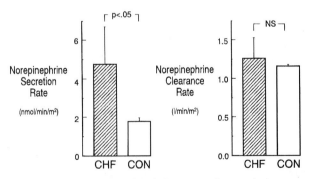

FIG. 84-3. Plasma norepinephrine secretion and clearance rates in patients with mild to moderate heart failure (CHF) and in normal control subjects (CON). The findings of increased norepinephrine secretion and normal norepinephrine clearance in the CHF patients are consistent with early activation of the sympathetic nervous system in cardiac failure. *NS,* not significant. (From: Abraham WT, Hensen J, Schrier RW. Elevated plasma noradrenaline concentrations in patients with low-output cardiac failure: dependence on increased noradrenaline secretion rates. *Clin Sci* 1990;79:429, with permission.)

(doxorubicin injection). In each experimental model, renal sodium or water excretion of an acutely administered oral or intravenous isotonic saline load was significantly less than that in control rats. Bilateral renal denervation in the experimental rats restored their renal excretory response to normal. Moreover, in response to the acute administration of a standard intravenous isotonic saline load, the decrease in efferent renal adrenergic nerve activity was significantly less in all three experimental models than control animals. These results support an increased basal efferent renal sympathetic nerve activity in heart failure and the other edematous disorders that fails to suppress normally in response to the isotonic saline load. These findings also are consistent with the aforementioned alterations in low-pressure baroreceptor function observed in human heart failure, where adrenergic activation is seen despite chronic increased loading of these cardiopulmonary receptors.

In dogs (133) and humans (100) with heart failure, α-adrenergic receptor blockade induces a natriuresis. Moreover, adrenergic blockade with either phenoxybenzamine or hexamethonium abolishes the sodium retention seen in acute TIVC constriction (21). On the other hand, sodium retention persists in dogs with denervated transplanted kidneys and chronic vena caval constriction (134). In addition, in dogs with pacing-induced heart failure, no differences in renal hemodynamic or electrolyte excretion between innervated or denervated kidneys in compensated or decompensated animals were observed (135). These latter observations implicate factors in addition to renal nerves in the sodium retention of heart failure. However, in these renal denervation experiments and in human heart failure, other hormonal factors (e.g., ANG II, aldosterone, and AVP) may play an important role in the sodium and water retention.

Experience with the partial β_1-adrenergic receptor agonist xamoterol in heart failure suggests a role for the renal β-receptor in modulating proximal tubular sodium reabsorption (136). Botker and colleagues (136) examined the acute renal effects of xamoterol in 12 patients with mild to moderate heart failure. Each patient was given xamoterol (0.2 mg/kg) or placebo in random order separated by 2 weeks of a clinically stable drug washout period. Renal clearance and excretion measurements were made with the patient in the supine position at 30- to 60-minute intervals before, during, and up to 6 hours after infusion. Lithium clearance was used as a measure of proximal tubular sodium handling (137). Blood pressure, heart rate, renal plasma flow, GFR, and urinary flow rate remained unchanged, whereas xamoterol significantly decreased renal sodium excretion by 30%. This acute decrease in sodium excretion with xamoterol was associated with an increase in proximal tubular sodium reabsorption, as indicated by decreased lithium clearance. Of note, plasma concentrations of ANG II and aldosterone were unaffected by xamoterol. These observations suggest a direct effect of acute xamoterol to enhance proximal tubular sodium reabsorption in heart failure. In patients with heart failure, the endogenous adrenergic receptor agonist and neurotransmitter

norepinephrine may exert a similar effect on the proximal renal tubule.

Finally, as noted, renal nerves have been implicated as a stimulus for renin release from the kidney (82). Thus, with heart failure, adrenergic activation may lead to activation of the renin–angiotensin–aldosterone system. Conversely, ß-adrenergic receptor blockade may decrease renin release and improve the neurohormonal milieu in heart failure patients. In this regard, Eichhorn and coworkers (138) showed that the third-generation ß-adrenergic receptor blocker bucindolol lowers PRA in patients with mild to moderate heart failure. The renal tubular effects of ANG II and aldosterone are discussed in the following.

Activation of the Renin–Angiotensin–Aldosterone System in Heart Failure

The renin–angiotensin–aldosterone system is usually activated in patients with heart failure, as assessed by PRA and plasma aldosterone (125,139,140). In the substudy report from the SOLVD investigators (124), PRA was increased not only in the patients with established heart failure but also in the subjects with asymptomatic left ventricular dysfunction. Of note, activation of the renin–angiotensin–aldosterone system is associated with hyponatremia and an unfavorable prognosis in patients with heart failure (72,141). Dzau and colleagues (72) first described the association of PRA and hyponatremia in a group of 15 heart failure patients. These data showed that normal or suppressed PRA is associated with a normal serum sodium level, whereas the highest PRA is associated with the lowest serum sodium concentrations. Lee and Packer (141) subsequently confirmed this association between PRA and hyponatremia in a larger cohort of heart failure patients. Moreover, these investigators demonstrated the association of this hyponatremic, hyperreninemic state with poor survival. Finally, the proven beneficial effects of ACE inhibition on symptoms, hemodynamics, exercise capacity, and survival in heart failure patients further underscore the deleterious effects of ANG II and aldosterone in these patients (142,143).

Recently, a positive feedback between the renin–angiotensin–aldosterone system and sympathetic activation was proposed (144). This interaction is based in part on the ability of ANG II to augment neuronal norepinephrine release at the presynaptic level (145). In humans, presynaptic facilitation of norepinephrine release by ANG II may play a role in the cardiorenal adrenergic activation of heart failure. Clemson and associates (146) demonstrated ANG II-mediated increases in norepinephrine spillover in the human forearm. In heart failure patients, we demonstrated increased neuronal norepinephrine release from the heart during ANG II infusion, whereas cardiac adrenergic activity was decreased by the bolus injection of the ACE inhibitor enalaprilat (147). In addition, Gilbert and associates (148) showed that chronic ACE inhibition with lisinopril lowers cardiac adrenergic activity in patients with chronic symptomatic heart failure. Thus, activation of renal nerves is a stimulus for renal renin release, thus activating the renin–angiotensin–aldosterone system, whereas activation of the renin–angiotensin–aldosterone system may further stimulate adrenergic activity at the presynaptic level.

Renal Tubular Effects of Angiotensin II and Aldosterone in Heart Failure

In animal models, ANG II has a direct effect on enhancing proximal tubular sodium reabsorption (149). In these studies of the rat proximal tubule, the administration of ANG II resulted in a marked increase in the rate of sodium chloride reabsorption, whereas the infusion of the ANG II receptor antagonist saralasin significantly reduced proximal tubular sodium chloride reabsorption. Moreover, in a study from Abassi and colleagues (150), administration of the ANG II receptor antagonist losartan to decompensated sodium-retaining rats with heart failure secondary to AV fistulae produced a marked natriuresis. Although proximal tubular sodium handling was not examined in this study, the observation that losartan restored renal responsiveness to ANP is consistent with a losartan-induced increase in the delivery of sodium to the distal tubular site of ANP action. The role of distal tubular sodium delivery in the renal sodium retention of heart failure is discussed in the following.

In humans with heart failure, the finding that urinary sodium excretion correlates inversely with PRA and urinary aldosterone excretion also supports a role for ANG II or aldosterone, or both, in the renal sodium retention (151). However, the administration of ACE inhibitors to patients with heart failure results in inconsistent effects on renal sodium excretion, despite a consistent fall in plasma aldosterone concentration (152). A simultaneous fall in blood pressure or decline in renal hemodynamics owing to decreased circulating ANG II concentrations, however, could obscure the beneficial renal effects of lowered ANG II and aldosterone concentrations. Support for this hypothesis may be found in a report from Motwani and coworkers (153). These investigators examined the hemodynamic and hormonal correlates of the initial effect of ACE inhibition with captopril on blood pressure, GFR, and natriuresis in 36 patients with moderate heart failure. In these subjects, a captopril-induced fall in GFR was predicted by a decrease in renal plasma flow, low pretreatment GFR, *and* low absolute posttreatment serum ANG II concentration. A decrease in urinary sodium excretion was related to this fall in GFR. On the other hand, Good and coworkers (154) showed in eight patients with chronic heart failure that long-term ANG II suppression with captopril enhances renal responsiveness to the loop diuretic furosemide. This observation also supports a role for ANG II in the renal sodium retention of heart failure.

The role of aldosterone in the renal sodium retention of heart failure has been debated for many years. In the presence of a high sodium intake, dogs with caval constriction retain sodium even after surgical removal of the adrenal source of aldosterone (155). Moreover, patients with heart failure do not always show increased urinary sodium excretion after the administration of the aldosterone antagonist spironolactone (156). In addition, Chonko and coworkers (157) showed that patients with heart failure may have edema without increased aldosterone secretion. However, a normal plasma aldosterone level in heart failure patients may be relatively high in the presence of excess total body sodium. A role for aldosterone in the renal sodium retention of human heart failure was demonstrated by our group (158). We examined the effect of spironolactone on urinary sodium excretion in patients with mild to moderate heart failure who were withdrawn from all medications prior to study. Sodium was retained in all subjects throughout the period prior to aldosterone antagonism (Fig. 84-4). With an average sodium intake of 97 ± 8 mmol/day, the average sodium excretion before spironolactone treatment was 76 ± 8 mmol/day. During therapy with spironolactone, all heart failure patients demonstrated a significant increase in urinary sodium excretion to 131 ± 13 mmol/day. Moreover, the urine sodium:potassium concentration ratio significantly increased during spironolactone administration, consistent with a decrease in aldosterone action in the distal nephron. Of note, norepinephrine concentration and PRA increased and ANP decreased during spironolactone administration, suggesting a possible explanation for the attenuation of the natriuretic effect of spironolactone in long-term studies. Thus, the combined use of spironolactone with other neurohormonal antagonists (e.g., ACE inhibitors)

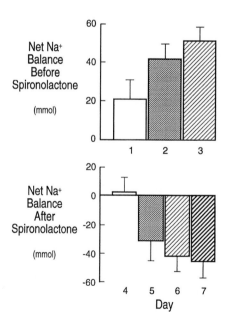

FIG. 84-4. Reversal of sodium retention with aldosterone antagonism in patients with heart failure. Net positive cumulative sodium balance, by day, for the period before spironolactone therapy *(upper panel)* and net negative cumulative sodium balance after the initiation of spironolactone, 400 mg/day *(lower panel)* are shown. (From: Hensen J, et al. Aldosterone in congestive heart failure: analysis of determinants and role in sodium retention. *Am J Nephrol* 1991;11:441, with permission of S. Karger AG, Basel.)

may result in optimal long-term benefit and is now under active investigation (159–161). In this regard, Pitt, on behalf of the Randomized Aldactone Evaluation Study (RALES) investigators (161), recently reported that in patients with heart failure, the addition of spironolactone (25 mg/day) to ACE inhibition decreased both hospitalizations and mortality by over 30% as compared to controls. Blocking the aldosterone-mediated cardiac fibrosis was proposed to explain this effect of spironolactone.

Nonosmotic Release of Vasopressin in Heart Failure

Plasma AVP is usually elevated in patients with advanced heart failure and correlates with the clinical and hemodynamic severity of disease and the serum sodium concentration (162–167). Several clinical and experimental observations indicate that nonosmotic mechanisms are responsible for increased AVP release in heart failure. A study from our laboratory (167) found plasma AVP concentrations to be inappropriately elevated in 30 of 37 hyponatremic patients with heart failure. The 30 patients with detectable plasma AVP levels had higher levels of blood urea nitrogen (BUN) and serum creatinine and higher ratios of BUN to serum creatinine than did the seven patients with undetectable plasma AVP levels. This latter finding could be dissociated from diuretic use because it was also observed in 14 patients who had never received diuretics. The presence of prerenal azotemia in these patients is consistent with diminished cardiac output as a mediator of the nonosmotic AVP release. Alternatively, this observation of prerenal azotemia in association with hyponatremia also supports an intrarenal component of the impaired water excretion.

Osmotically inappropriate elevations of plasma AVP in human heart failure were also reported by Riegger and coworkers (165), Rondeau and associates (166), and Goldsmith and associates (162). The study by Riegger and coworkers (165) demonstrated a decrease in the elevated plasma AVP levels after improvement in cardiac function by hemofiltration, whereas no change in plasma AVP was observed after decreasing left atrial pressure with prazosin. Moreover, the elevated plasma AVP levels seen in patients with heart failure often (164,168) but not always (8) failed to suppress normally in response to acute water loading. Taken together, these observations demonstrate that there is enhanced nonosmotic release of AVP in heart failure and support the hypothesis that diminished cardiac output, rather than alterations in atrial pressures, is responsible. As previously mentioned, baroreceptor activation of the sympathetic nervous system in response to arterial underfilling likely mediates this nonosmotic AVP release (81).

To shed further light on the mechanism of nonosmotic stimulation of AVP in heart failure patients and, more specifically, to determine the precise relationship between AVP release, cardiac hemodynamics, and the renin–angiotensin system, we studied 25 consecutive patients with severe heart failure (cardiac index 2.1 ± 0.1 L/minute per m^2 and

pulmonary capillary wedge pressure 27.5 ± 1.5 mm Hg) (91). These patients received two water loads of 15 mL/kg of body weight, the first load without drugs on day 1 and the second on day 3 after receiving vasodilator therapy with either captopril or prazosin for 2 days. Baseline and hourly hemodynamic, renal, and hormonal measurements were obtained for 5 hours following the water load. Basal plasma AVP was detectable (mean 3.0 ± 0.4 pg/mL) in 17 of the 25 patients (group 1) despite a diminished plasma sodium concentration (P_{Na}, 133.5 mmol/L) and low effective plasma osmolality (E_{osm}, 262 ± 3 mOsm/kg H_2O). The remaining eight patients (group 2) had appropriately suppressed plasma AVP (<0.5 pg/mL, undetectable) for their P_{Na} (136.5 ± 0.9 mol/L) and E_{osm} (268 ± 2 mOsm/kg H_2O). Cardiac index (1.9 versus 2.6 L/minute per m^2, $P < 0.005$) and the percentage of water load excreted (31.4% versus 57.1%, $P < 0.005$) were lower in group 1 than in group 2 patients, but GFR was similar (55 versus 54 mL/minute per 1.73 m^2). PRA and plasma aldosterone concentrations were higher in group 1 patients, suggesting arterial underfilling. In group 1 patients, vasodilators increased the cardiac index from 1.9 to 2.1 L/minute per m^2 and the percentage of water load excreted from 31% to 53% (both $P < 0.001$). In these same patients, plasma AVP decreased from 3.0 to 1.8 pg/mL ($P < 0.01$), platelet-associated AVP decreased from 8.6 to 5.1 pg/mL ($P < 0.005$), and minimal urinary osmolality decreased from 375 to 208 mOsm/kg H_2O ($P < 0.001$). There was no change in GFR. In group 1 patients in the control condition as well as after vasodilator therapy, plasma AVP decreased with plasma osmolality during the water load, suggesting some preservation of the osmoregulation of AVP, but with a lower osmotic threshold in these patients. Moreover, changes in the renin–angiotensin–aldosterone system were unrelated to changes in water excretion after vasodilator therapy. We consequently concluded that plasma and platelet AVP levels were the major determinants of the abnormal water excretion in many patients with heart failure. These results, therefore, favor a role of impaired cardiac function to cause arterial underfilling with resultant nonosmotic AVP release as a mediator of "resetting" the osmotic threshold for AVP in patients with heart failure. Improved cardiac function secondary to afterload reduction diminishes this resetting of the osmotic threshold. Of interest, our results are reminiscent of earlier studies that suggested that an occasional hyponatremic cardiac patient responds to a large water load by the prompt onset of a water diuresis (8). Also, more recently, AVP secretion was found to respond in exaggerated fashion to osmotic loading in patients with heart failure undergoing radiologic procedures with radiocontrast hyperosmolar agents (169). This latter finding also suggests a form of reset osmostat.

Renal Effects of Vasopressin in Heart Failure

Vasopressin, via stimulation of its renal V_2 receptor (170), induces insertion of the aquaporin-2 (AQP2) water channel into the collecting duct apical membrane with resultant water reabsorption. Elevations in plasma vasopressin concentration and AQP2 are believed to contribute to water retention in heart failure. In animal models of heart failure, the absence of a pituitary source of AVP is associated with normal or near-normal water excretion (171,172). For example, in intact dogs with diminished cardiac outputs owing to TIVC constriction, removal of the pituitary with glucocorticoid replacement results in normalization of the impaired water excretion (171). In these animals, acute constriction of the TIVC caused a significant fall in cardiac output associated with a marked increase in urinary osmolality and a decrease in solute-free water clearance. The effects of TIVC constriction were dissociated from renal hemodynamic changes and the presence or absence of renal sympathetic innervation. However, in hypophysectomized, steroid-replaced animals, both urinary osmolality and solute-free water clearance were maintained at basal levels during constriction of the TIVC. Impaired water excretion also occurs in rats with heart failure because of AV fistulae (172). Significantly, the impairment in water excretion seen in this high-output model of heart failure was not demonstrable in Brattleboro rats with central diabetes insipidus (i.e., AVP deficiency), supporting a role for persistent AVP release in the abnormality in water excretion associated with high-output cardiac failure. Similar results were obtained by Riegger and coworkers (173).

Further evidence implicating a role for AVP in the water retention of heart failure comes from studies using selective peptide and nonpeptide V_2 receptor AVP antagonists in several animal models of heart failure (174–177). Ishikawa and coworkers (174) assessed the antidiuretic effect of AVP in a low-output model of acute heart failure secondary to TIVC constriction in the rat. In these animals, plasma AVP concentrations were increased and a peptide antagonist of the V_2 receptor of AVP reversed the defect in solute-free water excretion. Yared and coworkers (175) showed a similar reversal of water retention using another peptide antagonist to the antidiuretic effect of AVP in rats with cardiac failure owing to coronary artery ligation. An orally active nonpeptide V_2 receptor AVP antagonist, OPC-31260, was described (178). Intravenous administration of OPC-31260 during a dose-ranging study in normal human subjects increased urine output to a similar extent as 20 mg of furosemide given intravenously (179). In these healthy volunteers, urine osmolality was significantly lower after administration of the V_2 receptor antagonist, thus indicating an increase in solute-free water clearance. Moreover, this agent reversed the impairment in renal water excretion in rats with experimental heart failure owing to myocardial infarction (176) and in dogs with pacing-induced heart failure (177), further supporting a role for AVP in the renal water retention of heart failure. This effect of the nonosmotic release of AVP to cause water retention in cardiac failure was associated with increased transcription of messenger RNA (mRNA) for the AVP preprohormone in the rat hypothalamus (180).

The effects of V_2 receptor antagonists on water metabolism in heart failure have now been studied at the molecular level.

Kidney AQP2 expression is increased in experimental heart failure. Rats with cardiac failure due to coronary ligation demonstrate an increase in renal AQP2 expression (181,182) that was reversed with nonpeptide V_2 receptor antagonism (182). V_2 receptor antagonism also reversed water retention in heart failure rats. Recent studies have been undertaken in hyponatremic heart failure patients treated with the V_2 receptor antagonist, VPA-985 (183). VPA-985 treatment resulted in a dose-related increase in water excretion, correction of hyponatremia, and a decrease in urinary AQP2 excretion. It is known that 3% to 6% of AQP2 water channels that traffic to the luminal membrane are excreted in the urine (184).

Endothelin in Heart Failure

Endothelin is a potent vasoconstrictor, and its concentration is increased in patients with heart failure (185). Results of a study from Teerlink and colleagues (186) suggest that endothelin plays an important role in the maintenance of arterial pressure in experimental heart failure, as shown by a significant decrease in blood pressure following the administration of the endothelin antagonist bosentan in rats with coronary artery ligation. In the kidney, mesangial cells, endothelial cells, epithelial glomerular cells, and inner-medullary collecting duct cells are capable of synthesizing endothelin (187). Unfortunately, the role of increased endothelin in the pathogenesis of the renal sodium and water retention of heart failure is currently unknown. In this regard, however, endothelin may be a potent mediator of renal vasoconstriction and thus influence renal sodium and water handling.

In summary, activation of the three major neurohormonal vasoconstrictor systems—the sympathetic nervous system, the renin–angiotensin–aldosterone system, and the nonosmotic release of AVP—is implicated in the renal sodium and water retention of heart failure. These neuroendocrine systems exert direct (tubular) and indirect (hemodynamic) effects on the kidneys to promote retention of sodium and water. Furthermore, these observations provide the rationale for the use of neurohormonal antagonists in the treatment of heart failure (see the following). In this regard, endogenous counterregulatory vasodilatory and natriuretic hormones may play an important attenuating role in heart failure, and the exogenous administration of these agents may be important in the treatment of heart failure.

Vasodilator Systems

Natriuretic Peptides in Heart Failure

The natriuretic peptides, including ANP and BNP, circulate at increased concentrations in patients with heart failure (188–194). These peptide hormones possess natriuretic, vasorelaxant, and renin, aldosterone, and possibly AVP and sympathetic-inhibiting properties (195–200). Both of these peptide hormones appear to be released primarily from the heart in response to increased atrial or ventricular end-diastolic pressure or to increased transmural cardiac pressure (201,202). In a recent study of ANP kinetics in patients with cardiac dysfunction, we demonstrated that increased ANP production rather than decreased metabolic clearance was the major factor contributing to the elevated plasma ANP concentrations in these patients (203). This finding is consistent with the observed increase in expression of both ANP and BNP mRNA in the cardiac ventricles of humans and animals with heart failure (204,205). However, given the peripheral vasoconstriction and sodium retention associated with heart failure, these elevated circulating natriuretic peptide levels must be inadequate to attenuate fully vasoconstrictor hormone activation. In this regard, volume expansion experiments performed in dogs with heart failure demonstrated a deficiency to further increase the elevated ANP levels (206). This relative deficiency of ANP secretion may contribute to the body's limited ability to maintain hemodynamic and renal function during the advanced stages of heart failure. In a coronary ligation model of heart failure in the rat, the infusion of a monoclonal antibody shown to specifically block endogenous ANP in vivo caused a significant rise in right atrial pressure, left ventricular end-diastolic pressure, and peripheral vascular resistance (207). Alternatively, a recent study by Colucci and associates found that a 6-hour infusion of the recombinant human BNP, nesiritide, significantly decreased pulmonary-capillary wedge pressure and improved symptoms in patients hospitalized with symptomatic heart failure (208). However, in a more chronic trial comparing the effects of nesiritide versus standard intravenous therapy on symptoms of heart failure, no significant differences were found (208).

Renal Effects of the Natriuretic Peptides in Heart Failure

In normal humans, ANP and BNP increase GFR and urinary sodium excretion with no change or only a slight fall in renal blood flow (201,209). The changes in renal hemodynamics are likely mediated by afferent arteriolar vasodilation with constriction of the efferent arterioles, as indicated by micropuncture studies in rats (210,211). In addition to increasing GFR and filtered sodium load as a mechanism of their natriuretic effect, ANP and BNP are specific inhibitors of sodium reabsorption in the collecting tubule (212–214). An important role for endogenous ANP in the renal sodium balance of heart failure was demonstrated by the aforementioned study of Lee and associates (25). However, the administration of synthetic ANP to patients with low-output heart failure results in a much smaller increase in renal sodium excretion and less significant changes in renal hemodynamics as compared to normal subjects (201). Like ANP, the natriuretic effect of BNP is blunted in rats with high-output heart failure produced by AV fistulae (215). Nevertheless, in hypertensive patients with mild to moderate heart failure and normal renal sodium excretory capacity, the natriuretic effect of BNP appears comparable to that in control subjects (216). Because ANP and BNP appear to share the same receptor sites (217), it is possible that the natriuretic effect of

BNP is also blunted in sodium-retaining patients with more advanced heart failure. Support for this hypothesis may be found in a recent report (218). In 16 patients with advanced decompensated New York Heart Association (NYHA) class III heart failure owing to either ischemic or idiopathic dilated cardiomyopathy (left ventricular ejection fraction $18 \pm 2\%$, cardiac index 1.84 ± 0.15 L/minute per m^2, pulmonary capillary wedge pressure 27 ± 3 mm Hg), the administration of BNP at either 0.025 or 0.050 μg/kg per minute for 4 hours produced a natriuresis in only four patients. The effect of BNP on GFR and renal blood flow was inconsistent in these patients and did not predict the natriuretic response. While the renal effects of BNP were blunted in some of these heart failure patients, BNP did produce a significant 50% decrease in pulmonary capillary wedge pressure. At the higher dose, BNP also significantly lowered peripheral vascular resistance and improved cardiac performance.

In contrast to the mentioned findings of ANP and BNP resistance in heart failure, Elsner and associates (219) recently suggested that renal responsiveness to urodilatin (ANP$_{95-126}$), a slightly extended form of ANP$_{99-126}$, is preserved in heart failure. Urodilatin appears to be produced in the kidney by different posttranslational processing of the ANP prohormone ANP$_{1-126}$ (220). Endogenous urodilatin appears to be confined to the kidney (221); that is, it is not a circulating hormone like ANP and BNP. In normal humans, exogenously administered urodilatin produces hemodynamic and renal effects similar to those of ANP (222). In the report from Elsner and associates (219), 12 patients with class II or III heart failure received urodilatin, 15 ng/kg per minute, or placebo (N = six in each group) for 10 hours. Although the urodilatin-treated patients did demonstrate a modest natriuresis during urodilatin infusion, it should be noted that (a) digoxin and furosemide were continued during the study, (b) the patients were maintained on an 8-g/day sodium intake, and (c) the patients received a 500-mL water load (300 mL orally and 200 mL intravenously) during the hour preceding study drug infusion. In the former instance, furosemide likely facilitated the delivery of sodium to the distal nephron. In the latter two cases, the high daily sodium intake and oral water load would be expected to diminish the degree of vasoconstrictor neurohormone activation. In fact, plasma vasoconstrictor hormone concentrations were, at most, mildly elevated in these patients. Thus, these findings do not exclude the existence of renal resistance to urodilatin in patients with heart failure and more advanced degrees of neurohormonal activation.

The mechanism of this relative resistance to the natriuretic effect of ANP (and possibly BNP and urodilatin) in heart failure remains controversial. Possible mechanisms include: (a) downregulation of renal ANP receptors (223,224), (b) secretion of inactive immunoreactive ANP (225), (c) enhanced renal neutral endopeptidase activity limiting the delivery of ANP to receptor sites (226), (d) hyperaldosteronism by an increased sodium reabsorption in the distal renal tubule (227), and (e) diminished delivery of sodium to the distal renal tubule site of ANP action (212–214). In sodium-retaining

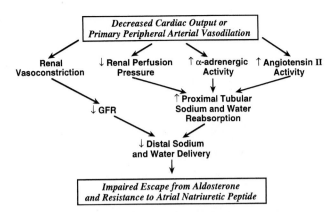

FIG. 84-5. Proposed mechanism of natriuretic peptide resistance and impaired aldosterone escape in states of arterial underfilling. (From: Schrier RW, Better OS. Pathogenesis of ascites formation. *Eur J Gastroenterol* 1991;3:721, with permission.)

patients with heart failure, we found a strong positive correlation between plasma ANP and urinary cyclic guanosine monophosphate (cGMP, the second messenger for the natriuretic effect of ANP, BNP, and urodilatin *in vivo*) (228,229). This observation supports the active biologic responsiveness of renal ANP receptors in heart failure and thus suggests that diminished distal tubular sodium delivery may be involved in the natriuretic peptide resistance observed in patients with cardiac failure. Further support for this hypothesis is found in our experience with cirrhosis, another edematous disorder associated with renal ANP resistance, where maneuvers that definitely increase distal tubular sodium delivery reversed the ANP resistance (230) (see the following). In addition, heart failure maneuvers that are expected to increase distal tubular sodium delivery, such as the administration of an ANG II receptor antagonist or furosemide, also improve the renal response to ANP (150,231). Finally, studies in rats with experimental heart failure demonstrated that renal denervation reverses the ANP resistance (232). Because proximal tubular sodium reabsorption is enhanced by adrenergic stimulation, this effect of renal denervation to enhance ANP sensitivity in experimental cardiac failure is also compatible with a role of distal sodium delivery. The proposed role of diminished distal tubular sodium delivery in natriuretic peptide resistance and impaired aldosterone escape is shown in Fig. 84-5.

Summary

As the heart begins to fail, the renal tubule reabsorbs sodium and water more avidly (Fig. 84-6). The afferent stimuli for this "compensatory" volume retention may involve aspects of both the forward and backward theories of heart failure. An acute fall in cardiac output may inactivate high-pressure baroreceptors located in the aortic arch, carotid sinus, and juxtaglomerular apparatus and thus activate the adrenergic nervous system. Diminished renal perfusion and increased renal sympathetic tone enhance the release of renin and thus activate the renin–angiotensin–aldosterone system. In acute

high-output heart failure, in which the cardiac output is insufficient to meet circulatory demands, the fall in peripheral vascular resistance provides the stimulus for arterial underfilling and deactivates high-pressure receptors. Although acute loading of the low-pressure receptors of the thorax may inhibit AVP release and stimulate the release of natriuretic peptides, this counterregulatory response to sodium and water retention may become ineffective because of progressive insensitivity of the cardiopulmonary receptors in the setting of chronic heart failure. Further cardiac compromise, resulting from either progression of the primary cardiac pathology or increased cardiac demand, results in further renal sodium and water retention, expansion of the ECF volume, and overt edema formation. The development of increased cardiac filling pressures with subsequent pulmonary or peripheral edema substantially contributes to the high morbidity and mortality of heart failure.

The efferent mechanisms for renal sodium and water retention in heart failure are multifactorial. Inactivation of receptors in the high-pressure circulation and blunting of receptors in the low-pressure system initiate reflexes in which renal sympathetic tone is augmented and renal vasoconstriction results. Renal blood flow decreases to a greater extent than GFR, and therefore the filtration fraction rises. This increase alters ultrafiltration of plasma and peritubular physical forces, which may in turn increase proximal tubular sodium reabsorption. Changes in cardiac output, ventricular filling pressures, and renal perfusion pressure also activate the renin–angiotensin–aldosterone system and nonosmotic stimulation of AVP, and increase the secretion or production, or both, of prostaglandins and the natriuretic peptides. At some point in the natural history of cardiac failure, the vasoconstrictive forces overcome the vasodilating effects of prostaglandins, natriuretic peptides, and other vasodilating substances, and peripheral vasoconstriction and renal sodium and water retention occur. Increases in ventricular preload and afterload ensue, resulting in a further deterioration in cardiac performance and further stimulation of neurohormonal vasoconstrictor systems.

Physiologic Basis for the Treatment of Sodium and Water Retention in Heart Failure

In heart failure, as in all of clinical medicine, effective therapy should be dictated by an understanding of the pathophysiologic process involved. Depressed ventricular function is associated with a vicious cycle of maladaptive responses, including increased neurohormonal activation, systemic vasoconstriction and renal sodium and water retention, and increased ventricular preload and afterload (Fig. 84-7). Treatment of heart failure should be directed at modifying the afferent and efferent factors responsible for the salt and water retention. Therefore, the primary goal in the treatment of cardiac failure is to improve the function of the heart as a pump. This increases the integrity of the arterial circulation and decreases the venous hypertension, thus interrupting two

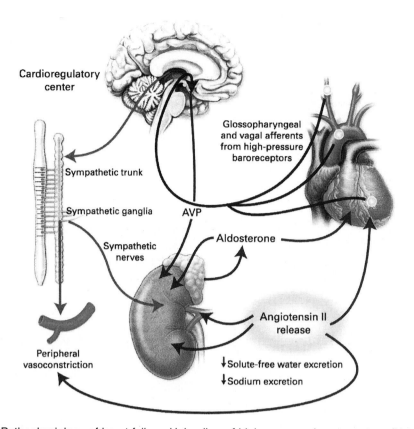

FIG. 84-6. Pathophysiology of heart failure. Unloading of high-pressure baroreceptors *(blue circles)* in the left ventricle, carotid sinus, and aortic arch generates afferent signals *(black)* that stimulate cardioregulatory centers in the brain, resulting in the activation of efferent pathways in the sympathetic nervous system *(green)*. The sympathetic nervous system appears to be the primary integrator of the neurohumoral vasoconstrictor response to arterial underfilling. Activation of renal sympathetic nerves stimulates the release of renin and angiotensin II, thus activating the renin–angiotensin–aldosterone system. Concomitantly, sympathetic stimulation of the supraoptic and paraventricular nuclei in the hypothalamus results in the nonosmotic release of arginine vasopressin (AVP). Sympathetic activation also causes peripheral and renal vasoconstriction, as does angiotensin II. Angiotensin II constricts blood vessels and stimulates the release of aldosterone from the adrenal gland, and it also increases tubular sodium reabsorption and causes remodeling of cardiac myocytes. Aldosterone may have direct cardiac effects, in addition to increasing the reabsorption of sodium and the secretion of potassium and hydrogen ions in the collecting duct. The blue lines designate circulating hormones. (From: Schrier RW, Abraham WT. Hormones and hemodynamics in heart failure. *N Engl J Med* 1999;341:577, copyright © 2000, Massachusetts Medical Society. All rights reserved.)

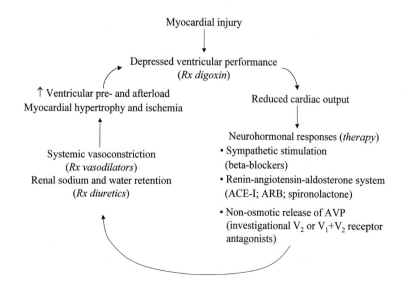

FIG. 84-7. Vicious cycle of depressed ventricular function. Potential therapies are in parentheses. *ACE-I,* angiotensin I converting enzyme inhibitors; *ARB,* angiotensin receptor blockers; *AVP,* arginine vasopressin. (From: Schrier RW, et al. Therapy of heart failure. *Kidney Int* 2000;57:1418, with permission of Blackwell Science, New York.)

of the major afferent mechanisms leading to sodium and water retention. Unfortunately, this goal of improving the contractile state of the heart is often difficult to accomplish. In certain cases of heart failure, however, left ventricular function may be improved by surgical intervention. For example, some patients with coronary artery disease and ischemic cardiomyopathy may exhibit improved cardiac function and less severe heart failure after surgical or percutaneous transluminal revascularization of the ischemic myocardium. A more classic example of surgically correctable heart failure is that seen in the setting of severe aortic stenosis. Patients with critical aortic stenosis often exhibit a severe degree of low-output heart failure with very avid renal sodium and water retention that is usually completely reversible following replacement of the stenotic aortic valve.

In other instances of heart failure, cardiac function may be augmented by the cardiac glycosides, such as digoxin, which modestly improve cardiac contractility and may favorably influence baroreceptor function (233). Vasodilators, such as nitrates and hydralazine, and the ACE inhibitors may improve cardiac function by decreasing cardiac preload and afterload (234). Investigational nonglycoside inotropic agents may acutely improve cardiac output but longer-term use has been shown to increase mortality (235–237). ß-Adrenergic receptor antagonists, once thought to be contraindicated in patients with low-output heart failure, can exhibit a favorable effect on cardiac function and outcome in patients with chronic heart failure. In fact, these agents improve the left ventricular ejection fraction to a greater extent than does any other form of heart failure therapy (128). Moreover, the commercially available second-generation selective $ß_1$-receptor blocker metoprolol improves left ventricular function and reduces the need for cardiac transplantation in patients with idiopathic dilated cardiomyopathy (129). In addition, carvedilol, a nonselective third-generation ß-blocker/vasodilator with α_1-adrenergic receptor-blocking properties, produces a dose-related improvement in ejection fraction and reduction in mortality in patients with class II to IV heart failure (130). In the U.S. Carvedilol Heart Failure Trials Program, this agent reduced all-cause mortality by 65% compared to placebo in patients with mild to moderate heart failure (238). Likewise, the Second Cardiac Insufficiency Bisoprolol Study demonstrated a 34% reduction in all-cause mortality versus placebo during treatment of heart failure with this $ß_1$ selective agent (239). In a randomized study of metoprolol CR/XL treatment of 3,991 patients with class II to IV heart failure, treatment with metoprolol CR/XL was associated with a 34% decrease in all-cause mortality, 38% decrease in cardiovascular mortality, 41% decrease in sudden death, and 49% decrease in death owing to progressive heart failure as compared to controls (240). These studies generally included patients with mild to moderate heart failure, as evident by annualized placebo mortality rates of 11% to 13%. Thus, ß-blockade has been recommended for the treatment of patients with NYHA class II to III heart failure (241,242). Most recently, the Carvedilol Prospective Randomized Cumulative Survival (COPERNICUS) Trial reported a 35%

reduction in all-cause mortality compared to placebo, when carvedilol was administered to patients with advanced heart failure (243). The Beta-Blocker Evaluation of Survival Trial (BEST) demonstrated no significant difference between the third-generation agent bucindolol and placebo on the primary endpoint of all-cause mortality (244).

As an improvement in pump function is a primary goal in the treatment of heart failure, agents that might further impair cardiac contractility should be avoided in this setting. Unfortunately, many medications that have been demonstrated to produce a negative effect on cardiac inotropy are commonly prescribed in cardiac disease patients. For example, most antiarrhythmic drugs and the commonly prescribed first-generation calcium channel antagonists exhibit some degree of negative inotropy *in vivo* (245). However, newer vascular-selective calcium channel blockers may be well tolerated in patients with heart failure. One of these agents, amlodipine, decreased mortality owing to sudden cardiac death by 38% and pump failure by 45% in patients with heart failure caused by nonischemic dilated cardiomyopathy, while exhibiting a neutral effect on outcome in patients with ischemic cardiomyopathy (246). However, in an adequately powered, large-scale, prospective, randomized, controlled trial, this effect was not replicated (247). In this later study, amlodipine was shown to be no better than placebo in the treatment of heart failure attributable to nonischemic causes.

The neuroendocrine activation in patients with heart failure provides another target for therapy. In fact, recent experience with various neurohormonal antagonists suggests that inhibition or antagonism of neurohormonal vasoconstrictor systems may be more beneficial than nonspecific diuretic or vasodilator therapy. ANG II is known to mediate myocardial hypertrophy, increase fibrosis and collagen deposition, and cause activation of the sympathetic nervous system. Thus, administration of ACE inhibitors would be anticipated to decrease myocardial remodeling and hypertrophy and decrease activation of the sympathetic nervous system. ACE inhibition also decreases the degradation of bradykinin, which is a well-known vasodilator that can reduce cardiac afterload. The proven beneficial effects of ACE inhibition on symptoms, hemodynamics, exercise capacity, and survival in heart failure patients support this hypothesis (142,143,236). Moreover, in the patients of the Cooperative North Scandinavian Enalapril Survival Study (CONSENSUS), all with class IV heart failure, significant reductions in mortality were consistently found in the patients treated with enalapril who had baseline hormone levels above median values (142). In the group of patients treated with the ACE inhibitor, there were significant reductions from baseline to 6 weeks in levels of ANG II, aldosterone, norepinephrine, and ANP but not epinephrine. These results suggest that the effect of enalapril on mortality was related to diminished hormonal activation in general and to the renin–angiotensin system in particular (248). In the SOLVD studies of less severe heart failure, the addition of enalapril to conventional therapy also significantly reduced mortality and hospitalization rates (143). In this regard, it should be noted that the recently published clinical practice guidelines for the treatment of heart failure from the Agency for Health Care Policy and Research recommend ACE inhibition as first-line therapy in nonedematous patients with heart failure (249). Other neurohormonal antagonists and various forms of vasodilator hormone therapy are under active investigation for the treatment of heart failure. Agents such as renin inhibitors and ANG II receptor antagonists may exhibit effects similar to the ACE inhibitors (250,251). ANG II type 1 (AT1) receptor antagonists are believed to achieve a more complete blockade of the action of ANG II than ACE inhibitors. In this regard, large multicenter randomized trials to compare the effects of AT1 receptor antagonists versus ACE inhibitors on cardiovascular morbidity and mortality are needed. The Evaluation of Losartan in the Elderly (ELITE) trial showed an association between the AT1 receptor antagonist losartan and an unexpected survival benefit in elderly heart failure patients as compared with captopril (252). This was a secondary endpoint, however. The losartan heart failure survival study (ELITE II) further examined the effects of losartan versus captopril on survival in 3,152 elderly patients with NYHA class II to IV heart failure (253). As primary endpoints, no significant differences in all-cause mortality or sudden cardiac death were noted between the two study groups. In fact, there was a nearly significant 12% trend favoring the ACE inhibitor in ELITE II. Importantly, the study was neither designed nor powered to show equivalency of the two regimens. Thus, ACE inhibitors remain the first-line agents in the management of systolic heart failure. Some investigators have suggested that combination ACE inhibition and AT1 receptor antagonism may be beneficial in the treatment of heart failure; however, such benefits have not been demonstrated in humans with heart failure. In the recent Randomized Evaluation of Strategies for Left Ventricular Dysfunction (RESOLVD) pilot study, no significant difference in rates of hospitalization or mortality were demonstrated among patients receiving candesartan, enalapril, or a combination of both (254). However, the study was not powered adequately to address these endpoints. Ongoing studies may clarify the role of AT1 receptor antagonists in the treatment of heart failure. Potential therapeutic roles for AVP receptor antagonists and the natriuretic peptides in the therapy of heart failure were mentioned already and are extensively reviewed elsewhere (255). The renal benefits of these newer investigational forms of antihormonal/hormonal therapy for heart failure remain to be proved.

Diuretics are indicated to restore the ECF volume toward normal as heart failure becomes more advanced and when edema formation occurs. Diuretic therapy is discussed extensively in Chapter 82, Mechanisms of Diuretic Action. Of note, although most patients with cardiac failure respond to a potent loop diuretic, for example, furosemide, and this agent can increase solute-free water clearance in patients with cardiac edema (117), cardiac output may actually decline during treatment (256). Volume depletion owing to overzealous diuretic treatment must be considered in any heart failure patient with worsening signs or symptoms of a low-output state. For example, diminished renal perfusion may occur in the setting of excessive diuretic treatment, resulting in elevations in BUN and serum creatinine concentrations. Alternatively, these signs of low cardiac output may result from progression of the pump dysfunction, and therefore an assessment of the volume status is of critical importance in the management of the heart failure patient. Diuretic resistance is not an uncommon finding in patients with advanced heart failure. Because intraluminal delivery of loop diuretics via tubular secretion is necessary for these agents to inhibit sodium chloride reabsorption in the thick ascending limb of Henle, renal vasoconstriction may play an important role in diuretic resistance associated with heart failure. Moreover, increased distal tubule sodium reabsorption further contributes to diuretic resistance in this condition. Thus, the addition of a more distal acting diuretic, such as metolazone or hydrochlorothiazide, may reverse resistance to loop diuretics.

Fluid removal by intermittent or continuous ultrafiltration has been suggested to have several advantages over diuretic therapy (257–260). In addition to the reduction of excess ECF volume in heart failure patients, it has been suggested that ultrafiltration of cytokines, which suppress myocardial contractility, may improve cardiac function. This remains to be proven, however. As compared to diuretics, fluid/electrolyte and acid–base disturbances may be more easily corrected and avoided with ultrafiltration. Furthermore, for the same amount of fluid removal, more sodium is removed with ultrafiltration than with diuretics, because the sodium concentration in the ultrafiltrate is equivalent to plasma, whereas with diuretic therapy the urinary sodium concentration is virtually always less than plasma. Although ultrafiltration provides an effective means of fluid removal, there are currently no data available to suggest that ultrafiltration prolongs life in patients with severe heart failure.

Water restriction remains the mainstay of therapy in patients with heart failure who are hyponatremic. Studies also suggested that in hyponatremic patients with heart failure receiving furosemide and captopril, plasma sodium values tended to normalize, whereas they did not in patients receiving other vasodilators (261,262). These data support the concomitant use of ACE inhibitors and loop diuretics in hyponatremic heart failure patients. Alternatively, a selective V_2-receptor AVP antagonist hopefully will be available in the future to correct the hyponatremia of heart failure.

Finally, other measures, including sodium restriction and oxygen administration, contribute to the overall management of patients with heart failure. Special emphasis should be placed on the salutary influence of bed rest, which increases osmolar and solute-free water clearances, cardiac output, renal plasma flow, and GFR and decreases plasma catecholamines and PRA (263). Such considerations lay the foundation for the physiologic basis of therapy in heart failure.

LIVER DISEASE

The association between edema formation and the presence of liver disease has captured the interest of many investigators during the past three decades and has inspired many detailed

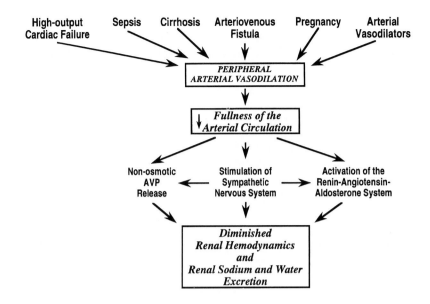

FIG. 84-8. Mechanism explaining the defect in renal sodium and water excretion in cirrhosis and in other states of arterial underfilling owing to peripheral arterial vasodilation.

reviews (19,264–273). It was first demonstrated that sodium and water were retained avidly in patients with decompensated (ascitic) cirrhosis (274). Furthermore, cirrhotic patients were shown to incompletely excrete an intravenous sodium load (275). In concert with these clinical observations, the control of renal sodium excretion has been intensively studied (45,276). Although Chapter 75 (Liver Disease and the Kidney) describes some of the important renal considerations in patients with hepatorenal syndrome, the following discussion addresses the afferent and efferent mechanisms of sodium and water reabsorption in decompensated cirrhosis. Specifically, the role of peripheral arterial vasodilation in initiating the renal sodium and water retention is reviewed, and the neurohormonal and other "effector" mechanisms for sodium and water retention in cirrhosis are discussed.

Afferent Mechanisms for Renal Sodium and Water Retention in Cirrhosis

Until recently, two competing theories attempted to explain the pathogenesis of sodium and water retention in cirrhosis (271,272). With the classic "underfill hypothesis," ascites formation secondary to portal hypertension was proposed to decrease plasma volume and cause secondary renal sodium and water retention (19). However, results of animal studies showed that sodium retention and water retention precede ascites formation in cirrhotic animals, thus contradicting the hypothesis (277). Subsequently, primary renal sodium and water retention, secondary to a hepatorenal reflex, was proposed to lead to plasma volume expansion of both the venous and arterial compartments and cause overflow ascites (277). This "overfill hypothesis" of ascites formation in cirrhotic patients, however, did not explain the progressive stimulation of the neurohumoral profile observed in cirrhotic patients and characteristic of arterial underfilling. Against this background, we proposed a primary role for peripheral arterial vasodilation in the initiation of renal sodium and water retention in cirrhosis (11–17,19,278) (Fig. 84-8). This mechanism of arterial underfilling and sodium and water retention explains the progressive increase in plasma volume and neurohormonal activation that occurs as cirrhotic subjects advance from compensated to decompensated cirrhosis to the hepatorenal syndrome (Table 84-2). According to the peripheral arterial vasodilation hypothesis, progressive arterial vasodilation is associated with progressive stimulation of neurohormonal vasoconstrictor systems, despite expansion of plasma volume.

The Peripheral Arterial Vasodilation Theory of Sodium and Water Retention in Cirrhosis

Table 84-2 shows the details whereby vasodilation-mediated arterial underfilling may account for the spectrum of compensated cirrhosis, decompensated cirrhosis, and hepatorenal

TABLE 84-2. *The range of pathophysiology from compensated to decompensated cirrhosis to the hepatorenal syndrome*

	Compensated cirrhosis (no ascites)	Decompensated cirrhosis (ascites)	Hepatorenal syndrome
Peripheral arterial vasodilation	↑	↑↑	↑↑↑
Plasma hormones (AVP, renin, aldosterone, NE)	↔	↑	↑↑
Plasma volume	↑	↑↑	↑↑↑

AVP, arginine vasopressin; *NE,* norepinephrine.

syndrome including stimulation of the neurohumoral response. It is known that several states of peripheral arterial vasodilation are accompanied by sodium and water retention. The degree of vasodilatation in each state dictates the degree of stimulation of the neurohumoral response to the arterial underfilling.

The primary site of arterial vasodilation in cirrhosis is the splanchnic circulation. Investigations in rats and dogs with experimental cirrhosis, as well as in rats with portal vein ligation, showed that portal hypertension is associated with a marked splanchnic arterial vasodilation (280–283). Furthermore, patients with cirrhosis usually have normal or increased hepatic blood flow and decreased mean transit times in the splanchnic circulation (284,285), supporting the presence of splanchnic arterial vasodilation in human cirrhosis. Of note, splanchnic vasodilation occurs prior to ascites formation, as required by the peripheral arterial vasodilation hypothesis. As cirrhosis progresses, vasodilation may occur at other sites, such as the skin, muscles, and lungs. However, whether arterial vasodilation occurs in other vascular territories in human cirrhosis remains controversial. Fernandez-Seara and coworkers (286) demonstrated that femoral artery blood flow, estimated by Doppler ultrasonography, was higher in a group of patients with cirrhosis and ascites than in a group of normal subjects. This finding is compatible with the presence of peripheral (femoral) arterial vasodilation in decompensated cirrhosis. However, other investigators reported decreased femoral blood flow using similar experimental techniques (287).

The mediators of this early splanchnic vasodilation in cirrhosis are unknown but may include opening of existing shunts, activation of various vasodilating substances, and ultimately the development of collaterals. Increased synthesis and release of the vasodilator nitric oxide, perhaps secondary to increased circulating levels of endotoxin in cirrhosis, has been proposed to account for the peripheral vasodilation and increased cardiac outputs seen in association with cirrhosis (288). Nitric oxide activity is difficult to measure *in vivo*, and therefore only indirect evidence supports a role for nitric oxide in the peripheral vasodilation of cirrhosis (289–294). For example, urinary cGMP, the second messenger of nitric oxide as well as the natriuretic peptides (289), is increased in patients with cirrhosis prior to the development of ascites and in some patients prior to an increase in circulating ANP concentrations (290). In addition, our laboratory has demonstrated a marked increase in endothelial nitric oxide synthase (eNOS) and cGMP concentrations in aortic and mesenteric arteries from rats with experimental cirrhosis (292). In these animals, aortic cGMP concentration correlated inversely with arterial pressure (r = 0.54, P < 0.0001). Significantly, chronic administration of the nitric oxide synthesis inhibitor N^G-nitro-L-arginine-methyl-ester (L-NAME, 10 mg/kg per day for 7 days) induced a marked reduction in mesenteric and aortic eNOS and aortic cGMP concentration and an increase in arterial blood pressure in cirrhotic

rats to similar levels obtained in L-NAME-treated control animals. These results indicate that the high aortic cGMP content and decreased arterial blood pressure in cirrhotic rats were due to increased nitric oxide synthesis (Fig. 84-9) (293). We also showed that normalization of vascular nitric oxide production by chronic nitric oxide synthesis inhibition corrects more than the systemic hemodynamic abnormalities in cirrhotic rats with ascites (295). These hemodynamic changes were accompanied by normalization of plasma renin, aldosterone, and AVP (Fig. 84-10) as well as either a profound decrease or complete resolution of ascites. Water retention and hyponatremia were also reversed with chronic nitric oxide inhibition in cirrhotic rats. In human studies, Guarner and associates (291) recently demonstrated elevated serum nitrite and nitrate levels, a crude index of *in vivo* nitric oxide generation, in 51 cirrhotic patients. Of note, in these patients, the elevated serum nitrite/nitrate levels significantly correlated with plasma endotoxin levels and decreased in response to a reduction in plasma endotoxin concentration following the administration of colistin (291). In addition, an enhanced sensitivity to mediators of endothelium-dependent vasodilation recently was demonstrated in human cirrhosis (294). Taken together, these observations are compatible with nitric oxide-induced vasodilation early in cirrhosis.

Endogenous opioids may also contribute to the peripheral vasodilation and renal salt and water retention of cirrhosis, because the administration of the opioid antagonist naloxone increases sodium and water excretion after water loading in patients with cirrhosis and ascites (296). Other factors that may possibly play a role in the splanchnic and peripheral vasodilation of cirrhosis include vasodilating prostaglandins, glucagon, platelet-activating factor, calcitonin gene-related peptide, substance P, and vasoactive intestinal peptide. However, definitive proof is lacking for all of these. Alternatively, impaired responsiveness of the peripheral vasculature to endogenous pressor agents could explain the peripheral vasodilation of cirrhosis. In cirrhosis, the reactivity of the vasculature to various vasoconstricting substances has yielded inconclusive results. For example, in experimental cirrhosis in the rat, normal or increased vascular sensitivity to infused norepinephrine has been demonstrated (297). On the other hand, other investigators reported impaired pressor reactivity to norepinephrine and ANG II in cirrhosis (298). As a result it is possible that both increased activity of vasodilating substances *and* decreased pressor sensitivity contribute to the peripheral vasodilation of cirrhosis.

In summary, the peripheral arterial vasodilation theory explains both the hemodynamic and neurohormonal alterations observed in cirrhosis and accounts for the mechanism of the renal sodium and water retention in cirrhotic subjects (see the following). Although the exact substance responsible for the early arterial vasodilation is unknown, the leading candidate appears to be nitric oxide. Neurohormonal activation and the effector mechanisms for renal sodium and water retention in cirrhosis are discussed in the following.

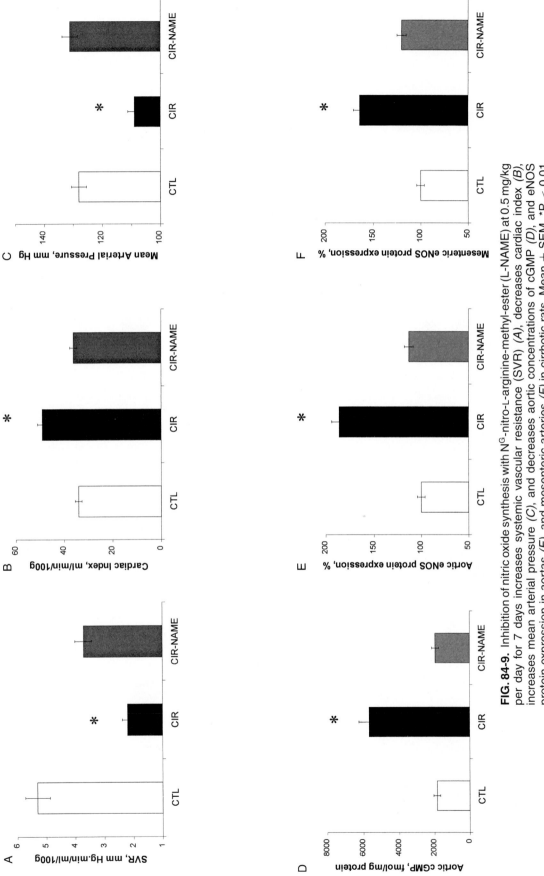

FIG. 84-9. Inhibition of nitric oxide synthesis with N^G-nitro-L-arginine-methyl-ester (L-NAME) at 0.5 mg/kg per day for 7 days increases systemic vascular resistance (SVR) (*A*), decreases cardiac index (*B*), increases mean arterial pressure (*C*), and decreases aortic concentrations of cGMP (*D*), and eNOS protein expression in aortas (*E*), and mesenteric arteries (*F*) in cirrhotic rats. Mean $\pm$ SEM. *P $<$ 0.01 versus CTL and *CIR-NAME* rats. *CIR*, untreated cirrhosis; *CIR-NAME*, cirrhosis with L-NAME treatment; *CTL*, control. (Adapted from: Niederberger M, et al. Normalization of nitric oxide production corrects arterial vasodilation and hyperdynamic circulation in cirrhotic rats. *Gastroenterology* 1995;109:1624, with permission.)

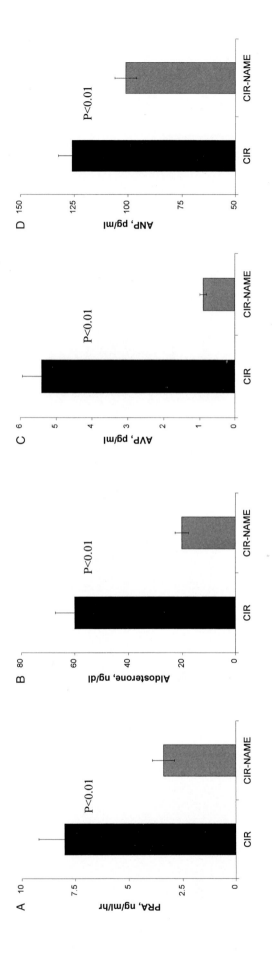
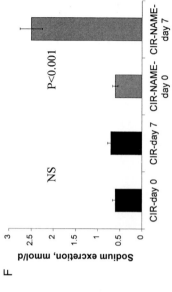
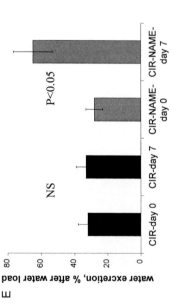

FIG. 84-10. PRA (*A*), aldosterone (*B*), AVP (*C*), and ANP (*D*) concentrations decrease in cirrhotic rats with ascites with seven days of L-NAME treatment. Water excretion (*E*) 3 hours following a water load of 30 mL/kg, and sodium excretion (*F*) were impaired in both treated and untreated cirrhotic rats at day 0. After 7 days of L-NAME, a significant improvement in water and sodium excretion occurred in rats treated with L-NAME, but not in untreated cirrhotic rats. Mean ± SEM. *ANP*, atrial natriuretic peptide; *AVP*, arginine vasopressin; *CIR*, untreated cirrhosis; *CIR-NAME*, cirrhosis with L-NAME treatment; *PRA*, plasma renin activity. (Adapted from: Martin PY, et al. Nitric oxide synthase inhibition for one week improves renal sodium and water excretion in cirrhotic rats with ascites. *J Clin Invest* 1998;101:235, with permission.)

Efferent Mechanisms for Renal Sodium and Water Retention in Cirrhosis

Similar to patients with heart failure, neurohormonal vasoconstrictor systems are activated in patients with cirrhosis. Furthermore, as mentioned already, the degree of activation of these neuroendocrine systems is related to the severity of the disease, with compensated cirrhotics demonstrating the mildest activation of these systems and patients with the hepatorenal syndrome demonstrating the highest circulating levels of plasma vasoconstrictor hormones. In this regard, it should be noted that normal circulating vasoconstrictor hormone levels may be inappropriately elevated in patients with early cirrhosis, given the degree of plasma volume expansion. As discussed here and in Chapter 75 (Liver Disease and the Kidney), neurohormonal activation has been implicated in the renal sodium and water retention of cirrhosis.

Nephron Sites of Sodium and Water Retention

There is indirect evidence for enhanced tubular reabsorption both proximally and distally in human cirrhotic subjects. The following findings support enhanced proximal tubular reabsorption in hepatic cirrhosis: (a) Maneuvers that expand plasma volume and increase distal nephron delivery of fluid (i.e., headout water immersion [HWI] and infusion of saline or mannitol) result in increased renal sodium excretion and solute-free water formation independent of changes in GFR (34,44,299–301); (b) in water-loaded cirrhotics with ascites and minimal urinary osmolalities, urine flow rates (an index of distal delivery of tubular fluid under these circumstances) are lower than in normal subjects (302,303); and (c) enhanced proximal reabsorption of tubular fluid has been found in micropuncture and clearance studies of dogs and rats with chronic bile duct ligation as well as rats with cirrhosis secondary to carbon tetrachloride exposure (304–306).

Evidence for enhanced distal nephron sodium reabsorption is based on the following observations: (a) Water-loaded patients with sodium retention and cirrhosis with minimal urine osmolalities often have urine flow rates (an index of proximal reabsorption) comparable to those of normal control subjects (307); (b) water-loaded cirrhotic patients with minimal urine osmolalities have increased calculated distal fractional sodium reabsorption after receiving hypotonic saline infusions (307); (c) acetazolamide, a diuretic acting in the proximal tubule, produces a significant natriuresis in cirrhotics only when there is concomitant distal nephron blockade of sodium reabsorption with ethacrynic acid (308); and (d) micropuncture studies in the dimethylnitrosamine model of cirrhosis demonstrate enhanced distal nephron sodium reabsorption (304,309). In summary, clinical and experimental studies suggest that both proximal and distal nephron sites participate in enhanced renal tubular sodium reabsorption in cirrhosis. The role of distal sodium delivery in the impaired aldosterone escape and ANP resistance of cirrhosis is discussed in the following.

Mechanisms of Enhanced Tubular Sodium and Water Reabsorption, Renal Blood Flow, Glomerular Filtration Rate, Filtration Fraction, and Peritubular Physical Factors

The mechanisms responsible for enhanced sodium reabsorption at both proximal and distal sites have not been clearly defined and may be multifactorial. A decrease in GFR is not observed in many sodium-retaining cirrhotic patients, suggesting that sodium and water retention can occur independent of a decrease in GFR (44). An increase in renal vascular resistance and in filtration fraction is often seen in decompensated cirrhosis (310). Thus, peritubular physical forces (decreased hydrostatic pressure, increased oncotic pressure) may enhance proximal tubular sodium and water reabsorption in cirrhosis. As with cardiac failure, both a fall in GFR and an increase in proximal tubular reabsorption may result in decreased fluid delivery to the distal diluting segment in the cirrhotic patient, thereby impairing water excretion. This mechanism is suggested by the findings that the hyponatremic cirrhotic patient excretes a hypotonic urine during the infusion of mannitol (34), saline (299), saline plus albumin (299), or ascitic fluid (300), and during water immersion to the level of the neck (310). However, because all these maneuvers expand ECF volume, these observations should not be considered to exclude a role for AVP in the pathogenesis of the renal water retention and hyponatremia. That the administration of furosemide appears to improve solute-free water excretion in cirrhotic subjects (117) may favor an intrarenal mechanism of water retention. A similar generation of hypotonic urine was, however, observed in cirrhotic subjects receiving an exogenous infusion of AVP. A role for persistent endogenous release of AVP in the diluting defect, therefore, could not be excluded (117), and as mentioned, recent studies suggested that furosemide may attenuate the renal effect of AVP (118). The role of AVP in cirrhosis is discussed in the following.

Vasoconstrictor Systems

Activation of the Sympathetic Nervous System and Circulating Catecholamines in Cirrhosis

Numerous studies have demonstrated elevated plasma norepinephrine concentrations in patients with decompensated cirrhosis (311–315). Both indirect and direct evidence suggests that these increased circulating plasma norepinephrine levels are due to activation of the sympathetic nervous system rather than to decreased norepinephrine clearance. In 1982, Ring-Larsen and associates (315) demonstrated normal hepatic norepinephrine clearances and increased renal norepinephrine release in patients with cirrhosis. In more recent experiments using tritiated norepinephrine, we demonstrated elevated norepinephrine spillover rates in cirrhotic patients compared to normal controls (1.5 ± 0.25 versus 0.26 ± 0.08 μg/minute m^2, $P < 0.001$), whereas norepinephrine clearance rates were comparable between the two groups (3.13 ± 0.5 versus 2.6 ± 0.3 L/minute, not significant) (316).

Taken together, these findings are compatible with the presence of systemic and renal adrenergic activation in cirrhosis. These observations were confirmed by Floras and colleagues (317) using the technique of peroneal nerve microneurography to directly measure sympathetic nerve activity to muscle in cirrhotic patients. In their cirrhotic patients with ascites, muscle sympathetic nerve activity was markedly increased and strongly correlated with plasma norepinephrine concentration.

Renal Effects of Adrenergic Activation in Cirrhosis

We measured high plasma norepinephrine levels in a series of patients with liver disease with variable degrees of compensation (312). Because plasma norepinephrine is an index of baroreceptor activity (318), we examined the hypothesis that in decompensated cirrhosis, arterial underfilling secondary to peripheral vasodilation, decreased oncotic pressure, and splanchnic venous pooling could induce a decrease in baroreceptor afferent traffic via the vagus and glossopharyngeal nerves to the pons and hypothalamus. This decrease in nervous afferent traffic could be associated with increased sympathetic efferent activity and nonosmotic stimulation of AVP, which might then contribute to the renal sodium and water retention. In the 26 cirrhotic patients studied, a positive correlation was indeed found between plasma AVP levels and plasma norepinephrine concentrations. Furthermore, nonexcretor patients (excretion <80% of water load in 5 hours) had higher norepinephrine, PRA, and aldosterone levels and lower plasma albumin levels compared with excretor patients (excretion of ≥80% of water load in 5 hours). We also demonstrated a positive correlation between norepinephrine and PRA as well as between norepinephrine and plasma aldosterone levels. Significantly, a negative correlation was found between plasma norepinephrine and urinary sodium excretion ($r = 0.76$, $P < 0.001$). These results suggest that increased renal sympathetic activity could directly increase proximal sodium reabsorption, thereby limiting the absolute quantity of sodium and water presented to the distal diluting site of the nephron (312). Moreover, increased renal sympathetic activity could stimulate the renin–angiotensin–aldosterone system, thus increasing distal sodium reabsorption. Of interest, Ring-Larsen and colleagues (319) demonstrated an inverse correlation between plasma norepinephrine and renal blood flow, suggesting an important renal hemodynamic role for enhanced renal sympathetic activity in cirrhosis. In addition, in the microneurographic study from Floras and colleagues (317), muscle sympathetic nerve activity was inversely correlated with 24-hour urinary sodium excretion in the patients with cirrhosis and ascites. Activation of renal nerves may also play a role in the blunted natriuretic response to ANP seen in cirrhosis (see the following).

Role of Aldosterone in Cirrhosis

The role of aldosterone in the renal sodium retention of cirrhosis has been controversial. Evidence supporting a role for aldosterone in the abnormal sodium retention characteristic of patients with liver disease comes from studies that either eliminated the adrenal source of aldosterone or pharmacologically antagonized its effect. For example, there have been reports of natriuresis occurring in cirrhosis either after surgical adrenalectomy or after the administration of spironolactone, a competitive inhibitor of aldosterone (320,321). In fact, in the majority of ascitic cirrhotic patients a diuresis can be established and ascites eliminated with a high dose (400 mg/day) of spironolactone. However, in some patients, inhibition of aldosterone synthesis with either aminoglutethimide (322) or adrenalectomy (319) did not restore renal sodium excretion completely to normal. Moreover, water immersion of patients with cirrhosis results in natriuresis, even in the presence of pharmacologic doses of mineralocorticoids (267). Furthermore, in one study of cirrhotic patients given excess sodium, four of 11 patients had suppressed levels of PRA and aldosterone, yet gained approximately 1 kg of weight per day (157). These five patients retained as much sodium as did the six patients who had persistently elevated plasma aldosterone levels (157). Thus, it seems that aldosterone is not the sole factor responsible for sodium retention in cirrhosis. However, the near-uniform response to spironolactone suggests that the high plasma levels of aldosterone frequently seen in cirrhotics contribute to the increased distal sodium reabsorption.

We further examined the role of aldosterone in the abnormal sodium retention seen in cirrhotic patients during control conditions (water loading) or during experimental maneuvers with increased centralization of blood volume with or without peripheral vasoconstriction (water immersion or immersion plus norepinephrine infusion) (323). All 13 patients studied were in positive sodium balance under baseline conditions, with a mean plasma aldosterone concentration of 79 ± 16 ng/dL. Regardless of the maneuver performed, no patient in whom plasma aldosterone exceeded 50 ng/dL achieved a negative sodium balance. Furthermore, only in those studies utilizing HWI, with or without norepinephrine infusion, was negative sodium balance observed. We concluded, therefore, that simultaneous expansion of central blood volume and relative suppression of plasma aldosterone were required to overcome the sodium avidity in decompensated cirrhosis (323). The central blood volume expansion may result in increased ANP release as well as increased distal sodium and fluid delivery.

Nonosmotic Release of Arginine Vasopressin in Cirrhosis

We demonstrated osmotically inappropriately elevated levels of AVP relative to their plasma osmolality in decompensated, hyponatremic cirrhotic patients (312,324). Twenty-six patients with alcoholic liver disease and variable degrees of ascites and edema received a water load of 20 mL/kg of body weight. Hourly blood and urine samples were then obtained during the next 5 hours for sodium, potassium, osmolality, inulin, *para*-aminohippurate, and hormonal measurements. Patients were then classified prospectively into excretor or nonexcretor groups by their capacity to excrete water according to the aforementioned criteria. Seven patients were excretors, excreting a mean of 82% of the water load in 5 hours; 19 patients were nonexcretors, excreting a mean of 29% of the water load in 5 hours. The nonexcretor patients had significantly higher minimal urinary osmolality (243 versus 72 mOsm/kg H_2O, $P < 0.001$), lower basal serum sodium (132.6 versus 140 mEq/L, $P < 0.001$), and lower serum osmolality (275 versus 282 mOsm/kg H_2O, $P < 0.05$) compared with excretor patients. Moreover, all of the 19 nonexcretor patients had ascites compared with only two of seven excretor patients. Plasma AVP was measured prior to and at regular intervals following the water load. Values in nonexcretors were significantly higher than those in excretors at 0, 1, 3, and 5 hours after the water load. Significantly, mean AVP values after the water load were higher in the nonexcretor group (2.06 versus 0.68 pg/mL, $P < 0.01$) despite a lower plasma osmolality. As discussed, nonexcretor patients also had significantly lower albumin and significantly higher PRA, plasma aldosterone, and plasma norepinephrine levels than did excretor patients (312,324). In spite of comparable sodium intakes for 5 days, nonexcretor patients also had lower urinary sodium excretions. Similar results were recently obtained by other investigators (313). Our findings are thus compatible with vasodilation-mediated arterial underfilling in decompensated cirrhotic patients that provided a nonosmotic (baroreceptor) stimulation of AVP release.

To further test this hypothesis, HWI was used to translocate peripheral fluid to the central blood volume in eight nonexcretor cirrhotic patients (36% of acute water load excreted) (44). Headout water immersion increased cardiac index, right atrial pressure, and capillary pulmonary wedge pressure and decreased systemic vascular resistance. Headout water immersion was associated with a diminution in AVP (1.0 ± 0.15 to 0.76 ± 0.08 pg/mL, $P < 0.05$) and with an increase in the percentage of water load excreted, which was inversely correlated with AVP levels ($r = 0.52$, $P < 0.05$) and directly correlated with right atrial pressure ($r = 0.74$, $P < 0.05$). Taken together, these observations are consistent with nonosmotic AVP release in cirrhosis.

Role of Vasopressin in the Renal Water Retention and Hyponatremia of Cirrhosis

Hyponatremia with impaired ability to excrete a water load occurs in a substantial number of patients with cirrhosis of the liver (274,302,313,314,323–329). It appears from previous studies that decompensated cirrhotic patients (i.e., those with ascites or edema) have an abnormal response to water administration, whereas cirrhotic patients without ascites or edema may excrete water normally (274,302,330). Although intrarenal mechanisms may contribute to this abnormal water retention (see the preceding), the mechanisms responsible for this defect in water excretion may also include nonosmotic stimulation of AVP and upregulation of the kidney water channel AQP2. In this regard, numerous abnormalities

encountered in cirrhosis, such as portal hypertension with increased splanchnic venous pooling, decreased total peripheral resistance, and diminished plasma oncotic pressure secondary to hypoalbuminemia, may all contribute to arterial underfilling and thus to baroreceptor-mediated nonosmotic AVP release.

A predominant role of AVP in the impairment of water excretion was demonstrated in four experimental models of altered liver function studied in our laboratory: (a) TIVC constriction in the dog as a model of hepatic congestion (171), (b) acute portal vein constriction in the dog as a model of portal hypertension (35), (c) chronic bile duct ligation in the rat as a model of obstructive jaundice (331), and (d) carbon tetrachloride (CCl_4)-induced liver disease in the rat as a model of chronic cirrhosis (332). In each case, however, there was also evidence that diminished fluid delivery to the distal diluting segment contributed to the abnormal water excretion. These observations in animals are consistent with the recent findings of Salerno and associates (333), who demonstrated a role for AVP in the renal water retention of some but not all of 19 cirrhotic patients studied during three separate maneuvers—60-degree leg elevation to expand central blood volume, 0.45% saline infusion to reduce plasma osmolality, and hypertonic sodium chloride injection to increase plasma osmolality. In the patients who were incapable of excreting the hypotonic saline load, the inability to improve solute-free water clearance was associated with high circulating AVP levels or with reduced distal delivery of the glomerular filtrate. This study also demonstrated a lower theoretical osmolar threshold for suppression of AVP release in the nonexcretor patients.

The administration of specific antagonists of the hydroosmotic effect of AVP to rats made cirrhotic after exposure to CCl_4 confirms that AVP hypersecretion is the predominant mechanism of the impairment of water excretion in experimental cirrhosis (334,335). Using the orally effective nonpeptide selective V_2-receptor AVP antagonist OPC-31260, Tsuboi and coworkers (335) normalized the defect in solute-free water excretion in this animal model of cirrhosis. Without the AVP antagonist, cirrhotic rats excreted 62.5% of a 30-mL/kg water load, whereas control animals excreted 102.1% ($P < 0.01$). Minimal urinary osmolality was 185.5 mOsm/kg H_2O in the cirrhotic rats, a value that was significantly greater than the minimal urinary osmolality of 125.5 mOsm/kg H_2O in the control rats ($P < 0.01$). In cirrhotic animals, oral administration of OPC-31260 (5 mg/kg of body weight) increased the percent water load excreted to 215.1% and decreased minimal urinary osmolality to 85.2 mOsm/kg H_2O ($P < 0.01$ for both, compared to pretreatment values), indicating that AVP was involved in the impaired water excretion in these animals.

Additional experimental data supporting a primary role for AVP in the impaired water excretion in cirrhosis comes from Fujita and coworkers (336). These investigators examined the effect of experimental cirrhosis on expression of the mRNA for the AVP-dependent collecting duct water channel, aquaporin-2, in the rat. Binding of AVP to the

V_2 receptor initiates a chain of intracellular signaling events that ultimately leads to the transient insertion of aquaporin-2 water channels into the apical membrane of collecting duct cells, thus rendering these cells permeable to water. Thus, a marker for the induction of these collecting duct water channels, such as expression of the aquaporin-2 mRNA, may serve as a biologic assay of AVP action in the collecting duct. In the cirrhotic rats studied by Fujita and coworkers (336), aquaporin-2 mRNA was markedly increased as compared to control animals. Moreover, an oral water load (30 mL/kg) did not reduce aquaporin-2 mRNA expression, but the blockade of AVP action by the V_2-receptor AVP antagonist OPC-31260 significantly diminished its expression in the cirrhotic animals. More recently, Fernandez-Llama and associates demonstrated an increase in aquaporin-2 trafficking to the apical membrane in rats with carbon tetrachloride-induced cirrhosis (337). This finding was accompanied by upregulation of aquaporin-1 in the proximal tubule, aquaporin-3 in the collecting duct basolateral membrane, and the Na-K-2Cl and NaCl cotransporters. In another study, renal expression of AQP2 in experimental cirrhosis owing to common bile duct ligation was associated with a decrease in aquaporin-2 despite water retention and hyponatremia (338). Studies in humans with cirrhosis, however, have demonstrated improved urinary dilution and solute-free water excretion with administration of a V_2 receptor antagonist (339). Thus, both experimental and clinical data suggest that AVP is a major determinant of the abnormality of water excretion observed in both experimental and clinical conditions associated with liver dysfunction.

In this regard, it is of interest that in nonexcretor cirrhotic patients, the severity of the defect in water excretion may have some prognostic significance. We prospectively examined two groups of nonexcretor cirrhotic patients (340). Group I patients, who excreted 25% or less of a water load, had 12 serious complications, including hepatorenal syndrome, hepatic encephalopathy, intractable ascites requiring a LeVeen shunt, and bacterial peritonitis, during a 36 patient-month observation period. By contrast, group II patients, who excreted more than 25% of a water load, had only five complications during a 225 patient-month observation period (340). These data suggest that cirrhotic patients with a very low water excretion capability have a poor prognosis. Prognostic factors in cirrhotic patients admitted to the hospital for the treatment of an episode of ascites also were studied by Llach and colleagues (341). In a series of 139 patients hospitalized between 1980 and 1985, mean arterial blood pressure and plasma norepinephrine concentrations were the variables that best predicted prognosis. Fernández-Esparrach and colleagues have recently developed and validated a regression model that predicts prognosis in cirrhotic patients with ascites (342). Predictive prognostic variables included diuresis after a water load, mean arterial pressure, Child-Pugh class, and serum creatinine. These findings suggest that impaired solute-free water excretion and abnormal renal function are important markers of early mortality. The utility of this model in the evaluation of candidates for liver transplantation remains to be proven.

In summary, like heart failure, baroreceptor activation of the three major neurohormonal vasoconstrictor systems is involved in the avid renal sodium and water retention of cirrhosis. Increased sympathetic nervous system activity in response to arterial underfilling also likely orchestrates the hormonal response to cirrhosis. Renal nerves, ANG II, aldosterone, and AVP may all play a role in the abnormal sodium and water retention of cirrhosis. Counterregulatory vasodilator substances may attenuate, to some degree, this neurohormonal vasoconstrictor activation (see the following).

Vasodilator Systems

Atrial Natriuretic Peptide in Cirrhosis

Some patients with cirrhosis exhibit elevated circulating ANP concentrations (343,344). However, the natriuretic effect of elevated endogenous and of exogenous ANP is blunted in patients with advanced cirrhosis (227,345). The possible mechanisms for ANP resistance in cirrhosis are identical to those in heart failure reviewed earlier. According to the diminished distal tubular sodium delivery hypothesis (Fig. 84-5) (11–17,346), arterial underfilling owing to peripheral vasodilation in cirrhosis results in renal vasoconstriction, decreased renal perfusion pressure, and activation of the sympathetic and renin–angiotensin systems. These renal hemodynamic and neurohormonal changes then decrease the GFR and increase proximal tubular sodium reabsorption, thereby resulting in diminished distal tubular sodium delivery, which impairs escape from the sodium-retaining effects of aldosterone and the natriuretic response to ANP. A report from Morali and colleagues (347) supports this hypothesis. In six of their 10 patients with cirrhosis and refractory ascites, high-dose mannitol, 80 g over 2 1/2-hours, produced a natriuresis, diuresis, and an increase in distal tubular sodium delivery, and restored partial renal responsiveness to infused ANP. However, in the responders, nearly half of the increase in urinary sodium excretion with ANP plus mannitol was attributable to mannitol alone. Moreover, compared to mannitol alone, there was no further increase in urinary volume excretion following the addition of ANP to mannitol. Thus, we examined the effects of a low-dose mannitol infusion, 12 g over 3 hours, on distal sodium delivery and urinary sodium and volume excretion in 12 patients with advanced decompensated cirrhosis (230). Distal tubular sodium delivery, as assessed by lithium clearance, was increased during the infusion of mannitol (13.8 ± 3.4 to 23.7 ± 5.7 mL/minute, $P < 0.05$) and during the ANP plus mannitol infusion (13.8 ± 3.4 to 28.5 ± 6.3 mL/minute, $P < 0.001$) in 6 patients, termed *responders*. Both responders and nonresponders were resistant to the natriuretic effect of ANP infused alone. Furthermore, mannitol alone did not produce an increase in urinary sodium excretion in any of the patients (responders or nonresponders). In responders, however, the mannitol-induced increase in distal tubular sodium

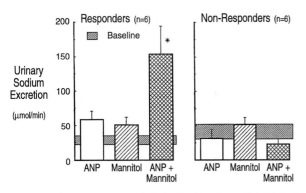

FIG. 84-11. Decompensated cirrhotics in whom distal tubular sodium delivery increases in response to mannitol (responders) exhibit a marked increase in urinary sodium excretion during treatment with mannitol plus atrial natriuretic peptide (ANP). *$P < 0.01$ versus baseline, ANP, mannitol, and nonresponders. (From: Abraham WT, et al. Reversal of atrial natriuretic peptide resistance by increasing distal tubular sodium delivery in patients with decompensated cirrhosis. *Hepatology* 1995;22:737, with permission.)

delivery produced a fivefold increase in urinary sodium excretion during the concomitant infusion of ANP (29 ± 6 to 154 ± 40 μmol/minute, $P < 0.01$) (Fig. 84-11). Similar increases in urinary cGMP excretion in responders and nonresponders confirmed the active biologic responsiveness of the renal ANP receptors in both groups of patients. These observations support the hypothesis that diminished distal tubular sodium delivery is a major factor contributing to ANP resistance in cirrhosis.

Evidence implicating renal nerves in the blunted natriuretic response to ANP may be found in studies of cirrhotic rats (348). In conscious control rats, ANP increased urine flow rate and urinary sodium excretion. In conscious cirrhotic rats, however, ANP had no effect on urine flow rate or urinary sodium excretion. Renal denervation reversed the blunted diuretic and natriuretic responses to ANP in the cirrhotic rats. Of interest, inhibition of the renin–angiotensin system with captopril had no effect on the diuretic or natriuretic responses to ANP in conscious control or cirrhotic rats. The authors concluded that increased renal sympathetic nerve activity, but not ANG II, mediates the blunted diuretic and natriuretic responses to ANP in conscious cirrhotic rats. This observation is also compatible with the diminished distal tubular sodium delivery hypothesis of ANP resistance in cirrhosis.

Role of Prostaglandins in Cirrhosis

Experiments have shown that prostaglandins with vasodilator properties are necessary to maintain renal blood flow and GFR in dogs with cirrhosis secondary to bile duct ligation (349). Similar conclusions about the importance of prostaglandins have been obtained in cirrhotic humans. Inhibition of prostaglandin synthesis in decompensated cirrhotic patients decreases renal blood flow, GFR, sodium excretion,

and solute-free water excretion and impairs the natriuretic response to furosemide or spironolactone (314,350). Infusion of PGE_1 reverses these diminutions in renal blood flow and GFR observed after prostaglandin inhibition (350). Inhibition of prostaglandin synthesis also could cause a syndrome that mimics hepatorenal syndrome (314). Moreover, vasodilating renal prostaglandins may play an important counterregulatory role in early or well-compensated cirrhosis. In 12 patients with biopsy-proved, ascites-free, Pugh grade A, alcoholic cirrhosis studied by Wong and coworkers (351), oral administration of 50 mg of indomethacin was followed by significant decreases in urinary excretion of both PGE_2 and $6ketoPGF_{1\alpha}$, GFR, renal blood flow, and urinary sodium and volume excretion. Of note, proximal tubular sodium reabsorption was substantially increased by indomethacin, as determined by the lithium clearance method. Thus, although inhibition of prostaglandin synthesis in cirrhotic patients also could have some beneficial effects, including decreases in PRA and plasma aldosterone and reversal of the vascular insensitivity to infused ANG II (352), these beneficial effects seem outweighed by the previously described adverse reactions of prostaglandin inhibition on renal blood flow, GFR, and sodium and water excretion. More recent research has focused on selective inhibition of the cyclooxygenase-2 (COX2) isoform. This isoform is induced by cytokines, mitogens, and endotoxin and is believed to account for increased prostaglandin release during inflammation. In contrast to nonselective cyclooxygenase inhibitors, COX2 inhibitors may not only decrease gastrointestinal complications (i.e., ulcers) but in cirrhosis may protect renal function. Recent studies in rats with carbon tetrachloride-induced cirrhosis support this idea (353). Nonselective cyclooxygenase inhibition with ketorolac was associated with significant decreases in urine volume and glomerular filtration rate, whereas selective COX2 inhibition did not produce any renal effects. In summary, in decompensated cirrhosis increases in prostaglandin synthesis could contribute to peripheral vasodilation and thus could be a factor in the arterial underfilling. Also, the enhanced intrarenal prostaglandin production could counteract the vasoconstrictive properties of renal nerve stimulation and circulating ANG II, norepinephrine, and AVP and thus may be an important factor in maintaining renal function.

Summary

Numerous afferent and efferent mechanisms are involved in the abnormal sodium and water excretion characteristic of patients with liver disease, and it now seems certain that these mechanisms are triggered by an arterial vasodilation-mediated arterial underfilling. Recent experimental data indicate that an overproduction of the endothelium-derived vasodilator nitric oxide plays a major role in the pathogenesis of the peripheral vasodilation of cirrhosis. The sympathetic nervous system, renin–angiotensin–aldosterone axis, and the nonosmotic release of AVP are the major effector components of this increased sodium and water reabsorption, which may also be modulated by the release of prostaglandins and natriuretic peptides. Other vasoconstrictor (e.g., endothelin) and vasodilator (e.g., kallikrein) substances may be implicated but data are currently lacking. In any event, a current understanding of these afferent and efferent mechanisms has implications for the treatment of cirrhosis.

Physiologic Basis for the Treatment of Sodium and Water Retention in Liver Disease

General Principles

In 1970, Shear and associates (354) measured ascitic fluid volume using the radioactive-iodinated serum albumin method. Patients with decompensated liver disease were studied during spontaneous diuresis and during the use of diuretic agents. Individual patients mobilized small amounts of ascitic fluid (300 mL/day) during spontaneous diuresis. Diuretic agents greatly exaggerated the disparity between the rates of ascitic and nonascitic fluid reabsorption that had been evident during spontaneous diuresis. With the use of diuretic agents, excretion of up to 4.7 kg of nonascitic fluid in 24 hours could be obtained, but ascitic absorption did not exceed 930 mL in 24 hours. From these results, it appears that ascitic fluid is a separate and relatively nonmobilizable compartment of ECF. Thus, it is essential that the nonedematous ascitic patient not be diuresed more than 0.5 kg in 24 hours. These findings were confirmed by other investigators (355,356).

Numerous investigators have shown that repeated large-volume paracentesis is a fast, effective, and safe therapy for ascites in patients with cirrhosis (166,357–360). The subsequent administration of diuretics avoids reaccumulation of ascites in the patients responding to these drugs. Of interest, contrary to the traditional concept of the potential danger of rapid and large paracentesis, the mobilization of ascites by paracentesis with the concomitant administration of intravenous albumin (8 g/L of ascites fluid removed) did not alter renal function or systemic hemodynamics, the latter being estimated either directly (by measuring plasma volume, cardiac output, or peripheral resistance) or indirectly (by measuring PRA, plasma norepinephrine, and plasma AVP concentrations) (360). Peritoneovenous (LeVeen) shunting is a reasonable therapy to relieve ascites in appropriately selected patients. Because of the frequency and severity of the complications, however, the procedure should be reserved for patients in whom more conservative forms of medical therapy are ineffective (361,362). According to Epstein (361), large-volume paracentesis, carefully performed, may prove to be preferable in many patients with refractory ascites. A recent multicenter randomized trial (363) compared large-volume paracentesis plus intravenous albumin with peritoneovenous shunting in patients with refractory ascites. During the first hospitalization, ascites was removed in all 41 patients in the paracentesis group and in 44 of the 48 patients in the peritoneovenous shunt group. The duration of this first hospitalization was longer (19 versus 11 days) in the LeVeen shunt group but there were no significant differences in the number of patients who had complications or died. During follow-up, 37 patients in each group were hospitalized again. The number of rehospitalizations was higher in the paracentesis group. Survival was similar in both groups. Ginès and colleagues (363) concluded that the LeVeen shunt and paracentesis are equally effective in relieving refractory ascites. The high occlusion rate of the shunt, however, has substantially decreased the use of this procedure.

Recently, the transjugular intrahepatic portosystemic shunt (TIPS) procedure was evaluated as a therapy for refractory ascites (364,365). The TIPS procedure and its efficacy and safety in the treatment of variceal bleeding are extensively reviewed elsewhere (366). Ochs and colleagues (364) performed the TIPS procedure in 50 of 62 consecutive patients with cirrhosis and medically refractory ascites. The shunt was successfully placed in all 50 patients, substantially reducing the pressure gradient between the portal vein and the inferior vena cava by an average of 63%. Forty-six patients (92%) responded to the procedure with either complete (N = 37) or partial (N = 9) resolution of the ascites. All of the patients who responded required low doses of diuretics to maintain their responses and treat peripheral edema. Of note, the TIPS was associated with an improvement in renal function at 6 months, as demonstrated by a significant fall in the serum creatinine (1.5 ± 0.9 to 0.9 ± 0.3 mg/dL, $P < 0.01$) and improvement in the creatinine clearance (41 ± 29 to 88 ± 62 mL/minute, $P < 0.05$). Whereas the procedure significantly lowered portal vein pressures in these patients, the effect of the TIPS on systemic hemodynamics and neurohormones was not determined in this study. Thus, the mechanism of the improved renal function cannot be fully ascertained. A more recent randomized trial by Rossle and associates compared large volume paracentesis with the TIPS procedure in 60 patients with alcoholic cirrhosis with ascites that was either refractory to diuretic therapy or recurrent (365). These investigators found that the rate of survival without liver transplantation was improved in patients who underwent the TIPS procedure. Moreover, significantly more patients in the TIPS group demonstrated resolution of ascites. It is important to note that these patients primarily had Child-Pugh class B liver disease and good renal function. Several investigators have reported that the hyperdynamic circulation characteristic of cirrhosis is exaggerated following the TIPS procedure (367–369). These effects appear to persist up to 3 months following the procedure, with cardiac output and systemic vascular resistance returning to pre-TIPS values by 1 year following the procedure.

General Principles for Therapy in Cirrhosis

A careful evaluation for reversible factors leading to hepatic dysfunction should be undertaken, and active diuretic therapy should be delayed until the clinical and biochemical stability of the patient is determined. This latter recommendation should be underlined in patients with acute alcoholic hepatitis. The goals of diuresis should be a daily weight loss of 1 to 2 pounds in patients with ascites and edema and 0.5 to 1.0 pound in patients with ascites but no edema. Large-volume paracentesis with strict aseptic conditions using a small 18-gauge catheter to avoid postparacentesis leak and with concomitant intravenous administration of albumin comprise an alternative treatment. The endpoint of therapy should be maximum patient comfort with minimal drug-induced complications. As noted previously, the total amount of ascitic fluid can be removed in one setting without complications if albumin 8 gm/L ascites is replaced. Albumin may be replaced by less expensive colloid if ascites removal is less than 5 L. Patients who demonstrate a rise in plasma renin with paracentesis in the absence of colloid replacement have a worse prognosis (358). Although paracentesis to treat ascites in cirrhotic patients has been shown to be associated with fewer and shorter hospitalizations than diuretic treatment, survival is not different (358). There does not appear to be any benefit of the LeVeen shunt over repeated paracentesis on total duration of hospitalization or mortality in cirrhotic patients (363). The vasopressin V_1 receptor agonist terlipressin may be beneficial in the treatment of hepatorenal syndrome and acute variceal bleeding (370–372). A recent study using albumin and terlipressin infusion was shown to improve renal function over a 15-day period in patients with hepatorenal syndrome (372). Such therapy is proposed to delay the need for liver transplantation. Whether NOS inhibition in patients with cirrhosis will have a beneficial effect, as has been shown in experimental cirrhosis (292,293,295), remains to be studied.

Moderate dietary sodium restriction remains the cornerstone of therapy, as 5% to 15% of decompensated cirrhotics can be successfully managed by a trial of bed rest and moderate dietary sodium restriction (373,374). Occasionally, slight liberalization of sodium intake at the expense of an increased dosage of diuretics and the maintenance of some residual ascites may be recommended in selected patients. The TIPS procedure may provide additional benefit in some patients with refractory ascites or the functional renal failure of advanced cirrhosis. An extensive review of the management of patients with cirrhosis and ascites has been published by Arroyo and colleagues (375).

Pharmacologic Agents

We recommend the use of diuretic agents to treat moderate to severe amounts of ascites in order to improve the decompensated cirrhotic patient's comfort and physical activities. Furthermore, the presence of ascites per se could induce severe potential complications. In this regard, it is recognized that ascites could increase portal pressure and also induce gastroesophageal reflux; both of these effects could facilitate bleeding esophageal varices. Spontaneous bacterial peritonitis also may occur in the presence of ascites.

We therefore propose that it is justified to hospitalize decompensated cirrhotic patients to perform large-volume repeated paracentesis with albumin infusions and, if indicated, to initiate a low-sodium diet and diuretic treatment. Spironolactone and spironolactone plus furosemide are the most widely used diuretic regimens in patients with decompensated liver disease (376,377). These diuretics decrease ascites and peripheral edema in the majority of patients treated. High-dose spironolactone (300 to 600 mg/day) used alone is almost uniformly effective in cirrhotic patients with relatively refractory ascites (378).

Prior to the large-volume paracentesis era, the efficacy of three commonly used diuretic regimens in the treatment of ascites was compared. Ninety patients were randomized to three treatment groups: sequential spironolactone (spironolactone followed by furosemide if necessary), combination treatment (spironolactone and furosemide together), and furosemide (furosemide given alone) (376). All diuretics were begun at a low dose by mouth, and the dosage was increased until a 0.4- to 0.8-kg daily diuresis was achieved. All three regimens produced a similar rate of diuresis, but larger doses of furosemide were necessary to achieve a significant diuresis in the furosemide-alone group. The incidence of encephalopathy, hepatorenal syndrome, and marked electrolyte abnormalities was comparable in the three treatment groups. Thus, this study clearly demonstrated the beneficial effect of spironolactone alone and spironolactone plus furosemide in cirrhotic ascites. Of interest, similar results were more recently obtained by Pérez-Ayuso and coworkers (377).

Treatment of Hyponatremia

Most cirrhotic patients appear to tolerate mild chronic hyponatremia without symptoms, and mild to moderate water restriction (<500 to 1,000 mL/day) usually results in either stabilization or a slight increase in plasma sodium. Demeclocycline, a pharmacologic agent that inhibits the renal hydroosmotic effect of AVP, may result in brisk decreases in GFR with potentially lethal side effects (379–382). In our opinion, this drug should not be used to treat the hyponatremia associated with decompensated liver disease. As noted, the use of V_2 receptor antagonists in animals and humans with cirrhosis is associated with increased urine volume and improved urinary dilution. These agents can improve hyponatremia in animals with experimentally induced syndrome of inappropriate antidiuretic hormone (SIADH) secretion and cirrhosis (336). Studies are ongoing to evaluate the role of chronic oral nonpeptide V_2 antagonists in the treatment of hyponatremia in patients with cirrhosis.

THE NEPHROTIC SYNDROME

In contrast to heart failure and cirrhosis of the liver, in which the kidneys are structurally normal, the nephrotic state is characterized by intrinsic renal damage often but not always with a substantial decrease in renal function. This parenchymal damage may be responsible for the elevated arterial blood pressure observed in some patients with the nephrotic

TABLE 84-3. *Similarities and contrasting clinical and biochemical features between "nonexcretor" cardiac, cirrhotic, and nephrotic patients*

	Cardiac failure patients ($N = 17$)	Cirrhotic patients ($N = 19$)	Nephrotic patients ($N = 16$)
Mean arterial blood pressure (mm Hg)	85.8 ± 2.7	86.3 ± 1.9	97.0 ± 3.0
Glomerular filtration rate (mL/min/1.73 m^2)	55.4 ± 4.9	70.0 ± 7.3	72.6 ± 7.0
Percent of water load excreted	31.4 ± 3.2	29.0 ± 3.4	43.3 ± 6.0
Urinary sodium excretion (mEq/5 hr)	5.5 ± 1.4	2.5 ± 0.7	13.5 ± 3.4
Plasma sodium (mEq/L)	133.5 ± 1.0	132.6 ± 1.4	139.8 ± 1.2
Minimal urinary osmolality during the water load (mOsm/kg H$_2$O)	371 ± 36	243 ± 37	205 ± 45

Patients were usually given a 50-mEq sodium diet for 3 days to 1 week prior to the water load procedure. Cardiac patients received a water load of 15 mL/kg of body weight; cirrhotic and nephrotic patients received a water load of 20 mL/kg of body weight. Most of the cirrhotic patients and all the nephrotic patients were ad libitum water intake; cardiac failure patients were limited to 800 mL of free water intake per 24 hours.

From Bichet DG, van Putten VJ, Schrier RW. Potential role of increased sympathetic activity in impaired sodium and water excretion in cirrhosis. *N Engl J Med* 1982;307:1552; Bichet D, Manzini C. Role of vasopressin (AVP) in the abnormal water excretion in nephrotic patients. *Kidney Int* 1984;25:160A, with permission.

syndrome. Other contrasting features among these three classic edematous states are described in Table 84-3, in which nonexcretor edematous patients with cardiac failure, liver disease, and nephrotic syndrome are compared. As shown in Table 84-3, nephrotic patients were characterized by a relatively higher arterial blood pressure, a higher GFR, and less impairment in sodium and water excretion.

The state of arterial filling and the pathogenesis of the renal sodium and water retention in patients with the nephrotic syndrome remains controversial (383). Two contrasting hypotheses have been proposed to explain the mechanism of the abnormal sodium and water reabsorption seen in nephrotic syndrome. In nephrotic syndrome, usually defined as the combination of a 24-hour urinary protein excretion in excess of 3.5 g/1.73 m^2 of body surface area, hypoalbuminemia, hyperlipidemia, and edema, the underfill theory of edema formation is as follows. Proteinuria results in hypoalbuminemia with decreased oncotic pressure causing fluid loss from the intravascular space, and reduced plasma and blood volume with resultant activation of homeostatic responses involving the sympathetic nervous system and the renin–angiotensin–aldosterone axis. This hypovolemia may also contribute to a reduction in GFR.

In contrast to this classic theory of edema formation in nephrotic syndrome, it has also been documented (384–386) that many patients with the nephrotic syndrome who retain sodium and water show elevated plasma volume and arterial blood pressure, whereas PRA and plasma aldosterone concentration are not elevated or are even decreased. In these patients, the overfill theory of edema formation might predominate, and the abnormal sodium and water retention might be related to an intrinsic renal abnormality associated with the renal disease. Of interest, it was originally thought that this hypervolemic state was a characteristic of patients with nephrotic syndrome and abnormal renal histology (273,387),

but it has been recognized that this hypervolemic state may also occur in patients with minimal change nephrotic syndrome (384–386,390). It is important, however, to note that the response to upright posture may be necessary to detect differences in plasma volume (see the following).

In the remainder of this chapter, we describe the potential afferent and efferent mechanisms of sodium and water reabsorption in the nephrotic syndrome. The arguments in favor of the underfill and overfill theories of edema formation in nephrotic syndrome are reviewed. In fact, both the underfill and overfill theories may be implicated, depending on the subset of nephrotic syndrome patients studied (i.e., hypovolemic versus hypervolemic). In the hypovolemic subset, as in heart failure and cirrhosis, activation of neurohormonal vasoconstrictor systems may in part mediate the renal sodium and water retention, whereas in the hypervolemic subset, intrarenal mechanisms also may be implicated. Finally, specific therapeutic modalities are discussed.

Afferent Mechanisms for Renal Sodium and Water Retention in the Nephrotic Syndrome

The Underfill Theory

The evidence supporting the traditional underfill view of edema formation in nephrotic syndrome includes the following factors. Plasma volume may be decreased in some nephrotic patients in the absence of diuretic therapy (389–393). Moreover, systemic arterial hypotension and diminished cardiac output, sometimes correctable by plasma volume expansion, have been observed in some patients with nephrosis (394–396). In addition, some nephrotic patients have "humoral markers" of arterial underfilling such as elevated plasma levels of renin, aldosterone, and catecholamines, suggesting a volume-contracted state (390,397,398). Finally,

HWI and intravascular infusion of albumin, maneuvers that increase plasma volume, may result in substantial increases in GFR and fractional excretion of sodium chloride and water in these patients (389,393,399). Of interest, the natriuresis observed during HWI was found to be directly related to the patient's estimated plasma volume (399).

Usberti and coworkers (400) described two groups of nephrotic syndrome patients distinguished on the basis of their plasma albumin concentrations. Patients in group 1 had a plasma albumin concentration of less than 1.7 g/dL associated with low blood volumes and plasma ANP levels, elevated plasma ANG II concentrations, and increased proximal tubular reabsorption of sodium (determined by lithium clearance). In contrast, group 2 patients with a plasma albumin concentration greater than 1.7 g/dL exhibited normal blood volumes and plasma hormone concentrations. In all patients blood volume was positively correlated with the plasma albumin concentration, and PRA was inversely correlated with both blood volume and plasma albumin. Of note, GFR was not different between group 1 and group 2 patients (100 ± 25 versus 101 ± 22 mL/minute, not significant), whereas urinary sodium excretion was substantially lower in group 1 patients (4.88 ± 5.53 versus 29.9 ± 9.3 mEq/4 hours, P < 0.001). Moreover, the acute expansion of blood volume in group 1 patients normalized PRA, plasma ANG II and aldosterone concentrations, fractional sodium excretion, and lithium clearance, while increasing circulating ANP concentrations. Taken together, all of these observations (389–400) support the traditional underfill view of the pathogenesis of edema formation in nephrotic syndrome.

The Overfill Theory

Dorhout-Mees and coworkers (384–386,388) and Meltzer and associates (387) challenged this traditional theory. Dorhout-Mees and coworkers (388) initially studied a group of 10 adult patients with 13 episodes of minimal change nephrotic syndrome. The patients were selected for the study because of increased blood volume and blood pressure. Each patient was studied prior to and following prednisone-induced remission. After remission, blood pressure fell in 12 cases, plasma volume fell in 10 cases, and PRA increased in eight cases. If total plasma volume and PRA are reliable indices of arterial circulatory integrity, these data could constitute powerful arguments against the traditional underfill theory of edema formation in the nephrotic syndrome. In contrast to this study, in which all patients with increased blood volume had minimal lesion nephrotic syndrome, Meltzer and coworkers (387) found that their hypervolemic patients tended to have more severe glomerular involvement, lower GFR, and hypertension.

The potential problems associated with plasma volume measurements in nephrotic syndrome patients have been extensively studied (384). Most investigators now normalize their plasma and blood volume values for lean body mass, and the dry weight of the patients is measured by diuresing them to an edema-free state shortly after plasma volume and blood volume are measured (384–388,401). No correction is needed for an increased albumin disappearance rate from the vascular tree (402). In addition to these measurements, hypertension and low PRA, two indices suggesting volume expansion, have been frequently observed in patients with nephrotic syndrome (387,388,398). As described, hypoalbuminemia in animal studies as well as in patients with analbuminemia does not necessarily lead to edema formation (6). Finally, it is important to note that a low filtration fraction is often observed in nephrotic patients either with minimal lesions or with histologically defined glomerular lesions (385). This is of interest because arterial underfilling usually leads to renal hypoperfusion with a relatively well-maintained GFR and thus to an increase in filtration fraction. Taken together, these observations are compatible with the overfill view of edema formation in the nephrotic syndrome.

Some explanations appear tenable in trying to reconcile the underfill and overfill theories of nephrotic edema formation (383). The method of plasma volume measurement must be considered. An analysis of 217 nephrotic patients from 10 studies found that only 25% had expanded plasma volumes, whereas 33% had reduced plasma volumes and 42% normal plasma volumes (384). The variability of current techniques for plasma volume measurement is ±10%; thus, plasma volume measurement may not be sufficiently sensitive to distinguish between underfill and overfill states. Moreover, it is important to recognize that the afferent stimulus for edema formation is likely to be a dynamic process (403). Most plasma and blood volume studies have been performed during the maintenance phase of edema after the patient has retained significant sodium and water and reached a new steady state of sodium balance. Thus, these normal values do not preclude a role for a contracted plasma or blood volume in the initiating phase of edema formation. As early as 1963, Eisenberg (404) compared plasma volume measured during the recumbent and standing positions in nephrotic patients and normal individuals. In the standing position, there was a 7% fall in plasma volume in control subjects and a 15% to 20% decrease in nephrotic patients, thereby demonstrating a dynamic process even in the maintenance phase of edema formation. Results of studies indeed favor the dynamic nature of edema formation in the nephrotic syndrome. Serial measurements of plasma volume, PRA, and plasma aldosterone were made during the edema-forming stage, the stage of diuresis, and the stage of remission in 11 patients with steroid-responsive minimal change nephrotic syndrome (390). Of interest, plasma volume decreased significantly at the edema-forming stage and increased during the stage of diuresis. Also, an inverse correlation was obtained between plasma volume and PRA. It is thus possible that the renin–angiotensin–aldosterone system may be a compensatory mechanism for hypovolemia in the edema-forming stage but has less importance in the chronic compensated stage of edema.

In summary, it is clear that the precise afferent stimulus of edema formation in nephrotic syndrome cannot be stated with certainty. However, it seems that edema in these patients frequently can not be explained entirely by intravascular hypovolemia. Furthermore, a "nephritic" or intrarenal mechanism, may be important in sodium retention not only in nephrotic syndrome with histologic glomerular lesions but also in minimal change nephrotic syndrome (385,386).

Efferent Mechanisms for the Renal Sodium and Water Retention of the Nephrotic Syndrome

Nephron Sites of Sodium and Water Retention

Micropuncture Studies

The nephron site of enhanced renal sodium and water retention in the nephrotic syndrome has been studied predominantly in animal models of glomerulonephritis. Bernard and collaborators (405) used micropuncture and clearance methodology to study the site of sodium retention in saline-loaded rats with autologous immune complex nephritis. These rats developed heavy proteinuria, hypoalbuminemia, and hypercholesterolemia. Histopathologic examination of kidneys from these animals revealed slight thickening of the basement membranes; uniform finely granular deposits of immunoglobulin, IgG, and complement distributed along the basement membranes of all glomeruli; and electron-dense subepithelial deposits. These findings are similar to those observed in human idiopathic membranous nephropathy. Arterial blood pressure, hematocrit, GFR, and renal plasma flow were comparable in control and experimental animals. Proximal sodium reabsorption was actually decreased in the nephrotic rats (35% versus 44%). Absolute sodium reabsorption along the loop of Henle and in the distal convoluted tubule was comparable in nephrotic and control animals. In spite of comparable or greater sites of sodium delivery beyond the late distal convoluted tubule, the fractional excretion of sodium was significantly lower in nephrotic (2.2%) than control (4.0%) animals. From these results, the authors concluded that nephron sites beyond the late distal convoluted tubule were responsible for the enhanced sodium reabsorption observed in this model of nephrotic syndrome. In this regard, Sonnenberg suggested that the collecting duct may be the nephron site concerned with final adjustments in renal sodium excretion (406). Alternatively, it remains possible that enhanced sodium reabsorption by deep nephrons (not accessible to micropuncture) also could contribute to the diminished sodium excretion. It should also be noted that in the experiments of Bernard and coworkers (405) the rats studied were markedly volume expanded; their conclusions thus may not clarify the mechanism of sodium retention in the hydropenic state.

Results different from those reported by Bernard and colleagues (405) were reported by Kuroda and coworkers utilizing a rat nephrotoxic serum model of nephrotic syndrome (407). In this model, proteinuria, hypoalbuminemia, and hypercholesterolemia also occurred. Histologic examination of the kidneys revealed mild glomerular hypercellularity, widely dilated proximal tubules, diffuse uniform glomerular linear immunofluorescence, and electron-dense subepithelial deposits. In contrast to the previous study (405), the animals were more actively retaining sodium. In micropuncture studies, single-nephron GFR was decreased, and the percentage of filtered water reabsorbed prior to late proximal and distal tubular convolutions was increased in the nephrotic rats. In addition, high proximal intratubular pressures were measured. From this study (407) and the study of Bernard and coworkers (405), it is clear that the nephron site of enhanced sodium reabsorption in nephrotic syndrome may vary, depending on the nature of the renal lesion and the stage of edema formation.

Ichikawa and coworkers (408) studied a unilateral version of the model of aminonucleoside-induced nephrosis in the rat and showed that proteinuria and diminished urinary sodium excretion were confined to the kidney treated with the puromycin aminonucleoside. A reduction of the glomerular capillary ultrafiltration coefficient was the major determinant of diminished single-nephron GFR in the superficial nephrons studied. Also, the absolute rate of reabsorption of sodium in the superficial proximal tubule was decreased on the affected side. Assuming that superficial nephrons are representative of the entire nephron population, it was concluded that renal sodium retention in this model of nephrotic syndrome was mainly owing to intrarenal factor(s) acting beyond the proximal convoluted tubule. Similar results were obtained when kidneys were taken from nephrotic rats (puromycin aminonucleoside) and studied over a range of perfusion pressures using the isolated perfused kidney technique (409). When perfused with medium containing 6.7 g of albumin per deciliter, the nephrotic kidneys performed differently from control kidneys, with a reduction of sodium excretion at all pressures. Renal vascular resistance, inulin clearance, fractional sodium excretion, and fractional lithium excretion were also reduced. When kidneys were perfused without oncotic agents, the differences between nephrotic and control kidneys remained. Also, captopril had no effect on the sodium retention or vascular resistance of nephrotic kidneys (409). Finally, the exact site within the distal nephron where increased sodium reabsorption takes place in nephrotic rats is not known, as puromycin-injected rats with a structurally altered inner renal medulla induced by bromoethylamine hydrobromide still demonstrated impaired sodium excretion (410).

Clearance Studies

Clearance studies have been undertaken in nephrotic patients in an attempt to clarify the nephron site of enhanced sodium and water reabsorption (386,411,412). These studies were undertaken in patients with a wide variety of primary renal diseases and GFRs. In 1979, Usberti and colleagues (413) measured tubular reabsorption of glucose in 21 patients with glomerulonephritis. Tubular glucose reabsorption was used as a marker of proximal tubular sodium reabsorption. The threshold for glucose reabsorption was reduced in the 10 nephrotic patients with edema, suggesting diminished proximal tubular reabsorption. In studies undertaken in five nephrotic patients, a similar conclusion was reached by Grausz and colleagues (411). In these clearance studies, blockade of sodium reabsorption in the distal nephron with ethacrynic acid and chlorothiazide was used to assess proximal sodium reabsorption. Proximal sodium reabsorption was lower in the nephrotic patients than in normal and in cirrhotic patients. On the other hand, the more recent study of Usberti and colleagues (400), using the more precise technique of lithium clearance, demonstrated increased proximal tubular sodium reabsorption in nephrotic syndrome patients with low serum albumin concentrations and blood volumes and elevated PRA.

Gur and coworkers (412) used maximal solute-free water clearance as a marker of distal sodium chloride reabsorption in pediatric patients. Their data, however, are inconclusive because secretion of AVP was not maximally suppressed during their experiments. More recently, Koomans et al. (386) also performed clearance studies in 10 patients with nephrotic syndrome before and after a single infusion of 75 g of albumin. Proximal fractional sodium chloride reabsorption was elevated before ($95 \pm 1.5\%$) and decreased after ($93 \pm 1.7\%$) the infusion. Distal fractional sodium chloride reabsorption was also elevated before ($93 \pm 6.4\%$) but was unaltered after the albumin infusion ($93 \pm 5.6\%$).

In summary, it appears from experimental and clinical studies that distal nephron sites are involved in avid sodium and water retention in the nephrotic state. However, it is likely that increased proximal tubular sodium reabsorption also may be operative in selected cases, depending on the nature of the underlying renal disease and the phase of sodium retention. Distal sodium reabsorption may be secondary to an intrinsic defect independent of intravascular hypovolemia, as suggested by the results from the unilateral aminonucleoside model. Nevertheless, in some nephrotic syndrome patients, the distal and possibly proximal sodium and water reabsorption may be owing to neurohormonal activation.

Mechanisms of Enhanced Tubular Sodium
and Water Reabsorption

Several studies have been undertaken to identify the mechanism underlying enhanced renal tubular sodium and water reabsorption in the nephrotic syndrome. Although a reduced GFR is frequently observed in nephrotic patients, many nephrotic patients with a normal GFR avidly retain sodium and water. Thus, factors in addition to a reduced filtered load of sodium are involved in most patients. However, the presence of a marked reduction in GFR often is associated with the most profound sodium retention in patients with nephrotic syndrome (387,414).

Peritubular physical forces (oncotic and hydrostatic pressures) are believed to exert a modulating influence on renal sodium and water reabsorption in the proximal tubule. On the other hand, the high renal plasma flow, normal renal vascular resistance, and diminished filtration fraction frequently observed in patients with nephrotic syndrome (385) suggest that factors other than peritubular physical forces are responsible for enhanced tubular sodium reabsorption. Several lines of evidence indicate a role for neurohormonal activation.

Vasoconstrictor Systems

The Sympathetic Nervous System
in the Nephrotic Syndrome

Many patients with nephrotic syndrome exhibit elevated peripheral venous plasma norepinephrine concentrations (398), a finding consistent with activation of the sympathetic nervous system and arterial underfilling in these patients. Confirmatory evidence of adrenergic activation and arterial underfilling in nephrotic syndrome patients may be found in a report from our laboratory (415). We assessed sympathetic nervous system activity by determining plasma norepinephrine spillover and clearance rates using the whole body steady-state radionuclide tracer method in six edematous patients with the nephrotic syndrome and in six normal control subjects in the supine position. Mean creatinine clearances and serum creatinine concentrations were normal in both nephrotic syndrome patients and control subjects. However, the nephrotic syndrome patients exhibited significant hypoalbuminemia (2.0 ± 0.4 versus 3.8 ± 0.1 g/dL, $P < 0.01$). The supine plasma norepinephrine level was elevated in the patients with the nephrotic syndrome as compared with the control subjects; in nephrotic syndrome patients, the spillover rate of norepinephrine was markedly increased (0.30 ± 0.07 versus 0.13 ± 0.02 μg/minute per m^2, $P < 0.05$), whereas the norepinephrine clearance rate was comparable to that in the normal subjects (2.60 ± 0.29 versus 2.26 ± 0.27 L/minute, not significant). Of note, PRA and plasma aldosterone, AVP, and ANP concentrations were not different in the nephrotic syndrome patients compared with control subjects. These findings indicate that the sympathetic nervous system is activated in patients with the nephrotic syndrome prior to a significant fall in GFR or a marked activation of either the renin–angiotensin–aldosterone system or the nonosmotic release of AVP. Furthermore, these data support the presence of arterial underfilling in these patients with the nephrotic syndrome. Although the role of the adrenergic nervous system in the sodium and water retention of nephrosis remains to be defined, the observation that renal denervation restores renal ANP responsiveness in experimental nephrotic syndrome demonstrates the potential influence of renal nerves on proximal tubular sodium reabsorption in the nephrotic syndrome (132) (see the following).

The Renin–Angiotensin–Aldosterone System
in the Nephrotic Syndrome

A role for the renin–angiotensin–aldosterone humoral axis in the pathogenesis of nephrotic sodium retention remains controversial. Early work in this area strongly suggested a pathogenetic role for aldosterone in nephrotic edema (416,417). In rats made nephrotic with aminonucleoside, Tobian and coworkers (417) found an increase in juxtaglomerular cell granularity during sodium retention. Moreover, Kalant and coworkers (416) found that adrenalectomy prevented the sodium retention of aminonucleoside nephrosis. However, marked saline loading of these adrenalectomized nephrotic animals did result in edema formation (416). Also, as described earlier in this chapter, sodium retention in aminonucleoside-induced nephrotic syndrome in the rat can occur secondary to intrarenal factors (408). Taken together, these experimental observations suggest a pathogenetic role for aldosterone as well as aldosterone-independent factors in experimental nephrotic edema.

Numerous studies have measured components of the renin–angiotensin–aldosterone system in nephrotic humans (57,100,386–388,390,403). These studies were undertaken in heterogeneous patient populations at a variety of stages of nephrotic syndrome, and a wide range of plasma hormone values varying from very high to very low were observed. Of interest, in 70 observations made in patients with nephrotic syndrome on a low-sodium diet there was a striking absence of correlation between the plasma albumin level and PRA or between blood volume and PRA. However, there was a significant negative correlation between plasma aldosterone concentration and sodium excretion ($R = 0.52$, $P < 0.001$) (385). In the aforementioned study from Usberti and coworkers (393); however, PRA and plasma aldosterone concentrations were correlated with plasma albumin concentrations, blood volume, and urinary sodium excretion in the hypovolemic subjects, whereas changes in the urinary excretion of aldosterone predicted the renal response in the nephrotic syndrome patients with normal blood volumes. The determinant of the stimulation of PRA in nephrotic patients is unclear. Similar conclusions were also obtained by other investigators; in spite of similar plasma volumes, PRA and plasma aldosterone were found to be significantly greater in nephrotic patients with minimal change disease than those in patients with other renal histopathology (397). It is thus possible that a specific intrarenal factor, independent of circulating blood volume, may stimulate the renin–angiotensin–aldosterone system in some nephrotic patients.

Brown and coworkers (418,419) and others (420) questioned the importance of aldosterone in the sodium retention of the nephrotic syndrome. This assertion is supported by studies involving the administration of either the angiotensin antagonist saralasin or the ACE inhibitor captopril to patients with the nephrotic syndrome. In the nephrotic syndrome patients studied by Brown and coworkers (418,419), plasma aldosterone concentrations were pharmacologically suppressed by means of the ACE inhibitor, with no associated increase in urinary sodium excretion. However, because blood pressure fell in these patients, the ACE inhibition must have reduced plasma ANG II concentrations, resulting in a decrease in renal perfusion pressure. This effect could have obscured the benefit of a decrease in plasma aldosterone concentration on urinary sodium excretion. A recent study by Shapiro and colleagues (421) supported this interpretation because the more specific inhibitor of aldosterone, spironolactone, allowed sodium-retaining patients with the nephrotic syndrome to attain sodium balance.

Arginine Vasopressin in the Nephrotic Syndrome

As described in Table 84-3 and in contrast to the two previously described clinical edematous entities (i.e., heart failure and decompensated cirrhosis), the nephrotic syndrome is less frequently associated with hyponatremia. In fact, serum sodium concentration is usually normal unless it is influenced by vigorous diuretic measures or an acute water load (388,411,422,423). Furthermore, in nephrotic patients, high serum lipid levels may induce pseudohyponatremia unless serum sodium concentration is measured by a direct ion-specific electrode (424). Nevertheless, abnormal water excretion was clearly demonstrated by Gur and colleagues (412) in six nephrotic children; their solute-free water clearance during water loading was only 0.9 ± 0.8 mL/minute compared with 3.6 ± 0.6 mL/minute after remission of their disease. Because HWI induces an increase in free water clearance in patients with nephrotic syndrome (389,399), this improvement may be secondary to the suppression of the nonosmotic release of AVP. Alternatively, HWI might improve intrarenal hemodynamics and increase the amount of solute-free water delivered to the distal site of the nephron, thereby improving water excretion. Usberti and coworkers (393) studied 16 nephrotic patients and 13 normal control subjects in basal conditions and following a water load or isoosmotic blood volume expansion with a 20% albumin infusion. The nephrotic patients had a delayed water excretion, and their plasma AVP levels were not suppressed by the water load procedure. Of interest, plasma AVP was inversely correlated with blood volume in nephrotic patients but not in normal control subjects. Furthermore, in the nephrotic patients the expansion of blood volume with 20% albumin, or HWI, was effective in reducing plasma levels of AVP and in promoting a water diuresis (393,425). Pedersen and coworkers (423) administered an oral water load of 20 mL/kg of body weight to 17 patients with nephrotic syndrome and 15 healthy control subjects. Creatinine clearance and the maximum increase in solute-free water clearance were significantly correlated in patients with nephrotic syndrome as well as in control subjects. Plasma AVP was reduced in both groups during water loading, but AVP was clearly elevated in nephrotic syndrome patients when compared with the control subjects both before and during the water load. The study by Shapiro and associates (414) also showed a close correlation between decrements in GFR and water excretion during a water load in nephrotic patients.

Bichet and Manzini also studied 24 consecutive stable adult patients with nephrotic syndrome (422). Of these 24 patients who received a 20 mL/kg water load, 16 displayed abnormal water excretion (nonexcretors, group I) as they excreted 43% ± 6% of the water load in 5 hours and had a minimal urinary osmolality of 205 ± 49 mOsm/kg H_2O. Eight patients (excretors, group II) had normal water excretion as they excreted 97 ± 5% of the water load in 5 hours and had a minimum urinary osmolality of 61 ± 4 mOsm/kg H_2O. Basal plasma sodium concentration and effective plasma osmolality were comparable in groups I and II (139.8 ± 1.2 versus 139.7 ± 0.5 mEq/L and 274 ± 2 versus 273 ± 1.2 mOsm/kg H_2O, respectively). Basal supine, upright, and mean plasma AVP values after the water load were significantly higher in group I than in group II (4.4 ± 1.0 versus 1.4 ± 0.3, $P < 0.01$; 9.3 ± 2.9 versus 1.8 ± 0.5, $P < 0.025$; and 2.9 ± 0.5 versus 1.25 ± 0.2 pg/mL, $P < 0.025$, respectively). Nonexcretor patients also had more urinary protein loss (12.4 versus 6.5 g/24 hours, $P < 0.05$) and a lower GFR (72.6 ± 7 versus 106 ± 5 mL/minute per 1.73 m², $P < 0.005$). Group I patients were also characterized by a lower fractional excretion of sodium (0.5 ± 0.1 versus 0.8 ± 0.1, $P < 0.05$) and higher PRA (3.4 versus 1.9 ng/mL per hours, $P < 0.025$), plasma aldosterone (15.5 versus 8.8 ng/dL, $P < 0.005$), plasma free norepinephrine (288 ± 48 versus 181 ± 50 pg/mL, $P < 0.005$), and plasma conjugated norepinephrine levels (2038 ± 564 versus 510 ± 93 pg/mL, $P < 0.02$) (385).

Analysis of these studies, therefore, indicates that the impaired water excretion in nephrotic patients may be related both to intrarenal factors, involving a fall in GFR and diminished distal fluid delivery, and to extrarenal factors, which primarily involve the nonosmotic release of AVP. In this regard, Pyo and associates (426) reported elevated circulating AVP concentrations and increased hypothalamic AVP mRNA levels in rats with puromycin aminonucleoside-induced nephrotic syndrome, thus supporting the notion that increased hypothalamic AVP biosynthesis and release occur in this model of the nephrotic syndrome.

Aquaporins in Nephrotic Syndrome

In contrast to heart failure and cirrhosis, aquaporin-2 expression appears to be decreased in experimental models of nephrotic syndrome. This occurs despite elevated plasma vasopressin concentrations and clinical edema. In rats with puromycin aminonucleoside-induced nephrotic syndrome, there was an 87% decrease in inner medulla aquaporin-2 expression and a 70% decrease in collecting duct basolateral aquaporin-3 expression as compared to control rats (427). Consistent with the finding of aquaporin-2 and -3 downregulation, rats with nephrotic syndrome also demonstrated decreased maximal urinary osmolality. Similar findings were also noted in an adriamycin-induced model of nephrotic syndrome (428). Little data exist regarding the role of aquaporin-2 in water metabolism in humans with nephrotic syndrome. The mechanism by which adriamycin and puromycin aminonucleoside induce nephrotic syndrome is unknown, but several accompanying tubular defects have been demonstrated (428). Thus, extrapolation of the results of these

studies to human nephrotic syndrome must be performed with caution. Studies of urinary aquaporin-2 excretion in humans with nephrotic syndrome are needed.

Vasodilator Systems

Natriuretic Peptides in the Nephrotic Syndrome

Plasma ANP and BNP concentrations are elevated in animals and humans with the nephrotic syndrome (429,430); however, the hemodynamic and renal responses to exogenous ANP or BNP are blunted in experimental nephrosis (430) and in patients with the nephrotic syndrome (429). Recently, Perico and Remuzzi (431) proposed tubular insensitivity to ANP as an initiating factor in the formation of edema in the nephrotic syndrome. According to their hypothesis, renal unresponsiveness to ANP results in distal tubular sodium and water retention with subsequent edema formation; this renal ANP resistance may be receptor-independent, because urinary cGMP responds appropriately to ANP infusion in nephrotic animals (432). Alternatively, this blunted natriuretic response to ANP and BNP may be a secondary phenomenon owing to neurohormonal vasoconstrictor activation. Our aforementioned observations of sympathetic activation and normal plasma ANP concentrations in edematous patients with the nephrotic syndrome support this latter hypothesis (415). Moreover, Koepke and DiBona (232) showed that renal denervation reversed the blunted diuretic and natriuretic responses to ANP in a rat model of the nephrotic syndrome. The exact role of the natriuretic peptides in the pathogenesis of the renal sodium and water retention observed in the nephrotic syndrome remains to be defined.

Other humoral factors such as kinins and prostaglandins may modulate renal sodium reabsorption in nephrotic patients. For example, inhibitors of prostaglandin synthesis reduce the GFR in patients with the nephrotic syndrome and may precipitate renal insufficiency (433). The role of these different humoral mechanisms in the sodium retention in nephrotic syndrome patients remains unanswered.

In summary, it appears that the effector mechanisms for sodium and water retention in the nephrotic syndrome may involve a fall in GFR, alterations in peritubular physical factors, and activation of the sympathetic nervous system, the renin–angiotensin–aldosterone system, and the nonosmotic release of AVP. Other still undefined factors may, however, also be involved in the enhanced renal tubular sodium and water reabsorption observed in nephrotic patients; some results suggest that a diminution in ANP sensitivity in nephrotic syndrome also may be involved in the sodium retention.

Physiologic Basis for Therapy of Sodium and Water Retention in the Nephrotic Syndrome

The treatment modalities in nephrotic patients have been reviewed (434,435). The first principle of therapy of nephrotic syndrome is to treat the primary disease process. Several histologic lesions that produce nephrotic syndrome appear to be favorably influenced by corticosteroid therapy (434). Obviously, if the lesion proves to be steroid responsive, the edematous state will improve and further modalities of treatment may be unnecessary.

In patients with hypoalbuminemia, it is reasonable to recommend the ingestion of 2 to 3 g of protein per kilogram of body weight provided the GFR is well maintained. However, there is no evidence that dietary protein supplementation consistently increases serum albumin concentration or lessens the edema (436).

When symptomatic edema develops, dietary salt restriction should be instituted. A sodium intake of between 2 and 3 g/day is generally a reasonable compromise between effectiveness and palatability. Water restriction need not be implemented unless the patient is hyponatremic with hypoosmolality. Although impaired water excretion often occurs in nephrotic patients, clinically significant hyponatremia occurs primarily in association with concomitant diuretic usage.

Diuretic agents, the mainstay of therapy in edematous states, should be utilized only if symptomatic edema persists in spite of salt restriction. A few prospective controlled trials compared the efficacy and frequency of adverse effects of different diuretic agents used in nephrotic patients. These studies focused on the use of furosemide, metolazone, and piretanide in the edematous nephrotic patient (437–439). In view of the experimental data demonstrating enhanced renal sodium reabsorption beyond the proximal tubule in nephrotic syndrome, diuretics that act in distal tubular segments would be expected to be most efficacious. Many nephrotic patients with well-maintained GFRs respond to thiazide diuretics alone.

In adult nephrotic patients, furosemide is usually an effective diuretic agent, and one study in children found furosemide to be safe and efficacious in the treatment of nephrotic edema (437). However, some children with low GFRs become resistant to as much as 5 mg/kg of furosemide (437). In this setting, both in children and in adults, the addition of a second distal blocker such as metolazone often produces a diuresis (438); severe hypokalemia, however, may be seen with this combination of diuretics.

The pharmacokinetic patterns of the "loop diuretics" have been evaluated extensively in nephrotic patients (440–442). Although the presence of nephrotic syndrome decreases protein binding of furosemide, it does not appear to induce major changes in furosemide disposition when renal function is well maintained (440–442). The efficacy of high doses of spironolactone, the specific aldosterone antagonist, in nephrotic patients has been demonstrated and correlates with the activation of the renin–angiotensin–aldosterone system. Spironolactone may also be effective as an additive diuretic effect when given with other agents (443).

Diuretic therapy of nephrotic syndrome often can be instituted in the outpatient setting. Patients should be instructed to weigh themselves daily and to diminish or discontinue the diuretic if weight loss exceeds 1 pound per day or when edema no longer becomes a source of discomfort. We also instruct our patients to reduce or discontinue the diuretic when orthostatic lightheadedness develops and when only a small amount of edema remains. One practical way to follow these patients' proteinuria is with single voided urine samples to estimate quantitative urinary protein loss; a protein:creatinine ratio of more than 3 to 5 can be taken to represent "nephrotic" proteinuria (444). Hospitalization may be required to initiate and monitor diuresis in patients with either severe edema or marked hypoalbuminemia, especially when a significant decrease in GFR is present.

Albumin infusions have been utilized in the treatment of edema in nephrotic patients since the 1950s (445). This form of therapy increases plasma volume and may increase GFR, urine flow, sodium excretion, and solute-free water clearance (386,393,443,445). Leutscher and collaborators (445) treated 13 adult nephrotics with 50 g/day of salt-poor albumin (200 mL of 25% albumin solution) for 4 consecutive days. A diuresis was observed in all patients, and five of the 13 patients became edema free. More recently, Davison and collaborators (443) used albumin in the management of diuretic-resistant nephrotic patients. Twelve nephrotic patients, referred for a diuretic-resistant state, were studied. Diverse glomerular diseases were present in these patients, and nine of 12 patients had a creatinine clearance rate of less than 40 mL/minute. All patients were treated with furosemide in increasing doses to 500 mg/day. Spironolactone with increasing doses to 200 mg/day was added if a diuresis did not occur with furosemide. Six of the 12 patients could be satisfactorily diuresed with the preceding regimen. In the remaining six patients, diuresis either was unsuccessful (two patients) or resulted in serious complications, including increasing blood urea nitrogen in three patients and hyponatremia in one patient. In the six responsive patients, 300 mL of a 15% solution of salt-poor albumin led to a significant diuresis and resolution of edema without worsening renal function.

Studies both in nephrotic patients (446) and in an experimental model of nephrotic syndrome in the rat (447) indicated that rather than compensating for urinary protein losses, ingestion of a high-protein diet results in an augmentation of urinary albumin excretion and a net decrease in serum albumin concentration and body albumin pools. Also, treatment with converting enzyme inhibitors reduced the rate of urinary protein loss (448,449) and retarded the progression of renal dysfunction (449) in nephrotic syndrome patients. Don and coworkers (451) studied the effects of dietary protein restriction or treatment with an ACE inhibitor on protein metabolism in 12 patients with the nephrotic syndrome. Protein metabolism was assessed by plasma amino acid levels and nitrogen balance. Reducing dietary protein intake decreased whereas treatment with enalapril increased nitrogen balance, although neither of these changes achieved a level of statistical significance. Moreover, Gansevoort and colleagues (452) recently showed comparable decreases in urinary protein excretion induced by either the ANG II receptor antagonist losartan or the ACE inhibitor enalapril in 11 nondiabetic nephrotic syndrome patients. This observation supports the notion that the antiproteinuric effect of ACE inhibition is mediated by the inhibition of ANG II rather than an ACE inhibitor-induced increase in bradykinin or prostaglandin levels. Further studies will be necessary to assess the potential value of changes in protein intake, converting enzyme inhibition, and ANG II receptor antagonism in the long-term treatment of nephrotic patients. As well, the potential beneficial effect of lipid-lowering agents on the progression and expression of nephrotic syndrome needs to be addressed (453,454).

Although albumin infusion remains an attractive therapeutic tool for the temporary treatment of patients with diuretic-resistant nephrotic syndrome, this form of therapy remains relatively expensive, and the diuretic effects of albumin infusion are usually short-lived (386). For example, in the study of Koomans and associates (386), 10 patients with the nephrotic syndrome received a 75 g hyperoncotic albumin infusion, and their urinary sodium excretion increased only minimally from 10 to 45 μEq/min. This rate would account for a loss of less than 1 kg of ECF volume in 24 hours. Nevertheless, albumin infusions may be beneficial in some diuretic-resistant nephrotic patients. Water immersion has also been used to treat nephrotic patients, with weight loss ranging from 0.5 to 2.0 kg observed after 4 hours of HWI (455). This form of therapy, although extremely interesting from a physiopathologic viewpoint, remains impractical.

Vasopressin V_2 receptor antagonists have been shown to be useful aquaretic agents in animals and humans with heart failure and cirrhosis. Similar studies have not been performed in nephrotic syndrome. In contrast to diuretics, these agents have the theoretical advantage of inducing solute-free water clearance without electrolyte losses. Further study in this area is indicated.

REFERENCES

1. Koppel MH, et al. Transplantation of cadaveric kidneys from patients with hepatorenal syndrome: evidence for the functional nature of renal failure in advanced liver disease. *N Engl J Med* 1969;280:1367.
2. Iwatsuki S, et al. Recovery from hepatorenal syndrome after orthotopic liver transplantation. *N Engl J Med* 1973;289:1155.
3. Nizet A. Quantitative influence of nonhormonal blood factors on the control of sodium excretion by the isolated dog kidney. *Kidney Int* 1972;1:27.
4. Starling EH. On the absorption of fluid from the connective tissue spaces. *J Physiol (Lond)* 1896;19:312.
5. Intaglietta M, Zweifach BW. Microcirculatory basis of fluid exchange. *Adv Biol Med Phys* 1974;15:11.
6. Bennhold H, Klaus D, Scheurlen PG. Volume regulation and renal function in analbuminemia. *Lancet* 1960;2:1169.
7. Braunwald E, Plauth WH, Morrow AG. A method for detection and quantification of impaired sodium excretion. *Circulation* 1965;32:223.
8. Takasu T, Lasker N, Shalhoub RJ. Mechanism of hyponatremia in chronic congestive heart failure. *Ann Intern Med* 1961;55:368.
9. Hope J. *A treatise on the diseases of the heart and blood vessels.* London: William Kidd, 1832.
10. Mackenzie J. *Disease of the heart,* 3rd ed. London: Oxford University Press, 1913.
11. Schrier RW. Pathogenesis of sodium and water retention in high-output and low-output cardiac failure, nephrotic syndrome, cirrhosis, and pregnancy. *N Engl J Med* 1988;319:1065.
12. Schrier RW. Body fluid volume regulation in health and disease: a unifying hypothesis. *Ann Intern Med* 1990;113:155.
13. Schrier RW. A unifying hypothesis of body fluid volume regulation. The Lilly Lecture 1992. *J Roy Coll Phys (Lond)* 1992;26:295.
14. Schrier RW. An odyssey into the milieu interieur: pondering the enigmas. *J Am Soc Nephrol* 1992;2:1549.
15. Abraham WT, Schrier RW. Edematous disorders: pathophysiology of renal sodium and water retention and treatment with diuretics. *Curr Opin Nephrol Hypertens* 1993;2:798.
16. Abraham WT, Schrier RW. Body fluid regulation in health and disease. In: Schrier RW, Abboud FM, Baxter JD, et al, eds. *Advances in internal medicine,* vol. 39. Chicago: Mosby Yearbook, 1994.
17. Schrier RW, Gurevich AK, Cadnapaphornchai MA. Pathogenesis and management of sodium and water retention in cardiac failure and cirrhosis. *Semin Nephrol* 2001;21:157.
18. Epstein FH, et al. Cardiac output and intracardiac pressure in patients with arteriovenous fistulas. *J Clin Invest* 1953;32:543.
19. Papper S. The role of the kidney in Laënnec's cirrhosis of the liver. *Medicine* 1958;37:299.
20. Lifshitz MD, Schrier RW. Alterations in cardiac output with chronic constriction of thoracic inferior vena cava. *Am J Physiol* 1964;225:1364.
21. Schrier RW, Humphreys MH. Factors involved in the antinatriuretic effects of acute constriction of the thoracic and abdominal inferior vena cava. *Circ Res* 1971;29:479.
22. Schrier RW, Humphreys MH, Ufferman RC. Role of cardiac output and autonomic nervous system in the antinatriuretic response to acute constriction of the thoracic superior vena cava. *Circ Res* 1971;29:490.
23. Migdal SE, Alexander EA, Levinsky NG. Evidence that decreased cardiac output is not the stimulus to sodium retention during acute constriction of the vena cava. *J Lab Clin Med* 1977;89:809.
24. Yaron M, Bennett CM. Renal sodium handling in acute right-sided heart failure in dogs. *Miner Electrolyte Metab* 1978;1:303.
25. Lee ME, et al. Role of endogenous atrial natriuretic factor in acute congestive heart failure. *J Clin Invest* 1989;84:1962.
26. Hostetter TH, et al. Cardiorenal hemodynamics and sodium excretion in rats with myocardial infarction. *Am J Physiol* 1983;245:H98.
27. Priebe HJ, Heimann JC, Hedley-White J. Effects of renal and hepatic venous congestion on renal function in the presence of low and normal cardiac output in dogs. *Circ Res* 1980;17:883.
28. Davis JO. The control of renin release. *Am J Med* 1973;55:333.
29. Guyton A, Scanlon CJ, Armstrong GG. Effects of pressoreceptor reflex and Cushing's reflex on urinary output. *Fed Proc* 1952;11:61.
30. Gilmore JP. Contribution of baroreceptors to the control of renal function. *Circ Res* 1964;14:301.
31. Gilmore JP, Daggett WM. Response of chronic cardiac denervated dog to acute volume expansion. *Am J Physiol* 1966;210:509.
32. Knox FG, Davis BB, Berliner RW. Effect of chronic cardiac denervation on renal response to saline infusion. *Am J Physiol* 1967;213:174.
33. Pearce JW, Sonnenberg H. Effects of spinal section and renal denervation on the renal response to blood volume expansion. *Can J Physiol Pharmacol* 1965;43:211.
34. Schedl HP, Bartter FC. An explanation for an experimental correction of the abnormal water diuresis in cirrhosis. *J Clin Invest* 1960;39:248.
35. Anderson RJ, et al. Mechanism of portal hypertension induced alterations in renal hemodynamics, renal water excretion and renin secretion. *J Clin Invest* 1976;58:964.
36. Schrier RW, et al. Nonosmolar control of renal water excretion. In: Andreoli T, Grantham J, Rector F, eds. *Disturbances in body fluid osmolality.* Bethesda, MD: American Physiological Society, 1977.
37. Tobian L, Tomboulian A, Janecek J. The effect of high perfusion pressure on the granulation of juxtaglomerular cells in an isolated kidney. *J Clin Invest* 1959;38:605.
38. Blaine EH, Davis JO, Witty RT. Renin release after hemorrhage and after suprarenal aortic constriction in dogs without sodium delivery to the macula densa. *Circ Res* 1970;27:1081.
39. Epstein FH, Post RS, McDowell M. The effects of an arteriovenous fistula on renal hemodynamics and electrolyte excretion. *J Clin Invest* 1953;32:233.
40. Gauer OH, Henry JP. Neurohormonal control of plasma volume. In: Guyton AC, Cowley AW Jr, eds. *Cardiovascular physiology II. International review of physiology,* vol 9. Baltimore: University Part, 1976.
41. Paintal AS. Vagal sensory receptors and their reflex effects. *Physiol Rev* 1973;53:159.

42. Coleridge HM, Coleridge JCG. Afferent innervation of lungs, airways, and pulmonary artery. In: Zucker IH, Gilmore JP, eds. *Reflex control of the circulation.* Boca Raton, FL: CRC Press, 1991.

43. Arborelius M, et al. Hemodynamic changes in man during immersion with the head above water. *Aerospace Med* 1972;43:592.

44. Bichet DG, Groves BM, Schrier RW. Mechanisms of improvement of water and sodium excretion by enhancement of central hemodynamics in decompensated cirrhotic patients. *Kidney Int* 1983;24:788.

45. Epstein FH. Renal excretion of sodium and the concept of a volume receptor. *Yale J Biol Med* 1956;29:282.

46. Epstein M, Duncan DC, Fishman LM. Characterization of the natriuresis caused in normal man by immersion in water. *Clin Sci* 1972;43:275.

47. Gauer OH, et al. The effect of negative pressure breathing on urine flow. *J Clin Invest* 1954;33:287.

48. Hulet WH, Smith HH. Postural natriuresis and urine osmotic concentration in hydropenic subjects. *Am J Med* 1961;30:8.

49. Epstein FH, et al. Studies of the antidiuresis of quiet standing: the importance of changes in plasma volume in glomerular filtration rate. *J Clin Invest* 1951;30:63.

50. Murdaugh HV Jr, Sieker HO, Manfredi F. Effect of altered intrathoracic pressure on renal hemodynamics, electrolyte excretion and water clearance. *J Clin Invest* 1959;38:834.

51. Gillespie DJ, Sandberg RL, Koike TI. Dual effect on left atrial receptors on excretion of sodium and water in the dog. *Am J Physiol* 1973;225:706.

52. Henry JP, Gauer OH, Reeves JL. Evidence of the atrial location of receptors influencing urine flow. *Circ Res* 1956;4:85.

53. Reinhardt HW, et al. Left atrial pressure and sodium balance in conscious dogs on a low sodium intake. *Pflugers Arch* 1977;370:59.

54. Bello-Reuss E, Trevino DL, Gottschalk CW. Effect of renal sympathetic nerve stimulation on proximal water and sodium reabsorption. *J Clin Invest* 1976;57:1104.

55. DiBona GF. Neurogenic regulation of renal tubular sodium reabsorption. *Am J Physiol* 1977;233:F73.

56. deTorrente A, et al. Mechanism of diuretic response to increased left atrial pressure in the anesthetized dog. *Kidney Int* 1975;8:355.

57. Gauer OH, Henry JP. Circulating basis of fluid volume control. *Physiol Rev* 1963;43:423.

58. Share L. Effects of carotid occlusion and left atrial distension on plasma vasopressin titer. *Am J Physiol* 1965;208:219.

59. Gupta PD, et al. Responses of atrial and aortic baroreceptors to nonhypotensive hemorrhage and to transfusion. *Am J Physiol* 1966;211:1429.

60. Henry JP, Gupta PD, Meehan R. The role of afferents from the low pressure system in the release of antidiuretic hormone during nonhypotensive hemorrhage. *Can J Physiol Pharmacol* 1968;46:287.

61. Goets KL, Hermeck AS, Slick GL. Atrial receptors and renal function in conscious dog. *Am J Physiol* 1970;219:1417.

62. Barger AC, Ytes FE, Rudolph AM. Renal hemodynamics and sodium excretion in dogs with graded valvular damage in congestive heart failure. *Am J Physiol* 1961;200:601.

63. Stitzer SO, Malvin RL. Right atrium and renal sodium excretion. *Am J Physiol* 1975;228:184.

64. Zucker IH, et al. Impaired atrial receptor modulation of renal nerve activity in dogs with chronic volume overload. *Cardiovasc Res* 1985;19:411.

65. Ferguson DW, Abboud FM, Mark AL. Selective impairment of baroreceptor-mediated vasoconstrictor responses in patients with ventricular dysfunction. *Circulation* 1984;69:451.

66. Mohanty PK, et al. Neurohormonal and hemodynamic effects of lower body negative pressure in patients with congestive heart failure. *Am Heart J* 1989;118:78.

67. Nishian K, Kawashima S, Iwasaki T. Paradoxical forearm vasodilation and hemodynamic improvement during cardiopulmonary baroreceptor unloading in patients with congestive heart failure. *Clin Sci* 1993;84:271.

68. Sandoval AB, et al. Hemodynamic correlates of increased cardiac adrenergic drive in the intact failing human heart. *J Am Coll Cardiol* 1989;13:245A.

69. Baker DG, et al. Search for a cardiac nociceptor: stimulation by bradykinin of sympathetic afferent nerve endings in the heart of the cat. *J Physiol* 1980;306:519.

70. Panzenbeck MJ, et al. PGE$_2$ and arachidonate inhibit the baroreflex in conscious dogs via cardiac receptors. *Am J Physiol* 1989;256:H999.

71. Zucker IH, et al. PGI$_2$ attenuates the baroreflex control of renal nerve activity by an afferent vagal mechanism. *Am J Physiol* 1988;254:R424.

72. Dzau VJ, et al. Prostaglandins in severe congestive heart failure: relation to activation of the renin–angiotensin system and hyponatremia. *N Engl J Med* 1984;310:347.

73. Daly JJ, Roe JW, Horrocks PA comparison of sodium excretion following the infusion of saline into systemic and portal veins in the dog: evidence for hepatic role in the control of sodium excretion. *Clin Sci* 1967;33:481.

74. Passo SS, Thornborough JR, Rothballer AB. Hepatic receptors in control of sodium excretion in anesthetized cats. *Am J Physiol* 1975;224:373.

75. Carey RM, Smith JR, Ortt EM. Gastrointestinal control of sodium excretion in sodium-depleted conscious rabbits. *Am J Physiol* 1976;230:1504.

76. Carey RM. Evidence for a splanchnic sodium input monitor regulating renal sodium excretion in man: lack of dependence upon aldosterone. *Circ Res* 1978;43:19.

77. Lennane RJ, et al. A comparison of natriuresis after oral and intravenous sodium loading in sodium depleted rabbits: evidence for a gastrointestinal or portal monitor of sodium intake. *Clin Sci Mol Med* 1975;49:433.

78. Potkay S, Gilmore JP. Renal response to vena caval and portal venous infusions of sodium chloride in unanesthetized dogs. *Clin Sci Mol Med* 1970;39:13.

79. Schneider EG, et al. Lack of evidence for a hepatic osmoreceptor in conscious dogs. *Am J Physiol* 1970;218:42.

80. Obika LFO, et al. Lack of evidence for gastrointestinal control of sodium excretion in unanesthetized rabbits. *Am J Physiol* 1981;240:F94.

81. Schrier RW Berl T, Anderson RJ. Osmotic and nonosmotic control of vasopressin release. *Am J Physiol* 1979;236:F321.

82. Berl T, et al. Prostaglandins in the beta adrenergic and baroreceptor-mediated secretion of renin. *Am J Physiol* 1979;235:F472.

83. de Wardener HE, et al. Studies on the efferent mechanism of the sodium diuresis which follows the intravenous administration of saline in the dog. *Clin Sci* 1961;21:249.

84. Merrill AJ. Mechanism of salt and water retention in heart failure. *Am J Med* 1949;6:357.

85. Kilcoyne MM, Schmidt DH, Cannon PJ. Intrarenal blood flow in congestive heart failure. *Circ Res* 1973;47:786.

86. Sparks HV, et al. Intrarenal distribution of blood flow with chronic congestive heart failure. *Am J Physiol* 1972;223:840.

87. Boudreau R, Mandin H. Cardiac edema in dogs. II. Distribution of glomerular filtrate in renal blood flow. *Kidney Int* 1976;10:578.

88. Stumpe KO, et al. Mechanism of sodium and water retention in rats with experimental heart failure. *Kidney Int* 1973;4:309.

89. Meyers BD, Deen WM, Brenner BM. Effects of norepinephrine and angiotensin II on the determinants of glomerular ultrafiltration and proximal tubule fluid reabsorption in the rat. *Circ Res* 1975;37:101.

90. Ichikawa I, et al. Role of angiotensin II in the altered renal function in congestive heart failure. *Circ Res* 1984;55:669.

91. Bichet DG, et al. Modulation of plasma and platelet vasopressin by cardiac function in patients with heart failure. *Kidney Int* 1986;29:1188.

92. Munger MA. Renal functional alterations induced by angiotensin-converting enzyme inhibitors in heart failure. *Ann Pharmacother* 1993;27:205.

93. Henrich WL, et al. Angiotensin, renal nerves and prostaglandins in renal hemodynamics during hemorrhage. *Am J Physiol* 1978;235:F46.

94. Blasingham MC, Nasjletti A. Differential renal effects of cyclooxygenase inhibition in sodium-replete and sodium-deprived dog. *Am J Physiol* 1980;239:F360.

95. Dunn MJ, Zambraski EJ. Renal effect of drugs that inhibit prostaglandin synthesis. *Kidney Int* 1980;18:609.

96. Riegger GA, et al. Effects of acetylsalicylic acid on renal function in patients with chronic heart failure. *Am J Med* 1991;90:571.

97. Walshe JJ, Venuto RC. Acute oliguric renal failure induced by indomethacin: possible mechanism. *Ann Intern Med* 1979;91:47.

98. Oliver JA, et al. Participation of the prostaglandins in the control of renal blood flow during acute reduction of cardiac output in the dog. *J Clin Invest* 1981;67:229.

99. Hasking GJ, et al. Norepinephrine spillover to plasma in patients with congestive heart failure: evidence of increased overall and cardiorenal sympathetic nervous activity. *Circulation* 1986;73:615.

100. Brod J, Fejfar Z, Fejfarova MH. The role of neurohumoral factors in the genesis of renal hemodynamic changes in heart failure. *Acta Med Scand* 1954;148:273.

101. Brenner BM, et al. The relationship between peritubular capillary protein concentration and fluid reabsorption by the renal proximal tubule. *J Clin Invest* 1969;48:1519.

102. Brenner BM, Galla HH. Influence of postglomerular hematocrit and protein concentration on rat nephron fluid transfer. *Am J Physiol* 1971;220:148.

103. Brenner BM, Troy JL. Postglomerular vascular protein concentration: evidence for causal role in governing fluid reabsorption in glomerular tubular balance by the renal proximal tubule. *J Clin Invest* 1971;50:336.

104. Brenner BM, Troy JL, Daugharty TM. Quantitative importance of changes in postglomerular colloid osmotic pressure in mediating glomerular tubular balance in the rat. *J Clin Invest* 1973;52:190.

105. Falchuk KH, Brenner BM, Tadokoro M. Oncotic and hydrostatic pressure in peritubular capillaries and fluid reabsorption of proximal tubule. *Am J Physiol* 1971;220:1427.

106. Auld RB, Alexander EA, Levinsky NG. Proximal tubular function in dogs with thoracic caval constriction. *J Clin Invest* 1971;50:2150.

107. Mandin H. Cardiac edema in dogs. I. Proximal tubular and renal function. *Kidney Int* 1976;10:591.

108. Rumrich G, Ullrich KJ. The minimum requirements for the maintenance of sodium chloride reabsorption in the proximal convolution of the mammalian kidney. *J Physiol (Lond)* 1968;197:69.

109. Lowitz HD, Stumpe KO, Ochwadt B. Micropuncture study of the action of angiotensin II on tubular sodium and water reabsorption in the rat. *Nephron* 1969;6:173.

110. Bank N, Aynedjian HS, Wada T. Effect of peritubular capillary perfusion rate on proximal sodium reabsorption. *Kidney Int* 1972;1:397.

111. Holzgreve H, Schrier RW. Effect of peritubular protein concentration on renal proximal tubular fluid reabsorption in the volume expanded rat. *Pflugers Arch* 1972;332:R32.

112. Conger JD, Bartoli E, Earley LE. A study of *in vivo* peritubular oncotic pressure and proximal tubular reabsorption in the rat. *Clin Sci Mol Med* 1976;51:379.

113. Ott CE, et al. Effect of increased peritubular protein concentration on proximal tubule reabsorption in the presence and absence of extracellular volume expansion. *J Clin Invest* 1975;55:612.

114. Schneider EG, Dresser TP, Lynch RF, et al. Sodium reabsorption by proximal tubules of dogs with experimental heart failure. *Am J Physiol* 1971;220:952.

115. Levy M. Effects of acute volume expansion and altered hemodynamics on renal tubular function in chronic caval dogs. *J Clin Invest* 1972;51:922.

116. Bell NH, Schedl HP, Bartter FC. An explanation for abnormal water retention and hypoosmolality in congestive heart failure. *Am J Med* 1964;36:351.

117. Schrier RW, et al. Effect of furosemide on free water excretion in edematous patients with hyponatremia. *Kidney Int* 1973;3:30.

118. Szatalowicz VL, et al. Comparative effect of diuretics on renal water excretion in hyponatremic edematous disorders. *Clin Sci* 1982;62:235.

119. Werko L, et al. Studies on the renal circulation and renal function in mitral valvular disease. I. Effect of exercise. *Circulation* 1954;9:687.

120. Thomas JA, Marks BH. Plasma norepinephrine in congestive heart failure. *Am J Cardiol* 1978;41:233.

121. Levine TB, et al. Activity of the sympathetic nervous system and renin–angiotensin system assessed by plasma hormone levels and their relation to hemodynamic abnormalities in congestive heart failure. *Am J Cardiol* 1982;49:1659.

122. Davis D, Baily R, Zelis R. Abnormalities in systemic norepinephrine kinetics in human congestive heart failure. *Am J Physiol* 1988;254: E760.

123. Abraham WT, Hensen J, Schrier RW. Elevated plasma noradrenaline concentrations in patients with low-output cardiac failure: dependence on increased noradrenaline secretion rates. *Clin Sci* 1990;79: 429.

124. Francis GS, et al. Comparison of neuroendocrine activation in patients with left ventricular dysfunction with and without congestive heart failure. A substudy of the Studies of Left Ventricular Dysfunction (SOLVD). *Circulation* 1990;82:1724.

125. Chidsey CA, Braunwald E, Morrow AG. Catecholamine excretion and cardiac stores of norepinephrine in congestive heart failure. *Am J Med* 1965;39:442.

126. Cody RJ, et al. Sympathetic responsiveness and plasma norepinephrine during therapy of congestive heart failure with captopril. *Am J Med* 1981;72:791.

127. Leimbach WN, et al. Direct evidence from intraneural recordings for increased central sympathetic outflow in patients with heart failure. *Circulation* 1986;73:913.

128. Lowes BD, Abraham WT, Bristow MR. Role of beta blockers in the treatment of heart failure. In: Braunwald E, ed. *Heart disease: a textbook of cardiovascular medicine—update summer 1994.* Philadelphia: WB Saunders, 1994.

129. Waagstein F, et al. Beneficial effects of metoprolol in idiopathic dilated cardiomyopathy. *Lancet* 1993;342:1441.

130. Bristow MR, et al. Multicenter oral carvedilol assessment (MOCHA): a six-month dose-response evaluation in class II to IV patients. *Circulation* 1995;92:I142.

131. Cohn JN, et al. Plasma norepinephrine as a guide to prognosis in patients with chronic congestive heart failure. *N Engl J Med* 1984; 311:819.

132. DiBona GF, Herman PJ, Sawin LL. Normal control of renal function in edema forming states. *Am J Physiol* 1988;254:R1017.

133. Gill JR, Mason DT, Bartter GC. Adrenergic nervous system in sodium metabolism: effects of guanethidine and sodium-retaining steroids in normal man. *J Clin Invest* 1964;43:177.

134. Carpenter CCJ, et al. Studies on the response of the transplanted kidney and transplanted adrenal gland to thoracic inferior vena caval constriction. *J Clin Invest* 1961;40:196.

135. Mizelle HL, Hall JE, Montani JP. Role of renal nerves in control of sodium excretion in chronic congestive heart failure. *Am J Physiol* 1989;256:F1084.

136. Botker HE, et al. Renal effects of xamoterol in patients with moderate heart failure. *Cardiovasc Drugs Ther* 1993;7:111.

137. Thomsen K. Lithium clearance: a new method for determining proximal and distal tubular reabsorption of sodium and water. *Nephron* 1984;37:217.

138. Eichhorn E, et al. Effects of bucindolol on neurohormonal activation in congestive heart failure. *Am J Cardiol* 1991;67:67.

139. Merrill AJ, Morrison JL, Brannon ES. Concentration of renin in renal venous blood in patients with chronic heart failure. *Am J Med* 1946;1:468.

140. Watkins L, et al. The renin–angiotensin–aldosterone system in congestive heart failure in conscious dogs. *J Clin Invest* 1976;57:1606.

141. Lee WH, Packer M. Prognostic importance of serum sodium concentration and its modification by converting-enzyme inhibition in patients with severe chronic heart failure. *Circulation* 1986;73:257.

142. The CONSENSUS Trial Study Group. Effects of enalapril on mortality in severe congestive heart failure: results of the Cooperative North Scandinavian Enalapril Survival Study (CONSENSUS). *N Engl J Med* 1987;316:1429.

143. The SOLVD Investigators. Effect of enalapril on survival in patients with reduced left ventricular ejection fractions and congestive heart failure. *N Engl J Med* 1991;325:293.

144. Bristow MR, Abraham WT. Antiadrenergic effects of angiotensin converting enzyme inhibitors. *Eur Heart J* 1995;16:37.

145. Hilgers KF, et al. Angiotensin II facilitates sympathetic transmission in rat hind limb circulation. *Hypertension* 1993;21:322.

146. Clemson B, et al. Prejunctional angiotensin II receptors: facilitation of norepinephrine release in the human forearm. *J Clin Invest* 1994;93:684.

147. Abraham WT, et al. Angiotensin II selectively increases cardiac adrenergic activity in patients with heart failure. *J Am Coll Cardiol* 1994;23:215A.

148. Gilbert EM, et al. Lisinopril lowers cardiac adrenergic drive and increases ß-receptor density in the failing human heart. *Circulation* 1993; 88:472.

149. Liu FY, Cogan MG. Angiotensin II: a potent regulator of acidification in the rat early proximal convoluted tubule. *J Clin Invest* 1987;80: 272.

150. Abassi ZA, et al. Losartan improves the natriuretic response to ANF in rats with high-output heart failure. *J Pharmacol Exper Ther* 1994;268:224.

151. Cody RJ, et al. Sodium and water balance in chronic congestive heart failure. *J Clin Invest* 1986;77:1441.

152. Pierpont GL, Francis GS, Cohn JN. Effect of captopril on renal function in patients with congestive heart failure. *Br Heart J* 1981;46:522.

153. Motwani JG, et al. Determinants of the initial effects of captopril on blood pressure, glomerular filtration rate, and natriuresis in mild-to-moderate chronic congestive heart failure secondary to coronary artery disease. *Am J Cardiol* 1994;73:1191.

154. Good JM, et al. Effect of intense angiotensin II suppression on the diuretic response to furosemide during chronic ACE inhibition. *Circulation* 1994;90:220.

155. Davis JO, et al. Accumulation of ascites during maintenance of adrenalectomized dogs with thoracic inferior vena cava constriction on a high sodium diet without hormone therapy. *Am J Physiol* 1956;185:230.

156. Gill JR. Edema. *Annu Rev Med* 1970;21:269.

157. Chonko AM, et al. The role of renin and aldosterone in the salt retention of edema. *Am J Med* 1977;63:881.

158. Hensen J, et al. Aldosterone in congestive heart failure: analysis of determinants and role in sodium retention. *Am J Nephrol* 1991;11:441.

159. Dahlstrom U, Karlsson E. Captopril and spironolactone therapy for refractory congestive heart failure. *Am J Cardiol* 1993;71:29A.

160. van Vliet AA, et al. Spironolactone in congestive heart failure refractory to high-dose loop diuretic and low-dose angiotensin-converting enzyme inhibitor. *Am J Cardiol* 1993;71:21A.

161. Pitt B, et al. The effect of spironolactone on morbidity and mortality in patients with severe heart failure. Randomized Aldactone Evaluation Study Investigators. *N Engl J Med* 1999;341:709.

162. Goldsmith SR, et al. Increased plasma arginine vasopressin levels in patients with congestive heart failure. *J Am Coll Cardiol* 1983;1:1385.

163. Preibisz JJ, et al. Plasma and platelet vasopressin in essential hypertension and congestive heart failure. *Hypertension* 1983;5:129.

164. Pruszczynski W, et al. Role of antidiuretic hormone in impaired water excretion of patients with congestive heart failure. *J Clin Endocrinol Metab* 1984;58:599.

165. Riegger GAJ, Liebau G, Kochsie K. Antidiuretic hormone in congestive heart failure. *Am J Med* 1982;72:49.

166. Rondeau E, et al. High plasma antidiuretic hormone in patients with cardiac failure: influence of age. *Miner Electrolyte Metab* 1982;8:267.

167. Szatalowicz VL, et al. Radioimmunoassay of plasma arginine vasopressin in hyponatremic patients with congestive heart failure. *N Engl J Med* 1981;305:263.

168. Goldsmith SR, Francis GS, Cowley AW Jr. Arginine vasopressin and the renal response to water loading in congestive heart failure. *Am J Cardiol* 1986;58:295.

169. Uretsky BF, et al. Plasma vasopressin response to osmotic and hemodynamic stimuli in heart failure. *Am J Physiol* 1985;248:H396.

170. Guillon G, et al. Kinetic and pharmacologic characterization of vasopressin membrane receptors from human kidney medulla: relation to adenylate cyclase activation. *Eur J Pharmacol* 1982;85:291.

171. Anderson RJ, et al. Mechanism of effect of thoracic inferior vena cava constriction on renal water excretion. *J Clin Invest* 1974;54:1473.

172. Handelman W, Lum G, Schrier RW. Impaired water excretion in high output cardiac failure in the rat. *Clin Res* 1979;27:173A.

173. Riegger GA, et al. Vasopressin and renin in high output heart failure of rats: hemodynamic effects of elevated plasma hormone levels. *J Cardiovasc Pharmacol* 1995;7:1.

174. Ishikawa S, et al. Effect of vasopressin antagonist on renal water excretion in rats with inferior vena cava constriction. *Kidney Int* 1986;30:49.

175. Yared A, et al. Role for vasopressin in rats with congestive heart failure. *Kidney Int* 1985;27:337.

176. Fujita H, et al. The effect of vasopressin V_1 and V_2 receptor antagonists on heart failure after myocardial infarction. *J Am Coll Cardiol* 1995;25:234A.

177. Naitoh M, et al. Effects of oral AVP receptor antagonists OPC-21268 and OPC-31260 on congestive heart failure in conscious dogs. *Am J Physiol* 1994;267:H2245.

178. Yamamura Y, et al. Characterization of a novel aquaretic agent, OPC-31260, as an orally effective, nonpeptide vasopressin V_2 receptor antagonist. *Br J Pharmacol* 1992;105:787.

179. Ohnishi A, et al. Potent aquaretic agent: a novel nonpeptide selective vasopressin 2 antagonist (OPC-31260) in men. *J Clin Invest* 1993;92:2653.

180. Kim JK, et al. Arginine vasopressin gene expression in chronic cardiac failure in rats. *Kidney Int* 1990;38:818.

181. Nielsen S, et al. Congestive heart failure in rats is associated with increased expression and targeting of aquaporin-2 water channel in collecting duct. *Proc Natl Acad Sci USA* 1997;94:5450.

182. Xu DL, et al. Upregulation of aquaporin-2 water channel expression in chronic heart failure rat. *J Clin Invest* 1997;99:1500.

183. Martin PY, et al. Selective V2-receptor vasopressin antagonism decreases urinary aquaporin-2 excretion in patients with chronic heart failure. *J Am Soc Nephrol* 1999;10:2165.

184. Rai T, et al. Urinary excretion of aquaporin-2 water channel protein in human and rat. *J Am Soc Nephrol* 1997;8:1357.

185. Good JM, et al. Elevated plasma endothelin concentrations in heart failure: an effect of angiotensin II? *Eur Heart J* 1994;15:1634.

186. Teerlink JR, et al. Role of endothelin in the maintenance of blood pressure in conscious rats with chronic heart failure: acute effects of the endothelin receptor antagonist Ro 470203 (bosentan). *Circulation* 1994;90:2510.

187. Nord EP. Renal actions of endothelin. *Kidney Int* 1993;44:451.

188. Bates ER, Shenker Y, Grekin RJ. The relationship between plasma levels of immunoreactive atrial natriuretic hormone and hemodynamic function in man. *Circulation* 1986;73:1155.

189. Burnett JC Jr, et al. Atrial natriuretic peptide elevation in congestive heart failure in the human. *Science* 1986;231:1145.

190. Girata Y, et al. Plasma concentration of a human atrial natriuretic polypeptide and cyclic GMP in patients with heart disease. *Am Heart J* 1987;113:1463.

191. Michel JB, Arnal JF, Corvol P. Atrial natriuretic factor as a marker in congestive heart failure. *Horm Res* 1990;34:166.

192. Nakaoka H, et al. Plasma levels of atrial natriuretic factor in patients with congestive heart failure. *N Engl J Med* 1985;313:892.

193. Raine AEG, et al. Atrial natriuretic peptide and atrial pressure in patients with congestive heart failure. *N Engl J Med* 1986;315:533.

194. Mukoyama M, et al. Increased human brain natriuretic peptide in congestive heart failure. *N Engl J Med* 1990;323:757.

195. Atlas SA, et al. Purification, sequencing, and synthesis of natriuretic and vasoactive rat atrial peptide. *Nature* 1984;309:717.

196. Currie MG, et al. Bioactive cardiac substances: potent vasorelaxant activity in mammalian atria. *Science* 1983;221:71.

197. Molina CR, et al. Hemodynamic, renal, and endocrine effects of atrial natriuretic peptide in severe heart failure. *J Am Coll Cardiol* 1988;12:175.

198. Atarashi K, et al. Inhibition of aldosterone production by an atrial extract. *Science* 1984;224:992.

199. Samson WK. Atrial natriuretic factor inhibits dehydration and hemorrhage-induced vasopressin release. *Neuroendocrinology* 1985;40:277.

200. Floras JS. Sympathoinhibitory effects of atrial natriuretic factor in normal humans. *Circulation* 1990;81:1860.

201. Cody RJ, et al. Atrial natriuretic factor in normal subjects and heart failure patients: plasma levels and renal, hormonal, and hemodynamic responses to peptide infusion. *J Clin Invest* 1986;78:1362.

202. Sato F, et al. Relationship between plasma atrial natriuretic peptide levels and atrial pressure in man. *J Endocrinol Metab* 1986;63:823.

203. Hensen J, et al. Atrial natriuretic peptide kinetic studies in patients with cardiac dysfunction. *Kidney Int* 1992;42:1333.

204. Saito Y, et al. Atrial natriuretic polypeptide (ANP) in human ventricle: increased gene expression of ANP in dilated cardiomyopathy. *Biochem Biophys Res Commun* 1987;148:211.

205. Hosoda K, et al. Expression of brain natriuretic peptide gene in human heart: production in the ventricle. *Hypertension* 1991;17:1152.

206. Redfield MM, et al. Failure of atrial natriuretic factor to increase with volume expansion in acute and chronic heart failure in the dog. *Circulation* 1989;80:651.

207. Drexler H, et al. Vasodilatory action of endogenous atrial natriuretic factor in a rat model of chronic heart failure as determined by monoclonal ANF antibody. *Circ Res* 1990;66:1371.

208. Colucci WS, et al. Intravenous nesiritide, a natriuretic peptide, in the treatment of decompensated congestive heart failure. The nesiritide study group. *N Engl J Med* 2000;343:246.

209. Biollaz J, et al. Four-hour infusion of synthetic atrial natriuretic peptide in normal volunteers. *Hypertension* 1986;8:II96.

210. Borenstein HB, et al. The effect of natriuretic atrial extract on renal hemodynamics and urinary excretion in anesthetized rats. *J Physiol* 1983;334:133.

211. Dunn BR, et al. Renal and systemic hemodynamic effects of synthetic atrial natriuretic peptide in the anesthetized rat. *Circ Res* 1986;58:237.

212. Kim JK, et al. Enzymatic and binding effects of atrial natriuretic factor in glomeruli and nephrons. *Kidney Int* 1989;35:799.

213. Koseki C, et al. Localization of binding sites for alpha-rat natriuretic polypeptide in rat kidney. *Am J Physiol* 1986;250:F210.
214. Healy DP, Fanestil DD. Localization of atrial natriuretic peptide binding sites within the rat kidney. *Am J Physiol* 1986;250:F573.
215. Hoffman A, Grossman E, Keiser HR. Increased plasma levels and blunted effects of brain natriuretic peptide in rats with congestive heart failure. *Am J Hypertens* 1991;4:597.
216. Yoshimura M, et al. Hemodynamic, renal, and hormonal responses to brain natriuretic peptide infusion in patients with congestive heart failure. *Circulation* 1991;84:1581.
217. Gelfand RA, et al. Brain and atrial natriuretic peptides bind to common receptors in brain capillary endothelial cells. *Am J Physiol* 1991;261:E183.
218. Abraham WT, et al. Systemic hemodynamic, neurohormonal, and renal effects of a steady-state infusion of human brain natriuretic peptide in patients with hemodynamically decompensated heart failure. *J Card Fail* 1998;4:37.
219. Elsner D, et al. Efficacy of prolonged infusion of urodilatin [ANP(95-126)] in patients with congestive heart failure. *Am Heart J* 1995;129:766.
220. Feller SM, Gagelmann M, Forssmann WG. Urodilatin: a newly described member of the ANP family. *Trends Pharmacol Sci* 1989;10:93.
221. Drummer C, et al. Urodilatin, a kidney-derived natriuretic factor, is excreted with a circadian rhythm and is stimulated by saline infusion in man. *J Am Soc Nephrol* 1991;2:1109.
222. Saxenhofer H, et al. Urodilatin, a natriuretic factor from kidneys can modify renal and cardiovascular function in men. *Am J Physiol* 1990;259:F832.
223. Levin ER, et al. Decreased atrial natriuretic factor receptors and impaired cGMP generation in glomeruli from the cardiomyopathic hamster. *Biochem Biophys Res Commun* 1989;159:807.
224. Schiffrin EL. Decreased density of binding sites for atrial natriuretic peptide on platelets of patients with severe congestive heart failure. *Clin Sci* 1988;74:213.
225. Gutkowska J, et al. Circulating forms and radioimmunoassay of atrial natriuretic factor. *Endocrinol Metab Clin North Am* 1987;16:183.
226. Wilkins MR, et al. Maximizing the natriuretic effect of endogenous atriopeptin in a rat model of heart failure. *Proc Natl Acad Sci USA* 1990;87:6465.
227. Salerno F, et al. Renal response to atrial natriuretic peptide in patients with advanced liver cirrhosis. *Hepatology* 1988;8:21.
228. Huang CL, Ives HE, Cogan MG. In vivo evidence that cGMP is the second messenger for atrial natriuretic factor. *Proc Natl Acad Sci USA* 1986;83:8015.
229. Abraham WT, et al. Atrial natriuretic peptide and urinary cyclic guanosine monophosphate in patients with congestive heart failure. *J Am Soc Nephrol* 1992;2:697.
230. Abraham WT, et al. Reversal of atrial natriuretic peptide resistance by increasing distal tubular sodium delivery in patients with decompensated cirrhosis. *Hepatology* 1995;22:737.
231. Connelly TP, et al. Interaction of intravenous atrial natriuretic factor with furosemide in patients with heart failure. *Am Heart J* 1994;127:392.
232. Koepke JP, DiBona GF. Blunted natriuresis to atrial natriuretic peptide in chronic sodium-retaining disorders. *Am J Physiol* 1987;252:F865.
233. Arnold SB, et al. Long-term digitalis therapy improves left ventricular function in heart failure. *N Engl J Med* 1980;303:1443.
234. Ader R, et al. Immediate and sustained hemodynamic and clinical improvement in chronic heart failure by an oral angiotensin-converting enzyme inhibitor. *Circulation* 1980;61:931.
235. Packer M, et al. Effect of oral milrinone on mortality in severe chronic heart failure. *N Engl J Med* 1991;325:1468.
236. Feldman AM, et al. Effects of vesnarinone on morbidity and mortality in patients with heart failure. *N Engl J Med* 1993;329:149.
237. Cohn JN, et al. A dose-dependent increase in mortality with vesnarinone among patients with severe heart failure. *N Engl J Med* 1998;339:1810.
238. Packer M, et al. The effect of carvedilol on morbidity and mortality in patients with chronic heart failure. *N Engl J Med* 1996;334:1349.
239. CIBIS-II Investigators and Committees. The Cardiac Insufficiency Bisoprolol Study II (CIBIS-II): a randomized trial. *Lancet* 1999;353:9.
240. Goldstein S, et al. The mortality effect of metoprolol CR/XL in patients with heart failure: results of the MERIT-HF Trial. *Clin Cardiol* 1999;22:V30.
241. Packer M, et al. Consensus recommendations for the management of heart failure. *Am J Cardiol* 1999;83:1A.
242. Adams KF Jr, et al. Heart Failure Society of America guidelines for management of patients with heart failure caused by left ventricular systolic dysfunction—pharmacological approaches. *J Card Fail* 1999;5:357.
243. Packer M, on behalf of the COPERNICUS Investigators. Preliminary results of the Carvedilol Prospective Randomized Cumulative Survival (COPERNICUS) Trial. Presented at the XXIInd Congress of the European Society of Cardiology, Amsterdam, The Netherlands, August 26–30, 2000.
244. Eichhorn E, on behalf of the BEST Investigators. Preliminary results of the Beta-Blocker Evaluation of Survival Trial (BEST). Presented at the 72nd Annual Scientific Sessions of the American Heart Association, Atlanta, Georgia, November 7–10, 1999.
245. Agostoni PG, et al. Afterload reduction: a comparison of captopril and nifedipine in dilated cardiomyopathy. *Br Heart J* 55:391, 1986.
246. O'Connor CM, et al. Effect of amlodipine on mode of death among patients with advanced heart failure in the trial. Prospective Randomized Amlodipine Survival Evaluation. *Am J Cardiol* 1998;82:881.
247. Packer M, on behalf of the PRAISE II Investigators. Preliminary results of the Second Prospective Randomized Amlodipine Survival Evaluation. Presented at the 49th Annual Scientific Session of the American College of Cardiology, Anaheim, California, March 11, 2000.
248. Swedberg K, et al. Hormones regulating cardiovascular function in patients with severe congestive heart failure and their relation to mortality. *Circulation* 1990;82:1730.
249. Konstam MA, Dracup K, Baker DW, et al. Heart Failure: Evaluation and Care of Patients with Left Ventricular Systolic Dysfunction. Clinical Practice Guideline Number 11. Rockville, MD: Agency for Health Care Policy and Research, 1994.
250. Neuberg GW, Kukin ML, Penn J, et al. Hemodynamic effects of renin inhibition by enalkiren in chronic congestive heart failure. *Am J Cardiol* 1991;67:63.
251. Christen Y, et al. Oral administration of DuP 753, a specific angiotensin II receptor antagonist, to normal male volunteers: inhibition of pressor response to exogenous angiotensin I and II. *Circulation* 1991;83:1333.
252. Pitt B, et al. Randomised trial of losartan versus captopril in patients over 65 with heart failure. *Lancet* 1997;349:747.
253. Pitt B, et al. Effect of losartan compared with captopril on mortality in patients with symptomatic heart failure: randomised trial—the Losartan Heart Failure Survival Study ELITE II. *Lancet* 2000;355:1582.
254. McKelvie RS, et al. Comparisons of candesartan, enalapril, and their combination in congestive heart failure: Randomized Evaluation of Strategies for Left Ventricular Dysfunction (RESOLVD) pilot study. The RESOLVD Pilot Study investigators. *Circulation* 1999;100:1056.
255. Abraham WT. New neurohormonal antagonists and natriuretic peptides in the treatment of congestive heart failure. *Coronary Artery Dis* 1994;5:127.
256. Francis GS, et al. Acute vasoconstrictor response to intravenous furosemide in patients with chronic congestive heart failure. Activation of the neurohumoral axis. *Ann Intern Med* 1985;103:1.
257. Dileo M, et al. Ultrafiltration in the treatment of refractory congestive heart failure. *Clin Cardiol* 1988;11:449.
258. Marenzi G, et al. Interrelation of humoral factors, hemodynamics, and fluid and salt metabolism in congestive heart failure: effects of extracorporeal ultrafiltration. *Am J Med* 1993;94:49.
259. Agostoni P, et al. Sustained improvement in functional capacity after removal of body fluid with isolated ultrafiltration in chronic cardiac insufficiency: failure of furosemide to provide the same result. *Am J Med* 1994;96:191.
260. Canaud B, et al. Slow continuous and daily ultrafiltration for refractory congestive heart failure. *Nephrol Dial Transplant* 1998;13:51.
261. Dzau VJ, Hollenberg NK. Renal response to captopril in severe heart failure: role of furosemide in natriuresis and reversal of hyponatremia. *Ann Intern Med* 1984;100:777.
262. Packer M, Medina M, Yushak M. Correction of dilutional hyponatremia in severe chronic heart failure by converting-enzyme inhibition. *Ann Intern Med* 1984;100:782.
263. Gauer OH, Henry JP, Behn C. The regulation of extracellular fluid volume. *Annu Rev Physiol* 1970;32:547.
264. Better OS, Schrier RW. Disturbed volume homeostasis in cirrhosis of the liver. *Kidney Int* 1983;23:303.

265. Epstein M. Pathogenesis of renal sodium handling in cirrhosis. *Am J Nephrol* 1983;3:287.
266. Epstein M. Renal sodium handling in cirrhosis. *Semin Nephrol* 1983;3:225.
267. Epstein M. Renal sodium handling in cirrhosis. In: Epstein M, ed. *The kidney in liver disease,* 2nd ed. New York: Elsevier, 1983.
268. Levinsky NG. Refractory ascites in cirrhosis. *Kidney Int* 1978;14:93.
269. Levy M. The kidney in liver disease. In: Brenner BM, Stein JH, eds. *Contemporary issues in nephrology,* vol 1. New York: Churchill Livingstone, 1978.
270. Levy M. Pathophysiology of ascites formation in the kidney. In: Epstein M, ed. *The kidney in liver disease,* 2nd ed. New York: Elsevier, 1983.
271. Levy M, Wexler MJ. Salt and water balance in liver disease. *Hosp Pract* 1984;19:57.
272. Paller MS, Schrier RW. Pathogenesis of sodium and water retention in edematous disorders. *Am J Kidney Dis* 1982;2:241.
273. Skorecki K, Brenner BM. Edema forming states: congestive heart failure, liver disease and nephrotic syndrome. In: Arieff AI, de Fronzo RA, ed. *Fluid, electrolyte and acid–base disorders.* New York: Churchill Livingstone, 1985.
274. Eisenmenger WJ, et al. Electrolyte studies on patients with cirrhosis of the liver. *J Clin Invest* 1950;292:1491.
275. Papper S, Saxon L. The influence of intravenous infusion of sodium chloride solutions on the renal excretion of sodium in patients with cirrhosis of the liver. *J Clin Invest* 1956;35:728.
276. Smith HW. Salt and water volume receptors. An exercise in physiologic apologetics. *Am J Med* 1957;23:623.
277. Lieberman FL, Denison EK, Reynolds TF. The relationship of plasma volume, portal hypertension, ascites and renal sodium retention in cirrhosis: the overflow theory of ascites formation. *Ann NY Acad Sci* 1970;170:202.
278. Schrier RW, et al. Peripheral arterial vasodilation hypothesis: a proposal for the initiation of renal sodium and water retention in cirrhosis. *Hepatology* 1988;8:1151.
279. Rahman SN, Abraham WT, Schrier RW. Peripheral arterial vasodilation hypothesis in cirrhosis. *Gastroenterol Int* 1992;5:192.
280. Vorobioff J, Bredfeldt JE, Groszmann RJ. Hyperdynamic circulation in portal-hypertensive rat model: a primary factor for maintenance of chronic portal hypertension. *Am J Physiol* 1983;244:G52.
281. Vorobioff J, Bredfeldt JE, Groszmann RJ. Increased blood flow through the portal system in cirrhotic rats. *Gastroenterology* 1984;87:1120.
282. Benoit JN, Granger DN. Splanchnic hemodynamics in chronic portal hypertension. *Semin Liver Dis* 1986;6:287.
283. Sugita S, et al. Splanchnic hemodynamics in portal hypertensive dogs with portal fibrosis. *Am J Physiol* 1987;252:G748.
284. Huet PM, et al. Intrahepatic circulation in liver disease. *Semin Liver Dis* 1986;6:277.
285. Kotelanski B, Groszmann R, Cohn JN. Circulation times in the splanchnic and hepatic beds in alcoholic liver disease. *Gastroenterology* 1972;63:102.
286. Fernandez-Seara J, et al. Systemic and regional hemodynamics in patients with liver cirrhosis and ascites with and without functional renal failure. *Gastroenterology* 1989;97:1304.
287. Maroto A, et al. Brachial and femoral artery blood flow in cirrhosis. *Hepatology* 1993;17:788.
288. Vallance P, Moncada S. Hyperdynamic circulation in cirrhosis: a role for nitric oxide? *Lancet* 1991;337:776.
289. Burton GA, et al. Cyclic GMP release and vasodilation induced by EDRF and atrial natriuretic factor in the isolated perfused kidney of the rat. *Br J Pharmacol* 1990;99:364.
290. Miyase S, et al. Atrial natriuretic peptide in liver cirrhosis with mild ascites. *Gastroenterol Jpn* 1990;25:356.
291. Guarner C, et al. Increased serum nitrite and nitrate levels in patients with cirrhosis: relationship to endotoxemia. *Hepatology* 1993;18:1139.
292. Niederberger M, et al. Increased aortic cyclic guanosine monophosphate concentration in experimental cirrhosis in rats: evidence for a role of nitric oxide in the pathogenesis of arterial vasodilation in cirrhosis. *Hepatology* 1995;250:1625.
293. Niederberger M, et al. Normalization of nitric oxide production corrects arterial vasodilation and hyperdynamic circulation in cirrhotic rats. *Gastroenterology* 1995;109:1624.
294. Albillos A, et al. Enhanced endothelium-derived vasodilation in patients with cirrhosis. *Am J Physiol* 1995;268:G459.
295. Martin PY, et al. Nitric oxide synthase (NOS) inhibition for one week improves renal sodium and water excretion in cirrhotic rats with ascites. *J Clin Invest* 1998;101:235.
296. Leehey DJ, et al. Naloxone increases water and electrolyte excretion after water loading in patients with cirrhosis and ascites. *J Lab Clin Med* 1991;118:484.
297. Villamediana LM, et al. Vascular reactivity to norepinephrine in rats with cirrhosis of the liver. *Can J Physiol Pharmacol* 1988;66:567.
298. Ryan J, et al. Impaired reactivity of the peripheral vasculature to pressor agents in alcoholic cirrhosis. *Gastroenterology* 1993;105:1167.
299. Vlachcevic ZR, et al. Renal effects of acute expansion of plasma volume in cirrhosis. *N Engl J Med* 1965;272:387.
300. Yamahiro HS, Reynolds TB. Effects of ascitic fluid infusion on sodium excretion, blood volume and creatinine clearance in cirrhosis. *Gastroenterology* 1961;40:497.
301. Epstein M. The peritoneovenous shunt in the management of ascites and the hepatorenal syndrome. *Gastroenterology* 1982;82:790.
302. Klinger EL Jr, et al. Renal function changes in cirrhosis of the liver. *Arch Intern Med* 1970;125:1010.
303. Laragh JH, et al. Angiotensin II, norepinephrine and renal transport of electrolytes and water in normal man and in cirrhosis with ascites. *J Clin Invest* 1963;42:1179.
304. Lopez-Nova JM, et al. A micropuncture study of salt and water retention in chronic experimental cirrhosis. *Am J Physiol* 1977;232:F315.
305. Bank N, Aynedjian HS. A micropuncture study of renal salt and water retention in chronic bile duct obstruction. *J Clin Invest* 1975;55:994.
306. Better OS, Massry SG. Effect of chronic bile duct obstruction on renal handling of salt and water. *J Clin Invest* 1972;51:402.
307. Chaimovitz C, et al. Mechanism of increased renal tubular sodium reabsorption in cirrhosis. *Am J Med* 1972;52:198.
308. Schubert J, Puschett J, Goldberg M. The renal mechanism of sodium reabsorption in cirrhosis. *Am Sci Nephrol* 1969;3:58A.
309. Levy M. Sodium retention and ascites formation in dogs with experimental portal cirrhosis. *Am J Physiol* 1977;233:F575.
310. Epstein M, et al. Determinants of deranged sodium and water homeostasis in decompensated cirrhosis. *J Lab Clin Med* 1976;87:822.
311. Henriksen JH, Christensen JJ, Ring-Larsen H. Noradrenaline and adrenaline concentrations in various vascular beds in patients with cirrhosis: relation to hemodynamics. *Clin Physiol* 1981;1:293.
312. Bichet DG, van Putten VJ, Schrier RW. Potential role of increased sympathetic activity in impaired sodium and water excretion in cirrhosis. *N Engl J Med* 1982;307:1552.
313. Pérez-Ayuso RM, et al. Evidence that renal prostaglandins are involved in renal water metabolism in cirrhosis. *Kidney Int* 1984;26:72.
314. Arroyo V, et al. Sympathetic nervous activity, renin–angiotensin system and renal excretion of prostaglandin E2 in cirrhosis. Relationship to functional renal failure and sodium and water excretion. *Eur J Clin Invest* 1983;13:271.
315. Ring-Larsen H, et al. Sympathetic nervous activity and renal and systemic hemodynamics in cirrhosis: plasma norepinephrine concentration, hepatic extraction and renal release. *Hepatology* 1982;2:304.
316. Nicholls KM, et al. Elevated plasma norepinephrine concentration in decompensated cirrhosis: association with increased secretion rates, normal clearance rates, and suppressibility by central blood volume expansion. *Circ Res* 1985;56:457.
317. Floras JS, et al. Increased sympathetic outflow in cirrhosis and ascites: direct evidence from intraneural recordings. *Ann Intern Med* 1991;114:373.
318. Grossman SH, et al. Plasma norepinephrine in the evaluation of baroreceptor function in humans. *Hypertension* 1982;4:566.
319. Ring-Larsen H, Henriksen JG, Christensen NJ. Increased sympathetic activity in cirrhosis. *N Engl J Med* 1983;308:1029.
320. Eggert RC. Spironolactone diuresis in patients with cirrhosis and ascites. *Br Med J* 1970;4:401.
321. Giuseffi J, et al. Effect of bilateral adrenalectomy in a patient with massive ascites and postnecrotic cirrhosis. *N Engl J Med* 1957;257:796.
322. Rosoff L, et al. Studies of renin and aldosterone in cirrhotic patients with ascites. *Gastroenterology* 1975;69:698.
323. Nicholls KM, et al. Sodium excretion in advanced cirrhosis: requirement for simultaneous expansion of central blood volume and relative suppression of plasma aldosterone. *Hepatology* 1986;6:253.
324. Bichet D, et al. Role of vasopressin in abnormal water excretion in cirrhotic patients. *Ann Intern Med* 1982;96:413.

325. Arroyo V, et al. Prognostic value of spontaneous hyponatremia in cirrhosis with ascites. *Dig Dis Sci* 1976;21:249.

326. Birchard WH, et al. Diuretic responses to oral and intravenous water loads in patients with hepatic cirrhosis. *J Lab Clin Med* 1956;48:26.

327. Ralli EP, et al. Studies of the serum and urine constituents in patients with cirrhosis of the liver during water tolerance tests. *Am J Med* 1951;11:157.

328. Reznick RK, et al. Hyponatremia and arginine vasopressin secretion in patients with refractory hepatic ascites undergoing peritoneovenous shunting. *Gastroenterology* 1983;84:713.

329. Schrier RW. Mechanisms of disturbed renal water excretion in cirrhosis. *Gastroenterology* 1983;84:870.

330. Madsen M, et al. Impaired renal water excretion in early hepatic cirrhosis. *Scand J Gastroenterol* 1986;21:749.

331. Better OS, et al. Role of antidiuretic hormone in impaired urinary dilution associated with chronic bile duct ligation. *Clin Sci* 1980;58:493.

332. Linas SL, et al. The role of vasopressin in the impaired water excretion in the conscious rat with experimental cirrhosis. *Kidney Int* 1981;20:173.

333. Salerno F, et al. Vasopressin release and water metabolism in patients with cirrhosis. *J Hepatol* 1994;21:822.

334. Claria J, et al. Blockade of the hydroosmotic effect of vasopressin normalizes water excretion in cirrhotic rats. *Gastroenterology* 1989;97:1294.

335. Tsuboi Y, et al. Therapeutic efficacy of the nonpeptide AVP antagonist OPC-31260 in cirrhotic rats. *Kidney Int* 1994;46:237.

336. Fujita N, et al. Role of water channel AQP-CD in water retention in SIADH and cirrhotic rats. *Am J Physiol* 1995;269:F926.

337. Fernandez-Llama P, et al. Dysregulation of renal aquaporins and Na-Cl cotransporter in CCl4-induced cirrhosis. *Kidney Int* 2000;58:216.

338. Fernandez-Llama P, et al. Renal expression of aquaporins in liver cirrhosis induced by chronic common bile duct ligation in rats. *J Am Soc Nephrol* 1999;10:1950.

339. Inoue T, et al. Therapeutic and diagnostic potential of a vasopressin-2 antagonist for impaired water handling in cirrhosis. *Clin Pharmacol Ther* 1998;63:561.

340. Cosby RL, Yee B, Schrier RW. New classification with prognostic value in cirrhotic patients. *Miner Electrolyte Metab* 1989;15:261.

341. Llach J, et al. Prognostic value of arterial pressure, endogenous vasoactive systems, and renal function in cirrhotic patients admitted to the hospital for the treatment of ascites. *Gastroenterology* 1988;94:482.

342. Fernández-Esparrach G, et al. A prognostic model for predicting survival in cirrhosis with ascites. *J Hepatol* 2001;34:46.

343. Fernández-Cruz A, et al. Plasma levels of atrial natriuretic peptide in cirrhotic patients. *Lancet* 1985;ii:1439.

344. Panos MZ, et al. Plasma atrial natriuretic peptide and renin-aldosterone in patients with cirrhosis and ascites: basal levels, changes during daily activity and nocturnal diuresis. *Hepatology* 1992;16:82.

345. Fyhrquist F, Tötterman KJ, Tikkanen I. Infusion of atrial natriuretic peptide in liver cirrhosis with ascites. *Lancet* 1985;ii:1439.

346. Schrier RW, Better OS. Pathogenesis of ascites formation: Mechanism of impaired aldosterone escape in cirrhosis. *Eur J Gastroenterol Hepatol* 1991;3:721.

347. Morali GA, et al. Refractory ascites: modulation of atrial natriuretic factor unresponsiveness by mannitol. *Hepatology* 1992;16:42.

348. Koepke JP, Jones S, DiBona GF. Renal nerves mediate blunted natriuresis to atrial natriuretic peptide in cirrhotic rats. *Am J Physiol* 1987;252:R1019.

349. Zambraski EJ, Dunn MJ. Importance of renal prostaglandins in control of renal function after chronic ligation of the common bile duct in dogs. *J Lab Clin Med* 1984;103:549.

350. Boyer TD, Zia P, Reynolds TB. Effect of indomethacin and prostaglandin A1 on renal function and plasma renin activity in alcoholic liver disease. *Gastroenterology* 1979;77:215.

351. Wong F, et al. Indomethacin-induced renal dysfunction in patients with well-compensated cirrhosis. *Gastroenterology* 1993;104:869.

352. Zipser RD, et al. Prostaglandins: modulators of renal function and pressor resistance in chronic liver disease. *J Clin Endocrinol Metab* 1979;48:895.

353. Bosch-Marce M, et al. Selective inhibition of cyclooxygenase-2 spares renal function and prostaglandin synthesis in cirrhotic rats with ascites. *Gastroenterology* 1999;116:1167.

354. Shear L, Ching S, Gabuzda GJ. Compartmentalization of ascites and edema in patients with hepatic cirrhosis. *N Engl J Med* 1970;282:1391.

355. Pockros PJ, Reynolds TB. Rapid diuresis in patients with ascites from chronic liver disease: the importance of peripheral edema. *Gastroenterology* 1986;90:1827.

356. Rocco UK, Ware AJ. Cirrhotic ascites. *Ann Intern Med* 1986;105:573.

357. Ginès P, et al. Comparison between paracentesis and diuretics in the treatment of cirrhotics with tense ascites. *Gastroenterology* 1987;93:234.

358. Ginès P, et al. Randomized comparative study of therapeutic paracentesis with and without intravenous albumin in cirrhosis. *Gastroenterology* 1988;94:1493.

359. Quintero E, et al. Paracentesis versus diuretics in the treatment of cirrhotics with tense ascites. *Lancet* 1985;1:611.

360. Tito L, et al. Total paracentesis associated with intravenous albumin management of patients with cirrhosis and ascites. *Gastroenterology* 1990;98:146.

361. Epstein M. Treatment of refractory ascites. *N Engl J Med* 1989;321:1675.

362. Stanley MM, et al. Peritoneovenous shunting as compared with medical treatment in patients with alcoholic cirrhosis and massive ascites. *N Engl J Med* 1989;321:1632.

363. Ginès P, et al. Paracentesis with intravenous infusion of albumin as compared with peritoneovenous shunting in cirrhosis with refractory ascites. *N Engl J Med* 1991;325:829.

364. Ochs A, et al. The transjugular intrahepatic portosystemic stent-shunt procedure for refractory ascites. *N Engl J Med* 1995;332:1192.

365. Rossle M, et al. A comparison of paracentesis and transjugular intrahepatic portosystemic shunting in patients with ascites. *N Engl J Med* 2000;342:1701.

366. Miller-Catchpole R. Transjugular intrahepatic portosystemic shunt (TIPS): diagnostic and therapeutic assessment (DATTA). *JAMA* 1995;272:1824.

367. Lotterer E, et al. Transjugular intrahepatic portosystemic shunt: short-term and long-term effects on hepatic and systemic hemodynamics in patients with cirrhosis. *Hepatology* 1999;29:632.

368. Colombato LA, et al. Haemodynamic adaptation two months after transjugular intrahepatic portosystemic shunt (TIPS) in cirrhotic patients. *Gut* 1996;39:600.

369. Rodriguez-Laiz JM, et al. Effects of transjugular intrahepatic portasystemic shunt (TIPS) on splanchnic and systemic hemodynamics, and hepatic function in patients with portal hypertension. Preliminary results. *Dig Dis Sci* 1995;40:2121.

370. Escorsell A, et al. Multicenter randomized controlled trial of terlipressin versus sclerotherapy in the treatment of acute variceal bleeding: the TEST study. *Hepatology* 2000;32:471.

371. Moller S, et al. Central and systemic haemodynamic effects of terlipressin in portal hypertensive patients. *Liver* 2000;20:51.

372. Uriz J, et al. Terlipressin plus albumin infusion: an effective and safe therapy of hepatorenal syndrome. *J Hepatol* 2000;33:43.

373. Davidson CS. Cirrhosis of the liver: treatment with prolonged sodium restriction. *JAMA* 1955;159:1257.

374. Reynolds TB, et al. Spontaneous decrease in portal pressure with clinical improvement in cirrhosis. *N Engl J Med* 1960;263:734.

375. Arroyo V, et al. Management of patients with cirrhosis and ascites. *Semin Liver Dis* 1986;6:353.

376. Fogel MR, et al. Diuresis in the ascitic patient: a randomized controlled trial of three regimens. *J Clin Gastroenterol* 1981;3:73.

377. Pérez-Ayuso RM, et al. Randomized comparative study of efficacy of furosemide versus spironolactone in nonazotemic cirrhosis with ascites. Relationship between the diuretic response and the activity of the renin-aldosterone system. *Gastroenterology* 1983;84:961.

378. Campra JL, Reynolds TB. Effectiveness of high-dose spironolactone therapy in patients with chronic liver disease and relatively refractory ascites. *Dig Dis Sci* 1978;23:1025.

379. Carrilho F, et al. Renal failure associated with demeclocycline in cirrhosis. *Ann Intern Med* 1977;87:195.

380. Miller PD, Linas SL, Schrier RW. Plasma demeclocycline levels and nephrotoxicity. Correlation in hyponatremic cirrhotic patients. *JAMA* 1980;243:2513.

381. Oster JR, Epstein M, Ulano HB. Deterioration of renal function with demeclocycline administration. *Curr Ther Res* 1976;20:794.

382. Pérez-Ayuso RM, et al. Effect of demeclocycline on renal function and urinary prostaglandin E2 and kallikrein in hyponatremic cirrhotics. *Nephron* 1984;36:30.

383. Schrier RW, Fassett RG. A critique of the overfill hypothesis of sodium and water retention in the nephrotic syndrome. *Kidney Int* 1998;53:1111.

384. Dorhout-Mees EJ, Geers HG, Koomans HA. Blood volume and sodium retention in the nephrotic syndrome: a controversial pathophysiological concept. *Nephron* 1984;36:201.

385. Geers AB, et al. Functional relationships in the nephrotic syndrome. *Kidney Int* 1984;26:324.

386. Koomans HA, et al. Effects of plasma volume expansion on renal salt handling in patients with nephrotic syndrome. *Am J Nephrol* 1984;4:227.

387. Meltzer JI, et al. Nephrotic syndrome: vasoconstriction and hypervolemic types indicated by renin-sodium profiling. *Ann Intern Med* 1979;91:688.

388. Dorhout-Mees EJ, et al. Observations on edema formation in the nephrotic syndrome in adults with minimal lesions. *Am J Med* 1979; 67:378.

389. Krishna GG, Danovitch GM. Effect of water immersion on renal function in the nephrotic syndrome. *Kidney Int* 1982;21:395.

390. Kumagai H, et al. Role of renin–angiotensin–aldosterone on minimal change nephrotic syndrome. *Clin Nephrol* 1985;25:229.

391. Metcoff J, Janaway CA. Studies on the pathogenesis of nephrotic edema. *J Pediatr* 1951;58:640.

392. Squire JR. The nephrotic syndrome. *Adv Intern Med* 1955;7:201.

393. Usberti M, et al. Role of plasma vasopressin in the impairment of water excretion in nephrotic syndrome. *Kidney Int* 1984;25:422.

394. Chamberlain MJ, Pringl A, Wrong OM. Oliguric renal failure in the nephrotic syndrome. *Q J Med* 1966;35:215.

395. Hopper JJ, et al. Lipoid nephrosis in 31 adult patients. *Medicine* 1970;49:321.

396. Yamauchi H, Hopper J. Hypovolemic shock and hypotension as a complication in the nephrotic syndrome. *Medicine* 1964;60:242.

397. Hammond TG, et al. Renin–angiotensin–aldosterone system in nephrotic syndrome. *Am J Kidney Dis* 1984;4:18.

398. Kelsch RC, Light GS, Oliver WJ. The effect of albumin infusion upon plasma norepinephrine concentration in nephrotic children. *J Lab Clin Med* 1972;79:516.

399. Berlyne GM, et al. Renal salt and water handling in water immersion in the nephrotic syndrome. *Clin Sci* 1981;61:605.

400. Usberti M, et al. Considerations on the sodium retention in nephrotic syndrome. *Am J Nephrol* 1995;15:38.

401. Brown EA, et al. Evidence that some mechanism other than the renin system causes sodium retention in the nephrotic syndrome. *Lancet* 1982;2:1237.

402. Geers AB, et al. Plasma and blood volumes in the nephrotic syndrome. *Nephron* 1984;38:170.

403. Epstein FH. Underfilling vs. overflow in hepatic ascites. *N Engl J Med* 1982;307:1577.

404. Eisenberg MD. Postural changes in plasma volume in hypoalbuminemia. *Arch Intern Med* 1963;112:544.

405. Bernard DB, et al. Renal sodium retention during volume expansion in experimental nephrotic syndrome. *Kidney Int* 1978;14:478.

406. Sonnenberg H. Medullary collecting duct function in antidiuretic and in salt- or water-diuretic rats. *Am J Physiol* 1974;226:501.

407. Kuroda S, Aynedjian HS, Bank N. A micropuncture study of renal sodium retention in nephrotic syndrome in rats: evidence for increased resistance to tubular fluid flow. *Kidney Int* 1979;16: 561.

408. Ichikawa I, et al. Role of intrarenal mechanisms in the impaired salt excretion in experimental nephrotic syndrome. *J Clin Invest* 1983; 71:91.

409. Firth JD, Raine AE, Ledingham JG. Abnormal sodium handling occurs in the isolated perfused kidney of the nephrotic rat. *Clin Sci* 1989;76:387.

410. Keeler R. Chemical medullectomy does not prevent sodium retention in nephrotic rats. *Miner Electrolyte Metab* 1989;15:241.

411. Grausz H, Lieberman R, Earley LE. Effect of plasma albumin on sodium reabsorption in patients with nephrotic syndrome. *Kidney Int* 1972;1:47.

412. Gur A, et al. A study of the renal handling of water in lipid nephrosis. *Pediatr Res* 1976;20:197.

413. Usberti M, et al. Relationship between serum albumin concentration and tubular reabsorption of glucose in renal disease. *Kidney Int* 1979;16:546.

414. Shapiro MD, et al. Role of glomerular filtration rate in the impaired sodium and water excretion of patients with the nephrotic syndrome. *Am J Kidney Dis* 1986;3:81.

415. Rahman SN, et al. Increased norepinephrine secretion in patients with the nephrotic syndrome and normal glomerular filtration rates: evidence for primary sympathetic activation. *Am J Nephrol* 1993;13:266.

416. Kalant N, et al. Mechanisms of edema formation in experimental nephrosis. *Am J Physiol* 1962;202:91.

417. Tobian L, Perry S, Mork J. The relationship of the juxtaglomerular apparatus to sodium retention in experimental nephrosis. *Ann Intern Med* 1962;57:382.

418. Brown A, et al. Is the renin–angiotensin–aldosterone system involved in the sodium retention in the nephrotic syndrome? *Nephron* 1982;32:102.

419. Brown EA, et al. Lack of effect of captopril on the sodium retention in nephrotic syndrome. *Nephron* 1984;37:43.

420. Dusing R, Vetter H, Kramer HJ. The renin–angiotensin–aldosterone system in patients with nephrotic syndrome. *Nephron* 1980;25:187.

421. Shapiro MD, et al. Role of aldosterone in the sodium retention of patients with nephrotic syndrome. *Am J Nephrol* 1990;10:44.

422. Bichet D, Manzini C. Role of vasopressin (AVP) in the abnormal water excretion in nephrotic patients. *Kidney Int* 1984;25:160.

423. Pedersen EB, et al. Defective renal water excretion in nephrotic syndrome: the relationship between renal water excretion and kidney function, arginine vasopressin, angiotensin II and aldosterone in plasma before and after water loading. *Eur J Clin Invest* 1985;15:24.

424. Ladenson JH, Apple FS, Koch DD. Misleading hyponatremia due to hyperlipemia: a method dependent on error. *Ann Intern Med* 1981;95:707.

425. Rascher W, et al. Diuretic and hormonal responses to head-out water immersion in nephrotic syndrome. *J Pediatr* 1986;109:609.

426. Pyo HJ, et al. Arginine vasopressin gene expression in rats with puromycin-induced nephrotic syndrome. *Am J Kidney Dis* 1995;25:58.

427. Apostol E, et al. Reduced renal medullary water channel expression in puromycin aminonucleoside-induced nephrotic syndrome. *J Am Soc Nephrol* 1997;8:15.

428. Fernandez-Llama P, et al. Impaired aquaporin and urea transporter expression in rats with adriamycin-induced nephrotic syndrome. *Kidney Int* 1998;53:1244.

429. Hisanaga S, et al. Plasma concentration and renal effect of human atrial natriuretic peptide in nephrotic syndrome. *Jpn J Nephrol* 1989;31:661.

430. Yokota N, et al. Increased plasma levels and effects of brain natriuretic peptide in experimental nephrosis. *Nephron* 1993;65:454.

431. Perico N, Remuzzi G. Renal handling of sodium in the nephrotic syndrome. *Am J Nephrol* 1993;13:413.

432. Abassi Z, et al. Effect of atrial natriuretic factor on renal cGMP production in rats with adriamycin-induced nephrotic syndrome. *J Am Soc Nephrol* 1992;2:1538.

433. Kleinknecht C, et al. Irreversible renal failure after indomethacin in steroid resistant nephrosis. *N Engl J Med* 1980;302:691.

434. Border WA, Glassock RJ. The management of the nephrotic syndrome. In: Suki WN, Massry RJ, eds. *Therapy of renal diseases and related disorders*. Boston: Martinus Nijhoff, 1984.

435. Strauss J, Freundlich M, Zilleruelo G. Nephrotic edema: etiopathogenic and therapeutic considerations. *Nephron* 1984;38:73.

436. Blainey JO. High protein diets in the treatment of nephrotic syndrome. *Clin Sci* 1964;13:567.

437. Engle ME, et al. The use of furosemide in the treatment of edema in infants and children. *Pediatrics* 1978;62:811.

438. Garin EH, Richard GA. Edema resistant to furosemide therapy in nephrotic syndrome: treatment with furosemide and metolazone. *Int J Pediatr Nephrol* 1981;2:181.

439. Marone C, Reubi FC. Effects of a new diuretic (piretanide) compared with furosemide on renal diluting and concentrating mechanisms in patients with nephrotic syndrome. *Eur J Clin Pharmacol* 1980;17: 165.

440. Keller E, Hoppe-Seyler G, Schollmeyer P. Disposition and diuretic effect of furosemide in the nephrotic syndrome. *Clin Pharmacol Ther* 1982;12:442.

441. Prandota J, Pruitt AW. Furosemide binding to human albumin and plasma of nephrotic children. *Clin Pharmacol Ther* 1975;17:159.

442. Rane A, et al. Plasma binding and disposition of furosemide in the nephrotic syndrome and in uremia. *Clin Pharmacol Ther* 1978;24:199.

443. Davison AM, et al. Salt-poor human albumin in management of nephrotic syndrome. *Br Med J* 1974;1:481.

444. Ginsberg JM, et al. Use of single voided urine samples to estimate quantitative proteinuria. *N Engl J Med* 1983;309:1543.
445. Luetscher JA, Hall AD, Kremer VL. Treatment of nephrosis with concentrated human serum albumin. II. Effects on renal function and on excretion of water and some electrolytes. *J Clin Invest* 1950;29:896.
446. Kaysen GA, et al. Effect of dietary protein intake on albumin homeostasis in nephrotic patients. *Kidney Int* 1986;29:572.
447. Kaysen GA, Kirkpatrick WG, Couser WG. Albumin homeostasis in the nephrotic rat: nutritional considerations. *Am J Physiol* 1984;247:F192.
448. Hutchison FN, Schambelan M, Kaysen GA. Modulation of albuminuria by dietary protein and converting enzyme inhibition. *Am J Physiol* 1987;53:F719.
449. Taguma Y, et al. Effect of captopril on heavy proteinuria in azotemic diabetics. *N Engl J Med* 1985;313:1617.
450. Bjorck S, et al. Beneficial effects of angiotensin converting enzyme inhibition on renal function in patients with diabetic nephropathy. *Br Med J* 1986;293:471.
451. Don BR, et al. Effect of dietary protein restriction and angiotensin converting enzyme inhibition on protein metabolism in the nephrotic syndrome. *Kidney Int* 1989;36:S163.
452. Gansevoort RT, De Zeeuw D, De Jong PE. Is the antiproteinuric effect of ACE inhibition mediated by interference in the renin–angiotensin system? *Kidney Int* 1994;45:861.
453. Rabelink AJ, et al. Partial remission of nephrotic syndrome in patients on long-term simvastatin. *Lancet* 1990;335:1045.
454. Thomas M, Moorhead JF. Nephrotic syndrome and simvastatin. *Lancet* 1990;335:1344.
455. Berlyne GM, et al. Water immersion in nephrotic syndrome. *Arch Intern Med* 1981;141:1275.

CHAPTER 85

The Syndrome of Inappropriate Antidiuretic Hormone Secretion and Other Hypoosmolar Disorders

The syndrome of inappropriate antidiuretic hormone secretion (SIADH) is produced when plasma levels of arginine vasopressin (AVP) are elevated at times when physiologic AVP secretion from the posterior pituitary would normally be suppressed. Because the only clinical abnormality known to result from increased secretion of AVP is a decrease in the osmotic pressure of body fluids, the hallmark of SIADH is hypoosmolality. This clinical finding led to the identification of the first well described cases of this disorder in 1957 (1) and the subsequent clinical investigations, which resulted in the delineation of the essential characteristics of the syndrome (2). It therefore not only is appropriate, but necessary, to begin this chapter with a summary of some general issues concerning hypoosmolality and hyponatremia before discussing details that are specific to SIADH and related disorders associated with dilutional hypoosmolality of body fluids. Although much has been learned over the last four decades about the pathophysiology of SIADH and hyponatremia, it remains surprising how rudimentary our understanding is of some of the most basic aspects of this disorder (3). One particularly striking example of this is the controversy in the last decade concerning the most appropriate rate of correction of hyponatremic patients (4). Nonetheless, recent and ongoing clinical and basic studies have begun to shed new light on many heretofore incompletely understood aspects of hypoosmolar disorders. In addition, we are on the verge of an exciting new era with regard to the therapy of these disorders using specific AVP receptor antagonists (5). Consequently, this chapter is written with the expectation that much of the specific information contained herein will be outdated at some future time. However, many of the basic concepts underlying the pathophysiology, differential diagnosis, and therapy of hypoosmolar disorders have withstood the tests of time and clinical utility, and consequently these will likely remain valid for some time to come.

HYPOOSMOLALITY AND HYPONATREMIA

Incidence

Hypoosmolality is one of the most common disorders of fluid and electrolyte balance encountered in hospitalized patients. The incidence and prevalence of hypoosmolar disorders depend both on the nature of the patient population being studied as well as on the laboratory methods and diagnostic criteria used to ascertain hyponatremia. Most investigators have used the serum sodium concentration ($[Na^+]$) to determine the clinical incidence of hypoosmolality. When hyponatremia is defined as a serum $[Na^+]$ of less than 135 mEq/L, incidences as high as 15% to 30% have been observed in studies of both acutely (6,7) and chronically (8) hospitalized patients. These high incidences in hospitalized patients are corroborated by frequency analysis of a large population of hospitalized patients, which demonstrated that serum $[Na^+]$ and chloride concentrations were approximately 5 mEq/L lower than those in a control group of healthy, nonhospitalized subjects (9). However, incidences decrease to the range of 1% to 4% when only patients with a serum $[Na^+]$ under 130 to 131 mEq/L are included (7,10–13), which represents a more appropriate level at which to define the occurrence of clinically significant cases of this disorder. Even using these more stringent criteria to define hypoosmolality, incidences from 7% to 53% have been reported in institutionalized geriatric patients (14–16). Perhaps most important, all studies to date have noted a high proportion of iatrogenic or hospital-acquired hyponatremia, which has accounted for as much as 40% to 75% of all patients studied (10,12). Therefore, although hyponatremia and hypoosmolality are exceedingly common, it is apparent that

J.G. Verbalis: Departments of Medicine and Physiology, Georgetown University School of Medicine and Georgetown University Medical Center, Washington, DC

most cases are relatively mild and most are acquired during the course of hospitalization.

These considerations could be interpreted to indicate that hypoosmolality is of relatively little clinical significance, but such a conclusion is unwarranted for several reasons. First, severe hypoosmolality (serum [Na$^+$] levels <120 mEq/L), although relatively uncommon, is associated with substantial morbidity and mortality rates (17,18). Second, even relatively mild hypoosmolality can quickly progress to more dangerous levels during the course of therapeutic management of other disorders. Third, overly rapid correction of hyponatremia can itself cause severe neurologic morbidity and mortality (19). Finally, it has been observed that mortality rates are much higher, from 3-fold (11,13) to 60-fold (12), in patients with even asymptomatic degrees of hypoosmolality compared with normonatremic patients. This probably is because hypoosmolality is more an indicator of the severity of many underlying illnesses than it is an independent contributing factor to mortality (20,21), but this presumption may not be true of all cases. These considerations therefore emphasize the importance of a careful evaluation of all hyponatremic patients, regardless of the clinical setting in which they present.

Osmolality, Tonicity, and Serum [Na$^+$]

As discussed in Chapter 3, the osmolality of body fluid normally is maintained within very narrow limits by osmotically regulated AVP secretion and thirst. Although basal plasma osmolality can vary appreciably among individuals, the range in the general population under conditions of normal hydration lies between 275 and 295 mOsm/kg H$_2$O. Plasma osmolality can be determined directly by measuring the freezing-point depression or the vapor pressure of plasma. Alternatively, it can be calculated indirectly from the concentrations of the three major solutes in plasma:

$$P_{osm} \, (mOsm/kg\,H_2O) = 2 \times [Na^+] \, (mEq/L)$$
$$+ \, glucose \, (mg/dL)/18$$
$$+ \, blood \, urea \, nitrogen \, (mg/dL)/2.8$$

Both methods produce comparable results under most conditions. However, although either of these methods produces valid measures of *total* osmolality, this is not always equivalent to the *effective* osmolality, which is commonly referred to as the tonicity of the plasma. Only cell membrane–impermeable solutes such as Na$^+$ and Cl$^-$ that remain relatively compartmentalized in the extracellular fluid (ECF) space are "effective" solutes, because these solutes create osmotic gradients across cell membranes and thus generate osmotic movement of water from the intracellular fluid (ICF) compartment into the ECF compartment. By contrast, solutes that readily permeate cell membranes (e.g., urea, ethanol, methanol) are not effective solutes because they do not create osmotic gradients across cell membranes and thus do

not generate water movement between body fluid compartments. Therefore, only the concentrations of effective solutes in plasma should be used to ascertain whether clinically significant hyperosmolality or hypoosmolality is present because these are the only solutes that directly affect cellular hydration (22).

Sodium and its accompanying anions represent the bulk of the major effective plasma solutes, so hyponatremia and hypoosmolality usually are synonymous. However, there are two important situations in which hyponatremia does not reflect true hypoosmolality. The first is pseudohyponatremia, which is produced by marked elevations of either lipids or proteins in plasma. In such cases, the concentration of Na$^+$ per liter of plasma water is unchanged, but the concentration of Na$^+$ per liter of plasma is artifactually decreased because of the larger relative proportion of plasma volume that is occupied by the excess lipids or proteins (23,24). However, the increased protein or lipid does not appreciably increase the total number of solute particles in solution, so the directly measured plasma osmolality is not significantly affected under these conditions. Fortunately, measurement of serum [Na$^+$] by ion-specific electrodes, which now is used commonly by most clinical laboratories, is less influenced by high concentrations of lipids or proteins than is measurement of serum [Na$^+$] by flame photometry (25), although such errors can nonetheless still occur.

The second situation in which hyponatremia does not reflect true plasma hypoosmolality occurs when high concentrations of effective solutes other than Na$^+$ are present in the plasma. The initial hyperosmolality produced by the additional solute causes an osmotic shift of water from the ICF to the ECF, which in turn produces a dilutional decrease in the serum [Na$^+$]. Once equilibrium between both fluid compartments is achieved, the total effective osmolality remains relatively unchanged. This situation most commonly occurs with hyperglycemia and represents a frequent cause of hyponatremia in hospitalized patients, accounting for up to 10% to 20% of all cases (12). Misdiagnosis of true hypoosmolality in such cases can be avoided by measuring plasma osmolality directly or, alternatively, by correcting the measured serum [Na$^+$] by 1.6 mEq/L for each 100 mg/dL increase in serum glucose concentration above normal levels (26) [recent studies have shown a more complex relation between hyperglycemia and serum [Na$^+$], and have suggested that a more accurate correction factor is closer to 2.4 mEq/L (27)]. However, when the plasma contains significant amounts of unmeasured solutes, such as osmotic diuretics, radiographic contrast agents, and some toxins (ethanol, methanol, and ethylene glycol), plasma osmolality obviously cannot be calculated accurately. In these situations, osmolality must be ascertained by direct measurement, although even this method does not yield an accurate measure of the true effective osmolality if the unmeasured solutes are noneffective solutes that freely permeate cell membranes (e.g., ethanol).

Because of the aforementioned considerations, it should be apparent that the determination of whether true hypoosmolality is present can sometimes be a difficult task. Nevertheless, a straightforward and relatively simple approach suffices in most cases:

1. The effective plasma osmolality should be calculated from the measured serum [Na$^+$] and glucose concentration ($2 \times$ [Na$^+$] + glucose/18); alternatively, the measured serum [Na$^+$] can simply be corrected by 1.6 to 2.4 mEq/L for each 100 mg/dL increase in serum glucose concentration above normal levels (100 mg/dL).

2. If the calculated effective plasma osmolality is less than 275 mOsm/kg H$_2$O, or if the corrected serum [Na$^+$] is less than 135 mEq/L, then significant hypoosmolality exists, providing that large concentrations of unmeasured solutes or pseudohyponatremia secondary to hyperlipidemia or hyperproteinemia are not present.

3. To eliminate the latter possibilities, plasma osmolality also should be measured directly in all cases in which the hyponatremia cannot be accounted for by elevated serum glucose levels. The absence of a discrepancy between the calculated and measured total plasma osmolality (<10 mOsm/kg H$_2$O) confirms the absence of significant amounts of unmeasured solutes, such as osmotic diuretics, radiocontrast agents, or alcohol; if a significant discrepancy between these measures is found (called an *osmolal gap*) (28), appropriate tests then must be conducted to rule out pseudohyponatremia or identify possible unmeasured plasma solutes (22,29,30). Whether significant hypoosmolality exists in the latter case depends on the nature of the unmeasured solutes; although this determination is not always possible, the clinician at least will be alerted to uncertainty about the diagnosis of true hypoosmolality.

Pathogenesis of Hypoosmolality

Because water moves freely between the ICF and ECF across most cell membranes, osmolality is always equivalent in both of these fluid compartments because water distributes between them in response to osmotic gradients. Consequently, total body osmolality must always be the same as both ECF and ICF osmolality. Because the bulk of body solute comprises electrolytes, namely, the exchangeable Na$^+$ (Na$_E^+$) in the ECF and the exchangeable K$^+$ (K$_E^+$) in the ICF along with their associated anions, total body osmolality is largely a function of these parameters (31):

$$\text{OSM}_{\text{ECF}} = \text{OSM}_{\text{ICF}} = \text{total body osmolality}$$

$$= (\text{ECF solute} + \text{ICF solute})/\text{body water}$$

$$= (2 \times \text{Na}_E^+ + 2 \times \text{K}_E^+$$

$$+ \text{nonelectrolyte solute})/\text{body water}$$

By definition, the presence of plasma hypoosmolality indicates a relative excess of water to solute in the ECF. From the preceding equations, it should be apparent that this can be

TABLE 85-1. *Pathogenesis of hypoosmolar disorders*

Depletion (primary decreases in total body solute + secondary water retention)
Renal solute loss
  Diuretic use
  Solute diuresis (glucose, mannitol)
  Salt-wasting nephropathy
  Mineralocorticoid deficiency or resistance
Nonrenal solute loss
  Gastrointestinal (diarrhea, vomiting, pancreatitis, bowel obstruction)
  Cutaneous (sweating, burns)
  Blood loss

Dilution (primary increases in total body water + secondary solute depletion)
Impaired renal free water excretion
  Increased proximal reabsorption
    Hypothyroidism
  Impaired distal dilution
    Syndrome of inappropriate antidiuretic hormone secretion
    Glucocorticoid deficiency
  Combined increased proximal reabsorption and impaired distal dilution
    Congestive heart failure
    Cirrhosis
    Nephrotic syndrome
  Decreased urinary solute excretion
    Beer potomania
    Very-low-protein diet
Excess water intake
  Primary polydipsia
  Dilute infant formula
  Fresh-water drowning

produced either by an excess of body water, resulting in a *dilution* of remaining body solute, or alternatively by a *depletion* of body solute, either Na$^+$ or K$^+$, relative to the remaining body water. Table 85-1 summarizes the potential causes of hyponatremia categorized according to whether the initiating event is dilution or depletion of body solute. Such a classification represents an obvious oversimplification because most clinical hypoosmolar states involve significant components of both solute depletion and water retention. Nonetheless, it is conceptually quite useful as a starting point for understanding the mechanisms underlying the pathogenesis of hypoosmolality and as a framework for discussions of therapy of hypoosmolar disorders.

Solute Depletion

Depletion of body solute can result from any significant losses of ECF. Whether through renal or nonrenal routes, body fluid losses by themselves rarely cause hypoosmolality because excreted or secreted body fluids usually are isotonic or hypotonic relative to plasma and therefore tend to increase plasma osmolality. Consequently, when hypoosmolality accompanies ECF losses it usually is the result of replacement of body fluid losses by more hypotonic solutions, thereby diluting the remaining body solutes. This often occurs when patients drink water or other hypotonic fluids in response to ongoing solute and water losses, and also when hypotonic intravenous fluids are administered to hospitalized patients. When the solute losses are marked, these patients can show all of the obvious signs of volume depletion (e.g., Addisonian crisis). However, such patients often have a more deceptive clinical presentation because their volume deficits may be partially replaced by subsequently ingested or infused fluids. Moreover, they may not manifest signs or symptoms of cellular dehydration because osmotic gradients draw water into the relatively hypertonic ICF. Therefore, clinical evidence of hypovolemia strongly supports solute depletion as the cause of plasma hypoosmolality, but absence of clinically evident hypovolemia never completely eliminates this as a possibility. Although ECF solute losses are responsible for most cases of depletion-induced hypoosmolality, ICF solute loss also can cause hypoosmolality as a result of osmotic water shifts from the ICF into the ECF (31). This mechanism likely contributes to some cases of diuretic-induced hypoosmolality in which depletion of total body K$^+$ often occurs (32–34).

Water Retention

Despite the obvious importance of solute depletion in some patients, most cases of clinically significant hypoosmolality are caused by increases in total body water rather than by primary loss of extracellular solute. This can occur because of either impaired renal solute-free water excretion or excessive free water intake. However, the former accounts for most hypoosmolar disorders because normal kidneys have sufficient diluting capacity to allow excretion of up to 20 to 30 L/day of solute-free water (see Chapter 3). Intakes of this magnitude are seen occasionally in a subset of psychiatric patients (35,36) but not in most patients, including patients with SIADH in whom fluid intakes average 2 to 3 L/day (37). Consequently, dilutional hypoosmolality usually is the result of an abnormality of renal solute-free water excretion. The renal mechanisms responsible for impairments in solute-free water excretion can be subgrouped according to whether the *major* impairment in solute-free water excretion occurs in proximal or distal parts of the nephron, or both (Table 85-1).

Any disorder that leads to a decrease in glomerular filtration rate (GFR) causes increased reabsorption of both Na$^+$ and water in the proximal tubule. As a result, the ability to excrete solute-free water is limited because of decreased delivery of tubular fluid to the distal nephron. Disorders causing solute depletion through nonrenal mechanisms (e.g., gastrointestinal fluid losses) also produce this effect. Disorders that cause a decreased GFR in the absence of significant ECF fluid losses are, for the most part, edema-forming states associated with decreased effective arterial blood volume (EABV) and secondary hyperaldosteronism (38–40). Even though these conditions are typified by increased proximal reabsorption of both Na$^+$ and fluid, it now is clear that in most cases water retention also results from increased distal reabsorption caused by nonosmotic, baroreceptor-mediated increases in plasma AVP levels (41,42), with the possible exception of hypothyroidism.

Distal nephron impairments in solute-free water excretion are characterized by an inability to dilute tubular fluid maximally. These disorders usually are associated with abnormalities in the secretion of AVP from the posterior pituitary. However, just as depletion-induced hypoosmolar disorders usually include an important component of secondary impairments of solute-free water excretion, so do most dilution-induced hypoosmolar disorders involve some degree of secondary solute depletion. This was recognized even before the first clinical description of SIADH from studies of the effects of posterior pituitary extracts on water retention, which demonstrated that renal salt wasting was predominantly a result of the ECF volume expansion produced by the retained water (43). Thus, after sustained increases in total body water secondary to inappropriately elevated AVP levels, sufficient secondary solute losses, predominantly as Na$^+$, occur and sometimes result in further lowering of plasma osmolality. The actual contribution of Na$^+$ losses to the hypoosmolality of SIADH is variable and depends in part on both the rate and volume of water retention (44). The major factor responsible for secondary Na$^+$ losses appears to be renal hemodynamic effects, and specifically the phenomenon of pressure natriuresis and diuresis induced by the volume expansion (45). However, volume-stimulated hormones such as atrial natriuretic peptide (ANP) also are elevated in response to the water retention of patients with SIADH (46,47), and it seems likely that these factors also contribute to the secondary natriuresis, possibly through interactions with intrarenal hemodynamic effects (48). Regardless of the actual mechanisms involved, the solute losses that occur secondarily to water retention can be understood best in the context of volume regulation of the ICF and ECF fluid compartments in response to induced hypoosmolality, which is discussed in the next section.

Some dilutional disorders do not fit well into either category. Chief among these is the hyponatremia that sometimes occurs in patients who ingest large volumes of beer with little food intake for prolonged periods, frequently called *beer potomania* (49,50). Even though the volume of fluid ingested may not seem sufficiently excessive to overwhelm renal diluting mechanisms, in these cases solute-free water excretion is limited by very low urinary solute excretion, thereby causing water retention and dilutional hyponatremia. A case in which hyponatremia occurred in an ovolactovegetarian with a very low protein intake but no beer ingestion is consistent with this pathophysiologic mechanism (51). However, because most such patients have very low salt intakes as well, it is likely that relative depletion of body Na$^+$ stores also is a contributing factor to the hypoosmolality in at least some cases.

Adaptation to Hyponatremia: Intracellular and Extracellular Fluid Volume Regulation

Many studies have indicated that the combined effects of water retention plus urinary solute excretion cannot adequately explain the degree of plasma hypoosmolality observed in patients (2,52,53). This observation originally led to the theory of "cellular inactivation of solute" (2). Simply stated, this theory suggested that as ECF osmolality falls, water moves into cells along osmotic gradients, thereby causing the cells to swell. At some point during this volume expansion, the cells osmotically "inactivate" some of their intracellular solutes as a defense mechanism to prevent continued cellular swelling with subsequent detrimental effects on cell function and survival. As a result of this decrease in intracellular osmolality, water then shifts back out of the ICF into the ECF, but at the expense of further worsening the dilution-induced hypoosmolality. Despite the appeal of this theory, its validity has never been demonstrated conclusively in either human or animal studies.

An appealing alternative theory has been suggested by studies of cellular volume regulation, in which cell volume is maintained under hypoosmolar conditions by extrusion of potassium rather than by osmotic inactivation of cellular solute (54,55). Whole-brain volume regulation through similar types of electrolyte losses was first described by Yannet in 1940 (56) and has long been recognized as the mechanism by which the brain was able to adapt to hyponatremia and limit brain edema to sublethal levels (57–59). After the recognition that low-molecular-weight organic compounds, called *organic osmolytes,* also constituted a significant osmotic component of a wide variety of cell types, studies demonstrated the accumulation of these compounds in response to hyperosmolality in both kidney (60) and brain (61) tissue. Multiple groups have now shown that the brain loses organic osmolytes in addition to electrolytes during the process of volume regulation to hypoosmolar conditions in experimental animals (62–65) and human patients (66). These losses occur relatively quickly (within 24 to 48 hours in rats) and can account for as much as one-third of the brain solute losses during hyponatremia (67). Such coordinate losses of both electrolytes and organic osmolytes from brain tissue enable very effective regulation of brain volume during chronic hyponatremia (Fig. 85-1). Consequently, it is now clear that cellular volume regulation *in vivo* in brain tissue occurs predominantly through depletion, rather than intracellular osmotic "inactivation," of a variety of intracellular solutes. Ongoing experimental studies will better define the many cellular and molecular mechanisms that underlie this profound adaptation to hypoosmolality (68–72).

Most recent studies have focused on volume regulation in the brain during hyponatremia, but all cells volume regulate to varying degrees (54), and there is little question that this process occurs throughout the body as whole organisms adapt to hypoosmolar conditions. As in the brain, unexplained components of hyponatremia, which led to previous speculation

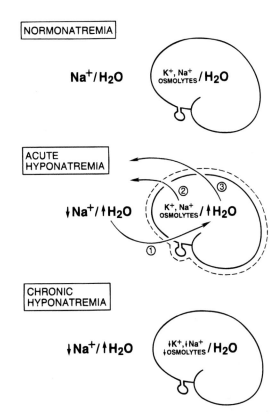

FIG. 85-1. Schematic diagram of brain volume adaptation to hyponatremia. Under normal conditions, brain osmolality and extracellular fluid (ECF) osmolality are in equilibrium (**top panel;** for simplicity, the predominant intracellular solutes are depicted as K^+ and organic osmolytes, and the extracellular solute as Na^+). After the induction of ECF hypoosmolality, water moves into the brain in response to osmotic gradients, producing brain edema (**middle panel,** no. 1). However, in response to the induced swelling the brain rapidly loses both extracellular and intracellular solutes (**middle panel,** no. 2). As water losses accompany the losses of brain solute, the expanded brain volume then decreases back toward normal (**middle panel,** no. 3). If hypoosmolality is sustained, brain volume eventually normalizes completely and the brain becomes fully adapted to the ECF hyponatremia (**bottom panel**).

about cellular inactivation of solute, are now better explained by cellular losses of both electrolyte and organic solutes as cells throughout the body volume regulate during hypoosmolar conditions. However, volume-regulatory processes are not limited to cells. Although most cases of hyponatremia clearly result from initial water retention induced by stimulated antidiuresis, it always has seemed likely that the resulting natriuresis served the purpose of regulating the volumes of the ECF and intravascular spaces. Many experimental and clinical observations are consistent with ECF volume regulation through secondary solute losses. First, dilutional decreases in concentrations of most blood constituents other than Na^+ and Cl^- do not occur in patients with SIADH (73), suggesting that their plasma volume is not nearly as expanded as would be predicted simply by the measured decreases in serum [Na$^+$]. Second, an increased incidence of hypertension never has been observed in patients with SIADH (74), again arguing against significant expansion of the arterial blood volume. Third, results of animal studies in both dogs (75) and rats (76) have clearly indicated that a component of chronic hyponatremia is attributable to secondary Na$^+$ losses rather than water retention. Furthermore, the relative contributions from water retention versus sodium loss vary with the duration and severity of the hyponatremia: water retention was found to be the major cause of decreased serum [Na$^+$] in the first 24 hours of induced hyponatremia in rats, but Na$^+$ depletion then became the predominant etiologic factor after longer periods (7 to 14 days) of sustained hyponatremia, particularly at very low (<115 mEq/L) serum [Na$^+$] levels (76). Finally, multiple studies have attempted to measure body fluid compartment volumes in hyponatremic patients, but without consistent results that indicate either plasma or ECF expansion (1,53,77,78). In particular, a recent report of body fluid space measurements using isotope dilution techniques in hyponatremic and normonatremic patients with small cell lung carcinoma showed no differences between the two groups with regard to exchangeable sodium space, ECF volume by ^{35}SO$_4$ distribution, or total body water (79). Such results traditionally have been explained by the relative insensitivity of isotope dilution techniques for measurement of body fluid compartment spaces, but an equally plausible possibility is that in the chronically adapted hyponatremic state, body fluid compartments have regulated their volumes back toward normal through a combination of extracellular (predominantly electrolyte) and intracellular (electrolyte and organic osmolyte) solute losses (80). Figure 85-2 schematically illustrates some of the volume-regulatory processes that likely occur in response to water retention induced by inappropriate antidiuresis. The degree to which solute losses versus water retention contribute to the resulting hyponatremia varies in association with many different factors, including the etiology of the hyponatremia, the rapidity of development of the hyponatremia, the chronicity of the hyponatremia, the volume of daily water loading and subsequent volume expansion, and undoubtedly some degree of individual variability as well. It therefore hardly seems surprising that studies of hyponatremic patients have failed to yield uniform results regarding the pathogenesis of hyponatremia in view of the marked diversity of hyponatremic patients and their presentation at different times during the adaptation to hypoosmolality through volume regulatory processes.

Differential Diagnosis of Hyponatremia and Hypoosmolality

Because of the multiplicity of disorders causing hypoosmolality and the fact that many involve more than one pathologic mechanism, a definitive diagnosis is not always possible at the time of initial presentation. Nonetheless, a relatively straightforward approach based on the commonly used parameters of ECF volume status and urine sodium concentration usually allows a sufficient categorization of the underlying etiology to permit appropriate decisions regarding initial therapy and further evaluation (Table 85-2).

Decreased Extracellular Fluid Volume

The presence of clinically detectable hypovolemia always signifies total body solute depletion. A low urinary [Na$^+$] indicates a nonrenal cause of solute depletion. If the urinary [Na$^+$] is high despite hypoosmolality, renal causes of solute depletion are likely responsible. Therapy with thiazide diuretics is the most common cause of renal solute losses (34), particularly in the elderly (81), but mineralocorticoid deficiency as a result of adrenal insufficiency (82) or mineralocorticoid resistance (83) must always be considered as well. Less commonly, renal solute losses may be the result of a salt-wasting nephropathy (e.g., polycystic kidney disease) (84), interstitial nephritis (85), or chemotherapy (86).

Increased Extracellular Fluid Volume

The presence of clinically detectable hypervolemia always signifies total body Na$^+$ excess. In these patients, hypoosmolality results from an even greater expansion of total body water caused by a marked reduction in the rate of water excretion (and sometimes an increased rate of water ingestion). The impairment in water excretion is secondary to a decreased EABV (38–40), which increases the reabsorption of glomerular filtrate not only in the proximal nephron but in the distal and collecting tubules by stimulating AVP secretion (41,42). These patients usually have a low urinary [Na$^+$] because of secondary hyperaldosteronism, which also is a product of decreased EABV. However, under certain conditions urinary [Na$^+$] may be elevated, usually secondary to concurrent diuretic therapy, but also sometimes because of a solute diuresis (e.g., glucosuria in diabetic patients) or after successful treatment of the underlying disease (e.g., inotropic therapy in patients with congestive heart failure). An additional disorder that can produce hypoosmolality and hypervolemia is acute or chronic renal failure with fluid overload (12) [although in early stages of renal failure polyuria from vasopressin resistance is more likely (87)]. Urinary [Na$^+$] in these cases usually is elevated, but it can be variable depending on the stage of renal failure. Primary polydipsia is not accompanied by signs of hypervolemia because water ingestion alone, in the absence of Na$^+$ retention, does not produce clinically apparent degrees of ECF volume expansion.

Normal Extracellular Fluid Volume

Many different hypoosmolar disorders can potentially present clinically with euvolemia, in large part because it is difficult to detect modest changes in volume status using standard methods of clinical assessment; in such cases measurement of urinary [Na$^+$] is an especially important first step (88).

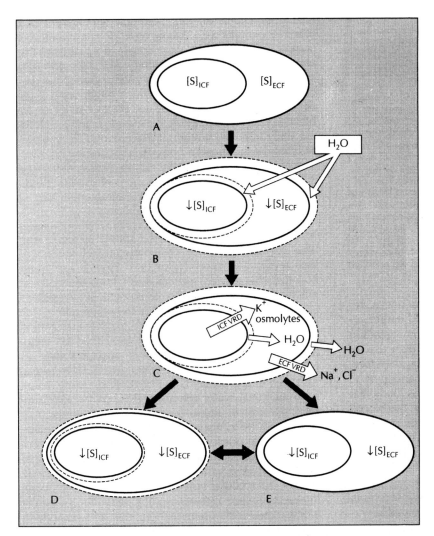

FIG. 85-2. Schematic illustration of potential changes in whole-body fluid compartment volumes at various times during adaptation to hyponatremia. Under basal conditions the concentration of effective solutes in the extracellular fluid ($[S]_{ECF}$) and the intracellular fluid ($[S]_{ICF}$) are in osmotic balance **(A)**. During the first phase of water retention resulting from inappropriate antidiuresis, the excess water distributes across total body water, causing expansion of both ECF and ICF volumes *(dotted lines)* with equivalent dilutional decreases in $[S]_{ICF}$ and $[S]_{ECF}$ **(B)**. In response to the volume expansion, compensatory volume regulatory decreases (VRD) occur to reduce the effective solute content of both the ECF (through pressure diuresis and natriuretic factors) and ICF (through increased electrolyte and osmolyte extrusion mediated by stretch activated channels and downregulation of synthesis of osmolytes and osmolyte uptake transporters) **(C)**. If both processes go to completion, such as under conditions of fluid restriction, a final steady state can be reached in which ICF and ECF volumes have returned to normal levels but $[S]_{ICF}$ and $[S]_{ECF}$ remain low **(E)**. In most cases, this final steady state is not reached, and moderate degrees of ECF and ICF expansion persist, but significantly less than would be predicted from the decrease in body osmolality **(D)**. Consequently, the degree to which hyponatremia is due to dilution from water retention versus solute depletion from volume-regulatory processes can vary markedly depending on which phase of adaptation the patient is in, and also on the relative rates at which the different compensatory processes occur (e.g., delayed ICF VRD can worsen hyponatremia due to shifts of intracellular water into the extracellular fluid as intracellular organic osmolytes are extruded and subsequently metabolized, likely accounting for some component of the hyponatremia unexplained by the combination of water retention and sodium excretion in previous clinical studies). (From Verbalis JG. Hyponatremia: epidemiology, pathophysiology, and therapy. *Curr Opin Nephrol Hypertens* 1993;2:636, with permission.)

TABLE 85-2. *Differential diagnosis of hyponatremia*

Extracellular fluid volume	Urinary [Na+][a]	Presumptive diagnosis
↓	Low	Depletion (nonrenal): gastrointestinal, cutaneous, or blood extracellular fluid loss
	High	Depletion (renal): diuretics, mineralocorticoid insufficiency (Addison's disease), salt-losing nephropathy
→	Low	Depletion (nonrenal): any cause + hypotonic fluid replacement
		Dilution (proximal): hypothyroidism, early decreased effective arterial blood volume
		Dilution (distal): SIADH + fluid restriction
	High	Dilution (distal): SIADH, glucocorticoid insufficiency
		Depletion (renal): any cause + hypotonic fluid replacement (especially diuretic treatment)
↑	Low	Dilution (proximal): decreased, effective arterial blood volume (congestive heart failure, cirrhosis, nephrosis)
	High	Dilution (proximal): any cause + diuretics or improvement in underlying disease, renal failure

SIADH, syndrome of inappropriate antidiuretic hormone secretion.
[a]Urinary [Na+] values <30 mEq/L are usually considered to be low and values ≥30 mEq/L to be high, based on studies of responses of hyponatremic patients to infusions of isotonic saline (88).

A high urinary [Na+] in euvolemic patients usually implies a distally mediated, dilution-induced hypoosmolality such as SIADH. However, glucocorticoid deficiency can mimic SIADH so closely that these two disorders often are indistinguishable in terms of water balance (89). Hyponatremia from diuretic use also can present without clinically evident hypovolemia, and the urinary [Na+] often is elevated in such cases because of the renal tubular effects of the diuretics (34). A low urinary [Na+] suggests a depletion-induced hypoosmolality from ECF losses with subsequent volume replacement by water or other hypotonic fluids. The solute loss often is nonrenal in origin, but an important exception is recent cessation of diuretic therapy because urinary [Na+] can quickly decrease to low values within 12 to 24 hours after discontinuation of the drug. The presence of a low serum [K+] is an important clue to diuretic use because few of the other disorders that cause hypoosmolality are associated with significant hypokalemia. However, even in the absence of hypokalemia, any hypoosmolar, clinically euvolemic patient taking diuretics should be assumed to have solute depletion and treated accordingly; subsequent failure to correct the hypoosmolality with isotonic saline administration and persistence of an elevated urinary [Na+] after discontinuation of diuretics then requires reconsideration of a diagnosis of dilution-induced hypoosmolality. A low urinary [Na+] also can be seen in some cases of hypothyroidism, in the early stages of decreased EABV before the development of clinically apparent salt retention and fluid overload, or during the recovery phase from SIADH. Hence, a low urinary Na+ is less meaningful diagnostically than a high value.

Because euvolemic causes of hypoosmolality represent the most challenging etiologies of this disease, both in terms of differential diagnosis as well as with regard to the underlying pathophysiologic process, the subsequent sections discuss the major causes of euvolemic hypoosmolality and hyponatremia in greater detail.

SYNDROME OF INAPPROPRIATE ANTIDIURETIC HORMONE SECRETION

The syndrome of inappropriate antidiuretic hormone secretion is the most common cause of euvolemic hypoosmolality. It also is the single most prevalent cause of hypoosmolality of all etiologies encountered in clinical practice, with prevalence rates ranging from 20% to 40% among all hypoosmolar patients (8,12,37,90). The clinical criteria necessary to diagnose SIADH remain basically as set forth by Bartter and Schwartz in 1967 (2). A modified summary of these criteria is presented in Table 85-3, along with several other clinical findings that support this diagnosis. Several points about each

TABLE 85-3. *Criteria for the diagnosis of syndrome of inappropriate antidiuretic hormone secretion*

Essential
Decreased effective osmolality of the extracellular fluid (P_{osm} < 275 mOsm/kg H_2O)
Inappropriate urinary concentration (U_{osm} > 100 mOsm/kg H_2O with normal renal function) at some level of hypoosmolality
Clinical euvolemia, as defined by the absence of signs of hypovolemia (orthostasis, tachycardia, decreased skin turgor, dry mucous membranes) or hypervolemia (subcutaneous edema, ascites)
Elevated urinary sodium excretion while on a normal salt and water intake
Absence of other potential causes of euvolemic hypoosmolality: hypothyroidism, hypocortisolism (Addison's disease or pituitary adrenocorticotropic hormone insufficiency), and diuretic use

Supplemental
Abnormal water load test (inability to excrete at least 90% of a 20 mL/kg water load in 4 hr or failure to dilute U_{osm} to <100 mOsm/kg H_2O)
Plasma arginine vasopressin level inappropriately elevated relative to plasma osmolality
No significant correction of serum [Na+] with volume expansion but improvement after fluid restriction

of these criteria deserve emphasis or qualification:

1. True hypoosmolality must be present and hyponatremia secondary to pseudohyponatremia or hyperglycemia alone must be excluded.
2. Urinary concentration (osmolality) must be inappropriate for plasma hypoosmolality. This does not mean that urine osmolality must be greater than plasma osmolality (a common misinterpretation of this criterion), but simply that the urine must be less than maximally dilute (i.e., urine osmolality > 100 mOsm/kg H_2O). In addition, urine osmolality need not be elevated inappropriately at all levels of plasma osmolality, because in the reset osmostat variant form of SIADH, AVP secretion can be suppressed with resultant maximal urinary dilution and solute-free water excretion if plasma osmolality is decreased to sufficiently low levels (91,92). Hence, to satisfy the classical criteria for the diagnosis of SIADH, it is necessary only that urine osmolality be inadequately suppressed at *some* level of plasma osmolality below 275 mOsm/kg H_2O.
3. Clinical euvolemia must be present to establish a diagnosis of SIADH because both hypovolemia and hypervolemia strongly suggest different causes of hypoosmolality. This does not mean that patients with SIADH cannot become hypovolemic or hypervolemic for other reasons, but in such cases it is impossible to diagnose the underlying inappropriate antidiuresis until the patient is rendered euvolemic and is found to have persistent hypoosmolality.
4. The criterion of renal salt wasting has probably caused the most confusion regarding diagnosis of SIADH. This criterion is included because of its utility in differentiating between hypoosmolality caused by a decreased EABV, in which case renal Na^+ conservation occurs, and distal dilution-induced disorders, in which urinary Na^+ excretion is normal or increased secondary to ECF volume expansion. However, two important qualifications limit the utility of urinary $[Na^+]$ measurement in the hypoosmolar patient: urinary $[Na^+]$ also is high when solute depletion is of renal origin, as seen with diuretic use or Addison's disease, and patients with SIADH can have low urinary Na^+ excretion if they subsequently become hypovolemic or solute depleted, conditions that sometimes follow severe salt and water restriction. Consequently, although a high urinary Na^+ excretion is the rule in most patients with SIADH, its presence does not guarantee this diagnosis, and, conversely, its absence does not rule out the diagnosis.
5. The final criterion emphasizes that SIADH remains a diagnosis of exclusion. Thus, the presence of other potential causes of euvolemic hypoosmolality always must be excluded. This includes not only thyroid and adrenal dysfunction, but diuretic use, because this also sometimes can present as euvolemic hypoosmolality.

Table 85-3 also lists several other criteria that support, but are not essential for a diagnosis of SIADH. The first of these, the water loading test, is of value when there is uncertainty regarding the etiology of modest degrees of hypoosmolality in euvolemic patients, but it does not add useful information if the plasma osmolality is less than 275 mOsm/kg H_2O. Inability to excrete a standard water load normally [with normal excretion defined as a cumulative urine output of at least 90% of the administered water load within 4 hours and suppression of urine osmolality to <100 mOsm/kg H_2O (93)] confirms the presence of an underlying defect in solute-free water excretion. Unfortunately, water loading is abnormal in almost all disorders that cause hypoosmolality, whether dilutional or depletion induced with secondary impairments in solute-free water excretion. Two exceptions are primary polydipsia, in which hypoosmolality rarely is secondary to excessive water intake alone, and the reset osmostat variant of SIADH, in which normal excretion of a water load can occur once plasma osmolality falls below the new set-point for AVP secretion. The water load test also may be used to assess water excretion after treatment of an underlying disorder thought to be causing SIADH. For example, after discontinuation of a drug associated with SIADH in a patient who has already achieved a normal plasma osmolality by fluid restriction, a normal water load test result can confirm the absence of persistent inappropriate antidiuresis much more quickly than simple monitoring of the serum $[Na^+]$ during a period of *ad libitum* fluid intake. Despite these limitations as a diagnostic clinical test, water loading remains an extremely useful tool in clinical research for quantitating changes in solute-free water excretion in response to physiologic or pharmacologic manipulations.

The second supportive criterion for a diagnosis of SIADH is an inappropriately elevated plasma AVP level in relation to plasma osmolality. At the time that SIADH was originally described, inappropriately elevated plasma levels of AVP (or "ADH") were postulated merely because the measurement of plasma levels of AVP was limited to relatively insensitive bioassays. With the development of sensitive AVP radioimmunoassays capable of detecting the small physiologic concentrations of this peptide that circulate in plasma (94), there was hope that measurement of plasma AVP levels might supplant the classic criteria and become the definitive test for diagnosing SIADH, as is the case for most syndromes of hormone hypersecretion. This has not occurred for several reasons. First, although plasma AVP levels are elevated in most patients with this syndrome, the elevations usually remain within the normal physiologic range and are abnormal only in relation to plasma osmolality (Fig. 85-3). Thus, plasma AVP levels can be interpreted only in conjunction with a simultaneous plasma osmolality and knowledge of the relation between AVP levels and plasma osmolality in normal subjects (see Chapter 3). Second, 10% to 20% of patients with SIADH do not have measurably elevated plasma AVP levels; as shown in Fig. 85-3, many such patients have AVP levels that are precisely at, or even below, the limits of detection by radioimmunoassay. Whether these cases are true examples of inappropriate antidiuresis in the absence of circulating AVP, or whether they simply represent inappropriate AVP levels that fall below the limits of detection by radioimmunoassay is not clear. For this reason, Zerbe et al. have proposed using the term "SIAD" (syndrome of inappropriate antidiuresis) rather than SIADH to describe this entire group of disorders

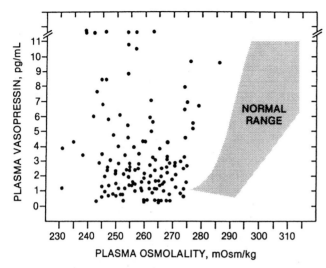

FIG. 85-3. Plasma arginine vasopressin (AVP) levels in patients with syndrome of inappropriate antidiuretic hormone secretion (SIADH) as a function of plasma osmolality. Each point depicts one patient at a single point in time. The *shaded area* represents AVP levels in normal subjects over physiologic ranges of plasma osmolality. The lowest measurable plasma AVP level using this radioimmunoassay was 0.5 pg/mL. (From Robertson GL, Aycinena P, Zerbe RL. Neurogenic disorders of osmoregulation. *Am J Med* 1982;72:339, with permission.)

(95). Third, just as water loading fails to distinguish among various causes of hypoosmolality, so do plasma AVP levels. Many disorders causing solute and volume depletion are associated with elevations of plasma AVP levels secondary to nonosmotic hemodynamic stimuli. For similar reasons, patients with disorders that cause decreased EABV, such as congestive heart failure and cirrhosis, also have elevated AVP levels (see Chapter 84). Even glucocorticoid insufficiency has been associated with inappropriately elevated AVP levels, as is discussed in the following section (96). Thus, multiple different disorders cause stimulation of AVP secretion through nonosmotic mechanisms, rendering this measurement of relatively limited differential diagnostic value.

Finally, an improvement in plasma osmolality with fluid restriction but not with volume expansion sometimes can be helpful in differentiating between disorders causing solute depletion and those associated with dilution-induced hypoosmolality. Infusion of isotonic NaCl in patients with SIADH provokes a natriuresis with little correction of osmolality, whereas fluid restriction allows such patients to achieve solute and water balance gradually through insensible free water losses (1). By contrast, isotonic saline is the treatment of choice in disorders of solute depletion because once volume deficits are corrected, the stimulus to continued AVP secretion and solute free water retention is eliminated. The diagnostic value of this therapeutic response is limited somewhat by the fact that patients with proximal types of dilution-induced disorders may show a response similar to that found in patients with SIADH. However, the major drawback is that this represents a retrospective test in a situation in which it would be preferable to establish a diagnosis before mak-

ing a decision regarding treatment options. Nonetheless, in difficult cases of euvolemic hypoosmolality, an appropriate therapeutic response sometimes can be helpful in confirming a diagnosis of SIADH.

Etiology

Although the list of disorders associated with SIADH is long, they can be divided into four major etiologic groups (Table 85-4).

Tumors

The most common association of SIADH is with tumors. Although many different types of tumors have been associated with SIADH (Table 85-4), bronchogenic carcinoma of

TABLE 85-4. *Common etiologies of syndrome of inappropriate antidiuretic hormone secretion*

Tumors
  Pulmonary/mediastinal (bronchogenic carcinoma; mesothelioma; thymoma)
  Nonchest (duodenal carcinoma; pancreatic carcinoma; ureteral/prostate carcinoma; uterine carcinoma; nasopharyngeal carcinoma; leukemia)

Central nervous system disorders
  Mass lesions (tumors; brain abscesses; subdural hematoma)
  Inflammatory diseases (encephalitis; meningitis; systemic lupus erythematosus; acute intermittent porphyria, multiple sclerosis)
  Degenerative/demyelinative diseases (Guillain-Barré syndrome; spinal cord lesions)
  Miscellaneous (subarachnoid hemorrhage; head trauma; acute psychosis; delirium tremens; pituitary stalk section; transsphenoidal adenomectomy; hydrocephalus)

Drug induced
  Stimulated AVP release (nicotine; phenothiazines; tricyclics)
  Direct renal effects or potentiation of AVP antidiuretic effects (desmopressin; oxytocin; prostaglandin synthesis inhibitors)
  Mixed or uncertain actions [angiotensin-converting enzyme inhibitors; carbamazepine and oxcarbazepine; chlorpropamide; clofibrate; clozapine; cyclophosphamide; 3,4-methylenedioxymethamphetamine ("ecstasy"); omeprazole; serotonin reuptake inhibitors; vincristine]

Pulmonary diseases
  Infections (tuberculosis; acute bacterial and viral pneumonia; aspergillosis; empyema)
  Mechanical/ventilatory (acute respiratory failure; chronic obstructive pulmonary disease; positive pressure ventilation)

Other
  Acquired immunodeficiency syndrome (AIDS) and AIDS-related complex
  Prolonged strenuous exercise (marathon; triathalon; ultramarathon; hot-weather hiking)
  Senile atrophy
  Idiopathic

AVP, arginine vasopressin.

the lung has been uniquely associated with SIADH since the first description of this disorder in 1957 (1). In virtually all cases, the bronchogenic carcinomas causing this syndrome have been of the small cell (or oat cell) variety; a few squamous cell types have been described, but these are rare. Incidences of hyponatremia as high as 11% of all patients with small cell carcinoma (97), or 33% of cases with more extensive disease (98), have been reported. The unusually high incidence of small cell carcinoma of the lung in patients with SIADH, together with the relatively favorable therapeutic response of this type of tumor, make it imperative that all adult patients presenting with an otherwise unexplained SIADH be investigated thoroughly and aggressively for a possible tumor. The evaluation should include a chest computed tomography (CT) or magnetic resonance imaging (MRI) scan and bronchoscopy with cytologic analysis of bronchial washings even if the results of routine chest radiography are normal, because several studies have reported hypoosmolality that predated any radiographically evident abnormality in patients who then were found to harbor bronchogenic carcinomas 3 to 12 months later (99,100). Head and neck cancers account for another group of malignancies associated with

relatively higher incidences of SIADH (101,102), and some of these tumors have been shown to have the ability to synthesize AVP ectopically (103). A report from a large cancer hospital showed an incidence of hyponatremia for all malignancies combined of 3.7%, with approximately one-third of these due to SIADH (13).

Central Nervous System Disorders

The second major etiologic group of disorders causing SIADH has its origins in the central nervous system (CNS). Despite the large number of different CNS disorders associated with SIADH, there is no obvious common denominator linking them. However, this actually is not surprising given the neuroanatomy of neurohypophysial innervation. The magnocellular AVP neurons receive excitatory inputs from osmoreceptive cells located in the anterior hypothalamus, but also a major innervation from brainstem cardiovascular regulatory and emetic centers (Fig. 85-4). Although various components of these pathways have yet to be elucidated fully, many of them appear to have inhibitory as well as excitatory components (104). Consequently, any diffuse

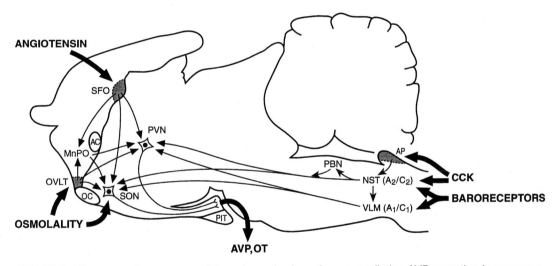

FIG. 85-4. Diagrammatic summary of the primary brain pathways mediating AVP secretion in response to the major factors that stimulate pituitary AVP secretion. Osmolality activates neurons throughout the anterior hypothalamus, including the SFO and MnPO, but the OVLT appears to be uniquely sensitive to osmotic stimulation and is essential for osmotically stimulated AVP and OT secretion; in addition, osmotic stimulation can act directly on magnocellular neurons, which themselves are intrinsically osmosensitive. Similarly, circulating angiotensin II activates cells throughout the OVLT and MnPO, but the SFO appears to be its major and essential site of action. For both of these stimuli, projections from the SFO and OVLT to the MnPO activate both excitatory and inhibitory interneurons that project to the SON and PVN and modulate the direct circumventricular inputs to these areas. Emetic stimuli act both on gastric vagal afferents that terminate in the NST and in some cases directly at the AP. Most of the AVP secretion appears to be a result of monosynaptic projections from catecholaminergic A2/C2 cells in the NST. Baroreceptor-mediated stimuli such as hypovolemia and hypotension are considerably more complex. Although they also arise from cranial nerves (IX and X) that terminate in the NST, most experimental data suggest that the major projection to magnocellular AVP neurons arises from catecholaminergic A1 cells of the VLM that are activated by excitatory interneurons from the NST, although some component might also arise from multisynaptic projections through other areas such as the PBN. *AC*, anterior commissure; *AP*, area postrema; *AVP*, arginine vasopressin; *MnPO*, median preoptic nucleus; *NST*, nucleus of the solitary tract; *OC*, optic chiasm; *OT*, oxytocin; *OVLT*, organum vasculosum of the lamina terminalis; *PBN*, parabrachial nucleus; *PIT*, anterior pituitary; *PVN*, paraventricular nucleus; *SFO*, subfornical organ; *SON*, supraoptic nucleus; *VLM*, ventrolateral medulla.

CNS disorder can potentially cause AVP hypersecretion either by nonspecifically exciting these pathways through irritative foci, or by disrupting them and thereby decreasing the level of inhibition impinging on the AVP neurons in the neurohypophysis. The wide variety of diverse CNS processes that can potentially cause SIADH stands in contrast to CNS causes of diabetes insipidus, which are for the most part limited to lesions of the hypothalamus or posterior pituitary that destroy the magnocellular vasopressin neurons (see Chapter 86).

Drugs

Drug-induced hyponatremia is one of the most common causes of hypoosmolality (105), and may soon replace tumors as the most common cause of SIADH. Table 85-3 lists some of the agents that have been associated with SIADH, and new drugs are being continually added to this list. In general, pharmacologic agents cause this syndrome by directly stimulating AVP secretion, by directly activating AVP renal receptors to cause antidiuresis, or by potentiating the antidiuretic effect of AVP on the kidney. However, not all of the drug effects associated with inappropriate antidiuresis are fully understood; indeed, many agents may work by means of a combination of mechanisms. For example, chlorpropamide appears to have both a direct pituitary as well as a renal stimulatory effect because it has been reported to increase urine osmolality even in some patients with complete central diabetes insipidus (106,107). Agents that cause AVP secretion through solute depletion, such as thiazide diuretics, are not listed here because these are generally considered to cause depletion-induced hypoosmolality rather than true SIADH. However, some studies have suggested that in some elderly patients the precipitous hyponatremia occasionally seen after administration of thiazide diuretics is caused by polydipsia and water retention more than by stimulated Na^+ excretion (108). Whether this represents true SIADH independent of prior ECF volume contraction, as well as whether such cases are typical of a significant portion of patients with diuretic-induced hyponatremia, remains to be determined. A particularly interesting, and clinically important, class of agents associated with SIADH are the selective serotonin reuptake inhibitors (SSRIs). Serotonergic agents have been found to increase AVP secretion in rats in some experimental studies (109), but most animal studies have suggested more direct effects on oxytocin rather than AVP secretion (110,111). Furthermore, studies of SSRIs in humans have in general failed to show significant effects on AVP secretion (112). However, hyponatremia after SSRI administration has been reported almost exclusively in the elderly, at rates as high as 22% to 28% in some studies (113–115), although larger series have suggested an incidence closer to 1 in 200 (116). This therefore suggests the possibility that elderly patients are uniquely hypersensitive to serotonin stimulation of AVP secretion. A similar effect also is likely responsible for reports of severe fatal hyponatremia caused by use of the recreational drug 3,4-methylenedioxymethamphetamine—"ecstasy" (117–120)—because this agent also possesses substantial serotonergic activity (121). Studies of cFos expression in rats indicate that ecstasy appears to activate hypothalamic magnocellular neurons (122), suggesting direct effects on AVP secretion as the etiology of the SIADH.

Pulmonary Disorders

Pulmonary disorders represent a relatively common but frequently misunderstood cause of SIADH. A variety of pulmonary disorders have been associated with this syndrome, but other than tuberculosis (123–125), acute pneumonia (126–129), and advanced chronic obstructive lung disease (130), the occurrence of hypoosmolality has been noted mainly in sporadic case reports. Although one case of pulmonary tuberculosis has been reported that suggested the possibility that tuberculous lung tissue might synthesize AVP ectopically (131), several other studies have reported that advanced pulmonary tuberculosis is associated with the reset osmostat form of SIADH (92,123), presumably from nonosmotic stimulation of posterior pituitary AVP secretion. Virtually all cases of nontuberculous pulmonary SIADH have occurred in the setting of respiratory failure. Although hypoxia clearly has been shown to stimulate AVP secretion in animals (132,133), it appears to be less effective as a stimulus in humans (134), in whom the stimulus to abnormal water retention appears to be hypercarbia more than hypoxia (135,136). When such patients were evaluated serially, the inappropriate AVP secretion was found to be limited to the initial days of hospitalization, when respiratory failure was most marked (127). Even the cases of tubercular SIADH uniformly occurred in patients with far-advanced, active pulmonary tuberculosis. Therefore, SIADH in non–tumor-related pulmonary disease usually conforms to the following characteristics: (a) the pulmonary disease always is obvious as a result of severe dyspnea or extensive radiographically evident infiltrates; and (b) the inappropriate antidiuresis usually is limited to the period of respiratory failure; once clinical improvement has begun, solute-free water excretion usually improves rapidly. Mechanical ventilation can cause inappropriate AVP secretion, or it can worsen any SIADH caused by other factors. This phenomenon has been associated most often with continuous positive-pressure ventilation (137), but it also can occur to a lesser degree with the use of positive end-expiratory pressure.

Other Causes

One of the most recently described causes of hypoosmolality is the acquired immunodeficiency syndrome (AIDS) or AIDS-related complex (ARC), in patients with human immunodeficiency virus infection, with incidences of hyponatremia reported as high as 30% to 38% in adults (138–140) and children (141). Although there are many potential etiologies for hyponatremia in patients with AIDS/ARC, including dehydration, adrenal insufficiency, and pneumonitis, from 12% to 68% of patients with AIDS in whom hyponatremia develops appear to meet criteria for a diagnosis of SIADH (138–140). Not unexpectedly, reports have implicated some of the medications used to treat these patients as the cause of the hyponatremia, either through direct renal tubular toxicity or SIADH (142,143).

Unexplained or idiopathic causes account for a relatively small proportion of all cases of SIADH. Although the etiology of the syndrome may not be diagnosed initially in many cases, the number of patients in whom an apparent cause cannot be established after consistent follow-up over time is relatively small. One exception to this appears to be elderly patients in whom SIADH sometimes develops without any apparent underlying etiology (144–146). Coupled with the significantly increased incidence of hyponatremia in geriatric patients (8,14,16,90,147), this suggests that the normal aging process may be accompanied by abnormalities of regulation of AVP secretion that predispose to SIADH. Such an effect could potentially account for the fact that virtually all causes of drug-induced hyponatremia occur much more frequently in elderly patients (148,149). In a series of 50 consecutive elderly patients meeting criteria for SIADH, 60% remained idiopathic despite rigorous evaluation, leading the authors to conclude that extensive diagnostic procedures were not warranted in such elderly patients if routine history, physical examination, and laboratory evaluation failed to suggest a diagnosis (150).

Some well known stimuli to AVP secretion are notable primarily because of their exclusion from Table 85-4. Despite unequivocal stimulation of AVP secretion by nicotine (151), cigarette smoking has been associated only rarely with SIADH, and primarily in psychiatric patients who have several other potential causes of inappropriate AVP secretion (35,152,153). This is in part because of chronic adaptation to the effects of nicotine, but also because the short half-life of AVP in plasma [approximately 15 minutes in humans (154)] limits the duration of antidiuresis produced by relatively short-lived stimuli such as smoking. Although nausea remains the most potent stimulus to AVP secretion known in humans (155), chronic nausea rarely is associated with hypoosmolality unless accompanied by vomiting with subsequent ECF solute depletion followed by ingestion of hypotonic fluids (156). Similar to smoking, this probably is attributable the short half-life of AVP, but also to the fact that most such patients are not inclined to drink fluids under such circumstances. However, hyponatremia can occur when such patients are infused with high volumes of hypotonic fluids. This is likely a contributing factor to the hyponatremia that often occurs in patients with cancer receiving chemotherapy (97). Finally, a causal relation between stress and SIADH often has been suggested, but never conclusively established. This underscores the fact that stress, independently of associated nausea, dehydration, or hypotension, is not a major stimulus causing sustained elevations of AVP levels in humans (157).

Pathophysiology

Sources of Arginine Vasopressin Secretion

Disorders that cause inappropriate antidiuresis secondary to elevated plasma AVP levels can be subdivided into those associated with either paraneoplastic ("ectopic") or pituitary AVP hypersecretion. Most ectopic production is from tumors, and there is conclusive, cumulative evidence that tumor tissue can, in fact, synthesize AVP: (a) tumor extracts have been found to possess antidiuretic hormone bioactivity and immunologically recognizable AVP and neurophysin, which is synthesized with AVP as part of a common precursor (158–160); (b) electron microscopy has revealed that many tumors possess secretory granules; and (c) cultured tumor tissue has been shown to synthesize not only AVP (161) but the entire AVP prohormone [propressophysin or provasopressin (162,163)]. Although it is clear that some tumors can produce AVP, it is not certain that all tumors associated with SIADH do so because only approximately half of small cell carcinomas have been found to contain AVP immunoreactivity (164), and many of the tumors listed in Table 85-3 have not been studied as extensively as have bronchogenic carcinomas. The only nonneoplastic disorder that possibly can cause SIADH by means of ectopic AVP production is tuberculosis. However, this is based on studies of a single patient in whom extracts of tuberculous lung tissue were shown by bioassay to possess antidiuretic activity (131).

Pituitary Arginine Vasopressin Secretion: Inappropriate Versus Appropriate

In most cases of SIADH, the AVP secretion originates from the posterior pituitary. However, this also is true of more than 90% of all cases of hyponatremia, including patients with hypovolemic and hypervolemic hyponatremia (12). This raises the question of what exactly constitutes "inappropriate" AVP secretion (80,165). It is well known that AVP secretion is most sensitively stimulated by increases in osmolality, but also occurs in response to a wide variety of nonosmotic stimuli, including hypotension, hypovolemia, nausea, hypoglycemia, angiotensin, and probably other stimuli yet to be discovered (166) (see Chapter 3). Consequently, AVP secretion in response to a hypovolemic stimulus such as hemorrhage clearly is physiologically "appropriate," but when it leads to symptomatic hyponatremia from secondary water retention it could easily be considered to be "inappropriate" for osmotic homeostasis. Despite such semantic difficulties, it is important that the criteria for diagnosing SIADH remain as originally described, specifically excluding other clinical conditions that cause known impairments in solute-free water excretion *even when* these are mediated by a secondary stimulation of AVP secretion through known physiologic mechanisms (e.g., hypovolemia, hypotension, hypocortisolism, edema-forming states, hypothyroidism). Without maintaining these distinctions, arguable as some of them may be, the definition of SIADH would become too broad to retain any degree of practical clinical usefulness.

Although measurable plasma AVP levels are found in most patients with SIADH, they rarely are elevated into pathologic ranges in the vast majority of cases, even those associated with ectopic AVP production from tumors. Rather, in most cases of SIADH, plasma AVP levels remain in "normal" physiologic ranges, which become abnormal only under hypoosmolar conditions when plasma AVP levels should be suppressed into unmeasurable ranges (Fig. 85-3). This is important for several reasons. First, the well known vasoconstrictive effects of AVP do not come into play until much higher plasma levels are achieved (30 to 80 pg/mL) (167), whereas maximal antidiuresis is achieved with much lower levels (5 to 10 pg/mL). Consequently, it is unlikely that any of the clinical manifestations of hyponatremia can be ascribed to vasopressor effects of AVP. In this regard, it is particularly worrisome that most animal models of induced hyponatremia have used pharmacologic doses of AVP, which usually elevate plasma AVP levels well into vasopressor ranges, raising the possibility that some results of previous studies of experimental hyponatremia were due to activation of AVP V_1 vascular and hepatic receptors. Results that demonstrate the absence of mortality when hyponatremia is induced in animals using the V_2-selective agonist desmopressin (dDAVP) (59), or using vasopressin infusions that maintain plasma AVP levels at lower ranges (168), emphasize the need to take potential vasopressor effects of vasopressin into consideration in the interpretation of past and future studies. Second, the presence of "normal" plasma AVP levels, or of only mildly elevated urine osmolalities, cannot be used as arguments against SIADH as an etiology for hyponatremia. Low but nonsuppressible levels of AVP clearly can cause sufficient impairment of solute-free water excretion to produce hypoosmolality when exogenous fluid intakes are high, as in psychiatric patients with polydipsia (169). Studies of patients with SIADH and hypopituitarism have measured high nonsuppressible levels of urinary aquaporin-2 excretion that correlated with their impaired water excretion, supporting persistent activation of AVP V_2 receptors as the cause of the water retention (170).

Patterns of Arginine Vasopressin Secretion

Studies of plasma AVP levels in patients with SIADH during graded increases in plasma osmolality produced by hypertonic saline administration have suggested four patterns of secretion (Fig. 85-5): (a) random hypersecretion of AVP; (b) a "reset osmostat" system, whereby AVP is secreted at an abnormally low threshold of plasma osmolality but otherwise displays a normal response to relative changes in osmolality; (c) inappropriate hypersecretion below the normal threshold for AVP release, but normal secretion in response to osmolar changes within normal ranges of plasma osmolality; and (d) low or undetectable plasma AVP levels despite classic clinical characteristics of SIADH (95,171). The first pattern

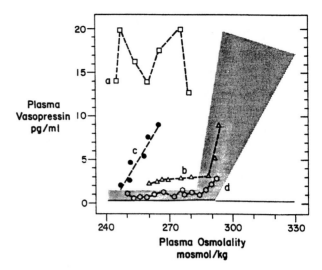

FIG. 85-5. Schematic summary of different patterns of arginine vasopressin (AVP) secretion in patients with syndrome of inappropriate antidiuretic hormone secretion. Each line *(a–d)* represents the relation between plasma AVP and plasma osmolality of individual patients in whom osmolality was increased by infusion of hypertonic NaCl. The *shaded area* represents plasma AVP levels in normal subjects over physiologic ranges of plasma osmolality. (From Robertson GL. Thirst and vasopressin function in normal and disordered states of water balance. *J Lab Clin Med* 1983;101:351, with permission.)

simply represents unregulated AVP secretion, which is often, but not always, observed in patients exhibiting paraneoplastic AVP production. Resetting of the osmotic threshold for AVP secretion has been well described with volume depletion (172,173) and also has been shown to occur in various edema-forming states, presumably as a result of decreases in EABV (38,42,174). However, most patients with a reset osmostat are clinically euvolemic (91,92). It has been suggested that chronic hypoosmolality itself may reset the intracellular threshold for osmoreceptor firing, but studies in animals have not supported a major role for this mechanism because chronic hyponatremia does not appear significantly to alter the osmotic threshold for AVP secretion (175,176). Perhaps the best known physiologic example of a reset osmostat for AVP secretion is the hypoosmolality and hyponatremia that occur during late pregnancy. Despite intensive studies over many years to identify potential hormonal factors that might be responsible for this resetting, a single factor has not yet been identified (177), although recent studies have indicated that the placental hormone relaxin causes a stimulation of AVP and oxytocin secretion that closely resembles the reset osmostat pattern of AVP secretion (178,179). Perhaps the most perplexing aspect of the reset osmostat pattern is its occurrence in patients with tumors, which suggests that some of these cases represent tumor-stimulated pituitary AVP secretion rather than paraneoplastic AVP secretion (95,171,180). The pattern of SIADH that occurs without measurable AVP secretion is not yet well understood. This form of the syndrome may be attributable to the secretion of AVP with some bioactivity but altered immunoreactivity, to the presence of other circulating antidiuretic factors, to increased renal sensitivity to very low circulating levels of AVP, or possibly in some cases to ANP-induced natriuresis. A sufficient number of patients with this form of the disorder has not been studied to form any basis for discrimination among these possibilities, but the positive response of one such patient to a vasopressin V_2 receptor antagonist suggests that this most likely represents increased renal sensitivity to low circulating levels of AVP (181). Despite these well described patterns of abnormal AVP secretion in SIADH, it is surprising that no correlation has been found between any of these four patterns and the various etiologies of the syndrome (95).

Stimuli to Arginine Vasopressin Secretion in Patients with SIADH

Regardless of the pattern of pituitary AVP secretion, and whether this represents an "inappropriate" or physiologically "appropriate" secretion, it is important to try to identify the cause of the continued AVP secretion in patients with this disorder. Because of the variety of stimuli that can stimulate AVP secretion independently of osmolality, it seems logical to hypothesize that SIADH can be caused by continued nonosmotic stimulation of AVP secretion despite the presence of plasma hypoosmolality. The effect of hypovolemia to lower the threshold and increase the sensitivity of osmotically stimulated AVP secretion is well known, and this mechanism almost certainly accounts for the elevated plasma AVP levels in patents with edema-forming disorders, in whom a decreased EABV activates baroreceptor-mediated AVP secretion (39,40). Tumor interference with vagal pathways to brainstem baroreceptive centers could conceivably mimic or exaggerate such hypovolemic conditions, potentially accounting for the occurrence of a reset osmostat pattern of AVP secretion found in some patients with lung cancer. Reports of a 3% to 4% incidence of SIADH in patients with advanced head and neck malignancies represent a group in which some, although clearly not all (182), of the hyponatremia also might be secondary to interference with vagal baroreceptor pathways (101). However, not all cases of SIADH can be comfortably ascribed to nonosmotic stimuli because it is difficult to identify any such possible stimuli in many patients. Another possibility is that brain pathways conveying afferent signals that actively inhibit AVP secretion from hypothalamic magnocellular neurons may somehow be impaired in some patients. Substantial data support the likelihood that hypoosmolality does not lead simply to decreased AVP secretion by virtue of absence of excitatory osmoreceptor inputs, but rather represents a state of active inhibition of the AVP-secreting neurons (183), possibly through endogenous opioid (184) or γ-aminobutyric acid pathways (104,185). In this case, it would be easy to imagine that impairments or alterations in the activity of these inhibitory pathways might allow continued AVP secretion despite hypoosmolality. Although such abnormalities have not yet been identified, there

is one situation in which a decreased inhibitory tone to AVP neurons clearly does lead to enhanced AVP secretion: elderly patients have decreased AVP responses to orthostasis but exaggerated responses to osmotic stimuli (186,187). The latter is presumably due to a diminution of inhibitory, as well as excitatory, inputs from brainstem baroreceptive centers to the hypothalamus, thereby producing an unopposed stimulation by osmotic stimuli from the anterior hypothalamus (Fig. 85-4). Similar phenomena could contribute to the high frequency of SIADH seen in elderly individuals (8,14–16). Despite our lack of precise information about the mechanisms responsible for osmotically inappropriate AVP secretion, it seems certain that this will prove to be a heterogeneous group of processes rather a single dominant cause.

Contribution of Natriuresis to the Hyponatremia of SIADH

Since the original cases studied by Schwartz and Bartter, increased renal Na$^+$ excretion has been one of the cardinal manifestations of SIADH, indeed one that later became embedded in the requirements for its diagnosis (2). However, next to the use of the term *inappropriate,* probably no other aspect of SIADH has been so widely misinterpreted. That the natriuresis accompanying administration of antidiuretic hormone is not due to AVP itself but rather to the volume expansion produced as a result of water retention was unequivocally shown by Leaf et al. even before the description of the clinical occurrence of this disorder (43). Subsequent metabolic balance studies demonstrated that excess urinary Na$^+$ excretion and a negative Na$^+$ balance occurred during the development of hyponatremia in patients with SIADH, but eventually urinary sodium excretion simply reflected daily sodium intake (1). Thus, patients appear to exhibit "renal sodium wasting" because they continue to excrete sodium despite being hyponatremic, but in reality they have simply achieved a new steady state in which they are in neutral sodium balance, albeit at a lower serum [Na$^+$]. Although this interpretation now is supported by abundant clinical and experimental evidence, several important questions remain unanswered regarding natriuresis and hyponatremia: What physiologic or pathophysiologic mechanisms underlie the natriuresis? Is natriuresis in SIADH always secondary to AVP-induced water retention, or is hyponatremia sometimes caused primarily by Na$^+$ losses? Even when it is secondary to water retention, can the natriuresis further aggravate the hyponatremia?

As described earlier, studies of long-term antidiuretic-induced hyponatremia in both dogs and rats have indicated that a larger proportion of the hyponatremia is attributable to secondary Na$^+$ losses rather than to water retention (75,76). However, it is important to appreciate that in these models the natriuresis actually did not worsen the hyponatremia, but rather allowed volume regulation of blood and ECF volumes to occur. Thus, over long periods, what begins as a "purely" dilutional hyponatremia from water retention becomes a mixed hyponatremia in which urinary solute losses allow maintenance of equivalent levels of hyponatremia but with lesser degrees of volume expansion due to water retention. Much of the past difficulty in consistently demonstrating expanded plasma or ECF volumes in patients with SIADH using tracer dilution techniques (77–79) can probably be ascribed to this process. It has become clear that intrinsic renal mechanisms are capable of producing both diuresis and natriuresis in response to increases in renal perfusion pressures (so-called pressure diuresis); this mechanism has been shown to underlie the renal escape from antidiuresis produced when AVP-infused animals are continually fluid loaded (45). However, it has not yet been proven whether this mechanism is sensitive enough to detect the relatively mild degrees of volume expansion that accompany dilutional hyponatremias. Another, not mutually exclusive, possibility is that the natriuresis is mediated by increases in circulating natriuretic peptides such as ANP. Most cases of SIADH have been shown to have elevated levels of these peptides into ranges that are capable of promoting renal sodium excretion (46,47,188). However, just as for all other potential effects of ANP, the lack of effective receptor antagonists for these peptides has frustrated attempts at proving the physiologic relevance of this mechanism. The degree to which hyponatremia occurs primarily as a result of natriuresis has remained controversial over many years. Cerebral salt wasting syndrome was first proposed by Peters et al. in 1950 (189) as an explanation for the natriuresis and hyponatremia that sometimes accompany intracranial disease, particularly subarachnoid hemorrhage (SAH), in which hyponatremia develops in up to one-third of patients. After the first clinical description of SIADH in 1957, such patients usually were assumed to have hyponatremia secondary to AVP hypersecretion with a secondary natriuresis (190). However, over the 1990s, clinical and experimental data have suggested that some patients with SAH and other intracranial diseases indeed have a primary natriuresis leading to volume contraction rather than SIADH (191–194), in which case the elevated measured plasma AVP levels actually may be physiologically appropriate for the degree of volume contraction present. The major clinical question as to whether cerebral salt wasting syndrome actually exists relates to the criteria used to assess the ECF volume status of these patients; opponents argue that there is insufficient evidence of true hypovolemia despite ongoing natriuresis (195), whereas proponents argue that the combined measures that traditionally have been used to estimate ECF volume do in fact support the presence of hypovolemia in many cases (196). With regard to the potential mechanisms underlying the natriuresis, both plasma and cerebrospinal fluid ANP levels clearly are elevated in many patients with SAH (194), and have been found to correlate variably with hyponatremia in patients with intracranial diseases (194,197). However, because SIADH also frequently is associated with elevated plasma ANP levels, this finding does not prove causality. Ample precedent certainly exists for hyponatremia due to Na$^+$ wasting with secondary antidiuresis in Addison's disease, as well as diuretic-induced hyponatremia. Characteristic of these disorders, normalization of ECF volume with isotonic NaCl infusions restores plasma tonicity to normal ranges by virtue of shutting off secondary AVP secretion. If hyponatremia in patients with SAH occurred through a similar mechanism, it also should respond to this therapy. However, recent studies indicate that it does not. Nineteen patients with SAH were treated with large volumes of isotonic saline sufficient to maintain plasma volume at normal or slightly elevated levels, but despite removal of any volemic stimulus to AVP secretion, 32% still had hyponatremia in association with nonsuppressed plasma AVP levels, an incidence equivalent to that found in previous studies of SAH (198). In contrast, other studies have demonstrated that mineralocorticoid therapy to inhibit natriuresis can reduce the incidence of hyponatremia in patients with SAH (199); such results are not unique to patients with intracranial diseases because a subset of elderly patients with SIADH also has been shown to respond favorably to mineralocorticoid therapy (200). Although seemingly disparate, these types of results support the existence of disordered AVP secretion as well as a coexisting stimulus to natriuresis in many such patients. It seems most likely that SAH and other intracranial diseases represent a mixed disorder in which some patients have *both* exaggerated natriuresis and inappropriate AVP secretion; which effect predominates in terms of the clinical presentation depends on their relative intensities as well as the effects of concomitant therapy. The possibility of ANP-induced natriuresis aggravating hyponatremia is not confined to intracranial diseases, and it has been suggested that ectopic ANP production might contribute to, or even cause, the hyponatremia accompanying some small cell lung cancers (201). In support of this possibility, several studies have analyzed tumor cell lines from patients with hyponatremia and small cell lung carcinoma and found that many produced ANP or ANP mRNA in addition to, or in some cases instead of, AVP (202–204). These data allow the possibility that some patients with tumors may also have hyponatremia as a result of ectopic ANP secretion. However, in clinical studies of such patients, the hyponatremia appears to correlate more with plasma AVP levels than plasma ANP levels (205). Consequently, it seems likely that such cases represent a mixture of inappropriate secretion of both hormones, analogous to patients with cerebral salt wasting, in which case the ANP further exacerbates the secondary natriuresis produced primarily by AVP-induced water retention.

ADRENAL INSUFFICIENCY

The frequent occurrence of hyponatremia in patients with adrenal insufficiency was appreciated well before the discovery of the role of AVP in hypoosmolar disorders (206). Incidences as high as 88% have been reported in patients with primary adrenal insufficiency, particularly during episodes of "Addisonian crisis" (207,208). This section summarizes the factors related to the development of hyponatremia in patients with adrenal insufficiency; a more complete description of many of the studies on which these conclusions are based can be found in an earlier edition of this textbook (209).

Etiology

The adrenal cortex produces many different types of corticosteroids, which can be broadly divided into three categories: glucocorticoids, mineralocorticoids, and androgens. Only the first two of these have been found to have significant effects on body fluid homeostasis. Disorders of impaired adrenal function can be divided into those in which the adrenal gland itself is damaged or destroyed, or *primary adrenal insufficiency,* and those in which the adrenal does not receive appropriate adrenocorticotropic hormone (ACTH) stimulation from the pituitary, or *secondary adrenal insufficiency.* Addison's disease is the major cause of primary adrenal insufficiency, and hypopituitarism is the best example of secondary adrenal insufficiency. The clinical presentation of these two types of adrenocortical insufficiency varies significantly because adrenal destruction causes loss of both mineralocorticoids and glucocorticoids, whereas pituitary insufficiency causes only glucocorticoid insufficiency, because pituitary ACTH is not necessary for mineralocorticoid secretion, which is controlled primarily through the renin–angiotensin system. To understand the fluid and electrolyte abnormalities that accompany these disorders, the pathophysiologic processes of hyponatremia due to mineralocorticoid and glucocorticoid deficiency must be considered separately.

Pathophysiology

Mineralocorticoid Deficiency

The absence of aldosterone impairs Na^+-K^+ exchange in the distal tubule. Because this defect occurs distally in the nephron, it cannot be completely compensated for by later Na^+ reabsorption, leading to the continued renal Na^+ wasting that is the hallmark of adrenal insufficiency (210). As long as sodium intake is sufficient to replace the ongoing renal losses, patients with mineralocorticoid insufficiency remain relatively stable. However, when sodium intakes are not sufficient, adrenally insufficient patients experience progressive hypovolemia, hyponatremia, and hyperkalemia, the classic fluid and electrolyte manifestations of addisonian crisis (207,208). Proof that these effects were indeed caused primarily by the renal Na^+ losses was documented long ago by studies in animals (210,211) and Addisonian patients (212), which demonstrated that all of these abnormalities could be prevented by volume expansion with NaCl. However, the water retention of mineralocorticoid deficiency has multiple potential causes: (a) the loss of aldosterone-mediated Na^+ reabsorption in the distal tubule impairs urinary dilution, similar to the use of thiazide diuretics; (b) the ECF volume contraction as a result of the Na^+ losses causes increased

fluid reabsorption in the proximal tubule with decreased delivery to the distal diluting segments of the nephron; and (c) the ECF volume contraction also stimulates baroreceptor-mediated (i.e., nonosmotic) AVP secretion with resultant antidiuresis.

Numerous experimental studies have documented elevated plasma AVP levels despite hypoosmolality in adrenalectomized animals with mineralocorticoid insufficiency (213–215), and the elevated AVP levels usually return to normal ranges after volume replacement with NaCl (213). Proof that the elevations in plasma AVP levels were causally related to the water retention was provided by studies in which adrenalectomized rats replaced only with glucocorticoids were given a vasopressin V_2 receptor antagonist (216) (Fig. 85-6); the antagonist significantly reduced urine osmolality in chronically, but not acutely, mineralocorticoid-deficient rats, consistent with hypovolemia-mediated stimulation of AVP secretion as a result of progressive Na^+ depletion over time. On the other hand, AVP-independent effects appear to play some role in the water retention as well. Studies in adrenalectomized homozygous Brattleboro rats, which cannot synthesize AVP, have demonstrated normalization of urine dilution, free water clearance, and solute clearance after physiologic aldosterone, but not glucocorticoid, replacement (217). These results demonstrate the contribution of factors such as impaired urinary dilution, due to the loss of aldosterone-mediated Na^+ reabsorption in the distal tubule, and increased proximal tubular fluid reabsorption, as a result of hypovolemia, to the impaired water excretion of mineralocorticoid deficiency. The latter factor would be predicted to be reversed by volume repletion, but not the former, possibly accounting for the observation that in some studies patients with primary adrenal insufficiency still maintained higher urine osmolalities even under conditions of volume expansion (218), although other studies in humans (212) and animals (219) have shown complete normalization of water excretion after volume expansion. Whatever the contribution of these additional factors, it nonetheless seems appropriate to conclude that the major mechanism responsible for the impaired water excretion of mineralocorticoid deficiency is hypovolemia-stimulated AVP secretion.

Glucocorticoid Deficiency

As described previously, isolated glucocorticoid deficiency usually occurs with pituitary disorders that impair normal ACTH secretion but leave other stimuli to aldosterone secretion intact. That glucocorticoid deficiency alone also could impair water excretion was recognized based on long-standing clinical observations that anterior pituitary insufficiency ameliorates, and sometimes even completely masks, the polyuria of patients with coexistent central diabetes insipidus (220,221). It is not surprising, therefore, that hyponatremia occurs relatively frequently in hypopituitary patients without diabetes insipidus (222–224). However, hypopituitary patients usually do not have ECF volume contraction

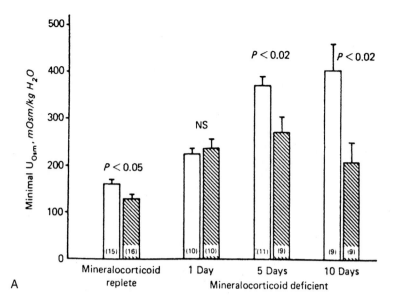

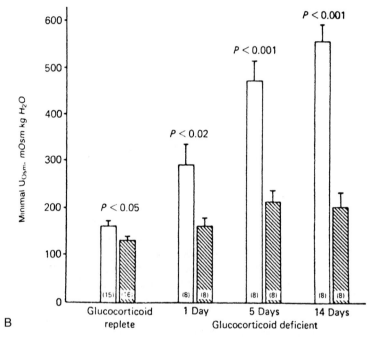

FIG. 85-6. Effect of an arginine vasopressin (AVP) V_2 receptor antagonist on urine osmolality after an acute water load in adrenalectomized rats selectively replaced with either mineralocorticoids or glucocorticoids. The *open bars* depict vehicle-treated rats and the *hatched bars* the AVP antagonist-treated rats. The mineralocorticoid-deficient rats **(top panel)** demonstrated an impaired urinary dilution that became progressively worse over the 10 days of study; treatment with the AVP receptor antagonist significantly reduced the minimum urine osmolality, but not until 5 days after the adrenalectomy, consistent with a hypovolemia-mediated stimulation of AVP secretion by this time. The glucocorticoid-deficient rats **(bottom panel)** demonstrated impaired urinary dilution that also became progressively worse over the 14 days of study, but in contrast to the mineralocorticoid-deficient rats, the minimum urine osmolality returned toward normal ranges after treatment with the AVP antagonist as early as 1 day after the adrenalectomy, indicating a different type of nonosmotic stimulation of AVP secretion in these rats. (From Ishikawa S, Schrier RW. Effect of arginine vasopressin antagonist on renal water excretion in glucocorticoid and mineralocorticoid deficient rats. *Kidney Int* 1982;22:587, with permission.)

because they maintain adequate aldosterone secretion to prevent renal Na^+ wasting. Consequently, volume replacement with NaCl does not reverse the impaired water excretion of patients with secondary adrenal insufficiency (218), as it does in primary adrenal insufficiency.

Despite the lack of an apparent hypovolemia-mediated stimulus to AVP secretion, nonosmotic AVP secretion has been strongly implicated in the impaired water excretion of glucocorticoid insufficiency. Elevated plasma AVP levels have been clearly documented in animals (225) and patients (96) with hypopituitarism (Fig. 85-7). Similarly, because primary adrenal insufficiency has components of both mineralocorticoid and glucocorticoid deficiency, adrenalectomized animals maintained only on physiologic replacement doses of mineralocorticoids also have been found to have

inappropriately elevated plasma AVP levels (226,227). That these elevated AVP levels were causally related to the impaired water excretion was again proven by studies using an AVP V_2 receptor antagonist, which demonstrated near normalization of urinary dilution in adrenalectomized mineralocorticoid-replaced rats (216) (Fig. 85-6). However, as with mineralocorticoid deficiency, AVP-independent mechanisms also have been suggested to play a role in the impaired water excretion of glucocorticoid deficiency, because Brattleboro rats maintained on aldosterone had somewhat decreased urine flow that increased after glucocorticoid replacement (217). Because ECF volume depletion usually is not a manifestation of glucocorticoid deficiency, other factors must therefore be responsible for the AVP-independent aspects of the water retention. The possibility that glucocorticoids exert

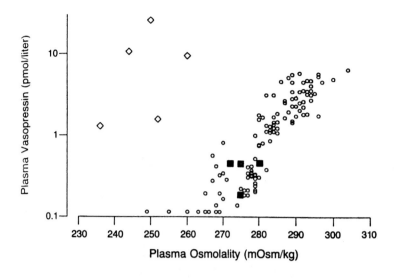

FIG. 85-7. Plasma arginine vasopressin (AVP) levels as a function of plasma osmolality in patients with hypopituitarism and adrenocorticotropic hormone insufficiency. The *diamonds* show patients with untreated hypopituitarism and the *solid squares* the same patients after hydrocortisone therapy. The *open circles* depict AVP levels in normal subjects over physiologic ranges of plasma osmolality. In comparison with Fig. 85-3, it is apparent that these patients would be indistinguishable from those with syndrome of inappropriate antidiuretic hormone secretion based on their plasma AVP–osmolality relation. (From Oelkers W. Hyponatremia and inappropriate secretion of vasopressin (antidiuretic hormone) in patients with hypopituitarism. *N Engl J Med* 1989; 321:492, with permission.)

direct effects on renal tubular epithelium, such that glucocorticoid insufficiency causes increased water permeability in the collecting tubules even in the absence of AVP, has been suggested (218). However, studies on isolated collecting tubules have failed to demonstrate any significant influence of glucocorticoids on water permeability of this tissue (228). Consequently, the AVP-independent effects of glucocorticoid insufficiency remain poorly defined.

Regardless of the etiology of the AVP-independent defect in water excretion, the major mechanism responsible for the impaired water excretion of glucocorticoid deficiency appears to be nonosmotically stimulated AVP secretion. However, the stimulus to AVP secretion under these conditions also remains unclear. Studies of prolonged glucocorticoid insufficiency in dogs have shown an increased pulse pressure and decreased cardiac stroke volume (226), and similar studies in rats have suggested decreases in cardiac index along with increased systemic vascular resistance (227). Although these findings differ somewhat, in both cases they raise the possibility of hemodynamically mediated effects on AVP secretion. Alternatively, glucocorticoid deficiency might directly stimulate AVP secretion through two possible mechanisms. First, both clinical (229) and experimental (230) studies have shown a modest but significant effect of glucocorticoids to inhibit pituitary AVP secretion. Presumably this is mediated by glucocorticoid receptors that have been localized in magnocellular neurons (231); recent studies have shown that these receptors are increased during induced hypoosmolality, suggesting that glucocorticoids may play a particularly important role in the inhibition of AVP secretion under hypoosmolar conditions (232). Second, in the absence of glucocorticoid feedback inhibition of the parvocellular AVP neurons that project to the median eminence rather than to the posterior pituitary, AVP content increases markedly in this area (233,234). This presumably reflects increased secretion of AVP into the pituitary portal blood system to stimulate pituitary ACTH secretion (235–238). Because the pituitary portal blood eventually drains into the systemic circulation, increased levels of AVP released from the median eminence

could increase plasma AVP levels sufficiently to produce inappropriate antidiuresis (such levels need not be very high, but simply inappropriate for the plasma osmolality, as shown in Fig. 85-7).

HYPOTHYROIDISM

Although hypothyroidism is considerably more common than adrenal insufficiency, hyponatremia secondary to hypothyroidism occurs much less frequently than hyponatremia from adrenal insufficiency. The infrequent occurrence of hyponatremia with hypothyroidism has led some investigators to question whether hypothyroidism is in fact causally related to hyponatremia (239), but this is simply a manifestation of the fact that impaired water excretion usually is seen only in more severely hypothyroid patients. Typically, such patients are elderly and meet criteria for myxedema "coma" as a result of their altered mental status (240–242). This section summarizes the factors related to the development of hyponatremia in patients with hypothyroidism; a more complete description of many of the studies on which these conclusions are based can be found in an earlier edition of this textbook (209).

Etiology

Similar to adrenal insufficiency, hypothyroidism can result from either dysfunction or damage to the thyroid gland itself, or *primary hypothyroidism,* or from inadequate thyroid-stimulating hormone (TSH) stimulation from the pituitary, or *secondary hypothyroidism.* Also like adrenal insufficiency, there can be significant differences in the presentation of these two disorders. However, because the only biologically active products of the thyroid gland are the hormones thyroxine (T_4) and triiodothyronine (T_3), in this case the clinical variations are due mainly to quantitative differences in the severity of the thyroid hormone deficiency rather than qualitative differences in the nature of the hormone deficits. With moderate degrees of hypothyroidism, patients with both primary and secondary disease have similar signs and symptoms of thyroid hormone deficiency (e.g., cold intolerance, increased fatigue, dry skin, constipation), but in general only patients with primary hypothyroidism progress to more severe degrees of myxedema, including the life-threatening metabolic and neurologic abnormalities of myxedema coma, whereas these extreme manifestations are virtually never seen with secondary hypothyroidism. This is because severe myxedema occurs only after plasma T_4 and T_3 levels have fallen to very low levels, often less than 1 μg/dL. This scenario can easily occur with primary hypothyroidism because in the absence of thyroid tissue, there is no alternative source of thyroid hormone production. However, T_4 and T_3 levels never decrease as severely in hypopituitary patients who simply lack TSH, and frequently plasma levels remain just at or slightly below the lower limits of normal (243). This likely reflects either some degree of constitutive thyroid hormone synthesis by the thyroid gland, or possibly low-grade stimulation of TSH receptors by other circulating substances, analogous to the thyrotoxicosis produced by thyroid-stimulating immunoglobulins in patients with Graves' disease. Because hyponatremia is seen only in hypothyroid patients who have progressed to severe degrees of myxedema, it follows that this manifestation mainly occurs in patients with primary hypothyroidism. When hyponatremia accompanies hypopituitarism it usually is a manifestation of secondary adrenal insufficiency from glucocorticoid deficiency rather than coexisting hypothyroidism (89,244).

Pathophysiology

Several studies have confirmed abnormalities of water excretion in hypothyroid patients. However, in almost all cases the abnormality was found to consist of a delayed excretion of water rather than major impairments in urinary dilution (245–247). This was best shown in the studies of DeRubertis et al., in which near-normal urinary dilution occurred after water loading in hypothyroid patients (Fig. 85-8), even though cumulative excretion of the water load in the hypothyroid patients lagged far behind that of euthyroid control subjects (39.8% ± 5.1% versus 78.7% ± 5.7%) after 2 hours (246). Similar results have been found in studies of hypothyroid rats (248,249). Experimental studies in hypothyroid animals have implicated decreases in renal blood flow and GFR as the primary factors responsible for the delayed water excretion. In particular, the relation between solute-free water clearance and distal tubular Na^+ delivery was found to be identical in hypothyroid and euthyroid rats, suggesting that the observed impairments in water excretion were likely secondary to reduced delivery of glomerular filtrate to the distal nephron in the hypothyroid rats (248). These results are consistent with findings of a decreased GFR in severely hypothyroid patients (246,247,250–252), which is most likely due to decreased renal blood flow as a result of the compromised cardiac output and increased peripheral vascular resistance known to occur in such patients (253–255). Experimental studies also have supported this hypothesis because a variety

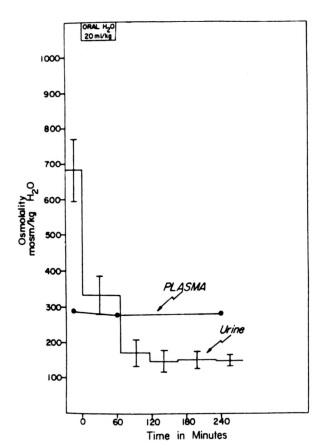

FIG. 85-8. Mean plasma and urine osmolalities in 16 patients with untreated myxedema for 6 hours after an oral water load (20 mL/kg body weight). Urine osmolalities decreased significantly to less than 200 mOsm/kg H_2O by 4 hours after the water load, indicating fairly intact renal diluting mechanisms in these patients. (From DeRubertis FR Jr, Michelis MF, Bloom ME, et al. Impaired water excretion in myxedema. *Am J Med* 1971;51:41, with permission.)

of maneuvers that increase distal tubular fluid delivery (e.g., carbonic hydrase inhibition, isotonic saline infusion, and unilateral nephrectomy) all markedly increase solute-free water clearance in hypothyroid rats (248,256,257). Thus, similar to patients with edema-forming states, hypothyroid patients have increased proximal Na^+ and water absorption as a result of decreased EABV with subsequent decreased delivery of tubular fluid to the distal diluting sites of the nephron, thereby accounting for much of their impaired rate of water excretion.

As noted earlier, patients with edema-forming states also have baroreceptor-mediated stimulation of AVP secretion that leads to further impairment of solute-free water excretion by preventing maximal urinary dilution (38). The results of some studies have supported a similar dual effect in hypothyroid patients as well. Fifteen of 20 patients studied by Skowsky and Kikuchi had elevated plasma AVP levels even after water loading, which then suppressed normally after the patients were made euthyroid (247). Similarly, other investigators have found frankly elevated plasma AVP levels (258,259), inappropriately normal levels despite plasma hypoosmolality (259), or a decreased osmotic threshold for

AVP secretion in hypothyroid patients (260). On the other hand, equal numbers of studies have failed to find evidence of inappropriately elevated plasma AVP levels, urine AVP secretion, or significantly altered osmotic thresholds for AVP secretion or urinary dilution in hypothyroid patients (246, 261–265). Consistent with these findings are several reported cases in which treatment with demeclocycline to antagonize renal AVP effects failed to increase serum [Na$^+$] or decrease urine osmolality in hyponatremic hypothyroid patients (261,266). Experimental studies also have shown variable results. Hypothyroid rats have been reported to manifest higher plasma AVP levels than euthyroid rats after water loading (249). However, hypothyroid Brattleboro rats appear to have similar defects in water excretion as rats with intact AVP secretion (248), supporting a major role for AVP-independent mechanisms of impaired free water excretion in hypothyroid animals. Studies of hypothalamic AVP gene expression have failed to demonstrate upregulation of AVP synthesis in hypothyroid rats (267), again arguing against a major stimulation of AVP secretion under these conditions, although the sensitivity of these methods for ascertaining small increases in hormone secretion and synthesis is limited. Perhaps the strongest argument against a major role for AVP-stimulated water retention in hypothyroidism has been the failure of any animal model of hypothyroidism to reproduce the degrees of hyponatremia commonly found in animal models of SIADH, adrenal insufficiency, and cardiac failure.

In light of the clinical and experimental observations to date, it has to be concluded that the major cause of impaired water excretion in hypothyroidism is an alteration in renal perfusion and GFR secondary to systemic effects of thyroid hormone deficiency on cardiac output and peripheral vascular resistance. However, severe hypothyroidism is a multisystem disease, and just as the presentation of patients with SIADH varies depending on the degree of volume adaptation that has occurred, it is hardly surprising that different results have been reported regarding the potential role of AVP in hypothyroidism depending on the individual characteristics of the cases studied. Thus, in uncomplicated hypothyroidism there appears to be little elevation of plasma AVP levels, and any defects in water excretion are due primarily to effects on renal hemodynamics. As the hypothyroidism becomes more severe, EABV can decrease sufficiently to stimulate AVP secretion secondarily through baroreceptive mechanisms. However, even in this case, the elevated AVP levels may not be causally related to the impaired water excretion because several studies have suggested that hypothyroid animals are resistant to the effects of AVP based on decreased medullary cyclic adenosine monophosphate generation in response to AVP (249,268). However, when cardiac function becomes severely compromised, as often occurs with advanced myxedema, plasma AVP can become elevated sufficiently to override any renal resistance and cause an antidiuresis, which then contributes to the hemodynamic impairments of water excretion. Whether hyponatremia develops at any stage of disease progression depends on the relative balance

between water intake and excretory capacity; because maximal solute-free water clearance decreases as these defects become more pronounced, this accounts for the increased incidence of hyponatremia as the severity of the underlying hypothyroidism worsens.

PRIMARY POLYDIPSIA

As discussed previously, excessive water intake is only rarely of sufficient magnitude to produce hyponatremia in the presence of normal renal function. However, it often is a significant contributing factor to hyponatremia in polydipsic patients, particularly those with underlying defects in solute-free water excretion. In addition, because a positive water balance is required for the production of hyponatremia even under conditions of maximal antidiuresis in humans and animals, an appreciation of the control mechanisms regulating water ingestion is important for understanding the development of hyponatremia in patients with SIADH and other hypoosmolar disorders.

Etiology

The most dramatic cases of primary polydipsia are seen in psychiatric patients, particularly with acute psychosis secondary to schizophrenia (269–276). The prevalence of this disorder based on hospital admissions for acute symptomatic hyponatremia may have been underestimated because studies of polydipsic psychiatric patients have shown a marked diurnal variation in serum [Na$^+$] (from 141 mEq/L at 7 AM to 130 mEq/L at 4 PM), suggesting that many such patients drink excessively during the daytime but then correct themselves through a water diuresis at night (277). This and other considerations have led to defining this disorder as the "psychosis-intermittent hyponatremia-polydipsia" (PIP) syndrome. Polydipsia has been observed in up to 20% of psychiatric inpatients (275), with incidences of intermittent hyponatremia ranging from 5% to 10% (275,278,279). Despite the frequent occurrence of polydipsia in psychiatric patients, not all polydipsia is caused by psychiatric disease; infiltrative diseases such as CNS sarcoidosis (280) or critically placed brain tumors also can be associated with increased thirst and fluid ingestion. Consequently, polydipsic patients should be evaluated with a CT or MRI scan of the brain before concluding that excessive water intake is due to a psychiatric cause.

Pathophysiology

There is little question that excessive water intake alone can sometimes be sufficient to override renal excretory capacity and produce severe hyponatremia (36,281). Although the water excretion rate of normal adult kidneys can exceed 20 L/day, maximum hourly rates rarely exceed 1,000 mL/hour. Because many psychiatric patients drink predominantly during the day or during intense drinking binges (271,277,282,283), they can transiently achieve symptomatic levels of hyponatremia with total daily volumes of water intake under 20 L if it is ingested sufficiently rapidly. This likely accounts for many of the cases in which such patients present with maximally dilute urine, accounting for as many as 50% of patients in some studies (284), and correct quickly by a solute-free water diuresis (285). However, many other cases have been found to meet the criteria for SIADH (272,284,286–288), suggesting nonosmotically stimulated AVP secretion. As might be expected, in the face of much higher than normal water intakes, virtually any impairment of urinary dilution and water excretion can exacerbate the development of a positive water balance and thereby produce hypoosmolality. Thus, hyponatremia has been reported in polydipsic patients taking thiazide diuretics (289,290) or drugs known to be associated with SIADH (152,275,278,291–294), in association with smoking and presumed nicotine-stimulated AVP secretion (295,296) [although a consistent relation with smoking has not been found (153)] and adrenal insufficiency (297). Acute psychosis itself also can cause AVP secretion (270,298), which often appears to take the form of a reset osmostat (169,271,287). It therefore is apparent that no single mechanism can completely explain the occurrence of hyponatremia in polydipsic psychiatric patients, but the combination of higher than normal water intakes plus modest elevations of plasma AVP levels from a variety of potential sources appears to account for a significant portion of such cases.

Although patients with SIADH do not in general manifest the water intakes of patients with primary polydipsia, nonetheless continued water intake in the face of plasma hypoosmolality is inappropriate for maintenance of osmotic homeostasis. Analysis of daily fluid intakes of 91 hyponatremic patients showed an average fluid intake of 2.4 ± 0.2 L/24 hours (37) (Fig. 85-9), which does not differ appreciably from earlier measured intakes of medical students or hospitalized cardiac patients (mean fluid intakes of 2.4 and 2.8 L/24 hours, respectively) (299), or studies of middle-aged subjects (mean fluid intake of 2.1 L/24 hours) (300). This consistent pattern of continued water intake in hyponatremic patients raises important questions as to its cause. Most, although not all, patients treated with dDAVP do not become hyponatremic because they limit their water intakes in the absence of stimulated thirst. This observation has suggested the possibility that patients with SIADH and other hypoosmolar disorders might have a coexisting defect in thirst regulation. A potential underlying mechanism could be stimulation of thirst by central AVP hypersecretion, but to date only relatively small effects of AVP to stimulate thirst have been seen in a single species (301). Alternatively, other animal studies have suggested that osmotic inhibition of thirst is a relatively weak phenomenon and easily overcome by a variety of nonhomeostatic stimuli causing drinking. Not only do rats increase intakes when fluids are made more palatable (302), but rats made antidiuretic with dDAVP continue to ingest such fluids to the point of extreme hypoosmolality, and the degree of hypoosmolality achieved is proportional to the palatability of the fluid (303). Analogous results have been obtained with schedule-induced

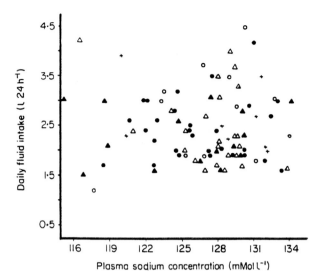

FIG. 85-9. Daily fluid intakes of 91 hospitalized patients with hyponatremia of varying degrees and etiologies. Each point represents a single patient: *open circles,* syndrome of inappropriate antidiuretic hormone secretion; *open triangles,* cardiac failure; *closed circles,* volume contraction; *closed triangles,* cirrhosis; *pluses,* undiagnosed. Despite widely different etiologies for the hyponatremia, mean fluid intakes were equivalent in all groups of patients. (From Gross PA, Pehrisch H, Rascher W, et al. Pathogenesis of clinical hyponatremia: observations of vasopressin and fluid intake in 100 hyponatremic medical patients. *Eur J Clin Invest* 1987;17:123, with permission.)

polydipsia in rats treated with AVP (304). In these examples, drinking continued despite the production of both osmotic dilution and volume expansion, and despite drinking behavior sufficient to activate both oropharyngeal and gastrointestinal inhibitory factors that modulate fluid ingestion (305). Obviously, drinking will not continue indefinitely in the absence of renal excretion until some factor causes inhibition of further intake, but before this happens it is possible to achieve plasma dilutions of 20% to 30%. In humans, similar to animals, there are many nonhomeostatic stimuli to drink fluids, including meal-associated drinking, oral habituation to various beverages, pleasurable sensations from palatable fluids, social interactions promoting fluid ingestion, and mouth dryness as a result of local factors, and these actually account for the major part of human fluid ingestion (300). By themselves, such stimuli are benign and simply lead to more frequent urination of dilute urine to excrete the increased fluids ingested. However, in the presence of pathologic conditions that impair renal water excretion, they can lead to hyponatremia. Therefore, although direct inhibitory physiologic stimuli to thirst and fluid ingestion clearly exist, they appear to be relatively weak compared with excitatory stimuli and can be overridden by a variety of nonhomeostatic stimuli that cause continued fluid ingestion despite plasma hypoosmolality (305). The extent to which such nonhomeostatic drinking versus disordered thirst regulation is responsible for the continued fluid ingestion in hypoosmolar disorders remains to be evaluated by more extensive clinical and experimental studies.

CLINICAL MANIFESTATIONS OF HYPOOSMOLAR DISORDERS

Regardless of the etiology of hypoosmolality, the clinical manifestations are similar. Nonneurologic symptoms are relatively uncommon, but a number of cases of rhabdomyolysis have been reported (306–310), presumably secondary to osmotically induced swelling of muscle fibers. Hypoosmolality is primarily associated with a broad spectrum of neurologic manifestations, ranging from mild, nonspecific symptoms (e.g., headache, nausea) to more significant disorders (e.g., disorientation, confusion, obtundation, focal neurologic deficits, and seizures) (20,311,312). This neurologic symptom complex has been termed *hyponatremic encephalopathy* (313) and primarily reflects brain edema resulting from osmotic water shifts into the brain because of decreased effective plasma osmolality (314). Significant neurologic symptoms usually do not occur until serum [Na^+] falls below 125 mEq/L, and the severity of symptoms can be roughly correlated with the degree of hypoosmolality (20,311). However, individual variability is marked, and for any single patient, the level of serum [Na^+] at which symptoms appear cannot be predicted with great accuracy. Much of this variability can be understood within the framework provided by the process of brain volume regulation (Fig. 85-1), as discussed earlier (67). Although most of the neurologic symptoms associated with acute hyponatremia are caused by brain edema as a result of osmotic water movement into the CNS, a potential exception is the development of seizure activity, which may possibly be caused or aggravated by increased brain ECF concentrations of the excitatory amino acids glutamate and aspartate as a result of cellular extrusion of these osmolytes during the process of brain volume regulation to hyponatremia (64). Once the brain has volume-adapted through solute losses, thereby reducing brain edema, neurologic symptoms are not as prominent and may even be virtually absent. This accounts for the fairly common finding of relatively asymptomatic patients despite severe levels of hyponatremia (17,311). It also is well known from animal studies that the rate of fall of serum [Na^+] is often more strongly correlated with morbidity and mortality than is the actual magnitude of the decrease (20). This is because the volume-adaptation process takes a finite time to complete; the more rapid the fall in serum [Na^+], the more brain edema will be accumulated before the brain is able to lose solute and along with it part of the increased water content. These effects are responsible for the much higher incidence of neurologic symptoms, as well as the higher mortality rates, in patients with acute hyponatremia than in those with chronic hyponatremia (20,315). This phenomenon also likely underlies the observation that the most dramatic cases of death due to hyponatremic encephalopathy have usually been reported in postoperative patients in whom hyponatremia often develops rapidly as a result of intravenous infusion of hypotonic fluids (18,316). In such cases, nausea and vomiting frequently are overlooked as potential early signs of increased intracranial pressure in acutely hypoosmolar patients.

Because hypoosmolality does not cause any known direct effects on the gastrointestinal tract, the presence of unexplained nausea or vomiting in a hypoosmolar patient should be assumed to be of CNS origin and the patient treated for symptomatic hypoosmolality, as described later. Similarly, critically ill patients with unexplained seizures should be rapidly evaluated for possible hyponatremia because as much as one-third of such patients have been found to have a serum [Na^+] of less than 125 mEq/L as the cause of the seizure activity (317). Underlying neurologic disease also affects the level of hypoosmolality at which CNS symptoms appear; moderate hypoosmolality is of little concern in an otherwise healthy patient but can cause morbidity in a patient with an underlying seizure disorder. Nonneurologic metabolic disorders [e.g., hypoxia (318), acidosis, hypercalcemia] similarly can affect the level of plasma osmolality at which CNS symptoms occur.

In the most severe cases of hyponatremic encephalopathy, death results from respiratory failure after tentorial cerebral herniation and brainstem compression. Studies of patients with severe postoperative hyponatremic encephalopathy have indicated a high incidence of patients with hypoxia, of whom one-fourth manifested hypercapnic respiratory failure, the expected result of brainstem compression, but three-fourths of whom had pulmonary edema as the apparent cause of the hypoxia (319). More recent studies of acute hyponatremia after marathon races have similarly shown hypoxia and pulmonary edema in association with brain edema (320). These results therefore suggest the possibility that hypoxia from noncardiogenic pulmonary edema may represent an early sign of developing cerebral edema even before the swelling progresses to the point of brainstem compression and tentorial herniation. Clinical studies also have suggested that menstruating women (316) and young children (321) may be particularly susceptible to the development of neurologic morbidity and mortality during hyponatremia, especially in the acute postoperative setting (313). However, other studies have failed to corroborate these findings (322,323). Consequently, the true clinical incidence as well as the underlying mechanisms responsible for these sometimes catastrophic cases remain to be determined.

THERAPY OF HYPOOSMOLAR DISORDERS

Despite some areas of continuing controversy concerning correction of osmolality in hypoosmolar patients, a relative consensus has evolved regarding the most appropriate treatment of this disorder. The following recommendations are summarized in the diagnostic and therapeutic flow diagram shown in Fig. 85-10.

Initial Evaluation

Once true hypoosmolality is verified, the ECF volume status of the patient should be assessed by careful clinical

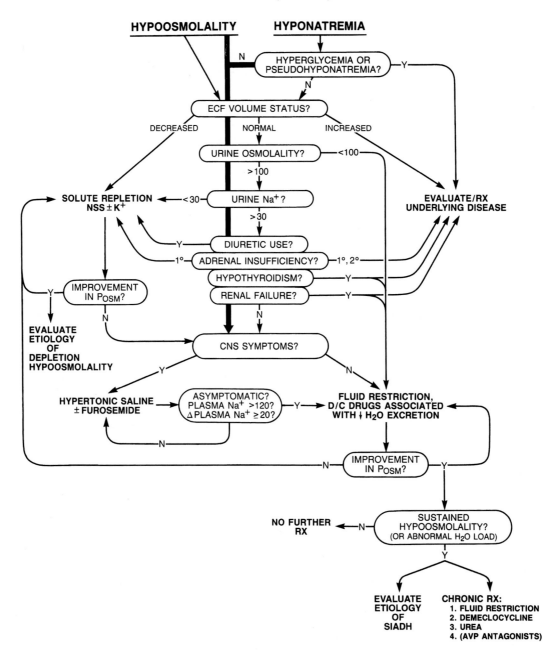

FIG. 85-10. Schematic summary of the evaluation and therapy of hypoosmolar patients. The *dark arrow* in the center emphasizes that the presence of central nervous system dysfunction due to hyponatremia always should be assessed immediately so that appropriate therapy can be started as soon as possible in symptomatic patients while the outlined diagnostic evaluation is proceeding. (From Verbalis JG. Inappropriate antidiuresis and other hypoosmolar states. In: Becker KL, ed. *Principles and practice of endocrinology and metabolism,* 2nd ed. Philadelphia: JB Lippincott, 1995:265, with permission.)

examination. If fluid retention is present, the treatment of the underlying disease should take precedence over correction of plasma osmolality. Often this involves treatment with diuretics, which should simultaneously improve plasma tonicity by virtue of stimulating excretion of hypotonic urine (see Chapter 84). If hypovolemia is present, the patient must be considered to have depletion-induced hypoosmolality, in which case volume repletion with isotonic saline (0.9% NaCl) at a rate appropriate for the estimated fluid deficit should be initiated. If diuretic use is known or suspected, the isotonic

saline should be supplemented with potassium (30 to 40 mEq/L) even if serum $[K^+]$ is not low because of the propensity of such patients to development of total-body potassium depletion. Most often, the hypoosmolar patient is clinically euvolemic, in which case the evaluation should then proceed to the measurement of urine osmolality and $[Na^+]$. However, several situations dictate a reconsideration of solute depletion as a potential diagnosis, even in the patient without clinically apparent hypovolemia. These include (a) a urine $[Na^+]$ less than 30 mEq/L (88), (b) a history of recent diuretic use, and (c) any suggestion of primary adrenal insufficiency. Whenever a possibility of depletion-induced, rather than dilution-induced, hypoosmolality exists, it is most appropriate to treat the patient initially with isotonic saline, regardless of whether signs of hypovolemia are present. An improvement in, and eventual correction of, the hyponatremia verifies solute and volume depletion. On the other hand, if the patient has SIADH rather than solute depletion, no harm is done by administration of a limited volume (e.g., 1 to 2 L) of isotonic saline because patients with SIADH simply excrete excess infused or ingested NaCl without significantly changing their plasma osmolality (1). However, in the absence of an initial positive response, continued infusion of isotonic saline should be avoided because over longer periods, sufficient solute-free water can be retained to lower the serum $[Na^+]$ further.

The approach to patients with euvolemic hypoosmolality varies according to the clinical situation. A patient who meets all the essential criteria for SIADH but has a low urine osmolality should be observed on a trial of modest fluid restriction. If the hypoosmolality is attributable to transient SIADH or severe polydipsia, the urine will remain dilute and the plasma osmolality will be fully corrected as solute-free water is excreted. If, however, the patient has the reset osmostat form of the disorder, then the urine will become concentrated at some point before the plasma osmolality and serum $[Na^+]$ return to normal ranges. If either primary or secondary adrenal insufficiency is suspected, glucocorticoid replacement should be initiated immediately after the completion of a rapid ACTH stimulation test (324,325). A prompt water diuresis after initiation of glucocorticoid treatment supports a diagnosis of glucocorticoid deficiency (223). However, the absence of a quick response does not necessarily negate this diagnosis because several days of glucocorticoid replacement sometimes are required for normalization of plasma osmolality (89). If hypothyroidism is suspected, thyroid function tests should be conducted and a plasma TSH level should be obtained; usually, however, replacement therapy is withheld pending these results unless the patient is obviously myxedematous. If renal failure is present in a patient with hypoosmolality, a more extensive evaluation of renal function is necessary before deciding what course of treatment is most appropriate (see Chapter 41).

Acute Treatment

In any significantly hyponatremic patient, the clinician must decide how quickly the plasma osmolality should be increased, and to what level. This decision in turn depends on knowledge about two basic questions: (a) what are the risks of uncorrected hyponatremia, and (b) what are the risks of the correction itself? As described in the previous section, hyponatremia is associated with a broad spectrum of neurologic symptoms (20), sometimes leading to death in severe cases (316,321). However, since the early 1980s it has become clear that correcting severe hyponatremia too rapidly also is dangerous because this sometimes can be associated with pontine and extrapontine myelinolysis, a brain demyelinating disease that also causes severe neurologic morbidity and death (19,326). Consequently, appreciation of the appropriate therapy of this disorder requires understanding this disease as well as the pathophysiologic process underlying hyponatremic encephalopathy.

Pontine and Extrapontine Myelinolysis

Despite the obvious survival advantages afforded by brain volume regulation in response to hyponatremia, every adaptation made by the body in response to a perturbation of homeostasis bears within it the potential to create a new set of problems, and this is true for brain volume regulation as well. Over the 1990s, it has become apparent that the demyelinating disease of central pontine myelinolysis (CPM) occurs with a significantly higher incidence in patients with hyponatremia (327–329), and in both animal (330–334) and human studies (19,326,335), brain demyelination has clearly been shown to be associated with the correction of existing hyponatremia rather than simply with the presence of severe hyponatremia itself. Although the mechanisms by which correction of hyponatremia leads to brain demyelination remain under investigation, this pathologic disorder likely is precipitated by the brain dehydration that has been demonstrated to occur after correction of serum $[Na^+]$ toward normal ranges in animal models of chronic hyponatremia. Because the degree of osmotic brain shrinkage is greater in animals that are maintained chronically hyponatremic than in normonatremic animals undergoing similar increases in plasma osmolality (175,332,336), by analogy the brains of human patients adapted to hyponatremia are likely to be particularly susceptible to dehydration after subsequent increases in osmolality, which in turn leads to pathologic demyelination in some patients. Recent magnetic resonance studies in animals have shown that chronic hypoosmolality predisposes rats to opening of the blood-brain barrier after rapid correction of hyponatremia (337), and that the disruption of the blood-brain barrier is highly correlated with subsequent demyelination (338); a potential mechanism by which blood-brain barrier disruption might lead to subsequent myelinolysis is through an influx of complement, which is toxic to the oligodendrocytes that manufacture and maintain myelin sheaths of neurons, into the brain (339).

Although there has been considerable debate in the literature regarding the parameters of correction of hyponatremia associated with an increased risk of myelinolysis, studies in both patients (340–342) and experimental animals (332–334) support the notion that both the rate of correction of hyponatremia and the total magnitude of the correction over the first few days likely represent significant factors that increase the risk of demyelination (Fig. 85-11). Studies in rats have shown that the initial rate of correction of hyponatremia may not be important for the development of demyelinative lesions as long as the total magnitude of the correction remains less

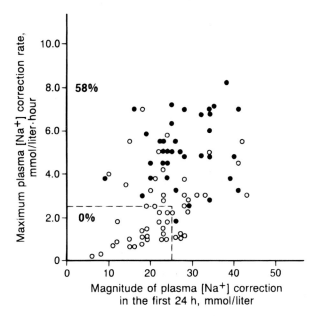

FIG. 85-11. Relation between the production of brain myelinolysis and the maximal rate and 24-hour magnitude of correction of hyponatremia in 87 rats with dDAVP-induced hyponatremia. ○, Rats with no brain lesions; ●, rats with demyelinative brain lesions. Different methods were used to correct the hyponatremia to produce varying initial rates and magnitudes of serum [Na+] correction. The *dashed lines* enclose the area within which no rats had demonstrable neuropathologic lesions, whereas 58% manifested lesions when their correction parameters were outside these ranges. (From Verbalis JG, Martinez AJ. Determinants of brain myelinolysis following correction of chronic hyponatremia in rats. In: Jamison RL, Jard S, eds. *Vasopressin.* Paris: John Libbey, 1991:539, with permission.)

than 20 mEq/L in 24 hours (343), which supports clinical data indicating that magnitude of correction represents the major risk factor related to subsequent neurologic morbidity and mortality, although there still is some disagreement as to the actual level at which patients are at risk for CPM; initial reports implicated increases in serum [Na+] greater than 25 mEq/L over the first 24 to 48 hours of treatment (340), whereas later studies suggested occurrence of CPM with even lesser increases in serum [Na+] of greater than 12 mEq/L in 24 hours or 18 mEq/h in 48 hours (344). Although overcorrection of hyponatremia to supranormal levels also clearly is a risk factor for neurologic deterioration, both clinical and experimental studies have found that demyelination occurred after corrections to serum [Na+] levels still below normal ranges. Regardless of the level of increase in serum [Na+] at which CPM occurs, the methods used to correct hyponatremia do not appear to have any significant bearing on the production of brain demyelination because both experimental studies (334) and clinical reports (19,345,346) have demonstrated that demyelination occurs independently of the method used to correct the hyponatremia.

Other factors also clearly can influence the susceptibility to demyelination after correction of hyponatremia. Perhaps most important are the severity and duration of the preexisting hyponatremia. Both of these risk factors likely relate to the degree of brain volume regulation that has occurred before the correction: the more severe the hyponatremia and the longer it has been maintained, the greater the degree of solute loss that will have occurred during the process of brain volume regulation. As larger amounts of solute are lost, the ability of the brain to buffer subsequent increases in plasma osmolality is impaired, resulting in greater degrees of brain dehydration as serum [Na+] is later raised, which in turn can lead to brain demyelination through mechanisms discussed earlier. Clinical implications of this pathophysiologic mechanism are that CPM should not occur in cases of either mild or very acute hyponatremia. Both of these findings have been found to be true. CPM has been reported only rarely in patients with a starting serum [Na+] greater than 120 mmol/L (19,344,347), and also does not appear to occur in most patients with psychogenic polydipsia, who are well known to develop hyponatremia acutely from episodes of massive water ingestion followed by rapid correction as they diurese the excess fluid (285). There also are some independent risk factors for the occurrence of CPM, particularly chronic alcoholism and malnutrition, which led to the original description of this disorder in 1959 (348). Although no studies to date have clearly documented interactive effects between these risk factors and CPM, it seems likely that the threshold for increases in serum [Na+] that increase the risk for CPM is lower in alcoholic and malnourished patients, and a case report of myelinolysis in a patient with beer potomania in whom the rate of correction stayed within the recommended guidelines supports this likelihood (349). One factor that appears to protect hyponatremic patients from myelinolysis after rapid correction of hyponatremia is uremia. Although uremic patients on dialysis frequently have large swings of serum [Na+], only very rare cases of osmotically induced demyelination have been reported in this group (350). A study in rats showed that azotemic rats were able to sustain large increases in serum [Na+] without brain damage, purportedly because the urea acts as an intracellular osmolyte to stabilize intracellular volume and thereby reduces the degree of brain dehydration produced after rapid correction of hyponatremia (351).

Several other aspects of this unique disease deserve emphasis. First, demyelination after correction of hyponatremia frequently occurs in white matter areas of the brain other than the pons; this has led to proposals that occurrence of the disorder in hyponatremic patients be called the *osmotic demyelination syndrome* (19). Alternatively, the term *pontine and extrapontine myelinolysis* (PEM) would be more accurate than CPM (329), which is historically correct but anatomically too limited. Second, apropos the widespread distribution of the neuropathologic lesions, a much broader range of neurologic disorders is now being reported in patients after correction of hyponatremia, including cognitive, behavioral, and neuropsychiatric disorders, presumably as a result of demyelination in subcortical, corpus callosal, and hippocampal white matter (352,353), and movement disorders, as a result of demyelination in the basal ganglia (354,355). Third, MRI scans often fail to demonstrate the characteristic demyelinative lesions in many cases because scans usually are negative until sufficient time has passed (usually 3 to 4 weeks) after the correction of hyponatremia and the onset of neurologic symptoms (356–358). Consequently, the presence of positive MRI findings strongly [although not unequivocally (359)] supports a diagnosis of PEM, but the absence of radiologic findings can never eliminate the possibility of this disorder. Third, although most cases of osmotically induced PEM have been associated with rapid correction of hyponatremia, the disorder also has been reported with severe hypernatremia in both animal models (360) and patients (361). This is consistent with the hypothesis that brain dehydration with subsequent disruption of the blood-brain barrier is related to the pathogenesis of the demyelinative process (338,339). Finally, it is clear that given our present knowledge, we cannot predict with any degree of certainty in which patients demyelination will develop regardless of the parameters used to correct hyponatremia. Many patients undergo very rapid and large corrections of their serum [Na$^+$] without subsequent neurologic complications (362), as is true of experimental animals as well (334,343) (Fig. 85-11). Consequently, overly rapid correction of hyponatremia should be viewed as a factor that puts patients *at risk* for PEM, but does not inevitably precipitate this disorder

Individualization of Therapy

Based on the previous discussions of hyponatremic encephalopathy and pontine and extrapontine myelinolysis, it follows that optimal treatment of hyponatremic patients must entail balancing the risks of hyponatremia against the risks of correction for each patient individually (Fig. 85-12). Although individual variability in response is great, and consequently one cannot always accurately predict which patients will experience neurologic complications from either hyponatremia or its correction, consensus guidelines for treating hypoosmolar patients allow a rational approach to minimizing the risks of both these complications. Implicit in these guidelines is the realization that treatment must be tailored to each patient's clinical presentation: appropriate therapy for one hyponatremic patient may be inappropriate for another despite equivalent degrees of hypoosmolality (4,363). To accomplish this, three factors should be taken into consideration when making a treatment decision in a hypoosmolar patient: (a) the severity of the hyponatremia, (b) the duration of the hyponatremia, and (c) the patient's neurologic symptomatology. The severity of the hypoosmolality is an important consideration because neither sequelae from hyponatremia itself nor myelinolysis after therapy are likely in patients whose serum [Na$^+$] remains 120 mEq/L or greater, although occasionally significant symptoms of hyponatremic encephalopathy can develop even at a higher serum [Na$^+$] if the rate of fall of plasma osmolality is particularly rapid.

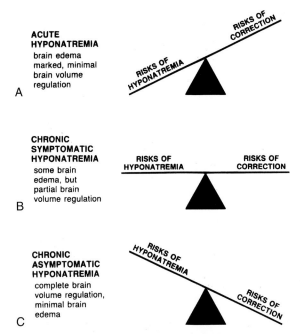

FIG. 85-12. Schematic summary of the balance between the relative risks of hyponatremia versus the risks of rapidly correcting the hyponatremia in patients with hyponatremia of varying durations and symptomatology. Treatment indications are clear for both acute (≤48 hours' duration) symptomatic hyponatremia **(top panel)** and chronic (>48 hours' duration) asymptomatic hyponatremia **(bottom panel).** However, cases of chronic symptomatic hyponatremia represent the greatest clinical challenge because some brain volume adaptation has occurred but the presence of symptoms indicates some residual degree of brain edema as well. Such patients are optimally treated using limited and carefully controlled corrections regardless of the methods by which the increases in serum [Na$^+$] occur. (From Verbalis JG. Hyponatremia: endocrinologic causes and consequences of therapy. *Trends Endocrinol Metab* 1992;3:1, with permission.)

The importance of duration and symptomatology both relate to how well the brain has adapted to the hyponatremia and consequently its degree of risk for subsequent demyelination with rapid correction.

Acute Hyponatremia

Cases of acute hyponatremia (arbitrarily defined as ≤48 hours in duration) usually are symptomatic if the hyponatremia is severe (i.e., ≤120 mEq/L). These patients are at greatest risk for neurologic complications from the hyponatremia, but rarely experience demyelination (285), presumably because sufficient brain volume regulation has not yet occurred to increase brain susceptibility to osmotic dehydration with the correction. Consequently, serum [Na$^+$] in such patients should be corrected to higher levels relatively quickly. Postoperative patients (18,364,365), and particularly young women and children in some studies (316,321,366), appear to be at somewhat greater risk for rapidly progressing hyponatremic encephalopathy and therefore should be treated especially promptly. Administration of hypotonic fluids should be avoided in such patients postoperatively (313), though this will not necessarily prevent the occurrence of postoperative hyponatremia in all surgical patients (367). The dark black arrow in Fig. 85-10 emphasizes that hypoosmolar patients should always be evaluated quickly for the presence of neurologic symptoms so that appropriate therapy can be initiated, if indicated, even while other results of the diagnostic evaluation are still pending.

Chronic Asymptomatic Hyponatremia

Conversely, patients with more chronic hyponatremia (arbitrarily defined as >48 hours in duration) who have minimal neurologic symptomatology are at little risk from complications of hyponatremia itself but can have demyelination after rapid correction because of greater degrees of brain volume regulation through electrolyte and osmolyte losses (67,175,332). There is no indication to correct these patients rapidly, regardless of the initial serum [Na$^+$], and they should be treated using slower-acting therapies, such as fluid restriction.

Chronic Symptomatic Hyponatremia

Although the first two extremes have clear treatment indications, most hypoosmolar patients have hyponatremia of indeterminate duration and varying degrees of neurologic symptomatology. This group represents the most challenging treatment decision because the hyponatremia has been present sufficiently long to allow some degree of brain volume regulation, but not enough to prevent some brain edema and neurologic symptomatology (Fig. 85-12). Such patients should be treated promptly because of their symptoms, but using methods that allow a *controlled and limited increase* of their hypoosmolality (363,368). Some studies have suggested that correction parameters should consist of a maximal rate of correction of serum [Na$^+$] in the range of 1 to 2 mEq/L/hour so long as the total magnitude of correction does not exceed 25 mEq/L over the first 48 hours (340), whereas others recommend that these parameters should be even more conservative, with maximal correction rates of 0.5 mEq/L/hour or less and magnitudes of correction that do not exceed 12 mEq/L in the first 24 hours and 18 mEq/L in the first 48 hours (344). A reasonable approach for treatment of individual patients therefore entails choosing correction parameters within these limits depending on their symptomatology: in patients who are only minimally symptomatic, the clinician should proceed at the lower recommended limits of 0.5 mEq/L/hour or less, whereas in those who manifest more severe neurologic symptoms, an initial correction at a rate of 1 to 2 mEq/L/hour, or even 3 to 5 mEq/L/hour in comatose or seizing patients who are at risk for imminent tentorial herniation and respiratory arrest, is more appropriate. Regardless of the initial rate of correction chosen, acute treatment should be interrupted once any of three endpoints is reached: (a) the patient's symptoms are abolished; (b) a safe serum [Na$^+$] (usually ≥120 mEq/L)

is achieved; or (c) a total magnitude of correction of 20 mEq/L is achieved. Once any of these endpoints is reached, the active correction should be stopped and the patient treated with slower-acting therapies, such as oral rehydration or fluid restriction, depending on the etiology of the hypoosmolality. It follows from these recommendations that serum [Na$^+$] levels must be carefully monitored at frequent intervals (at least every 4 hours) during the active phases of treatment to adjust therapy to keep the correction within these guidelines. A retrospective study of chronic symptomatic hyponatremia in 53 postmenopausal women has confirmed the safety and efficacy of using a controlled and limited correction of the hyponatremia with intravenous NaCl. Patients whose serum [Na$^+$] was corrected by 22 ± 10 mEq/L over 35 hours had significantly better neurologic outcomes than those corrected much more slowly, 3 ± 2 mEq/L over 41 hours, by fluid restriction (369).

The preceding recommendations do not preclude promptly treating hyponatremia when it is severe and symptomatic, and particularly when it is acute and of short duration. Such patients are indeed at significant risk of complications from hyponatremic encephalopathy (313). However, even for this group of high-risk patients, it has been argued that only very limited corrections actually are necessary (370). The reasoning on which this is based is the fact that the most brain edema that can be tolerated before tentorial herniation occurs is an approximately 8% to 10% increase in brain water. Therefore, decreasing brain water by this amount should have maximal therapeutic benefit, whereas exceeding this amount is more likely to produce brain dehydration with an increased risk of precipitating demyelination. By this reasoning, a 10% increase in plasma osmolality (i.e., a 10 mmol/L increase of serum [Na$^+$] in a patient with a starting serum [Na$^+$] of 100 mmol/L) should maximize potential benefit while minimizing potential risk. Although brain water content does not bear an exact relation to changes in plasma osmolality because of the complex nature of secondary adaptive processes, over short periods there is a relatively good relation between these parameters and therefore this argument has considerable merit. Anecdotal reports have been cited as evidence supporting the contention that small increases in serum [Na$^+$] are sufficient to reverse hyponatremic seizures and other aspects of hyponatremic encephalopathy, but as for many other treatment recommendations, no controlled studies exist to confirm the safety and efficacy of this approach.

Choice of Interventional (Active) Therapies for Acute Corrections

Controlled limited corrections can be accomplished with either isotonic or hypertonic saline infusions, depending on the etiology of the hypoosmolality. Patients with volume depletion hypoosmolality (e.g., clinical hypovolemia, diuretic use, or urine [Na$^+$] <30 mEq/L) usually respond well to isotonic (0.9%) NaCl (88). However, patients with diuretic-induced hyponatremia are especially prone to rapid corrections because (a) such patients usually are only minimally volume depleted; (b) they often are small, elderly women with correspondingly small plasma volumes; and (c) with cessation of diuretic therapy they often experience a solute-free water diuresis as their urinary diluting defect dissipates (371). Furthermore, the hypokalemia that frequently accompanies the hyponatremia in such patients appears to be an additional risk factor for demyelination after correction (347). Consequently, in the absence of marked neurologic symptomatology, such patients should simply be treated by institution of a regular sodium diet (4 to 8 g/day) and discontinuing the diuretics; if isotonic saline is infused it should be done so judiciously (e.g., 50 to 75 mL/hour), with K^+ replacement, while the serum $[Na^+]$ is monitored frequently to prevent overly rapid correction. Patients with euvolemic hypoosmolality (including patients with SIADH) usually do not respond to isotonic NaCl (1,88) and are best treated with hypertonic (3%) NaCl solution given by continuous infusion. An initial infusion rate can be estimated by multiplying the patient's body weight in kilograms by the desired rate of increase in serum $[Na^+]$ in milliequivalents per liter per hour (e.g., in a 70-kg patient an infusion of 3% NaCl at 70 mL/hour increases serum $[Na^+]$ by approximately 1 mEq/L/hour, whereas an infusion of 35 mL/hour increases serum $[Na^+]$ by approximately 0.5 mEq/L/hour). Furosemide should be used to treat volume overload, in some cases anticipatorily in patients with known cardiovascular disease (372). Regardless of the therapy or rate initially chosen, it cannot be emphasized too strongly that it is necessary only to correct the plasma osmolality acutely to a safe range rather than completely to normonatremia.

Spontaneous (Passive) Correction

Rarely, patients may spontaneously correct their hyponatremia by means of a water diuresis (341,345). If the hyponatremia is acute, such as water intoxication from psychogenic polydipsia, these patients appear to be at little risk for subsequent demyelination (285). However, in cases in which the hyponatremia has been chronic, patients are at risk for demyelination (345,373,374), and intervention (e.g., administration of dDAVP or intravenous infusion of hypotonic fluid) should be considered to limit the rate and magnitude of correction of serum $[Na^+]$, using the same endpoints as described previously for active corrections. A recent report of such a case demonstrates the utility of interrupting a spontaneous solute-free water diuresis with dDAVP (375). However, in some cases an overcorrection unfortunately occurs before it is noticed. Animal models of this situation have suggested that a delayed lowering of the serum $[Na^+]$ can prevent subsequent brain damage from occurring (376,377), and this would be consistent with the occurrence of a delayed immunologic demyelination as a result of complement influx into the brain after a sustained blood-brain barrier disruption (339). Once again, a recent clinical case in which delayed lowering of serum $[Na^+]$ was associated with a reversal of symptoms suggestive of early myelinolysis supports this as a potential therapy in similar cases (378).

Chronic Treatment

Fluid Restriction

If hyponatremia persists, then investigation of other potential causes of SIADH should be pursued (Table 85-3) and chronic therapy should be instituted. The treatment of chronic SIADH entails a choice among several suboptimal therapeutic regimens. Continued fluid restriction represents the least toxic treatment choice and is the preferred treatment for most cases of mild to moderate SIADH. Several points should be remembered when using this approach: (a) all fluids, not only water, must be included in the restriction; (b) the degree of restriction required depends on urine output plus insensible fluid loss [in general, discretionary, i.e., nonfood, fluids should be limited to 500 mL/day below the average daily urine volume (93)]; (c) several days of restriction usually are necessary before a significant increase in plasma osmolality occurs; and (d) only fluid, not salt, should be restricted. Because of the ongoing natriuresis, patients with chronic SIADH often have a negative total body $[Na^+]$ balance and therefore should be maintained on relatively high NaCl intakes unless otherwise contraindicated. However, just as failure to correct a presumed depletion-induced hyponatremia with isotonic saline should lead the clinician to consider the possibility of a dilution-induced hypoosmolality, so should the failure of significant fluid restriction after several days of confirmed negative fluid balance prompt reconsideration of other possible causes, including solute depletion and clinically inapparent hypovolemia (Fig. 85-10). When fluid restriction is initiated, any drugs known to be associated with SIADH should be discontinued or changed (e.g., newer-generation oral hypoglycemic agents, which in general have not been associated with hyponatremia, should be substituted for chlorpropamide).

Treatment of Polydipsia

Patients whose hyponatremia is caused primarily by polydipsia should ideally have therapy directed at reducing fluid intakes into normal ranges. Unfortunately, this has proven difficult to accomplish in many cases. Patients with a reset thirst threshold are resistant to fluid restriction because of the resulting thirst from stimulation of brain thirst centers at higher plasma osmolalities (379). In some cases, the use of alternative methods to ameliorate the sensation of thirst (e.g., wetting the mouth with ice chips or using sour candies to increase salivary flow) can help to reduce fluid intakes. Fluid intake in patients with psychogenic causes of polydipsia is driven by psychiatric factors that have responded variably to behavioral modification and pharmacologic therapy.

However, several reports have suggested the efficacy of the antipsychotic drug clozapine as a promising agent to reduce polydipsia and prevent recurrent hyponatremia in at least a subset of these patients (380–384).

Pharmacologic Therapy

Fluid restriction always should be tried as the initial therapy for patients with chronic SIADH, with pharmacological intervention reserved for refractory cases in which the degree of fluid restriction required to avoid hypoosmolality is so severe that the patient is unable, or unwilling, to maintain it. In such cases reasonable efforts should be made to ameliorate thirst, such as substituting hard candy or ice chips for drinking fluids. Pharmacologic intervention also should be avoided initially in patients with SIADH that is secondary to tumors because successful treatment of the underlying malignant lesion often eliminates or reduces the inappropriate AVP secretion (97). However, alternative pharmacologic management often is necessary. In such cases the preferred drug is the tetracycline derivative demeclocycline (385,386). This agent causes a nephrogenic form of diabetes insipidus (387), thereby decreasing urine concentration even in the presence of high plasma AVP levels. Appropriate dosages of demeclocycline range from 600 to 1,200 mg/day administered in divided doses. Treatment must be continued for several days to achieve maximal diuretic effects; consequently, the clinician should wait 3 to 4 days before deciding to increase the dose. Demeclocycline can cause reversible azotemia, and sometimes nephrotoxicity, especially in patients with cirrhosis (388). Renal function therefore should be monitored in patients treated with demeclocycline on a regular basis and the medication discontinued if increasing azotemia is noted.

Other agents, such as lithium, have similar renal effects, but are less desirable because of inconsistent results and significant side effects (389). Urea also has been described as an alternative mode of treatment for SIADH as well as other hyponatremic disorders (390–393). Although it has long been recognized that any osmotic diuretic can be used to treat hypoosmolality by virtue of increasing solute-free water excretion, such therapeutic modalities usually have proved impractical for chronic ambulatory use. Urea is an exception because it can be administered orally; furthermore, it corrects hypoosmolality not only by increasing solute-free water excretion but by decreasing urinary sodium excretion. Dosages of 30 g/day usually are effective; it is advisable to dissolve the urea in orange juice or some other strongly flavored liquid to camouflage the taste. Even if completely normal water balance is not achieved, it often is possible to allow the patient to maintain a less strict regimen of fluid restriction while receiving urea. The disadvantages associated with the use of urea include poor palatability, the development of azotemia at higher doses, and the unavailability of a convenient form of the agent. Several other drugs that have been described appear to decrease AVP hypersecretion in some cases (e.g., diphenylhydantoin, opiates, ethanol), but responses are erratic and unpredictable (171). One potential exception is the recent development of agonists selective for kappa opioid receptors, which appear to be more specific for inhibition of AVP hypersecretion in animal studies (394,395), and in clinical trials successfully produced an aquaresis in patients with cirrhosis (396).

Vasopressin Antagonists

Diseases caused by excess or inappropriate circulating levels of hormones can be treated by interfering with secretion of the hormone, interfering with the effects of the hormone at its target tissue, or indirectly counteracting the physiologic and pathophysiologic effects produced by the effects of the hormone. As described previously, all of these methods have been used with limited degrees of success in treating patients with SIADH. However, all of these therapies have significant limitations, and it has long been recognized that an antagonist of the kidney AVP V_2 receptors would be the ideal agent for treatment of patients with dilutional hyponatremia (397). Previous attempts at synthesizing peptide AVP receptor antagonists were frustrated by species variability with regard to partial agonistic effects of such compounds (398). More recently, several nonpeptide AVP V_2 receptor antagonists have been described that appear to overcome these problems (5,399,400). At the time this chapter was written, several of these compounds were already in clinical trials, with promising results (401). It therefore appears that we are poised to begin a new era in both the evaluation and treatment of patients with SIADH. When eventually approved for clinical use, clinical trials using selective AVP V_2, and also AVP V_1 (402), receptor antagonists will enable investigators to address some long-standing questions about the role of AVP receptor activation in producing antidiuresis, as well as other potential effects, in various disease states [e.g., hyponatremic patients without measurable AVP levels (181)]. Even more promising, therapy of patients with chronic hyponatremia will very likely be much easier and much more effective than at present. Caution will, of course, still be necessary in some situations. Because demyelination appears to be independent of the method used to correct hyponatremia, patients corrected too rapidly with AVP receptor antagonists also will be at risk for pontine and extrapontine myelinolysis, which already has been documented with the use of peptide AVP receptor antagonists to correct hyponatremia in animals (403). Nonetheless, appropriate dosing and monitoring should allow successful adherence to the same guidelines for limited controlled correction that apply to other correction methods. Furthermore, it seems reasonable to predict that single doses of such agents may prove to be the ideal method for achieving small controlled increases of serum [Na^+] that will satisfactorily reverse hyponatremic encephalopathy without producing dangerously large corrections that increase the risk of pontine and extrapontine myelinolysis.

REFERENCES

1. Schwartz WB, Bennett S, Curelop S, et al. A syndrome of renal sodium loss and hyponatremia probably resulting from inappropriate secretion of antidiuretic hormone. *Am J Med* 1957;23:529.
2. Bartter FC, Schwartz WB. The syndrome of inappropriate secretion of antidiuretic hormone. *Am J Med* 1967;42:790.
3. Verbalis JG. Hyponatremia: answered and unanswered questions. *Am J Kidney Dis* 1991;18:546.
4. Berl T. Treating hyponatremia: damned if we do and damned if we don't. *Kidney Int* 1990;37:1006.
5. Yamamura Y, Ogawa H, Yamashita H, et al. Characterization of a novel aquaretic agent, OPC-31260, as an orally effective, nonpeptide vasopressin V2 receptor antagonist. *Br J Pharmacol* 1992;105:787.
6. DeVita MV, Gardenswartz MH, Konecky A, et al. Incidence and etiology of hyponatremia in an intensive care unit. *Clin Nephrol* 1990; 34:163.
7. Flear CT, Gill GV, Burn J. Hyponatraemia: mechanisms and management. *Lancet* 1981;2:26.
8. Kleinfeld M, Casimir M, Borra S. Hyponatremia as observed in a chronic disease facility. *J Am Geriatr Soc* 1979;27:156.
9. Owen JA, Campbell DG. A comparison of plasma electrolyte and urea values in healthy persons and in hospital patients. *Clin Chim Acta* 1968; 22:611.
10. Natkunam A, Shek CC, Swaminathan R. Hyponatremia in a hospital population. *J Med* 1991;22:83.
11. Brunsvig PF, Os I, Frederichsen P. Hyponatremia: a retrospective study of occurrence, etiology and mortality. *Tidsskr Nor Laegeforen* 1990;110:2367.
12. Anderson RJ, Chung HM, Kluge R, et al. Hyponatremia: a prospective analysis of its epidemiology and the pathogenetic role of vasopressin. *Ann Intern Med* 1985;102:164.
13. Berghmans T, Paesmans M, Body JJ. A prospective study on hyponatraemia in medical cancer patients: epidemiology, aetiology and differential diagnosis. *Support Care Cancer* 2000;8:192.
14. Sorensen IJ, Matzen LE. Serum electrolytes and drug therapy of patients admitted to a geriatric department. *Ugeskr Laeger* 1993;155: 3921.
15. Misra SC, Mansharamani GC. Hyponatremia in elderly hospital inpatients. *Br J Clin Pract* 1989;43:295.
16. Miller M, Morley JE, Rubenstein LZ. Hyponatremia in a nursing home population. *J Am Geriatr Soc* 1995;43:1410.
17. Sterns RH. Severe symptomatic hyponatremia: treatment and outcome: a study of 64 cases. *Ann Intern Med* 1987;107:656.
18. Arieff AI. Hyponatremia, convulsions, respiratory arrest, and permanent brain damage after elective surgery in healthy women. *N Engl J Med* 1986;314:1529.
19. Sterns RH, Riggs JE, Schochet SS Jr. Osmotic demyelination syndrome following correction of hyponatremia. *N Engl J Med* 1986;314:1535.
20. Arieff AI, Llach F, Massry SG. Neurological manifestations and morbidity of hyponatremia: correlation with brain water and electrolytes. *Medicine (Baltimore)* 1976;55:121.
21. Oster JR, Materson BJ. Renal and electrolyte complications of congestive heart failure and effects of therapy with angiotensin-converting enzyme inhibitors. *Arch Intern Med* 1992;152:704.
22. Oster JR, Singer I. Hyponatremia, hyposmolality, and hypotonicity: tables and fables [see comments]. *Arch Intern Med* 1999;159:333.
23. Albrink MJ, Hald PM, Man EBPJP. The displacement of serum water by the lipids of hyperlipemic serum: a new method for the rapid determination of serum water. *J Clin Invest* 1955;34:1483.
24. Weisberg LS. Pseudohyponatremia: a reappraisal [Review]. *Am J Med* 1989;86:315.
25. Ladenson JH, Apple FS, Koch DD. Misleading hyponatremia due to hyperlipemia: a method-dependent error. *Ann Intern Med* 1981;95: 707.
26. Katz MA. Hyperglycemia-induced hyponatremia: calculation of expected serum sodium depression. *N Engl J Med* 1973;289:843.
27. Hillier TA, Abbott RD, Barrett EJ. Hyponatremia: evaluating the correction factor for hyperglycemia. *Am J Med* 1999;106:399.
28. Dorwart WV, Chalmers L. Comparison of methods for calculating serum osmolality form chemical concentrations, and the prognostic value of such calculations. *Clin Chem* 1975;21:190.
29. Gennari FJ. Current concepts. Serum osmolality: uses and limitations. *N Engl J Med* 1984;310:102.
30. Jacobsen D, Bredesen JE, Eide I, et al. Anion and osmolal gaps in the diagnosis of methanol and ethylene glycol poisoning. *Acta Med Scand* 1982;212:17.
31. Rose BD. New approach to disturbances in the plasma sodium concentration. *Am J Med* 1986;81:1033.
32. Abramow M, Cogan E. Clinical aspects and pathophysiology of diuretic-induced hyponatremia. *Adv Nephrol* 1984;13:1.
33. Fichman MP, Vorherr H, Kleeman CR, et al. Diuretic-induced hyponatremia. *Ann Intern Med* 1971;75:853.
34. Spital A. Diuretic-induced hyponatremia. *Am J Nephrol* 1999;19:447.
35. Vieweg WV, Karp BI. Severe hyponatremia in the polydipsia-hyponatremia syndrome. *J Clin Psychiatry* 1994;55:355.
36. Gillum DM, Linas SL. Water intoxication in a psychotic patient with normal renal water excretion. *Am J Med* 1984;77:773.
37. Gross PA, Pehrisch H, Rascher W, et al. Pathogenesis of clinical hyponatremia: observations of vasopressin and fluid intake in 100 hyponatremic medical patients. *Eur J Clin Invest* 1987;17:123.
38. Schrier RW. Body fluid volume regulation in health and disease: a unifying hypothesis. *Ann Intern Med* 1990;113:155.
39. Schrier RW. Pathogenesis of sodium and water retention in high-output and low-output cardiac failure, nephrotic syndrome, cirrhosis, and pregnancy (1). *N Engl J Med* 1988;319:1065.
40. Schrier RW. Pathogenesis of sodium and water retention in high-output and low-output cardiac failure, nephrotic syndrome, cirrhosis, and pregnancy (2). *N Engl J Med* 1988;319:1127.
41. Szatalowicz VL, Arnold PE, Chaimovitz C, et al. Radioimmunoassay of plasma arginine vasopressin in hyponatremic patients with congestive heart failure. *N Engl J Med* 1981;305:263.
42. Bichet D, Szatalowicz V, Chaimovitz C, et al. Role of vasopressin in abnormal water excretion in cirrhotic patients. *Ann Intern Med* 1982; 96:413.
43. Leaf A, Bartter FC, Santos RF, et al. Evidence in man that urinary electrolyte loss induced by pitressin is a function of water retention. *J Clin Invest* 1953;32:868.
44. Nolph KD, Schrier RW. Sodium, potassium and water metabolism in the syndrome of inappropriate antidiuretic hormone secretion. *Am J Med* 1970;49:534.
45. Hall JE, Montani JP, Woods LL, et al. Renal escape from vasopressin: role of pressure diuresis. *Am J Physiol* 1986;250:F907.
46. Kamoi K, Ebe T, Kobayashi O, et al. Atrial natriuretic peptide in patients with the syndrome of inappropriate antidiuretic hormone secretion and with diabetes insipidus. *J Clin Endocrinol Metab* 1990;70: 1385.
47. Cogan E, Debieve MF, Pepersack T, et al. Natriuresis and atrial natriuretic factor secretion during inappropriate antidiuresis. *Am J Med* 1988;84:409.
48. Mizelle HL, Hall JE, Hildebrandt DA. Atrial natriuretic peptide and pressure natriuresis: interactions with the renin-angiotensin system. *Am J Physiol* 1989;257:R1169.
49. Demanet JC, Bonnyns M, Bleiberg H, et al. Coma due to water intoxication in beer drinkers. *Lancet* 1971;2:1115.
50. Hilden T, Svendsen TL. Electrolyte disturbances in beer drinkers: a specific "hypo-osmolality syndrome." *Lancet* 1975;2:245.
51. Thaler SM, Teitelbaum I, Berl T. "Beer potomania" in non-beer drinkers: effect of low dietary solute intake. *Am J Kidney Dis* 1998;31: 1028.
52. Cooke CR, Turin MD, Walker WG. The syndrome of inappropriate antidiuretic hormone secretion (SIADH): pathophysiologic mechanisms in solute and volume regulation. *Medicine (Baltimore)* 1979;58:240.
53. Stormont JM, Waterhouse C. The genesis of hyponatremia associated with marked overhydration and water intoxication. *Circulation* 1961;24:191.
54. Grantham JJ. Pathophysiology of hyposmolar conditions: a cellular perspective. In: Andreoli TE, Grantham JJ, Rector FC, eds. *Disturbances in body fluid osmolality*. Bethesda, MD: American Physiological Society, 1977:217.
55. Grantham J, Linshaw M. The effect of hyponatremia on the regulation of intracellular volume and solute composition. *Circ Res* 1984;54: 483.
56. Yannet H. Changes in the brain resulting from depletion of extracellular electrolytes. *Am J Physiol* 1940;128:683.
57. Holliday MA, Kalayci MN, Harrah J. Factors that limit brain volume changes in response to acute and sustained hyper- and hyponatremia. *J Clin Invest* 1968;47:1916.

58. Melton JE, Patlak CS, Pettigrew KD, et al. Volume regulatory loss of Na, Cl, and K from rat brain during acute hyponatremia. *Am J Physiol* 1987;252:F661.

59. Verbalis JG, Drutarosky MD. Adaptation to chronic hypoosmolality in rats. *Kidney Int* 1988;34:351.

60. Garcia-Perez A, Burg MB. Renal medullary organic osmolytes. *Physiol Rev* 1991;71:1081.

61. Heilig CW, Stromski ME, Blumenfeld JD. Characterization of the major brain osmolytes that accumulate in salt-loaded rats. *Am J Physiol* 1989;257:F1108.

62. Thurston JH, Hauhart RE, Nelson JS. Adaptive decreases in amino acids (taurine in particular), creatine, and electrolytes prevent cerebral edema in chronically hyponatremic mice: rapid correction (experimental model of central pontine myelinolysis) causes dehydration and shrinkage of brain. *Metab Brain Dis* 1987;2:223.

63. Lien YH, Shapiro JI, Chan L. Study of brain electrolytes and organic osmolytes during correction of chronic hyponatremia: implications for the pathogenesis of central pontine myelinolysis. *J Clin Invest* 1991;88:303.

64. Verbalis JG, Gullans SR. Hyponatremia causes large sustained reductions in brain content of multiple organic osmolytes in rats. *Brain Res* 1991;567:274.

65. Sterns RH, Baer J, Ebersol S, et al. Organic osmolytes in acute hyponatremia. *Am J Physiol* 1993;264:F833.

66. Videen JS, Michaelis T, Pinto P, et al. Human cerebral osmolytes during chronic hyponatremia. *J Clin Invest* 1995;95:788.

67. Gullans SR, Verbalis JG. Control of brain volume during hyperosmolar and hypoosmolar conditions. *Annu Rev Med* 1993;44:289.

68. Strange K. Maintenance of cell volume in the central nervous system [Review]. *Pediatr Nephrol* 1993;7:689.

69. Emma F, McManus M, Strange K. Intracellular electrolytes regulate the volume set point of the organic osmolyte/anion channel VSOAC. *Am J Physiol* 1997;272:C1766.

70. Law RO. The role of taurine in the regulation of brain cell volume in chronically hyponatraemic rats. *Neurochem Int* 1998;33:467.

71. Glasgow E, Murase T, Zhang B, et al. Gene expression in the rat supraoptic nucleus induced by chronic hyperosmolality versus hypoosmolality. *Am J Physiol* 2000;279:R1239.

72. Vajda Z, Promeneur D, Doczi T, et al. Increased aquaporin-4 immunoreactivity in rat brain in response to systemic hyponatremia. *Biochem Biophys Res Commun* 2000;270:495.

73. Graber M, Corish D. The electrolytes in hyponatremia. *Am J Kidney Dis* 1991;18:527.

74. Padfield PL, Brown JJ, Lever AF, et al. Blood pressure in acute and chronic vasopressin excess: studies of malignant hypertension and the syndrome of inappropriate antidiuretic hormone secretion. *N Engl J Med* 1981;304:1067.

75. Smith MJ Jr, Cowley AW Jr, Guyton AC, et al. Acute and chronic effects of vasopressin on blood pressure, electrolytes, and fluid volumes. *Am J Physiol* 1979;237:F232.

76. Verbalis JG. Pathogenesis of hyponatremia in an experimental model of the syndrome of inappropriate antidiuresis. *Am J Physiol* 1994;267:R1617.

77. Jaenike JR, Waterhouse C. The renal response to sustained administration of vasopressin and water in man. *J Clin Endocrinol Metab* 1961;21:231.

78. Kaye M. An investigation into the cause of hyponatremia in the syndrome of inappropriate secretion of antidiuretic hormone. *Am J Med* 1966;41:910.

79. Southgate HJ, Burke BJ, Walters G. Body space measurements in the hyponatraemia of carcinoma of the bronchus: evidence for the chronic "sick cell" syndrome? *Ann Clin Biochem* 1992;29:90.

80. Verbalis JG. Hyponatremia: epidemiology, pathophysiology, and therapy. *Curr Opin Nephrol Hypertens* 1993;2:636.

81. Clark BA, Shannon RP, Rosa RM, et al. Increased susceptibility to thiazide-induced hyponatremia in the elderly. *J Am Soc Nephrol* 1994;5:1106.

82. Werbel SS, Ober KP. Acute adrenal insufficiency. *Endocrinol Metab Clin North Am* 1993;22:303.

83. Zennaro MC. Mineralocorticoid resistance. *Steroids* 1996;61:189.

84. D'Angelo A, Mioni G, Ossi E, et al. Alterations in renal tubular sodium and water transport in polycystic kidney disease. *Clin Nephrol* 1975;3:99.

85. Nzerue C, Schlanger L, Jena M, et al. Granulomatous interstitial nephritis and uveitis presenting as salt-losing nephropathy. *Am J Nephrol* 1997;17:462.

86. Hutchison FN, Perez EA, Gandara DR, et al. Renal salt wasting in patients treated with cisplatin. *Ann Intern Med* 1988;108:21.

87. Teitelbaum I, McGuinness S. Vasopressin resistance in chronic renal failure: evidence for the role of decreased V2 receptor mRNA. *J Clin Invest* 1995;96:378.

88. Chung HM, Kluge R, Schrier RW, et al. Clinical assessment of extracellular fluid volume in hyponatremia. *Am J Med* 1987;83:905.

89. Carroll PB, McHenry L, Verbalis JG. Isolated adrenocorticotrophic hormone deficiency presenting as chronic hyponatremia. *N Y State J Med* 1990;90:210.

90. Misra SC, Mansharamani GG. Hyponatremia in elderly hospital inpatients. *Br J Clin Pract* 1989;43:295.

91. Michelis MF, Fusco RD, Bragdon RW, et al. Reset of osmoreceptors in association with normovolemic hyponatremia. *Am J Med Sci* 1974;267:267.

92. DeFronzo RA, Goldberg M, Agus ZS. Normal diluting capacity in hyponatremic patients: reset osmostat or a variant of the syndrome of inappropriate antidiuretic hormone secretion. *Ann Intern Med* 1976;84:538.

93. Robertson GL. Posterior pituitary. In: Felig P, Baxter J, Broadus A, et al., eds. *Endocrinology and metabolism*, 2nd ed. New York: McGraw-Hill, 1987:338.

94. Robertson GL, Mahr EA, Athar S, et al. Development and clinical application of a new method for the radioimmunoassay of arginine vasopressin in human plasma. *J Clin Invest* 1973;52:2340.

95. Zerbe R, Stropes L, Robertson G. Vasopressin function in the syndrome of inappropriate antidiuresis. *Ann Rev Med* 1980;31:315.

96. Oelkers W. Hyponatremia and inappropriate secretion of vasopressin (antidiuretic hormone) in patients with hypopituitarism. *N Engl J Med* 1989;321:492.

97. List AF, Hainsworth JD, Davis BW, et al. The syndrome of inappropriate secretion of antidiuretic hormone (SIADH) in small-cell lung cancer. *J Clin Oncol* 1986;4:1191.

98. Maurer LH, O'Donnell JF, Kennedy S, et al. Human neurophysins in carcinoma of the lung: relation to histology, disease stage, response rate, survival, and syndrome of inappropriate antidiuretic hormone secretion. *Cancer Treat Rep* 1983;67:971.

99. Gschwantler M, Weiss W. Hyponatremic coma as the first symptom of a small cell bronchial carcinoma. *Dtsch Med Wochenschr* 1994;119:261.

100. Kamoi K, Kurokawa I, Kasai H, et al. Asymptomatic hyponatremia due to inappropriate secretion of antidiuretic hormone as the first sign of a small cell lung cancer in an elderly man [see comments]. *Intern Med* 1998;37:950.

101. Talmi YP, Hoffman HT, McCabe BF. Syndrome of inappropriate secretion of arginine vasopressin in patients with cancer of the head and neck. *Ann Otol Rhinol Laryngol* 1992;101:946.

102. Ferlito A, Rinaldo A, Devaney KO. Syndrome of inappropriate antidiuretic hormone secretion associated with head neck cancers: review of the literature. *Ann Otol Rhinol Laryngol* 1997;106:878.

103. Kavanagh BD, Halperin EC, Rosenbaum LC, et al. Syndrome of inappropriate secretion of antidiuretic hormone in a patient with carcinoma of the nasopharynx. *Cancer* 1992;69:1315.

104. Renaud L. Hypothalamic magnocellular neurosecretory neurons: intrinsic membrane properties and synaptic connections. *Prog Brain Res* 1994;100:133.

105. Moses AM, Miller M. Drug-induced dilutional hyponatremia. *N Engl J Med* 1974;291:1234.

106. Moses AM, Numann P, Miller M. Mechanism of chlorpropamide-induced antidiuresis in man: evidence for release of ADH and enhancement of peripheral action. *Metabolism* 1973;22:59.

107. Robertson GL. Posterior pituitary. In: Felig P, Baxter J, Frohman L, eds. *Endocrinology and metabolism*, 3rd ed. New York: McGraw-Hill, 1995:385.

108. Friedman E, Shadel M, Halkin H, et al. Thiazide-induced hyponatremia. Reproducibility by single dose rechallenge and an analysis of pathogenesis. *Ann Intern Med* 1989;110:24.

109. Gibbs DM, Vale W. Effect of the serotonin reuptake inhibitor fluoxetine on corticotropin-releasing factor and vasopressin secretion into hypophysial portal blood. *Brain Res* 1983;280:176.

110. Javed A, Kamradt MC, Van de Kar LD, et al. D-fenfluramine induces serotonin-mediated Fos expression in corticotropin-releasing factor and oxytocin neurons of the hypothalamus, and serotonin-independent

Fos expression in enkephalin and neurotensin neurons of the amygdala. *Neuroscience* 1999;90:851.

111. Mikkelsen JD, Jensen JB, Engelbrecht T, et al. D-fenfluramine activates rat oxytocinergic and vasopressinergic neurons through different mechanisms. *Brain Res* 1999;851:247.

112. Faull CM, Rooke P, Baylis PH. The effect of a highly specific serotonin agonist on osmoregulated vasopressin secretion in healthy man. *Clin Endocrinol (Oxf)* 1991;35:423.

113. Strachan J, Shepherd J. Hyponatraemia associated with the use of selective serotonin re- uptake inhibitors. *Aust N Z J Psychiatry* 1998;32:295.

114. Bouman WP, Pinner G, Johnson H. Incidence of selective serotonin reuptake inhibitor (SSRI) induced hyponatraemia due to the syndrome of inappropriate antidiuretic hormone (SIADH) secretion in the elderly. *Int J Geriatr Psychiatry* 1998;13:12.

115. Odeh M, Seligmann H, Oliven A. Severe life-threatening hyponatremia during paroxetine therapy. *J Clin Pharmacol* 1999;39:1290.

116. Wilkinson TJ, Begg EJ, Winter AC, et al. Incidence and risk factors for hyponatraemia following treatment with fluoxetine or paroxetine in elderly people. *Br J Clin Pharmacol* 1999;47:211.

117. Maxwell DL, Polkey MI, Henry JA. Hyponatraemia and catatonic stupor after taking "ecstasy" [see comments]. *BMJ* 1993;307:1399.

118. Parr MJ, Low HM, Botterill P. Hyponatraemia and death after "ecstasy" ingestion. *Med J Aust* 1997;166:136.

119. Holmes SB, Banerjee AK, Alexander WD. Hyponatraemia and seizures after ecstasy use. *Postgrad Med J* 1999;75:32.

120. O'Connor A, Cluroe A, Couch R, et al. Death from hyponatraemia-induced cerebral oedema associated with MDMA ("ecstasy") use. *N Z Med J* 1999;112:255.

121. Burgess C, O'Donohoe A, Gill M. Agony and ecstasy: a review of MDMA effects and toxicity. *Eur Psychiatry* 2000;15:287.

122. Stephenson CP, Hunt GE, Topple AN, et al. The distribution of 3,4-methylenedioxymethamphetamine "ecstasy"-induced c-fos expression in rat brain. *Neuroscience* 1999;92:1011.

123. Hill AR, Uribarri J, Mann J, et al. Altered water metabolism in tuberculosis: role of vasopressin. *Am J Med* 1990;88:357.

124. Shalhoub RJ, Antoniou LD. The mechanism of hyponatremia in pulmonary tuberculosis. *Ann Intern Med* 1969;70:943.

125. Weiss H, Katz S. Hyponatremia resulting from apparently inappropriate secretion of antidiuretic hormone in patients with pulmonary tuberculosis. *Am Rev Respir Dis* 1965;92:609.

126. Breuer R, Rubinow A. Inappropriate secretion of antidiuretic hormone and mycoplasma pneumonia infection. *Respiration* 1981;42:217.

127. Dhawan A, Narang A, Singhi S. Hyponatraemia and the inappropriate ADH syndrome in pneumonia. *Ann Trop Paediatr* 1992;12:455.

128. Pollard RB. Inappropriate secretion of antidiuretic hormone associated with adenovirus pneumonia. *Chest* 1975;68:589.

129. Rosenow EC, Segar WE, Zehr JE. Inappropriate antidiuretic hormone secretion in pneumonia. *Mayo Clin Proc* 1972;47:169.

130. Farber MO, Roberts LR, Weinberger MH, et al. Abnormalities of sodium and H_2O handling in chronic obstructive lung disease. *Arch Intern Med* 1982;142:1326.

131. Vorherr H, Massry SG, Fallet R, et al. Antidiuretic principle in tuberculous lung tissue of a patient with pulmonary tuberculosis and hyponatremia. *Ann Intern Med* 1970;72:383.

132. Raff H, Shinsako J, Keil LC, et al. Vasopressin, ACTH, and blood pressure during hypoxia induced at different rates. *Am J Physiol* 1983;245:E489.

133. Kelestimur H, Leach RM, Ward JP, et al. Vasopressin and oxytocin release during prolonged environmental hypoxia in the rat. *Thorax* 1997;52:84.

134. Baylis PH, Stockley RA, Heath DA. Effect of acute hypoxaemia on plasma arginine vasopressin in conscious man. *Clin Sci Mol Med* 1977;53:401.

135. Farber MO, Bright TP, Strawbridge RA, et al. Impaired water handling in chronic obstructive lung disease. *J Lab Clin Med* 1975;85:41.

136. Reihman DH, Farber MO, Weinberger MH, et al. Effect of hypoxemia on sodium and water excretion in chronic obstructive lung disease. *Am J Med* 1985;78:87.

137. Baratz RA, Ingraham RC. Renal hemodynamics and antidiuretic hormone release associated with volume regulation. *Am J Physiol* 1960;198:565.

138. Agarwal A, Soni A, Ciechanowsky M, et al. Hyponatremia in patients with the acquired immunodeficiency syndrome. *Nephron* 1989;53:317.

139. Cusano AJ, Thies HL, Siegal FP, et al. Hyponatremia in patients with acquired immune deficiency syndrome. *J Acquir Immune Defic Syndr* 1990;3:949.

140. Tang WW, Kaptein EM, Feinstein EI, et al. Hyponatremia in hospitalized patients with the acquired immunodeficiency syndrome (AIDS) and the AIDS-related complex. *Am J Med* 1993;94:169.

141. Tolaymat A, al-Mousily F, Sleasman J, et al. Hyponatremia in pediatric patients with HIV-1 infection. *South Med J* 1995;88:1039.

142. Noto H, Kaneko Y, Takano T, et al. Severe hyponatremia and hyperkalemia induced by trimethoprim-sulfamethoxazole in patients with *Pneumocystis carinii* pneumonia. *Intern Med* 1995;34:96.

143. Yeung KT, Chan M, Chan CK. The safety of i.v. pentamidine administered in an ambulatory setting. *Chest* 1996;110:136.

144. Goldstein CS, Braunstein S, Goldfarb S. Idiopathic syndrome of inappropriate antidiuretic hormone secretion possibly related to advanced age. *Ann Intern Med* 1983;99:185.

145. Hamilton DV. Inappropriate secretion of antidiuretic hormone associated with cerebellar and cerebral atrophy. *Postgrad Med J* 1978;54:427.

146. Miller M. Hyponatremia: age-related risk factors and therapy decisions. *Geriatrics* 1998;53:32.

147. Miller M, Hecker MS, Friedlander DA, et al. Apparent idiopathic hyponatremia in an ambulatory geriatric population. *J Am Geriatr Soc* 1996;44:404.

148. Pillans PI, Coulter DM. Fluoxetine and hyponatraemia: a potential hazard in the elderly. *N Z Med J* 1994;107:85.

149. Rault RM. Case report: hyponatremia associated with nonsteroidal antiinflammatory drugs. *Am J Med Sci* 1993;305:318.

150. Hirshberg B, Ben-Yehuda A. The syndrome of inappropriate antidiuretic hormone secretion in the elderly. *Am J Med* 1997;103:270.

151. Rowe JW, Kilgore A, Robertson GL. Evidence in man that cigarette smoking induces vasopressin release via an airway-specific mechanism. *J Clin Endocrinol Metab* 1980;51:170.

152. Ellinas PA, Rosner F, Jaume JC. Symptomatic hyponatremia associated with psychosis, medications, and smoking. *J Natl Med Assoc* 1993;85:135.

153. Vieweg WV, David JJ, Rowe WT, et al. Correlation of cigarette-induced increase in serum nicotine levels with arginine vasopressin concentrations in the syndrome of self-induced water intoxication and psychosis (SIWIP). *Can J Psychiatry* 1986;31:108.

154. Lausen HD. Metabolism of the neurohypophyseal hormones. In: Greep RO, Astwood EB, Knobil E, et al., eds. *Handbook of physiology.* Washington, DC: American Physiological Society, 1974:287.

155. Rowe JW, Shelton RL, Helderman JH, et al. Influence of the emetic reflex on vasopressin release in man. *Kidney Int* 1979;16:729.

156. Coslovsky R, Bruck R, Estrov Z. Hypo-osmolal syndrome due to prolonged nausea. *Arch Intern Med* 1984;144:191.

157. Edelson JT, Robertson GL. The effect of the cold pressor test on vasopressin secretion in man. *Psychoneuroendocrinology* 1986;11:307.

158. North WG, Friedmann AS, Yu X. Tumor biosynthesis of vasopressin and oxytocin. *Ann N Y Acad Sci* 1993;689:107.

159. Legros JJ, Geenen V, Carvelli T, et al. Neurophysins as markers of vasopressin and oxytocin release: a study in carcinoma of the lung. *Horm Res* 1990;34:151.

160. Ishikawa S, Kuratomi Y, Saito T. A case of oat cell carcinoma of the lung associated with ectopic production of ADH, neurophysin and ACTH. *Endocrinol Jpn* 1980;27:257.

161. George JM, Capen CC, Phillips AS. Biosynthesis of vasopressin in vitro and ultrastructure of a bronchogenic carcinoma: patient with the syndrome of inappropriate secretion of antidiuretic hormone. *J Clin Invest* 1972;51:141.

162. Rosenbaum LC, Neuwelt EA, Van Tol HH, et al. Expression of neurophysin-related precursor in cell membranes of a small-cell lung carcinoma. *Proc Natl Acad Sci USA* 1990;87:9928.

163. Yamaji T, Ishibashi M, Yamada N, et al. Biosynthesis of the common precursor to vasopressin and neurophysin in vitro in transplantable human oat cell carcinoma of the lung with ectopic vasopressin production. *Endocrinol Jpn* 1983;30:451.

164. Vorherr H, Massry SG, Utiger RD, et al. Antidiuretic principle in malignant tumor extracts from patients with inappropriate ADH syndrome. *J Clin Endocrinol Metab* 1968;28:162.

165. Schrier RW. "Inappropriate" versus "appropriate" antidiuretic hormone secretion [Editorial]. *West J Med* 1974;121:62.

166. Schrier RW, Berl T, Anderson RJ. Osmotic and nonosmotic control of vasopressin release. *Am J Physiol* 1979;236:F321.

167. Cowley AW, Jr. Vasopressin and cardiovascular regulation. *Int Rev Physiol* 1982;26:189.

168. Verbalis JG. Hyponatremia induced by vasopressin or desmopressin in female and male rats. *J Am Soc Nephrol* 1993;3:1600.

169. Goldman MB, Luchins DJ, Robertson GL. Mechanisms of altered water metabolism in psychotic patients with polydipsia and hyponatremia. *N Engl J Med* 1988;318:397.

170. Saito T, Ishikawa SE, Ando F, et al. Exaggerated urinary excretion of aquaporin-2 in the pathological state of impaired water excretion dependent upon arginine vasopressin. *J Clin Endocrinol Metab* 1998; 83:4034.

171. Robertson GL, Aycinena P, Zerbe RL. Neurogenic disorders of osmoregulation. *Am J Med* 1982;72:339.

172. Robertson GL, Athar S. The interaction of blood osmolality and blood volume in regulating plasma vasopressin in man. *J Clin Endocrinol Metab* 1976;42:613.

173. Robertson GL. The regulation of vasopressin function in health and disease. *Rec Prog Horm Res* 1976;33:333.

174. Kortas C, Bichet DG, Rouleau JL, et al. Vasopressin in congestive heart failure. *J Cardiovasc Pharmacol* 1986;8[Suppl. 7]:S107.

175. Verbalis JG, Baldwin EF, Robinson AG. Osmotic regulation of plasma vasopressin and oxytocin after sustained hyponatremia. *Am J Physiol* 1986;250:R444.

176. Verbalis JG, Dohanics J. Vasopressin and oxytocin secretion in chronically hypoosmolar rats. *Am J Physiol* 1991;261:R1028.

177. Lindheimer MD, Davison JM. Osmoregulation, the secretion of arginine vasopressin and its metabolism during pregnancy. *Eur J Endocrinol* 1995;132:133.

178. Weisinger RS, Burns P, Eddie LW, et al. Relaxin alters the plasma osmolality-arginine vasopressin relationship in the rat. *J Endocrinol* 1993;137:505.

179. Wilson BC, Summerlee AJ. Effects of exogenous relaxin on oxytocin and vasopressin release and the intramammary pressure response to central hyperosmotic challenge. *J Endocrinol* 1994;141:75.

180. Wall BM, Crofton JT, Share L, et al. Chronic hyponatremia due to resetting of the osmostat in a patient with gastric carcinoma. *Am J Med* 1992;93:223.

181. Kamoi K. Syndrome of inappropriate antidiuresis without involving inappropriate secretion of vasopressin in an elderly woman: effect of intravenous administration of the nonpeptide vasopressin V2 receptor antagonist opc-31260. *Nephron* 1997;76:111.

182. Kavanaugh BD, Halperin EC, Rosenbaum LC, et al. Syndrome of inappropriate secretion of antidiuretic hormone in a patient with carcinoma of the nasopharynx. *Cancer* 1992;69:1315.

183. Verbalis JG. Osmotic inhibition of neurohypophysial secretion. *Ann N Y Acad Sci* 1993;689:146.

184. Dohanics J, Verbalis JG. Naloxone disinhibits magnocellular responses to osmotic and volemic stimuli in chronically hypoosmolar rats. *J Neuroendocrinol* 1995;7:57.

185. Nissen R, Renaud LP. GABA receptor mediation of median preoptic nucleus-evoked inhibition of supraoptic neurosecretory neurones in the rat. *J Physiol* 1994;479:207.

186. Helderman JH, Vestal RE, Rowe JW, et al. The response of arginine vasopressin to intravenous ethanol and hypertonic saline in man: the impact of aging. *J Gerontol* 1978;33:39.

187. Rowe JW, Minaker KL, Sparrow D, et al. Age-related failure of volume-pressure-mediated vasopressin release. *J Clin Endocrinol Metab* 1982;54:661.

188. Manoogian C, Pandian M, Ehrlich L, et al. Plasma atrial natriuretic hormone levels in patients with the syndrome of inappropriate antidiuretic hormone secretion. *J Clin Endocrinol Metab* 1988;67: 571.

189. Peters JP, Welt KG, Sims EAH, et al. A salt-wasting syndrome associated with cerebral disease. *Trans Assoc Am Physiol* 1950;63:57.

190. Doczi T, Tarjanyi J, Huszka E, et al. Syndrome of inappropriate secretion of antidiuretic hormone (SIADH) after head injury. *Neurosurgery* 1982;10:685.

191. Nelson PB, Seif S, Gutai J, et al. Hyponatremia and natriuresis following subarachnoid hemorrhage in a monkey model. *J Neurosurg* 1984;60:233.

192. Wijdicks EF, Vermeulen M, Hijdra A, et al. Hyponatremia and cerebral infarction in patients with ruptured intracranial aneurysms: is fluid restriction harmful? *Ann Neurol* 1985;17:137.

193. Wijdicks EF, Ropper AH, Hunnicutt EJ, et al. Atrial natriuretic factor and salt wasting after aneurysmal subarachnoid hemorrhage. *Stroke* 1991;22:1519.

194. Diringer MN, Lim JS, Kirsch JR, et al. Suprasellar and intraventricular blood predict elevated plasma atrial natriuretic factor in subarachnoid hemorrhage. *Stroke* 1991;22:577.

195. Oh MS, Carroll HJ. Cerebral salt-wasting syndrome: we need better proof of its existence. *Nephron* 1999;82:110.

196. Maesaka JK, Gupta S, Fishbane S. Cerebral salt-wasting syndrome: does it exist? *Nephron* 1999;82:100.

197. Weinand ME, O'Boynick PL, Goetz KL. A study of serum antidiuretic hormone and atrial natriuretic peptide levels in a series of patients with intracranial disease and hyponatremia. *Neurosurgery* 1989;25: 781.

198. Diringer MN, Wu KC, Verbalis JG, et al. Hypervolemic therapy prevents volume contraction but not hyponatremia following subarachnoid hemorrhage. *Ann Neurol* 1992;31:543.

199. Mori T, Katayama Y, Kawamata T, et al. Improved efficiency of hypervolemic therapy with inhibition of natriuresis by fludrocortisone in patients with aneurysmal subarachnoid hemorrhage. *J Neurosurg* 1999;91:947.

200. Ishikawa S, Fujita N, Fujisawa G, et al. Involvement of arginine vasopressin and renal sodium handling in pathogenesis of hyponatremia in elderly patients. *Endocr J* 1996;43:101.

201. Kamoi K, Ebe T, Hasegawa A, et al. Hyponatremia in small cell lung cancer: mechanisms not involving inappropriate ADH secretion. *Cancer* 1987;60:1089.

202. Gross AJ, Steinberg SM, Reilly JG, et al. Atrial natriuretic factor and arginine vasopressin production in tumor cell lines from patients with lung cancer and their relationship to serum sodium. *Cancer Res* 1993;53:67.

203. Shimizu K, Nakano S, Nakano Y, et al. Ectopic atrial natriuretic peptide production in small cell lung cancer with the syndrome of inappropriate antidiuretic hormone secretion. *Cancer* 1991;68:2284.

204. Bliss DP Jr, Battey JF, Linnoila RI, et al. Expression of the atrial natriuretic factor gene in small cell lung cancer tumors and tumor cell lines. *J Natl Cancer Inst* 1990;82:305.

205. Johnson BE, Chute JP, Rushin J, et al. A prospective study of patients with lung cancer and hyponatremia of malignancy. *Am J Respir Crit Care Med* 1997;156:1669.

206. Thorn GW. *The diagnosis and treatment of adrenal insufficiency.* Springfield, IL: Charles C Thomas, 1951.

207. Knowlton AI. Addison's disease: a review of its clinical course and management. In: Christy NP, ed. *The human adrenal cortex.* New York: Harper & Row, 1971:329.

208. Nerup J. Addison's disease: clinical studies. *Acta Endocrinol (Copenh)* 1974;76:127.

209. Robinson AG, DeRubertis FR. Disorders of sodium and water balance associated with adrenal, thyroid, and pituitary disease. In: Schrier RW, Gottschalk CW, eds. *Diseases of the kidney,* 5th ed. Boston: Little, Brown, 1993:2539.

210. Loeb RF, Atchley DW, Benedict EM. Electrolyte balance studies in adrenalectomized dogs with particular reference to excretion of sodium. *J Exp Med* 1933;57:775.

211. Harrop GA, Soffer LJ, Ellsworth R. Studies on the suprarenal cortex: III. plasma electrolytes and electrolyte excretion during suprarenal insufficiency in the dog. *J Exp Med* 1933;58:17.

212. Gill JR Jr, Gann DS, Bartter FC. Restoration of water diuresis in addisonian patients by expansion of the volume of the extracellular fluid. *J Clin Invest* 1962;41:1078.

213. Share L, Travis RH. Plasma vasopressin concentration in the adrenally insufficient dog. *Endocrinology* 1970;86:196.

214. Seif SM, Robinson AG, Zimmerman EA, et al. Plasma neurophysin and vasopressin in the rat: response to adrenalectomy and steroid replacement. *Endocrinology* 1978;103:1009.

215. Boykin J, DeTorrente A, Robertson GL, et al. Persistent plasma vasopressin levels in the hypoosmolar state associated with mineralocorticoid deficiency. *Miner Electrolyte Metab* 1979;2:310.

216. Ishikawa S, Schrier RW. Effect of arginine vasopressin antagonist on renal water excretion in glucocorticoid and mineralocorticoid deficient rats. *Kidney Int* 1982;22:587.

217. Green HH, Harrington AR, Valtin H. On the role of antidiuretic hormone in the inhibition of acute water diuresis in adrenal insufficiency and the effects of gluco- and mineralocorticoids in reversing the inhibition. *J Clin Invest* 1970;49:1724.

218. Cutler RE, Kleeman CR, Koplowitz J, et al. Mechanisms of impaired water excretion in adrenal and pituitary insufficiency: III. the effect of extracellular or plasma volume expansion, or both, on the impaired diuresis. *J Clin Invest* 1962;41:1524.

219. Ufferman RC, Schrier RW. Importance of sodium intake and mineralocorticoid hormone in the impaired water excretion in adrenal insufficiency. *J Clin Invest* 1972;51:1639.

220. Richter CP. Experimental diabetes insipidus: its relation to the anterior and posterior lobes of the hypophysis. *Am J Physiol* 1934;110:439.

221. Ikkos D, Luft R, Olivecrona H. Hypophysectomy in man: effect on water excretion during the first two postoperative months. *J Clin Endocrinol Metab* 1955;15:553.

222. Bethune JE, Nelson DH. Hyponatremia in hypopituitarism. *N Engl J Med* 1965;272:771.

223. Davis BB, Bloom ME, Field JB, et al. Hyponatremia in pituitary insufficiency. *Metab Clin Exp* 1969;18:821.

224. Stacpoole PW, Interlandi JW, Nicholson WE. Isolated ACTH deficiency: a heterogeneous disorder. *Medicine (Baltimore)* 1982;61:13.

225. Mandell IN, DeFronzo RA, Robertson GL, et al. Role of plasma arginine vasopressin in the impaired water diuresis of isolated glucocorticoid deficiency in the rat. *Kidney Int* 1980;17:186.

226. Boykin J, DeTorrente A, Erickson A, et al. Role of plasma vasopressin in impaired water excretion of glucocorticoid deficiency. *J Clin Invest* 1978;62:738.

227. Linas SL, Berl T, Robertson GL, et al. Role of vasopressin in the impaired water excretion of glucocorticoid deficiency. *Kidney Int* 1980; 18:58.

228. Schwartz MJ, Kokko JP. Urinary concentrating defect of adrenal insufficiency: permissive role of adrenal steroids on the hydroosmotic response across the rabbit cortical collecting tubule. *J Clin Invest* 1980;66:234.

229. Aubry RH, Nankin HR, Moses AM, et al. Measurement of the osmotic threshold for vasopressin release in human subjects, and its modification by cortisol. *J Clin Endocrinol Metab* 1965;25:1481.

230. Raff H. Interactions between neurohypophysial hormones and the ACTH-adrenocortical axis. *Ann N Y Acad Sci* 1993;689:411.

231. Kiss JZ, Van Eckelen AM, Reul JMHM. Glucocorticoid receptor in magnocellular neurosecretory neurons. *Endocrinology* 1988;122:444.

232. Berghorn KA, Knapp LT, Hoffman GE, et al. Induction of glucocorticoid receptor expression in hypothalamic neurons during chronic hypoosmolality. *Endocrinology* 1995;136:804.

233. Stillman MA, Recht LD, Rosario SL, et al. The effects of adrenalectomy and glucocorticoid replacement on vasopressin and vasopressin-neurophysin in the zona externa of the rat. *Endocrinology* 1977;101:42.

234. Robinson AG, Seif SM, Verbalis JG, et al. Quantitation of changes in the content of neurohypophyseal peptides in hypothalamic nuclei after adrenalectomy. *Neuroendocrinology* 1983;36:347.

235. Recht LD, Hoffman DL, Haldar J, et al. Vasopressin concentrations in hypophysial portal plasma: insignificant reduction following removal of the posterior pituitary. *Neuroendocrinology* 1981;33:88.

236. Rivier C, Vale W. Modulation of stress-induced ACTH release by corticotropin-releasing factor, catecholamines and vasopressin. *Nature* 1983;305:325.

237. Antoni FA. Hypothalamic control of adrenocorticotropin secretion: advances since the discovery of 41-residue corticotropin-releasing factor. *Endocr Rev* 1986;7:351.

238. Verbalis JG, Baldwin EF, Ronnekleiv OK, et al. In vitro release of vasopressin and oxytocin from rat median eminence tissue. *Neuroendocrinology* 1986;42:481.

239. Hanna FW, Scanlon MF. Hyponatraemia, hypothyroidism, and role of arginine-vasopressin. *Lancet* 1997;350:755.

240. Curtis RH. Hyponatremia in primary myxedema. *Ann Intern Med* 1956; 44:376.

241. Kelley JI, Sherk HH. Myxedema coma. *Ann Intern Med* 1959;50:1303.

242. Chinitz A, Turner FL. The association of primary hypothyroidism and inappropriate secretion of the antidiuretic hormone. *Arch Intern Med* 1965;116:871.

243. Larsen PR, Ingbar SH. The thyroid gland. In: Wilson JD, Foster DW, eds. *Williams textbook of endocrinology,* 8th ed. Philadelphia: WB Saunders, 1992:357.

244. LeRoith D, Broitman D, Sukenik S, et al. Isolated ACTH deficiency and primary hypothyroidism: volume-dependent elevation of antidiuretic hormone secretion in the presence of hyponatremia. *Isr J Med Sci* 1980;16:440.

245. Crispell KR, Parson W, Sprinkle PA. A cortisone-resistant abnormality in the diuretic response to ingested water in primary myxedema. *J Clin Endocrinol Metab* 1954;14:640.

246. DeRubertis FR Jr, Michelis MF, Bloom ME, et al. Impaired water excretion in myxedema. *Am J Med* 1971;51:41.

247. Skowsky WR, Kikuchi TA. The role of vasopressin in the impaired water excretion of myxedema. *Am J Med* 1978;64:613.

248. Emmanouel DS, Lindheimer MD, Karz AI. Mechanism of impaired water excretion in the hypothyroid rat. *J Clin Invest* 1974;54:926.

249. Seif SM, Robinson AG, Zenser TV, et al. Neurohypophyseal peptides in hypothyroid rats: plasma levels and kidney response. *Metabolism* 1979;28:137.

250. Corcoran AC, Page IH. Specific renal functions in hyperthyroidism and myxedema. *J Clin Endocrinol Metab* 1947;7:801.

251. Hlad CJ, Bricker NS. Renal function and I^{125} clearance in hyperthyroidism and myxedema. *J Clin Endocrinol Metab* 1954;14:1539.

252. Ford RV, Owens JC, Curd GW. Kidney function in various thyroid states. *J Clin Endocrinol Metab* 1961;21:548.

253. Davies CE, Mackinnon J, Platts MM. Renal circulation and cardiac output in "low-output" heart failure and in myxedema. *BMJ* 1952;2:595.

254. Graettinger JS, Muenster JJ, Checchia CS, et al. A correlation of clinical and hemodynamic studies in patients with hypothyroidism. *J Clin Invest* 1958;37:502.

255. Amidi M, Leon DF, DeGroot WJ. Effect of the thyroid state on myocardial contractility and ventricular ejection rate in man. *Circulation* 1968;38:229.

256. Holmes EW, DiScala VA. Studies on the exaggerated natriuretic response to a saline infusion in the hypothyroid rat. *J Clin Invest* 1970; 49:1224.

257. Michael UF, Kelley J, Alpert H, et al. Role of distal delivery of filtrate in impaired renal dilution of the hypothyroid rat. *Am J Physiol* 1976;230:699.

258. Archambeaud-Mouveroux F, Dejax C, Jadaud JM, et al. Myxedema coma with hypervasopressinism: 2 cases. *Ann Med Intern* 1987;138: 114.

259. Salomez-Granier F, Lefebvre J, Racadot A, et al. Antidiuretic hormone levels (arginine-vasopressin) in cases of peripheral hypothyroidism: 26 cases. *Presse Med* 1983;12:1001.

260. Laczi F, Janaky T, Ivanyi T, et al. Osmoregulation of arginine-8-vasopressin secretion in primary hypothyroidism and in Addison's disease. *Acta Endocrinol (Copenh)* 1987;114:389.

261. Macaron C, Famuyiwa O. Hyponatremia of hypothyroidism: appropriate suppression of antidiuretic hormone levels. *Arch Intern Med* 1978; 138:820.

262. Waters AK. Increased vasopressin excretion in patients with hypothyroidism. *Acta Endocrinol (Copenh)* 1978;88:285.

263. Iwasaki Y, Oiso Y, Yamauchi K, et al. Osmoregulation of plasma vasopressin in myxedema. *J Clin Endocrinol Metab* 1990;70:534.

264. Koide Y, Oda K, Shimizu K, et al. Hyponatremia without inappropriate secretion of vasopressin in a case of myxedema coma. *Endocrinol Jpn* 1982;29:363.

265. Hochberg Z, Benderly A. Normal osmotic threshold for vasopressin release in the hyponatremia of hypothyroidism. *Horm Res* 1983;17: 128.

266. Caron C, Plante GE, Belanger R, et al. Hypothyroid hyponatremia: dilution defect non-correctable with demeclocycline. *CMAJ* 1980;123: 1019.

267. Howard RL, Summer S, Rossi N, et al. Short-term hypothyroidism and vasopressin gene expression in the rat. *Am J Kidney Dis* 1992;19:573.

268. Kim JK, Summer SN, Schrier RW. Cellular action of arginine vasopressin in the isolated renal tubules of hypothyroid rats. *Am J Physiol* 1987;253:F104.

269. Barlow ED, DeWardner HE. Compulsive water drinking. *QJM* 1959; 28:235.

270. Dubovsky SL, Grabon S, Berl T, et al. Syndrome of inappropriate secretion of antidiuretic hormone with exacerbated psychosis. *Ann Intern Med* 1973;79:551.

271. Hariprasad MK, Eisinger RP, Nadler IM, et al. Hyponatremia in psychogenic polydipsia. *Arch Intern Med* 1980;140:1639.

272. Kramer DS, Drake ME, Jr. Acute psychosis, polydipsia, and inappropriate secretion of antidiuretic hormone. *Am J Med* 1983;75:712.

273. Vieweg WV, Rowe WT, David JJ, et al. Evaluation of patients with self-induced water intoxication and schizophrenic disorders (SIWIS). *J Nerv Ment Dis* 1984;172:552.

274. Pavalonis D, Shutty M, Hundley P, et al. Behavioral intervention to reduce water intake in the syndrome of psychosis, intermittent hyponatremia, and polydipsia. *J Behav Ther Exp Psychiatry* 1992;23:51.

275. de Leon J, Verghese C, Tracy JI, et al. Polydipsia and water intoxication in psychiatric patients: a review of the epidemiological literature. *Biol Psychiatry* 1994;35:408.

276. Leadbetter RA, Shutty MS Jr, Higgins PB, et al. Multidisciplinary approach to psychosis, intermittent hyponatremia, and polydipsia. *Schizophr Bull* 1994;20:375.

277. Vieweg WV, Robertson GL, Godleski LS, et al. Diurnal variation in water homeostasis among schizophrenic patients subject to water intoxication. *Schizophr Res* 1988;1:351.

278. Gleadhill IC, Smith TA, Yium JJ. Hyponatremia in patients with schizophrenia. *South Med J* 1982;75:426.

279. Ohsawa H, Kishimoto T, Hirai M, et al. An epidemiological study on hyponatremia in psychiatric patients in mental hospitals in Nara Prefecture. *Jpn J Psychiatry Neurol* 1992;46:883.

280. Stuart CA, Neelon FA, Lebovitz HE. Disordered control of thirst in hypothalamic-pituitary sarcoidosis. *N Engl J Med* 1980;303:1078.

281. Kushnir M, Schattner A, Ezri T, et al. Schizophrenia and fatal self-induced water intoxication with appropriately-diluted urine. *Am J Med Sci* 1990;300:385.

282. Mendelson WB, Deza PC. Polydipsia, hyponatremia, and seizures in psychotic patients. *J Nerv Ment Dis* 1976;162:140.

283. Vieweg WV, Carey RM, Godleski LS, et al. The syndrome of psychosis, intermittent hyponatremia, and polydipsia: evidence for diurnal volume expansion. *Psychiatr Med* 1990;8:135.

284. Bouget J, Thomas R, Camus C, et al. Water intoxication in psychiatric patients: 13 cases of severe hyponatremia. *Rev Med Intern* 1989;10:515.

285. Cheng JC, Zikos D, Skopicki HA, et al. Long-term neurologic outcome in psychogenic water drinkers with severe symptomatic hyponatremia: the effect of rapid correction. *Am J Med* 1990;88:561.

286. Rosenbaum JF, Rothman JS, Murray GB. Psychosis and water intoxication. *J Clin Psychiatry* 1979;40:287.

287. Delva NJ, Crammer JL, Lawson JS, et al. Vasopressin in chronic psychiatric patients with primary polydipsia. *Br J Psychiatry* 1990;157:703.

288. Emsley R, Potgieter A, Taljaard F, et al. Water excretion and plasma vasopressin in psychotic disorders. *Am J Psychiatry* 1989;146:250.

289. Levine S, McManus BM, Blackbourne BD, et al. Fatal water intoxication, schizophrenia and diuretic therapy for systemic hypertension. *Am J Med* 1987;82:153.

290. Shah PJ, Greenberg WM. Water intoxication precipitated by thiazide diuretics in polydipsic psychiatric patients. *Am J Psychiatry* 1991;148:1424.

291. Kimelman N, Albert SG. Phenothiazine-induced hyponatremia in the elderly. *Gerontology* 1984;30:132.

292. Gossain VV, Hagen GA, Sugawara M. Drug-induced hyponatraemia in psychogenic polydipsia. *Postgrad Med J* 1976;52:720.

293. Tildesley HD, Toth E, Crockford PM. Syndrome of inappropriate secretion of antidiuretic hormone in association with chlorpromazine ingestion. *Can J Psychiatry* 1983;28:487.

294. Kastner T, Friedman DL, Pond WS. Carbamazepine-induced hyponatremia in patients with mental retardation. *Am J Ment Retard* 1992;96:536.

295. Blum A. The possible role of tobacco cigarette smoking in hyponatremia of long-term psychiatric patients. *JAMA* 1984;252:2864.

296. Allon M, Allen HM, Deck LV, et al. Role of cigarette use in hyponatremia in schizophrenic patients. *Am J Psychiatry* 1990;147:1075.

297. Lever EG, Stansfeld SA. Addison's disease, psychosis, and the syndrome of inappropriate secretion of antidiuretic hormone. *Br J Psychiatry* 1983;143:406.

298. Goldman MB, Robertson GL, Luchins DJ, et al. Psychotic exacerbations and enhanced vasopressin secretion in schizophrenic patients with hyponatremia and polydipsia. *Arch Gen Psychiatry* 1997;54:443.

299. Holmes JH. Thirst and fluid intake problems in clinical medicine. In: Wayner MJ, eds. *Thirst.* Oxford: Pergamon Press, 1964:57.

300. de Castro J. A microregulatory analysis of spontaneous fluid intake in humans: evidence that the amount of liquid ingested and its timing is mainly governed by feeding. *Physiol Behav* 1988;3:705.

301. Szczepanska-Sadowska E, Sobocinska J, Sadowski B. Central dipsogenic effect of vasopressin. *Am J Physiol* 1982;242:R372.

302. Ernits T, Corbit JD. Taste as a dipsogenic stimulus. *J Comp Physiol Psychol* 1973;83:27.

303. Verbalis JG. An experimental model of syndrome of inappropriate antidiuretic hormone secretion in the rat. *Am J Physiol* 1984;247:E540.

304. Stricker EM, Adair ER. Body fluid balance, taste, and postprandial factors in schedule-induced polydipsia. *J Comp Physiol Psychol* 1966;62:449.

305. Verbalis JG. Inhibitory controls of drinking. In: Ramsay DJ, Booth DA, eds. *Thirst: physiology and psychological aspects.* London: Springer-Verlag, 1991:313.

306. Browne PM. Rhabdomyolysis and myoglobinuria associated with acute water intoxication. *West J Med* 1979;130:459.

307. Mitnick PD, Bell S. Rhabdomyolysis associated with severe hyponatremia after prostatic surgery. *Am J Kidney Dis* 1990;16:73.

308. Tomiyama J, Kametani H, Kumagai Y, et al. Water intoxication and rhabdomyolysis. *Jpn J Med* 1990;29:52.

309. Putterman C, Levy L, Rubinger D. Transient exercise-induced water intoxication and rhabdomyolysis. *Am J Kidney Dis* 1993;21:206.

310. Trimarchi H, Gonzalez J, Olivero J. Hyponatremia-associated rhabdomyolysis. *Nephron* 1999;82:274.

311. Daggett P, Deanfield J, Moss F. Neurological aspects of hyponatraemia. *Postgrad Med J* 1982;58:737.

312. Arieff AI. Central nervous system manifestations of disordered sodium metabolism. *Clin Endocrinol Metab* 1984;13:269.

313. Fraser CL, Arieff AI. Epidemiology, pathophysiology, and management of hyponatremic encephalopathy. *Am J Med* 1997;102:67.

314. Adrogue HJ, Madias NE. Hyponatremia. *N Engl J Med* 2000;342:1581.

315. Kleeman CR. The kidney in health and disease: X. CNS manifestations of disordered salt and water balance. *Hosp Pract* 1979;14:59.

316. Ayus JC, Wheeler JM, Arieff AI. Postoperative hyponatremic encephalopathy in menstruant women. *Ann Intern Med* 1992;117:891.

317. Wijdicks EF, Sharbrough FW. New-onset seizures in critically ill patients. *Neurology* 1993;43:1042.

318. Vexler ZS, Ayus JC, Roberts TP, et al. Hypoxic and ischemic hypoxia exacerbate brain injury associated with metabolic encephalopathy in laboratory animals. *J Clin Invest* 1994;93:256.

319. Ayus JC, Arieff AI. Pulmonary complications of hyponatremic encephalopathy: noncardiogenic pulmonary edema and hypercapnic respiratory failure [see comments]. *Chest* 1995;107:517.

320. Ayus JC, Varon J, Arieff AI. Hyponatremia, cerebral edema, and noncardiogenic pulmonary edema in marathon runners. *Ann Intern Med* 2000;132:711.

321. Arieff AI, Ayus JC, Fraser CL. Hyponatraemia and death or permanent brain damage in healthy children. *BMJ* 1992;304:1218.

322. Wattad A, Chiang ML, Hill LL. Hyponatremia in hospitalized children. *Clin Pediatr* 1992;31:153.

323. Wijdicks EF, Larson TS. Absence of postoperative hyponatremia syndrome in young, healthy females. *Ann Neurol* 1994;35:626.

324. Lindholm J, Kehlet H, Blichert-Toft M, et al. Reliability of the 30-minute ACTH test in assessing hypothalamic-pituitary-adrenal function. *J Clin Endocrinol Metab* 1978;47:272.

325. May ME, Carey RM. Rapid adrenocorticotropic hormone test in practice. *Am J Med* 1985;79:679.

326. Karp BI, Laureno R. Pontine and extrapontine myelinolysis: a neurologic disorder following rapid correction of hyponatremia. *Medicine (Baltimore)* 1993;72:359.

327. Tomlinson BE, Pierides AM, Bradley WG. Central pontine myelinolysis: two cases with associated electrolyte disturbance. *QJM* 1976;45:373.

328. Burcar PJ, Norenberg MD, Yarnell PR. Hyponatremia and central pontine myelinolysis. *Neurology* 1977;27:223.

329. Wright DG, Laureno R, Victor M. Pontine and extrapontine myelinolysis. *Brain* 1979;102:361.

330. Kleinschmidt-DeMasters BK, Norenberg MD. Rapid correction of hyponatremia causes demyelination: relation to central pontine myelinolysis. *Science* 1981;211:1068.

331. Laureno R. Central pontine myelinolysis following rapid correction of hyponatremia. *Ann Neurol* 1983;13:232.

332. Sterns RH, Thomas DJ, Herndon RM. Brain dehydration and neurologic deterioration after rapid correction of hyponatremia. *Kidney Int* 1989;35:69.

333. Ayus JC, Krothapalli RK, Armstrong DL, et al. Symptomatic hyponatremia in rats: effect of treatment on mortality and brain lesions. *Am J Physiol* 1989;257:F18.

334. Verbalis JG, Martinez AJ. Neurological and neuropathological sequelae of correction of chronic hyponatremia. *Kidney Int* 1991;39:1274.

335. Norenberg MD, Leslie KO, Robertson AS. Association between rise in serum sodium and central pontine myelinolysis. *Ann Neurol* 1982;11:128.

336. Cserr H, DePasquale M, Patlak CS. Regulation of brain water and electrolytes during acute hyperosmolality. *Am J Physiol* 1987;253:F522.

337. Adler S, Verbalis JG, Williams D. Effect of rapid correction of hyponatremia on the blood brain barrier of rats. *Brain Res* 1995;679:135.

338. Adler S, Martinez J, Williams DS, et al. Positive association between blood brain barrier disruption and osmotically-induced demyelination. *Mult Scler* 2000;6:24.

339. Baker EA, Tian Y, Adler S, et al. Blood-brain barrier disruption and complement activation in the brain following rapid correction of chronic hyponatremia. *Exp Neurol* 2000;165:221.

340. Ayus JC, Krothapalli RK, Arieff AI. Treatment of symptomatic hyponatremia and its relation to brain damage: a prospective study. *N Engl J Med* 1987;317:1190.

341. Sterns RH. The management of symptomatic hyponatremia. *Semin Nephrol* 1990;10:503.

342. Kumar S, Berl T. Sodium. *Lancet* 1998;352:220.

343. Soupart A, Penninckx R, Stenuit A, et al. Treatment of chronic hyponatremia in rats by intravenous saline: comparison of rate versus magnitude of correction. *Kidney Int* 1992;41:1662.

344. Sterns RH, Cappuccio JD, Silver SM, et al. Neurologic sequelae after treatment of severe hyponatremia: a multicenter perspective. *J Am Soc Nephrol* 1994;4:1522.

345. Verbalis JG. Hyponatremia: endocrinologic causes and consequences of therapy. *Trends Endocrinol Metab* 1992;3:1.

346. Ellis SJ. Extrapontine myelinolysis after correction of chronic hyponatraemia with isotonic saline. *Br J Clin Pract* 1995;49:49.

347. Lohr JW. Osmotic demyelination syndrome following correction of hyponatremia: association with hypokalemia. *Am J Med* 1994;96:408.

348. Adams RD, Victor M, Mancall EL. Central pontine myelinolysis: a hitherto undescribed disease occurring in alcoholic and malnourished patients. *Arch Neurol Psychiatry* 1959;81:154.

349. Kelly J, Wassif W, Mitchard J, et al. Severe hyponatraemia secondary to beer potomania complicated by central pontine myelinolysis. *Int J Clin Pract* 1998;52:585.

350. Loo CS, Lim TO, Fan KS, et al. Pontine myelinolysis following correction of hyponatraemia. *Med J Malaysia* 1995;50:180.

351. Soupart A, Penninckx R, Stenuit A, et al. Azotemia (48 h) decreases the risk of brain damage in rats after correction of chronic hyponatremia. *Brain Res* 2000;852:167.

352. Price BH, Mesulam MM. Behavioral manifestations of central pontine myelinolysis. *Arch Neurol* 1987;44:671.

353. Vermetten E, Rutten SJ, Boon PJ, et al. Neuropsychiatric and neuropsychological manifestations of central pontine myelinolysis. *Gen Hosp Psychiatry* 1999;21:296.

354. Maraganore DM, Folger WN, Swanson JW, et al. Movement disorders as sequelae of central pontine myelinolysis: report of three cases. *Move Disord* 1992;7:142.

355. Sullivan AA, Chervin RD, Albin RL. Parkinsonism after correction of hyponatremia with radiological central pontine myelinolysis and changes in the basal ganglia. *J Clin Neurosci* 2000;7:256.

356. Brunner JE, Redmond JM, Haggar AM, et al. Central pontine myelinolysis after rapid correction of hyponatremia: a magnetic resonance imaging study. *Ann Neurol* 1988;23:389.

357. Brunner JE, Redmond JM, Haggar AM, et al. Central pontine myelinolysis and pontine lesions after rapid correction of hyponatremia: a prospective magnetic resonance imaging study. *Ann Neurol* 1990;27:61.

358. Kumar SR, Mone AP, Gray LC, et al. Central pontine myelinolysis: delayed changes on neuroimaging. *J Neuroimaging* 2000;10:169.

359. Miller GM, Baker HL, Jr., Okazaki H, et al. Central pontine myelinolysis and its imitators: MR findings. *Radiology* 1988;168:795.

360. Soupart A, Penninckx R, Namias B, et al. Brain myelinolysis following hypernatremia in rats. *J Neuropathol Exp Neurol* 1997;55:106.

361. McComb RD, Pfeiffer RF, Casey JH, et al. Lateral pontine and extrapontine myelinolysis associated with hypernatremia and hyperglycemia. *Clin Neuropathol* 1989;8:284.

362. Ayus JC, Olivero JJ, Frommer JP. Rapid correction of severe hyponatremia with intravenous hypertonic saline solution. *Am J Med* 1982;72:43.

363. Verbalis JG. Adaptation to acute and chronic hyponatremia: implications for symptomatology, diagnosis, and therapy. *Semin Nephrol* 1998;18:3.

364. Ayus JC, Arieff AI. Brain damage and postoperative hyponatremia: the role of gender. *Neurology* 1996;46:323.

365. Lane N, Allen K. Hyponatraemia after orthopaedic surgery [Editorial; see comments]. *BMJ* 1999;318:1363.

366. Paut O, Remond C, Lagier P, et al. Severe hyponatremic encephalopathy after pediatric surgery: report of seven cases and recommendations for management and prevention [in French]. *Ann Fr Anesth Reanim* 2000;19:467.

367. Steele A, Gowrishankar M, Abrahamson S, et al. Postoperative hyponatremia despite near-isotonic saline infusion: a phenomenon of desalination [see comments]. *Ann Intern Med* 1997;126:20.

368. Verbalis JG. Inappropriate antidiuresis and other hypoosmolar states. In: Becker KL, ed. *Principles and practice of endocrinology and metabolism,* 3rd ed. Philadelphia: JB Lippincott, 2001:293.

369. Ayus JC, Arieff AI. Chronic hyponatremic encephalopathy in postmenopausal women: association of therapies with morbidity and mortality [see comments]. *JAMA* 1999;281:2299.

370. Sterns RH. Severe hyponatremia: the case for conservative management. *Crit Care Med* 1992;20:534.

371. Sterns RH, Ocdol H, Schrier RW et al. Hyponatremia: pathophysiology, diagnosis, and therapy. In: Narins RG, ed. *Disorders of fluid and electrolytes,* 5th ed. New York: McGraw-Hill, 1994:583.

372. Hantman D, Rossier B, Zohlman R, et al. Rapid correction of hyponatremia in the syndrome of inappropriate secretion of antidiuretic hormone: an alternative treatment to hypertonic saline. *Ann Intern Med* 1973;78:870.

373. Tanneau R, Garre M, Pennec YL, et al. Brain damage and spontaneous correction of hyponatremia. *Lancet* 1988;2:1031.

374. Tanneau RS, Henry A, Rouhart F, et al. High incidence of neurologic complications following rapid correction of severe hyponatremia in polydipsic patients. *J Clin Psychiatry* 1994;55:349.

375. Goldszmidt MA, Iliescu EA. DDAVP to prevent rapid correction in hyponatremia. *Clin Nephrol* 2000;53:226.

376. Soupart A, Penninckx R, Crenier L, et al. Prevention of brain demyelination in rats after excessive correction of chronic hyponatremia by serum sodium lowering. *Kidney Int* 1994;45:193.

377. Soupart A, Penninckx R, Stenuit A, et al. Reinduction of hyponatremia improves survival in rats with myelinolysis-related neurologic symptoms. *J Neuropathol Exp Neurol* 1996;55:594.

378. Soupart A, Ngassa M, Decaux G. Therapeutic relowering of the serum sodium in a patient after excessive correction of hyponatremia. *Clin Nephrol* 1999;51:383.

379. Robertson GL. Abnormalities of thirst regulation. *Kidney Int* 1984;25:460.

380. Gupta S, Baker P. Clozapine treatment of polydipsia. *Ann Clin Psychiatry* 1994;6:135.

381. de Leon J, Verghese C, Stanilla JK, et al. Treatment of polydipsia and hyponatremia in psychiatric patients. Can clozapine be a new option? *Neuropsychopharmacology* 1995;12:133.

382. Fuller MA, Jurjus G, Kwon K, et al. Clozapine reduces water-drinking behavior in schizophrenic patients with polydipsia. *J Clin Psychopharmacol* 1996;16:329.

383. Spears NM, Leadbetter RA, Shutty MS, Jr. Clozapine treatment in polydipsia and intermittent hyponatremia. *J Clin Psychiatry* 1996;57:123.

384. Canuso CM, Goldman MB. Clozapine restores water balance in schizophrenic patients with polydipsia-hyponatremia syndrome. *J Neuropsychiatry Clin Neurosci* 1999;11:86.

385. Cherrill DA, Stote RM, Birge JR, et al. Demeclocycline treatment in the syndrome of inappropriate antidiuretic hormone secretion. *Ann Intern Med* 1975;83:654.

386. de Troyer A. Demeclocycline: treatment for syndrome of inappropriate antidiuretic hormone secretion. *JAMA* 1977;237:2723.

387. Dousa TP, Wilson DM. Effect of demethylchlortetracycline on cellular action of antidiuretic hormone in vitro. *Kidney Int* 1974;5:279.

388. Miller PD, Linas SL, Schrier RW. Plasma demeclocycline levels and nephrotoxicity: correlation in hyponatremic cirrhotic patients. *JAMA* 1980;243:2513.

389. Forrest JN Jr, Cox M, Hong C, et al. Superiority of demeclocycline over lithium in the treatment of chronic syndrome of inappropriate secretion of antidiuretic hormone. *N Engl J Med* 1978;298:173.

390. Decaux G, Genette F. Urea for long-term treatment of syndrome of inappropriate secretion of antidiuretic hormone. *BMJ* 1981;283:1081.
391. Decaux G, Unger J, Brimioulle S, et al. Hyponatremia in the syndrome of inappropriate secretion of antidiuretic hormone: rapid correction with urea, sodium chloride, and water restriction therapy. *JAMA* 1982;247:471.
392. Decaux G, Mols P, Cauchi P, et al. Use of urea for treatment of water retention in hyponatraemic cirrhosis with ascites resistant to diuretics. *BMJ* 1985;290:1782.
393. Cauchie P, Vincken W, Decaux G. Urea treatment for water retention in hyponatremic congestive heart failure. *Int J Cardiol* 1987;17:102.
394. Brooks DP, Valente M, Petrone G, et al. Comparison of the water diuretic activity of kappa receptor agonists and a vasopressin receptor antagonist in dogs. *J Pharmacol Exp Ther* 1997;280:1176.
395. Bosch-Marce M, Poo JL, Jimenez W, et al. Comparison of two aquaretic drugs (niravoline and OPC-31260) in cirrhotic rats with ascites and water retention. *J Pharmacol Exp Ther* 1999;289:194.
396. Gadano A, Moreau R, Pessione F, et al. Aquaretic effects of niravoline, a kappa-opioid agonist, in patients with cirrhosis. *J Hepatol* 2000;32:38.
397. Schrier RW. New treatments for hyponatremia. *N Engl J Med* 1978;298:214.
398. Kinter LB, Ileson BE, Caltabinol S et al. Antidiuretic hormone antagonism in humans: are there predictors? In: Jard S, Jamison R, eds. *Vasopressin.* Paris: John Libbey Eurotext, 1991:321.
399. Serradeil-Le Gal C, Lacour C, Valette G, et al. Characterization of SR 121463A, a highly potent and selective, orally active vasopressin V2 receptor antagonist. *J Clin Invest* 1996;98:2729.
400. Tahara A, Tomura Y, Wada KI, et al. Pharmacological profile of YM087, a novel potent nonpeptide vasopressin V1A and V2 receptor antagonist, in vitro and in vivo. *J Pharmacol Exp Ther* 1997;282:301.
401. Saito T, Ishikawa S, Abe K, et al. Acute aquaresis by the nonpeptide arginine vasopressin (AVP) antagonist OPC-31260 improves hyponatremia in patients with syndrome of inappropriate secretion of antidiuretic hormone (SIADH). *J Clin Endocrinol Metab* 1997;82:1054.
402. Yamamura Y, Ogawa H, Chihara T, et al. OPC-21268, an orally effective, nonpeptide vasopressin V1 receptor antagonist. *Science* 1991; 252:572.
403. Verbalis JG, Martinez AJ. Determinants of brain myelinolysis following correction of chronic hyponatremia in rats. In: Jamison RL, Jard S, eds. *Vasopressin.* Paris: John Libbey Eurotext, 1991:539.
404. Robertson GL. Thirst and vasopressin function in normal and disordered states of water balance. *J Lab Clin Med* 1983;101:351.

CHAPTER 86

Nephrogenic and Central Diabetes Insipidus

Daniel G. Bichet

Diabetes insipidus is a disorder characterized by the excretion of abnormally large volumes (greater than 30 mL/kg body weight/day for an adult patient) of dilute urine (less than 250 mmol/kg). Four basic defects can be involved. The most common, a deficient secretion of the antidiuretic hormone (ADH) arginine vasopressin (AVP), is referred to as neurogenic (or central, neurohypophyseal, cranial, or hypothalamic) diabetes insipidus. Diabetes insipidus can also result from renal insensitivity to the antidiuretic effect of AVP, which is referred to as nephrogenic diabetes insipidus. Excessive water intake can result in polyuria, which is referred to as primary polydipsia: it can be due to an abnormality in the thirst mechanism, referred to as dipsogenic diabetes insipidus; or it can be associated with a severe emotional cognitive dysfunction, referred to as psychogenic polydipsia. Finally, increased metabolism of vasopressin during pregnancy is referred to as gestational diabetes insipidus.

ARGININE VASOPRESSIN

Synthesis

The ADH in humans is AVP, a cyclic nonapeptide. AVP and its corresponding carrier, neurophysin II (NPII), are synthesized as a composite precursor by the magnocellular neurons of the supraoptic and paraventricular nuclei of the hypothalamus (1). The precursor is packaged into neurosecretory granules and transported axonally in the stalk of the posterior pituitary. On route to the neurohypophysis, the precursor is processed into the active hormone. Prepro-vasopressin has 164 amino acids and is encoded by the 2.5-kb *prepro-AVP-NPII* gene located in chromosome region 20p13 (2). Exon 1 of the *prepro-AVP-NPII* gene encodes the signal peptide, AVP, and the NH_2-terminal region of NPII. Exon 2 encodes the central region of NPII, and exon 3 encodes the COOH-terminal region of NPII and the glycopeptide. Provasopressin is generated by the removal of the signal peptide

from prepro-vasopressin and the addition of a carbohydrate chain to the glycopeptide. Additional posttranslation processing occurs within neurosecretory vesicles during transport of the precursor protein to axon terminals in the posterior pituitary, yielding AVP, NPII, and glycopeptide (Fig. 86-1). The AVP–NPII complex forms tetramers that can self-associate to form higher oligomers (3) (Fig. 86-2).

Immunocytochemical and radioimmunologic studies have demonstrated that oxytocin and vasopressin are synthesized in separate populations of the supraoptic nuclei and the paraventricular nuclei neurons (4,5), whose central and vascular projections have been described in great detail (6). Some cells express the *prepro-AVP-NPII* gene and other cells express the *prepro-OX-NPI* gene. Immunohistochemical studies have revealed a second vasopressin neurosecretory pathway that transports high concentrations of the hormone to the anterior pituitary gland from parvocellular neurons to the hypophyseal portal system. In the portal system, the high concentration of AVP acts synergistically with corticotropin-releasing hormone (CRH) to stimulate adrenocorticotropin hormone (ACTH) release from the anterior pituitary. More than half of parvocellular neurons coexpress both *CRH* and *prepro-AVP-NPII*. In addition, while passing through the median eminence and the hypophyseal stalk, magnocellular axons can also release AVP into the long portal system. Furthermore, a number of neuroanatomic studies have shown the existence of short portal vessels that allow communication between the posterior and anterior pituitary. Thus, in addition to parvocellular vasopressin, magnocellular vasopressin is able to influence ACTH secretion (7,8).

Osmotic and Nonosmotic Stimulation

The regulation of ADH release from the posterior pituitary is dependent primarily on two mechanisms involving the osmotic and nonosmotic pathways (9) (Fig. 86-3).

Vasopressin release can be regulated by changes in either osmolality (10) or cerebrospinal fluid (CSF) Na^+ concentration (11–14). More recently, Voisin and colleagues demonstrated coincident detection of CSF Na^+ and osmotic pressure

D. G. Bichet: Department of Medicine, Université de Montréal; and Clinical Research Unit, Hôpital du Sacré-Coeur de Montréal, Montreal, Quebec, Canada

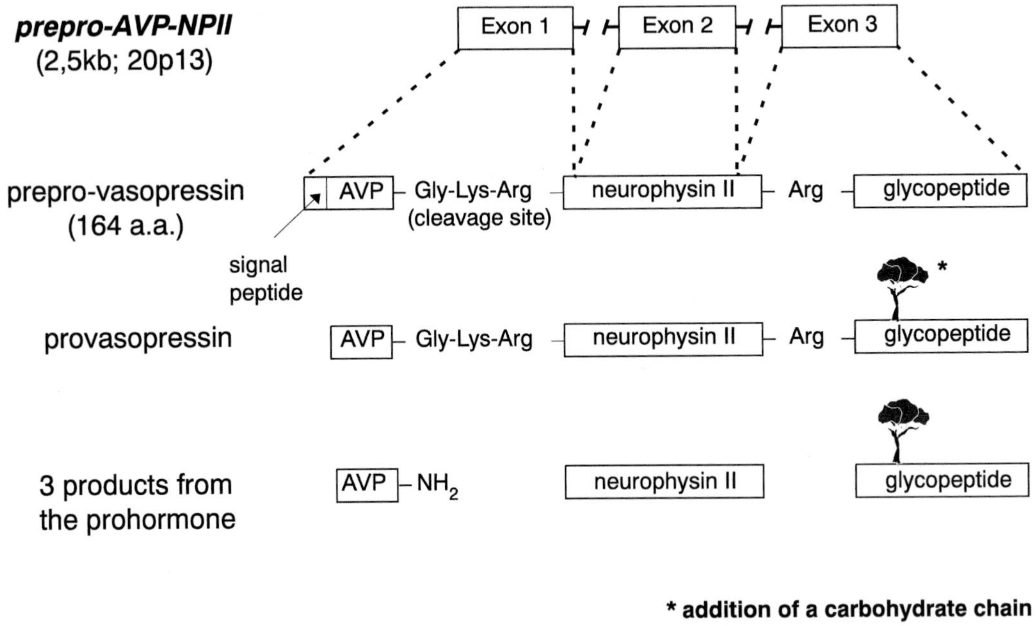

FIG. 86-1. Structure of the human vasopressin (AVP) gene and prohormone.

in magnocellular osmoregulatory neurons of the supraoptic nucleus (SON) (15).

The concept of cerebral osmoreceptors and their role in the control of vasopressin secretion derives from the classic studies of Verney (16). These osmoreceptors have been shown to respond to changes in blood osmolality of 1% or less, and all of the available evidence leads to the conclusion that they are located in the anterior part of the brain, presumably in the anterior hypothalamus.

Three criteria must be met for cells to be identified as osmoreceptive. First, increasing the osmolality of the perfusing fluid should result in an increase in firing frequency (a specific electrophysiologic property of vasopressin secreting magnocellular cells), but no response should be obtained if the osmolality is increased with solutes such as urea or glycerol, since these solutes are able to diffuse across the cell membrane. Furthermore, the osmoreceptor cells should display a sensitivity to changes in osmolality which approaches that observed *in vivo*. Second, the putative osmoreceptors must, if they are not the magnocellular neurons themselves, have neuroanatomic connections with the magnocellular neurons. Third, if the osmoreceptors are separated from the magnocellular neurons, alterations in vasopressin secretion secondary to changes in plasma osmolality should occur (17). The following candidates fulfill these criteria for osmoreceptors:

magnocellular cells which synthesize vasopressin in the SON and paraventricular nucleus (PVN);
the perinuclear zone around the SON;
cells in the subfornical organ (SFO) and organum vasculosum lamina terminalis (OVLT); and
cells in the lateral preoptic area.

Changes in excitatory synaptic drive, derived from osmosensitive neurons in the OVLT, combine with endogenously generated osmoreceptor potentials to modulate the firing rate of magnocellular cells and hence the release of AVP. The cellular basis for osmoreceptor potentials has been characterized using patch-clamp recordings and morphometric analysis in magnocellular cells isolated from the supraoptic nucleus of the adult rat (14). In these cells, stretch-inactivating cationic channels transduce osmotically evoked changes in cell volume into functionally relevant changes in membrane potential (Fig. 86-4). In addition, magnocellular neurons also operate as intrinsic Na^+ detectors (15).

A vanilloid receptor-related osmotically activated channel has been cloned and shown to be expressed in neurons of the circumventricular organs (18). However, a full biophysical characterization of this channel has not been published.

Vasopressin release can also be caused by the nonosmotic stimulation of AVP. Large decrements in blood volume or blood pressure (greater than 10%) stimulate ADH release (Fig. 86-3).

The osmotic stimulation of AVP release by dehydration, hypertonic saline infusion, or both is regularly used to determine the vasopressin secretory capacity of the posterior pituitary. This secretory capacity can be assessed *directly* by comparing the plasma AVP concentrations measured sequentially during the dehydration procedure with the normal values (19) and then correlating the plasma AVP values with the urine osmolality measurements obtained simultaneously (Fig. 86-5).

The AVP release can also be assessed *indirectly* by measuring plasma and urine osmolalities at regular intervals during the dehydration test (20). The maximal urine osmolality

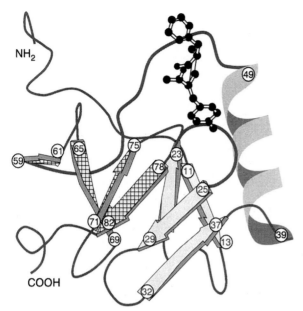

FIG. 86-2. Three-dimensional structure of a bovine peptide-neurophysin monomer complex. The structure of each chain is 12% helix and 40% β-sheet. The chain is folded into two domains as predicted by disulfide-pairing studies. The amino-terminal domain begins in a long loop (residues 1–10), then enters a four-stranded (residues 11–13, 19–23, 25–29, and 32–37) antiparallel β-sheet (sheet I; *four shaded arrows*), followed by a 3-turn 3_{10}-helix (residues 39–49) and another loop (residues 50–58). The carboxyl-terminal domain is shorter, consisting of only a four-stranded (residues 59–61, 65–69, 71–75, and 78–82) antiparallel β-sheet (sheet II; *four cross-hatched arrows*) (3). The arginine vasopressin molecule (balls and sticks model) is shown in the peptide-binding pocket of the neurophysin monomer. The strongest interactions in this binding pocket are salt-bridge interactions between the αNH_3^+ group of the peptide, the γ-COO$^-$ group of Glu^{NP47} (residue number 47 of the neurophysin molecule) and the side chain of Arg^{NP8}. The γ-COO$^-$ group of Glu^{NP47} plays a bifunctional role in the peptide-binding pocket: (a) it directly interacts with the hormone; and (b) it interacts with other neurophysin residues to establish the correct, local structure of the peptide–neurophysin complex. Arg^{NP8} and Glu^{NP47} are conserved in all neurophysin sequences from mammals to invertebrates.

obtained during dehydration is compared with the maximal urine osmolality obtained after the administration of vasopressin (Pitressin, 5 U s.c. in adults, 1 U s.c. in children) or 1-desamino-8-D-arginine vasopressin (desmopressin [d$_D$AVP], 1 to 4 μg i.v. over 5 to 10 minutes).

The nonosmotic stimulation of AVP release can be used to assess the vasopressin secretory capacity of the posterior pituitary in a rare group of patients with the essential hyponatremia and hypodipsia syndrome (21). Although some of these patients may have partial central diabetes insipidus, they respond normally to nonosmolar AVP release signals such as hypotension, emesis, and hypoglycemia (21). In all other cases of suspected central diabetes insipidus, these nonosmotic stimulation tests will not give additional clinical information (22).

Clinically Important Hormonal Influences on the Secretion of Vasopressin

Angiotensin is a well-known dipsogen and has been shown to cause drinking in all the species tested (23). Angiotensin II receptors have been described in the SFO and OVLT (reviewed in reference 24). However, knockout models for angiotensinogen (25) or for angiotensin-1A (AT1A) receptor (26,27) did not alter thirst or water balance. Disruption of the AT2 receptor only induced mild abnormalities of thirst postdehydration (28). Earlier reports suggested that the i.v. administration of atrial peptides inhibits the release of vasopressin (29), but this was not confirmed by Goetz and associates (30). Furthermore, Ogawa and coworkers (31) found no evidence that atrial natriuretic peptide, administered centrally or peripherally, was important in the physiologic regulation of plasma AVP release in conscious rats. A very rapid and robust release of AVP is seen in humans after cholecystokinin (CCK) injection (32). Nitric oxide is an inhibitory modulator of the hypothalamo-neurohypophyseal system in response to osmotic stimuli (33–36). Vasopressin secretion is under the influence of a glucocorticoid-negative feedback system (37) and the vasopressin responses to a variety of stimuli (hemorrhage, hypoxia, hypertonic saline) in normal humans and animals appear to be attenuated or eliminated by pretreatment with glucocorticoids. Finally, nausea and emesis are potent stimuli of AVP release in humans and seem to involve dopaminergic neurotransmission (38).

Cellular Actions of Vasopressin

The neurohypophyseal hormone AVP has multiple actions, including the inhibition of diuresis, contraction of smooth muscle, platelet aggregation, stimulation of liver glycogenolysis, modulation of ACTH release from the pituitary, and central regulation of somatic functions (thermoregulation, blood pressure) (39). These multiple actions of AVP could be explained by the interaction of AVP with at least three types of G protein-coupled receptors; the V_{1a} (vascular hepatic) and V_{1b} (anterior pituitary) receptors act through phosphatidylinositol hydrolysis to mobilize calcium (40), and the V_2 (kidney) receptor is coupled to adenylate cyclase (39).

The first step in the action of AVP on water excretion is its binding to AVP type 2 receptors (V_2 receptors) on the basolateral membrane of the collecting duct cells (Fig. 86-6). The human V_2 receptor gene, *AVPR2*, is located in chromosome region Xq28 and has three exons and two small introns (41,42). The sequence of the complementary DNA (cDNA) predicts a polypeptide of 371 amino acids with a structure typical of guanine nucleotide (G) protein-coupled receptors with seven transmembrane, four extracellular, and four cytoplasmic domains (43) (Fig. 86-7). The activation of the V_2 receptor on renal collecting tubules stimulates adenylate cyclase via the stimulatory G protein (G_s) and promotes the cyclic adenosine monophosphate (cAMP)-mediated incorporation of water channels (aquaporins) into the luminal

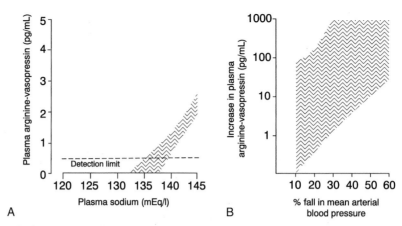

FIG. 86-3. Osmotic and nonosmotic stimulation of arginine vasopressin (AVP). **A:** The relationship between plasma AVP (P_{AVP}) and plasma sodium (P_{Na}) in 19 normal subjects is described by the area with *vertical lines*, which includes the 99% confidence limits of the regression line P_{Na}/P_{AVP}. The osmotic threshold for AVP release is about 280 to 285 mmol/kg or 136 mEq of Na/L. AVP secretion should be abolished when plasma sodium is lower than 135 mEq/L (223). **B:** Increase in plasma AVP during hypotension (*vertical lines*). Note that a large diminution in blood pressure in normal humans induces large increments in AVP. (From Vokes T, Robertson GL. Physiology of secretion of vasopressin. In: Czernichow P, Robinson AG, eds. *Diabetes insipidus in man*, Basel: S. Karger, 1985:134, with permission).

surface of these cells. This process is the molecular basis of the vasopressin-induced increase in the osmotic water permeability of the apical membrane of the collecting tubule. Aquaporin-1 (AQP1, also known as CHIP, channel-forming integral membrane protein of 28 kd) was the first protein shown to function as a molecular water channel (44) and is constitutively expressed in mammalian red cells, renal proximal tubules, thin descending limbs (45–48), and other water-permeable epithelia (47). At the subcellular level, AQP1 is localized in both apical and basolateral plasma membranes, which may represent entrance and exit routes for transep-

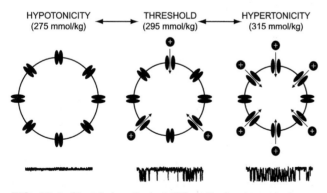

FIG. 86-4. Stretch inactivated (SI) cationic channels transduce osmoreception. Under resting osmotic conditions (**middle panel**) a portion of the SI cationic channels is active and allows the influx of positive charge (*diagram*). Hypotonic stimulation (**left**) provokes cell swelling and inhibits channel activity, thereby hyperpolarizing the cell. In contrast, hypertonic stimulation (**right**) causes cell shrinking. Activation of an increased number of channels under this condition augments charge influx and results in membrane depolarization. Traces representing changes in the activity of a single SI channel are shown below. (From Bourque CW, Oliet SHR. Osmoreceptors in the central nervous system. *Annu Rev Physiol* 1997;59:601, with permission.)

ithelial water transport. Murata and colleagues (49) have described an atomic model of AQP1 at 3.8 Å resolution from electron crystallographic data and solved a long-standing physiologic puzzle—how membranes can be freely permeable to water but impermeable to protons. They have confirmed the key importance of the two Asn-Pro-Ala motifs in the pore helices HB and HE (for a review on aquaporins see reference 50). The positive charge of a proton (H_3O^+) can move along a column of water by hydrogen bond exchange and this single-file, hydrogen-bonded chain of water molecules which conducts protons with great efficiency has been termed "proton wire" by Pomes and Roux (51). In the middle of the AQP1 pore, the oxygen atom of the water molecule will form hydrogen bonds with Asn 76 and/or Asn 192 by changing the hydrogen-bonding partner from the adjacent water molecule. This reorients the two hydrogen atoms of the water molecule at the pore constriction perpendicular to the channel axis (Fig. 86-8). Thus, the two hydrogen atoms of the water molecule are prevented from forming hydrogen bonds with adjacent water molecule in the single-file column.

AQP2 is the vasopressin-regulated water channel in renal collecting ducts. It is exclusively present in principal cells of inner medullary collecting duct cells and is diffusely distributed in the cytoplasm in the euhydrated condition, whereas apical staining of AQP2 is intensified in the dehydrated condition or after administration of d_DAVP, a synthetic structural analog of AVP. The short-term AQP2 regulation by AVP involves the movement of AQP2 from intracellular vesicles to the plasma membrane, a confirmation of the shuttle hypothesis of AVP action that was proposed two decades ago (52). In the long-term regulation, which requires a sustained elevation of circulating AVP levels for 24 hours or more, AVP increases the abundance of water channels. This is thought to be a consequence of increased transcription of the *AQP2*

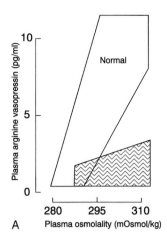

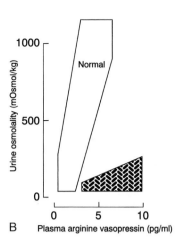

FIG. 86-5. A: Relationship between plasma arginine vasopressin (AVP) and plasma osmolality during infusion of hypertonic saline solution. Patients with primary polydipsia and nephrogenic diabetes insipidus have values within the normal range (*open area*) in contrast to patients with neurogenic diabetes insipidus, who show subnormal plasma antidiuretic hormone (ADH) responses (*cross-hatched area*). **B:** Relationship between urine osmolality and plasma ADH during dehydration and water loading. Patients with neurogenic diabetes insipidus and primary polydipsia have values within the normal range (*open area*) in contrast to patients with nephrogenic diabetes insipidus, who have hypotonic urine despite high plasma ADH (*stippled area*). (From Zerbe RL, Robertson GL. Disorders of ADH. *Med North Am* 1984;13:1570, with permission.)

gene (53). The activation of protein kinase A (PKA) leads to phosphorylation of AQP2 on serine residue 256 in the cytoplasmic carboxyl terminus. This phosphorylation step is essential for the regulated movement of AQP2-containing vesicles to the plasma membrane upon elevation of intracellular cAMP concentration (54,55). A second G-protein (the first being the cholera-toxin sensitive G-protein G_s) has also been shown to be essential for the AVP-induced shuttling of AQP2.

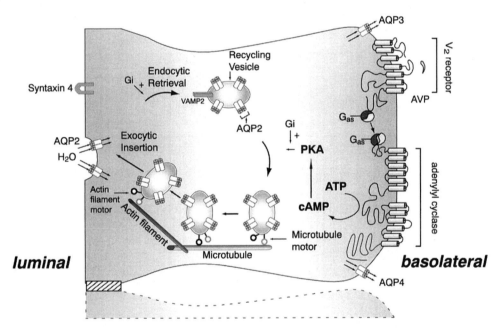

FIG. 86-6. Schematic representation of the effect of arginine vasopressin (AVP) to increase water permeability in the principal cells of the collecting duct. AVP is bound to the V_2 receptor (a G-protein-linked receptor) on the basolateral membrane. The basic process of G-protein-coupled receptor signaling consists of three steps: a hepta–helical receptor that detects a ligand (in this case, AVP) in the extracellular milieu; a G-protein that dissociates into α-subunits bound to GTP and $\beta\gamma$-subunits after interaction with the ligand-bound receptor; and an effector (in this case, adenylyl cyclase) that interacts with dissociated G-protein subunits to generate small-molecule second messengers. AVP activates adenylyl cyclase increasing the intracellular concentration of cyclic adenosine monophosphate (cAMP). The topology of adenylyl cyclase is characterized by two tandem repeats of six hydrophobic transmembrane domains separated by a large cytoplasmic loop and terminates in a large intracellular tail. Generation of cAMP follows receptor-linked activation of the heteromeric G-protein (G_s) and interaction of the free $G_{\alpha s}$-chain with the adenylyl cyclase catalyst. Protein kinase A (PKA) is the target of the generated cAMP. Cytoplasmic vesicles carrying the water channel proteins (represented as homotetrameric complexes) are fused to the luminal membrane in response to AVP, thereby increasing the water permeability of this membrane. Microtubules and actin filaments are necessary for vesicle movement toward the membrane. The mechanisms underlying docking and fusion of aquaporin-2 (AQP2)-bearing vesicles are not known. The detection of the small GTP binding protein Rab3a, synaptobrevin 2, and syntaxin 4 in principal cells suggests that these proteins are involved in AQP2 trafficking (56). When AVP is not available, water channels are retrieved by an endocytic process, and water permeability returns to its original low rate. AQP3 and AQP4 water channels are expressed on the basolateral membrane.

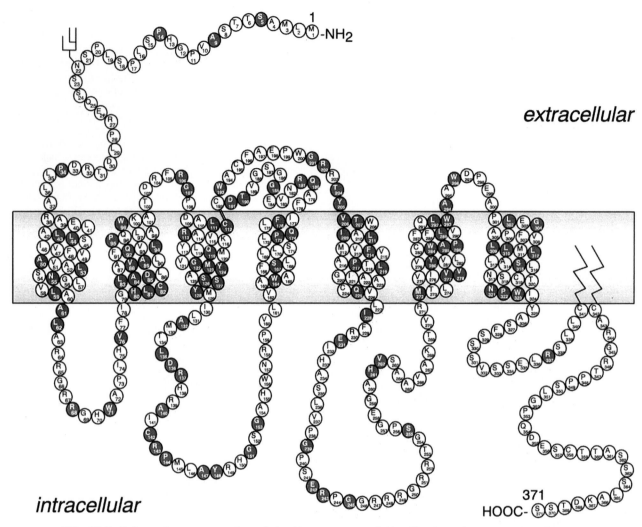

FIG. 86-7. Schematic representation of the V_2 receptor and identification of 155 putative disease-causing *AVPR2* mutations. Predicted amino acids are given as the one-letter code. A solid symbol indicates the location (or the closest codon) of a mutation; a number indicates more than one mutation in the same codon. The names of the mutations were assigned according to recommended nomenclature (236). The extracellular, transmembrane, and cytoplasmic domains are defined according to Mouillac and colleagues (240). The common names of the mutations are listed by type. **78 missense**: L43P, L44F, L44P, L53R, N55D, N55H, L59P, L62P, H80R, L81F, L83P, L83Q, A84D, D85N, V88L, V88M, Q92R, L94Q, P95L, W99R, R106C, G107E, C112R, R113W, G122R, M123K, S126F, S127F, Y128S, A132D, L135P, R137H, (C142W; R143G), R143P, A147V, W164S, S167L, S167T, Q174L, R181C, G185C, D191G, G201D, R202C, T204N, Y205C, V206D, T207N, I209F, F214S, P217T, L219P, L219R, M272K, V277A, Y280C, A285P, P286L, P286R, P286S, L289P, L292P, A294P, L309P, S315R (AGC > AGA), S315R (AGC > AGG), N317K, C319R, N321D, N321K, N321Y, P322H, P322S, W323R, W323S. **17 nonsense**: W71X, Q119X, Y124X, W164X, S167X, Q180X, W193X (TGG >TAG), W193X (TGG > TGA), Q225X, E231X, E242X, W284X, W293X, W296X, L312X, W323X, R337X. **42 frameshift**: in E$_I$—15delc, 27-54del, 46-47delct, 54-55ins28, 102delg; in TMI—137-138delta; in C$_I$—185-219del, 206-207insg, (225delc; 223C > A); in TM$_{II}$—247-248ins7, 268-269delCT, 295delT; in TM$_{III}$—331-332delCT, 335-336delGT, 340delg, 407-446del; in C$_{II}$—418delG, 430-442del, 442-443insG, 452delG, 457-463del, 460delG; in E$_{III}$—567-568insC, 572-575del, 612-613insC, 614-615delAT; in TM$_V$—631delC; C$_{III}$—682-683insC, 692delA, 717delG, 727-728delAG, 738delG, 738-739insG, 763delA, 784delG, 785-786insT; in TM$_{VI}$—838-839insT, 847-851del, 851-852ins5; in TM$_{VII}$—907delG, 930delC, 969delG; **6 inframe deletions or insertions**: in C$_I$—185-193del; in TM$_{II}$—252-253ins9; in TM$_{III}$—y128del; in TM$_{IV}$—f176del; in E$_{III}$—r202del; in TM$_{VI}$—v279del; **3 splice-site**: IVS2+1delG, IVS2+1G>A, IVS2-2A>G (149,152,153,155,164,165,241–268). Eight large deletions and one complex mutation are not shown (149,155,164,257,261).

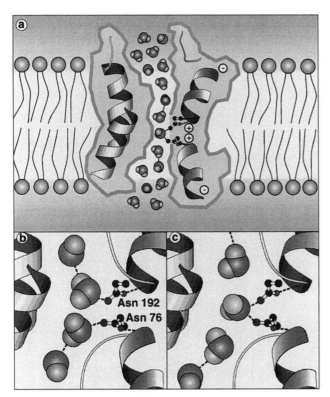

FIG. 86-8. Schematic representations explaining the mechanism for blocking proton permeation of aquaporin-1 (AQP1). **A:** Diagram illustrating how partial charges from the helix dipoles restrict the orientation of the water molecules passing through the constriction of the pore. **B & C:** Diagram illustrating hydrogen bonding of a water molecule with Asn 76 and/or Asn 192, which extends their amido groups into the constriction of the pore. The ribbon and ball-stick models in this figure were prepared with MOLSCRIPT (269). (Reprinted by permission from Murata K, et al. Structural determinants of water permeation through aquaporin-1. *Nature* 2000;407:599, © 2000 Macmillan Magazines, Ltd.)

This G-protein is sensitive to pertussis toxin and is involved in the pathway downstream of the cAMP/cAMP-dependent protein kinase signal (56). The molecular basis for the translocation of the AQP2 containing vesicles remains incompletely known, but it is thought to be analogous to neuronal exocytosis (57). This is supported by the identification in the vesicles of various proteins known to be involved in regulated exocytosis, for example, Rab3a and synaptobrevin II (VAMP2) or synaptobrevin II-like protein (58–60). In contrast to neuronal exocytosis, which is triggered by Ca^{2+}, cAMP and PKA appear to be crucial for the AQP2 translocation process (61,62). Vesicle trafficking probably involves the interaction of AQP2-containing vesicles with the cytoskeleton (63) (Fig. 86-6). Drugs that disrupt microtubules or actin filaments have long been known to inhibit the hormonally induced permeability response in target epithelia (64). More recently, Sabolic and coworkers have shown that microtubules are required for the apical polarization of AQP2 in principal cells (65). AQP3 and AQP4 are the constitutive water channels in the basolateral membranes of renal medullary collecting ducts.

AVP also increases the water reabsorptive capacity of the kidney by regulating the urea transporter UT1 which is present in the inner medullary collecting duct, predominantly in its terminal part (66). AVP also increases the permeability of principal collecting duct cells to sodium (67).

In summary, as stated elegantly by Ward and colleagues (67), in the absence of AVP stimulation, collecting duct epithelia exhibit very low permeabilities to sodium urea and water. These specialized permeability properties permit the excretion of large volumes of hypotonic urine formed during intervals of water diuresis. In contrast, AVP stimulation of the principal cells of the collecting ducts leads to selective increases in the permeability of the apical membrane to water (P_f), urea (P_{urea}, and Na (P_{Na}).

These actions of vasopressin in the distal nephron are possibly modulated by prostaglandin E_2 and by the luminal calcium concentration. High levels of E-prostanoid (EP_3) receptors are expressed in the kidney (68). However, mice lacking EP_3 receptors for prostaglandin E_2 were found to have quasi-normal regulation of urine volume and osmolality in response to various physiologic stimuli (68). An apical calcium/polycation receptor protein expressed in the terminal portion of the inner medullary collecting duct of the rat has been shown to reduce AVP-elicited osmotic water permeability when luminal calcium concentration rises (69). This possible link between calcium and water metabolism may play a role in the pathogenesis of renal stone formation (69).

The gene that codes for the water channel of the apical membrane of the kidney collecting tubule has been designated aquaporin-2 (*AQP2*) and was cloned by homology to the rat aquaporin of collecting duct (70–72). The human *AQP2* gene is located in chromosome region 12q13 and has four exons and three introns (71–73). It is predicted to code for a polypeptide of 271 amino acids that is organized into two repeats oriented at 180 degrees to each other and has six membrane-spanning domains, both terminal ends located intracellularly, and conserved Asn-Pro-Ala boxes (Fig. 86-9). These features are characteristic of the major intrinsic protein family (72). AQP2 is detectable in urine, and changes in urinary excretion of this protein can be used as an index of the action of vasopressin on the kidney (74–76).

KNOCKOUT MICE WITH URINARY CONCENTRATION DEFECTS

A useful strategy to establish the physiologic function of a protein is to determine the phenotype produced by pharmacologic inhibition of protein function or by gene disruption. Transgenic knockout mice deficient in AQP1, AQP2, AQP3, AQP4, AQP3 and AQP4, CLCNK1, NKCC2, AVPR2, or AGT have been engineered (77–85). Angiotensinogen (AGT)-deficient mice are characterized by both concentrating and diluting defects secondary to a defective renal papillary architecture (85).

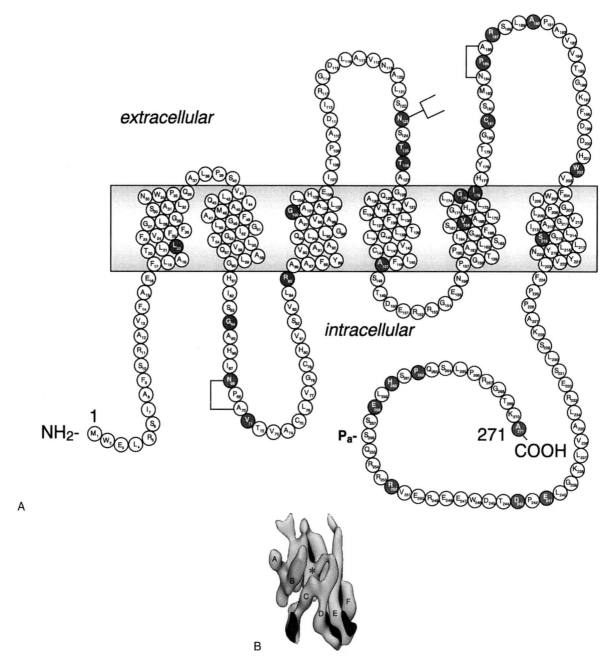

FIG. 86-9. A: Schematic representation of the aquaporin-2 (AQP2) protein and identification of 26 putative disease-causing *AQP2* mutations. A monomer is represented with six transmembrane helices. The location of the protein kinase A (PKA) phosphorylation site (P_a) is indicated. This site is possibly involved in the arginine vasopressin (AVP)-induced trafficking of AQP2 from intracellular vesicles to the plasma membrane and in the subsequent stimulation of endocytosis (54,55). The extracellular (*E*), transmembrane (*TM*), and cytoplasmic (*C*) domains are defined according to Deen and colleagues (71). As in Fig. 163-13, *solid symbols* indicate the location of the mutations. The common names of the mutations are listed by domain. TM_I: *L22V*; C_{II}: *G64R, N68S, V71M, R85X*; TM_{III}: *G100X*; E_{II}: *369delC, T125M, T126M*; TM_{IV}: *A147T*; TM_V: *V168M, G175R, IVS2-1G>A*; E_{III}: *C181W, P185A, R187C, A190T, W202C*; TM_{VI}: *S216P*; C_{IV}: *721delG, 727delG, 756-765del, E258K, 779-780insA, P262L, 812-816del* (71,88,191,258,263, 270–274 and Bichet DG and Sasaki S, unpublished data). **B:** A surface-shaded representation of the 6-helix barrel of the AQP1 protein viewed parallel to the bilayer; *black lines* indicate the approximate helix axes. (Modified from Cheng A, et al. Three-dimensional organization of a human water channel. *Nature* 1997;387:627, with permission.)

As reviewed by Rao and Verkman (86) extrapolation of data in mice to humans must be made with caution. For example, the maximum osmolality of mouse (greater than 3,000 mOsm/kg H_2O) is much greater than that of human urine (=1,000 mOsmol/kg H_2O) and normal serum osmolality in mice is 330 to 345 mOsmol/kg H_2O, substantially greater than that in humans (280 to 290 mOsm/kg H_2O). Protein expression patterns and thus the interpretation of phenotype studies may also be species-dependent. For example, AQP4 is expressed in both proximal tubule and collecting duct in the mouse but only in collecting duct in the rat and in humans (86).

The *Aqp3, Aqp4, Clcnk-1* and *Agt* knockout mice have no identified human counterparts. Of interest, *AQP1*-null individuals have no obvious symptoms (87). Yang and associates (84) have generated *AQP2-T126M* knock-in mutant mice to recapitulate the clinical features of the naturally occurring human *AQP2* mutation T126M (88). The mutant mice appeared normal at 2 to 3 days after birth, but failed to thrive and generally died by day 6 if not given supplemental fluid. These mice were characterized by an extremely severe concentrating defect with urine osmolality of 225 ± 9 mOsm/kg H_2O with concomitant serum osmolality of 450 ± 50 mOsm/kg H_2O and renal failure. Mice lacking the AVPR2 receptor (83) also failed to thrive and died within the first week after birth due to hypernatremic dehydration (83).

The absence of the gene coding for the NaK2Cl cotransport (NKCC2) in the luminal membrane of the thick ascending loop of Henle in the mouse also caused polyuria that was not compensated elsewhere in the nephron and recapitulated many features of the human classic Bartter's syndrome (82). The absence of transcellular NaCl transport via NKCC2 probably abolished the lumen positive transepithelial voltage that enables paracellular reabsorption of Na and K across the wall of the thick ascending tubule. The combined absence of transcellular and paracellular transport of salt across the thick ascending limb cells prevents the establishment of the normal osmotic gradient necessary for urine concentration.

THE BRATTLEBORO RAT WITH AUTOSOMAL-RECESSIVE NEUROGENIC DIABETES INSIPIDUS

The classic animal model for studying diabetes insipidus has been the Brattleboro rat with autosomal-recessive neurogenic diabetes insipidus. These *di/di* rats are homozygous for a 1-bp deletion (G) in the second exon that results in a frameshift mutation in the coding sequence of the carrier NPII (89) (Fig. 86-10). The polyuric symptoms are also observed in heterozygous *di/n* rats. Homozygous Brattleboro rats may still demonstrate some V_2 antidiuretic effect since the administration of a selective nonpeptide V_2 antagonist (SR121463A, 10 mg/kg i.p.) induced a further increase in urine flow rate (200 to 354 ± 42 mL/24 hours) and a decline in urinary osmolality (170 to 92 ± 8 mmol/kg) (90). Oxytocin which is present at enhanced plasma concentrations in Brattleboro rats, may be responsible for the antidiuretic activity observed (91,92). Oxytocin is not stimulated by increased plasma osmolality in humans. The Brattleboro rat model is therefore not strictly comparable with the rarely observed human cases of autosomal-recessive neurogenic diabetes insipidus (93,94).

```
deleted in Brattleboro rat
        ↓
GGA AGC GGA GGC CGC TGC GCT GCC
Gly Ser Gly Gly Arg Cys Ala Ala     Rat

GGG AGC GGG GGC CGC TGC GCC GCC
Gly Ser Gly Gly Arg Cys Ala Ala     Human
 62  63  64  65  66  67  68  69
```

FIG. 86-10. Neurophysin II genomic and amino acid sequence showing the 1 bp (G) deleted in the Brattleboro rat. The human sequence (GenBank entry M11166) is also shown. It is almost identical to the rat prepro sequence. In the Brattleboro rat, G1880 is deleted with a resultant frameshift after 63 amino acids (amino acid 1 is the first amino acid of neurophysin II).

QUANTITATING RENAL WATER EXCRETION

Diabetes insipidus is characterized by the excretion of abnormally large volumes of hypoosmotic urine (less than 250 mmol/kg). This definition excludes osmotic diuresis, which occurs when excess solute is being excreted, as with glucose in the polyuria of diabetes mellitus. Other agents that produce osmotic diuresis are mannitol, urea, glycerol, contrast media, and loop diuretics. Osmotic diuresis should be considered when solute excretion exceeds 60 mmol/hour. The quantification of water excretion (solute-free water clearance, osmolar clearance, free electrolyte water reabsorption, effective water clearance) is described in Chapter 85.

CLINICAL CHARACTERISTICS OF DIABETES INSIPIDUS DISORDERS

Central Diabetes Insipidus

Common Forms

Failure to synthesize or secrete vasopressin normally limits its maximal urinary concentration and, depending on the severity of the disease, causes varying degrees of polyuria and polydipsia. Experimental destruction of the vasopressin-synthesizing areas of the hypothalamus (supraoptic and paraventricular nuclei) causes a permanent form of the disease. Similar results are obtained by sectioning the hypophyseal–hypothalamic tract above the median eminence. Sections below the median eminence, however, produce only transient diabetes insipidus. Lesions to the hypothalamic–pituitary tract are often associated with a three-stage response both in experimental animals and in humans (95) which consists of:

1. An initial diuretic phase lasting from a few hours to 5 to 6 days.
2. A period of antidiuresis unresponsive to fluid administration. This antidiuresis is probably due to vasopressin release from injured axons and may last from a few hours to several days. Since urinary dilution is impaired during this phase, continued water administration can cause severe hyponatremia.
3. A final period of diabetes insipidus. The extent of the injury determines the completeness of the diabetes insipidus, and as already discussed, the site of the lesion determines whether the disease will or will not be permanent.

A detailed assessment of water balance following transsphenoidal surgery has been reported (96). One hundred and one patients who underwent transsphenoidal pituitary surgery at the National Institutes of Health Clinical Center were studied. Twenty-five percent of the patients developed spontaneous isolated hyponatremia, 20% developed diabetes insipidus, and 46% remained normonatremic. Normonatremia, hyponatremia, and diabetes insipidus were associated with increasing degrees of surgical manipulation of the posterior lobe and pituitary stalk during surgery.

The etiologies of central diabetes insipidus in adults and in children are listed in Table 86-1 (97–99). Rare causes of central diabetes insipidus include leukemia, thrombotic thrombocytopenic purpura, pituitary apoplexy, sarcoidosis, and Wegener's granulomatosis (100). A distinctive syndrome characterized by early diabetes insipidus with subsequent progressive spastic cerebellar ataxia has also been described (101). Five patients who all presented with central diabetes insipidus and hypogonadism as first manifestations of neurosarcoidosis have been reported (102).

Finally, circulating antibodies to vasopressin do not play a role in the development of diabetes insipidus (103). Antibodies to vasopressin occasionally develop during treatment with ADH and, when they do, almost always result in secondary resistance to its antidiuretic effect (103,104).

Maghnie and coworkers (99) studied 79 patients with central diabetes insipidus who were seen at 4 pediatric endocrinology units between 1970 and 1996. There were 37 male and 42 female patients whose median age at diagnosis was 7 years (range, 0.1 to 24.8). In 10 patients, central diabetes insipidus developed during an infectious illness or less than 2 months afterward (varicella in 5 patients, mumps in 3 patients, and measles, toxoplasmosis, and hepatitis B in 1 patient each). Deficits in anterior pituitary hormones were documented in 48 patients (61%) a median of 0.6 years (range, 0.1 to 18.0) after the onset of diabetes insipidus. The most frequent abnormality was growth hormone deficiency (59%), followed by hypothyroidism (28%), hypogonadism (24%), and adrenal insufficiency (22%). Seventy-five percent of the patients with histiocytosis of the Langerhans' cells had an anterior pituitary hormone deficiency that was first detected at a median of 3.5 years after the onset of diabetes insipidus. The frequency and progression of histiocytosis of the Langerhans' cells related to anterior pituitary and other nonendocrine hypothalamic dysfunction, and their response to treatment in 12 adult patients has also been recently reviewed (105). None of the patients with central diabetes insipidus secondary to *prepro-AVP-NPII* mutations developed anterior pituitary hormone deficiencies.

Rare Forms: Autosomal-Dominant Central Diabetes Insipidus and the DIDMOAD Syndrome

Lacombe (106) and Weil (107) described a familial non-X-linked form of diabetes insipidus without any associated mental retardation. The descendants of the family described by Weil were later found to have autosomal-dominant neurogenic diabetes insipidus (108–110).

Repaske and coworkers (111) reported in 1990 that the genetic locus for autosomal-dominant central diabetes insipidus (106–110) was within or near the gene encoding for AVP.

TABLE 86-1. *Etiology of hypothalamic diabetes insipidus in children and adults*

	Children (%)	Children and young adults (%)	Adults (%)
Primary brain tumor[a]	49.5	22	30
Before surgery	33.5	—	13
After surgery	16	—	17
Idiopathic (isolated or familial)	29	58	25
Histiocytosis	16	12	—
Metastatic cancer[b]	—	—	8
Trauma[c]	2.2	2.0	17
Postinfectious disease	2.2	6.0	—

[a]Primary malignancy: craniopharyngioma, dysgerminoma, meningioma, adenoma, glioma, astrocytoma.
[b]Secondary malignancy: metastasis from lung or breast, lymphoma, leukemia, dysplastic pancytopenia.
[c]Trauma could be severe or mild.
(Data from Czernichow, et al. (97), Greger, et al. (98), Maghnie, et al. (99), and Moses, et al. (100).)

Furthermore, they suggested that a defective *AVP-NPII* gene might be the basis for this disease.

Neurogenic diabetes insipidus (OMIM 125700, see Online Mendelian Inheritance in Man, http://www.ncbi.nlm.nih.gov/omim) (112) is a now well-characterized entity, secondary to mutations in the *prepro-AVP-NPII* (OMIM 192340) (112). This disorder is also referred to as central, cranial, pituitary, or neurohypophyseal diabetes insipidus. Patients with autosomal-dominant neurogenic diabetes insipidus retain some limited capacity to secrete AVP during severe dehydration, and the polyuro–polydipsic symptoms usually appear after the first year of life (113), when the infant's demand for water is more likely to be understood by adults. Thirty-four *prepro-AVP-NPII* mutations segregating with autosomal-dominant or autosomal-recessive neurogenic diabetes insipidus have been described (94,113–136) (Table 86-2). The mechanism(s) by which a mutant allele causes neurogenic diabetes insipidus could involve the induction of magnocellular cell death as a result of the accumulation of AVP precursors within the endoplasmic reticulum (132,137). This hypothesis could account for the delayed onset and autosomal mode of inheritance of the disease. In addition to the cytotoxicity caused by mutant AVP precursors, the interaction between the wild-type and the mutant precursors suggests that a dominant-negative mechanism may also contribute to the pathogenesis of autosomal-dominant diabetes insipidus (138). The absence of symptoms in infancy in autosomal-dominant central diabetes insipidus is in sharp contrast with nephrogenic diabetes insipidus secondary to mutations in *AVPR2* or in *AQP2* (*vide infra*) in which the polyuro–polydipsic symptoms are present during the first week of life. Of interest, errors in protein folding represent the underlying basis for a large number of inherited diseases (139,140) and are also pathogenic mechanisms for *AVPR2* and *AQP2* mutants responsible for hereditary nephrogenic diabetes insipidus (*vide infra*). Why *prepro-AVP-NPII* misfolded mutants are cytotoxic to AVP-producing neurons is an unresolved issue. The nephrogenic diabetes insipidus *AVPR2* missense mutations are likely to impair folding and to lead to the rapid degradation of the affected polypeptide and not to the accumulation of toxic aggregates since the other important function of the principal cells of the collecting ducts (where *AVPR2* is expressed) are entirely normal. Three families with autosomal-recessive neurogenic diabetes insipidus have been identified in which the patients were homozygotes or compound heterozygotes for *prepro-AVP-NPII* mutations (93,94). Two of these families are characterized phenotypically by severe and early onset in the first 3 months of life, polyuria, polydipsia, and dehydration. As a consequence, early hereditary diabetes insipidus can be neurogenic or nephrogenic.

The acronym DIDMOAD describes the following clinical features of a syndrome: *d*iabetes insipidus, *d*iabetes *m*ellitus, *o*ptic *a*trophy, sensorineural *d*eafness (141,142). An unusual incidence of psychiatric symptoms has also been described in these patients (143). These include paranoid delusions, auditory or visual hallucinations, psychotic behavior, violent behavior, organic brain syndrome typically in the late or preterminal stages of illness, progressive dementia, and severe learning disabilities or mental retardation or both. The syndrome is an autosomal-recessive trait, the diabetes insipidus is usually partial and of gradual onset (142), and the polyuria can be wrongly attributed to poor glycemic control. Furthermore, a severe hyperosmolar state can occur if untreated diabetes mellitus is associated with an unrecognized pituitary deficiency. The dilation of the urinary tract observed in the DIDMOAD syndrome may be secondary to chronic high urine flow rates and, perhaps, to some degenerative aspects of the innervation of the urinary tract (141). Wolfram syndrome (OMIM 222300) (112) is secondary to mutations in the *WFS1* gene (chromosome region 4p16), which codes for a transmembrane protein expressed in various tissues including brain and pancreas (144–146).

The Syndrome of Hypernatremia and Hypodipsia

Some patients with the hypernatremia and hypodipsia syndrome may have partial central diabetes insipidus (147). These patients also have persistent hypernatremia, which is not due to any apparent extracellular volume loss; absence or attenuation of thirst; or a normal renal response to AVP. In almost all of the patients studied to date, the hypodipsia has been associated with cerebral lesions in the vicinity of the hypothalamus. It has been proposed that in these patients there is a "resetting" of the osmoreceptor, because their urine tends to become concentrated or diluted at inappropriately high levels of plasma osmolality. However, by using the regression analysis of plasma AVP concentration versus plasma osmolality, it has been possible to show that in some of these patients the tendency to concentrate and dilute urine at inappropriately high levels of plasma osmolality is due solely to a marked reduction in sensitivity or a gain in the osmoregulatory mechanism. This finding is compatible with the diagnosis of partial central diabetes insipidus. In other patients, however, plasma AVP concentrations fluctuate randomly, bearing no apparent relationship to changes in plasma osmolality. Such patients often display large swings in serum sodium concentrations and often exhibit hypodipsia. It appears that most patients with essential hypernatremia fit one of these two patterns (Fig. 86-11). Both of these groups of patients consistently respond normally to nonosmolar AVP release signals, such as hypotension, emesis, hypoglycemia, or all three of these signals. These observations suggest that the osmoreceptor may be anatomically as well as functionally separate from the nonosmotic efferent pathways and neurosecretory neurons for vasopressin. Furthermore, a hypothalamic lesion may impair the osmotic release of AVP while the nonosmotic release of AVP remains intact, and the osmoreceptor neurons that regulate vasopressin secretion are not totally synonymous with those that regulate

TABLE 86-2. *Prepro–arginine vasopressin–neurophysin II mutations causing autosomal-dominant and autosomal-recessive human neurogenic diabetes insipidus*

Systematic name	Common name	Nucleotide change	Predicted amino acid change	Restriction-enzyme analysis	Comments and putative functional consequence	References
g.3delG	3delG (previously called 277delG)	Deletion of G of ATG, the first a.a. of the signal peptide	Frameshift starting with the first a.a. of the signal peptide	*Bam*HI site created	Retention in the ER, alternative ATG with production of truncated signal sequence	(114,129)
g.50C>T	S17F	TCC-to-TTC	Ser→Phe at codon 17	*Mbo*II site created		(113)
g.55G>A	A19T	GCG-to-ACG	Ala→Thr at codon 19	*Bst*UI site abolished, *Pml*II site created	CG→CA; alteration of the cleavage of the leader peptide	(116–119,130,132) (total of 7 families)
g.56C>T	A19V	GCG-to-GTG	Ala→Val at codon 19	*Bst*UI site abolished		(113,120,121) (3 independent families)
g.61T>C	Y21H	TAC-to-CAC	Tyr→His at codon 21		Substitution of the second a.a. in the antidiuretic hormone	(115)
g.77C>T	P26L	CCG-to-CTG	Pro→Leu at codon 26		Autosomal-recessive, substitution of the seventh a.a. in the antidiuretic hormone	(94)
g.1506>C	G45R	GGC-to-CGC	Gly→Arg at codon 45 (NP$_{14}$)	*Bsl*I site created		(113,121)
g.1516G>T	G48V	GGC-to-GTC	Gly→Val at codon 48 (NP$_{17}$)	*Bgl*I site abolished	Disruption of a β-turn in AVP–NPII precursor	(122)
g.1524C>T	R51C	CGC-to-TGC	Arg→Cys at codon 51 (NP$_{20}$)			(113)
g.1533G>A	G54R	GGG-to-GTG	Gly→Arg at codon 54 (NP$_{23}$)			(131)
g.1533G>C	G54R	GGG-to-CGG	Gly→Arg at codon 54 (NP$_{23}$)	*Bsp*120I site abolished		(121)
g.1534G>T	G54V	GGG-to-GTG	Gly→Val at codon 54 (NP$_{23}$)	*Apa*I site abolished		(123)
g.1537C>T	P55L	CCC-to-CTC	Pro→Leu at codon 55 (NP$_{24}$)	*Dde*I site created	*De novo* mutation, amino acid substitution in NPII	(119,124)
g.1605–1607del	E78del (previously called ΔE77)	Deletion of 3 nucleotides in region 1602–1607	Deletion of Glu (glutamic acid) at codon 77 (NP$_{46}$)	*Mnl*I site abolished	Two sets of staggered 3 bp tandem repeats; unable to form a salt bridge between AVP and NPII	(113,125)
g.1606A>G	E78G	GAG-to-GGG	Glu→Gly at codon 78 (NP$_{47}$)			(113)
g.1615T>C	L81P	CTG-to-CCG	Leu→Pro at codon 81 (NP$_{50}$)			(113)

Nucleotide change	a.a. change	Codon change	Amino acid	Restriction site	Functional effect	Reference
g.1633C>T	S87F	TCC-to-TTC	Ser→Phe at codon 87 (NP56)	MspI site abolished		(135)
g.1635G>C	G88R	GGC-to-CGC	Gly→Arg at codon 88 (NP57)	MspI and BglI sites abolished		(113)
g.1635G>A	G88S	GGC-to-AGC	Gly→Ser at codon 88 (NP57)	MspI and BglI sites abolished	Failure of dimerization of NPII, alteration of axonal transport or postranslation processing	(113,119,126) (3 families)
g.1648G>C	C92S	TGC-to-TCC	Cys→Ser at codon 92 (NP61)	HgaI site created		(113)
g.1648G>A	C92Y	TGC-to-TAC	Cys→Tyr at codon 92 (NP61)	RsaI site created		(135)
g.1649C>A	C92X	TGC-to-TGA	Cys→stop at codon 92 (NP61)	MnlI site created		(113)
g.1650G>T	G93W	GGG-to-TGG	Gly→Trp at codon 93 (NP62)	BpmI site created		(127)
g.1659G>T	G96C	GGC-to-TGC	Gly→Cys at codon 96 (NP65)			(113)
g.1660G>T	G96V	GGC-to-GTC	Gly→Val at codon 96 (NP65)			(128)
g.1662C>T	R97C	CGC-to-TGC	Arg→Cys at 97 (NP66)			(134)
g.1667C>A	C98X	TGC-to-TGA	Cys→Stop at codon 99 (NP68)	DdeI site created		(127)
g.1687G>A	C105Y	TGC-to-TAC	Cys→Tyr at codon 105 (NP74)			(133)
g.1870C>A	C110X	TGC-to-TGA	Cys→Stop at codon 110 (NP79)	BbvI site abolished		(113)
g.1877C>T	E113X	GAG-to-TAG	Glu→Stop at codon 113 (NP82)			(130)
g.1882C>G;		CCC-to-CCG;	Pro→Pro at 114 (NP83)			(113)
g.1883G>T	E115X	GAG-to-TAG	Glu→Stop at 115 (NP84)			
g.1886T>G	C116G	TGC-to-GGC	Cys→Gly at codon 116 (NP85)	Sau96I site created		(136)
G.1886T>C	C116R	TGC-to-CGC	Cys→Arg at codon 116 (NP85)	HaeII site created		(136)
g.1892G>T	E118X	GAG-to-TAG	Glu→Stop at 118 (NP87)	MaeI site created		(113)

a.a., amino acid; AVP, arginine vasopressin; ER, endoplasmic reticulum; NP, neurophysin

The nucleotides and amino acids are numbered according to GenBank accession number M11166 and modified according to corrections in reference 126. The nucleotides are numbered according to the recommendation for genomic DNA sequence and correspond to the numbers used in the systematic names of mutations (see reference 236). The codons corresponding to the moieties are: 1 to 19—signal peptide; 20 to 28—AVP; 29 to 31—cleavage site; 32 to 124—NPII; and 126 to 164—glycopeptide. NP14 indicates the 14th amino acid of the protein neurophysin, other superscript numbers with NP indicate corresponding amino acids.

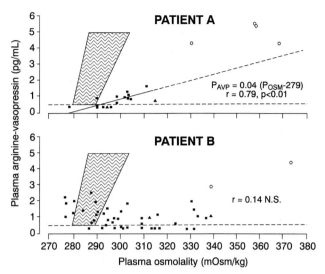

FIG. 86-11. Plasma vasopressin (P_{AVP}) as a function of "effective" plasma osmolality (P_{OSM}) in two patients with adipsic hypernatremia. *Open circles* indicate values obtained on admission; *filled squares* indicate those obtained during forced hydration; *filled triangles* indicate those obtained after 1 to 2 weeks of ad libitum water intake; *shaded areas* indicate range of normal values. (From Robertson GL. The physiopathology of ADH secretion. In: Tolis G, et al., eds. *Clinical neuroendocrinology: a pathophysiological approach.* New York: Raven Press, 1979:247, with permission.)

thirst, although they appear to be anatomically close if not overlapping.

Nephrogenic Diabetes Insipidus

X-Linked Nephrogenic Diabetes Insipidus and Mutations in the AVPR2 Gene

X-linked nephrogenic diabetes insipidus (NDI) (OMIM 304800) (112) is generally a rare disease in which affected male patients do not concentrate their urine after the administration of AVP (148). Because it is a rare, recessive X-linked disease, females are unlikely to be affected, but heterozygous females exhibit variable degrees of polyuria and polydipsia because of skewed X chromosome inactivation. X-linked NDI is secondary to *AVPR2* mutations that result in the loss of function or a dysregulation of the V_2 receptor.

Rareness and Diversity of AVPR2 Mutations

We estimated the incidence of X-linked NDI in the general population from patients born in the province of Quebec during the 10-year period 1988 to 1997 to be approximately 8.8 per million (SD = 4.4 per million) male live births (149). Thus, X-linked NDI is generally a rare disorder. By contrast, NDI was known to be a common disorder in Nova Scotia (150). Thirty affected males who reside mainly in two small villages with a total population size of 2,500 (151) are descendants of members of the Hopewell pedigree studied by Bode and Crawford (150) and carry the nonsense mutation,

W71X (152,153). This is the largest known pedigree with X-linked NDI and has been referred to as the Hopewell kindred, named after the Irish ship Hopewell, which arrived in Halifax in 1761 (150). The members of the Hopewell pedigree are descendants of Scottish Presbyterians, who migrated to the Ulster Province of Ireland in the seventeenth century, emigrated from Ireland in 1718, and settled in northern Massachusetts. A later group of immigrants were passengers on the ship Hopewell and settled in Colchester County, Nova Scotia. Members of the two groups were subsequently united in Colchester County (150). Thus, it is likely that Ulster Scot immigrants, perhaps on more than one occasion, brought the *W71X* mutation to North America. To date, we have identified the *W71X* mutation in 38 affected males who predominantly reside in the Maritime provinces of Nova Scotia and New Brunswick. We estimated the incidence in these two Maritime provinces to be 6 per 104,063 or approximately 58 per million (SD = 24 per million) male live births for the 10-year period, 1988 to 1997.

To date, 155 putative disease-causing *AVPR2* mutations have been identified in 239 NDI families (Fig. 86-7) (154) (additional information is available in the NDI Mutation Database at http://www.medcon.mcgill.ca/~nephros/). Of these, we identified 82 different mutations in 117 NDI families referred to our laboratory. Half of the mutations are missense mutations. Frameshift mutations due to nucleotide deletions or insertions (27%), nonsense mutations (11%), large deletions (5%), inframe deletions or insertions (4%), splice-site mutations (2%), and one complex mutation account for the remainder of the mutations. Mutations have been identified in every domain, but on a per nucleotide basis, about twice as many mutations occur in transmembrane domains compared to the extracellular or intracellular domains. We previously identified private mutations, recurrent mutations, and mechanisms of mutagenesis (155,156). The 10 recurrent mutations (*D85N, V88M, R113W, Y128S, R137H, S167L, R181C, R202C, A294P,* and *S315R*) were found in 35 ancestrally independent families (149). The occurrence of the same mutation on different haplotypes was considered as evidence for recurrent mutation. In addition, the most frequent mutations, *D85N, V88N, R113W, R137H, S167L, R181C,* and *R202C,* occurred at potential mutational hotspots (a C-to-T or G-to-A nucleotide substitution occurred at a CpG dinucleotide).

Benefits of Genetic Testing

The natural history of untreated X-linked NDI includes hypernatremia, hyperthermia, mental retardation, and repeated episodes of dehydration in early infancy (157–161). Mental retardation, a consequence of repeated episodes of dehydration, was prevalent in the Crawford and Bode study (160), in which only 9 of 82 patients (11%) had normal intelligence. Data from the Nijmegen group however suggest that this complication was overestimated in their group of NDI patients (161,162). Early recognition and treatment of X-linked NDI, with an abundant intake of water allows a normal life span with normal physical and mental development (163). Familial occurrence of males and mental retardation in untreated patients are two characteristics suggestive of X-linked NDI. Skewed X-inactivation is the most likely explanation for clinical symptoms of NDI in female carriers (149,164,165).

The identification of the molecular defect underlying X-linked NDI is of immediate clinical significance because early diagnosis and treatment of affected infants can avert the physical and mental retardation resulting from repeated episodes of dehydration. Diagnosis of X-linked NDI was accomplished by mutation testing of chorionic villous samples (n = 4), cultured amniotic cells (n = 5), or cord blood (n = 17). Three infants who had mutation testing done on amniotic cells (n = 1) or chorionic villous samples (n = 2) also had their diagnosis confirmed by cord blood testing. Of the 23 offspring tested, 12 were found to be affected boys, 7 were unaffected boys, and 4 were noncarrier girls (Bichet DG, et al., unpublished data). The affected boys were immediately treated with abundant water intake, a low-sodium diet, and hydrochlorothiazide. Following this treatment, no severe episodes of dehydration have yet to be reported. The boys' physical and mental development remains normal, however, their urinary output has only decreased by 30% and a normal growth curve has been difficult to reach during the first 2 to 3 years of life despite this treatments and intensive attention. Water should be offered every 2 hours day and night, and temperature, appetite, and growth should be monitored. Admission to the hospital may be necessary for continuous gastric feeding. The voluminous amounts of water kept in patients' stomachs will exacerbate physiologic gastrointestinal reflux as an infant and toddler, and many affected boys frequently vomit and have a strong positive "Tuttle test" (esophageal pH testing). These young patients often improve with an H-2 blocker treatment and with metoclopramide (which could induce extrapyramidal symptoms) or with domperidone, which seems to be better tolerated and more efficacious.

Most Mutant V$_2$ Receptors are not Transported to the Cell Membrane and are Retained in the Intracellular Compartments

The classification of the defects of mutant V$_2$ receptors is based on that of the low-density lipoprotein receptor where mutations have been grouped according to the function and subcellular localization of the mutant protein whose cDNA has been transiently transfected in an heterologous expression system (166). Following this classification, type 1 mutant receptors reach the cell surface but display impaired ligand binding and are consequently unable to induce normal cAMP production. The presence of mutant V$_2$ receptors on the surface of transfected cells can be determined pharmacologically. By carrying out saturation binding experiments using a tritiated AVP, the number of cell surface mutant receptors and their apparent binding affinity can be compared to that of the wild type receptor. In addition, the presence of cell surface receptors can be assessed directly by using immuno-detection strategies to visualize epitope-tagged receptors in whole-cell immunofluorescence assays.

Type 2 mutant receptors have defective intracellular transport. This phenotype is confirmed by carrying out, in parallel, immunofluorescence experiments on cells that are intact (to demonstrate the absence of cell surface receptors) or permeabilized (to confirm the presence of intracellular receptor pools). In addition, protein expression is confirmed by Western blot analysis of membrane preparations from transfected cells. It is likely that these mutant type 2 receptors accumulate in a pre-Golgi compartment since they are initially glycosylated but fail to undergo glycosyl trimming maturation.

Type 3 mutant receptors are ineffectively transcribed. This subgroup seems to be rare since Northern blot analysis of transfected cells reveals that most V$_2$ receptor mutations produce the same quantity and molecular size of receptor mRNA.

Of the 12 mutants that we tested (*N55H, L59P, L83Q, V88M, 497CC−>GG, ΔR202, I209F, 700delC, 908insT, A294P, P322H, P322S*) only three (*ΔR202, P322S, P322H*) were detected on the cell surface. Similarly, the 10 mutant receptors (*Y128S, E242X, 803insG, 834delA, ΔV278, Y280C, W284X, L292P, W293X, L312Y*) tested by Schöneberg and coworkers (167,168) did not reach the cell membrane and were trapped in the interior of the cell. Similar results for the following mutants were obtained: *L44F, L44P, W164S, S167L, S167T* (169); *R143P, ΔV278* (170); *Y280C, L292P, R333X* (171).

Other genetic disorders are also characterized by protein misfolding. *AQP2* mutations responsible for autosomal-recessive NDI are also characterized by misrouting of the misfolded mutant proteins and trapping in the endoplasmic reticulum (ER) (172). The *ΔF508* mutation in cystic fibrosis is also characterized by misfolding and retention in the ER of the mutated cystic fibrosis transmembrane conductance regulator (CFTCR), which is associated with calnexin and Hsp70 (for review see reference 173). The *C282Y* mutant HFE protein, which is responsible for 83% of hemochromatosis in the Caucasian population, is retained in the ER and middle Golgi compartment, fails to undergo late Golgi processing, and is subject to accelerated degradation (174). Mutants encoding other renal membrane proteins that are responsible for Gitelman's syndrome (175) and cystinuria (176) are also retained in the ER.

Missense mutations responsible for these various diseases are often situated in regions of the protein that are not part of either the active site, the binding site, or the site of interaction with other proteins. These mutations have been shown to decrease the half-life of the affected protein (139). Missense mutations and short inframe deletions or insertions that impair the propensity of the affected polypeptide to fold into its functional conformation and the term "conformational diseases" has been coined (177). The NDI missense mutations are likely to impair folding and to lead to rapid degradation of the affected polypeptide and not to accumulation of toxic aggregates since the other important functions of the principal cells of the collecting duct (where V_2 receptors are expressed) are entirely normal. These cells express the epithelial Na channel (ENaC). A decreased function of this channel will result in an Na-losing state (178). This has not been observed in patients with *AVPR2* mutations.

In Vitro Adenovirus-Mediated Gene Transfer Experiments have been Successful for a Limited Number of Mutations

Schöneberg and coworkers (167,168) genetically rescued truncated or missense V_2 receptors by coexpression of a polypeptide consisting of the last 130 amino acids of the V_2 receptor in COS-7 cells. Four of the six truncated receptors (E242X, 804delG, 834delA, and W284X) and the missense mutant *Y280C*, regained considerable functional activity, as demonstrated by an increase in the number of binding sites and stimulation of adenylyl cyclase activity, but the absolute number of expressed receptors at the cell surface remained low and the precise mechanism of the rescue phenomenon (dimerization) (179) was unclear. Most of the loss-of-function mutations secondary to *AVPR2* missense mutations are unlikely to be improved by this coexpression strategy and delivery of the gene transfer vehicle is a major unresolved problem.

Nonpeptide Vasopressin Antagonists Act as Pharmacologic Chaperones to Functionally Rescue Misfolded Mutant V_2 Receptors Responsible for X-Linked Nephrogenic Diabetes Insipidus

Several orally active, nonpeptide AVP receptor antagonists have been reported (180,181), and one, SR 121463, is a potent and selective V_2 receptor antagonist (90). This extremely stable molecule is highly selective for V_2 receptors from several species, including humans, and exhibits powerful intravenous and oral aquaretic effects (90). SR 121463 inhibits AVP-evoked cAMP formation in human kidney membranes and reverses extrarenal V_2 receptor antagonism of dDAVP-induced release of hemostatic factors in dogs (182). VPA-985 is a similar aquaretic compound (181). From a therapeutic point of view, V_2 receptor-specific antagonists able to block the action of AVP at the level of the renal collecting duct specifically promote water excretion.

We recently assessed whether these selective V_2 vasopressin receptor antagonists could facilitate the folding of mutant proteins that are responsible for NDI and are retained in the ER. We monitored the biosynthesis of mutant V_2 receptors in the presence of SR121463 and VPA-985. These cell-permeable antagonists were able to convert precursor forms of mutant V_2 receptor into fully glycosylated mature receptor proteins that were now targeted to the cell surface as determined by pulse-chase analysis and cell surface immunofluorescence microscopy. Once at their correct cellular location, these receptors were able to bind AVP and produce an intracellular cAMP response that was 15 times higher than that produced in cells not exposed to these antagonists

(183). This effect could not be mediated by nor compete with V_2 receptor antagonists that are membrane-impermeant, indicating that SR121463A was mediating its effects intracellularly.

On the basis of these data, we propose a model in which small nonpeptide V_2 receptor antagonists permeate into the cell and bind to incompletely folded mutant receptors. This would then stabilize a conformation of the receptor that allows its release from the ER quality control apparatus. The stabilized receptor would then be targeted to the cell surface, where upon dissociation from the antagonist it could bind vasopressin and promote signal transduction. Given that these antagonists are specific to the V_2 receptor and that they perform a chaperonelike function, we termed these compounds "pharmacologic chaperones" (140,183).

Autosomal-Recessive and Autosomal-Dominant Nephrogenic Diabetes Insipidus due to Mutations in the AQP2 Gene

On the basis of desmopressin infusion studies and phenotypic characteristics of both males and females affected with NDI, a non-X-linked form of NDI with a postreceptor (post-cAMP) defect was suggested (184–187). A patient who presented shortly after birth with typical features of NDI but who exhibited normal coagulation and normal fibrinolytic and vasodilatory responses to desmopressin was shown to be a compound heterozygote for two missense mutations (*R187C* and *S217P*) in the *AQP2* gene (71) (Fig. 86-9). To date, 26 putative disease-causing *AQP2* mutations have been identified in 25 NDI families (Fig. 86-9). By type of mutation, there are 65% missense, 23% frameshift due to small nucleotide deletions or insertions, 8% nonsense, and 4% splice-site mutations. Additional information is available in the NDI Mutation Database at http://www.medcor.mcgill.ca/~nephros/.

Reminiscent of expression studies done with AVPR2 proteins, misrouting of AQP2 mutant proteins has been shown to be the major cause underlying autosomal-recessive NDI (88,172,188). To determine if the severe AQP2 trafficking defect observed with the naturally occurring mutations *T126M*, *R187C*, and *A147T* is correctable, CHO and Madin-Darby canine kidney cells were incubated with the chemical chaperone glycerol for 48 hours. Using immunofluorescence, redistribution of AQP2 from the endoplasmic reticulum to the plasma membrane-endosome fractions was observed. This redistribution was correlated with improved water permeability measurements (172,189). It will be important to correct this defective AQP2 trafficking *in vivo*.

In contrast to the *AQP2* mutations in autosomal-recessive NDI, which are located throughout the gene, the dominant mutations are predicted to affect the carboxyl terminus of AQP2 (190). One dominant mutation, *E258K*, has been analyzed in detail *in vitro*; AQP2-E258K had reduced water permeability compared to wild-type AQP2 (191). In addition, AQP2-E258K was retained in the Golgi apparatus, which differs from mutant AQP2 in recessive NDI that is retained in the endoplasmic reticulum. The dominant action of *AQP2* mutations can be explained by the formation of heterotetramers of mutant and wild-type AQP2 that are impaired in their routing after oligomerization (191,192).

Acquired Nephrogenic Diabetes Insipidus

The acquired form of NDI is much more common than the congenital form of the disease, but it is rarely severe. The ability to elaborate a hypertonic urine is usually preserved despite the impairment of the maximal concentrating ability of the nephrons. Polyuria and polydipsia are therefore moderate (3 to 4 L/day). The more common causes of acquired NDI are listed in Table 86-3.

Lithium administration has become the most common cause of NDI. Boton and colleagues (193) reported that this abnormality was estimated to be present in at least 54% of 1,105 unselected patients on chronic lithium therapy. Nineteen percent of these patients had polyuria, as defined by a 24-hour urine output exceeding 3 L. Renal biopsy revealed a chronic tubulointerstitial nephropathy in all 24 patients with biopsy-proven lithium toxicity (194). The mechanism whereby lithium causes polyuria has been extensively studied. Lithium has been shown to inhibit adenylate cyclase in a number of cell types, including renal epithelia (195,196). The concentration of lithium in the urine of patients on well-controlled lithium therapy (i.e., 10 to 40 mmol/L) is sufficient to inhibit adenylate cyclase. Measurements of adenylate cyclase activity in membranes isolated from a cultured pig kidney cell line (LLC-PK$_1$) revealed that lithium in the concentration area of 10 mmol/L interfered with the hormone-stimulated guanyl nucleotide regulatory unit (G$_s$) (197). The effect of chronic lithium therapy has been studied in rat kidney membranes prepared from the inner medulla. It caused a marked downregulation of AQP2 and AQP3 (198), only partially reversed by cessation of therapy, dehydration, or dDAVP treatment, consistent with clinical observations of slow recovery from lithium-induced urinary concentrating defects (199). Downregulation of AQP2 has also been shown to be associated with the development of severe polyuria due to other causes of acquired NDI (hypokalemia [200,201], release of bilateral ureteral obstruction [202], and hypercalciuria [203]). Thus, AQP2 expression is severely downregulated in both congenital (74) and acquired NDI. More studies will be needed to determine whether nonpeptide vasopressin agonists, permeable cAMP-like compounds, or other signaling molecules will be able to restore AQP2 expression and function. In patients receiving long-term lithium therapy, amiloride has been proposed to prevent the uptake of lithium in the collecting ducts. Amiloride may thus prevent the inhibitory effect of intracellular lithium on water transport (204).

TABLE 86-3. *Acquired causes of nephrogenic diabetes insipidus*

Chronic renal disease
  Polycystic disease
  Medullary cystic disease
Pyelonephritis
  Ureteral obstruction
  Far-advanced renal failure
Electrolyte disorders
  Hypokalemia
  Hypercalcemia
Drugs
  Alcohol
  Phenytoin
  Lithium
  Demeclocycline
  Acetohexamide
  Tolazamide
  Glyburide
  Propoxyphene
  Amphotericin
  Foscarnet
  Methoxyflurane
  Norepinephrine
  Vinblastine
  Colchicine
  Gentamicin
  Methicillin
  Isophosphamide
  Angiographic dyes
  Osmotic diuretics
  Furosemide and ethacrynic acid
Sickle cell disease
Dietary abnormalities
  Excessive water intake
  Decreased sodium chloride intake
  Decreased protein intake
Miscellaneous
  Multiple myeloma
  Amyloidosis
  Sjögren's disease
  Sarcoidosis

Primary Polydipsia

Primary polydipsia is a state of hypotonic polyuria secondary to excessive fluid intake. Primary polydipsia was extensively studied by Barlow and de Wardener in 1959 (205); however, the understanding of the pathophysiology of this disease has made little progress over the past 30 years. Barlow and de Wardener (205) described seven women and two men who were compulsive water drinkers; their ages ranged from 48 to 59 years except for one patient who was 24. Eight of these patients had histories of previous psychological disorders, which ranged from delusions, depression, and agitation to frank hysterical behavior. The other patient appeared normal. The consumption of water fluctuated irregularly from hour to hour or from day to day; in some patients, there were remissions and relapses lasting several months or longer. In eight of the patients, the mean plasma osmolality was significantly lower than normal. Vasopressin tannate in oil made most of these patients feel ill; in one, it caused overhydration. In four patients, the fluid intake returned to normal after electroconvulsive therapy or a period of continuous narcosis; the improvement in three was transient, but in the fourth it lasted 2 years. Polyuric female subjects might be heterozygous for *de novo* or previously unrecognized *AVPR2* mutations or autosomal-dominant *AQP2* mutations (191) and may be classified as compulsive water drinkers (206). Therefore, the diagnosis of compulsive water drinking must be made with care and may represent our ignorance of yet undescribed pathophysiologic mechanisms. Robertson (206) has described under the term *dipsogenic diabetes insipidus* a selective defect in the osmoregulation of thirst. Three patients studied had under basal conditions of ad libitum water intake, thirst, polydipsia, polyuria, and high-normal plasma osmolality. They had a normal secretion of AVP, but osmotic threshold for thirst was abnormally low. Such cases of dipsogenic diabetes insipidus might represent up to 10% of all patients with diabetes insipidus (206).

Diabetes Insipidus and Pregnancy

Pregnancy in a Patient Known to have Diabetes Insipidus

An isolated deficiency of vasopressin without a concomitant loss of hormones in the anterior pituitary does not result in altered fertility, and with the exception of polyuria and polydipsia, gestation, delivery, and lactation are uncomplicated (207). Treated patients may require increasing dosages of desmopressin. The increased thirst may be due to a resetting of the thirst osmostat (208).

Increased polyuria also occurs during pregnancy in patients with partial NDI (209). These patients may be obligatory carriers of the NDI gene (210).

Syndromes of Diabetes Insipidus that Begin During Gestation and Remit After Delivery

Barron and associates (211) describe three pregnant women in whom transient diabetes insipidus developed late in gestation and subsequently remitted postpartum. In one of these patients, dilute urine was present in spite of high plasma concentrations of AVP. Hyposthenuria in all three patients was resistant to administered aqueous vasopressin. Since excessive vasopressinase activity was not excluded as a cause of this disorder, the Barron group labeled the disease vasopressin-resistant rather than NDI.

A well-documented case of enhanced activity of vasopressinase has been described in a woman in the third trimester of a previously uncomplicated pregnancy (212). She had massive polyuria and markedly elevated plasma vasopressinase activity. The polyuria did not respond to large intravenous doses of AVP but responded promptly to desmopressin, a vasopressinase-resistant analog of AVP. The polyuria disappeared with the disappearance of the vasopressinase. The incidence of vasopressinase-mediated, desmopressin-responsive diabetes insipidus is not known. However, a case of transient desmopressin-resistant diabetes

insipidus in a pregnant woman has been described recently (213). It is suggested that pregnancy may be associated with several different forms of diabetes insipidus, including central-, nephrogenic-, and vasopressinase-mediated (209).

DIFFERENTIAL DIAGNOSIS OF POLYURIC STATES

Plasma sodium and osmolality are maintained within normal limits (136 to 143 mmol/L for plasma sodium, 275 to 290 mmol/kg for plasma osmolality) by a thirst–ADH–renal axis. Thirst and ADH, both stimulated by increased osmolality, have been termed a "double-negative" feedback system (214). Thus, even when the ADH limb of this double-negative regulatory feedback system is lost, the thirst mechanism still preserves the plasma sodium and osmolality within the normal range but at the expense of pronounced polydipsia and polyuria. Thus, the plasma sodium concentration or osmolality of an untreated patient with diabetes insipidus may be slightly higher than the mean normal value, but since the values usually remain within the normal range, these small increases have no diagnostic significance.

Theoretically, it should be relatively easy to differentiate between central diabetes insipidus, NDI, and primary polydipsia. A comparison of the osmolality of urine obtained during dehydration from patients with central diabetes insipidus or NDI with that of urine obtained after the administration of AVP should reveal a rapid increase in osmolality only in the central diabetes insipidus patients. Urine osmolality should increase normally in response to moderate dehydration in primary polydipsia patients.

However, these distinctions may not be as clear as one might expect because of several factors (215). First, chronic polyuria of any etiology interferes with the maintenance of the medullary concentration gradient, and this "washout" effect diminishes the maximum concentrating ability of the kidney. The extent of the blunting varies in direct proportion to the severity of the polyuria and is independent of its cause. Hence, for any given level of basal urine output, the maximum urine osmolality achieved in the presence of saturating concentrations of AVP is depressed to the same extent in patients with primary polydipsia, central diabetes insipidus, and NDI (Fig. 86-12). Second, most patients with central diabetes insipidus maintain a small, but detectable capacity to secrete AVP during severe dehydration, and urine osmolality may then rise above plasma osmolality. Third, many patients with acquired NDI have an incomplete deficit in AVP action, and concentrated urine could again be obtained during dehydration testing. Finally, all polyuric states (whether central, nephrogenic, or psychogenic) can induce large dilations of the urinary tract and bladder (161,216,217) As a consequence, the urinary bladder of these patients may contain an increased residual capacity, and changes in urine osmolalities induced by diagnostic maneuvers might be difficult to demonstrate.

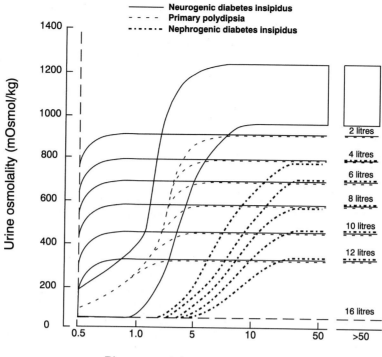

FIG. 86-12. The relationship between urine osmolality and plasma vasopressin in patients with polyuria of diverse etiology and severity. Note that for each of the three categories of polyuria (neurogenic diabetes insipidus, nephrogenic diabetes insipidus, and primary polydipsia), the relationship is described by a family of sigmoid curves that differ in height. These differences in height reflect differences in maximum concentrating capacity due to "washout" of the medullary concentration gradient. They are proportional to the severity of the underlying polyuria (indicated in L/day at the right end of each plateau) and are largely independent of the etiology. Thus, the three categories of diabetes insipidus differ principally in the submaximal or ascending portion of the dose-response curve. In patients with partial neurogenic diabetes insipidus, this part of the curve lies to the left of normal, reflecting increased sensitivity to the antidiuretic effects of very low concentrations of plasma AVP. In contrast, in patients with partial nephrogenic diabetes insipidus, this part of the curve lies to the right of normal, reflecting decreased sensitivity to the antidiuretic effects of normal concentrations of plasma arginine vasopressin (AVP). In primary polydipsia, this relationship is relatively normal. (From Robertson GL. Diagnosis of diabetes insipidus. In: Czernichow P, Robinson AG, eds. *Frontiers of hormone research*, vol 13, "Diabetes insipidus in man." Basel: Karger, 1985:176, with permission.)

Indirect Test

The measurements of urine osmolality after dehydration followed by vasopressin administration is usually referred to as "indirect testing" because vasopressin secretion is indirectly assessed through changes in urine osmolalities.

The patient is maintained on a complete fluid restriction regimen until urine osmolality reaches a plateau, as indicated by an hourly increase of less than 30 mmol/kg for at least 3 successive hours. After the plasma osmolality is measured, 5 U of aqueous vasopressin is administered subcutaneously. Urine osmolality is measured 30 and 60 minutes later. The last urine osmolality value obtained before the vasopressin injection and the highest value obtained after the injection are compared. The patients are then separated into five categories according to previously published criteria (20) (Table 86-4).

Direct Test

The two approaches of Zerbe and Robertson (19) are used. First, during the dehydration test, plasma is collected and assayed for vasopressin. The results are plotted on a nomogram depicting the normal relationship between plasma sodium or osmolality and plasma AVP in normal subjects (Fig. 86-5). If the relationship between plasma vasopressin and osmolality falls below the normal range, the disorder is diagnosed as central diabetes insipidus.

Second, partial NDI and primary polydipsia can be differentiated by analyzing the relationship between plasma AVP and urine osmolality at the end of the dehydration period (Figs. 86-5 and 86-12). However, a definitive differentiation between these two disorders might be impossible because a normal or even supranormal AVP response to increased plasma osmolality occurs in polydipsic patients. None of the

TABLE 86-4. *Urinary responses to fluid deprivation and exogenous vasopressin in recognition of partial defects in antidiuretic hormone secretion*

	No. of cases	Maximum U_{osm} with dehydration (mmol/kg)	U_{osm} after vasopressin (mmol/kg)	% Change (U_{osm})	U_{osm} increase after vasopressin (%)
Normal subjects	9	$1,068 \pm 69$	979 ± 79	-9 ± 3	<9
Complete central diabetes insipidus	18	168 ± 13	445 ± 52	183 ± 41	>50
Partial central diabetes insipidus	11	438 ± 34	549 ± 28	28 ± 5	>9 to <50
Nephrogenic diabetes insipidus	2	123.5	174.5	42	<50
Compulsive water drinking	7	738 ± 53	780 ± 73	5.0 ± 2.2	<9

(Data compiled from Miller M, et al. Recognition of partial defects in antidiuretic hormone secretion. *Ann Intern Med* 1970;73:721.)

patients with psychogenic or other forms of severe polydipsia studied by Robertson (215) have ever shown any evidence of pituitary suppression.

Zerbe and Robertson (19) found that in the differential diagnosis of polyuria, all seven of the cases of severe neurogenic diabetes insipidus diagnosed by the standard indirect test were confirmed when diagnosed by the plasma vasopressin assay. However, two of six patients diagnosed by the indirect test as having partial neurogenic diabetes insipidus had normal vasopressin secretion as measured by the direct assay; one was found to have primary polydipsia and the other NDI. Moreover, three of ten patients diagnosed as having primary polydipsia by the indirect test had clear evidence of partial vasopressin deficiency by the direct assay (19). These patients were thus wrongly diagnosed as primary polydipsic! A *combined* direct and indirect testing of the AVP function is described in Table 86-5.

Therapeutic Trial

In selected patients with an uncertain diagnosis, a closely monitored therapeutic trial of desmopressin (10 μg intranasally twice a day) may be used to distinguish partial NDI from partial neurogenic diabetes insipidus and primary polydipsia. If desmopressin at this dosage causes a significant antidiuretic effect, NDI is effectively excluded. If polydipsia as well as polyuria is abolished and plasma sodium does not fall below the normal range, the patient probably has central

TABLE 86-5. *Direct and indirect tests of arginine vasopressin function in patients with polyuria*

Measurements of arginine vasopressin (AVP) cannot be used in isolation but must be interpreted in light of four other factors:
    Clinical history
    Concurrent measurements of plasma osmolality, urine osmolality, and maximal urinary response to exogenous vasopressin in reference to the basal urine flow

(Data from Stern P, Valtin H. Verney was right, but . . . [Editorial]. *N Engl J Med* 1981;305:1581.)

diabetes insipidus. Conversely if desmopressin causes a reduction in urine output without a reduction in water intake and hyponatremia appears, the patient probably has primary polydipsia. Since fatal water intoxication is a remote possibility, the desmopressin trial should be carried out with close monitoring.

Recommendations

Table 86-6 lists recommendations for obtaining a differential diagnosis of diabetes insipidus (218).

TABLE 86-6. *Differential diagnosis of diabetes insipidus*

1. Measure plasma osmolality and/or sodium concentration under conditions of ad libitum fluid intake. If they are above 295 mmol/kg and 143 mmol/L, the diagnosis of primary polydipsia is excluded, and the workup should proceed directly to steps 5 and/or 6 to distinguish between neurogenic and nephrogenic diabetes insipidus. *Otherwise,*
2. Perform a dehydration test. If urinary concentration does not occur before plasma osmolality and/or sodium reach 295 mmol/kg or 143 mmol/L, the diagnosis of primary polydipsia is again excluded, and the workup should proceed to steps 5 and/or 6. *Otherwise,*
3. Determine the ratio of urine to plasma osmolality at the end of the dehydration test. If it is <1.5, the diagnosis of primary polydipsia is again excluded, and the workup should proceed to steps 5 and/or 6. *Otherwise,*
4. Perform a hypertonic saline infusion with measurements of plasma vasopressin and osmolality at intervals during the procedure. If the relationship between these two variables is subnormal, the diagnosis of diabetes insipidus is established. *Otherwise,*
5. Perform a vasopressin infusion test. If urine osmolality rises by more than 150 mOsm/kg above the value obtained at the end of the dehydration test, nephrogenic diabetes insipidus is excluded. *Alternately,*
6. Measure urine osmolality and plasma vasopressin at the end of the dehydration test. If the relationship is normal, the diagnosis of nephrogenic diabetes insipidus is excluded.

(Data from Robertson GL. Diseases of the posterior pituitary. In Felig D, et al., eds. *Endocrinology and metabolism.* New York: McGraw-Hill, 1981:251.)

Carrier Detection and Postnatal Diagnosis

As discussed earlier in this chapter, the identification, characterization, and mutation analysis of three different genes, namely, *prepro-AVP-NPII*, *AVPR2*, and the vasopressin-sensitive water channel gene (*AQP2*), provide the basis for the understanding of different hereditary forms of diabetes insipidus, autosomal-dominant and autosomal-recessive neurogenic diabetes insipidus, X-linked NDI, and autosomal-recessive or autosomal-dominant NDI, respectively. The identification of mutations in these three genes that cause diabetes insipidus enables the early diagnosis and management of at-risk members of families with identified mutations. Some patients with Bartter's syndrome secondary to mutations in the Na-K-2Cl cotransporter gene (*NKCC2*) may present with severe hypernatremia, hyperchloremia, and a low urine osmolality unresponsive to dDAVP (219). In these cases, the antenatal period is characterized by polyhydramnios. In my experience, perinatal polyuro–polydipsic patients with a mother's pregnancy characterized by polyhydramnios are likely not bearing *AVPR2* or *AQP2* mutations. We encourage physicians who follow families with X-linked NDI to recommend mutation analysis before the birth of a male infant because early diagnosis and treatment of male infants can avert the physical and mental retardation associated with episodes of dehydration. Diagnosis of X-linked NDI within 72 hours of birth was accomplished by mutation testing of a sample of cord blood (220). Early diagnosis of autosomal-recessive NDI is also essential for early treatment of affected infants to avoid repeated episodes of dehydration. Mutation detection in families with inherited neurogenic diabetes insipidus provides a powerful clinical tool for early diagnosis and management of subsequent cases, especially in early childhood when diagnosis is difficult and the clinical risks are the greatest (113).

RADIOIMMUNOASSAY OF ARGININE VASOPRESSIN AND OTHER LABORATORY DETERMINATIONS

Radioimmunoassay of Arginine Vasopressin

Three developments were basic to the elaboration of a clinically useful radioimmunoassay for plasma AVP (221,222): (a) the extraction of AVP from plasma with petrol-ether and acetone and the subsequent elimination of nonspecific immunoreactivity; (b) the use of highly specific and sensitive rabbit antiserum; and (c) the use of a tracer (^{125}I-AVP) with high specific activity. More than 25 years later, the same extraction procedures are widely used (223–226), and commercial tracers (^{125}I-AVP) and antibodies are available. AVP can also be extracted from plasma by using Sep-Pak C18 cartridges (227–229).

Blood samples collected in chilled 7-mL lavender-stoppered tubes containing ethylenediaminetetraacetic acid (EDTA) are centrifuged at 4°C, 1,000 g (3,000 rpm in a usual laboratory centrifuge), for 20 minutes. This 20-minute cen-

TABLE 86-7. *Arginine vasopressin measurements: sample preparation*

4°C—blood in EDTA tubes
Centrifugation 1,000 g × 20 min
Plasma frozen −20°C
Extraction:
    2 mL acetone + 1 mL plasma
    1,000 g × 30 min 4°C
    Supernatant + 5 mL of petrol-ether
    1,000 g × 20 min 4°C
    Freeze −80°C
    Throw nonfrozen upper phase
    Evaporate lower phase to dryness
    Store desiccated samples at −20°C

EDTA, ethylenediaminetetraacetic acid

trifugation is mandatory for obtaining platelet-poor plasma samples because a large fraction of the circulating vasopressin is associated with the platelets in humans (224,230). The tubes may be kept for 2 hours on slushed ice prior to centrifugation. Plasma is then separated, frozen at −20°C, and extracted within 6 weeks of sampling. Details for sample preparation (Table 86-7) and assay procedure (Table 86-8) can be found in writings by Bichet and colleagues (223,224). An AVP radioimmunoassay should be validated by demonstrating (a) a good correlation between plasma sodium or osmolality and plasma AVP during dehydration and infusion of hypertonic saline solution (Fig. 86-5) and (b) the inability to obtain detectable values of AVP in patients with severe central diabetes insipidus. Plasma AVP immunoreactivity may be elevated in patients with diabetes insipidus following hypothalamic surgery (231).

In pregnant patients, the blood contains high concentrations of cystine aminopeptidase, which can (*in vitro*) inactivate enormous quantities (ng $\times$ mL^{-1} $\times$ min^{-1}) of AVP. However, phenanthroline effectively inhibits these cystine aminopeptidases (Table 89-9).

Aquaporin-2 Measurements

Urinary AQP2 excretion could be measured by radioimmunoassay (74) or quantitative Western analysis (75) and could provide an additional indication of the responsiveness of the collecting duct to AVP (75,76).

TABLE 86-8. *Arginine vasopressin measurements: assay procedure*

Day 1	Assay setup
	400 µL/tube (200-µL sample or standard + 200 µL of antiserum or buffer)
	Incubation 80 h, 4°C
Day 4	^{125}I-AVP
	100 µL/tube
	1,000 cpm/tube
	Incubation 72 h, 4°C
Day 7	Separation dextran + charcoal

^{125}*I-AVP*, iodine 125 = arginine vasopressin

TABLE 86-9. *Measurements of arginine vasopressin levels in pregnant patients*

1,10-phenanthroline monohydrate (Sigma) 60 mg/mL–solubilized with several drops of glacial acetic acid 0.1 mL/10 mL of blood

Data from Davison JM, et al. Altered osmotic thresholds for vasopressin secretion and thirst in human pregnancy. *Am J Physiol* 1984;246:F105.

Plasma Sodium and Plasma and Urine Osmolality Measurements

Measurements of plasma sodium and plasma and urine osmolality should be immediately available at various intervals during dehydration procedures. Plasma sodium is easily measured by flame photometry or with a sodium-specific electrode (232). Plasma and urine osmolalities are also reliably measured by freezing point depression instruments with a coefficient of variation at 290 mmol/kg of less than 1%.

In our clinical research unit, plasma sodium and plasma and urine osmolalities are measured at the beginning of each dehydration procedure and at regular intervals (usually hourly) thereafter, depending on the severity of the polyuric syndrome explored.

In one case, an 8-year-old patient (31-kg body weight) with a clinical diagnosis of congenital NDI (later found to bear the *de novo AVPR2* mutant *274insG* [155]) continued to excrete large volumes of urine (300 mL/hour) during a short 4-hour dehydration test. During this time, the patient was suffering from severe thirst, his plasma sodium was 155 mEq/L, his plasma osmolality was 310 mmol/kg, and his urine osmolality was 85 mmol/kg. The patient received 1 μg of desmopressin intravenously and was allowed to drink water. Repeated urine osmolality measurements demonstrated a complete urinary resistance to desmopressin.

It would have been dangerous and unnecessary to prolong the dehydration further in this young patient. Thus, the usual prescription of overnight dehydration should not be used in patients, and especially children, with severe polyuria and polydipsia (more than 4 L/day). Great care should be taken to avoid any severe hypertonic state arbitrarily defined as a plasma sodium greater than 155 mEq/L.

At variance with published data (19,224), we have found that plasma and serum osmolalities are equivalent (i.e., similar values are obtained). Blood taken in heparinized tubes is easier to handle because the plasma can be more readily removed after centrifugation. The tube used (green-stoppered tube) contains a minuscule concentration of lithium and sodium, which does not interfere with plasma sodium or osmolality measurements. Frozen plasma or urine samples can be kept for further analysis of their osmolalities because the results obtained are similar to those obtained immediately after blood sampling, except in patients with severe renal failure. In the latter patients, plasma osmolality measurements are increased after freezing and thawing, but the plasma sodium values remain unchanged.

Plasma osmolality measurements can be used to demonstrate the absence of unusual osmotically active substances (e.g., glucose and urea in high concentrations, mannitol, ethanol) (233). With this information, plasma or serum sodium measurements are sufficient to assess the degree of dehydration and its relationship to plasma AVP. Nomograms describing the normal plasma sodium-plasma AVP relationship (Fig. 86-2) are equally as valuable as "classical" nomograms describing the relationship between plasma osmolality and effective osmolality (i.e., plasma osmolality minus the contribution of "ineffective" solutes: glucose and urea).

MAGNETIC RESONANCE IMAGING IN PATIENTS WITH DIABETES INSIPIDUS

Magnetic resonance imaging (MRI) permits visualization of the anterior and posterior pituitary glands and the pituitary stalk. The pituitary stalk is permeated by numerous capillary loops of the hypophyseal–portal blood system. This vascular structure also provides the principal blood supply to the anterior pituitary lobe, as there is no direct arterial supply to this organ. In contrast, the posterior pituitary lobe has a direct vascular supply. Therefore, the posterior lobe can be more rapidly visualized in a dynamic mode after administration of a gadolinium (gadopentetate dimeglumine) as contrast material during MRI. The posterior pituitary lobe is easily distinguished by a round, high-intensity signal (the posterior pituitary "bright spot") in the posterior part of the sella turcica on T1-weighted images. This round, high-intensity signal is usually absent in patients with central diabetes insipidus (99). MRI is reported to be "the best technique" with which to evaluate the pituitary stalk and infundibulum in patients with idiopathic polyuria. Thus, the absence of posterior pituitary hyperintensity, although nonspecific, is a cardinal feature of central diabetes insipidus. In the five patients who did have posterior pituitary hyperintensity at diagnosis, this feature invariably disappeared during follow-up (99). Thickening of either the entire pituitary stalk or just the proximal portion was the second most common abnormality on MRI scans (99).

Treatment

In most patients with complete hypothalamic diabetes insipidus, the thirst mechanism remains intact. Thus, these patients do not develop hypernatremia and suffer only from the inconvenience associated with marked polyuria and polydipsia. If hypodipsia develops or access to water is limited, then severe hypernatremia can supervene. The treatment of choice for patients with severe hypothalamic diabetes insipidus is desmopressin, a synthetic, long-acting vasopressin analog, with minimal vasopressor activity but a large antidiuretic potency. The usual intranasal daily dose is between 5 and 20 μg. To avoid the potential complication of dilutional hyponatremia, which is exceptional in these patients due to an intact thirst mechanism, desmopressin can be withdrawn at regular intervals to allow the patients to become polyuric. Aqueous vasopressin (Pitressin) or desmopressin (4.0 μg/1-mL ampule) can be used intravenously in acute situations such as after hypophysectomy or for the treatment of diabetes insipidus in the brain-dead organ donor. Pitressin tannate in oil and nonhormonal antidiuretic drugs are somewhat obsolete and rarely used. For example, chlorpropamide (250 to 500 mg daily) appears to potentiate the antidiuretic action of circulating AVP, but troublesome side effects of hypoglycemia and hyponatremia do occur.

The treatment of congenital NDI has been reviewed (161, 234,235). An abundant unrestricted water intake should always be provided, and affected patients should be carefully followed during their first years of life. Water should be offered every 2 hours day and night, and temperature, appetite, and growth should be monitored. The parents of these children easily accept setting their alarm clock every 2 hours during the night. Hospital admission may be necessary to allow continuous gastric feeding. A low-osmolar and low-sodium diet, hydrochlorothiazide (1 to 2 mg/kg/day) alone or with amiloride (20 mg/1.73 m^2 per day), and indomethacin (0.75 to 1.5 mg/kg) substantially reduce water excretion and are helpful in the treatment of children. Prostaglandin-synthetase inhibitors should only be used for short periods because of possible deleterious effects of their chronic administration. Initial nausea may occur in some patients who start on amiloride, but it is generally transient and rarely a reason to discontinue therapy (161). Many adult patients receive no treatment at all.

ACKNOWLEDGMENTS

The author work cited in this chapter is supported by the Canadian Institutes of Health Research, the Canadian Kidney Foundation, the Fonds de la Recherche en Santé du Québec and by la Fondation J. Rodolphe-La Haye. Dr. Daniel G. Bichet is a Career Investigator of le Fonds de la Recherche en Santé du Québec.

REFERENCES

1. Richter D. Molecular events in the expression of vasopressin and oxytocin and their cognate receptors. *Am J Physiol* 255:1988;F207.
2. Rao VV, et al. The human gene for oxytocin-neurophysin I (OXT) is physically mapped to chromosome 20p13 by in situ hybridization. *Cell Genet* 1992;61:271.
3. Chen L, et al. Crystal structure of a bovine neurophysin II dipeptide complex at 2.8 Angström determined from the single-wave length anomalous scattering signal of an incorporated iodine atom. *Proc Natl Acad Sci USA* 1991;88:4240.
4. Swaab DF, Pool CW, Nijveldt F. Immunofluorescence of vasopressin and oxytocin in the rat hypothalamo-neurohypophyseal system. *J Neural Transm* 1975;36:195.
5. Vandesande F, Dierickx K. Identification of the vasopressin producing and of the oxytocin producing neurons in the hypothalamic magnocellular neurosecretory system of the rat. *Cell Tissue Res* 1975;164:153.
6. Sofroniew MV. Morphology of vasopressin and oxytocin neurones and their central and vascular projections. In: Cross L, ed. *The neurohypophysis: structure, function, and control*, vol 60. New York: Elsevier, 1983:101.
7. Kalogeras KT, et al. Inferior petrosal sinus sampling in healthy human subjects reveals a unilateral corticotropin-releasing hormone-induced arginine vasopressin release associated with ipsilateral adrenocorticotropin secretion. *J Clin Invest* 1996;97:2045.
8. Yanovski JA, et al. Inferior petrosal sinus AVP in patients with Cushing's syndrome. *Clin Endocrinol (Oxf)* 1997;47:199.
9. Robertson GL, Berl T. Pathophysiology of water metabolism. In: Brenner BM, Rector FC, eds. *The kidney*, 5th ed. Philadelphia: WB Saunders, 1996:873.
10. Thrasher TN, et al. Thirst and vasopressin release in the dog: an osmoreceptor or sodium receptor mechanism? *Am J Physiol* 1980;238: R333.
11. Olsson K, Kolmodin R. Dependence of basic secretion of antidiuretic hormone on cerebrospinal fluid (Na+). *Acta Physiol Scand* 1974; 91:286.
12. Leng G, Dyball RE, Luckman SM. Mechanisms of vasopressin secretion. *Horm Res* 1992;37:33.
13. Bourque CW, Oliet SHR, Richard D. Osmoreceptors, osmoreception, and osmoregulation. *Front Neuroendocrinol* 1994;15:231.
14. Bourque CW, Oliet SHR. Osmoreceptors in the central nervous system. *Annu Rev Physiol* 1997;59:601.
15. Voisin DL, Chakfe Y, Bourque CW. Coincident detection of CSF Na+ and osmotic pressure in osmoregulatory neurons of the supraoptic nucleus. *Neuron* 1999;24:453.
16. Verney E. The antidiuretic hormone and the factors which determine its release. *Proc R Soc London Ser B* 1947;135: 25.
17. Thrasher TN, Ramsey DJ. Anatomy of osmoreception. In: Jard S, Jamison R, eds. *Vasopressin*, vol 208. Paris: Colloques INSERM/John Libbey Eurotext, 1991:267.
18. Liedtke W, et al. Vanilloid receptor-related osmotically activated channel (VR-OAC), a candidate vertebrate osmoreceptor. *Cell* 2000; 103:525.
19. Zerbe RL, Robertson GL. A comparison of plasma vasopressin measurements with a standard indirect test in the differential diagnosis of polyuria. *N Engl J Med* 1981;305:1539.
20. Miller M, et al. Recognition of partial defects in antidiuretic hormone secretion. *Ann Intern Med* 1970;73:721.
21. Bichet DG, et al. Hyponatremic states. In: Seldin DW, Giebisch G, eds. *The kidney: physiology and pathophysiology*, 2nd ed. New York: Raven Press, 1992:1727.
22. Baylis PH, Gaskill MB, Robertson GL. Vasopressin secretion in primary polydipsia and cranial diabetes insipidus. *Q J Med* 1981;50:345.
23. Rolls B, Rolls E. *Thirst: problems in the behavioural sciences*. Cambridge, UK: Cambridge University Press, 1982.
24. Fitzsimons JT. Angiotensin, thirst, and sodium appetite. *Physiol Rev* 1998;78:583.
25. Nimura F, et al. Gene targeting in mice reveals a requirement for angiotensin in the development and maintenance of kidney morphology and growth factor regulation. *J Clin Invest* 1995;96:2947.
26. Ito M, et al. Regulation of blood pressure by the type 1A angiotensin II receptor gene. *Proc Natl Acad Sci USA* 1995;92:3521.
27. Sugaya T, et al. Angiotensin II type 1a receptor-deficient mice with hypotension and hyperreninemia. *J Biol Chem* 1995;270:18719.
28. Hein L, et al. Behavioural and cardiovascular effects of disrupting the angiotensin II type-2 receptor gene in mice. *Nature* 1995;377:744.
29. Samson WK. Atrial natriuretic factor inhibits dehydration and hemorrhage-induced vasopressin release. *Neuroendocrinology* 1985; 40:277.
30. Goetz KL, et al. Effects of atriopeptin infusion versus effects of left atrial stretch in awake dogs. *Am J Physiol* 1986;250:R221.
31. Ogawa K, et al. Lack of effect of atrial natriuretic peptide on vasopressin release. *Clin Sci* 1987;72:525.
32. Abelson JL, Le Mellédo J-M, Bichet DG. Dose response of arginine vasopressin to the CCK-B agonist pentagastrin. *Neuropsychopharmacology* 2001;24:161.
33. Ota M, et al. Evidence that nitric oxide can act centrally to stimulate vasopressin release. *Neuroendocrinology* 1993;57:955.
34. Yasin S, et al. Nitric oxide modulates the release of vasopressin from rat hypothalamic explants. *Endocrinology* 1993;133:1466.
35. Kadowaki K, et al. Up-regulation of nitric oxide synthase (NOS) gene expression together with NOS activity in the rat hypothalamo-hypophyseal system after chronic salt loading: evidence of a neuromodulatory role of nitric oxide in arginine vasopressin and oxytocin secretion. *Endocrinology* 1994;134:1011.

36. Wang H, Morris JF. Constitutive nitric oxide synthase in hypothalami of normal and hereditary diabetes insipidus rats and mice: role of nitric oxide in osmotic regulation and its mechanism. *Endocrinology* 1996;137:1745.

37. Raff H. Glucocorticoid inhibition of neurohypophyseal vasopressin secretion. *Am J Physiol* 1987;252:R635.

38. Rowe JW, et al. Influence of the emetic reflex on vasopressin release in man. *Kidney Int* 1979;16:729.

39. Jard S, et al. Vasopressin and oxytocin receptors: an overview. In: Imura H, Shizume K, eds. *Progress in endocrinology.* Amsterdam: Elsevier Science Publishers B.V., 1988:1183.

40. Nathanson MH, et al. Mechanisms of subcellular cytosolic Ca2+ signaling evoked by stimulation of the vasopressin V1a receptor. *J Biol Chem* 1992;267:23282.

41. Birnbaumer M, et al. Molecular cloning of the receptor for human antidiuretic hormone. *Nature* 1992;357:333.

42. Seibold A, et al. Structure and chromosomal localization of the human antidiuretic hormone receptor gene. *Am J Hum Genet* 1992;51:1078.

43. Watson S, Arkinstall S. *The G protein linked receptor factsbook.* London: Academic Press, 1994.

44. Preston GM, et al. Appearance of water channels in *Xenopus* oocytes expressing red cell CHIP28 protein. *Science* 1992;256:385.

45. Denker BM, et al. Identification, purification, and partial characterization of a novel Mr 28,000 integral membrane protein from erythrocytes and renal tubules. *J Biol Chem* 1988;263:15634.

46. Sabolic I, et al. Localization of the CHIP28 water channel in rat kidney. *Am J Physiol* 1992;263:C1225.

47. Nielsen S, et al. CHIP28 water channels are localized in constitutively water-permeable segments of the nephron. *J Cell Biol* 1993;120:371.

48. Nielsen S, Agre P. The aquaporin family of water channels in kidney. *Kidney Int* 1995;48:1057.

49. Murata K, et al. Structural determinants of water permeation through aquaporin-1. *Nature* 2000;407:599.

50. Verkman AS, Mitra AK. Structure and function of aquaporin water channels. *Am J Physiol Renal Physiol* 2000;278:F13.

51. Pomes R, Roux B. Structure and dynamics of a proton wire: a theoretical study of H+ translocation along the single-file water chain in the gramicidin A channel. *Biophys J* 1996;71:19.

52. Wade JB, Stetson DL, Lewis SA. ADH action: evidence for a membrane shuttle mechanism. *Ann NY Acad Sci* 1981;372:106.

53. Knepper MA. Molecular physiology of urinary concentrating mechanism: regulation of aquaporin water channels by vasopressin. *Am J Physiol* 1997;272:F3.

54. Fushimi K, Sasaki S, Marumo F. Phosphorylation of serine 256 is required for cAMP-dependent regulatory exocytosis of the aquaporin-2 water channel. *J Biol Chem* 1997;272:14800.

55. Katsura T, et al. Protein kinase A phosphorylation is involved in regulated exocytosis of aquaporin-2 in transfected LLC-PK1 cells. *Am J Physiol* 1997;272:F817.

56. Valenti G, et al. A heterotrimeric G protein of the Gi family is required for cAMP-triggered trafficking of aquaporin 2 in kidney epithelial cells. *J Biol Chem* 1998;273:22627.

57. Mandon B, et al. Expression of syntaxins in rat kidney. *Am J Physiol* 1997;273:F718.

58. Jo I, et al. Rat kidney papilla contains abundant synaptobrevin protein that participates in the fusion of antidiuretic hormone-regulated water channel-containing endosomes in vitro. *Proc Natl Acad Sci USA* 1995;92:1876.

59. Liebenhoff U, Rosenthal W. Identification of Rab3-, Rab5a- and synaptobrevin II-like proteins in a preparation of rat kidney vesicles containing the vasopressin-regulated water channel. *FEBS Lett* 1995;365:209.

60. Nielsen S, et al. Expression of VAMP-2-like protein in kidney collecting duct intracellular vesicles. Colocalization with aquaporin-2 water channels. *J Clin Invest* 1995;96:1834.

61. Star RA, et al. Calcium and cyclic adenosine monophosphate as second messengers for vasopressin in the rat inner medullary collecting duct. *J Clin Invest* 1988;81:1879,.

62. Snyder HM, Noland TD, Breyer MD. cAMP-dependent protein kinase mediates hydroosmotic effect of vasopressin in collecting duct. *Am J Physiol* 1992;263:C147.

63. Brown D, Katsura T, Gustafson CE. Cellular mechanisms of aquaporin trafficking. *Am J Physiol* 1998;275:F328.

64. Taylor A, et al. Vasopressin: possible role of microtubules and microfilaments in its action. *Science* 1973;181:347.

65. Sabolic I, et al. The AQP2 water channel: effect of vasopressin treatment, microtubule disruption, and distribution in neonatal rats. *J Membr Biol* 1995;143:165,1995.

66. Shayakul C, Steel A, Hediger MA. Molecular cloning and characterization of the vasopressin-regulated urea transporter of rat kidney collecting ducts. *J Clin Invest* 1996;98:2580.

67. Ward DT, Hammond TG, Harris HW. Modulation of vasopressin-elicited water transport by trafficking of aquaporin-2-containing vesicles. *Annu Rev Physiol* 1999;61:683.

68. Fleming EF, et al. Urinary concentrating function in mice lacking EP3 receptors for prostaglandin E2. *Am J Physiol* 1998;275:F955.

69. Sands JM, et al. Apical extracellular calcium/polyvalent cation-sensing receptor regulates vasopressin-elicited water permeability in rat kidney inner medullary collecting duct. *J Clin Invest* 1997;99:1399.

70. Fushimi K, et al. Cloning and expression of apical membrane water channel of rat kidney collecting tubule. *Nature* 1993;361:549.

71. Deen PMT, et al. Requirement of human renal water channel aquaporin-2 for vasopressin-dependent concentration of urine. *Science* 1994;264:92.

72. Sasaki S, et al. Cloning, characterization, and chromosomal mapping of human aquaporin of collecting duct. *J Clin Invest* 1994;93:1250.

73. Deen PMT, et al. Assignment of the human gene for the water channel of renal collecting duct aquaporin 2 (AQP2) to chromosome 12 region q12->q13. *Cytogenet Cell Genet* 1994;66:260.

74. Kanno K, et al. Urinary excretion of aquaporin-2 in patients with diabetes insipidus. *N Engl J Med* 1995;332:1540.

75. Elliot S, et al. Urinary excretion of aquaporin-2 in humans: a potential marker of collecting duct responsiveness to vasopressin. *J Am Soc Nephrol* 1996;7:403.

76. Saito T, et al. Urinary excretion of aquaporin-2 in the diagnosis of central diabetes insipidus. *J Clin Endocrinol Metab* 1997;82:1823.

77. Ma T, et al. Generation and phenotype of a transgenic knockout mouse lacking the mercurial-insensitive water channel aquaporin-4. *J Clin Invest* 1997;100:957.

78. Ma T, et al. Severely impaired urinary concentrating ability in transgenic mice lacking aquaporin-1 water channels. *J Biol Chem* 1998;273:4296.

79. Matsumura Y, et al. Overt nephrogenic diabetes insipidus in mice lacking the CLC-K1 chloride channel. *Nat Genet* 1999;21:95.

80. Chou C-L, et al. Reduced water permeability and altered ultrastructure in thin descending limb of Henle in aquaporin-1 null mice. *J Clin Invest* 1999;103:491.

81. Ma T, et al. Nephrogenic diabetes insipidus in mice lacking aquaporin-3 water channels. *Proc Natl Acad Sci USA* 2000;97:4386.

82. Takahashi N, et al. Uncompensated polyuria in a mouse model of Bartter's syndrome. *Proc Natl Acad Sci USA* 2000;97:5434.

83. Yun J, et al. Generation and phenotype of mice harboring a nonsense mutation in the V2 vasopressin receptor gene. *J Clin Invest* 2000;106:1361.

84. Yang B, et al. Neonatal mortality in an aquaporin-2 knock-in mouse model of recessive nephrogenic diabetes insipidus. *J Biol Chem* 2000;276:2775.

85. Okubo S, et al. Angiotensinogen gene null-mutant mice lack homeostatic regulation of glomerular filtration and tubular reabsorption. *Kidney Int* 1998;53:617.

86. Rao S, Verkman AS. Analysis of organ physiology in transgenic mice. *Am J Physiol Cell Physiol* 2000;279:C1.

87. Preston GM, et al. Mutations in aquaporin-1 in phenotypically normal humans without functional CHIP water channels. *Science* 1994;265:1585.

88. Mulders SB, et al. New mutations in the AQP2 gene in nephrogenic diabetes insipidus resulting in functional but misrouted water channels. *J Am Soc Nephrol* 1997;8:242.

89. Schmale H, Richter D. Single base deletion in the vasopressin gene is the cause of diabetes insipidus in Brattleboro rats. *Nature* 1984;308:705.

90. Serradeil-Le Gal C, et al. Characterization of SR 121463A, a highly potent and selective, orally active vasopressin V2 receptor antagonist. *J Clin Invest* 1996;98:2729.

91. Balment RJ, Brimble MJ, Forsling ML. Oxytocin release and renal actions in normal and Brattleboro rats. *Ann NY Acad Sci USA* 1982;394:241.

92. Chou CL, et al. Oxytocin as an antidiuretic hormone II. Role of V2 vasopressin receptor. *Am J Physiol (Renal Fluid Electrolyte Physiol 38)* 1995;269:F78.

93. Bichet DG, et al. Hereditary central diabetes insipidus: autosomal dominant and autosomal recessive phenotypes due to mutations in the prepro-AVP-NPII gene. *J Am Soc Nephrol* 1998;9:386A.

94. Willcutts MD, Felner E, White PC. Autosomal recessive familial neurohypophyseal diabetes insipidus with continued secretion of mutant weakly active vasopressin. *Hum Mol Genet* 1999;8:1303.

95. Verbalis JG, Robinson AG, Moses AM. Postoperative and post-traumatic diabetes insipidus. In: Czernichow P, Robinson AG, eds. *Frontiers of hormone research*, vol 13, "Diabetes insipidus in man." Basel: Karger, 1985:247.

96. Olson BR, et al. Pathophysiology of hyponatremia after transsphenoidal pituitary surgery. *J Neurosurg* 1997;87:499.

97. Czernichow P, et al. Neurogenic diabetes insipidus in children. In: Czernichow P, Robinson AG, eds. *Frontiers of hormone research*, vol 13, "Diabetes insipidus in man." Basel: Karger, 1985:190.

98. Greger NG, et al. Central diabetes insipidus. 22 years' experience. *Am J Dis Child* 1986;140:551.

99. Maghnie M, et al. Central diabetes insipidus in children and young adults. *N Engl J Med* 2000;343:998.

100. Moses AM, Blumenthal SA, Streeten DHP. Acid-base and electrolyte disorders associated with endocrine disease: pituitary and thyroid. In: Arieff AI, de Fronzo RA, eds. *Fluid, electrolyte and acid-base disorders*. New York: Churchill Livingstone, 1985:851.

101. Birnbaum DC, et al. Idiopathic central diabetes insipidus followed by progressive spastic cerebral ataxia. Report of four cases. *Arch Neurol* 1989;46:1001.

102. Bullmann C, et al. Five cases with central diabetes insipidus and hypogonadism as first presentation of neurosarcoidosis. *Eur J Endocrinol* 2000;142:365.

103. Vokes TJ, Gaskill MB, Robertson GL. Antibodies to vasopressin in patients with diabetes insipidus. Implications for diagnosis and therapy. *Ann Intern Med* 1988;108:190.

104. Bichet DG, et al. A specific antibody to vasopressin in a man with concomitant resistance to treatment with Pitressin. *Clin Chem* 1986; 32:211.

105. Kaltsas GA, et al. Hypothalamo-pituitary abnormalities in adult patients with Langerhans' cell histiocytosis: clinical, endocrinological, and radiological features and response to treatment. *J Clin Endocrinol Metab* 2000;85:1370.

106. Lacombe UL. De la polydipsie [Thesis of Medicine, no. 99]. Imprimerie et Fonderie de Rignoux; Paris, 1841.

107. Weil A. Ueber die hereditare form des diabetes insipidus. Archives fur pathologische anatomie und physiologie and fur klinische medicine. *Virchow's Arch* 1884;95:70.

108. Weil A. Ueber die hereditare form des diabetes insipidus. *Deutches Archiv fur Klinische Medizin* 1908;93:180.

109. Camerer JW. Eine ergänzung des Weilschen diabetes-insipidus-stammbaumes. *Archiv för Rassen-und Gesellschaftshygiene Biologie* 1935;28:382.

110. Dölle W. Eine weitere ergänzung des weilschen diabetes-insipidus-stammbaumes. Zeitschrift für Menschliche Vererbungs-und Konstitutionslehre 1951;30:372.

111. Repaske DR, et al. Molecular analysis of autosomal dominant neurohypophyseal diabetes insipidus. *J Clin Endocrinol Metab* 1990;70: 752.

112. OMIM. Online Mendelian Inheritance in Man OMIM™. Baltimore: Center for Medical Genetics, Johns Hopkins University and Bethesda, MD: National Center for Biotechnology Information, National Library of Medicine, 1997. http://www.ncbi.nlm.nih.gov/omim/.

113. Rittig R, et al. Identification of 13 new mutations in the vasopressin–neurophysin II gene in 17 kindreds with familial autosomal dominant neurohypophyseal diabetes insipidus. *Am J Hum Genet* 1996;58: 107.

114. Rutishauser J, et al. A novel point mutation in the translation initiation codon of the pre- pro-vasopressin-neurophysin II gene: cosegregation with morphological abnormalities and clinical symptoms in autosomal dominant neurohypophyseal diabetes insipidus. *J Clin Endocrinol Metab* 1996;81:192.

115. Rittig S, et al. Familial neurohypophyseal diabetes insipidus due to mutation that substitutes histidine for tyrosine-2 in the antidiuretic hormone. *J Invest Med* 1996;44:387A.

116. Ito M, et al. Possible involvement of inefficient cleavage of preprovasopressin by signal peptidase as a cause for familial central diabetes insipidus. *J Clin Invest* 1993;91:2565.

117. Krishnamani MRS, Phillips JAI, Copeland KC. Detection of a novel arginine vasopressin defect by dideoxy fingerprinting. *J Clin Endocrinol Metab* 1993;77:596.

118. McLeod JF, et al. Familial neurohypophyseal diabetes insipidus associated with a signal peptide mutation. *J Clin Endocrinol Metab* 1993;77:599A.

119. Repaske DR, et al. Recurrent mutations in the vasopressin-neurophysin II gene cause autosomal dominant neurohypophyseal diabetes insipidus. *J Clin Endocrinol Metab* 1996;81:2328.

120. Repaske DR, et al. Heterogeneity in clinical manifestation of autosomal dominant neurohypophyseal diabetes insipidus caused by a mutation encoding Ala-1->Val in the signal peptide of the arginine vasopressin/neurophysin II/copeptin precursor. *J Clin Endocrinol Metab* 1997;82:51.

121. Heppner C, et al. Identification of mutations of the arginine vasopressin-neurophysin II gene in two kindreds with familial central diabetes insipidus. *J Clin Endocrinol Metab* 1998;83:693.

122. Bahnsen U, et al. A missense mutation in the vasopressin-neurophysin precursor gene cosegregates with human autosomal dominant neurohypophyseal diabetes insipidus. *EMBO J* 1992;11:19.

123. Gagliardi PC, Bernasconi S, Repaske DR. Autosomal dominant neurohypophyseal diabetes insipidus associated with a missense mutation encoding Gly23->Val in neurophysin II. *J Clin Endocrinol Metab* 1997;82:3643.

124. Repaske DR, Browning JE. A de novo mutation in the coding sequence for neurophysin-II (Pro24->Leu) is associated with onset and transmission of autosomal dominant neurohypophyseal diabetes insipidus. *J Clin Endocrinol Metab* 1994;79:421.

125. Yuasa H, et al. Glu-47, which forms a salt bridge between neurophysin-II and arginine vasopressin, is deleted in patients with familial central diabetes insipidus. *J Clin Endocrinol Metab* 1993;77:600.

126. Ito M, et al. A single base substitution in the coding region for neurophysin II associated with familial central diabetes insipidus. *J Clin Invest* 1991;87:725.

127. Nagasaki H, et al. Two novel mutations in the coding region for neurophysin-II associated with familial central diabetes insipidus. *J Clin Endocrinol Metab* 1995;80:1352.

128. Ueta Y, et al. A new type of familial central diabetes insipidus caused by a single base substitution in the neurophysin II coding region of the vasopressin gene. *J Clin Endocrinol Metab* 1996;81:1787.

129. Beuret N, et al. Mechanism of endoplasmic reticulum retention of mutant vasopressin precursor caused by a signal peptide truncation associated with diabetes insipidus. *J Biol Chem* 1999;274:18965.

130. Calvo B, et al. Identification of a novel nonsense mutation and a missense substitution in the vasopressin-neurophysin II gene in two Spanish kindreds with familial neurohypophyseal diabetes insipidus. *J Clin Endocrinol Metab* 1998;83:995.

131. Calvo B, et al. Molecular analysis in familial neurohypophyseal diabetes insipidus: early diagnosis of an asymptomatic carrier. *J Clin Endocrinol Metab* 1999;84:3351.

132. Siggaard C, et al. Clinical and molecular evidence of abnormal processing and trafficking of the vasopressin preprohormone in a large kindred with familial neurohypophyseal diabetes insipidus due to a signal peptide mutation. *J Clin Endocrinol Metab* 1999;84:2933.

133. Fujii H, Iida S, Moriwaki K. Familial neurohypophyseal diabetes insipidus associated with a novel mutation in the vasopressin-neurophysin II gene. *Int J Mol Med* 2000;5:229.

134. Rutishauser J, et al. A novel mutation (R97C) in the neurophysin moiety of prepro- vasopressin-neurophysin II associated with autosomal-dominant neurohypophyseal diabetes insipidus. *Mol Genet Metab* 1999;67:89.

135. Grant FD, et al. Two novel mutations of the vasopressin gene associated with familial diabetes insipidus and identification of an asymptomatic carrier infant. *J Clin Endocrinol Metab* 1998;83:3958.

136. Abbes AP, et al. Identification of two distinct mutations at the same nucleotide position, concomitantly with a novel polymorphism in the vasopressin-neurophysin II gene (AVP-NP II) in two Dutch families with familial neurohypophyseal diabetes insipidus. *Clin Chem* 2000;46:1699.

137. Ito M, Jameson JL, Ito M. Molecular basis of autosomal dominant neurohypophyseal diabetes insipidus. Cellular toxicity caused by the

accumulation of mutant vasopressin precursors within the endoplasmic reticulum. *J Clin Invest* 1997;99:1897.

138. Ito M, Yu RN, Jameson JL. Mutant vasopressin precursors that cause autosomal dominant neurohypophyseal diabetes insipidus retain dimerization and impair the secretion of wild- type proteins. *J Biol Chem* 1999;274:9029.

139. Bross P, et al. Protein misfolding and degradation in genetic diseases. *Hum Mutat* 1999;14:186.

140. Welch WJ, Howard M. Commentary: antagonists to the rescue. *J Clin Invest* 2000;105:853.

141. Peden NR, et al. Wolfram (DIDMOAD) syndrome: a complex long-term problem in management. *Q J Med* 1986;58:167.

142. Wolfram DJ. Diabetes mellitus and simple optic atrophy among siblings: report of four cases. *Mayo Clin Proc* 1938;13:715.

143. Swift RG, Sadler DB, Swift M. Psychiatric findings in Wolfram syndrome homozygotes. *Lancet* 1990;336:667.

144. Inoue H, et al. A gene encoding a transmembrane protein is mutated in patients with diabetes mellitus and optic atrophy (Wolfram syndrome). *Nature Genet* 1998;20:143.

145. Strom TM, et al. Diabetes insipidus, diabetes mellitus, optic atrophy and deafness (DIDMOAD) caused by mutations in a novel gene (wolframian) coding for a predicted transmembrane protein. *Hum Mol Genet* 1998;7:2021.

146. Hardy C, et al. Clinical and molecular genetic analysis of 19 Wolfram syndrome kindreds demonstrating a wide spectrum of mutations in WFS1. *Am J Hum Genet* 1999;65:1279.

147. Howard RL, Bichet DG, Schrier RW. Hypernatremic and polyuric states. In Seldin DW, Giebisch G, eds. *The kidney: physiology and pathophysiology*, 2nd ed. New York: Raven Press, 1992:1753.

148. Bichet DG. Nephrogenic diabetes insipidus. In: Cameronet JS, et al, eds. *Oxford textbook of clinical nephrology*. New York: Oxford University Press, 1992:789.

149. Arthus M-F, et al. Report of 33 novel *AVPR2* mutations and analysis of 117 families with X-linked nephrogenic diabetes insipidus. *J Am Soc Nephrol* 2000;11:1044.

150. Bode HH, Crawford JD. Nephrogenic diabetes insipidus in North America: the Hopewell hypothesis. *N Engl J Med* 1969;280:750.

151. Bichet DG, et al. X-linked nephrogenic diabetes insipidus: from the ship Hopewell to restriction fragment length polymorphism studies. *Am J Hum Genet* 1992;51:1089.

152. Bichet DG, et al. X-linked nephrogenic diabetes insipidus mutations in North America and the Hopewell hypothesis. *J Clin Invest* 1993; 92:1262.

153. Holtzman EJ, et al. A null mutation in the vasopressin V2 receptor gene (AVPR2) associated with nephrogenic diabetes insipidus in the Hopewell kindred. *Hum Mol Genet* 1993;2:1201.

154. Bichet DG, Fujiwara TM. Nephrogenic diabetes insipidus. In Scriver CR, et al., eds. *The metabolic and molecular bases of inherited disease*, 8th ed. New York: McGraw-Hill, 2001:4181.

155. Bichet DG, et al. Nature and recurrence of AVPR2 mutations in X-linked nephrogenic diabetes insipidus. *Am J Hum Genet* 1994;55:278.

156. Fujiwara TM, Morgan K, Bichet DG. Molecular analysis of X-linked nephrogenic diabetes insipidus. *Eur J Endocrinol* 1996;134:675.

157. Forssman H. On the mode of hereditary transmission in diabetes insipidus. *Nordisk Med* 1942;16:3211.

158. Waring AG, Kajdi L, Tappan V. Congenital defect of water metabolism. *Am J Dis Child* 1945;69:323.

159. Williams RM, Henry C. Nephrogenic diabetes insipidus transmitted by females and appearing during infancy in males. *Ann Int Med* 1947;27:84.

160. Crawford JD, Bode HH. Disorders of the posterior pituitary in children. In Gardner LI, ed. *Endocrine and genetic diseases of childhood and adolescence*, 2nd ed. Philadelphia: WB Saunders, 1975:126.

161. van Lieburg AF, Knoers NVAM, Monnens LAH. Clinical presentation and follow-up of 30 patients with congenital nephrogenic diabetes insipidus. *J Am Soc Nephrol* 1999;10:1958.

162. Hoekstra JA, et al. Cognitive and psychosocial functioning of patients with congenital nephrogenic diabetes insipidus. *Am J Med Genet* 1996;61:81.

163. Niaudet P, et al. Nephrogenic diabetes insipidus: clinical and pathophysiological aspects. *Adv Nephrol Necker Hosp* 1984;13:247.

164. van Lieburg AF, et al. Clinical phenotype of nephrogenic diabetes insipidus in females heterozygous for a vasopressin type 2 receptor mutation. *Hum Genet* 1995;96:70.

165. Nomura Y, et al. Detection of skewed X-inactivation in two female carriers of vasopressin type 2 receptor gene mutation. *J Clin Endocrinol Metab* 1997;82:3434.

166. Hobbs HH, et al. The LDL receptor locus in familial hypercholesterolemia: mutational analysis of a membrane protein. *Annu Rev Genet* 1990;24:133.

167. Schöneberg T, et al. Functional rescue of mutant V2 vasopressin receptors causing nephrogenic diabetes insipidus by a coexpressed receptor polypeptide. *EMBO J* 1996;15:1283.

168. Schöneberg T, et al. Reconstitution of mutant V2 vasopressin receptors by adenovirus-mediated gene transfer. *J Clin Invest* 1997;100:1547.

169. Oksche A, et al. Vasopressin V2 receptor mutants that cause X-linked nephrogenic diabetes insipidus: analysis of expression, processing, and function. *Mol Pharmacol* 1996;50:820.

170. Tsukaguchi H, et al. Binding-, intracellular transport-, and biosynthesis-defective mutants of vasopressin type 2 receptor in patients with X-linked nephrogenic diabetes insipidus. *J Clin Invest* 1995; 96:2043.

171. Wenkert D, et al. Functional characterization of five V2 vasopressin receptor gene mutations. *Mol Cell Endocrinol* 1996;124:43.

172. Tamarappoo BK, Verkman AS. Defective aquaporin-2 trafficking in nephrogenic diabetes insipidus and correction by chemical chaperones. *J Clin Invest* 1998;101:2257.

173. Kuznetsov G, Nigam SK. Folding of secretory and membrane proteins. *N Engl J Med* 1998;339:1688.

174. Waheed A, et al. Hereditary hemochromatosis: effects of C282Y and H63D mutations on association with beta2-microglobulin, intracellular processing, and cell surface expression of the HFE protein in COS-7 cells. *Proc Natl Acad Sci USA* 1997;94:12384.

175. Kunchaparty S, et al. Defective processing and expression of thiazide-sensitive Na-Cl cotransporter as a cause of Gitelman's syndrome. *Am J Physiol* 1999;277:F643.

176. Chillaron J, et al. An intracellular trafficking defect in type I cystinuria rBAT mutants M467T and M467K. *J Biol Chem* 1997;272:9543.

177. Carrell RW, Lomas DA. Conformational disease. *Lancet* 1997; 350:134.

178. Bonnardeaux A, Bichet DG. Inherited disorders of the renal tubule. In Brenner BM, ed. *The kidney*, 6th ed. Philadelphia: WB Saunders, 2000:1656.

179. Schulz A, et al. Structural implication for receptor oligomerization from functional reconstitution studies of mutant V2 vasopressin receptors. *J Biol Chem* 2000;275:2381.

180. Serradeil-Le Gal C. Nonpeptide antagonists for vasopressin receptors. Pharmacology of SR 121463A, a new potent and highly selective V2 receptor antagonist. *Adv Exp Med Biol* 1998;449:427.

181. Chan PS, et al. VPA-985 a nonpeptide orally active and selective vasopressin V2 receptor antagonist. *Adv Exp Med Biol* 1998;449: 439.

182. Bernat A, et al. V2 receptor antagonism of DDAVP-induced release of hemostasis factors in conscious dogs. J Pharmacol Exp Ther 282: 597, 1997.

183. Morello JP, et al. Pharmacological chaperones rescue cell-surface expression and function of misfolded V2 vasopressin receptor mutants. *J Clin Invest* 2000;105:887.

184. Brenner B, Seligsohn U, Hochberg Z. Normal response of factor VIII and von Willebrand factor to 1-deamino-8D-arginine vasopressin in nephrogenic diabetes insipidus. *J Clin Endocrinol Metab* 1988;67: 191.

185. Knoers N, Monnens LA. A variant of nephrogenic diabetes insipidus: V2 receptor abnormality restricted to the kidney. *Eur J Pediatr* 1991;150:370.

186. Langley JM, et al. Autosomal recessive inheritance of vasopressin-resistant diabetes insipidus. *Am J Med Genet* 1991;38:90.

187. Lonergan M, et al. Non-X-linked nephrogenic diabetes insipidus: phenotype and genotype features. *J Am Soc Nephrol* 1993;4:264A.

188. Deen PMT, et al. Water channels encoded by mutant aquaporin-2 genes in nephrogenic diabetes insipidus are impaired in their cellular routing. *J Clin Invest* 1995;95:2291.

189. Tamarappoo BK, Yang B, Verkman AS. Misfolding of mutant aquaporin-2 water channels in nephrogenic diabetes insipidus. *J Biol Chem* 1999;274:34825.

190. van Os CH, Deen PM. Aquaporin-2 water channel mutations causing nephrogenic diabetes insipidus. *Proc Assoc Am Physicians* 1998; 110:395.

191. Mulders SM, et al. An aquaporin-2 water channel mutant which causes autosomal dominant nephrogenic diabetes insipidus is retained in the Golgi complex. *J Clin Invest* 1998;102:57.

192. Kamsteeg EJ, et al. An impaired routing of wild-type aquaporin-2 after tetramerization with an aquaporin-2 mutant explains dominant nephrogenic diabetes insipidus. *EMBO J* 1999;18:2394.

193. Boton R, Gaviria M, Batlle DC. Prevalence, pathogenesis, and treatment of renal dysfunction associated with chronic lithium therapy. *Am J Kidney Dis* 1987;10:329.

194. Markowitz GS, et al. Lithium nephrotoxicity: a progressive combined glomerular and tubulointerstitial nephropathy. *J Am Soc Nephrol* 2000;11:1439.

195. Christensen S, et al. Pathogenesis of nephrogenic diabetes insipidus due to chronic administration of lithium in rats. *J Clin Invest* 1985;75:1869.

196. Cogan E, Svoboda M, Abramow M. Mechanisms of lithium–vasopressin interaction in rabbit cortical collecting tubule. *Am J Physiol* 1987;252:F1080.

197. Goldberg H, Clayman P, Skorecki K. Mechanism of Li inhibition of vasopressin-sensitive adenylate cyclase in cultured renal epithelial cells. *Am J Physiol* 1988;255:F995.

198. Kwon TH, et al. Altered expression of renal AQPs and Na(+) transporters in rats with lithium-induced NDI. *Am J Physiol Renal Physiol* 2000;279:F552.

199. Marples D, et al. Lithium-induced downregulation of aquaporin-2 water channel expression in rat kidney medulla. *J Clin Invest* 1995;95:1838.

200. Marples D, et al. Hypokalemia-induced downregulation of aquaporin-2 water channel expression in rat kidney medulla and cortex. *J Clin Invest* 1996;97:1960.

201. Amlal H, et al. Early polyuria and urinary concentrating defect in potassium deprivation. *Am J Physiol Renal Physiol* 2000;279:F655.

202. Frokiaer J, et al. Bilateral ureteral obstruction downregulates expression of vasopressin-sensitive AQP-2 water channel in rat kidney. *Am J Physiol* 1996;270:F657.

203. Sands JM, et al. Vasopressin-elicited water and urea permeabilities are altered in IMCD in hypercalcemic rats. *Am J Physiol* 1998;274:F978.

204. Batlle DC, et al. Amelioration of polyuria by amiloride in patients receiving long-term lithium therapy. *N Engl J Med* 1985;312:408.

205. Barlow ED, de Wardener HE. Compulsive water drinking. *Q J Med New Series* 1959;28:235.

206. Robertson GL. Dipsogenic diabetes insipidus: a newly recognized syndrome caused by a selective defect in the osmoregulation of thirst. *Trans Assoc Am Physicians* 1987;100:241.

207. Amico JA. Diabetes insipidus and pregnancy. In: Czernichow P, Robinson AG, eds. *Frontiers of hormone research*, vol 13, "Diabetes insipidus in man." Basel: Karger, 1985:266.

208. Davison JM, et al. Serial evaluation of vasopressin release and thirst in human pregnancy. Role of human chorionic gonadotrophin in the osmoregulatory changes of gestation. *J Clin Invest* 1988;81:798.

209. Iwasaki Y, et al. Aggravation of subclinical diabetes insipidus during pregnancy. *N Engl J Med* 1991;324:522.

210. Forssman H. On hereditary diabetes insipidus, with special regard to a sex-linked form. *Acta Med Scand* 1945;159:1.

211. Barron WM, et al. Transient vasopressin-resistant diabetes insipidus of pregnancy. *N Engl J Med* 1984;310:442.

212. Durr JA, et al. Diabetes insipidus in pregnancy associated with abnormally high circulating vasopressinase activity. *N Engl J Med* 1987;316:1070.

213. Ford SM Jr. Transient vasopressin-resistant diabetes insipidus of pregnancy. *Obstet Gynecol* 1986;68:288.

214. Leaf A. Neurogenic diabetes insipidus. *Kidney Int* 1979;15:572.

215. Robertson GL. Diagnosis of diabetes insipidus. In: Czernichow P, Robinson AG, eds. *Frontiers of hormone research*, vol 13, "Diabetes insipidus in man." Basel: Karger, 1985:176.

216. Boyd SD, Raz S, Ehrlich RM. Diabetes insipidus and nonobstructive dilatation of urinary tract. *Urology* 1980;16:266.

217. Gautier B, Thieblot P, Steg A. Mégauretère, mégavessie et diabète insipide familial. *Sem Hop* 1981;57:60.

218. Robertson GL. Diseases of the posterior pituitary. In Felig D, et al., eds. *Endocrinology and metabolism.* New York: McGraw-Hill, 1981:251.

219. Bettinelli A, et al. Phenotypic variability in Bartter syndrome type I. *Pediatr Nephrol* 2000;14:940.

220. Bichet DG. Nephrogenic diabetes insipidus. *Semin Nephrol* 1994;14:349.

221. Robertson GL, et al. Immunoassay of plasma vasopressin in man. *Proc Natl Acad Sci USA* 1970;66:1298.

222. Robertson GL, et al. Development and clinical application of a new method for the radioimmunoassay of arginine vasopressin in human plasma. *J Clin Invest* 1973;52:2340.

223. Bichet DG, et al. Modulation of plasma and platelet vasopressin by cardiac function in patients with heart failure. *Kidney Int* 1986;29:1188.

224. Bichet DG, et al. Human platelet fraction arginine-vasopressin. *J Clin Invest* 1987;79:881.

225. Davison JM, et al. Altered osmotic thresholds for vasopressin secretion and thirst in human pregnancy. *Am J Physiol* 1984;246:F105.

226. Vokes TP, Aycinena PR, Robertson GL. Effect of insulin on osmoregulation of vasopressin. *Am J Physiol* 252: E538, 1987.

227. Hartter E, Woloszczuk W. Radioimmunological determination of arginine vasopressin and human atrial natriuretic peptide after simultaneous extraction from plasma. *J Clin Chem Clin Biochem* 1986;24:559.

228. LaRochelle FT Jr, North WG, Stern P. A new extraction of arginine vasopressin from blood: the use of octadecasilyl-silica. *Pflugers Arch* 1980;387:79.

229. Ysewijn-Van Brussel KA, De Leenheer AP. Development and evaluation of a radioimmunoassay for Arg8-vasopressin, after extraction with Sep-Pak C18. *Clin Chem* 1985;31:861.

230. Preibisz JJ, et al. Plasma and platelet vasopressin in essential hypertension and congestive heart failure. *Hypertension* 1983;5:I129.

231. Seckl JR, et al. Vasopressin antagonist in early postoperative diabetes insipidus. *Lancet* 1990;355:1353.

232. Maas AH, et al. Ion-selective electrodes for sodium and potassium: a new problem of what is measured and what should be reported. *Clin Chem* 1985;31:482.

233. Gennari FJ. Current concepts. Serum osmolality. Uses and limitations. *N Engl J Med* 1984;310:102.

234. Knoers N, Monnens LA. Nephrogenic diabetes insipidus: clinical symptoms, pathogenesis, genetics and treatment. *Pediatr Nephrol* 1992;6:476.

235. Kirchlechner V, et al. Treatment of nephrogenic diabetes insipidus with hydrochlorothiazide and amiloride. *Arch Dis Child* 1999;80:548.

236. Antonarakis S, and the Nomenclature Working Group. Recommendations for a nomenclature system for human gene mutations. Nomenclature Working Group. *Hum Mutat* 1998;11:1.

237. Stern P, Valtin H. Verney was right, but . . . [Editorial]. *N Engl J Med* 1981;305:1581.

238. Vokes T, Robertson GL. Physiology of secretion of vasopressin. In: Czernichow P, Robinson AG, eds. *Diabetes insipidus in man*. Basel: Karger, 1985:127.

239. Zerbe RL, Robertson GL. Disorders of ADH. *Med North Am* 1984;13:1570.

240. Mouillac B, et al. The binding site of neuropeptide vasopressin V1a receptor. Evidence for a major localization within transmembrane regions. *J Biol Chem* 1995;270:25771.

241. Pan Y, et al. Mutations in the V2 vasopressin receptor gene are associated with X-linked nephrogenic diabetes insipidus. *Nat Genet* 1992;2:103.

242. Rosenthal W, et al. Molecular identification of the gene responsible for congenital nephrogenic diabetes insipidus. *Nature* 1992;359:233.

243. van den Ouweland AM, et al. Mutations in the vasopressin type 2 receptor gene (AVPR2) associated with nephrogenic diabetes insipidus. *Nat Genet* 1992;2:99.

244. Holtzman EJ, et al. Brief report: a molecular defect in the vasopressin V2-receptor gene causing nephrogenic diabetes insipidus. *N Engl J Med* 1993;328:1534.

245. Merendino JJJ, et al. Brief report: a mutation in the vasopressin V2-receptor gene in a kindred with X-linked nephrogenic diabetes insipidus. *N Engl J Med* 1993;328:1538.

246. Tsukaguchi H, et al. Two novel mutations in the vasopressin V2 receptor gene in unrelated Japanese kindreds with nephrogenic diabetes insipidus. *Biochem Biophys Res Comm* 1993;197:1000.

247. Faa V, et al. Mutations in the vasopressin V2-receptor gene in three families of Italian descent with nephrogenic diabetes insipidus. *Hum Mol Genet* 1994;3:1685.

248. Friedman E, et al. Nephrogenic diabetes insipidus: an X chromosome-linked dominant inheritance pattern with a vasopressin type 2 receptor gene that is structurally normal. *Proc Natl Acad Sci USA* 1994;91:8457.

249. Holtzman EJ, et al. Mutations in the vasopressin V2 receptor gene in two families with nephrogenic diabetes insipidus. *J Am Soc Nephrol* 1994;5:169.
250. Knoers NV, et al. Inheritance of mutations in the V2 receptor gene in thirteen families with nephrogenic diabetes insipidus. *Kidney Int* 1994;46:170.
251. Oksche A, et al. Two novel mutations in the vasopressin V2 receptor gene in patients with congenital nephrogenic diabetes insipidus. *Biophys Biochem Res Comm* 1994;205:552.
252. Pan Y, Wilson P, Gitschier J. The effect of eight V2 vasopressin receptor mutations on stimulation of adenylyl cyclase and binding to vasopressin. *J Biol Chem* 1994;269:31933.
253. Wenkert D, et al. Novel mutations in the V2 vasopressin receptor gene of patients with X-linked nephrogenic diabetes insipidus. *Hum Mol Genet* 1994;3:1429.
254. Wildin RS, et al. Heterogeneous AVPR2 gene mutations in congenital nephrogenic diabetes insipidus. *Am J Hum Genet* 1994;55:266.
255. Yuasa H, et al. Novel mutations in the V2 vasopressin receptor gene in two pedigrees with congenital nephrogenic diabetes insipidus. *J Clin Endocrinol Metab* 1994;79:361.
256. Tsukaguchi H, Matsubara H, Inada, M. Expression studies of two vasopressin V2 receptor gene mutations, R202C and 804insG, in nephrogenic diabetes insipidus. *Kidney Int* 1995;48:554.
257. Jinnouchi H, et al. Analysis of vasopressin receptor type II (V2R) gene in three Japanese pedigrees with congenital nephrogenic diabetes insipidus: identification of a family with complete deletion of the V2R gene. *Eur J Endocrinol* 1996;134:689.
258. Oksche A, et al. Two novel mutations in the aquaporin-2 and the vasopressin V2 receptor genes in patients with congenital nephrogenic diabetes insipidus. *Hum Genet* 1996;98:587.
259. Tajima T, et al. Three novel AVPR2 mutations in three Japanese families with X-linked nephrogenic diabetes insipidus. *Pediatr Res* 1996;39:522.
260. Yokoyama K, et al. A low-affinity vasopressin V2-receptor gene in a kindred with X-linked nephrogenic diabetes insipidus. *J Am Soc Nephrol* 1996;7:410.
261. Cheong HI, et al. Six novel mutations in the vasopressin V2 receptor gene causing nephrogenic diabetes insipidus. *Nephron* 1997;75: 431.
262. Sadeghi H, et al. Biochemical basis of partial NDI phenotypes. *Mol Endocrinol* 1997;11:1806.
263. Vargas-Poussou R, et al. Mutations in the vasopressin V2 receptor and aquaporin-2 genes in 12 families with congenital nephrogenic diabetes insipidus. *J Am Soc Nephrol* 1997;8:1855.
264. Ala Y, et al. Functional studies of twelve mutant V2 vasopressin receptors related to nephrogenic diabetes insipidus: molecular basis of a mild clinical phenotype. *J Am Soc Nephrol* 1998;9:1861.
265. Szalai C, Triga D, Czinner A. C112R, W323S, N317K mutations in the vasopressin V2 receptor gene in patients with nephrogenic diabetes insipidus. Mutations in brief no. 165. Online. *Hum Mutat* 1998;12: 137.
266. Schöneberg T, et al. V2 vasopressin receptor dysfunction in nephrogenic diabetes insipidus caused by different molecular mechanisms. *Hum Mutat* 1998;12:196.
267. Shoji Y, et al. Mutational analyses of AVPR2 gene in three Japanese families with X-linked nephrogenic diabetes insipidus: two recurrent mutations, R137H and delta V278, caused by the hypermutability at CpG dinucleotides. *Hum Mutat* 1998;[Suppl 1]:S278.
268. Wildin RS, Cogdell DE, Valadez V. AVPR2 variants and V2 vasopressin receptor function in nephrogenic diabetes insipidus. *Kidney Int* 1998;54:1909.
269. Kraulis PJ. MOLSCRIPT-a program to produce both detailed and schematic plots of proteins. *J Appl Crystallogr* 1991;24:946.
270. van Lieburg AF, et al. Patients with autosomal nephrogenic diabetes insipidus homozygous for mutations in the aquaporin 2 water-channel gene. *Am J Hum Genet* 1994;55:648.
271. Canfield MC, et al. Identification and characterization of aquaporin-2 water channel mutations causing nephrogenic diabetes insipidus with partial vasopressin response. *Hum Mol Genet* 1997;6:1865.
272. Hochberg Z, et al. Autosomal recessive nephrogenic diabetes insipidus caused by an aquaporin-2 mutation. *J Clin Endocrinol Metab* 1997;82:686.
273. Goji K, et al. Novel mutations in aquaporin-2 gene in female siblings with nephrogenic diabetes insipidus: evidence of disrupted water channel function. *J Clin Endocrinol Metab* 1998;83:3205.
274. Kuwahara M. Aquaporin-2, a vasopressin-sensitive water channel, and nephrogenic diabetes insipidus. *Int Med* 1998;37:215.
275. Cheng A, et al. Three-dimensional organization of a human water channel. *Nature* 1997;387:627.
276. Robertson GL. The physiopathology of ADH secretion. In: Tolis G, et al., eds. *Clinical neuroendocrinology: a pathophysiological approach.* New York: Raven Press, 1979:247.

CHAPTER 87

Disorders of Potassium and Acid–Base Metabolism in Association with Renal Disease

Mark A. Perazella and Asghar Rastegar

In this chapter we review disturbances in potassium and acid–base homeostasis seen in patients with renal disease. Our discussion is, however, limited to disorders of potassium and acid–base homeostasis seen in (a) patients with progressive chronic renal failure, and (b) patients with renal insufficiency and defects in the renin–aldosterone axis or in the tubular response to aldosterone. To provide a background, we briefly review potassium and acid–base homeostasis in normal humans before focusing on patients with underlying renal disease. We do not, however, discuss normal renal handling of potassium and only briefly review renal handling of hydrogen ion. These two topics are extensively reviewed in Chapter 5, Tubular Potassium Transport, and Chapter 6, Renal Acid–Base Transport, respectively.

POTASSIUM HOMEOSTASIS

Potassium is the most abundant cation in the body. The distribution of potassium is such that 90% of total body potassium is intracellular, whereas only 2% is extracellular (1). The high intracellular to extracellular potassium ratio (K_i/K_o) is crucial to the normal cell function, as it is the major determinant of the resting membrane potential. The body is able to maintain this distribution in a highly regulated and efficient fashion through hormonal modulation of Na-K-ATPase pump activity. This enzyme is composed of two subunits and is found in highest density in skeletal muscle (2,3). Functional activity of the Na-K-ATPase pump is restricted to the catalytic α subunit, whereas the ß(glycoprotein) subunit acts to ensure α subunit assembly and maintain its stability. The α subunit contains binding sites for sodium, potassium, magnesium, ATP, Pi, and the inhibitor ouabain. Several hormones acutely modulate Na-K-ATPase pump activity by altering the phosphorylation status of the catalytic subunit and/or

transporting pumps from subcellular locations to the cellular membrane where sodium and potassium transport occurs (2,3). For example, insulin and catecholamines regulate the phosphorylation status of the Na-K-ATPase pump through modulation of certain phosphatases and kinases. Rapid recruitment of inactive pump units from a preformed pool of pumps is also stimulated by both insulin and aldosterone. These Na-K-ATPase pumps are then deposited in the cell membrane and converted to an activated state (2,3). In contrast, chronic and sustained changes in Na-K-ATPase enzyme activity are achieved through regulation of the total number of active pump units available in the cell membrane. Chronic control occurs at the transcriptional and posttranscriptional levels, regulated through the effects of hormones such as aldosterone and insulin. Hence, the overall abundance of pump subunits is controlled at the levels of transcription, transcript stability, translation, and protein stability (2,3).

Large potassium loads continuously challenge humans, who are carnivorous intermittent eaters. On a long-term basis, this challenge is met primarily by the renal excretion of potassium load; however, on a short-term basis, a significant amount of potassium is shifted intracellularly (4). This shift temporarily buffers the expected change in K_i/K_o ratio until potassium intake is balanced by comparable output.

Internal Potassium Homeostasis

The kidney is able to excrete only about 50% of the administered potassium during the first 4 hours after intravenous or oral intake of potassium. Approximately 80% of the retained potassium is shifted intracellularly, and only 20% (or 10% of the total intake) remains in the extracellular space (5–7). The retained potassium will be excreted completely over the next 24 hours (8). The major regulators of this internal redistribution are: (a) insulin, (b) catecholamines, (c) mineralocorticoids, and possibly (4) parathyroid hormone. These hormones induce cellular movement of potassium primarily through the modulation of Na-K-ATPase pumps and

M. A. Perazella and A. Rastegar: Department of Internal Medicine, Yale University School of Medicine; and Department of Nephrology, Yale–New Haven Hospital, New Haven, Connecticut

potassium channels located in cellular membranes (see the preceding).

Insulin

The ability of insulin to shift potassium intracellularly has been known for over 70 years (9) and has been used therapeutically for the treatment of hyperkalemia. Several investigators have shown that pancreatectomized dogs tolerate exogenous potassium loads poorly (10). This is reversed by exogenous replacement of insulin (11,12). To study the role of endogenous insulin, DeFronzo and coworkers (6) examined potassium tolerance in dogs by intravenous potassium chloride infusion before and after inhibition of endogenous insulin secretion with somatostatin. Inhibition of endogenous insulin by 50% results in a twofold rise in serum potassium compared to controls (Fig. 87-1). If physiologic doses of insulin were added to the somatostatin infusion, potassium tolerance returned to normal. In healthy volunteers, somatostatin infusion in the postabsorptive state led to a 50% decline in the plasma insulin concentration and a 0.5 to 0.7 mEq/L rise in serum potassium that was reversed by a physiologic infusion of exogenous insulin (6). A similar phenomenon was observed in maturity-onset diabetics, who have normal or increased fasting plasma insulin levels, but not insulin-deficient juvenile diabetics (13).

The effect of hyperkalemia on endogenous insulin concentration is more complex. A 1.0- to 1.5-mEq rise in serum potassium is uniformly associated with a severalfold rise in serum insulin level (10,12,14,15), whereas a more physiologic

rise of less than 1.0 mEq has no effect. Hiatt and associates (14) noted a significant rise in portal insulin level with a more modest rise of 0.3 to 1.0 mEq in serum potassium; however, in a more recent report, the rise in portal insulin could only be shown if serum potassium was increased by 2.0 mEq/L (16); therefore, the presence of a classic negative feedback loop at physiologic potassium concentration remains controversial. The primary sites of insulin-mediated potassium uptake include muscle and liver, although adipose tissue uptake of potassium is also enhanced (17–21). DeFronzo and colleagues (21), using variable doses of insulin in normal volunteers, have shown that during the first hour, liver is the primary site of potassium uptake. However, during the second hour, despite continued drop in serum potassium, there is net release of potassium from the portal and splanchnic bed, indicating a shift of potassium uptake to the peripheral tissue, especially muscle.

At the cellular level insulin reacts with specific receptors on the plasma membrane (22), increasing the activity of the Na-K-ATPase pump in the skeletal and heart muscle, epithelial cells of the kidney and bladder, as well as liver and fat cells (23). This augmentation is blocked by ouabain, which binds to the α subunit. As shown in animals (opossum and rat), it appears that insulin induces phosphorylation of the α-1 subunit of the Na-K-ATPase pump at the level of tyrosine 10 (24). Phosphorylation of this enzyme increases the activity of pumps, thereby facilitating sodium and potassium transport (2,24). Additionally, insulin also acutely triggers the translocation of previously unavailable pumps from intracellular pools to the plasma membrane in skeletal muscle, liver cells, and adipocytes (2,24). Ultimately, insulin's effect on the Na-K-ATPase pump stimulates a series of intracellular events leading to hyperpolarization of cell membranes (19,20,23). The time course for this interaction is consistent with both an increase in enzyme activity as well as the rapid recruitment of Na-K-ATPase pumps to the cellular membrane. In contrast, chronic stimulation by insulin probably increases the total number of available pump sites. This occurs through regulation of the Na-K-ATPase pump at the transcriptional and posttranscriptional levels, by inducing the synthesis of new α and ß subunits (2). Several *in vitro* studies have shown that insulin-driven potassium uptake by both muscle and liver is independent of glucose uptake (19,21). In addition, Cohen and coworkers (25), using euglycemic clamp in humans, have provided strong evidence that effect of insulin on potassium uptake is independent of its effect on glucose entry into the cell.

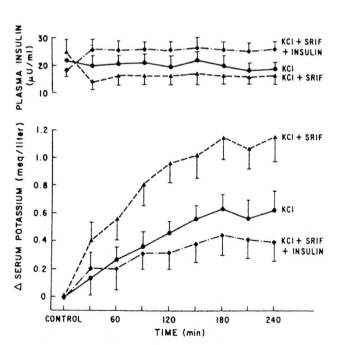

FIG. 87-1. The effect of potassium chloride infusion on the plasma potassium concentration in the control state, with somatostatin (STS), which inhibits insulin secretion, or with somatostatin plus insulin. (From: DeFronzo RA, et al. *JCI* 1978;61:472, with permission.)

Catecholamines

D'Silva, beginning in 1934, first observed a biphasic response of plasma potassium to epinephrine injection (26,27). Plasma potassium rose during the first 1 to 3 minutes, but with continued infusion fell and remained lower than baseline. Other investigators have shown increased potassium tolerance in animals infused with pharmacologic doses of epinephrine

(28,29) despite pancreatectomy (11) or nephrectomy (30). Brown and coworkers (31) have shown that infusion of stress-level doses of epinephrine resulted in a decrease in serum potassium by 0.4 to 0.6 mEq/L. Because epinephrine inhibits the renal excretion of potassium (32,33), the decline in potassium concentration is entirely accounted for by enhanced cellular potassium uptake.

Specific receptors are involved in the cellular disposal of potassium by catecholamines. α Stimulation in humans by phenylephrine (41) significantly impairs cellular potassium tolerance, which is reversed by the α-antagonist phentolamine. This phenomenon may explain the initial rise in serum potassium after infusion of catecholamine (32,33). ß Blockade impairs the catecholamine-induced shift of potassium into extrarenal tissues (42–45) and causes hyperkalemia despite increase in renal excretion of this ion (Fig. 87-2). In normal volunteers who exercise while taking ß-adrenergic blocking agents, the serum potassium level is raised 2- to 2.5-fold higher than during similar exercise performed without ß blockade (4,46,47). The effect of nonspecific ß-blockers such as propranolol on serum potassium is mimicked by specific β_2-blockers (38,46,48,49) but not β_1-blockers (34). Although an important role for catecholamine-stimulated uptake of potassium by muscle has been demonstrated (43,50–52), the role of the liver remains controversial (34,53). The effect of potassium on catecholamine levels is less clear. In humans, physiologic changes in plasma potassium did not affect plasma epinephrine or norepinephrine levels (54). However, because the majority of catecholamines are locally released and rapidly retaken up by nerve endings, it is possible that changes in catecholamine secretion are not reflected in the serum concentration of these mediators.

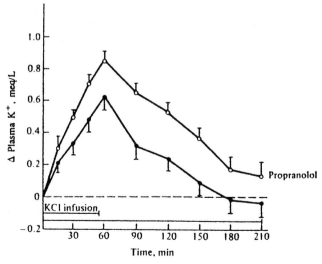

FIG. 87-2. Changes in plasma potassium concentration after a potassium chloride infusion in the presence and absence of the nonselective ß-adrenergic blocker propranolol. (From: Rosa, Silva P, Young JB, et al. Adrenergic modulation of extrarenal potassium disposal. *NEJM* 1980;302:431, with permission.)

At the cellular level epinephrine binds to the β_2-receptor resulting in the stimulation of adenyl cyclase, and conversion of adenosine triphosphate to cyclic 3′,5′-adenosine monophosphate (cAMP). It is postulated that cAMP then activates protein kinase A, which then phosphorylates the Na-K-ATPase pump, increasing its activity and promoting potassium influx into the cell and Na^+ efflux (1,43,46,47). Binding of catecholamines to the α receptor decreases cellular potassium uptake through inhibiting adenylate cyclase activity and decreasing Na-K-ATPase pump activity (48). In addition, activation of the α-1 receptor alters cytoplasmic calcium, thereby increasing intracellular calcium concentration and opening calcium-activated potassium channels, which allow potassium to exit the cell (48). Interestingly, the effect of insulin and epinephrine on plasma potassium is additive, confirming separate mechanisms of action (47). In insulin-induced hypoglycemia, hypokalemia is therefore due to the combined effect of both insulin and the hypoglycemia-induced rise in catecholamines (49).

Mineralocorticoids

The role of mineralocorticoids in external potassium homeostasis is of critical importance because aldosterone influences potassium excretion by the kidney (50), colon (51), salivary (52), and sweat glands (53). However, aldosterone's role in internal potassium homeostasis is unclear (54,55). Anephric rats adapted to high potassium intake handle an acute potassium load more efficiently than do nonadapted rats. This adaptation is lost by prior adrenalectomy and restored by exogenous mineralocorticoid replacement (56). However, Spital and Stern (57,58) observed that during the 20 hours of fasting before nephrectomy and acute potassium loading, these rats became potassium depleted owing to marked kaliuresis resulting from high-serum potassium coupled with a high aldosterone level. In adrenalectomized dogs, Young and Jackson (59) have shown that plasma potassium concentration at any exchangeable potassium level was a function of aldosterone replacement dose. High-dose aldosterone in anephric rabbits delays death owing to hyperkalemia (60). Similarly, baseline potassium was significantly higher in hormonally deficient adrenalectomized rats, despite negative potassium balance, compared to exogenously replaced controls, supporting a defect in cellular uptake of the potassium (6,61). This impairment was corrected by either aldosterone or epinephrine replacement. In rat studies, aldosterone has been shown to increase Na-K-ATPase pump activity by inducing the synthesis of new α- and ß-subunits in heart and vascular smooth muscle (2). This effect presumably represents the action of aldosterone on Na-K-ATPase pump gene expression and supports a role for aldosterone in cellular potassium homeostasis. In anephric humans treated with deoxycorticosterone acetate (DOCA), spironolactone, or placebo for 3 days, the baseline potassium was similar; however, the DOCA-treated subjects showed greater tolerance to acute potassium load than did the other two groups

(62). In addition, high-dose spironolactone (300 mg/day) induced a significant rise in plasma potassium (0.5 mEq/L) and caused hyperkalemia after 3 weeks of therapy in nine chronically hemodialyzed end-stage renal disease (ESRD) patients (three anephrics) (63). In this study, it is difficult to dissect out the actual effect of spironolactone on impairment of cell potassium uptake and gastrointestinal potassium excretion.

Parathyroid Hormone and Intracellular Calcium

It is known that intracellular calcium has a significant effect on the permeability of cellular membrane to potassium. Sugarman and Kahn evaluated the role of parathyroid hormone (PTH) (a calcium ionophore) (64) and calcium channel blockers (65) in potassium tolerance in an acutely nephrectomized rat model. Infusion of PTH in acutely nephrectomized rats results in a greater rise in serum potassium following challenge with a standard potassium load (3.0 versus 2.0 mEq/L at 90 minutes) (64). The difference could not be explained by changes in serum insulin, aldosterone, catecholamine, calcium, or bicarbonate levels. Rats with intact parathyroid glands and chronic renal failure have a higher basal potassium level and an attenuated response to potassium loading, which improves by the addition of verapamil or nifedipine (66). A potential explanation for this observation is based on the effect of intracellular calcium concentration on high conductance calcium-activated potassium channels. A rise in intracellular calcium opens K channels, allowing potassium to leak out of cells and increasing serum potassium concentration (48). Furthermore, administration of a calcium channel blocker (diltiazem) to seven subjects with ESRD decreased the rise in interdialytic plasma potassium levels (0.37 ± 0.07 mmol/L versus 0.72 ± 0.14 mmol/L), suggesting enhanced internal potassium disposal (67). Diltiazem may act by reducing intracellular calcium concentration, thereby preventing opening of potassium channels and decreasing potassium exit from cells (67). Although PTH worsens and calcium channel blockers improve potassium tolerance, the clinical importance of these interesting observations remains speculative.

Acid–Base Balance

The role of acid–base balance on the internal distribution of potassium (68–70) is based on the concept that during the development of acute acidemia hydrogen ion enters the cell in exchange for potassium and that the reverse occurs during the development of alkalemia (70–74). This dynamic interrelationship has been simplified clinically to a general rule that for each 0.1 U change in serum pH, the serum potassium changes in the opposite direction by 0.6 mEq/L. However, the relationship between serum potassium and serum pH is much more complex and depends on the type of acid–base problem, the anion accompanying hydrogen, the duration of acidosis, changes in plasma bicarbonate concentration

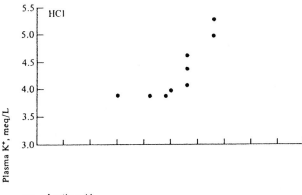

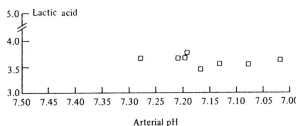

FIG. 87-3. The effect of arterial pH on plasma potassium concentration in experimentally induced mineral acidosis (hydrochloric acid-HCl) and lactic acidosis in dogs. (From: Perez GO, Oster JR, Vaamonde CA. Serum potassium concentration in acidemic states. *Nephron* 1981;27:233, with permission.)

independent of changes in pH and the extent of intracellular buffering, and so on. The following generalizations are clinically useful nevertheless.

1. On the whole, acidosis is accompanied by a greater change in serum potassium than is alkalosis (54,75,76).
2. Mineral acidosis (Fig. 87-3) causes the greatest shift (0.24–1.7 mEq/L for each 0.1 U pH change), whereas organic acidosis has a much smaller effect (74,77–80).
3. The amounts of potassium shifted into the cell in metabolic and respiratory alkalosis are approximately similar (0.1–0.4 mEq/L for each 0.1 U pH change). Respiratory acidosis shifts a similar amount of potassium out of the cell (71).
4. Changes in serum bicarbonate, independent of serum pH, have an inverse effect on the serum potassium concentration.
5. In chronic acidosis and alkalosis, the final serum potassium is a function of the effect of acid–base disturbance on the renal handling of potassium, as well as on the transcellular distribution of this ion. In dogs with ammonium chloride-induced acidosis, Magner and associates (81) noted a fall in serum potassium below baseline by days 3 to 5, owing to severe kaliuresis (81).

Osmolality

The acute hyperkalemic effect of a sudden rise in plasma osmolality is probably caused by the shift of potassium-rich intracellular fluid by solvent drag (82,83). Clinically, this

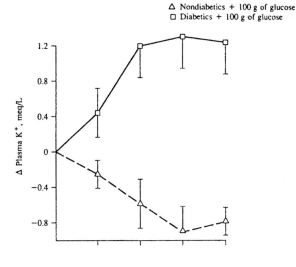

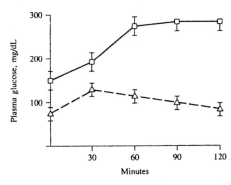

△ Nondiabetics + 100 g of glucose
□ Diabetics + 100 g of glucose

FIG. 87-4. Effect of glucose infusion on plasma potassium and glucose concentrations in diabetics *(squares)* and normal subjects *(triangles)*. The plasma potassium rises in diabetics owing to the development of hyperosmolality (hyperglycemia) but falls in normal subjects as a result of the glucose-induced release of endogenous insulin. (From: Nicolis GL, Kahn T, Sanchez A, et al. Glucose-induced hyperkalemia in diabetic subjects. *Arch Intern Med* 1981;141:49, with permission.)

phenomenon is most commonly observed in hyperosmolar diabetics (Fig. 87-4), with or without ketoacidosis (84–89) when insulin deficiency augments the rise in potassium. Although, chronic hyperkalemia in diabetics is multifactorial, a sudden rise in plasma osmolality seems to play a contributory role. Infusion of hypertonic mannitol in normal humans (90) or hypertonic saline in patients with chronic renal failure (91) results in a modest rise in serum potassium (0.4 to 0.6 mEq/L). These clinical observations support an independent role of sudden osmolar shifts in the regulation of serum potassium.

POTASSIUM HOMEOSTASIS IN RENAL FAILURE

Patients with renal failure are able to maintain a near-normal serum potassium concentration despite a marked decrease in glomerular filtration rate (GFR) (92,93). However, under certain conditions, hyperkalemia may occur in patients with

TABLE 87-1. *Etiologies of hyperkalemia in patients with renal insufficiency*

GFR <20 mL/min
Defects in the renin–angiotensin–aldosterone axis
Tubular defects in potassium secretion
High potassium input (e.g., rhabdomyolysis, hemolysis, severe catabolic states, gastrointestinal bleeding, exogenous potassium administration)
Shift of potassium from intracellular compartment
Drugs that interfere with renal and extrarenal potassium homeostasis

mild to moderate renal failure (Table 87-1). Although hyperkalemia could be due to increased potassium intake and/or rapid shifts of potassium from the cell, renal failure is the most important cause of hyperkalemia accounting for 77% of the cases reported by Acker and coworkers (94). This is often compounded by treatment with drugs that interfere with potassium handling (see the following).

In this section we initially discuss total body potassium content in patients with renal failure before treatment with dialysis and then review internal and external potassium homeostasis in these patients. In the subsequent section, we discuss hyperkalemia seen in patients with renal insufficiency with a defect in the renin–angiotensin–aldosterone axis or in the tubular responsiveness to aldosterone.

Total Body and Cellular Potassium Content in Renal Failure

Total body potassium content is a reflection of the balance between potassium intake and potassium output, whereas the cellular content reflects the distribution of potassium between the intracellular and the extracellular compartments. Exchangeable potassium (K_e) in pre-ESRD patients has been generally reported as lower than normal (95,96). However, Berlyne and associates (97), after excluding patients with intercurrent problems (such as vomiting, diarrhea, or malnutrition), reported a normal value. As Patrick has pointed out (98), the normal range for K_e is not well defined and depends on age, sex, and the reference points used (e.g., total body weight, lean body weight, or intracellular water). These reference points may be distorted in patients with chronic renal failure. Measurement of total body potassium by the use of a naturally occurring isotope (^{40}K) also has given normal values (99).

Cellular potassium content has been estimated by the use of muscle biopsy (100–105). Bergstrom and colleagues (100) extensively studied 102 patients with serum creatinine levels ranging from 4.8 to 25.0 mg/dL before therapy. In this and other studies, the intracellular potassium concentration was low owing to an increase in intracellular water, despite normal intracellular potassium content (100,103). However, Bilbrey and coworkers (106) and Montanari and coworkers (105) have reported normal intracellular potassium concentrations. Importantly, the intracellular potassium content was either low or normal (but not increased) in all four studies

(100,103,105,106). The low intracellular potassium (and high intracellular sodium content) has also been reported in erythrocytes (102,107,108) and leukocytes (96,109) from these patients. This bespeaks a decrease in the number and/or the activity of the Na-K-ATPase pumps in the cell membrane. In chronic dialysis patients, the pump transport rate is higher immediately after fluid removal (110), and the abnormal levels of intracellular sodium and potassium in uremic patients return to normal following several weeks of dialysis (108,111). Because the number of pump sites inversely correlates with intracellular sodium, and a change in their number requires the production of new cells with lower intracellular sodium, the acute effect of fluid removal by dialysis may result from the removal of a volume-sensitive pump inhibitor (112). In contrast, the long-term effect of dialysis reflects the production of new cells with lower intracellular sodium and a higher number of pump sites (for a detailed discussion, refer to the article by Kaji and Kahn [112]).

Internal Potassium Homeostasis in Chronic Renal Failure

The role of cellular uptake of potassium in renal failure has been studied in both humans (92,93,113) and animals (114–117). Schon and associates (116) have shown that the cellular uptake of potassium in rats with remnant kidney is similar to that in normal rats maintained on a comparable diet but is lower than normal when both groups consume a high potassium diet. In contrast, in two different models of renal failure in rats, Bia and DeFronzo (114) showed impairment in the cellular disposal of an acute potassium load. Bourgoignie and associates (115) challenged chronically uremic dogs (remnant kidney model) who were adapted to different potassium intakes with an acute potassium load. Whereas the percentage of retained potassium that was shifted into the intracellular compartment was greater in normal dogs (90%), the absolute amount was significantly less than that in dogs with remnant kidney (9.0 versus 20.5 mEq, respectively). They concluded that extrarenal cellular uptake was normal in the dogs with renal failure. Gonick and colleagues (92) challenged patients with moderate renal failure with an oral potassium load. Whereas serum potassium 5 hours postchallenge was slightly higher in patients than in controls (5.2 versus 4.7 mEq/L), this result was entirely because of a lower urinary excretion. Perez and associates (113) studied patients with tubulointerstitial disease and showed that, whereas the absolute amount of potassium shifted into the cell was greater in patients compared with controls, the relative amount (expressed as percentage of total potassium retained) was similar. In contrast, Kahn and colleagues (93) observed a significantly greater rise in serum potassium in patients compared with controls when dietary potassium was increased by 50 mEq/day. The study by Kahn and colleagues cannot be strictly compared with others because they relied on 24-hour urinary potassium measurements and their study reflects long-term adaptation

to a high-potassium diet in patients with chronic renal failure. In dialysis patients, serum potassium rose significantly more in patients than in controls challenged with acute potassium load (1.06 versus 0.39 mEq/L). However, the baseline potassium was significantly higher in patients than controls (5.17 versus 3.59 mEq/L), making the interpretation of this study difficult (118). More recently, Allon and colleagues (119) noted similar response in these patients with lower baseline potassium. In summary, extrarenal cellular uptake of an acute potassium load in patients with chronic renal failure is near normal; however, it may be impaired in patients on hemodialysis with higher baseline plasma potassium.

As discussed previously, internal potassium homeostasis is regulated by insulin, catecholamines, and, to a lesser extent, aldosterone and PTH. Although the serum insulin level is increased in renal failure (120,121), three studies provide strong support for normal insulin-stimulated potassium uptake (121,122) by the splanchnic as well as by peripheral tissues (122). Alvestrand and coworkers (122), using the euglycemic insulin clamp technique, demonstrated a similar uptake of potassium by both splanchnic and leg tissues in patients with chronic renal failure. Inhibition of endogenous insulin by somatostatin results in a significantly greater rise in serum potassium in uremic rats than in controls (1.0 versus 0.2 mEq/L at 60 minutes) (123). Administration of glucose with potassium stimulates insulin secretion and attenuates the rise in potassium in patients on dialysis as well as normal controls (119).

Serum catecholamine levels have been reported to be high in chronic renal failure (124,125). Yang and coworkers (126) noted higher mean potassium in patients on a nonspecific ß-blocker, propranolol. Infusion of epinephrine resulted in two different responses: In four of 10 patients, serum potassium did not fall; in the remaining six, an exaggerated response was noted. The authors felt that the latter group of patients are those who have a propensity to develop hyperkalemia while on propranolol. Gifford and associates (127), using a much lower epinephrine dose, could not show a hypokalemic response in patients with ESRD. Plasma aldosterone is normal or high in most patients with chronic renal failure (93,128–131). As noted, patients with ESRD who are taking DOCA, spironolactone, or placebo have similar baseline potassium levels; however, patients on DOCA can dispose an acute potassium load more promptly than the other groups (62). In addition, high dose spironolactone for 3 weeks in ESRD patients can result in a significant rise in serum potassium (63). These two studies would support a minor role for aldosterone in internal potassium homeostasis in ESRD patients. The role of osmolality, as well as PTH and calcium channel blockers, has been discussed previously. In summary, the major cellular defect in potassium disposal seems to be an abnormal response to catecholamines seen in a subgroup of patients on dialysis. The role of hyperparathyroidism, a common accompaniment of renal failure, while intriguing, is still speculative in humans and requires more studies.

External Potassium Homeostasis in Severe Renal Failure

Renal Adaptation

Patients with a marked decrease in GFR are able to excrete the ingested dietary potassium load and maintain near normal potassium balance. This adaptive process is reflected by an increase in the fractional excretion of potassium (FE_K) modulated by an increase in secretory rate per functioning nephron. However, this adaptive response is limited and a sudden increase in potassium intake may result in life-threatening hyperkalemia. The quantitative aspects as well as the anatomic and functional characteristics of this adaptive response are briefly reviewed herein.

In conscious dogs with a 10% remnant kidney, Schultze and coworkers (132) showed that potassium excretion by the remnant kidney increased fourfold by 18 hours and approached 85% of the control value by seventh day. Kunau and Whinnery (133) and Wilson and Sonnenberg (117) reported similar data in rats. In experiments by Schultze and associates (132) and Finkelstein and Hayslett (134), animals with remnant kidney manifested an exaggerated kaliuresis following a potassium load. In contrast to these data and independent of previous potassium intake, dogs with 25% remnant kidney were only able to excrete 30% to 37% of the load in 5 hours compared with 70% to 90% in the control animals (115). There is no easy resolution to the differences in these two studies (115,132).

Gonick and colleagues (92) documented that human subjects with chronic renal failure were able to excrete only 20% of an oral potassium load in 6 hours compared with 46% in normal controls. Similar data have been reported by Perez and colleagues (113) in patients with tubulointerstitial disease. Kahn and colleagues (93), in 10 patients with chronic stable renal failure, showed that renal adaptation to increased dietary potassium occurs in these patients. In summary, it can be concluded that residual renal tissue is able to maintain external potassium homeostasis in the postabsorptive state. However, the initial phase of this adaptation is impaired when an acute potassium load is administered.

The nephron sites involved in this adaptation have been studied utilizing a variety of techniques in both rats and rabbits and appear to include both the distal convoluted tubule and the collecting duct (117,133–137). The discrepancies reported in the literature are most likely owing to interspecies and intraspecies differences as well as the anatomic definition of different distal tubular segments.

The mechanisms involved in this renal adaptation have been partially defined. In both humans (128) and rodents (138), aldosterone has been shown to play an important role in the adaptive ability of the diseased kidney to maintain a normal rate of potassium excretion. This renal adaptation has been shown to be independent of dietary sodium intake (139). Schultze and coworkers (132) argued that aldosterone is not important in the renal potassium adaptation that

occurs following a reduction in renal mass, since uremic dogs maintained on constant aldosterone replacement maintained normal rates of potassium excretion (132). However, the replacement dose of aldosterone in this study was in the high pharmacologic range. Serum potassium concentration itself may directly or indirectly augment urinary potassium excretion and play a role in renal adaptation following a reduction in kidney mass. Bourgoignie and colleagues (115) found a direct relationship between serum potassium and both the absolute and fractional potassium excretion. The slope of the curve relating serum potassium to the absolute rate of urinary potassium excretion was much steeper in normal dogs than in dogs with a remnant kidney. However, the slope of the curve relating serum potassium to the FE_K was similar in control and uremic dogs.

Microperfusion studies by Fine and associates (136) indicate that adaptation is an inherent characteristic of the renal tubular cells of uremic animals and once learned can be retained *in vitro,* at least for short periods of time. Schon and associates (116) showed that augmented potassium excretion is associated with an increase in Na-K-ATPase in the outer medulla in animals subjected to three-quarter nephrectomy. This increase is quite specific to this enzyme and occurs only in the kidney (116) and colon (140). Other mechanisms may include a higher rate of potassium delivery and an increase in tubular flow rate in the distal nephron (133).

Intestinal Potassium Excretion in Renal Failure

Patients with renal failure secrete more potassium in the stool than do normal controls (128,141,142). Net colonic secretion of potassium is increased significantly above control levels in rats with renal insufficiency (141). This increase is associated with an increase in Na-K-ATPase activity in colonic mucosa and is functionally similar to the increase seen with the administration of DOCA, glucocorticoids, or high dietary potassium (143). Although the rise in fecal potassium concentration is significant, the absolute amount of K^+ lost through this route in patients with mild to moderate chronic renal failure is small and contributes only minimally to the external K^+ homeostasis. In patients with advanced renal insufficiency (GFR < 5 to 10 mL/minute); however, up to 30% to 40% of the ingested potassium load may be excreted in the stool (142).

Acid–Base Homeostasis

The kidney through its ability to excrete nonvolatile (fixed) acid produced by combustion of foodstuff, chiefly proteins, plays a major role in hydrogen ion homeostasis. This is done by reclamation of filtered buffers (primarily bicarbonate) and regeneration of buffers lost in daily titration of ingested acids. Although the total fixed acid generated from combustion of foodstuff is relatively small, estimated at 1 mEq/kg body weight/day, unless this is excreted it can deplete the total buffer reserve, estimated at 600 to 700 mEq, in days to weeks.

Bicarbonate reclamation occurs by hydrogen secretion through Na-H antiporter in the proximal tubules as well as H-ATPase pump in both proximal and distal tubules. This process accounts for reabsorption of approximately 4,000 to 5,000 mEq of base per day, resulting in acid urine devoid of bicarbonate. The bicarbonate regeneration occurs primarily in the distal tubules through protonation of urinary buffers made up of titratable acids (primarily phosphates) and ammonia. The proximal tubule is therefore responsible for 85% to 90% of bicarbonate reclamation, whereas the distal tubule is responsible for the remaining 10% to 15%. In addition, the distal tubule is also responsible for regeneration of 60 to 80 mEq of new bicarbonate. When faced with an additional acid load, the kidney increases H^+ secretion (and bicarbonate regeneration) primarily through an increase in ammonium production by the deamination of circulating glutamine. The ability of the kidney to increase ammonium secretion is limited and is estimated at three to five times baseline production (143–145). (See Chapter 6, Renal Acid–Base Transport, for a detailed discussion.)

Acid–Base Homeostasis in Renal Failure

The ability of the kidney to excrete hydrogen ion is progressively diminished with the diminution of GFR. Although it is commonly stated that a significant decrease in serum bicarbonate does not occur until GFR falls below 25 to 30 mL/minute, this is not strictly true. Widmer and colleagues (146) noted a serum bicarbonate reduction from 28 to 22 mEq/L in patients with a creatinine of 2 to 4 mg/dL and further reduction to 19 mEq/L in patients with a creatinine of 4 to 14 mg/dL (146). The anion gap remained unchanged in the first group and rose significantly with a further decrease in GFR. The concept of orderly progression of metabolic acidosis of renal failure from hyperchloremic to anion gap acidosis, however, occurs in the minority of patients. Wallia and colleagues (147) studied the electrolyte pattern in 70 patients with ESRD just before dialytic therapy was begun. Five patterns were found: 14 patients with normal electrolytes; 14 with anion gap metabolic acidosis; 21 with hyperchloremic acidosis; 11 with mixed hyperchloremic and anion gap acidosis; and 10 with normal serum chloride, low serum bicarbonate, and normal anion gap. This last group, however, had the lowest serum sodium and therefore were relatively hyperchloremic. Therefore, among these 70 patients with ESRD, 31 (44%) had hyperchloremic acidosis, only 14 (20%) had classic anion gap acidosis, and interestingly another 14 (20%) had normal electrolytes. Patients with increased anion gap, however, had a slight but significantly higher serum creatinine than patients with pure hyperchloremic acidosis or with normal electrolytes (13.2 versus 10.0 versus 9.0 mg/dL, respectively). In addition, these two studies did not support the common impression that hyperchloremic acidosis occurs more often in patients with

tubulointerstitial than glomerular disease (146,147). Interestingly, diabetic patients with moderately severe renal failure (GFR < 30 mL/minute) have recently been reported to have milder metabolic acidosis than nondiabetics with similar renal function (148).

Renal tubular acidosis (RTA) defines a group of disorders characterized by the presence of metabolic acidosis out of proportion to the decrease in GFR. The hallmark of these disorders is the presence of significant metabolic acidosis with hyperchloremia and normal anion gap. Renal tubular acidosis in patients with mild to moderate renal insufficiency is often associated with significant hyperkalemia and is discussed later in this chapter.

Pathophysiology of Metabolic Acidosis in Chronic Renal Failure

Many studies have shown that acid production in renal failure is normal, and therefore uremic acidosis reflects a decrease in net acid excretion, defined as the difference between proton excretion in the form of titratable acid and ammonium ion (NH_4^+) and bicarbonate excretion (149–151). Careful metabolic studies by Goodman and colleagues (151) documented that patients with chronic renal failure have a daily bicarbonate deficit of approximately 13 to 19 mEq. It is notable that despite this persistent deficit, serum bicarbonate in patients with chronic renal failure, after an initial drop, remains stable over long periods of time (152,153). This is chiefly owing to the buffering of excess hydrogen ion by bone buffers including calcium carbonate (152).

Renal Excretion of Bicarbonate

Several studies in humans have shown that some patients with severe renal failure have significant bicarbonate wasting (149,154–158). In an early study by Schwartz and coworkers (149), three out of four patients with renal failure had significant bicarbonaturia, which disappeared only after the fall of serum bicarbonate to below 20 mEq/L. In a more detailed study in 17 uremic patients (serum creatinine of 5.6 to 18.9 mg/dL), the majority had significant bicarbonate wasting (fractional excretion of HCO_3 of 0% to 17.56%) despite the presence of metabolic acidosis (serum HCO_3 of 16 to 23 mEq/L). After NH_4Cl loading, serum bicarbonate decreased to below 14 mEq/L, and bicarbonaturia disappeared in all but four patients (158). Interestingly, the bicarbonate wasting in these four patients also disappeared with institution of a low-sodium diet. These two studies support the presence of a diminished maximal tubular reabsorption (T_m) for bicarbonate in the majority of patients with renal failure. Further, they demonstrate that the low T_m is partly responsive to volume status.

Arruda and colleagues (157) and Wong and associates (159), working with a remnant kidney model in dogs with variable levels of volume expansion and serum bicarbonate, noted that the ratio of absolute bicarbonate to sodium reabsorption was increased in chronic renal failure. In addition Wong and associates (159), using micropuncture method, showed that this ratio was also higher at the beginning of the distal tubule, indicating avid bicarbonate absorption by the proximal tubule of the remnant kidney. Although absolute absorption was higher, the absolute amount of bicarbonate delivered to the distal tubule was also higher, reflecting the marked increase in filtered load per nephron owing to an increase in single nephron GFR (159). In summary, the whole-kidney T_m for bicarbonate is in general diminished in chronic renal failure despite an absolute increase in bicarbonate resorption at the single nephron. The discrepancy in these findings may reflect the variation in the experimental designs and the role of nonvolume regulators in bicarbonate handling by the kidney.

Renal Excretion of Titratable Acid

Excretion of titratable acids chiefly reflects the amount of urinary phosphate and the urinary pH. Most patients with chronic renal failure are able to maximally acidify their urine (149,160), and urine-serum PCO_2, as a measure of hydrogen pump activity in the distal tubule, is normal (161). The amount of titratable acids in these patients is normal (151,152–164). This is primarily owing to an increase in fractional excretion of phosphate initiated by secondary hyperparathyroidism. It should be noted, however, that urinary phosphate does decrease with severe renal failure. This reflects both a decrease in dietary phosphate as well as the effect of phosphate binders commonly used in these patients.

Renal Excretion of Ammonium

Although bicarbonaturia may contribute to metabolic acidosis, the major abnormality is a decrease in renal excretion of ammonium. Ammonium is primarily produced by the deamination of amino acids, chiefly glutamine, in the proximal tubule and to a much lesser extent in the loop of Henle and distal convoluted tubule (144,145) (Chapter 6, Renal Acid–Base Transport). The production of ammonium in the proximal tubule is increased significantly by acidosis and inhibited by alkalosis (165). This pathway is regulated by two key enzymes, glutaminase and phosphoenolpyruvate carboxylase. In metabolic acidosis there is an increase activity of both enzymes in association to increase in their respective messenger RNA (166). The majority of ammonium produced is reabsorbed in the ascending limb of the loop of Henle by both active and passive processes and is added to the medullary interstitium. The active transport involves substitution of ammonium instead of potassium on Na+-2Cl-K+ transporter in the TALH, which is inhibited by hyperkalemia (167). In the medullary interstitium, ammonium ion exists in dynamic equilibrium with ammonia gas. The latter diffuses chiefly into the collecting duct, where it is protonated by hydrogen secreted by the H-ATPase pump, located in the luminal membrane of the intercalated cells, and is trapped intralu-

minally and finally excreted. However, some ammonia gas enters into the descending limb of the loop of Henle, creating a countercurrent mechanism for ammonium. The final urinary ammonium is therefore a reflection of production of ammonium in the proximal tubule, its transport into the loop of Henle, accumulation in the renal interstitium, and finally secretion of ammonia and its entrapment in the collecting duct (144,145).

In chronic renal failure, fractional renal ammonium excretion initially increases by severalfold, thereby resulting in the maintenance of a normal absolute excretion rate (168). However, as the GFR decreases below 20 mL/minute, despite maximal increase in fractional excretion of ammonium, the absolute excretory rate decreases significantly, thus resulting in progressive metabolic acidosis. This decrease in the rate of ammonium excretion also reflects a decreased ability of the kidney to trap ammonia in the collecting duct (160). Warnock (153) has suggested that the decrease in ammonia trapping in the remnant kidney model may be secondary to excess delivery of bicarbonate to the collecting duct, thereby resulting in an unfavorable environment for the diffusion and trapping of ammonia.

The role of aldosterone in ammonium excretion is complex. Aldosterone increases the rate of Na^+-dependent and Na^+-independent H^+ secretion in the cortical and medullary collecting duct (169,170). Hypoaldosteronism is associated with a decrease in the rate of H^+ secretion, while the ability to maintain a steep H^+ gradient between urine and plasma, as measured by urinary pH and urine minus blood PCO_2 in alkaline urine, is not affected (171,172). The decrease in the rate of H^+ secretion is associated with a decrease in the availability of ammonium buffer in the urine that is not augmented appropriately in response to sodium sulfate infusion (173,174). Hypoaldosteronism is universally associated with a decreased potassium excretion and hyperkalemia. Hyperkalemia decreases renal ammonium excretion significantly. This is owing to a decrease in accumulation of ammonium in the renal interstitium despite normal production by the proximal tubule (175). In the syndrome of hyperkalemic renal tubular acidosis, this mechanism probably plays the major role in the production of hyperchloremic acidosis seen early in the course of renal failure. Reversal of hyperkalemia with sodium binding resin (176), mineralocorticoids (177), or low-potassium diet (178) ameliorates the metabolic acidosis by increasing ammonium secretion.

HYPERKALEMIC RENAL TUBULAR ACIDOSIS OWING TO A DEFECT IN RENIN–ANGIOTENSIN–ALDOSTERONE AXIS OR TUBULAR UNRESPONSIVENESS TO ALDOSTERONE

Although a decrease in GFR may be associated with the development of significant hyperkalemia and hyperchloremic (HCA) or anion gap metabolic acidosis, this usually occurs only with severe reductions in GFR, below 15 to

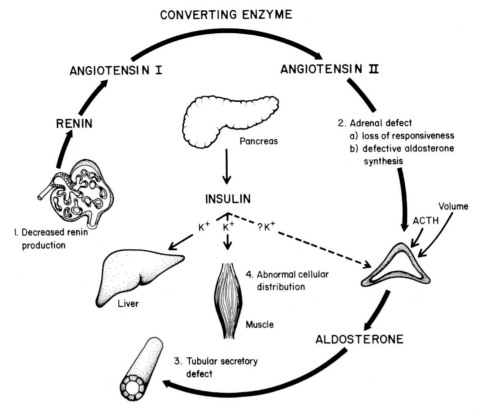

FIG. 87-5. Schematic representation of potential hormonal, renal, and extrarenal defects resulting in hyperkalemia. Hyperkalemia may result from one of the following conditions: (a) decreased renin production, (b) decreased aldosterone production despite normal renin secretion (adrenal defect), (c) a renal tubular secretory defect, or (d) an abnormal distribution of potassium between intracellular and extracellular fluid compartments. (From: DeFronzo RA, et al. Nonuremic hypokalemia: a possible role for insulin deficiency. *Arch Intern Med* 1979;137:842, with permission.)

20 mL/minute. However, some patients with underlying renal disease and mild to moderate azotemia present with striking hyperkalemia with or without HCA. The elevated serum potassium in these patients is primarily owing to a disturbance in the renin–angiotensin–aldosterone axis or to renal tubular responsiveness to aldosterone (Fig. 87-5; Table 87-2). Since the report by Hudson and associates (179) numerous cases have been described in which hyperkalemia with or without HCA developed in the presence of only mild to moderate renal insufficiency (180–191). In the majority of these cases, the underlying renal disease has been diabetic or hypertensive nephropathy or chronic interstitial nephritis (181). In 1972 Schambelan and colleagues (192) presented evidence linking hypoaldosteronism with hyporeninism in six patients with this syndrome. This association was verified in subsequent reports (193–196), and the entity became known as hyporeninemic hypoaldosteronism (HHA). However, it became quickly clear that a significant minority of these patients had normal renin levels. DeFronzo (197) in 1980, after reviewing 81 published cases, came to the conclusion that in 20% of cases the low plasma aldosterone levels could not be explained by renin deficiency, and therefore a primary abnormality in aldosterone synthesis had to be postulated. At the same time, some patients with sickle cell disease (7,198,199),

systemic lupus erythematosus (200,201), and renal transplantation (202,203) have a renal tubular secretory defect resulting in hyperkalemia despite a normal renin–aldosterone axis. Therefore, at the present time these patients can be divided into two large categories: (1) hyperkalemia resulting from hypoaldosteronism with or without hyporeninism; and (2) hyperkalemia resulting from a primary renal tubular potassium secretory defect. One could consider this entity as a spectrum ranging from pure aldosterone deficiency with normal tubular responsiveness to severe tubular resistance with normal aldosterone secretion. Between these two extremes there are many overlapping presentations in which either the defect in the hormonal axis or tubular responsiveness dominates. Although Table 87-2 summarizes all the hormonal or tubular defects that can lead to hyperkalemia, often with HCA our discussion is limited to the disturbances associated with renal insufficiency.

Hyperkalemic Renal Tubular Acidosis Owing to a Defect in Renin–Angiotensin–Aldosterone Axis

This group (Fig. 87-5, Table 87-2) comprises approximately 80% of the patients with renal insufficiency and hyperkalemia (197,204–206). The hallmark of this group is a low plasma

TABLE 87-2. *Etiology of chronic hyperkalemia due to disturbances in renal potassium excretion*

I. Decrease in GFR
  A. Acute renal failure
  B. Chronic renal failure (GFR <15–20 mL/min)
II. Defect in renal tubular secretion of potassium
  A. Disturbance in the renin–angiotensin–aldosterone axis
    1. Hyporeninism: associated with renal insufficiency (diabetes mellitus, interstitial nephritis)
    2. Disturbance in angiotensin II activation or function (captopril, saralasin)
    3. Hypoaldosteronism
      a. With glucocorticoid deficiency (Addison's disease, enzyme deficiency)
      b. Block in aldosterone synthesis (heparin, 18-methyloxidase deficiency)
      c. Primary hypoaldosteronism
  B. Tubular resistance to the action of aldosterone (renal tubular hyperkalemia)
    1. Pseudohypoaldosteronism
    2. Hyperkalemia, hypertension, and normal renal function
    3. Hyperkalemia with mild to moderate renal insufficiency and variable plasma aldosterone levels (sickle cell disease, systemic lupus erythematosus, renal transplant, obstructive uropathy, miscellaneous)
    4. Pharmacologic inhibition of the tubular action of aldosterone (spironolactone, triamterene, amiloride, pentamidine, trimethoprim) in distal nephron

GFR, glomerular filtration rate.

aldosterone concentration. The majority (80%) of this group also has low plasma renin activity (PRA) and therefore represents the classic syndrome of HHA. However, 20% have a normal PRA. Clinically and physiologically, these patients present with fairly uniform features. Several large (192,207) as well as smaller series (252,255–260), have defined the characteristics of these patients first summarized in a review by DeFronzo (197). These include: (a) mean age of about 60 years, (b) presence of diabetes mellitus in about 50%, (c) presence of mild to moderate renal failure in the majority, and (d) lack of symptoms referable to hyperkalemia in 75%. Physiologic features include: (a) low or low-normal baseline and/or stimulated aldosterone levels, (b) normal plasma cortisol, (c) low baseline and/or stimulated renin values in 80%, (d) normal aldosterone response to angiotensin or ACTH stimulation in the minority, (e) presence of hyperchloremic acidosis in well over 50%, and (f) lack of significant salt wasting.

To gain an understanding of the physiologic basis of this syndrome, we initially review the defect in renin secretion and then summarize our present understanding of aldosterone deficiency in this syndrome.

Hyporeninism

At present no single abnormality can explain the low PRA seen in 80% of these patients (197,205,206). Evidence has been presented in support of a defect in one or more phy-

siologic regulators of renin secretion including volume, autonomic nervous system, serum potassium concentration, and prostaglandins.

Oh and colleagues (195), Perez and colleagues (212), and others (213,214) have demonstrated that long-term sodium and volume depletion in these patients is associated with a significant increase in the PRA. However, comparable data in normal controls with the same degree of volume depletion were not provided. In the report of Oh and colleagues (195), after 3 to 6 weeks of salt depletion, the PRA rose into the normal range, but plasma aldosterone remained subnormal. In the study by Chan and coworkers, eight of the 12 patients with hyporeninism responded to 2 weeks of furosemide with increase in PRA without similar response in plasma aldosterone (214). In a study of four patients with acute postinfectious glomerulonephritis (181), plasma renin and aldosterone concentrations were low during the acute phase, but returned to normal following recovery from acute nephritis. Interestingly, in two patients, the renin and aldosterone levels remained low during the acute phase despite an excellent response to diuretics. These two patients, however, responded appropriately to physiologic doses of fludrocortisone. This study (181), coupled with previous studies of acute glomerulonephritis (215,216), supports the concept that although physiologic suppression of the renin–aldosterone axis by volume expansion may play a significant role in certain patients with glomerular disease, hypertension, and edema, other factors such as decreased GFR and damage to the juxtaglomerular apparatus play an important contributory role. Gordon and colleagues (217) have described a patient with hypertension, acidosis, hyperkalemia, and normal renal function associated with HHA. Prolonged sodium restriction resulted in correction of these abnormalities. A similar pathophysiologic mechanism has been postulated in hypertensive patients with hyperkalemia and renal insufficiency (218).

The autonomic nervous system plays an important physiologic role in the regulation of renin secretion. Sympathetic nerve terminals are known to innervate the juxtaglomerular apparatus, and renin secretion is stimulated by epinephrine (219,220). Therefore, autonomic insufficiency could result in a state of hyporeninemia. This hypothesis has been investigated primarily in diabetic patients, in whom autonomic neuropathy is common and circulating catecholamine levels are often low (221). In five diabetic patients with autonomic neuropathy Tuck and colleagues (222) reported low basal PRA as well as diminished plasma aldosterone and norepinephrine concentrations. In addition, infusion of isoproterenol, a ß-adrenergic agonist, did not increase PRA, indicating a possible block at or beyond the receptor level. In contrast, normal circulating catecholamine levels have previously been reported in diabetic patients with the syndrome of hypoaldosteronism (180,193,223,224). Fernandez-Cruz and coworkers (225) compared stimulated PRA in 16 normotensive diabetic patients without overt nephropathy and nine age-matched controls. The simulated PRA was significantly lower in these patients and correlated directly with the degree of autonomic dysfunction as measured by the velocity of esophageal peristalsis. De Chatel and colleagues (226), however, were unable to demonstrate in a large group of diabetic individuals any correlation between the plasma epinephrine concentration and abnormalities in the renin–aldosterone axis. Therefore, although autonomic neuropathy may play a role in the development of hypoaldosteronism in some diabetics, it is not a uniform finding and certainly cannot explain the occurrence of this syndrome in nondiabetic patients.

Hyperkalemia is known to inhibit PRA (227); consequently, one could hypothesize that hyporeninemia is not a primary defect but is secondary to hyperkalemia. In two studies (192,196), short-term normalization of serum potassium did not increase PRA significantly; however, long-term studies have not been undertaken to examine this very important question.

Prostaglandins E_2, I_2, and D_2 are known stimulators of renin release (228,229), whereas prostaglandins E_1 and E_2 directly increase aldosterone biosynthesis *in vitro* (230). Furthermore, hyperkalemia has been reported following treatment with indomethacin, a potent prostaglandin inhibitor (231). These observations raise the possibility that a defect in prostaglandin synthesis may play a role in the development of HHA in some hyperkalemic patients. Consistent with this, Tan and colleagues (232) found a strong correlation between urinary PGE_2 level and the ratio of active to inactive renin in normal controls and in patients with the syndrome of hypoaldosteronism. In four of the nine patients, low urinary PGE_2 was associated with a low ratio of active to inactive renin. In normal controls, inhibition of prostaglandin synthesis with indomethacin resulted in a similar decrease in this ratio. These authors postulated that prostaglandins may play a critical role in the activation of renin, and therefore hypoaldosteronism in these patients may be secondary to a prostaglandin deficiency. In two patients with diabetes mellitus and hypoaldosteronism, the total renin concentration was normal, whereas PRA was low (233). Fractionation of the plasma yielded an inactive renin precursor (prorenin or "big renin"); unfortunately, prostaglandin levels were not measured in these diabetic patients. It should be noted, however, that other investigators have failed to find an association between prostaglandin deficiency and the development of HHA (234).

Another hypothesis that links chronic renal insufficiency with hyporeninism is fibrosis of the juxtaglomerular apparatus owing to intrinsic renal disease. Although occasional reports of juxtaglomerular apparatus fibrosis have appeared (213), this is a rare finding. Besides, the presence of juxtaglomerular apparatus damage alone does not explain the development of hypoaldosteronism.

Hyperfiltration hypothesis has been linked to the development of HHA in both diabetic and nondiabetic patients with renal insufficiency (235). According to this hypothesis, as the number of nephrons is reduced, there is an adaptive increase in the renal plasma flow and GFR by the remaining functioning glomeruli. These alterations in renal hemodynamics serve to inhibit renin synthesis and release, leading secondarily to the development of hypoaldosteronism.

Hypoaldosteronism

The hallmark of the syndrome of HHA is a low basal or low stimulated plasma aldosterone level in spite of normal levels of glucocorticoids and other ACTH-dependent steroids such as DOCA or corticosterone. Aldosterone secretion is primarily stimulated by the renin–angiotensin system. However, ACTH and serum potassium, as well as other regulators, play independent roles.

As stated previously, hyporeninemia is present in 80% of patients with hypoaldosteronism (197,205,206), and therefore it is logical to consider that the primary defect in these patients lies in renin synthesis or release. Schambelan and colleagues (206) showed that stimulation of renin by volume contraction resulted in a rise in plasma aldosterone that was appropriate for the increase in PRA. The slope of the curve relating plasma renin and aldosterone was similar in patients with HHA and normal controls. Surprisingly, for any given level of PRA, the plasma aldosterone concentration was disproportionately elevated, probably because of the independent stimulatory effect of plasma potassium on aldosterone secretion. Nevertheless, the highest levels of renin and aldosterone achieved in these patients were comparable only to the basal levels in control subjects. In contrast, as indicated, other investigators have found a clear disconnect between renin and aldosterone level after stimulation with volume depletion (212–214) and captopril (214). In all studies, however, the response of aldosterone was significantly blunted despite increase renin and persistent hyperkalemia. In addition, most investigators have reported a marked impairment in the ability of angiotensin II to stimulate aldosterone secretion (197,206). This finding, coupled with a subnormal aldosterone response to ACTH stimulation (197,206), and the failure of hyperkalemia to stimulate aldosterone secretion, has strengthened the possibility of a primary adrenal defect in some patients with hypoaldosteronism. This is further supported by the observation that 20% of patients with hypoaldosteronism have normal PRA (197,205,206). One should also consider the possibility that the poor response of aldosterone to ACTH, angiotensin II, and hyperkalemia may be secondary to long-term atrophy of the zona glomerulosa of the adrenal gland rather than to a specific enzymatic defect in aldosterone production. Consistent with this possibility, Fredlund and colleagues (236) provided evidence in isolated adrenal glomerulosa cells that the aldosterone response to hyperkalemia is dependent on the circulating angiotensin level. However, no study so far has evaluated response of adrenal gland to prolonged stimulation by angiotensin II in patients.

The serum potassium concentration is an important regulator of the plasma aldosterone level (237–239). In nephrectomized patients, a significant correlation between serum potassium and plasma aldosterone exists (240), and this relationship is independent of renin or ACTH. Therefore, in interpreting a given plasma aldosterone level, the effect of serum potassium must be considered. Schambelan and colleagues (206) categorized 31 patients into two groups based on the ratio of urinary aldosterone excretion to serum potassium concentration. Group A (23 patients) had a low ratio and was considered to have hypoaldosteronism. Group B (eight patients) had a normal ratio and was considered to have a primary tubular defect in potassium secretion. Twenty percent of group A had a normal PRA. Therefore, hypoaldosteronism in this group, in spite of normal PRA and high plasma potassium, is probably owing to a defect in aldosterone synthesis.

Another regulator of aldosterone secretion and plasma volume is atrial natriuretic factor (ANF). Atrial natriuretic factor has been shown to be a strong inhibitor of baseline as well as stimulated aldosterone in humans (241,242). In normal humans, ANF also prevents potassium-stimulated rise in aldosterone level (243). In addition, ANF level is markedly elevated 10- to 50-fold in patients with hypoaldosteronism (243). Although the rise in ANF (and suppression of aldosterone) could be secondary to volume expansion, ANF also suppresses potassium, angiotensin and ACTH-stimulated aldosterone secretion supporting presence of a common cellular mechanism for its action possibly through stimulation of cGMP (244).

Several investigators have explored the possibility of an enzymatic defect in aldosterone biosynthesis (212,224,227), and an enzymatic block involving the conversion of 18-hydroxycorticosterone to aldosterone has been postulated, but these findings have not been supported by other studies (192,245,246).

As indicated, diabetic patients constitute a large percentage of patients with HHA. To explain this high incidence, two other postulates have been presented. Insulin is an important regulator of potassium uptake by a variety of tissues, and chronic hypoinsulinemia (absolute or relative) might be expected to result in a state of intracellular potassium deficiency. Furthermore, it is known that the intracellular potassium concentration is an important regulator of aldosterone synthesis (197). Potassium-deficient cultured zona glomerulosa cells have a blunted response to angiotensin II and ACTH (236,247). Insulinopenia, by decreasing intracellular potassium, may lead to a defect in aldosterone synthesis and the syndrome of hypoaldosteronism (13). A second hypothesis is offered by Smith and DeFronzo (248) and involves the concept of tubuloglomerular feedback. Normal tubuloglomerular balance is disrupted in the presence of osmotic agents in the renal tubule (249,250), including glucose (251–253). It is postulated that, in diabetics with a high filtered glucose load, sodium chloride delivery out of the proximal tubule is enhanced, leading to increased delivery of solute to the loop of Henle. Enhanced chloride reabsorption by the thick ascending limb of Henle's loop may inhibit renin secretion (254), which secondarily leads to the development of hypoaldosteronism.

In summary, at present a unified etiologic hypothesis cannot be formulated to explain the occurrence of the syndrome of HHA in different patients. It is likely that this syndrome is quite heterogeneous and can be explained only by multiple etiologic abnormalities. In a given patient, the role of different regulatory systems (i.e., volume status, prostaglandins, ANF, autonomic nervous system, structural damage to the juxtaglomerular apparatus, enzymatic defects in aldosterone and renin biosynthesis, and intracellular adrenal potassium deficiency) should be considered and evaluated.

Hyperkalemic Renal Tubular Acidosis Owing to a Renal Tubular Secretory Defect

This group of disorders (Table 87-2 and Fig. 87-5) includes patients who have hyperkalemia out of proportion to the degree of renal failure or hypoaldosteronism. The primary defect is a partial resistance to the physiologic effect of aldosterone to promote potassium secretion. Perez and coworkers (255) named this syndrome renal tubular hyperkalemia and divided it into three groups: group I, patients with pseudohypoaldosteronism; group II, patients with hyperkalemia, hypertension, and normal renal function; and group III, patients with hyperkalemia, mild to moderate renal insufficiency, and normal-plasma aldosterone (group IIIa), low-plasma aldosterone (group IIIb), or high-plasma aldosterone (IIIc) (Table 87-2).

Groups I and II represent examples of a pure tubular secretory defect without renal insufficiency and is not discussed here. In this section we deal only with group III patients, who present with mild to moderate renal insufficiency, hyperkalemia, hyperchloremic acidosis, variable plasma renin and aldosterone levels, and resistance to physiologic doses of mineralocorticoids. This clinical entity has been described in patients with sickle cell disease, systemic lupus erythematosus, renal transplant, obstructive uropathy, acquired immunodeficiency syndrome (AIDS), and a group of miscellaneous diseases including lead nephropathy and chronic interstitial nephritis.

Sickle Cell Disease

A renal tubular potassium secretory defect in sickle cell disease was first reported in patients with normal renal function and normal serum electrolyte concentrations (7) and later in patients with sickle cell nephropathy (197,256), sickle cell trait (198), and sickle C disease (199). Although basal and stimulated aldosterone levels were normal in all subjects, these patients were unable to excrete a potassium load normally. Infusion of potassium chloride, sodium sulfate, and furosemide failed to augment potassium secretion normally. This defect is thought to result from ischemic damage to the collecting tubules and medullary area by sickle cells. An immunologic reaction against a renal tubular antigen also has been suggested. It should be noted that the syndrome of HHA also occurs in sickle cell disease (197,256).

Systemic Lupus Erythematosus

A defect in potassium secretion, similar to the defect in sickle cell disease, has been reported in several patients with systemic lupus erythematosus (SLE) (200,201). The defect is often accompanied by a defect in hydrogen ion secretion (200,201,257). In two patients, an increase in sodium and bicarbonate delivery (by furosemide, acetazolamide, and bicarbonate) to the distal sites of potassium exchange did not augment potassium secretion. High-dose fludrocortisone therapy also failed to increase potassium excretion in these two patients (200). Recently, a single patient has been reported in whom fludrocortisone was successful in controlling hyperkalemia (258). In a study of two patients with SLE and hyperkalemic RTA, Bastani and associates showed presence of autoantibodies to collecting duct cells in one patient. The serum from this patient labeled the intercalated cell in rat kidney section. However, the serum from both patients did not react with affinity-purified bovine H(+)-ATPase or human H(+)-ATPase B subunit (259). This is in contrast to the finding in a single patient with Sjögren's syndrome who had absence of vacuolar H(+)-ATPase in intercalated cells (260). These findings support the concept that cellular and molecular mechanisms in these patients probably are heterogeneous in nature.

Obstructive Uropathy

Hyperkalemic RTA, as a complication of obstructive uropathy, is common and best described in a report of 13 patients by Batlle and associates (204). Two patterns were noted: (a) Five patients had normal plasma aldosterone levels but failed to increase urinary potassium excretion after administration of acetazolamide, fludrocortisone, and sodium sulfate. The primary defect in this group is renal tubular unresponsiveness to aldosterone. (b) Eight patients had low plasma aldosterone levels but failed to augment renal potassium excretion with mineralocorticoid administration. As noted, this reflects a combined defect in this group. Furthermore, urinary acidification in response to systemic acidosis and sodium sulfate infusion was abnormal in eight of 13 patients. In a rat model of acute ureteral obstruction, no change in the number or tubular distribution of vacuolar H+ATPase was noted; however, the intracellular distribution was changed with a significant decrease in plasma membrane bound pumps in intercalated cells (261). This finding may explain HMA commonly noted in these patients.

Renal Transplantation

In the precyclosporine era, hyperkalemia was a relatively unusual phenomenon following successful renal transplantation (202,203,262). However, two large series from Australia and the United States (202,203) and a small series from Israel (263) have reported the occurrence of renal tubular hyperkalemia in this group. In the largest series, 23 of 75 patients with a successful kidney transplant had hyperkalemia unrelated to rejection episodes, renal failure, oliguria, or acidosis (202). The renin–angiotensin–aldosterone axis was normal in these patients, and hyperkalemia did not respond to furosemide. The hyperkalemia was transient, disappearing spontaneously, and did not correlate with clinical or laboratory evidence of rejection. In contrast, in two patients studied by Battle and coworkers (262), hyperkalemia was associated with very low levels of aldosterone, which did not respond to volume contraction. Urinary potassium was low and did not respond to infusion of sodium sulfate or acetazolamide. The etiology of this disorder is not clear, but immunologic damage to the renal tubular cells is postulated (202). In the cyclosporine era, hyperkalemia is more common in kidney transplant recipients (264,265). The role of cyclosporine and tacrolimus (FK-506) in the development of hyperkalemia is discussed in the following section, which outlines drugs that exacerbate hyperkalemia.

Hyperkalemic Renal Tubular Acidosis Associated with Acquired Immunodeficiency Syndrome

Acid–base and electrolyte disturbances, with or without renal failure, are common in patients with AIDS. As reviewed by Perazella and Brown, the incidence varies from 5% to 53% and is owing to a variety of causes including adrenal insufficiency, renal failure, type IV RTA, and finally as a complication of drugs used in these patients (266,267). The syndrome of hyporenin-hypoaldosteronism is relatively uncommon and usually is associated with AIDS nephropathy. Patients with AIDS are exposed to a variety of drugs that could result in hyperkalemia, often associated with HCA and/or renal insufficiency. These culprit drugs are discussed further in the section that outlines those medications that most often exacerbate hyperkalemia in patients with impaired potassium handling.

Miscellaneous Conditions

Renal tubular hyperkalemia has been reported in a variety of other renal diseases. These include chronic interstitial nephritis of unknown etiology (268), nephrosclerosis (207), diabetes mellitus (206), postinfectious glomerulonephritis (181,215,216), lead nephropathy (269), and drug-induced acute interstitial nephritis (270). Although in our experience this entity seems to be relatively common in nonspecific interstitial nephritis, no incidence or prevalence data are available.

TABLE 87-3. *Common drugs that cause hyperkalemia and mechanism of action*

Medication	Mechanism of action
Potassium supplement	Increase intake
Salt substitutes	Increase intake
Nutritional/herbal supplements	Increase intake
Beta-blocking agents	Decrease potassium movement into cells, decrease renin/aldosterone
Digoxin intoxication	Decrease Na^+-K^+ ATPase activity
Lysine, arginine and epsilon-aminocaproic acid	Shift of potassium out of cells
Succinylcholine	Shift of potassium out of cells
Potassium-sparing diuretics	
Spironolactone	Aldosterone antagonism
Triamterene	Block Na^+ channels in principal cells
Amiloride	Block Na^+ channels in principal cells
NSAIDs	Decrease renin/aldosterone
	Decrease RBF and GFR
ACE inhibitors and AII receptor antagonists	Decrease aldosterone synthesis
	Decrease RBF and GFR
Heparin	Decrease aldosterone synthesis
Trimethoprim and pentamidine	Block Na^+ channels in principal cells
Cyclosporine and tacrolimus (FK506)	Decrease aldosterone synthesis
	Decrease Na^+-K^+ ATPase activity
	Decrease K^+ channel activity

NSAIDs, nonsteroidal antiinflammatory drugs; *ACE,* angiotensin converting enzyme; *AII,* angiotensin II.

Drugs Associated with Hyperkalemia in Patients with Renal Disease

In patients with underlying renal insufficiency, prescribed drugs or over the counter medications and supplements play an increasingly dominant role in development of hyperkalemia. It is therefore important to recognize that a variety of products are capable of elevating serum potassium concentration through multiple mechanisms (Table 87-3). Hyperkalemia, depending on the criteria used, has been reported to develop in anywhere from 1.3% to 10% of patients and is often multifactorial. Of the many factors involved, culprit medications, either alone or in association with other disturbances in potassium homeostasis, were a contributing cause of hyperkalemia in 35% to 75% of hospitalized patients (271–275). Of note, renal insufficiency and older age (>60 years) were important predisposing risk factors in many studies (271–273).

Increased Potassium Input

Enteral and parenteral input of potassium are very common causes of hyperkalemia in hospitalized patients. Nonetheless, chronic hyperkalemia does not occur with these products unless an underlying defect in potassium homeostasis also is present. Deliberate potassium intake often lies at the root of hyperkalemia, although unsuspected potassium delivery also occurs. A 3.6% incidence of hyperkalemia among 4,921 patients taking physician-prescribed potassium supplements was documented in the Boston Collaborative Drug

Surveillance Program (271). The mean peak potassium concentration in these patients was 6.0 mEq/L, whereas a level greater than 7.5 mEq/L was noted in 13 of the 179 patients (7.3%). Azotemia and older age were more frequent among those with hyperkalemia (7). In addition, several other studies reveal that potassium supplements cause or contribute to hyperkalemia in 15% to 40% of hospitalized patients (272–275).

Salt substitutes and salt alternatives, recommended for patients with hypertension and edematous disorders, provide yet another rich source of potassium (276,277). Some "no-salt" salt substitutes contain 10 to 13 mEq of potassium per gram (277). A number of nutritional supplements contain as much as 49 to 54 mEq of potassium per liter, whereas foods prepared as "low sodium" contain greater amounts of potassium (because potassium replaces sodium in these foods). As a result, enteral feeds employing these products and some herbal remedies, such as noni juice (potassium, 56.3 mEq/L) can deliver excessive amounts of potassium to patients with impaired potassium homeostasis (278).

Another unsuspected source of potassium excess in the hospital includes the antibiotic penicillin G potassium (1.7 mEq of potassium per 1 million units), which can cause hyperkalemia if administered in sufficiently high doses (279). The urinary alkalinizing agent potassium citrate (2 mEq of potassium per 1 mL), and packed red blood cells transfused after 10 or more days of storage (7.5 to 13 mEq of potassium per L) can precipitate hyperkalemia in at risk patients (280,281). Potassium-containing cardioplegia solution employed during cardiac surgery may also cause hyperkalemia in patients with a defect in potassium handling.

Impaired Cellular Potassium Homeostasis

As discussed previously, cellular uptake of a potassium load is the primary mechanism by which the body acutely prevents the development of hyperkalemia. Several commonly prescribed drugs can impair this protective cellular response. ß-Adrenergic blocking drugs through inhibition of renin secretion as well as cellular uptake of potassium have been associated with the development of mild and, on rare occasions, life-threatening hyperkalemia (38,45,282,283). Hyperkalemia often develops rapidly, as one would expect with disruption of cellular potassium homeostasis, but rarely develops in the absence of heavy exercise or other risk factors for hyperkalemia (4,284). As an example, three renal transplant recipients developed severe hyperkalemia (potassium range 6.0 to 8.3 mEq/L) within hours of treatment with intravenous labetalol (285). Most studies evaluating hyperkalemia in hospitalized patients have shown that ß-adrenergic blockers have caused or at least contributed to hyperkalemia in anywhere from 4% to 17% of patients (94,275,286–288). Not unexpectedly, the hyperkalemic potential of ß-adrenergic blockers is increased by underlying renal insufficiency, the coexistence of diabetes mellitus or hypoaldosteronism, and concurrent therapy with other medications that reduce renal potassium secretion (45,282,283).

Digoxin by blocking Na-K-ATPase pump function has also been demonstrated to disrupt potassium homeostasis (289). As a result of this effect, impaired cellular uptake of potassium as well as reduced renal potassium excretion occurs. In general, therapeutic digoxin levels do not lead to hyperkalemia but in rare circumstances can be a contributing factor (289). Nonetheless, digoxin intoxication will result in hyperkalemia, which at times is fatal (289,290).

Both natural (lysine, arginine) and synthetic (ϵ-aminocaproic acid) amino acids have been associated with hyperkalemia (291–295). This is owing to the shift of potassium out of cells (291–295). Levinsky and colleagues demonstrated lysine uptake into isolated rat muscle within 1 hour in an amount equivalent to the potassium lost from the muscle tissue (291). In intact animals, infusion of lysine was associated with hyperkalemia, with a 1.0- to 1.5-mEq/L rise in plasma potassium concentration noted for every 10-mEq/L increase in plasma lysine concentration (292). Hyperkalemia has also been described with intravenous arginine administration (293–295). In normal humans, serum potassium increased by approximately 1 mEq/L following infusion of 30 to 60 g of arginine, whereas patients with end-stage renal disease developed a mean increase in serum potassium of 1.5 mEq/L at 2 hours after 30 g of intravenous arginine (293,294). In two patients with mild renal insufficiency and liver disease, potassium concentrations were 7.5 and 7.1 mmol/L, respectively, after infusion of arginine (295). Serum potassium concentrations increased as early as 45 minutes after arginine infusion and

peaked between 2 to 6 hours following injection, bespeaking a disturbance in cellular potassium homeostasis (294,295). Hyperkalemia can also develop in subjects treated with the synthetic amino acid, ϵ-aminocaproic acid, which is structurally similar to both lysine and arginine (296). A study in nephrectomized dogs demonstrated a significant rise in serum potassium in animals administered intravenous ϵ-aminocaproic acid as either a constant infusion (2 or 4 g/hour) or a bolus injection of 2.5 g (296). Clinical relevance in humans was demonstrated in a case report where hyperkalemia (potassium 6.7 mEq/L) developed acutely in a patient with chronic renal insufficiency treated with ϵ-aminocaproic acid (three boluses of 10 g) to reduce perioperative blood loss during cardiac surgery (297). The rapid onset of hyperkalemia following ϵ-aminocaproic acid therapy in this patient suggested that cellular release of potassium was the cause of this electrolyte disturbance. In addition, Perazella and coworkers in a retrospective study in patients undergoing cardiac surgery noted higher intraoperative serum potassium concentrations (potassium, 5.9 mEq/L) in 232 patients treated with intravenous ϵ-aminocaproic acid as compared with 371 well-matched controls (potassium, 5.5 mEq/L) who did not receive this medication (298). Other possible confounding factors did not explain the rapid development of hyperkalemia in these patients. It is therefore likely that intravenous ϵ-aminocaproic acid causes hyperkalemia through the cellular release of potassium in exchange for this synthetic amino acid.

The anesthetic agent succinylcholine by depolarization of cell membrane can cause hyperkalemia (299–301). A rapid cellular potassium leak induced by these agents, resulting in the abrupt onset of hyperkalemia, has been demonstrated in muscle preparations in intact animals and humans (299–301). Plasma potassium increased by 0.5 mEq/L within 3 to 5 minutes in patients with normal muscle, whereas increases as high as 3.0 mEq/L occurred in patients afflicted by trauma or nervous system disease (4,300). In 12 patients with renal insufficiency, plasma potassium concentration rose by 1.2 mEq/L in one patient and up to 0.7 mEq/L in the rest (301).

Impaired Renal Potassium Excretion

Although an increase in potassium intake can contribute to hyperkalemia, impaired renal excretion almost always plays the dominant role in this process. Potassium-sparing diuretics are used to enhance renal sodium losses and diminish potassium excretion in patients with hypertension and edematous states (302,303). Two basic mechanisms underlie the pharmacologic actions of these diuretics, which act to modulate principal cells residing in the distal nephron (304). The aldosterone antagonist, spironolactone, competes with aldosterone binding to cytoplasmic aldosterone receptors, thereby preventing nuclear uptake of the receptor and blunting aldosterone's effects on the principal cell (305,306). Amiloride and triamterene directly block sodium channel activity in the luminal membrane of the principal cell, effectively inhibiting sodium reabsorption through the epithelium and decreasing the driving force for potassium secretion (307,308). Moderate to severe hyperkalemia has been reported in 4% to 19% of patients treated with these medications (94,287,305–317). In one small study, treatment with the combination of triamterene and hydrochlorothiazide resulted in hyperkalemia in 26% of the patients (308). In a retrospective chart review, five patients were noted to develop severe hyperkalemia (potassium concentrations in the 9.4 to 11 mEq/L range) within 8 to 18 days of combination therapy with amiloride/hydrochlorothiazide and an ACE inhibitor (311). All of these patients were diabetics and three had underlying chronic renal insufficiency. The combination of spironolactone and losartan increased plasma potassium by 0.8 mEq/L (up to 5.0 mEq/L) and decreased urinary potassium excretion (from 108 to 87 mEq/L) in eight normal subjects studied (313). Hyperkalemia occurred most frequently in patients with preexisting renal insufficiency or diabetes mellitus, and those taking potassium supplements or another medication that also impairs potassium excretion (310,311,314–317).

Nonsteroidal antiinflammatory drugs (NSAIDs) are widely prescribed for a variety of inflammatory diseases and pain syndromes. Hyperkalemia is one of the many renal complications associated with NSAID therapy and over the counter availability of these agents further increases the risk of drug toxicity (318). Nonsteroidal antiinflammatory drugs disturb potassium homeostasis via inhibition of renal prostaglandin synthesis, especially PGE2 and PGI2 (319). Inhibition of prostaglandin synthesis decreases potassium secretion through (a) lack of activation of renin–angiotensin system, (b) direct inhibition of potassium channels in principal cells, and (c) decreased renal blood flow and diminished delivery of sodium to the distal nephron (231,318–324). Several reports have confirmed the hyperkalemic complication of NSAIDs prescribed to normal subjects, diabetics, and patients with underlying renal insufficiency (277,321–328). This is especially problematic in patients with reduced effective renal perfusion such as those with intravascular fluid depletion, CHF, and third-spacing of intravascular fluid (318–320). Predictably NSAID-induced hyperkalemia occurs more often in patients with preexisting hyporeninemic hypoaldosteronism, renal insufficiency, and concomitant therapy with potassium-sparing diuretics and ACE inhibitors (318–328).

Angiotensin-converting enzyme inhibitors indirectly reduce renal potassium excretion by inducing a state of hypoaldosteronism (277,329,330). These drugs may additionally impair renal potassium excretion by reducing effective GFR in patients with volume depletion, renal artery stenosis, and/or moderate to severe chronic renal insufficiency. In these conditions, ACE inhibitors interfere with angiotensin II production and blunt the postglomerular arteriolar constriction induced by this hormone, thereby lowering effective filtration pressure and glomerular filtration rate. Ultimately, a reduction in distal nephron delivery of sodium and water results, together with decreased aldosterone production, may precipitate hy-

perkalemia (329). In hospitalized patients, ACE inhibitors have been noted to be the culprit drug in 9% to 38% of patients who developed hyperkalemia (94,287,288,331). In outpatients treated with an ACE inhibitor for 1 year, 10% developed a serum potassium concentration greater than 6.0 mEq/L (332). In this study, patients with renal impairment and age over 70 years were at highest risk. Most studies suggest that the risk of ACE inhibitor-induced hyperkalemia is directly proportional to the existing degree of renal insufficiency (94,287,288,329–331). However, serum potassium concentrations can rise significantly in patients with only modest renal insufficiency (329,330,333). For example, a rise in serum potassium concentration, a positive cumulative potassium balance, and a reduction in both plasma and urinary aldosterone were demonstrated in 22 of 23 patients treated with high-dose captopril for 10 days despite a creatinine clearance greater than 50 mL/minute (330). In addition, another study noted a fall in aldosterone excretion and a rise in serum potassium concentration (mean rise 0.8 mEq/L) in 23 of 33 hypertensive patients after 1 week of captopril therapy (329). In this study, all but three of the patients had a creatinine clearance above 60 mL/minute and peak serum potassium concentration was not predicted by the pretherapy serum creatinine concentration (329). In contrast, Memon and colleagues demonstrated a significant positive correlation of hyperkalemia with serum creatinine and negative correlation with creatinine clearance, emphasizing the importance of the underlying level of renal function (331). In patients with renal impairment, reducing the dose of ACE inhibitor and initiating a low-potassium diet has been shown to decrease the development of hyperkalemia in a significant percentage of patients (331,333). Unfortunately, as many as one-third of patients still require discontinuation of this medication because of ongoing hyperkalemia (331). Predictably, combination therapy with an ACE inhibitor and other medications capable of altering potassium homeostasis can increase plasma potassium and precipitate hyperkalemia in patients with only modest renal impairment (277,329,330,334–340). Other notable risk factors include hypoaldosteronism, and states of effective volume depletion such as CHF and cirrhosis (277,329,330, 341,342).

Angiotensin-II receptor antagonists are a relatively new class of drugs marketed for the treatment of hypertension. Their action to block binding of angiotensin-II (A-II) to its receptor ultimately decreases A-II-driven adrenal synthesis of aldosterone, causing hyperkalemia through the induction of hypoaldosteronemia in a manner similar to ACE inhibitors. Current data are conflicting with regard to the effect of this class of drugs on the development of hyperkalemia. In healthy patients with essential hypertension, the A-II receptor blocker, losartan (100 mg) and the ACE inhibitor, enalapril (20 mg) similarly depressed plasma aldosterone levels (50% decrease) and 24-hour urinary aldosterone excretion (343). The effect of these two drugs on the RAAS did not include evaluation of serum potassium concentrations in these patients (343). Data pooled from 16 double-blind clinical trials evaluating the safety of therapy with losartan as compared with ACE inhibitors in healthy patients with hypertension demonstrated no significant difference in the development of hyperkalemia (potassium > 5.5 mEq/L) between the two drug classes (1.3% versus 1.5%) (344). It is important to remember that the patients evaluated in these studies were healthy and at very low risk of developing hyperkalemia (344). Evaluation of the effect of losartan in elderly patients demonstrated a significant rise in serum potassium (>0.5 mEq/L) in 19% of patients, whereas hyperkalemia actually developed in 7% of patients (345). A clinical history of diabetic nephropathy and a serum creatinine greater than 1.3 mg/dL were predictors of a significant increase in serum potassium. Bakris and colleagues compared the effects of the ACE inhibitor, lisinopril to the A-II blocker, valsartan on serum potassium concentration, urinary potassium excretion, and plasma aldosterone in 35 subjects with a mean GFR of approximately 71 mL/minute per 1.73 m^2 (346). After 4 weeks of therapy with lisinopril, serum potassium increased (0.2 mEq/L), whereas plasma aldosterone and urinary potassium excretion also decreased. In contrast, serum potassium, plasma aldosterone, and urinary potassium excretion were essentially unchanged in the valsartan group (346).

Trimethoprim and pentamidine are antimicrobial agents employed to treat infections in both HIV-infected patients as well as other hosts. Hyperkalemia evolves through a reduction in renal potassium secretion, the result of competitive inhibition of sodium transport channels in the luminal membranes of the distal nephron by these drugs (347,348). Blockade of epithelial sodium channel transport indirectly inhibits potassium secretion (Fig. 87-6) (348), because potassium movement into the distal nephron lumen is electrogenically linked to the movement of sodium out of the lumen (303,304,348). This action is identical to that exhibited by amiloride, which has a molecular structure very similar to both trimethoprim and pentamidine (348). Hyperkalemia was first described in a patient treated with "high-dose" trimethoprim (20 mg/kg per day) for *Pneumocystis carinii* pneumonia (349). Subsequently, a 50% incidence of mild hyperkalemia (K+ > 5.0 mEq/L) and 10% to 12% incidence of severe hyperkalemia (K+ > 6.0 mEq/L) was observed in HIV-infected patients receiving high-dose trimethoprim (347,348). Shortly thereafter, 21% of hospitalized non-HIV patients treated with standard dose trimethoprim (360 mg/day) developed hyperkalemia (K+ > 5.5 mEq/L) (350). Mild renal impairment (serum creatinine ≥ 1.2 mg/dL) was significantly associated with the development of a higher serum potassium concentration (350). More recently, a prospective, randomized controlled study in healthy outpatients treated with standard-dose trimethoprim revealed that 18% (9/51) and 6% (3/51) of trimethoprim-treated patients developed serum potassium concentrations greater than 5.0 and 5.5 mEq/L, respectively (351). Older age, diabetes mellitus, and higher serum creatinine level appeared to predispose to more severe hyperkalemia. Additionally, therapy with pentamidine also has been complicated by hyperkalemia (352,353). A retrospective study in 32 patients with AIDS noted a significant increase in mean serum potassium from 4.2 to 4.7 mEq/L, with 24% of the patients developing severe hyperkalemia (352). All cases of hyperkalemia were associated with renal insufficiency, providing an underlying risk factor in these patients.

Heparin and its congeners have been shown to inhibit adrenal aldosterone production and precipitate hyperkalemia in approximately 8% of patients treated with at least 10,000 U per day (354). This drug reduces both the number and affinity of angiotensin II receptors in the adrenal zona glomerulosa, thus decreasing the principal stimulus for aldosterone synthesis (354). Heparin also directly inhibits the final enzymatic steps of aldosterone formation (18-hydroxylation) and promotes atrophy of the zona glomerulosa in rats following prolonged administration, further reducing aldosterone production (354). Finally, excess anticoagulation with heparin may rarely precipitate adrenal hemorrhage and induce frank adrenal insufficiency (354). Although heparin-associated hyperkalemia has been reported in normal subjects, patients with preexisting hypoaldosteronism, renal insufficiency, or diabetes mellitus, and patients treated with other medications that disrupt potassium homeostasis more commonly develop hyperkalemia (354).

Cyclosporine and tacrolimus (FK506) have been associated with the development of hyperkalemia in organ transplant recipients. In the precyclosporine era, 31% (23/75) of renal transplant patients were noted to develop transient hyperkalemia because of an underlying disturbance in potassium excretion (355). Not unexpectedly, therapy with cyclosporine and tacrolimus increases risk of this disorder in

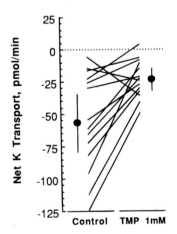

FIG. 87-6. Net potassium transport during perfusion of 14 distal tubules with control and trimethoprim (TMP) solutions. Lines connect measurements in the same tubules. Black circles and vertical lines indicate means and confidence intervals. Positive values indicate absorption; negative values indicate secretion. (From: Velazquez H, et al. Renal mechanism of trimethoprim-induced hyperkalemia. *Ann Intern Med* 1993;119:296, with permission.)

these patients (356). Heering and Grabensee (264) documented the presence of incomplete RTA in eight of 35 recipients on cyclosporine compared with none of the 15 on azathioprine. Four of the former group also had HHA syndrome. In a detailed study of 12 cadaveric recipients with hyperkalemia on cyclosporine, Kamel and colleagues (265) documented the presence of low urinary potassium excretion that did not respond to 0.2 mg of fludrocortisone. Renal potassium excretion, however, responded to bicarbonaturia initiated by acetazolamide, suggesting a defect in generating a favorable electrochemical gradient in the distal tubule, leading to hyperkalemia and varying degrees of hyperchloremic acidosis. Recently, Yu and coworkers demonstrated higher serum potassium concentrations and lower TTKGs in 35 renal transplant recipients receiving cyclosporine as compared with matched normal controls, supporting a disturbance in renal potassium excretion (357). Tacrolimus has similarly caused hyperkalemia in solid organ transplant patients. Hyperkalemia was noted in 26 of 49 (53%) pediatric heart transplant recipients treated with tacrolimus (358). Of note, the majority of subjects who developed hyperkalemia had impaired renal function. The reduction in renal potassium excretion that occurs with these two drugs is likely owing to a dose-dependent decrease in the activity of the basolateral Na-K-ATPase pumps in principal cells in the distal nephron (359,360). Calcineurin, which modulates sodium pump function through its regulation of phosphatase activity, is inhibited by both cyclosporine and tacrolimus (360). *In vitro* inhibition of calcineurin by these two drugs has been shown to decrease Na-K-ATPase pump activity and probably explains the observed reduction in renal potassium excretion. Ling and Eaton have also demonstrated the inhibition of apical secretory potassium channels by cyclosporine, providing yet another possible mechanism of decreased renal potassium excretion and hyperkalemia (361). Cyclosporine also impairs cellular potassium homeostasis and cause transient hyperkalemia by acutely increasing potassium efflux from cells (362). Although the mechanism is currently unknown, cyclosporine may cause hyperkalemia through the impairment of Na-K-ATPase pumps in muscle and liver cell membranes.

Acute Treatment of Serious Hyperkalemia

Severe hyperkalemia is a potentially life-threatening disorder because of its toxic effect on cardiac and other excitable neuromuscular tissues. Importantly, patients with underlying renal disease and disturbances in potassium homeostasis can develop serious hyperkalemia. It is therefore imperative that this electrolyte disturbance is rapidly recognized and aggressively treated. Symptoms of hyperkalemia are sometimes impressive and quite obvious; however, serious hyperkalemia also may present with only very subtle symptoms or signs. Rarely, patients may have absolutely no clinical evidence of this disorder, the presence of renal impairment

or other disturbances in potassium homeostasis providing the only clues to hyperkalemia. Nonspecific muscle weakness and generalized malaise are common, but severe muscle weakness, paresthesias, and ascending paralysis may rarely be seen in these patients with extreme elevations in serum potassium levels (363). The cardiac toxicity of hyperkalemia may manifest as weakness or dizziness from arrhythmias that induce hypotension and cerebral hypoperfusion (363). Cardiac monitoring or a 12-lead electrocardiogram (ECG) may reveal a rhythm suspicious of hyperkalemia. These include tenting of the T waves (K+, 5.5 to 6.0 mEq/L), lengthening of the P-R interval and widening of the QRS complex (K+, 6.0 to 7.0 mEq/L), disappearance of the P waves (K+, 7.0 to 7.5 mEq/L), and finally the sine wave pattern (K+, 8.0 mEq/L or greater). These ECG changes may occur at different concentrations (higher or lower) of potassium, depending on underlying heart disease and acuity of hyperkalemia (363). The presence of hypocalcemia, hypomagnesemia, and hyponatremia potentiate the toxic effects of hyperkalemia on the cardiac conduction system and potassium concentrations in the 6.0 to 6.5 mEq/L range can precipitate life-threatening arrhythmias (363). Additionally, patients with underlying cardiac disease may deteriorate directly to a ventricular arrhythmia in the absence of other ECG changes (363).

Once the clinician judges that hyperkalemia warrants treatment (plasma K+ >6.0 to 6.5 mEq/L, clinical manifestations, or ECG changes), immediate therapy should be commenced. Stabilization of excitable cell membranes, in particular cardiac tissue, is the most urgent priority in the treatment of hyperkalemia. Intravenous calcium, as either calcium gluconate (10% solution, calcium ion at 3 mEq/mL) or calcium chloride (10% solution, calcium ion at 13 mEq/mL), is the treatment of first choice and should be administered in a monitored setting (Table 87-4). Calcium acts within 1 to 3 minutes, and the effect persists for approximately one-half hour (363). If no effect is noted within 5 minutes following the first dose, repeated administration may provide benefit. Patients who have been treated with digoxin should receive a slower infusion of calcium (calcium mixed in 100 mL of 5% dextrose) over 10 to 20 minutes (363).

Intravenous administration of regular insulin as a 10-unit bolus followed by 50 mL of intravenous 50% dextrose (Table 87-4) should be the next therapeutic choice (364,365). The beneficial effect of insulin is observed within 15 minutes and lasts approximately 3 to 6 hours (364,365). Dextrose is given to prevent hypoglycemia in nondiabetic patients. However, because a high incidence of hypoglycemia occurs even with this regimen, it is prudent to monitor blood glucose levels and redose dextrose based on levels (364,365). Dextrose should not be infused before insulin because an acute worsening of hyperkalemia can occur with hyperglycemia, through a shift of potassium out of cells (364,365). Glucose levels should be checked prior to administration of dextrose to diabetic patients (364,365).

TABLE 87-4. *Acute treatment of serious hyperkalemia*

Stabilize excitable tissues (cardiac and neuromuscular)
Calcium gluconate (10% solution), given as a 10- to 20-mL intravenous bolus. Calcium chloride (10% solution), given as a 5-mL intravenous bolus. Each may be repeated every 5 min, if ECG appearance does not improve. Calcium gluconate should be mixed in 100 mL of 5% and infused over 10–20 min if the patient has been treated with digoxin.

Shift potassium into cells
Regular insulin, 10 units plus 50% dextrose (50 mL), given as an intravenous bolus, followed by 10% dextrose at 50 mL/min until definitive therapy. Check glucose levels at 1- to 2-hr intervals.
Albuterol (5 mg/mL), 10–20 mg, nebulized over approximately 10 min.
Combination therapy of insulin/dextrose and nebulized albuterol.

Remove potassium from the body
Acute hemodialysis (low potassium dialysate) to remove potassium in patients with severe renal insufficiency.
Sodium polystyrene sulfonate (15–30 g) plus sorbital (15–30 mL), oral ingestion or rectal administration (without sorbital).

High-dose nebulized albuterol (10 to 20 mg), which is fourfold to eightfold higher than used to treat asthma, also effectively lowers potassium concentrations in patients with hyperkalemia (Table 87-4) (366,367). However, the potassium-lowering effect of albuterol is less reliable in ESRD patients, and as many as 40% of these patients are resistant to the potassium-lowering effect of this ß agonist (366,367). In general, the plasma potassium concentration declines significantly at 30 minutes following albuterol inhalation and remains depressed for approximately 2 hours (366,367). To date, no adverse cardiovascular effects from albuterol have been documented in ESRD patients (366,367). Therefore, nebulized albuterol is useful to acutely lower plasma potassium concentration in most hyperkalemic patients; however, it should not replace insulin as the most important therapy to move potassium into cells.

Combined therapy with intravenous insulin and nebulized albuterol has been shown to be additive in the reduction of plasma potassium concentrations (367). Plasma potassium decreases approximately 0.6 mEq/L with 10 units of insulin, whereas 20 mg of nebulized albuterol lowers plasma potassium to a similar degree (367); however, the combination of these agents lowers plasma potassium by approximately 1.2 mEq/L (274). As a result it is worthwhile to combine these two agents to treat severe hyperkalemia (Table 87-4).

Although sodium bicarbonate is listed as a useful treatment for hyperkalemia, critical evaluation of the literature suggests that this agent is ineffective as an isolated therapy to acutely lower plasma potassium (368,369). In studies where bicarbonate infusion successfully lowered plasma potassium concentrations in ESRD patients, the effect was not observed until at least 4 hours after treatment. Similarly, other studies have confirmed the utility of sodium bicarbonate therapy in the chronic (not acute) lowering of plasma potassium concentrations (368,369). In contrast, patients with severe metabolic acidosis and concurrent hyperkalemia should receive bicarbonate to correct pH and stabilize cardiac tissue. In this setting, sodium bicarbonate (50 mEq) may be given intravenously to correct pH and serum bicarbonate levels in patients who are normocalcemic and can tolerate the sodium load (368,369).

WORKUP AND MANAGEMENT OF CHRONIC HYPERKALEMIC RENAL TUBULAR ACIDOSIS

Although acute hyperkalemia with or without significant HCA requiring immediate treatment occurs in patients with impaired potassium handling, the major challenge is the workup and treatment of chronic hyperkalemia seen in this setting. Given the frequency of this syndrome and lack of individualized treatment for specific subgroups, most patients can be adequately managed without complex workups. However, in certain patients it may be important to make a more specific pathophysiologic diagnosis. Although hyperchloremic metabolic acidosis is the dominant finding in some patients, hyperkalemia is the prominent presentation requiring workup and treatment.

Figure 87-7 summarizes a simple pathophysiologic approach to chronic hyperkalemia in these patients. The first

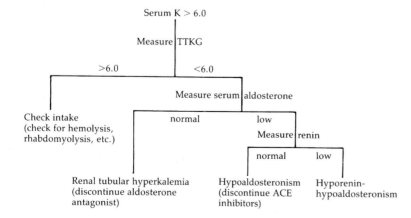

FIG. 87-7. Pathophysiologic approach to chronic hyperkalemia. *ACE,* angiotensin converting enzyme; *TTKG,* transtubular potassium gradient.

question to be answered is, "Is the hyperkalemia owing to an increase in intake or a decrease in output?" Although dietary history and pertinent clinical data may be helpful, a specific laboratory test that would answer this question could simplify the workup. Urinary potassium concentration and the urinary to serum potassium ratio do not account for the variability in the urinary potassium concentration as a function of water reabsorption in the collecting duct. The FE_{K^+} normalizes potassium excretion for GFR; however, as potassium is primarily secreted (and therefore, less dependent on filtration), its clinical utility is questionable.

Halperin and colleagues (81,370–372) have suggested correcting the urinary (U_K) to serum potassium (S_K) concentration by the ratio of urine (U_{Osm}) to serum osmolality (S_{Osm}) to normalize the data for water reabsorption. This ratio ($U_K^+/S_K^+ \times S_{Osm}/U_{Osm}$), called the *transtubular potassium gradient* (TTKG), attempts to approximate the gradient across potassium-secreting cells in the distal nephron. Despite several pitfalls (urine more diluted than the plasma or very low urinary sodium), a value less than 6 in patients with hyperkalemia suggests a lack of aldosterone or response to aldosterone; a value above 6 is in favor of an increase in potassium intake, with or without renal abnormality in potassium handling. It should, however, be noted that the published clinical experience with the use of TTKG is still very limited and therefore the values given here may be modified as further information becomes available. If the TTKG is normal, one should search for excessive potassium intake, either externally (e.g., potassium supplements or salt substitutes) or internally (e.g., severe hemolysis, rhabdomyolysis, or acidosis). In general, given the renal ability to handle a large oral potassium load (e.g., serum potassium rising by less than 1.0 mEq/L on a 400-mEq diet), a significant increase in serum potassium is indicative of either a major internal shift of potassium or a decrease in urinary excretion output. If the TTKG is low in the face of hyperkalemia, the aldosterone level should be measured to separate the group with tubular unresponsiveness from that with low aldosterone. Patients also can be challenged with exogenous mineralocorticoids (0.05 mg of fludrocortisone). If the TTKG increases to 7 or above, hypoaldosteronism is probably the major factor in the development of hyperkalemia (372). The role of renin–angiotensin in patients with hypoaldosteronism can be evaluated by measuring the renin level. A low renin associated with low aldosterone is the hallmark of the most common subgroup (i.e., hyporenin-hypoaldosteronism). If the renin level is normal, then either generation of angiotensin II is abnormal (e.g., in patients on ACE inhibitors) or the synthesis and secretion of aldosterone are abnormal. The adrenal response to angiotensin II infusion would provide appropriate answers to this question.

In practice, this type of workup should be reserved for unusual patients who do not represent the commonly recognized groups with this syndrome (e.g., diabetics, hypertensives), or as part of a research protocol. In addition, it should be noted

that this approach does not lead to an etiologic diagnosis, but only a pathophysiologic one. The etiologic diagnosis (as discussed elsewhere in this chapter) should depend on other diagnostic evaluations.

Some patients with type IV RTA present primarily with HCA. In these patients, the diagnostic workup should focus on the pathogenesis and etiology of this abnormality. The major defect leading to HCA is either loss of bicarbonate, often through the gastrointestinal tract, or a decrease in regeneration of bicarbonate by the kidney through stimulation of ammoniogenesis. Urinary ammonium should be high in the former and low in the latter group. However, urinary ammonium is not commonly measured in clinical laboratories. Clinicians are forced to rely on measurements of surrogates for urinary ammonium excretion. The most commonly used surrogate is urinary anion gap, which is the difference between major urinary cations (Na + K) and urinary anions (Cl + HCO₃). As the amount of bicarbonate is very small in acid urine (urine pH < 6.5), the difference between urinary Na + K and Cl reflects the major missing ion (i.e., ammonium). Using this formula, one can demonstrate an inverse relationship between the urinary anion gap and the amount of ammonium in the urine (373,374) (Fig. 87-8). In the presence of extrarenal acidosis, the urinary ammonium excretion should increase severalfold, resulting in a very negative anion gap value. In contrast, in distal RTA, the urinary ammonium will remain low, resulting in a positive anion gap. The amount of ammonium in the urine also can be deduced from

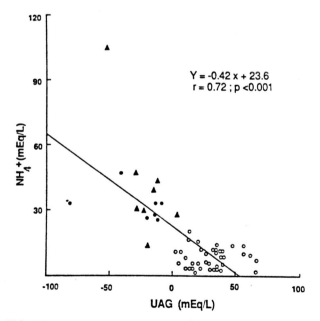

FIG. 87-8. Urinary ammonium (NH_4^+) in relation to the urinary anion gap (UAG). The 38 patients with altered distal urinary acidification are represented by open circles; the seven normal subjects receiving ammonium chloride, by closed circles; and the eight patients with hyperchloremic metabolic acidosis associated with diarrhea, by triangles. (From: Battle DC, et al. The use of urinary anion gap in the diagnosis of hyperchloremic metabolic acidosis. *N Engl J Med* 1988;318:594, with permission.)

a modified urinary osmolar gap using the following formula:

$$\text{urinary ammonium} = 1/2(\text{urine osmolality}$$
$$-2(Na + K) + \text{urea} + \text{glucose})$$

This is based on the concept that NH_4^+ with its accompanying anion is the major missing osmole accounting for the osmolar gap (375). It should be noted that neither calculation predicts the exact amount of ammonium in the urine but rather provides a qualitative estimate of it. This is still helpful if utilized to answer the appropriate question in a patient with HCA.

The major utility of urinary anion or osmolar gap is to differentiate renal from extrarenal causes of hyperchloremic acidosis such as diarrhea or ingestion of hydrochloric acid or its equivalent where the gap is negative. However, a low or negative anion gap in itself does not establish the diagnosis of type IV RTA, as this is also seen in classic RTA as well as uremic acidosis. Batlle and colleagues (374) studied a group of patients with classic RTA, hyperkalemic RTA, and selective aldosterone deficiency and compared the results to controls with a serum pH 7.30 to 7.35. These investigators noted a urinary anion gap of -20 ± 5.7 in controls and $+23 \pm 4.1$, $+30 \pm 4.2$, and $+39 \pm 4.2$ mEq/L in patients, respectively. The major pitfall in using urinary anion gap is the presence of a significant amount of bicarbonate or an unexpected charged molecule, such as penicillin or ketoacids, in the urine. In summary, urinary anion gap is a physiologic concept that indirectly assesses the amount of urinary ammonium. This measurement in conjunction with other data is helpful in establishing the pathogenesis of HCA in selected patients (376).

In patients with hyperkalemic RTA, treatment of chronic hyperkalemia should be instituted only when absolutely necessary (i.e., when clinical signs of hyperkalemia are present or plasma potassium is over 6.0 mEq/L). If therapy is deemed necessary, simple modalities should be tried first before more complex therapies with their associated side effects are instituted.

Discontinuation of Drugs that Cause Hyperkalemia

As these patients have an intrinsic difficulty in the excretion of potassium, any drugs that can cause hyperkalemia should be immediately discontinued. The list of drugs that should be stopped includes those discussed in the previous section.

Dietary Intervention

The next step in patients with mild to moderate hyperkalemia is to decrease potassium intake to less than 60 mEq/day. This can be done by the elimination of potassium-rich foods. This may be difficult if the patient is on a low-sodium diet because such a diet, by definition, contains foods that are high in potassium content.

Treatment of Acidemia

Because hyperchloremic acidosis is commonly associated with hyperkalemia, correction of the acidosis by sodium bicarbonate decreases the serum potassium concentration. The effect of bicarbonate is partly related to a change in H^+ concentration and is partly independent of pH change. As acidemia is corrected, H^+ moves out of cells in exchange for potassium. The inhibitory effect of acidemia on renal potassium secretion also is removed. In addition, sodium bicarbonate, through volume expansion and delivery of both sodium and bicarbonate to the distal potassium exchange site, may also increase renal excretion of potassium.

In some patients with significant metabolic acidosis (HCO_3 < 16 mEq/L and/or pH < 7.30), it is important to treat acidosis with base replacement to prevent mobilization of bone calcium and protein catabolism. Bone provides a buffer sink for hydrogen ion, resulting in release of calcium and its loss in the urine (151,377). This phenomenon is independent of Vitamin D, parathyroid hormone, and calcitonin (378,379). In addition, there is increasing evidence for a catabolic role for metabolic acidosis independent of uremia in patients with chronic renal failure (380). Both effects can be reversed by alkali therapy. The bicarbonate needed in these patients is close to 0.5 to 0.75 mEq/kg per day and can be easily supplied as citric acid-sodium citrate (Shohl's) solution, which contains 1 mEq of bicarbonate equivalent per milliliter.

Volume Expansion

Volume expansion may enhance potassium excretion by increasing distal fluid and sodium delivery. This therapy is especially effective in patients with chronic volume depletion owing to mild sodium wastage.

Diuretic Therapy

Use of most diuretics, especially loop blockers and thiazides, results in hypokalemic, hypochloremic metabolic alkalosis. In patients with hyperkalemia, the previously mentioned side effects may ameliorate hyperkalemia and, when present, metabolic acidosis. To prevent volume depletion with its resultant decrease in distal tubular sodium and fluid delivery, a high salt intake can be added to the diuretic regimen. Thiazide diuretics have proved effective in some patients with renal tubular hyperkalemia despite the failure of loop blockers such as furosemide.

Mineralocorticoids

Mineralocorticoid replacement represents the most logical approach to therapy in these patients. DeFronzo (197) reported an 84% success rate with this therapy; however, the effective dose of fludrocortisone (up to 0.4 to 1.0 mg per day) was much higher than the true physiologic dose. This observation suggests that most of these patients possess some degree of tubular resistance to the potassium stimulatory effect of mineralocorticoids. Surprisingly, although such high doses were needed to augment renal potassium excretion and normalize serum potassium levels, the sodium-retaining effects of aldosterone remained intact in some patients, resulting in marked edema formation, hypertension, and congestive heart failure. In general, if the dose of fludrocortisone required to maintain normokalemia exceeds 0.2 mg per day, side effects are common, and these drugs probably should be combined with diuretics or not employed at all. Use of mineralocorticoids should be limited to patients who have not responded to other maneuvers and continue to have clinically significant hyperkalemia.

Sodium-Potassium Exchange Resins

Sodium-potassium exchange resins are quite effective in reducing the plasma potassium concentration but have a low patient acceptability. This therapy should be used orally with an osmotic cathartic. The dose should be titrated against the decline in serum potassium level.

REFERENCES

1. Edelman IS, Liebman J. Anatomy of body water and electrolytes. *Am J Med* 1959;27:256.
2. Ewart HS, Klip A. Hormonal regulation of the Na+-K+-ATPase: mechanisms underlying rapid and sustained changes in pump activity. *Am J Physiol* 1995;269:C295.
3. Yang S, Curtis B, Thompson J, et al. Extrarenal regulation of potassium homeostasis: muscle Na, K-ATPase and NKCCl subcellular distribution. *J Am Soc Nephrol* 1999;10:49A.
4. Bia MJ, DeFronzo RA. Extrarenal potassium homeostasis. *Am J Physiol* 1981;240:F257.
5. DeFronzo RA, et al. Effect of insulinopenia and adrenal hormone deficiency on acute potassium tolerance. *Kidney Int* 1980;17:586.
6. DeFronzo RA, et al. Influence of basal insulin and glucagon secretion on potassium and sodium metabolism. *J Clin Invest* 1978;61:472.
7. DeFronzo RA, et al. Impaired renal tubular potassium secretion in sickle cell disease. *Ann Intern Med* 1979;90:310.
8. Brown RS. Extrarenal potassium homeostasis. *Kidney Int* 1986;30:116.
9. Briggs AP, et al. Some changes in the composition of blood due to the injection of insulin. *J Biol Chem* 1924;58:721.
10. Hiatt N, Yamakawa T, Davidson MB. Necessity for insulin in transfer of excess infused K to intracellular fluid. *Metabolism* 1974;23:43.
11. Pettit GW, Vick RL. Contribution of pancreatic insulin to extrarenal potassium homeostasis: a two compartment model. *Am J Physiol* 1974;226:319.
12. Santeusanio F, et al. Evidence for a role of endogenous insulin and glucagon in the regulation of potassium homeostasis. *J Lab Clin Med* 1973;81:809.
13. DeFronzo RA, et al. Nonuremic diabetic hypokalemia: a possible role of insulin deficiency. *Arch Intern Med* 1977;137:842.
14. Hiatt N, Davidson MB, Bonorris G. The effect of potassium chloride infusion on insulin secretion *in vivo*. *Horm Metab Res* 1972;4:64.
15. Pettit GW, Vick RL, Swander AM. Plasma K+ and insulin: changes during KCl infusion in normal and nephrectomized dogs. *Am J Physiol* 1975;228:107.
16. Martinez R, et al. Effect of hyperkalemia on insulin secretion. *Experientia* 1991;47:270.
17. Clausen T, Hansen O. Active Na-K transport and the rate of ouabain binding. The effect of insulin and other stimuli on skeletal muscle and adipocytes. *J Physiol* 1977;270:415.
18. Zierler KL. Effect of insulin on potassium efflux from rat muscle in the presence and absence of glucose. *Am J Physiol* 1968;198:1066.
19. Zierler KL. Hyperpolarization of muscle by insulin in a glucose-free environment. *Am J Physiol* 1959;197:524.
20. Zierler KL, Rabinowitz D. Effect of very small concentrations of insulin on forearm metabolism. Persistence of its action on potassium and free fatty acids without its effect on glucose. *J Clin Invest* 1964;43:950.
21. DeFronzo RA, et al. Effect of graded doses of insulin on splanchnic and peripheral potassium metabolism in man. *Am J Physiol* 1980;238:E421.
22. Kahn CR. The molecular mechanism of insulin action. *Ann Rev Med* 1985;36:429.
23. Moore RD. Effects of insulin upon ion transport. *Biochim Biophys Acta* 1983;737:1.
24. Feraille E, et al. Insulin-induced stimulation of Na+, K-ATPase activity in kidney proximal tubule cells depends on phosphorylation of the α subunit at Tyr-10. *Mol Biol Cell* 1999;10:2847.
25. Cohen P, et al. Insulin effects on glucose and potassium metabolism *in vivo*: evidence for selective insulin resistance in humans. *J Clin Endocrinol Metab* 1991;73:564.
26. D'Silva JH. The action of adrenaline on serum potassium. *J Physiol (Lond)* 1934;82:393.
27. D'Silva JH. The action of adrenaline on serum potassium. *J Physiol (Lond)* 1935;86:219.
28. Lockwood RH, Lum BK. Effects of adrenergic agonists and antagonists on potassium metabolism. *J Pharmacol Exp Ther* 1974;189:119.
29. Lockwood RH, Lum BK. Effects of adrenalectomy and adrenergic antagonists on potassium metabolism. *J Pharmacol Exp Ther* 1977;203:103.
30. Hiatt N, Chapman LW, Davidson MB. Influence of epinephrine and propranolol on transmembrane K transfer in anuric dogs with hyperkalemia. *J Pharmacol Exp Ther* 1979;209:282.
31. Brown MJ, Brown DC, Murphy MB. Hypokalemia from ß2 receptor stimulation by circulating epinephrine. *N Engl J Med* 1983;309:1414.
32. DeFronzo RA, et al. Inhibitory effect of epinephrine on renal potassium secretion: a micropuncture study. *Am J Physiol* 1983;245:F303.
33. Katz L, D'Avella J, DeFronzo RA. Effect of epinephrine on renal potassium excretion in the isolated perfused rat kidney. *Am J Physiol* 1984;247:F331.
34. Williams ME, et al. Impairment of extrarenal potassium disposal by α-adrenergic stimulation. *N Engl J Med* 1984;311:145.
35. Brown MJ, Brown DC, Murphy MB. Adrenaline associated hypokalemia and tachycardia are selectively antagonized by low dose B-receptor blockade in man. *Clin Sci* 1983;64:71P.
36. Clausen T, Flatman JA. ß2 adrenoceptors mediate the stimulating effect of adrenaline on active electrogenic Na-K transport in rat soleus muscle. *Br J Pharmacol* 1980;68:749.
37. DeFronzo RA, Birkhead G, Bia M. Effect of epinephrine on potassium homeostasis in man. *Kidney Int* 1979;16:917A.
38. Rosa RM, et al. Adrenergic modulation of extrarenal potassium disposal. *N Engl J Med* 1980;302:431.
39. Carlsson E, et al. ß-adrenoceptor blockers, plasma potassium, and exercise. *Lancet* 1978;2:424.
40. Williams M, et al. Catecholamine modulation of rapid potassium shifts during exercise. *N Engl J Med* 1985;312:823.
41. Berend N, Marlin GE. Characterization of ß-adrenoreceptor subtype mediating the metabolic actions of salbutamol. *Br J Clin Pharmacol* 1978;5:207.
42. Bia MJ, et al. ß adrenergic control of extrarenal potassium disposal. A ß-2 mediated phenomenon. *Nephron* 1986;43:117.
43. Clausen T. Adrenergic control of Na+-K+ homeostasis. *Acta Med Scand* 1983;672:111.
44. Vick RL, Todd EP, Leudke DW. Epinephrine-induced hypokalemia: relation to liver and skeletal muscle. *J Pharmacol Exp Ther* 1972;181:139.
45. DeFronzo RA, Bia M, Birkhead G. Epinephrine and potassium homeostasis. *Kidney Int* 1981;20:83.
46. Cheng LC, Rogus EM, Zierler K. Catechol, a structural requirement for (Na+-K+)-ATPase stimulation in rat skeletal muscle membrane. *Biochim Biophys Acta* 1977;464:338.
47. Flatman JA, Clausen T. Combined effects of adrenaline and insulin on active electrogenic Na+-K+ transport in rat soleus muscle. *Nature* 1979;281:580.
48. Antes LM, Kujubu TA, Fernandex PC. Hypokalemia and the pathology of ion transport molecules. *Sem Nephrol* 1998;18:31.
49. Peterson KG, Shuter KJ, Kemp L. Regulation of serum potassium during insulin-induced hypoglycemia. *Diabetes* 1982;31:615.

50. Wright FS. Potassium transport by successive segments of the mammalian nephron. *Fed Proc* 1981;40:2398.

51. Hayslett JP, et al. Demonstration of net potassium absorption in mammalian colon. *Am J Physiol* 1982;242:G209.

52. Simpson SAS, Tait JF. Recent progress on methods of isolation, chemistry, and physiology of aldosterone. *Recent Prog Horm Res* 1955; 11:183.

53. Conn JW. Aldosteronism in man. Some clinical and climatological aspects. *JAMA* 1963;183:775.

54. Adler S. An extrarenal action of aldosterone on mammalian skeletal muscle. *Am J Physiol* 1970;218:616.

55. Lim VS, Webster GD. The effect of aldosterone on water and electrolyte composition of incubated rat diaphragms. *Clin Sci* 1967;33:261.

56. Alexander EA, Levinsky NG. An extrarenal mechanism of potassium adaptation. *J Clin Invest* 1968;47:740.

57. Spital A, Sterns RH. Extrarenal potassium adaptation: the role of aldosterone. *Clin Sci* 1989;76:213.

58. Spital A, Sterns RH. Paradoxical potassium depletion: a renal mechanism for extrarenal potassium adaptation. *Kidney Int* 1986;30:532.

59. Young DB, Jackson TE. Effects of aldosterone on potassium distribution. *Am J Physiol* 1982;243:R526.

60. Ross EJ. *Aldosterone and aldosteronism.* London: The Whitefriars, 1975.

61. Bia MJ, Tyler KA, DeFronzo RA. Regulation of extrarenal potassium homeostasis by adrenal hormones in rats. *Am J Physiol* 1982;242:F641.

62. Sugarman A, Brown RS. The role of aldosterone in potassium tolerance: studies in anephric humans. *Kidney Int* 1988;34:397.

63. Papadimitriou M, et al. The effect of spironolactone in hypertensive patients on regular haemodialysis and after renal allotransplantation. *Life Support Systems* 1983;1:197.

64. Sugarman A, Kahn T. Parathyroid hormone impairs extra-renal potassium tolerance in the rat. *Am J Physiol* 1988;254:F385.

65. Sugarman A, Kahn T. Calcium channel blockers enhance extrarenal potassium disposal in the rat. *Am J Physiol* 1986;250:F695.

66. Soliman AR, Akmal M, Massry SG. Parathyroid hormone interferes with extrarenal disposition of potassium in chronic renal failure. *Nephron* 1989;52:262.

67. Solomon R, Dubey A. Diltiazem enhances potassium disposal in subjects with end-stage renal disease. *Am J Kidney Dis* 1992;19:420.

68. Burnell JM, Villamil MF, Uyeno BJ, et al. Effect in humans of extracellular pH change in relationship between serum potassium concentration and intracellular potassium. *J Clin Invest* 1956;35:935.

69. Keating RE, Weichselbaum TE, Alanis M, et al. The movement of potassium during experimental acidosis and alkalosis in the nephrectomized dog. *Surg Gynecol Obstet* 1953;96:323.

70. Simmons DH, Avedon M. Acid base alterations and plasma potassium concentrations. *Am J Physiol* 1959;197:319.

71. Adler S, Fraley DS. Potassium and intracellular pH. *Kidney Int* 1977; 11:433.

72. Arbus GS, et al. Characterization and clinical application of the significance band for acute respiratory alkalosis. *N Engl J Med* 1969;280: 117.

73. Giebisch G, Berger L, Pitts RF. The extrarenal response to acute acid–base disturbances of respiratory origin. *J Clin Invest* 1955;34:231.

74. Perez GO, Oster JR, Vaamonde CA. Serum potassium concentration in acidemic states. *Nephron* 1981;27:233.

75. Adrogue HJ, Madias NE. Changes in plasma potassium concentration during acute acid–base disturbances. *Am J Med* 1981;71:456.

76. Liebman J, Edelman IS. Interrelationship of plasma potassium concentration, plasma sodium concentration, arterial pH and total exchangeable potassium. *J Clin Invest* 1959;38:2176.

77. Fulop M. Serum potassium in lactic acidosis and ketoacidosis. *N Engl J Med* 1979;300:1087.

78. Orringer CE, et al. Natural history of lactic acidosis after grand-mal seizures. A model for the study of an anion-gap acidosis not associated with hyperkalemia. *N Engl J Med* 1977;297:796.

79. Oster JR, et al. Plasma potassium response to metabolic acidosis induced by mineral and nonmineral acids. *Miner Electrolyte Metab* 1980;4:28.

80. Oster JR, Perez GO, Vaamonde CA. Relationship between blood pH and potassium and phosphorus during acute metabolic acidosis. *Am J Physiol* 1978;235:F345.

81. Magner PO, et al. The plasma potassium concentration in metabolic acidosis: a re-evaluation. *Am J Kidney Dis* 1988;11:220.

82. Moreno M, Murphy C, Goldsmith C. Increase in serum potassium resulting from the administration of hypertonic mannitol and other solutions. *J Lab Clin Med* 1969;73:291.

83. Tarail R, Seldin DW, Goodyer AVN. Effects of injection of hypertonic glucose on metabolism of water and electrolytes in patients with edema. *J Clin Invest* 1951;30:1111.

84. Goldfarb S, et al. Acute hyperkalemia induced by hyperglycemia: hormonal mechanisms. *Ann Intern Med* 1976;84:426.

85. Ammon RA, May WS, Nightingale SD. Glucose induced hyperkalemia with normal aldosterone levels. Studies in a patient with diabetes mellitus. *Ann Intern Med* 1978;89:349.

86. Goldfarb S, et al. Paradoxical glucose-induced hyperkalemia. Combined aldosterone-insulin deficiencies. *Am J Med* 1975;59:744.

87. Nicolis GL, et al. Glucose-induced hyperkalemia in diabetic subjects. *Arch Intern Med* 1981;141:49.

88. Rado JP. Glucose-induced paradoxical hyperkalemia in patients with suppression of the renin–aldosterone system: prevention by sodium depletion. *J Endocrinol Invest* 1979;2:401.

89. Viberti GC. Glucose-induced hyperkalemia: a hazard for "diabetics?" *Lancet* 1978;1:690.

90. Bratusch-Marrain PR, DeFronzo RA. Impairment of insulin-mediated glucose metabolism by hyperosmolality in man. *Diabetes* 1983;32:1028.

91. Conte G, et al. Acute increase in plasma osmolality as a cause of hyperkalemia in patients with renal failure. *Kidney Int* 1990;38: 301.

92. Gonick HC, et al. Functional impairment in chronic renal disease. 3. Studies of potassium excretion. *Am J Med Sci* 1971;261:281.

93. Kahn T, et al. Factors related to potassium transport in chronic stable renal disease in man. *Clin Sci Mol Med* 1978;54:661.

94. Acker CG, et al. Hyperkalemia in the hospital. *J Am Soc Nephrol* 1996;7:1346.

95. Adesman J, et al. Simultaneous measurement of body sodium and potassium using Na^{22} and K^{42}. *Metabolism* 1960;9:561.

96. Patrick J, et al. Leucocyte potassium in uraemia: comparisons with erythrocyte potassium and total exchangeable potassium. *Clin Sci* 1972;43:669.

97. Berlyne GM, Van Laethem L, Ben Ari J. Exchangeable potassium and renal potassium handling in advanced chronic renal failure in man. *Nephron* 1971;8:264.

98. Patrick J. The assessment of body potassium stores. *Kidney Int* 1977;11:476.

99. Boddy K, et al. Exchangeable and total body potassium in patients with chronic renal failure. *Br Med J* 1972;1:140.

100. Bergstrom J, et al. Muscle intracellular electrolytes in patients with chronic uremia. *Kidney Int* 1983;24:S-153.

101. Bergstrom J, Hultman E. Water, electrolyte and glycogen content of muscle tissue in patients undergoing regular dialysis therapy. *Clin Nephrol* 1974;2:24.

102. Ericsson F, Carlmark B. Potassium in whole body, skeletal muscle and erythrocytes in chronic renal failure. *Nephron* 1983;33:173.

103. Graham JA, Lawson DH, Linton AL. Muscle biopsy water and electrolyte contents in chronic renal failure. *Clin Sci* 1970;38:583.

104. Montanari A, et al. Studies on cell water and electrolytes in chronic renal failure. *Clin Nephrol* 1978;9:200.

105. Montanari A, et al. Skeletal muscle water and electrolytes in chronic renal failure. Effects of long-term regular dialysis treatment. *Nephron* 1985;39:316.

106. Bilbrey GL, et al. Potassium deficiency in chronic renal failure. *Kidney Int* 1973;4:423.

107. Cole CH. Decreased ouabain-sensitive adenosine triphosphatase activity in the erythrocyte membrane of patients with chronic renal disease. *Clin Sci* 1973;45:775.

108. Welt LG, Sachs JR, McManus TJ. An ion transport defect in erythrocytes from uremic patients. *Trans Assoc Am Phys* 1964;77:169.

109. Patrick J, Jones NF. Cell sodium, potassium and water in uraemia and the effects of regular dialysis as studied in the leucocyte. *Clin Sci* 1974;46:583.

110. Cole CH, Balfe JW, Welt LG. Induction of an ouabain-sensitive ATPase defect by uremic plasma. *Trans Assoc Am Phys* 1968;81:213.

111. Edmondson RP, et al. Leucocyte sodium transport in uraemia. *Clin Sci Mol Med* 1975;49:213.

112. Kaji D, Kahn T. Na^+-K^+ pump in chronic renal failure. *Am J Physiol* 1987;252:F785.

113. Perez GO, et al. Blunted kaliuresis after an acute potassium load in patients with chronic renal failure. *Kidney Int* 1983;24:656.

114. Bia MJ, DeFronzo RA. The medullary collecting duct (MCD) does not play a primary role in potassium (K) adaptation following decreased GFR. *Clin Res* 1978;26:457A.

115. Bourgoignie JJ, et al. Renal handling of potassium in dogs with chronic renal insufficiency. *Kidney Int* 1981;20:482.

116. Schon DA, Silva P, Hayslett JP. Mechanism of potassium excretion in renal insufficiency. *Am J Physiol* 1974;227:1323.

117. Wilson DR, Sonnenberg H. Medullary collecting duct function in the remnant kidney before and after volume expansion. *Kidney Int* 1979;15:487.

118. Fernandez J, Oster JR, Perez GO. Impaired extrarenal disposal of an acute oral potassium load in patients with endstage renal disease on chronic hemodialysis. *Miner Electrolyte Metab* 1986;12:125.

119. Allon M, Dansby L, Shanklin N. Glucose modulation of the disposal of an acute potassium load in patients with end-stage renal disease. *Am J Med* 1993;94:475.

120. DeFronzo RA, et al. The effect of insulin on renal handling of sodium, potassium, calcium, and phosphate in man. *J Clin Invest* 1975;55: 845.

121. Westervelt FB. Insulin effect in uremia. *J Lab Clin Med* 1969;74:79.

122. Alvestrand A, et al. Insulin-mediated potassium uptake is normal in uremic and healthy subjects. *Am J Physiol* 1984;246:E174.

123. Goecke IA, et al. Enhanced insulin sensitivity in extrarenal potassium handling in uremic rats. *Kidney Int* 1991;39:39.

124. Atuk NO, Westervelt FB, Peach M. Altered catecholamine metabolism, plasma renin activity and hypertension in renal failure. *Int Cong Nephrol* 1975;475A.

125. Henrich WL, et al. Competitive effects of hypokalemia and volume depletion on plasma renin activity, aldosterone and catecholamine concentrations in hemodialysis patients. *Kidney Int* 1977;12:279.

126. Yang W, et al. ß-adrenergic-mediated extrarenal potassium disposal in patients with end-stage renal disease: effect of propranolol. *Miner Electrolyte Metab* 1986;12:186.

127. Gifford JD, et al. Control of serum potassium during fasting in patients with end-stage renal disease. *Kidney Int* 1989;35:90.

128. Schrier RW, Regal EM. Influence of aldosterone on sodium, water and potassium metabolism in chronic renal disease. *Kidney Int* 1972;1:156.

129. Weidmann P, et al. Control of aldosterone responsiveness in terminal renal failure. *Kidney Int* 1975;7:351.

130. Weidmann P, et al. Role of the renin–angiotensin–aldosterone system in the regulation of plasma potassium in chronic renal disease. *Nephron* 1975;15:35.

131. Williams GH, et al. Studies on the metabolism of aldosterone in chronic renal failure and anephric man. *Kidney Int* 1973;4:280.

132. Schultze RG, et al. On the adaptation of potassium excretion associated with nephron reduction in the dog. *J Clin Invest* 1971;50:1061.

133. Kunau RT, Whinnery MA. Potassium transfer in distal tubule of normal and remnant kidneys. *Am J Physiol* 1978;235:F186.

134. Finkelstein FO, Hayslett JP. Role of medullary structures in the functional adaptation of renal insufficiency. *Kidney Int* 1974;6:419.

135. Bank N, Aynedjian HS. A micropuncture study of potassium excretion by the remnant kidney. *J Clin Invest* 1973;52:1480.

136. Fine LG, et al. Functional profile of the isolated uremic nephron: potassium adaptation in the rabbit cortical collective tubule. *J Clin Invest* 1979;64:1033.

137. Rocha A, Marcondes M, Malnic G. Micropuncture study in rats with experimental glomerulonephritis. *Kidney Int* 1973;3:14.

138. Bia MJ, Tyler K, DeFronzo RA. Role of glucocorticoids and mineralocorticoids in potassium adaptation after decreased GFR. *Kidney Int* 1983;23:211A.

139. Espinel CH. Effect of proportional reduction of sodium intake on the adaptive increase in glomerular filtration rate/nephron and potassium and phosphate excretion in chronic renal failure in the rat. *Clin Sci Mol Med* 1975;49:193.

140. Charney AN, et al. Na+-K+-activated adenosine triphosphatase and intestinal electrolyte transport. Effect of adrenal steroids. *J Clin Invest* 1975;56:653.

141. Bastl C, Hayslett JP, Binder HJ. Increased large intestinal secretion of potassium in renal insufficiency. *Kidney Int* 1977;12:9.

142. Hayes CP, MacLeod ME, Robinson RR. An extrarenal mechanism for the maintenance of potassium balance in severe chronic renal failure. *Trans Assoc Am Phys* 1964;80:207.

143. Pitts RF. Symposium on acid–base homeostasis. Control of renal production of ammonia. *Kidney Int* 1972;1:297.

144. Knepper MA, Packer R, Good DW. Ammonium transport in the kidney. *Physiol Rev* 1989;69:179.

145. DuBose TD, et al. Ammonium transport in the kidney: new physiological concepts and their clinical implications. *J Am Soc Nephrol* 1991;1:1193.

146. Widmer B, et al. Serum electrolyte and acid–base composition. The influence of graded degrees of chronic renal failure. *Arch Intern Med* 1979;139:1099.

147. Wallia R, et al. Serum electrolyte patterns in end-stage renal disease. *Am J Kidney Dis* 1986;8:98.

148. Caravaca F, et al. Metabolic acidosis in advanced renal failure: differences between diabetic and nondiabetic patients. *Am J Kidney Dis* 1999;33:892.

149. Schwartz WB, et al. On the mechanism of acidosis in chronic renal disease. *J Clin Invest* 1959;38:39.

150. Relman AS, Lennon EJ, Lemann J Jr. Endogenous production of fixed acid and measurement of the net balance acid in normal subject. *J Clin Invest* 1961;40:1621.

151. Goodman AD, et al. Production, excretion, and net balance of fixed acid in patient with renal acidosis. *J Clin Invest* 1965;44:495.

152. Litzow JR, Lemann J Jr, Lennon EJ. The effect of treatment of acidosis on calcium balance in patients with chronic azotemic renal disease. *J Clin Invest* 1967;46:280.

153. Warnock DG. Uremic acidosis. *Kidney Int* 1988;34:278.

154. Wrong O, Davies HEF. The excretion of acid in renal disease. *Q J Med* 1959;28:259.

155. Slatopolsky E, et al. On the influence of extracellular fluid volume expansion and uremia of bicarbonate reabsorption in man. *J Clin Invest* 1970;49:988.

156. Muldowney F, et al. Parathyroid acidosis in uremia. *Q J Med* 1972; 41:321.

157. Arruda JA, et al. Bicarbonate reabsorption in chronic renal failure. *Kidney Int* 1976;9:481.

158. Lameire N, Matthys E. Influence of progressive salt restriction on urinary bicarbonate wasting in uremic acidosis. *Am J Kidney Dis* 1986; 8:151.

159. Wong NL, Quamme GA, Dirks JH. Tubular handling of bicarbonate in dogs with experimental renal failure. *Kidney Int* 1984;25:912.

160. Buerkert J, et al. Effect of reduced renal mass on ammonium handling and net acid formation by the superficial and juxtamedullary nephron of the rat. *J Clin Invest* 1983;71:1661.

161. Oster JR. Renal acidification in patients with chronic renal insufficiency. PCO2 of alkaline urine and response to ammonium chloride. *Miner Electrolyte Metab* 1978;1:253.

162. Brigg AP, et al. Pathophysiology of uremic acidosis as indicated by urinary acidification on a controlled diet. *Metabolism* 1961;10: 749.

163. Gonick HC, et al. Functional impairment in chronic renal disease. II. Studies of acid excretion. *Nephron* 1969;6:28.

164. Simpson DP. Control of hydrogen ion homeostasis and renal acidosis. *Medicine* 1971;50:503.

165. Good DW, Burg MB. Ammonia production in individual segments of the rat nephron. *J Clin Invest* 1984;73:602.

166. Hwang JJ, Curthoys NP. Effect of acute alteration in acid–base balance on rat renal glutaminase and phosphoenolpyruvate carboxykinase gene expression. *J Biol Chem* 1991;266:9392.

167. Good DW. Ammonium transport by the thick ascending limb of loop of rat kidney. *Ann Rev Physiol* 1994;56:623.

168. MacClean AJ, Hayslett JP. Adaptive change in ammonia excretion in renal insufficiency. *Kidney Int* 1980;17:595.

169. Stone DK, et al. Mineralocorticoid modulation of rabbit medullary collecting duct acidification. A sodium-independent effect. *J Clin Invest* 1983;72:77.

170. Koeppen BM, Helmann SI. Acidification of luminal fluid by the rabbit cortical collecting tubule perfused *in vitro*. *Am J Physiol* 1982; 242:F521.

171. Al-Awqati Q, et al. Characteristics of stimulation of H$^+$ transport by aldosterone in turtle urinary bladder. *J Clin Invest* 1976;58:351.

172. Kurtzman NA. Acquired distal renal tubular acidosis. *Kidney Int* 1983; 24:807.

173. DiTella PJ, et al. Mechanism of the metabolic acidosis of selective mineralocorticoid deficiency. *Kidney Int* 1978;14:466.

174. Hulter HN, et al. Impaired renal H$^+$ secretion and NH^3 production in mineralocorticoid-deficient glucocorticoid-replete dogs. *Am J Physiol* 1977;232:F136.

175. Good DW. Active absorption of NH^{4+} by rat medullary thick ascending limb: inhibition by potassium. *Am J Physiol* 1988;255:F78.

176. Szylman P, et al. Role of hyperkalemia in the metabolic acidosis of isolated hypoaldosteronism. *N Engl J Med* 1976;294:361.

177. Sebastian A, et al. Amelioration of metabolic acidosis with fludrocortisone therapy in hyporeninemic hypoaldosteronism. *N Engl J Med* 1977;297:576.

178. Matsuda O, et al. Primary role of hyperkalemia in the acidosis of hyporeninemic hypoaldosteronism. *Nephron* 1988;49:203.

179. Hudson J, Chobanian A, Relman A. Hypoaldosteronism. A clinical study of a patient with an isolated adrenal mineralocorticoid deficiency, resulting in hyperkalemia and Stokes-Adams attacks. *N Engl J Med* 1957;257:529.

180. Christlieb AR, et al. Hypertension with inappropriate aldosterone stimulation. *N Engl J Med* 1969;281:128.

181. Don BR, Schambelan M. Hyperkalemia in acute glomerulonephritis due to transient hyporeninemic hypoaldosteronism. *Kidney Int* 1990;38:1159.

182. Ferrara E, et al. Selective hypoaldosteronism with blunted renin-activity responsiveness. *Clin Res* 1970;18:602.

183. Gerstein AR, et al. Aldosterone deficiency in chronic renal failure. *Nephron* 1968;5:90.

184. Hill S, et al. Studies in man on hyper- and hypoaldosteronism. *Arch Intern Med* 1959;104:982.

185. Lambrew C, et al. Hypoaldosteronism as a cause of hyperkalemia and syncopal attacks in a patient with complete heart block. *Am J Med* 1961;31:81.

186. Posner J, Jacobs D. Isolated antialdosteronism. I. Clinical entity, with manifestations of persistent hyperkalemia, periodic paralysis, salt-losing tendency, and acidosis. *Metabolism* 1964;13:513.

187. Skanse B, Hokfelt B. Hypoaldosteronism with otherwise intact adrenocortical function, resulting in a characteristic clinical entity. *Acta Endocrinol* 1958;28:29.

188. Stockigt J, et al. Subordinate hypoaldosteronism. *Clin Res* 1971;19:174.

189. Ulick S, et al. An aldosterone biosynthetic defect in a salt-losing disorder. *J Clin Endocrinol Metab* 1964;24:669.

190. Vagnucci A. Selective aldosterone deficiency in chronic pyelonephritis. *Nephron* 1970;7:524.

191. Wilson I, Goetz F. Selective hypoaldosteronism after prolonged heparin administration. *Am J Med* 1964;36:635.

192. Schambelan M, Stockigt JR, Biglieri EG. Isolated hypoaldosteronism in adults. A renin-deficiency syndrome. *N Engl J Med* 1972;287:573.

193. Brown J, et al. Recurrent hyperkalemia due to selective aldosterone deficiency: correction by angiotensin infusion. *Br Med J* 1973;1:650.

194. Perez G, Siegel L, Schreiner G. Selective hypoaldosteronism with hyperkalemia. *Ann Intern Med* 1972;76:757.

195. Oh MS, et al. A mechanism for hyporeninemic hypoaldosteronism in chronic renal disease. *Metabolism* 1974;23:1157.

196. Weidmann P, et al. Syndrome of hyporeninemic hypoaldosteronism and hyperkalemia in renal disease. *J Clin Endocrinol Metab* 1973;36:965.

197. DeFronzo RA. Hyperkalemia and hyporeninemic hypoaldosteronism. *Kidney Int* 1980;17:118.

198. Rosansky SJ, Kennedy M. Sickle cell trait with episodic acute renal failure and Type IV renal tubular acidosis. *Ann Intern Med* 1980;93:643.

199. Roseman MK, et al. Studies on the mechanism of hyperkalemic distal renal tubular acidosis (dRTA): gradient type dRTA in SC hemoglobinopathy. *Kidney Int* 1977;12:473.

200. DeFronzo RA, et al. Impaired renal tubular potassium secretion in systemic lupus erythematosus. *Ann Intern Med* 1977;86:268.

201. Hadler NM, Gill JR, Gardner JD. Impaired renal tubular secretion of potassium, elevated sweat sodium chloride concentration and plasma inhibition of erythrocyte sodium outflux as complications of systemic lupus erythematosus. *Arthritis Rheum* 1972;15:515.

202. DeFronzo RA, et al. Investigations into the mechanisms of hyperkalemia following renal transplantation. *Kidney Int* 1977;11:357.

203. Gyory AZ, et al. Renal tubular acidosis, acidosis due to hyperkalemia, hypercalcemia, disordered citrate metabolism and other tubular dysfunctions following human renal transplantation. *Q J Med* 1969;38:231.

204. Batlle DC, Arruda JA, Kurtzman NA. Hyperkalemic distal renal tubular acidosis associated with obstructive uropathy. *N Engl J Med* 1981;304:373.

205. Glassock RJ, et al. Diabetes mellitus, moderate renal insufficiency and hyperkalemia. *Am J Nephrol* 1983;3:233.

206. Schambelan M, Sebastian A, Biglieri EG. Prevalence, pathogenesis, and functional significance of aldosterone deficiency in hyperkalemic patients with chronic renal insufficiency. *Kidney Int* 1980;17:89.

207. Arruda JA, et al. Hyperkalemia and renal insufficiency: role of selective aldosterone deficiency and tubular unresponsiveness to aldosterone. *Am J Nephrol* 1981;1:160.

208. Christlieb AR, et al. Aldosterone responsiveness in patients with diabetes mellitus. *Diabetes* 1978;27:732.

209. Perez G, et al. Hyporeninemia and hypoaldosteronism in diabetes mellitus. *Arch Intern Med* 1977;137:852.

210. Saruta T, et al. Renin, aldosterone and other mineralocorticoids in hyperkalemic patients with chronic renal failure showing mild azotemia. *Nephron* 1981;29:128.

211. Sunderlin FS, Anderson GH Jr, Streeten DH, et al. The renin–angiotensin–aldosterone system in diabetic patients with hyperkalemia. *Diabetes* 1981;30:335.

212. Perez GO, et al. Effect of alterations of sodium intake in patients with hyporeninemic hypoaldosteronism. *Nephron* 1977;18:259.

213. Phelps KR, et al. Pathophysiology of the syndrome of hyporeninemic hypoaldosteronism. *Metabolism* 1980;29:186.

214. Chan R, et al. Renin–aldosterone system can respond to furosemide in patients with hyperkalemic hyporeninism. *J Lab Clin Med* 1998;132:229.

215. Birkenhager WH, et al. Interrelations between arterial pressure, fluid-volumes, and plasma-renin concentration in the course of acute glomerulonephritis. *Lancet* 1970;1:1086.

216. Powell HR, et al. Plasma renin activity in acute post streptococcal glomerulonephritis and the haemolytic-uraemic syndrome. *Arch Dis Child* 1974;49:802.

217. Gordon RD, et al. Hypertension and severe hyperkalemia associated with suppression of renin and aldosterone and completely reversed by dietary sodium restriction. *Aust Ann Med* 1970;4:287.

218. Rado JP, et al. Outpatient hyperkalemia syndrome in renal and hypertensive patients with suppressed aldosterone production. *J Med* 1979;10:145.

219. DeChamplain J, et al. Factors controlling renin in man. *Arch Intern Med* 1966;117:355.

220. Wagermark J, Ungerstedt U, Ljungqvist A. Sympathetic innervation of the juxtaglomerular cells of the kidney. *Circ Res* 1968;22:149.

221. Christensen NJ. Plasma catecholamines in long-term diabetes with and without neuropathy and in hypophysectomized subjects. *J Clin Invest* 1972;51:779.

222. Tuck ML, Sambhi MP, Levin L. Hyporeninemic hypoaldosteronism in diabetes mellitus. Studies of the autonomic nervous system's control of renin release. *Diabetes* 1979;28:237.

223. Gossain VV, et al. Impaired renin responsiveness with secondary hypoaldosteronism. *Arch Intern Med* 1973;132:885.

224. Vagnucci AH. Selective aldosterone deficiency. *J Clin Endocrinol Metab* 1969;29:279.

225. Fernandez-Cruz A, et al. Low plasma renin activity in normotensive patients with diabetes mellitus: relationship to neuropathy. *Hypertension* 1981;3:87.

226. de Chatel R, et al. Sodium, renin, aldosterone, catecholamines, and blood pressure in diabetes mellitus. *Kidney Int* 1977;12:412.

227. Tuck ML, Mayes DM. Mineralocorticoid biosynthesis in patients with hyporeninemic hypoaldosteronism. *J Clin Endocrinol Metab* 1980;50:341.

228. Dunn MJ, Zambraski EJ. Renal effects of drugs that inhibit prostaglandin synthesis. *Kidney Int* 1980;18:609.

229. Yun J, et al. Role of prostaglandins in the control of renin secretion in the dog. *Circ Res* 1977;40:459.

230. Saruta T, Kaplan NM. Adrenocortical steroidogenesis: the effects of prostaglandins. *J Clin Invest* 1972;51:2246.

231. Tan SY, et al. Indomethacin-induced prostaglandin inhibition with hyperkalemia. A reversible cause of hyporeninemic hypoaldosteronism. *Ann Intern Med* 1979;90:783.

232. Tan SY, Antonipillai I, Mulrow PJ. Inactive renin and prostaglandin production in hyporeninemic hypoaldosteronism. *J Clin Endocrinol Metab* 1980;51:849.

233. deLeiva A, et al. Big renin and biosynthetic defect of aldosterone in diabetes mellitus. *N Engl J Med* 1976;295:639.

234. Farese RV, Rodriguez-Colome M, O'Malley BC. Urinary prostaglandins following furosemide treatment and salt depletion in normal subjects with diabetic hyporeninemic hypoaldosteronism. *Clin Endocrinol* 1980;13:447.

235. Brenner BM, Meyer TW, Hostetter TH. Dietary protein intake and the progressive nature of kidney disease. (The role of hemodynamically mediated glomerular injury in the pathogenesis of progressive glomerular sclerosis in aging, renal ablation, and intrinsic renal disease.) *N Engl J Med* 1982;307:652.

236. Fredlund P, et al. Aldosterone production by isolated glomerulosa cells: modulation of sensitivity to angiotensin II and ACTH by extracellular potassium concentration. *Endocrinology* 1977;100:481.

237. Dluhy RG, et al. Studies of the control of plasma aldosterone concentration in normal man. II. Effect of dietary potassium and acute potassium infusion. *J Clin Invest* 1972;51:1950.

238. Himathongkam T, Dluhy RG, Williams GH. Potassium-aldosterone-renin interrelationships. *J Clin Endocrinol Metab* 1975;41:153.

239. Walker WG, Cooke CR. Plasma aldosterone regulation in anephric man. *Kidney Int* 1973;3:1.

240. Bayard F, et al. The regulation of aldosterone secretion in anephric man. *J Clin Invest* 1971;50:1585.

241. Williams TDM, et al. Atrial natriuretic peptide inhibits postural release of renin and vasopressin in humans. *Am J Physiol* 1988;255:R368.

242. Tuchelt H, et al. Role of atrial natriuretic factor in changes in the responsiveness of aldosterone to angiotensin II secondary to sodium loading and depletion in man. *Clin Sci* 79:57,1990.

243. Clark BA, et al. Effect of atrial natriuretic peptide on potassium-stimulated aldosterone secretion: potential relevance to hypoaldosteronism in man. *J Clin Endocrinol Metab* 1992;75:399.

244. Barret PQ, Isales CM. The role of cyclic nucleotides in atrial natriuretic peptide-mediated inhibition of aldosterone secretion. *Endocrinology* 1988;122:799.

245. McGiff JC, et al. Interrelationships of renin and aldosterone in a patient with hypoaldosteronism. *Am J Med* 1970;48:247.

246. Mellinger RC, Petermann FL, Jurgenson JC. Hyponatremia with low urinary aldosterone occurring in an old woman. *J Clin Endocrinol Metab* 1972;34:85.

247. Tait JF, Tait, SA. The effect of changes in potassium concentration on the maximal steroidogenic response of purified zona glomerulosa cells to angiotensin II. *J Steroid Biochem* 1976;7:687.

248. Smith JD, DeFronzo RA. *Clinical disorders of potassium metabolism, fluid, electrolyte and acid–base disorders.* New York: Churchill Livingstone, 1985.

249. Schnermann J, Persson AE, Agerup B. Tubuloglomerular feedback. Nonlinear relation between glomerular hydrostatic pressure and loop of Henle perfusion rate. *J Clin Invest* 1973;52:862.

250. Schnermann J, et al. Regulation of superficial nephron filtration rate by tubuloglomerular feedback. *Pflugers Arch* 1970;318:147.

251. Blantz RC, Konnen KS. Relation of distal tubular delivery and reabsorptive rate to nephron filtration. *Am J Physiol* 1977;233:F315.

252. Blantz RC, et al. Effect of modest hyperglycemia on tubulo-glomerular feedback activity. *Kidney Int* 1982;22:S206.

253. Tucker BJ, et al. Mechanism of diuresis with modest hyperglycemia. *Clin Res* 1981;29:478A.

254. Wright FS, Briggs JP. Feedback control of glomerular blood flow, pressure, and filtration rate. *Physiol Rev* 1979;59:958.

255. Perez GO, Pelleya R, Oster JR. Renal tubular hyperkalemia. *Am J Nephrol* 1982;2:109.

256. Battle DC, et al. Hyperkalemic hyperchloremic metabolic acidosis in sickle cell hemoglobinopathies. *Am J Med* 1982;72:188.

257. Morris RC, McSherry E. Symposium on acid–base homeostasis. Renal acidosis. *Kidney Int* 1972;1:322.

258. Dreyling KW, Wanner C, Schollmeyer P. Control of hyperkalemia with fludrocortisone in a patient with systemic lupus erythematosus. *Clin Nephrol* 1990;33:179.

259. Bastani B, et al. Preservation of intercalated cell H(+)-ATPase in two patients with lupus nephritis and hyperkalemic distal renal tubular acidosis. *J Am Soc Nephrol* 8:1109,1997.

260. Cohen EP, et al. Absence of H(+)-ATPase in cortical collecting tubules of a patient with Sjogren's syndrome and distal renal tubular acidosis. *J Am Soc Nephrol* 1992;3:264.

261. Purcell H, et al. Cellular distribution of H(+)-ATPase following acute unilateral ureteral obstruction in rats. *Am J Physiol* 1991;261:F365.

262. Battle DC, et al. The pathogenesis of hyperchloremic metabolic acidosis associated with kidney transplantation. *Am J Med* 1981;70:786.

263. Roll D, et al. Transient hypoaldosteronism after renal allotransplantation. *Isr J Med Sci* 1979;15:29.

264. Heering P, Grabensee B. Influence of cyclosporine A on renal tubular function after kidney transplantation. *Nephron* 1991;59:66.

265. Kamel SK, et al. Studies to determine the basis of hyperkalemia in recipients of a renal transplant who are treated with cyclosporine. *J Am Soc Nephrol* 1992;2:1279.

266. Perazella MA, Brown E. Electrolyte and acid–base disorders associated with AIDS: an etiologic review. *J Gen Int Med* 1994;9:232.

267. Peter SA. Electrolyte disorders and renal dysfunction in acquired immuno-deficiency syndrome patients. *J Natl Med Assoc* 1991;83:889.

268. Popovtzer MM, et al. Hyperkalemia in salt-wasting nephropathy. Study of the mechanisms. *Arch Intern Med* 1973;132:203.

269. Morgan JM. Hyperkalemia and acidosis in lead nephropathy. *South Med J* 1976;69:881.

270. Cogan MC, Arieff AI. Sodium-wasting, acidosis and hyperkalemia induced by methicillin interstitial nephritis. Evidence for selective distal tubular dysfunction. *Am J Med* 1978;64:500.

271. Lawson DH. Adverse reactions to potassium chloride. *Q J Med* 1974;43:433.

272. Lawson DH, et al. Drug attributed alterations in potassium handling in congestive cardiac failure. *Eur J Clin Pharmacol* 1982;23:21.

273. Paice B, et al. Hyperkalemia in patients in hospital. *Br Med J* 1983;286:1189.

274. Shapiro S, et al. Fatal drug reactions among medical inpatients. *J Am Med Assoc* 1971;216:467.

275. Shemer J, et al. Incidence of hyperkalemia in hospitalized patients. *Isr J Med Sci* 1983;19:659.

276. McCaughan D. Hazards of non-prescription potassium supplements. *Lancet* 1984;1:513.

277. Ponce SP, et al. Drug-induced hyperkalemia. *Medicine* 1985;64:357.

278. Mueller BA, et al. Noni juice (Morinda citrifolia): hidden potential for hyperkalemia? *Am J Kidney Dis* 2000;35:310.

279. Mercer CW, Logic JR. Cardiac arrest due to hyperkalemia following intravenous penicillin administration. *Chest* 1973;64:358.

280. Browning JJ, Channer KS. Hyperkalaemic cardiac arrhythmia caused by potassium citrate mixture. *Br Med J* 1981;283:1366.

281. Michael JM, et al. Potassium load in CPD-preserved whole blood and two types of packed red blood cells. *Transfusion* 1975;15:144.

282. Bethune DW, McKay R. Paradoxical changes in serum potassium during cardiopulmonary bypass in association with non-cardioselective ß-blockade. *Lancet* 1978;2:380.

283. Lundborg P. The effect of adrenergic blockade on potassium concentrations in different conditions. *Acta Med Scand* 1983;672:121.

284. Traub YM, et al. Elevation of serum potassium during ßblockade: absence of relationship to the renin–aldosterone system. *Clin Pharmacol Ther* 1980;28:765.

285. Arthur S, Greenberg A. Hyperkalemia associated with intravenous laßlol therapy for acute hypertension in renal transplant recipients. *Clin Nephrol* 1990;33:269.

286. Borra S, et al. Hyperkalemia in an adult hospitalized population. *Mt Sinai J Med* 1988;55:226.

287. Rimmer JM, et al. Hyperkalemia as a complication of drug therapy. *Arch Intern Med* 1987;147:867.

288. Ahmed EU, et al. Etiology of hyperkalemia in hospitalized patients: an answer to Harrinton's question. *J Am Soc Nephrol* 1999;10:103A.

289. Smith TW, Willerson JT. Suicidal and accidental digoxin ingestion. Report of five cases with serum digoxin level correlations. *Circulation* 1971;44:29.

290. Reza MJ, et al. Massive intravenous digoxin overdosage. *N Engl J Med* 1974;291:777.

291. Levinsky NG, et al. The relationship between amino acids and potassium in isolated rat muscle. *J Clin Invest* 1962;41:480.

292. Dickerman HW, Walker WG. Effect of cationic amino acid infusion on potassium metabolism *in vivo. Am J Physiol* 1964;206:403.

293. Alberti KGM, et al. Effect of arginine on electrolyte metabolism in man. *Clin Res* 1967;15:476A.

294. Hertz P, Richardson JA. Arginine-induced hyperkalemia in renal failure patients. *Arch Intern Med* 1972;130:778.

295. Bushinsky DA, Gennari FJ. Life-threatening hyperkalemia induced by arginine. *Ann Intern Med* 1978;89:632.

296. Carroll HJ, Tice DA. The effects of epsilon amino-caproic acid upon potassium metabolism in the dog. *Metabolism* 1966;15:449.

297. Perazella MA, Biswas P. Acute hyperkalemia associated with intravenous epsilon-aminocaproic acid therapy. *Am J Kidney Dis* 1999; 33:782.

298. Perazella MA, et al. Hyperkalemia associated with IV epsilon-aminocaproic acid. *J Am Soc Nephrol* 1999;10:123A.

299. Weintraub HD, et al. Changes in plasma potassium concentration after depolarizing blockers in anaesthetized man. *Br J Anaesth* 1969; 41:1048.

300. Yentis SM. Suxamethonium and hyperkalaemia. *Anaesth Intens Care* 1990;18:92.

301. Gronert GA, Theye RA. Pathophysiology of hyperkalemia induced by succinylcholine. *Anesthesiology* 1975;43:89.

302. Laragh JH. Amiloride, a potassium-conserving agent new to the USA: mechanisms and clinical relevance. *Curr Ther Res* 1982;32:173.

303. Ramsay LE, et al. Amiloride, spironolactone, and potassium chloride in thiazide-treated hypertensive patients. *Clin Pharmacol* 1980;4:533.

304. Good DW, Wright FS. Luminal influences on potassium secretion: sodium concentration and fluid flow rate. *Am J Physiol* 1979;236:F192.

305. Udezue FU, Harrold BP. Hyperkalaemic paralysis due to spironolactone. *Postgrad Med* 1980;56:254.

306. Greenblatt DJ, Koch-Weser J. Adverse reactions to spironolactone. A report from Boston Collaborative Drug Surveillance Program. *JAMA* 1973;225:40.

307. Whiting GF, et al. Severe hyperkalaemia with Moduretic. *Med J Aust* 1979;1:409.

308. Petersen AG. Letter: dyazide and hyperkalemia. *Ann Intern Med* 1976; 84:612.

309. Feinfeld DA, Carvounis CP. Fatal hyperkalemia and hyperchloremic acidosis. Association with spironolactone in the absence of renal impairment. *J Am Med Assoc* 1978;240:1516.

310. Jaffey L, Martin A. Malignant hyperkalemia after amiloride/hydrochlorothiazide treatment. *Lancet* 1981;1:1272.

311. Chiu TF, et al. Rapid life-threatening hyperkalemia after addition of amiloride HCl/hydrochlorothiazide to angiotensin-converting enzyme inhibitor therapy. *Ann Emerg Med* 1997;30:612.

312. Maddox RW, et al. Extreme hyperkalemia associated with amiloride. *South Med J* 1985;78:365.

313. Henger A, et al. Acid–base effects of inhibition of aldosterone and angiotensin II action in chronic metabolic acidosis in humans. *J Am Soc Nephrol* 1999;10:121A.

314. McNay JL, Oran E. Possible predisposition of diabetic patients to hyperkalemia following administration of potassium-retaining diuretic, amiloride (MK-870). *Metabolism* 1970;19:58.

315. Mor R, et al. Indomethacin- and Moduretic-induced hyperkalemia. *Isr J Med Sci* 1983;19:535.

316. Walker BR, et al. Hyperkalemia after triamterene in diabetic patients. *Clin Pharmacol Ther* 1972;13:643.

317. Wan HH, Lye MDW. Moduretic-induced metabolic acidosis and hyperkalemia. *Postgrad Med J* 1980;56:348.

318. Schlondorff D. Renal complications of nonsteroidal anti-inflammatory drugs. *Kidney Int* 1993;44:643.

319. Garella S, Matarese RA. Renal effects of prostaglandins and clinical adverse effects of nonsteroidal anti-inflammatory agents. *Medicine* 1984;63:165.

320. Goldszer RC, et al. Hyperkalemia associated with indomethacin. *Arch Intern Med* 1981;141:802.

321. Miller KP, et al. Severe hyperkalemia during piroxicam therapy. *Arch Intern Med* 1984;144:2414.

322. Mactier RA, Khanna R. Hyperkalemia induced by indomethacin and naproxen and reversed by fludrocortisone. *South Med J* 1988;81:799.

323. Kimberly RP, et al. Reduction of renal function by newer non-steroidal anti-inflammatory drugs. *Am J Med* 1978;64:799.

324. Meier DE, et al. Indomethacin-associated hyperkalemia in the elderly. *J Am Ger Soc* 1983;31:371.

325. Corwin HL, Bonventre JV. Renal insufficiency associated with nonsteroidal anti-inflammatory agents. *Am J Kidney Dis* 1984;4:147.

326. Frais MA, et al. Piroxicam-induced renal failure and hyperkalemia. *Ann Intern Med* 1983;99:129.

327. Galler M, et al. Reversible acute renal insufficiency and hyperkalemia following indomethacin therapy. *J Am Med Assoc* 1981;246:154.

328. Nicholls MG, Espiner EA. Indomethacin-induced azotaemia and hyperkalemia. *NZ Med J* 1981;94:377.

329. Textor SC, et al. Hyperkalemia in azotemic patients during angiotensin-converting enzyme inhibition and aldosterone reduction with captopril. *Am J Med* 1982;73:719.

330. Atlas SA, et al. Interruption of the renin–angiotensin system in hypertensive patients by captopril induces sustained reduction in aldosterone secretion, potassium retention and natriuresis. *Hypertension* 1979;1:274.

331. Memon A, et al. Incidence and predictors of hyperkalemia in patients with chronic renal failure on angiotensin converting enzyme inhibitors. *J Am Soc Nephrol* 1999;10:294A.

332. Reardon LC, Macpherson DS. Hyperkalemia in outpatients using angiotensin-converting enzyme inhibitors. How much should we worry? *Arch Intern Med* 1998;158:26.

333. Keilani T, et al. A subdepressor low dose of ramipril lowers urinary protein excretion without increasing plasma potassium. *Am J Kidney Dis* 1999;33:450.

334. Russo D, et al. Additive antiproteinuric effect of converting enzyme inhibitor and losartan in normotensive patients with IgA nephropathy. *Am J Kidney Dis* 1999;33:851.

335. Heeg JE, et al. Additive antiproteinuric effect of the NSAID indomethacin and the ACE inhibitor lisinopril. *Am J Nephrol* 1990;10:94.

336. White WB, Aydelotte ME. Clinical experience with labetalol and enalapril in combination in patients with severe essential and renovascular hypertension. *Am J Med Sci* 1988;296:187.

337. Dahlstrom U, Karlsson E. Captopril and spironolactone therapy for refractory congestive heart failure. *Am J Cardiol* 1993;71:29A.

338. Hannedouche T, et al. Randomised controlled trial of enalapril and ßblockers in non-diabetic chronic renal failure. *Br Med J* 1994;309:833.

339. Apperloo AJ, et al. Differential effects of enalapril and atenolol on proteinuria and renal haemodynamics in non-diabetic renal disease. *Br Med J* 1991;303:821.

340. Bugge JF. Severe hyperkalaemia induced by trimethoprim in combination with an angiotensin-converting enzyme inhibitor in a patient with transplanted lungs. *J Intern Med* 1996;240:249.

341. Ferder L, et al. Angiotensin converting enzyme inhibitors versus calcium antagonists in the treatment of diabetic hypertensive patients. *Hypertension* 1992;19:II237.

342. Kjekshus J, Swedberg K. Tolerability of enalapril in congestive heart failure. *Am J Cardiol* 1988;62:67A.

343. Goldberg MR, et al. Biochemical effects of losartan, a nonpeptide angiotensin II receptor antagonist, on the renin–angiotensin–aldosterone system in hypertensive patients. *Hypertension* 1995;25:37.

344. Goldberg AI, et al. Safety and tolerability of losartan potassium, an angiotensin II receptor antagonist, compared with hydrochlorothiazide, atenolol, felodipine ER, and angiotensin-converting enzyme inhibitors for the treatment of systemic hypertension. *Am J Cardiol* 1995;75:793.

345. Savoy A, et al. Losartan effects on serum potassium in an elderly population. *J Am Soc Nephrol* 1998;9:111A.

346. Bakris GL, et al. Differential effects of valsartan and lisinopril on potassium homeostasis in hypertensive patients with nephropathy. *J Am Soc Nephrol* 1999;10:68A.

347. Greenberg S, et al. Trimethoprim-sulfamethoxazole induces reversible hyperkalemia. *Ann Intern Med* 1993;119:291.

348. Velázquez H, et al. Renal mechanism of trimethoprim-induced hyperkalemia. *Ann Intern Med* 1993;119:296.

349. Kaufman AM, et al. Renal salt wasting and metabolic acidosis with trimethoprim-sulfamethoxazole therapy. *Mt Sinai J Med* 1983;50:238.

350. Alappan R, Perazella MA, Buller GK. Hyperkalemia in hospitalized patients treated with trimethoprim-sulfamethoxazole. *Ann Intern Med* 1996;124:316.

351. Alappan R, Buller GK, Perazella MA. Trimethoprim-sulfamethoxazole therapy in outpatients: is hyperkalemia a significant problem? *Am J Nephrol* 1999;19:389.

352. Briceland LL, Bailie GR. Pentamidine-associated nephrotoxicity and hyperkalemia in patients with AIDS. *DICP* 1991;25:1171.

353. Kleyman TR, Roberts C, Ling BN. A mechanism for pentamidine-induced hyperkalemia: inhibition of distal nephron sodium transport. *Ann Intern Med* 1995;122:103.

354. Oster JR, Singer I, Fishman LM. Heparin-induced aldosterone suppression and hyperkalemia. *Am J Med* 1995;98:575.

355. Batlle DC, et al. The pathogenesis of hyperchloremic metabolic acidosis associated with kidney transplantation. *Am J Med* 1981;70:786.

356. DeFronzo RA, et al. Investigations into the mechanisms of hyperkalemia following renal transplantation. *Kidney Int* 1977;11:357.

357. Yu HS, et al. Change of transtubular potassium gradient (TTKG) in renal transplant recipients. *J Am Soc Nephrol* 1999;10:14A.

358. Asante-Korang A, et al. Experience of FK506 immune suppression in pediatric heart transplantation: a study of long term adverse effects. *J Heart Lung Transplant* 1996;15:415.

359. Tumlin JA, Sands JM. Nephron segment-specific inhibition of Na+/K(+)-ATPase activity by cyclosporin A. *Kidney Int* 1993;43:246.

360. Lea JP, et al. Evidence that the inhibition of Na+/K(+)-ATPase activity by FK506 involves calcineurin. *Kidney Int* 1994;46:647.

361. Ling BN, Eaton DC. Cyclosporin A inhibits apical secretory K+ channels in rabbit cortical collecting tubule principal cells. *Kidney Int* 1993;44:974.

362. Pei Y, et al. Extrarenal effect of cyclosporine A on potassium homeostasis in renal transplant recipients. *Am J Kidney Dis* 1993;22:314.

363. DeFronzo RA, Smith JD. Disorders of potassium metabolism-hyperkalemia. In: Arieff AI, DeFronzo RA, eds. *Fluid, electrolyte and acid–base disorders.* New York: Churchill-Livingstone, 1995:319.

364. Moore RD. Stimulation of Na:H exchange by insulin. *Biophys J* 1981; 33:203.

365. Gourley DRH. Effect of insulin on potassium exchange in normal and ouabain-treated skeletal muscle. *J Pharmacol Exp Ther* 1965;148:339.

366. Allon M, Dunlay R, Copkney C. Nebulized albuterol for acute hyperkalemia in patients on hemodialysis. *Ann Intern Med* 1989;110:426.

367. Allon M, Copkney C. Albuterol and insulin for treatment of hyperkalemia in hemodialysis patients. *Kidney Int* 1990;38:869.

368. Spital A. Bicarbonate in the treatment of severe hyperkalemia. *Am J Med* 1989;86:511.

369. Blumberg A, et al. Effect of various therapeutic approaches on plasma potassium and major regulating factors in terminal renal failure. *Am J Med* 1988;85:507.

370. Ethier JH, et al. The transtubular potassium concentration in patients with hypokalemia and hyperkalemia. *Am J Kidney Dis* 1990;15:309.

371. Kamel KS, et al. Urine electrolytes and osmolality: when and how to use them. *Am J Nephrol* 1990;10:89.

372. Zettle RM, et al. Renal potassium handling during states of low aldosterone bio-activity: a method to differentiate renal from non-renal causes. *Am J Nephrol* 1987;7:360.

373. Goldstein MB, et al. The urine anion gap: a clinically useful index of ammonium excretion. *Am J Med Sci* 1986;292:198.

374. Batlle DC, et al. The use of urinary anion gap in the diagnosis of hyperchloremic metabolic acidosis. *N Engl J Med* 1988;318:594.

375. Dyck RF, et al. A modification of the urine osmolal gap: an improved method for estimating urine ammonium. *Am J Nephrol* 1990;10: 359.

376. Halperin ML, et al. Urine ammonium: the key to the diagnosis of distal renal tubular acidosis. *Nephron* 1988;50:1.

377. Dominguez JH, Raisz LG. Effects of changing hydrogen ion, carbonic acid, and bicarbonate concentrations on bone resorption *in vitro. Calcif Tissue Int* 1979;29:7.

378. Adams ND, Gray RW, Lemann J Jr. The calciuria of increased fixed acid production: evidence against a role for parathyroid hormone and 1, 25(OH)2-vitamin D. *Calcif Tiss Int* 1979;28:233.

379. Kraut JA, Mishler DR, Kurokawa K. Effect of colchicine and calcitonin on calcemic response to metabolic acidosis. *Kidney Int* 1984;25:608.

380. Greiber S, Mitch WE. Catabolism in uremia: metabolic acidosis and activation of specific pathways. *Contrib Nephrol* 1992;98:20.

CHAPTER 88

Disorders of Phosphorus, Calcium, and Magnesium Metabolism

Eduardo Slatopolsky and Keith A. Hruska

PHOSPHORUS

Phosphorus is a common anion ubiquitously distributed throughout the body. Approximately 80% to 85% of the phosphorus is present in the skeleton. The rest is widely distributed in the form of organic phosphate compounds that play fundamental roles in several aspects of cellular metabolism. The energy required for many cellular reactions including biosynthesis derives from hydrolysis of adenosine triphosphate (ATP). Organic phosphates are important components of cell membrane phospholipids. Changes in serum phosphorus influence the dissociation of oxygen from hemoglobin through regulation of 2,3-diphosphoglycerate concentrations. The concentration of phosphorus influences the activity of several metabolic pathways such as ammoniagenesis, glycolysis, gluconeogenesis, parathyroid hormone (PTH) secretion, and phosphate reabsorption, as well as the formation of 1,25-dihydroxycholecalciferol [$1,25(OH)_2D_3$] from 25-hydroxycholecalciferol [$25(OH)D_3$]. In the extracellular fluid (ECF), phosphorus is present predominantly in the inorganic form (P_i). The physiologic concentration of serum phosphorus ranges from 2.5 to 4.5 mg/dL (0.9 to 1.45 mmol/L) in adults (1). In serum, phosphorus exists mainly as the free ion, and only a small fraction (less than 15%) is protein bound (2,3). There is a diurnal variation in serum phosphorus of 0.6 to 1.0 mg/dL, with the nadir occurring between 8 AM and 11 AM. Ingestion of meals rich in carbohydrate decreases serum phosphorus concentrations as a result of the movement of phosphorus from the extracellular to the intracellular space.

E. Slatopolsky: Department of Medicine, Renal Division, Washington University School of Medicine and Barnes-Jewish Hospital, St. Louis, Missouri

K. A. Hruska: Department of Internal Medicine, Washington University School of Medicine and Barnes-Jewish Hospital, St. Louis, Missouri

Gastrointestinal Absorption of Phosphorus

Approximately 1 g of phosphorus is ingested daily in an average diet in the United States. About 300 mg is excreted in the stool, and 700 mg is absorbed (Fig. 88-1). Most of the phosphorus is absorbed in the duodenum and jejunum, with minimal absorption occurring in the ileum (4). Phosphorus transport in proximal segments of the small intestine appears to involve both passive and active components and to be under the influence of Vitamin D. The movement of phosphorus from the intestinal lumen to the blood requires (a) transport across the luminal brush-border membrane of the intestine; (b) transport through the cytoplasm; and (c) transport across the basolateral plasma membrane of the epithelium. The rate-limiting step and the main driving force of absorption is the luminal membrane step (1).

Luminal Membrane Transport

The mechanism of transport across the intestinal brush-border epithelial membrane involves a sodium–phosphate cotransport system, as suggested by Berner et al. (5) and confirmed by the identification of the responsible molecular mechanism, a type IIb sodium–phosphate (NaPi) cotransporter, NPT2 (6). The NaPi cotransporters are a secondary active form of ion transport using the energy of the Na gradient from outside to inside the cell to move phosphate ion uphill against an electrochemical gradient (Fig. 88-2). The role of 1,25-dihydroxycholecalciferol and 25-hydroxycholecalciferol in this transport system has been studied by several investigators (7–10). Murer and Hildman showed that *in vivo* administration of 1,25-dihydroxycholecalciferol to rabbits affects *in vitro* uptake of phosphorus by intestinal brush-border membrane vesicles (8). Reduction of endogenous 1,25-dihydroxycholecalciferol decreases uptake of phosphorus by approximately 65% in brush-border membrane vesicles. This uptake increased threefold after injection of high

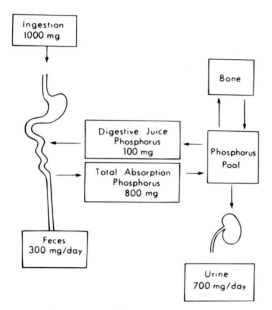

FIG. 88-1. Summary of phosphorus metabolism in humans. Approximately 1 g of phosphorus is ingested daily, of which 300 mg is excreted in the stool and 700 mg in the urine. The gastrointestinal tract, bone, and kidney are the major organs involved in phosphorus homeostasis.

doses of 1,25-dihydroxycholecalciferol. These studies are in agreement with those of Fuchs and Peterlik, who found similar results using chick intestinal epithelial brush-border membrane vesicles (4). Vitamin D seems to stimulate phosphorus absorption by two mechanisms—a calcium-dependent duodenal process and a calcium-independent jejunal system. In the rat, the major effect of 1,25-dihydroxycholecalciferol on phosphorus absorption appears to involve increased active transport.

Studies of phosphorus accumulation by rat intestinal brush-border vesicles have demonstrated that at physiologic pH levels, phosphorus uptake is dependent on luminal sodium, and that it is affected by the transmembrane potential, indicating that like the renal type II cotransporter, NaPi-2, the intestinal type IIb cotransporter, NaPi-2b, is electrogenic (6).

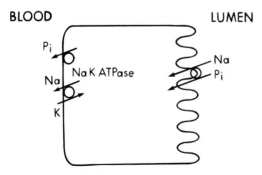

FIG. 88-2. The apical membrane Na^+–inorganic phosphate (P_i) cotransport proteins utilize the electrochemical driving force for Na^+ to move P_i into the cell. The electrochemical Na^+ gradient is maintained by active Na^+ extrusion across the basolateral membrane through the action of Na^+-K^+-ATPase.

The $K_m(P_i)$ of NaPi-2b is approximately 50 μm, a finding that is consistent with the renal transport protein. In contrast to the renal NaPi-2a isoform, the intestinal NaPi-2b cotransporter is less dependent on the pH level and is slightly more active at acid pH values. PTH may influence phosphorus absorption in the gut but does so indirectly by stimulating the renal synthesis of 1,25-dihydroxycholecalciferol. PTH does not directly affect the activity of NaPi-2b. Low-phosphorus diets increase the absorption of phosphorus from the intestine but may do so also by stimulating the formation of 1,25-dihydroxycholecalciferol. In animals fed a high-phosphorus diet, suppression of 1,25-dihydroxycholecalciferol may result in decreased intestinal absorption of phosphorus.

Transcellular Movement of Phosphorus

The second component of transcellular intestinal phosphorus transport involves the movement of phosphorus from the luminal to the basolateral membrane. Although little is known about the cellular events that mediate this transcellular process, evidence suggests a role for the microtubular microfilament system of intestinal cells (4). Microfilaments in the cell may be important in conveying phosphorus from the brush-border membrane to the basolateral membrane and may be involved in the extrusion of phosphorus at the basolateral membrane from the epithelial cell.

Phosphate Exit at Basolateral Membrane

Little is known about the mechanisms of phosphorus extrusion at the basolateral membrane of intestinal epithelial cells. The electrochemical gradient for phosphorus favors movement from the intracellular to the extracellular compartment because the interior of the cell is electrically negative compared with the basolateral external surface (8). Thus, it has been presumed that the exit of phosphorus across the basolateral membrane represents a mode of passive transport (11).

Renal Reabsorption of Phosphorus

Most of the inorganic phosphorus in serum (90% to 95%) is ultrafilterable at the level of the glomerulus. At physiologic levels of serum phosphorus, approximately 7 g of phosphorus is filtered daily by the kidney, of which 80% to 90% is reabsorbed by the renal tubules and the remainder is excreted in the urine (about 700 mg on a 1-g phosphorus diet) equal to absorption (12). Thus, at steady-state, adults are in a state of balance between intake and excretion of phosphorus (Fig. 88-1). Micropuncture studies have demonstrated that 60% to 70% of the filtered phosphorus is reabsorbed in the proximal tubule. However, there is also evidence that a significant amount of filtered phosphorus is reabsorbed in distal segments of the nephron (13). When serum phosphorus levels increase and the filtered load of phosphorus increases, the capacity to reabsorb phosphorus also increases. However, a maximum rate of transport (Tm) for phosphorus reabsorption is obtained usually at serum phosphorus concentrations of 6 mg/dL. There is a direct correlation between Tm phosphorus values and glomerular filtration rate (GFR) even when the GFR is varied over a broad range. Micropuncture studies suggest two different mechanisms responsible for phosphorus reabsorption in the proximal tubule. In the first third of the proximal tubule, in which only 10% to 15% of the filtered sodium and fluid is reabsorbed, the ratio of tubular fluid (TF) phosphorus to plasma ultrafilterable (UF) phosphorus falls to values of approximately 0.6. This indicates that the first third of the proximal tubule accounts for approximately 50% of the total amount of phosphorus reabsorbed in this segment of the nephron. In the last two-thirds of the proximal tubule, the reabsorption of phosphorus parallels the movement of salt and water. In the remaining 70% of the pars convoluta, the TF : UF phosphorous ratio remains at a value of 0.6 to 0.7, whereas fluid reabsorption increases to approximately 60% to 70% of the filtered load. Thus, in the last two-thirds of proximal tubule, the TF : UF phosphorus reabsorption ratio is directly proportional to sodium and fluid reabsorption. A significant amount of phosphorus, perhaps on the order of 20% to 30%, is reabsorbed beyond the portion of the proximal tubule that is accessible to micropuncture. There is little phosphorus transport within the loop of Henle (14), with most transport distal to micropuncture accessibility occurring in the distal convoluted tubule. In this location, Pastoriza-Munoz et al. (13) found that approximately 15% of filtered phosphorus is reabsorbed under baseline conditions in animals subjected to parathyroidectomy, but that the value falls to about 6% after administration of large doses of PTH. The collecting duct is a potential site for distal nephron reabsorption of phosphorus (15–17). Transport in this nephron segment may explain the discrepancy between the amount of phosphorus delivered to the late distal tubule in micropuncture studies and the considerably smaller amount of phosphorus that appears in the final urine of the same kidney. Phosphorus transport in the cortical collecting tubule is independent of regulation by PTH. This is in agreement with the absence of PTH-dependent adenylate cyclase in the cortical collecting tubule (17).

Comparison of Superficial and Deep Nephron Transport

The contribution of superficial nephrons and deep nephrons of the kidney to phosphorus homeostasis differs. Nephron heterogeneity in phosphorus handling has been evaluated under a number of conditions by puncture of the papillary tip and the superficial early distal tubule, with the recorded fractional delivery representing deep and superficial nephron function, respectively. Using this technique, Haramati et al. (18,19) demonstrated that in thyroparathyroidectomized (TPTX) rats fed a normal phosphorus diet, phosphorus reabsorption was greater in deep nephrons than in superficial nephrons, and this heterogeneous handling of phosphorus can be mitigated by both PTH infusion (19) and a low-phosphorus diet (18).

Studies in TPTX rats fed a normal phosphorus diet have presented *in vivo* measurements of maximum tubular reabsorptive capacities for phosphorus of deep and superficial nephrons. Deep nephron values (5.05 pmol/mL per minute) were significantly greater than the values obtained in superficial nephrons (3.38 pmol/mL per minute). These results suggest that the juxtamedullary nephrons are more responsive to body phosphorus requirements than the superficial nephrons. Also, microinjection of phosphorus tracer into thin ascending and descending limbs of loops of Henle reveals that only 80% of phosphorus was recovered in the urine, whereas 88% to 100% of phosphorus was recovered when the tracer was injected into the late superficial distal tubule. It was concluded that a significant amount of phosphorus must be reabsorbed by juxtamedullary distal tubules or by segments connecting the juxtamedullary distal tubules to the collecting ducts to account for the discrepancy between the results of superficial nephron injection and injection into the juxtamedullary ascending limb of loops of Henle. These data seem to support an increased reabsorptive capacity for phosphorus in deep as opposed to superficial nephrons.

In summary, phosphorus transport occurs in the distal nephron, particularly in the distal convoluted tubule and cortical collecting tubular system. This transport may be considerable under certain experimental conditions, but the importance of the terminal nephron system in day-to-day phosphorus homeostasis remains to be defined. It is also evident from data obtained from various micropuncture and microinjection studies that juxtamedullary and superficial nephrons have different capacities for phosphorus transport. The increased responsiveness of the deep nephrons to phosphorus intake suggests a key regulatory role for this system in phosphorus homeostasis.

Cellular Mechanisms of Phosphate Reabsorption in the Kidney

The apical membrane of renal tubular cells is the initial barrier across which phosphorus and other solutes present in the tubular fluid must pass to be transported into the peritubular capillary network. Because the electrical charge of the cell interior is negative to the exterior, and phosphorus concentrations are higher in the cytosol, phosphorus must move against an electrochemical gradient into the cell interior, whereas at the antiluminal membrane, the transport of phosphorus into the peritubular capillary is favored by the high intracellular phosphorus concentration and the electronegativity of the cell interior. Studies with apical membrane vesicles have demonstrated cotransport of Na^+ with phosphate across the brush-border membrane, whereas the transport of phosphorus across the basolateral membrane is independent of that of Na^+ (20). The apical membrane Na^+-phosphate cotransport protein (NPT2a) energizes the uphill transport of phosphate across the brush-border membrane by the movement of Na^+ down its electrochemical gradient. The latter gradient is established and maintained by active extrusion of Na^+ across the basolateral cell membrane into the peritubular capillary through the action of Na^+-K^+-ATPase (Fig. 88-2) (21).

Three families of NaPi cotransport proteins of the proximal tubule (types I, II, and III) have been cloned using Xenopus RNA expression strategies (22,23). The DNA clones encode 80- to 95-kd proteins that reconstitute Na^+-dependent concentrative, or "uphill," transport of phosphate upon chromosomal RNA injection in oocytes (23) or transfection of sf9 cells (24). The type I cotransporter, NPT1, is expressed predominantly in the renal proximal tubule, and it accounts for about 13% of the known NaPi cotransporter mRNA in the mouse kidney (25). NPT1 is not regulated by dietary P_i, and studies in NPT1-cRNA–injected oocytes revealed that it may function not only as an NaPi cotransporter but also as a chloride and organic anion channel (26).

The NPT2 proteins are similar between several species including humans (22) and several isoforms have been described (27). Nephron localization of NPT2 proteins has been limited to the proximal tubule of superficial and deep nephrons (greatest in the latter, concordant with physiologic studies) (22). Immunolocalization studies in renal epithelial cells demonstrated apical membrane and subapical membrane vesicle staining (22), suggesting that a functional pool of transporters is available for insertion into or retrieval from the brush-border membrane itself. This has been postulated to be a major mechanism of P_i transport regulation in response to acute changes in phosphorus and PTH levels (22,28,29). The NPT2 family is upregulated at message and protein levels by chronic feeding of low-P_i diets (27,30,31) and regulated at message and protein levels by PTH (30–32).

The type III NaPi cotransporters were originally identified as retroviral receptors for gibbon ape leukemia virus (Glvr1) and rat amphotropic virus (Ram1) (33). They are ubiquitously expressed, and they comprise about 1% of the known NaPi cotransporter mRNAs in the mouse kidney (25). Their levels and activity adapt to dietary phosphate changes, but they are felt to represent mainly "housekeeping" NaPi cotransporters.

Studies of phosphorus exit across the basolateral membrane suggest that it is accompanied by the net transfer of a negative charge and occurs down a favorable electrochemical gradient via sodium-independent mechanisms (34).

Factors that Affect the Urinary Excretion of Phosphorus

Several factors are known to affect the urinary excretion of phosphorus. Of the multiplicity of factors that regulate phosphate transport in the kidney, the most important are phosphate delivery and PTH.

Effects of PTH on Phosphorus Reabsorption by the Kidney. Parathyroidectomy decreases urinary phosphorus excretion, whereas administration of PTH rapidly increases phosphorus excretion (34–36). Micropuncture studies indicate that PTH inhibits phosphorus transport in the proximal tubule (37,38) and probably in segments of the nephron located beyond the proximal tubule (13). TF : UF phosphorus ratio reaches a value of 0.6 by the S_2 segment of the proximal tubule, and

once achieved, this equilibrium ratio is maintained along the accessible portion of the proximal tubule. Within 6 to 24 hours of parathyroidectomy, the proximal TF : UF phosphorus ratio falls to a value of 0.2 to 0.4, indicating an increase in phosphorus reabsorption (38–40). TF phosphorus falls progressively with continuous fluid absorption along the length of the tubule, so by the end of the proximal tubule, the reabsorption of phosphorus is 70% to 85% of the filtered load, resulting in decreased phosphorus delivery to distal segments of the nephron. Because decreased delivery of phosphorus out of the proximal tubule complicates the evaluation of any distal effects of PTH on phosphorus excretion, maneuvers have been designed to increase phosphorus delivery to the distal nephron to study distal effects of parathyroidectomy on phosphorus reabsorption [e.g., phosphorus loading by intravenous infusion (41,42)]. In the nonphosphorus-loaded, acutely parathyroidectomized animal, virtually all the distal load of phosphorus is reabsorbed by the distal nephron, reducing urinary phosphorus excretion to very low levels (43,44). In the phosphorus-loaded animal, the distal reabsorption of phosphorus increases until saturation is approached and urinary phosphorus excretion begins to rise. Acute administration of PTH to phosphorus-loaded parathyroidectomized dogs sharply lowers the distal reabsorption. These experiments indicate that PTH inhibits reabsorption of phosphorus in the distal and the proximal nephron.

Administration of PTH *in vivo* results in decreased rates of Na^+-dependent phosphorus transport in brush-border membrane vesicles isolated from the kidneys of treated rats (45,46). The uptakes of D-glucose and Na^+ were not affected by administration of PTH. Intravenous infusion of dibutyryl cyclic adenosine monophosphate (cAMP) also decreased Na^+-dependent phosphorus uptake in isolated brushborder vesicles, but neither PTH nor dibutyryl cAMP decreased phosphate transport when added directly to membrane vesicles (45). These observations suggest that the effects of PTH on renal phosphate transport were mediated through altered functional characteristics (decreased V_{max}) of the renal brush-border membrane Na^+-dependent phosphate transporter (46).

PTH stimulates two signaling pathways in proximal tubule cells: adenylate cyclase and phospholipase C (PLC), resulting in activation of protein kinase A (PKA) and protein kinase C (PKC) (47). The first pathway, activation of the adenylate cyclase, differs from that of PKC. Studies in OK cells show that PKA activation by PTH decreases the expression of NaPi-2 cotransporter (Lederer), likely due to internalization and degradation of the transporter. Binding of PTH to its receptor leads to activation of PLC with the subsequent hydrolysis of phosphatidylinositol 4,5-bisphosphate to inositol 1,4,5-trisphosphate (IP_3) and 1,2-diacylglycerol (DAG). IP_3 generation leads to the release of intracellular calcium stores. DAG activates PKC (47). In addition to its direct effect on NaPi-2, PTH inhibits PO_4 transport indirectly by inhibiting the Na^+-K^+-ATPase by decreasing the favorable gradient for PO_4 entry into the cell (48).

Measurement studies of *in vivo* renal reabsorption of phosphorus and calculations of kinetic parameters of Na^+-dependent phosphorus transport in membrane vesicles isolated from the renal brush-border membranes of normal dogs, parathyroidectomized dogs, dogs fed a low-phosphorus diet, and dogs receiving human growth hormone were performed (Table 88-2) (46,49). The latter three groups of dogs had greater baseline values for absolute tubular reabsorption of phosphorus compared with normal dogs. Na^+-dependent phosphate transport in brush-border membrane vesicles isolated from kidneys of these dogs was significantly increased compared with transport in brush-border vesicles from kidneys of normal dogs. Administration of PTH decreased significantly the apparent V_{max} for Na^+-dependent phosphorus transport in brush-border membrane vesicles isolated from kidneys of each of the four groups of dogs (Table 88-2). The apparent K_m (intrinsic binding affinity) for Na^+-dependent phosphorus transport was not significantly changed by experimental maneuvers. Absolute tubular reabsorption of phosphorus measured *in vivo* was decreased by administration of PTH in each group of dogs with the exception of the dogs fed a low-phosphorus diet (46,49). Thus, alterations in phosphorus reabsorption measured *in vivo* were paralleled by alterations in Na^+-dependent phosphorus transport in isolated membrane vesicles, and the administration of PTH *in vivo* resulted in altered transport characteristics of the isolated brush-border membranes.

The cloning of the NPT2 cotransport proteins has not completely elucidated the mechanisms of PTH action on phosphate transport. Because the phosphaturic effect of PTH can be reproduced by analogs of cAMP, the intracellular mechanism of phosphate transport regulation is thought to involve the cAMP/PKA signal pathway. However, the NaPi transport proteins are not characterized by a PKA–mediated phosphorylation site (50). Phosphorylation of brush-border membrane proteins *in vitro* occurs in parallel with inhibition with NPT2 cotransport (46). Parathyroidectomy of rats causes a twofold to threefold increase in the NPT2 protein content of brush-border membrane vesicles (32). Immunocytochemistry reveals the increase in protein exclusively in apical brush-border membranes of proximal tubules. PTH treatment of parathyroidectomized rats for 2 hours decreased protein levels and decreased the abundance of NPT2-specific messenger RNA (mRNA) by 31% (51). Parathyroidectomy did not affect NPT2 mRNA levels. The effects of PTH were apparent within 2 hours of administration and indicate that PTH regulation of NPT2 is determined in part by changes in the expression of NPT2 protein in the renal brush-border membranes. In addition, PTH may decrease the NPT2 protein content of the apical membrane in part by a mechanism that results in endocytic withdrawal of NPT2 into a cytoplasmic pool (32).

Effects of Changes in Acid–Base Balance on Phosphate Excretion. The effect of acid–base status on the renal excretion and transport of phosphate is complex. Acute respiratory acidosis increases and acute respiratory alkalosis decreases

phosphate excretion (51). These effects occur independent of PTH and plasma or luminal bicarbonate levels (51). However, other studies suggest that the effects of respiratory acid–base changes may be mediated by changes in plasma phosphate (51).

Acute metabolic acidosis has minimal effects on phosphate excretion; however, the phosphaturic effect of PTH is blunted (39). Acute metabolic alkalosis causes an increase in phosphate excretion independently of PTH (52–56). This effect is due, in part, to volume expansion produced by the infusion of bicarbonate (53,54).

Chronic acidosis increases phosphate excretion, again independent of PTH or changes in ionized Ca^{2+} (56–59). The effect appears to be directly on the sodium-dependent phosphate transport mechanism (60). Chronic alkalosis decreases phosphate excretion, probably by the same mechanism as acidosis, operating in the opposite direction (52,61). It has been shown (62) that acute and chronic acidosis in rats decreases the proximal tubule cell luminal membrane expression of the NPT2 cotransporter. It will seem that in acute acidosis, the transporter is internalized because the total cortical homogenate cotransporter expression is unchanged. The effects of acid–base perturbations are complex and depend on antecedent dietary intake, the chronicity of the change, and whether the change affects luminal or intracellular pH, or both.

Adrenal Hormones. Administration of pharmacologic amounts of cortisol leads to phosphaturia. Acute adrenalectomy reduces the GFR and increases the reabsorption of phosphorus in the proximal tubule. Frick and Durasene (63) concluded that glucocorticoid hormones could play an important role in the regulation of fractional reabsorption of phosphorus. The current notion of an important role for cellular metabolism in regulating the proximal tubular reabsorption of phosphorus is relevant to these observations. An effect of glucocorticoid hormones in altering carbohydrate metabolism within the proximal tubular cells could underlie the effects described.

Vitamin D. Controversy still surrounds the regulatory role of Vitamin D in renal phosphorus handling. Several studies have demonstrated that the chronic administration of Vitamin D to parathyroidectomized animals is phosphaturic (64–66). Conversely, other investigators reported that Vitamin D acutely stimulates proximal tubular phosphorus transport in both parathyroidectomized and Vitamin D–depleted rats (67). A unifying interpretation of these studies was hampered by the fact that the dosages of Vitamin D administered and the status of the serum calcium, phosphorus, and PTH varied considerably from study to study.

Liang et al. (68) administered 1,25-dihydroxycholecalciferol to Vitamin D–deficient chicks and subsequently examined the transport characteristics of isolated renal tubule cells. Three hours after the *in vivo* administration of Vitamin D, phosphorus uptake by the cells was significantly increased, whereas 17 hours after the administration of Vitamin D, phosphorus uptake was reduced. The serum phosphorus concentration, however, was significantly increased at 17 hours after administration, and administration of phosphorus to Vitamin D–depleted animals so their serum phosphorus levels were comparable to those of the 17-hour Vitamin D–replenished group resulted in a similar decrease in phosphorus uptake (68). In response to *in vitro* preincubation with as little as 0.01 pm of 1,25-dihydroxycholecalciferol, renal cells isolated from Vitamin D–deficient chicks demonstrated a specific increase in sodium-dependent phosphorus uptake, which was blocked by pretreatment with actinomycin D. The stimulatory effect was relatively specific for 1,25-dihydroxycholecalciferol, and kinetic analysis indicated that the V_{max} of the phosphorus transport system was increased, whereas the affinity of the system for phosphorus was unaffected (68).

Kurnik and Hruska (69) also examined the relationship between Vitamin D and renal phosphorus excretion in a normocalcemic, normophosphatemic weanling rat model fed a Vitamin D–deficient diet. The animals were mildly Vitamin D deficient (92 pg/mL of 1,25-dihydroxycholecalciferol versus 169 pg/mL in controls) but had no evidence of secondary hyperparathyroidism. Clearance studies performed in the basal partially Vitamin D–deficient state showed an increase in both absolute and fractional phosphorus excretion compared with controls. Animals that were replenished with 1,25-dihydroxycholecalciferol and maintained on diets designed to protect against the development of hyperphosphatemia demonstrated a significant decrease in urinary phosphorus excretion. Other animals were similarly replenished with Vitamin D but did not receive dietary adjustment; and in this group, both the serum phosphorus and the urinary phosphorus excretion level increased significantly. A third group was fed a normal diet and received smaller doses of 1,25-dihydroxycholecalciferol (15 pmol/g of body weight) for shorter periods, and although this dose had no effect on the serum phosphorus concentration, the phosphaturia was completely resolved.

Studies on brush-border membrane vesicles prepared from these animals revealed that in the partially Vitamin D–deficient state, sodium-dependent phosphorus uptake was significantly reduced compared with control animals. Animals that were replenished with Vitamin D and fed a controlled diet had a greater sodium-dependent phosphorus uptake than both Vitamin D–depleted and Vitamin D–replenished animals not maintained on controlled diets.

The results of this series of studies suggest that the primary action of 1,25-dihydroxycholecalciferol is to increase tubular phosphorus reabsorption. Long-term administration of Vitamin D, however, represents a more complex situation, and here, phosphaturia may occur secondary to changes in the filtered load of phosphorus, in the body distribution of phosphorus, or in intracellular phosphorus activity.

Growth Hormone. An increase in serum phosphorus and a rise in renal phosphorus transport are characteristics of growth hormone excess during the period of rapid growth in the child, during acromegaly, or during exogenous growth hormone administration to experimental animals.

Hammerman et al. reexamined this phenomenon in the brush-border membrane vesicle preparation in the dog (46) and demonstrated that growth hormone treatment resulted in an increased sodium-dependent phosphorus transport. These data reassert the importance of brush-border membrane phosphorus uptake in regulating overall renal phosphorus reabsorptive capacity. The actin of growth hormone is likely mediated by insulin-like growth factor-1 (70).

Alterations in Dietary Phosphorus Intake. The mechanism by which the kidney conserves phosphorus when dietary phosphorus is reduced or increased continues to be intriguing. Earlier micropuncture studies suggested that the most striking adaptive increase in phosphorus transport occurs in the proximal tubule. Later studies (38) suggested that the entire nephron participates in the reduction of phosphorus excretion during dietary phosphorus deprivation. It has been shown that isolated perfused tubules obtained from rabbits that were fed a normal or low-phosphorus diet differ in their capacity to reabsorb phosphate. In normal animals, the proximal convoluted tubule (PCT) is capable of reabsorbing 7.2 ± 0.8 pmol/mL per minute, whereas tubules obtained from phosphorus-deprived animals reabsorb 11.1 ± 1.3 pmol/mL per minute. Conversely, animals that are fed a high-phosphorus diet show reduced phosphorus reabsorption when the proximal tubules are perfused *in vitro* (2.7 ± 2.6 pmol/mL per minute).

Based on renal brush-border membrane preparations, it has been suggested that the effect of reduced dietary phosphorus to stimulate renal phosphorus transport is intrinsic to the renal tubular epithelium and occurs specifically at the brush-border membrane Na^+-phosphate cotransporter. Considerable evidence has accrued from studies performed in cell lines isolated from mammalian kidneys, indicating that the adaptation to phosphate supply by the sodium–phosphate cotransporter is biphasic (71–73). These studies demonstrated that incubation of cells in a low-phosphate medium results in a twofold increase in Na^+-independent phosphate cotransport. The first phase of adaptation is observed rapidly (within 10 minutes) and is characterized by an increase in the V_{max} of the transporter. This initial phase is independent of new protein synthesis. A slower phase resulting in a doubling of the phosphate transport rate, again through an increase in V_{max}, occurs over several hours (maximum of about 15 hours) and is inhibited by blocking new protein synthesis. These studies have been interpreted to indicate that the immediate response to reduced phosphate availability is the insertion of new transport units into the brush-border membrane from an intracellular store. Secondly, through gene transcription and increased NaPi protein synthesis, additional units are produced and inserted into the brush border.

The cloning of the NPT2 NaPi cotransport proteins has enabled further confirmation of results of the above-mentioned P_i transport studies. As discussed already, chronic feeding of low-P_i diet increases steady-state mRNA levels of NPT6 in rabbits and NPT2 in rats (27,74). Acute P_i deprivation does not affect NPT2 family mRNA levels, compatible with a protein synthesis–independent action related to insertion of new transport proteins from subapical vesicles into the brush-border membrane (28,75).

Stanniocalcin. Stanniocalcin is a new calcium-regulating hormone recently found in serum and the kidney (76). Its name derives from its synthesis by the corpuscles of Stannius, which are endocrine glands found in the kidneys of bony fish. In mammals, stanniocalcin lowers calcium transport and increases phosphate reabsorption. Bony fish use this action to increase phosphate deposition into bone and scales. The role of stanniocalcin in human physiology requires elucidation, as does the regulation of its secretion.

Diuretics. Acetazolamide inhibits phosphate reabsorption by its effects on proximal tubule decreases in Na^+-dependent bicarbonate transport, essential for the maintenance of the Na^+ gradient. Furosemide inhibits carbonic anhydrase activity and thus decreases phosphate transport. Similar effects have been demonstrated with the administration of large doses of thiazide diuretics (77).

Hypophosphatemia

Hypophosphatemia refers to serum phosphorus concentrations of less than 2.5 mg/dL. Hypophosphatemia usually results from one or a combination of the following factors (78,79): (a) increased excretion of phosphorus in the urine; (b) decreased gastrointestinal absorption of phosphorus; or (c) translocation of phosphorus from the extracellular to the intracellular space. The major causes of hypophosphatemia are listed in Table 88-1.

TABLE 88-1. *Causes of hypophosphatemia*

I. Increased excretion of phosphorus in the urine
  A. Primary hyperparathyroidism
  B. Secondary hyperparathyroidism
  C. Renal tubular defects
  D. Diuretic phase of acute tubular necrosis
  E. Postobstructive diuresis
  F. After renal transplantation
  G. Extracellular fluid volume expansion
  H. Familial
    1. X-linked hypophosphatemia
    2. McCune-Albright syndrome

II. Decrease in gastrointestinal absorption of phosphorus
  A. Malabsorption
  B. Malnutrition-starvation
  C. Administration of phosphate binders
  D. Abnormalities of Vitamin D metabolism
    1. Vitamin D deficiency—rickets
    2. Familial
      a. Vitamin D–dependent rickets
      b. X-linked hypophosphatemia

III. Miscellaneous causes/translocation of phosphorus
  A. Diabetes mellitus: during treatment for ketoacidosis
  B. Severe respiratory alkalosis
  C. Recovery phase of malnutrition
  D. Alcohol withdrawal
  E. Toxic shock syndrome
  F. Leukemia, lymphoma
  G. Severe burns

Increased Excretion of Phosphorus in the Urine

Several pathophysiologic conditions may increase excretion of phosphorus in the urine. Some of these conditions are characterized by elevated levels of circulating PTH. Because PTH decreases phosphorus reabsorption by the kidney, modest to marked elevations of this hormone may increase urinary excretion of this anion. Decreased tubular reabsorption of phosphorus may also occur without increased levels of PTH and may be due to changes in the reabsorption of salt and water or to renal tubular defects specific for the reabsorption of certain solutes or phosphorus. Hypophosphatemia may also occur in the diuretic phase of acute tubular necrosis or in postobstructive diuresis, presumably due to a combination of high levels of PTH and decreased tubular reabsorption of salt and water.

Primary Hyperparathyroidism

Primary hyperparathyroidism is a common entity in clinical medicine (80). PTH is secreted in excess of the physiologic needs for mineral homeostasis due to either adenomas or hyperplasia of the parathyroid glands (81). This results in decreased phosphorus reabsorption by the kidney. The losses of phosphorus in the urine result in hypophosphatemia. The degree of hypophosphatemia may vary considerably among patients because mobilization of phosphorus from bone will in part mitigate the hypophosphatemia. Moreover, if the patient ingests large amounts of dietary phosphorus, the degree of hypophosphatemia observed may be mild. Because these patients also have elevated levels of serum calcium, the diagnosis is made relatively easy in most cases by the finding of elevated levels of immunoreactive PTH.

Secondary Hyperparathyroidism

Although secondary hyperparathyroidism is present in most patients with chronic renal disease, hyperphosphatemia rather than hypophosphatemia occurs in such patients because of decreased phosphorus excretion in the urine resulting from the fall in GFR. However, certain conditions characterized by malabsorption of calcium from the gastrointestinal tract may produce hypocalcemia, leading to development of secondary hyperparathyroidism (82). The elevated levels of PTH will decrease phosphorus reabsorption by the kidney, resulting in hypophosphatemia. Thus, patients with gastrointestinal tract abnormalities resulting in calcium malabsorption and secondary hyperparathyroidism will have low levels of serum calcium and phosphorus. In these patients, the hypocalcemia is responsible for the increased release of PTH. In addition, decreased intestinal absorption of phosphorus as a result of the primary gastrointestinal tract disease may also contribute to the decrement in the levels of serum phosphorus. In general, these patients have urinary losses of phosphorus that are out of proportion to the hypophosphatemia in contrast to patients with predominant phosphorus malabsorption and no secondary hyperparathyroidism in whom urinary excretion of phosphorus is low.

Renal Tubular Defects

Several conditions characterized by single or multiple tubular defects have been described in which phosphorus reabsorption is decreased (83). In the Fanconi syndrome (83), patients excrete not only increased amounts of phosphorus in the urine but also increased quantities of amino acids, uric acid, and glucose, resulting in hypouricemia and hypophosphatemia. Rare familial forms of hypercalciuria are often associated with one or more of the components of the Fanconi syndrome including hypophosphatemia or hyperphosphaturia (84–86). Interestingly, these familial syndromes, Dent's disease, and its variants have been found to be caused by a mutation in the CLCN5 chloride channel (84,87), which is an intracellular vesicular channel, perhaps related to the vesicles that harbor the NaPi cotransport proteins (88,89). There are other conditions in which an isolated defect in the renal tubular transport of phosphorus has been found—for example, fructose intolerance, which is an autosomal-recessive disorder (90). After renal transplantation, an acquired renal tubular defect may be responsible for the persistence of hypophosphatemia in some patients (91), although current evidence suggests that an abnormality in PHEX (gene encoding for neutral endopeptidase activity; see later discussion) activity or increased production of phosphatonin is the likely cause of persistent posttransplantation hypophosphatemia, rather than an intrinsic renal tubular transport defect.

Diuretic Phase of Acute Tubular Necrosis

Most patients with acute renal failure develop secondary hyperparathyroidism and hyperphosphatemia during the oliguric phase. During the recovery phase of acute renal failure, the combined occurrence of a profound diuresis, secondary hyperparathyroidism, and continued use of phosphate binders may lead to severe hypophosphatemia. This hypophosphatemia is usually short lived, and serum phosphorus levels return to within the normal range as the diuretic phase of acute tubular necrosis subsides.

Postobstructive Diuresis

A marked phosphaturia may develop in some patients after relief of urinary tract obstruction. This phosphaturia may be severe enough in a few patients to lead to hypophosphatemia (92).

Postrenal Transplantation

Hypophosphatemia, sometimes severe, is common in patients after renal transplantation (91,93). Patients undergoing renal transplantation usually have severe secondary hyperparathyroidism (91,93). Because the GFR is restored after placement of the graft, the high levels of PTH acting on the transplanted kidney markedly increase phosphorus excretion in the urine. However, in some patients after renal transplantation, a persistent phosphaturia that is out of proportion to the levels of serum phosphorus has been observed, even after the levels of PTH have returned to within the normal range. In these patients, it appears that either a defect in PHEX activity or an excessive level of phosphatonin is present. Thus, hypophosphatemia in the first few days after renal transplantation may result from a combination of factors: (a) ingestion of phosphate binders that has continued even after the transplant has adequate function; (b) secondary hyperparathyroidism in the presence of near-normal GFR; and (c) an abnormality in PHEX activity or phosphatonin production. When phosphate binders are decreased or discontinued and hyperparathyroidism subsides, phosphorus levels usually return to within the normal range in most patients with a renal graft. When this fails to occur, either PHEX or phosphatonin appears to be implicated (91). Prolonged periods of severe hypophosphatemia may cause bone disease characterized by severe osteomalacia in some of these patients.

Extracellular Fluid Volume Expansion

Expansion of the ECF volume by the administration of solutions containing sodium increases the urinary excretion of phosphorus. An important mechanism by which ECF volume expansion produces phosphaturia consists of a fall in ionized calcium and subsequent release of PTH (94). This condition is probably of minor importance in clinical medicine, and restoration of the ECF volume to within the normal range results in the return of phosphorus reabsorption to physiologic levels.

X-Linked Hypophosphatemic Rickets

This X-linked dominant disorder is characterized by hypophosphatemia, decreased reabsorption of phosphorus by the renal tubule, decreased absorption of calcium and phosphorus from the gastrointestinal tract, and varying degrees of rickets or osteomalacia. Patients with this disorder exhibit normal levels of 1,25-dihydroxycholecalciferol and reduced Na-phosphate transport in the proximal tubule in the face of severe hypophosphatemia. The gene for X-linked hypophosphatemia is not the P_i transport protein itself, which maps to chromosome 5 (95) in humans, and which exhibits normal function in isolated brush-border membrane preparations from animal models of X-linked hypophosphatemic rickets. The genetic defect for this disorder is in a gene termed *PHEX*, which encodes for a neutral endopeptidase presumed to be responsible for the degradation of an unidentified systemic phosphaturic hormone, "phosphatonin" (96). The defective *PHEX* gene product in X-linked hypophosphatemic rickets permits "phosphatonin" to inhibit renal phosphate absorption, despite persistent hypophosphatemia. Phosphatonin remains to be discovered, but candidate proteins have been suggested (97).

The roles of alterations in Vitamin D sensitivity or synthesis in the defective transport of phosphorus observed in both the gut and the kidney have been investigated in the murine homolog of X-linked hypophosphatemia (Hyp) (98). Tenenhouse and Scriver found that administration of small doses of 1,25-dihydroxycholecalciferol to healthy animals significantly increased plasma calcium, plasma phosphorus, and fractional calcium excretion without a change in fractional phosphorus excretion or phosphorus transport as measured in proximal tubular brush-border membrane vesicles (99). However, there was no response to this dose of 1,25-dihydroxycholecalciferol in the Hyp mice. At a fivefold higher dose of Vitamin D, the familial hypophosphatemic mice did show increased plasma calcium and fractional calcium excretion, as well as increased plasma phosphorus levels, but again there was no change in fractional phosphorus excretion or in sodium-dependent phosphorus transport in brush-border membrane vesicles. Although 1,25-dihydroxycholecalciferol increased phosphorus transport in the intestine, there was no defect of phosphorus transport in the intestine of untreated hypophosphatemic mice. The conclusion from these studies is that Vitamin D influences phosphorus homeostasis in Hyp mice by stimulation of phosphorus absorption from the gastrointestinal tract. The defect in renal phosphorus reabsorption was unchanged despite high levels of Vitamin D. These observations are consistent with those of studies performed in humans with familial hypophosphatemia, in whom the renal reabsorptive defect persists despite correction of growth by administration of Vitamin D and oral phosphate supplements (100,101). There is, however, evidence of defective or altered metabolism of Vitamin D_3 in Hyp mice. Meyer et al. found that on a normal diet, plasma 1,25-dihydroxycholecalciferol levels were the same in Hyp and healthy mice (95), although 25-hydroxycholecalciferol levels were reduced in Hyp mice. Because hypophosphatemia increases plasma 1,25-dihydroxycholecalciferol levels, the hypophosphatemic mice were resistant to the stimulatory effect of hypophosphatemia. To test this possibility, these authors fed the animals a low-phosphorus diet and found a paradoxical reduction in 1,25-dihydroxycholecalciferol levels in hypophosphatemic mice. They concluded that Hyp mice have a defective control system for plasma 1,25-dihydroxycholecalciferol that is unresponsive to a low-phosphate diet stimulus. The issue is further complicated by studies by Beamer et al. (102), who studied the effect of various preparations of Vitamin D_3 on intestinal transport of phosphorus. The Hyp mice responded to 1α-hydroxycholecalciferol but not to 1,25-dihydroxycholecalciferol, suggesting that intestinal phosphorus transport responsiveness is not genetically absent in this model but does not respond to normal endogenous levels of 1,25-dihydroxycholecalciferol. Thus, mice with familial hypophosphatemia appear to have impaired metabolism of Vitamin D, but this impairment does not cause the renal phosphate transport defect. There is also evidence suggesting that the decreased tubular reabsorption of phosphorus is not due to increased PTH levels (102). The component of renal phosphorus transport, which is PTH-independent, is abnormal and responsible for the increased phosphaturia.

Tenenhouse et al. (103) have shown that tissue phosphate levels were normal in Hyp mice, whereas these levels tended to be low in animals that have hypophosphatemia secondary to reduction in dietary phosphorus. It would seem, therefore, that X-linked hypophosphatemia is a selective disorder of the transepithelial transport of phosphate. However, there is no correlation between the degree of hypophosphatemia and the severity of bone disease. Moreover, alterations in Vitamin D metabolism cannot be explained solely by the presence of hypophosphatemia. Therefore, an undefined pathologic mechanism related to PHEX function involves both abnormal phosphate transport and renal 1-hydroxylase function.

Tenenhouse et al. (104) have extended their studies in Hyp mice to demonstrate that the message levels for the NPT2 cotransport protein are reduced by 50% in the renal cortex, similar to the reduction in apical membrane vesicle NPT2 protein levels. However, the mapping of NPT2 and NPT1 to chromosomes 5 and 6, respectfully (95,105), indicated that these genes were not candidates for the genetic defects leading to X-linked hypophosphatemia or Hyp. X-linked hypophosphatemia and Hyp are due to abnormal levels of a circulating hormonal factor. Results of the cross-perfusion studies of Meyer et al. (106) and the cross-transplantation studies of Nesbitt et al. (107) were interpreted to indicate the presence of a circulating factor. Furthermore, Nesbitt et al. (107) were unable to demonstrate transmission of the Hyp renal defect by transplanting a Hyp kidney into a healthy recipient. Likewise, transplantation of a normal kidney into a Hyp recipient failed to correct the Hyp phenotypic abnormalities. These studies, in addition to studies in oncogenic osteomalacia, suggest that the presence of a circulating humoral factor could be capable of producing the Hyp and X-linked hypophosphatemia phenotype. The substance has been named phosphatonin before its discovery (108).

The circulating humoral factor hypothesis for the etiology of X-linked hypophosphatemia was supported by the discovery of the defective gene, *PHEX*, through positional cloning (96). The PHEX gene product encodes a neutral endopeptidase of the same family as endothelin-converting enzyme, and it is characterized by zinc regulation and a single transmembrane spanning domain. The model proposed by this result suggests that a circulating phosphaturic factor is normally catabolized by the PHEX gene product. When *PHEX* is mutated, the phosphaturic factor levels are increased and hypophosphatemia results.

An interesting aspect of the Hyp phenotype is the presence of a normal Na-dependent phosphate cotransport in osteoblasts (109). However, the osteoblasts of Hyp have been shown to be defective in models of endochondral bone formation (110,111). Defective mineralization is an important aspect of osteomalacia, and mineralization is controlled by calcium, phosphate, and bone matrix proteins. We recently demonstrated defective phosphorylation of a key bone matrix protein, osteopontin, in Hyp mice and abnormal low activity of a protein kinase (casein kinase II–like activity) responsible for osteopontin phosphorylation (112,113). Thus, multiple proteins appear to be defective in the Hyp phenotype. This is compatible with multiple targets of the *PHEX* gene such as phosphatonin and an inhibitor of casein kinase II, which achieve greater activity when *PHEX* is defective (106,107,112,114).

From a therapeutic point of view, the combination of neutral phosphate and 1,25-dihydroxycholecalciferol has lead to an improvement in the bone disease of some patients with X-linked hypophosphatemia and in the Hyp mice (115,116). The administration of phosphorus in X-linked hypophosphatemia is usually divided into four doses, with the total amount ranging between 1 to 4 g per day. Pharmacologic doses of 1,25-dihydroxycholecalciferol on the order of 1 to 3 μg per day may be necessary to correct the skeletal alterations. 1,25-Dihydroxycholecalciferol does not correct the increased fractional excretion of phosphate. The enthusiasm for this regimen is tempered by a high incidence of nephrocalcinosis and occasional renal failure (115–117).

Autosomal-Dominant Hypophosphatemic Rickets

This is a rare condition that clinically resembles X-linked hypophosphatemia except in its inheritance. It has recently become critically important because of the positional cloning of the gene responsible for the disorder, fibroblast growth factor 23 (FGF23) (97) on chromosome 12p13. FGF23 is not known to regulate phosphate transport, but it is an attractive candidate for being the PHEX substrate, phosphatonin, which is normally inactivated. The possibility is that because of mutations, FGF23 is resistant to the PHEX endopeptidase and circulates in an active form. This is totally speculative, and the discovery of the gene now provides the opportunity to investigate how this new factor regulates P_i transport.

McCune-Albright's Syndrome

McCune-Albright's syndrome is characterized by the clinical triad of polyostotic fibrous dysplasia, café au lait skin pigmentation, and endocrine/metabolic disorders. The endocrine disorders include autonomous secretion of various hormones such as growth hormone, thyroid hormone, cortisol, estradiol, and testosterone. Rickets and osteomalacia due to hyperphosphaturic hypophosphatemia are prominent components of the syndrome. The disorders of the syndrome share in common excessive function of cells whose actions are normally regulated by hormones that induce cAMP generation. The molecular basis for the phenotype is an activating mutation of the $G_{S\alpha}$ protein (the α component of the stimulatory heterotrimeric guanosine triphosphate binding protein) in cells from affected tissues from patients with the syndrome (118). Kidney tissue, presumably proximal tubule, from patients has been reported to contain cells with the mutation (118).

Abnormalities of Vitamin D Metabolism

Vitamin D and its metabolites play an important role in phosphorus homeostasis (119). Vitamin D promotes the intestinal absorption of calcium and phosphorus and is necessary to maintain the normal mineralization of bone. Dietary deficiencies of Vitamin D increase the amount of osteoid tissue in the skeleton and decrease normal mineralization. Bone mineralization is a complex process that is not completely understood. Normally, the osteoblast is responsible for laying down normal collagen that is well organized and distributed in a lamellar fashion. Between the recently deposited collagen and the old bone, there is an area called the mineralization front. Initially, amorphous calcium phosphate is deposited in the mineralization front and eventually matures into hydroxyapatite $[Ca_{10}(PO_4)_6(OH)_2]$. Thus, the osteoid tissue changes into bone. Optimal mineralization requires the following: (a) normal bone cell activity; (b) normal supply of minerals; (c) the appropriate pH level (7.4 to 7.6); (d) normal synthesis and composition of the matrix; and (e) control of inhibitors of calcification.

The appositional growth rate in normal bone is about 1 μm per day and complete mineralization of the osteoid requires 13 to 21 days. Thus, the thickness of the osteoid usually does not exceed 20 μm. Less than 20% of the surface of the bone is normally covered by osteoid. When a biopsy is performed in a healthy subject who has previously ingested two doses of tetracycline separately and 3 weeks apart, one usually detects two fluorescent rings or bands, indicating the locations of the mineralization front. In a patient with osteomalacia, usually a single band, no band, or an irregular and spotty uptake of tetracycline is seen. In rickets or osteomalacia, there is a quantitative and qualitative defect in bone mineralization.

Vitamin D–Deficient Rickets

Diets deficient in Vitamin D lead to the metabolic disorder known as rickets when it occurs in children or osteomalacia when it appears in adults (120). Vitamin D deficiency in childhood results in severe deformities of bone because of rapid growth. These deformities are characterized by soft loose areas in the skull known as *craniotabes* and costochondral swelling or bending (known as *rachitic rosary*). The chest usually becomes flattened, and the sternum may be pushed forward to form the so-called *pigeon chest.* Thoracic expansion may be greatly reduced with impairment of respiratory function. Kyphosis is a common finding. There is remarkable swelling of the joints, particularly the wrists and ankles, with characteristic anterior bowing of the legs, and fractures of the "greenstick" variety may also be seen. In adults, the symptoms are not as striking and are usually characterized by bone pain, weakness, radiolucent areas, and pseudofractures. Pseudofractures represent stretch fractures in which the normal process of healing is impaired because of a mineralization defect. Mild hypocalcemia may be present; however, hypophosphatemia is the most frequent biochemical alteration. This metabolic abnormality responds well to administration of small amounts of Vitamin D.

Vitamin D–Dependent Rickets

These are recessively inherited forms of Vitamin D–refractory rickets. The conditions are characterized by hypophosphatemia, hypocalcemia, elevated levels of serum alkaline phosphatase, and sometimes, generalized aminoaciduria and severe bone lesions. Currently, two main forms of Vitamin D–dependent rickets have been characterized. The serum concentrations of 1,25-dihydroxycholecalciferol serve to differentiate the two types of Vitamin D–dependent rickets. Type I is caused by a mutation in the gene converting 25(OH)D to 1,25-dihydroxycholecalciferol, the renal 1α-hydroxylase enzyme (121,122). This condition responds to very large doses of Vitamin D_2 and D_3 (100 to 300 times the normal requirement of physiologic doses), however, 0.5 to 1.0 μg per day of 1,25-dihydroxycholecalciferol. Type II is characterized by an end-organ resistance to 1,25-dihydroxycholecalciferol. Plasma levels of 1,25-dihydroxycholecalciferol are elevated. This finding, in association with radiographic and biochemical signs of rickets, implies resistance to the target tissue to 1,25-dihydroxycholecalciferol. Cellular defects found in patients with Vitamin D–resistant rickets type II are heterogeneous, providing in part an explanation for the different clinical manifestations of this disorder. Among the cellular defects are (a) decreased number of cytosolic receptors, (b) deficient maximal hormonal binding, (c) deficient hormone binding affinity, (d) normal hormonal binding but undetectable nuclear localization, and (e) abnormal DNA binding domain for the 1,25-dihydroxycholecalciferol receptor (123).

Numerous studies (124–131) have demonstrated that hereditary type II Vitamin D–resistant rickets is a genetic disease affecting the Vitamin D receptor (VDR). Defects in the hormone binding domain (124,125) and the DNA binding domain (126,127) have been defined. In addition, several cases of human Vitamin D–resistant rickets have been studied and no abnormality in the coding region of the VDR has been found (128), suggesting a defect elsewhere in the hormone action pathway. An unexplained feature of this disease in adolescents is the tendency for calcium levels to normalize and for the radiographic abnormalities of rickets to improve, thus giving the appearance that they outgrow the disease. Human Vitamin D–resistant rickets as a genetic defect in the VDR varies significantly from other genetic diseases of steroid hormone receptors caused by resistance to thyroid hormone, androgens, and estrogens (129–131). For instance, individuals heterozygous for VDR mutations are apparently completely healthy. Secondly, no dominant negative mutations, which are prominent in thyroid hormone resistance, have been identified as a cause of human Vitamin D–resistant rickets. Thus, much remains to be learned from the genetic analysis of this disease. The treatment of this condition requires large pharmacologic doses of calcium, which overcome the receptor defects and maintain bone remodeling (127). Studies in mice with targeted disruption of the *VDR* gene, an animal model of Vitamin D–dependent rickets type II, confirm that many aspects of the clinical phenotype are due to decreased intestinal ion transport and can be overcome by adjustments of dietary intake (132).

Oncogenic Osteomalacia

Oncogenic osteomalacia is a rare syndrome characterized by hypophosphatemia associated with tumors. It was described initially in association with benign mesenchymal tumors; however, recent reports emphasized the association of this syndrome with malignant tumors (133–135). The other characteristics of this syndrome are increased phosphate excretion, low plasma 1,25-dihydroxycholecalciferol concentrations, and osteomalacia. All of the biochemical and pathologic abnormalities disappear when the tumor is resected. The tumors associated with this syndrome are thought to secrete a substance that inhibits the renal tubular reabsorption of phosphate and suppresses 25-hydroxycholecalciferol 1α-hydroxylase activity. Whether this factor interacts directly with renal tubular cells is unknown. Studies by Cai et al. (114) have investigated the ability of media in which sclerosing hemangioma cells from a patient with osteogenic osteomalacia were cultured to affect Na-dependent phosphate transport. They found that the medium inhibited sodium-dependent phosphate transport, without increasing cellular concentrations of cAMP. The medium had PTH-like immunoreactivity but no PTH-related protein immunoreactivity. And the action of the tumor medium was not blocked by a PTH antagonist. The plasma 1,25-dihydroxycholecalciferol concentrations are low in patients with oncogenic osteomalacia despite the presence of hypophosphatemia (136–138), which usually increases plasma 1,25-dihydroxycholecalciferol concentrations by stimulating the renal 25-hydroxycholecalciferol 1α-hydroxylase in a PTH-independent manner (139). Besides the hypophosphatemia, deficient production of 1,25-dihydroxycholecalciferol is a factor contributing to the pathogenesis of the osteomalacia in these patients. Miyauchi et al. (140) have reported that 25-hydroxycholecalciferol 1α-hydroxylase activity of cultured renal tubular cells was decreased by incubating the cells with tumor extracts. This supports the concept that the tumor extracts contain a substance that inhibits the formation of 1,25-dihydroxycholecalciferol in the proximal tubule.

Various studies of oncogenic osteomalacia and some studies associated with X-linked hypophosphatemic rickets support the possibility that a hormone primarily responsible for the regulation of renal phosphate reabsorption is abnormally produced in these conditions. Econs and Drezner (108) have termed the substance *phosphatonin*. The similarity between oncogenic osteomalacia and X-linked hypophosphatemia raises the possibility that phosphatonin is the factor normally degraded by the PHEX gene product that causes abnormal phosphate transport in X-linked hypophosphatemia and in the Hyp mouse.

Malabsorption

Because most of the absorption of phosphorus from the gastrointestinal tract occurs in the duodenum and jejunum, gastrointestinal tract disorders such as celiac disease, tropical and nontropical sprue, and regional enteritis may decrease the absorption of phosphorus (82). Phosphorus malabsorption has also been described in patients who have undergone surgical bypass procedures for morbid obesity. The degree of hypophosphatemia varies among patients with intestinal malabsorption, being extremely mild in some and severe in others.

Malnutrition

Most of the phosphorus ingested in the diet is present in protein, particularly meat, cheese, milk, and eggs. In many parts of the world where protein consumption is extremely low, hypophosphatemia occurs predominantly in children. Overall growth is retarded and a series of metabolic abnormalities are present (141).

Administration of Phosphate Binders

Certain compounds, mainly aluminum salts (aluminum hydroxide, aluminum carbonate gel) and calcium carbonate, are used in the treatment of hyperphosphatemia (142). However, when these compounds are given in excess, they may produce profound hypophosphatemia. These gels trap phosphorus in the small intestine and increase the amount of phosphorus in the stool. Patients ingesting large amounts of phosphate binders and not followed closely may develop phosphate depletion. With time, such individuals may develop severe weakness, bone pain, and osteomalacia.

Other Causes of Hypophosphatemia

Recent reviews of the causes of hypophosphatemia in hospitalized patients (143,144) attributed most instances to *intravenous administration of carbohydrate*. However, many other causes were found, including *diuretic usage, hyperalimentation, alcoholism, respiratory alkalosis, and use of phosphate binders* (145). A 31% incidence of hypophosphatemia was seen in patients admitted to a general medical ward, and a further fall in serum concentrations occurred in all patients with *acute alcoholism* between the second and fifth day after admission to a medical ward (146). Hypophosphatemia is also seen frequently during treatment of *diabetic ketoacidosis* (147). When diabetic patients develop ketoacidosis, they usually have an increase in phosphate excretion in the urine; however, the serum phosphate level may be slightly elevated due to acidosis. During the administration of insulin, there

is a rapid decrease in the level of glucose with translocation of phosphate from the extracellular to the intracellular space, resulting in hypophosphatemia.

Acute respiratory alkalosis decreases urinary phosphate excretion but produces marked hypophosphatemia (148). In contrast, patients who receive sodium bicarbonate excrete large amounts of phosphate in the urine; however, the hypophosphatemia that may develop is only moderate in nature. It has been postulated that in respiratory alkalosis, there is an increase in the intracellular pH level with activation of glycolysis and increased formation of phosphate-containing sugars, leading to a precipitous fall in the concentration of serum phosphorus. The mild hypophosphatemia that may be seen during administration of sodium bicarbonate is probably secondary to increased renal phosphate excretion due to a decrease in ionized calcium and release of PTH, as well as to the consequences of ECF volume expansion (54).

In addition, new clinical disorders have been identified in which hypophosphatemia is an important aspect of the pathologic condition. Marked hypophosphatemia has been associated with acute leukemia or with *lymphomas in the leukemic phase* (149–151). These individuals typically present with hypophosphatemia, normocalcemia, and no evidence of excess PTH activity. Urinary phosphate concentration is typically extremely low. Although kinetic studies have not been performed in this setting, the facts that serum phosphate concentration correlates with a growth phase of the tumors and that hyperphosphatemia is seen when cells are destroyed by chemotherapy or radiotherapy strongly suggest that serum phosphorus was initially used in the rapid growth of new cells. Because these patients are often severely ill and under treatment with glucose infusions, as well as antacids and other drugs known to induce hypophosphatemia, they may be at great risk of developing severe acute phosphorus depletion.

Another clinical condition in which hypophosphatemia has been a prominent feature is the *toxic shock syndrome*. Chesney et al. (152) described 22 women with this disorder who showed hypocalcemia and hypophosphatemia as prominent manifestations. Whether respiratory alkalosis or staphylococcal sepsis induced release of substances that were responsible for acute phosphorus shifts into cells is unknown. Lindquist et al. (153) studied in a prospective fashion the importance of hypophosphatemia in patients with *severe burns*. In 33 patients studied for 2 weeks after injury, transient hypophosphatemia was seen in the second to tenth day in all these individuals. Five of seven patients who died from complications of the terminal injury had severe hypophosphatemia. Because urinary phosphorus excretion was not increased, tissue uptake seems to be the predominant mechanism responsible for the hypophosphatemia. Levy (154) reported the occurrence of severe hypophosphatemia during the *rewarming phase in a profoundly hypothermic patient*. In this individual, urinary excretion of phosphorus was minimal, suggesting that a shift of phosphate into the cells occurred as a result of rewarming. Finally, the development of hypophosphatemia resulting from refeeding clinically starved patients has been emphasized. Silvis et al. (155) showed that the classic phosphorus-depletion syndrome, consisting of paresthesias, weakness, seizures, and hypophosphatemia, can occur in individuals who receive oral caloric supplements after a prolonged period of starvation. To further evaluate this issue, they performed studies in normal dogs who had been starved or had received normal diets and found that the infusion of calories through an intragastric catheter to previously starved animals resulted in a fall in serum phosphorus concentration from an average of 4.8 mg/dL to 1.6 mg/dL. Nearly 50% of starved animals developed clinical signs of phosphate depletion after oral refeeding. Weinsier and Krumdiek (156) reported two patients who developed the phosphorus-depletion syndrome in association with cardiopulmonary decompensation following overzealous hyperalimentation after prolonged caloric deprivation (156).

Clinical and Biochemical Manifestations of Hypophosphatemia

The manifestations of hypophosphatemia are presented in Table 88-2. It has been suggested that the clinical manifestations of hypophosphatemia and severe phosphorus depletion are related to disturbances in cellular energy and metabolism. Studies have examined the effects of phosphate depletion on cellular energetics and other components of cell function. A study of glycolytic intermediates and adenine nucleotides during insulin treatment of patients with diabetic ketoacidosis emphasized the important effects of insulin-induced cellular phosphate depletion on cell metabolism (157). These results demonstrated that the reduced level of 2,3-diphosphoglycerate (2,3-DPG) seen during insulin treatment of diabetes is due to intracellular phosphorus depletion, producing a decrease in glyceraldehyde 3-phosphate dehydrogenase activity rather than inhibition of the phosphofructokinase enzyme system. Ditzel (158) has suggested that repeated transient decreases in red cell oxygen delivery due to reduced 2,3-DPG with insulin-induced hypophosphatemia could contribute over many years to the microvascular disease seen in diabetic patients. Patients with mild degrees of hypophosphatemia are usually asymptomatic. However, if hypophosphatemia is severe—that is, if serum phosphorus levels are less than 1.5 mg/dL—a series of hematologic, neurologic, and metabolic disorders may develop. In general, the patients become anorectic and weak, and mild bone pain may be present if the hypophosphatemia persists for several months (Table 88-2).

Cardiovascular and Skeletal Muscle Manifestations. Severe cardiomyopathy with decreased cardiac output has been described in patients and animals with severe hypophosphatemia (159,160). Studies revealed that the resting muscle membrane potential fell, sodium chloride and water content of the tissue increased, and potassium content decreased in severe hypophosphatemia (161). These values returned

TABLE 88-2. *Clinical and biochemical manifestations of marked hypophosphatemia*

I. Cardiovascular and skeletal muscle
   A. Decreased cardiac output
   B. Muscle weakness
   C. Decreased transmembrane resting potential
   D. Rhabdomyolysis
II. Carbohydrate metabolism
   A. Hyperinsulinemia
   B. Decreased glucose metabolism
III. Hematologic alterations
   A. Red blood cells
      1. Decreased adenosine triphosphate (ATP) content
      2. Decreased 2,3-DPG
      3. Decreased P_{50}
      4. Increased oxygen affinity
      5. Decreased lifespan
      6. Hemolysis
      7. Spherocytosis
   B. Leukocytes
      1. Decreased phagocytosis
      2. Decreased chemotaxis
      3. Decreased bactericidal activity
   C. Platelets
      1. Impaired clot retraction
      2. Thrombocytopenia
      3. Decreased ATP content
      4. Megakaryocytosis
      5. Decreased lifespan
IV. Neurologic manifestations
   A. Anorexia
   B. Irritability
   C. Confusion
   D. Paresthesias
   E. Dysarthria
   F. Ataxia
   G. Seizures
   H. Coma
V. Skeletal abnormalities
   A. Bone pain
   B. Radiolucent areas (x-ray)
   C. Pseudofractures
   D. Rickets or osteomalacia
VI. Biochemical and renal manifestations
   A. Low parathyroid hormone levels
   B. Increased $1,25(OH)_2D_3$
   C. Hypercalciuria
   D. Hypomagnesemia
   E. Hypermagnesuria
   F. Hypophosphaturia
   G. Decreased glomerular filtration rate
   H. Decreased T_m for bicarbonate
   I. Decreased renal gluconeogenesis
   J. Decreased titratable acid excretion
   K. Increased creatinine phosphokinase
   L. Increased aldolase

Source: From Slatopolsky E. Pathophysiology of calcium, magnesium, and phosphorus. In: Klahr S, ed. *The kidney and body fluids in health and disease.* New York: Plenum Press, 1983:269, with permission.

to within the normal range after phosphate was administered. Skeletal muscle weakness and electromyographic abnormalities are associated with chronic hypophosphatemia and phosphate depletion. Dogs that were fed low-phosphate diets for several months developed changes in muscle, rhabdomyolysis, and characteristic increases in their levels of creatinine kinase and aldolase in blood (162). Rhabdomyolysis has been observed in alcoholic patients with hypophosphatemia (163). Knochel et al. (162) showed that myopathy associated with phosphate depletion in dogs did lead to changes in cell water content, sodium concentration, and transmembrane potential difference. Kretz et al. (164) examined the possibility that changes in calcium transport in the sarcoplasmic reticulum of muscle were responsible for the clinical myopathy seen in acute phosphate depletion. Despite significant hypophosphatemia and a reduction in muscle phosphorus concentration, they found no significant changes in the rate of calcium uptake of calcium-concentrating ability in vesicles prepared from muscle sarcoplasmic reticulum of phosphate-depleted rats. Thus, the role of altered transcellular calcium movements in phosphate-depleted tissues is yet to be completely resolved.

Effects on Carbohydrate Metabolism. Hyperinsulinemia and abnormal glucose metabolism suggesting insulin resistance have been described in phosphate depletion. DeFronzo and Lange (165) have used the glucose and insulin clamp technique to study the kinetics of glucose metabolism in patients with various chronic hypophosphatemic conditions including Vitamin D–resistant rickets. When glucose was infused to maintain constant glycemia at 125 mg/dL, hypophosphatemic individuals required 36% less glucose to maintain these glycemic levels than controls. Also when euglycemic was achieved by combined insulin and glucose infusion, the hypophosphatemic individuals required 40% less glucose to maintain euglycemia than controls. Insulin catabolism was apparently unaffected in these hypophosphatemic individuals. These data indicate that hypophosphatemia is associated with impaired glucose metabolism in both hyperglycemic and euglycemic patients.

Hematologic Manifestations. Hematologic abnormalities of hypophosphatemia are a major manifestation of this syndrome (166–168). In addition to defects in affinity of oxyhemoglobin leading to generalized tissue hypoxia, there may be increased hemolysis (169,170). Quantitative and functional defects have also been described in platelets and leukocytes (171). These defects lead to diminished platelet aggregation and abnormalities in chemotaxis and phagocytosis of white blood cells. The latter may contribute to the increased risk of Gram-negative sepsis reported in hypophosphatemic patients (172). This is of particular concern in immunosuppressed patients receiving phosphate-poor alimentation through a central venous line.

Neurologic Manifestations. Manifestations at the level of the central nervous system, resulting in generalized anorexia and malaise or more severe disturbances such as ataxia, seizures, and coma, have been described in hypophosphatemia

(173–175). Neuromuscular abnormalities include paresthesias and weakness, the result of both myopathic changes and diminished nerve conduction (176).

Skeletal Abnormalities. The skeletal abnormalities associated with hypophosphatemia, particularly in Vitamin D–resistant rickets, may be quite marked. In addition, bony abnormalities, including osteomalacia and pathologic fractures, have been described in antacid-induced phosphate depletion (177,178), as well as in hypophosphatemic patients undergoing hemodialysis who did not receive phosphate binding gels (179). A rheumatic syndrome resembling ankylosing spondylitis also has been reported in hypophosphatemic patients (180).

Gastrointestinal Disturbances. These manifestations include anorexia, nausea, and vomiting (174). It has been speculated that hypophosphatemia in the alcoholic patient may further impair hepatic function through hypoxic insult.

Renal Manifestations. There is decreased phosphorus excretion and decreased tubular reabsorption of calcium, magnesium, bicarbonate, and glucose (181–186). The renal conservation of phosphorus occurs early in the syndrome and is the result of a primary increase in the tubular reabsorption of the anion and a decrease in the GFR and consequently in the filtered load of phosphorus (186,187). This mechanism results in complete renal conservation of phosphorus, with net losses representing only a small fraction of total body phosphorus stores (174). The increase in phosphorus reabsorption seen with phosphorus depletion is independent of several hormones known to influence phosphorus transport under other circumstances, including PTH, Vitamin D, calcitonin, and thyroxine (188). The possibility that serum phosphorus concentration per se (or intracellular phosphorus) may in some manner regulate its absorption along the nephron seems plausible. Hypercalciuria of enough magnitude to produce a negative calcium balance is seen commonly in hypophosphatemic patients. Several factors contribute to this increase in calcium excretion including increased calcium mobilization from bone, enhanced gastrointestinal tract calcium absorption, and inhibition of renal tubular calcium reabsorption (181,186). These effects appear to be independent of PTH activity and may be the result of a direct effect of phosphate on these transport processes.

Acid–Base Disturbances. Renal bicarbonate wasting, diminished titratable acid excretion, and decreased ammoniagenesis have been reported in hypophosphatemia (182,189). However, these defects are counterbalanced to some extent by the mobilization of alkali from bone. Thus, steady-state pH may be near normal at the expense of skeletal buffers (183).

Differential Diagnosis of Hypophosphatemia

In general, the cause of hypophosphatemia can be determined either from the medical history or from the clinical setting in which it occurs. When the cause is in doubt, measurement of the urinary phosphorus excretion level may be helpful. If the urinary phosphorus concentration is less than 4 mg/dL when the serum phosphorus level is less than 2 mg/dL, renal losses may be excluded (190). Of the three major extrarenal causes including diminished phosphorus intake, increased extrarenal losses (gastrointestinal tract), and translocation into the intracellular space, the last is the most common, particularly in the hospitalized patient (143,191). When the urinary phosphorus excretion level is high, the differential diagnosis includes hyperparathyroidism, a primary renal tubular abnormality, or Vitamin D–dependent or –resistant renal rickets. Measurements of serum calcium, PTH, and Vitamin D and its metabolites, as well as urinary excretion of other solutes (glucose, amino acids, and bicarbonate) will usually elucidate the underlying disturbance that is responsible for the hypophosphatemia.

Treatment of Hypophosphatemia

There are several general principles that apply to the treatment of hypophosphatemic patients. As with any predominantly intracellular ion (e.g., potassium), the state of total body phosphorus stores, as well as the magnitude of phosphorus losses, cannot be readily assessed by measurement of the concentrations in serum. In fact, under conditions in which a rapid shift of phosphorus has resulted from glucose infusion or hyperalimentation, total body stores of phosphorus may be normal, although with diminished intake and renal losses, there may be severe phosphorus depletion. Furthermore, the volume of distribution of phosphorus may vary widely, reflecting in part the intensity and duration of the underlying cause (192).

In clinical situations in which hypophosphatemia is to be expected (e.g., glucose infusion or hyperalimentation in the alcoholic or nutritionally compromised patient during treatment of diabetic ketoacidosis), careful monitoring of the concentration of serum phosphorus is crucial. In these situations, addition of phosphorus supplementation to prevent the development of severe hypophosphatemia may prove very helpful. Certainly, other contributing causes of hypophosphatemia in this setting should be identified and treated. This is particularly true of the use of phosphate binding antacids (aluminum and magnesium hydroxide) for peptic ulcer disease, which may be replaced by aluminum phosphate antacids (Phosphagel) or cimetidine (Tagamet). It is now generally recommended that hyperalimentation solutions contain a phosphorus concentration of 12 to 15 mmol/L (37 to 46.5 mg/dL) to provide an appropriate amount of phosphorus in the patient in whom renal impairment is absent (192). Phosphorus supplementation during glucose infusion or during the treatment of ketoacidosis is usually withheld until the serum phosphorus levels decrease to less than 1 mg/dL. Phosphorus may be given orally to these patients and others with mild asymptomatic hypophosphatemia in the form of skim milk, which contains 0.9 mg/mL, Neutra-phos (3.3 mg/mL), or phosphorus soda (129 mg/mL). However, intestinal absorption is quite variable, and diarrhea often complicates the oral adminis-

tration of phosphate-containing compounds. For these reasons, parenteral administration is usually recommended in the hospitalized patient. If oral therapy is permissible, Fleet Phospho-soda may be given at a dosage of 60 mmol daily in three doses (21 mmoL/5 mL or 643 mg/5 mL). A convenient method is to provide the phosphorus together with potassium replacement in these patients. Addition of 5 mL of potassium phosphate (K phosphate) into 1 L of intravenous fluid provides 22 mEq of potassium and 15 mmol (466 mg) of phosphorus (192). However, because potassium losses may greatly exceed the phosphorus deficit, the repletion of potassium should not be totally linked to phosphorus therapy. In patients with severe phosphate depletion, it is difficult to determine the magnitude of the total deficit of phosphorus and to calculate a precise initial dose. It is usually prudent to proceed with caution and repair the deficit slowly. The most frequently recommended regimen is 0.08 mmol/kg of body weight (2.5 mg/kg body weight) given over 6 hours for severe but uncomplicated hypophosphatemia and 0.016 mmol/kg of body weight (5 mg/kg of body weight) in symptomatic patients (192). Parenteral administration should be discontinued when the serum phosphorus concentration is greater than 2 mg/dL.

Calcium administration may be needed during phosphate repletion to prevent severe hypocalcemia. Calcium must not be added to bicarbonate- or phosphate-containing solutions because of the potential precipitation of calcium salts. Intravenous infusion of calcium gluconate or calcium chloride may be given until tetany abates. In addition to hypocalcemia, metastatic calcification, hypotension, hyperkalemia, and hypernatremia are potential side effects of parenteral infusion of phosphorus. These problems can be prevented by judicious use of therapy and frequent monitoring of serum electrolyte concentrations.

Hyperphosphatemia

Hyperphosphatemia is said to occur when the serum phosphorus concentration exceeds 5 mg/dL in adults. It should be remembered that in children and adolescents, serum levels of phosphorus of up to 6 mg/dL may be physiologic. The most frequent cause of hyperphosphatemia is decreased excretion of phosphorus in the urine as a result of a fall in the GFR. However, increases in serum phosphorus concentration can also occur as a result of increased entry into the ECF due to excessive intake of phosphorus or increased release of phosphorus from tissue breakdown. The major causes of hyperphosphatemia are listed in Table 88-3.

Causes of Hyperphosphatemia

Decreased Excretion of Phosphorus in Urine. Decreased Renal Function. In progressive renal failure, phosphorus homeostasis is maintained by a progressive increase in phosphorus excretion per nephron (193,194). As a result of this increased phosphorus excretion, it is unusual to see marked hyperphosphatemia until GFRs decrease to less than 25 mL per

TABLE 88-3. *Causes of hyperphosphatemia*

I. Decreased renal excretion of phosphate
  A. Renal insufficiency
    1. Chronic
    2. Acute
  B. Hypoparathyroidism
  C. Pseudohypoparathyroidism
    1. Type I
    2. Type II
  D. Abnormal circulating parathyroid hormone
  E. Acromegaly
  F. Tumoral calcinosis
  G. Administration of bisphosphonates
II. Increased entrance of phosphorus into the extracellular fluid
  A. Neoplastic diseases
    1. Leukemia
    2. Lymphoma
  B. Increased catabolism
  C. Respiratory acidosis
III. Administration of PO_4 salts or Vitamin D
  A. Pharmacologic administration of Vitamin D metabolites
  B. Ingestion and/or administration of phosphate salts
IV. Miscellaneous
  A. Cortical hyperostosis
  B. Intermittent hyperphosphatemia
  C. Artifacts

Source: From Slatopolsky E. Pathophysiology of calcium, magnesium, and phosphorus. In: Klahr S, ed. *The kidney and body fluids and disease.* New York: Plenum Press, 1983:269, with permission.

minute (195). Under physiologic conditions with a GFR of 120 mL per minute, a fractional excretion of 5% to 15% of the filtered load of phosphorus is adequate to maintain phosphorus homeostasis. However, as renal insufficiency progresses and the number of nephrons decreases, fractional excretion of phosphorus may increase to as high as 60% to 80% of the filtered load. This progressive phosphaturia per nephron, as renal disease progresses, serves to maintain the concentration of phosphorus within normal limits in plasma. However, when the number of nephrons is greatly diminished, if the dietary intake of phosphorus remains constant, phosphorus homeostasis can no longer be maintained and hyperphosphatemia develops. This usually occurs when the GFR falls to less than 25 mL per minute. As hyperphosphatemia develops, the filtered load of phosphorus per nephron increases, phosphorus excretion rises, and phosphorus balance is reestablished but at higher concentrations of serum phosphorus. Hyperphosphatemia is a usual finding in patients with far-advanced renal insufficiency unless phosphorus intake in the diet has decreased through dietary manipulations or the patient is receiving phosphate binders such as calcium carbonate or aluminum-containing salts that will decrease the absorption of phosphate from the gastrointestinal tract (196). In patients with acute renal failure, hyperphosphatemia is a usual finding (197). The degree of hyperphosphatemia in patients with acute renal failure varies considerably. It is quite marked in patients with renal insufficiency secondary to severe trauma

or known traumatic rhabdomyolysis, as frequently occurs in patients ingesting large amounts of alcohol or in heroin addicts (198). The degree of hyperphosphatemia depends on the amount of phosphorus released from damaged tissue because phosphorus intake and decreased GFR, to less than 2 mL per minute, are constant across different forms of oliguric acute renal failure. In most patients with acute renal failure, hyperphosphatemia is transitory, and serum phosphorus values return toward the normal range as renal function improves. However, in some of these patients, infection or tissue destruction resulting from many causes may maintain relatively high serum phosphorus values even during the recovery phase of renal function.

Decreased or Absent Levels of Circulating PTH. Hypoparathyroidism is characterized by low or absent levels of PTH, low levels of serum calcium, and hyperphosphatemia (199). The most common cause of hypoparathyroidism results from injury to the parathyroid glands or their blood supply during thyroid, parathyroid, or radical neck surgery. Idiopathic hypoparathyroidism is a rare disease. Because PTH normally inhibits the renal reabsorption of phosphorus, its absence leads to an elevation in the Tm for phosphorus and a decrease in the excretion of the anion in the urine. Balance is reestablished when the serum phosphorus concentration rises to 6 to 8 mg/dL. At this concentration of serum phosphorus, the filtered load of phosphate is increased, exceeding the Tm for phosphorus reabsorption, and a new steady-state is reestablished. Patients with hypoparathyroidism are easily diagnosed by the findings of a low level of serum calcium, hyperphosphatemia, and undetectable levels of circulating immunoreactive PTH. After several years of hypoparathyroidism, other signs may become manifest such as cataracts and bilateral symmetrical calcification of the basal ganglia on x-ray films of the skull. The most striking symptoms in patients presenting with hypoparathyroidism are related to an increase in neuromuscular excitability resulting from a decrease in the levels of ionized calcium in serum. Some patients may not develop hypocalcemia and severe tetany, but increased neuromuscular excitability may be demonstrated by contraction of facial muscles in response to stimulus over the facial nerve (Chvostek's sign) or by carpal spasm (Trousseau's sign) occurring 2 or 3 minutes after inflating a blood pressure cuff around the arm above systolic blood pressure. In other patients, psychiatric disturbances, paresthesias, numbness, muscle cramps, and dysphagia may be presenting symptoms.

Pseudohypoparathyroidism. This is a relatively rare condition characterized by end-organ resistance to the action of PTH (200). Characteristically, the kidney and skeleton do not respond appropriately to the action of PTH. Some patients with pseudohypoparathyroidism may have specific somatic characteristics such as short stature, round face, short metacarpal bones and phalanges, and some degree of mental retardation. Biochemically, these patients, like those with hypoparathyroidism, have low concentrations of serum calcium and hyperphosphatemia. However, there are two important points in the differential diagnosis. First, in most patients with pseudohypoparathyroidism, the circulating levels of immunoreactive PTH are elevated, whereas in patients with true hypoparathyroidism PTH levels are low or absent. Second, patients with pseudohypoparathyroidism do not respond to the administration of exogenous PTH with phosphaturia. Patients with true hypoparathyroidism demonstrate a heightened phosphaturic response to administration of exogenous PTH. Two major types of pseudohypoparathyroidism have been described. In type I, patients fail to increase the excretion of cAMP or phosphate in the urine in response to the administration of exogenous PTH. This abnormal response seems to be related, at least in some of these patients, to a defect in the guanosine triphosphate (GTP) binding protein, G_S, of the adenylate cyclase complex (201,202). In other patients, there is an increase in cAMP in response to the administration of exogenous PTH but no phosphaturic response. This condition has been termed *pseudohypoparathyroidism* type II (203).

Abnormal Circulating PTH. This syndrome is characterized by hyperphosphatemia, hypocalcemia, chronic tetany, and cataracts. These manifestations, as described previously, are those observed in patients with hypoparathyroidism, but these patients have normal or high serum levels of PTH. However, in contrast to patients with pseudohypoparathyroidism, they do respond to the exogenous administration of PTH, with an increase in the excretion of cAMP and phosphaturia. It has been postulated that the defect in these patients relates to an abnormal form of endogenous PTH that is devoid of physiologic effects (204). However, this postulate has not been substantiated by characterization and analysis of the circulating PTH in these patients.

Acromegaly. Growth hormone decreases the urinary excretion of phosphorus and increases the Tm for phosphorus (205). Hypersecretion of growth hormone may lead to development of gigantism if the increased secretion occurs before the closure of the epiphysis or to acromegaly if the excessive secretion occurs after puberty. Hyperphosphatemia has been described in patients with acromegaly. It is known that serum phosphorus concentrations are higher in children (5 to 8 mg/dL) than in adults. This may be related in part to increased levels of circulating growth hormone in children.

Tumoral Calcinosis. Although the etiology of this entity is not completely characterized, its pathogenesis is probably related to a primary increase in phosphorus reabsorption by the kidney (206). This condition, which is seen more frequently in young African Americans, is characterized by hyperphosphatemia, ectopic calcification around large joints, normal levels of circulating immunoreactive PTH, and a normal response to administration of exogenous PTH (207,208). The extensive calcification of soft tissues observed in patients with this condition is most likely due to an elevated phosphorus–calcium product in blood. Despite the development of hyperphosphatemia, patients with tumoral calcinosis do not develop secondary hyperparathyroidism. This may be due to the fact that circulating levels of 1,25-dihydroxycholecalciferol remain within the normal range in these patients despite hyperphosphatemia. These normal levels of 1,25-dihydroxycholecalciferol maintain a normal gastrointestinal tract absorption of calcium. This, combined with the decreased urinary calcium observed in these patients, may serve to maintain normal serum calcium values and prevent the development of secondary hyperparathyroidism.

Administration of Bisphosphonates. Administration of bisphosphonates, which are used in the treatment of Paget's disease and osteoporosis, may result in the development of hyperphosphatemia (209). The mechanisms by which bisphosphonates increase serum phosphorus are not completely clear but may involve an alteration in phosphate distribution between different cellular compartments and a decrease in renal phosphorus excretion. It appears that the levels of both circulating PTH and the urinary excretion of cAMP after administration of exogenous PTH are within the normal range in patients receiving bisphosphonates.

Redistribution of Phosphorus Between Intracellular and Extracellular Pools: Tumor Lysis Syndrome. Various syndromes of tissue breakdown may result in the development of hyperphosphatemia and subsequent hypocalcemia. Hyperphosphatemia has been described in patients with several types of lymphomas. Patients receiving treatment for lymphoblastic leukemia may develop hyperphosphatemia with a concomitant decrease in serum calcium concentration (210). The phosphorus load originates primarily from the destruction of lymphoblasts, which have about four times the concentration of organic and inorganic phosphorus present in mature lymphocytes.

Similar findings have been described during treatment of Burkitt's lymphoma. Cohen et al. (211) reviewed the acute tumor lysis syndrome associated with the treatment of Burkitt's lymphoma. In 37 patients with American Burkitt's lymphoma, azotemia occurred in 14 patients and preceded chemotherapy in 8. Pretreatment of azotemia was associated with elevated levels of lactate dehydrogenase (LDH) and uric acid and sometimes extrinsic ureteral obstruction by the tumor. After chemotherapy, major metabolic complications related to tumor lysis were associated with large tumors and high LDH levels and were manifested by hyperkalemia, hyperphosphatemia, and hyperuricemia. Elevated phosphorus levels were seen in 31% of nonazotemic patients and in all azotemic patients. Hemodialysis was required in three patients for control of azotemia, hyperuricemia, hyperphosphatemia, or hyperkalemia.

Tsokos et al. (212) studied the renal metabolic complications of other undifferentiated lymphomas and lymphoblastic lymphomas. These workers found that serum LDH concentration before chemotherapy correlated well with the stage of disease and predicted the serum levels of creatinine, uric acid, and phosphorus in the posttreatment period. Patients with LDH values of more than 2,000 IU were likely to develop severe hyperphosphatemia. When azotemia developed in the postchemotherapy period, it was attributed to hyperuricemia or hyperphosphatemia. Some of these patients had elevated serum phosphorus levels in the range of 20 to 30 mg/dL, which may contribute to the development of renal insufficiency due to calcium deposition in the kidney and other tissues.

Thus, there is a great risk of hyperphosphatemia in patients undergoing chemotherapy for rapidly growing malignant lymphomas. The best method of prevention of this complication, as well as the best therapeutic intervention, has not been well defined. Initially, it appears useful to attempt to increase the renal excretion of phosphate during the induction of remission by chemotherapy in these patients. This requires infusion of large amounts of saline and possibly bicarbonate, which has been shown to increase renal phosphorus excretion above and beyond the mere effects of volume expansion. Acetazolamide, a potent phosphaturic agent, might also be beneficial in these individuals. The general recommendation of hemodialysis as the prime therapeutic modality for hyperphosphatemia and acute renal insufficiency resulting from tumor lysis is not based on experimental data. Although hemodialysis no doubt rapidly lowers serum phosphorus levels, the mass of phosphorus continually presented to the extracellular space from ongoing tissue breakdown is not continuously treated by this modality. Thus, it is possible that combined hemodialysis and peritoneal dialysis, or even peritoneal dialysis alone, might be as, if not more, beneficial and safer in individuals with tumor lysis syndrome.

Increased Catabolism. Conditions characterized by increased protein breakdown (e.g., severe tissue muscle damage and severe infections) may sometimes be accompanied by hyperphosphatemia. Although the hyperphosphatemia may be related simply to translocation of phosphorus into the extracellular space, other factors seem to play a role. Hyperphosphatemia has been described in patients with ketoacidosis before treatment. After administration of intravenous fluids and insulin therapy, the entrance of glucose into the cells is usually followed by movement of phosphorus back into the intracellular space, and some patients now may develop hypophosphatemia. Thus, the combination of dehydration, acidosis, and tissue breakdown in different catabolic states may lead to hyperphosphatemia.

Respiratory Acidosis. Acute respiratory acidosis may lead to a marked increase in serum phosphorus concentration (213). By contrast, chronic respiratory acidosis is usually not manifested by sustained elevated levels of serum phosphorous. Acute rises in PCO_2 in experimental animals have been shown to lead to increased serum phosphorus levels. The modest degree of hyperphosphatemia seen in chronic respiratory acidosis is probably related to renal compensation and increased phosphorus excretion via the kidney to maintain phosphorus homeostasis.

Administration of Phosphate Salts or Vitamin D or its Metabolites. Administration of Vitamin D_3 or its metabolites, particularly 1,25-dihydroxycholecalciferol, may result in increases in serum phosphorus, particularly in uremic patients. These compounds very likely may result in hyperphosphatemia in uremic individuals by increasing phosphorus absorption from the gut and perhaps by potentiating the effect of PTH on the skeleton with increased release of phosphorus from bone. Decreased renal function limits the compensatory mechanism of the kidney to excrete the increased load

of phosphate entering the extracellular space. In addition to elevating serum phosphorus levels, Vitamin D metabolites may result in hypercalcemia. An increase in the phosphorus–calcium product may result in tissue deposition of calcium, particularly in the kidney, leading to further renal functional deterioration.

Ingestion or Administration of Salts Containing Phosphate. Hyperphosphatemia has been observed in adults ingesting laxative-containing phosphate salts or after administration of enemas containing large amounts of phosphate (214,215). Intravenous phosphate administration has been used in the treatment of hypercalcemia of malignancy. The administration of 1 to 2 g of phosphate intravenously decreases the concentration of serum calcium. Unfortunately, the severe hyperphosphatemia induced by administration of large amounts of phosphorus intravenously may lead to calcium phosphate precipitation in important organs such as the heart and kidney, and several deaths resulting from this form of therapy have been reported. Hyperphosphatemia may develop in newborn infants who are fed cow's milk, which is higher in phosphorus content than human milk. This may be an important factor in the genesis of neonatal tetany.

Clinical Manifestations of Hyperphosphatemia

Most of the clinical effects of hyperphosphatemia are related to secondary changes of calcium metabolism. Hyperphosphatemia produces hypocalcemia by several mechanisms (Fig. 88-3), including decreased production of 1,25-dihydroxycholecalciferol (119), precipitation of calcium (216), and decreased absorption of calcium from the gastrointestinal tract, presumably due to a direct effect of phosphorus on calcium absorption (217). In addition to the manifestations by hypocalcemia, which are described elsewhere in this chapter, ectopic calcification is one of the important manifestations of hyperphosphatemia. The association of hyperphosphatemia and ectopic calcification has been observed in

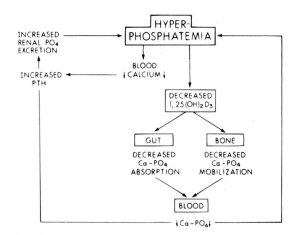

FIG. 88-3. Pathophysiologic changes occurring during the development of hyperphosphatemia. These changes tend to increase the urinary excretion of phosphorus and to correct the hyperphosphatemia.

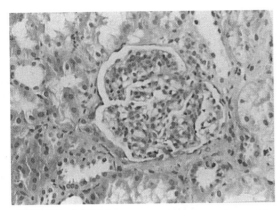

COLOR FIGURE 79-12. Axial mesangial proliferation in early schistosomal glomerulopathy. (hematoxylin and eosin stain, magnification ×200) (From Barsoum RS. Schistosomal glomerulopathies. *Kidney Int* 1993;44:1, with permission.)

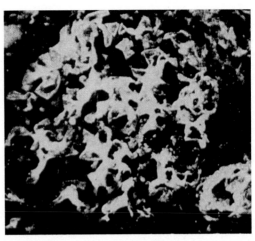

COLOR FIGURE 79-13. Mesangial deposits of schistosomal Guy antigens in early schistosomal glomerulopathy.

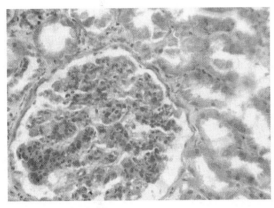

COLOR FIGURE 79-14. Exudative glomerulonephritis in the nephrotic syndrome associated with combined *Schistosoma-Salmonella* infection. Note the abundance of neutrophils and monocytes in the glomerular capillaries and mesangium. (hematoxylin and eosin stain, magnification ×200) (From Barsoum RS. Schistosomal glomerulopathies. *Kidney Int* 1993;44:1, with permission.)

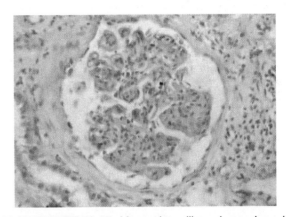

COLOR FIGURE 79-15. Mesangiocapillary glomerulonephritis in advanced schistosomal glomerulopathy. Note the mesangial matrix expansion and the thickening of the glomerular basement membrane. (hematoxylin and eosin stain, magnification ×200) (From Barsoum RS. Schistosomal glomerulopathies. *Kidney Int* 1993;44:1, with permission.)

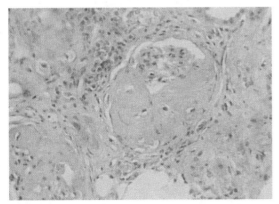

COLOR FIGURE 79-16. Focal segmental glomerulosclerosis in advanced schistosomal glomerulopathy. (Masson trichrome stain, magnification ×200)

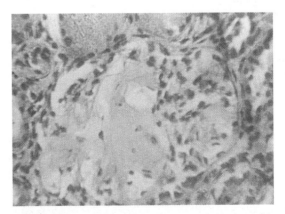

COLOR FIGURE 79-17. Glomerular amyloid deposition in mixed *Schistosoma haematobium* and *Schistosoma mansoni* infection. (hematoxylin and eosin stain, magnification ×200) (From Barsoum RS, et al. Renal amyloidosis and schistosomiasis. *Trans R Soc Trop Med Hyg* 1979;73:367, with permission.)

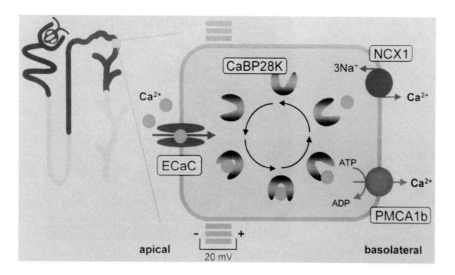

COLOR FIGURE 88-9. Model of transcellular Ca^{2+} transport by cells lining the distal part of the nephron. Entry of Ca^{2+} is facilitated by the apical epithelial Ca^{2+} channel (ECaC). Subsequently, the ion binds to calbindin-D_{28K} (CaBP28K) and diffuses through the cytosol to the basolateral membrane. Here, Ca^{2+} ions are extruded by a Na^+-Ca^{2+} exchanger (NCX1) and a Ca^{2+}-ATPase (PMCA1b). (From Hoenderop JGJ, Willems PHGM, Bindels RJM. Toward a comprehensive molecular model of active calcium reabsorption. *Am J Physiol Renal* 2000; 278:F352, with permission.)

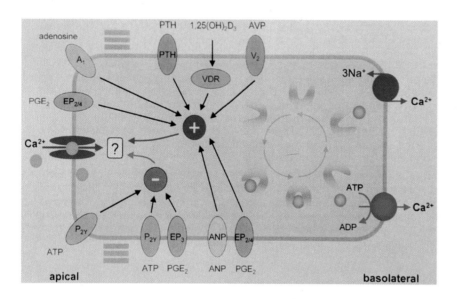

COLOR FIGURE 88-10. Schematic model for hormonal regulation of transcellular Ca^{2+} transport in distal nephron. Parathyroid hormone (PTH), V_2, atrial natriuretic peptide (ANP), and EP_3 receptors are localized in the basolateral membrane, whereas A_1 is present in the apical membrane. $EP_{2/4}$ and P_{2Y} are present in both membranes 1,25-dihydroxycholecalciferol passes plasma membranes and binds to the intracellular Vitamin D receptor (VDR). Hormones can be divided into stimulatory hormones, including PTH, arginine vasopressin, ANP, prostaglandin E_2 (PGE_2) (via $EP_{2/4}$), and adenosine, and inhibitory hormones such as adenosine triphosphate and PGE_2 (via EP_3). (From Hoenderop JGJ, Willems PHGM, Bindels RJM. Toward a comprehensive molecular model of active calcium reabsorption. *Am J Physiol Renal* 2000;278:F352, with permission.

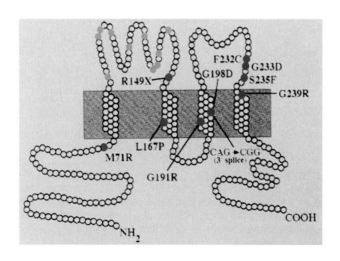

COLOR FIGURE 88-14. Structure of the paracellin-1 (PCLN1) human gene. *Red dots* indicate mutations in PCLN1 in patients with recessive renal hypomagnesemia. (From Simon DB, Lu Y, Chaote KA, et al. Paracellin-1, a renal tight junction protein required for paracellular Mg^{2+} resorption. *Science* 1999;285: 103, with permission.)

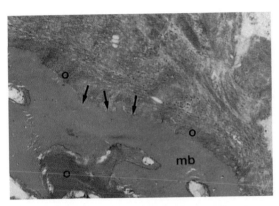

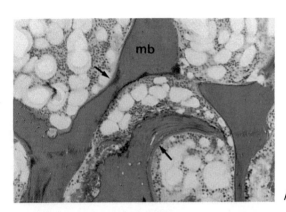

A

COLOR FIGURE 92-7. Subperiosteal resorption *(arrows)* of mineralized bone *(mb)* filled in with unmineralized osteoid *(O)* in a patient on dialysis with osteomalacia. (Goldner's stain, magnification ×115.)

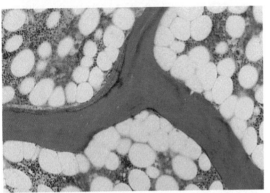

B

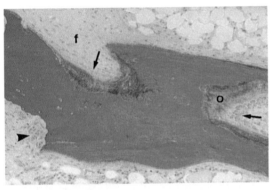

COLOR FIGURE 92-12. Osteitis fibrosa. Osteoid *(O)* is a mixture of woven and lamellar collagen. Plump osteoblasts *(arrows)* and multinucleated osteoclasts *(arrowhead)* are numerous. Fibrosis *(f)* is present. (Goldner's stain, magnification ×115.)

COLOR FIGURE 92-11. A: Histologic section of bone from a patient on dialysis with mild hyperparathyroidism. Length of unmineralized osteoid *(arrow)* is increased. Width of osteoid seam and volume of mineralized bone *(mb)* are normal. **B:** Bone section from a normal subject. (**A** and **B,** Goldner's stain, magnification ×115.)

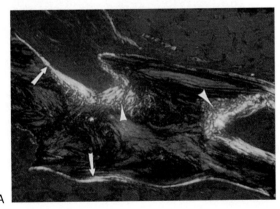

A

B

COLOR FIGURE 92-13. A: Polarized light section showing woven *(arrowheads)* and lamellar *(arrows)* collagen in osteitis fibrosa. **B:** Polarization of normal bone showing only lamellar collagen. (**A** and **B,** magnification ×115)

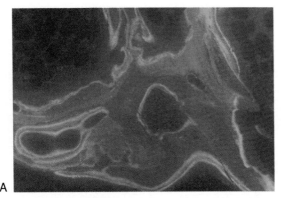
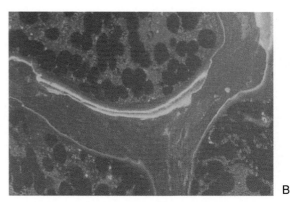

A

B

COLOR FIGURE 92-14. A: Double tetracycline labels in a patient with severe osteitis fibrosa. The distance between labels and the total length of the double labels is increased, demonstrating a high formation rate. **B:** Tetracycline labels from a normal subject. (**A** and **B,** unstained fluorescent micrographs, magnification ×115.)

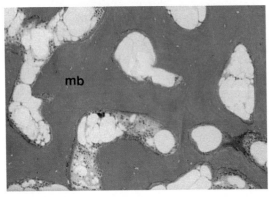

COLOR FIGURE 92-15. Osteosclerosis. The amount of mineralized bone *(mb)* is increased. (Goldner's stain, magnification ×115.)

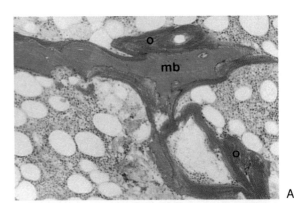

A

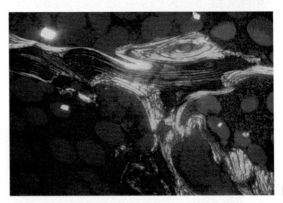

B

COLOR FIGURE 92-17. Osteomalacia. **A:** The unmineralized osteoid *(O)* is increased in width and total volume; *mb,* mineralized bone. **B:** Polarized section showing predominantly lamellar orientation of collagen in osteomalacia. (**A** and **B,** magnification ×115.)

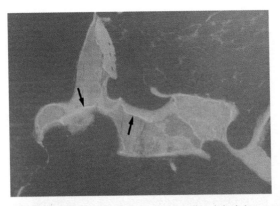

COLOR FIGURE 92-18. Single tetracycline label *(arrows)* in bone from a patient on dialysis with osteomalacia given two time-spaced doses of tetracycline. Absence of double labels indicates abnormally low bone formation. (Unstained fluorescent micrograph, magnification ×115.)

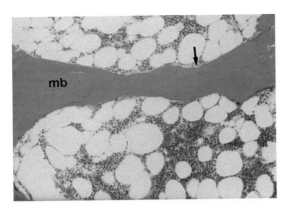

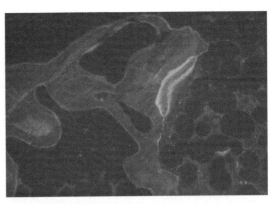

COLOR FIGURE 92-19. Aplastic (adynamic) bone disease. Marked decrease in amount of unmineralized osteoid *(arrows); mb,* mineralized bone. Osteoblasts are flat when present. (Goldner's stain, magnification ×115.)

COLOR FIGURE 92-20. Aplastic (adynamic) bone disease. The total amount of tetracycline uptake is decreased, as is the number of double tetracycline labels. When present, the double label is shorter than normal, demonstrating reduced bone formation. (Unstained fluorescent micrograph, magnification ×115.)

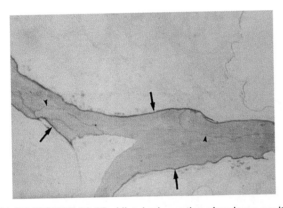

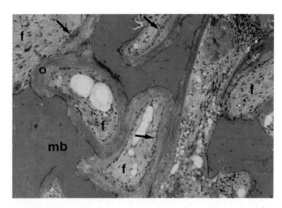

COLOR FIGURE 92-22. Histologic section showing a positive stain for aluminum on the surface *(arrows)* of mineralized bone and within cement lines *(arrowheads).* (Aurin-tricarboxylic acid, magnification ×115.)

COLOR FIGURE 92-25. Mixed bone disease in a patient on dialysis. Width and total volume of unmineralized osteoid *(O)* are increased; *mb,* mineralized bone. The number of osteoblasts *(arrows)* also is increased, and fibrosis *(f)* is present in most of the marrow space. (Goldner's stain, magnification ×115.)

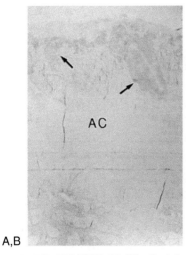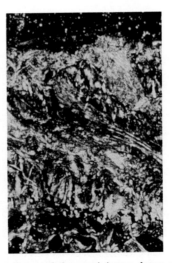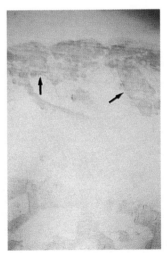

A,B   C

COLOR FIGURE 92-26. Serial sections of femoral bone from a patient on dialysis. **A:** Congo red–stained amyloid deposits *(arrows)* are seen in the superficial articular cartilage *(AC).* **B:** The same seen under polarized light. Congo red–stained amyloid deposits demonstrate green birefringence. **C:** Immunohistochemical staining with anti-β_2-microglobulin. Amyloid deposits *(arrows)* stain brown for β_2-microglobulin. (From Onishi S, et al. Beta-2 microglobulin deposition in bone in chronic renal failure. *Kidney Int* 1991;39:990, with permission.)

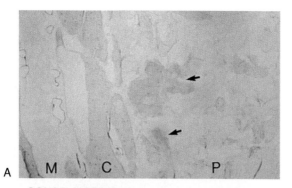
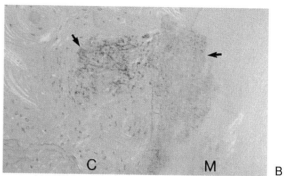

COLOR FIGURE 92-27. A: Iliac crest bone biopsy with anti-β_2-microglobulin and hematoxylin counterstain. β_2-Microglobulin deposits *(arrows)* are located in the iliac periosteum. B: Bone section from the tibia with anti-β_2-microglobulin and methylene blue counterstain. β_2-Microglobulin deposits *(arrows)* appear to invade the cortical bone *(C)* from the marrow *(M)*. (From Onishi S, et al. Beta-2-microglobulin deposition in bone in chronic renal failure. *Kidney Int* 1991;39:990, with permission.)

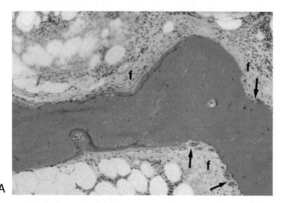
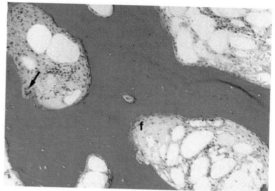

COLOR FIGURE 92-29. A: Osteitis fibrosa in a patient on dialysis refractory to treatment with oral calcitriol. B: Histologic section from the same patient after treatment with intravenous calcitriol. Amount of fibrosis *(f)* and number of osteoclasts *(arrows)* are decreased after treatment. (A and B, Goldner's stain, magnification ×115.)

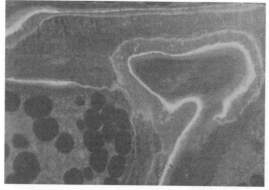
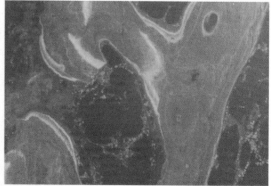

COLOR FIGURE 92-31. A: Tetracycline labels in a patient on dialysis with osteitis fibrosa and high bone formation. B: Tetracycline labels in the same patient after treatment with intravenous calcitriol. The reductions in the interlabel distance and the length of double labels after treatment indicate a decrease in bone formation to normal. (A and B, Unstained fluorescent micrographs, magnification ×115.)

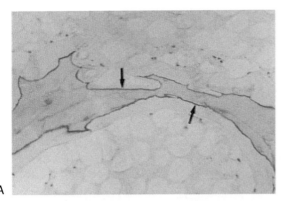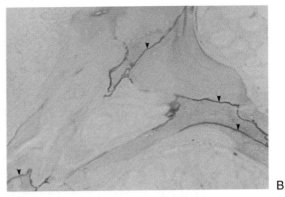

A

B

COLOR FIGURE 92-33. **A:** Aluminum-associated bone disease in a patient on dialysis. Aluminum deposits *(arrows)* cover the mineralized bone surface. **B:** Aluminum stain in the same patient after treatment with intravenous deferoxamine. Most of the aluminum is now within the mineralized bone *(arrowheads),* indicating that new bone formation occurred despite the presence of aluminum at the mineralization front. (**A** and **B,** Aurin-tricarboxylic acid stain, magnification ×115.)

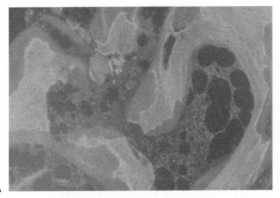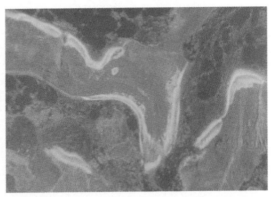

A

B

COLOR FIGURE 92-34. **A:** Absence of tetracycline labels in a patient on dialysis with aluminum-associated osteomalacia. **B:** Tetracycline labels in the same patient after treatment with intravenous deferoxamine. The calculated bone formation rate is normal. (**A** and **B,** Unstained fluorescent micrographs, magnification ×115.)

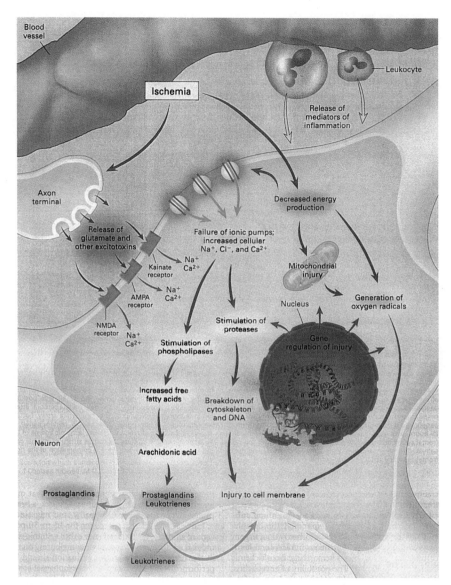

COLOR FIGURE 93-6. The molecular events initiated in brain tissue by acute cerebral ischemia. Interruption of cerebral blood flow results in decreased energy production, which in turn causes failure of ionic pumps, mitochondrial injury, activation of leukocytes (with release of mediators of inflammation), generation of oxygen radicals, and release of excitotoxins. Increased cellular levels of sodium, chloride and calcium ions result in stimulation of phospholipases and proteases, followed by generation and release of prostaglandins and leukotrienes, breakdown of DNA and the cytoskeleton, and ultimately, breakdown of the cell membrane. Alteration of genetic components regulates elements of the cascade to alter the degree of injury. AMPA denotes α-amino-3-hydroxy-5-methyl-4-isoxazole propionic acid and N-methyl-D-aspartate. (From: Brott T, Bogousslavsky J. Treatment of acute ischemic stroke. *N Engl J Med* 2000;343:710, with permission.)

several clinical settings including in patients with chronic renal failure, hypoparathyroidism, and tumoral calcinosis. It appears that when the calcium–phosphorus product exceeds 70, the likelihood for calcium precipitation is greatly increased. In addition to the calcium–phosphorus product, local tissue factors may play an important role in calcium deposition. For example, regional changes in pH (local alkalosis) may favor calcification in tissue such as cornea and lungs. In patients with severe calcification (calciphylaxis), it appears that high levels of circulating PTH may also aggravate this condition. Hyperphosphatemia plays a key role in the development of secondary hyperparathyroidism in patients with renal insufficiency. It has been observed that when phosphate ingestion is decreased and hyperphosphatemia is prevented in experimental animals with induced renal insufficiency, hyperparathyroidism can be prevented (218). The mechanisms presumably relate to maintenance of serum calcium levels with prevention of hyperphosphatemia and, at the same time, continued synthesis of 1,25-dihydroxycholecalciferol, the circulating levels of which may directly influence the secretion of PTH (219,220). In the past decade, several investigators (221–224) have demonstrated that dietary phosphate markedly influences the rate of parathyroid cell proliferation and PTH synthesis and secretion independent of changes in ionized calcium or 1,25-dihydroxycholecalciferol. It will seem that the mechanism by which phosphorus increases PTH synthesis and secretion is posttranscriptional. Moreover, in experimental uremic rats, it has been shown that phosphate restriction suppresses parathyroid cell growth by inducing p21, a repressor of the cell cycle. On the other hand a high-phosphate intake rapidly (3 to 5 days) induces significant parathyroid cell hyperplasia by inducing an increase in transforming growth factor α (TGFα) (225). TGFα, which is known to promote growth not only in malignant transformation but also in normal tissues (226,227), is enhanced in hyperplastic and adenomatous human parathyroid glands (228). In patients on chronic hemodialysis, the degree of hyperparathyroidism correlates well with the concentration of serum phosphorus. Patients who do not adhere to their therapeutic prescriptions requiring ingestion of phosphate binders seem to develop more severe and persistent hyperphosphatemia with marked secondary hyperparathyroidism and bone disease than patients who adhere carefully to dietary and therapeutic prescriptions. Vascular calcification has been observed in some patients with chronic renal insufficiency and severe calcification, hyperphosphatemia, and hyperparathyroidism, leading to necrosis and gangrene of extremities. Slit-lamp examination may show ocular calcification, and some patients may develop acute conjunctivitis, the so-called red eye syndrome of uremia. Precipitation of calcium in the skin may be in part responsible for pruritus, a symptom that is usually seen in patients with far-advanced uremia. It has been reported that parathyroidectomy in such patients may alleviate the symptoms. From the therapeutic point of view, the most efficacious way of controlling hyperphosphatemia is through the use of phosphate binders that decrease the absorption of phosphorus from the gastrointestinal tract. In patients with adequate renal function, expansion of the ECF with saline will greatly increase phosphorus excretion in the urine and contribute to correction of the hyperphosphatemia.

Treatment of Hyperphosphatemia

Decreased absorption of phosphate from the gastrointestinal tract is a cornerstone of treatment of hyperphosphatemia. Phosphate absorption from the gastrointestinal tract can be markedly decreased by decreasing the amount of phosphorus in the diet, by administering phosphate binding agents capable of decreasing absorption of phosphorus, or both. Because protein requirements limit the amount of phosphorus restriction that can be achieved through dietary manipulation, from a practical point of view, administration of agents capable of decreasing phosphorus absorption from the gastrointestinal tract is the mainstay of treatment. Administration of calcium salts has replaced aluminum salts as the traditional treatment to control hyperphosphatemia. Most of these preparations require the administration of two to four tablets or capsules three or four times daily. If the patient develops constipation, one of the complications of such medications, magnesium salts may be incorporated into these preparations. However, if the patient has hyperphosphatemia secondary to severe renal insufficiency, magnesium should not be given because of the likelihood of producing severe hypermagnesemia, which may lead to magnesium intoxication, muscle paralysis, and death.

The elucidation of aluminum toxicity, which results from prolonged administration of aluminum-containing salts, as phosphate binders to patients with chronic renal insufficiency, has led to diminished use of these agents or their elimination (229,230). Several studies indicate that calcium carbonate (231–233) is an effective agent for control of hyperphosphatemia in chronic renal failure. However, in the past 10 years, numerous investigators have demonstrated an increase in the number of aortic and mitral valve calcifications in patients on dialysis when compared with the general population. Cardiovascular events are responsible for a 40% to 60% mortality rate of patients on dialysis (234–237). Morbidity and mortality rates increase as the Ca–PO$_4$ product raises to more than 60. Currently, Braun et al. (238), with the use of the electron beam computed tomography, demonstrated a significant deposition of calcium in the coronary arteries of patients on dialysis. Although coronary artery calcifications worsen with age, this abnormality has been demonstrated in young patients (239). In fact, postmortem examination of children with renal failure demonstrated that 60% to 70% had calcification of the heart, lungs, and blood vessels (240). Positive calcium balances of 500 to 900 mg daily were demonstrated in uremic patients receiving large doses of calcium carbonate (233). Thus, it is critical not only to reduce the Ca–PO$_4$ product to less than 60, but also to significantly decrease the calcium load that patients receive to control serum phosphorus.

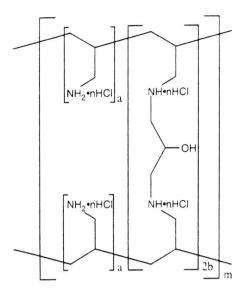

FIG. 88-4. Structure of sevelamer hydrochloride (Renagel), cross-linked poly(allylamine hydrochloride).

To avoid these deleterious side effects, a well-tolerated calcium albumin–free phosphate binder was developed, sevelamer hydrochloride (Renagel). This new phosphate binder is a hydrogel of cross-linked poly(allylamine hydrochloride) that is resistant to digestive degradation and is not absorbed from the gastrointestinal tract (Fig. 88-4). Its mechanism of action relates to the presence of partially protonated amines spaced one carbon from the polymer backbone, which interact with phosphate ions by ionic and hydrogen bonding. Several short-term clinical studies in patients with end-stage renal disease have established that sevelamer hydrochloride is an effective phosphate binder without increasing the calcium load to the patients (241,242) (Fig. 88-5). In addition, sevelamer hydrochloride decreases low-density lipoprotein cholesterol by 30% to 40%, and in long-term studies increases high-density lipoprotein cholesterol by 20% to 30%; it does not affect triglycerides (243). Studies in progress will provide critical information on its potential efficacy in reducing morbidity and mortality rates in patients on dialysis.

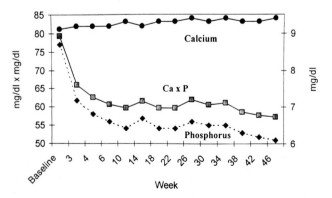

FIG. 88-5. Effects of sevelamer hydrochloride (Renagel) on serum calcium, phosphorus, and calcium–phosphate product in a group of 192 patients on hemodialysis. (From Chertow GM, et al. *Nephrol Dial Transplantation* 1999;14:2907, with permission.)

Although decreased gastrointestinal absorption of phosphorus is an effective way to control hyperphosphatemia in patients with renal insufficiency, excretion of phosphorus through the kidney is also an important mechanism. Thus expansion of the ECF volume may markedly increase phosphorus excretion by the kidney. This result is presumably related both to direct effects of volume expansion on the kidney, which decreases salt and water reabsorption and hence phosphorus reabsorption, and to increased PTH release, particularly as a consequence of decreased ionized calcium during volume expansion. In patients with marked renal insufficiency or with marked degrees of hyperphosphatemia due to tumor lysis or chemotherapy, peritoneal dialysis or hemodialysis may be used to remove large quantities of phosphorus from the extracellular space. Redistribution of phosphorus from the intracellular to the extracellular space can sometimes be rapidly corrected by the administration of glucose and insulin. In general, mild degrees of hyperphosphatemia can be tolerated, particularly if calcium levels are not markedly elevated. The goal in patients with chronic renal insufficiency is to keep phosphorus levels at less than 4.5 mg/dL to avoid falls in serum ionized calcium and marked development of severe hyperparathyroidism.

CALCIUM

Calcium, the most abundant cation of the body and the principal mineral of the human skeleton, is essential to the integrity and function of cell membranes, neuromuscular excitability, transmission of nerve impulses, multiple enzymatic reactions, and regulation of hormones such as PTH, calcitonin, and 1,25-dihydroxycholecalciferol. The primary factor in the regulation of extracellular calcium is PTH. It acts on the skeleton, small intestine (indirectly), and kidney and interrelates with Vitamin D and calcitonin to maintain the extracellular calcium concentration within narrow limits.

Distribution of Calcium

The total amount of calcium in the human body ranges from 1,000 to 1,200 g or 20 to 25 g/kg of fat-free body tissue. Approximately 99% of body calcium resides in the skeleton; the other 1% is present in the extracellular and intracellular spaces. About 1% of the calcium in the skeleton is freely exchangeable with calcium in the ECF. Together, these two fractions are known as the miscible pool of calcium and account for 2% of total body calcium. Calcium in bone is found primarily in the form of small crystals similar to hydroxyapatite, although some calcium exists as amorphous crystals in combination with phosphate. The normal calcium : phosphate ratio in bone is 1.5 : 1.

Extracellular Calcium

In humans, the serum calcium concentration is kept remarkably constant, between 9.0 and 10.4 mg/dL, or 4.5 to 5.2 mEq/L, or 2.25 to 2.6 mmol/L. About 50% of serum calcium is ionized and 10% is complexed with citrate, phosphate, bicarbonate, and lactate. These two fractions, ionized plus complexed calcium ("ultrafilterable calcium"), make up approximately 60% of the total serum calcium. The rest, 40%, is protein bound, mainly to albumin. In hypoproteinemic states, such as the nephrotic syndrome or cirrhosis, although total serum calcium may be low, the ionized fraction may be within the normal range. Five percent to 10% of the calcium is bound to globulins. It is unusual for total serum calcium concentrations to change because of alterations in the levels of serum globulins. However, in severe hyperglobulinemia, such as may occur in patients with multiple myeloma or other dysproteinemias, elevations of total serum calcium concentrations may be observed.

One gram of albumin binds approximately 0.8 mg of calcium; thus, at the normal plasma albumin concentration of 4.0 to 4.5 g/dL, only 10% to 15% of the binding sites for calcium are occupied. Consequently, when excess calcium is added to blood *in vitro* or *in vivo,* all the fractions increase in the same proportion, and the ultrafilterable fraction as a percentage of the total calcium concentration does not change. The binding of calcium by albumin, therefore, acts as a buffer that reduces by about half the potential changes in ionized calcium that may result from acute gains or losses of calcium by the blood. The most important factor modifying the binding of calcium to albumin is the pH of plasma. Alkalosis increases the binding of free calcium, resulting in a fall in ionized calcium concentration; acidosis has the opposite effect. This is due not only to competition between H^+ and Ca^{2+} for binding sites on albumin but also to changes in the conformation of the albumin molecule. Changes in PcO_2 do not affect calcium binding other than through changes in pH. In the past, ionized calcium was difficult to measure. This difficulty has been overcome by the use of sensitive flow-through electrodes, which can measure changes in ionized calcium of as small as 0.1 mg/dL.

Intracellular Calcium

Calcium is the major intracellular ionic messenger for the activation of many biologic processes (244). The intracellular concentration of calcium is approximately 150 nmol/L. Cells extrude calcium via pumps or exchangers, sequester it in intracellular organelles, or use low-affinity binding sites with large capacities to maintain free calcium, Ca^{2+}, at the 150-nmol/L level (245,246). Intracellular calcium is complexed with ions such as orthophosphate or pyrophosphate and is bound to organic molecules such as ATP and proteins. Three major cellular calcium pools exist: (a) bound to multiple diverse sites, (b) sequestered in intracellular organelles, and (c) bound or free within the cytosol (244).

Extrusion of Ca^{2+} from the cell and sequestration in intracellular organelles are transport functions generally carried out by two mechanisms, Na^+-Ca^{2+} exchange and Ca-ATPase (247—250). In cardiac muscle, nerve, brain, and kidney, calcium extrusion is directly coupled to sodium transport (247,251). The Na^+-Ca^{2+} transport system depends on the asymmetric distribution of Na^+ across the plasma membrane. The Na-K-ATPase of the plasma membrane is involved in the metabolic process necessary to maintain the Na^+ gradient. Thus, the movement of Na^+ into the cell is coupled to the flux of Ca^{2+} out of the cell. This Na^+-Ca^{2+} antiport system is electrogenic with a stoichiometry of three Na^+ per Ca^{2+} (251,252). A second and more ubiquitous mechanism of calcium efflux energizes uphill transport of calcium by the hydrolysis of high-energy–yielding phosphate bonds of ATP (250).

In the kidney, considerable progress has been made in clarifying the physiologic role of these transporters responsible in Ca^{2+} efflux from renal epithelial cells. In addition to involvement in regulating cytosolic Ca^{2+}, these exchangers may participate in the extrusion of Ca^{2+} on stimulation of transcellular Ca^{2+} absorption. Such an action would more likely be expected in cortical thick ascending limbs (TALs), distal convoluted tubules, or (rabbit) connecting tubules, that is, those segments in which transcellular Ca^{2+} absorption is found. The cloning of cardiac (247), renal (251), and other forms of the Na^+-Ca^{2+} exchanger, NCX, has led to improved information regarding the role of this transporter. Three genes encoding NCX, designated *NCX1, NCX2,* and *NCX3,* have been identified in mammals. Only *NCX1* is found in the kidney, where it is mainly localized to the distal nephron along the basolateral membrane (253). This is in concordance with evidence for ATP-dependent Ca^{2+} extrusion, but not for Na^+-Ca^{2+} exchange in rabbit cortical TALs (254). In contrast, removal of basolateral Na^+ inhibited Ca^{2+} absorption and increased cytosolic Ca^{2+} in rabbit distal convoluted tubules and connecting tubules, consistent with the presence of Na^+-Ca^{2+} exchange in these nephron segments (255–258). Such observations are compatible with the view that basolateral membrane Ca^{2+}-ATPase may mediate cellular Ca^{2+} extrusion in cortical TALs, whereas Na^+-Ca^{2+} exchange and Ca^{2+}-ATPase may be responsible for Ca^{2+} efflux in distal convoluted tubules and connecting tubules. Na^+-Ca^{2+} exchanger transport activity increases in response to PTH (259–261).

The plasma membrane Ca^{2+}-ATPase (PMCA) is a P-type ATPase (262–264). In human kidneys, all four known isoforms (265) have been found with the highest staining for immunoreactive Ca^{2+}-ATPase along basolateral membranes of the distal convoluted tubules (266). These observations and others demonstrating PMCA1B transcripts in rabbit connecting tubule and cortical collecting duct suggest that human distal convoluted tubules express the Ca^{2+}-ATPase immunologically similar to that of human erythrocyte membranes. Immunologically distinct epitopes of the Ca^{2+}-ATPase are probably expressed on proximal tubule membranes and in other nephron segments. Magocsi et al. (267) have studied the localization of mRNAs encoding isozymes of plasma membrane Ca^{2+}-ATPases in rat kidney. Message for the first isoform of the rat plasma membrane Ca^{2+}-ATPase (RPMCA1) was found in the cortex and outer and inner medulla. Whereas, RPMCA2 was abundant in the cortex and outer medulla. Transcripts for the third isoform, RPMCA3, were conspicuous in the outer medulla. mRNA for RPMCA2 was detected in the distal convoluted tubules and in the cortical TALs by *in situ* reverse transcription polymerase chain reaction. This is discordant with the rabbit, but it is possible that RPMCA2 may be specifically related to epithelial cells that are engaged in active Ca^{2+} absorption (267).

The cytosolic calcium concentration is also maintained by an active transport into mitochondria and the endoplasmic reticulum. It has been shown that mitochondria accumulate Ca^{2+} through a Ca-uniporter, with Ca^{2+} moving down an electrochemical gradient. The K_m for Ca^{2+} of the uniporter is about 1 μmmol/L. Mitochondria also contain an Na^+-Ca^{2+} exchange mechanism. In the mitochondria, calcium and phosphate ions form insoluble amorphous tricalcium phosphate, a reaction that releases hydrogen ions into the cytosol. Cell injury may lead to a rise in intracellular calcium sufficient for Ca^{2+} to be sequestered in the mitochondria (268). Ca^{2+} is sequestered in the endoplasmic reticulum by the action of a Ca-ATPase, which differs in properties from that found on the plasma membrane and Golgi apparatus. During the early response of cells to certain stimuli, production of IP_3 and cyclic adenosine diphosphate ribose stimulates the opening of Ca^{2+} channels in the endoplasmic reticulum, serving to transiently increase cytosolic Ca^{2+} and allow the ion to act as an intracellular signal.

Skeletal Calcium

More than 99% of the total body calcium is found in the skeleton. Bone consists of approximately 40% mineral, 30% organic matrix, and 30% water. Bone mineral exists in two physical forms, the amorphous and the crystalline. The amorphous form consists mainly of brushite and tricalcium phosphate; the crystalline form is composed mainly of hydroxyapatite. More than 90% of the organic material of the bone matrix is in the form of collagen fibers that are arranged in bundles with specific interaction with hydroxyapatite. The nature of the freely exchangeable calcium pool in bone is unknown, but it is unlikely to be collagen-associated hydroxyapatite.

A coupled process of bone resorption and formation (remodeling) is responsible for exit of calcium from the exchangeable pool (bone formation) and release of skeletal calcium (bone resorption) into the exchangeable pool, but remodeling probably contributes little to minute-to-minute control of serum calcium. Pathologic states in which bone resorption is greatly increased (i.e., when bone resorption is greater than bone formation) produce profound changes in calcium homeostasis. Bone remodeling is a coupled process because the activation of a remodeling unit sets two cell differentiation programs into operation–that of the osteoblast and that of the osteoclast. Bone marrow stromal cells, the osteoprogenitors that will become osteoblasts, harbor the receptors that are recognized by the factors capable of activating bone remodeling. Their stimulation results in the synthesis of a cell-attached ligand for RANK (receptor for activation of nuclear factor kappa b) on osteoclast progenitors, variously known as osteoprotegerin ligand (OPGL), rank ligand (RANKL), or osteoclast differentiation factor (ODF) (269–271). OPGL and macrophage colony-stimulating factor (MCSF-1) are the critical osteoclast differentiation factors, and these local bone marrow factors are sufficient to direct osteoclast formation. The osteoclasts responsible for bone resorption are multinucleated giant cells lying in irregular indentations of the bone surface known as Howship's lacunae. Bone resorption depends on the number and activity of osteoclasts. The process of bone resorption performed by the osteoclasts includes the production of an acidic environment by proton secretion and matrix degradation by cathepsin K. The osteoblasts, on the other hand, are the cells responsible for the repair process after bone resorption (bone formation). Differentiation of the cells in the osteoblast lineage begins with specification of mesenchymal stromal cells to the lineage by expression of osteoblast-specific transcription factors—one of which has been identified and is Cbfa1/Osf2 (272). Cbfa1 expression is stimulated by the bone morphogenetic protein subfamily of the $TGF\beta$ superfamily responsible for the direction of osteoblast differentiation and bone formation. Cells early in the process of osteoblast differentiation initiate bone matrix production by the biosynthesis of collagen. Thereafter, the matrix is mineralized by the deposition of calcium and phosphate, with formation of amorphous material initially and then development of hydroxyapatite. The deposition of mineral occurs along a well-defined front ("mineralization front"), outside of which there is an osteoid border or seam. The osteoid begins to calcify about 10 days after deposition. From the architectural point of view, the skeleton is composed of two types of bone: (a) compact cortical bone, which surrounds the marrow cavity and forms the shaft of the long bones, and (b) cancellous or trabecular bone, which is the main component of flat bone and vertebra.

A differentiation between two other general types of bone is critical in the diagnosis of metabolic bone disease. The first, called *woven bone* (immature bone) (273), is a loosely organized, highly mineralized bone in which the collagen fibers are coarsely arranged and the osteocytes are large and irregular in size and shape. Woven bone is formed by simultaneous and unorganized actions of many cells. The calcification of the tissue is patchy, occurring in a speckled pattern and independent of the presence of Vitamin D activity. Woven bone is present in the fetus but after age 14 is no longer found in the human skeleton, except with pathologic conditions such as Paget's disease and hyperparathyroidism and during rapid bone turnover, as in the presence of healing fractures (273,274). The second general type of bone is lamellar bone (mature bone), which is the major component of the normal adult skeleton. It is a highly organized tissue in which the collagen bundles are arranged in successive layers, between which are cells called *osteocytes*. Lamellar bone is the product of synchronized activity by the osteoblast depositing collagen materials at a specific cell surface. Another difference between woven bone and lamellar bone relates to the relation of mineral to collagen. In lamellar bone, the relative amounts of collagen and minerals are closely related, making hypermineralization in these bones difficult. Mineralization of woven bone is disorderly, and the degree of mineralization varies enormously; thus, hypermineralization may occur in this type of bone (273,274). PTH, in conjunction with PTH-related peptide (PTHrP), other locally produced cytokines, and Vitamin D, plays a key role in bone turnover. At physiologic doses, PTH has an anabolic effect, increasing bone formation. Thus, PTH, by increasing calcium reabsorption by the kidney and gut and through stimulation of the osteoblast, affects the rate of bone formation. However, in pathologic conditions (e.g., hyperparathyroidism), the concentration of PTH in serum may be increased 10- to 50-fold. At this high concentration, PTH increases the activity and number of osteoclasts; thus, bone resorption predominates over bone formation, and minerals and organic matrix are removed from bone and enter the ECF. Not only PTH but also other hormones such as PTH-related proteins, thyroxine, interleukin-1 (IL-1), and tumor necrosis factor can produce severe hypercalcemia by increasing the activity of osteoclasts.

Calcium Balance

Approximately 700 to 1,000 mg of calcium is ingested daily in the diet. However, this amount may vary depending on the amount of milk consumed. Milk and cheese are the major sources of calcium, contributing 50% to 70% of the total amount ingested in the diet. In the United States, 1 L of milk contains approximately 800 to 900 mg of calcium. About 10 to 15 mg of calcium per kilogram of body weight is the recommended daily intake. However, during the last trimester of pregnancy, there is an increased requirement for calcium because approximately 20 to 30 g of calcium enters the fetus. With age, intestinal calcium absorption declines; thus, an increase in calcium intake may be necessary to maintain calcium homeostasis. When 1 g of calcium is ingested in the diet, approximately 800 mg is excreted in the feces and 200 mg in the urine. With a normal calcium intake (700 to 1,000 mg per day), approximately 30% to 40% of ingested calcium is absorbed in the intestine (Fig. 88-6). However, on lower calcium diets, the percentage of calcium absorbed increases, and the percentage of calcium absorbed decreases when the diet has a high calcium content (more than 1,500 mg per day). The mechanisms responsible for this adaptation have been partially characterized and require the participation of PTH, Vitamin D, and perhaps calcitonin. With low-calcium diet feeding, mild transient hypocalcemia activates the parathyroid gland chief cell Ca sensor and the release of PTH, which increases the conversion of 25-hydroxycholecalciferol to 1,25-dihydroxycholecalciferol in the renal cortex. 1,25-Dihydroxycholecalciferol is the hormonal metabolite of Vitamin D, and it increases the intestinal absorption of calcium and mobilizes calcium from bone, synergistically with PTH. Thus, serum calcium levels return to normal. On the other hand, if the patient is fed a

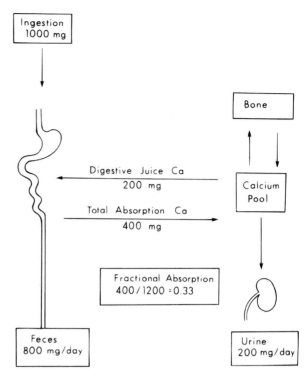

FIG. 88-6. Diagrammatic representation of calcium metabolism in humans showing the contribution of the gastrointestinal tract, the kidney, and bone to the maintenance of the calcium pool.

high-calcium diet, the mild hypercalcemia inhibits the chief cell Ca sensor, suppressing PTH, and stimulates the release of calcitonin from the C cells of the thyroid. In the absence of PTH, the activity of the 1α-hydroxylase is diminished and the 24-hydroxylase is activated; thus, the kidney makes preferentially 24,25-dihydroxycholecalciferol [24,25(OH)$_2$D$_3$], which is less efficient than 1,25-dihydroxycholecalciferol in promoting calcium absorption from the gastrointestinal tract and mobilizing calcium from the skeleton. Fecal calcium consists of the fraction of ingested calcium that is not absorbed plus 100 to 200 mg of calcium secreted by the intestine daily. The secreted digestive juice calcium is known as *endogenous fecal calcium*. The amount of calcium secreted by the intestine is fairly constant and is not greatly influenced by hypercalcemia.

Intestinal Calcium Absorption

The mechanisms of calcium transport across the intestinal mucosa are complex, but our understanding of the physiology is rapidly progressing. Intestinal calcium absorption occurs by two general mechanisms: active and passive transport (275). The passive process involves paracellular movement of calcium in some intestinal segments, and active transport involves movement through mucosal epithelial cells. When the intestine is perfused *in vitro* with increasing calcium concentrations, the rate of movement of calcium from the mucosa to the serosa increases without evidence of saturation or a maximum transport rate. An active transport process would be expected to be saturable. It has been estimated that at luminal calcium concentrations of more than 7.0 mmol/L, calcium is transported primarily by a diffusional process. This suggests that in regions of the intestine such as the ileum, where the calcium concentration is high, the passive transport process predominates. In the duodenum and jejunum, where the luminal calcium concentration is lower than 6.0 mmol/L, the active transport process assumes a predominant role.

Active intestinal calcium transport involves three steps: (a) the transport of calcium from the lumen into the cell; (b) the movement of calcium within the cell; and (c) the movement of calcium from the cell into the interstitial fluid. Insulation of the cell interior from the millimolar Ca concentrations of plasma suggests that a brush-border component is instrumental in the transfer of calcium into the epithelial cell. The transfer of calcium across the intestinal brush-border surface is modulated by Vitamin D (276). The early effects of 1,25-dihydroxycholecalciferol on calcium transport are mediated by changes in the structure of the luminal membrane of the intestine (277). Administration of 1,25-dihydroxycholecalciferol leads to an increase in *de novo* synthesis and total content of phosphatidylcholine of the brush-border membrane. These changes in lipid structure precede or occur simultaneously with the change in calcium transport rate (277). However, the major mechanism of calcium entry across the intestinal enterocyte brush border of the duodenum, proximal jejunum, and cecum is through a channel, CaT1 (278), which shares high homology (75%) with the renal tubular epithelial calcium channel (ECaC). Different from the ECaC, CaT1 is not regulated by 1,25-dihydroxycholecalciferol (278). CaT1 is voltage-dependent and permeant to Sr and Ba but not Mg. It is inhibited by the trivalent cations Gd and La, and the divalent Cd and Co.

Less is known about the movement of calcium within the intestinal cell. When calcium enters the cell, it either diffuses or is carried across the cell to the basolateral membrane, where it is pumped out into the serosal medium. Studies suggest that calcium entering through the apical membrane is accumulated in subcellular organelles within the terminal web of the microvillus. This process is stimulated by 1,25-dihydroxycholecalciferol through nongenomic mechanisms (279,280). Calmodulin is the major calcium binding protein in the microvillus (281,282). Its concentration in the microvillus is increased by 1,25-dihydroxycholecalciferol by redistribution from the cytosol. No new calmodulin synthesis is required or observed after 1,25-dihydroxycholecalciferol administration (282). Calmodulin is thought to play a major role in calcium transport within the microvillus, whereas calbindin is thought to be the dominant calcium binding protein in the cytoplasm. The hypothesis put forth by Bikle et al. (281,282) is that calmodulin and myosin 1 regulate calcium movement within the microvillus to where calcium accumulates within intracellular organelles through the action of calbindin. Movement in the intracellular organelle provides

calcium access to the efflux mechanisms. Thus, calcium is transported across the cell without affecting cytoplasmic calcium levels. Specific calcium binding proteins have been demonstrated in the mucosal cells of the intestine of many species (283–286). Their molecular weights are 8,000 to 25,000 and they are referred to as calbindins. Calbindins are transcriptionally regulated by Vitamin D, and calbindin-$_{9K}$ is present in intestinal mucosal cells, whereas calbindin-$_{25K}$ is present in distal renal tubular cells involved in active transepithelial Ca^{2+} transport and the brain, but not in bone or other cells. The time course of the calbindins' appearance after Vitamin D treatment is similar to the time course of changes in calcium transport; and they are localized in the glycocalyx surface of the brush border of the mucosal intestinal cells. The exact role of these proteins in calcium transport by mucosal cells is still unknown, but it appears to be related to movement of calcium from the entry channel to a shuttle mechanism delivering it to the cell exit mechanism. Increased intestinal calcium absorption is accompanied by an increase in calbindin levels without changes in their intrinsic binding affinity (K_m) for calcium.

Calcium movement from the mucosa to the serosal surface of the intestinal epithelia occurs against a concentration gradient. This suggests that the intestinal cells contain a "pump" capable of moving calcium against an electrochemical gradient. The basolateral membrane of intestinal cells has a calcium-dependent ATPase that serves this pump function and whose activity is increased by Vitamin D. The increase in calcium ATPase parallels the change in calcium transport after Vitamin D repletion. Delivery of intracellular calcium to the exit pump is a process largely unknown but appears to involve calbindins.

Many factors regulate intestinal calcium absorption including (a) dietary calcium intake; (b) Vitamin D intake; (c) age of the patient; (d) the general state of calcium balance; and (e) circulating levels of PTH, which all affect active transport. In addition to PTH and Vitamin D, other factors such as phosphate influence calcium absorption. High-phosphate diets decrease calcium absorption, possibly due to decreased 1,25-dihydroxycholecalciferol synthesis secondary to hyperphosphatemia and to the formation of relatively insoluble calcium–phosphate complexes that decrease the availability of calcium for transepithelial uptake. Experimentally, large concentrations of lactose or other sugars (mannose, xylose) or certain amino acids (lysine, arginine) inhibit intestinal calcium absorption. The physiologic significance of these observations is unknown. The decreased calcium absorption produced by glucocorticoids has therapeutic implications in the management of hypercalcemic disorders associated with excessive intake or increased sensitivity to Vitamin D.

Renal Handling of Calcium

In humans who have a GFR of 170 L per 24 hours and serum ultrafilterable calcium concentrations of 6 mg/dL, roughly 10 g of calcium is filtered per day. The amount of calcium

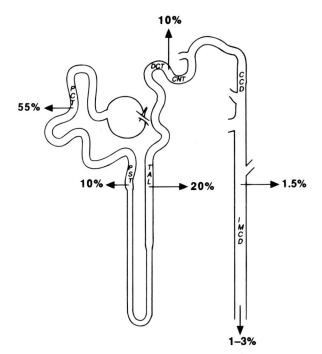

FIG. 88-7. Schematic illustration of the reabsorption of calcium by different segments of the nephron. CCD, cortical collecting duct; CNT, connecting tubule; DCT, distal convoluted tubule; IMCD, intermedullary collecting duct; PCT, proximal convoluted tubule; PST, proximal straight tubule; TAL, thick ascending limb. (From Friedman P, Gesek F. Calcium transport in renal epithelial cells. *Am J Physiol* 1993;264:F181, with permission.)

excreted in the urine usually ranges from 100 to 200 mg per 24 hours; hence, 98% to 99% of the filtered load of calcium is reabsorbed by the renal tubular intestine (Fig. 88-6). There are remarkable similarities in the handling of calcium and sodium by the kidney. Less than 2% of their filtered load is excreted normally, and there is no evidence of tubular secretion of either calcium or sodium in the mammalian nephron. Urinary excretion of either sodium or calcium is controlled by adjustments in tubular reabsorption. Approximately 60% of the filtered calcium is reabsorbed in the PCT (Fig. 88-7), 20% to 30% in the loop of Henle, 10% by the distal convoluted tubule, and 5% by the collecting system. The terminal nephron (connecting segment, distal tubule, and collecting duct), although responsible for the reabsorption of only 5% to 10% of the filtered calcium load, is the major site for regulation of calcium excretion.

Calcium in the Glomerular Filtrate

Micropuncture studies of the kidney in the Munich-Wistar rat with surface glomeruli have demonstrated that the ratio of calcium in fluid of Bowman's space to plasma (TF/P calcium) is 0.6, indicating that only the serum calcium not bound to protein is filterable (191). Thus, approximately 60% of the total calcium, which is the ultrafilterable calcium, is filtered across the glomerulus.

Proximal Convoluted Tubule

Potential factors regulating calcium reabsorption in the PCT include convection (solvent drag), concentration (increased calcium concentration in tubular fluid due to absorption of sodium and water), and transepithelial potential difference. Microperfusion studies of the rabbit PCT *in vitro* (287,288) and micropuncture of the rat *in vivo* (289) indicate that fluid absorption and solvent drag, as well as diffusion along an electrochemical gradient, contribute to net calcium flux. The reabsorption of calcium in the PCT parallels that of sodium and water: The ratio of tubular fluid to plasma ultrafilterable calcium in the earliest portion of the PCT rises to 1.1 and remains at this value along the rest of the PCT. This is compatible with passive calcium reabsorption secondary to sodium and water reabsorption along most of the PCT. The transepithelial movement occurs through the paracellular pathway across the tight junction. Although the passive movement of calcium through a paracellular pathway accounts for most of the calcium transport across the proximal tubule, there is evidence of an active transport component in this segment of the nephron (Fig. 88-7) (287,289–291). During stop-flow microperfusion experiments measuring net PCT efflux, Ullrich et al. demonstrated that the tubular fluid calcium concentration was lower than that in the capillary (289). They calculated the active transport rate as 3.4×10^{-13} mol/cm per second, which is in the range of 20% to 30% of the total reabsorptive rate for this segment.

The reabsorption of calcium transcellularly rather than through intercellular channels is a multistep process in which calcium enters the cell across apical membrane and exits across basolateral plasma membranes. Calcium-permeable channels in PCT cells have been described (292–295). However, these are activated by membrane stretch and therefore are thought to participate in cell volume regulation (295). Basolateral efflux of calcium PCTs may be mediated in whole or in part by Na^+-Ca^{2+} exchange (289,296–299).

Proximal Straight Tubule (Pars Recta)

Calcium is transported in the pars recta by a process that is not inhibited by ouabain (300). Because ouabain abolishes water and sodium transport, this suggests that the sodium–calcium exchange is not the major mechanism for calcium extrusion across the basolateral membrane in this segment of the nephron. Approximately one-third of the calcium transported can be attributed to sodium and water, and thus, it would seem that an active transport component plays an important role in the reabsorption of calcium in the proximal straight tubule.

Loop of Henle

Neither the thin descending limb nor the thin ascending limb of Henle's loop plays an important role in calcium reabsorption (300). In contrast, *in vitro* studies have shown that the TAL of Henle's loop reabsorbs calcium from lumen to bath

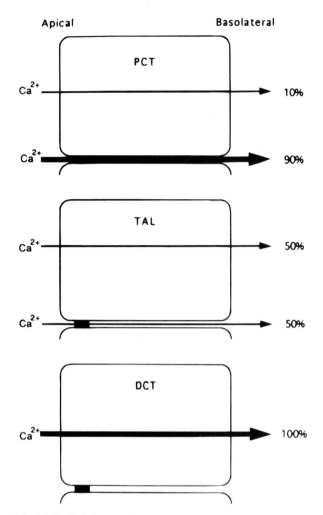

FIG. 88-8. Cellular and paracellular calcium transport pathways along the nephron. Relative percentage of calcium absorbed by cellular or paracellular pathways in the proximal convoluted tubule (PCT), thick ascending limb (TAL), and distal convoluted tubule (DCT). (From Friedman P, Gesek F. Calcium transport in renal epithelial cells. *Am J Physiol* 1993;264:F181, with permission.)

in the absence of water movement. About 20% of the filtered calcium is reabsorbed in this segment of the nephron. The transepithelial flux of calcium is proportional to the positive transepithelial potential gradient generated by sodium chloride transport mechanisms (301–303). Much of this flux is probably paracellular. Studies of the TAL suggest that the flux ratio for calcium may be greater than can be accounted for by the positive intraluminal potential; thus, an additional active transport process for calcium is present in this segment (304–306), and it accounts for up to 50% of the total calcium transported (Fig. 88-8). This transcellular component is regulated by PTH (307,308) and calcitonin in the cortical and medullary TALs, respectively (309).

Under resting conditions, Ca^{2+} transport is passive in the TAL. Changes in the electrochemical drive for Ca^{2+} determine the magnitude of passive, paracellular absorption. Under these circumstances, the transepithelial voltage is the primary determinant of the driving force, and the magnitude of the voltage, oriented electropositive in the lumen, is set by the rate of Na^+ absorption. As Na^+ absorption increases, transepithelial voltage increases (310,311) and Ca^{2+} flux increases. Peptide hormones that enhance Na^+ transport and thereby increase the transepithelial voltage in medullary TALs would be expected to stimulate passive Ca^{2+} absorption. Extensive evidence consistent with this model has been provided (312–314). Inhibition of Na^+ absorption reduces the transepithelial voltage and would be expected to decrease passive calcium absorption. Furosemide, bumetanide, and ethacrynic acid, which block sodium transport in the TAL of Henle's loop, also block calcium transport. Paracellin-1 (PCLN1) is a member of the claudin family of epithelial tight junction proteins (315), and mutations in the *PCLN1* gene produce a syndrome of renal magnesium wasting, hypercalciuria, and nephrocalcinosis (316). This proves that the tight junction of the TAL has a specific permeability for calcium that participates in the voltage-dependent paracellular flux of the cation.

Distal Convoluted Tubule, Connecting Tubule, and Collecting Tubule

Calcium transport in these segments is an active process. It occurs against an electrochemical gradient, and the epithelium is "tight," with very little fluid or electrolyte flux through the paracellular route. Free flow micropuncture studies in the rat demonstrate that TF_{Ca2+}/UF_{Ca2+} falls from a value of 0.6 in the early PCT to 0.3 by the early portion of the cortical collecting duct. This is consistent with active transcellular calcium movement.

Active transcellular Ca^{2+} absorption in the distal convoluted tubule and connecting tubule is a three-step process. Ca^{2+} enters the cell across apical plasma membranes, diffuses across the cytosol bound to calcium binding proteins, and is actively extruded from the cell across basolateral membranes (Fig. 88-9). The mechanism of Ca^{2+} entry into the cells was defined with the expression cloning of the ECaC (317), (Fig. 88-10). Apical influx is considered the rate-limiting step in transcellular calcium transport, and therefore, the regulatory target of stimulatory and inhibitory hormones (318). Evidence suggests that hormonal stimuli of Ca^{2+} transport produce an insertion of calcium channels into the apical membrane (319). Furthermore, thiazide diuretics stimulate Ca^{2+} transport in this segment (320,321). Thiazides produce their diuretic action by inhibiting a, Na^+-Cl^- cotransport mechanism of the apical membrane (320–322). How this is translated into a stimulation of Ca^{2+} transport was elucidated by Shimizu et al. (321) and Bordeau and Lau (255) (Fig. 88-11). In the presence of inhibited apical Na^+ entry, there is increased Na^+ flux into the cell across the basolateral membranes, which is coupled to Ca^{2+} extrusion, in other words actuation of a basolateral Na^+-Ca^{2+} exchanger. This nephron segment is also characterized by a hormonally regulated isoform of the Ca-ATPase, PMCA1B, found only in epithelia

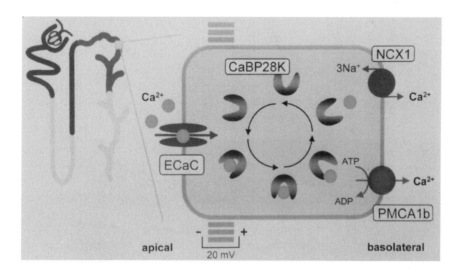

FIG. 88-9. Model of transcellular Ca^{2+} transport by cells lining the distal part of the nephron. Entry of Ca^{2+} is facilitated by the apical epithelial Ca^{2+} channel (ECaC). Subsequently, the ion binds to calbindin-D_{28K} (CaBP28K) and diffuses through the cytosol to the basolateral membrane. Here, Ca^{2+} ions are extruded by a Na^+-Ca^{2+} exchanger (NCX1) and a Ca^{2+}-ATPase (PMCA1b). (From Hoenderop JGJ, Willems PHGM, Bindels RJM. Toward a comprehensive molecular model of active calcium reabsorption. *Am J Physiol Renal* 2000;278:F352, with permission.) (See Color Figure 88-9 following page 2624.)

involved in active Ca^{2+} transport (266) (Fig. 88-9). In addition, the Vitamin D–regulated calcium binding protein, calbindin-$_{28K}$, associated with Ca^{2+} transport is also localized in the distal tubule (323) (Fig. 88-9).

The apical Na-Cl cotransport, which is thiazide sensitive, appears mainly in the connecting tubule. In the distal tubule and the collecting duct, Na^+ entry occurs through an apical, amiloride-sensitive Na^+ channel (322,324). Amiloride also stimulates Ca^{2+} reabsorption in these segments. The mechanism appears to be, as for thiazides, a limitation of apical Na^+ entry stimulating basolateral Na^+ entry through an Na^+-Ca^{2+} exchange, activating Ca^{2+} efflux (Fig. 88-11).

Factors that Regulate Calcium Transport

Maneuvers such as administration of PTH (17,325,326), cAMP (303), and calcitonin (327), ECF volume expansion (190), insulin administration (328,329), and phosphate depletion (4,330,331) have all been shown to inhibit proximal tubular reabsorption of calcium and increase the delivery of calcium to the more distal nephron segments. The effect of these maneuvers on urinary calcium excretion, however, may be a decrease, no change, or an increase in calcium excretion, emphasizing again the critical role of the distal tubule in the final regulation of calcium excretion. Both metabolic acidosis (332) and phosphate depletion (40,330,331) are accompanied

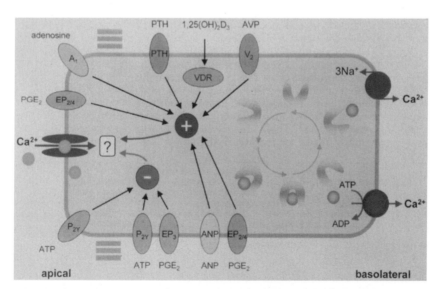

FIG. 88-10. Schematic model for hormonal regulation of transcellular Ca^{2+} transport in distal nephron. Parathyroid hormone (PTH), V_2, atrial natriuretic peptide (ANP), and EP_3 receptors are localized in the basolateral membrane, whereas A_1 is present in the apical membrane. $EP_{2/4}$ and P_{2Y} are present in both membranes 1,25-dihydroxycholecalciferol passes plasma membranes and binds to the intracellular Vitamin D receptor (VDR). Hormones can be divided into stimulatory hormones, including PTH, arginine vasopressin, ANP, prostaglandin E_2 (PGE_2) (via $EP_{2/4}$), and adenosine, and inhibitory hormones such as adenosine triphosphate and PGE_2 (via EP_3). (From Hoenderop JGJ, Willems PHGM, Bindels RJM. Toward a comprehensive molecular model of active calcium reabsorption. *Am J Physiol Renal* 2000;278:F352, with permission.) (See Color Figure 88-10 following page 2624.)

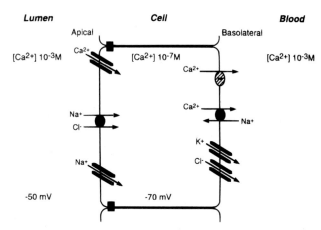

Lumen **Cell** **Blood**

Apical Basolateral

$[Ca^{2+}]$ $10^{-3}M$ Ca^{2+} $[Ca^{2+}]$ $10^{-7}M$ $[Ca^{2+}]$ $10^{-3}M$

Ca^{2+}

Ca^{2+}

Na^+ Na^+
Cl^-

K^+

Na^+ Cl^-

-50 mV   -70 mV

FIG. 88-11. Model of Ca^{2+} transport in distal convoluted tubule, connecting tubule, and cortical collecting duct cells. Transport mechanisms involved in apical Ca^{2+} entry (channels) and basolateral efflux (Ca^{2+}-ATPase and Na^+-Ca^{2+} exchange) are depicted. Other transport proteins whose action impinges on Ca^{2+} absorption (apical Na^+-Cl cotransport, Na^+ channels, basolateral Cl channels, and basolateral K^+ channels) are shown. The apical Na^+-Cl cotransport is inhibited by thiazide diuretics, whose action on Ca^{2+} transport is thought to be a limitation of Na^+ availability, leading to increased activity of the basolateral Na^+-Ca^{2+} exchange, causing increased Ca^{2+} efflux. This would assume basal activity of Ca^{2+} channel activity. The dependency of the thiazide effect on the presence of parathyroid hormone (PTH) would be expected because PTH stimulates insertion of Ca^{2+} channels into the apical membrane. (From Friedman P, Gesek F. Calcium transport in renal epithelial cells. *Am J Physiol* 1993;264:F181, with permission.)

by increased calcium excretion in the urine. Experimental studies in animals suggest that the "defect" in calcium reabsorption in metabolic acidosis (332) and phosphate depletion (331) is located in the distal tubule and probably through an effect on the ECaC (333), although phosphate depletion may also affect calcium transport in the proximal tubule. The administration of sodium bicarbonate, which rapidly corrects acidosis, increases calcium reabsorption in the late distal tubule. Similar results are found when phosphate is given to an animal that has been previously phosphate depleted.

PTH plays an important role in the regulation of calcium transport and reduces urinary calcium excretion. In humans, the status of the parathyroid gland greatly influences the amount of calcium excreted in the urine. At equal filtered loads of calcium, patients with high levels of circulating PTH have less calcium in the urine than those in whom the levels of PTH in serum are low. Experimental evidence indicates the main effect of PTH is in the connecting tubule (258,321,334) and is mediated through the adenylate cyclase system. Although PTH inhibits proximal tubular reabsorption of sodium and calcium, the main action of PTH is localized in more distal segments of the nephron.

Studies in rabbits have shown a PTH-sensitive calcium transport mechanism in the cortical TAL (325,326). Little is known about how PTH affects the paracellular pathway for Na^+ and Ca^{2+} reabsorption of the PCT. Studies in

isolated renal cortical brush-border membrane vesicles indicate that PTH mimics the effect of membrane phosphorylation on calcium binding and translocation (335). Phosphorylation of brush-border membrane vesicles produces an increase in membrane-bound calcium due to production of negatively charged phospholipids (336). Aminoglycosides compete for the binding of calcium to phospholipids. In the presence of a chemical potential for calcium, PTH also stimulates calcium binding that is aminoglycoside inhibitable, as well as an increase in the brush-border membrane content of the acidic phospholipids produced by phosphorylation (336). The control of calcium efflux across the basolateral membrane of the PCT by PTH involves the Na^+-Ca^{2+} exchange. Scoble et al. (299) and Jayakumar et al. (337) demonstrated sodium gradient (outside > inside) dependent of calcium efflux stimulated by PTH in basolateral membrane vesicles from dog and rat renal cortex. These studies were thought to use membranes from the proximal tubule. However, more recent studies suggested that the Na^+-Ca^{2+} exchange activity is the highest in the distal tubule and the earlier studies may have been affected by contaminants from these segments (338).

PTH stimulation of Ca^{2+} transport in the TAL of Henle's loop is localized to the cortical portion, whereas the calcitonin effect is exerted in the medullary portion. Because PTH does not stimulate Na^+ or Cl^- transport, it is unlikely that it works to increase the lumen-positive transepithelial electrical driving force. Rather, its main action has been suggested to be at the level of the permeability to Ca^{2+} of the paracellular pathway (339,340) and to be related to the function of PCLN1. Recent thought indicates that an effect on transcellular transport may be involved (341).

Significant progress has been made in the understanding of PTH actions on Ca^{2+} transport in the connecting tubule and the cortical collecting duct. Here, Ca^{2+} reabsorption is transcellular and an active energy consuming process. Studies (341,342) suggest that PTH hyperpolarizes the epithelium and produces insertion of voltage-operated Ca^{2+} channels in the apical membrane (319,341). Patch clamp studies of PTH-stimulated distal convoluted tubule cells (341,343) demonstrated an increase in open time of apical membrane channels with increasing membrane voltage (342). However, these findings remain controversial (341–343), and the mechanism of anomalous function of the apical calcium entry channel remains to be elucidated. Voltage-operated calcium channels are complex heteromultimers consisting of $\alpha 1$, $\alpha 2$, δ, γ, and β subunits. Identification of the distal nephron calcium entry channel, ECaC (317,333) (Fig. 88-10), which is insensitive to membrane potential, failed to shed light on the mechanism of calcium entry associated with hyperpolarization (344).

Plasma Calcium Concentrations

Hypocalcemia

Hypocalcemia decreases the renal excretion of calcium, secondary to a decrease in the filtered load of calcium and enhanced tubular reabsorption of calcium. Hypocalcemia triggers the release of PTH, which increases calcium reabsorption in the TAL and distal tubule. The effects on the TAL could also be observed in TPTX (345). Recent studies have indicated that the calcium sensor receptor (CaSR) plays an important role in the enhancement of calcium transport in the TAL during hypocalcemia (346,347).

Hypercalcemia

In general, patients with hypercalcemia have increased amounts of calcium in the urine, partly due to an increase in the filtered load of calcium and partly to suppression of PTH secretion. Activation of the CaSR also may increase the excretion of calcium by decreasing the activity of the apical K^+ channel and decreasing the positive potential difference (PD). Thus, less calcium and magnesium are reabsorbed via the paracellular pathway in the TAL (348).

Volume Status

Volume contraction decreases and volume expansion increases the renal excretion of sodium and calcium. Volume expansion decreases tubular reabsorption of both sodium and calcium even if the filtered load is reduced (349), clearly demonstrating that the regulation of these ions is primarily by changes in tubular reabsorption.

Diuretics

Furosemide produces a significant increase in Na^+ and Ca^{2+} excretion by inhibiting the reabsorption of both ions in the TAL (350). Furosemide decreases the PD in the TAL. Because the reabsorption of calcium in this segment of the nephron is passive, a decrease in the positive voltage of the lumen diminishes the movement of calcium through the paracellular pathway. Thiazide, on the other hand, produces dissociation between sodium and calcium excretion. A mild natriuresis is usually accompanied by a decrease in calcium excretion. Micropuncture studies have shown that this mechanism occurs in the distal portion of the nephron. Thiazide stimulates calcium entry through the apical Ca^{2+} channel by activating Cl channels (351). These effects are independent of PTH, although PTH is important in the presence of ECaC in the apical membrane of the connecting tubule. The chronic administration of thiazide produces significant decrease in calcium excretion secondary to volume contraction, since this effect can be reversed by the administration of NaCl.

Vitamin D

The acute administration of 1,25-dihydroxycholecalciferol increases transepithelial calcium transport by its effects on the distal, connecting, and collecting duct system. In these segments of the nephron, the transport of calcium is mainly active. 1,25-Dihydroxycholecalciferol has a positive transcriptional effect on ECAC gene transcription. In addition,

an increase in calbindin-$_{28K}$ and on the calcium ATPase in the basolateral side of the cell is also transcriptionally regulated by 1,25-dihydroxycholecalciferol (Fig. 88-9) (333).

The chronic administration of 1,25-dihydroxycholecalciferol increases the excretion of calcium secondary to an increase in the filtered load of calcium. This is due to an increase in calcium absorption in the gut and calcium resorption in the skeleton.

Hypocalcemia

The clinical manifestations of hypocalcemia vary greatly among patients (352). Patients who suddenly become hypocalcemic, such as those with postsurgical hypoparathyroidism, may develop profound symptomatology, including tetany, even after a moderate decrease in serum calcium levels. On the other hand, patients with chronic renal insufficiency adjust well to low levels of serum calcium and seldom become symptomatic. Before the pathophysiologic mechanisms responsible for the hypocalcemia can be correlated with the clinical symptomatology, it is critical to determine whether both total and ionized calcium levels are low. In conditions such as the nephrotic syndrome and cirrhosis with severe hypoalbuminemia, total serum calcium may be decreased, but ionized calcium levels may be within the normal range or only slightly decreased, and the patient remains asymptomatic.

Clinical Symptoms

Patients with significant hypocalcemia have increased neuromuscular irritability. The hallmark of hypocalcemia is tetany. Latent tetany may be detected by tapping over the facial nerves, which results in contraction of the facial muscles (Chvostek's sign), or by occluding the arterial blood supply to the forearm, which produces carpal spasm (Trousseau's sign). The symptomatology depends on the rapidity of onset of hypocalcemia. Patients with chronic renal failure occasionally have marked hypocalcemia; however, tetany is extremely rare. This may be due in part to the presence of metabolic acidosis. However, the changes in ionized calcium produced by metabolic acidosis in the majority of patients with profound hypocalcemia are not sufficient to bring the ionized calcium level back too normal. On the other hand, respiratory alkalosis due to hyperventilation can precipitate tetany. Clinically, the patient may complain of tingling in the tips of the fingers, stiff muscles, and cramps and may develop convulsions or impaired mental function. Children may develop mental retardation, and dementia may occur in adults. Extrapyramidal disorders also have been found in some patients. Psychiatric manifestations are characterized by confusion and hallucinations. Proximal muscle weakness is more frequently seen when the hypocalcemia is secondary to Vitamin D deficiency.

Severe complications include development of cataracts (353), papilledema, and rarely, optic neuritis. In general, the skin may be dry and puffy, and the patient may develop dermatitis. Hypocalcemia may produce hypotension and a delay in ventricular repolarization, thus increasing the QT interval and ST segment. Ventricular arrhythmias and atrial fibrillation refractory to digoxin (354) have been seen in patients with hypocalcemia. Because calcium, as mentioned previously, has an inotropic effect, hypocalcemia may be responsible in part for a decrease in cardiac output (355).

The pathogenetic mechanisms responsible for the development of hypocalcemia are described in Table 88-4 and

TABLE 88-4. *Causes of hypocalcemia*

I. Hypocalcemia secondary to low or absent levels of parathyroid hormone in blood
  A. Hypoparathyroidism
    1. Congenital
    2. Idiopathic
    3. DiGeorge's syndrome
    4. Postsurgical
    5. Infiltration of parathyroid glands by malignancy or amyloidosis
  B. Transient hypoparathyroidism
    1. Neonatal
    2. Postsurgical (for parathyroid adenoma)
II. Hypocalcemia secondary to a decrease in calcium mobilization from bone
  A. Vitamin D deficiency
    1. Decreased ingestion
    2. Decreased absorption (gastrointestinal disorders)
      a. Partial gastrectomy
      b. Intestinal bypass
      c. Sprue
      d. Pancreatic insufficiency
  B. 25(OH)D$_3$ deficiency
    1. Severe liver disease
      a. Biliary cirrhosis
      b. Amyloidosis
    2. Ingestion of anticonvulsant medication
    3. Nephrotic syndrome
  C. 1,25(OH)$_2$D$_3$ deficiency
    1. Advanced renal failure
    2. Severe hyperphosphatemia
    3. Hypoparathyroidism
  D. Pseudohypoparathyroidism types I and II
  E. Magnesium deficiency
III. Hypocalcemia secondary to reduced calcium absorption in the gastrointestinal tract
  A. Deficiency of Vitamin D or its metabolites
IV. Hypocalcemia secondary to translocation of calcium into different compartments
  A. Hyperphosphatemia
  B. Administration of citrate
  C. Administration of ethylenediaminetetraacetic acid
V. Miscellaneous conditions
  A. Pancreatitis
  B. Colchicine intoxication
  C. Pharmacologic dose of calcitonin
  D. Administration of mithramycin

Source: From Slatopolsky E. Pathophysiology of calcium, magnesium, and phosphorus. In: Klahr S, ed. *The kidney and body fluids in health and disease.* New York: Plenum Press, 1983:269, with permission.

include (a) absence of PTH; (b) abnormalities of Vitamin D metabolism or decreased magnesium levels that may make the bones resistant to the action of PTH; (c) a genetic disorder, "pseudohypoparathyroidism," in which the target organs do not respond to the action of PTH; (d) decreased absorption of calcium from the gut; (e) translocation of calcium between different compartments of the body; (f) increased urinary excretion of calcium; and (g) Ca-receptor gene mutations.

Hypocalcemia Secondary to Low or Absent Levels of PTH in Blood

A decrease or absence of PTH will have significant effects on calcium metabolism (1,356,357). Because PTH plays a key role in regulation osteoclasts, which are the cells responsible for bone resorption, through the production of OPGL, a decrease in the activity or in the number of these cells will eventually reduce the efflux of calcium from bone. In the absence of PTH, the capacity of the ascending portion of the loop of Henle and distal nephron to transport calcium is decreased; thus, at any filtered load of calcium, a greater amount of calcium will be excreted in the urine. Moreover, the absence of PTH decreases the activity of 1α-hydroxylase in the kidney and leads to decreased formation of 1,25-dihydroxycholecalciferol and a reduction in calcium absorption from the gastrointestinal tract. Thus, decreased mobilization of calcium from bone, excretion of larger amounts of calcium in the urine, and decreased absorption of calcium from the gut lead to profound hypocalcemia. The most common cause of hypoparathyroidism is excision or damage to the parathyroid glands at surgery. This may be secondary to thyroid or parathyroid surgery or to radical neck dissection performed for the treatment of cancer (358,359). Some patients might develop transient hypocalcemia. This phenomenon is observed in patients who have one adenoma of the parathyroid gland. The hypercalcemia produced by the excessive secretion of PTH by the adenoma usually suppresses secretion from the other glands, and the removal of the adenoma may produce a transient period of hypoparathyroidism and hypocalcemia. However, the remaining glands, if they are intact, will respond to the hypocalcemia, and this abnormality will be reversible in a relatively short period of time.

Idiopathic hypoparathyroidism is a rare disease, and tetany may occur soon after birth. Idiopathic hypoparathyroidism may be associated with congenital absence of the thymus (DiGeorge's syndrome) (360,361). These patients have depressed cell immunity and many other malformations; they frequently have mucosal candidiasis and usually die in early childhood of severe hypocalcemia or severe infections. The parathyroid gland may be suppressed at birth as a result of maternal hypercalcemia; thus, neonatal tetany should be looked for in the presence of hypercalcemia of any cause in the mother. The fetal parathyroid glands are suppressed by maternal hypercalcemia when the infant is stressed; for example, with a phosphate load (cow's milk), tetany may result.

Another factor that plays a key role in the secretion of PTH is magnesium (362–365). As will be discussed in a subsequent section, profound hypomagnesemia may decrease the release of PTH. In this syndrome, administration of magnesium to correct the hypomagnesemia increases the release of PTH within minutes.

Hypocalcemia Secondary to Decreased Calcium Mobilization from Bone

Vitamin D has a synergistic effect with PTH that increases the mobilization of calcium from bone. The mechanism by which Vitamin D and its metabolites increase bone resorption is not fully understood. Both hormones are key factors in the differentiation of osteoclasts (366,367), and both factors regulate the osteoblast through differentiation of osteoblast precursors and direct regulation of bone matrix protein gene transcription (366,367). Many disorders can alter the metabolism of Vitamin D, and different Vitamin D metabolites could be responsible for decreased mobilization of calcium from bone. In Vitamin D–deficient rickets, a nutritional condition observed in children, the lack of Vitamin D is responsible for hypocalcemia, hypophosphatemia, and mild secondary hyperparathyroidism. Disorders of the gastrointestinal tract such as partial gastrectomy, intestinal bypass, tropical and nontropical sprue, and Crohn's disease may impair the absorption of Vitamin D from the diet. Pathologic processes that involve the liver, such as hepatobiliary cirrhosis, may decrease the production of 25-hydroxycholecalciferol (368). The lack of this metabolite greatly diminishes the mineralization front, and adults with low levels of 25-hydroxycholecalciferol may develop osteomalacia. Although there may be an increase in the level of PTH, osteoclasts are unable to remove calcium because the osteoid material lacks minerals; therefore, there is decreased mobilization of calcium from bone. Administration of anticonvulsant medication may also result in low serum levels of 25-hydroxycholecalciferol, possibly due to the enhanced microsomal activity in the liver with increased catabolism of 25-hydroxycholecalciferol (369–371).

Pseudohypoparathyroidism

Another important condition is pseudohypoparathyroidism, which is a genetic disorder characterized by skeletal and somatic defects including short stature, rounded face, brachydactyly, subcutaneous calcification, and subnormal intelligence (372,373). The secretion of PTH is increased as assessed by elevated levels of immunoreactive PTH; thus, the hypocalcemia in pseudohypoparathyroidism is felt to represent a bone resistance to the effects of PTH. This syndrome is collectively referred to as Albright's hereditary osteodystrophy (AHO) (374). Many patients also have renal resistance to the action of the hormone because administration of exogenous PTH does not lead to increased urinary excretion of cAMP and phosphate. The syndrome has been subclassi-

fied as pseudohypoparathyroidism type Ia, in which there is neither a cAMP nor a phosphaturic response to exogenous PTH. These patients have approximately a 50% reduction in the guanine nucleotide binding protein G_S, which is the molecular switch between the PTH receptor and adenylate cyclase (375,376). The mRNA for G_S is also reduced about 50% in these patients (376). Heterozygous mutations of the $G_{S\alpha}$ gene have been identified in families of subjects with AHO, providing molecular confirmation that transmission of the $G_{S\alpha}$ gene defects accounts for the autosomal-dominant inheritance of AHO (377,378).

Some subjects with pseudohypoparathyroidism type I lack features of AHO. Patients with this subtype, termed pseudohypoparathyroidism type Ib, typically show hormone resistance that is limited to PTH target organs and have normal $G_{S\alpha}$ activity (379). This variant has not been defined, but it may be due to a defect in the receptor for PTH (374,380). Although patients with pseudohypoparathyroidism type Ib fail to show a nephrogenous cAMP response to PTH, they often manifest skeletal lesions similar to those that occur in patients with hyperparathyroidism (381). These observations suggest that at least one intracellular signaling pathway coupled to the PTH receptor may be intact in patients with pseudohypoparathyroidism type Ib. The molecular basis for reduced PTH receptor activity in pseudohypoparathyroidism type Ib has not been defined.

Pseudohypoparathyroidism type II, in which there is no phosphaturia despite a normal cAMP excretion rate in response to PTH (2,203,382–385), is a heterogeneous disorder. Some of these patients have low levels of 1,25-dihydroxycholecalciferol, perhaps representing renal resistance to PTH-stimulated 1α-hydroxylase activity. Thus, the high levels of PTH and the lack of response to the exogenous administration of PTH differentiate this syndrome from true hypoparathyroidism. The hyperphosphatemia that is present in this syndrome also may be partly responsible for the low levels of 1,25-dihydroxycholecalciferol. Pseudohypoparathyroidism is a heterogeneous disorder; some patients have resistance to PTH at the renal level only, others at the skeletal level, and still others in both organs.

Chronic renal failure is characterized by moderate hypocalcemia. Serum calcium seldom falls to less than 7.0 mg/dL. The pathogenesis of hypocalcemia in chronic renal failure is multifactorial. However, phosphate retention and low levels of 1,25-dihydroxycholecalciferol play a key role in its genesis (386). In patients with profound hypomagnesemia, the skeleton becomes resistant to the action of PTH, and there is decreased calcium mobilization from bone (364).

Hypocalcemia Secondary to Reduced Intestinal Calcium Absorption

A healthy individual who ingests a low-calcium diet usually does not develop hypocalcemia or develops it to a minimal degree because compensatory secondary hyperparathyroidism will correct mild hypocalcemia. Hypocalcemia is usually associated with pathologic processes of the gastrointestinal tract that affect the absorption of Vitamin D. Under these circumstances, the low absorption of calcium, plus abnormalities in Vitamin D metabolism, greatly affects calcium homeostasis, and the patient may develop profound hypocalcemia. Growing animals fed a low-calcium diet develop severe hypocalcemia.

Hypocalcemia Secondary to Translocation of Calcium into Different Compartments

Precipitation of ionized calcium is seen in disorders in which there is retention of phosphorus. Patients with advanced renal insufficiency, malignancies (151), or severe rhabdomyolysis and hyperphosphatemia (198) may precipitate calcium rapidly and may develop symptoms characterized by tremors, muscular irritability, and tetany. In the neonate, administration of cow's milk, which is high in phosphorus content compared with human milk, may produce severe hyperphosphatemia and hypocalcemia. Neonatal parathyroid function is not adequate to cope with this challenge, and the neonate may develop severe symptoms secondary to hypocalcemia. When large amounts of blood containing citrate are given to patients (open heart surgery, exchange transfusions for neonatal hyperbilirubinemia), the ionized calcium is complexed by citrate and hypocalcemia leading to tetany may develop.

Hypocalcemia Secondary to Increased Urinary Excretion of Calcium

This condition is rare and self limited. The expansion of the ECF compartment produces a remarkable decrease in the reabsorption of sodium and calcium, and large amounts of these cations may be excreted in the urine. However, these are transitory mechanisms that are rapidly corrected by the release of PTH. Thus, if the PTH, Vitamin D, and skeletal axis is intact, an increase in urinary calcium excretion should not result in significant hypocalcemia. Diuretics such as furosemide or ethacrynic acid, which block the reabsorption of calcium in the thick ascending portion of Henle's loop, are effective drugs in the treatment of hypercalcemia. However, very seldom do patients ingesting these drugs develop hypocalcemia.

Ca Receptor Gene Mutations

Defects in the human CaSRs have been shown to cause familial hypocalciuria, hypercalcemia, and neonatal severe hyperparathyroidism (387–389). Recently, Pollak et al. (390) demonstrated that a missense mutation (GLU128 Ala) in this gene causes familial hypocalcemia in affected membranes of one family. In this syndrome, an alteration in the CaSR shifts the "set point" for calcium to the left, and the parathyroid glands are hyperresponsive to extracellular calcium.

Miscellaneous Conditions

Approximately 10% to 20% of patients with acute pancreatitis develop some degree of hypocalcemia. The hypocalcemia is related to deposition of calcium salts in areas of lipolysis and tissue necrosis (391). Some investigators have postulated that proteolytic digestion of PTH may explain the lack of elevated levels of PTH in the serum of patients with acute pancreatitis. Some drugs such as calcitonin, mithramycin (used for testicular carcinoma), and colchicine (used in gout) can produce profound hypocalcemia by decreasing bone resorption. A series of disorders are characterized by increased bone formation in which the uptake of calcium by the skeleton is greatly increased. Such patients may develop profound hypocalcemia. A disorder known as "hungry bone syndrome" is seen in patients with chronic renal insufficiency and severe secondary hyperparathyroidism. The removal of the parathyroid glands in these uremic patients produces profound hypocalcemia, which sometimes is difficult to correct even with pharmacologic doses of 1,25-dihydroxycholecalciferol. Under these conditions, when the factors producing bone resorption have been removed and the osteoblastic activity is greatly increased, there is a remarkable increase in bone formation, and the greater uptake of minerals by the skeleton may produce profound hypocalcemia.

Hypercalcemia

Hypercalcemia is an elevation of total serum calcium levels to more than 10.5 mg/dL (when serum protein values are within the normal range). The manifestations of hypercalcemia differ among patients. Mild hypercalcemia may be totally asymptomatic and may be detected during routine blood chemistry tests; however, hypercalcemia may be severe enough to produce lethargy, disorientation, coma, and death.

Clinical Symptoms of Hypercalcemia

Patients with mild hypercalcemia may be totally asymptomatic; however, as serum calcium increases, usually more than 11.5 mg/dL, numerous symptoms may be present and practically every organ of the body is affected. The most common symptoms are nausea, vomiting, polyuria, polydipsia, lack of concentration, fatigue, somnolence, mental confusion, and even death (Table 88-5).

Renal Effects

Hypercalcemia may cause either an acute and reversible decrement in the GFR or a chronic nephropathy. There are numerous mechanisms by which hypercalcemia decrease the GFR (392–394). Hypercalcemia may lead to vasoconstriction of the afferent arterioles and decreased renal blood flow. It can decrease ultrafiltration across glomerular capillaries. In addition, acute hypercalcemia may produce natriuresis and ECF volume contraction. In chronic hypercalcemic nephropathy,

TABLE 88-5. *Clinical manifestations of hypercalcemia*

I. General: Apathy, lethargy, weakness
II. Cardiovascular: Cardiac arrhythmias, hypertension, vascular calcification
III. Renal: Polyuria, hypercalciuria, stones, nephrocalcinosis-impaired concentration of urine renal insufficiency
IV. Gastrointestinal: Anorexia, nausea, vomiting, polydipsia, constipation, abdominal pain, gastric ulcer, pancreatitis
V. Neuropsychiatric and muscular: Headache, impaired concentration, loss of memory, confusion, hallucination, coma, myalgia, muscle weakness, arthralgia
VI. Metastatic calcification: Band keratopathy, conjunctival irritation, vascular calcification, periarticular calcification

Source: From Slatopolsky E. Pathophysiology of calcium, magnesium, and phosphorus. In: Klahr S, ed. *The kidney and body fluids in health and disease.* New York: Plenum Press, 1983:269, with permission.

there is a fall in the GFR and a decrease in the maximum urinary concentrating capacity, and the urine is free of cells or casts, although mild proteinuria may be observed. The findings are similar to those seen in patients with interstitial nephritis. The characteristic abnormality of hypercalcemic nephropathy is an inability to concentrate the urine (395–397). This abnormality persists even after the administration of antidiuretic hormone (ADH) (398). The mechanisms by which hypercalcemia impairs concentration of the urine are multiple (399–401). The osmotic gradient of the medulla is decreased, partly because of decreased sodium transport in the thick ascending portion of the loop of Henle. Moreover, hypercalcemia decreases the permeability of the collecting duct to water by inhibiting the adenylate cyclase activity and generation of cAMP in response to ADH. There is some evidence to suggest that increased prostaglandin synthesis may mediate part of this effect. Prostaglandin E_2 (PGE_2) enhances medullary blood flow, inhibits sodium chloride transport in the loop of Henle, and antagonizes the effect of ADH on the collecting duct (402). It is possible that several of the effects of hypercalcemia on the concentrating mechanism are related to increased prostaglandin synthesis in the medulla. Thus, a salt-wasting nephropathy and the inability to concentrate the urine may explain some of the symptoms such as polyuria and polydipsia seen in patients with hypercalcemia. Chronic persistent hypercalcemia eventually leads to the development of nephrocalcinosis, most commonly localized to the medulla of the kidney.

Gastrointestinal Manifestations

Anorexia, nausea, and vomiting are frequently seen in patients with hypercalcemia. Occasionally, abdominal pain, distention, and ileus may be present (403). There is an increased incidence of peptic ulcer in patients with primary hyperparathyroidism, and it has been shown that calcium increases the release of gastrin and hydrochloric acid in the stomach. Moreover, the incidence of pancreatitis is also greatly increased. Several mechanisms have been implicated in the

development of pancreatitis. Usually, hypercalcemia increases pancreatic enzyme secretion, and intraductal proteins may cause obstruction of the pancreatic duct. Enhanced conversion of trypsinogen to trypsin due to elevated calcium levels may contribute to the inflammatory process.

Cardiovascular Effects

Calcium has an inotropic effect on the cardiovascular system. Calcium increases peripheral resistance, and hypertension occurs in 20% to 30% of patients with chronic hypercalcemia (404–406). Renal parenchymal damage with elevated levels of renin, increased cardiac output, and severe vasoconstriction may participate in the development of hypertension. The most significant change in the electrocardiogram is a shortening of the QT interval. Because the positive inotropic effect of digitalis is enhanced by calcium, digitalis toxicity may be aggravated by hypercalcemia.

Neurologic and Psychiatric Effects of Hypercalcemia

Patients with hypercalcemia are frequently admitted to psychiatric wards because of nonspecific complaints characterized by lethargy, apathy, depression, and decreased memory. Patients with hypercalcemia secondary to increased PTH levels have electroencephalographic changes that are reversible after removal of the parathyroid adenoma. Moreover, the administration of large doses of PTH to dogs results in increased brain calcium and changes in the electroencephalogram (407).

Metastatic Calcification

Patients with hypercalcemia may develop band keratopathy, which is the appearance of corneal calcification. The changes in the cornea are usually permanent. However, conjunctival irritation disappears after correction of the hypercalcemia. Arterial and periarticular calcifications are observed more frequently in patients who have some degree of renal insufficiency, especially those who also have hyperphosphatemia.

Hypercalcemia

Pathologically, three general mechanisms may lead to the development of hypercalcemia (Table 88-6): (a) increased mobilization of calcium from bone, by far the most common and important mechanism, (b) increased absorption of calcium from the gastrointestinal tract, and (c) decreased urinary excretion of calcium (of minor importance). In some clinical disorders, although one or more of these mechanisms may be operative, compensatory adaptations develop and hypercalcemia may not occur. For example, in idiopathic hypercalciuria due to increased calcium absorption from the gastrointestinal tract, increased urinary excretion of calcium may prevent the development of hypercalcemia. On the other hand, in hyperparathyroidism, all three mechanisms (increased bone resorption, augmented gastrointestinal absorption of

TABLE 88-6. *Causes of hypercalcemia*

I. Hypercalcemia secondary to increased calcium mobilization from bone
  A. Malignancy
    1. Metastatic
    2. Nonmetastatic
      a. Osteoclastic-activating factor
      b. Prostaglandin E_2
      c. Ectopic hyperparathyroidism
  B. Hyperparathyroidism
    1. Primary
      a. Adenoma
      b. Hyperplasia
      c. Neoplastic
    2. Secondary
    3. Multiple endocrine neoplasias
      a. Type I with pituitary and pancreatic tumors
      b. Type II with medullary carcinoma of thyroid and pheochromocytoma
  C. Immobilization
  D. Hyperthyroidism
  E. Vitamin D intoxication
  F. Renal disease
    1. Chronic renal failure
    2. After renal transplantation
    3. Diuretic phase of acute renal failure
  G. Vitamin A intoxication
II. Hypercalcemia secondary to an increase in calcium absorption from the gastrointestinal tract
  A. Sarcoidosis
  B. Vitamin D intoxication
  C. Milk-alkali syndrome
III. Hypercalcemia secondary to a decrease in urinary calcium excretion
  A. Thiazide diuretics
  B. Familial hypocalciuric hypercalcemia
IV. Miscellaneous
  A. Adrenal insufficiency
  B. Tuberculosis
  C. Berylliosis
  D. Dysproteinemias
  E. Hemoconcentration
  F. Hyperalimentation regimens

Source: From Slatopolsky E. Pathophysiology of calcium, magnesium, and phosphorus. In: Klahr S. *The kidney and body fluids in health and disease.* New York: Plenum Press, 1983:269, with permission.

calcium, and decreased urinary calcium excretion) lead to the development of hypercalcemia.

Hypercalcemia Secondary to Increased Calcium Mobilization from Bone

Hypercalcemia Secondary to Malignancies/Humoral Hypercalcemia of Malignancy

Malignancy is the most common cause of hypercalcemia. Multiple mechanisms underlie the development of hypercalcemia of malignancy, but in general, it is due to a combined disorder of increased mobilization of calcium from the skeleton secondary to increased bone resorption by osteoclasts and variable decreases in the renal excretion of calcium. This increased resorption could be due to the action of malignant cells that have metastasized to bone from tumors of such organs as the breast, prostate, kidney, lung, and thyroid (408–411). The tumor cells in the bone metastasis produce locally active cytokines that stimulate production of active osteoclasts. However, on some occasions, hypercalcemia occurs with no evidence of bone metastasis, and generally, the removal of the tumor results in correction of the hypercalcemia. In these cases, humoral agents are involved. The major humoral osteoclast-stimulating factor is PTH-related peptide (PTHrP) (412,413). This factor, which is an endogenous paracrine of the mammary glands, oviduct, fibroblasts, and vascular smooth muscle, has sufficient homology with PTH in its amino terminal region to act through PTH receptors on PTH target cells such as the osteoblast and the distal connecting tubule. Thus, its production by tumors mimics the action of high PTH levels in stimulating bone resorption and renal calcium retention. PTHrP accounts for about 80% of the hypercalcemia associated with malignancies. Other mechanisms of hypercalcemia due to tumors include secretion of PGE_2 (414–417), especially by solid tumors, the production of tumor necrosis factor β, as in patients with multiple myeloma and lymphosarcoma (418–421), and the secretion of IL-1 and TGFβ The latter factors are often produced in association with PTHrP. TGFβ works through epidermal growth factor receptors and stimulates bone resorption. Its production is highly prevalent (40%) in tumors associated with hypercalcemia, and it may play a secondary role in association with many cases in which PTHrP is being produced. In metastatic bone disease, there are usually two effects: (a) an increase in bone resorption and (b) an increase in woven bone formation. If the osteoblastic process (bone formation) predominates, hypercalcemia may not develop. However, if the osteolytic process predominates, the patient develops severe hypercalciuria and hypercalcemia. In contrast to tumors that produce a "parathyroid-like material," the serum phosphorus level or the tubular reabsorption of phosphate usually is not decreased in metastatic bone disease. However, the patient may develop hypophosphatemia when the disease progresses and malnutrition becomes evident. Although many tumors may secrete PTHrP (59 of 72 cases with hypercalcemia) (422), the two most important ones are the epidermoid squamous cell carcinoma of the lung and renal cell carcinoma. About 10% of patients with hypercalcemia of malignancy have elevated levels of circulating immunoreactive PTH (422). Most often this is due to coexistent parathyroid disease and malignancy (422).

Primary Hyperparathyroidism

Primary hyperparathyroidism is the most common endocrine disorder causing hypercalcemia. It is probably the major cause of asymptomatic hypercalcemia in young people. A single adenoma of the parathyroid gland is the most common cause of primary hyperparathyroidism. In contrast, chief cell hyperplasia is the lesion seen in practically all patients with secondary hyperparathyroidism caused by renal insufficiency. The incidence of primary hyperparathyroidism increases substantially in both men and women older than 50 years but is two to four times more common in women. The mechanism of hypercalcemia is related to the effects of PTH. The levels of PTH measurable by radioimmunoassay are elevated in primary hyperparathyroidism. The percentage of positive results to confirm the diagnosis depends on the type of antibody used and the sensitivity of each particular radioimmunoassay for PTH. Sensitive assays, using a carboxyterminal antibody, demonstrate elevated levels of PTH in 90% to 95% of patients with primary hyperparathyroidism. As PTH increases the activity and number of osteoclasts, bone resorption is seen on bone histology. X-ray films of the phalanges show subperiosteal bone resorption. The increased calcium mobilization from bone raises the filtered load of calcium and leads to the development of hypercalciuria despite the effect of PTH in increasing the reabsorption of calcium in the distal nephron. Moreover, the hypercalcemia is aggravated by increased calcium absorption from the gut secondary to high levels of 1,25-dihydroxycholecalciferol in response to high levels of PTH in blood. PTH decreases the renal reabsorption of phosphorus in the proximal and distal tubules, resulting in hypophosphatemia. Patients with primary hyperparathyroidism have a high incidence of peptic ulcer, renal stones, soft tissue calcification, neuromuscular disease, and psychiatric disorders. Because hypercalcemia interferes with the renal countercurrent mechanism responsible for the concentration of the urine, the patient develops polyuria and polydipsia. By measuring ionized calcium and immunoreactive PTH, some laboratories have been able to establish the diagnosis of primary hyperparathyroidism in more than 95% of cases (423). The treatment of this condition is surgery (parathyroidectomy), except in mild cases of asymptomatic hypercalcemia (plasma calcium concentration of less than 11 mg/dL), especially in older adults (424,425).

Immobilization

Patients who are immobilized for several days develop some degree of hypercalciuria. However, some of these patients may develop hypercalcemia (404). This occurs in diseases involving increased bone turnover such as Paget's disease. Hypercalcemia is seen frequently in immobilized patients with multiple fractures. It seems that prolonged periods of immobilization disrupt the balance between bone resorption and formation. The resorptive process predominates because of the depression of osteoblastic activity, and calcium mobilization occurs.

Hyperthyroidism

Serum calcium concentration may increase in thyrotoxicosis. Usually the increment is mild and does not produce severe symptoms. Bone histology reveals an increase in osteoclastic bone resorption and fibroblastic proliferation resembling osteitis fibrosa cystica. Moreover, patients with thyrotoxicosis who present with hypercalcemia usually have low or undetectable levels of PTH in blood.

Vitamin D Intoxication

Vitamin D increases both calcium absorption from the gastrointestinal tract and bone resorption. Metabolites of Vitamin D have been shown to increase the efflux of calcium from bone *in vitro*. Moreover, administration of 1,25-dihydroxycholecalciferol to dogs fed low-calcium diets leads to hypercalcemia, suggesting that the effect on bone was responsible for the rise in extracellular calcium. The manifestations of Vitamin D intoxication are probably secondary to high levels of 25-hydroxycholecalciferol in blood, because the circulating levels of 1,25-dihydroxycholecalciferol remain within the normal range. Of course, if a patient receives pharmacologic doses of 1,25-dihydroxycholecalciferol, this metabolite of Vitamin D may produce toxic effects and the characteristic hypercalcemia.

Renal Disease

Hypercalcemia is rare in patients with *chronic renal failure* (426). Most patients with renal disease have hypocalcemia, which leads to the development of secondary hyperparathyroidism. However, hypercalcemia has been described in patients with chronic renal failure. The mechanism is not fully understood. Potentially, the extreme hyperplasia of the parathyroid glands, which may develop in these patients, progresses to a point at which they no longer respond to normal feedback mechanisms. Thus, a greater degree of hypercalcemia may be necessary to suppress PTH secretion by such enlarged glands. In some patients, hypercalcemia may be seen after significant reductions of serum phosphorus levels or after ingestion of large amounts of calcium carbonate.

More recently, a mineralization defect has been described in a substantial number of patients maintained on chronic hemodialysis (3,426). It has been shown that aluminum deposition in the interface between osteoid and mineralized bone is responsible for this defect. Many of these patients have mild hypercalcemia and relatively low levels of PTH.

Hypercalcemia occurs more frequently *after a successful renal transplantation* than in patients with chronic renal insufficiency (426). Because patients receiving kidney transplants usually have severe secondary hyperparathyroidism, the amount of 1,25-dihydroxycholecalciferol produced by the new kidney, if the graft is successful, is greatly increased due to both high levels of PTH and decreased serum phosphate levels due to the marked phosphaturia after the transplantation. Synergistically, 1,25-dihydroxycholecalciferol and PTH would increase calcium mobilization from bone, leading to hypercalcemia. Obviously, 1,25-dihydroxycholecalciferol also increases calcium absorption from the gastrointestinal tract. In most patients, the hypercalcemia does not require specific treatment and subsides after 3 to 4 weeks. However, in some patients, specific measures should be taken to prevent nephrocalcinosis, and if the hypercalcemia is severe and persists for several months or years, the patient may require surgical parathyroidectomy.

Vitamin A Intoxication

This is a very rare cause of hypercalcemia and is seen more frequently in children than adults (427,428).

Hypercalcemia Secondary to Increased Calcium Absorption from the Gastrointestinal Tract

There are several clinical entities such as sarcoidosis, Vitamin D intoxication, and milk alkali syndrome that are characterized by increased calcium absorption from the gut and positive calcium balance. Some patients also have widespread soft tissue calcification and nephrocalcinosis. Most of these patients have low or undetectable levels of PTH.

Sarcoidosis

About 10% to 20% of patients with sarcoidosis have mild hypercalcemia (429). Although this abnormality is secondary to an increase in calcium absorption, controversy still exists about the mechanism responsible for the increased calcium absorption. Serum levels of 1,25-dihydroxycholecalciferol may be elevated in sarcoidosis, but this is not uniform (430, 431). Recent studies in an anephric patient with sarcoidosis with high levels of 1,25-dihydroxycholecalciferol (430) clearly indicate an extrarenal production of 1,25-dihydroxycholecalciferol in sarcoidosis. Adams et al. (432) demonstrated that alveolar macrophages obtained by bronchial lavage from a patient with sarcoidosis and hypercalcemia converted 25-hydroxy-cholecalciferol to 1,25-dihydroxycholecalciferol. In general, patients with sarcoidosis are sensitive to small doses of Vitamin D and exposure to ultraviolet radiation of the skin. It is possible that not only are the concentrations of Vitamin D metabolites, especially 1,25-dihydroxycholecalciferol, increased, but also target cells in the intestine responsible for calcium transport may have an increased sensitivity to Vitamin D or an increased rate of calcium transport independent of Vitamin D. The administration of corticosteroids in these patients decreases intestinal calcium absorption and corrects the hypercalcemia. Hypercalcemia also has been demonstrated in patients with histoplasmosis (433), tuberculosis (434), disseminated coccidioidomycosis (435), and berylliosis (436).

Vitamin D Intoxication

Vitamin D and its metabolites, especially 1,25-dihydroxycholecalciferol, increase intestinal calcium absorption. Thus, high concentrations of Vitamin D metabolites (mainly 25-hydroxycholecalciferol) in blood are responsible for the hypercalcemia observed in Vitamin D intoxication. As described already, Vitamin D metabolites may also have a direct effect on bone resorption, which contributes to the development of hypercalcemia.

Milk Alkali Syndrome

This syndrome was seen frequently in patients with peptic ulcer disease who ingested large amounts of sodium and calcium bicarbonate (437,438). Calcium carbonate contains 40% of elemental calcium. Some patients who ingested up to 20 g of calcium carbonate in 24 hours developed severe hypercalcemia. Moreover, alkalosis increases renal calcium reabsorption in the distal tubule and reduces bone turnover, thus decreasing calcium uptake by bone.

Hypercalcemia Secondary to Decreased Urinary Calcium Excretion

The decrease in urinary excretion of calcium may be secondary to a fall in the filtered load of calcium or to an increase in the tubular reabsorption of calcium. The fall in the filtered load of calcium may be secondary to a decrease in serum calcium level or the GFR. By definition, if the patient has a disorder that produces hypocalcemia with a decrease in urinary calcium excretion, he or she cannot be at the same time hypercalcemic; thus, such disorders can be excluded. A fall in the GFR may decrease calcium delivery to the distal tubule, and less calcium may be excreted in the urine. This situation, which may occur in profound dehydration, is self limited and the hypercalcemia does not persist for a prolonged time. Moreover, dehydration or other conditions that decrease GFR may also modify the transport of sodium and water and affect the reabsorption of calcium by the nephron.

Thiazide Diuretics

Patients taking thiazide diuretics may develop moderate hypercalcemia (439–442). The mechanisms for the hypercalcemia are not fully understood, and a number of factors are involved. Thiazides decrease urinary excretion of calcium by increasing calcium resorption in the distal tubule. This reduction in urinary calcium seems to require some degree of ECF volume contraction and the presence of PTH, because patients with hypoparathyroidism do not greatly reduce the amount of calcium in the urine after the administration of thiazides. Thus, in patients with increased calcium mobilization from bone, the administration of thiazides may blunt the expected hypercalciuria and potentially raise serum calcium. However, thiazides also have a direct effect on the skeleton (440). Administration of thiazides intravenously produces a mild change in ionized calcium. This effect is apparently potentiated by PTH because the effect is greater in patients with hyperparathyroidism than in healthy subjects (442). Finally, there is controversy about whether thiazides per se increase the release of PTH. Most of the evidence indicates that this is not the case.

Familial Hypocalciuric Hypercalcemia and Neonatal Severe Hyperparathyroidism

Marx et al. (443,444) described a syndrome characterized by hypocalciuria and mild hypercalcemia. Usually several members of the same family are affected. Familial hypocalciuric hypercalcemia is characterized by autosomal dominant transmission and generally follows a benign course. Some patients may have a mild degree of hyperparathyroidism; however, the hypercalcemia persists after subtotal parathyroidectomy. The main characteristic of this syndrome is a decrease in urinary calcium. Thus, the calcium : creatinine ratio provides an important diagnostic tool to differentiate familial hypocalciuric hypercalcemia from primary hyperparathyroidism. The development of hypercalcemia in young members of the family also favors this diagnosis. The pathogenesis of this syndrome is due to mutations in the calcium sensor of the parathyroid gland chief cells and the TAL/distal nephron epithelia (445,446). As a result, these cells do not downregulate PTH secretion and calcium transport with the correct sensitivity to the plasma calcium. Mutations in the calcium sensor are also responsible for neonatal primary hyperparathyroidism. Two abnormal alleles for calcium sensor mutations produce the primary hyperparathyroidism, whereas single abnormal alleles produce familial hypocalciuric hypercalcemia (447).

Treatment of Disorders of Calcium Metabolism

Hypocalcemia

The treatment of severe hypocalcemia and tetany is a medical emergency. Administration of calcium intravenously is mandatory to prevent severe complications and even death in these patients. If the patient has severe hypocalcemia and tetany in the absence of hypomagnesemia, the symptoms can be easily relieved by administration of 1 or 2 ampules of calcium gluconate given intravenously over 10 minutes (1 ampule of calcium gluconate has approximately 100 mg of elemental calcium). This initial treatment can be followed by administration of 1.0 g of elemental calcium dissolved in 500 mL of dextrose in water and given intravenously over 4 to 6 hours. If the condition responsible for the hypocalcemia cannot be corrected (e.g., hypoparathyroidism), a program for the chronic treatment of hypocalcemia should be instituted. The amount of calcium in the diet should be supplemented by 1 to 3 g of elemental calcium. Calcium carbonate has roughly 40% of elemental calcium; commercial preparations such as 3M Titralac or Os-Cal can be used in this situation. However, in many circumstances, administration of

large amounts of calcium may not be sufficient to increase absorption by the intestine; therefore, different metabolites of Vitamin D should be used. In chronic situations, 1,25-dihydroxycholecalciferol could be used. The dosage used ranges from 0.5 to 2 μg per 24 hours. Most patients eventually require 0.5 μg per day. If this metabolite of Vitamin D is not available, Vitamin D_2 or D_3, about 50,000 U three times a week, could be used instead. The dosage can be gradually increased up to 50,000 to 100,000 units daily. The serum calcium should be carefully monitored to prevent severe hypercalcemia, nephrocalcinosis, and potentially irreversible renal disease.

Hypercalcemia

A useful maneuver to correct hypercalcemia is to increase urinary calcium excretion (Table 88-7). As discussed previously, only 1% to 2% of the filtered load of calcium is excreted by the kidney. This percentage can be greatly increased, and the kidney may thus become an excellent excretory organ for calcium. Because most patients with hypercalcemia develop dehydration and volume contraction with a consequent decrease in GFR, one of the first therapeutic maneuvers is the expansion of the ECF space. Expansion with saline requires several liters per day; therefore, it is mandatory that strict records be kept to maintain accurate determination of the intake and output of fluids. In most patients, it is convenient to determine the central venous pressure (CVP), which will allow volume expansion and prevent the potential risk of overexpansion and heart failure. Thus, after a CVP line is inserted, volume expansion with saline should be instituted until the venous pressure increases to 10 to 14 mm Hg. This maneuver alone will increase the GFR and decrease the reabsorption of calcium in the proximal tubule and in the ascending portion of the loop of Henle. Thus, fractional excretion of calcium will be greatly increased. This effect can be enhanced by administration of diuretics such as furosemide, bumetanide, or ethacrynic acid. The administration of 40 to 120 mg of furosemide every 4 hours is recommended in most patients. Using these maneuvers, fractional excretion of calcium can be increased to 10% of the filtered load. Thus, 1 g of calcium can be easily excreted in the urine in 24 hours. The administration of large amounts of saline and diuretics usually increases the excretion of potassium. To prevent arrhythmias, serum potassium should be maintained between 3.5 and 5.0 mEq/L. This can be achieved by adding 10 to 30 mEq of potassium to each liter of saline.

Although expansion of the ECF may control the hypercalcemia, this effect is temporary, and because in most circumstances, hypercalcemia is secondary to increased mobilization of calcium from bone, the physician may be forced to add a second line of medications to decrease the efflux of calcium from bone. In addition, many patients with hypercalcemia have renal failure and are not responsive to diuretics.

TABLE 88-7. *Treatment of hypercalcemia*

Agent	Dosage	Route of administration	Effect	Mechanism of action	Side effects
I. Measurements directed to enhance renal excretion of calcium					
Saline	1–3 L	IV	4–8 hr	GFR; tubular reabsorption of Ca	Heart failure; electrolyte imbalance
Furosemide	40–20 mg every 2–4 hr	IV	2–4 hr	Tubular reabsorption of Ca	Hypokalemia
II. Measurements directed to decrease calcium efflux from bone					
Biphosphonates					
Paminodrate	60–90 mg	IV	24–72 hr	DBR, effect on osteoclasts	Hypocalcemia
Alendronate	5–10 mg daily	PO	2–3 d	DBR effect on osteoclasts	Gastrointestinal disorders
Risedronate	30 mg daily	PO	2–3 d	DBR effect on osteoclasts	Gastrointestinal disorders
Calcitonin	2–5 MRC/kg every 4–8 hr	IM	4–12 hr	DBR effect on osteoclasts	Allergic reaction, nausea, flushing
Mithramycin	25 μg/kg in 500 mL saline	IV	24–72 hr	DBR (marked)	Thrombocytopenia, bleeding
Indomethacin	75 mg q12h	PO	2–4 d	DBR secondary to prostaglandins	Gastrointestinal disorders
Aspirin	1 g q6h	PO	2–4 d	DBR secondary to prostaglandins	Gastrointestinal disorders, allergic
III. Measurements directed to decrease calcium absorption in gastrointestinal tract					
Prednisone	20–30 mg q12h	PO	2–4 d	Decreased gastrointestinal absorption	Acute toxic steroid effects
IV. Measurements directed to decrease serum calcium					
Hemodialysis	Low dialysate calcium		$\frac{1}{2}$ hr	Direct removal from serum	

IV, intravenous; IM, intramuscular; PO, by mouth; MRC, Medical Research Council; DBR, decreased bone resorption; GFR, glomerular filtration rate.

A derivative of the bisphosphonates, disodium dichloro-methylene diphosphonate (448), was originally used with success on an experimental basis in patients with tumors and bone metastases and severe hypercalcemia (449). Pamidronate and ibandronate, a second- and third-generation bisphosphonate, respectively, have become the standard of therapy for hypercalcemia of malignancy (450,451) and other causes of hypercalcemia requiring inhibition of bone resorption. One or two doses of 30 to 60 mg intravenously are usually effective. Potent bisphosphonates, including alendronate and risedronate, have become available and are effective as oral agents for hypercalcemia.

Calcitonin produces hypocalcemia by decreasing the activity of osteoclasts. The dose commonly used ranges from 2 to 5 MRC U/kg of body weight every 6 to 12 hours. The degree of hypocalcemia produced by this drug is mild, and the decrease is usually 1 to 3 mg/dL (452). Calcitonin can be given either intramuscularly or intravenously in a concentration of 5 MRC U/kg dissolved in 500 mL of 5% dextrose in water to be given over 6 hours. Calcitonin is also available as a nasal spray. Unfortunately, in most patients, there is an escape from the hypocalcemic effect of calcitonin after 6 to 10 days of administration.

Mithramycin is an antibiotic originally introduced for the treatment of testicular tumors. Mithramycin blocks the activity of osteoclasts and may result in severe hypocalcemia (453,454). It is usually given intravenously over 3 to 4 hours in a dose of 25 μg/kg of body weight dissolved in 500 mL of 5% dextrose in water or saline. Mithramycin is an effective drug. However, the effects may be seen only after 48 to 72 hours. One of the toxic effects of the drug is severe thrombocytopenia and bleeding. In general, the drug should not be given more than once every 4 or 5 days, and its use has been almost eliminated by development of effective less toxic agents such as the bisphosphonates (449).

There are rare tumors that produce prostaglandins that have resulted in the development of hypercalcemia. The use of aspirin in a dosage of 1 g four times daily or indomethacin 75 mg twice daily has ameliorated the hypercalcemia (455–457).

If hypercalcemia is mainly due to increased absorption of calcium from the gastrointestinal tract, such as in sarcoidosis, it is obviously important to decrease the amount of calcium in the diet and to administer corticosteroids, which will result in decreased absorption (418,458). Usually prednisone (20 mg twice daily) has been effective in conditions such as sarcoidosis, which is characterized by increased 1,25-dihydroxycholecalciferol production by macrophages in the granulomas. The dose of corticosteroid should be titrated down to the lowest dose required to maintain normocalcemia.

Phosphate has been used in the treatment of hypercalcemia (459). However, the presence of a normal or slightly elevated serum phosphorus level or decreased renal function precludes the use of this medication. Phosphorus should be given only when the serum phosphorus level is low, and its use is generally discouraged. If an elevation of the serum phosphorus level is achieved and the serum calcium level decreases, the patient may deposit calcium phosphate in soft tissues.

There are some general measures that are important in the treatment of hypercalcemia. Immobilization should be avoided as much as possible, especially in patients with rapid bone turnover such as those with Paget's disease. Because most patients with hypercalcemia have an underlying tumor that is causing the hypercalcemia, physicians should be aware of this pathogenetic mechanism and join efforts with oncologists in the diagnosis and treatment of the malignancy. Finally, when the hypercalcemia is very severe and the patient has advanced renal insufficiency, acute hemodialysis is an effective method of correcting the hypercalcemia (Table 88-7).

MAGNESIUM

General Considerations

Magnesium is the second most abundant intracellular cation (after potassium) and the fourth most abundant cation of the body. Magnesium has an essential role as a cofactor for various enzymes, most of which use ATP. Mg^{2+} increases the stimulus threshold in nerve fibers and in pharmacologic doses has a curare-like action on neuromuscular function, probably inhibiting the release of acetylcholine at the neuromuscular junction. Mg^{2+} decreases peripheral resistance and lowers blood pressure. Like Ca^{2+}, Mg^{2+} plays a role in the regulation of PTH secretion. Hypermagnesemia suppresses the release of PTH. Acute hypomagnesemia has the opposite effect; however, profound magnesium depletion decreases the release of PTH. *In vitro*, magnesium increases the solubility of both calcium and phosphorus.

Body Stores of Magnesium

The total body magnesium concentration is approximately 2,000 mEq, or 25 g. As with calcium, only a small fraction (about 1%) of the body magnesium is present in the ECF compartment. Approximately 60% of the total body magnesium is found in bone. Most of the magnesium in bone is associated with apatite crystals, and a significant amount is present as a surface-limited ion on the bone crystal and is freely exchangeable. Approximately 20% of the total body magnesium is localized in the muscle. The remaining 20% is localized in other tissues of the body; the liver has a high magnesium content. The concentration of magnesium in blood is maintained within narrow limits, ranging between 1.5 and 1.9 mEq/L. Approximately 75% to 80% of the magnesium in serum is ultrafilterable, and the rest is protein bound (460,461). Most of the ultrafilterable magnesium is present in the ionized form. Red cell magnesium concentration is approximately 5 mEq/L.

Intracellular free Mg^{2+} levels in renal tubular cells are in the range of 500 μmol/L (462). High-performance liquid chromatography and fluorescent methods have been used to ascertain intracellular Mg^{2+} levels. Mitochondrial inhibitors that deplete intracellular ATP produce modest increases in intracellular Mg^{2+} and Ca^{2+}. The effects of these inhibitors are due to the changes in ATP levels (462). Another agent, antimycin, diminishes ATP levels and decreases intracellular Mg^{2+} to 430 μmol/L but increases cytosolic Ca^{2+}, indicating that Mg^{2+} movements can be distinguished from those of Ca^{2+} by fluorescent techniques. Also, these studies indicate that intracellular regulation of Mg^{2+} is distinctive from that of Ca^{2+}. The role of intracellular Mg^{2+} in the control of cell function remains poorly understood (463). However, intracellular Mg^{2+} levels are rapidly changed through a number of different influences that have important effects on cell function.

Magnesium Balance

Approximately 300 mg, or 25 mEq, of magnesium is ingested daily in the diet. A large portion of dietary magnesium is provided by the ingestion of green vegetables. A minimal magnesium intake of 0.3 mEq/kg of body weight is apparently necessary to maintain magnesium balance in the average person. Of the total amount of magnesium ingested in the diet, about one-third is eliminated in urine and the rest in feces (Fig. 88-12). Thus, on a normal diet containing approximately 300 mg of magnesium, 30% to 40% of the ingested magnesium is absorbed (Fig. 88-12). Small amounts of magnesium, on the order of 15 to 30 mg per day, are secreted by the gastrointestinal tract. Many studies have shown that animals fed low-magnesium diets can excrete urine that is very low in magnesium (460,463,464). However, the gastrointestinal tract continues to secrete small amounts of magnesium, and the animal becomes magnesium depleted. Most of the magnesium is absorbed in the upper

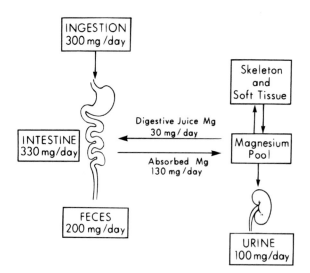

FIG. 88-12. Diagrammatic representation of magnesium metabolism in humans showing the contribution of the gastrointestinal tract, the kidney, bone, and soft tissues to the magnesium pool. (From Slatopolsky E, et al. The hypocalcemia of magnesium depletion. In: Massry S, Ritz E, Rapado A, eds. *Homeostasis of phosphate and other minerals.* New York: Plenum Publishing, 1978:263, with permission.)

gastrointestinal tract. Magnesium shares with calcium similar pathways for absorption in the intestine, but whereas most of the evidence suggests that calcium is actively absorbed from the gastrointestinal tract, magnesium is absorbed mainly by ionic diffusion and "solvent drag" resulting from the bulk flow of water. A carrier mechanism also may be involved in this process (465,466). There is no good evidence to indicate that magnesium is actively transported. The factors controlling the absorption of magnesium from the bowel are not fully understood. Although there is some evidence to suggest that Vitamin D may influence the absorption of magnesium, this role seems to be less important for magnesium than for the absorption of calcium (467,468). It is known that patients with severe renal insufficiency and low levels of 1,25-dihydroxycholecalciferol may develop profound hypermagnesemia by slightly increasing the amount of magnesium in the diet without modifying the metabolites of Vitamin D in serum. The sigmoid colon has the capability of absorbing magnesium, and there are several reports in the literature of patients who developed magnesium toxicity after receiving enemas containing magnesium; most of these patients also had renal insufficiency. Experimental evidence in different species suggests an interrelationship between magnesium and calcium absorption from the gastrointestinal tract. Diets high in calcium decrease the absorption of magnesium, and diets low in magnesium increase the absorption of calcium.

Renal Handling of Magnesium

Approximately 2 g of magnesium is filtered daily by the kidney, and about 100 mg appears in the urine. Thus, 95% of the filtered load of magnesium is reabsorbed, and 5% is excreted in the urine (Fig. 88-13) (463,469). In states of magnesium deficiency, the kidney can reduce the amount of magnesium excreted in the urine to less than 0.5% of the filtered load. On the other hand, during magnesium infusion (Fig. 88-13) or in patients with far-advanced renal insufficiency, as is commonly seen, the kidney can excrete 40% to 80% of the filtered load of magnesium (470). The proximal tubule is poorly permeable to magnesium (460,469–473), and probably no more than 20% to 30% is reabsorbed in this segment. This is in contrast to the amount of sodium and calcium (60%) reabsorbed in this segment of the nephron. The tubular fluid magnesium is usually 1.5-fold greater than the plasma magnesium. Studies by Quamme and Dirks (474) using microperfusion techniques in the proximal tubule indicated that the absolute magnesium concentration increased along the perfused tubule in a linear manner, with net water reabsorption. This study (474) confirmed the low permeability of the superficial proximal tubule to magnesium. Further studies indicated a low level of back-flux from peritubular membrane into the lumen (475,476). In the descending limb of the loop of Henle, the magnesium concentration is raised severalfold over the ultrafilterable serum concentration due to water removal. The TAL of the loop of Henle seems to play a critical role in the

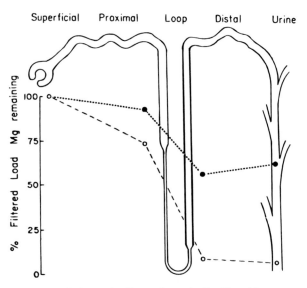

FIG. 88-13. Schematic illustration of ultrafilterable magnesium remaining in different segments of the nephron in normal hydropenic conditions (o–o) and after acute $MgCl_2$ loading (•–•). The results observed emphasize the importance of the thick ascending loop of Henle on magnesium reabsorption. (From Dirks JH, Quamme GA. Renal handling of magnesium. In: Massry S, Ritz E, Rapado A, eds. *Homeostasis of phosphate and other minerals.* New York: Plenum Publishing, 1978:51, with permission.)

reabsorption of magnesium. Early studies by LeGrimellec et al. (477) and by Morel et al. (478) demonstrated that the loop of Henle was the major site for magnesium reabsorption. Approximately 50% to 60% of the filtered magnesium was reabsorbed between the last accessible portion of the proximal tubule and the early distal tubule. Studies by Quamme and Dirks (474) further characterized the behavior of the loop of Henle. These investigators demonstrated that in the presence of a normal plasma magnesium concentration, magnesium absorption increased with intraluminal magnesium concentration. There was no indication of a T_{max} for magnesium when the luminal magnesium concentration increased from 0 to 5 mmol/L. On the other hand, an increase in plasma magnesium concentration (i.e., on the basolateral membrane) resulted in a significant depression of magnesium absorption, suggesting that hypermagnesemia decreases magnesium absorption in the loop of Henle by inhibiting magnesium transport at the basolateral membrane. Thus, the permeability of the TAL to magnesium is quite different from that of the proximal tubule. Two mechanisms have been proposed to explain magnesium transport in the TAL of the loop of Henle: (a) passive, secondary to the potential difference generated by the active transport of sodium chloride, which facilitates paracellular movement of Mg^{2+} (302); and (b) active (304–306), because the chemical concentration of magnesium in the cells is higher than that in the lumen, and the potential gradient may not be great enough to explain the entry of magnesium into cells. Diets deficient in magnesium or the administration of PTH enhances

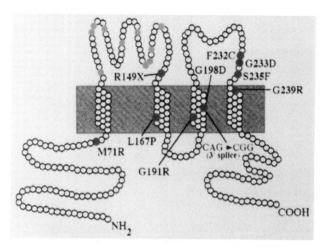

FIG. 88-14. Structure of the paracellin-1 (PCLN1) human gene. Red dots indicate mutations in PCLN1 in patients with recessive renal hypomagnesemia. (From Simon DB, Lu Y, Chaote KA, et al. Paracellin-I, a renal tight junction protein required for paracellular Mg²⁺ resorption. *Science* 1999;285:103, with permission.) (See Color Figure 88-14 following page 2624.)

the reabsorption of magnesium in the TAL of the loop of Henle. On the other hand, diets containing large amounts of magnesium or factors that decrease the reabsorption of sodium chloride in this portion of the nephron (ECF volume expansion, administration of diuretics such as furosemide, bumetanide, or ethacrynic acid) also decrease the reabsorption of magnesium.

Recently a protein, PCLN1 was detected in the TAL and in the distal tubule (316). PCLN1 a member of the claudin family of high-junction proteins. PCLN1 is a highly negative-charged protein, with 10 negatively charged residues and a net charge of -5 (316) (Fig. 88-14). Mutations in the protein can induce renal Mg²⁺ wasting, hypercalciuria, nephrocalcinosis, and renal failure. PCLN1 plays an important role in the conductance of the TAL: The negative charges may contribute to the cationic selectivity of the paracellular pathway for the reabsorption of calcium and magnesium (316).

The terminal segment of the nephron (late distal tubule and collecting duct) appears to play a minor role in the reabsorption of magnesium under normal conditions (474,479,480). However, more recent studies by the same investigators indicate that the distal tubule also plays an important role in magnesium conservation (481).

Chronic administration of mineralocorticoids increases magnesium excretion. Several interrelationships between calcium and magnesium reabsorption have been demonstrated. The administration of one of these two elements decreases the reabsorption of the other. When large amounts of magnesium are given intravenously, there is a remarkable decrease in the renal reabsorption of calcium and vice versa. Alcohol also affects the handling of magnesium by the kidney. A remarkable short-lived hypermagnesuria is seen after alcohol is given to experimental animals or humans. The intravenous administration of glucose has a similar effect.

Recently, Bapty et al. (482) further characterized the role of the distal convoluted tubule in the regulation of magnesium. These investigators demonstrated that an immortalized cell line possesses a polyvalent action-sensing mechanism responsive to extracellular magnesium and calcium. The responses are unlike those observed for the calcium sensor (CaSR) in the parathyroid gland (482).

In summary, in contrast to calcium, it seems that the thick ascending portion of the loop of Henle is the most important portion of the nephron in the regulation of magnesium reabsorption. Magnesium reabsorption in the loop occurs within the cortical TAL primarily by passive means driven by the transepithelial voltage through the paracellular pathway. On the other hand, magnesium reabsorption in the distal tubule is transcellular and active in nature. Moreover, the reabsorption of magnesium in the proximal tubule, in contrast to that of sodium, calcium, and phosphate, is rather limited.

Hypermagnesemia

By far the most common cause of hypermagnesemia is chronic renal insufficiency (483). The kidney can excrete large amounts of magnesium in the urine. Thus, hypermagnesemia is seldom seen in patients with normal renal function, even if the patient ingests large amounts of magnesium such as antacids containing magnesium or laxatives such as milk of magnesia. Mild hypermagnesemia may be seen in patients with GFRs of approximately 10 mL per minute. However, moderate hypermagnesemia is usually seen in patients with GFRs of less than 5 mL per minute. As renal insufficiency progresses, the fractional excretion of magnesium in the urine significantly increases. Patients with a GFR of 120 mL per minute excrete approximately 5% of the filtered load of magnesium. However, patients with far-advanced renal failure (GFR of less than 10 mL per minute) may excrete up to 40% to 80% of the filtered load of magnesium (483). Thus, patients with chronic renal failure may not be able to increase magnesium excretion further after ingestion of large amounts of magnesium. Therefore, if magnesium ingestion is increased (after administration of laxatives or antacids containing magnesium) in patients with advanced renal failure, profound hypermagnesemia and death may occur. In obstetric wards, magnesium is still used for the treatment of eclampsia (484). In some of these patients, the GFR is decreased, and the administration of large amounts of magnesium sulfate may result in hypermagnesemia. Although most of the magnesium is absorbed in the small intestine, the sigmoid colon can also absorb magnesium. Healthy subjects receiving large amounts of magnesium sulfate per rectum have been found to have serum magnesium levels of more than 10 mEq/L (485).

Symptoms and Signs of Hypermagnesemia

Profound hypermagnesemia blocks neuromuscular transmission and depresses the conduction system of the heart. The neuromuscular effects of magnesium are antagonized by the administration of calcium. Mild hypermagnesemia is well tolerated. However, if serum magnesium levels increase to 5 to 6 mg/dL, there may be a decrease in tendon refluxes (486) and some degree of mental confusion. If the serum magnesium level increases to 7 to 9 mg/dL, the respiratory rate slows and the blood pressure falls. If serum magnesium levels increase to about 10 to 13 mg/dL, there is usually profound hypotension and severe mental depression. When the levels increase further to about 15 mg/dL, death may occur (485–487). In uremic patients, the adverse effect of hypermagnesemia may be worsened by the presence of hypocalcemia. Acute hypermagnesemia may also produce mild hypocalcemia. This may be due to (a) suppression of the release of PTH and (b) competition for tubular reabsorption between calcium and magnesium, leading to decreased calcium reabsorption and hypercalciuria, which aggravates the hypocalcemia produced by decreased release of PTH. In chronic renal insufficiency, there is probably an increase in red cell magnesium and muscle magnesium, but the results are controversial. The amount of magnesium in bone is apparently increased in cortical and trabecular bone (487).

Hypomagnesemia

Hypomagnesemia is defined as a decrease in serum magnesium to levels less than 1.5 mg/dL. Diseases involving the small intestine may decrease magnesium absorption and are the most common cause of hypomagnesemia (Table 88-8). It is difficult to predict the degree of total body magnesium deficiency by determining only serum magnesium concentration. Because only 1% of magnesium is present in the ECF compartment, changes in intracellular magnesium and skeletal magnesium can modify the concentration of serum magnesium, and it may not be possible to assess precisely the degree of magnesium deficiency by determining serum magnesium level. Probably the determination of skeletal or muscle magnesium may provide a better index of magnesium deficiency. However, these determinations are not practical in clinical medicine. In patients with magnesium deficiency, the administration of 50 to 100 mEq of magnesium per day usually corrects the hypomagnesemia after a short time. Magnesium depletion can also produce changes in other electrolytes. Usually there is an increase in potassium excretion in the urine, and patients may develop hypokalemia (488). In several experimental studies, it has been shown in humans (489) and animals (490) that magnesium depletion is accompanied by urinary potassium losses. Potassium alone did not increase muscle potassium unless magnesium replacement was given as well to patients receiving diuretics (491). It has been suggested that the effect of magnesium on intracellular potassium is a result of magnesium stimulating Na-K-ATPase activity, allowing the cell to maintain a potassium gradient (492). However, the most important manifestation of hypomagnesemia is the development of hypocalcemia and tetany.

TABLE 88-8. *Causes of hypomagnesemia*

I. Decreased intestinal absorption
  A. Severe diarrhea
  B. Intestinal bypass
  C. Surgical resection
  D. Tropical and nontropical sprue
  E. Celiac disease
  F. Invasive and infiltrative process; lymphomas
  G. Prolonged gastrointestinal suction
II. Decrease intake
  A. Starvation
  B. Protein energy malnutrition
  C. Chronic alcoholism
  D. Prolonged therapy with intravenous fluids lacking magnesium
III. Excessive urinary losses
  A. Diuretic phase of acute tubular necrosis
  B. Postobstructive diuresis
  C. Diuretic therapy
  D. Diabetic ketoacidosis (during treatment)
  E. Chronic alcoholism
  F. Hypercalcemic states
  G. Primary aldosteronism
  H. Inappropriate antidiuretic hormone secretion
  I. Aminoglycoside toxicity
  J. Idiopathic renal magnesium wasting
  K. Cisplatinum
  L. Cyclosporin
  M. Gitelman's syndrome

Source: From Slatopolsky E. Pathophysiology of calcium, magnesiuum, and phosphorus. In: Klahr S, ed. *The kidney and body fluids in health and disease.* New York: Plenum Press, 1983:269, with permission.

Experimental animals fed a low-magnesium diet develop hypocalcemia (493–496). However, the rat becomes hypercalcemic. The pathogenesis of hypocalcemia in magnesium depletion is multifactorial. Hypomagnesemia has profound effects on PTH metabolism and bone physiology. It is known that mild hypomagnesemia increases acutely the levels of PTH *in vivo* (497) or *in vitro* (498); on the other hand, profound hypomagnesemia decreases the levels of PTH in blood (362). It seems that neither the biosynthesis nor the conversion of pro-PTH to PTH is greatly affected by the concentration of magnesium (499,500). However, the release of PTH is influenced by the serum magnesium concentration (501). Several investigators have demonstrated that the administration of magnesium to patients with severe hypomagnesemia who have low levels of immunoreactive PTH in serum increases the release of PTH a few minutes after magnesium administration. Also, there is evidence to indicate that during hypomagnesemia, the skeleton is resistant to the action of PTH (502,503), and in general, the administration of mildly pharmacologic doses of PTH does not elicit a normal calcemic response in patients with magnesium depletion. Studies by Freitag et al. (504) have further clarified this abnormality. The uptake of PTH by bones obtained from dogs with experimental magnesium depletion was greatly diminished, and the release of cAMP by bone was also blunted in hypomagnesemia. In addition to a decrease in the release of PTH and skeletal resistance to this hormone, in magnesium depletion, there is evidence that the ionic exchange from the hydration shell of bone between calcium and magnesium also is decreased (505); thus, on a physicochemical basis, less calcium is mobilized from bone in hypomagnesemia. Thus, the decrease in the release of PTH, the low uptake of PTH by bone, and the decreased heteroionic exchange of calcium for magnesium in bone are all pathogenetic factors responsible for the hypocalcemia observed in patients with profound magnesium depletion.

Clinical Manifestations of Hypomagnesemia

Patients with severe hypomagnesemia usually develop some degree of anorexia, mental confusion, and vomiting. In general, there is increased neuromuscular irritability, and tremors and seizures are usually observed in these patients. Muscle fasciculation and positive Trousseau's and Chvostek's signs can be observed. Nodal or sinus tachycardia and premature atrial or ventricular contractions may occur. The electrocardiogram may show prolongation of the QT interval and broadening and flattening or even inversion of the T waves. Magnesium deficiency potentiates the action of digitalis, and there is an enhanced sensitivity to the toxic effects of digitalis. Because magnesium plays a key role in regulating the activity of Na-K-ATPase, which is the enzyme responsible for the maintenance of intracellular potassium concentration, severe alterations in skeletal muscle and myocardial function are observed. Sometimes it is difficult to decide whether the changes in the electrocardiogram are related to magnesium or potassium depletion. Most of these patients also have profound hypocalcemia, and sometimes it is difficult to determine whether the symptoms are due to magnesium deficiency or to the concomitant hypocalcemia. Other neurologic manifestations may include vertigo, ataxia, nystagmus, and dysarthria. Changes in personality, depression, and sometimes hallucinations and psychosis have been observed. Patients also may show some degree of hypophosphatemia. In the rat, it has been shown that magnesium deficiency promotes renal phosphate excretion (506).

Mechanisms Responsible for the Development of Hypomagnesemia

From the pathogenetic point of view, three main mechanisms are responsible for the development of hypomagnesemia: (a) decreased intestinal absorption, (b) decreased intake, and (c) excessive urinary losses.

Hypomagnesemia Secondary to Decreased Intestinal Absorption of Magnesium

By far the most common causes responsible for the development of hypomagnesemia are pathologic entities affecting the small bowel. In these conditions, the kidney adapts to the hypomagnesemia and decreases the urinary excretion of magnesium. However, the amount of magnesium in the stool does not decrease appropriately (probably the secretion of magnesium is not greatly reduced), and the patient develops hypomagnesemia. Severe magnesium depletion is associated with steatorrheic syndromes (507). Pathologic processes such as celiac disease, tropical and nontropical sprue, malignancies (characteristically lymphoma), surgical resection, intestinal bypass, and profound diarrhea have all been considered responsible for the development of hypomagnesemia. From 1960 to 1975, when the number of surgical bypass procedures for the treatment of obesity increased greatly, it was noted that many of these patients developed profound hypomagnesemia and tetany. Hypomagnesemia is especially prominent in patients with idiopathic steatorrhea and diseases affecting the terminal ileum.

Hypomagnesemia Secondary to Decreased Magnesium Intake

Magnesium depletion has been described in children with protein-calorie malnutrition (508). The hypomagnesemia results from a combination of decreased intake and gastrointestinal losses due to diarrhea or severe vomiting. In a hospital setting, perhaps the most common cause of hypomagnesemia is prolonged therapy with intravenous fluids lacking magnesium. Often, when surgical patients require intestinal suction, they are given intravenous fluid, sometimes for several weeks, and seldom is magnesium added to the intravenous fluids. Alcoholism is probably the most common cause of hypomagnesemia in the United States (509–511). The chronic ingestion of alcohol produces hypomagnesemia. The mechanisms are multifactorial. Usually patients with chronic alcoholism ingest diets poor in magnesium. Alcohol increases the urinary excretion of magnesium (512). From the point of view of differential diagnosis, the clinical history, evidence of malnutrition, the presence of diarrhea and vomiting, or a history of surgery may help to differentiate individuals with decreased absorption of magnesium due either to a primary gastrointestinal disease or to decreased intake from individuals with increased urinary excretion of magnesium. As mentioned previously, when there is decreased intake or absorption of magnesium from the gastrointestinal tract, the amount of magnesium excreted in the urine is greatly reduced, on the order of 10 to 15 mg per day.

Hypomagnesemia Secondary to Increased Urinary Losses of Magnesium

Because 60% to 70% of magnesium is absorbed in the TAL of the loop of Henle, any factor that blocks the reabsorption of sodium chloride in this part of the nephron will also promote the urinary excretion of magnesium. In conditions in which the ECF volume is increased and in entities characterized by profound diuresis (diuretic phase of acute tubular necrosis, postobstructive diuresis), the patient may excrete 20% to 30% of the filtered load of magnesium and may develop profound hypomagnesemia. Administration of large amounts of diuretics such as ethacrynic acid, bumetanide, or furosemide has a significant effect on renal magnesium excretion. Patients with ketoacidosis may develop hypomagnesemia. Serum magnesium, phosphorus, and potassium concentrations may be elevated during periods of ketoacidosis; however, the levels usually fall after the administration of insulin and fluid replacement. Increased excretion of magnesium has been seen after the treatment of diabetic ketoacidosis (513) and in metabolic conditions characterized by an excess of mineralocorticoids (514) such as primary aldosteronism. A specific defect has been described in patients receiving aminoglycosides (515) or cisplatin (an antitumoral agent) (516). The usual lesions produced by aminoglycosides are acute tubular necrosis, renal insufficiency, and hypermagnesemia; however, several patients have developed a specific tubular defect characterized by profound hypermagnesuria and hypomagnesemia that may persist for several weeks after the drug is discontinued. Some of these patients also developed hypokalemia.

Patients with chronic hypokalemia and a phenotype other than that of Bartter's syndrome, who have hypomagnesemia and excess urinary magnesium, are described as having Gitelman's syndrome (517). Gitelman's syndrome is actually more common than Bartter's syndrome and is characterized as follows. The patients may be children or adults with primary renal tubular hypokalemic metabolic alkalosis with magnesium deficiency, hypocalciuria, and skin lesions. Hyperreninemic hyperaldosteronism is present, as are the other features of Bartter's syndrome. The inheritance is autosomal recessive, and linkage analysis to the locus encoding the renal thiazide–sensitive Na-Cl cotransporter is uniform (518). Thus, reduced sodium chloride reabsorption in the diluting segment is the pathogenesis of the disease, and it further leads to abnormalities in magnesium transport.

Treatment of Alterations in Magnesium Metabolism

Hypermagnesemia

Hypermagnesemia is seen very seldom in clinical medicine. In general, it is observed in patients with far-advanced renal insufficiency, usually with a GFR of less than 10 mL per minute. The treatment is similar to that for hypercalcemia (i.e., volume expansion with saline and administration of furosemide). However, care is required because this therapeutic regimen will also increase the excretion of calcium in the urine and potentiate the toxic effects of hypermagnesemia. Thus, if expansion with saline and furosemide is used, calcium should be added to the solutions, approximately 1 to 3 ampules of calcium gluconate per liter of saline, to prevent hypocalcemia. If the patient's GFR is extremely low, and volume expansion with saline and diuretics is not effective, dialysis with a low or zero magnesium dialysate should be instituted. Hypermagnesemia is also seen clinically when large amounts of magnesium are given intravenously to patients. A decrease in the dose administered will rapidly correct the condition.

Hypomagnesemia

Profound magnesium depletion may be accompanied by hypocalcemia and tetany. Thus, the treatment of severe hypomagnesemia may constitute a medical emergency. Profound hypomagnesemia can be easily corrected by administration of magnesium intravenously, provided that the patient has fairly normal renal function. In patients with compromised renal function, magnesium should be given cautiously, and serum magnesium should be closely monitored. Fifty to 75 mEq of magnesium sulfate or magnesium chloride should be mixed in 500 mL of dextrose in water and given intravenously over 6 to 8 hours. The next morning, serum magnesium should be measured, and if hypomagnesemia persists, the amount of magnesium should be increased to 100 mEq dissolved in the same type of solution and given over 8 hours. In some circumstances, this procedure should be repeated two or three times until the serum magnesium level increases to 2.5 mg/dL. If the patient requires magnesium orally over a prolonged period, magnesium salts can be given to these patients. One gram of magnesium oxide has roughly 50 mEq, or 600 mg, of magnesium. Thus, magnesium oxide in a dose of 250 to 500 mg can be given to patients two to four times daily. Larger doses are not well tolerated, and most patients will develop diarrhea. It is important to emphasize that a normal diet provides approximately 25 mEq, or 300 mg, of magnesium.

ACKNOWLEDGMENTS

This work was supported by grant nos. R01 AR41677-08, RO1-DK49728-02, R01 DK09976-33, R01 AR32087-17, and R01 AR 39561-07 by the National Institutes of Health.

REFERENCES

1. Levine BS, Kleeman CR. Hypophosphatemia and hyperphosphatemia: clinical and pathophysiologic aspects. In: Maxwell MH, Kleeman CR, eds. *Clinical disorders of fluid and electrolyte metabolism.* New York: McGraw-Hill, 1994:1040.
2. Hopkins T, Howard JE, Eisenberg H. Ultrafiltration studies on calcium and phosphorus in human serum. *Bull Johns Hopkins Hosp* 1952;91:1.
3. Walser M. Ion association. VI. Interactions between calcium, magnesium, inorganic phosphate, citrate and protein in normal human plasma. *J Clin Invest* 1961;40:723.
4. Fuchs R, Peterlik M. Intestinal phosphate transport. In: Massry SG, Ritz E, Jahn H, eds. *Phosphate and minerals in health and disease.* New York: Plenum Publishing, 1980:380.
5. Berner W, Kinne R, Murer H. Phosphate transport into brush border membrane vesicles isolated from rat small intestine. *Biochem J* 1976;160:467.
6. Hilfiker H, Hattenhauer O, Traebert M, et al Characterization of a murine type II sodium-phosphate cotransporter expressed in mammalian small intestine. *Proc Natl Acad Sci* 1998;95:14564.

7. Matsumoto T, Fontaine O, Rasmussen H. Effect of 1,25(OH)$_2$ vitamin D$_3$ on phosphate uptake into chick intestinal brush border membrane vesicles. *Biochim Biophys Acta* 1980;599:13.

8. Murer H, Hildmann B. Transcellular transport of calcium and inorganic phosphate in the small intestinal epithelium. *Am J Physiol* 1981;240:G409.

9. Norman AW. Calcium and phosphorus absorption. In: Lawson DEM, ed. *Vitamin D.* New York: Academic Press, 1978:90.

10. Peterlik M, Wasserman RH. Effect of Vitamin D on transepithelial phosphate transport in chick intestine. *Am J Physiol* 1978;234:E379.

11. Kikuchi K, Ghishan FK. Phosphate transport by basolateral plasma membranes of human small intestine. *Gastroenterology* 1987;93:106.

12. Knox FG, Osswald H, Marchand GR, et al. Phosphate transport along the nephron. *Am J Physiol* 1977;233:F261.

13. Pastoriza-Munoz E, Colindres RE, Lassiter WE, et al. Effect of parathyroid hormone on phosphate reabsorption in rat distal convolution. *Am J Physiol* 1978;235:F321.

14. Jamison RL, Arrascue JF. Calcium and phosphate reabsorption by the loop of Henle. *Miner Electrolyte Metab* 1980;4:90.

15. Peraino RA, Suki WN. Phosphate transport by isolated rabbit cortical collecting tubule. *Am J Physiol* 1980;238:F358.

16. Shareghi GR, Agus ZS. Phosphate transport in the light segment of the rabbit cortical collecting tubule. *Am J Physiol* 1982;242:F379.

17. Chabardes D, Imbert M, Clique A, et al. PTH sensitive adenyl cyclase activity in different segments of the rabbit nephron. *Pflugers Arch (Eur J Physiol)* 1975;354:229.

18. Haramati A, Haas JA, Knox FG. Adaptation of deep and superficial nephrons to changes in dietary phosphate intake. *Am J Physiol* 1983;244:F265.

19. Haramati A, Haas JA, Knox FG. Nephron heterogeneity of phosphate reabsorption: effect of parathyroid hormone. *Am J Physiol* 1984;246:F155.

20. Hoffmann N, Thees M, Kinne R. Phosphate transport by isolated renal brush border vesicles. *Pflugers Arch (Eur J Physiol)* 1976;362:147.

21. Sacktor B. Transport in membrane vesicles isolated from the mammalian kidney and intestine. In: Sanadi R, ed. *Current topics in bioenergetics.* New York: Academic Press, 1977:30.

22. Murer H, Biber J. Molecular mechanisms of renal apical Na phosphate cotransport. *Annu Rev Physiol* 1996;58:607.

23. Werner A, Moore ML, Mantei N, et al. Cloning and expression of cDNA for a Na/P$_i$ cotransport system of kidney cortex. *Proc Natl Acad Sci USA* 1991;88:9608.

24. Fucentese M, Murer H, Biber J. Expression of rat renal Na cotransport of phosphate and sulfate in Sf9 insect cells. *J Am Soc Nephrol* 1994;5:860.

25. Tenenhouse HS, Roy S, Martel J, et al. Differential expression, abundance, and regulation of Na$^+$-phosphate cotransporter genes in murine kidney. *Am J Physiol* 1998;275:F527.

26. Busch AE, Schuster A, Waldegger S. Expression of a renal type I sodium/phosphate transporter (NaPi-1) induces a conductance in Xenopus oocytes permeable for organic and inorganic anions. *Proc Natl Acad Sci USA* 1996;93:5347.

27. Verri T, Markovich D, Perego C, et al. Cloning of a rabbit renal Na-Pi cotransporter which is regulated by dietary phosphate. *Am J Physiol* 1995;268:F626.

28. Murer H, Werner A, Reshkin S, et al. Cellular mechanisms in proximal tubular reabsorption of inorganic phosphate. *Am J Physiol* 1991;260:C885.

29. Keusch I, et al. Parathyroid hormone and dietary phosphate provoke a lysosomal routing of the proximal tubular Na/Pi-cotransporter type II. *Kidney Int* 1998;54:1224.

30. Levi M, Kempson SA, Lotscher M, et al. Molecular regulation of renal phosphate transport. *J Membr Biol* 1996;154:1.

31. Lotscher M, Wilson P, Nguyen S, et al. New aspects of adaptation of rat renal Na-Pi cotransporter to alterations in dietary phosphate. *Kidney Int* 1996;49:1012.

32. Kempson SA, Lotscher M, Kaissling B, et al. Parathyroid hormone action on phosphate transporter mRNA and protein in rat renal proximal tubules. *Am J Physiol* 1995;268:F784.

33. Kavanaugh MP, Miller DG, Zhang W, et al. Cell-surface receptors for gibbon ape leukemia virus and amphotropic murine retroviruses are inducible sodium-dependent phosphate symporters. *Proc Natl Acad Sci USA* 1994;91:7071.

34. Schwab SJ, Hammerman MR. Mechanisms of phosphate exit across the basolateral membrane of the renal proximal tubule cell. *Clin Res* 1984;32:530.

35. Beutner EH, Munson PL. Time course of urinary excretion of inorganic phosphate by rats after parathyroidectomy and after injection of parathyroid extract. *Endocrinology* 1960;66:610.

36. Pullman TN, Lavender AR, Aho I, et al. Direct renal action of a purified parathyroid extract. *Endocrinology* 1960;67:570.

37. Agus ZS, Gardner LB, Beck LH, et al. Effects of parathyroid hormone on renal tubular reabsorption of calcium, sodium and phosphate. *Am J Physiol* 1973;224:1143.

38. Wen SF. Micropuncture studies of phosphate transport in the proximal tubule of the dog. The relationship of sodium reabsorption. *J Clin Invest* 1974;53:143.

39. Beck N: Effect of metabolic acidosis on renal response to parathyroid hormone in phosphorus-deprived rats. *Am J Physiol* 1981;241:F23.

40. Beck LH, Goldberg M. Effects of acetazolamide and parathyroidectomy on renal transport of sodium, calcium and phosphate. *Am J Physiol* 1973;224:1136.

41. Amiel C, Kuntziger H, Richet G. Micropuncture study of handling of phosphate by proximal and distal nephron in normal and parathyroidectomized rat. Evidence for distal reabsorption. *Pflugers Arch (Eur J Physiol)* 1970;317:93.

42. Goldfarb S, Beck LH, Agus ZS, et al. Dissociation of tubular sites of action of saline, PTH and DbCAMP on renal phosphate reabsorption. *Nephron* 1978;21:221.

43. Knox FG, Preiss J, Kim JK, et al. Mechanism of resistance to the phosphaturic effect of the parathyroid hormone in the hamster. *J Clin Invest* 1977;59:675.

44. Le Grimellec C, Roinel N, Morel F. Simultaneous Mg, Ca, P, K and Cl analysis in rat tubular fluid. IV. During acute phosphate plasma loading. *Pflugers Arch (Eur J Physiol)* 1974;346:189.

45. Evers C, Murer H, Kinne R. Effect of parathyrin on the transport properties of isolated renal brush-border vesicles. *Biochem J* 1978;172:49.

46. Hammerman MR, Hruska KA. Cyclic AMP-dependent protein phosphorylation in canine renal brush-border membrane vesicles is associated with decreased P$_i$ transport. *J Biol Chem* 1982;257:992.

47. Dunlay R, Hruska KA. Parathyroid hormone receptor coupling to phospholipase C is an alternate pathway of signal transduction in the bone and kidney. *Am J Physiol* 1990;258:F223.

48. Ribeiro CP, Mandel LJ. Parathyroid hormone inhibits proximal tubule. *Am J Physiol* 1992;262:F209.

49. Hruska KA, Hammerman MR. Parathyroid hormone inhibition of phosphate transport in renal brush border vesicles from phosphate-depleted dogs. *Biochim Biophys Acta* 1981;645:351.

50. Hayes G, Busch AE, Lang F, et al. Protein kinase C consensus sites and the regulation of renal Na/Pi-cotransport (NaPi-2) expressed in Xenopus laevis oocytes. *Pflugers Arch (Eur J Physiol)* 1995;430:819.

51. Hoppe A, Metler M, Berndt TJ, et al. Effect of respiratory alkalosis on renal phosphate excretion. *Am J Physiol* 1982;243:F471.

52. Fulop M, Brazeau P. The phosphaturic effect of sodium bicarbonate and acetazolamide in dogs. *J Clin Invest* 1968;47:983.

53. Quamme GA. Urinary alkalinization may not result in an increase in urinary phosphate excretion. *Kidney Int* 1984;25:150(abst).

54. Mercado A, Slatopolsky E, Klahr S. On the mechanisms responsible for the phosphaturia of bicarbonate administration. *J Clin Invest* 1975;56:1386.

55. Puschett JB, Goldberg M. The relationship between the renal handling of phosphate and bicarbonate in man. *J Lab Clin Med* 1969;73:956.

56. Kuntziger HE, Amiel C, Couette S, et al. Localization of parathyroid-hormone-independent sodium bicarbonate inhibition of tubular phosphate reabsorption. *Kidney Int* 1980;17:749.

57. Cuche JL, Ott CE, Marchand GR, et al. Intrarenal calcium in phosphate handling. *Am J Physiol* 1976;230:790.

58. Pitts RF, Alexander RS. The renal reabsorptive mechanism for inorganic phosphate in normal and acidotic dogs. *Am J Physiol* 1944;142:648.

59. Guntupalli J, Eby B, Lau K. Mechanism for the phosphaturia of NH$_4$Cl: dependence on acidemia but not on diet PO$_4$ or PTH. *Am J Physiol* 1982;242:F552.

60. Kempson SA. Effect of metabolic acidosis on renal brush border membrane adaptation to low phosphorus diet. *Kidney Int* 1982;22:225.

61. Quamme GA, Mizgala CL, Wong NLM, et al. Effects of intraluminal pH and dietary phosphate on phosphate transport in the proximal convoluted tubule. *Am J Physiol* 1985;249:F759.

62. Ambuhl PM, Zajicek HK, Wang H, et al. Regulation of renal phosphate transport by acute and chronic metabolic acidosis in the rat. *Kidney Int* 1998;53:1288.

63. Frick A, Durasin I. Proximal tubular reabsorption of inorganic phosphate in adrenalectomized rats. *Pflugers Arch (Eur J Physiol)* 1980;385:189.

64. Bonjour JP, Preston C, Fleisch H. Effect of 1,25-dihydroxyvitamin D₃ on renal handling of Pᵢ in thyroparathyroidectomized rats. *J Clin Invest* 1977;60:1419.

65. Muhlbauer RC, Bonjour J-P, Fleisch H. Tubular handling of Pᵢ: localization of effects of 1,25(OH)₂D₃ and dietary Pᵢ in TPTX rats. *Am J Physiol* 1981;241:F123.

66. Stoll R, Kinne R, Murer H, et al. Phosphate transport by rat renal brush border membrane vesicles: influence of dietary phosphate, thyroparathyroidectomy, and 1,25-dihydroxyvitamin D₃. *Pflugers Arch (Eur J Physiol)* 1979;380:47.

67. Gekle DJ, Stroder J, Rostock D. The effect of Vitamin D on renal inorganic phosphate reabsorption on normal rats, parathyroidectomized rats, and rats with rickets. *Pediatr Res* 1971;5:40.

68. Liang CT, Barnes J, Cheng L, et al. Effects of 1,25(OH)₂D₃ administered in vivo on phosphate uptake by isolated chick renal cells. *Am J Physiol* 1982;242:C312.

69. Kurnik BR, Hruska KA. Effects of 1,25-dihydroxycholecalciferol on phosphate transport in Vitamin D-deprived rats. *Am J Physiol* 1984; 247:F177.

70. Caverzasio J, Montessuit C, Bonjour J-P. Stimulatory effect of insulin-like growth factor-1 on renal Pᵢ transport and plasma 1,25-dihydroxyvitamin D₃. *Endocrinology* 1990;127:453.

71. Biber J, Murer H. Na-Pi cotransport in LLC-PK₁ cells: fast adaptive response to Pᵢ deprivation. *Am J Physiol* 1985;249:C430.

72. Brown CD, Bodmer M, Biber J, et al. Sodium-dependent phosphate transport by apical membrane vesicles from a cultured renal epithelial cell line (LLC-PK₁). *Biochim Biophys Acta* 1984;769:471.

73. Caverzasio J, Brown CD, Biber J, et al. Adaptation of phosphate transport in phosphate-deprived LLC-PK₁ cells. *Am J Physiol.* 1985; 248:F122.

74. Werner A, Kempson SA, Biber J, et al. Increase of Na/Pi-cotransport encoding mRNA in response to low Pᵢ diet in rat kidney cortex. *J Biol Chem* 1994;269:6637.

75. Levi M, Lotscher M, Sorribas V, et al. Cellular mechanisms of acute and chronic adaptation of rat renal P(i) transporter to alterations in dietary P(i). *Am J Physiol* 1994;267:F900.

76. Olsen HS, Cepeda MA, Zhang Q-Q, et al. Human stanniocalcin: a possible hormonal regulator of mineral metabolism. *Proc Natl Acad Sci USA* 1996;93:1792.

77. Haas JA, Larson MV, Marchand GR, et al. Phosphaturic effect of furosemide: role of TH and carbonic anhydrase. *Am J Physiol* 1977; 232:F105.

78. Knochel JP. The pathophysiology and clinical characteristics of severe hyperphosphatemia. *Arch Intern Med* 1977;137:203.

79. Kreisberg RA. Phosphorus deficiency and hypophosphatemia. *Hosp Pract* 1977;12:121.

80. Arnaud CD, Clar OH. Primary hyperparathyroidism. In: Krieger DT, Bardin CW, eds. *Current therapy in endocrinology 1983–1984.* Philadelphia: Marcel Dekker Inc, 1983:270.

81. Berson SA, Yalow RS. Parathyroid hormone in plasma in adenomatous hyperparathyroidism, uremia and bronchogenic carcinoma. *Science* 1966;154:907.

82. Glikman RM. Malabsorption. Pathophysiology and diagnosis. In: Wyngaarden JB, Smith LHJ, eds. *Cecil's textbook of medicine.* Philadelphia: WB Saunders, 1985:710.

83. Roth KS, Foreman JW, Segal S. The Faconi syndrome and mechanisms of tubular dysfunction. *Kidney Int* 1981;20:705.

84. Lloyd SE, Pearce SHS, Fisher SE, et al. A common molecular basis for three inherited kidney stone diseases. *Nature* 1996;379: 445.

85. Tieder M. Hereditary hypophosphatemic rickets with hypercalciuria. *N Engl J Med* 1985;312:611.

86. Gazit D, Tieder M, Liberman UA, et al. Osteomalacia in hereditary hypophosphatemic rickets with hypercalciuria: a correlative clinical-histomorphometric study. *J Clin Endocr Metab* 1991;72:229.

87. Scheinman SJ. X-linked hypercalciuric nephrolithiasis: clinical syndromes and chloride channel mutations. *Kidney Int* 1998;53:3.

88. Gunther W, Luchow A, Cluzeaud F, et al. ClC-5, the chloride channel mutated in Dent's disease, colocalizes with the proton pump in endocytotically active kidney cells. *Proc Natl Acad Sci USA* 1998;95: 8075.

89. Jentsch TJ, Gunther W. Chloride channels: an emerging molecular picture. *BioEssays* 1997;19:117.

90. Howell RR. Essential fructosuria and hereditary fructose intolerance. In: Wyngaarden JB, Smith LHJ, eds. *Cecil's textbook of medicine.* Philadelphia: WB Saunders, 1985:1108.

91. Rosenbaum RW, Hruska KA, Korkor A, et al. Decreased phosphate reabsorption after renal transplantation: evidence for a mechanism independent of calcium and parathyroid hormone. *Kidney Int* 1981;19: 568.

92. Falls WFJ, Stacey WK. Postobstructive diuresis. Studies in a dialyzed patient with a solitary kidney. *Am J Med* 1973;54:404.

93. Moorhead JF, Wills MR, Ahmed KY, et al. Hypophosphatemic osteomalacia after cadaveric renal transplantation. *Lancet* 1974;1:694.

94. Beck LH, Goldberg M. Mechanism of the blunted phosphaturia in saline-loaded thyroparathyroidectomized dogs. *Kidney Int* 1974; 6:18.

95. Kos CH, Lemieux N, Tihy F, et al. The renal specific Na⁺-phosphate cotransporter cDNA maps to human chromosome 5q35. *J Am Soc Nephrol* 1993;4:810(abst).

96. The Hyp Consortium. A gene (PEX) with homologies to endopeptidases is mutated in patients with X-linked hypophosphatemic rickets. *Nat Genetics* 1995;11:130.

97. White KE, Lorenz B, Evans WE, et al. Autosomal dominant hypophosphatemic rickets is caused by mutations in a novel gene, FGF23, that shares homology with the fibroblast growth factor family. *J Bone Miner Res* 2000;15:S153(abst).

98. Eicher EM, Southard JL, Scriver CR, et al. Hypophosphatemia: mouse model for human familial hypophosphatemic (Vitamin D-resistant) rickets. *Proc Natl Acad Sci USA* 1976;73:4667.

99. Tenenhouse HS, Scriver CR. Effect of 1,25-dihydroxyvitamin D₃ on phosphate homeostasis in the X-linked hypophosphatemic (Hyp) mouse. *Endocrinology* 1981;109:658.

100. Brickman AS, Coburn JW, Kurokawa K, et al. Actions of 1,25-dihydroxycholecalciferol in patients with hypophosphatemic, Vitamin D-resistant rickets. *N Engl J Med* 1973;289:495.

101. Russell RG, Smith R, Preston C, et al. The effect of 1,25-dihydroxycholecalciferol on renal tubular reabsorption of phosphate, intestinal absorption of calcium and bone histology in hypophosphataemic renal tubular rickets. *Clin Sci Mol Med* 1975;48:177.

102. Beamer WG, Wilson MD, DeLuca HF. Successful treatment of genetically hypophosphatemic mice by 1-alpha-hydroxy Vitamin D₃ but not 1,25-dihydroxyvitamin D₃. *Endocrinology* 1980;106:1949.

103. Tenenhouse HS, Scriver CR, McInnes RR, et al. Renal handling of phosphate in vivo and in vitro by the X-linked hypophosphatemic male mouse: evidence for a defect in the brush border membrane. *Kidney Int* 1978;14:236.

104. Tenenhouse HS, Werner A, Biber J, et al. Renal Na⁺-phosphate cotransport in murine X-linked hypophosphatemic rickets: molecular characterization. *J Clin Invest* 1994;93:671.

105. Chong SS, Kristjansson K, Zoghbi HY, et al. Molecular cloning of the cDNA encoding a human renal sodium phosphate transport protein and its assignment to chromosome 6p21.3-p23. *Genomics* 1993;18:355.

106. Meyer RAJ, Tenenhouse HS, Meyer M, et al. The renal phosphate transport defect in normal mice parabiosed to X-linked hypophosphatemic mice persists after parathyroidectomy. *J Bone Miner Res* 1989;4: 523.

107. Nesbitt T, Coffman TM, Griffiths R, et al. Crosstransplantation of kidneys in normal and Hyp mice. Evidence that the Hyp mouse phenotype is unrelated to an intrinsic renal defect. *J Clin Invest* 1992;89:1453.

108. Econs MJ, Drezner MK. Tumor-induced osteomalacia: unveiling a new hormone. *N Engl J Med* 1994;330:1645.

109. Rifas L, Dawson LL, Halstead LH, et al. Phosphate transport in osteoblasts from normal and X-linked hypophosphatemic mice. *Calcif Tissue Int* 1995;54:505.

110. Ecarot B, Glorieux FH, Desbarats M, et al. Defective bone formation by Hyp mouse bone cells transplanted into normal mice: evidence in favor of an intrinsic osteoblast defect. *J Bone Miner Res* 1992;7: 215.

111. Ecarot B, Glorieux FH, Desbarats M, et al. Effect of dietary phosphate deprivation and supplementation of recipient mice on bone formation by transplanted cells from normal and X-linked hypophosphatemic mice. *J Bone Miner Res* 1992;7:523.

112. Hruska KA, Rifas L, Cheng S-L, et al. X-linked hypophosphatemic rickets and the murine *Hyp* homologue. *Am J Physiol* 1995;268:F357.

113. Rifas L, Avioli LV, Cheng SL. 1,25(OH)$_2$D$_3$ Corrects underphosphorylation of osteopontin in the Hyp/Y mouse osteoblast. In: Bouillon R, Norman AW, Thomasset M, eds. *Vitamin D, a pluripotent steroid hormone: structural studies, molecular endocrinology and clinical applications.* New York: de Gruyter, 1994:700.

114. Cai Q, Hodgson SF, Kao PC, et al. Brief report: inhibition of renal phosphate transport by a tumor product in a patient with oncogenic osteomalacia. *N Engl J Med* 1994;330:1645.

115. Glorieux FH, Marie PJ, Pettifor JM, et al. Bone response to phosphate salts, ergocalciferol, and calcitriol in hypophosphatemic Vitamin D-resistant rickets. *N Engl J Med* 1980;303:1023.

116. Verge CF, Lam A, Simpson JM, et al. Effect of therapy in X-linked hypophosphatemic rickets. *N Engl J Med* 1991;325:1875.

117. Friedman NE, Lobaugh B, Drezner MK. Effects of calcitriol and phosphorus therapy on the growth of patients with X-linked hypophosphatemia. *J Clin Endocrinol Metab* 1993;76:839.

118. Weinstein LS, Shenker A, Gejman PV, et al. Activation mutations of the stimulatory G protein in the McCune-Albright syndrome. *N Engl J Med* 1991;325:1688.

119. Gray RW, Wilz DR, Caldas AE, et al. The importance of phosphate in regulating plasma 1,25-(OH)$_2$-vitamin D levels in human: studies in healthy subjects, in calcium-stone formers and in patients with primary hyperparathyroidism. *J Clin Endocrinol Metab* 1977;45:299.

120. Frame B, Parfitt AM. Osteomalacia current concepts. *Ann Intern Med* 1978;89:966.

121. Eberle M, Traynor-Kaplan AE, Sklar LA, et al. Is there a relationship between phosphatidylinositol triphosphate and F-actin polymerization in human neutrophils? *J Biol Chem* 1990;265:16725.

122. Fu GK, Lin D, Zhang MY, et al. Cloning of human 25-hydroxyvitamin D-1 alpha-hydroxylase and mutations causing Vitamin D-dependent rickets type 1. *Mol Endocrinol* 1997;11:1961.

123. Liberman UA, Eil C, Marx SJ. Resistance of 1,25-dihydroxyvitamin D. Associated with heterogeneous defects in cultured skin fibroblasts. *J Clin Invest* 1983;71:192.

124. Feldman D, Chen T, Cone C, et al. Vitamin D resistant rickets with alopecia: cultured skin fibroblasts exhibit defective cytoplasmic receptors and unresponsiveness to 1,25(OH)$_2$D$_3$. *J Clin Endocrinol Metab* 1982;55:1020.

125. Chen TL, Hirst MA, Cone CM, et al. 1,25-dihydroxyvitamin D resistance, rickets and alopecia: analysis of receptors and bioresponse in cultured fibroblasts from patients and parents. *J Clin Endocrinol Metab* 1984;59:383.

126. Malloy PJ, Hochberg Z, Pike JW, et al. Abnormal binding of Vitamin D receptors to deoxyribonucleic acid in a kindred with Vitamin D-dependent rickets, type II. *J Clin Endocrinol Metab* 1989;68:263.

127. Hochberg Z, Weisman Y. Calcitriol-resistant rickets due to Vitamin D receptor defects. *Trends Endocrinol Metab* 1995;6:216.

128. Hewison M, Rut AR, Kristjansson K, et al. Tissue resistance to 1,25-dihydroxyvitamin D without a mutation of the Vitamin D receptor gene. *Clin Endocrinol* 1993;39:663.

129. Refetoff S, Weiss RE, Usala SJ. The syndromes of resistance to thyroid hormone. *Endocr Rev* 1993;14:348.

130. McPhaul MJ, Marcelli M, Zoppi S, et al. Genetic basis of endocrine disease. 4. The spectrum of mutations in the androgen receptor gene that causes androgen resistance. *J Clin Endocrinol Metab* 1993;76:17.

131. Smith EP, Boyd J, Frank GR, et al. Estrogen resistance caused by a mutation in the estrogen receptor gene in a man. *N Engl J Med* 1994;331:1088.

132. Li YC, Amling M, Pirro AE, et al. Normalization of mineral ion homeostasis by dietary means prevents hyperparathyroidism, rickets, and osteomalacia, but not alopecia in Vitamin D receptor-ablated mice. *Endocrinology* 1998;139:4391.

133. Parker MS, Klein I, Haussler MR, et al. Tumor-induced osteomalacia: evidence of a surgically correctable alteration in Vitamin D metabolism. *JAMA* 1981;245:492.

134. Rowe PSN, Ong ACM, Cockerill FJ, et al. Candidate 56 and 58 kDa protein(s) responsible for mediating the renal defects in oncogenic hypophosphatemic osteomalacia. *Bone* 1996;18:159.

135. Nemere I, Norman AW. The rapid, hormonally stimulated transport of calcium (transcaltachia). *J Bone Miner Res* 1987;2:167.

136. Weidner N. Review and update: oncogenic osteomalacia-rickets. *Ultrastruct Pathol* 1991;15:317.

137. Sweet RA, Males JL, Hamstra AJ, et al. Vitamin D metabolite-levels in oncogenic osteomalacia. *Ann Intern Med* 1980;93:270.

138. Drezner MK, Feinglos MN. Osteomalacia due to 1alpha,25-dihydroxycholecalciferol deficiency. Association with a giant cell tumor of bone. *J Clin Invest* 1977;60:1046.

139. Ribovich ML, DeLuca HF. Effect of dietary calcium and phosphorus on intestinal calcium absorption and Vitamin D metabolism. *Arch Biochem Biophys* 1978;188:145.

140. Miyauchi A, Fukase M, Tsutsumi M, et al. Hemangiopericytoma-induced osteomalacia: tumor transplantation in nude mice causes hypophosphatemia and tumor extracts inhibit renal 25-hydroxyvitamin D 1-hydroxylase activity. *J Clin Endocrinol Metab* 1988;67:46.

141. Klahr S, Davis TA. Changes in renal function with chronic protein-calorie malnutrition. In: Mitch WE, Klahr S, eds. *Nutrition and the kidney.* Boston: Little, Brown and Company, 1988:59.

142. Shields HM. Rapid fall of serum phosphorus secondary to antacid therapy. *Gastroenterology* 1978;75:1137.

143. Juan D, Elrazak MA. Hypophosphatemia in hospitalized patients. *JAMA* 1979;242:163.

144. Larsson L, Rebel K, Sorbo B. Severe hypophosphatemia-a hospital survey. *Acta Med Scand* 1983;214:221.

145. Betro MG, Pain RW. Hypophosphatemia and hyperphosphatemia in a hospital population. *Br Med J* 1972;1:273.

146. Ryback RS, Eckardt MJ, Pautler CP. Clinical relationships between serum phosphorus and other blood chemistry values in alcoholics. *Arch Intern Med* 1980;140:673.

147. Seldin DW, Tarail R. The metabolism of glucose and electrolytes in diabetic acidosis. *J Clin Invest* 1950;29:552.

148. Mostellar ME, Tuttle EPJ. Effects of alkalosis on plasma concentration and urinary excretion of urinary phosphate in man. *J Clin Invest* 1964;43:138.

149. Aderka D, Shoenfeld Y, Santo M, et al. Life-threatening hypophosphatemia in a patient with acute myelogenous leukemia. *Acta Haematol* 1980;64:117.

150. Matzner Y, Prococimer M, Polliack A, et al. Hypophosphatemia in a patient with lymphoma in leukemic phase. *Arch Intern Med* 1981;141:805.

151. Zamkoff KW, Kirshner JJ. Marked hypophosphatemia associated with acute myelomonocytic leukemia: indirect evidence of phosphorus uptake by leukemic cells. *Arch Intern Med* 1980;140:1523.

152. Chesney PJ, Davis JP, Purdy WK, et al. Clinical manifestations of toxic shock syndrome. *JAMA* 1981;246:741.

153. Lennquist S, Lindell B, Nordstrom H, et al. Hypophosphatemia in severe burns: a prospective study. *Acta Chir Scand* 1979;145:1.

154. Levy LA. Severe hypophosphatemia as a complication of the treatment of hypothermia. *Arch Intern Med* 1980;140:128.

155. Silvis SE, DiBartolomeo AG, Aaker HM. Hypophosphatemia and neurologic changes secondary to oral caloric intake: a variant of hyperalimentation syndrome. *Am J Gastroenterol* 1980;73:215.

156. Weinsier RL, Krumdiek CL. Death resulting from overzealous total parenteral nutrition: the refeeding syndrome revisited. *Am J Clin Nutr* 1981;34:393.

157. Kono N, Kuwajima M, Tarui S. Alteration of glycolytic intermediary metabolism in erythrocytes during diabetic ketoacidosis and its recovery phase. *Diabetes* 1981;30:346.

158. Ditzel J. Changes in red cell oxygen release capacity in diabetes mellitus. *Fed Proc* 1979;38:2484.

159. Nutter DO, Glenn JF. Reversible severe congestive cardiomyopathy in three cases of hypophosphatemia [retraction of Darsee JR, Nutter DO. In: *Ann Intern Med* 1978;89:867]. *Ann Intern Med* 1983;99:275.

160. Zazzo JF, Troche G, Ruel P, et al. High incidence of hypophosphatemia in surgical intensive care patients: efficacy of phosphorus therapy on myocardial function. *Intensive Care Med* 1995;21:826.

161. Fuller TJ, Nichols WW, Brenner BJ, et al. Reversible depression in myocardial performance in dogs with experimental phosphorus deficiency. *J Clin Invest* 1978;62:1190.

162. Knochel JP, Barcenas C, Cotton JR, et al. Hypophosphatemia and rhabdomyolysis. *J Clin Invest* 1978;62:1240.

163. Knochel JP, Bilbrey GL, Fuller TJ. The muscle cell in chronic alcoholism: the possible role of phosphate depletion in alcoholic myopathy. *Ann N Y Acad Sci* 1975;252:274.

164. Kretz J, Sommer G, Boland R, et al. Lack of involvement of sarcoplasmic reticulum in myopathy of acute phosphorus depletion. *Klin Wochenschr* 1980;58:833.

165. DeFronzo RA, Lang R. Hypophosphatemia and glucose intolerance: evidence for tissue insensitivity to insulin. *N Engl J Med* 1980;303:1259.

166. Bellingham AJ, Detter JC, Lenfant C. The role of hemoglobin affinity for oxygen and red cell 2,3-diphosphoglycerate in the management of diabetic ketoacidosis. *Trans Assoc Am Physicians* 1970;83:113.

167. Lichtman MA, Miller DR, Cohen J, et al. Reduced red cell glycolysis, 2,3-diphosphoglycerate and adenosine triphosphate concentration and increased hemoglobin-oxygen affinity caused by hypophosphatemia. *Ann Intern Med* 1971;74:562.

168. Travis SF, Sugarman HJ, Ruberg RL, et al. Alterations of red-cell glycolytic intermediates and oxygen transport as a consequence of hypophosphatemia in patients receiving intravenous hyperalimentation. *N Engl J Med* 1971;285:763.

169. Jacob HS, Amsden T. Acute hemolytic anemia and rigid red cells in hypophosphatemia. *N Engl J Med* 1971;285:1446.

170. Klock JC, Williams HE, Mentzer WC. Hemolytic anemia and somatic cell dysfunction in severe hypophosphatemia. *Arch Intern Med* 1974;134:360.

171. Craddock PR, Yawata Y, Van Santen L, et al. Acquired phagocyte dysfunction: a complication of the hypophosphatemia of parental hyperalimentation. *N Engl J Med* 1974;290:1403.

172. Riedler GF, Scheitlin WA. Hypophosphatemia in septicemia: higher incidence in Gram-negative than in Gram-positive infections. *Br Med J* 1969;1:753.

173. Lotz M, Ney R, Bartter FC. Osteomalacia and debility resulting from phosphorus depletion. *Trans Assoc Am Physicians* 1964;77:281.

174. Lotz M, Zisman E, Bartter FC. Evidence for a phosphorus-depletion syndrome in man. *N Engl J Med* 1968;278:409.

175. Prins JG, Schrijver H, Staghouwer JM. Hyperalimentation, hypophosphatemia and coma. *Lancet* 1973;1:1253.

176. Boelens PA, Norwood W, Kjellstrand C, et al. Hypophosphatemia with muscle weakness due to antacids and hemodialysis. *Am J Dis Child* 1970;120:350.

177. Baker LRI, Ackrill P, Cattell WR, et al. Iatrogenic osteomalacia and myopathy due to phosphate depletion. *Br Med J* 1974;3:150.

178. Cooke N, Teitelbaum S, Avioli LV. Antacid-induced osteomalacia and nephrolithiasis. *Arch Intern Med* 1978;138:1007.

179. Ahmed KY, Varghese Z, Willis MR, et al. Persistent hypophosphatemia and osteomalacia in dialysis patients not on oral phosphate-binders: response to dihydrotachysterol therapy. *Lancet* 1976;1:439.

180. Moser CR, Fessel WJ. Rheumatic manifestations of hypophosphatemia. *Arch Intern Med* 1974;134:674.

181. Coburn JW, Massry SG. Changes in serum and urinary calcium during phosphate depletion: studies on mechanisms. *J Clin Invest* 1970;49:1073.

182. Dominguez JH, Gray RW, Lemann JJ. Dietary phosphate deprivation in women and men: effects on mineral and acid balances, parathyroid hormone and the metabolism of 25-OH-Vitamin D. *J Clin Endocrinol Metab* 1976;43:1056.

183. Emmett M, Goldfarb S, Agus ZS, et al. The pathophysiology of acid-base changes in chronically phosphate-depleted rats: bone-kidney interactions. *J Clin Invest* 1977;59:291.

184. Gold LW, Massry SG, Arieff AI, et al. Renal bicarbonate wasting during phosphate depletion: a possible cause of altered acid-base homeostasis in hyperparathyroidism. *J Clin Invest* 1973;52:2556.

185. Gold LW, Massry SG, Friedler RM. Effect of phosphate depletion on renal tubular reabsorption of glucose. *J Lab Clin Med* 1977;89:554.

186. Goldfarb S, Westby GR, Goldberg M, et al. Renal tubular effects of chronic phosphate depletion. *J Clin Invest* 1977;59:770.

187. Muhlbauer RC, Bonjour JP, Fleisch H. Tubular localization to dietary phosphate in rats. *Am J Physiol* 1978;234:E290.

188. Steele TH, Stromberg BA, Larmore CA. Renal resistance to parathyroid hormone during phosphorus deprivation. *J Clin Invest* 1976;58:1461.

189. O'Donovan DJ, Lotspeich WD. Activation of kidney mitochondrial glutaminase by inorganic phosphate and organic acids. *Nature* 1966;212:930.

190. Agus ZS, Goldfarb S, Wasserstein A. Disorders of calcium and phosphate balance. In: Brenner BM, Rector FCJ, eds. *The kidney.* Philadelphia: WB Saunders, 1981:940.

191. Harris CA, Bauer PG, Chirito E, et al. Composition of mammalian glomerular filtrate. *Am J Physiol* 1974;227:972.

192. Lentz RD, Brown DM, Kjellstrand CM. Treatment of severe hypophosphatemia. *Ann Intern Med* 1978;89:941.

193. Slatopolsky E, Gradowska L, Kashemsant C. The control of phosphate excretion in uremia. *J Clin Invest* 1966;45:672.

194. Slatopolsky E, Robson AM, Elkan I, et al. Control of phosphate excretion in uremic man. *J Clin Invest* 1968;47:1865.

195. Goldman R, Bassett SH. Phosphorus excretion in renal failure. *J Clin Invest* 1954;33:1623.

196. Rutherford E, Mercado A, Hruska K, et al. An evaluation of a new and effective phosphate binding agent. *Trans Am Soc Artif Intern Organs* 1973;19:446.

197. Massry SG, Arieff AI, Coburn JW, et al. Divalent ion metabolism in patients with acute renal failure: studies on the mechanism of hypocalcemia. *Kidney Int* 1974;5:437.

198. Koffler A, Friedler RM, Massry SG. Acute renal failure due to nontraumatic rhabdomyolysis. *Ann Intern Med* 1976;85:23.

199. Parfitt AM. The spectrum of hypoparathyroidism. *J Clin Endocrinol Metab* 1972;34:152.

200. Albright F, Burnett CH, Smith PH, et al. Pseudohypoparathyroidism—an example of "Seabright-Bantam syndrome." *Endocrinology* 1942;30:922.

201. Bourne HR, Kaslow HR, Brickman AS, et al. Fibroblast defect in pseudohypoparathyroidism, type I: reduced activity of receptor-cyclase coupling protein. *J Clin Endocrinol Metab* 1981;53:636.

202. Farfel Z, Brickman AS, Kaslow HR, et al. Defect of receptor-cyclase coupling protein in pseudohypoparathyroidism. *N Engl J Med* 1980;303:237.

203. Drezner M, Neelon FA, Lebovitz HE. Pseudohypoparathyroidism type II: a possible defect in the reception of the cyclic AMP signal. *N Engl J Med* 1973;289:1056.

204. Connors MH, Irias JJ, Golabi M. Hypo-hyperparathyroidism: evidence for a defective parathyroid hormone. *Pediatrics* 1977;60:343.

205. Lambert PP, Corvilan J. Site of action of parathyroid hormone and role of growth hormone in phosphate excretion. In: Williams PC, ed. *Hormones and the kidney (memoirs of the Society of Endocrinology, no. 13).* New York: Academic Press, 1963:130.

206. Mitnick PD, Goldbarb S, Slatopolsky E, et al. Calcium and phosphate metabolism in tumoral calcinosis. *Ann Intern Med* 1980;92:482.

207. Lufkin EG, Wilson DM, Smith LH, et al. Phosphorus excretion in tumoral calcinosis: response to parathyroid hormone and acetazolamide. *J Clin Endocrinol Metab* 1980;50:648.

208. Zerwekh JE, Sanders LA, Townsend J, et al. Tumoral calcinosis: evidence for concurrent defects in renal tubular phosphorus transport and in 1alpha,25-dihydroxycholecalciferol synthesis. *Calcif Tissue Int* 1980;32:1.

209. Walton RJ, Russell RG, Smith R. Changes in the renal and extrarenal handling of phosphate induced by disodium etidronate (EHDP) in man. *Clin Sci Mol Med* 1975;49:45.

210. Zusman J, Brown DM, Nesbit ME. Hyperphosphatemia, hyperphosphaturia and hypocalcemia in acute lymphoblastic leukemia. *N Engl J Med* 1973;289:1335.

211. Cohen LF, Balow JE, Magrath IT, et al. Acute tumor lysis syndrome. A review of 37 patients with Burkitt's lymphoma. *Am J Med* 1980;68:486.

212. Tsokos GC, Balow JE, Spiegel RJ, et al. Renal and metabolic complications of undifferentiated and lymphoblastic lymphomas. *Medicine* 1981;60:218.

213. Giebisch G, Berger L, Pitts RF. The extra-renal response to acute acid-base disturbances of respiratory origin. *J Clin Invest* 1955;34:231.

214. Honig PJ, Holtzapple PG. Hypocalcemic tetany following hypertonic phosphate enemas. *Clin Pediatr* 1975;14:678.

215. McConnell TH. Fatal hypocalcemia from phosphate absorption from laxative preparation. *JAMA* 1971;216:147.

216. Payne JW, Walser M. Ion association. II. The effect of multivalent ions on the concentration of free calcium ions as measured by the frog heart method. *Bull Johns Hopkins Hosp* 1959;105:298.

217. Morgan DB. Calcium and phosphorus transport across the intestine. In: Girdwood RM, Smith AW, eds. *Malabsorption.* Baltimore: Williams & Wilkins, 1969.

218. Slatopolsky E, Caglar S, Gradowska L, et al. On the prevention of secondary hyperparathyroidism in experimental chronic renal disease using "proportional reduction" of dietary phosphorus intake. *Kidney Int* 1972;2:147.

219. Golden P, Mazey R, Greenwalt A, et al. Vitamin D: a direct effect on the parathyroid gland. *Miner Electrolyte Metab* 1979;2:1.

220. Slatopolsky E, Weerts C, Thielan J. Marked suppression of secondary hyperparathyroidism by intravenous administration of 1,25-dihydroxycholecalciferol in uremic patients. *J Clin Invest* 1984;74:2136.

221. Parfitt AM. The hyperparathyroidism of chronic renal failure: a disorder of growth. *Kidney Int* 1997;52:3.

222. Slatopolsky E, Finch J, Denda M, et al. Phosphorus restriction prevents parathyroid gland growth. High phosphorus directly stimulates PTH secretion in vitro. *J Clin Invest* 1996;97:2534.

223. Silver J, Sela SB, Naveh-Man T. Regulation of parathyroid cell proliferation. *Curr Opinion Nephrol Hypertens* 1997;6:321.

224. Denda M, Finch J, Slatopolsky E. Phosphorus accelerates the development of parathyroid hyperplasia and secondary hyperparathyroidism in rats with renal failure. *Am J Kidney Dis* 1996;28:596.

225. Dusso AS, Lu Y, Pavlopoulos T, et al. A role of enhanced expression of transforming growth factor alpha (TGF-alpha) in the mitogenic effect of high dietary phosphorus on parathyroid cell growth in uremia. *J Am Soc Nephrol* 1999;10:617(abst).

226. Kumar V, Bustin SA, McKay IA. Transforming growth factor alpha. *Cell Biol Int* 1995;19:373.

227. Driman DK, Kobrin MS, Kudlow JE, et al. Transforming growth factor-alpha in normal and neoplastic human endocrinal tissues. *Hum Pathol* 1992;23:1360.

228. Gogusev J, Duchambon P, Stoermann-Chopard C, et al. De novo expression of transforming growth factor-alpha in parathyroid gland tissue of patients with primary or secondary uraemic hyperparathyroidism. *Nephrol Dial Transplantation* 1996;11:2155.

229. Berlyne GM, Ben-Ari J, Pest D, et al. Hyperaluminaemia from aluminum resins in renal failure. *Lancet* 1970;2:494.

230. Ward MK, Feest TG, Ellis HA. Osteomalacic dialysis osteodystrophy: evidence for a water-borne aetiological agent, probably aluminum. *Lancet* 1978;1:841.

231. Moriniere PH, Roussel A, Tahira Y, et al. Substitution of aluminum hydroxide by high doses of calcium carbonate in patients on chronic hemodialysis: disappearance of hyperaluminaemia and equal control of hyperparathyroidism. *Proc Eur Dial Transplant Assoc* 1982;19:784.

232. Slatopolsky E, Weerts C, Lopez-Hilker S, et al. Calcium carbonate as a phosphate binder in patients with chronic renal failure undergoing dialysis. *N Engl J Med* 1986;315:157.

233. Slatopolsky E, Weerts C, Norwood K, et al. Long-term effects of calcium carbonate and 2.5 mEq/liter calcium dialysate on mineral metabolism. *Kidney Int* 1989;36:897.

234. Ribeiro S, Ramos A, Brandao A, et al. Cardiac valve calcification in hemodialysis patients: role of calcium-phosphate metabolism. *Nephrol Dial Transplantation* 1988;13:2037.

235. Rostand SG, Sanders C, Kirk KA, et al. Myocardial calcification and cardiac dysfunction in chronic renal failure. *Am J Med* 1988;85:651.

236. London GM, Dannier B, Marchais SJ, et al. Calcification of the aortic valve in the dialyzed patient. *J Am Soc Nephrol* 2000;11:778.

237. Guerin AP, London GM, Marchais SJ, et al. Arterial stiffening and vascular calcifications in end-stage renal disease. *Nephrol Dial Transplantation* 2000;13:2037.

238. Braun J, Oldendorf M, Moshage W, et al. Electron beam computed tomography in the evaluation of cardiac calcification in chronic dialysis patients. *Am J Kidney Dis* 1996;27:394.

239. Goodman WG, Goldin J, Kuizon BD, et al. Coronary-artery calcification in young adults with end-stage renal disease who are undergoing dialysis. *N Engl J Med* 2000;342:1478.

240. Milliner DS, Zinsmeister AR, Lieberman L, et al. Soft tissue calcification in pediatric patients with end-stage renal disease. *Kidney Int* 1990;38:931.

241. Chertow GM, Burke SK, Lazarus JM, et al. Poly(allylamine hydrochloride) (Renagel): a noncalcemic phosphate binder for the treatment of hyperphosphatemia in chronic renal failure. *Am J Kidney Dis* 1997;29:66.

242. Slatopolsky E, Burke SK, Dillon MA. Renagel, a nonabsorbed calcium and aluminum-free phosphate-binder, lowers serum phosphorus and parathyroid hormone. *Kidney Int* 1999;55:299.

243. Chertow GM, Burke SK, Dillon MA, et al Long-term effects of sevelamer hydrochloride on the calcium × phosphate product and lipid profile of haemodialysis patients. *Nephrol Dial Transplantation* 1999;14:2907.

244. Humes HD. Regulation of intracellular calcium. *Semin Nephrol* 1984;4(2):110.

245. Carafoli E. Calcium pump of the plasma membrane. *Physiol Rev* 1991;71:129.

246. Jencks WP. How does a calcium pump pump calcium? *J Biol Chem* 1989;264:18855.

247. Nicoll DA, Longoni S, Philipson KD. Molecular cloning and functional expression of the cardiac sarcolemmal Na^+-Ca^{2+} exchanger. *Science* 1990;250:562.

248. Dominguez JH, Juhaszova M, Feister HA. The renal sodium-calcium exchanger. *J Lab Clin Med* 1992;119:640.

249. Windhager EE, Frindt G, Milovanovic S. The role of Na-Ca exchange in renal epithelia: an overview. *Ann N Y Acad Sci* 1991;639:577.

250. Schatzmann HJ. The red cell calcium pump. *Annu Rev Physiol* 1983;45:303.

251. Reilly RF, Shugrue CA. cDNA cloning of a renal Na^+/Ca^{2+} exchanger. *Am J Physiol* 1992;262:F1105.

252. Caroni P, Reinlib L, Carafoli E. Charge movements during the Na^+-Ca^{++} exchange in heart sarcolemmal vesicles. *Proc Natl Acad Sci USA* 1980;77:6350.

253. Yu ASL, Hebert SC, Lee S-L, et al. Identification and localization of renal Na^+/Ca^{2+} exchanger by polymerase chain reaction. *Am J Physiol* 1992;263:F680.

254. Hanaoka K, Imai M, Yoshitomi K. Evidence for pH-dependent active Ca^{2+} transport in the basolateral membrane of rabbit cortical thick ascending limb (CTAL). *J Am Soc Nephrol* 1990;1:570(abst).

255. Bourdeau JE, Lau K. Basolateral cell membrane Ca-Na exchange in single rabbit connecting tubules. *Am J Physiol* 1990;258:F1490.

256. Lau K, Bourdeau JE. Evidence of luminal and peritubular (Na) on cytosolic free (Ca) (Ca$_i$) in single connecting tubules (CNTs): evidence for a basolateral membrane (BLM) Ca-Na exchanger. *Kidney Int* 1990;37:450(abst).

257. Shimizu T, Yamasaki F, Imai M, et al. Regulation of calcium transport in the distal nephron segments. *Kidney Int* 1990;37:460(abst).

258. Shimizu T, Yoshitomi K, Nakamura M, et al. Effects of PTH, calcitonin, and cAMP on calcium transport in rabbit distal nephron segments. *Am J Physiol* 1990;259:F400.

259. Bouhtiauy I, Lajeunesse D, Brunette MG. The mechanism of parathyroid hormone action on calcium reabsorption by the distal tubule. *Endocrinology* 1991;128:251.

260. Hanai H, Ishida M, Liang CT, et al. Parathyroid hormone increases sodium/calcium exchange activity in renal cells and the blunting of the response in aging. *J Biol Chem* 1986;261:5410.

261. Hanai H, Liang CT, Cheng L, et al. Desensitization to parathyroid hormone in renal cells from aged rats is associated with alterations in G-protein activity. *J Clin Invest* 1989;83:260.

262. Carafoli E. The Ca^{2+} pump of the plasma membrane. *J Biol Chem* 1992;267:2110.

263. Strehler EE. Recent advances in the molecular characterization of plasma membrane Ca^{2+} pumps. *J Membr Biol* 1991;120:1.

264. Villalobo A. Reconstitution of ion-motive transport ATPases in artificial lipid membranes. *Biochim Biophys Acta* 1990;1017:1.

265. Gonzalez JM, Dalmeida W, Abramowitz J, et al. Evidence for a fourth rat isoform of the plasma membrane calcium pump in the kidney. *Biochem Biophys Res Com* 1992;184:380.

266. Borke JL, Minami J, Verma A, et al. Monoclonal antibodies to human erythrocyte membrane Ca^{++}-Mg^{++} adenosine triphosphatase pump recognize an epitope in the basolateral membrane of human kidney distal tubule cells. *J Clin Invest* 1987;80:1220.

267. Magocsi M, Yamaki M, Penniston JT, et al. Localization of mRNAs coding for isozymes of plasma membrane Ca^{2+}-ATPase pump in rat kidney. *Am J Physiol* 1992;263:F0.

268. Weinberg JM. Calcium as a mediator of renal tubule cell injury. *Semin Nephrol* 1984;4:170.

269. Burgess TL, Qian Y, Kaufman S, et al. The ligand for osteoprotegerin (OPGL) directly activates mature osteoclasts. *J Cell Biol* 1999;145:527.

270. Lacey DL, Timms E, Tan H-L, et al. Osteoprotegerin ligand is a cytokine that regulates osteoclast differentiation and activation. *Cell* 1998;93:165.

271. Kong Y-Y, Yoshida H, Sarosi I, et al. OPGL is a key regulator of osteoclastogenesis, lymphocyte development and lymph-node organogenesis. *Nature* 1999;397:315.

272. Ducy P, Zhang R, Geoffroy V, et al. Osf2/Cbfa1: a transcriptional activator of osteoblast differentiation. *Cell* 1997;89:747.

273. Rasmussen H, Bordier P. *The physiological and cellular basis of metabolic bone disease.* Baltimore: Williams & Wilkins, 1974.

274. Eriksen EF, Axelrod DW, Melsen F. *Bone histomorphometry.* New York: Raven Press, 1994.

275. Wasserman RH. Intestinal absorption of calcium and phosphorus. *Fed Proc* 1981;40:60.

276. Fleet JC, Wood RJ. Specific 1,25(OH)$_2$D$_3$-mediated regulation of transcellular calcium transport in Caco-2 cells. *Am Physiol Soc* 1999;276:G958.

277. Rasmussen H, Fontaine O, Max EE, et al. Effect of 1alpha-hydroxyvitamin D$_3$ administration on calcium transport in chick intestine brush border membrane vesicles. *J Biol Chem* 1979;254:2990.

278. Szerencsei RT, Tucker JE, Cooper CB, et al. Minimal domain requirement for cation transport by the potassium-dependent Na/Ca-K exchanger. *J Biol Chem* 2000;275:669.

279. Denhardt DT, Chambers AF. Overcoming obstacles to metastasis—defenses against host defenses: osteopontin as a shield against attack by cytotoxic host cells. *J Cell Biochem* 1994;56:48.

280. Behrend EI, Craig AM, Wilson SM, et al. Reduced malignancy of ras-transformed NIH3T3 cells expressing antisense osteopontin RNA. *Cancer Res* 1994;54:832.

281. Bikle DD, Munson S, Chafouleas J. Calmodulin may mediate 1,25-dihydroxyvitamin D-stimulated calcium transport. *FEBS Lett* 1984;174:30.

282. Bikle DD, Munson S. 1,25-dihydroxyvitamin D increases calmodulin binding to specific proteins in the chick duodenal brush border membrane. *J Clin Invest* 1985;76:2310.

283. Taylor AN, Wasserman RH. Immunofluorescent localization of Vitamin D-dependent calcium-binding proteins. *J Histochem Cytochem* 1970;18:100.

284. Wasserman RH, Corradino RA, Taylor AN. Vitamin D-dependent calcium binding protein: purification and some properties. *J Biol Chem* 1968;243:3970.

285. Wasserman RH, Taylor AN. Evidence for a Vitamin D$_3$-induced calcium-binding protein in new world primates. *Proc Soc Exp Biol Med* 1970;136:20.

286. Wasserman RH, Taylor AN. Vitamin D$_3$-induced calcium binding protein in chick intestinal mucosa. *Science* 1966;152:790.

287. Bomsztyk K, Wright FS. Effects of transepithelial fluid flux on transepithelial voltage and transport of calcium, sodium, chloride and potassium by renal proximal tubule. *Kidney Int* 1982;21:260.

288. Murphy E, Mandel JL. Cytosolic free calcium levels in rabbit proximal kidney tubules. *Am J Physiol* 1982;242:6120.

289. Ullrich KJ, Rumrich G, Kloss S. Active Ca^{2+} reabsorption in the proximal tubule of the rat kidney. Dependence on sodium and buffer transport. *Pflugers Arch (Eur J Physiol)* 1976;364:220.

290. Lassiter WE, Gottschalk CW, Mylle M. Micropuncture study of tubular reabsorption of calcium in normal rodents. *Am J Physiol* 1963;204:770.

291. Duarte CG, Watson JG. Calcium reabsorption in proximal tubule of the dog nephron. *Am J Physiol* 1967;212:1350.

292. Filipovic D, Sackin H. A calcium-permeable stretch-activated cation channel in renal proximal tubule. *Am J Physiol* 1991;260:F119.

293. McCarty NA, O'Neil RG. Dihydropyridine-sensitive cell volume regulation in proximal tubule: the calcium window. *Am J Physiol* 1990;259:950.

294. McCarty NA, O'Neil RG. Calcium-dependent control of volume regulation in renal proximal cells. I. Swelling-activated Ca^{2+} entry and release. *J Membr Biol* 1991;123:149.

295. McCarty NA, O'Neil RG. Calcium-dependent control of volume regulation in renal proximal cells. II. Roles of dihydropyridine-sensitive and insensitive Ca^{2+} entry pathways. *J Membr Biol* 1991;123:161.

296. Dominguez JH, Mann C, Rothrock JK, et al. Na$^+$-Ca^{2+} exchange and Ca^{2+} depletion in proximal tubules. *Am J Physiol* 1991;261:F328.

297. Friedman PA, Figueiredo JF, Maack T, et al. Sodium-calcium interactions in renal proximal convoluted tubule of the rabbit. *Am J Physiol* 1981;240:F558.

298. Yang JM, Lee CO, Windhager EE. Regulation of cytosolic free calcium in isolated perfused proximal tubules of Necturus. *Am J Physiol* 1988;255:F787.

299. Scoble J, Mills S, Hruska KA. Calcium transport (Ca^{2+}) in renal basolateral vesicles (BLMV): effects of parathyroid hormone (PTH). *J Clin Invest* 1985;75:1096.

300. Rouse D, Ng RCK, Suki WN. Calcium transport in the pars recta and thin descending limb of Henle of the rabbit, perfused in vitro. *J Clin Invest* 1980;65:37.

301. Bourdeau JE, Burg MB. Voltage dependence of calcium transport in the thick ascending limb of Henle's loop. *Am J Physiol* 1979;236:F357.

302. Shareghi GR, Agus ZS. Magnesium transport in the cortical thick ascending limb of Henle's loop of the rabbit. *J Clin Invest* 1982;69:759.

303. Shareghi GR, Stoner LC. Calcium transport across segments of the rabbit distal nephron in vitro. *Am J Physiol* 1978;235:F367.

304. Imai M. Calcium transport across the rabbit thick ascending limb of Henle's loop perfused in vitro. *Pflugers Arch* 1978;374:255.

305. Rocha AS, Magaldi JB, Kokko JP. Calcium and phosphate transport in isolated segments of rabbit Henle's loop. *J Clin Invest* 1977;59:975.

306. Suki WN. Calcium transport in the thick ascending limb of Henle: heterogeneity of function in the medullary and cortical segments. *J Clin Invest* 1980;66:1004.

307. Friedman PA. Renal calcium transport: sites and insights. *News Physiol Sci* 1988;3:17.

308. Friedman PA. Basal and hormone-activated calcium absorption in mouse renal thick ascending limbs. *Am J Physiol* 1988;254:F62.

309. Suki WN, Rouse D, Ng RCK, et al. Calcium transport in the thick ascending limb of Henle: heterogeneity of function in the medullary and cortical segments. *J Clin Invest* 1980;68:1004.

310. Friedman PA, Andreoli TE. CO$_2$-stimulated NaCl absorption in the mouse renal cortical thick ascending limb of Henle. Evidence for synchronous Na$^+$/H$^+$ and Cl/HCO$_3$-exchange in apical plasma membranes. *J Gen Physiol* 1982;80:683.

311. Hebert SC, Culpepper RM, Andreoli TE. NaCl transport in mouse medullary thick ascending limbs. I. Functional nephron heterogeneity and ADH-stimulated NaCl co-transport. *Am J Physiol* 1981;241:F412.

312. DeRouffignac C, DiStefano A, Wittner M, et al. Consequences of different effects of ADH and other peptide hormones on thick ascending limb of mammalian kidney. *Am J Physiol* 1991;260:R1023.

313. DiStefano A, Wittner M, Nitschke R, et al. Effects of glucagon on Na$^+$, Cl$^−$, K$^+$, Mg^{2+}, and Ca^{2+} transports in cortical medullary thick ascending limbs of mouse kidney. *Pflugers Arch* 1989;414:640.

314. Elalouf JM, Roinel N, DeRouffignac C. ADH-like effects of calcitonin on electrolyte transport by Henle's loop of rat kidney. *Am J Physiol* 1984;246:F213.

315. Furuse M, Fujita K, Hiiragi T, et al. Claudin-1 and -2: novel integral membrane proteins localizing at tight junctions with no sequence similarity to occludin. *J Cell Biol* 1998;141:1539.

316. Simon DB, Lu Y, Chaote KA, et al. Paracellin-I, a renal tight junction protein required for paracellular Mg^{2+} resorption. *Science* 1999;285:103.

317. Hoenderop JGJ, vanderKemp AWCM, Hartog A, et al. Molecular identification of the apical Ca^{2+} channel in 1,25-dihydroxyvitamin D$_3$-responsive epithelia. *J Biol Chem* 1999;274:8375.

318. Friedman PA, Gesek FA. Cellular calcium transport in renal epithelia: measurement, mechanisms, and regulation. *Physiol Rev* 1995;75:429.

319. Bacskai BJ, Friedman PA. Activation of latent Ca^{2+} channels in renal epithelial cells by parathyroid hormone. *Nature* 1990;347:388.

320. Constanzo LS. Localization of diuretic action in microperfused rat distal tubules; Ca and Na transport. *Nature* 1990;347:388.

321. Shimizu T, Nakamura M, Yoshitomi K. Interaction of trichlormethiazide or amiloride with PTH in stimulating calcium absorption in the rabbit connecting tubule. *Am J Physiol* 1991;261:F36.

322. Terada Y, Knepper MA. Thiazide-sensitive NaCl absorption in rat cortical collecting duct. *Am J Physiol* 1990;259:F519.

323. Borke JL, Caride A, Verma AK. Plasma membrane calcium pump and 28-kDa calcium protein in cells of rat kidney distal tubules. *Am J Physiol* 1989;257:F842.

324. Palmer LG, Frindt G. Amiloride-sensitive Na channels from the apical membrane of the rat cortical collecting tubule. *Proc Natl Acad Sci USA* 1986;83:2767.

325. Morel F. Sites of hormone action in the mammalian nephron. *Am J Physiol* 1981;240:F159.

326. Morel F, Chabardes D, Imbert M. Functional segmentation of the rabbit distal tubule by microdetermination of hormone dependent adenylate cyclase activity. *Kidney Int* 1976;9:264.

327. Chabardes D, Imbert-TeBoule M, Clique A. Distribution of calcitonin-sensitive adenylate cyclase along the rabbit kidney tubule. *Proc Natl Acad Sci USA* 1976;73:3608.

328. DeFronzo RA, Cooke CR, Andres R. The effect of insulin on renal handling of sodium, potassium, calcium and phosphate in man. *J Clin Invest* 1975;55:845.

329. DeFronzo RA, Goldberg M, Agus ZS. The effects of glucose and insulin on renal electrolyte transport. *J Clin Invest* 1976;58:83.

330. Lau YK, Goldfarb S, Goldberg M. Effects of phosphate administration on tubular calcium transport. *J Lab Clin Med* 1982;99:317.

331. Wong NL, Quamme GA, O'Callaghan TJ. Renal tubular transport and phosphate depletion: a micropuncture study. *Can J Physiol Pharmacol* 1980;58:1063.

332. Sutton RAL, Wong NLM, Dirks JH. Effects of metabolic acidosis and alkalosis on sodium transport in the dog kidney. *Kidney Int* 1979;15:520.

333. Hoenderop JGJ, Willems PHGM, Bindels RJM. Toward a comprehensive molecular model of active calcium reabsorption. *Am J Physiol–Renal* 2000;278:F352.

334. Shimizu T, Yoshitomi K, Nakamura M. Effect of parathyroid hormone on the connecting tubule from the rabbit kidney: biphasic response of transmural voltage. *Pflugers Arch* 1990;416:257.

335. Khalifa S, Mills SC, Hruska K. Stimulation of calcium uptake by parathyroid hormone in renal border membrane vesicles. *J Biol Chem* 1983;258:400.

336. Hruska KA, Mills SC, Khalifa S. Phosphorylation of renal brush border membrane vesicles of calcium uptake and membrane content of polyphosphoinositides. *J Biol Chem* 1983;258:2501.

337. Jayakumar A, Liang CT, Sacktor B. Na^+ gradient-dependent Ca^{2+} transport in rat renal cortex basolateral membrane vesicles. *Fed Proc* 1982;41:1366A(abst).

338. Ramachandran C, Brunette MG. Renal Na/Ca^{2+} exchange system is located exclusively in the distal tubule. *Biochem J* 1989;257:259.

339. Bourdeau JE. Calcium transport across the cortical thick ascending limb of Henle's loop. In: Bronner F, Peterlik M, eds. *Calcium and phosphate transport across biomembranes*. New York: Academic Press, 1981.

340. Bourdeau JE, Burg MB. Effect of PTH on calcium transport across the thick ascending limb of Henle's loop. *Am J Physiol* 1980;239:F121.

341. Friedman PA, Gesek FA. Calcium transport in renal epithelial cells. *Am J Physiol* 1993;264:F181.

342. Gesek FA, Friedman PA. On the mechanism of parathyroid hormone stimulation of calcium uptake by mouse distal convoluted tubule cells. *J Clin Invest* 1992;90:749.

343. Gesek FA, Friedman PA. Calcitonin stimulates calcium transport in distal convoluted tubule cells. *Am J Physiol* 1993;264:F744.

344. Yu ASL, Hebert SC, Brenner BM, et al. Molecular characterization and nephron distribution of a family of transcripts encoding the pore-forming subunit of Ca^{2+} channels in the kidney. *Proc Natl Acad Sci USA* 1992;89:10494.

345. Quamme GA. Effect of hypercalcemia on renal tubular handling of calcium and magnesium. *Can J Physiol Pharmacol* 1982;60:1275.

346. Brown EM, Hebert SC. A cloned Ca^{2+}-sensing receptor; a mediator of direct effects of extracellular Ca^{2+} on renal function? *J Am Soc Nephrol* 1995;6:1530.

347. Hebert SC, Brown EM. The scent of an ion: calcium-sensing and its roles in health and disease. *Curr Opinion Nephrol Hypertens* 1996;5:45.

348. Hebert SC. Extracellular calcium-sensing receptor: implications for calcium and magnesium handling in the kidney. *Kidney Int* 1996;50:129.

349. Massry SG, Coburn JW, Chapman LW, et al. Effect of NaCl infusion on urinary Ca^{++} and Mg^{++} during reduction in their filtered loads. *Am J Physiol* 1967;213:1218.

350. Edwards BR, Baer PG, Sutton RA, et al. Micropuncture study of diuretic effects on sodium and calcium reabsorption in the dog nephron. *J Clin Invest* 1973;52:2418.

351. Gesek FA, Friedman PA. Mechanism of calcium transport stimulated by chlorothiazide in mouse distal convoluted tubule cells. *J Clin Invest* 1992;90:429.

352. Schneider AB, Sherwood LM. Pathogenesis and management of hypoparathyroidism and hypocalcemic disorders. *Metabolism* 1975;24:871.

353. Ireland AW, Hornbrook HW, Neale FC. The crystalline lens in chronic surgical hypoparathyroidism. *Arch Intern Med* 1968;122:408.

354. Chopra D, Janson P, Sawin CT. Insensitivity to digoxin associated with hypocalcemia. *N Engl J Med* 1977;296:917.

355. Connor TB, Rosen BL, Blaustein MP. Hypocalcemia precipitating congestive heart failure. *N Engl J Med* 1982;307:869.

356. Nagant de Deuxchaisnes C, Krane SM. Hypoparathyroidism. In: Avioli LV, Krane SM, eds. *Metabolic bone disease*. New York: Academic Press, 1978:217.

357. Sherwood LM, Santora AC. Hypoparathyroid states in the differential diagnosis of hypocalcemia. In: Bilezikian JP, Marcus R, Levine MA, eds. *The parathyroids: basic and clinical concepts*. New York: Raven Press, 1994:747.

358. Davis RH, Fourman P, Smith JWG. Prevalence of parathyroid insufficiency after thyroidectomy. *Lancet* 1961;2:1432.

359. Salander H, Tisell LE. Incidence of hypoparathyroidism after radical surgery for thyroid carcinoma and autotransplantation of parathyroid glands. *Am J Surg* 1977;134:358.

360. DiGeorge AM. Congenital absence of the thymus and its immunologic consequence: concurrence with congenital hypoparathyroidism. *Birth Defects* 1968;4:16.

361. Miller MJ, Frame B, Poyanski A. Branchial anomalies in idiopathic hypoparathyroidism: branchial dysembryogenesis. *Henry Ford Hosp Med J* 1972;20:3.

362. Anast CW, Mohs JM, Kaplan SL. Evidence for parathyroid failure in magnesium deficiency. *Science* 1972;177:606.

363. Chase LR, Slatopolsky E. Secretion and metabolic efficacy of parathyroid hormone in patients with severe hypomagnesemia. *J Clin Endocrinol Metab* 1974;38:363.

364. Levi J, Massry SG, Coburn JW. Hypocalcemia in magnesium depleted dogs: evidence for reduced responsiveness to parathyroid hormone and relative failure of parathyroid gland function. *Metabolism* 1974;23:323.

365. Suh SM, Tashjian AH, Matsuo N. Pathogenesis of hypocalcemia in primary hypomagnesemia: normal end-organ responsiveness to parathyroid hormone, impaired parathyroid gland function. *J Clin Invest* 1973;52:153.

366. Stein GS, Lian JB. Molecular mechanisms mediating proliferation/differentiation interrelationships during progressive development of the osteoblast phenotype. *Endocr Rev* 1993;14:424.

367. Watson P, Lazowski D, Han V, et al. Parathyroid hormone restores bone mass and enhances osteoblast insulin-like growth factor I gene expression in ovariectomized rats. *Bone* 1995;16:357.

368. Bordier P, Rasmussen H, Marie P. Vitamin D metabolites and bone mineralization in man. *Clin Endocrinol Metab* 1978;46:284.

369. Breslau NA, Zerwekh JE. Pharmacology of Vitamin D preparations. In: Feldman D, Glorieux FH, Pike JW, eds. *Vitamin D*. San Diego: Academic Press, 1997:607.

370. Habener JL, Mahaffey JE. Osteomalacia and disorders of Vitamin D metabolism. *Annu Rev Med* 1978;29:327.

371. Silver J, Neale G, Thompson GR. Effect of phenobarbitone treatment on Vitamin D metabolism in mammals. *Clin Sci Mol Med* 1974;46:433.

372. Albright F, Forbes AP, Hinneman PH. Pseudopseudohypoparathyroidism. *Trans Assoc Am Physicians* 1952;65:337.

373. Mann JB, Alterman S, Hills AG. Albright's hereditary osteodystrophy comprising pseudohypoparathyroidism. *Ann Intern Med* 1962;36:315.

374. Levine MA, Schwindinger WF, Downs RW Jr, et al. Pseudohypoparathyroidism: clinical, biochemical, and molecular features. In: Bilezikian JP, Marcus R, Levine MA, eds. *The parathyroids: basic and clinical concepts*. New York: Raven Press, 1994:781.

375. Levine MA, Jap TS, Mauseth RS, et al. Activity of the stimulatory guanine nucleotide-binding protein is reduced in erythrocytes from patients with pseudohypoparathyroidism and pseudopseudohypoparathyroidism: biochemical, endocrine, and genetic analysis of Albright's hereditary osteodystrophy in six kindreds. *J Clin Endocrinol Metab* 1986;62:497.

376. Patten JL, Levine MA. Immunochemical analysis of the α-subunit of the stimulatory G-protein of adenylyl cyclase in patients with Albright's hereditary osteodystrophy. *J Clin Endocrinol Metab* 1986;76:1208.

377. Miric A, Vechio JD, Levine MA. Heterogeneous mutations in the gene encoding the alpha subunit of the stimulatory G protein of adenylyl cyclase in Albright hereditary osteodystrophy. *J Clin Endocrinol Metab* 1993;76:1560.

378. Weinstein LS. Mutations of the Gs alpha-subunit gene in Albright hereditary osteodystrophy detected by denaturing gradient gel electrophoresis. *Proc Natl Acad Sci USA* 1990;87:8287.

379. Levine MA. Resistance to multiple hormones in patients with pseudohypoparathyroidism: association with deficient activity of guanine nucleotide regulatory protein. *Am J Med* 1983;74:545.

380. Silve C, Suarez F, el Hessni A, et al. The resistance to parathyroid hormone of fibroblasts from some patients with type Ib pseudohypoparathyroidism is reversible with dexamethasone. *J Clin Endocrinol Metab* 1990;71:631.

381. Kidd GS, Schaaf M, Adler RA, et al. Skeletal responsiveness in pseudohypoparathyroidism: a spectrum of clinical disease. *Am J Med* 1980;68:772.

382. Chase LR, Melson GL, Aurbach GD. Pseudohypoparathyroidism: defective excretion of 3'-5'-AMP in response to parathyroid hormone. *J Clin Invest* 1969;48:1832.

383. Klahr S, Slatopolsky E. Urinary phosphate and cyclic AMP in pseudohypoparathyroidism. In: Massry SG, Ritz E, Rapado A, eds. *Homeostasis of phosphate and other minerals*. New York: Plenum Publishing, 1977:173.

384. Nusynowitz ML, Frame B, Kolb FO. The spectrum of the hypoparathyroid states: a classification based on physiologic principles. *Medicine* 1976;55:105.

385. Rodriguez HJ, Villareal H, Klahr S. Pseudohypoparathyroidism type II: restoration of normal renal responsiveness to parathyroid hormone by calcium administration. *J Clin Endocrinol Metab* 1974;39:693.

386. Coburn J, Slatopolsky E. Vitamin D, PTH and renal osteodystrophy. In: Brenner B, Rector F, eds. *The kidney*. Philadelphia: WB Saunders, 1981:2213.

387. Pollak MR, Brown EM, Chou YH, et al. Mutations in the human Ca^{2+}-sensing receptor gene cause familial hypocalciuric hypercalcemia and neonatal severe hyperparathyroidism. *Cell* 1993;75:1297.

388. Pearce SHS, Brown EM. Calcium-sensing receptor mutations: insights into a structurally and functionally novel receptor. *J Clin Endocrinol Metab* 1996;81:1309.

389. Chou YH, Pollak MR, Brandi ML, et al. Mutations in the human Ca^{2+}-sensing-receptor gene that cause familial hypocalciuric hypercalcemia. *Am J Hum Genetics* 1995;56:1075.

390. Pollak MR, Brown EM, Estep HL, et al. Autosomal dominant hypocalcaemia caused by a Ca^{2+}-sensing receptor gene mutation. *Nat Genetics* 1994;8:303.

391. Haldiman B, Goldstein DA, Akmal M. Renal function and blood levels of divalent ions in acute pancreatitis: a prospective study in 99 patients. *Miner Electrolyte Metab* 1980;3:190.

392. Humes HD, Ichikawa I, Troy JL. Influence of calcium on the determinants of glomerular ultrafiltration. *Trans Assoc Am Physicians* 1977;90:228.

393. Levitt MF, Halpern MH, Polimeros DP. The effect of abrupt changes in plasma calcium concentrations on renal function and electrolyte excretion in man and monkey. *J Clin Invest* 1958;37:294.

394. Poulos PP. The renal tubular reabsorption and urinary excretion of calcium by the dog. *J Lab Clin Med* 1957;49:253.

395. Beck D, Levitin H, Epstein FH. The effect of intravenous infusion of calcium on renal concentrating ability. *Am J Physiol* 1959;197:1118.

396. Carone FA. The effects upon the kidney of transient hypercalcemia induced by parathyroid extract. *Am J Pathol* 1960;36:77.

397. Gill JR, Bartter FC. On the impairment of renal concentrating ability in prolonged hypercalcemia and hypercalciuria in man. *J Clin Invest* 1961;49:16.

398. Beck N, Singh H, Reed SW. Pathogenic role of cyclic AMP in the impairment of urinary concentrating ability in acute hypercalcemia. *J Clin Invest* 1974;54:1049.

399. Guignard JP, Jones NF, Barraclough MA. Effect of brief hypercalcemia on free water reabsorption during solute diuresis: evidence for impairment of sodium transport in Henle's loop. *Clin Sci* 1970;39:337.

400. Manitius A, Levitin H, Beck D. On the mechanism of impairment of renal concentrating ability in hypercalcemia. *J Clin Invest* 1960;39:693.

401. Suki WN, Eknoyan G, Rector FC. The renal diluting and concentrating mechanisms in hypercalcemia. *Nephron* 1969;6:50.

402. Lipschitz MD, Stein JH. Renal vasoactive hormones. In: Brenner B, Rector F, eds. *The kidney*. Philadelphia: WB Saunders, 1981:650.

403. Neer RM, Potts JT Jr. Medical management of hypercalcemia and hyperparathyroidism. In: DeGroot LJCGF, Martini L, eds. *Endocrinology*. New York: Grune & Stratton, 1979:725.

404. Berliner BC, Shenker IR, Weinstock MS. Hypercalcemia associated with hypertension due to prolonged immobilization (an unusual complication of extensive burns). *Pediatrics* 1972;49:92.

405. Coburn JW, Massry SG, DePalma JR. Rapid appearance of hypercalcemia with initiation of hemodialysis. *J Am Med Assoc* 1969;210:2276.

406. Mallette LE, Bilezikian JP, Heath DA. Primary hyperparathyroidism: clinical and biochemical features. *Medicine* 1974;83:127.

407. Arieff AI, Massry SG. Calcium metabolism of brain in acute renal failure. *J Clin Invest* 1974;53:387.

408. Gardner B. The relation between serum calcium and tumor metastases. *Surg Gynecol Obstet* 1969;12:369.

409. Jessiman AG, Emerson K Jr, Shah RC. Hypercalcemia in carcinoma of the breast. *Ann Surg* 1963;157:377.

410. Myers WPL. Hypercalcemia in neoplastic disease. *Arch Surg* 1960;80:308.

411. Spencer H, Lewin I. Derangements of calcium metabolism in patients with neoplastic bone involvement. *J Chronic Dis* 1963;16:713.

412. Grill V, Martin TJ. Parathyroid hormone-related protein as a cause of hypercalcemia in malignancy. In: Bilezikian JP, Marcus R, Levine MA, eds. *The parathyroids: basic and clinical concepts*. New York: Raven Press, 1994:295.

413. Wysolmerski JJ, Broadus AE. Hypercalcemia of malignancy: the central role of parathyroid hormone-related protein. *Annu Rev Med* 1994;45:189.

414. Atkins D, Ibbotson KJ, Hillier K. Secretion of prostaglandins as bone resorbing agents by renal cortical carcinoma in culture. *Br J Cancer* 1971;36:601.

415. Cummings KB, Robertson RP. Prostaglandin: increased production by renal cell carcinoma. *J Urol* 1977;118:720.

416. Jaffe BM, Parker CW, Philpott GW. Immunochemical measurement of prostaglandin or prostaglandin-like activity from normal and neoplastic cultured tissue. *Surg Forum* 1971;22:90.

417. Klein DC, Raisz LA. Prostaglandin stimulation of bone resorption in tissue culture. *Endocrinology* 1970;86:1436.

418. Mundy GR, Luben RA, Raisz LG. Evidence for the secretion of an osteoclast stimulating factor in myeloma. *N Engl J Med* 1974;291:1041.

419. Mundy GR, Raisz LG. Big and little forms of osteoclast activating factor. *J Clin Invest* 1977;60:122.

420. Mundy GR, Rick ME, Turcotte R. Pathogenesis of hypercalcemia in lymphosarcoma cell leukemia: role of an osteoclast activating factor-like substance and a mechanism of action for glucocorticoid therapy. *Am J Med* 1978;65:600.

421. Mundy GR. Evaluation and treatment of hypercalcemia. *Hosp Pract* 1994;29:79.

422. Walls J, Ratcliffe WA, Howell A, et al. Parathyroid hormone and parathyroid-hormone related protein in the investigation of hypercalcemia in two hospital populations. *Clin Endocrinol* 1994;41:407.

423. Benson RC Jr, Riggs BL, Pickard BM. Immunoreactive forms of circulating parathyroid hormone in primary and ectopic hyperparathyroidism. *J Clin Invest* 1974;54:175.

424. Norton JA, Brennan MF, Wells SA Jr. Surgical management of hyperparathyroidism. In: Bilezikian JP, Marcus R, Levine MA, eds. *The parathyroids: basic and clinical concepts*. New York: Raven Press, 1994:531.

425. Stock JL, Marcus R. Medical management of primary hyperparathyroidism. In: Bilezik JP, Marcus R, Levine MA, eds. *The parathyroids: basic and clinical concepts*. New York: Raven Press, 1994:519.

426. Slatopolsky E. Pathophysiology of calcium, magnesium and phosphorus. In: Klahr S, ed. *The kidney and body fluids in health and disease*. New York: Plenum Publishing, 1984:269.

427. owsey J, Riggs BL. Bone changes in a patient with hypervitaminosis. *J Clin Endocrinol Metab* 1968;28:1833.

428. Katz CM, Tzagournis M. Chronic adult hypervitaminosis A with hypercalcemia. *Metabolism* 1972;21:1171.

429. Mayock RL, Bertrand P, Morrison CE. Manifestations of sarcoidosis: analysis of 145 patients, with review of nine selected from the literature. *Am J Med* 1963;35:67.

430. Barbour GL, Coburn JW, Slatopolsky E. Hypercalcemia in an anephric patient with sarcoidosis: evidence for extra-renal generation of 1,25-dihydroxyvitamin D. *N Engl J Med* 1982;305:440.

431. Bell HH, Stern PH, Pantzer E. Evidence that increased circulating 1α,25-dihydroxyvitamin D is the probable cause for abnormal calcium metabolism in sarcoidosis. *J Clin Invest* 1979;64:218.

432. Adams JS, Sharma OP, Singer FR. Metabolism of 25-hyperoxyvitamin D₃ by alveolar macrophages in sarcoidosis. *Clin Res* 1983;31:499A.

433. Walker JV, Baran D, Yakub DN. Histoplasmosis with hypercalcemia, renal failure, and papillary necrosis: confusion with sarcoidosis. *JAMA* 1977;237:1350.

434. Abassi AA, Chemplavil JK, Farah S. Hypercalcemia in active tuberculosis. *Ann Intern Med* 1979;90:324.

435. Lee JC, Catanzaro A, Parthemore JG. Hypercalcemia in disseminated coccidioidomycosis. *N Engl J Med* 1977;297:431.

436. Stoeckle JD, Hardy HL, Weber AL. Chronic beryllium disease: long-term follow up of sixty cases and selective review of the literature. *Am J Med* 1969;46:545.

437. McMillan DE, Freeman RB. The milk alkali syndrome: a study of the acute disorder with comments on the development of the chronic condition. *Medicine* 1965;44:485.

438. Orwoll ES. The milk-alkali syndrome: current concepts. *Ann Intern Med* 1982;97:242.

439. Brickman AS, Massry SG, Coburn JW. Changes in serum and urinary calcium during treatment of hydrochlorothiazide Studies on mechanisms. *J Clin Invest* 1972;51:945.

440. Malluche HH, Meyer-Sabellek WA, Singer FR. Evidence for a direct effect of thiazides on bone. *Miner Electrolyte Metab* 1980;4:89.

441. Parfitt AM. The interactions of thiazide diuretics with parathyroid hormone and Vitamin D: studies in patients with hypoparathyroidism. *J Clin Invest* 1972;51:1879.

442. Popovtzer MM, Subryan VL, Alfrey AC. The acute effect of chlorothiazide on serum ionized calcium: evidence for a parathyroid hormone-dependent mechanism. *J Clin Invest* 1975;55:1295.

443. Marx SJ, Spiegel AM, Brown EM. Divalent cation metabolism: familial hypocalciuric hypercalcemia versus typical primary hyperparathyroidism. *Am J Med* 1978;65:235.

444. Marx SJ, Stock JL, Attie MF. Familial hypocalciuric hypercalcemia: recognition among patients referred after unsuccessful parathyroid exploration. *Ann Intern Med* 1980;92:351.

445. Riccardi D, Park J, Lee WS, et al. Cloning and functional expression of a rat kidney extracellular calcium/polyvalent cation-sensing receptor. *Proc Natl Acad Sci USA* 1995;92:131.

446. Brown EM, Gamba G, Riccardi D, et al. Cloning and characterization of an extracellular Ca²⁺-sensing receptor from bovine parathyroid. *Nature* 1993;366:575.

447. Pollak MR, Brown EM, Chou YH, et al. Mutations in the human Ca²⁺-sensing receptor gene cause familial hypocalciuric hypercalcemia and neonatal severe hyperparathyroidism. *Cell* 1993;75:1297.

448. Siris ES, Sherman WH, Baguiran DC. Effects of dichloromethylene-diphosphonate on skeletal mobilization of calcium in multiple myeloma. *N Engl J Med* 1980;302:310.

449. Singer FR, Ritch PS, Lad TE. Treatment of hypercalcemia of malignancy with intravenous etidronate. *Arch Intern Med* 1991;151:471.

450. Gucalp R, Theriault R, Gill I, et al. Treatment of cancer-associated hypercalcemia: double-blind comparison of rapid and slow intravenous infusion regimens of pamidronate disodium and saline alone. *Arch Intern Med* 1994;154:1935.

451. Body JJ, Dumon JC. Treatment of tumor-induced hypercalcemia with the bisphosphonate pamidronate: dose-response relationship and influence of tumor type. *Ann Oncol* 1994;5:359.

452. Kammerman S, Canfield RE. Effect of porcine calcitonin on hypercalcemia in man. *J Clin Endocrinol* 1970;31:70.

453. Singer FR, Neer RM, Murray JM. Mithramycin treatment of intractable hypercalcemia due to parathyroid adenomas. *N Engl J Med* 1970;283:634.

454. Singer FR, Sharp CF, Rude RK. Pathogenesis of hypercalcemia in malignancy. *Miner Electrolyte Metab* 1979;2:161.

455. Seyberth HW, Segre GV, Hamet P. Characterization of the group of patients with hypercalcemia of cancer who respond to treatment with prostaglandin synthesis inhibitors. *Trans Assoc Am Physicians* 1976;89:92.

456. Brereton HD, Halushka PV, Alexander RW. Indomethacin-responsive hypercalcemia in a patient with renal cell adenocarcinoma. *N Engl J Med* 1974;291:83.

457. Ito H, Sanada T, Katayama T. Indomethacin-responsive hypercalcemia. *N Engl J Med* 1975;293:558.

458. Winnacker JL, Becker KL, Katz S. Endocrine aspects of sarcoidosis. *N Engl J Med* 1968;278:427.

459. Massry SG, Mueller E, Silverman AG. Inorganic phosphate treatment of hypercalcemia. *Intern Med* 1968;12:307.

460. Brunette MG, Vigneault N, Carriere S. Micropuncture study of renal magnesium transport in magnesium-loaded rats. *Am J Physiol* 1975;229:1695.

461. Massry SG, Coburn JW, Kleeman CR. Renal handling of magnesium in the dog. *Am J Physiol* 1969;216:1460.

462. Li HY, Dai LJ, Quamme GA. Effect of chemical hypoxia on intracellular ATP and cytosolic levels. *J Lab Clin Med* 1993;122:232.

463. DeRouffignac C, Quamme G. Renal magnesium handling and its hormonal control. *Phys Rev* 1994;74:305.

464. Dudley HR, Ritchie AC, Schilling A. Pathological changes associated with the use of sodium ethylene diamine tetra-acetate in the treatment of hypercalcemia. *N Engl J Med* 1955;252:331.

465. Aikawa JK, Rhoades EL, Gordon GS. Urinary and fecal excretion of orally administered Mg²⁺. *Proc Soc Exp Biol Med* 1958;98:29.

466. Granam LACJJ, Burger ASV. Gastrointestinal absorption and excretion of Mg²⁸ in man. *Metabolism* 1960;9:646.

467. Meintzer RB, Steenbock H. Vitamin D and magnesium absorption. *J Nutr* 1955;56:285.

468. Miller ER, Ullrey DE, Zutaut CL. Effect of dietary Vitamin D₂ levels upon calcium, phosphorus and magnesium balance. *J Nutr* 1965;85:255.

469. DeRouffignac C, Mandon B, Wittner M, et al. Hormonal control of renal magnesium handling. *Miner Electrolyte Metab* 1993;19:226.

470. Steele TH, Weng SF, Evenson MA. The contributions of the chronically diseased kidney to magnesium homeostasis in man. *J Lab Clin Med* 1968;71:455.

471. Brunette MMG, Vigneault N, Carriere S. Micropuncture study of magnesium transport along the nephron in the young rat. *Am J Physiol* 1974;227:891.

472. Harris CA, Burnatowska MA, Seely JF. Effects of parathyroid hormone on electrolyte transport in the hamster nephron. *Am J Physiol* 1979;236:342.

473. Wong NLM, Quamme GA, Dirks JH. Tubular reabsorptive capacity for magnesium in the dog kidney. *Am J Physiol* 1983;224:62.

474. Guamme GA, Dirks JH. Effect of intraluminal and contraluminal magnesium on magnesium and calcium transfer in the rat nephron. *Am J Physiol* 1980;238:187.

475. Quamme GA. Influence of volume expansion on Mg influx into the superficial proximal tubule. *Kidney Int* 1980;17:721A.

476. Shirley Dg, Pooujeol P, LeGrimellec C. Phosphate, calcium and magnesium fluxes into the lumen of the rat proximal convoluted tubule. *Pflugers Arch* 1976;362:247.

477. LeGrimellec C, Roinel N, Morel F. Simultaneous Mg, Ca, P, K, Na, and Cl analysis in rat tubular fluid: I. During perfusion of either insulin or ferrocyanide. *Pflugers Arch* 1973;340:181.

478. Morel F, Roinel N, LeGrimellec C. Electron probe analysis of tubular fluid composition. *Nephron* 1969;6:350.

479. Quamme GA. Effect of calcitonin and magnesium transport in the rat nephron. *Am J Physiol* 1980;238:573.

480. Quamme GA, Carney SC, Wong NLM. Effect of parathyroid hormone on renal calcium and magnesium reabsorption in magnesium deficient rats. *Pflugers Arch* 1980;58:1.

481. Quamme GA. Renal magnesium handling: new insights in understanding old problems. *Kidney Int* 1997;52:1180.

482. Bapty BW, Dai LJ, Ritchie G, et al. Extracellular Mg²⁺ and Ca²⁺-sensing in mouse distal convoluted tubule cells. *Kidney Int* 1998;53:583.

483. Randall RE Jr, Chen MD, Spray CC. Hypermagnesemia in renal failure. *Ann Intern Med* 1949;61:73.

484. Pritchard JA. The use of magnesium ion in the management of eclamptogenic toxemias. *Surg Gynecol Obstet* 1955;100:131.

485. Ditzler JW. Epsom salts poisoning and a review of magnesium-ion physiology. *Anesthesiology* 1970;32:378.

486. Welt LG, Gitelman H. Disorders of magnesium metabolism. *Dis Mon* 1965;1:1.

487. Alfrey AC, Miller NL. Bone magnesium pools in uremia. *J Clin Invest* 1973;52:3019.

488. Whang R, Oei TO, Hamiter T. Frequency of hypomagnesemia associated with hypokalemia in hospitalized patients. *Am J Clin Pathol* 1979;71:610.

489. Shils ME. Experimental human magnesium depletion. *Medicine* 1969;48:61.
490. Whang R, Welt LG. Observations in experimental magnesium depletion. *J Clin Invest* 1963;42:305.
491. Dyckner T, Webster PO. Ventricular extrasystoles and intracellular electrolytes before and after potassium and magnesium infusions in patients on diuretic therapy. *Am Heart J* 1979;97:12.
492. Seller RH, Cangiano J, Kim EE. Digitalis toxicity and hypomagnesemia. *Am Heart J* 1970;79:57.
493. Chiemchaisri H, Phillips PH. Certain factors including fluoride which affect magnesium calcinosis in the dog and rat. *J Nutr* 1965;86:23.
494. Dunn MJ. Magnesium depletion in the rhesus monkey: induction of magnesium-dependent hypocalcaemia. *Clin Sci Mol Med* 1971;41:333.
495. L'Estrange JL, Axford RFE. A study of magnesium and calcium metabolism in lactating ewes semi-purified diet low in magnesium. *J Agric Sci* 1964;62:353.
496. Miller ER, Ullrey DE, Zutaut CL. Magnesium requirement of the baby pig. *J Nutr* 1965;85:13.
497. Buckle RH, Care AD, Cooper CW. The influence of plasma magnesium concentration on parathyroid hormone secretion. *J Endocrinol* 1968;42:529.
498. Habener JF, Potts JT Jr. Regulation of parathyroid hormone secretion in vitro. Quantitative aspects of calcium and magnesium ion control. *Endocrinology* 1971;88:1477.
499. Habener JF, Potts JT Jr. Relative effectiveness of magnesium and calcium on the secretion and biosynthesis of parathyroid hormone in vitro. *Endocrinology* 1976;98:197.
500. Hamilton JW, Spierto FW, MacGregor RR. Studies on the biosynthesis in vitro of parathyroid hormone. II. The effect of calcium and magnesium on synthesis of parathyroid hormone isolated from bovine parathyroid tissue and incubation medium. *J Biol Chem* 1971;246:3224.
501. Anast CA, Winnocker JL, Forte LR. Impaired release of parathyroid hormone in magnesium deficiency. *J Clin Endocrinol Metab* 1976;42:707.
502. Connor TBP, Toskes J, Mahaffey LG. Parathyroid function during chronic magnesium deficiency. *Johns Hopkins Med J* 1972;131:100.
503. Rude RK, Oldham SB, Singer FR. Functional hypoparathyroidism and parathyroid hormone organ resistance in human magnesium deficiency. *Clin Endocrinol* 1976;5:209.
504. Freitag J, Martin K, Conrades M. Evidence for skeletal resistance to parathyroid hormone magnesium depletion. *J Clin Invest* 1979; 64:1238.
505. MacManus J, Heaton FW. The influence of magnesium of calcium release from bone in vitro. *Biochim Biophys Acta* 1970;215: 360.
506. Kreusser WJ, Kurokawa K, Aznar E. Effect of phosphate depletion on magnesium homeostasis in rats. *J Clin Invest* 1978;61:573.
507. Booth CC, Babouris N, Hanna S. Incidence of hypomagnesemia in intestinal malabsorption. *Med J* 1963;2:141.
508. Caddell JL, Goddard DR. Studies in protein-calorie malnutrition 1. Chemical evidence for magnesium deficiency. *N Engl J Med* 1967; 275:533.
509. Flilnk EB, Stutzman FL, Anderson AR. Magnesium deficiency after prolonged parenteral fluid administration and after chronic alcoholism, complicated by delirium tremens. *J Lab Clin Med* 1954;43: 169.
510. Jones JE, Shane SR, Jacobs WH. Magnesium balance studies in chronic alcoholism. *N Y Acad Sci* 1969;162:934.
511. Mendelsoh JH, Barnes B, Mayman C. The determination of exchangeable magnesium in alcoholic patients. *Metabolism* 1965;14:88.
512. Kalbfleish JM, Lindeman RD, Ginn HE. Effects of ethanol administration on urinary excretion of magnesium and other electrolytes in alcoholic and normal subjects. *J Clin Invest* 1963;42:1471.
513. Butler AM, Talbot NB, Burnett CH. Metabolic studies in diabetic coma. *Trans Assoc Am Physicians* 1947;60:102.
514. Horton R, Biglieri EG. Effect of aldosterone on the metabolism of magnesium. *J Clin Endocrinol Metab* 1962;22:1187.
515. Keating MJ, Sethi MR, Bodey GP. Hypocalcemia with hypoparathyroidism and renal tubular dysfunction associated with aminoglycoside therapy. *Cancer* 1977;39:1410.
516. Schilsky RL, Anderson T. Hypomagnesemia and renal magnesium wasting in patients receiving cisplatin. *Ann Intern Med* 1979;90: 926.
517. Gitelman HJ, Graham JB, Welt LG. A new familial disorder characterized by hypokalemia and hypomagnesemia. *Trans Assoc Am Physicians* 1966;79:221.
518. Simon DB. Gitelman's variant of Bartter's syndrome, inherited hypokalemic alkalosis caused by mutations in the thiazide-sensitive Na-Cl cotransporter. *Nat Genetics* 1966;12:24.

CHAPTER 89

Fluid–Electrolyte and Acid–Base Disorders Complicating Diabetes Mellitus

Horacio J. Adrogué

Diabetes mellitus, the most prevalent endocrine illness, is a most challenging condition responsible for the development of severe abnormalities in whole body composition and target damage of critical functions. The deranged metabolic pathways lead to defects in the normal fluid–electrolyte and acid–base homeostasis, which are reviewed in this chapter. We first examine the essentials of energy metabolism to better understand the basic defects of diabetes mellitus, and then describe each of the various disturbances of water, electrolyte, and acid–base composition observed in association with this disease.

INTRODUCTORY CONCEPTS

Humans are able to utilize energy from carbohydrates, fats, or proteins, and the energy-rich foods consumed during times of plenty can be stored as the complex carbohydrate glycogen, or as the energy-dense triacylglycerols. The biochemical systems that regulate these processes rely on the availability of insulin, which represents one of the most prominent regulators of tissue metabolism (1–4).

Complex carbohydrates are broken down into simple sugars and absorbed by the gastrointestinal tract, with glucose being the predominant sugar added to body fluids. Glucose is taken into cells and can be metabolized to pyruvate by glycolysis, generating 2 moles of adenosine triphosphate (ATP) from each mole of glucose. The maximum ATP yield can be realized, however, only if pyruvate can be metabolized all the way to carbon dioxide and water through the citric acid cycle and the cytochrome oxidase chain, yielding 38 moles of ATP. Should the cell's energy stores be replete, glucose is not oxidized but rather is converted to glycogen, a complex polysaccharide that acts as a compact storage form for carbohydrate. Glycogen synthesis occurs primarily in the liver

and muscle, and is stimulated when insulin is present. If serum glucose is low and consequently, insulin secretion is depressed, as for example during fasting, glycogen is broken down into glucose. Alternatively, lactate, which is produced during anaerobic glycolysis, can be converted back to pyruvate and ultimately into glucose by the liver and renal cortex. Amino acids and glycerol can also yield glucose in these tissues, as described.

Proteins can be utilized either as a structural component for cell growth and repair or as an energy substrate. Reductions in serum insulin (as after an overnight fast) enhance the breakdown of protein and the mobilization of amino acids. In the liver and renal cortex, these amino acids are converted into pyruvate or oxaloacetate and enter the gluconeogenic route. The final product of this pathway, glucose, is then returned to the circulation and utilized to support energy metabolism of other tissues, notably muscle and brain. Thus, from the point of view of energy utilization, protein may be transformed into and subsequently used as glucose, the basic cell nutrient.

Fatty acids held in the form of triacylglycerols are the primary energy storage metabolite in humans: They are dense because of the anhydrous nature of this compound and contain approximately twice the energy per gram that carbohydrates do. These lipids are stored in the fat cells of adipose tissue. When insulin levels are low and epinephrine, norepinephrine, glucagon, and cortisol levels are relatively elevated, the stored triacylglycerol is hydrated, forming glycerol and free fatty acids, which are released into the circulation. In the liver under these conditions, glycerol is converted into pyruvate and ultimately to glucose. The free fatty acids can be used by many cells as an energy substrate. After uptake by cells, fatty acids may be transported to the mitochondria, where they are converted into acetyl coenzyme A (CoA) and enter the citric acid cycle, where they are broken down ultimately into carbon dioxide and water by the cytochrome oxidase chain, generating ATP. Free fatty acids derived from adipose stores represent the main substrate for the production of ketone bodies. The development of ketosis, as explained in

H. J. Adrogué: Department of Medicine, Baylor College of Medicine; and Renal Section, Department of Veterans Affairs Medical Center, Houston, Texas

more detail thereafter, requires elevated plasma levels of free fatty acids, a process that results from insulin deficiency, and accelerated fatty acid oxidation, the latter largely resulting from high glucagon levels. The effects of glucagon are mediated via the carnitine palmitoyltransferase system of enzymes responsible for the transport of fatty acids into the mitochondria. In the absence of glucagon, free fatty acids delivered to the liver are reesterified and stored as hepatic triglyceride or converted into very low density lipoproteins and transported back into the circulation. If free fatty acids are in great excess with respect to the availability of glucose for tissue oxidation, the surplus fatty acids are converted into acetoacetic acid. Acetoacetic acid is in equilibrium with ß-hydroxybutyric acid and acetone, with the final concentration of ß-hydroxybutyric acid being generally three times those of acetoacetic acid. These ketone bodies circulate in the blood and are the preferential energy sources for myocardium and the renal cortex; during prolonged fasting they can be used by the central nervous system as well. Thus fatty acids, glycerol, and ketoacids are versatile and widely used metabolic substrates that reach maximum serum levels during periods of fasting when the availability of glucose for oxidation is reduced.

INSULIN ACTION AND DIABETES MELLITUS

In the normal state, insulin is continuously secreted by the ß-cells of the pancreas at a low rate that maintains plasma levels of about 10 μU/mL, the so-called basal insulin secretion. Although the stimulus for this basal release is not totally known, factors other than plasma glucose level must play a role, as basal secretion of insulin persists during hypoglycemia. Glucose loading triggers a significant rise in basal insulin secretion and diurnal variations in insulin secretion also occur independently of glucose surplus, with peaks in early morning and trough levels in early afternoon. Food intake or hyperglycemia, or both, trigger additional bursts of insulin secretion that are mediated by gastrointestinal hormones and neural factors. An anticipatory rise in serum insulin normally develops in response to feeding prior to an increase in serum glucose and this rise in serum insulin blunts postabsorptive hyperglycemia. In a comparable manner, insulin secretion decreases as serum glucose begins to fall (while the patient is still hyperglycemic), thereby preventing a late fall in blood glucose.

Amino acids also stimulate insulin release, possibly through the action of gastrointestinal secretagogues such as gastric inhibitory polypeptide that enhances the effects of glucose on insulin release. The autonomic nervous system also plays a major role in the control of insulin secretion. ß-Adrenergic effects of catecholamines amplify the glucose-induced insulin release, whereas the opposite result occurs with α-adrenergic stimulation; the latter also enhances glycogenolysis. The parasympathetic nervous system, acting on the pancreas through the vagus nerve, stimulates glucose-mediated insulin secretion. The preceding information points out the existence of a complex system involved in the control of insulin secretion.

The liver, muscles, and adipose tissue represent the primary targets for insulin action and the abnormalities observed in these tissues in a state of diabetic ketoacidosis are depicted in Fig. 89-1. Because diabetes mellitus is characterized by insufficient insulin action on target tissues and excessive

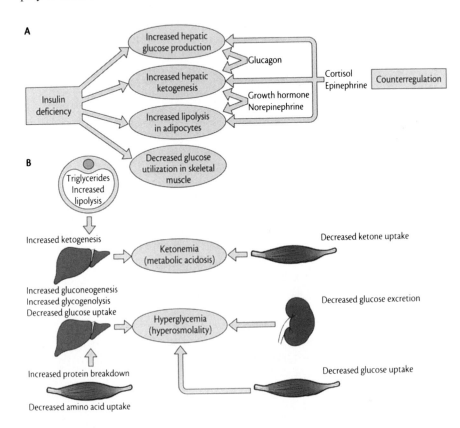

FIG. 89-1. Role of insulin deficiency and the counterregulatory hormones, and their respective site of action, in the pathogenesis of hyperglycemia and ketosis in diabetic ketoacidosis (DKA). (From: Adrogué HJ, Madias NE. *Disorders of acid–base balance.* In: Berl T, Bonventre JV, eds. *Atlas of diseases of the kidney.* Boston: Blackwell Scientific, 1999, with permission.)

TABLE 89-1. *Major fluid–electrolyte and acid–base disorders complicating diabetes mellitus*

Condition	Defect in homeostasis of	Specific entity
Single dominant disturbance	Glucose	Hyponatremia (hypertonic or translocational)
		Hypernatremia
	Lipids	Pseudohyponatremia
	Water	Hyponatremia (hypotonic)
		Hypernatremia
	Sodium	Volume depletion
		Volume expansion
	Potassium	Hypokalemia, K^+ depletion
		Hyperkalemia
	Acid–base balance	Ketoacidosis
		Hyperchloremic acidosis
		Renal tubular acidosis
		Lactic acidosis
Combination of multiple major disturbances	Glucose, fluid, and acid–base balance	Diabetic ketoacidosis
		Hyperosmolar nonketotic syndrome
		Renal failure

counterregulatory hormones, hyperglycemia, ketosis, and fluid–electrolyte disturbances may develop, the latter being largely secondary to the metabolic derangements. Excessive hepatic production of glucose and impaired glucose utilization by most tissues account for the development of hyperglycemia. As previously indicated, ketosis occurs largely as a combined effect of insulin deficiency and glucagon excess. The role of insulin is exerted on adipocytes, hepatocytes, and myocytes. In the adipose tissue, insulin inhibits lipolysis, thus decreasing the transfer of fatty acids and glycerol to the hepatocyte; in the liver, insulin enhances esterification rather than oxidation of free fatty acids; and in peripheral tissues, this hormone stimulates the oxidation of ketones. Consequently, insulin deficit promotes ketosis as a result of increased production and decreased consumption of ketoacids. An increase in the glucagon:insulin ratio activates the carnitine palmitoyltransferase system, thereby promoting the transport of fatty acids into the mitochondria by two mechanisms. First, glucagon depresses malonyl-CoA, the first committed intermediate in the synthesis of fatty acids from glucose, and a fall in its concentration activates the enzyme that transfers fatty acyl CoA into the mitochondria. Second, glucagon causes an increase in hepatic carnitine levels, which then activates by mass action the carnitine palmitoyltransferase system. Hepatic overproduction of ketones is the central event responsible for ketotic states with peripheral underutilization playing a smaller role. The insufficient tissue insulin action observed in diabetes mellitus might be caused by an absolute insulin deficiency as in type 1 diabetes, also known as insulin-dependent diabetes mellitus (IDDM), or by a combination of a relative insulin deficiency and insulin resistance as in type 2 diabetes mellitus, also known as non–insulin-dependent diabetes mellitus (NIDDM).

DISTURBANCES IN BODY COMPOSITION

The major fluid–electrolyte and acid–base disorders complicating diabetes mellitus are conveniently classified as single dominant disturbances and combinations of multiple disturbances (Table 89-1). Each of the single dominant disturbances, including defects in homeostasis of glucose, lipids, water, sodium, potassium, and acid–base balance, is characterized by unique features that are reviewed in this section. A combination of multiple disturbances comprising the simultaneous presence of defects in the homeostasis of glucose, fluid, electrolyte, and acid–base balance, are responsible for the development of the full-blown clinical pictures of diabetic ketoacidosis (DKA), hyperosmolar nonketotic syndrome (HONKS), and renal failure complicating diabetes mellitus. These combined disturbances are examined thereafter, with the exception of renal failure, which is discussed elsewhere.

Single Dominant Disturbances

Defect in Glucose Homeostasis

Plasma glucose levels in the normal state can be as low as 60 mg/dL during fasting and exercise and as high as 160 mg/dL after eating. As is well known, plasma glucose levels are determined by the opposing influences of glucose utilization (removal from the circulation) and glucose availability (addition to the circulation). Glucose, of course, is derived from both endogenous and exogenous sources. Insulin deficiency, either absolute or relative, results in hyperglycemia because of an impairment in glucose utilization by most tissues and the excessive hepatic production of glucose. The defect in glucose homeostasis might lead to either hyponatremia or hypernatremia, as described in the following (5–7).

The increase in effective osmolality of the extracellular fluid (ECF) consequent to the elevated plasma glucose level in the insulin-deficient or -resistant state causes a shift of water out of cells, most prominently from skeletal muscle, leading to the development of hyponatremia (5). Effective osmolality or tonicity refers to the contribution to osmolality of solutes, such as sodium and glucose, that cannot move freely across cell membranes, thereby inducing transcellular shifts in water. Each 100-mg/dL (5.6 mmol/L) increment in plasma glucose above normal decreases $[Na^+]_p$ (sodium concentration in plasma) by about 1.7 mEq/L, with the end result a rise in serum osmolality of approximately 2.0 mOsm/kg water. In fact, hyperglycemia is the most common cause of translocational hyponatremia, a form of nonhypotonic hyponatremia in which serum osmolality is increased, as is tonicity, the latter causing dehydration of cells. Consequently, a patient with plasma glucose of about 1,000 mg/dL is expected to have a $[Na^+]_p$ of approximately 125 mEq/L; complete correction to about 100 mg/dL of this patient's hyperglycemia will bring $[Na^+]_p$ from 125 to 140 mEq/L (normal level), in the absence of measures aimed at correcting any abnormality in external water balance (difference between water intake and excretion). Retention of hypertonic mannitol is a less common cause of translocational hyponatremia, having features that resemble the hyponatremia of uncontrolled diabetes mellitus. On the other hand, dilutional (hypotonic) hyponatremia, by far the most common form of the disorder (hyponatremia is defined as a decrease in the serum sodium concentration to a level below 136 mEq/L) is characterized by the presence of hypotonicity. Hypotonicity, in turn, can lead to cerebral edema, a potentially life-threatening complication.

Hyperglycemia might also lead to hypernatremia, the opposite disorder of serum $[Na^+]$, by its renal effects on water and electrolyte handling (6). The increased filtered load of glucose owing to hyperglycemia exceeds the renal tubular reabsorptive capacity, resulting in glucosuria. During this osmotic diuresis, urinary water losses are disproportionately greater than the accompanying electrolyte losses, an event that may lead to hypernatremia and further aggravate the progressive rise in serum osmolality. Thus, in the absence of intake, osmotic diuresis might increase serum sodium and chloride, thereby counterbalancing the dilution of these electrolytes caused by hyperglycemia.

Because sustained hypernatremia caused by hyperglycemia (osmotic diuresis caused by glucosuria) or other mechanisms can occur only when thirst or access to water is impaired, the groups at highest risk are patients with altered mental status, intubated patients, infants, and elderly persons. Thirst impairment may occur in elderly patients. Frail nursing home residents and hospitalized patients are prone to hypernatremia because they depend on others for their water requirements.

Hyperlipidemia

Diabetes mellitus is commonly associated with hyperlipidemia, which in turn may reduce measured serum sodium concentration, causing the so-called pseudohyponatremia or false hyponatremia. This electrolyte disorder is characterized by a normal $[Na^+]$ in plasma water in spite of a diminished $[Na^+]$ in a plasma or serum sample. The decreased $[Na^+]$ arises from an increased solid phase of plasma owing to severe hypertriglyceridemia or hyperproteinemia (e.g., myeloma). If $[Na^+]$ is measured directly (without dilution of the sample) with ion-sensitive electrodes instead of flame photometry (the latter being the classic method), a normal value will be found; thus, this type of hyponatremia is false because: (a) the $[Na^+]$ in plasma water is normal, and (b) its detection is dependent on the method used for measurement of $[Na^+]$. It should be evident that pseudohyponatremia does not produce any of the symptoms that classically occur with hypotonic hyponatremia. Furthermore, measured plasma osmolality is normal in pseudohyponatremia, because the solute concentration in plasma water is not altered in this condition.

Let us compare the hyponatremia owing to hyperglycemia or hypertonic infusions (e.g., mannitol) with that caused by hyperlipidemia. The decreased $[Na^+]$ owing to hyperglycemia or hypertonic infusions is not a form of pseudohyponatremia because $[Na^+]$ in plasma water also is diminished. The extracellular fluid (ECF) accumulation of solutes of relatively small molecular size, observed with hyperglycemia or hypertonic infusions, increases extracellular tonicity, which in turn osmotically pulls water from the intracellular fluid (ICF), diluting the $[Na^+]$ in ECF. By contrast, high plasma levels of large-molecular-size solutes (e.g., hypertriglyceridemia) fail to alter extracellular tonicity; therefore, not causing a shift of water from the ICF to the ECF. Thus, pseudohyponatremia is a spurious form of isoosmolar and isotonic hyponatremia identified when severe hypertriglyceridemia or paraproteinemia increases substantially the solid phase of plasma and the sodium concentration is measured by means of flame photometry. The increasing availability of direct measurement of serum sodium with ion-specific electrode has all but eliminated this laboratory artifact.

Defect in Water Homeostasis

Examination of the defect in water homeostasis that accompanies diabetes mellitus requires a brief overview of this topic (5–7). The disorders of salt and water balance may be classified into three major categories: (a) abnormalities in the size of body fluid compartments, (b) disturbances in the tonicity of body fluids, and (c) a selective deficit or excess of chloride with respect to sodium. The first group of disorders comprises an enlargement ("volume expansion") and a reduction ("volume depletion or contraction") in the size of body fluid compartments, which are produced by a combined salt and water excess and a combined salt and water deficit, respectively. Disturbances in the tonicity of body fluids include increases (e.g., hypernatremia) and decreases (e.g., hyponatremia) in the effective osmolality of body fluids. As opposed to disturbances in the size of body fluids in which salt and water excess or deficit develops in proportion to the relationship found in the normal state, a discordant abnormality in salt and water balance occurs in disorders of body fluid tonicity. Thus, a disproportion between salt and water content of body fluids explains the development of hypernatremia (water content in body fluids is relatively small for the concomitant salt content) and hyponatremia (water content in body fluids is relatively large for the concomitant salt content). The third group of salt and water disorders is characterized by an abnormal relationship between the $[Na^+]_p$ and $[Cl^-]_p$ (chloride concentration in plasma). Although the $[Na^+]_p$ is generally maintained within normal limits in these disorders because it is dependent on overall water homeostasis, the $[Cl^-]_p$ is either abnormally low or high. The major representatives of a selective deficit or excess of chloride with respect to sodium are hypochloremic metabolic alkalosis and hyperchloremic metabolic acidosis, respectively. These acid–base disorders are reviewed in the section dealing with such abnormalities.

An important concept that must be understood relates to the identification of the basic abnormality responsible for the disturbances in the volume of body fluids and that responsible for altered tonicity. Disturbances in salt balance are the primary causes of volume excess and depletion, whereas disorders in water balance are responsible for the development of the tonicity disorders, hypertonicity (hypernatremia) and hypotonicity (hyponatremia). Because sodium chloride (NaCl) excess only transiently increases tonicity, leading to augmented antidiuretic hormone (ADH) (i.e., arginine vasopressin secretion and secondary water retention), hypernatremia is not clinically observed. Expansion of the ECF volume, instead, is the hallmark of a primary salt excess. In a comparable fashion, NaCl deficit only transiently decreases tonicity, inhibiting ADH secretion with secondary increase in water excretion, so that hyponatremia is not observed, whereas volume depletion becomes the major manifestation of this electrolyte imbalance. A primary and exclusive disturbance in water balance, deficit and excess, causes hypertonicity (hypernatremia) and hypotonicity (hyponatremia), respectively, but does not produce a major alteration in the size of the fluid compartments because the latter are primarily determined by the osmolar content in the compartment (NaCl content in the ECF, which is unaltered in exclusive disturbances of water balance).

Dysnatremias in Diabetes Mellitus

A defect in water homeostasis in patients with diabetes mellitus might lead to either hypotonic hyponatremia or hypernatremia in response to positive or negative water balance, respectively. Water and electrolyte losses caused by vomiting or diarrhea are commonly encountered in uncontrolled diabetes and in patients with this disease experiencing target organ damage in the alimentary tract (e.g., gastroparesis, nocturnal diarrhea). In addition, excessive urinary fluid losses may develop as a result of osmotic diuresis, use of diuretics, adrenal insufficiency, or other causes. Whether hypotonic hyponatremia or hypernatremia develops is dependent on the concomitant water intake. Hypernatremia might be observed if water intake is insufficient, whereas a large salt-free fluid intake might lead to hyponatremia. Long-standing diabetes mellitus commonly predisposes or leads to heart failure or renal failure, or both, thereby impairing renal water excretion that may lead to hypotonic hyponatremia. Concomitant medication, including diuretics, might also play a role in the development of hyponatremia.

Abnormal $[Na^+]_p$ can produce signs and symptoms of disease owing to central nervous system dysfunction and the clinical manifestations elicited by opposite changes in tonicity are remarkably similar, except for seizures that are mostly caused by cerebral edema secondary to dilutional hyponatremia. When the patient's osmoregulating mechanisms (thirst, changes in water intake and ADH levels, renal water retention, or excretion) fail, an increase in plasma tonicity and $[Na^+]_p$, or conversely a decrease in plasma tonicity and $[Na^+]_p$, develops. Plasma hypertonicity induces brain water loss and hypotonicity produces water gain in this organ, accompanied in both cases by parallel volume changes. As a defense mechanism to correct brain volume changes, the intracellular osmolytes of this organ increase in hypernatremia and decrease in hyponatremia. The adaptive increase in brain osmolytes is owing to a modest increase in cellular K^+ and to the accumulation of organic solutes (e.g., glutamine, glutamate, and other organic metabolites). Conversely, the adaptive decrease in brain osmolytes is owing to a decrease in cellular K^+ accompanied by a diminished concentration of organic solutes. These secondary responses of the brain to altered extracellular tonicity can be demonstrated within a few hours of the initiation of abnormal tonicity and are complete within a few days. *Idiogenic osmoles* is the name given to the cerebral organic osmolytes detected in response to the adaptation of the brain to increases in extracellular tonicity.

Hypotonic Hyponatremia

Hypotonic (dilutional) hyponatremia represents an excess of water in relation to existing sodium stores, which can be decreased, essentially normal, or increased. Retention of water most commonly reflects the presence of conditions that impair renal excretion of water, in a minority of cases, it is caused by excessive water intake, with a normal or nearly normal excretory capacity.

Conditions of impaired renal excretion of water are categorized according to the characteristics of the ECF volume, as determined by clinical assessment. Decreased ECF volume can result from renal sodium loss (e.g., glucosuria-induced osmotic diuresis) or extrarenal sodium loss (e.g., vomiting). Conditions with essentially normal ECF volume include thiazide diuretics, syndrome of inappropriate secretion of antidiuretic hormone, decreased intake of solutes, hypothyroidism, and adrenal insufficiency. Increased ECF volume can be observed in pregnancy, renal failure, congestive heart failure, cirrhosis, and nephrotic syndrome. With the exception of renal failure, these conditions are characterized by high plasma concentrations of arginine vasopressin despite the presence of hypotonicity because arterial underfilling induces baroreceptor-mediated nonosmotic release of ADH overriding the osmotic regulation of the hormone, thereby impairing urinary dilution and causing hyponatremia. Depletion of potassium accompanies many of these disorders and contributes to hyponatremia, since the sodium concentration is determined by the ratio of the "exchangeable" (i.e., osmotically active) portions of the body's sodium and potassium content to total body water. Patients with hyponatremia induced by thiazides can present with variable hypovolemia or apparent euvolemia, depending on the magnitude of the sodium loss and water retention.

Excessive water intake can cause hyponatremia by overwhelming normal water excretory capacity (e.g., primary polydipsia). Frequently, however, psychiatric patients with excessive water intake have plasma arginine vasopressin concentrations that are not fully suppressed and urine that is not maximally dilute, thus contributing to water retention.

The optimal treatment of hypotonic hyponatremia requires balancing the risks of hypotonicity against those of therapy. The presence of symptoms and their severity largely determine the pace of correction. Patients with symptomatic hyponatremia and dilute urine (osmolality, <200 mOsm/kg water) but with less serious symptoms usually require only water restriction and close observation. Severe symptoms (e.g., seizures or coma) call for infusion of hypertonic saline. On the other hand, patients who have symptomatic hyponatremia with concentrated urine (osmolality = 200 mOsm/kg water) in association with a hypovolemic state are best treated with isotonic saline; those having clinical euvolemia or hypervolemia require infusion of hypertonic saline.

There is no consensus about the optimal treatment of symptomatic hyponatremia (5). Nevertheless, correction should be of a sufficient pace and magnitude to reverse the manifestations of hypotonicity but not be so rapid and large as to pose a risk of the development of central pontine myelinolysis. Osmotic demyelination is serious and can develop one to several days after aggressive treatment of hyponatremia by any method, including water restriction alone. Shrinkage of the brain triggers demyelination of pontine and extrapontine neurons that can cause neurologic dysfunction, including quadriplegia, pseudobulbar palsy, seizures, coma, and even death. Hepatic failure, potassium depletion, and malnutrition increase the risk of the complication. Physiologic considerations indicate that a relatively small increase in the serum sodium concentration, on the order of 5%, should substantially reduce cerebral edema in patients with symptomatic hypotonic hyponatremia. Even seizures induced by hyponatremia can be stopped by rapid increases in the serum sodium concentration that average only 3 to 7 mEq/L. Most reported cases osmotic demyelination occurred after rates of correction that exceeded 12 mEq/L per day were used, but isolated cases occurred after corrections of only 9 to 10 mEq/L in 24 hours or 19 mEq/L in 48 hours. After weighing the available evidence and the all-too-real risk of overshooting the mark, we recommend a targeted rate of correction that does not exceed 8 mEq/L on any day of treatment. Remaining within this target, the initial rate of correction can still be

1 to 2 mEq/L per hour for several hours in patients with severe symptoms.

The rate of infusion of the selected solution can be derived expediently by applying the following formulas.

1. $\Delta[Na^+]_s$
$$= \frac{[Na^+]_{inf} - [Na^+]_s}{TBW + 1}$$; this formula projects the impact of 1 liter of any infusate on the patient's $[Na^+]_s$

2. $\Delta[Na^+]_s$
$$= \frac{([Na^+]_{inf} + [K^+]_{inf}) - [Na^+]_s}{TBW + 1}$$; this formula is a simple derivative of Formula #1, which projects the impact of 1 liter of any infusate containing sodium and potassium on the patient's $[Na^+]_s$

The preceding formulas project the change in serum sodium elicited by the retention of 1 L of any infusate (5). Dividing the change in serum sodium targeted for a given treatment period by the output of this formula determines the volume of infusate required, and hence the rate of infusion. Although water restriction ameliorates all forms of hyponatremia, as explained, it is not the optimal therapy in all cases.

Corrective measures for nonhypotonic hyponatremia are directed at the underlying disorder rather than at the hyponatremia itself. Administration of insulin is the basis of treatment for uncontrolled diabetes, but deficits of water, sodium, and potassium also should be corrected.

Hypernatremia

Hypernatremia (defined as a rise in the $[Na^+]_p$ to a value exceeding 145 mEq/L) represents a deficit of water in relation to the body's sodium stores, which can result from a net water loss or a hypertonic sodium gain (6). Net water loss accounts for the majority of cases of hypernatremia. It can occur in the absence of a sodium deficit (pure water loss) or in its presence (hypotonic fluid loss). Net water loss can result from pure water (e.g., hypodipsia, diabetes insipidus) or hypotonic fluid loss, the latter secondary to renal, gastrointestinal, or cutaneous causes.

Hypertonic sodium gain usually results from clinical interventions (e.g., sodium bicarbonate infusion, hypertonic enemas) or accidental sodium loading. Signs and symptoms of hypernatremia largely reflect central nervous system dysfunction and are prominent when the increase in the serum sodium concentration is large or occurs rapidly (i.e., over a period of hours). Most outpatients with hypernatremia are either very young or very old. Common symptoms in infants include hyperpnea, muscle weakness, restlessness, a characteristic high-pitched cry, insomnia, lethargy, and even coma. Convulsions are typically absent except in cases of inadvertent sodium loading or aggressive rehydration. Brain shrinkage induced by hypernatremia can cause vascular rupture, with cerebral bleeding, subarachnoid hemorrhage, and permanent neurologic damage or death. Brain shrinkage is countered by an adaptive response that is initiated promptly and consists of solute gain by the brain that tends to restore lost water.

Proper treatment of hypernatremia requires a two-pronged approach: addressing the underlying cause and correcting the prevailing hypertonicity. Managing the underlying cause may mean stopping gastrointestinal fluid losses; controlling pyrexia, hyperglycemia, and glucosuria; with holding lactulose and diuretics; treating hypercalcemia and hypokalemia; moderating lithium-induced polyuria; or correcting the feeding preparation. In patients with hypernatremia that has developed over a period of hours (e.g., those with accidental sodium loading) rapid correction improves the prognosis without increasing the risk of cerebral edema, because accumulated electrolytes are rapidly extruded from brain cells. In such patients reducing the $(Na^+)_p$ by 1 mEq/L per hour is appropriate. A slower pace of correction is prudent in patient with hypernatremia of longer or unknown duration, because the full dissipation of accumulated brain solutes occurs over a period of several days. In such patients, reducing the $(Na^+)_p$ at a maximal rate of 0.5 mEq/L per hour prevents cerebral edema and convulsions. Consequently, we recommend a targeted fall in the $(Na^+)_p$ of 10 mEq/L per day for all patients with hypernatremia except those in whom the disorder has developed over a period of hours. The goal of treatment is to reduce the $(Na^+)_p$ to 145 mEq/L. Because ongoing losses of hypotonic fluids, whether obligatory or incidental, aggravate the hypernatremia, allowance for these losses must also be made.

The preferred route for administering fluids is the oral route or a feeding tube; if neither is feasible, fluids should be given intravenously. Only hypotonic fluids are appropriate, including pure water, 5% dextrose, 0.2% sodium chloride (referred to as one-quarter isotonic saline), and 0.45% sodium chloride (one-half isotonic saline). The more hypotonic the infusate, the lower the infusion rate required. The volume should be restricted to that required to correct hypertonicity because the risk of cerebral edema increases with the volume of the infusate. Except in cases of frank circulatory compromise, 0.9% sodium chloride (isotonic saline) is unsuitable for managing hypernatremia.

After selecting the appropriate infusate, the physician must determine the rate of infusion. This can be easily calculated with the use of a formula that estimates the change in the serum sodium concentration caused by the retention of 1 L of any infusate.

The formulas for use in managing hypernatremia (6) are identical to those previously presented for managing hyponatremia and include:

1. $\Delta[Na^+]_s$

$$= \frac{[Na^+]_{inf} - [Na^+]_s}{TBW + 1}$$

; this formula projects the impact of 1 liter of any infusate on the patient's $[Na^+]_s$

2. $\Delta[Na^+]_s$

$$= \frac{([Na^+]_{inf} + [K^+]_{inf}) - [Na^+]_s}{TBW + 1}$$

; this formula is a simple derivative of Formula #1, which projects the impact of 1 liter of any infusate containing sodium and potassium on the patient's $[Na^+]_s$

The required volume of infusate, and hence the infusion rate, is determined by dividing the change in the $[Na^+]_p$ targeted for a given treatment period by the value obtained from the formula. The sole indication for administering isotonic saline to a patient with hypernatremia is a depletion of ECF volume sufficient to cause substantial hemodynamic compromise. Even in this case, after a limited amount of isotonic saline has been administered to stabilize the patient's circulatory status, a hypotonic fluid (i.e., 0.2% or 0.45% sodium chloride) should be substituted in order to restore normal hemodynamic values while correcting the hypernatremia. If a hypotonic fluid is not substituted for isotonic saline, the ECF volume may become seriously overloaded.

Defect in Sodium Homeostasis

The quantity of solutes in each of the main compartments determines its size, so that deficit or excess of solutes in a particular space will shrink or swell that space in comparison with the other compartments (7). The partition of water is determined by the osmotic activity of the solutes confined to each body compartment. One major solute is responsible for the size of each fluid compartment. These solutes are potassium, sodium, and proteins, for the intracellular, extracellular, and intravascular spaces, respectively. Because the hydraulic permeability of most cell membranes is very high, solute-free water freely and rapidly moves among all body compartments.

Body stores of salt (NaCl) are determined by the balance of its intake and excretion. Under normal circumstances, salt intake is derived from the diet and its excretion occurs by urinary loss. A positive NaCl balance (intake exceeds excretion) increases salt stores, whereas a negative one (excretion exceeds intake) decreases salt stores. The effect of increased NaCl stores is expansion of ECF volume, while decreased NaCl stores lead to a reduced ECF volume. Thus, a NaCl deficit in body fluids (e.g., vomiting, diarrhea) reduces ECF volume, including the intravascular compartment. By contrast, NaCl excess (e.g., congestive heart failure) expands ECF volume and produces overt peripheral edema and accumulation of fluid in major body cavities (pleural effusion, ascites). A major decrease in serum protein concentration (mostly albumin) diminishes intravascular volume and promotes expansion of the interstitial compartment (e.g., nephrotic syndrome, hepatic cirrhosis). Diabetes mellitus is a common cause of both volume depletion and volume expansion. The former disturbance is characteristically observed in the course of severe metabolic complications of this disease, namely, DKA and HONKS. Conversely, volume expansion is observed in patients having long-term diabetic complications including congestive heart failure, nephrotic syndrome, and renal failure.

Volume Depletion

Volume depletion in diabetic patients can result from fluid loss (e.g., renal and/or extrarenal) or from fluid sequestered into a "third space" (e.g., acute pancreatitis). Renal losses may occur in the presence of normal intrinsic renal function (e.g., osmotic diuresis caused by glucosuria or urea diuresis, adrenal insufficiency, diuretics) or in acute and chronic renal disease (e.g., acute tubular necrosis, diabetic glomerulosclerosis). Osmotic diuresis owing to renal excretion of glucose can produce a large natriuresis, leading to volume depletion. Patients with significant hyperglycemia, including those with DKA or nonketotic coma, may have a fluid deficit of 10% or more of body weight. Extrarenal losses include those from the gastrointestinal tract (e.g., vomiting, diarrhea, gastrointestinal suction, fistulas) and those from the skin (sweat, burns, extensive skin lesions). Fluid sequestration into a third space occurs with abdominal accumulation (e.g., intestinal obstruction, pancreatitis, peritonitis), bleeding, skeletal fractures, and obstruction of a major venous system.

The patient's history, physical examination, and laboratory data are critical elements in the evaluation of volume depletion, allowing the physician to (a) assess the severity of the deficit, and (b) establish its cause. Immediate recognition of hypovolemic shock is of utmost importance, because rapid intravascular volume expansion might prevent tissue injury and death. Evaluation of its severity allows establishment of the rate of infusion and the total fluid requirements. Recognition of the factors responsible for fluid loss permits initiation of specific therapeutic measures to correct the volume depletion.

Patients with volume depletion have signs and symptoms related to (a) the process responsible for volume depletion, and (b) the hemodynamic consequences of fluid loss. Through the first group of manifestations it is possible to recognize the cause of volume depletion, such as loss or sequestration of fluid. The second group of signs and symptoms includes hypotension, decreased cardiac output, and tachy-cardia owing to intravascular volume depletion. In addition, diminished tissue perfusion produces altered mental status, generalized weakness, and occasionally severe organ damage (e.g., acute tubular necrosis, cerebral ischemia, myocardial infarction).

The severity of volume deficit may be estimated through evaluation of blood pressure, heart rate, neck veins and venous pressure, skin turgor, moistness of mucous membranes, changes in body weight, and blood and urine samples. If volume depletion results from mechanisms other than hemorrhage, the fluid loss produces hemoconcentration with increased hematocrit (Hct). The ECF volume deficit can be estimated in states of a primary extravascular fluid loss from the rise in Hct as follows:

$$\text{ECV volume deficit} = 0.25 \times \text{body weight (kg)}$$
$$\times (\text{actual Hct/normal Hct} - 1)$$

where *0.25* represents the fraction of ECF per kilogram of body weight (250 mL/kg). Because the normal range of Hct is relatively wide (38% to 45%), the patient's baseline Hct usually is unknown, and blood loss may have occurred, the reliability of changes in Hct is only modest. Therefore, a precise estimation of volume deficit is difficult. The loss of body weight from its baseline level (body weight prior to the episode of volume depletion) is a clinically useful index to estimate volume deficit, as follows:

$$\Delta \text{body weight (kg)} = \text{fluid deficit (liters)}$$

The change in body weight is unreliable for the estimation of fluid deficit in patients with "third space" sequestration. If $[Na^+]_p$ remains within normal limits, the weight loss in kilograms truly represents loss of isotonic fluid. Volume deficit accompanied by hypernatremia or hyponatremia indicates the existence of a disproportionate water loss compared to Na^+ loss. (The water loss is larger for the former and smaller for the latter, compared to Na^+ loss.)

Pertinent data obtained from a blood specimen that are most useful in the diagnosis and management of volume depletion include: (a) BUN and serum creatinine levels; (b) Hct, total plasma protein, and/or albumin values; and (c) levels of serum electrolytes including Na^+, K^+, Cl^-, and total carbon dioxide (almost identical to plasma $[HCO_3^-]$). In volume depletion, BUN and plasma creatinine increase because of an overall depression of renal function, manifested in oliguria, reduced glomerular filtration rate (GFR), and renal plasma flow. Increased plasma creatinine is caused by a reduced GFR (when muscle necrosis, which could release this substance into the circulation, is absent). Conversely, an elevated BUN, not accompanied by increased plasma creatinine and reduced GFR, reflects enhanced renal reabsorption of urea accompanied by increased salt and water reabsorption. Consequently, the BUN : plasma creatinine ratio increases from its normal value of 10 : 1 to 15 : 1 or more. Hct and concentration of plasma proteins also can increase in volume depletion, a process referred to as hemoconcentration. Alterations in serum electrolytes are commonly observed and they depend on the composition of the fluid lost (e.g., vomiting produces hypokalemia and metabolic alkalosis) as well as the concomitant water and electrolyte intake.

With respect to fluid therapy in volume depletion, considering that oral intake is the physiologic pathway for the entry of fluids, this route should be always considered. In addition, oral replacement therapy is effective, relatively inexpensive, and noninvasive; does not require hospitalization; and saves several million patients (mostly children in developing nations) each year from death owing to volume depletion. Nevertheless, the presence of vomiting, ileus, or altered mental status precludes its use, mandating intravenous administration of fluid. Most frequently, however, volume repletion in hospitalized patients is performed by the parenteral (intravenous) route.

Volume repletion should be promptly secured because severe volume depletion frequently produces a major reduction in intravascular volume and hypovolemic shock. The type of fluid to be used depends on the cause of volume depletion. Hypovolemia caused by bleeding (e.g., peptic ulcer, rupture of aortic aneurysm) must be treated with blood products or plasma volume expanders (e.g., packed red cells, albumin, or dextran solutions), whereas the one resulting from renal or extrarenal losses and fluid sequestration in body cavities (e.g., ileus, ascites) must be treated with saline or dextrose in saline or Ringer's solution. Plasma volume expanders can be used in the initial phase of treatment to secure a more rapid restoration of hemodynamic status in all patients with shock.

Various intravenous solutions can be selected in fluid therapy. The most commonly used intravenous fluids consist of a NaCl-containing solution (NaCl 0.23%, 0.45%, and 0.9%, known as *1/4 normal saline, 1/2 normal saline,* and *normal saline,* respectively) with or without 5% dextrose. The term normal used in reference to intravenous solutions does not imply "normality" (chemical notation) but simply refers to the isotonicity of intravenous solutions with respect to body fluids. It is more proper to refer to these solutions as 1/4 isotonic saline, 1/2 isotonic saline, and isotonic saline. Although 5% dextrose in water is isotonic with body fluids (i.e., 50,000 mg/L glucose divided by its molar weight of 180 mg/mmol equals 278 mmol/L), the glucose is metabolized so that this solution provides solute-free water without effective long-lasting osmoles (yet providing some caloric intake). The NaCl added to intravenous solutions provides effective osmoles that are preferentially retained in ECF. The efficacy of the various solutions with respect to volume deficit correction is a function of their NaCl concentration, with normal saline as the most effective one and dextrose in water without NaCl, the least effective. The selection of intravenous solution is also determined by the patient's $[Na^+]_p$; hypernatremic patients are most frequently treated with NaCl-free solutions (e.g., 5% dextrose in water) whereas those with hyponatremia are usually given isotonic saline or hypertonic (e.g., NaCl 3.0%) saline solutions. It is important to realize the expected changes in the volume of

ECF and ICF in response to an infusion of isotonic saline, 1/2 isotonic saline, and salt-free water. The infusion of a normal saline solution expands the ECF exclusively (ECF volume increment is identical to the volume infused); thus, ICF volume remains unaltered. The infusion of a 1/2 isotonic saline solution expands both the ECF and ICF, with the former receiving 40% and the latter 60% of the volume load. Finally, a salt-free water infusion (e.g., 5% dextrose in water) will also expand both the ECF and ICF, but in this case, the latter receives 60% of the volume load. In summary, a pure water infusion expands all body compartments but predominantly the ICF, whereas isotonic saline expands the ECF exclusively.

With respect to the rate of intravenous fluid infusion in the therapy of volume depletion, because patients in hypovolemic shock are at immediate risk of death or ischemic tissue injury, the initial fluid infusion should be at the maximal flow allowed by the intravenous catheter ("wide open"); once blood pressure and tissue perfusion return to acceptable levels, the rate must be diminished to approximately 100 mL/hour to minimize the risk of pulmonary edema, owing to rapid intravascular expansion, even when the state of volume depletion has not yet achieved full correction. Patients with acceptable hemodynamic parameters should receive fluid at the initial rates of 100 to 200 mL/hour, with subsequent reduction after 6 to 12 hours to rates of about 100 mL/hour, to secure gradual repletion of all fluid compartments without imposing undue stress on the circulation. Exceptions to these rules are patients with extreme volume depletion (e.g., DKA, hyperosmolar nonketotic [HONKS] coma syndrome) or large ongoing fluid losses (e.g., continuous drainage of large volume of gastrointestinal secretions, postobstructive diuresis, and diabetes insipidus) who might require fluids at a higher rate of infusion as described in the corresponding section of this chapter.

Proper monitoring of fluid replacement therapy is accomplished by evaluation of arterial blood pressure, presence of collapsed or distended neck veins, and urine output, to establish the optimum rate of fluid replacement. Additional information might be necessary in critically ill patients, including monitoring of left- and right-sided heart filling pressures, blood pressure measurement through an intraarterial line, arterial and/or venous blood gas analysis, and sequential chest x-ray films to detect pulmonary venous congestion and interstitial edema.

Volume Expansion

A syndrome of volume expansion caused by overt salt and water retention is commonly observed in long-standing diabetes mellitus (7,9). Both forms of generalized edema, the so-called primary as well as the secondary types, are encountered. In primary edema, renal retention of salt and water is the initial event that leads to expansion of plasma and ECF volume (e.g., diabetic glomerulosclerosis with reduced GFR and avid tubular reabsorption of salt and water). In secondary edema, also called *underfill edema,* the presence of renal hypoperfusion, owing to decreased "effective arterial circulating blood volume" initiates salt and water retention by the kidney (e.g., diabetes mellitus with congestive heart failure). Thus, the kidney is always involved in the development of positive salt and water balance that leads to generalized edema (in patients with and those without diabetes mellitus), yet the renal dysfunction might result from abnormalities initiated within it (primary edema) or be a response to "effective" intravascular arterial volume depletion (secondary edema). It must be recognized that salt and water retention, owing to primary renal disease and congestive heart failure, is the main cause of generalized edema and normal or near-normal serum albumin. Absence of proteinuria argues against renal disease as the primary cause of fluid retention. Patients with heart failure usually have either minimal or mild urinary protein excretion (1+ or 2+ on dipstick determination), whereas those with nephrotic syndrome have, as a rule, severe proteinuria (4+ dipstick). The fluid retention observed in nephrotic syndrome appears to occur as a combination of primary and secondary edema. It is common for physicians to incorrectly diagnose congestive heart failure on the basis of bilateral lower extremity edema, without realizing that a similar syndrome is observed in patients with salt and water retention owing to a primary renal disease.

The management of localized and generalized edema must be directed, if possible, at the primary cause of fluid accumulation. Effective treatment of the primary cause leads to resolution of the edema. Therapy of the primary process in congestive heart failure can involve the use of afterload-reducing agents, digoxin, and diuretics. Patients with generalized edema most frequently require treatment of the fluid overload in addition to that directed at the primary disease. Correction of fluid overload involves restriction of dietary NaCl, and if this is unsuccessful, the use of diuretic therapy. In addition, all forms of edema, localized and generalized, inflammatory and noninflammatory, are ameliorated by bed rest and elevation of the edematous body area (e.g., placement of swollen body region above the heart level, such as the head for facial phlegmon following dental surgery, and the lower extremity for thrombophlebitis of the calf). The benefits derived from bed rest and elevation of the edematous body region derive from: (a) facilitation of fluid exit from the edematous region owing to the salutary effect on the Starling forces, as reduction in arterial and increment in venous blood flow accompany the decreased metabolic demands of resting tissues, and the hydrostatic effect of elevation of the edematous region; (b) bed rest diminishes venous blood pooling, increasing venous return to the heart, which augments the atrial natriuretic factor that promotes renal vasodilation and increased NaCl excretion; and (c) bed rest suppresses the renin–angiotensin–aldosterone system and α-adrenergic-mediated vasoconstrictor influences, which in turn increase renal excretion of salt. Bed rest, extended for several days or intermittently (a few hours of daytime bed rest in addition to nocturnal sleep), helps to mobilize the dependent edema. The management of generalized edema caused by congestive heart failure, nephrotic syndrome, and diabetic glomerulosclerosis is examined in detail in other chapters.

Defect in Potassium Homeostasis

The levels of total body K^+ stores are established by the external K^+ balance, which is in turn determined by the difference between K^+ intake and excretion. The internal K^+ balance refers to the control mechanisms for the distribution of total body K^+ stores between the ICF and the ECF. Thus, internal K^+ balance refers to the internal exchanges of K^+. On the other hand, external K^+ balance refers to the determinants of total body K^+ stores, without any consideration for the distribution of K^+ among body compartments. The major factors that alter internal K^+ balance include hormones (insulin, catecholamines), the acidity of body fluids, the levels of other electrolytes, the tonicity of body fluids, and drugs (10).

Insulin is a major modulator of extrarenal K^+ homeostasis and promotes K^+ uptake in many cell types, including those from skeletal muscle and liver. The hypokalemic action occurs at very low concentrations of insulin and is independent of the effect of insulin on glucose uptake. The precise mechanism of this action remains to be fully defined but appears to involve the activation of several transport proteins (11) (Table 89-2). The cellular mechanisms of insulin-mediated K^+ loading include: (a) stimulation of the Na^+-K^+-ATPase,

TABLE 89-2. *Insulin-mediated cellular K^+ uptake*

Primary action	Immediate effect	Secondary effect
Stimulation of Na^+-K^+-ATPase	Hyperpolarization of cell membrane	New electrical gradient favors K^+ entry
		Deactivation of some K^+ channels may prevent K^+ exit
Stimulation of Na^+-H^+ exchanger	Cytosolic alkalinization	Increased K^+-binding capacity of intracellular proteins
		Stimulation of Na^+-K^+-ATPase
	Increased cell $[Na^+]$	Stimulation of Na^+-K^+-ATPase
K^+ channels (inward rectifier)	Increased K^+ conductance when cell membrane is hyperpolarized	Exaggeration of the inward rectifying properties

From: Adrogué HJ. Mechanisms of transcellular potassium shifts in acid-base disorders. In: Hatano M, ed., *Proceedings XIth International Congress of Nephrology, Tokyo, Japan.* Tokyo: Springer, 1991:259.

(b) stimulation of the Na^+-H^+ exchanger, and (c) changes in ionic conductance of some K^+ channels. The hypokalemic effect of insulin resulting from stimulation of the Na^+-K^+-ATPase occurs as follows. Direct stimulation of the Na^+-K^+ pump by insulin induces the translocation of K^+ to the cell interior (entry of two K^+ and exit of three Na^+). In addition, substantial changes occur in the transport of electrolytes across the cell. The immediate result of insulin-mediated stimulation of Na^+-K^+-ATPase on the electrical properties of the cell membrane is hyperpolarization of the membrane potential (a more negative cell interior). The secondary effects promoted by insulin-induced hyperpolarization of the cell membrane are: (a) a new electrical gradient, which favors cellular K^+ entry, and (b) deactivation of K^+ channels, which inhibits cellular K^+ exit. Thus, the secondary effects of insulin on the membrane potential increase the hypokalemic action of this hormone.

The hypokalemic effect of insulin results also from stimulation of the Na^+-H^+ exchanger in the cell membrane. Insulin promotes the cellular entry of Na^+ and the cellular exit of H^+ by stimulation of this exchanger. The entry of Na^+ increases the $[Na^+]_i$ (intracellular concentration of sodium), which further stimulates the Na^+-K^+-ATPase. The cellular exit of H^+ results in cytosolic alkalinization, which in turn: (a) increases the K^+-binding capacity of intracellular anions, and (b) stimulates the Na^+-K^+ pump, therefore favoring cellular K^+ loading.

A third mechanism for the hypokalemic effect of insulin is mediated from its action on K^+ channels. Insulin controls gating of the inward rectifier K^+ channel of skeletal muscle. This type of K^+ channel is of significant relevance because it is responsible for most of the K^+ conductance of the skeletal muscle in the resting state. This channel allows K^+ to flow into cells much more easily than it exits from them. Consequently, when the cell membrane is hyperpolarized, the high inward conductance facilitates cellular K^+ entry, whereas when the cell membrane is depolarized, the low outward conductance reduces K^+ exit from cells. Insulin exaggerates the inward rectifying properties of this class of K^+ channel by a dual effect of stimulation of K^+ entry and depression of K^+ exit.

Glucagon also has significant effects on internal K^+ balance and plasma potassium levels. Glucagon induces glycogen breakdown in the hepatocytes, releasing glucose and K^+; therefore, high glucagon levels can elicit a transient increase in $[K^+]_p$. An increase in plasma glucagon in acute metabolic acidosis has been described and this hormonal response might play a role in acidosis-induced hyperkalemia (11).

K^+ Depletion with Hyperkalemia

The development of uncontrolled diabetes, including DKA, is usually accompanied by varying degrees of total body potassium depletion, which results from multiple causes, including massive kaliuresis secondary to glucosuria, decreased intake, and frequent vomiting. Yet plasma potassium levels are rarely low at the time of hospitalization, ranging in most instances from normal to high levels and occasionally attaining dangerously elevated values. This paradoxical relationship has been classically attributed to the concomitant changes in blood acidity that would effect a shift in potassium out of the cells in exchange for hydrogen ions moving intracellularly (12). However, several of the metabolic derangements observed in patients presenting with DKA are known to alter potassium metabolism and may contribute to the development of hyperkalemia. Endogenous ketoacidemia and hyperglycemia correlate with increased plasma potassium concentration on admission in patients with DKA (13). However, exogenous ketoacidemia and hyperglycemia in the otherwise normal experimental animal fails to increase plasma potassium levels (14,15), so it would seem that the insulin deficit per se is the major cause of the hyperkalemia that develops in DKA (13).

Serum pH and bicarbonate levels are known to alter plasma potassium levels. Whereas some studies indicated that the changes in plasma potassium concentration observed during acute acid–base disorders are consequent to the attendant changes in plasma pH, others showed that a low plasma bicarbonate concentration, under isohydric conditions, may induce hyperkalemia (16,17). Increased effective serum osmolality is another abnormality characteristic of DKA that may affect serum potassium; extracellular hypertonicity resulting from the infusion of saline, mannitol, or glucose results in the translocation of potassium-rich cell water to the extracellular compartment (18). Hyperglycemia of either endogenous or exogenous origin unaccompanied by ketoacidosis results in hyperkalemia in insulin-deficient diabetics, especially when hypoaldosteronism also is present (15).

As previously described, glucagon may also play a role in the hyperkalemia of DKA. This hormone may cause an increased potassium output from the liver, an effect that is usually transient because of the counterregulatory enhancement of insulin secretion. However, in the presence of an impaired insulin secretion, as in patients with DKA, increments in plasma glucagon levels may result in uncontrolled hyperkalemia (19).

An additional mechanism that may be involved in the deranged potassium homeostasis observed in diabetes mellitus is the sympathetic system. Potassium tolerance has been found to be markedly impaired in chemically sympathectomized animals, but is improved in animals given a simultaneous infusion of epinephrine (20). The effects of the adrenergic agents on the internal potassium balance are mediated by their effect on the plasma levels of insulin and glucagon, and a direct cellular effect on K^+ transport. Therefore, any physiologic condition or pharmacologic maneuver that blocks the ß-adrenergic system could result in hyperkalemia, particularly during states of increased potassium load. It is possible then that diabetics may have a suboptimal epinephrine response or altered peripheral sympathetic activity, resulting in potassium movement from the intracellular to the extracellular space as well as an impairment in cellular entry of potassium.

In summary, acidemia with a decrease in serum bicarbonate, plasma hyperosmolality, high glucagon levels, and sympathetic nervous system dysfunction might induce a hyperkalemic response in states of insulin deficiency (13), thereby explaining the development of hyperkalemia in DKA. Overall, insulin deficiency is probably the major protagonist of the complex hormonal disarray that is responsible for the hyperkalemia in decompensated diabetes.

K^+ Depletion with Hypokalemia

Hypokalemia can result from the redistribution or depletion of K^+ stores. The hypokalemia that results from redistribution is caused by cellular uptake of K^+ from the ECF; K^+ redistribution can occur simultaneously with K^+ depletion so that the two processes leading to hypokalemia can have additive effects. The hypokalemia observed with K^+ depletion is characterized by a reduction in the K^+ content of all body fluids.

Potassium depletion can occur with diabetes mellitus when dietary K^+ intake is very low and therefore fails to counterbalance the obligatory urinary K^+ losses associated with glucosuria. Potassium depletion also can occur if K^+ losses are abnormally high and might develop in association with a normal dietary K^+ intake. Potassium losses may be renal or extrarenal as diarrhea in origin, yet a combination of losses from both routes is commonly encountered. It is of interest to compare the alteration in K^+ content in the ICF and ECF in the presence of K^+ depletion. Total body K^+ deficit results in a greater absolute reduction of K^+ content in ICF than in ECF. Nevertheless, the percent deviation in K^+ content is considerably smaller in ICF than in ECF. In a similar fashion, the decrease in $[K^+]_i$ with K^+ depletion is significantly smaller than the decrease in $[K^+]_p$. With respect to the relationship between $[K^+]_p$ and the degree of K^+ deficit, a linear relationship having a slope of 0.3 mEq/L per 100 mEq of K^+ deficit $[\Delta[K^+]_p/\Delta K^+$ stores] has been described for patients with K^+ depletion in the absence of redistribution of K^+ stores. According to this relationship, a K^+ depletion of 10% of total body K^+ stores (350 mEq) produces a decrease in $[K^+]_p$ of approximately 1 mEq/L.

Diabetic gastroparesis is a common cause of vomiting leading to fluid and electrolyte losses. Protracted vomiting leads to hypokalemia that is largely caused by increased renal K^+ excretion. The increased kaliuresis is owing to HCO_3^- excretion consequent of HCl depletion (metabolic alkalosis) and to secondary hyperaldosteronism resulting from ECF volume depletion. The direct loss of K^+ as a result of vomiting is relatively small, considering that $[K^+]$ in gastric juice is about 15 mEq/L (mean value). Diuretic therapy for the management of hypertension and congestive heart failure in patients with diabetes mellitus is a common additional cause of potassium depletion. Within a week from the start of diuretic therapy, a mild decrease (0.3 to 0.6 mEq/L) in $[K^+]_p$ occurs, and this new $[K^+]_p$ remains constant thereafter unless an intercurrent illness that decreases K^+ intake (vomiting) or increases K^+ loss (diarrhea) develops. Hypokalemia is most commonly observed with thiazides (5% of patients) than with

loop diuretics (1% of patients). The decrease in $[K^+]_p$ is directly proportional to the daily dosage and duration of action of the diuretic; thus, daily administration and high-dosage regimens of chlorthalidone, a long-acting thiazide, are more likely to produce severe K^+ depletion and hypokalemia. The antihypertensive effect of thiazides is achieved with small dosages (6.25 to 25.0 mg daily), which have a small effect on K^+ balance; consequently, high dosages of thiazides in the treatment of hypertension are not warranted because they will result in K^+ depletion without better blood pressure control. Insulin administration in the therapy of DKA, a condition in which K^+ depletion is usually present, can result in profound and symptomatic hypokalemia.

K^+ Overload with Hyperkalemia

Potassium overload leading to hyperkalemia can occur because of an increased K^+ intake or because of decreased renal K^+ excretion. The high K^+ intake-induced hyperkalemia occurs when the adaptive increase in renal K^+ excretion is insufficient to match the larger-than-normal K^+ intake. Salt substitutes are K^+ salts (KCl) that mimic the taste of NaCl and their use may lead to hyperkalemia. Whenever a patient is told to reduce his or her NaCl intake because of hypertension, heart failure, or another cause, these salt substitutes are often recommended. As these products are available over the counter, patients frequently use them whether they are recommended by physicians or not. A low NaCl intake reduces the ability of the kidney to excrete K^+ to its maximum; simultaneous ingestion of salt substitutes (K^+ salts) can lead to hyperkalemia owing to the combination of increased K^+ intake and reduced renal K^+ excretion. In fact, a low NaCl intake is the single most commonly observed contributing factor in the development of hyperkalemia in clinical practice. Removing the salt restriction promotes increased kaliuresis, which might partially or fully correct the hyperkalemia.

In addition to the previously discussed impairment in internal K^+ balance leading to hyperkalemia, diabetes mellitus commonly damages the renal mechanisms of potassium excretion (10). Such abnormality that limits renal K^+ excretion might result from: (a) oliguria or anuria of any cause, (b) decreased GFR, (c) decreased tubular secretion of K^+, (d) hypoaldosteronism or pseudohypoaldosteronism, or (e) drugs. In the absence of generalized renal failure (normal GFR), a diminished renal K^+ excretion can be owing to either a defect in the renin–angiotensin–aldosterone axis or renal resistance to aldosterone.

Renin deficiency leads to a low plasma aldosterone level that might reduce renal K^+ excretion. Renin deficiency occurs in certain physiologic states (advanced age, expansion of ECF volume), with the use of various drugs (ß-adrenergic blockers, inhibitors of prostaglandin synthesis, methyldopa), with certain toxins (lead), in some systemic diseases (diabetes mellitus), and in some renal diseases (obstructive uropathy, interstitial nephritis). A common cause of renin deficiency is the so-called type 4 renal tubular acidosis, characterized by impaired excretion of both K^+ and H^+. Perhaps its most common presentation is in elderly diabetic patients. Angiotensin converting enzyme (ACE) inhibitor deficiency leads to hypoaldosteronism, which reduces renal K^+ excretion. The widely used antihypertensive agents (e.g., captopril, enalapril, fosinopril, and lisinopril), belong to this category of drugs that can increase $[K^+]_p$ levels by this mechanism.

One or more of the various syndromes of diminished aldosterone activity may be observed in diabetes mellitus. A diminished aldosterone activity can occur as a result of:

1. A primary defect in the adrenal synthesis of aldosterone owing to a disease or defect in the adrenal cortex. This adrenal abnormality is the cause or initial event that might lead to the defect in K^+ homeostasis.
2. A secondary defect in the adrenal synthesis of aldosterone owing to failure in the production, release, or action of the various components in the cascade leading to stimulation of the adrenal synthesis of aldosterone (i.e., renin deficiency).
3. End-organ resistance to aldosterone, owing to either drugs acting on the kidney (e.g., spironolactone) or renal disease.

Drug-induced mechanisms of hypoaldosteronism leading to hyperkalemia are commonly encountered in diabetic patients. Hyperkalemia induced by hypoaldosteronism can be elicited or accentuated in these patients with the administration of prostaglandin synthetase inhibitors, cyclosporine, or heparin. Prostaglandin synthetase inhibitors such as the nonsteroidal antiinflammatory drugs (NSAIDs) (e.g., indomethacin) and cyclosporine inhibit renin secretion, producing hyporeninemic hypoaldosteronism. ACE inhibitors decrease plasma levels of angiotensin II. Finally, heparin acts directly on the adrenal gland, inhibiting aldosterone secretion. Increased $[K^+]_p$ can occur with heparin administration in approximately 5% of hospitalized patients. The mechanism of K^+ retention by NSAIDs includes their inhibitory effect on prostaglandins of renal origin, which in turn might diminish GFR and renin release (which leads to decreased aldosterone secretion). NSAIDs can also have a direct nephrotoxic effect leading to renal failure, thereby causing additional renal K^+ retention.

Diabetes mellitus is also associated with end-organ resistance to aldosterone, leading to hyperkalemia, a syndrome known as *pseudohypoaldosteronism*. This entity, characterized by a renal resistance to aldosterone effects, can develop as a result of drug administration or renal diseases. Hyperkalemia caused by spironolactone, triamterene, and amiloride, collectively known as *K^+-sparing diuretics,* exemplifies drug-induced pseudohypoaldosteronism. Renal diseases that primarily damage the renal tubules and spare the glomeruli (or compromise the GFR only mildly), collectively known as *tubulointerstitial renal diseases,* elicit this hyperkalemic syndrome. Diabetes mellitus is the single major cause of end-stage renal disease (ESRD), and therefore commonly leads to hyperkalemia because of decreased renal function (diminished GFR). It must be recognized that in the presence of renal insufficiency, potassium balance might be maintained within normal limits until the GFR decreases to less than 25% of normal. The ability of the kidney with decreased GFR to maintain K^+ balance depends on the development of compensatory mechanisms, collectively known as *K^+ adaptation,* that increase the fractional K^+ excretion (FE_K) by the kidney. The augmented FE_K in renal insufficiency allows these patients to remain normokalemic in spite of a major reduction in GFR. Because $[K^+]_p$ might remain within normal limits in patients with only 25% of overall renal function (GFR), whereas K^+ intake is unchanged, a fourfold increase in FE_K^+ must be present. As the calculated FE_K in normal individuals amounts to approximately 10%, the estimated FE_K in a patient with this degree of renal insufficiency is about 40%.

Management of Hyperkalemia

The management of K^+ retention should be initiated even in the presence of a mild degree of hyperkalemia (10). Several measures should be undertaken at once in patients who have high-normal $[K^+]_p$ (i.e., 5.0 mEq/L) and a disease that predisposes to hyperkalemia such as diabetes mellitus with renal dysfunction. Severe restriction of dietary NaCl intake should be avoided because it impairs renal K^+ excretion; dietary NaCl intake should be at least 4 g/day. Restriction of dietary K^+ must be enforced. Medications that impair the renal excretion of K^+, including ACE inhibitors and K^+-sparing diuretics (i.e., triamterene, amiloride, spironolactone) should be discontinued. Metabolic acidosis, if present, should be treated with alkali therapy.

Proper management of simultaneous retention of Na^+ and K^+ in patients with diabetes mellitus and a salt-retaining disease (hypertension, congestive heart failure, nephrotic syndrome, renal insufficiency) who have an elevated $[K^+]_p$ or even a high-normal $[K^+]_p$ (i.e., 5.0 mEq/L), is effectively achieved by avoiding severe restriction of dietary NaCl intake while concomitantly administering diuretics (e.g., furosemide, thiazides). This recommendation with respect to the dietary NaCl intake should be instituted once a large ECF volume excess is no longer present. A moderate dietary NaCl intake of about 4 g/day will not result in ECF volume expansion if increased urine excretion of NaCl is achieved with the use of diuretics. This strategy of enhancing salt (NaCl) intake and excretion secures adequate kaliuresis (delivery of salt to the distal nephron is reduced with a salt-restricted diet and predisposes to hyperkalemia). Thus, to correct hyperkalemia by promoting increased kaliuresis, all patients, except those with ESRD or physical signs of fluid overload or pulmonary edema, must have substantial NaCl intake via an oral or parenteral route. In addition, the renal excretion of K^+ can be increased by the administration of a single diuretic agent (e.g., furosemide, thiazides) or a combination of these agents. Diuretics should not be administered to patients with ESRD because a meaningful kaliuretic response is not expected. A negative external K^+ balance is achieved in all patients with ESRD by: (a) the utilization of cation exchange resins (such as Kayexalate, a sodium polystyrene sulfonate) that promote the excretion of K^+ in the stools, and (b) dialysis (hemodialysis or peritoneal dialysis).

Hyperkalemia is the major threat to life in patients with type 4 renal tubular acidosis; therefore, the main focus of attention should be placed on correcting this electrolyte abnormality. That is the reason why dietary K^+ restriction, diuretics (furosemide, thiazides), and K^+-binding resins are so valuable in these patients. The intake of NaCl should be encouraged, because the availability of Na^+ salts in the collecting tubules is a major determinant of renal K^+ excretion. The administration of fludrocortisone (Florinef) in daily doses of 0.1 to 0.3 mg helps in the correction of hyperkalemia and acidosis (enhances distal acidification), yet the associated volume expansion may induce hypertension or increase its severity. Alkali therapy (1 to 2 mEq/kg per day) is useful to ensure correction of hyperkalemia and acidosis.

The following three strategies must be considered whenever severe hyperkalemia is present in any patient:

1. To counterbalance the effect of hyperkalemia on the excitability of myocardial and skeletal muscle with the administration of drugs. This modality is not aimed at reducing the increased $[K^+]_p$.
2. To modify internal K^+ balance, promoting the translocation of K^+ from ECF to ICF. This modality will not alter the total body K^+ stores.
3. To modify external K^+ balance, inducing a net K^+ loss from the body.

The treatment of hyperkalemia with agents that ameliorate the effects of hyperkalemia on myocardial and skeletal muscle excitability involves the administration of Ca^{2+} salts (chloride or gluconate), which diminish tissue excitability by widening the difference between resting and threshold potentials. When Ca^{2+} salts are provided, the resting membrane potential will remain depolarized by the hyperkalemia, whereas the threshold membrane potential will be depolarized by the Ca^{2+} infusate, enlarging the difference between resting and threshold membrane potentials, thereby reducing tissue excitability. Calcium gluconate (20 mL of a 10% solution) can be infused intravenously over a 10-minute period. The intravenous administration of Ca^{2+} salts is definitely indicated when $[K^+]_p$ reaches 7.0 mEq/L or when significant electrocardiographic abnormalities (absence of P waves, prolongation of QRS complexes, etc.) are present. The effects of Ca^{2+} infusion are short lasting, with peak effect noted about 5 minutes after infusion.

The most important therapeutic agent that promotes cellular K^+ entry is insulin. Insulin leads to tissue uptake of K^+ as well as glucose; therefore, the latter must be infused to prevent hypoglycemia in patients presenting without hyperglycemia. Considering that hyperglycemia of endogenous and exogenous origin can result in hyperkalemia (especially in diabetics), caution should be exercised as to the rate of glucose infusion. Consequently, a situation that mimics a euglycemic insulin clamp (providing exogenous glucose in adequate amount to maintain normal plasma glucose level during insulin administration) must be instituted. A less important strategy that might translocate K^+ from ECF to ICF is sodium bicarbonate ($NaHCO_3$) infusion.

Achievement of a net K^+ loss is the most effective therapeutic modality to reduce and sustain a normal $[K^+]_p$ in patients with severe and persistent hyperkalemia. The first two modalities in the therapy of hyperkalemia, namely, the use of Ca^{2+} salts (to ameliorate the effect of hyperkalemia on the excitability of myocardial and skeletal muscle) and the administration of insulin and glucose, $NaHCO_3$, and albuterol (to modify internal K^+ translocation from ECF to ICF), are only temporary measures that remove the immediate threat to life resulting from hyperkalemia. Consequently, treatment of severe and persistent hyperkalemia must combine all three modalities.

The presence of associated clinical and laboratory abnormalities can prevent use of one or more treatment modalities of hyperkalemia. The use of K^+ exchange resins by oral or rectal routes is contraindicated in patients with significant gastrointestinal symptoms. Calcium infusions are contraindicated in patients with hypercalcemia. Sodium bicarbonate infusions are contraindicated in patients with alkalemia, patients with high $[HCO_3^-]_p$, those with hypernatremia, or in patients at a significant risk of developing pulmonary edema or with significant ECF volume expansion. Severe hyperkalemia accompanied by preserved renal function usually can be corrected without dialysis. Potassium removal can be achieved in these patients by inducing an enhanced kaliuresis with the administration of fluids containing NaCl or $NaHCO_3$, or both, and with the use of diuretics (acting on the proximal tubule, loop of Henle, and distal tubule, such as acetazolamide, furosemide, and thiazides, respectively). The majority of patients who develop severe hyperkalemia, however, have renal failure, and dialysis is the treatment of choice for this condition.

Defect in Acid–Base Balance

Ketoacidosis and Hyperchloremic Metabolic Acidosis

During the development of DKA, ketoacids released into the ECF are titrated by bicarbonate and other body buffers. This buffering process results in an increase of plasma unmeasured anions and accounts for the classic pattern of acid–base composition, namely, metabolic acidosis associated with an increased anion gap (1,21–24). This latter term refers to those plasma anions, other than chloride and bicarbonate, that balance the positive charge of sodium:

$$\text{Anion gap} = [Na^+] - ([Cl^-]_p + [HCO_3^-]_p)$$

It has been stated that in DKA, each increase in the plasma anion gap from the retained ketoacids should be mirrored by an identical decrease in the plasma bicarbonate concentration.

TABLE 89-3. *Acid–base patterns of patients with diabetic ketoacidosis*

	Pure high anion gap acidosis	Mixed forms	Pure hyperchloremic acidosis
Associated clinical features before start of therapy			
Fluid intake	Poor	⇔	Adequate
Extrarenal fluid loss	Present	⇔	Absent
ECF volume deficit	Severe	⇔	Mild
Impairment of renal function	Severe	⇔	Mild
Associated laboratory features before start of therapy			
Hematocrit, hemoglobin, serum proteins	Higher	⇔	Lower
BUN, creatinine, uric acid	Higher	⇔	Lower
Cause of changes in $\Delta AG/\Delta HCO_3^-$ after initiation of therapy[a]	Bicarbonate administration	⇔	Infusion of chloride-rich solutions

AG, anion gap; $AG = [Na^+]_p - ([Cl^-]_p + [HCO_3^-]_p)$
[a]Excess AG (mEq/L) equals measured AG minus normal AG, and bicarbonate deficit (mEq/L) equals normal plasma bicarbonate minus measured plasma bicarbonate. Expected value of $\Delta AG/\Delta HCO_3^-$ is 1.0 as the bicarbonate deficit is the result of its titration by ketoacids.

Thus, in uncomplicated DKA the increment in anion gap above its normal value should be approximately equal to the decrement in plasma bicarbonate. Thus, the ratio of excess anion gap to bicarbonate deficit should be about 1:

$$\text{Excess anion gap bicarbonate deficit} = 1.0$$

where *excess anion gap* (mEq/L) equals measured anion gap minus normal anion gap, and *bicarbonate deficit* (mEq/L) equals normal plasma bicarbonate minus measured plasma bicarbonate. This contention is only partly correct for several reasons (25–28). First, a stoichiometric substitution of 1 mmol of retained plasma ketoacids per liter for 1 mmol of bicarbonate per liter could take place only if plasma bicarbonate were the exclusive anion accepting hydrogen ions during the buffering process. The plasma proteins also buffer strong acids and thereby bring about a decrease in their net negative charge (26,27). Thus, the increased level of plasma ketoacids should be identical to the combined decrement of both bicarbonate and nonbicarbonate buffers. Nevertheless, because the plasma anion gap accounts for both ketoacids and nonbicarbonate buffers, the excess anion gap should still be identical to the bicarbonate deficit. Second, the retained ketoacids also titrate intracellular buffers by exchanging intracellular sodium and potassium for extracellular hydrogen ion. The sodium exchange transfers fluid from the intracellular to the extracellular milieu, diluting the other serum electrolytes (29). Third, contraction of ECF volume owing to osmotic diuresis or vomiting frequently accompanies DKA, thereby resulting in an increment in the concentration of unmeasured anions, mostly the plasma proteins, that is independent of the altered acid–base status. Fourth, vomiting (which frequently accompanies DKA) and exogenous bicarbonate therapy ameliorate the bicarbonate deficit without correcting the excess anion gap.

Patients admitted with DKA often have a metabolic acidosis with an excess anion gap-HCO_3^- deficit ratio quite different from 1 (30–32) (Table 89-3). Causes for an increase above unity of the ratio of excess anion gap to bicarbonate deficit include vomiting, exogenous bicarbonate therapy, renal acid excretion, hyperproteinemia, and tissue titration (Na^+-H^+ exchange). A decrease of this ratio to below unity may result from the renal excretion of sodium salts of ketones, infusion of chloride-containing fluids, suppression of bicarbonate reabsorption along the nephron owing to hypocapnia, and the possible presence of renal tubular acidosis. Plasma bicarbonate levels are always reduced (usually to <15 mEq/L) in DKA that is not complicated with metabolic alkalosis or respiratory acidosis. Acidemia is also present with blood pH values less than 7.30 unless metabolic alkalosis is superimposed on DKA.

With respect to the role of the kidney in the acid–base homeostasis of patients with DKA, its efficiency to restore the cation of the ketone salts to the blood is such that for each millimole of ß-hydroxybutyric acid excreted, the kidney could salvage only about half a milliequivalent of potential base (33–35). As the renal threshold for plasma ketones is low and the production of ketoacids can reach levels as high as 1,000 to 2,000 mEq/day, the urinary excretion of the sodium salts of the ketoacids may be enormous (36). The low renal threshold of ketoacids results in significant urinary excretion of ketones at plasma concentrations only slightly above normal (37,38). In addition, ß-hydroxybutyric and acetoacetic acids are relatively strong acids (pK$_a$ of 4.70 and 3.58, respectively) so that at the urine pH found in patients with DKA, they are excreted to a significant extent as sodium and potassium salts, which represents a loss of bicarbonate precursors. This renal "wasting" of ketone salts will result in a contraction of the ECF volume, which will signal the kidney to retain dietary or infused NaCl. As the urinary losses of ketones are replenished with chloride, the net effect will be the development of a hyperchloremic acidosis owing to replacement with chloride for the excreted or metabolized ketones (31). Therapy of DKA with isotonic saline to correct the state of volume depletion promotes within a few hours the development of hyperchloremic acidosis in most patients, because of the retention of chloride in excess of sodium and the excretion of ketones by the kidney. Reevaluation of the role of the kidney in the development of and recovery from DKA indicates that maximal stimulation of renal acidification may not suffice to compensate for the massive urinary loss of bicarbonate precursors in the form of ketone salts other than ammonium. Therefore, the end result may be a nonhomeostatic role for the kidney in the defense of the acid—base equilibrium in the early phase of DKA (39).

The level of renal function in patients admitted with DKA appears to be the major determinant of the type of metabolic acidosis (31). Patients having a major impairment of renal function and a severe ECF volume deficit on admission for DKA typically have a ratio of excess anion gap to that of HCO_3^- deficit above 1. In contrast, patients having mild ECF volume deficit, minor impairment of renal function, and lower values of Hct, hemoglobin, BUN, serum proteins, creatinine, and uric acid characteristically have a ratio of excess anion gap to HCO_3^- deficit below 1. The hyperchloremic acidosis observed before admission in some patients with DKA is usually brief, and it is considered to have no adverse clinical consequences. Because the development of this variety of acidosis results from the renal loss of bicarbonate precursors (ketone salts other than ammonium) accompanied by the retention of chloride, these patients should theoretically have a slower recovery from the acid—base disturbance. Indeed, prospective studies demonstrated that patients admitted with a greater component of hyperchloremic acidosis had, at any given time after admission, a smaller increment above their admission levels in their plasma bicarbonate. It appears that the more rapid recovery from metabolic acidosis in patients with DKA presenting with anion gap acidosis is consequent to the equimolar conversion of the retained ketone salts to bicarbonate after insulin administration.

Lactic Acidosis

Patients with diabetes mellitus may develop lactic acidosis, which represents a potentially serious condition (40). Its diagnosis is warranted in the presence of a high anion gap metabolic acidosis associated with blood lactate levels equal to or higher than 4 mEq/L. This acid—base disorder results from the imbalance between production and utilization of lactate; thus, lactic acidosis might result from increased production, decreased utilization, or a combination of these two mechanisms. The skeletal muscle and gut are the organs involved in the development of lactic acidosis because of overproduction. The liver and, to a lesser degree the kidney, are the organs playing the major role in lactate removal. Diabetes mellitus has been shown to be associated with type A as well as type B lactic acidosis. However, this classification has lost its appeal in clinical practice because patients frequently display features of type A as well as type B lactic acidosis simultaneously. Type A includes clinical conditions associated with impaired tissue oxygenation, which causes hyperlactatemia. Examples of type A lactic acidosis are clinical states with either reduced oxygen delivery (shock, cardiac arrest, severe hypoxemia, and sepsis) or those with increased oxygen demand (vigorous exercise, shivering, and generalized seizures). Type B includes clinical conditions in which there is no apparent oxygenation defect to explain the hyperlactatemia. Although patients with type A acidosis develop clinical signs of tissue hypoxia or underperfusion, patients with type B lactic acidosis lack these manifestations. Examples of type B acidosis include congenital defects in glucose or lactate metabolism and many acquired conditions (e.g., diabetes mellitus, malignancies, toxins, and liver disease). Lactic acidosis caused by metabolic defects comprises: (a) disorders of glucoregulation, including hypoglycemia and diabetes mellitus; (b) major organ failure, involving hepatic, renal, or multiple-organ failure; and (c) neoplasias, especially lymphomas, leukemias, sarcomas, and lung carcinomas.

Several drugs and toxins might cause lactic acidosis in diabetics and nondiabetics. Ethanol abuse is probably the most common cause within this group. The oral hypoglycemic agents of the biguanides group (phenformin and metformin) used to be a major cause of lactic acidosis, particularly in patients with impaired renal function; the limited worldwide use of these drugs, at the present time, explains their diminishing importance in the etiology of lactic acidosis, particularly in patients with impaired renal function. Many other drugs, including salicylates, methanol, ethylene glycol, propylene glycol, nitroprusside, and isoniazid, might cause this condition.

Correction of the underlying cause of lactic acidosis is the cornerstone of treatment of this condition. The high mortality associated with lactic acidosis can be reduced by securing adequate support of vital functions. The hemodynamic status and tissue perfusion might improve with correction of volume deficit, enhancing cardiac output and avoiding vasoconstricting drugs (e.g., norepinephrine). Tissue oxygenation must be optimized by correcting anemia or providing a higher inspired oxygen mixture with or without mechanical ventilation. Energy stores must be replenished to prevent the development of hypoglycemia. If drugs or toxins are responsible for the lactic acidosis, it is mandatory to remove these agents promptly from the patient's tissues by whatever means available (i.e., hemodialysis or hemoperfusion, if necessary). Sepsis must be treated aggressively. Other measures in the management of lactic acidosis might include alkali therapy as well as the use of dichloroacetate (DCA), which enhances the oxidation of pyruvate, as described in the following.

The utilization of alkali therapy in the treatment of lactic acidosis is controversial because the rising pH associated with this treatment tends to further increase hyperlactatemia. It has been known for years that acidosis inhibits glycolysis, whereas alkalosis stimulates it and consequently results in elevated plasma lactate levels; this effect, however, is generally mild and usually results in an increase in plasma lactate of only 1 to 3 mEq/L. This pH feedback control is not unique to lactic acid but also occurs with other organic acids, including ketoacids, whose production is inhibited by acidosis and stimulated by alkalosis (40). Additionally, HCO_3^- therapy neither alters the natural course of the deranged metabolism leading to lactic acidosis nor diminishes the mortality of this condition. Yet, most experts advise HCO_3^- therapy in lactic acidosis in the presence of extreme acidemia (blood pH < 7.20) or $[HCO_3^-]_p$ lower than 10 to 12 mEq/L. Bicarbonate administration, however, has several potential adverse effects that are described elsewhere in this chapter.

Other therapeutic measures include the administration of Carbicarb (0.33 mol/L sodium carbonate and 0.33 mol/L sodium bicarbonate) and DCA. The alkalinizing capacity of Carbicarb is identical to that of $NaHCO_3$, but Carbicarb produces less carbon dioxide. Thus, the potential risk of tissue acidosis owing to H_2CO_3 accumulation, associated with alkali therapy, appears to be lower, by comparison, when Carbicarb is used instead of pure $NaHCO_3$. However, the use of Carbicarb in clinical practice is not universally accepted. DCA limits lactate production by stimulating pyruvate dehydrogenase activity, resulting in oxidation of pyruvate to acetyl CoA. The usual dose in adults with lactic acidosis is 50 mg/kg of body weight, diluted in 50 mL of isotonic saline for intravenous infusion over a 30-minute period. This dose might be repeated if plasma lactate levels remain substantially elevated. Limited experience with DCA indicates that this therapy can be beneficial in some instances of lactic acidosis.

Renal Tubular Acidosis

A normal anion gap acidosis, also known as hyperchloremic acidosis, might develop either from a primary loss of HCO_3^- or from a failure to replenish HCO_3^- stores depleted by the daily production of fixed acids. These two defects are commonly encountered in patients with diabetes mellitus (41). A primary loss of HCO_3^- might result from intestinal (e.g., diarrhea) or urinary losses of alkali or its precursors (e.g., ketone salts of sodium and potassium). Hyperchloremic metabolic acidosis that results from failure to replace HCO_3^- stores that have been depleted by the daily production of fixed acids is observed in diabetics with distal tubular acidosis. In this condition, the daily net acid excretion by the kidney falls short of the daily acid production, leading to metabolic acidosis owing to depletion of HCO_3^- stores. Another example is adrenal insufficiency, in the form of diminished mineralocorticoid activity (selective hypoaldosteronism, aldosterone

resistance, and the administration of the K^+-sparing diuretic spironolactone) as well as diminished glucocorticoid activity. The major causes of distal renal tubular acidosis accompanied with hyperkalemia (type 4 renal tubular acidosis) include diabetic renal disease, hypoaldosteronism, obstructive uropathy, sickle cell nephropathy, and renal transplant rejection. The management of type 4 renal tubular acidosis has been described in this chapter.

Combination of Multiple Major Disturbances

The full-blown forms of DKA and HONKS represent the most frequently observed and clinically relevant acute metabolic complications of uncontrolled diabetes mellitus (42,43). Clinicians generally consider that each of these two entities illustrates a distinct condition that develops in isolation from the other in the course of diabetes mellitus. In addition, major textbooks of internal medicine commonly describe DKA and HONKS as different processes having little in common, thereby perpetuating such a notion. These conditions, however, are in fact closely interrelated and truly represent two different expressions of a remarkably similar pathophysiologic process (42–45). In fact, mixed forms having features of DKA and HONKS are observed as or even more frequently than the pure forms of each of these disturbances. As depicted in Fig. 89-2, insulin deficiency or resistance and excessive counterregulation are present in DKA as well as HONKS, yet the severity of these abnormalities differs in the two clinical conditions. The profound ketosis characteristic of DKA is caused by severe insulin deficiency or resistance in association with a mild degree of excessive counterregulation. Conversely, the profound hyperglycemia observed in HONKS is owing to mild insulin deficiency or resistance in association with a severe activation of counterregulatory hormones as well as superimposed renal failure (see the following).

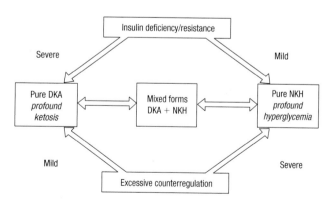

FIG. 89-2. Diabetic ketoacidosis (DKA) and nonketotic hyperglycemia (NKH or HONKS) are the most important acute metabolic complications of patients with uncontrolled diabetes mellitus. These disorders share the same overall pathogenesis that includes insulin deficiency and resistance and excessive counterregulation; however, the importance of each of these endocrine abnormalities differs significantly in DKA and HONKS.

The pathogenesis of ketosis and hyperglycemia in diabetes mellitus always involves the presence of either absolute or relative insulin deficiency. Such insulin deficit might occur because of augmented body requirements of insulin while receiving a fixed insulin dosage, withdrawal from insulin therapy, or failure of the pancreatic ß-cells. Resistance to insulin action also participates in the ketosis and hyperglycemia. Factors that contribute to insulin resistance include counterregulatory hormones, deficiency of electrolytes (mostly potassium), increased tonicity of body fluids, and acidemia. Counterregulatory hormones play a major role in the development of hyperglycemia, as follows. Elevated levels of cortisol, growth hormone, and epinephrine depress insulin-mediated glucose uptake in peripheral tissues (e.g., skeletal muscle) and promote the release of gluconeogenic precursors from myocytes and adipocytes. The latter effects combined with augmented glucagon levels contribute to enhanced gluconeogenesis by the liver and kidney (less important role).

Figure 89-1 depicts the dominant derangements observed in the liver and peripheral tissues that are responsible for the ketonemia and hyperglycemia in decompensated diabetes. Triglycerides stored in adipocytes are decomposed into free fatty acids and glycerol by activation of a "hormone-sensitive" lipase within these cells. Whereas insulin inhibits this lipase, growth hormone, glucagon, and epinephrine stimulate its activity. Consequently, the hormonal disarray of uncontrolled diabetes augments the release of ketone precursors. The increased plasma levels of free fatty acids promote their uptake by hepatocytes where fatty acids are activated to their fatty acyl CoA derivative. The long-chain fatty acyl CoA may be consumed in the cytosol for the synthesis of fatty acids (including malonyl CoA), triglycerides, and phospholipids (dominant pathway in the normal state) or transported by the carnitine shuttle into the mitochondria where it undergoes ß-oxidation producing acetyl CoA (dominant pathway in uncontrolled diabetes mellitus). Within the mitochondria of healthy individuals, the acetyl CoA condenses mostly with oxaloacetate for oxidation in Krebs tricarboxylic acid cycle forming carbon dioxide. The alternative pathway of acetyl CoA within the mitochondria is that two molecules of this compound combine with each other to form the "ketone bodies," acetoacetate and D-3-hydroxybutyrate (ketoacids). The latter route is greatly stimulated in uncontrolled diabetes mellitus because oxaloacetate is in short supply (being removed from the mitochondria for the augmented gluconeogenesis) and excessive acetyl CoA cannot be accommodated through the Krebs cycle so that it overflows through the ketogenic pathway (46). The carnitine shuttle, also known as the *carnitine carrier system,* which allows long-chain fatty acids to cross the inner mitochondrial membrane, consists of carnitine/acyl carnitine translocase and two carnitine-palmitoyl transferases (CPT), an outer CPT I and an inner CPT II. The carnitine shuttle is inhibited by cytosolic malonyl CoA, which is produced during fatty acid synthesis, ensuring that newly formed fatty acids are not immediately transported into the mitochondria and broken down. Because insulin augments, whereas glucagon and catecholamines diminish, the concentration of malonyl CoA, the hormonal imbalance of uncontrolled diabetes produces low cytosolic levels of malonyl CoA, enhancing fatty acid transport toward the mitochondria and thereby stimulating ketogenesis. In summary, synthesis of ketones in the liver largely depends on transfer of fatty acyl CoA into the mitochondria by CPT I. In the fed state of normal individuals, CPT activity is inhibited by cytoplasmic malonyl CoA. During fasting and in patients with ketoacidosis, malonyl CoA synthesis is suppressed, allowing for increased transfer of fatty acyl CoA into the mitochondria and increased ketogenesis. Decreased consumption of ketone bodies by peripheral tissues also contributes to the high levels of plasma ketones in DKA.

Renal Dysfunction and Hyperglycemia

Renal dysfunction must be present to initiate and sustain the extreme hyperglycemia observed in most patients with a full-blown syndrome of hyperglycemic hyperosmolar encephalopathy (47). The predisposing conditions of HONKS include the simultaneous presence of uncontrolled diabetes mellitus and renal failure. A simple calculation demonstrates the virtual impossibility of maintaining plasma glucose levels substantially higher than 400 mg/dL in the presence of normal renal function because of the magnitude of obligatory glucosuria. The difference between the patient's plasma glucose and the renal "threshold" of approximately 180 mg/dL, multiplied by the daily rate of renal ultrafiltration, allows estimation of the expected level of glucosuria. Assuming a normal GFR, the amount of glucose that escapes reabsorption at a plasma level of 400 mg/dL is approximately 400 g/day. Whole-body glucose utilization is approximately 200 g/day under euglycemic conditions, but during an acute elevation of blood glucose this rate increases in proportion to the glucose concentration, in the presence or absence of insulin. This effect is substantially intensified, of course, in the presence of high insulin levels. Doubling the plasma glucose concentration in the presence of physiologic levels of insulin doubles glucose consumption. Hyperglycemia increases both oxidative and nonoxidative glucose disposal. Glucose transport increases acutely in tissues having high transport capacity relative to metabolic capacity (brain and red cells) and in those having low transport capacity relative to their metabolic capacity (muscle, heart, adipose tissue). It follows that in patients with severe hyperglycemia and adequate renal function, substantial glucose removal (600 to 1,000 g/day) results from glucosuria plus internal disposal. An equal amount of glucose must enter the circulation to satisfy these demands in steady-state, severe hyperglycemia. However, endogenous glucose production by the liver is suppressed by hyperglycemia, even in the absence of inhibitory effects of the associated changes in insulin and glucagon levels. The inhibitory effect of hyperglycemia on the hepatic release of glucose is secondary to reduction of both glycogenolysis and

TABLE 89-4. *Fluid deficit and glucose load as precipitating factors of hyperosmolar nonketotic syndrome (HONKS) in diabetes mellitus*

Condition	Physiologic derangement	Clinical entity
Fluid deficit	Poor water intake	
	Relatively preserved CNS function	Elderly/nursing home patients
	Major CNS abnormality	Cerebrovascular accident, subdural hemorrhage
	Increased urinary fluid loss	Large osmotic diuresis, diuretics
	Extrarenal fluid loss	
	Gastrointestinal	Gastroenteritis, peptic ulcer disease, gastrointestinal bleeding, pancreatitis
	Skin	Heat stroke, burns
Glucose load	Increased glucose intake	Highly sweetened drinks, enteral or parenteral force-feeding, hyperalimentation, peritoneal dialysis
	Increased endogenous glucose production	
	Stress	Psychological/physical trauma
	Infection	Pneumonia, pyelonephritis, sepsis
	Major illness	Myocardial infarction
	Medication	Corticosteroids, phenytoin, calcium channel blockers[a]

[a]Phenytoin and calcium channel blockers may decrease insulin release and precipitate the HONKS.

gluconeogenesis. Thus, unless an extremely large exogenous source of glucose is present, severe hyperglycemia will not be sustained in the absence of renal failure. A possible exception to the obligatory presence of renal failure is the patient with decompensated diabetes who has an exceptionally high level of endogenous glucose production, that is, in excess of three times the normal value observed in the fasting state.

The diminished or absent urinary excretion of glucose at plasma glucose levels higher than the renal threshold plays a critical role in generating and maintaining severe hyperglycemia in patients with severe oliguric renal failure. In contrast to this mechanism of glucose retention owing to lack of renal glucose excretion, the so-called uremic pseudodiabetes of chronic renal insufficiency predisposes to only moderate hyperglycemia. Therefore, the most important precipitating factors of HONKS in patients with diabetes mellitus are fluid deficit leading to prerenal azotemia and glucose load of exogenous and endogenous origin (Table 89-4). The HONKS is often observed in patients with poor fluid intake (patients who are weak and unable to perceive or respond to thirst because of sedation, stroke, or other causes) and abnormal fluid losses owing to osmotic diuresis, vomiting, diarrhea, fever, or diuretics. Patients receiving tube feeding solutions, parenteral hyperalimentation, and peritoneal dialysis with a high glucose concentration in the dialysate also are prone to developing HONKS. The major determinant of marked hyperglycemia in the presence of abnormal glucoregulation in these patients is the impaired renal function, owing in most cases to volume depletion, which limits or prevents glucosuria. Thus, whenever a major derangement in glucoregulation develops, the overall level of renal function plays a critical role in determining disturbances in the electrolyte (13,31,39) and nonelectrolyte composition of the plasma, including the blood glucose levels.

Considering that BUN is consistently high in patients with HONKS, measured plasma osmolality overestimates the abnormal serum tonicity (effective osmolality) in these patients. Consequently, it is most important to calculate the effective osmolality (7) in patients with HONKS by multiplying serum sodium levels times two and adding the contribution of serum glucose (i.e., glucose in mg/dL divided by 18). Not infrequently, a comatose diabetic patient is found to have a measured osmolality of approximately 350 mOsm/kg but the calculated effective osmolality is lower, about 310 mOsm/kg; in this condition, the patient's coma is most likely owing to conditions other than a hyperosmolar encephalopathy (i.e., alcohol, uremia, cerebrovascular accident) because the deviation in effective osmolality is less severe than that expected to produce a comatose state. Consequently, the diagnosis of HONKS requires evaluation of calculated osmolality in addition to measurement of serum osmolality, allowing one to rule out the presence of hidden osmoles (e.g., alcohol, ethylene glycol, methanol).

Absence of Ketosis in Hyperosmolar Nonketotic Syndrome

Several theories account for the absence of significant ketosis in HONKS (48–50). It has been proposed that in HONKS there is sufficient insulin to inhibit lipolysis but not enough to stimulate adequate peripheral glucose uptake (Fig. 89-2). This explanation is based on the presumably less severe insulin deficit of patients with HONKS in comparison with DKA, and the inhibition of ketosis by relatively low insulin levels. The generally lower free fatty acid levels in HONKS than in DKA supports the theory that lipolysis is better controlled in the former condition. However, the plasma levels of glucoregulatory hormones are not consistently different in these two metabolic disorders. It has been also proposed that the liver is "insulinized" in HONKS (49), whereas the peripheral tissues (i.e., adipocytes) are not "insulinized"; consequently, peripheral lipolysis proceeds unrestrained, producing large amounts of nonesterified fatty acids (NEFAs) that reach the "insulinized" hepatocytes wherein the gluconeogenic pathway transforms them to glucose instead of being oxidized to ketone bodies. Because hyperosmolality inhibits lipolysis in vitro (52), it is also possible that this mechanism might be partly responsible for the absence of significant ketoacidosis in HONKS.

Clinical Manifestations and Diagnosis of Diabetic Ketoacidosis

Intense thirst, polydipsia, polyuria, tiredness, general malaise, and weight loss are classic symptoms of DKA (53,55). Nausea, vomiting, and abdominal pain secondary to ketosis are commonly observed; many of these patients are mistakenly triaged to surgery. Patients may describe experiencing the taste and smell of ketones, and the examiner might notice a pear drop (rotten pear) odor caused by ketones in the subject's breath. Depression of sensorium might be observed and the central nervous system dysfunction is caused by the hypertonicity of body fluids secondary to hyperglycemia (8,55). Severe obtundation, coma, and/or convulsions are rarely seen in pure DKA but are prominent manifestations of a severe hyperosmolar state (HONKS). Dyspnea with increased rate and depth of respirations, the so-called Kussmaul breathing, may be recognized in DKA. Signs of volume depletion including orthostatic hypotension, tachycardia, decreased skin turgor, and soft eyeballs might be evident on physical examination. Osmotic diuresis owing to massive glucosuria and extrarenal fluid losses are responsible for the signs and symptoms of volume depletion. The presence of fever usually indicates a concomitant infection that might have precipitated the severe metabolic derangement. The differential diagnosis includes conditions with signs and symptoms related to the neurologic, gastrointestinal, and respiratory systems. Entities in the differential diagnosis having neurologic symptoms include metabolic disorders (e.g., hypoglycemia, uremia, nonketotic hyperglycemia, lactic acidosis), toxic encephalopathies (e.g., ethanol, methanol, ethylene glycol, opium derivatives, narcotics), head trauma, cerebrovascular accidents, meningitis, and encephalitis. Conditions that might also resemble DKA include gastroenteritis (abdominal pain, nausea, vomiting) and pneumonia (dyspnea).

It is most important to identify the initiating events leading to the development of DKA. Infection is the most commonly observed precipitating cause of DKA worldwide (i.e., tuberculosis, malaria) followed by failure of insulin administration and intercurrent illness. Acute infectious illnesses very often precipitate DKA and must be aggressively treated if the ketoacidosis is to be controlled. Common etiologies include seemingly trivial viral infections as well as pneumonia, pyelonephritis, mucormycosis, and septicemia. Omission or reduction of the insulin dosage and dietary indiscretions (especially the consumption of alcoholic beverages) also are commonly implicated, especially in adolescent diabetic patients. Pregnancy, myocardial infarction, cerebrovascular accident, intraabdominal catastrophes, pancreatitis, potassium depletion, and drugs such as corticosteroids may also precipitate ketoacidosis in diabetic patients. Emotional stress can trigger DKA in some individuals with diabetes mellitus. Furthermore, ketoacidosis may be the initial manifestation of previously undiagnosed diabetes, and occasionally the precipitating cause for the DKA may not be found. A common denominator of many initiating events is the development of significant insulin deficit associated with a fasting state. Salt and water depletion accentuates the release of stress hormones and ultimately might lead to DKA. Ketoacidosis can be the initial manifestation of diabetes mellitus in some patients with type I disease (insulin-dependent clinical form).

Diagnosis of DKA is made on recognition of signs and symptoms of this disease, and biochemical features that include hyperglycemia and ketosis. Commonly used but more restrictive criteria of DKA include a triad of hyperglycemia (blood glucose >250 mg/dL), ketosis (serum or urine ketones positive by the nitroprusside reaction in a dilution >1 : 2), and acidosis (plasma bicarbonate <15 mEq/L, blood pH < 7.30). The diminished plasma bicarbonate level as well as acidemia might be absent in DKA if metabolic alkalosis is superimposed, because of persistent vomiting or other causes. Plasma glucose levels in DKA range most frequently between 350 and 750 mg/dL, yet substantially lower and higher levels are occasionally observed. Values below 200 mg/dL (euglycemic DKA) might be seen, especially in alcoholics or pregnant insulin-dependent diabetics. Values above 1,000 mg/dL might be seen, especially in patients with severe volume contraction leading to renal failure with loss of glucosuria (hyperglycemic hyperosmotic syndrome might develop concomitantly). There is no relationship between the severity of DKA and the magnitude of the hyperglycemia.

There are some potential pitfalls in the interpretation of plasma levels of ketones, creatinine, and enzymes that are indicative of tissue injury in patients with DKA. The nitroprusside reagent, utilized for the assessment of blood ketones, reacts almost exclusively with acetoacetate but not with ß-hydroxybutyrate. Consequently, elevated plasma ß-hydroxybutyrate levels might be undetected with the use of this assay. The presence of high levels of acetoacetate interferes with the colorimetric methods used to quantify creatinine and tissue injury enzymes (alanine aminotransferase, aspartate aminotransferase, lactate dehydrogenase, and creatine kinase), resulting in spurious elevation of these substances.

Clinical Manifestations and Diagnosis of Hyperosmolar Nonketotic Syndrome

The severe hyperglycemia of HONKS increases plasma osmolality, which is responsible for the characteristic functional

TABLE 89-5. *Comparison of salient clinical features of pure and mixed forms of diabetic ketoacidosis (DKA) and hyperosmolar nonketotic syndrome (HONKS)*

Feature	Pure DKA	Mixed forms	Pure HONKS
Incidence	5–10 times higher	⇔	5–10 times lower
Mortality	5%–10%	⇔	10%–60
Onset	Rapid (<2 days)	⇔	Slow (>5 days)
Age of patient	Usually <40 yr	⇔	Usually >40 yr
Type 1 diabetes	Common	⇔	Rare
Type 2 diabetes	Rare	⇔	Common
First indication of diabetes	Often	⇔	Often
Volume depletion	Mild/moderate	⇔	Severe
Renal failure (most commonly of prerenal nature)	Mild/not constant	⇔	Always present
Subsequent therapy with insulin	Always	⇔	Not always

abnormalities of the central nervous system (44,56). Depression of the sensorium, somnolence, obtundation, and coma are prominent manifestations of HONKS. The degree of obtundation correlates with the severity of serum hypertonicity owing to hyperglycemia (55). It is believed that the extracellular hyperosmolality might cause a shift of water from ICF to ECF, producing brain shrinkage with the consequent alteration in mental status. Such water loss from the brain has been documented within 1 hour of inducing severe hyperglycemia in experimental animals, but disappears at 4 to 6 hours. It must be recognized that neither ketosis nor metabolic acidosis, features that are consistently present in DKA but absent in HONKS produce major depression of the sensorium (55). Thus, hyperglycemia with hyperosmolality is the main determinant of the neurologic manifestations. Consequently, a comatose diabetic patient admitted with hyperglycemia (for whom other causes of coma have been ruled out) has a hyperosmolar nonketotic encephalopathy in almost all instances. Depending on the age of the patient, a level of effective osmolality or tonicity in the ECF of 340 mOsm/kg or higher appears to be necessary for the development of hyperosmolar coma (42,55).

Profound volume depletion leading to prerenal azotemia (47,57,58) and not uncommonly to circulatory collapse is observed in HONKS. All other symptoms and signs previously described for patients with DKA except for dyspnea might be evident in hyperosmolar nonketotic states. Dyspnea and Kussmaul respiration are owing to the metabolic acidosis observed in DKA but absent in hyperosmolar nonketotic states (59–62). Consequently, these respiratory manifestations are not observed HONKS. Diagnosis of the

"pure" HONKS is based on the presence of severe hyperglycemia (glucose levels >800 mg/dL) and hyperosmolality (>340 mOsm/kg), absence of significant ketosis (nitroprusside reaction of <2+ in a 1:1 dilution of plasma), and profound volume depletion (see Table 89-6). Patients with pure HONKS are generally older and have a milder form of diabetes mellitus as compared to those with pure DKA. Type II diabetes is most commonly the underlying disease of HONKS, and volume depletion and prerenal azotemia is characteristically present. Comparisons of the most salient clinical and biochemical features that allow one to distinguish the pure forms of DKA and HONKS are displayed in Tables 89-5 and 89-6. It must be recognized that many patients exhibit a mixed pattern with clinical and biochemical features of DKA as well as those of HONKS. These patients presenting with a mixed pattern should be diagnosed as having a DKA-HONKS. Thus, the physician should not choose either DKA or HONKS in such patients but should diagnose the patient's condition as a mixed pattern.

The initial bedside evaluation of the patient having uncontrolled diabetes mellitus must be thoroughly, yet expediently performed and should include determination of body weight, a chest roentgenogram, and testing of blood and urine for glucose and ketones. The diagnosis must be made promptly, and the precipitating event or underlying illness clearly delineated. It is of critical importance to rule out hypoglycemia; if this diagnosis is seriously entertained, glucose administration should be considered. The laboratory examination should focus on the patient's serum glucose, serum electrolytes, blood acid–base composition, serum osmolality, BUN, and serum creatinine. Complete white blood cell count

TABLE 89-6. *Comparison of salient biochemical features of pure and mixed forms of diabetic ketoacidosis (DKA) and hyperosmolar nonketotic syndrome (HONKS)*

Plasma levels	Pure DKA	Mixed forms	Pure HONKS
Glucose	<800 mg/dL	⇔	>800 mg/dL
Ketone bodies	$\geq 2+$ in 1:1 dilution	⇔	<2+ in 1:1 dilution
Effective osmolality	<340 mOs/kg	⇔	>340 mOsm/kg
pH	Decreased	⇔	Normal
$[HCO_3^-]_p$	Decreased	⇔	Normal
$[Na^+]_p$	Normal or low	⇔	Normal
$[K^+]_p$	Variable	⇔	Normal or high
			Variable

and differential, as well as cultures of blood and other body fluids must be obtained to rule out an infectious process. Arterial blood gas analysis and an electrocardiogram should also be obtained.

Therapy of Diabetic Ketoacidosis and Hyperosmolar Nonketotic Syndrome

The concepts previously discussed with respect to the therapy of each single dominant disturbance in body composition are applicable to that of combined disturbances examined in this section. The general management of DKA and HONKS is identical. The basic therapeutic goals may be summarized as follows: (a) repletion of intravascular volume and maintenance of an adequate circulation, (b) reversal with insulin of the altered intermediate metabolism, (c) correction of the electrolyte and acid–base imbalance, and (d) treatment of the initiating event (63–65). To accomplish these objectives, a number of requirements must be fulfilled: the continuous presence of a competent, responsible physician; 24-hour availability of laboratory facilities; equipment and drugs for handling medical emergencies, and those specific for DKA and HONKS including regular insulin, 0.9% and 0.45% saline, 5% glucose in water, sodium bicarbonate for intravenous infusion, potassium chloride, and potassium phosphate solutions; and maintenance of a flowchart with hourly evaluation of vital signs, mental condition, urine including output, serum chemistries, insulin intake, fluid administration (intravenous and oral), electrolyte intake, and other medications.

Patients who are comatose, obtunded, or in shock require admission to an intensive care unit. When an alteration in mental status is part of the picture, hypoglycemia, trauma, and meningitis must be quickly ruled out. Patients in shock require arterial and central venous pressure monitoring, close evaluation of urine output, and timely administration of plasma volume expanders. The airway must be protected in all patients, with endotracheal intubation if necessary. If abdominal distention or vomiting occurs, a nasogastric tube should be placed and the stomach drained to prevent pulmonary aspiration of gastric contents.

Insulin Administration

Because insulin is central to the regulation of ketone production and glucose utilization, adequate plasma insulin levels must be present if DKA or HONKS is to be reversed (66,67). Patients with HONKS are not more sensitive to insulin than are those with DKA, in spite of the commonly expressed opinion that the former have greater sensitivity to this hormone (43,68). A precipitous fall in extracellular tonicity might trigger cerebral edema with secondary worsening of the patient's condition; therefore, blood glucose should not decrease with treatment with more than 200 mg/dL per hour. Currently, the accepted practice is to give regular insulin (43) as a low-dose continuous intravenous infusion or if not possible, intramus-

cularly (e.g., deltoid muscle) at small intervals. Typically an initial intravenous bolus of 5 to 10 units of regular insulin is given and an intravenous drip of 0.1 U/kg per hour (or 5 to 10 U/hour) is started. Serum glucose will fall at approximately 5% to 10%/hour. As the serum glucose approaches 250 mg/dL, 5% dextrose in water should be included in the intravenous fluids and the blood glucose should be followed closely. Glucose administration is needed in this condition to prevent hypoglycemia. The intravenous insulin rate is thereafter decreased to 1 or 2 U/hour so that the patient's blood glucose level remains between 100 and 200 mg/dL. Subcutaneous insulin (regular or long-acting) is started when the patient can take oral nourishment and ketosis, if present, has stopped. Occasionally, patients with DKA exhibit marked insulin resistance (69). Should the blood glucose level not decrease at an insulin dose of 0.1 U/kg per hour, doubling or tripling that dosage may be needed. Care must be taken to decrease the dosage as the patient's blood glucose approaches 250 or 300 mg/dL.

Fluid Therapy

Hyperglycemia and glucosuria lead to significant cellular and ECF volume depletion such that water losses of 4 to 8 L might be present on admission. Fluid therapy must correct the actual volume deficit as well as replace ongoing sensible and insensible losses. Consequently, infusion of 5 L of fluid or more might be necessary within the first 24 hours (58,70–72). Because volume depletion triggers the release of counterregulatory hormones and substantially contributes to morbidity and mortality, fluid therapy is a cornerstone in the management of DKA and HONKS.

Administration of fluids repairs salt and water losses and the clinical consequences of such deficiencies, including the altered hemodynamic status and the renal dysfunction; in addition, it decreases the level of counterregulatory hormones and enhances glucosuria (73). At admission, the patient with DKA or HONKS should immediately undergo a clinical assessment of vascular volume and cardiovascular function. Although volume repletion is the usual finding on admission for DKA, the severity of this derangement varies widely. The choice of the replacement fluid is critical, as it may or may not be necessary to expand rapidly the intravascular volume.

The first consideration in planning fluid therapy of DKA and HONKS is to stabilize the patient hemodynamically by means of albumin-containing solutions if shock is present. Thereafter, isotonic saline (0.9% NaCl) should be infused (58,70–76). Although the estimated water and salt losses in these patients demonstrate the hypotonic nature of overall fluid deficit, other considerations including prevention of cerebral edema mandate the use of isotonic saline instead of half-isotonic saline during the initial several hours of treatment (70–74). The volume of distribution of the various solutions for intravenous infusion was described previously in this chapter.

Isotonic saline stands out as the best solution for the initial intravenous fluid therapy of DKA and HONKS, except for patients in severe circulatory collapse in whom infusions containing albumin, plasma fractions, or colloids might be indicated for prompt expansion of intravascular volume. Isotonic saline corrects the depleted ECF volume and prevents the rapid reduction of extracellular osmolality resulting from the progressive decrease in glucose levels owing to insulin therapy and to increasing glucosuria, as ECF volume depletion is corrected. It has been suggested that the brain swelling that might occur in the recovery phase of DKA and HONKS is causally related to a decrement in extracellular osmolality and that hypotonic solutions, such as 0.45% NaCl, may aggravate this process, whereas isotonic saline may exert a protective effect. Complete agreement has not been reached, however, with respect to the use of isotonic or hypotonic solutions (0.9% versus 0.45% NaCl) as the initial fluid in the therapy of DKA and HONKS.

A large-volume infusion might require that the patient be carefully monitored for signs of pulmonary edema. Central venous or pulmonary artery catheterization may be required in some patients to correctly monitor vascular volume. Although efforts should be made to avoid bladder catheterization in order to prevent the initiation or exacerbation of a urinary tract infection, a catheter may be inserted if the patient is stuporous or urine output cannot be monitored. An intravenous infusion of 1,000 to 2,000 mL/hour ($\sim$14 to 28 mL/kg per hour) has been recommended for the first few hours of treatment, but lower rates of 500 to 1,000 mL/hour ($\sim$7 to 14 mL/kg per hour) have been advised by others (54,73). However, the optimal rate of intravenous fluid administration necessary to replenish intravascular volume, restore normal hemodynamic status, and correct cellular and interstitial volume losses remains undefined. Theoretically, a slow correction of volume deficit may prolong the ketoacidotic state in patients with DKA as a result of continued catecholamine release, while overcorrection may enhance urinary losses of HCO_3^- precursors (ketone salts), leading to prolonged normal anion gap metabolic acidosis. In extreme cases, an inappropriately restricted regimen of fluid replacement may contribute substantially to prolonged circulatory failure with its multiple complications, including stroke; an overly generous supply of fluids, on the other hand, has been implicated in the pathogenesis of symptomatic brain swelling and pulmonary edema. Recent studies indicated that a regimen of isotonic saline infused at 500 mL/hour (approximately 7 mL/kg per hour) during the initial 4 hours, and 250 mL/hour (about 3.5 mL/kg per hour) during the subsequent 4 hours, promptly restores volume deficits without untoward effects (73).

Four hours after treatment with isotonic saline solutions is started, the initial infusion rate should be decreased to one-half, unless hemodynamic instability persists; the solution should be changed to 0.45% NaCl only if hypernatremia develops and signs of cerebral edema (i.e., aggravation of mental status, papilledema) are absent; 5% dextrose in water should be started when blood glucose decreases to 250 mg/dL; 0.45% or 0.9% NaCl should be also administered with the 5% dextrose solution if significant ECF volume deficit, hyponatremia, or cerebral edema is present; urine output should be at least 30 to 60 mL/hour. Clear liquids might be given orally (up to 100 to 200 mL/hour if tolerated) after 4 hours from either the last episode of vomiting or when therapy with gastric suction has been stopped; the rate of intravenous fluids should be reduced accordingly. The patient might be allowed to eat a solid meal 8 to 12 hours after clear liquids are started. Because fluid deficit is generally severe in patients with HONKS, many of whom have preexisting heart disease and are relatively old, close monitoring of intravascular volume during fluid replacement requires measurements of central venous pressure or pulmonary capillary wedge pressure, or both.

Alkali Administration

Considering that metabolic acidosis is generally absent in HONKS, bicarbonate therapy is not indicated in these patients. Conversely, clinicians have long thought that expedient correction of the metabolic acidosis was beneficial to the patient with DKA. Accordingly, bicarbonate was often given within the first few hours of treatment. However, bicarbonate administration should theoretically be unnecessary because ketones, when finally metabolized to carbon dioxide and water, regenerate bicarbonate. Indeed, the early administration of bicarbonate in patients with DKA may actually be harmful, leading to a worsening of the central nervous system acidosis and hypokalemia, and causing metabolic alkalosis after the DKA has resolved. Furthermore, some studies found that bicarbonate administration did nothing to improve the recovery of patients with DKA who presented with an arterial pH of 6.90 to 7.10 (77,78). The controversy in terms of the usefulness and indications of bicarbonate administration is based on differences in the appreciation of risks and benefits by different workers (42,79–83). It should be recognized that in the presence of severe hypobicarbonatemia (i.e., TCO_2 (total carbon dioxide content in plasma) <5 mM), relatively small increments in carbon dioxide tension (PCO_2) or in plasma organic acids may profoundly decrease blood pH to dangerously low levels (41,80,84–86). Bicarbonate should not be given by intravenous bolus in DKA patients unless hyperkalemia is present, because of the risk of lethal hypokalemia. After the arguments for and against the use of bicarbonate are weighed, it appears that the careful administration of bicarbonate to severely acidemic patients, especially those with hyperchloremic metabolic acidosis, to support their arterial pH at 7.10 or 7.20 and serum bicarbonate at approximately 10 mEq/L is more beneficial than harmful.

Potassium and Phosphate Supplementation

The typical patient with DKA has a potassium deficit of 4 to 8 mEq/kg of body weight at the time of admission, yet the initial serum potassium often is normal or elevated. On the other hand, K^+ depletion is of less importance in HONKS. Insulin therapy promotes a rapid decrease in serum potassium as this ion shifts intracellularly; therefore, potassium supplementation is required (42,42,45,53,54). Specifically, after the initial fluid challenge has restored the urinary output and if serum potassium is below 3.5 mEq/L, intravenous administration of 10 to 20 mEq/L of infusate is started and continued until the DKA is controlled and the serum potassium is 4.0 to 5.0 mEq/L. Serum potassium should be monitored periodically and the potassium infusion rate adjusted as needed.

Serum phosphate levels fluctuate widely in patients with DKA and HONKS in spite of the likely presence of phosphorus depletion in these patients. The osmotic diuresis caused by glucosuria leads to decreased renal reabsorption of phosphate, accounting for its depletion from body stores. Several studies demonstrated elevated serum phosphate in DKA at initial examination (2,87), but with insulin and fluid therapy the concentration decreased to normal or low levels (87–90). The initial serum phosphate was found to positively correlate with the serum effective osmolality, glucose, and anion gap (87). This finding suggests that in states of insulin deficit leading to metabolic acidosis, elevated serum glucose, and hyperosmolality, phosphate is shifted from cells into the interstitial and vascular spaces. Insulin therapy shifts phosphate back into cells, rapidly lowering the serum levels. Early research suggested that the relative phosphate depletion of DKA was harmful because phosphate replacement seemed to decrease mortality. More recent studies, however, were unable to document that phosphate replacement made any difference in the recovery from DKA (91). Consequently, it is difficult to make unequivocal recommendations regarding phosphorus replacement therapy. The actual consequences of phosphate shifts are not known. Because phosphorus replacement is of unproved clinical significance and potentially dangerous (i.e., it may result in hypocalcemia, hypomagnesemia, or both), it should not be infused unless the serum phosphate is below 1.5 mg/dL and serum calcium is normal or high; in those circumstances 10 to 30 mmol of potassium phosphate may be added to the intravenous infusion and repeated if necessary to correct persistent hypophosphatemia. The hypophosphatemia that accompanies DKA may have serious consequences (e.g., impaired myocardial or skeletal muscle contractility) in undernourished patients such as chronic alcoholics. In this population, parenteral phosphate replacement of 60 to 120 mmol administered over a 24-hour period might be recommended.

Cerebral Edema and Complications of Therapy

Patients with DKA may be admitted with a relatively normal mental status and become unconscious within the first 12 hours of therapy (92), in spite of a partial or complete correction of the hyperglycemia and ketoacidosis. These patients are typically but not exclusively children or young adults, and the morbidity and mortality of this group are relatively high (93). Often, the deaths of these patients are unexpected, as they do not have the underlying vascular, cardiac, and renal abnormalities found in older diabetics. At autopsy, cerebral edema is consistently present (93). The pathogenesis of this condition remains poorly understood (94–97). Osmotic disequilibrium between brain cells and cerebrospinal fluid (CSF) is often cited as a determinant of cerebral edema. In response to hyperglycemia, brain cells develop an increase in their osmolality to match that of the CSF and thus defend themselves against cell shrinkage. A sudden decrease in CSF osmolality owing to fluid infusions or a fall in blood glucose then cause brain swelling. The effects of rapid crystalloid volume loading in diabetics with DKA have been studied, and some degree of brain swelling or increase in CSF pressure was found (92,98–100). Clinically, patients in DKA with hyponatremia who receive insulin and more than 4 L of fluid per square meter within 24 hours may have an increased risk of developing cerebral edema (100). Alterations in CSF pH (82,98) and oxygen tension (83) following bicarbonate administration may also contribute to the development of cerebral edema. After bicarbonate therapy, the CSF pH may decrease acutely, as carbon dioxide but not bicarbonate can rapidly cross the blood-brain barrier. Also, oxygen tension in the central nervous system may decrease, possibly owing to acute shifts in the hemoglobin-oxygen dissociation curve with changes in pH; brain swelling may be secondary to either of these two factors as well (100). It must be emphasized that the proposed mechanisms are only hypotheses; the pathogenesis of cerebral edema in DKA is not definitively known (43,101–103) because it is not consistently associated with bicarbonate therapy, hyponatremia, hypoosmolality, plasma glucose levels, or excessive hypotonic fluid replacement. Nonetheless, it seems prudent in the therapy of DKA (and HONKS) to avoid excessively aggressive volume replacement, sudden changes in the patient's serum glucose and sodium concentration, and excessive use of bicarbonate. Fortunately, the development of clinically apparent cerebral edema associated with the therapy of DKA is not common; however, the fact that it occurs in young otherwise healthy patients pinpoints the importance of careful observation of all patients receiving therapy for DKA and HONKS for the earliest signs of mental deterioration.

A number of life-threatening complications may develop in the course of DKA and HONKS in spite of adequate medical care (42). Shock of cardiac origin or resulting from sepsis or volume depletion, as well as cerebral thrombosis and edema, are among the most prominent complications (103). Cerebral edema leading to death or responsible for chronic sequelae (104) fortunately is rare, yet milder forms may be regularly found with the standard treatment of DKA (100) and HONKS (101). Mortality from DKA has declined from more than 40% in the 1930s to less than 5% in some institutions, as the result of improvements in medical technology and appreciation of the seriousness of the disease. Yet, the prognosis of patients with HONKS is substantially worse, as evidenced by the higher mortality associated with this metabolic complication (43).

ACKNOWLEDGMENTS

The author is indebted to Linda Sue Seals for skillful assistance in preparing the manuscript.

REFERENCES

1. Foster DW, McGarry JD. The metabolic derangements and treatment of diabetic ketoacidosis. *N Engl J Med* 1983;309:159.
2. Kreisberg RA. Diabetic ketoacidosis: new concepts and trends in pathogenesis and treatment. *Ann Intern Med* 1978;88:681.
3. Karam JH, Salber PR, Forsham PH. Pancreatic hormones and diabetes mellitus. In: Greenspan FS, Forsham PH, eds. *Basic and clinical endocrinology*. East Norwalk, CT: Lange Medical, 1986.
4. Skillman TG. Diabetes mellitus. In: Mazzaferri EL, ed. *Endocrinology*. New York: Medical Exam, 1986.
5. Adrogué HJ, Madias NE. Hyponatremia. *N Engl J Med* 2000;342:1581.
6. Adrogué HJ, Madias NE. Hypernatremia. *N Engl J Med* 2000;342: 1493.
7. Adrogué HJ, Wesson DE. *Salt & water. Blackwell's basics of medicine series*. Boston: Blackwell Scientific, 1994.
8. Adrogué HJ, Barrero J, Dolson GM. Diabetic ketoacidosis. In: Suki WN, Massry SG, eds. *Therapy of renal diseases and related disorders*, 2nd ed. Boston: Martinus Nijhoff, 1991.
9. Narins RG, Krishna GG, Kopyt NP. Fluid–electrolyte and acid–base disorders complicating diabetes mellitus. In: Schrier RW, Gottschalk CW, eds. *Diseases of the kidney*, 5th ed. Boston: Little, Brown, 1993.
10. Adrogué HJ, Wesson DE. *Potassium. Blackwell's basics of medicine series*. Boston: Blackwell Scientific, 1994.
11. Adrogué HJ. Mechanisms of transcellular potassium shifts in acid–base disorders. In: Hatano M, ed. *Proceedings of the XIth International Congress on Nephrology, Tokyo, Japan*. Tokyo: Springer, 1991.
12. Adrogué HJ, Madias NE. Changes in plasma potassium concentration during acute acid–base disturbances. *Am J Med* 1981;71:456.
13. Adrogué HJ, et al. Determinants of plasma potassium levels in diabetic ketoacidosis. *Medicine* 1986;65:163.
14. Adrogué HJ, et al. Role of the endocrine pancreas in the kalemic response to acute metabolic acidosis in conscious dogs. *J Clin Invest* 1985;75:798.
15. Goldfarb S, et al. Acute hyperkalemia induced by hyperglycemia: hormonal mechanisms. *Ann Intern Med* 1976;84:426.
16. Fraley DS, Adler S. Isohydric regulation of plasma potassium by bicarbonate in the rat. *Kidney Int* 1976;9:333.
17. Fraley DS, Adler S. Correction of hyperkalemia by bicarbonate despite constant blood pH. *Kidney Int* 1977;12:354.
18. Makoff DL, et al. Hypertonic expansion: acid–base and electrolyte changes. *Am J Physiol* 1970;218:1201.
19. Massara F, et al. Influence of glucagon on plasma levels of potassium in man. *Diabetologia* 1980;19:414.
20. Silva P, Spokes K. Sympathetic system in potassium homeostasis. *Am J Physiol* 1981;241:F151.
21. Peters JP, et al. The nature of diabetic acidosis. *J Clin Invest* 1933; 12:377.
22. Oh MS, Carroll HJ. The anion gap. *N Engl J Med* 1977;297:814.
23. Emmett M, Narins RG. Clinical use of the anion gap. *Medicine* 1977; 56:38.
24. Narins RG, Emmet M. Simple and mixed acid–base disorders: a practical approach. *Medicine* 1980;59:161.
25. Adrogué HJ, et al. Pathogenesis of hyperchloremic acidosis during recovery from diabetic ketoacidosis. *Clin Res* 1980;28:434A.
26. Adrogué HJ, Brensilver J, Madias NE. Changes in the plasma anion gap during chronic metabolic acid–base disturbances. *Am J Physiol* 1978;235:F291.
27. Madias NE, Ayus JC, Adrogué HJ. Increased anion gap in metabolic alkalosis: the role of plasma-protein equivalency. *N Engl J Med* 1979; 300:1421.
28. Narins RG, Bastl CP, Rudnick MR. Anion gap and serum bicarbonate. *N Engl J Med* 1980;303:161.
29. Madias NE, et al. Hypochloremia as a consequence of high anion gap metabolic acidosis. *Clin Res* 1982;30:458A.
30. Oster JR, Epstein M. Acid–base aspects of ketoacidosis. *Am J Nephrol* 1984;4:137.
31. Adrogué HJ, et al. Plasma acid–base patterns in diabetic ketoacidosis. *N Engl J Med* 1982;307:1603.
32. Gamblin GT, et al. Diabetic ketoacidosis presenting with a normal anion gap. *Am J Med* 1986;80:758.
33. Guest GM, Rapoport S. Electrolytes of blood plasma and cells in diabetic acidosis and during recovery. *Proc Am Diabetes Assn* 1947; 7:97.
34. Pitts RF. The renal regulation of acid base balance with special reference to the mechanism for acidifying the urine. *Science* 1945; 102:49.
35. Pitts RF. Acid–base regulation by the kidneys. *Am J Med* 1950;9:356.
36. Daughaday WH. Hydrogen ion metabolism in diabetic acidosis. *Arch Intern Med* 1961;107:63.
37. Pitts RF. Production and excretion of ammonia in relation to acid–base regulation. In: Orloff J, Berliner RW, eds. *Handbook of physiology*. Washington, DC: American Physiological Society, 1972.
38. Pitts RF. Tubular reabsorption. In: *Physiology of the kidney and body fluids*. Chicago: Year Book, 1974.
39. Adrogué HJ, Eknoyan E, Suki WN. Diabetic ketoacidosis: role of the kidney in the acid–base homeostasis re-evaluated. *Kidney Int* 1984; 25:591.
40. Adrogué HJ, Tannen RL. Ketoacidosis, hyperosmolar states, and lactic acidosis. In: Tannen RL, Kokko JP, eds. *Fluids and electrolytes*, 3rd ed. Philadelphia: WB Saunders, 1995.
41. Adrogué HJ, Wesson DE. *Acid–base. Blackwell's basics of medicine series*. Boston: Blackwell Scientific, 1994.
42. Alberti KGMM. Diabetic acidosis, hyperosmolar coma, and lactic acidosis. In: Becker KL, ed. *Principles and practice of endocrinology and metabolism*. Philadelphia: JB Lippincott, 1990.
43. Marshall SM, Walker M, Alberti KGMM. Diabetic ketoacidosis and hyperglycaemic non-ketotic coma. In: Alberti KGMM, et al, eds. *International textbook of diabetes mellitus*. Chichester, England: Wiley, 1992.
44. Davidson MB. Diabetic ketoacidosis and hyperosmolar nonketotic syndrome. In: Davidson MB, ed. *Diabetes mellitus, diagnosis and treatment*. New York: Churchill Livingstone, 1991.
45. Genuth SM. Diabetic ketoacidosis and hyperglycemic hyperosmolar coma. In: Bardin CW, ed. *Current therapy in endocrinology and metabolism*. Philadelphia: BC Decker, 1991.
46. Salway JG. *Metabolism at a glance*. Oxford: Blackwell Scientific, 1994.
47. Adrogué HJ. Glucose homeostasis and the kidney. *Kidney Int* 1992; 42:1266.
48. Schade DS, Eaton RP. Dose response to insulin in man: differential effects on glucose and ketone body regulation. *J Clin Endocrinol Metab* 1977;44:1038.
49. Joffe BI, et al. Pathogenesis of nonketotic hyperosmolar diabetic coma. *Lancet* 1975;i:1069.
50. Whittaker J, et al. The effects of metabolic acidosis in vivo on insulin binding to isolated rat adipocytes. *Metabolism* 1982;31:553.
51. Lindsey CA, Faloona GR, Unger RH. Plasma glucagon in nonketotic hyperosmolar coma. *JAMA* 1974;229:1171.
52. Gerich J, et al. Effect of dehydration and hyperosmolarity on glucose free fatty acid and ketone body metabolism in the rat. *Diabetes* 1973;22:264.
53. Matz R. Uncontrolled diabetes mellitus. In: Bergman M, ed. *Diabetic ketoacidosis and hyperosmolar coma, principles of diabetes management*. New York: Medical Exam, 1987.
54. Adrogué HJ, et al. Diabetic ketoacidosis: a practical approach. *Hosp Pract* 1989;24:83.
55. Fulop M, et al. Hyperosmolar nature of diabetic coma. *Diabetes* 1975; 24:594.
56. Matz R. Coma in the nonketotic diabetic. In: Ellenberg M, Rifkin H, eds. *Diabetes mellitus*. New York: Medical Exam, 1983.
57. Gerich JE, Martin MM, Recant L. Clinical and metabolic characteristics of hyperosmolar nonketotic coma. *Diabetes* 1971;20:228.
58. Khardori R, Soler NG. Hyperosmolar hyperglycemic nonketotic syndrome. *Am J Med* 1984;77:899.
59. Danowski TS, Nabarro JDN. Hyperosmolar and other types of nonketoacidotic coma in diabetes. *Diabetes* 1965;14:162.

60. Jackson WPU, Forman R. Hyperosmolar nonketotic diabetic coma. *Diabetes* 1966;15:714.

61. Johnson RD, et al. Mechanisms and management of hyperosmolar coma without ketoacidosis in the diabetic. *Diabetes* 1969;18:111.

62. Arieff AI, Carroll HJ. Nonketotic hyperosmolar coma with hyperglycemia: clinical features, pathophysiology, renal function, acid–base balance, plasma-cerebrospinal fluid equilibria and the effects of therapy in 37 cases. *Medicine* 1972;51:73.

63. Adrogué HJ, Madias NE. Management of life-threatening acid–base disorders (first of two parts). *N Engl J Med* 1998;338:26.

64. Kreisberg RA. Diabetic ketoacidosis in adults. In: DeFronzo RA, ed. *Current therapy of diabetes mellitus.* St. Louis: Mosby-Year Book, 1998.

65. Marshall SM, Alberti KGMM. Hyperosmolar hyperglycemic nonketotic coma. In: DeFronzo RA, ed. *Current therapy of diabetes mellitus.* St. Louis: Mosby-Year Book, 1998.

66. Kitabchi AE, et al. Diabetic ketoacidosis. Reappraisal of therapeutic approach. *Ann Rev Med* 1979;30:339.

67. Kozak GP, Rolla AR. Diabetic comas. In: Kozak GP, ed. *Clinical diabetes mellitus.* Philadelphia: WB Saunders, 1982.

68. Rosenthal NR, Barrett EJ. An assessment of insulin action in hyperosmolar hyperglycemic nonketotic diabetic patients. *J Clin Endocrinol Metab* 1985;60:607.

69. Pedersen O, Beck-Nielsen H. Insulin resistance and insulin-dependent diabetes mellitus. *Diabetes Care* 1987;10:516.

70. Kandel G, Aberman A. Selected developments in the understanding of diabetic ketoacidosis. *Can Med Assoc J* 1983;128:392.

71. Brown RH, et al. Caveat on fluid replacement in hyperglycemic, hyperosmolar, nonketotic coma. *Diabetes Care* 1978;1:305.

72. Fulop M. The treatment of severely uncontrolled diabetes mellitus. *Adv Intern Med* 1984;29:327.

73. Adrogué HJ, Barrero J, Eknoyan G. Salutary effects of modest fluid replacement in the treatment of adults with diabetic ketoacidosis. *JAMA* 1989;262:2108.

74. Gundersen HJG, Christensen NJ. Intravenous insulin causing loss of intravascular water and albumin and increased adrenergic nervous activity in diabetics. *Diabetes* 1977;26:551.

75. Foster DW, McGarry JD. The metabolic derangements and treatment of diabetic ketoacidosis. *N Engl J Med* 1983;309:159.

76. Nattrass M, Hale PJ. Clinical aspects of diabetes ketoacidosis. In: Nattras M, Santiago JV, eds. *Recent advances in diabetes* Edinburgh: Churchill Livingstone, 1984.

77. Lever E, Jaspan JB. Sodium bicarbonate therapy in severe diabetic ketoacidosis. *Am J Med* 1983;75:263.

78. Morris LR, Murphy MB, Kitabchi AE. Bicarbonate therapy in severe diabetic ketoacidosis. *Ann Intern Med* 1986;105:836.

79. Levine SN, Loewenstein JE. Treatment of diabetic ketoacidosis. *Arch Intern Med* 1981;141:713.

80. Narins RG, Arieff A. I. Alkali therapy of metabolic acidosis owing to organic acids. *Nephrol Lett* 1985;2:13.

81. Adrogué HJ, et al. Acidosis-induced glucose intolerance is not prevented by adrenergic blockade. *Am J Physiol* 1988;255:E812.

82. Assal JP, et al. Metabolic effects of sodium bicarbonate in the management of diabetic ketoacidosis. *Diabetes* 1974;23:405.

83. Bureau MA, et al. Cerebral hypoxia from bicarbonate infusion in diabetic acidosis. *J Pediatr* 1980;96:968.

84. Madias NE, Adrogué HJ. Influence of chronic metabolic acid–base disorders on the acute CO_2 titration curve. *J Appl Physiol* 1983;55:1187.

85. Madias NE, Bossert WH, Adrogué HJ. Ventilatory response to chronic metabolic acidosis and alkalosis in the dog. *J Appl Physiol* 1984;56:1640.

86. Adrogué HJ, et al. Influence of steady-state alterations in acid–base equilibrium on the fate of administered bicarbonate in the dog. *J Clin Invest* 1983;71:867.

87. Kebler R, McDonald FD, Cadnapaphornchai P. Dynamic changes in serum phosphorus levels in diabetic ketoacidosis. *Am J Med* 1985;79:571.

88. Fisher JN, Shahshahani MN, Kitabchi AE. Diabetic ketoacidosis: low-dose insulin therapy by various routes. *N Engl J Med* 1977;297:238.

89. Pfeifer MA, et al. Low-dose versus high-dose insulin therapy for diabetic ketoacidosis. *South Med J* 1979;72:149.

90. Carroll P, Matz R. Uncontrolled diabetes mellitus in adults: experience in treating diabetic ketoacidosis and hyperosmolar nonketotic coma with low-dose insulin and a uniform treatment regimen. *Diabetes Care* 1983;6:579.

91. Clerbaux T, et al. Effect of phosphate on oxygen-hemoglobin affinity, diphosphoglycerate and blood gases during recovery from diabetic ketoacidosis. *Int Care Med* 1989;15:495.

92. Clements RS, et al. Increased cerebrospinal-fluid pressure during treatment of diabetic ketosis. *Lancet* 1971;2:671.

93. Young E, Bradley RF. Cerebral edema with irreversible coma in severe diabetic ketoacidosis. *N Engl J Med* 1967;276:665.

94. Arieff AI, Kleeman CR. Studies on mechanisms of cerebral edema in diabetic comas. *J Clin Invest* 1973;52:571.

95. Arieff AI, Kleeman CR. Cerebral edema in diabetic comas. II. Effects of hyperosmolality, hyperglycemia and insulin in diabetic rabbits. *J Clin Endocrinol Metab* 1974;38:1057.

96. Guisado R, Arieff AI. Neurologic manifestations of diabetic comas: correlation with biochemical alterations in the brain. *Metabolism* 1975;24:665.

97. Winegrad AI, Kern EFO, Simmons DA. Cerebral edema in diabetic ketoacidosis. *N Engl J Med* 1985;312:1184.

98. Ohman JL, et al. The cerebrospinal fluid in diabetic ketoacidosis. *N Engl J Med* 1971;284:283.

99. Fein IA, et al. Relation of colloid osmotic pressure to arterial hypoxemia and cerebral edema during crystalloid volume loading of patients with diabetic ketoacidosis. *Ann Intern Med* 1982;96:570.

100. Krane EJ, et al. Subclinical brain swelling in children during treatment of diabetic ketoacidosis. *N Engl J Med* 1985;312:1147.

101. Maccario M, Messis CP. Cerebral edema complicating treated nonketotic hyperglycemia. *Lancet* 1969;2:352.

102. Beigelman PM. Severe diabetic ketoacidosis (diabetic coma). *Diabetes* 1971;20:490.

103. Halmos PB, Nelson JK, Lowry RD. Hyperosmolar nonketoacidotic coma in diabetes. *Lancet* 1966;2:675.

104. Keller RJ, Wolfsdorf JI. Isolated growth hormone deficiency after cerebral edema complicating diabetic ketoacidosis. *N Engl J Med* 1987;316:857.

SECTION XII

Uremic Syndrome

CHAPTER 90

Pathophysiology and Nephron Adaptation in Chronic Renal Failure

Radko Komers, Timothy W. Meyer, and Sharon Anderson

Two million functioning nephrons collectively ultrafilter some 180 liters of fluid each day in the healthy human. Successive nephron segments modify the glomerular ultrafiltrate, so that the final urine volume and composition are appropriate for the daily ingested water and solute load. That we are endowed with a surfeit of nephrons, above that needed to maintain normal homeostasis, is clearly demonstrated by the ability of a single kidney following uninephrectomy to carry out the functions previously performed by two. This surplus is even more apparent in the setting of chronic progressive renal failure. Patients who have lost 75% of their renal function are asymptomatic, and those whose glomerular filtration rate (GFR) is only 10% of the normal value remain able to excrete their dietary loads of water and solutes.

This chapter first reviews the compensatory changes in function and structure that occur when functioning nephron number is reduced and that make possible the prominent adaptations that maintain homeostasis. Alterations in handling of individual solutes and water are then described. Finally, the evidence that some of these compensatory changes are in fact ultimately maladaptive, in that they accelerate loss of the remaining nephrons, is presented.

PRINCIPLES AND PATTERNS OF NEPHRON ADAPTATION: "INTACT NEPHRONS" AND GLOMERULOTUBULAR BALANCE

The ability of a reduced number of functioning nephrons to excrete a full day's load implies that as GFR declines, the fraction of the filtered load of water and solutes that is excreted

R. Komers: Division of Nephrology and Hypertension, Oregon Health Sciences University, Portland, Oregon

T. W. Meyer: Department of Medicine, Stanford University School of Medicine; and Nephrology Section, Palo Alto VA Medical Center, Palo Alto, California

S. Anderson: Division of Nephrology, Oregon Health Sciences University; and Nephrology Section, Portland VA Medical Center, Portland, Oregon

must increase. An increase in the whole kidney fractional excretion is an expression of increased fractional water and solute excretion by each remaining functional nephron. In 1952, Robert Platt (1) reasoned that although the total effective renal function may be reduced because of loss of tissue, the work of each remaining unit is increased, making an analogy with the remaining workers in a factory putting in overtime when their numbers are reduced by illness. This concept was further developed by Bricker and colleagues (2–4), who noted that the functional capacity of the residual nephrons determines the degree to which homeostasis is preserved, and that maintenance of homeostasis implies preservation (or even enhancement) of normal glomerular and tubular function in the remaining nephrons. In the absence of any adaptive changes in kidney function and in the presence of a continued dietary load, the consequence of continued ingestion of the daily diet would result in retention of water and all solutes cleared by the kidney, with rapid development of uremia and all of its complications. That homeostasis is maintained during progressive nephron loss until the very late stages indicates substantial adaptation in the remaining nephrons, which now manage to do the job formerly performed by the full complement.

Reasoning that globally hypofunctioning nephrons could not maintain homeostasis, Bricker and associates (2–4) coined the "intact nephron hypothesis" to explain the preserved ability of the remnant nephrons to excrete the required load of water and solutes. This hypothesis does not imply an all-or-nothing condition, whereby nephrons are either fully functional or dead. Rather, GFR may be reduced in some nephrons, whereas compensatory mechanisms elevate the GFR and enlarge the tubules of the less damaged nephrons (5,6). As reviewed by Bricker and Fine (4), the original studies examining this question were performed in experimental models of unilateral renal disease (7). Using clearance methods, GFR in the affected and unaffected contralateral kidneys was compared to the values simultaneously determined for tubular transport functions. When the ratio of glomerular to individual tubular functions in the diseased kidney was compared to the normal kidney, comparable values were found. These data were interpreted to indicate that for any given volume of glomerular filtrate, the diseased nephrons excrete exactly the same amount of the measured solute as do the nephrons of the contralateral kidney (4). Each remnant nephron presumably transports water and solutes in proportion to its individual GFR, whether reduced by disease processes or elevated by compensatory hypertrophy. Mechanisms by which these adaptations occur are further discussed later.

Another essential component of adaptation is the maintenance of glomerulotubular balance (8). Studies in experimental models confirm that glomerulotubular balance is maintained in both tubulointerstitial and glomerular diseases (5,9). In chronic experimental membranous glomerulonephritis, despite a wide range of single nephron GFR (SNGFR) values, proximal fluid reabsorption was correlated closely with SNGFR in individual nephron units, so that fractional reabsorption was the same in hypofiltering and hyperfiltering nephrons (10). Presumably, structural changes in the proximal tubule and peritubular capillary network act together with alterations in Starling forces to perpetuate glomerulotubular balance. In the glomerulonephritis studies, the net hydraulic permeability of the peritubular capillary network surrounding severely damaged nephrons is reduced, suggesting loss of capillary surface area available for fluid reabsorption (10). Morphologic studies have further shown that nephrons whose glomeruli are severely damaged by experimental immune injury exhibit proximal tubule atrophy, presumably associated with decreased tubule reabsorptive capacity. In contrast, proximal tubules of less damaged nephrons increase in diameter and length (and presumably in reabsorptive capacity). As recently reviewed, glomerulotubular balance appears to be maintained in tubulointerstitial diseases as well (8).

Functional Adaptations

The remarkable ability of the remaining nephrons to enlarge and augment function in response to a reduction in their number has long been recognized. The simplest and most extensively used example of this process is afforded by surgical ablation of renal tissue, which is used to mimic the more gradual loss of nephrons that occurs in renal disease. Experimentally, this model has been in use since the last century, and it remains the most commonly used model for study of compensatory mechanisms. Clinically, the most common example is unilateral nephrectomy, performed for such purposes as kidney transplantation, solitary tumor, or trauma. It should be emphasized that although discussed separately, functional and structural adaptations to reduced nephron number are closely interrelated, often sharing common pathophysiologic mediators. The exact scenario of events following the nephron loss still remains to be established. Yet, current evidence discussed in the following indicates that, at least in the

glomeruli, functional adaptations may precede changes in structure.

Compensatory Hyperfiltration

Remaining nephrons compensate for nephron loss by increased perfusion and filtration rates. Studies of renal transplant donors (in whom the remaining nephrons are considered to be normal) indicate that within the first weeks after nephrectomy, GFR and renal plasma flow (RPF) rates in the remaining kidney increase by about 40%, so that the GFR is about 70% of the prenephrectomy value (11,12). In general, long-term studies have indicated that this single kidney hyperfiltration is maintained for at least two decades and that renal function may be maintained reasonably well for up to 50 years after childhood nephrectomy (13) and for decades after nephrectomy in adulthood (14).

Studies in experimental models have provided insight into the mechanisms of compensatory hyperfiltration. New nephrons are not formed in mature animals; the increased remnant kidney GFR following nephrectomy is entirely owing to increases in the SNGFR in the remaining nephrons (15–17). Micropuncture studies have elucidated the magnitude and determinants of the single nephron compensatory hyperfiltration response. The SNGFR increases within 15 hours after nephrectomy in rats (18); by 2 weeks, the whole kidney and single nephron GFR values have increased by about 40% (19,20). Comparable changes are seen in the whole kidney and single nephron plasma flow rates. Vascular resistance is reduced in the afferent and efferent arterioles, allowing the increase in the glomerular capillary plasma flow rate (Q_A). Because the decrease in afferent arteriolar resistance (R_A) is proportionally greater than that in efferent arteriolar resistance (R_E), the hydraulic pressure in the glomerular capillary increases. Together, these increases in glomerular plasma flow and glomerular capillary hydraulic pressure (P_{GC}) account for the increase in SNGFR in the remnant nephrons. Further studies have shown that the magnitude of these increases in glomerular capillary pressures and flows correlates with the amount of renal tissue excised. Thus, unilateral nephrectomy in the rat leads to a 40% to 50% increase in the SNGFR (20); this rate more than doubles after removal of three-fourths of the renal mass (21–24). In moderate degrees of renal ablation (e.g., uninephrectomy), the increase in SNGFR is largely accounted for by a similar increase in QA. However, in more extensive renal ablation, substantial increases in P_{GC} occur, so that both hyperperfusion and glomerular capillary hypertension contribute to the observed increases in SNGFR. In rats with extensive renal mass removal (two-thirds to five-sixths of total renal mass), the magnitude of the adaptive increase in SNGFR is similar in superficial and juxtamedullary nephrons (25,26). The tubuloglomerular feedback mechanism remains intact, with its setpoint altered in a way that permits remnant nephron hyperfiltration (27,28).

Unilateral nephrectomy does not usually result in an increase in blood pressure, whereas more extensive renal ablation is generally accompanied by substantial and progressive systemic hypertension (21,29–31). In part owing to the afferent arteriolar vasodilatation, the higher systemic pressure is transmitted into the glomerular capillary network, further contributing to glomerular capillary hypertension. Because tubule pressure increases little if at all following renal ablation, increasing P_{GC} results in an increase in the glomerular transcapillary hydraulic pressure gradient, ΔP. Most, although not all, studies indicate that the glomerular capillary ultrafiltration coefficient (K_f) does not increase following renal ablation (21–23,29,30). The apparent stability of K_f in the setting of prominent glomerular hypertrophy is rather surprising, as is discussed in the following. The hemodynamic determinants of remnant nephron hyperfiltration in the dog differ somewhat from those in the rat. In the dog, extensive ablation of renal mass is not accompanied by systemic hypertension, and ΔP is only modestly elevated, whereas K_f is markedly increased (32,33).

Mechanisms of Glomerular Hemodynamic Adaptations

Many factors and mediators influence glomerular hemodynamics, and alterations in the levels and/or activity of a number of these have been proposed to contribute to the adaptive hemodynamic changes that characterize nephron loss.

Altered Autoregulation of Glomerular Blood Flow

Glomerular hypertension has been attributed to impaired afferent arteriolar autoregulation by remnant nephrons, with reduced ability to constrict in the setting of systemic hypertension (34–36). The observation that the dihydropyridine calcium channel blockers cause additional impairment of renal autoregulation in 5/6 nephrectomized rats emphasizes the importance of preglomerular resistance as a major determinant of the susceptibility to glomerular sclerosis (GS) for any blood pressure elevation (37).

Renin–Angiotensin–Aldosterone System

Angiotensin II (Ang II), the major effector peptide of the renin–angiotensin–aldosterone system (RAAS), causes vasoconstriction of afferent and efferent arterioles, mesangial contraction, and a rise in P_{GC} (38,39). The finding that chronic angiotensin converting enzyme (ACE) inhibition normalizes P_{GC} in remnant kidney rats (21,23) suggests that Ang II helps to sustain glomerular capillary hypertension in this setting. This effect has been attributed to the inhibition of the efferent arteriolar action of the peptide (21). However, the question whether acute Ang II blockade can rapidly reduce remnant P_{GC} is not settled (40–42). It is possible that Ang II increases remnant glomerular P_{GC} by promoting sodium retention and

causing systemic hypertension, rather than by direct action on the renal microcirculation (42). Several studies have sought to localize the source of the Ang II activity and components of the RAAS that contribute to glomerular hemodynamic adaptations. After uninephrectomy, renin mRNA increases in proximal tubules and glomeruli of the remnant kidney (43). In rats with nephron number reduced by partial renal infarction, renin activity is concentrated in areas adjacent to the infarcted tissue (44,45). Renin production by hypoperfused nephrons adjacent to the infarcted tissue could explain why blood pressure is not increased when nephron number is halved by uninephrectomy (46) and why blood pressure tends to be higher when ablation is accomplished by infarction than when it is accomplished by surgical removal of renal tissue (47,48). More recently, generalized renin overexpression in tubular cells has been reported in rats with reduced renal mass, further supporting the notion of the indirect effect of Ang II in mediating increased P_{GC} in this model (49). In contrast, Ang II AT_1 receptor mRNA is decreased in remnant kidneys, likely as a result of increased tissue levels of Ang II (50).

Another effector molecule of the RAAS, aldosterone, has been implicated in the pathogenesis of nephropathy after renal ablation, including the hemodynamic changes. Plasma aldosterone levels are high in this model (51), corresponding to the levels in patients with chronic renal failure (CRF) (52,53). Adrenalectomy ameliorates renal injury in 5/6 nephrectomized rats (54). The nephroprotective effects of ACE inhibitors and Ang II receptor blockers, commonly associated with suppression of aldosterone secretion, are offset by concomitant infusion of the hormone (51). Furthermore, Wistar-Furth rats, which are resistant to mineralocorticoid actions, have been shown to be strikingly resistant to renal injury after renal ablation. Glomerular capillary pressure was not measured in these studies. However, the fact that P_{GC} is increased in mineralocorticoid salt models of hypertension (55) suggests a possible contribution of aldosterone in remnant kidneys. These observations also further support previous notions about indirect effects of Ang II inhibition on P_{GC}.

Atrial Natriuretic Peptide

In contrast to its ability to control glomerular hypertension, blockade of Ang II activity does not reduce remnant kidney plasma flow or GFR (21,23,56); therefore, other mediators must contribute to remnant hyperperfusion and hyperfiltration. One such mediator appears to be atrial natriuretic peptide (ANP). In addition to its natriuretic actions, ANP is a potent afferent dilator. Plasma ANP levels are increased following renal ablation (57) and hyperfiltration is reversed with administration of an ANP receptor antagonist (58). Further supporting the role of this peptide in renal adaptations to nephron loss, ANP mRNA expression in the remnant kidney is significantly increased (59).

Endothelin

Endothelin (ET) infusion increases glomerular pressure in the normal kidney (60), and is therefore a possible player in the development of renal hemodynamic changes in the remnant kidney. Renal ET-1 activity rises after the first week following renal ablation (61,62). Several studies have shown that long-term treatment with ET receptor blockers is associated with better preservation of renal function, and amelioration of proteinuria and structural changes in rat with reduced nephron mass (63–65). To our knowledge, micropuncture studies exploring renal microvascular effects of treatment with endothelin receptor antagonists in animals with reduced renal mass are not available. Therefore, it is difficult to judge whether nephroprotective effects of ET receptor blockers are rather owing to inhibition of hemodynamic or growth actions (see the following). However, in other models of progressive renal injury and glomerulosclerosis, ET receptor blockade reduces P_{GC} (66).

Prostaglandins

A strong dependence of renal hemodynamics on prostaglandins (PG) in chronic renal failure can be derived simply from clinical observations of increased susceptibility to reduction in GFR by treatment with nonspecific nonsteroidal antiinflammatory drugs (NSAIDs). Synthesis of PGE2, PGI2, and thromboxane A2 are increased in glomeruli isolated from subtotally nephrectomized rats, and per nephron excretion of PGE2 and thromboxane A2 is increased in these animals (30,67,68). Acute inhibition of PG synthesis reduces remnant nephron plasma flow and GFR without reducing P_{GC} in remnant kidney rats, whereas chronic thromboxane synthesis inhibition decreases vascular resistance and increases plasma flow and GFR (30,69). PG synthesis inhibition reduces RPF and GFR in rabbits with renal ablation (70) and patients with renal insufficiency (71,72). Fujihara and coworkers (73) have reported mild reduction of P_{GC} and significant nephroprotection in subtotally nephrectomized rats after chronic treatment with nitroflurbiprofen, a compound combining nonselective cyclooxygenase (COX) inhibition and a nitric oxide-donating moiety, preventing critical depression of renal function. The possibility of species variation is again raised, however, because PG synthesis inhibitors had no effect on RPF or GFR in dogs with renal ablation (74).

Cyclooxygenase is a key enzyme in the synthesis of prostaglandins and thromboxanes from arachidonic acid. Two isoforms of COX have been identified, constitutive COX-1 and inducible COX-2. Although considered to be an inducible enzyme, COX-2 is constitutively expressed in the thick ascending limb and in the macula densa (MD) region of the rat kidney (75,76). Recent evidence has suggested that COX-2–derived prostaglandins play a role in physiologic regulations in the normal kidney, being involved in modulation of afferent arteriolar vasoconstriction and myogenic afferent responses

to increases in renal perfusion pressure (77), and stimulation of renin release (78,79). Wang and coworkers (76) have recently demonstrated overexpression of COX-2 in MD of remnant kidneys. Further studies by the same group and others have implicated increased activity of the enzyme with the pathogenesis of renal hemodynamic alterations in this model (81,82).

Nitric Oxide

In view of its renal hemodynamic actions (83), as well as reports suggesting the shear-stress activation of nitric oxide (NO) generation (84), NO would be a good candidate for mediating hyperfiltration associated with reduced nephron mass. There are, however, striking differences between studies exploring renal NO activity in uninephrectomized models, and models with more radical nephron reduction. Uninephrectomized rats demonstrate greater renal vasoconstrictor responses to inhibition of NO synthesis, and increased inducible NO synthase (NOS) protein expression, as compared with sham-operated controls (85). In contrast, in rats with 5/6 nephrectomy, several groups have noted decreased renal expression and enzymatic activity of all three NOS isoforms (86–88). Furthermore, treatment with L-arginine, a NO precursor, or the NO donor molsidomine, ameliorated increases in P_{GC} or renal injury in the same model (89,90). A blunted response to nonspecific NOS inhibition has also been shown in 5/6 nephrectomized rats (91). Because chronic inhibition of NO production with L-arginine analogs causes severe glomerular injury associated with an increase in P_{GC} (92,93), suppression of NO synthesis in glomeruli and vasculature of the remnant kidney could contribute to the development of glomerulosclerosis.

Insulin-like Growth Factor-1

Evidence that insulin-like growth factor-1 (IGF-I) increases renal perfusion and filtration in normal rats (94) and that levels of IGF-I increase in the remnant kidney (95,96) suggests a potential role for that hormone, also. This assumption has been recently confirmed by Haylor and colleagues (97) in a study showing an amelioration of hyperfiltration in remnant kidney following unilateral nephrectomy with IGF-I inhibition.

Alterations in Glomerular Permeability

Another index of glomerular function is the ability to restrict passage of macromolecules into the urinary space (98,99). The normal glomerular capillary wall is extremely permeable to water and small solutes, yet imposes a barrier to passage of plasma proteins. Permselectivity is characterized by examining the extent to which the glomerular capillary wall discriminates among molecules of different size, charge, and configuration. The most extensively used method for quantitation of glomerular permselectivity involves measurement of fractional clearances of test macromolecules, compared to clearance of inulin. Substances such as dextrans and Ficoll may be used in a neutral state, allowing assessment of size selectivity or, in a charged (anionic or cationic) state, allowing assessment of charge selectivity (99). The other major determinant of protein passage, molecular shape or configuration, has been less extensively studied. In the normal kidney, the fractional clearance of negatively charged dextran sulfate is lower than that for neutral dextran at any given molecular radius. Conversely, positively charged molecules pass through more freely (98,99).

Increased glomerular permselectivity to proteins is a component of adaptation to reduced nephron number, although magnitude and expression vary widely among diseases. Uninephrectomy alone is associated with a modest, late development of proteinuria in the rat (100) and, in some cases, humans (101). However, in the setting of a predisposition to proteinuria, the course can be accelerated. For example, in a rat strain predisposed to spontaneous proteinuria, uninephrectomy induces a defect in charge selectivity (102). With more extensive renal ablation, even in previously normal kidneys, permselectivity studies indicate that proteinuria results from defects in both size selectivity and charge selectivity (103–105), with increased flux through the shunt pathway. As discussed in the following, this phenomenon can be associated with lesser capability of podocytes to adapt to the loss of nephron mass (106).

SOLUTE HOMEOSTASIS: TUBULAR ADAPTATIONS TO NEPHRON LOSS

When functioning nephron number is reduced, adaptive increases in excretion of water and solutes by each remaining nephron must occur if homeostasis is to be maintained. The adaptive changes in SNGFR and in proximal tubular reabsorptive capacity are accompanied by specific mechanisms that augment the ability to excrete a constant load of a particular solute in the face of a dwindling number of functioning nephrons. In general, the adaptive mechanisms are not unique to renal insufficiency; rather, they are the same mechanisms that allow the normal kidney to excrete an excessive load. There are limits to the adaptive capability, however; when that capability is exceeded, the patient suffers from the well-known complications of renal failure.

As has been elucidated by Bricker and Fine (4), there are three major patterns of adaptation to advancing chronic renal disease (Fig. 90-1). According to this formulation, the pattern of adaptation is reflected by the change in serum concentration of specific solutes with the fall in GFR. If there is no regulation or adaptation, the plasma concentration will increase, as depicted in curve A of Fig. 90-1. Examples of this class of solutes are urea and creatinine, in which the rate of excretion depends on the filtered load, and tubular reabsorption and secretion mechanisms fail to adapt sufficiently to prevent net elevation of the serum concentration. Curve B represents "regulation with limitation" (i.e., maintenance of normal plasma concentration until the late stages of renal

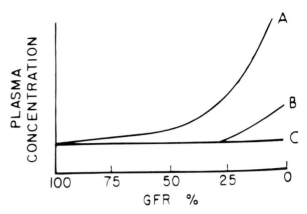

FIG. 90-1. Patterns of adaptation for different solutes in chronic progressive renal disease. **A:** No regulation or adaptation. **B:** Regulation with limitation. **C:** Complete regulation. See text for discussion. (From: Bricker NS, Fine LG. The renal response to progressive nephron loss. In: Brenner BM, Rector FC Jr, eds. *The kidney.* Philadelphia: WB Saunders, 1981:1058, with permission.)

insufficiency), when GFR falls below a critical level, excretion can no longer keep up with intake, and the plasma concentration rises. Solutes in this class are excreted by filtration and either tubule reabsorption, tubule secretion, or a combination. Examples of this class include phosphate and urate. The third pattern, curve C, is termed "complete regulation." The serum concentration is maintained in the normal range until the terminal stages of renal insufficiency. Examples include sodium, potassium, and magnesium. For normal serum levels to be maintained, increased single nephron excretion results from altered tubular transport patterns; specific mechanisms for these adaptations are discussed subsequently.

Prominent adaptations in proximal tubular function occur early after loss of renal mass (8,107). As single nephron GFR increases, so does the proximal absolute reabsorptive rate (108,109), with relative preservation of glomerulotubular balance (12,110). Tabei and coworkers found that fluid reabsorption in the proximal straight tubule increases within a day after nephrectomy, in concert with the increase in GFR (111). In addition, proximal reabsorptive rates for various solutes increase proportionally to the increase in filtered load (112–114) (Fig. 90-2). Functional studies in the rat indicate that reabsorption of fluid in the loop of Henle and distal nephron also increases proportionally with the increase in SNGFR (115,116). Mechanisms are unclear, although increased activity of Na-K-ATPase has been found in some but not all studies of this segment (117–119). Regarding transport functions in the distal tubule, increased distal K+ secretion accompanies nephron number reduction (120,121), accompanied by increased sodium reabsorption and associated with an increase in the basolateral membrane surface area of principal cells and with a local increase in Na-K-ATPase activity (117–119,122–126).

Changes in individual solute handling in renal failure have been reviewed extensively elsewhere (4,8), and are briefly summarized in this chapter.

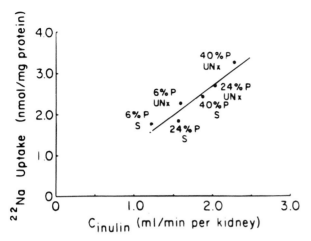

FIG. 90-2. Correlation of Na+ uptake in rat brush-border membrane vesicles and inulin clearance (Cinulin), showing a linear relationship in sham-operated (S) and uninephrectomized (Unx) rats on 6%, 24%, or 40% protein (P) diets. (From: Harris RC, Seifter JL, Brenner BM. Adaptation of Na+-H+ exchange in renal microvillus membrane vesicles: role of dietary protein and uninephrectomy. *J Clin Invest* 1984;74:1979, with permission.)

Sodium Excretion and the Regulation of Extracellular Fluid Volume

Extracellular fluid (ECF) volume is maintained remarkably close to normal in patients with chronic renal insufficiency, until the very late stages (127). Although the absolute sodium reabsorption in the proximal tubule is increased in parallel with the rise in SNGFR (108,109), fractional excretion of sodium and water increases (128–130). These alterations result in a marked increase in distal sodium delivery to the thick ascending limb of Henle and distal nephron (25). Mechanisms controlling adaptive changes in sodium handling in uremia remain incompletely understood. Earlier in this century, it was postulated that decreased aldosterone formation or effect might play a role (9). However, subsequent observations that serum aldosterone levels are normal or high (52,53,131), that responsiveness to aldosterone antagonist therapy is present (53), and that exogenous mineralocorticoid therapy does not cause sodium retention (128,132,133) in uremic patients have cast doubt on a significant role for such a mechanism.

Later, the discovery of ANP turned attention toward that hormone as a potential mediator of sodium excretion in renal insufficiency. Rats subjected to renal ablation exhibit increased ANP levels, which are related to dietary sodium intake and fractional sodium excretion (57,134). Similar increases in ANP levels in patients with renal insufficiency have been related to increased blood volume and to increased blood pressure (135,136). Interpretation of these studies may be complicated by the presence of heart failure and errors in the assay of plasma ANP caused by related peptides that are retained in renal failure. However, studies with a recently developed ANP antagonist confirm that increased ANP levels

make a major contribution to increased fractional sodium excretion in experimental renal insufficiency (58). Similarly, administration of a monoclonal anti-ANP antibody prevents the diuresis that follows uninephrectomy in the rat, by blunting both proximal and distal tubular reabsorption of sodium (137).

Hypertension may contribute to increased fractional sodium excretion in renal insufficiency, as has been suggested by Guyton and coworkers (138,139). According to this view, maintenance of constant sodium intake in the setting of fewer nephrons leads to sodium retention and expansion of ECF and blood volumes; the consequent increase in blood pressure in turn causes a higher fractional sodium excretion. However, blood pressure is higher in uremic patients than in normal subjects whose blood volumes have been increased by salt loading, and reducing dietary salt intake does not prevent hypertension in rats with reduced nephron number (140). Thus, blood pressure alone is not the sole factor regulating sodium excretion in chronic renal insufficiency.

Recent studies explored the molecular basis for sodium transport after reduction in nephron number. Terzi and colleagues (119), using microdissected tubule segments of 5/6 nephrectomized rats, found increased Na-K-ATPase activity along the nephron when expressed per unit of nephron length. Enzymatic activity correlated with the degree of tubular hypertrophy. However, when expressed per tubule surface unit, no changes were found, suggesting that the density of pumps remained stable during compensatory tubular hypertrophy. Addressing this issue, Kwon and associates (141) explored protein expression of sodium transporters and Na-K-ATPase along the nephron in rats 2 weeks after subtotal nephrectomy. They found a decrease in total kidney Na/H exchanger, a major sodium transporter in this segment, Na-phosphate cotransporter, and basolateral Na-K-ATPase in remnant kidneys as compared to controls. Densities of these transporters did not increase proportionally to the nephron hypertrophy and GFR. These findings reflected mainly changes in the proximal tubule and were associated with increased sodium excretion in remnant nephrons. In contrast, expression of bumetanide-sensitive channels in thick ascending limb and thiazide-sensitive channels in distal tubules was increased, and Na-K-ATPase expression maintained in these segments. These changes indicate compensatory increases in distal segments, partly because of elevated vasopressin and aldosterone levels associated with chronic renal failure (CRF).

Although chronic adaptations enable maintenance of normal sodium balance until the late stages of renal insufficiency, the immediate natriuretic response to a large sodium challenge may be impaired (32,142,143). The natriuresis evoked by sodium loading is generally reduced less than is the GFR (74,142,143), so acute volume expansion causes a greater increase in fractional sodium excretion in uremic animals than in normal controls, a "magnification" phenomenon (7,142, 144,145). In renal insufficiency, ability to conserve sodium is also compromised, so that most patients with advanced renal disease are unable to lower sodium excretion below 20 to 30 mEq/day (a phenomenon referred to as a "salt floor") (4,146,147). With high sodium intakes, the smaller number of functioning nephrons may not be able to increase sodium excretion enough to maintain sodium balance and thus may be termed as having a low "salt ceiling." As renal failure progresses, the distance between "floor" and "ceiling" increases, and maintenance of sodium balance becomes more difficult (4). However, in some cases, slowly reducing sodium intake may lead to more efficient reductions in sodium excretion, or reversal of the "salt-losing" tendency (148).

Potassium Homeostasis in Chronic Renal Failure

The failing kidney exhibits a remarkable ability to maintain potassium homeostasis and normal serum potassium levels until the GFR reaches about 10% of normal. Potassium secretion per nephron must increase to maintain potassium balance; in fact, in experimental animals, fractional excretion of potassium may exceed 100% of the filtered load (7), and this adaptation occurs within a day of uninephrectomy (149). Similar to sodium handling in CRF, animal studies show significant negative correlation between fractional excretion of potassium and GFR. The major factors responsible for increased potassium excretion per nephron appear to be elevation of plasma and intracellular potassium concentrations following potassium ingestion, particularly early in the course; later, an adaptive tubule process also augments potassium secretion (149–152). In uninephrectomized rats, secretion of potassium occurs within hours after nephrectomy being mediated by amiloride-sensitive channels (121). In addition, reduced potassium reabsorption by the loop of Henle may facilitate excretion of acute potassium loads in renal failure (153).

Following ingestion of a potassium load, serum potassium increases by about the same increment both in normal subjects and patients with moderate renal insufficiency, inducing an increase in distal potassium secretion (154). When factored for GFR, the kaliuresis in patients with moderate renal insufficiency is the same as normal subjects (154,155). However, because the patient with renal failure excretes potassium more slowly than the normal subject, there is prolonged elevation of serum potassium following an oral load.

Later in the course, distal tubular adaptations, specifically, increased activity of Na-K-ATPase and basolateral surface area in principal cells of the cortical collecting duct promote potassium excretion (122–126). As another adaptation, as renal failure progresses, intestinal excretion of potassium also increases in concert with increased colonic Na-K-ATPase activity (125,156). Administration of the aldosterone antagonist spironolactone to patients with renal failure often results in dangerous hyperkalemia (157), and hyperkalemia frequently is observed when aldosterone synthesis is reduced by ACE inhibition (158). Thus, it appears that adequate aldosterone levels are required to facilitate increased potassium secretion per nephron. Hyperkalemia may occur relatively early in the course of renal failure in patients who have low plasma aldosterone levels (159,160). Damage to the juxtaglomerular apparatus may be severe in patients with diabetic nephropathy, explaining the prevalence of hyperkalemic metabolic acidosis associated with low plasma renin and aldosterone levels in these patients.

Water Homeostasis in Chronic Renal Failure

The capacity to generate solute-free water (expressed as a fraction of the GFR) is remarkably well maintained when renal function is impaired (4,8,12,161–164). However, the reduction in GFR impairs the water excretory capacity, which is reflected in a reduction in the minimum urine osmolality that can be attained. Reduction in the ability to excrete solute-free water puts renal patients at risk for water intoxication when challenged with an excessive water load. In contrast to the somewhat preserved diluting mechanisms, the ability to concentrate the urine begins to fail relatively early in the course of renal insufficiency, resulting in marked decrease in fractional reabsorption of free H_2O. In CRF patients, severe dehydration is usually avoided because intact thirst mechanisms allow the patient to compensate for the urinary water losses. Accordingly, nocturia is the predominant symptom because of this impairment.

Concentration of the urine requires maintenance of hypertonicity of the medullary interstitium and normal water transport across distal nephron segments in response to antidiuretic hormone (ADH). Maintenance of medullary interstitial hypertonicity in turn requires structural preservation of the countercurrent system. Part of the defect in urinary concentration in patients with chronic renal disease may be attributed to the high solute load imposed on each nephron. However, diseases that profoundly disturb the medullary architecture (e.g., tubulointerstitial disease) may cause disproportionate impairment of concentrating ability (164–168). However, inability to concentrate urine is not limited to tubulointerstitial diseases because most glomerular diseases eventually result in accompanying tubulointerstitial injury as well. The presence of a concentration defect despite elevated ADH levels in plasma in CRF suggests distal tubular defect. Limited ADH responsiveness (25,169,170) may be caused by two factors. First, ADH-stimulated adenylate cyclase activity and water permeability in the distal nephron may be impaired in uremia (171). Also, increased tubular flow rates may limit the fraction of water that can be reabsorbed by the distal nephron in response to ADH (172). Several molecular mechanisms underlying concentration defect in CRF have been recently suggested. Teitelbaum and colleagues (173) described the absence of ADH V2 receptor mRNA in the inner medulla of CRF rats. Kwon and coworkers (174) studied protein expression of aquaporins (AQP) in rat remnant kidneys. Aquaporins are membrane proteins acting as water-selective channels. AQP1 is found mainly in proximal tubule and descending limb of the loop of Henle, whereas AQP2 and 3 localize in apical and basolateral membranes of collecting ducts. They reported marked reduction in all three channels. Furthermore, decreased AQP expression was resistant to treatment with ADH (174).

Acid–Base Homeostasis

Metabolic acidosis is the predominant acid–base disorder in CRF, due to a reduced renal ability to excrete acid (171,172, 175–177). This disorder is caused by a reduction in the renal capacity to excrete acid. With the initial fall in GFR, hydrogen balance is maintained by increased ammonium excretion per functioning nephron (172,177,178). However, later in the course, this adaptation proves insufficient, and the acidosis is maintained primarily owing to reduced ammonia synthetic capacity. Ammonium excretion per total GFR rises to three to four times normal (179,180), but this increase is insufficient to counteract the profound reduction in functioning nephron number (172,178). Studies in animals with CRF have shown that urinary ammonia excretion is impaired even before ammonia synthetic capacity is exhausted (180). Impaired excretion of ammonia was originally attributed to impairment of countercurrent mechanisms, which were thought to increase ammonium concentration in the medulla and facilitate "trapping" of ammonia by acidified luminal fluid in the collecting duct. However, this explanation may require modification in light of the discovery that ammonia enters tubule fluid by active secretion as well as by "trapping."

Renal acid excretion also requires reabsorption of filtered bicarbonate, and generation of a large hydrogen ion gradient in the distal nephron. Following uninephrectomy, stimulation of proximal tubular bicarbonate reabsorption occurs, as a result of a doubled transport rate. An increase in Na/H exchange contributes to this phenomenon (181). Some (129,182,183), although not all (180), micropuncture studies of rats with more radical nephron reduction have found slight increases in fractional reabsorption of bicarbonate. and studies of proximal tubule brush-border vesicles from rats with renal ablation have shown increases in V_{max} of the Na-H antiporter (130). However, clinically, Schwartz and coworkers (184,185) have presented evidence that a decrease in bicarbonate reabsorptive ability develops corresponding to more recent findings of reduced NHE-3 in proximal tubules of rat remnant kidneys (141). In severe renal insufficiency, the threshold for bicarbonate reabsorption may also be reduced (186,187), an effect enhanced by the actions of various stimuli including hyperkalemia, hyperparathyroidism, and ECF volume expansion (188–191).

In general, distal acidification is better maintained than proximal bicarbonate reabsorption in CRF, except in patients with distal renal tubular acidosis (192,193). However, patients with renal failure are unable to lower pH as completely as are normal subjects with experimental acidemia (172), and so a relative decrease in distal hydrogen ion pump capacity may also contribute to acidosis. Failure to attain normal minimal pH prevents optimal titration of nonammonia buffers and thus reduces the excretion of the titratable acid. Restriction of dietary phosphate intake may further contribute to reduced excretion of titratable acid in uremic patients.

Phosphate and Calcium Homeostasis in Chronic Renal Failure

Abnormalities of phosphate and calcium metabolism and their contributions to renal osteodystrophy are discussed elsewhere in this book. The intrarenal adaptations that contribute to calcium and phosphate homeostasis in CRF are discussed here.

Phosphate

A progressive increase in the fractional excretion of phosphate maintains phosphate balance early in the course of CRF (194–197). In more advanced disease, phosphate excretion is maintained by a further increase in the fractional excretion of phosphate, along with an increase in serum phosphate levels. Studies by Slatopolsky and coworkers (195,198–201) suggested that increased parathyroid hormone (PTH) caused the increase in fractional phosphate excretion. In dogs subjected to renal ablation, fractional excretion of phosphorus increased, and the magnitude of the increased fractional excretion correlated with the magnitude of the increase in circulating PTH levels. Restricting phosphate intake prevented increases in both PTH levels and fractional phosphate excretion (199–201). These observations formed the basis for the Bricker's "trade-off hypothesis" (202), which postulated that one or more of the major stigmata of the uremic state may occur as indirect consequences of the adaptations in nephron function (4). According to this hypothesis, the adverse consequences of hyperparathyroidism represented the biologic price paid to maintain excretion of a constant dietary phosphate load when nephron number was reduced. With each decrement in GFR, a transient period of phosphate retention would stimulate PTH synthesis and secretion, and the increased PTH activity would act to partially restore phosphate balance by augmented phosphate excretion (203) (Fig. 90-3). This adverse "trade-off" could be avoided by reducing phosphate intake as renal function declined.

Although intellectually compelling, the details of this trade-off scenario have been questioned by more recent studies showing that the increased fractional phosphate excretion does not depend on an increase in PTH levels or tubule responsiveness to PTH (204–208). The data suggest that the increased fractional excretion is achieved by the same mechanism responsible for this effect in intact animals fed a high-phosphate diet, that is, decreased phosphate reabsorption in the proximal nephron (209,210). Phosphate uptake per unit tubule mass is reduced in proximal nephron segments isolated from uremic rabbits, and sodium-phosphate cotransport activity is reduced in brush-border membrane vesicles from uremic dogs (113,211) and rats (141), but these reductions are not sufficient to fully account for the reduction in proximal phosphate reabsorption observed *in vivo*. Although

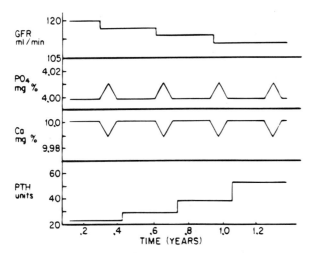

FIG. 90-3. Hypothetical treatment for the genesis of secondary hyperparathyroidism in chronic renal failure: the "trade-off hypothesis." *Ca*, calcium; *GFR*, glomerular filtration rate; *PO4*, phosphate; *PTH*, parathyroid hormone. (From: Bricker NS, et al. Calcium, phosphorus, and bone in renal disease and transplantation. *Arch Intern Med* 1969;123:543, with permission.)

reduced proximal reabsorption accounts for most of the increase in fractional phosphate excretion, there is also some evidence of altered distal phosphate transport (or reabsorption) (209,210).

Calcium

As renal disease advances, the production of the active Vitamin D [1,25(OH)2D$_3$] is impaired, leading to reduced intestinal calcium reabsorption and renal calcium excretion (196,197,212). As renal insufficiency advances, fractional excretion of calcium increases. In contrast to clinical studies, animal studies have shown that urinary calcium excretion remains constant, whereas fractional excretion of calcium increases when the GFR is reduced to about one-third of normal (213,214). The mechanism responsible for the increase in fractional calcium excretion in advanced CRF remains unclear. Possible factors include acidosis, suppression of Vitamin D production, increased distal nephron flow rates, and ECF volume expansion. Studies in rats with renal ablation suggest that the increase in remnant nephron calcium excretion associated with ECF expansion may be mediated by ANP (214).

STRUCTURAL ADAPTATIONS

An early hypothesis to explain compensatory hypertrophy was that of Addis (215), who reasoned that the excretion of urea required energy and that renal enlargement was a reflection of the need for added renal "work." Although Addis subsequently disproved his hypothesis in regard to urea, the notion that the kidney grows in response to the need for some other form of work remains. Despite ingenious experimen-

tation over the years, the question of whether hyperfiltration drives hypertrophy, or vice versa, remains unanswered (8).

Compensatory Renal Hypertrophy

The adaptive response to loss of renal mass includes the early development of renal hypertrophy (216–218). These changes are expressed as an increase in kidney weight and morphologically as an increase in the cross-sectional surface area of the kidney. The increase in kidney size is owing to enlargement of the glomeruli and, most prominently, the proximal convoluted tubules (115), resulting in disproportionate enlargement of the cortex in comparison to the relatively unaffected medulla.

Glomerular Hypertrophy

Although contributing relatively little to overall renal growth, the glomeruli undergo progressive enlargement (19,108,116, 217,219–222). Unilateral nephrectomy in the rat results in an average increase in tuft volume of 48%, 68%, and 75% at 3, 5, and 9 weeks, respectively (55,221). In more exuberant hypertrophic states, as occur with more extensive ablation or deoxycorticosterone acetate (DOCA)-salt hypertension, the degree of glomerular enlargement is even greater (46,55,223–227). Increased glomerular size does not necessarily parallel increased whole kidney size. For example, in young rats, one study found that remnant kidney growth and glomerular growth proceeded proportionally for 12 weeks, but thereafter kidney growth ceased, whereas glomerular size continued to increase (226). Serial structure-function studies in the rat have shown that glomerular volume and SNGFR increase in parallel following uninephrectomy (218,222). The contribution of constituent parts of the glomerulus to its expansion following nephrectomy remains controversial and incompletely characterized. Morphometric studies demonstrate an increase in the total volume occupied by cellular constituents in the remnant glomeruli of nephrectomized rats (46,221,224,228–230). Overall, these studies indicate that the fractions of the glomerulus occupied by different structural components (mesangium, capillary lumina, endothelium, and epithelial cells) remain constant as the glomerulus enlarges, at least in the early phases of adaptation. However, long-term adaptation may follow a different pattern. Schwartz and Bidani (229) found no change in the relative volume of the mesangium and its individual components at 6 weeks after ablation, but they subsequently found in studies at 26 weeks (about one-quarter of the life span) that the mesangial volume fraction, as well as the percentage of the mesangium occupied by cells and matrix, increased (224).

It remains uncertain to what extent different glomerular cell types increase in number and volume following renal ablation. An early study found a prominent increase in the number of glomerular endothelial, mesangial, and epithelial cells following uninephrectomy in very young rats (228). Subsequent studies, however, have found that visceral epithelial cell number remains constant when the glomerulus grows following loss of renal mass (46,225,226). The effect of glomerular hypertrophy on endothelial cell number has not been evaluated in detail, although one study found an early, transient increase in proliferation of peritubular endothelial cells after uninephrectomy in mice (231).

A number of investigators have noted increases in glomerular capillary length (223–226) and radius (140,218,221,232), so that capillary surface area increases (223,224,230). Diameters of the afferent and efferent arterioles increase as well (230). Morphometric measurements also have been used to try to estimate the filtering capacity of the enlarged remnant glomeruli. The glomerular capillary ultrafiltration coefficient (K_f) is the product of the surface area available for filtration (S) and the hydraulic permeability of the glomerular capillary wall (k). It is not clear which anatomic boundary constitutes the surface corresponding to S. As estimated by measuring the glomerular capillary area in direct apposition to epithelial foot processes, S increases following nephrectomy, albeit to a slightly lesser degree than total glomerular volume (221,222). Despite this potential increase in the filtration surface area, most functional studies have not found an increase in K_f of remnant glomeruli after extensive renal ablation (21–23,29,30). After uninephrectomy alone, some (233) but not all (20) studies have noted modest increases in K_f.

It is conceivable that k is reduced because a decrease in S cannot be involved to explain the fall in K_f. In theory, an increase in average foot process width would cause a decrease in the length of filtration slit overlying each unit area of peripheral capillary surface and thereby could decrease k in remnant glomeruli. In fact, morphometric studies have revealed an increase in the average width of epithelial cell foot processes in rats subjected to extensive renal ablation (222). Alternatively, it is possible that the filtering surface estimated by morphologic techniques in remnant glomeruli does not represent effective area available for filtration *in vivo*. Theoretic studies suggest that much of the glomerular capillary network is relatively underperfused in rats subjected to extensive renal ablation (234). It is notable that no increase in S was found following uninephrectomy in rats when infusion of glomerular basement membrane antibody was used to estimate capillary surface area *in vivo* (235). Alternatively, it is possible that the decrease in Kf in remnant glomeruli is more functional than structural, as ACE inhibitor therapy in remnant kidney rats routinely raises K_f to supranormal levels (21,23).

Tubular Hypertrophy

Quantitatively, the proximal convoluted tubule enlarges by approximately 15% in luminal and outside diameter and by 35% in length after uninephrectomy in the rat (115). Slightly larger increases in the diameter and length of the proximal convoluted tubule, along with lesser increases in the diameter of thick ascending limb and collecting duct segments, occur in uninephrectomized rabbits (219,236). The increase

in remnant proximal tubule size is proportional to the extent of nephron number reduction (237). Tabei and coworkers (111) found that an increase in tubule size follows the increase in fluid reabsorption by segments of isolated proximal straight tubule. Later in the course, the increased reabsorptive rate approximates the increase in proximal tubular size and protein content (108,109,238). Distal convoluted tubule enlarges by approximately 10% in luminal and outside diameter and by 17% in length in the rat (115), although studies in the rabbit found little change in size in the thick ascending limb after uninephrectomy (219). In the distal convoluted tubules and collecting ducts, cross-sectional area of both lumen and epithelium is increased, but by lesser magnitude than occurs in the proximal tubule (115,120,219). The cross-sectional area of the medullary collecting duct is increased following renal ablation in the rabbit but not in the rat; the length of the remnant medullary collecting duct has not been measured (239,240). Tubular cells do not enlarge symmetrically. Enlargement of basolateral portions of cells is more prominent as compared to luminal surface (236).

Mechanisms of Renal Hypertrophy

Renal hypertrophy has long fascinated investigators. The term compensatory renal hypertrophy generally has been used to describe the aggregate changes in nephron structure and function, including both cellular hypertrophy and hyperplasia, which follow loss of renal mass. Extensive work in this area has been the subject of several reviews (8,241–247) and is briefly summarized here.

General Principles of Renal Cell Growth Responses

Renal cells react to physical and biochemical stimuli imposed by reduction of nephron number with coordinate expression of a number of growth factors, their receptors, cellular signaling molecules, protooncogenes, and proteins involved in the regulation of cell cycle. It is apparent that the border between adaptive and maladaptive responses is murky. For example, uninephrectomy does not progress to renal failure, whereas more radical reduction of nephron mass results in progressive renal damage. These distinctions occur despite initial activation of similar growth promoting pathways. The degree of nephron loss that represents a point of no return has not been identified. This theoretic point is, however, likely to vary depending on species, underlying cause of nephron loss, and a wide spectrum of risk factors discussed in the following.

The role of growth factors in initiating compensatory renal growth has been suspected for over a century. A circulating factor has been suggested since at least 1896, when Sacerdotti (248) infused blood from bilaterally nephrectomized dogs into normal dogs and induced renal growth in the recipients. Observations of growth of transplanted kidneys placed in anephric humans, dogs, or rats further support this notion (249–251), and because transplanted kidneys are denervated, these data indicate that compensatory renal hypertrophy does not require renal innervation. In the 1950s, Braun Menèndez (252) postulated the existence of a humoral renal growth factor, termed renotropin. Fractions of urine, serum, and liver from uninephrectomized animals, and urine and serum from humans, stimulate biochemical changes (such as incorporation of radiolabeled nucleotides into DNA) in isolated renal tissue preparations, and stimulate growth in cultures of kidney-derived cells (253–258). Such studies have been proposed as further evidence for the existence of renotropin (259). These properties do not establish that these fractions induce whole kidney growth, however, and no truly "renotropic hormone" has been isolated.

Growth factors typically bind to their membrane tyrosine-kinase receptors and activate protein-kinase cascades involving mitogen-activated protein kinase (MAPK). Activated MAPK is translocated into the nucleus and phosphorylates transcription factors such as Elk-1, c-jun, and c-myc. Phosphorylated Elk-1 activates transcription of c-fos. c-fos then stimulates expression of further target genes after forming a complex with c-jun (246). Such genes include those coding for cell cycle regulatory proteins. Detailed description of this complex system is beyond the scope of this chapter and recently has been the subject of an excellent review (260). However, basic information about cell cycle proteins is useful for understanding structural adaptive and maladaptive responses after nephron loss.

Positive regulation (i.e. stimulation of transition from quiescent cell phase to ultimate cell division by mitosis) is carried out by cyclins and their partner molecules, cyclin-dependent kinases (CDK). Although CDK are constitutively expressed, cyclins are transcriptionally regulated and their levels are increased by specific mitogens such as growth factors. Negative regulation of the cell cycle is accomplished by CDK inhibitors, which bind to cyclin-CDK complexes and inhibit their activity. Two families of CDK inhibitors have been identified. The CIP/KIP family consists of inhibitors p21, p27, and p57; the INK4 family includes p15, p16, p18, p19, and p20.

In addition to the preceding processes, the cell also may be engaged in apoptosis, programmed cell death. The total number of cells in a particular organ reflects the balance between proliferation and apoptosis. Apoptotic cells exit from the cell cycle. Initiation of apoptosis also is regulated by cyclin-CDK complexes, and the progression of the cell into mitosis or apoptosis seems to be determined by the level of CDK inhibitor p27 (260).

Hyperplasia Versus Hypertrophy

In general, hyperplasia is a result of an increase in cell number associated with DNA replication and cell division, whereas hypertrophy is defined as cell enlargement owing to increases in protein and RNA content without DNA replication (218). Both processes are involved in renal compensatory growth. During hyperplasia the cells progress through the whole cell cycle. In contrast, hypertrophy occurs when the cells are engaged in the cycle but cannot progress to later stages.

Interaction of the cell with a variety of growth factors that modulate activity of either positive or negative regulators of the cell cycle then determines whether the cell will engage in hyperplasia or hypertrophy. For example, stimulation of the cell with platelet-derived growth factor (PDGF), a typical mitogen, results in activation of all cyclins and formation of cyclin-CDK complexes, and ultimately to cell division. Nevertheless, this process can be modulated by antimitogens (e.g., transforming growth factor-ß [TGF-ß]), which suppress cyclins and stimulate CDK inhibitors, resulting in cell hypertrophy, rather than division.

Biochemical Changes

"Dry" (desiccated) kidney weight increases in proportion to the "wet" (fresh) kidney weight following nephrectomy, implying an increase in the mass of tissue solids, primarily protein (261). The ratio of kidney protein to kidney wet weight remains constant during renal hypertrophy, although the increase in the rate of renal protein synthesis is increased as early as 3 hours after uninephrectomy in the mouse (262). Synthesis of new RNA precedes new protein synthesis. The quantity of RNA is notably increased within 12 hours after uninephrectomy, and radiolabeled nucleotide incorporation studies have noted an increased rate of RNA synthesis within 1 to 4 hours after nephrectomy (242,262,263). The early increase in RNA synthesis reflects largely increased production of ribosomal RNA (264), owing at least in part to an increase in the transcription rate (265), although decreased RNA degradation may also contribute to the increase in RNA levels (263,266). The peak in the RNA content of individual cells is reached within 2 days after uninephrectomy (242).

DNA content begins to increase later, at about 9 to 18 hours after nephrectomy, whereas a notable increase in mitotic figures, largely among proximal tubule cells, is apparent only after 1 to 2 days (262,267–269). Like the rate of protein synthesis, the prevalence of tubule mitotic figures declines to normal levels over 1 to 2 weeks following uninephrectomy (26). The lag of DNA synthesis behind RNA synthesis may reflect stimulation of mitosis by increases in cell size (262). According to this scenario, the renal hypertrophic stimulus causes cell enlargement, and cells reaching the largest size are stimulated to divide.

The ratio of increases in protein and DNA content has been used to estimate the relative contributions of cellular hypertrophy and hyperplasia to compensatory renal hypertrophy. In uninephrectomized adult animals, an increase in cell number of 10% to 25% accounts for up to half of the net increase in remnant kidney size (262,270,271). In very young animals and adult animals subjected to more extensive renal ablation, remnant nephron enlargement is more pronounced, and in these circumstances, cellular hyperplasia plays a proportionally greater role (272–275). In addition, biochemical changes also include enhanced activity of enzymes involved in tubular transport, as discussed, and enzymes involved in renal cell growth (276–281).

Factors Implicated in Compensatory Renal Hypertrophy

In this section we focus only on those factors that contribute to compensatory renal growth and hypertrophy following unilateral nephrectomy (i.e., in an adaptive process not usually associated with progressive renal injury) (282).

Physical Forces

As demonstrated by Cortes and coworkers (283,284), glomeruli are able to enlarge as perfusion pressure raises. In the remnant kidney, transmission of pressure fluctuations into the glomerular capillary tuft is not prevented by myogenic autoregulatory control, resulting in glomerular distension and enlargement. Glomerular volume is determined by capillary wall tension, size of the glomerulus, and glomerular stiffness. Glomerular compliance is increased in remnant kidneys. This process is independent of humoral or biochemical factors, least initially. Indeed, an increase in the glomerular capillary radius is the earliest morphologic finding after uninephrectomy (225,226). However, it should be noted that chronic mechanical stress imposed on glomerular cells may later trigger mechanisms leading to the development of glomerulosclerosis.

Growth Factors

Original evidence for the role of various peptide and non–peptide growth factors in structural adaptations to nephron loss was based on in vitro observations in cultured proximal tubule or mesangial cells (218,279,285–288). In general, however, these factors promote growth in many cell types; therefore, it seems likely that they participate in compensatory renal hypertrophy in a nonspecific manner, after growth has been triggered by some renal-specific signal. Moreover, factors that cause growth of kidney cells in vitro may not necessarily contribute importantly in vivo following nephron loss. For example, Ang II induces growth of proximal tubule and mesangial cells in culture (289), but Ang II blockade does not prevent compensatory hypertrophy in rats subjected to renal ablation (21,290), although, as discussed in the following, it may be effective in amelioration of interstitial fibrosis (291). Here we focus on those factors that have been implicated in structural adaptation or maladaptation by using several experimental approaches, including in vivo studies.

Insulin-like Growth Factors

This system consists of growth hormone (GH), IGFs, which mediate some GH actions including negative feedback, and IGF binding proteins (IGFBPs), which control IGF availability in plasma and tissues. Of these, IGF-I has been implicated in compensatory renal hypertrophy. Administration of IGF-I increases GFR and kidney weight in intact rats, although it is not clear whether the kidneys grow disproportionately to body weight (292–295). Following surgical reduction in renal mass, there is an increase in renal levels of IGF-I, whereas IGF-I receptor levels remain constant (95,292,296–299). An increase in IGF-I peptide is independent from GH, because it has been detected in dwarf rats lacking GH (300). There is disagreement, however, concerning the time course of the increase in IGF-I activity, and some studies have found that renal IGF-I levels begin to increase only after compensatory hypertrophy is already detectable (292,296–298). Age of an animal at the time of nephrectomy may be an important determinant, as suggested by Mulroney and coworkers (301). Remnant kidney IGF-I mRNA was increased in weanling rats already 1 to 6 hours after nephrectomy, whereas it was not detected in adult animals. Whether the increase in remnant kidney IGF-I activity is associated with an increase in IGF-I message is also controversial. Early reports suggesting an increase in IGF-I mRNA (297,302) were not confirmed by others showing no change in the mRNA for IGF-I (292,301,303), IGF-I receptor (303), and IGFBPs (299,303). Attempts to identify changes in IGF-I activity following more extensive ablation have been complicated by the finding that partial renal infarction increases IGF-I activity in the adjacent renal tissue (96). Thus, the data suggest that IGF-I participates in, but does not initiate, compensatory renal growth.

Interestingly, some studies suggest that IGF may even be protective against glomerulosclerosis. In contrast to GH and growth hormone releasing factor (GHRF) overexpressing rats, IGF-I transgenic mice do not develop glomerulosclerosis despite similar glomerular hypertrophy (304). Furthermore, IGFBP-1 transgenic mice, characterized by decreased availability of IGF-1, develop glomerulosclerosis without concomitant glomerular hypertrophy (305).

Less is known regarding the participation of other growth factors in compensatory renal hypertrophy. The distal nephron produces a large amount of the precursor protein for epidermal growth factor (EGF). Renal content of EGF, distribution of EGF, and receptor levels for EGF, however, all remain constant over the first few days following uninephrectomy (306–308). An increase in EGF content and a reduction in EGF receptor levels have been observed only after compensatory renal hypertrophy is established (308,309). In contrast, there is a very early increase in remnant kidney hepatocyte growth factor (HGF) and HGF messenger RNA (mRNA) following uninephrectomy (309). However, uninephrectomy and operative stress also increase HGF expression in distant organs such as the lung (310). Thus, evidence indicates that HGF is an important morphogen for growing tubule cells, but the significance of the early rise in HGF after nephrectomy is unclear (311).

Role of Gender

It was originally suggested that the magnitude of compensatory hypertrophy is not influenced by androgens or gender (312–315). However, despite the generally benign course after uninephrectomy (282), some clinical studies reported increased risk for renal abnormalities in uninephrectomized males as compared to females (101,316). More recent experimental evidence demonstrates effects of gender on renal compensatory growth following uninephrectomy. Although initial accelerated growth of rat remnant kidneys is comparable between the sexes, later in the course, kidney growth is greater in the males (317). Accelerated growth in males is accompanied by significant glomerular hypertrophy and glomerular and tubular lesions, and associated with the presence of testosterone. No morphologic lesions were found in remnant kidneys of female rats. Further studies demonstrated that, in contrast to males, early renal growth in uninephrectomized female rats, is not associated with enhanced GH secretion, although IGF-I receptor mRNA is upregulated. Furthermore, females showed more hyperplastic response than males (318). Thus, uninephrectomy in the female rat theoretically can be viewed as a model of "true" adaptation with a minimal risk for development of renal injury. Further studies, better defining differences between the sexes in terms of renal responses to nephron loss, may be crucial for understanding of progressive nature of renal injury.

Changes in Gene Expression

The activation of early response genes or protooncogenes, whose protein products regulate transcriptional control of large numbers of other genes, is an early step in cell proliferation and differentiation evoked by mitogens and growth factors. Thus far, studies of the expression of early response genes in the remnant kidney following uninephrectomy have not provided unequivocal information (263,264,319–323). For example, renal activity of protooncogenes, such as c-fos, c-myc, c-egr1, c-jun, and c-H-ras, following uninephrectomy has been found to increase in some studies, but not in others (265,321,322,324). Altogether, however, these studies suggest that protooncogene activation after uninephrectomy is modest or absent, consistent with the low risk of deterioration of renal function in this modest degree of nephron loss.

As recently suggested, compensatory renal growth may have a genetic component. Pravenec and colleagues (325) studied effects of uninephrectomy in inbred strains derived from spontaneously hypertensive rats (SHR) and Brown Norway rats. They found that heritability of compensatory renal growth approached 40% and genome wide scan analysis showed significant linkage to Crg 1 region of chromosome 4. This region contains genes encoding for such proteins as L-type Ca channel and TGF-ß superfamily.

Age

Probably the least controversial modifier of compensatory renal hypertrophy is age. Age at nephrectomy clearly affects the magnitude of compensatory renal growth, with greater responses being seen in the younger kidneys (15,326–328). The increased magnitude of compensatory renal hypertrophy in youth may reflect generally greater responsiveness of young tissue to stimuli responsible for organ growth, as similar increases occur in compensatory growth of other organs.

Dietary Factors

Feeding a low protein diet to rats subjected to renal ablation limits remnant kidney GFR and weight, whereas feeding a high-protein diet augments hypertrophy (100,329–332). These observations suggest that the stimuli to hyperfiltration and hypertrophy associated with nephrectomy and protein feeding are additive. Restriction of other dietary components also may influence the renal hypertrophic response. As compared to values for kidney weights in nephrectomized animals receiving normal diets, kidney weights are lower in nephrectomized rats ingesting diets that are restricted in sodium (140,333), phosphate (334), total calories (95), or carbohydrates (335), or are high in water (336).

Endocrine Factors

Manipulation of endogenous levels of various hormones has been used to examine the influence of these factors on compensatory renal hypertrophy. Although early, incompletely controlled studies concluded otherwise, the most convincing data appear to exclude an important modulating effect of pituitary ablation (277,338,339) thyroidectomy (340), adrenalectomy (341), or congenital growth hormone deficiency (342–344).

THE PRICE OF ADAPTATION: CONTRIBUTIONS TO PROGRESSIVE RENAL DISEASE

Once chronic renal insufficiency begins, deterioration of renal function often continues, eventually leading to end-stage renal disease (ESRD). Progressive loss of function occurs after initial injury from a number of causes, including vesicoureteral reflux (345,346), bilateral renal cortical necrosis (347), analgesic nephropathy (348), after initial recovery from acute poststreptococcal glomerulonephritis (349), or acute renal failure (350,351) and with a congenital reduction in nephron number, as in the case of oligomeganephronia (352) or a congenital solitary kidney (353). In addition to the extent and severity of the primary renal disease, other factors influence the rate of progression to ESRD. Well-recognized contributing factors include poorly controlled hypertension, urinary tract infection, obstruction, administration of nephrotoxic drugs, and intrarenal deposition of calcium and urate salts. Frequently, however, renal insufficiency progresses despite spontaneous resolution or therapeutic control of the initial disease and attention to the risk factors for disease progression cited in the preceding.

Experimentally, reduction in functioning nephron number leads to systemic hypertension, proteinuria, glomerular sclerosis, tubulointerstitial fibrosis, and progressive renal insufficiency. After surgical extirpation of renal mass, whole kidney filtration function is initially maintained by structural hypertrophy, hyperfiltration, and hyperperfusion, as discussed. However, with extensive renal mass reduction, these adaptations eventually prove inadequate, and the kidney fails. These observations suggest that, after a certain point, reduction in functioning nephron number leads to failure of the remaining units; that is, the compensatory adaptations in renal function and perhaps size themselves contribute to further nephron destruction (22,352,353).

Systemic Hypertension

An important risk factor contributing to acceleration of renal disease is systemic hypertension, which may be both cause and consequence of chronic renal disease. Patients with chronic renal failure (354), including diabetic nephropathy (355), exhibit not only higher blood pressure but also loss of the usual nocturnal blood pressure decline, so that the mechanisms of hypertensive injury are more continuously operable in these patients at risk. Once present, hypertension is associated with faster loss of renal function in patients with acquired renal disease, as well as acceleration of the more moderate loss of renal function associated with normal aging (356,357).

Studies in various experimental hypertensive renal disease models have helped to delineate mechanisms of hypertensive injury. Although certain recurring hemodynamic patterns are found, specific patterns are related in large part to changes in the arterial perfusion pressure and the accompanying patterns of glomerular arteriolar resistances. Impaired autoregulation leads to enhanced transmission of systemic pressure into the glomerular capillary network and thereby to glomerular capillary hypertension. Experimentally, the pace of remnant glomerular injury, like the magnitude of remnant hemodynamic change, is correlated with the amount of renal mass excised (100). These observations suggest that the adaptive increases in glomerular capillary pressures and flows, although serving to maintain whole kidney function in the short term, in themselves contribute to the development of glomerular morphologic injury. To examine this hypothesis, Hostetter and coworkers (100) subjected rats to 85% to 90% nephrectomy. Glomerular hemodynamic adaptations were apparent as early as 1 week after ablation. Untreated rats exhibited elevations in the SNGFR, owing to elevations in both P_{GC} and Q_A. These hemodynamic adaptations were subsequently shown to be associated with proteinuria and extensive focal and segmental glomerular sclerosis (FSGS) (103). Dietary protein restriction was used to blunt the adaptive hyperfiltration following renal ablation. In animals fed a low-protein diet, values for SNGFR, Q_A, and P_{GC} were nearly normalized, despite equally extensive ablation. Limitation of Q_A and P_{GC} with dietary protein restriction is associated with slowing of the development of proteinuria and FSGS in this and a number of other experimental models of renal disease (358).

Of the glomerular hemodynamic determinants of adaptive hyperfiltration, glomerular capillary hypertension appears to be the crucial cause of eventual structural injury. In various models, ACE inhibition results in control of glomerular capillary hypertension, without affecting the supranormal single nephron filtration and perfusion rates; this selective reduction of P_{GC} prevents development of proteinuria and FSGS (21,23,89,358,359). Conversely, antihypertensive therapy that lowers systemic but not intraglomerular pressure may not protect the kidney at risk.

Accordingly, the relative roles of systemic and glomerular capillary hypertension may be clearly dissociated in studies of experimental renal disease. That glomerular rather than systemic hypertension is the critical determinant of injury has been shown by demonstrating that therapeutic interventions may affect these pressures independently. For example, systemic hypertension need not lead to glomerular hypertension, as is demonstrated in the SHR, a model of human essential hypertension. These animals exhibit high systemic pressures but fairly normal glomerular pressures, and little renal injury (360). Alternatively, glomerular hypertension may occur in the absence of systemic hypertension. Uninephrectomy in the rat does not result in systemic hypertension; nevertheless, the moderate increases in Q_A and P_{GC} are associated with acceleration of age-related FSGS in the rat (100). Similar changes are found in other normotensive models of glomerulonephritis (361,362). An extremely important example of this relationship is found in experimental diabetes mellitus. In the insulin-treated diabetic rat, systemic blood pressure is normal, but elevations of Q_A and P_{GC} result in single nephron hyperfiltration (359). In this model as well, intraglomerular hyperperfusion and hypertension lead to FSGS.

RENAL STRUCTURAL INJURY

Glomerulosclerosis

Rennke (216) summarized the glomerular morphological changes associated with transition from glomerular hypertrophy to glomerular obsolescence (glomerulosclerosis). Expansion of mesangial elements (i.e., disproportionate increase in fractional volume of the glomerulus occupied by the mesangium) is a typical feature observed in situations associated with sustained hyperfiltration. Both mesangial hypercellularity and increased synthesis of extracellular matrix contribute to the expansion. In advanced stages, mesangial expansion leads to the obliteration of capillaries and glomerular obsolescence. The process is linked to the filtration of molecules into the mesangium due to increased glomerular pressure, and local generation of growth factors by intrinsic renal (endothelial and mesangial) and blood-borne (platelets and leukocytes) cells. Subendothelial hyalin deposition occurs in association with increased glomerular pressure and podocyte changes. A greatly hypertrophied or stretched visceral epithelial cell may no longer maintain an efficient attachment to the underlying basement membrane and capillary loop, resulting in formation of areas with high hydraulic conductivity. Large macromolecules are filtered into these areas, forming aggregates that may ultimately occlude the capillary lumen. Formation of microthrombi is another feature often associated with hyperfiltering states. This process is most likely a consequence of glomerular endothelial injury and local production of proclotting factors. Finally, capillary microaneurysms may occur, in particular in conditions characterized by a rapid rise in P_{GC} (216).

Tubulointerstitial Injury

Critical reduction of nephron number ultimately leads to profound tubulointerstitial changes that involve tubule atrophy and loss, and interstitial expansion and fibrosis, also referred as tubulointerstitial scarring (21,330,363). The importance of this observation is highlighted by the fact that the best histologic predictor of progression of renal diseases in general, is not glomerular changes, but the degree of involvement of the tubulointerstitial compartment (364,365). As extracellular matrix production increases, tubules and peritubular capillaries disappear. Loss of these structures explains the close association with the decline of renal function. Human studies have shown a negative correlation between renal interstitial and tubular renal function in various renal diseases (366). As summarized by Eddy (363), the interstitial "scar" is composed of normal interstitial matrix proteins (collagens, fibronectin, tenascin), basement membrane proteins (collagen IV, laminin), proteoglycans, and glycoproteins (hyaluronan, thrombospondin and SPARC). α-Integrins (367) may be involved in binding fibronectin in insoluble matrix. The various matrix proteins which accumulate in the interstitium are assembled into a complex three-dimensional scaffold supported by cross-linking of protein chains. Studies exploring the cellular origin of proteins involved in interstitial scarring identified tubular epithelial cells and interstitial fibroblasts. Importantly, later studies demonstrated an ability of normal tubular and renal cells to transdifferentiate into other cell types with less predictable patterns, and atypical regulation of protein synthesis (368,369). In addition to resident renal cells, interstitial macrophages and infiltrating monocytes represent an important source of growth factors involved in fibroproduction, vasoactive molecules, and matrix proteins (291,370,371). The role of these cells has been further supported by several observations showing that renal injury in 5/6 nephrectomized rats is ameliorated by treatment with immunosuppressive agents such as mycophenolate mofetil (372–375).

Humoral and Biochemical Mediators of Renal Injury

Most of these mediators are implicated in the development of both glomerular and interstitial injury. Therefore, they are presented and discussed together.

Renin–Angiotensin System

Ang II can be viewed as a central molecule in several of the processes involved in chronic renal injury. In addition to

TABLE 90-1. *Mechanisms of angiotensin II-mediated renal injury*

Renal hemodynamic and vascular effects
    Constriction of afferent and efferent arterioles with predominantly efferent actions, increase in P_{GC}, decrease in K_f
    Increased activity of tubuloglomerular feedback
    Increased mesangial influx of macromolecules
    Proteinuria owing to impaired glomerular sieving function
    Formation of superoxide anions
Tubular effects
    Sodium reabsorption
    Bicarbonate reabsorption
    Increased ammonia production
Growth-promoting and inflammatory effects
    Stimulation of protooncogenes (*fos, myc, jun*)
    Stimulation of growth and prosclerotic factors (TGF-ß, PDGF, FGF)
    ECM accumulation owing to increased synthesis (fibronectin, collagen, laminin, osteopontin) and inhibition of degradation (PAI, metalloproteinase)
    Activation of nuclear factor κ-B
    Simulation of MCP-1
    Upregulation of VCAM-1, TNF-α
Interactions with other local and circulating renal humoral systems
    Nitric oxide and endothelin
    Eicosanoids
    Sympathetic nervous system
    Stimulation of aldosterone secretion
    Atrial and brain natriuretic peptides

P_{GC}, glomerular pressure; K_f, ultrafiltration coefficient; *TGF-ß*, transforming growth factor-ß; *PDGF*, platelet-derived growth factor; *FGF*, fibroblast growth factor; *ECM*, extracellular matrix; *PAI*, plasminogen activator inhibitor; *MCP-1*, monocyte chemoattractant protein-1; *VCAM-1*, vascular cell adhesion molecule-1; *TNF-α*, tumor necrosis factor-α.

its hemodynamic and tubular effects, Ang II exerts a number of actions that influence renal morphology. These effects have been a subject of excellent reviews during the past decade (376–378), and are briefly reviewed here (Table 90-1). These processes have been directly or indirectly involved in the pathogenesis of renal chronic injury after reduction of nephron mass, or have been shown to contribute to its progression.

Transforming Growth Factor-ß

Transforming growth factor-ß (TGF-ß), a multifunctional prosclerotic growth cytokine, has been shown to be involved in a wide array of physiologic and pathophysiologic processes. In the kidney, TGF-ß stimulates production of extracellular matrix (ECM) components, such as fibronectin, laminin, and collagen IV, by inducing their synthesis and inhibiting their degradation (379–381). It acts also as a chemotactic factor for mononuclear cells and macrophages, and stimulates fibroblasts, and epithelial-myofibroblast transdifferentiation, which accelerate fibrotic process (291,382). Further studies showed that the effects of TGF-ß include a reduction of plasminogen activator activity, upregulation of plasminogen activator inhibitor (PAI) (382–384), and synthesis of ß1-integrins (385). TGF-ß stimulates endothelin production (386). It is apparent that a number of actions of TGF-ß mimic the actions of Ang II. Indeed, the activity of TGF-ß is linked to the RAAS. The trophic effects of Ang II are, at least in part, mediated by TGF-ß, postulating the existence of a renin–angiotensin–TGF-ß axis (291,387). Activation of TGF-ß early after renal ablation has been described and implicated in the development of renal structural damage (29,379,388). Furthermore, involvement of the renin–angiotensin–TGF-ß axis has been documented by studies showing that amelioration of renal injury in rats with reduced renal mass, achieved by treatment with ACE inhibitors or AT₁ receptor blockers, is associated with a reduction of renal TGF-ß expression (291,388).

Endothelin

The renal hemodynamic actions and expression of ET-1 in rats with reduced nephron number have been mentioned in the preceding. Importantly, ET-1 is a potent mitogen and fibrogenic molecule, which can contribute to interstitial fibrosis by causing ischemia due to its vasoconstrictor effects. However, ET-1 has also been shown to have direct *in vitro* effects on matrix production (389), tubular cell proliferation (390), and upregulation of TGF-ß (391). *In vivo,* long-term studies in rats with reduced nephron mass treated with ET-1 receptor blockers found that prevention of renal fibrosis was part of the nephroprotective effect (73,87,88). Further support for the role of ET-1 in renal structural injury was provided by studies with ET-1 transgenic mice. This model develops renal interstitial fibrosis and cysts, and renal failure associated with normal blood pressure (392).

Platelet-Derived Growth Factor

Platelet-derived growth factor (PDGF) is a potent mitogen acting on glomerular cells (393). Furthermore, its involvement in tubulointerstitial injury is likely because of its ability to transform fibroblasts to myofibroblasts (394). Similar to TGF-ß, PDGF is stimulated by Ang Ii (395). TGF-ß can be stimulated by PDGF resulting in a transition from cell proliferation to hypertrophy and fibroproduction (396). PDGF is upregulated in kidneys after 5/6 nephrectomy in the rat (397) and has been found in biopsies of diseased human kidneys (398). Its role in maladaptive rather than in adaptive processes after nephron reduction is underscored by the fact that overexpression of PDGF is detectable only from the second week after renal ablation (397). A pathophysiologic role of this factor in the development of FSGS is further supported by studies with PDGF transgenic rats (399).

Growth Hormone and Hepatocyte Growth Factor

A possible role of these factors in renal injury has been suggested by studies with transgenic models. Mice transgenic for GH display progressive FSGS and renal failure, whereas mice transgenic for a mutant form of GH which acts as an GH antagonist, seem to be protected against FSGS associated with experimental diabetes (304,400). The role of hepatocyte growth factor (HGF) in the development of renal injury is controversial. Mice overexpressing HGF develop renal cysts, FSGS and renal failure associated with prominent cellular proliferation (401). However, in a spontaneous model of renal injury developing FSGS, tubular atrophy and renal failure, treatment with recombinant HGF suppresses expression of TGF-ß and PDGF, as well as myofibroblast formation. These molecular changes were associated with amelioration of FSGS and tubulointerstitial fibrosis (402).

Cyclooxygenase Products

Recent studies demonstrated nephroprotective effects of treatment with a nonspecific cyclooxygenase inhibitor combined with a NO donor (72) or with a COX-2-specific inhibitor (81,82). In addition to possible hemodynamic mechanisms, Wang and associates (81) showed that the nephroprotective effect of specific COX-2 inhibition may be mediated via suppression of TGF-ß. (81). Because thromboxane A2 is a product of the COX pathway, the authors hypothesized that thromboxanes contribute to the development of injury by stimulating TGF-ß.

Protooncogenes and Transcription Factors

Expression of growth promoting systems is accompanied by increased expression of protooncogenes and transcription factors. Expression of c-fos and c-jun genes and proteins may be detected 2 weeks following extensive renal ablation (151). Unlike the situation after uninephrectomy, protooncogenes have been implicated in the pathogenesis of renal injury in the remnant model. Data indicate that nephroprotection achieved by different treatment modalities may be accompanied by suppressed renal c-fos overexpression (47,63). AP-1, a transcription factor formed by heterodimerization of fos and jun proteins, is also increased in remnant kidneys, and downregulated by nephroprotective treatment (403). Another transcription factor, nuclear factor-κB (NF-κB) (404), has not been specifically studied in rats with reduced renal mass; however, studies with other nonimmunologic models of renal injury suggest involvement of this factor in renal fibrosis. Mirza and coworkers (405) reported an important function of NF-κB in regulating of the enzyme transglutaminase, which is an activator of latent TGF-ß. Transglutaminase also cross-links matrix proteins, possibly contributing to interstitial fibrosis in the remnant kidney model (406). The activation of NF-κB may have an important role in mediating cortical interstitial monocyte infiltration and tubular injury in nonimmune proteinuric tubulointerstitial inflammation (407,408).

Alterations of Matrix Turnover

Extracellular matrix (ECM) accumulation, a hallmark of glomerulosclerosis and interstitial fibrosis, cannot be viewed merely as a result of increased production. In the normal kidney there is a delicate balance between ECM production and degradation. Extracellular matrix proteins are being constantly degraded by connective tissue proteases, such as cathepsins or metalloproteinases (MMP). Activity of these enzymes is further controlled by their tissue inhibitors. The balance between proteinases and their tissue inhibitors is regulated by growth factors such as Ang II, TGF-ß, PDGF, and others (409,410). Downregulation of MMP has been described in the remnant kidney (411). More information is available about the alterations of protease inhibitors, in particular, of the plasminogen activator inhibitor-1 (PAI-1) in progressive renal disease. In the radiation nephropathy, a model of FSGS, PAI-1 mRNA expression was colocalized with sites of glomerular injury (412). Mutant mice lacking PAI-1 do not develop FSGS after irradiation (410). The amelioration of sclerosis in 5/6 nephrectomized rats treated with ACE inhibitors or AT_1 receptor blockers is associated with marked inhibition of PAI-1 (410).

Cell Cycle Proteins

Recent studies provide compelling evidence for the role of cell cycle regulating proteins in the development of renal injury following nephron loss. Compensatory hypertrophy after renal ablation is associated with cyclin E and CDK2 expression coinciding with the early proliferative response (413). However, it appears that the key role in subsequent development of renal injury is played by CDK inhibitors. These molecules are regulated by factors that have been implicated in the pathogenesis of renal injury after nephron loss, such as Ang II or TGF-ß (414,415).

Although the renal expression of CDK inhibitors has not been investigated directly in remnant kidneys, increased expression has been found in other models of FSGS or interstitial fibrosis, such as diabetic nephropathy and ureteral obstruction (416,417). However, a recent study by Megyesi and associates (418) in p21 knockout mice has shown the major importance of this CDK inhibitor in the remnant kidney model as well. p21 knockout mice subjected to renal ablation demonstrated striking resistance to the development of FSGS, as compared to wild-type animals. In the absence of the p21 gene, the growth response in the remnant kidney was relatively more hyperplastic that hypertrophic. The authors alluded to a proposal, made by Goss (419) over 30 years ago, suggesting that when an organ accommodates increases in work by hypertrophy rather than hyperplasia, it is at a serious physiologic disadvantage and is more likely to undergo regression of structure and function.

In this context, the special role of podocytes should be noted. As mentioned, adult podocytes possess diminished ability to divide in response to immune, metabolic, and hemodynamic (nephron loss) stimuli including mesangial cells (106). Several groups have implicated the fact that podocytes undergo exaggerated stress as glomeruli enlarge, resulting in their dysfunction and possibly destruction, in the pathogenesis of glomerulosclerosis (46,225,420). As suggested by Shankland and Wolf (260), this phenomenon can be explained by the unique expression of CDK inhibitors in podocytes.

TRIGGERS OF MALADAPTIVE STRUCTURAL RESPONSES

Glomerular Injury

Glomerular Hemodynamics

A number of studies have addressed the hypothesis that increased glomerular capillary pressures and/or plasma flow rates alter the growth and activity of glomerular component cells, inducing the elaboration or expression of cytokines and other mediators, which then stimulate mesangial matrix production and promote structural injury. Hemodynamic physical forces, such as shear stress or changes in blood flow, are well recognized to influence activity of endothelial cells in extrarenal systems, and it seems likely that such forces exert cellular actions in the glomerulus as well. For instance, growing cultured endothelial cells under conditions of increased shear stress increases the activity or expression of such mediators as endothelin (421,422), nitric oxide (84,423), TGF-ß (424), basic fibroblast growth factor (425), and intercellular adhesion molecule-1 (ICAM-1) (426), and modulates levels and/or activity of PDGF mRNA (425,427). Indeed, even without shear stress, growing endothelial cells under conditions of increased pressure can increase endothelin release (428). Altered hemodynamics may also influence activity of mesangial cells. In support of this notion, it has been postulated that expansion of the glomerular capillaries and stretching of the mesangium in response to hypertension might be a force that translates high P_{GC} into increased mesangial matrix formation (429). Evidence for this mechanism comes from observations in microperfused rat glomeruli, in which increased P_{GC} was associated with increased glomerular volume; and in cultured mesangial cells, where cyclic stretching resulted in enhanced synthesis of protein, total collagen, collagen IV, collagen I, laminin, fibronectin, and TGF-ß (429–431). Additionally, growing mesangial cells under pulsatile conditions has been reported to stimulate protein kinase C, calcium influx, and protooncogene expression (432) and Ang II receptor and angiotensinogen mRNA levels (430), as well as altered extracellular matrix protein processing enzymes (432,433). In vivo, Shankland and coworkers (434) observed that increases in P_{GC} induced by uninephrectomy in SHR were associated with glomerular expression of TGF-ß and PDGF. Normalization of P_{GC} with an ACE inhibitor decreased glomerular TGF-ß and PDGF. Similar to that observation, Griffin and associates (435) compared glomerular pressure in relation to glomerular TGF-ß and PDGF expression between the excision and infarction models of renal ablation. The rats subjected to renal infarction demonstrated higher systemic and glomerular pressures, and markedly higher expression of TGF-ß and PDGF mRNA in glomeruli.

It should be noted in this context that although deleterious for long-term prognosis of renal function, even maladaptive changes in renal hemodynamics after nephron loss are likely to be life-saving in the short term. This contention is based on observations in mice lacking vimentin (Vim −/−), an intermediate filament protein necessary for appropriate vasomotor functions (436). Although the Vim −/− mice display a normal phenotype as compared to Vim +/+ animals, they suffer 100% early mortality after 3/4 renal mass reduction. This phenomenon is associated with impaired flow-induced dilation in renal arteries, and imbalance in renal ET/NO synthesis.

Glomerular Hypertrophy

Glomerular hypertrophy can be viewed as a consequence of renal hemodynamic alterations. However, it has been also proposed as an important condition in triggering FSGS. Studies in a number of experimental models have noted a strong association between increased glomerular size and development of proteinuria and FSGS (46,55,140,437,438). Conversely, a protective effect of low glomerular volume could account for the observations that a strain of rats with unusually small glomeruli exhibits less glomerular injury following uninephrectomy than a strain with larger glomeruli (439,440). Miller and colleagues (290) compared the rate of development of proteinuria and FSGS in normal and uninephrectomized rats treated long-term with a pressor dose of Ang II, a maneuver known to increase P_{GC}. Despite the fact that the Ang II dose was halved in uninephrectomized rats, these rats demonstrated markedly faster development of renal injury. There were no differences in P_{GC} between those groups; however, the groups differed in the glomerular volume, which was increased in uninephrectomized animals.

The combination of increases in both glomerular capillary intraluminal pressure and capillary radius is postulated to exert increased tension on the glomerular capillary wall (following Laplace's law), thus contributing to disruption of capillary wall integrity, activation of growth factors and FSGS. The potential additive deleterious effects of glomerular capillary hypertension and glomerular enlargement have also prompted speculation that injury may be mediated by detrimental effects on the glomerular visceral epithelial cells (46,226,420,437) and their lower ability to adapt. The important question of whether increases in glomerular pressure and/or flow stimulate glomerular growth requires further investigation. Available studies suggest that normalizing P_{GC} may limit but cannot prevent glomerular hypertrophy following renal ablation. Importantly, recent studies comparing two models of renal ablation showed differences in systemic and glomerular blood pressure, expression of prosclerotic factors, and the rate of development of renal injury, but similar degree

of glomerular hypertrophy (435). These studies indicate that the protective effect of reducing P_{GC} cannot be attributed to reduction in glomerular volume.

Tubular Injury

Proteins of Glomerular Origin

The appearance of protein casts suggests that remnant nephron proteinuria causes tubule obstruction and dilatation. Proteins of glomerular origin trigger tubular maladaptive processes by several mechanisms. First, tubular and interstitial cells can be activated by a number of growth-promoting factors that have been generated by glomerular cells. These factors can be reabsorbed from the tubular fluid and further transported into interstitium (441), or they can reach the tubulointerstitial compartment via the postglomerular vasculature. Second, Remuzzi's group (442) has suggested that glomerular proteinuria per se can exert deleterious effects on the tubulointerstitial compartment. As protein traffic across the glomerular barrier increases, the protein concentration in Bowman's capsule and tubules also increases. Proximal tubular cells actively reabsorb filtered proteins by phagocytosis. Increasing protein loads in tubular cells cause organelle congestion, lysosomal swelling and rupture, exposing the tubular cells and interstitium to lysosomal enzymes. Furthermore, protein may upregulate genes involved in tubulointerstitial infiltration and injury (442). For example, proximal tubular cells exposed to increased concentration of proteins such as albumin or immunoglobulin may respond with an increase in ET-1 production. The release is primarily basolateral, suggesting the link with the development of interstitial injury (443). In addition to these injurious effects of glomerular protein leakage, primary tubulointerstitial processes may contribute to remnant nephron destruction following renal ablation (445).

Hypoxia Theory

This theory, pioneered by Fine and coworkers (446), introduced hypoxia of tubular and interstitial cells as a major trigger of events resulting in tubulointerstitial injury. It is assumed that the blood flow and oxygen delivery to the interstitial and peritubular capillary network is limited owing to glomerular injury, or that the tubulointerstitial capillary network suffers the same hemodynamic injury as glomeruli. Peritubular capillaries may be compressed by hypertrophic tubules (447). An alternative mechanism of tubular hypoxia relates to increased metabolic demands caused by enhanced reabsorptive work (448–454). Hypoxia leads to expression of growth factors, vasoactive molecules, cytokines, adhesion molecules and other mediators involved in pathogenesis glomerular injury (455–459). Hypoxia acts both at transcriptional and posttranscriptional levels, altering gene expression and mRNA stability (455). At the level of gene transcription, hypoxia response elements (HRE) have been identified in a number of genes forming a binding site for the hypoxia-inducible transcription factor (HIF-1) (460,461). Hypoxia-inducible transcription factor-1 acts in concert with other transcription factors, such as NF-κB and the fos and jun families, to induce gene expression (460).

Changes in Interstitial Osmolarity

Bouby and associates (336) demonstrated a nephroprotective effect of high water intake in rats with subtotal nephrectomy, and ascribed those effects to inhibition of the process of urinary concentration. More recent studies provided insight into molecular mechanisms of this intervention. *In vitro,* hypertonicity activates latent TGF-ß into the biologically active form (462). *In vivo,* reduction of interstitial osmolality by high water intake in 5/6 nephrectomized rats results in a decrease in TGF-ß and fibronectin mRNA expression, and amelioration of predominantly tubulointerstitial, but also glomerular, injury (463).

Increased Ammoniagenesis

Increased ammonia production by remnant nephrons has been associated with intrarenal complement activation and interstitial inflammation (464). Administration of sodium bicarbonate, which reduces remnant nephron ammonia production, also limits tubulointerstitial injury in rats subjected to renal ablation (464).

OTHER FACTORS CONTRIBUTING TO NEPHRON INJURY

Hyperlipidemia and Glomerular Lipid Deposition

It has been suggested that glomerular deposition of circulating lipids contributes to progressive glomerular injury in renal disease (465). This area of research has been summarized in several recent reviews (466–468). In numerous animal models of progressive renal disease, feeding a high-cholesterol diet accelerates injury, whereas hypolipidemic therapy slows progression (465). Mechanisms of lipid-induced injury include a proliferative response of mesangial cells to low-density lipoproteins (LDL) (469,470); synergistic interactions among LDL, endothelin, PDGF, and IGF-I (469); aggravation of glomerular macrophage influx and stimulation of monocyte chemoattractant protein (MCP-1) (471); effects on mesangial type IV collagen synthesis (466); and increased TGF-ß expression by infiltrating macrophages (472). Hypolipidemic therapy with lovastatin has been shown to influence mesangial cell metabolism, by inhibiting serum-induced proliferation (473), inhibiting PDGF-induced mesangial cell mitogenesis (474), and inhibiting MCP-1 and interleukin-6 mRNA expression and protein secretion (475). Furthermore, lovastatin decreases membrane-bound p21 ras in proximal tubular cells and inhibits serum-induced c-fos and c-jun protein and AP1 activity (476). As in atherosclerosis, hyperlipidemia may act synergistically with other risk factors, such as hypertension, in promoting glomerular injury (477).

Glomerular Capillary Thrombosis

It has been suggested that capillary thrombosis is precipitated by early endothelial cell injury in the remnant glomeruli, and that capillary microthrombi contribute to FSGS by direct occlusion of capillary lumina and by release of platelet-derived factors that aggravate glomerular injury (216,478,479). This hypothesis has prompted evaluation of anticoagulant drugs in experimental renal disease. For example, heparin has proven protective in the remnant kidney model (480,481). The protective effect afforded by thromboxane synthesis inhibition has also been attributed to lessening thrombosis, whereas warfarin sodium (Coumadin) and aspirin have been shown to be less effective than heparin in preventing remnant glomerular injury (69,482,483). Heparin, may also protect remnant glomeruli by other mechanisms, including reduction of blood pressure (480,481,484,485), suppression of endothelin (444,486) and mesangial matrix accumulation (487), and inhibition of mesangial cell expression of basic fibroblast growth factor and PDGF, and of extracellular matrix proteins (488).

Altered Phosphate Metabolism and Renal Calcium Deposition

Studies by Alfrey and coworkers (489,490) provided the first evidence that intrarenal calcium deposition contributes to progressive loss of renal function in experimental renal disease. These studies showed that restricting phosphate intake reduced renal calcium content, preserved renal function, and prolonged life span in rats with renal ablation or nephrotoxic serum nephritis. It is not clear, however, that phosphate restriction protects the remnant kidney by preventing intrarenal deposition of calcium phosphate salts. Phosphorus restriction may protect remnant nephrons by lowering circulating lipid levels, reducing tubule energy consumption, altering remnant glomerular hemodynamic function, or reducing glomerular volume (491–494). Likewise, the beneficial effects of parathyroidectomy and hypocalcemia may result from reduction of lipid levels and prevention of remnant growth (394). Recent studies also have shown that increased parathyroid hormone contributes to suppression of NO generation in the remnant kidney (87).

PATHOPHYSIOLOGY OF PROGRESSIVE RENAL INJURY AFTER NEPHRON LOSS: UNIFYING SCENARIO

The different mechanisms proposed to account for remnant injury should not be regarded as mutually exclusive; indeed, there are most likely extensive interactions among them (216,217). Given the close apposition and functional interdependency of glomerular cell types, such interaction among

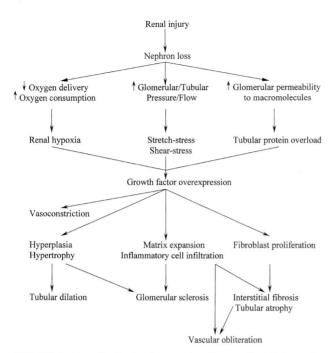

FIG. 90-4. Hypothetical schema of pathways that link nephron reduction to the development of renal lesions via hemodynamic forces and growth factor overexpression. (From: Terzi F, et al. *Kidney Int* 1998;53:S68, with permission.)

mechanisms of glomerular injury should be expected. The foregoing studies suggest that the progression of renal injury associated with systemic hypertension is mediated by the resultant adaptive increase in P_{GC}, which then contributes to structural injury. The sequence of events whereby alterations in hemodynamics, oxygen delivery, and glomerular permeability initiate growth factor overexpression and subsequent cellular injury is schematized in Fig. 90-4 (247). In addition to the better characterized effects on endothelial and mesangial cells, epithelial cell injury also participates. Glomerular hypertension and hypertrophy also may cause glomerular sclerosis by promoting movement of circulating macromolecules through the glomerular capillary wall. The development of proteinuria in rats subjected to renal ablation results from defects in both the charge- and size-selective properties of the glomerular capillary wall (105,496). These permselective defects are associated with abnormalities of epithelial cell structure including retraction of epithelial cell foot processes and focal detachment of epithelial cells from the underlying basement membrane. Epithelial cell injury in remnant glomeruli may reflect increased capillary wall tension and the inability of highly differentiated epithelial cells to replicate as glomerular volume increases following reduction in nephron number (46,225). Subendothelial deposition of large macromolecules in areas where macromolecule passage through the capillary wall is increased may result in hyalinosis, eventually proceeding to occlusion of capillary lumina (216). Together, damage to these cellular elements results in FSGS.

Meanwhile, tubulointerstitial injury develops owing to a primary interstitial process or secondary to glomerular events.

The cells in the tubulointerstitial compartment are being injured by hypoxia, resulting from high metabolic demands imposed by increased burden of molecules they process, impaired blood flow owing to obstruction in diseased glomeruli, or vascular injury of interstitial capillary network. Increased protein trafficking secondary to leakage from affected glomeruli causes direct tubular toxicity and includes humoral mediators of tubulointerstitial injury. Under these pathophysiologic stimuli, the cells in the tubulointerstitial compartment generate a large array of prosclerotic and profibrotic mediators and transdifferentiate to more primitive cell types, that further contribute to progressive injury. Tubulointerstitial injury then perpetuates nephron loss by creating atubular glomeruli (497). Progressive nephron destruction in turn contributes to systemic and glomerular hypertension, thus perpetuating the cycle.

THE PROGRESSION OF HUMAN RENAL INSUFFICIENCY: THERAPEUTIC IMPLICATIONS

The major clinical trials evaluating therapeutic interventions in slowing progression of renal disease are discussed elsewhere in this volume. The wide spectrum of pathophysiologic mechanisms described in the preceding suggests that the problem can be approached from many different directions. Indeed, during the past several decades, dozens of treatment possibilities have been tested experimentally and clinically. With respect to their role in the development of renal injury, systemic and glomerular hypertension represent the most attractive targets for intervention. Moreover, the same interventions can also ameliorate renal growth abnormalities resulting in beneficial effects in the tubulointerstitial as well as glomerular compartments. Considering the variety of actions of Ang II (Table 90-1), and its key position in the renal pathophysiology, inhibition of the RAAS still represents the major pharmacologic therapy of progressive renal injury. ACE inhibitors and AT_1 receptor blockers are not only effective in reducing blood pressure. Based on experimental studies, these agents are effective in reducing glomerular pressure and growth abnormalities in the kidney. In clinical studies, ACEI are the class of antihypertensive agents most often associated with nephroprotection. However, reduction of blood pressure per se seems to afford some protection in most nephropathies, regardless to the class of agent used (with some exceptions to the rule). This is not surprising with respect to the role of impaired autoregulation of renal blood flow in transmitting the systemic blood pressure into glomeruli.

Other therapeutic maneuvers also may prove helpful, as discussed elsewhere in this volume. One possible therapy is restriction of dietary protein intake, implemented early in the course of intrinsic renal disease. Anticoagulant agents have been shown in some studies to retard the progression of membranoproliferative glomerulonephritis. The protective effect of agents that lower serum lipid levels remains to be assessed. Finally, the efficacy of specific pharmaceutical blockers, such as those which limit the action of endothelin, TGF-ß, and other mediators, is likely to undergo clinical testing in the coming years.

REFERENCES

1. Platt R. Structural and functional adaptation in renal failure. *Br Med J* 1952;6/21/52:1313.
2. Bricker NS, Morrin PAF, Kime SW Jr. The pathologic physiology of chronic Bright's disease: an exposition of the "intact nephron hypothesis." *Am J Med* 1960;28:77.
3. Bricker NS. On the meaning of the intact nephron hypothesis. *Am J Med* 1969;46:1.
4. Bricker NS, Fine LG. The renal response to progressive nephron loss. In: Brenner BM, Rector FO Jr, eds. *The kidney,* 2nd ed. Philadelphia: WB Saunders, 1981:1056.
5. Allison MEM, Wilson CB, Gottschalk CW. Pathophysiology of experimental glomerulonephritis in rats. *J Clin Invest* 1974;53:1402.
6. Reiss E, Bricker NS, Lime SW Jr, et al. Observations on phosphate transport in experimental renal disease. *J Clin Invest* 1962;41:1303.
7. Wagnild JP, Gutmann FD, Rieselbach RE. Functional characterization of chronic unilateral glomerulonephritis in the dog. *Kidney Int* 1987; 5:422.
8. Meyer TW, Baboolal K, Brenner BM. Nephron adaptation to renal injury. In: Brenner BM, Rector FC Jr, eds. *The kidney,* 5th ed. Philadelphia: WB Saunders, 1996:2011.
9. Kramp RA, MacDowell M, Gottschalk CW, et al. A study by microdissection and micropuncture of the structure and function of the kidneys and the nephrons of rats with chronic renal damage. *Kidney Int* 1974;5:147.
10. Ichikawa I, Hoyer JR, Seiler MW, et al. Mechanism of glomerulotubular balance in the setting of heterogeneous glomerular injury: preservation of a close functional linkage between individual nephrons and surrounding microvasculature. *J Clin Invest* 1982;69:185.
11. Krohn AG, Ogden DA, Holmes JH. Renal function in 29 healthy adults before and after nephrectomy. *JAMA* 1966;196:322.
12. Pabico RC, McKenna BA, Freeman RB. Renal function before and after unilateral nephrectomy in renal donors. *Kidney Int* 1975;8:166.
13. Baudoin P, Provoost AP, Molenaar JC. Renal function up to 50 years after unilateral nephrectomy in childhood. *Am J Kidney Dis* 1993;21:603.
14. Narkun-Burgess DM, Nolan CR, Norman JE, et al. Forty-five year follow-up after uninephrectomy. *Kidney Int* 1993;43:1110.
15. Hayslett JP. Effect of age on compensatory renal growth. *Kidney Int* 1983;23:599.
16. Kaufman JM, Hardy R, Hayslett JP. Age-dependent characteristics of compensatory renal growth. *Kidney Int* 1975;8:21.
17. Larsson L, Aperia A, Wilton P. Effect of normal development on compensatory renal growth. *Kidney Int* 1980;18:29.
18. Diezi J, Michoud-Hausel P, Nicolas-Buxcel N. Studies on possible mechanisms of early functional compensatory adaptation in the remaining kidney. *Yale J Biol Med* 1978;51:265.
19. Meyer TW, Rennke HG. Progressive glomerular injury after limited renal infarction in the rat. *Am J Physiol* 1988;254:F856.
20. Deen WM, Maddox DA, Robertson CR, et al. Dynamics of glomerular ultrafiltration in the rat: VII. Response to reduced renal mass. *Am J Physiol* 1974;227:F556.
21. Anderson S, Meyer TW, Rennke HG, et al. Control of glomerular hypertension limits glomerular injury in rats with reduced renal mass. *J Clin Invest* 1985;76:612.
22. Hostetter TH, Olson JL, Rennke HG, et al. Hyperfiltration in remnant nephrons: a potentially adverse response to renal ablation. *Am J Physiol* 1981;241:F85.
23. Meyer TW, Anderson S, Rennke HG, et al. Reversing glomerular capillary hypertension stabilizes established glomerular injury. *Kidney Int* 1987;31:752.
24. Hayslett JP. Functional adaptation to reduction in renal mass. *Physiol Rev* 1979;59:137.
25. Buerkert J, Martin D, Prasad J, et al. Response of deep nephrons and the terminal collecting duct to a reduction in renal mass. *Am J Physiol* 1979;236:F454.
26. Pennell JP, Bourgoignie JJ. Adaptive changes of juxtamedullary glomerular filtration in the remnant kidney. *Pflugers Arch* 1981;389:131.
27. Salmond R, Seney FD Jr. Reset tubuloglomerular feedback permits and sustains glomerular hyperfunction after extensive renal ablation. *Am J Physiol* 1991;260:F395.
28. Pollock CA, Bostrom TE, Dyne M, et al. Tubular sodium handling and tubuloglomerular feedback in compensatory renal hypertrophy. *Pflugers Arch* 1992;420:159.
29. Kasiske BL, O'Donnell MP, Garvis WJ, et al. Pharmacologic treatment of hyperlipidemia reduces glomerular injury in rat 5/6 nephrectomy model of chronic renal failure. *Circ Res* 1988;62:367.
30. Nath KA, Chmielewski DH, Hostetter TH. Regulatory role of prostanoids in glomerular microcirculation of remnant nephrons. *Am J Physiol* 1987;252:F829.
31. Purkerson ML, Hoffsten PE, Klahr S. Pathogenesis of the glomerulopathy associated with renal infarction in rats. *Kidney Int* 1976;9:407.
32. Langston JB, Guyton AC, Douglas BH, et al. Effect of changes in salt intake on arterial pressure and renal function in nephrectomized dogs. *Circ Res* 1963;12:508.
33. Brown SA, Finco DR, Crowell WA, et al. Single-nephron adaptations to partial renal ablation in the dog. *Am J Physiol* 1990;258:F495.
34. Pelayo JC, Westcott JY. Impaired autoregulation of glomerular capillary hydrostatic pressure in the rat remnant nephron. *J Clin Invest* 1991;88:101.
35. Bidani AK, Schwartz MM, Lewis EJ. Renal autoregulation and vulnerability to hypertensive injury in remnant kidneys. *Am J Physiol* 1987;252:F1003.
36. Brown SA, Finco DR, Navar LG. Impaired renal autoregulatory ability in dogs with reduced renal mass. *J Am Soc Nephrol* 1995;5:1768.
37. Griffin KA, Picken MM, Bakris GL, et al. Class differences in the effects of calcium channel blockers in the rat remnant kidney model. *Kidney Int* 1999;55:1849.
38. Blantz RC, Konnen KS, Tucker BJ. Angiotensin II effects upon the glomerular microcirculation and ultrafiltration coefficient of the rat. *J Clin Invest* 1976;57:419.
39. Myers BD, Deen WM, Brenner BM. Effects of norepinephrine and angiotensin II on the determinants of glomerular ultrafiltration and proximal tubule fluid reabsorption in the rat. *Circ Res* 1975;37:101.
40. Rosenberg ME, Kren SM, Hostetter TH. Effect of dietary protein on the renin-angiotensin system in subtotally nephrectomized rats. *Kidney Int* 1990;38:240.
41. Pelayo JC, Quan AH, Shanley PF. Angiotensin II control of the renal microcirculation in rats with reduced renal mass. *Am J Physiol* 1990;258:F414.
42. Baboolal K, Meyer TW. The effect of acute angiotensin II blockade on renal function in rats with reduced renal mass. *Kidney Int* 1994;46:980.
43. Tank JE, Moe OW, Star RA, et al. Differential regulation of rat glomerular and proximal tubular renin mRNA following uninephrectomy. *Am J Physiol* 1996;270:F776.
44. Rosenberg ME, Correa-Rotter R, Inagami T, et al. Glomerular renin synthesis and storage in the remnant kidney in the rat. *Kidney Int* 1991;40:677.
45. Pupilli C, Chevalier RL, Carey RM, et al. Distribution and content of renin and renin mRNA in remnant kidney of adult rat. *Am J Physiol* 1992;263:F731.
46. Fries JWU, Sandstrom DJ, Meyer TW, et al. Glomerular hypertrophy and epithelial cell injury modulate progressive glomerulosclerosis in the rat. *Lab Invest* 1989;60:205.
47. Terzi F, Beaufils H, Laouari D, et al. Renal effect of anti-hypertensive drugs depends on sodium diet in the excision remnant kidney model. *Kidney Int* 1992;42:354.
48. Griffin KA, Picken M, Bidani AK. Method of renal mass reduction is a critical modulator of subsequent hypertension and glomerular injury. *J Amer Soc Nephrol* 1994;4:2023.
49. Gilbert RE, Wu LL, Kelly DJ, et al. Pathological expression of renin and angiotensin II in the renal tubule after subtotal nephrectomy. Implications for the pathogenesis of tubulointerstitial fibrosis. *Am J Pathol* 1999;155:429.
50. Wang DH, Yao A, Zhao H, et al. Regulation of ANG II receptor in hypertension: role of ANG II. *Am J Physiol* 1996;271:H120.
51. Greene EL, Kren S, Hostetter TH. Role of aldosterone in the remnant kidney model in the rat. *J Clin Invest* 1996;98:1063.

52. Berl T, Katz FH, Henrich WL, et al. Role of aldosterone in the control of sodium excretion in patients with advanced chronic renal failure. *Kidney Int* 1978;14:228.

53. Hene RJ, Boer P, Koomans HA, et al. Plasma aldosterone concentrations in chronic renal disease. *Kidney Int* 1982;21:98.

54. Quan ZY, Walser M, Hill GS. Adrenalectomy ameliorates ablative nephropathy in the rat independently of corticosterone maintenance level. *Kidney Int* 1992;41:326.

55. Dworkin LD, Hostetter TH, Rennke HG, et al. Hemodynamic basis for glomerular injury in rats with desoxycorticosterone-salt hypertension. *J Clin Invest* 1984;73:1448.

56. Lafayette RA, Mayer G, Park SK, et al. Angiotensin II receptor blockade limits glomerular injury in rats with reduced renal mass. *J Clin Invest* 1992;90:766.

57. Smith S, Anderson S, Ballermann BJ, et al. Role of atrial natriuretic peptide in the adaptation of sodium excretion with reduced renal mass. *J Clin Invest* 1986;77:1395.

58. Zhang PL, Mackenzie HS, Troy JL, et al. Effects of natriuretic peptide receptor inhibition on remnant kidney function in rats. *Kidney Int* 1994;46:414.

59. Totsune K, Mackenzie HS, Totsune H, et al. Upregulation of atrial natriuretic peptide gene expression in remnant kidney of rats with reduced renal mass. *J Am Soc Nephrol* 1998;9:1613.

60. King AJ, Brenner BM, Anderson S. Endothelin: a potent renal and systemic vasoconstrictor peptide. *Am J Physiol* 1989;256:F1051.

61. Benigni A, Perico N, Gaspari F, et al. Increased renal endothelin production in rats with reduced renal mass. *Am J Physiol* 1991;260:F331.

62. Orisio S, Benigni A, Bruzzi I, et al. Renal endothelin gene expression is increased in remnant kidney and correlates with disease progression. *Kidney Int* 1993;43:354.

63. Benigni A, Zoja C, Corna D, et al. A specific endothelin subtype A receptor antagonist protects against injury in renal disease progression. *Kidney Int* 1993;44:440.

64. Nabokov A, Amann K, Wagner J, et al. Influence of specific and non-specific endothelin receptor antagonists on renal morphology in rats with surgical renal ablation. *Nephrol Dial Transplant* 1996;11:514.

65. Orth SR, Esslinger JP, Amann K, et al. Nephroprotection of an ET(A)-receptor blocker (LU 135252) in salt-loaded uninephrectomized stroke-prone spontaneously hypertensive rats. *Hypertension* 1998;31:995.

66. Qiu C, Baylis C. Endothelin and angiotensin mediate most glomerular responses to nitric oxide inhibition. *Kidney Int* 1999;55:2390.

67. Stahl RA, Kudelka S, Paravicini M, et al. Prostaglandin and thromboxane formation in glomeruli from rats with reduced renal mass. *Nephron* 1986;42:252.

68. Griffin KA, Bidani AK, Picken M, et al. Prostaglandins do not mediate impaired autoregulation or increased renin secretion in remnant rat kidneys. *Am J Physiol* 1992;263:F1057.

69. Purkerson ML, Joist JH, Yates J, et al. Inhibition of thromboxane synthesis ameliorates the progressive kidney disease of rats with subtotal ablation. *Proc Natl Acad Sci USA* 1985;82:193.

70. Kirschenbaum MA, Serros ER. Effect of prostaglandin inhibition on glomerular filtration rate in normal and uremic rabbits. *Prostaglandins* 1981;22:245.

71. Arisz L, Donker AJM, Brentjens JRH, et al. The effect of indomethacin on proteinuria and kidney function in the nephrotic syndrome. *Acta Med Scand* 1976;199:121.

72. Ciabattoni G, Cinotti GA, Pierucci A, et al. Effects of sulindac and ibuprofen in patients with chronic glomerular disease: evidence for the dependence of renal function on prostacyclin. *N Engl J Med* 1984;310:279.

73. Fujihara CK, Malheiros DM, Donato JL, et al. Nitroflurbiprofen, a new nonsteroidal anti-inflammatory, ameliorates structural injury in the remnant kidney. *Am J Physiol* 1998;274:F573.

74. Altsheler P, Klahr S, Rosenbaum R, et al. Effects of inhibitors of prostaglandin synthesis on renal sodium excretion in normal dogs and dogs with decreased renal mass. *Am J Physiol* 1978;235:F338.

75. Harris RC, McKanna JA, Akai Y, et al. Cyclooxygenase-2 is associated with the macula densa of rat kidney and increases with salt restriction. *J Clin Invest* 1994;94:2504.

76. Wang J-L, Cheng H-F, Zhang M-Z, et al. Selective inhibition of cyclooxygenase-2 expression in a model of renal ablation. *Am J Physiol* 1998;275:F613.

77. Ichihara A, Imig JD, Navar LG. Cyclooxygenase-2 modulates afferent arteriolar responses to increases in pressure. *Hypertension* 1999;34:843.

78. Harding P, Sigmon DH, Alfie ME, et al. Cyclooxygenase-2 mediates increased renal renin content by low-sodium diet. *Hypertension* 1997;29:297.

79. Wang J-L, Cheng H-F, Harris RC. Cyclooxygenase-2 inhibition decreases renin content and lowers blood pressure in a model of renovascular hypertension. *Hypertension* 1999;34:96.

80. Traynor TR, Smart A, Briggs JP, et al. Inhibition of macula densa-stimulated renin secretion by pharmacological blockade of cyclooxygenase-2. *Am J Physiol* 1999;277:F706.

81. Wang JL, Cheng HF, Shappell S, et al. A selective cyclooxygenase-2 inhibitor decreases proteinuria and retards progressive renal injury in rats. *Kidney Int* 2000;57:2334.

82. Sanchez PL, Salgado LM, Ferreri NR, et al. Effect of cyclooxygenase-2 inhibition on renal function after renal ablation. *Hypertension* 1999;34:848.

83. Deng A, Baylis C. Locally produced EDRF controls preglomerular resistance and ultrafiltration coefficient. *Am J Physiol* 1993;264:F212.

84. Buga GM, Gold ME, Fukuto JM, et al. Shear stress-induced release of nitric oxide from endothelial cells grown on beads. *Hypertension* 1991;17:187.

85. Valdivielso JM, Perez-Barriocanal F, Garcia-Estan J, et al. Role of nitric oxide in the early renal hemodynamic response after unilateral nephrectomy. *Am J Physiol* 1999;276:R1718.

86. Aiello S, Remuzzi G, Noris M. Nitric oxide/endothelin balance after nephron reduction. *Kidney Int* 1998;65:S63.

87. Vaziri ND, Ni Z, Wang XQ, et al. Downregulation of nitric oxide synthase in chronic renal insufficiency: role of excess PTH. *Am J Physiol* 1998;274:F642.

88. Roczniak A, Fryer JN, Levine DZ, et al. Downregulation of neuronal nitric oxide synthase in the rat remnant kidney. *J Am Soc Nephrol* 1999;10:704.

89. Katoh T, Takahashi K, Klahr S, et al. Dietary supplementation with L-arginine ameliorates glomerular hypertension in rats with subtotal nephrectomy. *J Am Soc Nephrol* 1994;4:1690.

90. Benigni A, Zoja C, Noris M, et al. Renoprotection by nitric oxide donor and lisinopril in the remnant kidney model. *Am J Kidney Dis* 1999;33:746.

91. Tapia E, et al. Role of nitric oxide on glomerular dynamics in arterial hypertension with renal ablation. *J Am Soc Nephrol* 1991;2:484A.

92. Baylis C, Mitruka B, Deng A. Chronic blockade of nitric oxide synthesis in the rat produces systemic hypertension and glomerular damage. *J Clin Invest* 1992;90:278.

93. Ribeiro MO, Antunes E, de Nucci G, et al. Chronic inhibition of nitric oxide synthesis. A new model of arterial hypertension. *Hypertension* 1992;20:298.

94. Hirschberg R, Kopple JD. The growth hormone insulin-like growth factor I axis and renal glomerular function. *J Am Soc Nephrol* 1992;2:1417.

95. Kobayashi S, Venkatachalam MA. Differential effects of caloric restriction on glomeruli and tubules of the remnant kidney. *Kidney Int* 1992;42:710.

96. Rogers SA, Miller SB, Hammerman MR. Enhanced renal IGF-I expression following partial kidney infarction. *Am J Physiol* 1993;264:F963.

97. Haylor JL, McKillop IH, Oldroyd SD, et al. IGF-I inhibitors reduce compensatory hyperfiltration in the isolated rat kidney following unilateral nephrectomy. *Nephrol Dial Transplant* 2000;15:87.

98. Maddox DA, Deen WM, Brenner BM. Glomerular filtration. In: Windhager EE, ed. *Handbook of physiology: Section 8. Renal physiology*. New York: Oxford University, 1992:545.

99. Anderson S, Kennefick TM, Brenner BM. Systemic and renal manifestations of glomerular disease. In: Brenner BM, Rector FC Jr, eds. *The kidney*, 5th ed. Philadelphia: WB Saunders, 1996:1981.

100. Hostetter TH, Meyer TW, Rennke HG, et al. Chronic effects of dietary protein on renal structure and function in the rat with intact and reduced renal mass. *Kidney Int* 1986;30:509.

101. Hakim RM, Goldszer RC, Brenner BM. Hypertension and proteinuria: long-term sequelae of uninephrectomy in humans. *Kidney Int* 1984;25:930.

102. Oliver JD III, et al. Proteinuria and impaired glomerular permselectivity in uninephrectomized fawn-hooded rats. *Am J Physiol* 1994;267:F917.

103. Olson JL, et al. Altered glomerular permselectivity and progressive sclerosis following extreme ablation of renal mass. *Kidney Int* 1982;22:112.

104. Yoshioka T, et al. "Intact nephrons" as the primary origin of proteinuria in chronic renal disease: study in the rat model of subtotal nephrectomy. *J Clin Invest* 1988;82:1614.

105. Mayer G, et al. Effects of angiotensin II receptor blockade on remnant glomerular permselectivity. *Kidney Int* 1993;43:346.

106. Kriz W. Progressive renal failure—inability of podocytes to replicate and the consequences for development of glomerulosclerosis. *Nephrol Dial Transplant* 1996;11:1738.

107. Fine LG, Bradley T. Adaptation of proximal tubular structure and function: insights into compensatory renal hypertrophy. *Fed Proc* 1985;44:2723.

108. Fine LG, Trizna W, Bourgoignie JJ, et al. Functional profile of the isolated uremic nephron: Role of compensatory hypertrophy in the control of fluid reabsorption by the proximal straight tubule. *J Clin Invest* 1978;60:1508.

109. Trizna W, et al. Functional profile of the isolated uremic nephron: evidence of proximal tubular "memory" in experimental renal disease. *J Clin Invest* 1981;68:760.

110. Hayslett JP, Kashgarian M, Epstein FH. Mechanism of change in the excretion of sodium per nephron when renal mass is reduced. *J Clin Invest* 1969;48:1002.

111. Tabei K, Levenson DJ, Brenner BM. Early enhancement of fluid transport in rabbit proximal straight tubules after loss of contralateral renal excretory function. *J Clin Invest* 1983;72:871.

112. Mitchell AD, Valk WL. Compensatory renal hypertrophy. *J Urol* 1962;88:11.

113. Hruska KA, Klahr S, Hammerman MR. Decreased luminal membrane transport of phosphate in chronic renal failure. *Am J Physiol* 1982;242:F17.

114. Harris RC, Seifter JL, Brenner BM. Adaptation of Na+-H+ exchange in renal microvillus membrane vesicles: the role of dietary protein and uninephrectomy. *J Clin Invest* 1984;74:1979.

115. Hayslett JP, Kashgarian M, Epstein FH. Functional correlates of compensatory renal hypertrophy. *J Clin Invest* 1968;47:774.

116. Bank N, Aynedjian HS. Individual nephron function in experimental bilateral pyelonephritis. II. Distal tubular sodium and water reabsorption and the concentrating defect. *J Lab Clin Med* 1966;68:728.

117. Mujais SK, Kurtzman NA. Regulation of renal Na-K-ATPase in the rat: effect of uninephrectomy. *Am J Physiol* 1986;251:F506.

118. Scherzer P, Wald H, Czaczkes JW. Na-K-ATPase in isolated rabbit tubules after unilateral nephrectomy and Na+ loading. *Am J Physiol* 1985;248:F565.

119. Terzi F, Cheval L, Barlet-Bas C, et al. Na-K-ATPase along rat nephron after subtotal nephrectomy: effect of enalapril. *Am J Physiol* 1996;270:F997.

120. Fine LG, et al. Functional profile of the isolated uremic nephron: potassium adaptation in the rabbit cortical collecting tubule. *J Clin Invest* 1979;64:1033.

121. Aizman RI, Rabinowitz L, Mayer-Harnisch C. Early effects of uninephrectomy on K homeostasis in unanesthetized rats. *Am J Physiol* 1996;270:R434.

122. Kaissling B. Structural aspects of adaptive changes in renal electrolyte excretion. *Am J Physiol* 1982;243:F211.

123. Stanton BA, Biemesderfer D, Wade JB, et al. Structural and functional study of the rat distal nephron: effects of potassium adaptation and depletion. *Kidney Int* 1981;19:36.

124. Zalups RK, Stanton BA, Wade JB, et al. Structural adaptation in initial collecting tubule following reduction in renal mass. *Kidney Int* 1985;27:636.

125. Schon DA, Silva P, Hayslett JP. Mechanism of potassium excretion in renal insufficiency. *Am J Physiol* 1974;227:F1323.

126. Finkelstein FO, Hayslett JP. Role of medullary Na-K-ATPase in renal potassium adaptation. *Am J Physiol* 1975;229:F524.

127. Mitch WE, Wilcox CS. Disorders of body fluids, sodium and potassium in chronic renal failure. *Am J Med* 1982;72:536.

128. Slatopolsky E, Elkan IO, Weerts C, et al. Studies on the characteristics of the control system governing sodium excretion in uremic man. *J Clin Invest* 1968;47:521.

129. Wong NLM, Quamme GA, Dirks JH. Tubular handling of bicarbonate in dogs with experimental renal failure. *Kidney Int* 1984;25:912.

130. Lubowitz H, et al. Effect of nephron loss on proximal tubular bicarbonate reabsorption in the rat. *Am J Physiol* 1971;220:457.

131. Schrier RW, Regal EM. Influence of aldosterone on sodium, water and potassium metabolism in chronic renal disease. *Kidney Int* 1972;1:156.

132. Hene RJ, Koomans HA, Boer P, et al. Effect of high-dose aldosterone infusions on renal electrolyte excretion in patients with renal insufficiency. *Am J Nephrol* 1987;7:33.

133. Schmidt RW, Bourgoignie JJ, Bricker NS. On the adaptation in sodium excretion in chronic uremia: The effects of "proportional reduction" of sodium intake. *J Clin Invest* 1974;53:1736.

134. Jackson B, Hodsman P, Johnston CI. Changes in the renin-angiotensin system, exchangeable body sodium, and plasma and atrial content of atrial natriuretic factor during evolution of chronic renal failure in the rat. *Am J Hypertens* 1988;1:298.

135. Yamamoto Y, et al. Plasma concentration of human atrial natriuretic polypeptide in patients with impaired renal function. *Clin Nephrol* 1987;27:84.

136. Suda S, et al. Atrial natriuretic factor in mild to moderate chronic renal failure. *Hypertension* 1988;11:483.

137. Valentin J-P, et al. Effect of monoclonal anti-ANP antibodies on the acute functional adaptation to unilateral nephrectomy. *Kidney Int* 1993;43:1260.

138. Langston JB, Guyton AC, Douglas BH, et al. Effect of changes in salt intake on arterial pressure and renal function in partially nephrectomized dogs. *Circ Res* 1966;12:508.

139. Guyton AC, et al. Salt balance and long-term blood pressure control. *Annu Rev Med* 1980;31:15.

140. Daniels BS, Hostetter TH. Adverse effects of growth in the glomerular microcirculation. *Am J Physiol* 1990;258:F1409.

141. Kwon TH, Frokiaer J, Fernandez-Llama P, et al. Altered expression of Na transporters NHE-3, NaPi-II, Na-K-ATPase, BSC-1, and TSC in CRF rat kidneys. *Am J Physiol* 1999;277:F257.

142. Wen S-F, et al. Micropuncture studies of sodium transport in the remnant kidney of the dog. *J Clin Invest* 1973;52:386.

143. Bourgoignie JJ, Kaplan M, Gavellas G, et al. Sodium homeostasis in dogs with chronic renal insufficiency. *Kidney Int* 1982;21:820.

144. Schultze RG, Shapiro HS, Bricker NS. Studies on the control of sodium excretion in experimental uremia. *J Clin Invest* 1969;48:869.

145. Gutmann FD, Rieselbach RE. Disproportionate inhibition of sodium reabsorption in the unilaterally diseased kidney of dog and man after an acute saline load. *J Clin Invest* 1971;50:422.

146. Coleman AJ, et al. The mechanism of salt wastage in chronic renal disease. *J Clin Invest* 1966;45:116.

147. Gonick HC, Maxwell MH, Rubini ME, et al. Functional impairment in chronic renal disease. I. Studies on sodium conserving ability. *Nephron* 1966;3:137.

148. Danovitch GM, Bourgoignie JJ, Bricker NS. Reversibility of the "salt-losing" tendency of chronic renal failure. *N Engl J Med* 1977;296:14.

149. Schultze RG, et al. On the adaptation in potassium excretion associated with nephron reduction in the dog. *J Clin Invest* 1971;50:1061.

150. Leaf A, Camara AA. Renal tubular secretion of potassium in man. *J Clin Invest* 1949;28:1526.

151. Bank N, Aynedjian HS. A micropuncture study of potassium excretion by the remnant kidney. *J Clin Invest* 1973;52:1480.

152. Bengele HH, Evan A, McNamara ER, et al. Tubular sites of potassium regulation in the normal and uninephrectomized rat. *Am J Physiol* 1978;234:F146.

153. Milanes CL, Jamison RL. Effect of acute potassium load on reabsorption in Henle's loop in chronic renal failure in the rat. *Kidney Int* 1985;27:919.

154. Gonick HC, Kleeman CR, Rubini ME, et al. Functional impairment in chronic renal disease: III. Studies of potassium excretion. *Am J Med Sci* 1971;261:281.

155. Perez GO, et al. Blunted kaliuresis after an acute potassium load in patients with chronic renal failure. *Kidney Int* 1983;24:656.

156. Bastl CP, Hayslett JP, Binder HJ. Increased large intestinal secretion of potassium in renal insufficiency. *Kidney Int* 1977;12:9.

157. Greenblatt DJ, Koch-Weser J. Adverse reactions to spironolactone: a report from the Boston Collaborative Drug Surveillance Program. *JAMA* 1973;225:40.

158. Rimmer JM, Horn JF, Gennari FJ. Hyperkalemia as a complication of drug therapy. *Arch Intern Med* 1987;147:867.

159. Schambelan M, Sebastian A, Biglieri EG. Prevalence, pathogenesis, and functional significance of aldosterone deficiency in hyperkalemic patients with chronic renal insufficiency. *Kidney Int* 1980;17:89.

160. Batlle DC, Arruda JAL, Kurtzman NA. Hyperkalemic distal renal tubular acidosis associated with obstructive uropathy. *N Engl J Med* 1981; 304:373.

161. Emmanouel DS, Lindheimer MD, Katz AI. Urinary concentration and dilution after unilateral nephrectomy in the rat. *Clin Sci Mol Med* 1975; 49:563.

162. Bricker NS, et al. Observations on the concentrating and diluting mechanisms of the diseased kidney. *J Clin Invest* 1959;38:516.

163. Kleeman CR, Adams DA, Maxwell MH. An evaluation of maximal water diuresis in chronic renal disease. 1. Normal solute intake. *J Lab Clin Med* 1961;58:169.

164. Martinez-Maldonado M, Yium JJ, Eknoyan G, et al. Adult polycystic kidney disease: studies of the defect in urine concentration. *Kidney Int* 1972;2:107.

165. Keitel HG, Thompson D, Itano HA. Hyposthenuria in sickle cell anemia: a reversible renal defect. *J Clin Invest* 1956;35:998.

166. Dubach UC, et al. Relationship between regular intake of phenacetin-containing analgesics and laboratory evidence for urorenal disorders in a working female population of Switzerland. *Lancet* 1975;1:539.

167. Arruda JAL. Obstructive uropathy. In: Cotran RS, Brenner BM, Stein JH, eds. *Tubulo-interstitial nephropathy.* New York: Churchill Livingstone, 1983:243.

168. Finkelstein FO, Hayslett JP. Role of medullary structures in the functional adaptation of renal insufficiency. *Kidney Int* 1974;6:419.

169. Fine LG, et al. Functional profile of the isolated uremic nephron: impaired water permeability and adenylate cyclase responsiveness of the cortical collecting tubule to vasopressin. *J Clin Invest* 1978;61: 1519.

170. Wilson DR, Sonnenberg H. Medullary collecting duct function in the remnant kidney before and after volume expansion. *Kidney Int* 1979; 15:487.

171. Pennell JP, Bourgoignie JJ. Water reabsorption by papillary collecting ducts in the remnant kidney. *Am J Physiol* 1982;242:F657.

172. Wrong O, Davies HEF. Excretion of acid in renal disease. *Q J Med* 1959;28:259.

173. Teitelbaum I, McGuinness S. Vasopressin resistance in chronic renal failure. Evidence for the role of decreased V2 receptor mRNA. *J Clin Invest* 1995;96:378.

174. Kwon TH, Frokiaer J, Knepper MA, et al. Reduced AQP1, -2, and -3 levels in kidneys of rats with CRF induced by surgical reduction in renal mass. *Am J Physiol* 1998;275:F724.

175. Elkington JR. Hydrogen ion turnover in health and in renal disease. *Ann Intern Med* 1962;57:660.

176. Simpson DP. Control of hydrogen ion homeostasis and renal acidosis. *Medicine* 1971;50:503.

177. Widmer B, Gerhardt RE, Harrington JT, et al. Serum electrolyte and acid base composition: The influence of graded degrees of chronic renal failure. *Arch Intern Med* 1979;139:1099.

178. Dorhout-Mees EJ, et al. The functional adaptation of the diseased kidney. III. Ammonium excretion. *J Clin Invest* 1966;45:289.

179. Schoolwerth AC, Sandler RS, Hoffsten PM, et al. Effects of nephron reduction and dietary protein content on renal ammoniagenesis in the rat. *Kidney Int* 1975;7:397.

180. Buerkert J, Martin D, Trigg D, et al. Effect of reduced renal mass on ammonium handling and net acid formation by the superficial and juxtamedullary nephron of the rat: evidence of impaired re-entrapment rather than decreased production of ammonium in the acidosis of uremia. *J Clin Invest* 1983;71:1661.

181. Ohno A, Beck FX, Pfaller W, et al. Effects of chronic hyperfiltration on proximal tubule bicarbonate transport and cell electrolytes. *Kidney Int* 1995;48:712.

182. Maddox DA, Horn JF, Famiano FC, et al. Load dependence of proximal tubule fluid and bicarbonate reabsorption in the remnant kidney of the Munich-Wistar rat. *J Clin Invest* 1986;77:1639.

183. Bank N, Su W-S, Aynedjian HS. A micropuncture study of HCO3 reabsorption by the hypertrophied proximal tubule. *Yale J Biol Med* 1978;51:275.

184. Schwartz WB, et al. On the mechanism of acidosis in chronic renal failure. *J Clin Invest* 1959;38:39.

185. Schwartz WB, Relman AS. Acidosis in renal disease. *N Engl J Med* 1957;256:1184.

186. Arruda JAL, Nascimento L, Arevelo G, et al. Bicarbonate reabsorption in chronic renal failure; studies in man and the rat. *Pflugers Arch* 1978;376:193.

187. Muldowney FP. Renal acidosis. In: Black D, Jones NF, eds. *Renal disease,* 4th ed. Oxford: Blackwell Scientific, 1979:588.

188. Slatopolsky E, Hoffsten P, Purkerson M, et al. On the influence of extracellular fluid volume expansion on bicarbonate reabsorption in the rat. *J Clin Invest* 1969;48:1754.

189. Sastrasinh S, Tanenn RL. Effect of potassium on renal NH3 production. *Am J Physiol* 1983;244:F383.

190. Muldowney FP, et al. Parathyroid acidosis in uremia. *Q J Med* 1972; 41:321.

191. Dennis VW. Influence of bicarbonate on parathyroid hormone-induced changes in fluid absorption by the proximal tubule. *Kidney Int* 1976; 10:373.

192. Wilson DR, Siddiqui AA. Renal tubular acidosis after kidney transplantation. *Ann Intern Med* 1973;79:352.

193. Shioji R, et al. Sjögren's syndrome and renal tubular acidosis. *Ann J Med* 1970;48:456.

194. Goldman R, Bassett SH. Phosphorous excretion in renal failure. *J Clin Invest* 1954;33:1623.

195. Slatopolsky E, Robson AM, Elkan I, et al. Control of phosphate excretion in uremic man. *J Clin Invest* 1968;47:1865.

196. Coburn JW, Popovtzer MM, Massry SG, et al. The physicochemical state and renal handling of divalent ions in chronic renal failure. *Arch Intern Med* 1969;124:302.

197. Popovtzer MM, Schainuck LI, Massry SG, et al. Divalent ion excretion in chronic kidney disease: relation to degree of renal insufficiency. *Clin Sci* 1970;38:297.

198. Slatopolsky E, et al. The control of phosphate excretion in uremia. *J Clin Invest* 1966;45:672.

199. Slatopolsky E, et al. On the pathogenesis of hyperparathyroidism in chronic experimental renal insufficiency in the dog. *J Clin Invest* 1971; 50:492.

200. Slatopolsky E, et al. On the prevention of secondary hyperparathyroidism in experimental chronic renal disease using "proportional reduction" of dietary phosphorous intake. *Kidney Int* 1972;2:147.

201. Kaplan MA, et al. Reversal of hyperparathyroidism in response to dietary phosphorus restriction in the uremic dog. *Kidney Int* 1979;15:43.

202. Bricker NS. On the pathogenesis of the uremic state: an exposition of the "trade off hypothesis." *N Engl J Med* 1972;286:1093.

203. Bricker NS, et al. Calcium, phosphorus, and bone in renal disease and transplantation. *Arch Intern Med* 1969;123:543.

204. Milanes CL, et al. Altered response of adenylate cyclase to parathyroid hormone during compensatory renal growth. *Kidney Int* 1989;36:802.

205. Caverzasio J, Gloor HJ, Fleisch H, et al. Parathyroid hormone-independent adaptation of the renal handling of phosphate in response to renal mass reduction. *Kidney Int* 1982;21:471.

206. Kraus E, et al. Phosphate excretion in uremic rats: effects of parathyroidectomy and phosphate restriction. *Am J Physiol* 1985;248:F175.

207. Swenson RS, Weisinger JR, Ruggeri JL, et al. Evidence that parathyroid hormone is not required for phosphate homeostasis in renal failure. *Metabolism* 1975;24:199.

208. Isaac J, et al. Catecholamines and phosphate excretion by the remnant kidney. *Kidney Int* 1993;43:1021.

209. Bank N, Su W-S, Aynedjian HS. A micropuncture study of renal phosphate transport in rats with chronic renal failure and secondary hyperparathyroidism. *J Clin Invest* 1978;61:884.

210. Wen S-F, Stoll RW. Renal phosphate adaptation in uraemic dogs with a remnant kidney. *Clin Sci* 1981;60:273.

211. Yanagawa N, et al. Functional profile of the isolated uremic nephron: intrinsic adaptation of phosphate transport in the rabbit proximal tubule. *Kidney Int* 1983;23:674.

212. Better OS, et al. Renal handling of calcium, magnesium and inorganic phosphate in chronic renal failure. *Isr J Med Sci* 1967;3:60.

213. Finkelstein FO, Kliger AS. Medullary structures in calcium reabsorption in rats with renal insufficiency. *Am J Physiol* 1977;233:F197.

214. Ortola FV, Ballermann BJ, Brenner BM. Endogenous ANP augments fractional excretion of Pi, Ca, and Na in rats with reduced renal mass. *Am J Physiol* 1988;255:F1091.

215. Addis T. The ratio between the urea content of the urine and of the blood after the administration of large quantities of urea: an approximate index of the quantity of actively functioning kidney tissue. *J Urol* 1917;1:263.

216. Rennke HG. Pathology of glomerular hyperfiltration. In: Mitch WE, Brenner BM, Stein JH, eds. *The progressive nature of renal disease.* New York: Churchill Livingstone, 1986:111.

217. Rennke HG, Anderson S, Brenner BM. Structural and functional correlations in the progression of renal disease. In: Tisher CC, Brenner BM, eds. *Renal pathology,* 2nd ed. Philadelphia: JB Lippincott, 1994:116.

218. Fine LG. The biology of renal hypertrophy. *Kidney Int* 1986;29:619.

219. Oliver J. The regulation of renal activity. X. The morphologic study. *Arch Intern Med* 1924;34:258.

220. Addis T, Meyers BA, Oliver J. The regulation of renal activity. IX. The effect of unilateral nephrectomy on the function and structure of the remaining kidney. *Arch Intern Med* 1924;34:243.

221. Olivetti G, et al. Morphometry of the renal corpuscle during normal postnatal growth and compensatory hypertrophy: a light microscope study. *J Cell Biol* 1977;75:573.

222. Shea SM, Raskova J, Morrison AB. A stereologic study of glomerular hypertrophy in the subtotally nephrectomized rat. *Am J Pathol* 1978;90:201.

223. Bidani AK, et al. Absence of glomerular injury or nephron loss in a normotensive rat remnant kidney model. *Kidney Int* 1990;38:28.

224. Schwartz MM, Evans J, Bidani AK. The mesangium in the long-term remnant kidney model. *J Lab Clin Med* 1994;124:644.

225. Nagata M, Kriz W. Glomerular damage after uninephrectomy in young rats. I. Hypertrophy and distortion of capillary architecture. *Kidney Int* 1992;42:136.

226. Nagata M, Schärer K, Kriz W. Glomerular damage after uninephrectomy in young rats. II. Mechanical stress on podocytes as a pathway to sclerosis. *Kidney Int* 1992;42:148.

227. Seyer-Hansen K, Hansen J, Gundersen HJG. Renal hypertrophy in experimental diabetes: a morphometric study. *Diabetologia* 1980;18:501.

228. Olivetti G, Anversa P, Melissari M, et al. Morphometry of the renal corpuscle during postnatal growth and compensatory hypertrophy. *Kidney Int* 1980;17:438.

229. Schwartz MM, Bidani AK. Mesangial structure and function in the remnant kidney. *Kidney Int* 1991;40:226.

230. Nyengaard JR. Number and dimensions of rat glomerular capillaries in normal development and after nephrectomy. *Kidney Int* 1993;43:1049.

231. Kanda S, et al. Peritubular endothelial cell proliferation in mice during compensatory renal growth after unilateral nephrectomy. *Am J Physiol* 1993;265:F712.

232. Lax DS, Benstein JA, Tolbert E, et al. Effects of salt restriction on renal growth and glomerular injury in rats with remnant kidneys. *Kidney Int* 1992;41:1527.

233. Oliver JD III, et al. Proteinuria and impaired glomerular permselectivity in uninephrectomized fawn-hooded rats. *Am J Physiol* 1994;267:F917.

234. Shea SM, Raskova J. Glomerular hemodynamics and vascular structure in uremia: a network analysis of glomerular path lengths and maximal blood transit times computed for a microvascular model reconstructed from serial ultrathin sections. *Microvasc Res* 1984;28:37.

235. Knutson DW, Chieu F, Bennett CM, et al. Estimation of relative glomerular capillary surface area in normal and hypertrophic rat kidneys. *Kidney Int* 1978;14:437.

236. Salehmoghaddam S, et al. Hypertrophy of basolateral Na-K pump activity in the proximal tubule of the remnant kidney. *Lab Invest* 1985;53:443.

237. Oliver J. New direction in renal morphology: a method, its results and its future. *Harvey Lecture Series* 1945;XL:102.

238. Johnston JR, Brenner BM, Hebert SC. Uninephrectomy and dietary protein affect fluid absorption in rabbit proximal straight tubules. *Am J Physiol* 1987;253:F222.

239. Vehaskari VM, Hering-Smith KS, Klahr S, et al. Increased sodium transport by cortical collecting tubules from remnant kidneys. *Kidney Int* 1989;36:89.

240. Zalups RK, Henderson DA. Cellular morphology in outer medullary collecting duct: effect of 75% nephrectomy and K+ depletion. *Am J Physiol* 1992;263:F1119.

241. Preuss HG, ed. Symposium on compensatory renal growth. *Kidney Int* 1983;23:569.

242. Malt R. Compensatory growth of the kidney. *N Engl J Med* 1969;280:1446.

243. Wesson LG. Compensatory growth and other growth responses of the kidney. *Nephron* 1989;51:149.

244. Norman JT, Fine LG. Renal growth and hypertrophy. In: Massry SG, Glassock RJ, eds. *Textbook of nephrology.* Baltimore: Williams & Wilkins, 1995:146.

245. Fine LG, Norman J. Cellular events in renal hypertrophy. *Annu Rev Physiol* 1989;51:19.

246. Wolf G. Cellular mechanisms of tubule hypertrophy and hyperplasia in renal injury. *Miner Electrolyte Metab* 1995;21:303.

247. Terzi F, Burtin M, Friedlander G. Early molecular mechanisms in the progression of renal failure: role of growth factors and protooncogenes. *Kidney Int* 1998;53:S68.

248. Sacerdotti C. Über die compensatorische hypertrophie der nieren. *Virchows Arch Pathol Anat* 1896;146:267.

249. Flanigan WS, Burns RO, Takacs FJ, et al. Serial studies of glomerular filtration rate and renal plasma flow in kidney transplant donors, identical twins and allograft recipients. *Am J Surg* 1968;116:788.

250. Gazdiar AF, Dammin GJ. Neural degeneration and regeneration in human renal transplants. *N Engl J Med* 1970;283:222.

251. Malt RA. Humoral factors in regulation of compensatory renal hypertrophy. *Kidney Int* 1983;23:611.

252. Braun Menéndez E. Hypertension and relation between kidney and body weight. *Stanford Med Bull* 1952:10:65.

253. Lowenstein LM, Stern A. Serum factor in renal compensatory hyperplasia. *Science* 1963;142:1479.

254. Preuss HG, Goldin H. A renotropic system in rats. *J Clin Invest* 1976;57:94.

255. Gaydos DS, et al. Partial characterization of a renotropic factor. *Renal Physiol* 1983;6:139.

256. Harris RH, Hise MK, Best CF. Renotropic factors in urine. *Kidney Int* 1983;23:616.

257. Yamamoto H, Kanetake H, Yamada J. In vitro evidence from tissue cultures to prove existence of rabbit and human renotropic growth factor. *Kidney Int* 1983;23:624.

258. Kanda S, et al. A study of growth regulators of renal cortical tubular cells in the rabbit liver. *Kidney Int* 1990;37:875.

259. Preuss HG. Does renotropin have a role in the pathogenesis of hypertension? *Am J Hypertens* 1989;2:65.

260. Shankland SJ, Wolf G. Cell cycle regulatory proteins in renal disease: role in hypertrophy, proliferation, and apoptosis. *Am J Physiol* 2000;278:F515.

261. Nowinski WW. Early history of renal hypertrophy. In: Nowinski WW, Goss RJ, eds. *Compensatory renal hypertrophy.* New York: Academic, 1969:1.

262. Johnson HA, Roman JMV. Compensatory renal enlargement: hypertrophy versus hyperplasia. *Am J Pathol* 1966;49:1.

263. Ouellette AJ. Messenger RNA regulation during compensatory renal growth. *Kidney Int* 1983;23:575.

264. Ouellette AJ, Moonka R, Zelenetz AD, et al. Regulation of ribosome synthesis during compensatory renal hypertrophy in mice. *Am J Physiol* 1987;253:C506.

265. Ouellette AJ, Malt RA, Sukhatme VP, et al. Expression of two "immediate early" genes, Egr-1 and c-fos, in response to renal ischemia and during compensatory renal hypertrophy in mice. *J Clin Invest* 1990;85:766.

266. Melvin WT, Kumar A, Malt RA. Conservation of ribosomal RNA during compensatory renal hypertrophy: a major mechanism in RNA accretion. *J Cell Biol* 1976;69:548.

267. Goss RJ, Rankin M. Physiological factors affecting compensatory renal hyperplasia in the rat. *J Exp Zool* 1960;145:209.

268. Williams GEG. Effect of starvation and of adrenalectomy on compensatory hyperplasia of the kidney. *Nature* 1962;196:1221.

269. Argyris TS, Trimble ME, Janicki R. Control of induced kidney growth. In: Nowinski WW, Goss RJ, eds. *Compensatory renal hypertrophy.* New York: Academic, 1969:45.

270. Halliburton IW, Thomson RY. Chemical aspects of compensatory renal hypertrophy. *Cancer Res* 1967;25:1882.

271. Threlfall G, Taylor DM, Buck AT. Studies of changes in growth and DNA synthesis in the rat kidney during experimentally induced renal hypertrophy. *Am J Pathol* 1967;50:1.

272. Dicker SE, Shirley DG. Compensatory renal growth after unilateral nephrectomy in the newborn rat. *J Physiol* 1973;228:193.

273. Barrows CH Jr. Aging in the kidney. In: Nowinski WW, Goss RJ, eds. *Compensatory renal hypertrophy.* New York: Academic, 1969:283.

274. Zumoff B, Pachter MR. Studies of rat kidney and liver growth using total nuclear counts. *Am J Anat* 1964;114:479.

275. Celsi G, Jakobsson B, Aperia A. Influence of age on compensatory renal growth in rats. *Pediatr Res* 1986;20:347.

276. Austin HA, Goldin H, Gaydos D, et al. Polyamine metabolism in compensatory renal growth. *Kidney Int* 1983;23:581.

277. Humphreys MH, et al. Renal ornithine decarboxylase activity, polyamines, and compensatory renal hypertrophy in the rat. *Am J Physiol* 1988;255:F270.

278. Schlondorff D, Weber H. Cyclic nucleotide metabolism in compensatory renal hypertrophy and neonatal kidney growth. *Proc Natl Acad Sci USA* 1976;73:524.

279. Caramelo C, Tsai P, Okada K, et al. Protein kinase C activity in compensatory renal growth. *BBRC* 1988;152:315.

280. Toback FG. Phosphatidylcholine metabolism during renal growth and regeneration. *Am J Physiol* 1984;246:F249.

281. Hise MK, Harris RH, Mansbach CM II. Regulation of de novo phosphatidylcholine biosynthesis during renal growth. *Am J Physiol* 1984;247:F260.

282. Kasiske BL, Ma JZ, Louis TA, et al. Long-term effects of reduced renal mass in humans. *Kidney Int* 1995;48:814.

283. Cortes P, Riser BL, Zhao X, et al. Glomerular volume expansion and mesangial cell mechanical strain: mediators of glomerular pressure injury. *Kidney Int* 1994;45:S11.

284. Cortes P, Zhao X, Riser BL, et al. Regulation of glomerular volume in normal and partially nephrectomized rats. *Am J Physiol* 1996; 270:F356.

285. Igawa T, et al. Hepatocyte growth factor is a potent mitogen for cultured rabbit renal tubular epithelial cells. *Biochem Biophys Res Commun* 1991;174:831.

286. Fine LG, Hammerman MR, Abboud HE. Evolving role of growth factors in the renal response to acute and chronic disease. *J Am Soc Nephrol* 1992;2:1163.

287. Mendley SR, Toback FG. Cell proliferation in the end-stage kidney. *Am J Kidney Dis* 1990;16:80.

288. Kujubu DA, Fine LG. Polypeptide growth factors and their relation to renal disease. *Am J Kidney Dis* 1989;14:61.

289. Wolf G, Neilson EG. Angiotensin II as a renal growth factor. *J Am Soc Nephrol* 1993;3:1531.

290. Miller PL, Rennke HG, Meyer TW. Glomerular hypertrophy accelerates hypertensive glomerular injury in rats. *Am J Physiol* 1991; 261:F459.

291. Wu LL, Cox A, Roe CJ, et al. Transforming growth factor beta 1 and renal injury following subtotal nephrectomy in the rat: role of the renin-angiotensin system. *Kidney Int* 1997;51:1553.

292. Lajara R, et al. Dual regulation of insulin-like growth factor I expression during renal hypertrophy. *Am J Physiol* 1989;257:F252.

293. Miller SB, Hansen VA, Hammerman MR. Effects of growth hormone and IGF-I on renal function in rats with normal and reduced renal mass. *Am J Physiol* 1990;259:F747.

294. Quaife CJ, et al. Histopathology associated with elevated levels of growth hormone and insulin-like growth factor I in transgenic mice. *Endocrinology* 1989;124:40.

295. Mehls O, et al. Effects of rhGH and rhIGF-1 on renal growth and morphology. *Kidney Int* 1993;44:1251.

296. Stiles AD, Sosenko IR, Dercole AJ, et al. Relation of kidney tissue somatomedin-C/insulin-like growth factor I to postnephrectomy renal growth in the rat. *Endocrinology* 1985;117:2397.

297. Fagin JA, Melmed S. Relative increase in insulin-like growth factor I messenger ribonucleic acid levels in compensatory renal hypertrophy. *Endocrinology* 1987;120:718.

298. Flyvbjerg A, et al. Kidney tissue somatomedin C and initial renal growth in diabetic and uninephrectomized rats. *Diabetologia* 1988; 31:310.

299. Hise MK, et al. Insulin-like growth factor-I receptor and binding proteins in rat kidney after nephron loss. *J Am Soc Nephrol* 1993;4:62.

300. El Nahas AM, Le Carpentier JE, Bassett AH. Compensatory renal growth: role of growth hormone and insulin-like growth factor-I. *Nephrol Dial Transplant* 1990;5:123.

301. Mulroney SE, Koenig JI, Csikos T, et al. Temporal changes in insulin-like growth factor I, c-fos, and c-jun gene expression during hyperplastic kidney growth in weanling rats. *Endocrinology* 1996;137:839.

302. Evan AP, Henry DP, Connors BA, et al. Analysis of insulin-like growth factors (IGF)-I, and -II, type II IGF receptor and IGF-binding protein-2 mRNA and peptide levels in normal and nephrectomized rat kidney. *Kidney Int* 1995;48:1517.

303. Hise MK, Li L, Mantzouris N, Rohan RM. Differential mRNA expression of insulin-like growth factor system during renal injury and hypertrophy. *Am J Physiol* 1995;269:F817.

304. Doi T, Striker LJ, Quaife C, et al. Progressive glomerulosclerosis develops in transgenic mice chronically expressing growth hormone and growth hormone releasing factor but not in those expressing insulinlike growth factor-1. *Am J Pathol* 1988;131:398.

305. Doublier S, Seurin D, Fouqueray B, et al. Glomerulosclerosis in mice transgenic for human insulin-like growth factor-binding protein-1. *Kidney Int* 2000;57:2299.

306. Behrens MT, Corbin AL, Hise MK. Epidermal growth factor receptor regulation in rat kidney: two models of renal growth. *Am J Physiol* 1989;257:F105.

307. Sack EM, Arruda JA. Epidermal growth factor binding to cortical basolateral membranes in compensatory renal hypertrophy. *Regul Peptides* 1991;33:339.

308. Miller SB, Rogers SA, Estes CE, et al. Increased distal nephron EGF content and altered distribution of peptide in compensatory renal hypertrophy. *Am J Physiol* 1992;262:F1032.

309. Nagaike M, et al. Renotropic functions of hepatocyte growth factor in renal regeneration after unilateral nephrectomy. *J Biol Chem* 1991;266:22781.

310. Yanagita K, et al. Lung may have an endocrine function producing hepatocyte growth factor in response to injury of distal organs. *BBRC* 1992;182:802.

311. Montesano R, Matsumoto K, Nakamura T, et al. Identification of a fibroblast-derived epithelial morphogen as hepatocyte growth factor. *Cell* 1991;67:901.

312. Schlondorff D, Trizna W, DeRosis E, et al. Effect of testosterone on compensatory renal hypertrophy in the rat. *Endocrinology* 1977; 101:1670.

313. Blantz RC, Peterson OW, Blantz ER, et al. Sexual differences in glomerular ultrafiltration: effect of androgen administration in ovariectomized rats. *Endocrinology* 1988;122:767.

314. Shukla A, Shukla GS, Radin NS. Control of kidney size by sex hormones: possible involvement of glucosylceramide. *Am J Physiol* 1992;262:F24.

315. Silbiger SR, Neugarten J. The impact of gender on the progression of chronic renal disease. *Am J Kidney Dis* 1995;25:515.

316. Liu PL, Gallery ED, Grigg R, et al. Renal function in unilateral nephrectomy subjects. *J Urol* 1992;147:337.

317. Mulroney SE, Woda C, Johnson M, et al. Gender differences in renal growth and function after uninephrectomy in adult rats. *Kidney Int* 1999;56:944.

318. Mulroney SE, Pesce C. Early hyperplastic renal growth after uninephrectomy in adult female rats. *Endocrinology* 2000;141:932.

319. Norman JT, et al. Patterns of mRNA expression during early cell growth differ in kidney epithelial cells destined to undergo compensatory hypertrophy versus regenerative hyperplasia. *Proc Natl Acad Sci USA* 1988;85:6768.

320. Beer DG, Zweifel KA, Simpson DP, et al. Specific gene expression during compensatory renal hypertrophy in the rat. *J Cell Physiol* 1987; 131:29.

321. Sawczuk IS, Olsson CA, Hoke G, et al. Immediate induction of c-fos and c-myc transcripts following unilateral nephrectomy. *Nephron* 1990;55:193.

322. Nakamura T, et al. Gene expression of growth-related proteins and ECM constituents in response to unilateral nephrectomy. *Am J Physiol* 1992;262:F389.

323. Kujubu DA, Norman JT, Herschman HR, et al. Primary response gene expression in renal hypertrophy and hyperplasia: evidence for different growth initiation processes. *Am J Physiol* 1991;260:F823.

324. Terzi F, et al. Subtotal but not unilateral nephrectomy induces hyperplasia and protooncogene expression. *Am J Physiol* 1995;268: F793.

325. Pravenec M, Zidek V, Musilova A, et al. Chromosomal mapping of a major quantitative trait locus regulating compensatory renal growth in the rat. *J Am Soc Nephrol* 2000;11:1261.

326. Galla JH, Klein-Robbenhaar T, Hayslett JP. Influence of age on the compensatory response in growth and function to unilateral nephrectomy. *Yale J Biol Med* 1974;47:218.

327. MacKay EM, Mackay LL, Addis T. The degree of compensatory renal hypertrophy following unilateral nephrectomy. I. The influence of age. *J Exp Med* 1932;56:225.

328. O'Donnell MP, Kasiske BL, Raij L, et al. Age is a determinant of the glomerular morphologic and functional responses to chronic nephron loss. *J Lab Clin Med* 1985;106:308.

329. Dicker SE, Shirley DG. Mechanism of compensatory renal hypertrophy. *J Physiol* 1971;219:507.

330. Kenner CH, et al. Effect of protein intake on renal function and structure in partially nephrectomized rats. *Kidney Int* 1985;27:739.

331. Kaysen GA, Rosenthal C, Hutchison FN. GFR increases before renal mass or ODC activity increase in rats fed high protein diets. *Kidney Int* 1989;36:441.

332. Jarusiripipat C, Shapiro JI, Chan L, et al. Reduction of remnant nephron hypermetabolism by protein restriction. *Am J Kidney Dis* 1991;18:367.

333. Benstein JA, Feiner HD, Parker M, et al. Superiority of salt restriction over diuretics in reducing renal hypertrophy and injury in uninephrectomized SHR. *Am J Physiol* 1990;258:F1675.

334. Klahr S, Buerkert J, Purkerson ML. Role of dietary factors in the progression of chronic renal disease. *Kidney Int* 1983;24:579.

335. Kleinknecht C, et al. Role of amount and nature of carbohydrates in the course of experimental renal failure. *Kidney Int* 1986;30:687.

336. Bouby N, Bachmann S, Bichet D, et al. Effect of water intake on the progression of chronic renal failure in the 5/6 nephrectomized rat. *Am J Physiol* 1990;258:F973.

337. Dicker SE, Greenbaum AL, Morris CA. Compensatory renal hypertrophy in hypophysectomized rats. *J Physiol* 1977;273:241.

338. Poffenbarger PL, Prince MJ. The role of serum nonsuppressible insulin-like activity (NSILA) in compensatory renal growth. *Growth* 1976;40:83.

339. Torres VE, et al. The progression of vesicoureteral reflux. *Ann Intern Med* 1980;92:776.

340. Bradley SE, Coelho JB. Glomerulotubular dimensional readjustments during compensatory renal hypertrophy in the hypothyroid rat. *Yale J Biol Med* 1978;51:327.

341. Reiter RJ. The endocrines and compensatory renal enlargement. In: Nowinski WW, Gross RJ, eds. *Compensatory renal hypertrophy.* New York: Academic, 1969:183.

342. Basinger GT, Gittes RF. Compensatory renal hypertrophy in male dwarf mice. *Invest Urol* 1975;13:165.

343. Hutson JM, et al. Compensatory renal growth in the mouse. II. The effect of growth hormone deficiency. *Pediatr Res* 1981;15:1375.

344. Cotran R. Glomerulosclerosis in reflux nephropathy. *Kidney Int* 1982;21:528.

345. Kleinknecht D, et al. Diagnostic procedures and long-term prognosis in bilateral renal cortical necrosis. *Kidney Int* 1973;4:390.

346. Kincaid-Smith P. Analgesic nephropathy. *Kidney Int* 1978;13:1.

347. Baldwin DS. Chronic glomerulonephritis: nonimmunologic mechanisms of progressive glomerular damage. *Kidney Int* 1982;21:109.

348. Finn WF. Recovery from acute renal failure. In: Brenner BM, Lazarus JM, eds. *Acute renal failure,* 2nd ed. New York: Churchill Livingstone, 1988:875.

349. Georgaki-Angelaki HN, Steed DB, Chantler C, et al. Renal function following acute renal failure in childhood: a long term follow-up study. *Kidney Int* 1989;35:84.

350. Royer P, Habib R, Leclerc F. L'hypoplasie renale bilaterale avec oligomeganephronie. In: Schreiner GE, ed. *Proceedings of the 3rd International Congress on Nephrology,* vol 2. Basel: Karger, 1967:251.

351. Kiprov DD, Colvin RB, McCluskey RT. Focal and segmental glomerulosclerosis and proteinuria associated with unilateral renal agenesis. *Lab Invest* 1982;46:275.

352. Brenner BM, Meyer TW, Hostetter TH. Dietary protein intake and the progressive nature of kidney disease. *N Engl J Med* 1982;307:652.

353. Anderson S, Brenner BM. The role of nephron mass and of intraglomerular pressure in initiation and progression of experimental hypertensive-renal disorders. In: Laragh JH, Brenner BM, eds. *Hypertension: pathophysiology, diagnosis and management,* 2nd ed. New York: Raven, 1995:1553.

354. Portaluppi F, et al. Loss of nocturnal decline of blood pressure in hypertension due to chronic renal failure. *Am J Hypertens* 1991;4:20.

355. Nielsen FS, Rossing P, Bang LE, et al. On the mechanisms of blunted nocturnal decline in arterial blood pressure in NIDDM patients with diabetic nephropathy. *Diabetes* 1995;44:783.

356. Brazy PC, Stead WW, Fitzwilliam JF. Progression of renal insufficiency: role of blood pressure. *Kidney Int* 1989;35:670.

357. Lindeman RD, Tobin JD, Shock NW. Association between blood pressure and the rate of decline in renal function with age. *Kidney Int* 1984;26:861.

358. El Nahas AM, Mallick NP, Anderson S, eds. *Prevention of chronic renal failure.* Oxford: Oxford University, 1993.

359. Zatz R, et al. Prevention of diabetic glomerulopathy by pharmacological amelioration of glomerular capillary hypertension. *J Clin Invest* 1986;77:1925.

360. Dworkin LD, Feiner HD. Glomerular injury in uninephrectomized spontaneously hypertensive rats: a consequence of glomerular capillary hypertension. *J Clin Invest* 1986;77:797.

361. Anderson S, Diamond JR, Karnovsky MJ, et al. Mechanisms underlying transition from acute glomerular injury to glomerulosclerosis in a rat model of nephrotic syndrome. *J Clin Invest* 1988;82:1757.

362. Gabbai FB, Gushwa LC, Wilson CB, et al. An evaluation of the development of experimental membranous nephropathy. *Kidney Int* 1987;31:1267.

363. Eddy AA. Molecular insights into renal interstitial fibrosis. *J Am Soc Nephrol* 1996;7:2495.

364. Diamond JR, Anderson S. Irreversible tubulointerstitial damage associated with chronic aminonucleoside nephrosis. Amelioration by angiotensin I enzyme inhibition. *Am J Pathol* 1990;137:1323.

365. Bohle A, Strutz F, Muller GA. On the pathogenesis of chronic renal failure in primary glomerulopathies: a view from the interstitium. *Exp Nephrol* 1994;2:205.

366. Mackensen-Haen S, Bohle A, Christensen J, et al. The consequences for renal function of widening of the interstitium and changes in the tubular epithelium of the renal cortex and outer medulla in various renal diseases. *Clin Nephrol* 1992;37:70.

367. Roy-Chaudhury P, Hillis G, McDonald S, et al. Importance of the tubulointerstitium in human glomerulonephritis. II. Distribution of integrin chains beta 1, alpha 1 to 6 and alpha V. *Kidney Int* 1997;52:103.

368. Muller GA, Rodemann HP. Characterization of human renal fibroblasts in health and disease: I. Immunophenotyping of cultured tubular epithelial cells and fibroblasts derived from kidneys with histologically proven interstitial fibrosis. *Am J Kidney Dis* 1991;17:680.

369. Ng YY, Huang TP, Yang WC, et al. Tubular epithelial-myofibroblast transdifferentiation in progressive tubulointerstitial fibrosis in 5/6 nephrectomized rats. *Kidney Int* 1998;54:864.

370. Diamond JR, Pesek-Diamond I. Sublethal X-irradiation during acute puromycin nephrosis prevents late renal injury: role of macrophages. *Am J Physiol* 1991;260:F779.

371. Saito T, Atkins RC. Contribution of mononuclear leucocytes to the progression of experimental focal glomerular sclerosis. *Kidney Int* 1990;37:1076.

372. Fujihara CK, Malheiros DM, Zatz R, et al. Mycophenolate mofetil attenuates renal injury in the rat remnant kidney. *Kidney Int* 1998;54:1510.

373. Remuzzi G, Zoja C, Gagliardini E, et al. Combining an antiproteinuric approach with mycophenolate mofetil fully suppresses progressive nephropathy of experimental animals. *J Am Soc Nephrol* 1999;10:1542.

374. Romero F, Rodriguez-Iturbe B, Parra G, et al. Mycophenolate mofetil prevents the progressive renal failure induced by 5/6 renal ablation in rats. *Kidney Int* 1999;55:945.

375. Fujihara CK, De Lourdes Noronha I, Malheiros, et al. Combined mycophenolate mofetil and losartan therapy arrests established injury in the remnant kidney. *J Am Soc Nephrol* 2000;11:283.

376. Ichikawa I, Harris RC. Angiotensin actions in the kidney: renewed insight into the old hormone. *Kidney Int* 1991;40:583.

377. Harris RC, Martinez-Maldonado M. Angiotensin II-mediated renal injury. *Miner Electrolyte Metab* 1995;21:328.

378. Taal MW, Brenner BM. Renoprotective benefits of RAS inhibition: from ACEI to angiotensin II antagonists. *Kidney Int* 2000;57:1803.

379. Border WA, Brees D, Noble NA. Transforming growth factor-beta and extracellular matrix deposition in the kidney. *Contrib Nephrol* 1994;107:140.

380. Basile DP, Martin DR, Hammerman MR. Extracellular matrix-related genes in the kidney after ischemic injury: potential role for TGF-beta in repair. *Am J Physiol* 1998;275:F894.

381. Lee LK, Meyer TW, Pollock AS, et al. Endothelial cell injury initiates glomerular sclerosis in the rat remnant kidney. *J Clin Invest* 1995;96:953.

382. Sporn MB, Roberts AB. Transforming growth factor-beta. Multiple actions and potential clinical implications. *JAMA* 1989;262:938.

383. Tomooka S, Border WA, Marshall BC, et al. Glomerular matrix accumulation is linked to inhibition of the plasmin protease system. *Kidney Int* 1992;42:1462.

384. Kagami S, Kuhara T, Okada K, et al. Dual effects of angiotensin II on the plasminogen/plasmin system in rat mesangial cells. *Kidney Int* 1997;51:664.

385. Baricos WH, Cortez SL, Deboisblanc M, et al. Transforming growth factor-beta is a potent inhibitor of extracellular matrix degradation by cultured human mesangial cells. *J Am Soc Nephrol* 1999;10:790.

386. Kagami S, Border WA, Ruoslahti E, et al. Coordinated expression of ß1 integrins and transforming growth-factor-ß-induced matrix proteins in glomerulonephritis. *Lab Invest* 1993;69:68.

387. Schnermann JB, Zhu XL, Shu X, et al. Regulation of endothelin production and secretion in cultured collecting duct cells by endogenous transforming growth factor-beta. *Endocrinology* 1996;137:5000.

388. Junaid A, Hostetter TH, Rosenberg ME. Interaction of angiotensin II and TGF-ß1 in the rat remnant kidney. *J Am Soc Nephrol* 1997;8:1732.

389. Gomez-Garre D, Largo R, Liu XH, et al. An orally active ETA/ETB receptor antagonist ameliorates proteinuria and glomerular lesions in rats with proliferative nephritis. *Kidney Int* 1996;50:962.

390. Ong AC, Jowett TP, Firth JD, et al. An endothelin-1 mediated autocrine growth loop involved in human renal tubular regeneration. *Kidney Int* 1995;48:390.

391. Egido J. Vasoactive hormones and renal sclerosis. *Kidney Int* 1996;49:578.

392. Hocher B, Thone-Reineke C, Rohmeiss P, et al. Endothelin-1 transgenic mice develop glomerulosclerosis, interstitial fibrosis, and renal cysts but not hypertension. *J Clin Invest* 1997;99:1380.

393. Huwiler A, Stabel S, Fabbro D, et al. Platelet-derived growth factor and angiotensin II stimulate the mitogen-activated protein kinase cascade in renal mesangial cells: comparison of hypertrophic and hyperplastic agonists. *Biochem J* 1995;305:777.

394. Tang WW, Ulich TR, Lacey DL, et al. Platelet-derived growth factor-BB induces renal tubulointerstitial myofibroblast formation and tubulointerstitial fibrosis. *Am J Pathol* 1996;148:1169.

395. Johnson RJ, Alpers CE, Yoshimura A, et al. Renal injury from angiotensin II-mediated hypertension. *Hypertension* 1992;19:464.

396. Throckmorton DC, Brogden AP, Min B, et al. PDGF and TGF-beta mediate collagen production by mesangial cells exposed to advanced glycosylation end products. *Kidney Int* 1995;48:111.

397. Kliem V, Johnson RJ, Alpers CE, et al. Mechanisms involved in the pathogenesis of tubulointerstitial fibrosis in 5/6-nephrectomized rats. *Kidney Int* 1996;49:666.

398. Gesualdo L, Di Paolo S, Milani S, et al. Expression of platelet-derived growth factor receptors in normal and diseased human kidney. An immunohistochemistry and in situ hybridization study. *J Clin Invest* 1994;94:50.

399. Isaka Y, Fujiwara Y, Ueda N, et al. Glomerulosclerosis induced by in vivo transfection of transforming growth factor-beta or platelet-derived growth factor gene into the rat kidney. *J Clin Invest* 1993;92:2597.

400. Liu ZH, Striker LJ, Phillips C, et al. Growth hormone expression is required for the development of diabetic glomerulosclerosis in mice. *Kidney Int* 1995;51:S37.

401. Takayama H, LaRochelle WJ, Sabnis SG, et al. Renal tubular hyperplasia, polycystic disease, and glomerulosclerosis in transgenic mice overexpressing hepatocyte growth factor/scatter factor. *Lab Invest* 1997;77:131.

402. Mizuno S, Kurosawa T, Matsumoto K, et al. Hepatocyte growth factor prevents renal fibrosis and dysfunction in a mouse model of chronic renal disease. *J Clin Invest* 1998;101:1827.

403. Terzi F, Burtin M, Hekmati M, et al. Sodium restriction decreases AP-1 activation after nephron reduction in the rat: role in the progression of renal lesions. *Exp Nephrol* 2000;8:104.

404. Baeuerle PA, Henkel T. Function and activation of NF-kappa B in the immune system. *Annu Rev Immunol* 1994;12:141.

405. Mirza A, Liu SL, Frizell E, et al. A role for tissue transglutaminase in hepatic injury and fibrogenesis, and its regulation by NF-kappaB. *Am J Physiol* 1997;272:G281.

406. Johnson TS, Griffin M, Thomas GL, et al. The role of transglutaminase in the rat subtotal nephrectomy model of renal fibrosis. *J Clin Invest* 1997;99:2950.

407. Morrissey J, Klahr S. Transcription factor NF-kappaB regulation of renal fibrosis during ureteral obstruction. *Semin Nephrol* 1998;18:603.

408. Rangan GK, Wang Y, Tay YC, et al. Inhibition of nuclear factor-kappaB activation reduces cortical tubulointerstitial injury in proteinuric rats. *Kidney Int* 1999;56:118.

409. Gomez DE, Alonso DF, Yoshiji H, et al. Tissue inhibitors of metalloproteinases: structure, regulation and biological functions. *Eur J Cell Biol* 1997;74:111.

410. Fogo AB. The role of angiotensin II and plasminogen activator inhibitor-1 in progressive glomerulosclerosis. *Am J Kidney Dis* 2000;35:179.

411. Schaefer L, Meier K, Hafner C, et al. Protein restriction influences glomerular matrix turnover and tubular hypertrophy by modulation of renal proteinase activities. *Miner Electrolyte Metab* 1996;22:162.

412. Oikawa T, Freeman M, Lo W, et al. Modulation of plasminogen activator inhibitor-1 in vivo: a new mechanism for the anti-fibrotic effect of renin-angiotensin inhibition. *Kidney Int* 1997;51:164.

413. Shankland SJ, Hamel P, Scholey JW. Cyclin and cyclin-dependent kinase expression in the remnant glomerulus. *J Am Soc Nephrol* 1997;8:368.

414. Wolf G, Mueller E, Stahl RA, et al. Angiotensin II-induced hypertrophy of cultured murine proximal tubular cells is mediated by endogenous transforming growth factor-beta. *J Clin Invest* 1993;92:1366.

415. Wolf G, Stahl RA. Angiotensin II-stimulated hypertrophy of LLC-PK1 cells depends on the induction of the cyclin-dependent kinase inhibitor p27Kip1. *Kidney Int* 1996;50:2112.

416. Al-Douahji M, Brugarolas J, Brown PA, et al. The cyclin kinase inhibitor p21WAF1/CIP1 is required for glomerular hypertrophy in experimental diabetic nephropathy. *Kidney Int* 1999;56:1691.

417. Morrissey JJ, Ishidoya S, McCracken R, et al. Control of p53 and p21 (WAF1) expression during unilateral ureteral obstruction. *Kidney Int* 1996;57:S84.

418. Megyesi J, Price PM, Tamayo E, et al. The lack of a functional p21(WAF1/CIP1) gene ameliorates progression to chronic renal failure. *Proc Natl Acad Sci USA* 1999;96:10830.

419. Goss RJ. Hypertrophy versus hyperplasia. *Science* 1966;153:1615.

420. Pagtalunan ME, Miller PL, Jumping-Eagle S, et al. 1997. Podocyte loss and progressive glomerular injury in type II diabetes. *J Clin Invest* 1997;99:342.

421. Yoshizumi M, Kurihara H, Sugiyama T, et al. Hemodynamic shear stress regulates endothelin production by cultured endothelial cells. *Biochem Biophys Res Commun* 1989;161:859.

422. Kuchan MJ, Frangos JA. Shear stress regulates endothelin-1 release via protein kinase C and cGMP in cultured endothelial cells. *Am J Physiol* 1993;264:H150.

423. Noris M, et al. Nitric oxide synthesis by cultured endothelial cells is modulated by flow conditions. *Circ Res* 1995;76:536.

424. Ohno M, Cooke JC, Dzau VJ, et al. Fluid shear stress induces endothelial transforming growth factor beta-1 transcription and production: modulation by potassium-channel blockade. *J Clin Invest* 1995;95:1363.

425. Malek AM, Gibbons GH, Dzau VJ, et al. Fluid shear stress differentially modulates expression of genes encoding basic fibroblast growth factor and platelet-derived growth factor B chain in vascular endothelium. *J Clin Invest* 1993;92:2013.

426. Nagel T, et al. Shear stress selectively upregulates intercellular adhesion molecule-1 expression in cultured human vascular endothelial cells. *J Clin Invest* 1994;94:885.

427. Ott MJ, Ballermann BJ. Shear stress augments glomerular endothelial cell PDGF mRNA expression and mitogen production. *J Am Soc Nephrol* 1992;3:476A.

428. Hishikawa K, et al. Pressure enhances endothelin-1 release from cultured human endothelial cells. *Hypertension* 1995;25:449.

429. Riser BL, et al. Intraglomerular pressure and mesangial stretching stimulate extracellular matrix formation in the rat. *J Clin Invest* 1992;90:1932.

430. Becker BN, Yasuda T, Kondo S, et al. Mechanical stretch/relaxation stimulates a cellular renin-angiotensin system in cultured rat mesangial cells. *Exp Nephrol* 1998;6:57.

431. Harris RC, Haralson MA, Badr KF. Continuous stretch-relaxation in culture alters rat mesangial cell morphology, growth characteristics, and metabolic activity. *Lab Invest* 1992;66:548.

432. Yasuda T, Kondo S, Homma T, et al. Regulation of extracellular matrix by mechanical stress in rat glomerular mesangial cells. *J Clin Invest* 1996;98:1991.

433. Harris RC, Akai Y, Yasuda T, et al. The role of physical forces in alterations of mesangial cell function. *Kidney Int* 1995;45:S17.

434. Shankland SJ, Ly H, Thai K, et al. Increased glomerular capillary pressure alters glomerular cytokine expression. *Circ Res* 1994;75:844.

435. Griffin KA, Picken MM, Churchill M, et al. Functional and structural correlates of glomerulosclerosis after renal mass reduction in the rat. *J Am Soc Nephrol* 2000;11:497.

436. Terzi F, Henrion D, Colucci-Guyon E, et al. Reduction of renal mass is lethal in mice lacking vimentin. Role of endothelin-nitric oxide imbalance. *J Clin Invest* 1997;100:1520.

437. Miller PL, Scholey JW, Rennke HG, et al. Glomerular hypertrophy aggravates epithelial cell injury in nephrotic rats. *J Clin Invest* 1990;85:1119.

438. Yoshida Y, et al. Effects of antihypertensive drugs on glomerular morphology. *Kidney Int* 1989;36:626.

439. Grond J, et al. Analysis of renal structural and functional features in two rat strains with a different susceptibility to glomerular sclerosis. *Lab Invest* 1986;54:77.

440. Grond J, Muller EW, van Goor H, et al. Differences in puromycin nephrosis in two rat strains. *Kidney Int* 1988;33:524.

441. Wang SN, Hirschberg R. Growth factor ultrafiltration in experimental diabetic nephropathy contributes to interstitial fibrosis. *Am J Physiol* 2000;278:F554.

442. Remuzzi G, Ruggenenti P, Benigni A. Understanding the nature of renal disease progression. *Kidney Int* 1997;51:2.

443. Zoja C, Morigi M, Figliuzzi M, et al. Proximal tubular cell synthesis and secretion of endothelin-1 on challenge with albumin and other proteins. *Am J Kidney Dis* 1995;26:934.

444. Yokokawa K, et al. Heparin suppresses endothelin-1 peptide and mRNA expression in cultured endothelial cells of spontaneously hypertensive rats. *J Am Soc Nephrol* 1994;4:1683.

445. Fine LG, Norman JT, Ong A. Cell-cell cross-talk in the pathogenesis of renal interstitial fibrosis. *Kidney Int* 1995;47:S48.

446. Fine LG, Orphanides C, Norman JT. Progressive renal disease: the chronic hypoxia hypothesis. *Kidney Int* 1998;65:S74.

447. Bohle A, Wehrmann M, Bogenschutz O, et al. The long-term prognosis of the primary glomerulonephritides. A morphological and clinical analysis of 1747 cases. *Pathol Res Pract* 1992;88:908.

448. Nath KA, Croatt AJ, Hostetter TH. Oxygen consumption and oxidant stress in surviving nephrons. *Am J Physiol* 1990;258:F1354.

449. Harris DCH, Chan L, Schrier RW. Remnant kidney hypermetabolism and progression of chronic renal failure. *Am J Physiol* 1988;254:F267.

450. Schrier RW, et al. Tubular hypermetabolism as a factor in the progression of chronic renal failure. *Am J Kidney Dis* 1988;12:243.

451. Fine A. Remnant kidney metabolism in the dog. *J Am Soc Nephrol* 1991;2:70.

452. Culpepper RM, Schoolwerth AC. Remnant kidney oxygen consumption: hypermetabolism or hyperbole? *J Am Soc Nephrol* 1992;3:151.

453. Harris DCH, Hammond WS, Burke TJ, et al. Verapamil protects against progression of experimental chronic renal failure. *Kidney Int* 1987;33:41.

454. Shapiro JI, Harris DCH, Schrier RW, et al. Attenuation of hypermetabolism in the remnant kidney by dietary phosphate restriction in the rat. *Am J Physiol* 1990;258:F183.

455. Kramer BK, Bucher M, Sandner P, et al. Effects of hypoxia on growth factor expression in the rat kidney in vivo. *Kidney Int* 1997;51:444.

456. Gleadle JM, Ebert BL, Firth JD, et al. Regulation of angiogenic growth factor expression by hypoxia, transition metals and chelating agents. *Am J Physiol* 1995;268:C1362.

457. Kourembas S, Morita T, Liu Y, et al. Mechanisms by which oxygen regulates gene expression in cell-cell interaction in the vasculature. *Kidney Int* 1997;51:438.

458. Combe C, Burton CJ, Dufourcq P, et al. Hypoxia induces intercellular adhesion molecule-1 on cultured human tubular cells. *Kidney Int* 1997;51:1703.

459. Falanga V, Matrin TA, Tagaki H, et al. Low oxygen tension increases mRNA levels of alphal(I) procollagen in human dermal fibroblasts. *J Cell Physiol* 1993;157:408.

460. Bunn HF, Poyton RO. Oxygen sensing and molecular adaptation to hypoxia. *Physiol Rev* 1996;76:839.

461. Semenza GL, Agani F, Booth G, et al. Structural and functional analysis of hypoxia-inducible factor 1. *Kidney Int* 1997;51:553.

462. Sugiura T, Yamauchi A, Kitamura H, et al. Effects of hypertonic stress on transforming growth factor-beta activity in normal rat kidney cells. *Kidney Int* 1998;53:1654.

463. Sugiura T, Yamauchi A, Kitamura H, et al. High water intake ameliorates tubulointerstitial injury in rats with subtotal nephrectomy: possible role of TGF-beta. *Kidney Int* 1999;55:1800.

464. Nath KA, Hostetter MK, Hostetter TH. Pathophysiology of chronic tubulo-interstitial disease in rats: Interactions of dietary acid load, ammonia, and complement component C3. *J Clin Invest* 1985;76:667.

465. Keane WF, Kasiske BL, O'Donnell MP. Hyperlipidemia and the progression of renal disease. *Am J Clin Nutr* 1988;47:157.

466. Keane WF. Lipids and the kidney. *Kidney Int* 1994;46:910.

467. Walli AK, et al. Role of lipoproteins in progressive renal disease. *Am J Hypertens* 1993;6:358S.

468. Schlondorff D. Cellular mechanisms of lipid injury in the glomerulus. *Am J Kidney Dis* 1993;22:82.

469. Gröne EF, et al. Actions of lipoproteins in cultured human mesangial cells: modulation by mitogenic vasoconstrictors. *Am J Physiol* 1992;263:F686.

470. Keane WF, O'Donnell MP, Kasiske BL, et al. Oxidative modification of low density lipoproteins by mesangial cells. *J Am Soc Nephrol* 1993;4:187.

471. Rovin BH, Tan LC. LDL stimulates mesangial fibronectin production and chemoattractant expression. *Kidney Int* 1993;43:218.

472. Ding GH, Pesek-Diamond I, Diamond JR. Cholesterol, macrophages, and gene expression of TGF-b1 and fibronectin during nephrosis. *Am J Physiol* 1993;264:F577.

473. O'Donnell MP, et al. Lovastatin inhibits proliferation of rat mesangial cells. *J Clin Invest* 1993;91:83.

474. O'Donnell MP, Massy ZA, Guijarro C, et al. Isoprenoids, Ras and proliferative glomerular disease. *Contrib Nephrol* 1997;120:219.

475. Kim SY, Guijarro C, O'Donnell MP, et al. Human mesangial cell production of monocyte chemoattractant protein-1: modulation by lovastatin. *Kidney Int* 1995;48:363.

476. Vrtovsnik F, Couette S, Prie D, et al. Lovastatin-induced inhibition of renal epithelial tubular cell proliferation involves a p21ras activated, AP-1-dependent pathway. *Kidney Int* 1997;52:1016.

477. Mulec H, Johnsen SA, Wiklund O, et al. Cholesterol: a renal risk factor in diabetic nephropathy? *Am J Kidney Dis* 1993;22:196.

478. Ganz MB, Boron WF. Long-term effects of growth factors on pH and acid–base transport in rat glomerular mesangial cells. *Am J Physiol* 1994;266:F576.

479. Floege J, et al. Glomerular cell proliferation and PDGF expression precede glomerulosclerosis in the remnant kidney model. *Kidney Int* 1992;41:297.

480. Olson JL. Role of heparin as a protective agent following reduction of renal mass. *Kidney Int* 1984;25:376.

481. Purkerson ML, Tollefsen DM, Klahr S. N-desulfated/acetylated heparin ameliorates the progression of renal disease in rats with subtotal renal ablation. *J Clin Invest* 1988;81:69.

482. Purkerson ML, et al. Inhibition of anticoagulant drugs of the progressive hypertension and uremia associated with renal infarction in rats. *Thromb Res* 1982;26:227.

483. Zoja C, et al. Selective inhibition of platelet thromboxane generation with low-dose aspirin does not protect rats with reduced renal mass from the development of progressive disease. *Am J Pathol* 1989;134:1027.

484. Castello JJ Jr, Hoover RL, Harper PA, et al. Heparin and glomerular epithelial cell-secreted heparin-like species inhibit mesangial-cell proliferation. *Am J Pathol* 1985;120:427.

485. Mandal AK, Lyden TW, Saklayen MG. Heparin lowers blood pressure: biological and clinical perspectives. *Kidney Int* 1995;47:1017.

486. Kohno M, et al. Heparin inhibits endothelin-1 production in cultured rat mesangial cells. *Kidney Int* 1994;45:137.

487. Tang WW, Wilson CB. Heparin decreases mesangial matrix accumulation after selective antibody-induced mesangial cell injury. *J Am Soc Nephrol* 1992;3:921.

488. Floege J, et al. Heparin suppresses mesangial cell proliferation and matrix expansion in experimental mesangioproliferative glomerulonephritis. *Kidney Int* 1993;43:369.

489. Ibels LS, Alfrey AC, Haut L, et al. Preservation of function in experimental renal disease by dietary restriction of phosphate. *N Engl J Med* 1978;298:122.

490. Karlinsky ML, et al. Preservation of renal function in experimental glomerulonephritis. *Kidney Int* 1982;17:293.

491. Lumlertgul D, et al. Phosphate depletion arrests progression of chronic renal failure independent of protein intake. *Kidney Int* 1986;29:658.

492. Lau K. Phosphate excess and progressive renal failure: the precipitation-calcification hypothesis. *Kidney Int* 1989;36:918.

493. Harris DC, Chan L, Schrier RW. Remnant kidney hypermetabolism and progression of chronic renal failure. *Am J Physiol* 1988;254:F267.

494. Carter HR, et al. Effects of phosphate depletion and parathyroid hormone on glucose reabsorption. *Am J Physiol* 1974;227:1422.

495. Shigematsu T, Caverzasio J, Bonjour J-P. Parathyroid removal prevents the progression of chronic renal failure induced by high protein diet. *Kidney Int* 1993;44:173.

496. Mayer G, et al. Effects of angiotensin II receptor blockade on remnant glomerular permselectivity. *Kidney Int* 1993;43:346.

497. Gandhi M, Olson JL, Meyer TW. Contribution of tubular injury to loss of remnant kidney function. *Kidney Int* 1998;54:1157.

CHAPTER 91

Anemia in Renal Disease

Anatole Besarab

In addition to excreting toxic substances in urine and regulating blood solute concentrations, the kidney performs a variety of metabolic processes and produces hormones. Symptoms in chronic renal failure result from the deleterious effects of solute retention and from the absence of renally produced hormones, particularly erythropoietin (EPO), which leads to anemia. Anemia persists as a significant problem in many patients receiving adequate dialysis prescriptions. This chapter reviews the pathogenesis of the anemia associated with kidney disease and discusses its therapy.

PHYSIOLOGY OF ERYTHROPOIETIN AND ERYTHROPOIESIS

Bone marrow erythropoiesis in response to hypoxia was proposed in 1823 (1). Richard Bright (2) commented on the pallor of patients with renal disease in 1836. For the next 150 years, anemia remained an important clinical manifestation of progressive renal disease. In 1922, Brown and Roth (3) determined that the anemia of chronic nephritis resulted from reduced bone marrow production. Although cloning and production of recombinant human EPO is a recent development, the concept of a "hemopoietine" that stimulates marrow erythropoiesis dates from 1906 (4) and was quickly integrated into a hypoxia-induced feedback mechanism involving a hematopoietin (5). In 1953, Erslev (6) described this "erythropoietic stimulating factor" that is now known as EPO. In 1957, Jacobson and colleagues (7) demonstrated that this factor was lacking in bilaterally nephrectomized animals. Subsequent studies showed that it was absent in anephric humans (8). In general, there is a direct, although imperfect, relation between the degree of renal insufficiency and the degree of anemia (5,9).

Physiologic studies were hampered until EPO could be measured. The first bioassay measured the polycythemic mouse's utilization of ^{59}Fe after infusion of a serum sample

(10). In 1968, feedback control of erythropoiesis dependent on oxygen delivery to the EPO secretory site in the kidney was demonstrated for normal subjects. Urinary and plasma EPO increased logarithmically as hematocrit was lowered by phlebotomy, whereas these decreased with hypertransfusion (11). Erslev (12) in 1974 proved involvement of the kidney in erythropoiesis by showing that the perfusion of hypoxic rabbit kidneys *in vitro* with a serum-free solution resulted in the production of preformed EPO. Under normal conditions, the kidneys produce over 90% of EPO; the rest is produced largely by hepatocytes (with an insignificant contribution by macrophages) (13). Extensive physiologic and clinical studies became possible after development of a radioimmunoassay (RIA) with a highly purified protein (14).

Understanding of erythropoiesis progressed even though neither the intrarenal production site nor the biochemical composition of the EPO molecule was known. Miyake and coworkers (15) purified and Lai et al. (16) sequenced the amino acids of EPO, making it possible to identify and clone the EPO gene (16,17). Recombinant human EPO (rHuEPO, EPO, or epoetin) can now be mass produced for clinical use by transfection of the human gene into mammalian cells (16) or by gene activation (18).

The human EPO gene, located on the long arm of chromosome 7, consists of five exons and four introns (19). Its upstream promoter is not directly responsive to hypoxia; this responsiveness is found in an enhancer located immediately downstream from the gene (20,21). Hypoxia induces the production of a protein, hypoxia-inducible factor or HIF-1 (20,21), that binds to the oxygen-sensitive enhancer to induce gene transcription of messenger RNA (mRNA) (22,23). The EPO gene encodes for a 193-amino-acid prohormone. The first 27 amino acids are cleaved before secretion. Circulating EPO exists as a 166-amino-acid peptide containing 2 sulfide bridges and 4 sites of carbohydrate attachment (24). Four complex carbohydrate chains containing sialic acids are linked to the protein and constitute 40% of its molecular weight of 34,000 daltons (34 kd). The terminal arginine at position 166 is removed before secretion. The disulfide cross-links form two loops that are needed for biologic

A. Besarab: Section of Nephrology, West Virginia University School of Medicine; and Department of Medicine, West Virginia University Hospital Inc., Morgantown, West Virginia

activity (24). Glycosylation is necessary for cellular secretion (25) and for the hormone's biologic activity *in vivo* because the sialic acid moieties allow EPO to circulate long enough to reach the bone marrow. Rapid receptor-mediated endocytosis when galactose residues are exposed reduces the half-time of desialated EPO to minutes (25). The fully sialated hormone has, in humans, a half-time varying from 4 to 12 hours (26). The sialoglycoprotein released into the circulation is highly heat and pH resistant. The carbohydrate sialic acid moieties are not essential for EPO action on bone marrow progenitor cells through receptor binding (27). Despite some differences in carbohydrate structure among available rHuEPO products, the biologic activity appears to be the same. The amino acid sequence has been modified to permit the addition of two additional sialic acid residues (28), producing a molecule with a much longer pharmacologic half-life (29).

Erythropoietin regulates the number of committed erythroid precursors and causes them to mature into erythrocytes (30). The kidney, through its synthesis of EPO, controls such erythropoiesis (13). The release of EPO is regulated by feedback mechanisms involving tissue oxygenation. A decrease in the oxygen tension or content of the blood perfusing the kidneys produces "tissue" hypoxia. Several studies suggest that the oxygen-sensing mechanism depends on a heme protein (31) that is located in the cortex (32). In the presence of decreased oxygen delivery, activation of this sensor leads to the synthesis of a protein that binds to the active site on the enhancer region of the EPO gene, leading to increased EPO production (23). The ensuing rise in red blood cell production returns the oxygen-carrying capacity toward normal. This normal negative biofeedback system responsive to tissue hypoxia is reflected by the plasma EPO concentration (33). The initial renal response to tissue hypoxia is similar whether the tissue hypoxia reflects hypoxemia (low PO_2), reduced oxygen-carrying capacity (anemia), a hemoglobinopathy characterized by increased affinity for oxygen, or ischemia.

In situ hybridization studies have localized the EPO-producing cells to the peritubular area near the base of proximal tubular cells in the renal cortex (34). Studies using transgenic mice suggest that a population of interstitial fibroblasts (also known as the type I interstitial cell) is the source of renal EPO synthesis (35), and that these cells are limited to the deep cortex and outer medulla in the unstimulated kidney. With increasing anemia, the number of EPO-specific mRNA–positive cells increases and spreads into the superficial cortex. "Appropriate" compensation during severe anemia requires an approximately 100-fold increase in kidney EPO production. EPO-producing cells are recruited in an on-off fashion (36); increased production of EPO in response to hypoxia results from the recruitment of additional EPO-synthesizing cells (13,37). The number of EPO-producing cells increases exponentially as PO_2 decreases. Synthesis of EPO occurs *de novo*, secretion is rapid, and there is no significant intracellular accumulation (38). The short half-life of EPO mRNA provides a mechanism for rapidly

modulating EPO production in response to variations in tissue oxygen tension. Maintenance of "normal" plasma levels of 8 to 24 mU/mL in humans requires the daily continuous synthesis of approximately 2 to 3 U/kg body weight.

The pluripotent hematopoietic stem cell is capable of forming erythrocytes, leukocytes, and megakaryocytes (36). These primitive cells have the capacity for both self-renewal and differentiation into committed progenitor cells under appropriate stimuli. Renewal appears to occur by chance—"stochastically" (36)—and is initiated primarily by lineage-nonspecific cytokines such as interleukin (IL)-3, stem cell factor, insulin-like growth factor-1 (IGF-1), and granulocyte–macrophage colony-stimulating factor. The transformation of a multipotential stem cell into a mature red blood cell occurs in two morphologically distinct stages. Only the first stage is responsive to EPO. This first stage begins with small mononuclear cells displaying a specific glycophosphoprotein, CD34, on their surface (39), and then sequentially includes the committed erythroid progenitor, the primitive and mature burst-forming unit—erythroid (BFU-E), and the colony-forming unit—erythroid (CFU-E). In the second, precursor stage, the cells appear as morphologically recognizable erythroblasts that mature into pronormoblasts and daughter erythrocytes.

Peripheral demands for red cell production can be met only after a multipotential stem cell has transformed into a unipotential progenitor cell. During the progressive maturation from primitive BFU-E through CFU-E, the precursors become increasingly dependent on as well as sensitive to the effects of EPO (40), to the point that CFU-E can survive and differentiate into a pronormoblast only in the presence of EPO. Insulin or IGF-1 also is required for CFU-E growth (41). The observation that EPO is critical to the sustenance, multiplication, and differentiation of the committed erythroid progenitors and needs to be constantly present is a key concept with regard to clinical dosing practices.

Several other hormones such as androgens, thyroid-stimulating hormone, somatomedin, and catecholamines appear to augment the growth of CFU-E but are not absolute requirements (42). Other cytokines, including IL-1α, IL-1β, IL-2, tumor necrosis factor-α, and transforming growth factor-β, have a negative effect on erythropoiesis (43,44). These cytokines are significant mediators in the anemia of chronic diseases, may be activated by certain types of dialysis, and are invariably present during acute infection or inflammation. Their inhibitory effects produce resistance to exogenous EPO in patients with renal failure.

Erythropoietin exerts its signal through the EPO receptor, a 55-kd transmembrane protein (45). Phosphorylation of intracellular proteins results in the release of second messengers (46). The exact signals transmitted by these messengers are poorly understood. It is unlikely that the signals are transcription factors for genes involved in the synthesis of globin or other mature erythroid proteins; it is more likely that these signals maintain the viability of progenitor cells (47). In the absence of EPO, such cells undergo apoptosis and die before they reach the precursor cell stage. In the presence of EPO, they proliferate and eventually transform into precursor cells. The EPO–EPO receptor complex appears to require only a small number of contact points for full effect. A study evaluating a number of short peptides as possible agonists of the EPO receptor (48) showed that peptides whose sequence matched a minimum consensus sequence of only 14 amino acids bound to and activated the EPO receptor.

At a certain level of maturation, the CFU-E becomes activated and the cells are transformed into hemoglobin-synthesizing, morphologically recognizable erythroblasts. Further proliferation and maturation of these cells appears to be unaffected by EPO and proceeds at a fixed rate in the presence of adequate supplies of iron, folate, vitamin B_{12}, pyridoxine, ascorbic acid, and trace elements.

INTEGRATION OF THE ERYTHROPOIESIS CONTROL SYSTEM

The chief characteristic of the EPO–erythropoiesis system is that an error signal, reduced tissue oxygenation, defines the presence of an "inadequate erythron," leading to the production of EPO. Erythropoietin production rate is determined primarily by the ratio of the oxygen requirements at or near the site of production to its oxygen supply (49). Factors that decrease the supply of oxygen to the kidneys increase the production of EPO, and vice versa (the feedback control loop). However, the ratio of tissue oxygen demand to supply, through its effects on EPO production, is only a "coarse" regulator of the rate of erythropoiesis. Other modulators must fine-tune the system because the red cell mass (total number of erythrocytes) would oscillate owing to the prolonged life span of the erythrocytes and the lag time between exposure of CFU-E to elevated levels of EPO and the delivery of the mature reticulocyte to the bloodstream.

These fine-tuning mechanisms are incompletely understood but may depend on various combinations of the following:

1. The maximum response of the bone marrow to markedly elevated EPO levels is limited. In severe anemias, EPO increases 100- to 1,000-fold, but the maximum red cell production rate increases only 4- to 6-fold above basal (50).
2. For any level of anemia, the negative correlation between the logarithm of EPO concentration and blood hemoglobin is shifted to higher levels in individuals with hypoplastic marrows compared to those without hyperplastic marrows (51).
3. A decrease in EPO levels is observed before a noticeable change in red cell mass occurs in chronically hypoxic rats (52). Similarly, EPO levels in normal humans peak within 24 hours after phlebotomy but rapidly decrease within the next 24 hours, although the red cell deficit remains uncorrected (53). This rapid return in EPO levels toward normal may result from intrarenal and systemic hemodynamic

changes or in part from an expansion of progenitors that remove circulating EPO by receptor binding.

In normal people, levels of EPO are remarkably constant under steady-state conditions (range, 8 to 25 mU/mL) in both adults (8) and children (54). No differences in plasma immunoreactive EPO exist between the sexes in humans (55). Prolonged nocturnal hypoxia increases (56), whereas significant protein deprivation decreases (57) baseline EPO levels. Increased production of EPO results from the exponential recruitment of additional EPO-synthesizing cells (14,35) as the hypoxic stimulus increases. This exponential recruitment of EPO-producing cells produces the inverse relationship between circulating EPO levels and hematocrit. A negative feedback system resulting from the subsequent increase in oxygen-carrying capacity (increased hematocrit) turns off EPO production (58).

PATHOPHYSIOLOGY OF THE ANEMIA OF RENAL DISEASE

Clinical Aspects

The normal negative biofeedback system induces an increase in EPO production that is reflected by plasma EPO concentrations (8). In the absence of renal disease, plasma EPO levels increase from normal values of less than 25 to approximately 100 mU/mL as hematocrit decreases to mildly anemic levels of 27% to 33%. In severe anemia, EPO increases more than 100-fold (50). Levels in excess of 1,000 mU/mL are reached at hematocrits below 20% (50) (Fig. 91-1).

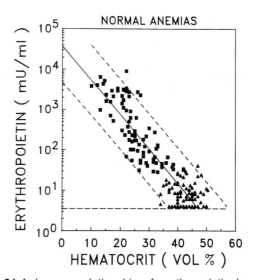

FIG. 91-1. Inverse relationship of erythropoietin levels to hematocrit. Normal subjects are depicted by *triangles* and patients with various anemias (but excluding those with kidney disease, malignancy, or rheumatoid arthritis) by *squares*. *Dashed horizontal line* represents limits of detection of the radioimmunoassay for erythropoietin. (Adapted from Erslev AJ. Erythropoietin. *N Engl J Med* 1991;324:1339, with permission.)

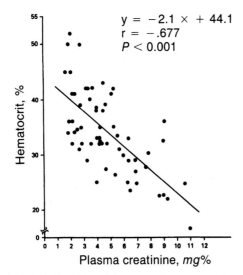

FIG. 91-2. Relationship of hematocrit to creatinine. (From McGonigle RSR, et al. Erythropoietin deficiency and erythropoiesis in renal insufficiency. *Kidney Int* 1984;25:437, with permission.)

In progressive renal insufficiency, the degree of anemia is in general proportional to the severity of azotemia (59). Among patients, the correlation of hematocrit with glomerular filtration rate (GFR), blood urea nitrogen, or serum creatinine is imprecise (60) (Fig. 91-2). However, as renal function approaches that requiring replacement therapy, the hematocrit tends to plateau at a level that varies little thereafter in the absence of complications or institution of rHuEPO therapy. Most patients on early dialysis have hematocrit values between 15% and 25%. In nephric anemic patients with end-stage renal disease (ESRD) on dialysis, the mean baseline values of EPO (19 to 30 mU/mL) are much lower than those observed in normal subjects at the same degrees of anemia. Thus, although the end-stage kidney continues to produce some EPO despite effective cessation of excretory function, it is incapable of augmenting EPO production in response to an appropriate anemic hypoxic stimulus. Yet an acute blood loss can transiently increase EPO levels (53). Although little data are available on sequential EPO levels with progressive renal failure, EPO production in such anemic patients probably also is inadequate. The bilaterally nephrectomized patient with no renal EPO production invariably had much lower levels of hematocrit (61) and depended on blood transfusions before the advent of rHuEPO.

Uncomplicated anemia of renal disease is normocytic and normochromic (62). The presence of echinocytes, or burr cells, is the most frequently observed morphologic change in red blood cells (63). Presence of normal cellularity and maturation sequence in the bone marrow of patients on dialysis is misleading inasmuch as erythropoiesis should be increased. After acute blood loss or prolonged hypoxia, erythropoiesis in the marrow does increase to higher levels, but not to the extent seen in nonuremic subjects.

Anemia develops during acute renal failure from tubular necrosis, interstitial nephritis, and glomerulonephritis, with the hematocrit gradually falling to 25% to 30% in the absence of excessive blood losses. The anemia results from deficient EPO production (which does not reverse until excretory function recovers) (64), from shortened red cell survival (65), and from hemodilution (66). As renal function recovers, erythropoiesis gradually improves, with the red cell mass normalizing over several months.

Anemia may be more severe than anticipated in some forms of acute renal failure (Goodpasture's syndrome, Henoch-Schönlein glomerulonephritis). Multiple myeloma often presents with a disproportionately severe anemia because erythropoiesis is further compromised by plasma cell infiltration and marrow replacement. Erythropoietin production relative to renal function may be reduced more than usual in radiation nephritis (67). Hemolysis may be significant in systemic lupus erythematosus, scleroderma, and other vasculitides associated with acute renal failure. Hemolysis with grossly deformed cells (fragmented red cells on peripheral smear) formed in the microcirculation occurs in the hemolytic-uremic syndrome. The hematologic features include a red cell production index that usually is greater than three times normal despite azotemia or acute renal failure.

Specific and sensitive RIA can measure even subnormal serum EPO levels. The persistent observations of many investigators of "inappropriately" low EPO levels in virtually all cases of chronic renal failure (8,50) indicate that the primary factor in the anemia of renal failure is the inadequate production of endogenous EPO by diseased kidneys. Patients with autosomal-dominant polycystic kidney disease are the exception and typically have higher EPO levels with less severe anemia (68). High EPO concentrations have been found in the fluid of cysts originating from proximal tubules with EPO mRNA identified in their interstitial cells (69). Shortened red blood cell survival (hemolysis or chronic blood loss) also may play a role but probably is more instrumental in determining the severity of anemia. Renal disease thus affects the red cell mass by interfering with both red cell production and red cell life span through disruption of the kidney's endocrine and exocrine functions. Other factors such as iron and other nutritional deficiencies and the putative effects of uremic inhibitors, if left unattended, will influence the severity of anemia and the outcome of rHuEPO treatment in any patient with progressive renal failure or ESRD.

Inadequate Erythropoietin Production

The steady-state relationship between plasma RIA EPO levels and hematocrit (Fig. 91-1) reflects the operation of a negative feedback system and the homeostatic attempt of normal kidneys to correct the anemia (70). In patients with ESRD, this biofeedback mechanism is impaired. In stable patients on dialysis, hematocrit correlates directly rather than inversely with EPO levels (Fig. 91-3). Plasma EPO levels

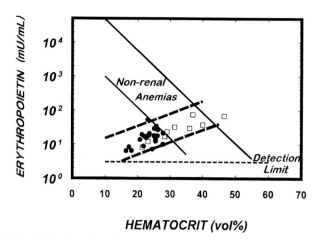

HEMATOCRIT (vol%)

FIG. 91-3. Relationship of erythropoietin levels to hematocrit in end-stage renal disease (ESRD). The 95% confidence range for erythropoietin values of patients without renal disease is given by the *solid lines.* The two *heavy dashed lines* represent 95% confidence range of patients just before renal transplantation (76). The *solid circles* and *open squares* represent erythropoietin levels of two cohorts of hemodialysis patients. Note the direct relationship between erythropoietin levels and hematocrit in patients with ESRD.

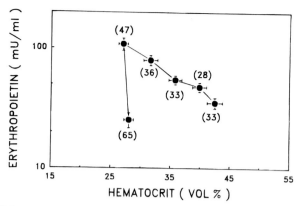

HEMATOCRIT (VOL %)

FIG. 91-4. Changes in erythropoietin levels and hematocrit after renal transplantation, illustrating the negative biofeedback system of erythropoiesis after establishment of normal renal function by renal transplantation. Numbers in parentheses reflect number of subjects. The peak response occurred at 16 days postimplantation and always followed resumption of excretory function by the graft. The subsequent values represent average values at 31, 50, 75, and 109 days postimplantation. (From Besarab A, et al. Dynamics of erythropoiesis following renal transplantation. *Kidney Int* 1987;32:526, with permission.)

among different patients with ESRD vary five- to tenfold; within a given patient, EPO levels tend to be similar over time. Patients with ESRD with acute blood loss or hemolysis can increase their plasma RIA EPO levels two- to fivefold (53), but normal subjects sustaining equivalent degrees of blood loss increase their levels 10- to 100-fold. These observations indicate that basal EPO production is disordered in a variable way but that the feedback loop between EPO and tissue oxygen delivery is still present. EPO production per unit weight of remaining "unscarred" kidney tissue may be above normal but limited by functional renal mass.

The importance of adequate renal mass is best illustrated by the correction of anemia after successful transplantation in patients with ESRD (71). After such transplantation, levels increase and are sustained severalfold as excretory function recovers (Fig. 91-4). With increased production of red blood cells, anemia corrects and EPO levels progressively decrease.

Shortened Erythrocyte Survival

The life span of red cells in patients with chronic renal disease usually is shorter than normal (72,73) (Fig. 91-5), typically decreasing from a normal value of 120 days to average values of 70 to 80 days. However, as first pointed out by Chaplin and Mollison in 1953 (72), a normal marrow should easily compensate for such mild decreases in red cell survival with sufficient circulating EPO. In renal failure, both metabolic and mechanical factors may shorten survival of red blood cells. Activities of transketolase (74) and adenosine triphosphatase (75), which supports the Na^+-K^+ membrane pumps, are decreased. The decreased activity of the Na^+-K^+ pumps

influences changes in red cell shape and rigidity that favor hemolysis. The observations that uremic red cells survive normally when transfused into healthy recipients (76), that normal red cells may have a shortened life span in uremic recipients (73,77), and that red cell life span can be normalized after intensive dialysis (78) suggest retention of one or more uremic solutes in the plasma as the primary cause of the mild hemolysis. No definite uremic solute has been incriminated yet as the cause of such hemolysis.

In patients with ESRD on hemodialysis, the "apparent" red cell life span can be further shortened by external blood losses associated with the procedure. Measurement of red cell life span in patients on hemodialysis measures both removal of senescent cells by the reticuloendothelial system

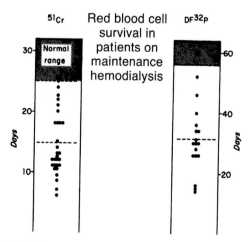

FIG. 91-5. Red cell survival in patients on maintenance dialysis as assessed by ^{51}Cr or DF ^{32}P half-lives.

and extracorporeal premature exit of erythrocytes from the circulation. The latter results from blood losses due to vascular access puncture, residual blood left in dialyzers, occasional blood leaks, and clotted dialyzers. Red cell life span can approach normal in well dialyzed patients with particular attention given to minimizing blood sampling for studies (79).

In patients on dialysis, decreased activity of the hexose monophosphate shunt renders hemoglobin and the red cell membrane sensitive to oxidant drugs or chemicals (80). Substances with strong oxidizing potential such as primaquine, quinidine, sulfones, and nitrofurantoin should be avoided. Hemolysis has resulted from inadequate removal of chloramine from dialysate water originating from municipal water sources (81). Acute hemolysis also must be avoided by removal of copper (82), zinc (83), aluminum (84), and nitrates (85) in the water supply, and formaldehyde (86) from reprocessed dialyzer equipment. Aluminum (87) and zinc (88) also impair erythropoiesis by interfering with heme synthesis. The dialysis process can induce hemolysis even without an underlying susceptibility of the "uremic" red blood cell. Hypotonic dialysate (89), overheated dialysate (90), malocclusion of the roller pump (91), and mechanical disruption from dialysis needles (92) can produce hemolysis. Hypophosphatemia, although uncommon in patients with ESRD, increases susceptibility to hemolysis (93).

Rarely, and now even less frequently, patients on long-term hemodialysis have splenomegaly with augmented erythrocyte destruction documented by radioisotope studies (94). Splenectomy should be reserved for those with either coexistent neutropenia or thrombocytopenia (95), or anemia resistant to rHuEPO. The pathogenesis of hypersplenism in chronic renal failure is multifactorial and includes chronic hepatitis (95), marrow fibrosis (96), and silicone splaying (97) arising from dialysis blood line tubing stressed by roller pumps.

Blood Loss

Blood loss may contribute to the anemia in patients with advanced renal failure before dialysis. As many as 25% of such patients may be iron deficient because of chronic blood loss (62).

Bleeding associated with renal insufficiency (98) has been known for decades. Common manifestations include telangiectasia and gastrointestinal angiodysplastic lesions (99). Functional abnormalities of platelets characterized by prolonged bleeding times, abnormal platelet aggregation and adhesiveness, and reduced platelet factor 3 release are well recognized (100). A reversible abnormality in the activation-dependent binding activity of glycoprotein (GP) IIb-IIIa occurs in uremia (100,101). Two adhesive proteins, fibrinogen and von Willebrand factor, and two adhesion receptors, the GP Ib-IX-V complex and GP IIb-IIIa complex, are crucial for the initiation of platelet thrombi at the site of vascular injury (102). Other defects include abnormalities in the

multimeric structure of von Willebrand factor (101), and acquired platelet storage pool deficiencies of adenosine diphosphate and serotonin (103). Removal of components present in uremic plasma, either *in vitro* by washing or *in vivo* by dialysis, markedly improves the GP IIb-IIIa defect (100), but not to normal. Uremic plasma also induces nitric oxide synthesis by cultured endothelial cells, which inhibits platelet function (104). This inhibitor has been shown to be a guanidine derivative (105).

All these factors notwithstanding, anemia itself appears to be a major factor in sustaining the bleeding tendency because prolonged bleeding times are corrected by both red cell transfusions (106) and the rise in hematocrit that occurs with therapeutic use of rHuEPO (107).

Marrow Inhibitors of Erythropoiesis

In the absence of significant overt blood loss, decreases in red cell survival of 30% to 40% alone cannot fully account for the degree of anemia in renal failure. Whereas EPO levels are comparable, red cell production in patients with renal failure is only one-half of normal (Fig. 91-6). Since the late 1960s, numerous *in vitro* studies have implicated an inhibitory effect of uremic serum on growth of erythroid precursors or on heme synthesis (108). Intensive dialysis can increase iron utilization and hematocrit without altering the level of circulating EPO (73,109). Older studies tried to identify polar lipids, arsenic, vitamin A, spermine, spermidine, and parathyroid hormone (110–117) as specific uremic inhibitors. More recent studies indicate that their role in the genesis of the anemia of renal failure is of lesser importance (118–121). In humans, acute ferrokinetic responses to rHuEPO do not differ among patients on hemodialysis, normal subjects, or patients with chronic renal failure restored to normal by

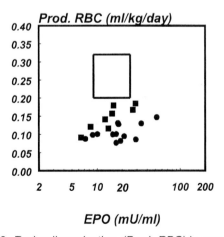

FIG. 91-6. Red cell production *(Prod. RBC)* in normal subjects and patients on maintenance hemodialysis. Normal range is shown by the area within the box. Dialysis patients are segregated into those with red cell survival greater than 100 days *(circles)* and less than 100 days *(squares)*. The erythropoietic *(EPO)* response is shifted down and to the right in patients on dialysis.

transplantation (119). The improvement of anemia demonstrated after parathyroidectomy is due to the resolution of marrow fibrosis rather than the removal of erythropoietic inhibition (121). Despite the clinical experience showing that exogenous EPO easily overcomes the effects of any such putative inhibitors, studies on uremic inhibitors continue because control of such factors could reduce the amount of rHuEPO needed to correct anemia. Recent studies have focused on effects of albumin-bound furancarboxylic acid (122) and activated monocyte and polymorphonuclear leukocyte products (123) on erythropoiesis. T cells from uremic subjects may be unable to release general growth cytokines needed for optimal erythropoiesis (124). In addition, urea-derived cyanate carbamylates EPO and decreases its biologic activity (125)

Nutritional Factors Contributing to Anemia

The patient with chronic renal failure or on maintenance dialysis is prone to anorexia, intercurrent illnesses, and dietary restrictions. Dialysis also can produce dialysate nutrient losses. All patients should be observed for malnutrition and vitamin deficiency syndromes. Of these, borderline or frank iron deficiency is the most common. It occurs to a lesser extent in patients with progressive renal failure and in those on continuous ambulatory peritoneal dialysis (CAPD). It is a major impediment to the cost-effective use of rHuEPO in patients on hemodialysis. Lindsay et al. (126) showed that blood losses of up to 20 mL per dialysis could occur with each hemodialysis treatment. The nontransfused patient on hemodialysis is prone to iron deficiency because of such repetitive blood losses. At a target hematocrit of 30% to 36%, such losses of red cells equate to an additional 6- to 7-mg iron loss per dialysis above normal obligatory daily iron losses of 1 to 2 mg/day. With the additional losses from periodic laboratory tests, the yearly iron losses can exceed normal total body stores of iron of approximately 1200 mg. Most regular hemodialysis programs require iron supplementation, averaging 2 to 3 g/year, usually parenterally, to prevent iron deficiency.

Folate deficiency is uncommon (127) in patients on dialysis because of the routine use of supplements. Because of the water solubility of thiamine, pyridoxine, and vitamin B_{12}, deficiencies in one or more of these vitamins could develop from dialytic removal, but no cases have been reported in patients on dialysis. Currently, only pyridoxine supplementation is recommended: 5 mg/day for those with progressive renal failure and 10 mg/day for patients on dialysis (128).

WORKUP AND MANAGEMENT OF ANEMIA, IRON DEFICIENCY/OVERLOAD, AND ERYTHROCYTOSIS

The treatment of the anemia of chronic renal failure has assumed greater clinical importance given the increasing age of

the ESRD population, which has more frequent and greater degrees of ischemic heart and peripheral vascular disease and is increasingly composed of diabetic patients with both microvascular and macrovascular disease. Many symptoms previously attributed to "uremia," such as fatigue, cold intolerance, and mental sluggishness, respond to correction of anemia. With the advent of rHuEPO therapy, nonspecific therapies such as transfusions and anabolic steroids are of historic interest only. Because rHuEPO therapy takes weeks to months to correct significant degrees of anemia, symptomatic patients with ischemic heart or cerebrovascular disease should receive transfusions. Similarly, treatment of symptomatic acute blood loss requires transfusions. If major surgery is anticipated, autologous blood donation for intraoperative use is possible if enough epoetin is used (129), thus avoiding the need for homologous red cell transfusions. Patients with sickle cell disease remain transfusion dependent despite very high doses of rHuEPO and continue to experience iron overload. Transfusions still have a risk of infection and can result in sensitization of potential transplant recipients.

The initial evaluation of the anemic patient with chronic renal failure should include a complete blood count, including red cell indices, a reticulocyte count, and determination of the serum iron, total iron-binding capacity, and ferritin (collectively referred to as *iron indices*). If the anemia is normochromic and normocytic with a normal or low reticulocyte index, the peripheral smear shows no abnormalities, and the iron indices are normal, then no further workup of the anemia is necessary. Several studies correlating serum ferritin, serum transferrin, and stainable bone marrow iron indicate that ferritin levels greater than 100 ng/mL cannot exclude iron deficiency in patients on dialysis (130). These parameters likely apply to the patient with progressive renal failure as well. Transferrin saturation and ferritin levels should exceed 25% and 200 ng/mL, respectively, in the iron-replete patient with renal insufficiency to optimize erythropoiesis (131). Periodic monitoring of the iron indices is mandatory to detect functional iron deficiency. Anemic patients with iron indices minimally greater than those enumerated become iron deficient during rHuEPO therapy unless supplemented with iron. The most common etiology for microcytosis remains iron deficiency. Low serum iron with elevated ferritin suggests systemic infection, inflammatory disease, or occult malignancy. Normal or high serum iron with normal ferritin but microcytic indices points to thalassemia or aluminum toxicity. Macrocytosis is unusual in the well dialyzed patient receiving a vitamin supplement and consuming a recommended protein diet of 1.0 to 1.4 g/kg.

Periodic monitoring of the complete blood count and red cell and iron indices in patients on dialysis detects variance from the patient's steady-state values. The nomogram of VanWyck et al. (132) is helpful in estimating the amount of exogenous iron needed during induction therapy to attain the target hemoglobin of 11 to 12 g/dL. A rough rule of thumb is to administer 1 mg of iron intravenously for each 1 mL of red blood cells to be formed. Most patients require maintenance parenteral iron to maintain optimal erythropoiesis. Patients allergic to iron dextran can receive some of the newer agents (133,134). Iron also can be delivered to patients on hemodialysis by adding ferric pyrophosphate to conventional dialysate (135).

The complication of iron overload from multiple transfusions has virtually disappeared after the widespread application of epoetin therapy. Some have even used the strategy of periodic phlebotomy to reduce iron deposition in epoetin-treated patients (136).

Absence of anemia or amelioration of preexisting anemia in patients with progressive renal failure or on dialysis requires a search for potential causes. Possible etiologies include (a) contracted predialysis plasma volume, (b) decreased hemoglobin oxygen saturation from cardiac or pulmonary disease, (c) hereditary or acquired cystic kidneys, and (d) conditions that cause decreased blood flow to the kidneys or liver. Increased endogenous EPO production (137) can occur in the last three circumstances, indicating that even anuric diseased kidneys can increase their production of EPO under some circumstances. Hypoxemia or conditions producing reduced renal blood flow can increase EPO production, but hematocrit seldom increases above normal levels. In some patients on dialysis with acquired renal cystic disease, erythrocytosis associated with "increased" endogenous EPO levels develops. Increasing tissue pressure on remaining renal parenchyma by the cysts probably produces *worsening local hypoxia.* Alternatively, *autonomous production* of EPO by proliferating epithelial cells in the cyst wall can occur (138).

Very rarely, polycythemia develops in patients with chronic renal failure, either coincidentally due to polycythemia rubra vera or secondary to processes known to cause secondary polycythemia. Marked increases in the red cell mass can occur in states associated with paraneoplastic EPO production. In most instances, high hematocrits (>48%) in uremic patients cannot be explained but occur in association with increased EPO levels. Erythrocytosis of renal origin can be distinguished from polycythemia vera by EPO levels because EPO is below normal in the latter condition. On occasion, hematocrit increases in a patient with ESRD and hepatitis. This increase usually is transient and follows an increase in EPO levels during the period of increased aminotransferases (139).

THERAPY OF RENAL ANEMIA

Clinical trials of rHuEPO were initiated in 1985, and replacement therapy with rHuEPO quickly became the most rational therapy for anemia of chronic renal failure (140,141). These initial clinical trials convincingly demonstrated that the hematocrit could be increased by up to ten points or more and maintained at a level above 30% in more than 90% of patients. Dialysis-treated patients increased their hematocrit in a dose-dependent manner (140), as shown in Fig. 91-7. Maintenance intravenous doses needed thrice weekly to maintain steady-state hematocrits greater than 31% varied significantly

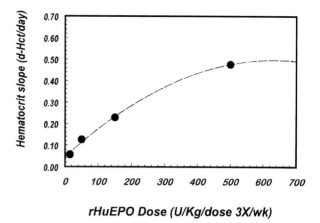

FIG. 91-7. Dose-response curve to intravenous epoetin alfa [recombinant human erythropoietin (rHuEPO)] administered three times a week. The linear part of the response curve extends up to 150 U/kg/dose. (Adapted from Eschbach JW, et al. Correction of the anemia of end-stage renal disease with recombinant human erythropoietin: results of combined phase I and II clinical trials. *N Engl J Med* 1987;316:73, with permission.)

among study patients: 15% required more than 150 U/kg, 20% less than 40 U/kg. Similar results have been observed worldwide (141). In patients on dialysis, correction of anemia with rHuEPO therapy improves quality-of-life indices, including those assessing global well-being and depression (142). Correction of anemia also improves cognition (143), and other aspects of quality of life (144). Improvement in aerobic capacity or cardiac function also have been demonstrated (145). Indeed, it was this global success in patients on dialysis that expanded the use of rHuEPO to patients with progressive renal failure.

Published reports on the effects of rHuEPO in predialysis patients are limited compared with those in patients with ESRD. Initial concern about accelerating renal failure from animal studies regarding correcting anemia in patients with progressive renal failure have not been substantiated by clinical experience. No significant alteration in the progression of renal disease (as assessed by the slope of the reciprocal of plasma creatinine or by direct measurement of GFR) secondary to changes in systemic hemodynamics or blood volume (146–152) has been noted in carefully conducted clinical trials. Direct measurements of renal hemodynamics during rHuEPO treatment are sparse (147,150,152). In one study, a significant increase in filtration fraction was noted after 4 weeks of therapy, but mean blood pressure had increased from 119 to 134 mm Hg (150). In another study, GFR, renal blood flow, and filtration fraction did not change from baseline after correction of anemia from a hematocrit of 24% to 39% (152). All investigators emphasize the *importance of blood pressure control* in preventing deterioration in renal function. The absence of adverse effects on residual renal function in many of the studies indicates the careful monitoring of blood pressure (146) and early use of additional antihypertensive agents (148–150) during rHuEPO therapy.

If increases in blood pressure during rHuEPO therapy are controlled, correction of anemia does not appear to alter renal hemodynamics or accelerate progression of renal insufficiency. This undoubtedly reflects the clinical experience gained from earlier clinical trials in patients on dialysis.

Benefits and Outcomes of Recombinant Human Erythropoietin Therapy

Transfusion Avoidance

Before epoetin therapy, up to 25% of patients on hemodialysis were transfusion dependent (153). Most patients with transfusional iron overload had hemosiderosis, a state with minimal organ dysfunction (154), and not hematochromatosis. With epoetin therapy, repeated transfusions have been virtually eliminated and the risk for development of hemochromatosis has vanished. In fact, the major problem for patients with ESRD on maintenance epoetin therapy is the development of iron deficiency. Given the infectious risks of transfusion (human immunodeficiency virus, hepatitis C, and perhaps hepatitis G) and the sensitization of potential transplant recipients, transfusions should be used prudently. Elimination of transfusions with epoetin produces a marked reduction in the percentage panel reactive antibody as well as in anti-human leukocyte antigen–specific antibody titers (155). In situations of gastrointestinal bleeding, postoperative blood loss, or hemolysis, transfusions must be used and remain the mainstay of therapy.

Quality of Life and Cognitive Functions

Correction of anemia to a hematocrit of 30% to 36% with rHuEPO therapy improves quality-of-life indices, including those assessing global well-being and depression, in patients on hemodialysis (142) and CAPD (156), and in those with progressive renal disease (144). Whether quality-of-life indicators could be improved further by raising the hematocrit above a level of 36% is debated. Improvement in cognition is highly sensitive to the hematocrit level and improves when anemic hematocrits are increased into the 32% to 36% range (143). Increasing the hematocrit to 42% with epoetin further improves brain and cognitive function (157).

Endocrine and Metabolic Changes

Uremic men manifest a variety of biochemical hormonal abnormalities as well as sexual dysfunction. Sexual function in younger uremic men treated with EPO improves (158), but the mechanism producing this improvement is not clear. Epoetin therapy also produces positive nitrogen balance (159) and improves diabetic retinopathy (160).

Immune/Granulocyte Function

Since the early 1980s, the incidence of life-threatening infection in patients with ESRD has remained unchanged. Correction of anemia produces the following effects: (a) an increase in the number of natural killer cells and in helper/suppresser T-cell ratios (161); (b) improvement in immunoglobulin production by peripheral mononuclear cells (162) and specifically in antibody titers after hepatitis B vaccine immunization (163); and (c) correction of deficient phagocytic functions (164). Cytokine secretion is decreased in anemia and is corrected by increasing the hematocrit, whether by transfusion or epoetin treatment (165).

Exercise Tolerance and Rehabilitation

In patients on hemodialysis, improvements in exercise and cardiorespiratory performance after correction of anemia to a hematocrit of 30% to 36% are maintained but not augmented on repeated testing out to 1 year (144,145). These findings suggest that poor physical performance in patients with chronic renal failure is not entirely due to anemia but that factors such as deconditioning, neuropathy, and cardiovascular disease also contribute. Changes in well-being and physical performance have not in general translated into greater employment.

Effects on Survival and Hospitalization

In adults undergoing hemodialysis, the overall mortality rate is reduced if hemoglobin is maintained above 10 g/dL with EPO therapy (166,167). Other studies demonstrate a reduction in overall hospitalization in EPO-treated patients (168,169). Use of epoetin may reduce long-term total costs for ESRD care (170).

Hazards of Recombinant Human Erythropoietin Therapy

Hypertension

Uncorrected anemia produces a hyperdynamic state that along with hypertension contributes to the development of left ventricular hypertrophy (LVH) in renal failure. De novo or worsening hypertension occurs in 20% to 40% of epoetin-treated patients predialysis (146,147) and in approximately 30% (171) of patients on dialysis. A number of risk factors for this epoetin-induced hypertension have been proposed, including preexisting hypertension, severe anemia at initiation, rapid increase in hematocrit, high recombinant human EPO doses given intravenously, and, in patients on dialysis, the presence of native kidneys.

The mechanisms producing hypertension during epoetin therapy are multifactorial. Anemia produces a hyperdynamic state characterized by increased cardiac output and a decrease in peripheral vascular resistance both in normal subjects (172) and in patients before dialysis (152) and those on dialysis (173). The decreased peripheral resistance results from both hypoxic vasodilatation as well as lower blood viscosity. An increase in whole-blood viscosity (174) and loss of hypoxic vasodilatation are potential causes of increased blood pressure in EPO-treated patients as the degree of anemia lessens. However, other factors must be important because the increase in blood pressure does not correlate with the rise in hematocrit (175).

The increase in peripheral resistance after therapy does not correlate with plasma renin activity, with concentrations of angiotensin I or II (175), or with catecholamines (176). EPO at pharmacologic concentrations (i.e., >1,000 mU/mL) achieved after intravenous injection can increase endothelin-1 release from endothelial cells (177). However, several studies have found no changes or decreases in endothelin-1 levels during chronic EPO therapy (178). EPO therapy may impair the vasodilatory response to nitric oxide (179). Nitric oxide activity is increased in rHuEPO-treated rats, perhaps as a counterregulatory mechanism that limits the pressor effect (180).

Whatever the exact role of vasoactive substances in the genesis of EPO-induced hypertension, it appears to be specific to those with renal failure. This hypertensive response has not been observed in other anemias or in nonrenal patients treated with epoetin for short or long periods (181). In experimental models, rHuEPO produces hypertension in a remnant model of renal failure but not in sham control animals (182). Also, blood pressure remains unchanged in iron-deficient patients on hemodialysis whose hematocrits are increased from 25% to 32% with simple iron repletion (183). The increase in blood pressure occurs primarily in patients with chronic renal failure in whom blood volume changes occur or in whom maladaptive cardiovascular changes persist.

A number of studies emphasize the importance of adequate control of body fluid and fluid gains in maintaining blood pressure control during epoetin therapy. Hemodynamic changes in patients predialysis are influenced by changes in total blood volume. In studies in which blood volume increased after rHuEPO correction of anemia, cardiac output also increased (184); cardiac output remained unchanged or decreased if blood volume remained unchanged (185). Maintenance of normal blood volume requires equivalent decreases in plasma volume as red cell mass is increased to avoid changes in preload to the heart. Lim et al. (186) achieved a constant blood volume of approximately 59 to 60 mL/kg during correction of anemia, as did Abrahams and coworkers (185). Mean blood pressure remained constant in both studies. The importance of blood volume control is emphasized by Anastassiades and coworkers (187). Blood pressure remained unchanged in patients on peritoneal dialysis but increased by 8 mm Hg in patients not on dialysis as anemia was corrected. Despite equal expansion of the red cell mass, plasma volume decreased in patients on peritoneal dialysis but not in those predialysis. Patients in the predialysis stage may need more aggressive diuresis to maintain constant blood volume to avoid hypertension.

Patients who become hypertensive or have worsening hypertension during epoetin therapy appear to have an inadequate decrease in cardiac output in response to the EPO-induced increase in peripheral vascular resistance (188). The increase in blood pressure after epoetin therapy usually occurs during the early phases of treatment when hematocrit is increasing rapidly (189); however, some patients become hypertensive months after the hematocrit has stabilized. No predictable relationship exists between the rate of hematocrit increase and blood pressure (187). Because of this hypertensive tendency and the inability to predict which patients might become significantly hypertensive, diastolic blood pressure must be controlled before initiating epoetin therapy. By contrast, patients with low blood pressure actually may benefit from the rise in diastolic blood pressure associated with the increase in red cell mass.

Cardiovascular Disease

Hypertension and LVH are known risk factors for cardiovascular disease. In patients on hemodialysis, partial regression of LVH and some degree of reduction in left ventricular volume (190,191) follow correction of anemia. Improvement in exercise-induced ST segment depression during exercise (192,193) also occurs. However, a major trial of the effect of normalizing hematocrit in patients with ESRD with coronary artery disease or congestive heart failure was halted for safety reasons without evidence of benefit (194).

Effects on Coagulation

Improvement in the bleeding time without change in routine coagulation test results is due primarily to the improvement in red blood cell mass. Up to 11% of patients experience clotting of dialyzers or lines after rHuEPO therapy (144) and require a 50% increase in heparin requirements at final target hematocrits of 30% to 38% (195). An increased risk of access thrombosis was noted in large clinical trials (196,197). The risk appears to be greater in patients with synthetic bridge grafts (197) and in patients with previously known access dysfunction (196).

Dialysis Efficiency

In vivo studies have found changes in dialyzer urea clearances because of a decrease in water flow as red cell mass increases. After correction of anemia, serum potassium, phosphate, and creatinine increase (198), but the magnitude of such changes is small. The effects on the urea kinetic modeling parameter, Kt/V, are easily corrected by changing the dialysis prescription. (199) During high-flux hemodialysis, treatment time needed to be increased from a mean of 140 to 169 minutes as hematocrit increased from 24% to 36% (200). Dialyzer reuse efficiency decreases despite 15% to 40% increases in heparin dosing (201). With peritoneal dialysis, clearances of sodium, potassium, and urea and levels of protein loss or glucose absorption do not change after EPO therapy (202).

Other Side Effects

Flu-like reactions have been reported in less than 1% of patients (195). Correction of anemia to hematocrits over 30% is associated with painless conjunctival injection, so-called *red eye* (146,195). It is of cosmetic concern only. Frequency of headache varies from 3% to 33%, but the incidence does not differ from that in untreated or placebo-treated patients (195). In the initial trials, development of encephalopathy or seizures was not uncommon (146,195) and resulted from suboptimal control of blood pressure.

Dosing, Pharmacokinetics, and Route of Administration

An optimal "target" hemoglobin/hematocrit cannot be defined *a priori* for each patient because sedentary, older patients differ from younger, more active or working patients. The currently recommended DOQI Work Group target hematocrit value for patients with ESRD is between 33% and 36%. A recent study has shown that it is not desirable to attain higher, "more normal" hematocrit values in patients on hemodialysis with congestive heart failure or coronary artery disease (194). Whether the target hematocrit may be extended to near-normal values among noncardiac patient groups is unknown. Higher target values may be safe and beneficial among younger (<65 years of age) patients on dialysis without diabetes, heart failure, coronary heart disease, or cerebrovascular disease, as shown by a prospective Spanish study that assessed outcomes in 156 stable patients on dialysis as the mean hematocrit was raised with epoetin therapy from 30.9% to 38.4% (203). At 6 months, decreased hospitalization and increased functional status and quality of life were noted.

The predialysis hematocrit is not an accurate measure of red cell mass because it may increase by 5 points postdialysis owing to removal of large intradialytic weight gains. In addition, red blood cell swelling during transport of samples to central laboratories results in further errors. To circumvent these problems, a target hemoglobin value of 11 to 12 g/dL is recommended for monitoring of efficacy.

Several principles govern the administration of EPO (204): (a) the response to epoetin is dose dependent, but with a variable subject response; (b) the response depends on the route of administration—intravenous versus subcutaneous—and the frequency of administration—daily, twice weekly, three times weekly; and (c) the response may be limited by inadequate iron stores, bone marrow fibrosis, and inflammation The ideal dose in a given patient is one that permits attainment of the target hematocrit over the life span of the erythrocyte because it satisfies both the initiation and maintenance requirements (205). During maintenance, new red blood cells should be formed at a rate comparable with the removal rate. Drug dosage should not be drastically lowered after reaching the target hematocrit because this produces a

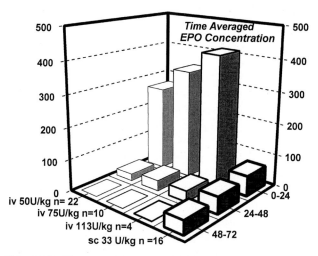

FIG. 91-8. Pharmacokinetic profiles comparing intravenous with subcutaneous doses of epoetin. Although time-averaged erythropoietin *(EPO)* concentrations after subcutaneous doses are lower in the first 24 hours, concentrations are higher in the next two 24-hour periods despite lower doses than for intravenous administration.

"yo-yo" or "ping-pong" effect. The reasons for the extreme variability among patients in dosage needs for epoetin (40 to 450 U/kg/week) are not known.

Subcutaneous injections are the most effective route of administration. Dosage requirements using the subcutaneous route are lower by approximately 30% than those using the intravenous route (26,206,207), providing greater cost efficiency. With subcutaneous dosing, EPO levels are sustained in the interdialytic period (26), decreasing apoptosis and permitting more sustained erythropoiesis (Fig. 91-8). Novel erythropoiesis-stimulating protein has an even greater half-life after subcutaneous administration and should allow dosing at a frequency of once a week or less. Studies have shown the safety of subcutaneously injected epoetin at home (148). Patients on CAPD respond better to equivalent weekly doses than patients on hemodialysis, perhaps because of lower ongoing blood losses (148,208).

Resistance to epoetin is defined either by the requirement for large doses during initiation (>150 U/kg) or by the development of refractoriness to a previously efficacious dose for maintaining the desired hemoglobin. In approximately 15% of subjects, a dose greater than 150 U/kg/week is needed in the absence of any "known" state producing resistance and probably represents differences in sensitivity to epoetin or red cell survival among individuals. However, the most common cause for EPO resistance is iron deficiency. Enhanced iron utilization due to EPO-enhanced red blood cell formation can quickly deplete iron stores in the presence of poor medical compliance, occult gastrointestinal blood loss, or dialysis-related blood losses. The U.S. Renal Data System Dialysis Morbidity and Mortality Study showed that 50% of patients receiving epoetin were iron deficient (209).

A number of studies have indicated that iron-replete patients receiving regular parenteral iron require less rHuEPO than patients receiving no parenteral iron supplementation or regular oral iron alone (209–211). On average, hematocrit increases by 14% and the epoetin dose decreases by 38% after administration of a prorated weekly dose of iron (212). We have an arbitrary ceiling for ferritin of 1,000 ng/mL, above which parenteral iron is not used. Transferrin saturations of less than 16% and less than 20% define absolute and relative iron deficiency, respectively. Other techniques have been sought to evaluate functional iron deficiency, including protoporphyrins (213) and the percentage of hypochromic cells (214). A new method that measures the hemoglobin content of reticulocytes holds greater promise (215) because the reticulocyte reflects bone marrow events affecting hemoglobin synthesis within the previous several days. Today, sequential automated measurements give early warning of impending iron deficiency and trigger appropriately intensified iron therapy.

Other unusual causes for refractoriness to rHuEPO include inadequate amounts of other essential nutrients such as folate, vitamin B$_{12}$, and pyridoxine. The red cell, not serum, folate concentration is the most reliable assay for evaluating a patient for possible folate deficiency (216). Inflammation blunts the response to epoetin. If iron deficiency is excluded, inflammation is the most common cause of *secondary* failure to respond to epoetin and is associated with increased levels of tumor necrosis factor-α, IL-2, and γ-interferon (217). Although less of a problem now because other agents have been developed to control hyperphosphatemia, aluminum overload produces resistance to epoetin (218). Hyperparathyroidism has reemerged as a cause of resistance to rHuEPO, requiring higher or increasing doses of rHuEPO owing to bone marrow fibrotic disease (121). Finally, angiotensin-converting enzyme inhibitors or angiotensin II receptor antagonists may impair erythropoiesis and produce relative EPO resistance (219,220).

REFERENCES

1. Remuzzi G, Rossi EC. Hematologic consequences of renal failure. In: Brenner BM, Rector FC, eds. *The kidney.* Philadelphia: WB Saunders, 1995:2170.
2. Bright R. Cases and observations, illustrative of renal disease accompanied with the secretion of albuminous urine. *Guys Hosp Rep* 1836;1:338.
3. Brown GE, Roth GM. The anemia of chronic nephritis. *Arch Intern Med* 1922;30:817.
4. Carnot P, Deflandre C. Sur l'activite hematopoietique de serum au cours de la regeneration du sang. *C R Seances Acad Sci (Paris)* 1906;143:384.
5. Erslev AJ. Blood and mountains. In: Wintrobe MM, ed. *Blood, pure and eloquent.* New York: McGraw-Hill, 1980:257.
6. Erslev AJ. Humoral regulation of red cell production. *Blood* 1953;8:349.
7. Jacobson LO, Goldwasser E, Fried W, et al. Role of the kidney in erythropoiesis. *Nature* 1957;179:633.
8. Caro J, et al. Erythropoietin levels in uremic nephric and anephric patients. *J Lab Clin Med* 1979;93:449.
9. Erslev A. Anemia of chronic renal disease. *Arch Intern Med* 1970;126:774.
10. Cotes PM, Baugham DR. Bioassay of erythropoietin in mice made plethoric by exposure to air at reduced pressure. *Nature* 1961;191:1065.
11. Adamson JW. The erythropoietin/hematocrit relationship in normal and polycythemic man: implications of marrow regulation. *Blood* 1968;32:597.
12. Erslev AJ. In vitro production of erythropoietin by kidneys perfused with a serum-free solution. *Blood* 1974;44:77.
13. Jelkmann W. Erythropoietin: structure, control of production, and function. *Physiol Rev* 1992;72:449.
14. Garcia JE, Sherwood JB, Goldwasser E. Radioimmunoassay of erythropoietin. *Blood Cells* 1979;5:405.
15. Miyake T, Kung CKH, Goldwasser E. Purification of human erythropoietin. *J Biol Chem* 1977;252:5558.
16. Lai P-H, et al. Structural characterization of human erythropoietin. *J Biol Chem* 1986;261:3116.
17. Lin FK, et al. Cloning and expression of the human erythropoietin gene. *Proc Natl Acad Sci USA* 1985;82:7580.
18. Ptashne M, Gann A. Transcriptional activation by recruitment. *Nature* 1997;386:569.
19. Egrie JC, Browne JK. The molecular biology of erythropoietin. In: Erslev AJ, Adamson JW, Eschbach JW, et al., eds. *Erythropoietin: molecular, cellular, and clinical biology.* Baltimore: The Johns Hopkins University Press, 1991:21.
20. Beck I, Ramirez S, Weinmann R, et al. Enhancer element at the 3′ flanking region controls transcriptional response to hypoxia in the human erythropoietin gene. *J Biol Chem* 1991;266:15563.
21. Semenza GL, Nejfelt MK, Chi SM, et al. Hypoxia-inducible nuclear factors bind to an enhancer element located 3′ to the human erythropoietin gene. *Proc Natl Acad Sci USA* 1991;88:5680.
22. Madan A, Custin PT. A 24-base-pair sequence 3′ to the human erythropoietin gene contains a hypoxia-responsive transcriptional enhancer. *Proc Natl Acad Sci USA* 1993;90:3928.
23. Beck I, Weinmann R, Caro J. Characterization of the hypoxia-responsive enhancer in the human erythropoietin gene shows presence of a hypoxia-inducible 120 KD nuclear DNA-binding protein in erythropoietin-producing and non-producing cells. *Blood* 1993;82:704.
24. Wang FF, Kung CKF, Goldwasser E. Some chemical properties of human erythropoietin. *Endocrinology* 1985;116:2286.
25. Dube S, Fisher JW, Powell JS. Glycosylation at specific sites of erythropoietin is essential for biosynthesis, secretion, and biological function. *J Biol Chem* 1988;263:17516.
26. Besarab A, et al. Clinical pharmacology and economics of recombinant human erythropoietin in end-stage renal disease: the case for subcutaneous administration. *J Am Soc Nephrol* 1992;2:1405.
27. Smith-Dordal M, Wang FF, Goldwasser E. The role of carbohydrate in erythropoietin action. *Endocrinology* 1985;116:2293.
28. Egrie JC, Dwyer E, Lykos M, et al. Novel erythropoiesis stimulating protein (NESP) has a longer serum half-life and greater in vivo biological activity compared to recombinant human erythropoietin (rHuEPO). *Blood* 1997;90:56a(abstr).
29. MacDougall IC, Gray SJ, Elston O, et al. Pharmacokinetics of novel erythropoiesis stimulating protein compared with epoetin alfa in dialysis patients. *J Am Soc Nephrol* 1999;10:2392.
30. Spivack JL. The mechanism of action of erythropoietin. *Int J Cell Cloning* 1986;4:139.
31. Goldberg MA, Dunning SP, Bunn HF. Regulation of the erythropoietin gene: evidence that the oxygen sensor is a heme protein. *Science* 1988;242:1412.
32. Ratcliffe PJ. Molecular biology of erythropoietin. *Kidney Int* 1993;44:887.
33. Erslev AJ, Wilson J, Caro J. Erythropoietin titers in anemic nonuremic patients. *J Lab Clin Med* 1987;109:429.
34. Eckard K, et al. Distribution of erythropoietin producing cell in rat kidneys during hypoxic hypoxia. *Kidney Int* 1993;43:815.
35. Maxwell PH, Osmond MK, Pugh CW, et al. Identification of the renal erythropoietin-producing cells using transgenic mice. *Kidney Int* 1993;44:1149.
36. Ogawa M. Differentiation and proliferation of hematopoietic stem cells. *Blood* 1993;81:2844.
37. Koury ST, et al. Quantitation of erythropoietin producing cells in kidneys of mice by in situ hybridization: correlation with hematocrit, renal erythropoietin mRNA, and serum erythropoietin concentration. *Blood* 1989;74:645.

38. Schuster S, Wilson JH, Erslev AJ, et al. Physiologic regulation and tissue localization of renal erythropoietin messenger RNA. *Blood* 1988;70:316.

39. Krause DS, Fackler MJ, Civin CI, et al. CD34: structure, biology, and clinical utility. *Blood* 1996;87:1.

40. Gregory CJ. Erythropoietin sensitivity as a differentiation marker in the hemapoietic system: studies of three erythropoietic colony responses in cell culture. *J Cell. Physiol* 1976;89:289.

41. Sawada K, Krantz SB, Dessypris EN, et al. Human colony-forming units-erythroid do not require accessory cells but do require direct interaction with insulin-like growth factors 1 and/or insulin for erythroid development. *J Clin Invest* 1989;83:1701.

42. Krantz SB. Erythropoietin. *Blood* 1991;77:419.

43. Faquin WC, Schneider TJ, Goldberg MA. Effect of inflammatory cytokines on hypoxia-induced erythropoietin production. *Blood* 1992; 79:1987.

44. Means RT, Krantz SB. Inhibition of human erythroid colony-forming units by tumor necrosis factor requires beta interferon. *J Clin Invest* 1992;91:416.

45. D'Andrea AD, Lodish HF, Wong GG. Expression cloning of the murine erythropoietin receptor. *Cell* 1989;57:277.

46. Klingmüller U, Lorenz U, Cantley LC, et al. Specific recruitment of SH-PTP1 to the erythropoietin receptor causes inactivation of JAK2 and termination of proliferative signals. *Cell* 1995;80:729.

47. Koury MJ, Bondurant MC. Erythropoietin retards DNA breakdown and prevents programmed death in erythroid progenitor cells. *Science* 1990;248:378.

48. Wrighton NC, Farrell FX, Chang R, et al. Small peptides as potent mimetics of the protein hormone erythropoietin. *Science* 1996;273: 458.

49. Tan CC, Eckard K-U, Firth JD, et al. Feedback modulation or renal and hepatic erythropoietin mRNA in response to graded anemia and hypoxia. *Am J Physiol* 1992;263:F474.

50. Erslev AJ. Erythropoietin. *N Engl J Med* 1991;324:1339.

51. Jelkmann W, Wiedemann G. Serum erythropoietin level: relationship to blood hemoglobin concentrations and erythrocytic activity of the bone marrow. *Klin Wochenschr* 1990;68:403.

52. Fried W, Barone-Varelas J. Regulation of the plasma erythropoietin level in hypoxic rats. *Exp Hematol* 1984;12:706.

53. Ross R, McCrea JB, Besarab A. Erythropoietin response to blood loss in hemodialysis patients is blunted but preserved. *ASAIO J* 1994; 40:M880.

54. Müller-Wiefel D, Schärer K. Serum erythropoietin levels in children with chronic renal failure. *Kidney Int* 1983;24[Suppl 15]:S70.

55. Garcia JF, et al. Radioimmunoassay of erythropoietin circulating levels in normal and polycythemic human being. *J Lab Clin Med* 1982; 99:624.

56. Cahan C, et al. Diurnal variations in serum erythropoietin levels in healthy subjects and sleep apnea patients. *J Appl Physiol* 1992;72:2112.

57. Catchatourian R, Eckerling G, Fried W. Effect of short term protein deprivation on hemapoietic functions of healthy volunteers. *Blood* 1980;55:625.

58. Fried W, Heller P, Johnson C. Observations on the regulation of erythropoietin production and of erythropoiesis during prolonged exposure to hypoxia. *Blood* 1970;36:607.

59. Radtke HW, et al. Serum erythropoietin concentration in chronic renal failure: relationship to degree of anemia and excretory renal function. *Blood* 1979;54:877.

60. McGonigle RSR, Wallin JD, Shadduck RK, et al. Erythropoietin deficiency and erythropoiesis in renal insufficiency. *Kidney Int* 1984; 25:437.

61. Naets JP, et al. Radioimmunoassay of erythropoietin in chronic uraemia of anephric patients. *Scand J Haematol* 1986;37:390.

62. Loge JP, Lange RD, Moore CV. Characterization of the anemia associated with chronic renal insufficiency. *Am J Med* 1958;24:4.

63. Aherne WA. The "burr" red cell and azotemia. *J Clin Pathol* 1957;10: 252.

64. Nielson OJ, Thaysen JH. Erythropoietic deficiency in acute tubular necrosis. *J Intern Med* 1990;227:373.

65. Pastermack A, Wahlberg P. Bone marrow in acute renal failure. *Acta Med Scand* 1967;181:505.

66. Emerson CP. The pathogenesis of anemia in acute glomerulonephritis: estimations of blood production and blood destruction in a case receiving massive transfusions. *Blood* 1948;4:363.

67. Frenkel EP, Douglas CC, McCall MS. Hypoerythropoietinemia and anemia. *Arch Intern Med* 1970;125:1050.

68. Chandra M, Miller ME, Garcia JF, et al. Serum immunoreactive erythropoietin levels in patients with polycystic kidney disease as compared with other hemodialysis patients. *Nephron* 1985;39:26.

69. Eckard K-U, Möllmann M, Neumann R, et al. Erythropoietin in polycystic kidneys. *J Clin Invest* 1989;84:1160.

70. Caro J, Schuster S, Besarab A, et al. Renal biogenesis of erythropoietin. In: Rich IN, ed. *Molecular and cellular aspects of erythropoietin and erythropoiesis.* NATO ASI series vol. H8. Berlin: Springer-Verlag, 1987.

71. Besarab A, et al. Dynamics of erythropoiesis following renal transplantation. *Kidney Int* 1987;32:526.

72. Chaplin H, Mollison PL. Red cell life-span in nephritis and in hepatic nephrosis. *Clin Sci* 1953;12:351.

73. Eschbach JW, et al. Erythropoiesis in patients with renal failure undergoing chronic dialysis. *N Engl J Med* 1967;276:653.

74. Lonergan ET, et al. Erythrocyte transketolase activity in dialyzed patients: a reversible metabolic lesion of uremia. *N Engl J Med* 1971; 284:1399.

75. Cole CH. Decreased ouabain-sensitive adenine triphosphatase activity in the erythrocyte membrane of patients with chronic renal disease. *Clin Sci* 1973;45:775.

76. Joske RA, McAlister JM, Prankerd TAJ. Isotope investigations of red cell production and destruction in chronic renal disease. *Clin Sci* 1956;15:511.

77. Ragen PA, Hagedorn AB, Owen CA. Radioisotope study of anemia in chronic renal disease. *Arch Intern Med* 1960;105:518.

78. Berry ER, Rambach WA, Alt HL, et al. Effect of peritoneal dialysis on erythrokinetics and ferrokinetics of azotemic anemia. *Trans Am Soc Artif Intern Organs* 1965;10:415.

79. Erslev A, Besarab A. The rate and control of baseline red cell production in hematologically stable uremic patients. *J Lab Clin Med* 1995; 126:283.

80. Rosenwund A, Binswanger U, Straub PW. Oxidative injury to erythrocytes, cell rigidity, and splenic hemolysis in hemodialyzed uremic patients. *Ann Intern Med* 1975;82:460.

81. Tipple MA, et al. Illness in hemodialysis patients after exposure to chloramine contaminated dialysate. *ASAIO Trans* 1991;37:588.

82. Manzler AD, Schreiner AW. Copper-induced acute hemolytic anemia: a new complication of home dialysis. *Ann Intern Med* 1970;73:409.

83. Petrie JJB, Row PG. Dialysis anaemia caused by sub acute zinc toxicity. *Lancet* 1977;1:1178.

84. Short AIK, Winney RJ, Robson JS. Reversible microcytic hypochromic anemia in dialysis patients due to aluminum intoxication. *Proc Eur Dial Transplant Assoc* 1980;17:233.

85. Carlson DJ, Shapiro FL. Methemoglobinemia from well water nitrates: a complication of home dialysis. *Ann Intern Med* 1970;73:757.

86. Orringer EP, Mattern WD. Formaldehyde-induced hemolysis during chronic hemodialysis. *N Engl J Med* 1976;294:1416.

87. Kaiser L, Schwartz KA, Burnatowska-Hledin A, et al. Microcytic anemia secondary to intraperitoneal aluminum in normal and uremic rats. *Kidney Int* 1984;26:269.

88. Gallery EDM, Blomfield J, Dixon SR. Acute zinc toxicity in haemodialysis. *BMJ* 1972;4:331.

89. Said R, Quintanilla A, Levin N, et al. Acute hemolysis due to profound hypo-osmolality: a complication of hemodialysis. *J Dial* 1977;1:447.

90. Schuett H, Port FK. Hemolysis in hemodialysis patients. *Dial Trans* 1980;9:345.

91. Keshaviah P, Leuhmann D, Shapiro F, et al. *Investigation of the risks and hazards associated with hemodialysis systems.* Silver Springs, MD: U.S. Department of Health and Human Services, Public Health Service/Food and Drug Administration/Bureau of Medical Devices, 1980.

92. Francos GC, et al. An unsuspected cause of acute hemolysis during hemodialysis. *Trans Am Soc Artif Intern Organs* 1983;24:140.

93. Iacob HS, Amsden T. Acute hemolytic anemia with rigid red cells in hypophosphatemia. *N Engl J Med* 1971;285:1146.

94. Hartley RA, Morgan TO, Innis MD, et al. Splenectomy for anemia in patients on regular dialysis. *Lancet* 1971;2:1343.

95. Bischel MD, et al. Hypersplenism in the uremic hemodialyzed patient. *Nephron* 1972;9:146.

96. Weinberg SG, et al. Myelofibrosis and renal osteodystrophy. *Am J Med* 1977;63:755.

97. Bommer J, Ritz E, Waldherr R. Silicone induced splenomegaly: treatment of pancytopenia by splenectomy in a patient on hemodialysis. *N Engl J Med* 1981;305:1077.

98. Hassanein AA, McNicol GP, Douglass AS. Relationship between platelet function tests in normal and uraemic subjects. *J Clin Invest* 1970;23:402.

99. Clouse RE, et al. Angiodysplasia as a cause of upper gastrointestinal bleeding in uremia. *Arch Intern Med* 1985;145:458.

100. Benigni A, et al. Reversible activation defect of the platelet glycoprotein IIb-IIIa complex in patients with uremia. *Am J Kidney Dis* 1993;22:668.

101. Gralnick HR, McKeown LP, Williams SB, et al. Plasma and platelet von Willebrand factor defects in uremia. *Am J Med* 1988;85:806.

102. Savage B, Shattil SJ, Ruggeri ZM. Modulation of platelet function through adhesion receptors: a dual role glycoprotein IIb-IIIa (integrin aIIbb3) mediated by fibrinogen and glycoprotein Ib-von Willebrand factor. *J Biol Chem* 1992;267:11300.

103. Di Minno G, et al. Platelet dysfunction in uremia: multifaceted defect partially corrected by dialysis. *Am J Med* 1985;79:552.

104. Noris M, et al. Enhanced nitric oxide synthesis in uremia: implications for platelet dysfunction and dialysis hypotension. *Kidney Int* 1993;44:445.

105. Norris M, Remuzzi G. Uremic bleeding: closing the circle after 30 years of controversies. *Blood* 1999;94:2569.

106. Fernandez F, Goudable C, Sie P, et al. Low hematocrit and prolonged bleeding time in uraemic patients: effect of red cell transfusion. *Br J Haematol* 1985;59:139.

107. Cases A, et al. Recombinant human erythropoietin treatment improves platelet function in uremic patients. *Kidney Int* 1992;42:668.

108. Fisher JW. Mechanism of the anemia of chronic renal failure [Editorial review]. *Nephron* 1980;25:106.

109. Zappacosta AR, Caro J, Erslev A. The normalization of hematocrit in end-stage renal disease patients on continuous ambulatory peritoneal dialysis: the role of erythropoietin. *Am J Med* 1982;72:53.

110. Ohne Y, Rege AB, Fisher JW, et al. Inhibitors of erythroid colony-forming cells (CFU-E and BFU-E) in sera of azotemic patients with anemia of renal disease. *J Lab Clin Med* 1978;92:916.

111. Radtke HW, et al. Identification of spermine as an inhibitor of erythropoiesis in patients with chronic renal failure. *J Clin Invest* 1980; 67:1623.

112. Segal GM, Stuere T, Adamson JW. Spermine and spermidine are non-specific inhibitors of in vitro hematopoiesis. *Kidney Int* 1987;31:72.

113. Pershagen G, Mast R, Lins LE, et al. Increased arsenic concentration in the bone marrow in chronic renal failure: a contribution to anemia? *Nephron* 1982;30:250.

114. Cambell RA. Anemia, uremia, and polyamines. *Nephron* 1985;41:299.

115. Ono K, Waki Y, Takeda K. Hypervitaminosis A: a contributing factor to anemia in regular dialysis patients. *Nephron* 1984;38:44.

116. Meytes D, Bogin E, Ma A, et al. Effect of parathyroid hormone on erythropoiesis. *J Clin Invest* 1981;67:1263.

117. Wallner SF, Vantrin RM. The anemia of chronic renal failure: studies of the affect of organic solvent extraction of the serum. *J Lab Clin Med* 1978;92:363.

118. Eschbach JW, et al. The anemia of chronic renal failure in sheep: the response to erythropoietin-rich plasma in vivo. *J Clin Invest* 1984;74:434.

119. Eschbach JW, Haley NR, Eagrie JC, et al. A comparison of the responses to recombinant erythropoietin in normal and uremic subjects. *Kidney Int* 1992;42:407.

120. Delwechi F, et al. High levels of the circulating form of parathyroid hormone do not inhibit in vivo erythropoiesis. *J Lab Clin Med* 1983;102:613.

121. Rao DS, Shih M-S, Mohini R. Effect of serum parathyroid hormone and bone marrow fibrosis on the response to erythropoietin in uremia. *N Engl J Med* 1993;328:171.

122. Niwa T, Yazawa T, Kodama T, et al. Efficient removal of albumin-bound furancarboxylic acid, an inhibitor of erythropoiesis, by continuous ambulatory peritoneal dialysis. *Nephron* 1990;56:241.

123. Himmelfarber J, Lazarus M, Hakim R. Reactive oxygen species production by monocytes and polymorphonuclear leukocytes during dialysis. *Am J Kidney Dis* 1991;3:271.

124. Morra L, Ponassi A, Gurreri G, et al. Inadequate ability of T-lymphocytes from chronic uremic subjects to stimulate the in vivo growth of committed erythroid progenitors (BFU-E). *Acta Haematol* 1988;79: 187.

125. Mun KC, Golper TA. Impaired biological activity of erythropoietin by cyanate carbamylation. *Blood Purif* 2000;18:13.

126. Lindsay RM, Burton JA, Edward N. Dialyzer blood loss. *Clin Nephrol* 1973;1:20.

127. Whitehead VM, Comty CH, Posen GA, et al. Homeostasis of folic acid in patients undergoing maintenance hemodialysis. *N Engl J Med* 1968;279:970.

128. Wolfson M. Use of water-soluble vitamins in patients with chronic renal failure. *Semin Dial* 1988;1:28.

129. Goodnough LT, et al. Increased preoperative collection of autologous blood with recombinant human erythropoietin therapy. *N Engl J Med* 1989;321:1163.

130. Birgegard G, Nilsson P, Wide L. Regulation of iron therapy by S-ferritin estimations in patients on chronic hemodialysis. *Scand J Nephrol* 1981;15:69.

131. Besarab A, Amin N, Ahsan M, et al. Optimization of epoetin therapy with intravenous iron therapy in hemodialysis patients. *J Am Soc Nephrol* 2000;11:530.

132. Van Wyck DB, et al. Iron status in patients receiving erythropoietin for dialysis-associated anemia. *Kidney Int* 1989;35:165.

133. Nissenson AR, Lindsay RM, Swan S, et al. Sodium ferric gluconate complex in sucrose is safe and effective in hemodialysis patients: North American Clinical Trial. *Am J Kidney Dis* 1999;33:471.

134. Silverberg DS, Blum M, Peer G, et al. Intravenous ferric saccharate as an iron supplement in dialysis patients. *Nephron* 1996;72:413.

135. Gupta A, Amin NB, Besarab A, et al. Dialysate iron therapy: infusion of soluble ferric pyrophosphate via the dialysate during hemodialysis. *Kidney Int* 1999;55:1891.

136. Lazarus JM, Hakim RM, Newell J. Recombinant human erythropoietin and phlebotomy in the treatment of iron overload in chronic hemodialysis patients. *Am J Kidney Dis* 1990;16:101.

137. Shalhoub RJ, Rajan U, Kim VV, et al. Erythrocytosis in patients on long-term hemodialysis. *Ann Intern Med* 1982;97:986.

138. Goldsmith HJ, et al. Association between rising haemoglobin concentration and renal cyst formation in patients on long term regular dialysis treatment. *Proc Eur Dial Assoc* 1982;19:313.

139. Pololi-Anagnostou L, Wastenfelder C, Anagnostou A. Marked improvement of erythropoiesis in an anephric patient. *Nephron* 1981; 29:277.

140. Eschbach JW, et al. Correction of the anemia of end-stage renal disease with recombinant human erythropoietin: results of combined phase I & II clinical trials. *N Engl J Med* 1987;316:73.

141. Erslev AJ, Adamson JW, Eschbach JW, et al., eds. *Erythropoietin: molecular, cellular, and clinical biology.* Baltimore: The Johns Hopkins University Press, 1991.

142. Evans RW. Recombinant human erythropoietin and the quality of life of end-stage renal disease patients: a comparative analysis. *Am J Kidney Dis* 1991;18[Suppl 1]:S62.

143. Temple RM, Langan SJ, Deary IJ. Recombinant human erythropoietin improves cognitive function in chronic haemodialysis patients. *Nephrol Dial Transplant* 1992;7:240.

144. Canadian Erythropoietin Study Group. Association between recombinant human erythropoietin and quality of life and exercise capacity of patients receiving haemodialysis. *BMJ* 1990;300:573.

145. Lundin AP, et al. Exercise in hemodialysis patients after treatment with recombinant human erythropoietin. *Nephron* 1991;58:315.

146. Eschbach JW, et al. Treatment of the anemia of progressive renal failure with recombinant human erythropoietin. *N Engl J Med* 1989;321:158.

147. U. S. Recombinant Human Erythropoietin Predialysis Group. Double-blind, placebo-controlled study of the therapeutic use of recombinant human erythropoietin for anemia associated with chronic renal failure in predialysis patients. *Am J Kidney Dis* 1991;14:50.

148. Austrian Multicenter Study Group of r-HuEPO in Predialysis Patients. Effectiveness and safety of recombinant human erythropoietin in predialysis patients. *Nephron* 1991;61:399.

149. Keinman KS, et al. The use of recombinant human erythropoietin: I. the correction of anemia in predialysis patients and its effects on renal function: a double blind, placebo-controlled trial. *Am J Kidney Dis* 1989;14:486.

150. Abraham PA, et al. Renal function during therapy for anemia in predialysis chronic renal failure patients. *Am J Nephrol* 1990;10:128.

151. Koene RA, Frenken LAM. Does treatment of predialysis patients with recombinant human erythropoietin compromise renal function? *Contrib Nephrol* 1990;87:105.

152. Frenken LAM, Wetzels JFM, Sluitter HE, et al. Evidence for renal vasodilatation in pre-dialysis patients during correction of anemia by erythropoietin. *Kidney Int* 1992;41:384.

153. Eschbach JW. The anemia of chronic renal failure: pathophysiology and the effects of recombinant erythropoietin [Review]. *Kidney Int* 1989;35:134.

154. Goldman M, Vangerweghen J-L. Multiple blood transfusions and iron overload in patients receiving haemodialysis. *Nephrol Dial Transplant* 1987;2:316.

155. Barany P, Fehrman I, Godoy C. Long term effects on lymphocytotoxic antibodies and immune reactivity in hemodialysis patients treated with recombinant human erythropoietin. *Clin Nephrol* 1992;37:90.

156. Auer J, et al. Quality of life improvements in CAPD patients treated with subcutaneously administered erythropoietin for anemia. *Perit Dial Int* 1992;12:40.

157. Pickett JL, Theberge DC, Brown WS, et al. Normalizing hematocrit in dialysis patients improves brain function. *Am J Kidney Dis* 1999; 33:1122.

158. Schaefer RM, Kokot F, Wirnze H, et al. Improved sexual function in hemodialysis patients on recombinant erythropoietin: a possible role for prolactin. *Clin Nephrol* 1989;33:1.

159. Garibotto G, et al. Erythropoietin treatment and amino acid metabolism in hemodialysis patients. *Nephron* 1993;65:533.

160. Friedman EA, Brown CD, Berman DH. Erythropoietin in diabetic macular edema and renal insufficiency. *Am J Kidney Dis* 1995;26: 202.

161. Collart FE, Dratwa M, Wittek M, et al. Effect of recombinant human erythropoietin on T-cell lymphocyte subsets in hemodialysis patients. *ASAIO Trans* 1990;36:M219.

162. Schaefer RM, Paczek L, Berthold G, et al. Improved immunoglobulin production in dialysis patients treated with recombinant erythropoietin. *Int J Artif Organs* 1992;3:71.

163. Sennasael JJ, Van der Niepen P, Verbeelen DL. Treatment with recombinant human erythropoietin increases antibody titers after hepatitis B vaccination in dialysis patients. *Kidney Int* 1990;40:121.

164. Veys N, Vanholder R, Ringoir S. Correction of deficient phagocytosis during erythropoietin treatment in maintenance dialysis patients. *Am J Kidney Dis* 1992;19:358.

165. Gafter U, Kalechman Y, Orlin JB, et al. Anemia of uremia is associated with reduced in vitro cytokine secretion: immunopotentiating activity of red blood cells. *Kidney Int* 1994;45:224.

166. Lowrie EC, et al. The relative contributions of measured variables to death risk among hemodialysis patients. In: Friedman EA, ed. *Death on hemodialysis: preventable or inevitable?* Dordrecht: Kluwer Academic Publishers, 1995:121.

167. Ma JZ, Ebben J, Xia H, et al.. Hematocrit level and associated mortality in hemodialysis patients. *J Am Soc Nephrol* 1999;10:610.

168. Churchill DN, et al. Effect of recombinant human erythropoietin on hospitalization of hemodialysis patients. *Clin Nephrol* 1995;43: 184.

169. Xia H, Ebben J, Ma JZ, et al. Hematocrit levels and hospitalizations risks in hemodialysis patients. *J Am Soc Nephrol* 1999;10:1309.

170. Powe NR, et al. Effect of recombinant erythropoietin on hospital admissions, readmissions, length of stay, and costs of dialysis patients. *J Am Soc Nephrol* 1994;4:1455.

171. Eschbach JW, et al. Recombinant human erythropoietin in anemic patients with end-stage renal disease: results of a phase III multicenter clinical trial. *Ann Intern Med* 1989;111:992.

172. Richardson TQ, Guyton AC. Effects of polycythemia and anemia on cardiac output and other circulatory factors. *Am J Physiol* 1959; 197:1167.

173. Neff MS, et al. Hemodynamics of uremic anemia. *Circulation* 1971; 43:876.

174. Brown CD, et al. Treatment of azotemic, nonoliguric, anemic patients with human recombinant erythropoietin raises whole blood viscosity proportional to hematocrit. *Nephron* 1991;59:394.

175. Stephen HM, et al. Peripheral hemodynamics, blood viscosity, and the renin-angiotensin system in hemodialysis patients under therapy with recombinant human erythropoietin. *Contrib Nephrol* 1989;76:292.

176. Portoles J, et al. Cardiovascular effects of recombinant human erythropoietin in predialysis patients. *Am J Kidney Dis* 1997;29:541.

177. Carlini R, Dusso AS, Chamberlain I, et al. Recombinant human erythropoietin (rHuEPO) increases endothelin-1 release by endothelial cells. *Kidney Int* 1993;43:1010.

178. Brunet P, et al. Plasma endothelin in haemodialysis patients treated with recombinant human erythropoietin. *Nephrol Dial Transplant* 1994; 9:650.

179. Vaziri ND, et al. Role of nitric oxide resistance in erythropoietin-induced hypertension in rats with chronic renal failure. *Am J Physiol* 1996;271:E113.

180. del Castillo D, Raij L, Shultz PJ, et al. The pressor effect of recombinant human erythropoietin is not due to decreased activity of the endogenous nitric oxide system. *Nephrol Dial Transplant* 1995;10:505.

181. Eschbach JW. Erythropoietin-associated hypertension. *N Engl J Med* 1990;323:999.

182. Poux JM, Lartigue M, Chaisemartin RA, et al. Uraemia is necessary for erythropoietin-induced hypertension in rats. *Clin Exp Pharmacol Physiol* 1995;22:769.

183. Kaupke CJ, Kim S, Vaziri ND. Effect of erythrocyte mass on arterial blood pressure in dialysis patients receiving maintenance erythropoietin therapy. *J Am Soc Nephrol* 1994;4:1874.

184. Onoyama, K, et al. Effects of human recombinant erythropoietin on anaemia, systemic haemodynamics and renal function in pre-dialysis renal failure patients. *Nephrol Dial Transplant* 1989;4:966.

185. Abraham PA, Macres MG. Blood pressure in hemodialysis patients during amelioration of anemia with erythropoietin. *J Am Soc Nephrol* 1991;2:927.

186. Lim VS, et al. The safety and efficacy of maintenance therapy of recombinant human erythropoietin treatment in patients with renal insufficiency. *Am J Kidney Dis* 1989;14:496.

187. Anastassiades E, et al. Influence of blood volume on the blood pressure of predialysis and peritoneal dialysis patients treated with erythropoietin. *Nephrol Dial Transplant* 1993;8:621.

188. Fellner SK, et al. Cardiovascular consequences of the correction of the anemia of renal failure with erythropoietin. *Kidney Int* 1993;44: 1309.

189. Creutzig A, et al. Skin microcirculation and regional peripheral resistance in patients with chronic anaemia treated with recombinant human erythropoietin. *Eur J Clin Invest* 1990;20:219.

190. Cannella G, et al. Reversal of left ventricular hypertrophy following recombinant human erythropoietin of anemic dialyzed uremic patients. *Nephrol Dial Transplant* 1991;6:31.

191. Goldberg N, et al. Changes in left ventricular size, wall thickness, and function in anemic patients treated with recombinant human erythropoietin. *Am Heart J* 1992;124:424.

192. Wizemann V, Kaufman N, Kramer W. Effect of erythropoietin on ischemic tolerance in anemic hemodialysis patients with confirmed coronary artery disease. *Nephron* 1992;62:161.

193. MacDougall IC, et al. Long-term cardiopulmonary effects of amelioration of renal anemia by erythropoietin. *Lancet* 1990;1:489.

194. Besarab A, et al. The effects of normal versus anemic hematocrit on hemodialysis patients with cardiac disease. *N Engl J Med* 1998;339: 584.

195. Sundal E, Kaeser U. Correction of anaemia of chronic renal failure with recombinant human erythropoietin: safety and efficacy of one year's treatment in a European multicentre study of 150 haemodialysis-dependent patients. *Nephrol Dial Transplant* 1989;4:979.

196. Sabota JT. Recombinant human erythropoietin in patients with anemia due to end-stage renal disease. *Contrib Nephrol* 1989;76:166.

197. Churchill DN, et al. Probability of thrombosis of vascular access among hemodialysis patients treated with recombinant human erythropoietin. *J Am Soc Nephrol* 1994;4:1809.

198. Acchiardo SR, et al. Evaluation of hemodialysis patients treated with erythropoietin. *Am J Kidney Dis* 1991;17:290.

199. Baur T, Lundberg M. Secondary effects of erythropoietin treatment on metabolism and dialysis efficiency in stable hemodialysis patients. *Clin Nephrol* 1990;34:230.

200. Lippi A, et al. Recombinant human erythropoietin and high flux haemodiafiltration. *Nephrol Dial Transplant* 1995;10[Suppl 6]:51.

201. Veys N, Vanholder R, De Guyper K, et al. Influence of erythropoietin on dialyzer re-use, heparin needs, and urea kinetics in maintenance hemodialysis patients. *Am J Kidney Dis* 1994;23:52.

202. Ksiazek A, Baranowska-Daca E. Hematocrit influence on peritoneal dialysis effectiveness during recombinant human erythropoietin treatment in patients with chronic renal failure. *Perit Dial Int* 1993;13[Suppl 2]:S550.

203. Moreno F, et al. Increasing the hematocrit has a beneficial effect on quality of life and is safe in selected hemodialysis patients: Spanish

Cooperative Renal Patients Quality of Life Study Group of the Spanish Society of Nephrology. *J Am Soc Nephrol* 2000;11:335.

204. Muirhead N, et al. Evidence-based recommendations for the clinical use of recombinant erythropoietin. *Am J Kidney Dis* 1995; 26[Suppl]:S1.

205. Uehlenger DE, Gotch FA, Steiner CB. A pharmacodynamic model of erythropoietin therapy for uremic anemia. *Clin Pharmacol Ther* 1992; 51:76.

206. Albitar S, et al. Subcutaneous versus intravenous administration of erythropoietin improves its efficacy for the treatment of anaemia in haemodialysis patients. *Nephrol Dial Transplant* 1995;10:40.

207. Kaufman JS, et al. Subcutaneous compared to intravenous epoetin in patients receiving hemodialysis: Department of Veterans Affairs Cooperative Study Group on Erythropoietin in Hemodialysis Patients. *N Engl J Med* 1998;339:578.

208. Besarab A, Golper TA. Response of continuous peritoneal dialysis patients to subcutaneous rHuEPO differs from that of hemodialysis patients. *ASAIO Trans* 1991;37:M395.

209. U.S. Renal Data Systems. The USRDS Dialysis Morbidity and Mortality Study (Wave 1). In: *U.S. Renal Data Systems annual report*. Bethesda, MD: National Institutes of Health, National Institutes of Diabetes and Digestive and Kidney Diseases, 1996:45.

210. Fishbane S, Frei GL, Maesaka J. Reduction in recombinant human erythropoietin doses by the use of chronic intravenous iron supplementation. *Am J Kidney Dis* 1995;26:41.

211. Besarab A, Kaiser JW, Frinak S. A study of parenteral iron regimens in hemodialysis patients. *Am J Kidney Dis* 1999;34:21.

212. Besarab A, Frinak S, Yee J. An indistinct balance: safety and efficacy of parenteral iron. *J Am Soc Nephrol* 1999;10:2029.

213. Fishbane S, Lynn RI. The utility of zinc protoporphyrin for predicting the need for intravenous iron therapy in hemodialysis patients. *Am J Kidney Dis* 1995;25:426.

214. Horl WH, Cavill I, Macdougall IC, et al. How to diagnose and correct iron deficiency during r-huEPO therapy: a consensus report [Review]. *Nephrol Dial Transplant* 1996;11:246.

215. Fishbane S, Galgano C, Langley RC, et al. Reticulocyte hemoglobin content in the evaluation of iron status of hemodialysis patients. *Kidney Int* 1997;52:217.

216. Bamonti-Catena F, et al. Folate measurements in patients on regular hemodialysis treatment. *Am J Kidney Dis* 1999;33:492.

217. Druecke TB. Modulating factors in the hematopoietic response to erythropoietin. *Am J Kidney Dis* 1991;18[Suppl 1]:87.

218. Bia MJ, et al. Aluminum induced anemia: pathogenesis and treatment in patients on chronic hemodialysis. *Kidney Int* 1989;36:852.

219. Albitar S, et al. High dose enalapril impairs the response to erythropoietin treatment in haemodialysis patients. *Nephrol Dial Transplant* 1998;13:1206.

220. Schwarzbeck A, Wittenmeier KW, Hallfrizsch U. Anaemia in dialysis patients as a side-effect of sartanes. *Lancet* 1998;352:286.

CHAPTER 92

The Osteodystrophy of Chronic Renal Failure

Dennis L. Andress and Donald J. Sherrard

Normal bone is a unique tissue in the body, involving a combination of organic and inorganic material under the control of two kinds of cells, osteoblasts and osteoclasts. These cells perform their contrasting but coordinated functions to maintain skeletal mass and modulate calcium balance. It is, in fact, alterations in calcium metabolism that commonly lead to metabolic bone disease. As calcium is removed from or prevented from entering bone to maintain the circulating level, structural consequences result in failure of bone strength. In the conflict between bone's function as a calcium reservoir and its function as a structural support system, the reservoir function almost always predominates.

The organic matrix of bone is produced by the osteoblast and is mainly composed of type I collagen (1). In the disorders in which bone formation is decreased, collagen (osteoid) production also is decreased, but it is not known to be abnormal qualitatively. On the other hand, in the high-bone-formation states associated with secondary hyperparathyroidism, an abnormal-appearing "woven" osteoid may contribute to defective mineralization in the bone that is formed (1,2). Osteoblasts also synthesize several noncollagenous proteins that become constituents of the osteoid and may be important in the mineralization process. Two of these, alkaline phosphatase and osteocalcin (3), are secreted by osteoblasts and are elevated in serum during certain high-turnover bone states, such as Paget's disease and hyperparathyroid bone disease. Although the exact role of these osteoblast-derived proteins in mineralization is unknown, they are useful clinically in the longitudinal assessment of bone turnover.

The inorganic material (largely calcium and phosphate salts) that deposits on the interlinking collagen strands of the osteoid forms apatite crystals of varying sizes. There is a link between osteoid maturation and crystal deposition in

that the mineral does not deposit until the osteoid reaches a certain maturational state. The mineralization lag time is a commonly determined measurement that expresses the time it takes before newly formed osteoid accepts mineral deposition. Variations in this measurement reflect abnormalities in the process of bone mineralization (4).

Of the cells that control bone remodeling, relatively little is precisely known. The osteoblast is involved in the formation of the osteoid and presumably controls the entry of the mineral (5). At sites of bone formation, the cell assumes a cuboidal shape and begins to make the osteoid. After a delay of 2 to 3 weeks, the osteoid begins to mineralize, and after a few months this bone-forming unit turns off, cells become quiescent, and bone formation moves to another site (6). Although the controls for osteoblast growth and differentiation are unknown, growth factors present in bone matrix may have a role (7–10). Perhaps more important are the cytokines and growth factors secreted by marrow precursor cells and osteoblasts. These include interleukin-1 (IL-1) and IL-6 (7), tumor necrosis factor α, transforming growth factor β (11), fibroblast growth factor (10), bone morphogenetic proteins (12), the insulin-like growth factors (IGFs) (13,14), and IGF-binding proteins (IGFBPs) (15,16), all of which stimulate either osteoblast proliferation or various differentiated cell functions (17,18). In addition to their probable autocrine function, they may be the primary mediators of hormonal stimulation of bone cell growth. This could be particularly important in the hyperparathyroidism of uremia because parathyroid hormone (PTH) is known to stimulate osteoblast proliferation (19) as well as the osteoblast production of transforming growth factor β (20), IL-6 (21), IGF-1 (22), and IGFBPs (23). Moreover, the elevated circulating levels of IL-6 (24), IL-1, tumor necrosis factor α (25), and IGF-1 (26) in some patients on dialysis also may significantly influence bone turnover.

Osteoclasts resorb bone. It is not clear why osteoclasts, which are derived from marrow macrophage precursors (27), choose to resorb bone at a particular site and time. Osteoclasts and osteoblasts are functionally linked such that when one is stimulated or suppressed, the other responds in the same

D.L. Andress: Department of Medicine, University of Washington; and VA Puget Sound Health Care System, Seattle, Washington

D.J. Sherrard: Department of Medicine, University of Washington; and Department of Medicine, Seattle VA Medical Center, Seattle, Washington

direction and magnitude (28). This balanced response allows the bone to modulate calcium metabolism for a few weeks until counterregulatory processes come into play. At that point, a new equilibrium is achieved between bone resorption and bone formation, protecting against major alterations in skeletal mass.

In the normal subject, bone is a dynamic organ, with approximately 400 mg of calcium entering and leaving the skeleton each day (29). Lesser amounts of other minerals as well as bicarbonate and phosphate accompany this movement of calcium. Deficiencies in calcium, phosphate, and bicarbonate both inhibit bone formation and enhance resorption. Other circulating factors that affect bone dynamics include PTH and vitamin D. Although calcitonin also may play a role, it appears to be only a weak and transient (effects lasting a few days) inhibitor of bone resorption (30). Other hormones, such as thyroid hormone and adrenal corticoids, may have permissive effects or lead to skeletal disorders when deficient or excessive, but usually are not primary offenders in metabolic bone disease and do not play major roles in renal osteodystrophy.

Although the hyperparathyroidism of renal failure is one of the most important biochemical derangements affecting bone remodeling, several other factors also are important in renal osteodystrophy. For example, uremia and its attendant acidosis inhibit some cellular processes that are important in bone remodeling (31,32), including cartilage production (33,34) and osteoblast function (35). Magnesium abnormalities may affect PTH metabolism (36,37) or have a direct impact on apatite formation (38). Heparin given in a continuous high dose is well described as a cause of osteoporosis (39), but its role in causing bone loss during intermittent use in patients on dialysis has not been determined.

PATHOGENESIS

High-Turnover Bone Disease

Historically, high-turnover bone disease is the predominant bone lesion in patients with renal failure. The lesion begins in a mild form and progresses to typical osteitis fibrosa (hyperparathyroid bone disease) (Table 92-1). This lesion is mediated by a steady rise in serum PTH (40). For many years it was thought that the trade-off hypothesis adequately explained PTH changes in renal failure (41–43). According to this hypothesis, the rise in phosphate, which occurs as renal failure advances, lowers serum calcium levels, which stimulates PTH secretion. Although considerable clinical and experimental data seemed to support this theory, many

TABLE 92-1. *Types of renal osteodystrophy*

I. High turnover
  A. Mild disease (mild hyperparathyroidism)
  B. Osteitis fibrosa (severe hyperparathyroidism)
II. Low turnover
  A. Aplastic (adynamic) disorder
  B. Osteomalacia
III. Mixed osteodystrophy

---

patients did not follow this proposed pattern. Other investigators suggested that the "set point" for PTH inhibition by calcium was altered in patients with renal failure (44,45). Later, it was proposed that this alteration in set point might be due to the lack of 1,25-dihydroxyvitamin D_3 (46,47). This seemed logical because one function of PTH in normal subjects is to stimulate renal synthesis of 1,25-dihydroxyvitamin D_3; it would be appropriate physiologically for 1,25-dihydroxyvitamin D_3 to inhibit its trophic hormone (48–50). Data from patients with moderate renal failure show that serum 1,25-dihydroxyvitamin D_3 levels decline before serum calcium decreases and that serum 1,25-dihydroxyvitamin D_3 correlates inversely with the rise in PTH levels (51). The demonstration that intravenous calcitriol suppresses PTH independent of its effect on the calcium level appears to provide the final proof that calcitriol is a direct inhibitor of PTH secretion *in vivo* (52–54). Other important factors that likely contribute to hyperparathyroidism in renal failure include a decrease in 1,25-dihydroxyvitamin D_3 receptors in parathyroid cells (55), the prolonged half-life of PTH in renal failure (56), the direct effect of high phosphate concentrations to stimulate PTH secretion, and decreased activity of the calcium-sensing receptor (57) (Fig. 92-1).

Hyperphosphatemia had been suspected of having more than an indirect role in promoting hyperparathyroidism (58), but convincing evidence for a direct stimulatory effect of phosphate on parathyroid metabolism has been shown only recently. High concentrations of phosphate in the media of parathyroid cultures stimulate PTH secretion (59,60), and phosphate administration to uremic rats increases PTH levels without changing serum calcium or 1,25-dihydroxyvitamin D_3 (59,61). Moreover, serum phosphate is directly correlated with serum PTH in patients with mild to moderate chronic renal failure (62) (Fig. 92-2). The stimulatory effect of phosphate has been attributed to enhanced parathyroid cell

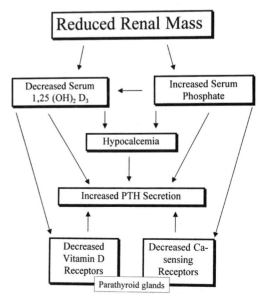

FIG. 92-1. Pathogenesis of secondary hyperparathyroidism in chronic renal failure.

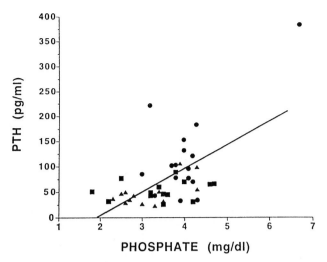

FIG. 92-2. Relationship between serum parathyroid hormone and serum phosphate in 44 patients with mild to moderate chronic renal failure (serum creatinine <3.0 mg/dL); r = 0.62, P < 0.01. (From Kates DM, Sherrard DJ, Andress DL. Evidence that serum phosphate is independently associated with serum PTH in patients with chronic renal failure. *Am J Kidney Dis* 1997;30:809, with permission.)

proliferation (61) and to decreased calcium-sensing receptor expression (63). How these two pathways are linked remains to be established. It is clear, however, that the calcium-sensing receptor in the parathyroid glands of uremic patients is down-regulated (64,65), and the use of calcium receptor agonists (calcimimetics) is effective in suppressing PTH secretion in patients on dialysis (66) (Fig. 92-3). Whether calcimimetics are capable of suppressing parathyroid gland hyperplasia in uremic patients (67) remains to be determined.

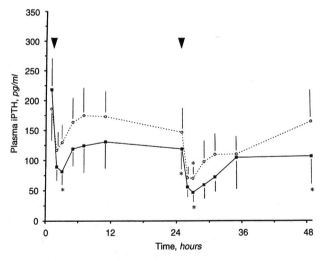

FIG. 92-3. Plasma parathyroid hormone levels in patients on dialysis receiving the calcimimetic, NPS R-568. *Arrowheads* indicate the time of a single oral dose. *Open symbols* indicate low dose and *closed symbols* indicate high dose. (From Antonsen JE, Sherrard DJ, Andress DL. A calcimimetic agent acutely suppresses parathyroid hormone levels in patients with chronic renal failure. *Kidney Int* 1998;53:223, with permission.)

Low-Turnover Bone Disease

The recognition that fracturing osteodystrophy and dialysis dementia occurred in the same epidemiologic setting led to the identification of aluminum toxicity (68). In early reports, it was evident that aluminum was entering the body through the dialysate. It has since become clear that aluminum also crosses the gut mucosa. In the normal subject, the small amount of aluminum that is absorbed (0.1% of the total) is rapidly eliminated by the kidney (69); only 10 to 30 mg is present in the normal body (69). In renal failure, gastrointestinal aluminum absorption is enhanced (70) and accumulations become significant when high oral doses are administered chronically (69,71). Consequently, uremic patients not yet on dialysis may have elevated serum aluminum (72), and aluminum bone disease develops in some of them (73). In other patients, residual renal function may offer protection against aluminum accumulation (74).

Aluminum deposition on bone surfaces usually is associated with a depressed rate of bone formation. However, this is not always true and the fact that aluminum often is present deep within mineralized bone suggests that its mere presence does not inhibit bone formation (75–77). Probably the amount of aluminum on bone surfaces is in part an indication of the level and chronicity of exposure.

In addition to aluminum, two other metals, iron and strontium, have been implicated as a cause of low-turnover bone disease (78–81). Iron has been found at bone surfaces in patients with osteomalacia and aplastic bone disease. Although the prevalence of iron-related bone disease is unknown, it probably is low. It may be that iron, therefore, occasionally simulates the toxicity usually attributed to aluminum. When treatment of iron overload is necessary, deferoxamine is efficacious (82). Increased bone strontium levels have been identified in patients on dialysis who have osteomalacia (81). Strontium is abundant in the earth's crust and is found in trace amounts in most foods, with grains and seafood containing the highest concentrations. In some regions, strontium levels in the water are quite high and can cause elevated serum levels in patients with moderate renal insufficiency and in patients receiving hemodialysis (83). The role of strontium in causing osteomalacia probably relates to its direct inhibition of the mineralization process (84) rather than a decrease in osteoblast number because the adynamic lesion cannot be induced by strontium in uremic rats (85). Adequate purification of dialysate water and use of strontium-free concentrates (83) appear to be the best way to prevent strontium overload.

Whether there are other specific uremic toxins that cause low-turnover bone disease remains to be seen. We have now observed a large number of patients with the adynamic lesion in whom neither iron nor aluminum could be found (86). In some, diabetes likely has a role by inducing a relative hypoparathyroid state (87,88), possibly because of hyperglycemia-induced PTH suppression (89). In others who are not diabetic, low PTH levels are thought to result from excessive therapeutic parathyroid gland suppression (86,90).

In others, an unidentified circulating low-molecular-weight inhibitor of osteoblast proliferation (35) may be important.

Aluminum seems to be able to produce this low-bone-formation picture by itself, and a marked reduction in PTH, as occurs with parathyroidectomy or aggressive medical therapy, accelerates its development (91). Thus, it is extremely important to be certain of the need for parathyroidectomy because such surgery, probably by the marked slowing of bone formation that results, potentiates the accumulation of aluminum at bone surfaces (91–93). The mechanism by which aluminum leads to depressed bone formation is unclear, but there are several possibilities. Aluminum deposits in the parathyroid gland (94) and appears to suppress PTH secretion (95). It also enters the osteoblast and may inhibit its activity (96). Aluminum deposits in the mineral itself and may impair apatite crystal development (97) and collagen cross-linking (98). All these possibilities are discussed in greater detail subsequently. Iron also apparently can lead to hypoparathyroidism in the hemochromatosis syndrome (99,100). Whether it deposits in the parathyroid gland in iron overload states associated with renal failure is unknown.

Mixed Uremic Osteodystrophy

The mixed lesion, as the name implies, combines features of both high- and low-turnover bone disease. This appearance can develop in at least two ways. First, if severe secondary hyperparathyroidism is associated with low calcium or low phosphate (as occurs in some poorly nourished patients), the high PTH stimulates both fibrous proliferation and osteoid production. Lacking calcium, phosphate, or both, however, this osteoid is slow to mineralize. Hypocalcemia was probably the major cause of this lesion in earlier reports. Second, if either hyperparathyroidism is being suppressed or osteomalacia is being treated by aluminum removal, a transitional state may occur in which a combination of both lesions is found.

CLINICAL FEATURES

Clinical and laboratory features that distinguish high- and low-turnover disease are extraordinarily subtle. Pain, weakness, and muscle wasting may be present in both. Similarly, hypercalcemia, increased alkaline phosphatase, and high PTH levels can occur in either disorder. Finally, the pathognomonic radiographic feature of hyperparathyroidism, subperiosteal resorption, is commonly noted in patients who have severe osteomalacia histologically with no histologic findings at all of hyperparathyroidism (101). Therefore, as the clinical features of these entities are discussed, the focus will be on distinguishing the two different processes.

Early Manifestations

As renal failure begins, few symptoms occur as a result of musculoskeletal problems. Most patients in the azotemic phase have biochemical abnormalities and some may have early histologic changes, but overt skeletal disease is rare. An exception to this general rule can be seen in certain tubular disorders, particularly distal renal tubular acidosis (type I) and proximal renal tubular acidosis (type II) associated with phosphate wasting. In these conditions, osteomalacia may occur even before the glomerular filtration rate (GFR) declines (102). Correction of the phosphate depletion in type II renal tubular acidosis and the acidosis of type I renal tubular acidosis improves mineralization remarkably (102). In children, adults with very slow progression of renal failure, or in anyone with marginal nutrition, musculoskeletal problems may occur of a severity not usually seen until several years of dialysis have elapsed. In children, the superimposition of growth requirements may make the skeleton more sensitive to excessive PTH. The aluminum problem certainly appears commonly in children before dialysis (103), which may be due to better compliance with medications or to increased gut permeability.

In adults with advanced but stable renal failure, all the factors are in place that lead to osteodystrophy. Thus, if there is enough time, it seems inevitable that bone disease will occur. Dietary innovations that may permit uremic patients to survive many years without dialysis require careful monitoring for this problem (104).

High-Turnover Bone Disease

Almost every symptom of uremia has been ascribed to elevated PTH (105). Although this may yet prove to be true, controlling PTH does not seem to alleviate the entire uremic syndrome. Perhaps the earliest symptom related to high-turnover bone disease is itching. This is particularly difficult to manage because pruritus in the uremic patient has such a variety of causes, including dry skin, uremia itself, disordered porphyrin metabolism, and abnormal calcium metabolism. With respect to the calcium abnormalities, most pruritic patients have high calcium × phosphate products and elevated PTH levels (106,107).

Frequently associated with or following appearance of pruritus, metastatic calcifications develop in some patients. Such calcifications usually occur in conjunction with high calcium × phosphate products, and patients present with a variety of patterns. Tumorous masses may appear, particularly adjacent to joints, which can reach 20 cm in diameter and weigh up to 10 kg (Fig. 92-4). The masses interfere with joint function and can become infected. Similar to those associated with foreign bodies, these infections are almost impossible to eliminate.

Deposits in other sites may be even more problematic. Myocardial calcification (108) can result in refractory arrhythmias or myocardial rupture. Diffuse pulmonary deposits in the alveolar–capillary basement membrane result in a restrictive lung disease with progressive pulmonary insufficiency (109). Vascular deposits likely contribute to the atherosclerosis to which these patients are prone, the most severe form

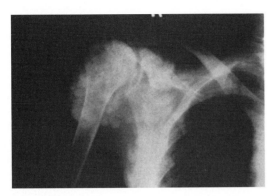

FIG. 92-4. Periarticular soft tissue calcification in a patient receiving dialysis.

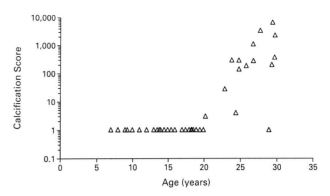

FIG. 92-6. Coronary artery calcification scores in 39 children and young adults with end-stage renal disease on dialysis, according to age. (From Goodman WG, et al. Coronary-artery calcification in young adults with end-stage renal disease who are undergoing dialysis. *N Engl J Med* 2000;342:1478, with permission.)

of which is calciphylaxis (Fig. 92-5). The finding of enhanced mortality rates in patients on dialysis who have a calcium × phosphate product greater than 65 or a phosphate concentration greater than 6.5 mg/dL (110) attests to the importance of fluctuating serum phosphate and the difficulty in ascribing a safe phosphate level for patients on dialysis. More recently, Goodman et al. have shown that coronary artery calcifications, as detected by electron beam computed tomography, are detectable in young patients within the first few years of commencing dialysis (Fig. 92-6). The calcifications were noted to occur in those with higher calcium intakes and higher calcium × phosphate products (111).

Bone pain and proximal muscle weakness usually go hand in hand. It often is hard to tell whether the muscle weakness is disuse atrophy (disuse because of skeletal pain and the patient's reluctance to move) or whether there is a specific muscle lesion. Occasionally, it is clear that proximal muscle atrophy and weakness, as occur in many other endocrine and metabolic disorders, develop before overt bone symptoms.

Bone symptoms usually are associated with weight-bearing activity. Pain occurs mostly in the lower extremities, particularly in the heels, knees, and hips. Less frequently, the ankles and feet hurt as well. Fractures are uncommon and usually are of smaller bones, although a patient may fracture a large bone through a cystic lesion. In general, fractures heal rather quickly with brisk callus formation.

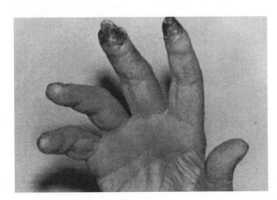

FIG. 92-5. Ischemic necrosis from severe vascular calcifications in a patient with chronic renal failure.

Enervation may occur with more severe hyperparathyroidism. Patients complain of a loss of enthusiasm, inability to "get started" with anything, and a vague depression. Obviously, all of these symptoms could be reactive depression, not uncommon in patients who feel overwhelmed by their disease. Changes in the electroencephalogram, brain calcium, and peripheral nerve conduction have been associated with the PTH elevation in uremia and may respond to its correction (112). The improvement with correction of the metabolic abnormality makes it likely that this is often a metabolic and not an emotional reaction.

A variety of arthropathies occur in patients with renal failure. Several may develop in conjunction with the bone disease. Pain with weight bearing in the hyperparathyroid patient often is felt in the joints, but there usually is little ancillary evidence of joint disease such as swelling, heat, tenderness, or limitation of motion. On the other hand, with a high calcium × phosphate product, a painful, crystal-induced arthritis can occur. This is particularly common in patients with large calcific deposits. In this setting, calcium pyrophosphate crystals may be seen in the joint. In the same patients, for unclear reasons, apatite crystals may form in the joint fluid and lead to a similar picture (113).

Low-Turnover Bone Disease

Many of the symptoms usually associated with high-turnover bone disease can be seen with low-turnover bone disease as well. Itching, metastatic calcification, and the crystal-induced arthropathies in general seem to correlate with the high phosphate levels. However, although these laboratory abnormalities are much more common in patients with secondary hyperparathyroidism, selective noncompliance in other patients can lead to similar laboratory abnormalities (see later) and hence similar symptoms.

Muscle weakness and proximal muscle wasting accompanying low-turnover bone disease are much more common and more severe (114). Although patients with

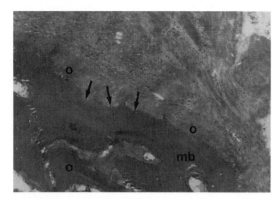

FIG. 92-7. Subperiosteal resorption *(arrows)* of mineralized bone *(mb)* filled in with unmineralized osteoid *(O)* in a patient on dialysis with osteomalacia. (Goldner's stain, magnification ×115.) (See Color Fig. 92-7 following page 2624.)

hyperparathyroidism may complain of decreased strength and have modest quadriceps wasting, patients with low-turnover bone disease often have severe weakness and atrophy and are unable to walk.

Similarly, bone pain, which usually is relatively mild and only minimally limiting with hyperparathyroidism, is much more severe with low-turnover bone disease. Also, in contrast to high-turnover bone disease, patients very frequently experience fractures (115). A fracture with little or no trauma or involving the ribs should make the clinician highly suspicious of this type of disease.

Mixed-Transitional Bone Disease

Depending more on the biochemistry and aluminum levels and the course the lesion is taking (e.g., does the patient have aluminum toxicity or PTH excess?), the symptoms of this disorder may be any of the foregoing symptoms of either of the two more common lesions. Bone deformity, however, is much more common with this condition than with either of the other two. If deformity is present, then bone pain, muscle weakness (often severely incapacitating), and fractures commonly occur as well.

Radiographs and Magnetic Resonance Imaging

Conventional radiographic studies are of limited value in distinguishing the different bone lesions of renal osteodystrophy. If radiographs reveal sclerotic bones of high density, the patient is more likely to have high-turnover bone disease. On the other hand, the pseudofractures typical of osteomalacia–rickets in the patient without renal failure also

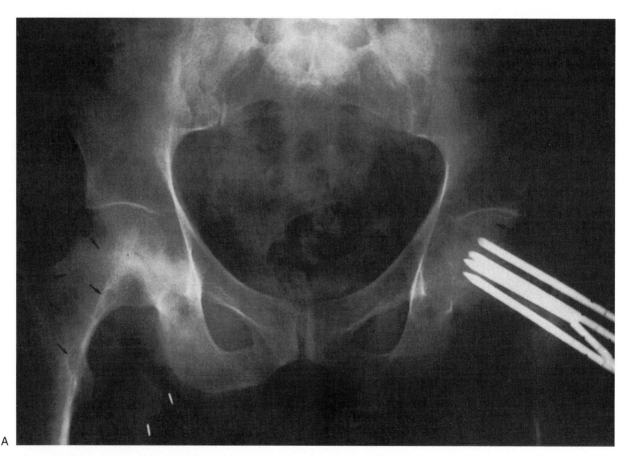

A

FIG. 92-8. Cystic bone lesions and erosions *(arrows)* from β_2-microglobulin amyloid deposition in a patient on long-term dialysis. **A:** Femoral head and neck.

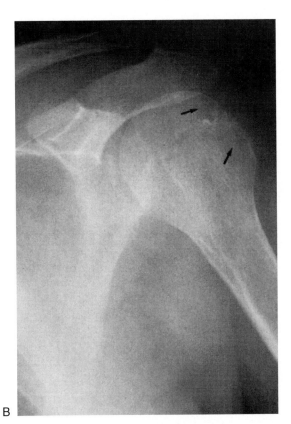

FIG. 92-8. *(continued)* **B:** Humeral head.

are characteristic of osteomalacia with low bone turnover in patients with renal failure. Other than these two findings, radiographs are of little value and may even be misleading. This is especially true for subperiosteal resorption (101). Said to be pathognomonic of hyperparathyroidism, this picture may be seen very frequently in patients with osteomalacia. The reason for this is clarified in Fig. 92-7. In the normal course of bone remodeling, bone is first resorbed by osteoclasts and the eroded area is filled in by active osteoblasts that produce osteoid. Normally, this osteoid is promptly mineralized and radiographs do not detect the eroded area. In hyperparathyroidism, however, the high level of osteoclastic bone resorbing activity makes this a common radiographic feature. It also is common in renal osteomalacia because the osteoblasts often fill in the resorption cavities with osteoid, but this osteoid takes up mineral slowly or not at all. The radiograph, then, being able to "see" only the calcified tissue, cannot distinguish the active resorption cavity of hyperparathyroidism from the inactive erosion of osteomalacia (101). Cystic bone lesions (Fig. 92-8), particularly in the patient on long-term dialysis, would be found with β_2-microglobulin (B$_2$M) amyloid deposition perhaps even more frequently than with hyperparathyroidism. Common sites for cystic changes are the femoral head, humerus, carpal bones, tibia, and pubic symphysis.

Although femoral fracture is a major complication of B$_2$M amyloid deposition, the more common complaint is shoulder pain. Secondary to deposition of B$_2$M amyloid in the synovium and tendon sheath around the humerus, the pain characteristically is continuous and worse with movement. Shoulder joint fluid usually can be detected early by magnetic resonance imaging (MRI), often in conjunction with other characteristic findings such as supraspinatus tendon thickening and cystic lesions of the humerus (116) (Fig. 92-9). The use of MRI in the early detection of B$_2$M amyloid lesions has made it easier to make early referrals for renal transplantation.

Bone Mass Measurements

The most common radiographic finding in uremic patients is osteopenia (reduced bone density). Because this finding has no specificity, most physicians have discontinued the use of conventional radiographs to monitor bone disease in renal patients. Newer techniques, however, that evaluate bone mass or bone mineral density (BMD) directly may be beneficial for long-term monitoring. Quantitative computed tomography and dual-energy x-ray absorptiometry (DEXA) are the two most commonly used methods that quantify bone density. The former technique is used less often because of its higher radiation dosage and its inability to image the hip. DEXA scans, on the other hand, have good precision and low radiation exposure and therefore are good for longitudinal evaluation. Unfortunately, only a limited number of DEXA studies have been performed in patients with chronic renal failure, so it is unclear what role this type of imaging should have in the current management of renal osteodystrophy. Low values for femoral neck BMD have been observed in patients receiving peritoneal dialysis and hemodialysis (117,118), consistent with the high hip fracture rate documented in the dialysis population (119). Amenorrhea and prior transplantation were significant risk factors for reduced femoral neck BMD in one study of 250 patients on dialysis (118). Femoral neck bone loss actually begins before dialysis is started. Rix et al. demonstrated that patients with a mean GFR as high as 58 mL/minute have significantly reduced femoral neck BMD and a sixfold higher prevalence of osteoporosis compared with normal control subjects (120) (Fig. 92-10). Moreover, in the group whose mean GFR was 16 mL/minute, 42% had osteoporosis of the femoral neck (120). More studies with larger populations and longitudinal evaluations of hip BMD are needed to identify other potential risk factors and answer questions regarding the role of PTH, androgens, estrogens, and vitamin D therapy in the preservation of bone mass.

BIOCHEMICAL STUDIES

Serum Chemistries

Serum calcium and phosphate levels are not particularly helpful in distinguishing the various bone lesions. High values are possible in either low or high bone turnover states. Low values for calcium or values below 45 for the calcium × phosphate product are more consistent with the mixed uremic

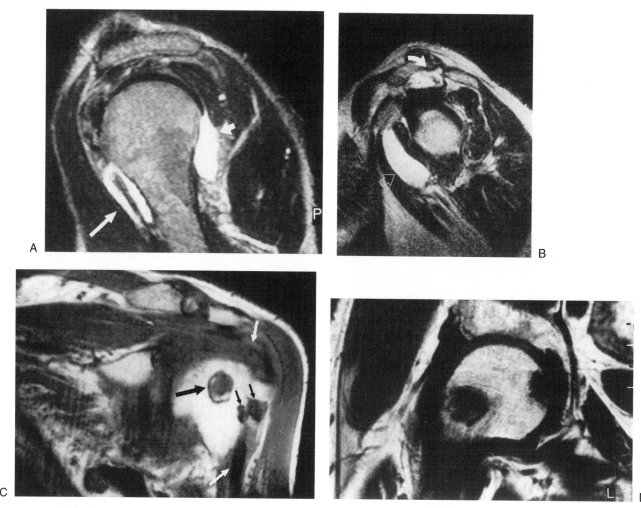

FIG. 92-9. Magnetic resonance images in patients on dialysis with β_2-microglobulin amyloid deposition. **A:** Sagittal T2-weighted image of the shoulder showing a large fluid collection in the biceps tendon *(long arrow)* with associated joint effusion *(short arrow)*. **B:** Sagittal T2-weighted image of the shoulder demonstrating a subcoracoid bursal effusion *(open arrow)* and subacromial bursal fluid *(curved arrow)*. **C:** T1-weighted image of the left shoulder demonstrating three focal lesions in the humeral head *(large black arrow)* and bicipital groove *(small black arrows)*. Note thickening of the supraspinatus and biceps tendon *(white arrows)*. **D:** Coronal T1-weighted image showing two periarticular lesions in the femoral head. (From Escobedo EM, et al. Magnetic resonance imaging of dialysis-related amyloidosis of the shoulder and hip. *Skeletal Radiol* 1996;25:41, with permission.)

osteodystrophy, although a wide range of values is seen in each group (121).

Although alkaline phosphatase levels also are nonspecific, they do show good correlations with bone histologic parameters of osteoblast function (122). Marked elevation (more than twice the upper limit of normal) is very unlikely in low-turnover bone disease and suggests either osteitis fibrosa or mixed uremic osteodystrophy. Normal values are unlikely with high-turnover bone disease. In low-turnover disorders, values usually are normal. For unclear reasons, some patients on dialysis have had a paradoxical increase in alkaline phosphatase levels after parathyroidectomy (123).

Serum immunoreactive osteocalcin may be a more specific parameter for bone cell activity than alkaline phosphatase. Osteocalcin levels are elevated in uremia and show good correlations with bone histologic parameters in patients on dialysis (124). Serum osteocalcin becomes elevated early in renal failure and its rise mirrors the progressive elevation of PTH. To what extent the osteocalcin level reflects osteoblast production of this protein or its release from mineralized matrix during bone resorption is unclear.

Parathyroid Hormone

Immunoreactive PTH is varyingly elevated depending on the assay used. The physician must be familiar with the assays used to see which provides the best information (Table 92-2). Available assays are specific for the carboxyl terminal, amino terminal, or a midregion of the PTH molecule. Results of carboxy-terminal and midregion PTH assays are almost

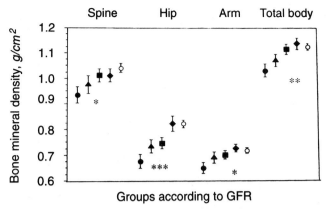

FIG. 92-10. Bone mineral density *(BMD)* in patients with chronic renal failure. *Closed circles* indicate mean glomerular filtration rate (GFR) of 16 mL/minute, *triangles* indicate mean GFR 39 mL/minute, *squares* indicate mean GFR 58 mL/minute, *diamonds* indicate mean GFR 83 mL/minute, and *open circles* indicate normal control subjects with a mean GFR of 144 mL/minute. (From Rix M, et al. Bone mineral density and biochemical markers of bone turnover in patients with predialysis chronic renal failure. *Kidney Int* 1999;56:1084, with permission.)

invariably elevated in renal failure, no matter what the actual size of the patient's parathyroid gland. This is because these assays measure not only the active hormone, but many inactive metabolites that are normally excreted by the kidney (125). Thus, carboxy-terminal or midregion assays in patients without parathyroid overactivity may be ten times the upper limit of normal in some laboratories. Indeed, a normal value implies decreased parathyroid activity (56).

Values for the amino-terminal or intact PTH assays seem more relevant to the true parathyroid status of patients with renal failure (126,127). Using these assays, the clinician can more reliably predict what is occurring at the skeletal level. Values up to three times normal are fairly typical for the well managed patients. Serum values above this raise concern about significant hyperparathyroid bone disease. Normal and particularly low normal values in a patient with advanced

TABLE 92-2. *Parathyroid hormone assay characteristics*

I. Carboxyterminal PTH
  A. Oldest assay
  B. Measures intact and inactive metabolites
  C. Values unpredictably elevated in renal failure
II. Midregion PTH
  A. Measures inactive region
  B. Values unpredictably elevated in renal failure
III. Aminoterminal PTH
  A. Measures active end of molecule
  B. Values correlated with bone histology in renal failure
IV. Intact PTH
  A. Measures intact hormone only
  B. Values correlated with bone histology in renal failure
  C. Only assay that can detect "low" values

PTH, parathyroid hormone.

renal failure should raise concern about low-turnover lesions (86,128) (Table 92-3).

Bioactive PTH measurements also correlate with some bone histologic parameters in patients on dialysis (129). However, they do not appear to be more discriminatory than intact or amino-terminal immunoreactive PTH assays in this patient group (129).

Whatever assay is used, low PTH values are of even greater concern if they do not rise with hypocalcemic stress. When a patient is given a calcium-free dialysate for the first hour of dialysis and the PTH fails to rise substantially, the diagnosis of low-turnover bone disease due to aluminum must be strongly suspected (130). It has been shown that patients with the aplastic lesion not due to aluminum respond with an increase in PTH and bone formation when challenged by hypocalcemia (86).

Aluminum Assays

As with PTH measurements, many commercial laboratories seem to be promoting their aluminum assays. Although some of these undoubtedly are accurate, many are not. Until further information is available, the physician is best advised to be wary of many of the current assays. Assuming an assay is properly carried out (131), the basal serum aluminum value can be of considerable help in assessing the possibility of excess aluminum accumulation (Table 92-3). Serum values below 20 μg/L (approximately five times the level in normal subjects) essentially exclude aluminum toxicity, whereas values above 300 μg/L confirm the diagnosis (132).

Deferoxamine Challenge

In the wide range between these values, additional studies may be helpful. The deferoxamine challenge test often is useful (133) (Table 92-4). In this test, 40 mg/kg of deferoxamine is administered intravenously over a 2-hour period at the end of dialysis. The baseline aluminum level is compared with the postdeferoxamine peak value 24 or 48 hours later. An increase greater than 150 μg/L confirms the presence of biologically significant aluminum accumulation (133). Because a negative deferoxamine challenge test does not always exclude aluminum toxicity, we have found that combining this test with serum PTH levels improves the diagnostic accuracy (132) (Table 92-4).

Parathyroid Hormone Stimulation

When basal serum PTH levels are borderline, the PTH stimulation test using calcium-free dialysate for 1 hour may provide further help. Aluminum accumulates in the parathyroid gland and inhibits responsiveness (130). If the calcium declines by at least 1.5 mg/dL, as it should in this test, the PTH value should double. An increase of less than 20% strongly suggests the diagnosis of excess aluminum.

TABLE 92-3. *Distinctions between hyperparathyroidism and bone aluminum intoxication in patients with renal failure*

	Hyperparathyroidism	Aluminum toxicity
Bone pain	Mild	Severe
Weakness	Mild to moderate	Severe
Fracture	Rare, heal readily	Frequent, poor healing
Radiography	Osteopenia, erosions, patchy osteosclerosis rare	Osteopenia, erosions, pseudofractures rare
Calcium	10–12 mg/dL	10–12 mg/dL
Alkaline phosphatase	2–8× normal	NL to 2× normal
PTH intact or N-terminal	>4× normal	<2× normal
C-terminal[a]	>5–20× normal[a]	>2–5× normal[a]
Stimulated PTH[b]	Doubles	Rise <20%
Basal aluminum	<300 μg/L	>300 μg/L
Stimulated aluminum (deferoxamine test)	Increases <150 μg/L	Increases >150 μg/L

PTH, parathyroid hormone.
[a]Marked variation between assays.
[b]See text.

β_2-Microglobulin Assays

Serum B$_2$M is elevated in uremic patients, but levels do not discriminate patients with B$_2$M amyloid deposition (134). B$_2$M measurements may be more helpful when evaluating B$_2$M clearance from blood during dialysis (135). Radionuclide scans using ^{131}I-labeled B$_2$M have proved to be impractical owing to the high dose of radiation (136).

Bone Biopsy

Bone biopsy sometimes is necessary to confirm or exclude aluminum toxicity. For this procedure to be helpful, the physician needs to obtain careful instructions from the histology laboratory that will process the specimens. Few hospitals are capable of properly processing such specimens. In addition to proper handling, it is important that time-spaced tetracycline labeling be given in the month before the biopsy. Normally, a patient receives a single dose of tetracycline 3 weeks and 1 week before the biopsy (137). In special circumstances, the labeling interval or the interval between the last label and the biopsy can be altered, but this should be discussed with the laboratory that will handle the specimen. The site of the biopsy also is important. The anterior superior iliac crest (between 2 and 5 cm posterior to the anterior superior iliac spine) is the preferred site because most studies have used bone from this region. In addition, it is a particularly benign area to sample because there are no vital structures nearby and this bone is non-weight bearing. The biopsy must contain trabecular bone and usually can be obtained with local anesthesia. There is minimal morbidity with such a procedure.

BONE HISTOLOGY

In patients with chronic renal insufficiency, histologic abnormalities of bone invariably develop (138–148). The type of pathologic process observed is determined by a variety of factors that relate to the duration of dialysis as well as to previous treatment. In general, the most common histologic findings are those associated with increased bone turnover, especially if the biopsy specimen is taken during the first few years of dialysis. Although a minority of patients beginning dialysis have low bone turnover, this type of bone lesion develops in increasing numbers of patients after long-term dialytic therapy.

High-Turnover Bone Disease

The earliest bone histologic change is an increase in the amount of unmineralized osteoid that covers the bone surface (Fig. 92-11). Although the osteoid width usually is not increased at this stage (149), the osteoid area (149) or osteoid volume exceeds normal values. In addition, the bone formation rate is either normal or increased (149,150). These changes in osteoid and bone formation parallel what has been described in early primary hyperparathyroidism (151,152) and in rats given excess PTH parenterally (153). Thus, bone histologic evidence of mild hyperparathyroidism usually is apparent before dialysis commences (154) and is the predominant type of bone lesion in patients who have had renal disease less than 5 years (149,155).

As serum levels of PTH continue to increase, a more severe form of hyperparathyroid bone disease, osteitis fibrosa, is observed (Fig. 92-12). Osteoclasts increase in number and size (156) and endosteal fibrosis becomes prominent. Osteoblasts lining the unmineralized osteoid also increase in number and become cuboidal or "plump" in appearance. The direct correlations between PTH levels and osteoblast number observed on bone histologic studies (126) agree with the known stimulatory effect of PTH on osteoblast proliferation *in vitro* (19). Osteoid area as well as osteoid width increase substantially, reflecting increased osteoblast activity (149). In some cases the excess osteoid resembles osteomalacia. Without tetracycline labeling (tetracycline deposits in newly forming bone as a fluorescent line), it may be quite difficult to

TABLE 92-4. *Diagnosis of aluminum toxicity*

I. Clinical features
  A. Bone pain/fracture
    1. Weight-bearing bones involved
    2. Fractures heal slowly
  B. Dementia
    1. Symptoms often appear first just during dialysis
    2. Sequential worsening
      a. Stuttering/halting speech
      b. Myoclonus
      c. Mutism
      d. Depressed consciousness
      e. Seizures
  C. Anemia
    1. Hypochromic, microcytic
    2. Normal iron levels
    3. May be erythropoietin resistant
II. Laboratory features
  A. Random serum aluminum >100 μg/L
    1. Most patients have some evidence of toxicity
    2. At least 30% are not toxic
  B. Deferoxamine challenge test
    1. A rise in aluminum level >300 μg/L
      a. Specificity—35%
      b. Sensitivity—90%
    2. A negative test—even with no increase—does not
      exclude aluminum toxicity
  C. PTH
    1. Random N-PTH within the upper limit of normal
      a. Specificity—76%
      b. Sensitivity—70%
    2. Random PTH normal and random aluminum
      >100 μg/L
      a. Specificity—88%
      b. Sensitivity—80%
    3. Stimulated PTH (N-PTH or intact PTH)
      a. Zero calcium dialysis for 1 hr
      b. <1.5-fold increase in PTH indicates decreased
        secretion
III. Bone biopsy
  A. Gold standard for bone toxicity
  B. Should include tetracycline labeling
  C. Diagnosis positive if >25% surface aluminum, and
    bone formation rate is less than normal (possible if
    15%–25% surface aluminum)
IV. Electroencephalogram
  A. Specific pattern said to be "diagnostic" of aluminum-
    related dementia
  B. False-positive rate unknown

PTH, parathyroid hormone; *N-PTH,* aminoterminal PTH.

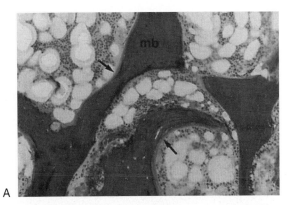

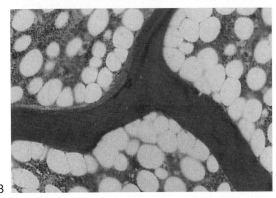

FIG. 92-11. **A:** Histologic section of bone from a patient on dialysis with mild hyperparathyroidism. Length of unmineralized osteoid *(arrow)* is increased. Width of osteoid seam and volume of mineralized bone *(mb)* are normal. **B:** Bone section from a normal subject. (**A** and **B,** Goldner's stain, magnification ×115.) (See Color Fig. 92-11 following page 2624.)

distinguish osteitis fibrosa from osteomalacia. Usually, some of the osteoid has a normal lamellar pattern, but this often is mixed with a large amount of woven osteoid, identified by its random arrangement of collagen fibers (Fig. 92-13). Woven osteoid is not found in normal bone but is characteristic of accelerated bone turnover states such as primary hyperthyroidism, Paget's disease, or fracture repair. Woven osteoid in uremic osteodystrophy is present during early renal failure and increases with declining renal function (154). It has been suggested that woven osteoid results when the osteoprogenitor cells revert to a more primitive form in the presence of

excess PTH, leading to the deposition of irregularly oriented collagen fibers (29).

Mineralization of osteoid in osteitis fibrosa is not impaired (149). This is determined by giving two time-spaced doses of tetracycline. In fact, the bone formation rate is markedly increased in the more severe forms of osteitis fibrosa

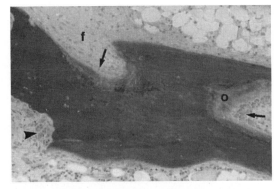

FIG. 92-12. Osteitis fibrosa. Osteoid *(O)* is a mixture of woven and lamellar collagen. Plump osteoblasts *(arrows)* and multinucleated osteoclasts *(arrowhead)* are numerous. Fibrosis *(f)* is present. (Goldner's stain, magnification ×115.) (See Color Fig. 92-12 following page 2624.)

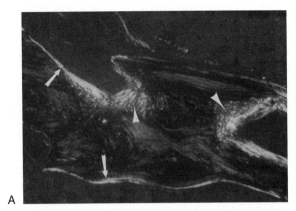
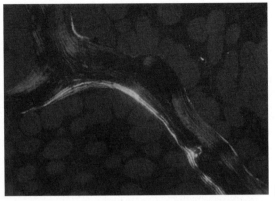

FIG. 92-13. A: Polarized light section showing woven *(arrowheads)* and lamellar *(arrows)* collagen in osteitis fibrosa. **B:** Polarization of normal bone showing only lamellar collagen. (**A** and **B,** magnification ×115.) (See Color Fig. 92-13 following page 2624.)

(149), as evidenced by the increased uptake of tetracycline (Fig. 92-14). Earlier reports of low bone formation in chronic renal failure (157) are most likely attributable to the coexistent hypocalcemia that was present in most of those patients studied.

Despite the fact that osteoclastic bone resorption is increased in osteitis fibrosa, the total bone area often is above normal (149), implying that bone formation and resorption are no longer in balance and that the increase in bone formation is of a greater magnitude than the increase in resorption. The term *osteosclerosis* is reserved for the most severe examples of increased bone mass as a result of hyperparathyroidism (158). Histologically, all trabeculae appear thickened and the boundary between cortical and trabecular bone is obscured (Fig. 92-15). Usually, the other histologic features of osteitis fibrosa also are present in osteosclerosis, although the amount of marrow fibrosis does not parallel the large increase in mineralized bone.

As would be expected, parathyroid gland activity correlates with many of the parameters of bone histology in osteitis fibrosa. Uremic patients with osteitis fibrosa have more

significant parathyroid hypertrophy than do patients without osteitis fibrosa (148,159), and positive correlations between serum PTH and bone histologic findings have been clearly demonstrated (160–162). Studies in our laboratory comparing bone histology with different PTH assays suggest that an amino-terminal–specific PTH assay may be a better predictor of osteitis fibrosa in patients on dialysis (126) (Fig. 92-16). This presumably is due to its measurement only of active intact PTH. In that study, it was noted that the correlation coefficient between PTH and bone formation was substantially lower ($r = 0.46$) when patients with aluminum-related bone disease were excluded from analysis (126). Because this suggested that circulating factors other than PTH might be involved in regulating bone formation, we examined plasma IGFs in patients on dialysis who did not have aluminum bone disease (163). The correlation of bone formation with plasma IGF-1 was slightly better than with plasma PTH. Moreover, all of the parameters of bone mineralization were better correlated with IGF-1, whereas the parameter for osteoblast number correlated better with PTH. This suggested that the mechanisms by which elevated IGF-1 and PTH

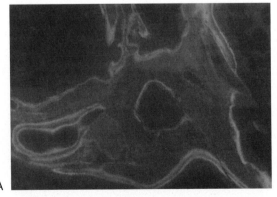
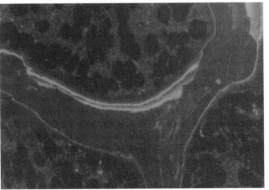

FIG. 92-14. A: Double tetracycline labels in a patient with severe osteitis fibrosa. The distance between labels and the total length of the double labels is increased, demonstrating a high formation rate. **B:** Tetracycline labels from a normal subject. (**A** and **B,** unstained fluorescent micrographs, magnification ×115.) (See Color Fig. 92-14 following page 2624.)

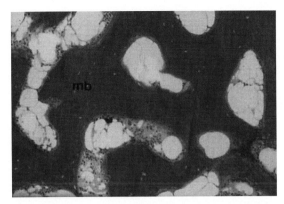

FIG. 92-15. Osteosclerosis. The amount of mineralized bone *(mb)* is increased. (Goldner's stain, magnification×115.) (See Color Fig. 92-15 following page 2624.)

enhance bone formation in uremia probably are different (163). A more recent study by Jehle et al. examined circulating IGF and IGFBP levels in 319 patients with varying levels of chronic renal insufficiency, half of whom were on chronic dialysis (164). They found that free IGF-1 levels were not elevated in most of the patients on dialysis but that IGFBP-2, -3, -4, and -6 were markedly elevated, suggesting that these inhibitory IGFBPs may act to suppress IGF action at the osteoblast level. In addition, serum IGFBP-5 was uniformly low in patients on dialysis, and it was lower in the subgroup with low-turnover bone disease than in those with high bone turnover. These data suggest that a deficiency in IGFBP-5, an osteoblast-stimulatory IGFBP, may contribute to the adynamic bone lesion (164), which is consistent with the known *in vitro* and *in vivo* effects of recombinant IGFBP-5 to stimulate osteoblast activity (16,165,166).

Low-Turnover Bone Disease

Osteomalacia, which is characterized by an excess accumulation of osteoid and an increase in osteoid seam width (Fig. 92-17), is the best-known type of low-turnover bone disease encountered in patients with chronic renal failure. Qualitatively, the osteoid usually is lamellar, although woven osteoid occasionally is present. Osteoblasts are typically flat or fusiform and decreased in number. Fibrosis is absent and the number of osteoclasts is decreased. In general, all bone cells appear active. The dynamic assessment of bone function as determined by tetracycline uptake confirms this impression (167). Double labels of tetracycline rarely are found in osteomalacic bone. More often, no tetracycline is evident, although sometimes a single label can be discerned as a short, thin line at the mineralization front (Fig. 92-18). Thus, bone formation is either greatly reduced or absent.

Not all patients on dialysis with low bone formation have excess osteoid accumulation typical of osteomalacia. Rather, a normal or reduced amount of unmineralized osteoid (Fig. 92-19) may be seen along with tetracycline evidence of decreased bone formation. Ott et al. used the term *aplastic bone disease* to differentiate this lesion from typical osteomalacia (168). Although some patients on dialysis with aplastic (or adynamic) disease have no bone uptake of tetracycline, many have at least a single tetracycline label, whereas others show normally separated double labels that are markedly reduced in total length (Fig. 92-20). Thus, even though the bone apposition rate (determined by the distance between the two labels) may be normal, the bone formation rate at the tissue level is reduced. When this situation occurs, it can be inferred that the total number of osteoblasts is decreased but that a normal rate of mineralization of osteoid continues in the few that remain.

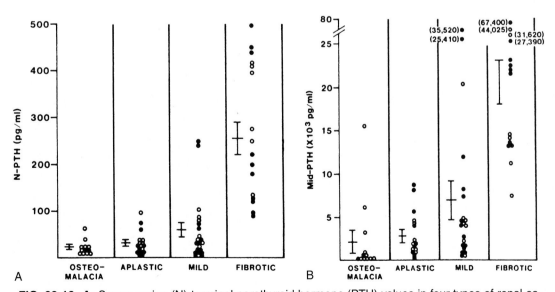

FIG. 92-16. A: Serum amino (N)-terminal parathyroid hormone (PTH) values in four types of renal osteodystrophy. **B:** Serum midregion PTH values in the same patients. (From Andress DL, et al. Comparison of parathyroid hormone assays with bone histomorphometry in renal osteodystrophy. *J Clin Endocrinol Metab* 1986;63:1163, with permission.)

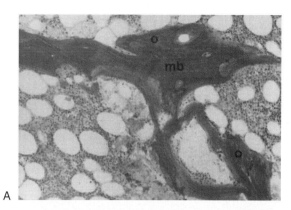

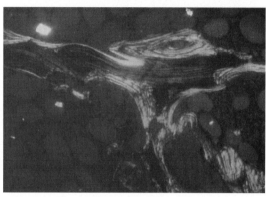

FIG. 92-17. Osteomalacia. **A:** The unmineralized osteoid (O) is increased in width and total volume; mb, mineralized bone. **B:** Polarized section showing predominantly lamellar orientation of collagen in osteomalacia. (**A** and **B,** magnification ×115.) (See Color Fig. 92-17 following page 2624.)

The etiology of osteomalacia and aplastic bone disease was an enigma until recently. The fact that patients on dialysis with osteomalacia failed to respond therapeutically to vitamin D treatment (114) was equally difficult to explain. It was not until researchers in the United Kingdom discovered that aluminum contamination of the water supply was

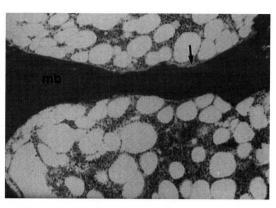

FIG. 92-19. Aplastic (adynamic) bone disease. Marked decrease in amount of unmineralized osteoid (arrows); mb, mineralized bone. Osteoblasts are flat when present. (Goldner's stain, magnification ×115.) (See Color Fig. 92-19 following page 2624.)

linked to a severe form of fracturing osteomalacia (68,169) that the association of aluminum and bone disease in the United States was made. Subsequently, a retrospective analysis of bone biopsy specimens from patients with osteomalacia revealed that significant aluminum deposition was present in most of the specimens studied (168). Figure 92-21 shows the relative frequency of positive aluminum staining in bone biopsy specimens from patients with osteomalacia as well as those with other types of uremic bone disease. More than 80% of the specimens that had osteomalacia showed either heavy or moderate staining for aluminum (168), as evidenced by a precipitation line on the mineralized bone surface (77). Usually the aluminum was located at the interface of osteoid and mineralized bone, although it was also found on "neutral" surfaces of bone without overlying osteoid (Fig. 92-22). Although most of the positive stains for aluminum were seen in patients with osteomalacia, aluminum was detected in some patients with osteitis fibrosa and mild bone disease as well (168). Aluminum accumulation in

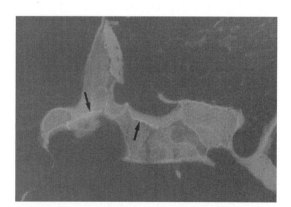

FIG. 92-18. Single tetracycline label (arrows) in bone from a patient on dialysis with osteomalacia given two time-spaced doses of tetracycline. Absence of double labels indicates abnormally low bone formation. (Unstained fluorescent micrograph, magnification ×115.) (See Color Fig. 92-18 following page 2624.)

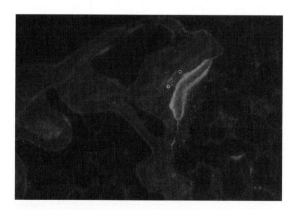

FIG. 92-20. Aplastic (adynamic) bone disease. The total amount of tetracycline uptake is decreased, as is the number of double tetracycline labels. When present, the double label is shorter than normal, demonstrating reduced bone formation. (Unstained fluorescent micrograph, magnification ×115.) (See Color Fig. 92-20 following page 2624.)

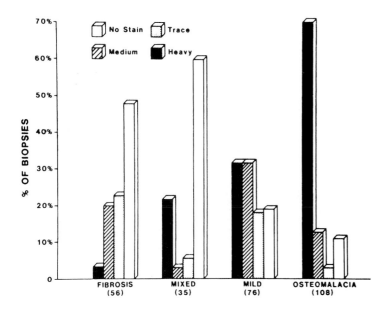

FIG. 92-21. Distribution of aluminum stain in bone among the histologic groups of uremic bone disease. (From Ott SM, et al. The prevalence of bone aluminum deposition in renal osteodystrophy and its relation to calcitriol therapy. *N Engl J Med* 1982;307:709, with permission.)

osteitis fibrosa has since been shown to be highly variable (157,170,171).

Until 1981, it was thought that only a small minority of patients on dialysis acquired aluminum-associated bone disease (114). However, several studies have demonstrated a relatively high prevalence of bone aluminum accumulation in this patient population (172–174), many of whom progress to symptomatic bone disease. In a study from our laboratory, prospective bone biopsy specimens from asymptomatic patients who had received dialysis for at least 8 years revealed a 37% prevalence of aluminum bone disease (172). In this study, aluminum bone disease was defined by an amount of aluminum on the bone surface that equaled at least 25% of the total mineralized bone surface in the presence of a bone formation rate below normal. This was done to distinguish patients with osteitis fibrosa who had small amounts of bone surface aluminum from those patients with low-turnover bone disease. Because both the tap water and dialysate were low in aluminum, it was inferred that the high prevalence of low bone formation was a result of the chronic ingestion of aluminum-containing phosphate binders (172). Subsequent studies showed that patients with the osteomalacic lesion had greater total-body aluminum stores than did those with the aplastic lesion (175).

There is other evidence to support the role of oral aluminum loading in bone aluminum deposition. Bone aluminum accumulation (174) and aluminum-associated bone disease (73,103) can occur in uremic patients before dialysis has been initiated. Moreover, diabetic patients on dialysis have been shown to have accelerated bone aluminum accumulation that is directly related to the cumulative oral intake of aluminum and to whole-body aluminum stores (176) (Fig. 92-23). Whether diabetic patients are also "hyperabsorbers" of aluminum remains to be evaluated.

The observation that serum PTH levels often are normal in patients on dialysis with heavy bone aluminum deposition (114,128) suggests that functional hypoparathyroidism probably has an important role in the pathogenesis of aluminum bone disease. Aluminum in the parathyroid glands of humans, as measured by neutron activation analysis, can be related to the ingestion of aluminum (94). *In vitro* studies using parathyroid gland slices have shown that aluminum inhibits PTH secretion, but not production, in a dose-dependent manner (95,177). Moreover, correction of aluminum contamination of the dialysate results in increased PTH levels in some patients (178). Because patients on dialysis with high levels of bone aluminum are more likely to have suppressed PTH levels during an acute hypocalcemic challenge than are patients with low levels of bone aluminum (130), a PTH stimulation test has been advocated as one method to screen for aluminum bone disease. While dialyzing patients using a calcium-free dialysate, we found that the serum amino-terminal PTH levels after 1 or 2 hours accurately discriminated patients who had documented aluminum bone disease. Further supporting the

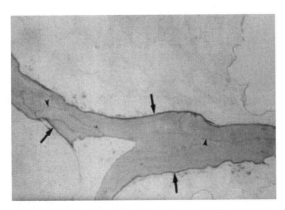

FIG. 92-22. Histologic section showing a positive stain for aluminum on the surface *(arrows)* of mineralized bone and within cement lines *(arrowheads).* (Aurin-tricarboxylic acid, magnification ×115.) (See Color Fig. 92-22 following page 2624.)

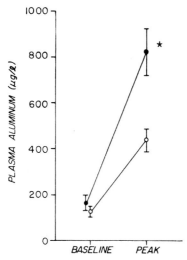

FIG. 92-23. Comparison of plasma aluminum response to a single deferoxamine infusion in matched diabetic and nondiabetic patients on dialysis. *Open circles* denote patients whose cumulative oral aluminum intake was more than 0. 5 kg and *closed circles* denote patients whose cumulative oral aluminum intake was less than 0. 5 kg. (From Andress DL, et al. Early deposition of aluminum in bone in diabetic patients on hemodialysis. *N Engl J Med* 1987;316:292, with permission.)

role of hypoparathyroidism in the development of aluminum bone disease is the observation that bone aluminum accumulation is markedly enhanced after parathyroidectomy (91) (Fig. 92-24). The decreased bone formation after parathyroidectomy was attributed to the decline in circulating levels of PTH. To what extent aluminum on the bone surface also contributed to the decreased bone formation could not be determined. It did appear, however, that the high rates of bone formation before parathyroidectomy protected against bone surface aluminum accumulation (91). Functional hypoparathyroidism also is likely to be important in causing reduced bone formation and increasing bone aluminum in the diabetic uremic patient (87,176). In this situation, high glucose concentrations in parathyroid cells may decrease PTH secretion (89).

The exact mechanism by which aluminum inhibits bone mineralization in humans has not been identified. Studies in rats (179–184) and dogs (185) have clearly shown that osteomalacia can be produced by the parenteral administration of aluminum. Moreover, the mineralization defect is enhanced when chronic renal failure also is present (179,181,184,185), is made worse by parathyroidectomy (186), and is ameliorated by PTH infusions (187,188). Studies performed by Plachot et al. (96) support the idea that PTH may protect osteoblast function when aluminum is deposited on bone. Using electron microscopy and x-ray microanalysis, they discovered aluminum in the mitochondria of osteoblasts in patients with osteitis fibrosa. Because the number of osteoblasts was increased, the authors suggested that the high serum PTH was responsible for stimulating osteoblast growth as well as

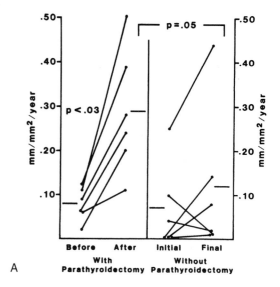

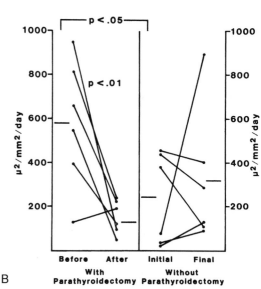

FIG. 92-24. A: Rates of bone surface aluminum accumulation in six patients on dialysis before and after parathyroidectomy **(left panel)** and in six control patients on dialysis **(right panel). B:** Rates of bone formation in the same patients. (From Andress DL, et al. Effect of parathyroidectomy on bone aluminum accumulation in chronic renal failure. *N Engl J Med* 1985;312:468, with permission.)

the cellular uptake and release of aluminum into the organic matrix (96). The fact that PTH administration is known to increase the bone aluminum content in rats (189) supports this hypothesis. However, most patients with osteitis fibrosa have a lower trabecular bone aluminum content than do patients with osteomalacia (190). Thus, it is possible that differences in the distribution of aluminum in bone may partially explain these discrepant findings. For example, the location of much of the aluminum in osteomalacia or aplastic bone disease is on the surface of the mineralized bone interfaced with the overlying unmineralized osteoid, as determined by electron microprobe analysis (76). In contrast, very little aluminum is seen on the bone surface in osteitis fibrosa (166); rather, it is more diffusely distributed throughout the mineralized compartment (170).

Whether aluminum in the osteoblast is responsible for inducing a mineralization defect characteristic of osteomalacia or aplastic disease has not been decided. However, *in vitro* studies involving aluminum incubation with osteoblasts indicate that aluminum has an adverse effect on bone cell function. Lieberherr et al. (191) have shown that the bone phosphatase activity in rat bone cells is inhibited at high aluminum concentrations (6×10^{-6} mol/L). In addition, aluminum decreased the stimulatory action of PTH on bone phosphatase activity (191). In other experiments, aluminum has been shown to suppress osteoblast proliferation *in vitro* (192,193), supporting clinical studies that show an inverse relationship between osteoblast number and bone surface aluminum (172,194). The adverse effect of aluminum on osteoblast function may also be mediated by alterations in osteoblast synthesis of 1,25-dihydroxyvitamin D_3 (195) and bone PTH receptors (196).

It is possible, of course, that aluminum also may inhibit mineralization by a mechanism that is not osteoblast mediated. Aluminum chloride reduces amorphous calcium phosphate transformation and hydroxyapatite crystal growth *in vitro* at concentrations of 0.25 to 0.50 mmol/L (87). Although these concentrations are in general higher than those found in the serum of patients on dialysis, they approximate the levels found in mineralized bone in aluminum-intoxicated animals (179) and humans (76,190).

Aluminum has been the cause of low-turnover bone disease in most of the patients with that lesion up to now (197). However, in an increasing number of patients identified with aplastic bone disease, neither aluminum nor iron is the cause. Although diabetes (87,88) or low-molecular-weight inhibitors (35) may be involved in some, in many the lesion is associated with excessive PTH suppression (86). Whether this condition is a disease state is not, in fact, clear. Based on aforementioned considerations, such excessive suppression of PTH may predispose to aluminum toxicity even if, by itself, it causes no problems. For these reasons it appears that bone in uremic patients requires a modest PTH elevation to maintain normal bone turnover. This form of low-turnover bone disease requires considerable additional investigative work before we understand its place in the spectrum of renal osteodystrophy.

Mixed and Transitional Bone Histology

Although most of the bone histologic changes in uremic osteodystrophy can be classified as mild disease, osteitis fibrosa, osteomalacia, or aplastic disease, a minority of patients do not fit into any of these categories. Rather, mixed histologic changes sometimes are seen in which aspects of both osteomalacia and osteitis fibrosa are present (198). Woven

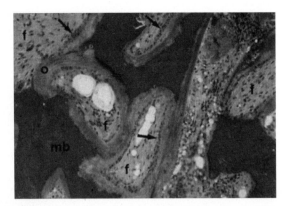

FIG. 92-25. Mixed bone disease in a patient on dialysis. Width and total volume of unmineralized osteoid *(O)* are increased; *mb,* mineralized bone. The number of osteoblasts *(arrows)* also is increased, and fibrosis *(f)* is present in most of the marrow space. (Goldner's stain, magnification ×115.) (See Color Fig. 92-25 following page 2624.)

osteoid, marked fibrosis, and excess unmineralized osteoid, with or without low bone formation, are the distinguishing features of mixed osteodystrophy (Fig. 92-25). The pathogenesis and evolution of this bone lesion are unclear, but it may represent a transitional state to a more clear-cut form of either osteomalacia or osteitis fibrosa. Because serum PTH levels often are high and woven osteoids invariably are present, we regard osteoblast function in the mixed lesion to be enhanced with respect to osteoid production. The histologic finding of cuboidal or "plump," active-appearing osteoblasts supports this hypothesis. The mineralization defect, when present, can be attributed to coexistent hypocalcemia. Once the hypocalcemia is corrected, mineralization proceeds normally and the amount of unmineralized osteoid diminishes while bone formation increases. Correction of the hypocalcemia also results in a lowering of the PTH levels, although serum PTH usually remains elevated. Thus, the new bone histologic picture more often resembles osteitis fibrosa after correction of hypocalcemia.

Other transitional states in bone histology have been noted but are relatively rare. Sometimes the histologic picture shows a significant accumulation of bone surface aluminum in the presence of fibrosis, normal osteoid volume, and low-normal bone formation, suggesting a transition from osteitis fibrosa to mild or aplastic bone disease. At other times, a lesser amount of bone aluminum is present, whereas fibrosis and a slightly higher bone formation rate are noted, suggesting a transition to osteitis fibrosa. Because most bone histologic studies in uremic patients are cross-sectional, it is difficult to know how a bone lesion is evolving without a previous biopsy.

β_2-Amyloid

The deposition of B_2M has been implicated as a cause of femoral fractures in patients on long-term dialysis (108,199). Already known for its role in causing carpal tunnel syndrome

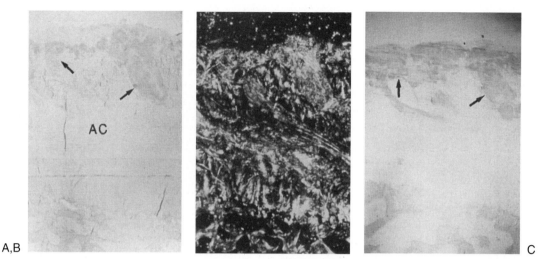

A,B   C

FIG. 92-26. Serial sections of femoral bone from a patient on dialysis. **A:** Congo red–stained amyloid deposits *(arrows)* are seen in the superficial articular cartilage *(AC).* **B:** The same seen under polarized light. Congo red–stained amyloid deposits demonstrate green birefringence. **C:** Immunohistochemical staining with anti-β_2-microglobulin. Amyloid deposits *(arrows)* stain brown for β_2-microglobulin. (From Onishi S, et al. Beta-2 microglobulin deposition in bone in chronic renal failure. *Kidney Int* 1991;39:990, with permission.) (See Color Fig. 92-26 following page 2624.)

(200), this circulating 11.8-kd protein, which forms amyloid fibrils spontaneously (201), has been found in cystic lesions of long bones, particularly in the femoral and humeral heads (134,202). The cystic radiolucency of this bone lesion has been mistaken for the "brown tumor" of hyperparathyroidism.

In a retrospective analysis of bone specimens from 224 patients on dialysis, we found that B_2M deposits were absent in patients on dialysis for less than 6 years but progressively increased with time, reaching a prevalence of 19% in those on dialysis longer than 10 years (203). In femoral head specimens, B_2M deposits were localized to synovium (Fig. 92-26), cartilage, and bone marrow. Its location in the iliac crest was predominantly in the periosteum (Fig. 92-27),

although bone marrow deposition of B_2M occurred occasionally. In patients with B_2M localized to the iliac periosteum, there was a 62% prevalence of femoral fracture, in contrast to only 4% in matched patients without B_2M at that location (P < 0.001). Although the pathogenesis of bone B_2M deposition could not be determined, B_2M deposits were not associated with aluminum or iron overload but were more common in patients with osteitis fibrosa (203). It is unknown whether B_2M has a role in promoting high-turnover bone disease. This is intriguing because B_2M can stimulate osteoblast proliferation *in vitro* (8). However, using an *in vitro* bone mineralization model, Kataoka et al. have shown that B_2M inhibits calcification (204). Moreover, Moe et al. have shown that B_2M stimulates osteoclastic bone

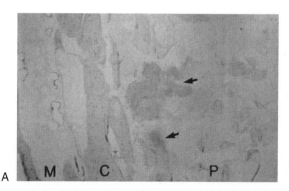
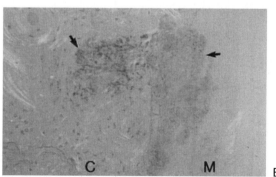

A   M   C   P   C   M   B

FIG. 92-27. **A:** Iliac crest bone biopsy with anti-β_2-microglobulin and hematoxylin counterstain. β_2-Microglobulin deposits *(arrows)* are located in the iliac periosteum. **B:** Bone section from the tibia with anti-β_2-microglobulin and methylene blue counterstain. β_2-Microglobulin deposits *(arrows)* appear to invade the cortical bone *(C)* from the marrow *(M).* (From Onishi S, et al. Beta-2-microglobulin deposition in bone in chronic renal failure. *Kidney Int* 1991;39:990, with permission.) (See Color Fig. 92-27 following page 2624.)

resorption (205). Thus, it may be that B_2M deposition in the femoral head stimulates bone turnover but inhibits bone mineralization, thereby causing predominant bone resorption and cyst formation.

In summary, the bone histologic changes of uremic osteodystrophy depend on the state of parathyroid gland function, the presence or absence of hypocalcemia, and the extent of aluminum accumulation. Mild hyperparathyroid bone disease is the most common finding in uremic patients, particularly during moderate renal failure and shortly after beginning dialytic therapy. The severity of osteitis fibrosa and accelerated bone turnover increases with increasing parathyroid gland activity. In some patients, enhanced bone formation is associated with elevated levels of IGF-1, and depressed bone formation is associated with the serum accumulation of inhibitory IGFBPs. In patients with a mixed bone histologic picture (osteitis fibrosa plus osteomalacia), hypocalcemia usually is present and, when corrected, results in normalization of the mineralization defect. Bone aluminum accumulation is associated with the low bone formation of osteomalacia and aplastic bone disease. Decreased PTH secretion, which often is present in aluminum-associated bone disease, probably has a major role in the development of low bone formation. Although bone fractures are the major complications of low-turnover bone disease, femoral fractures may be caused more often by B_2M deposition, particularly in patients on dialysis longer than 10 years.

UNIQUE PEDIATRIC FEATURES

Although much of the foregoing material certainly is true of children as well, there are some differences in the pediatric population. One of these relates to growth. Attention to maintaining appropriate levels of calcium and phosphate and judicious use of vitamin D appear to enhance bone growth and improve metabolic bone disease (206–211). Normalization of height is uncommon in uremic children, possibly because of the serum accumulation of IGFBPs, which inhibit IGF-1 stimulation of cartilage (212), and because of low-molecular-weight inhibitors of cartilage (33) and osteoblast (35) activity. Recent studies with recombinant growth hormone (rGH) have demonstrated its benefit in stimulating growth in these patients (213,214). Interestingly, serum levels of free IGF-1, IGFBP-3, and IGFBP-5 were elevated after rGH therapy, whereas IGFBP-1 and IGFBP-2 levels were reduced (215), suggesting that rGH treatment shifted the balance between potential growth promoters (IGF-1, IGFBP-3, IGFBP-5) and growth inhibitors (IGFBP-1 and IGFBP-2).

A second problem relates to aluminum toxicity, which at one time was relatively common in children who were taking aluminum-containing phosphate binders (216). Children with serum creatinine levels as low as 2 mg/dL have been found with serious aluminum-related bone disease. Even dementia has been reported (217). Whether this is due to enhanced gastrointestinal absorption or better compliance with aluminum gels for phosphate control is not clear. One prospective study documented that even low doses of aluminum-containing phosphate binders result in substantial aluminum accumulation (218). It is clear that aluminum levels must be monitored in children and other approaches to phosphate control must be attempted (e.g., calcium carbonate, calcium acetate, or sevelamer).

SPECIAL DIAGNOSTIC PROBLEMS

Hypercalcemia

Elevated calcium can occur in a patient on dialysis for the same reasons that cause it in a patient without renal disease. Too often, the physician faced with this problem ignores the possibility of these common disorders because the patient is on dialysis or has renal failure. Before attempting to assess the specific renal failure–dialysis-related causes, these better-known etiologies should be considered.

In the patient on chronic dialysis, there are four major causes of hypercalcemia: hyperparathyroidism, aluminum intoxication, vitamin D intoxication, and bed rest. Hyperparathyroidism occurs for reasons described previously and causes hypercalcemia because of excessive osteoclastic bone resorption, usually in the setting of intact PTH levels greater than 1,000 pg/mL.

Vitamin D intoxication is common because of the frequency of vitamin D use in these patients and the fact that therapeutic doses are close to toxic ones. For this reason, a short-acting vitamin D preparation, such as calcitriol, is preferable when vitamin D deficiency is present. Calcitonin may be particularly useful in controlling transient hypercalcemia from vitamin D excess.

Aluminum excess causes hypercalcemia in part by blocking bone formation and perhaps by stimulating osteoclast-mediated bone resorption. When patients receive calcium orally or intravenously, it enters the extracellular fluid compartment. The calcium level in this compartment normally is buffered by the huge bone reservoir. If aluminum prevents entry of calcium into the bone, then administered calcium quickly leads to hypercalcemia (114). Because most dialysate calcium levels are high and result in calcium transfer to the patient, persistent hypercalcemia is a frequent finding. Lowering the calcium dialysate (e.g., 2.5 mEq/L) may help with this problem (219). Perhaps the most confusing element of aluminum-induced hypercalcemia is the accompanying finding of modestly elevated PTH levels. This usually is due to renal failure and retention of PTH metabolites. The physician must be very wary of this problem and be certain that PTH elevation is sufficiently high to make the diagnosis of "renal hyperparathyroidism." An incorrect decision to remove the parathyroids in such patients is an invitation to disaster because this can worsen the bone disease (91,92,219,220), possibly as a result of accelerated bone surface aluminum accumulation (91).

Bed rest, in some ways, is physiologically similar to aluminum from the bone's point of view because bone formation ceases and bone resorption continues. In normal subjects, bone resorption continues and the calcium lost from bone disappears into the urine. This "bed rest" hypercalciuria may be severe enough to cause renal stones (221). Without kidney function, there is no route for the excess calcium to escape, so it accumulates in the extracellular fluid. Temporarily, low-calcium dialysate may be used, but in the long run the patient should increase his or her activity as soon as possible because low-calcium dialysate (<2.5 mEq/L) depletes total-body calcium.

Bone Pain and Fracture

The differential diagnosis of bone pain and fracture is, in general, the distinction of hyperparathyroidism from aluminum intoxication (Table 92-3). Clinically, the pain usually is very severe, often immobilizing, with aluminum intoxication, whereas the hyperparathyroid patient complains, but carries on. Where data are available, the PTH level is normal to moderately elevated with aluminum excess, but very high with hyperparathyroidism (114,126,128). Aluminum levels, either basal or after deferoxamine challenge and hypocalcemic stimulation of PTH, as described previously, may be useful. If the diagnosis is not absolutely clear after these studies, bone biopsy should be done before therapy is instituted. In patients on long-term (>6 years) dialysis with hip fractures, the possibility of B_2M disease must be considered. Radiographic or MRI evidence of bone cysts should not be assumed to be "brown tumors" of hyperparathyroidism. In the older dialysis population, osteoporosis also may play a role (119).

PREVENTIVE THERAPY

Hyperphosphatemia

A major emphasis has been placed on normalizing serum phosphate levels (Table 92-5) because of the importance of phosphate retention in causing decreased 1,25-dihydroxyvitamin D_3 synthesis, hypocalcemia (222), and secondary hyperparathyroidism (223,224). Although excellent control of serum phosphate helps prevent metastatic calcification, prevention of hyperphosphatemia during moderate renal failure also enhances 1,25-dihydroxyvitamin D_3 production (225) and further assists in PTH suppression (226). Reduction of dietary phosphorus intake (227) and use of aluminum-containing phosphate binders during meals have been the most effective forms of treatment. The increasing concern about aluminum toxicity, however, has led to the use of calcium salts as preferred alternatives to aluminum hydroxide (228). Both calcium carbonate (229–231) and calcium acetate (232) are useful phosphate binders when taken with meals. Calcium citrate, although an excellent phosphate binder, must be avoided because it markedly enhances aluminum absorption

TABLE 92-5. *Sequential treatment of hyperparathyroidism in renal failure*

I. Prophylactic measures
  A. Phosphate control (keep serum phosphate <5.5 mg/dL)
  B. Calcium supplementation
  C. Calcitriol (daily oral dosing to correct hypocalcemia)
II. With bone pain or fractures
  A. Hypocalcemic patients
    1. Institute prophylactic measures
    2. Increase calcitriol dose rapidly (every 2 wk) to achieve high normal calcium
    3. Monitor calcium weekly
  B. Normocalcemic patients
    1. Institute prophylactic measures
    2. Titrate daily oral calcitriol slowly to achieve high normal calcium (≤10.5 mg/dL)
    3. Consider
      a. Intravenous calcitriol
      b. Intravenous paricalcitol
      c. Oral intermittent doxercalciferol
  C. Hypercalcemic patients
    1. Trial of intermittent intravenous paricalcitol or oral doxercalciferol
    2. Switch to low-calcium dialysate (2.0 mEq/L calcium)
    3. Parathyroidectomy
III. Hypercalcemia without bone symptoms
  A. If calcium × phosphate product >70—consider parathyroidectomy
  B. If calcium × phosphate product <55—trial of intravenous paricalcitol or intermittent oral doxercalciferol
  C. Parathyroidectomy if the preceding measures fail to suppress intact parathyroid hormone to 300 pg/mL

(233,234), a complication that has not been observed with calcium acetate (235). Because some patients continue to require aluminum hydroxide in addition to calcium salts, calcium citrate in this setting can be lethal. Citrate and other organic acids present in food (236) also may enhance intestinal aluminum absorption.

Because hypercalcemia has become more of a problem since calcium salts became the phosphate binder of choice, there has been a renewed interest in identifying calcium- and aluminum-free binders. Magnesium, which has been available since the late 1980s, effectively lowers phosphate levels (237). Delmez et al. showed that the combination of magnesium carbonate with calcium acetate was effective in controlling phosphate levels. It also allowed the use of higher intravenous calcitriol dosages compared with patients receiving calcium acetate alone (238). A potential limitation of magnesium as a binder is the need to lower the dialysate magnesium to prevent hypermagnesemia. A metal-free compound recently approved for binding dietary phosphate is sevelamer. This nonabsorbable, cross-linked polyallylamine gel not only effectively lowers serum phosphate in patients on dialysis but decreases serum low-density lipoprotein cholesterol (239). Lanthanum, another new phosphate binder, is undergoing clinical trials.

Calcium Supplementation

The decreased intestinal calcium absorption of uremic patients can be attributed for the most part to the decreased production of calcitriol. When replaced in the diet, calcitriol improves calcium absorption and increases serum calcium levels (240). However, simply increasing the dietary intake of calcium also can improve calcium balance in uremia (241,242). Intestinal calcium absorption is especially enhanced when calcium salts are taken in combination with oral calcitriol. Thus, the high-calcium dialysates formerly recommended to maintain calcium balance (243,244) now are inappropriate. Although a dialysate calcium of 2.5 mEq/L may be the preferred concentration (219), some flexibility (2.0 to 2.5 mEq/L) is needed for individual patient variability when high doses of calcium are prescribed.

Calciferol (Vitamin D_3)

Treatment with vitamin D metabolites has been shown to ameliorate defects in calcium homeostasis in chronic renal failure. In 1943, Liu and Chu reported that physiologic doses of calciferol were ineffective in normalizing calcium homeostasis in uremic patients (245). Larger doses of calciferol, however, usually have been helpful in promoting positive calcium balance (142), resulting in a decrease in serum PTH (246). In addition, osteitis fibrosa can be ameliorated after treatment with calciferol (246). The major limitation of calciferol is the prolonged hypercalcemia that sometimes occurs (247,248).

Calcifediol (25-Hydroxyvitamin D_3)

One of the natural metabolites of calciferol is calcifediol. Produced in the liver by 25-hydroxylation of calciferol, 25-hydroxyvitamin D_3 has a pharmacologic half-life of approximately 30 days (249). Oral maintenance doses of calcifediol in the range of 200 μg thrice weekly are effective in increasing intestinal calcium absorption in uremic patients (250). Although high serum PTH levels are decreased in some patients after treatment with calcifediol (251,252), other studies have not shown this effect (253). In general, the bone histologic picture improves after calcifediol treatment (161,251,253). Bordier et al. described decreases in osteoclast number, bone resorption, and fibrosis and increased calcification front activity in those patients who had a decrease in serum PTH (251). Teitelbaum et al. reported similar changes in five patients treated for 3 to 9 months (161). Most agree that the bone histologic improvements are related to the degree of suppression of the hyperparathyroidism. This in turn depends on the extent of increased calcium absorption and correction of hypocalcemia. Because most patients on dialysis have normal circulating levels of 25-hydroxyvitamin D_3 (45,250), treatment with this substance results in a marked elevation of serum 25-hydroxyvitamin D_3 (250) and prolonged

hypercalcemia is a potential hazard of this long-lived metabolite also.

Calcitriol (1,25-Dihydroxyvitamin D_3)

In 1970, Fraser and Kodicek discovered that the most potent form of vitamin D, 1,25-dihydroxyvitamin D_3, is synthesized in the kidney from 25-hydroxyvitamin D_3 (254). Since that time, numerous studies have been conducted exploring the use of calcitriol in the treatment of renal osteodystrophy (255–258). Oral calcitriol causes a marked increase in intestinal calcium absorption (239) that is more pronounced than with any of the other vitamin D metabolites. Because of its relatively short plasma half-life (12 to 16 hours), episodes of hypercalcemia can be quickly corrected, usually within 1 week of stopping treatment. The incidence of hypercalcemia seems to depend on the underlying bone disease. In general, patients with osteitis fibrosa respond better to calcitriol and have fewer episodes of hypercalcemia initially than patients with pure osteomalacia (255,259,260). Amelioration of hyperparathyroidism is particularly apparent when hypocalcemia is present before treatment (261). Patients with mild hypercalcemia at the start of calcitriol therapy have a tendency to become hypercalcemic early during treatment compared with patients with pretreatment serum calcium levels in the low-normal range.

Alfacalcidol (1α-Hydroxyvitamin D_3)

A synthetic analog of calcitriol, 1α-hydroxyvitamin D_3, has a half-life two to three times longer than calcitriol (262) and must undergo hepatic hydroxylation at the 25 position to become activated. Thus, larger doses of 1α-hydroxyvitamin D_3 are necessary for comparable effects and hypercalcemia, when it occurs, lasts longer (263). Because of the need for hepatic hydroxylation, the effectiveness of 1α-hydroxyvitamin D_3 can be negated by the concomitant use of anticonvulsants because both compete for the same hydroxylation enzymes (264).

The biologic effects of alfacalcidol and calcitriol are indistinguishable (121,265). Most patients on dialysis with mild to moderate osteitis fibrosa or mixed bone disease have shown bone histologic improvement after treatment with alfacalcidol (266–268). However, poor responses to treatment were observed in patients with severe osteitis fibrosa or osteomalacia (267,269). Thus, treatment failures with alfacalcidol, like calcitriol, seem to occur in patients in whom hypercalcemia limits therapeutic dosing. The dose required to maintain serum calcium may be lower in those patients maintained on bicarbonate-supplemented dialysis (270).

Successful use of calcitriol or alfacalcidol in patients with moderate renal failure has been described. Both have caused declines in serum PTH and improvement in trabecular fibrosis (271–273). Massry et al. have shown healing of osteitis fibrosa and lowering of serum PTH levels at calcitriol doses of 0.5 to 1.0 μg/day for 1 year (274). More recently, it was shown that lower doses are effective (275,276), although in some patients abnormally low rates of bone formation have resulted. Although concern over premature declines in renal function during calcitriol or alfacalcidol therapy has been expressed (277,278), other studies have not shown this association (274,279,280).

Doxercalciferol (1α-Hydroxyvitamin D$_2$)

Studies in vitamin D–deficient rats have shown that 1α-hydroxyvitamin D$_2$ is equipotent to 1α-hydroxyvitamin D$_3$ in stimulating intestinal calcium transport and in healing rickets (281). The former compound, however, was found to be less toxic in normal rats because higher doses were required to produce a similar level of hypercalcemia (282). Because of these findings, Frazao et al. evaluated the efficacy of oral intermittent doxercalciferol in suppressing PTH levels in patients on dialysis (283). Using initial doses of 10 μg with each dialysis and then adjusting the dose to maintain intact PTH levels within a target range of 150 to 300 pg/mL, they demonstrated a 55% reduction in the mean serum PTH over a 16-week treatment period, with few episodes of hypercalcemia or hyperphosphatemia (Fig. 92-28). Although its use in patients with moderate renal failure has not been fully described, pilot studies suggest that it effectively suppresses hyperparathyroidism in this population without affecting GFR (J. Coburn, personal communication). Future studies should evaluate the bone histologic response to doxercalciferol to determine whether it carries the risk of inducing adynamic bone disease with long-term treatment.

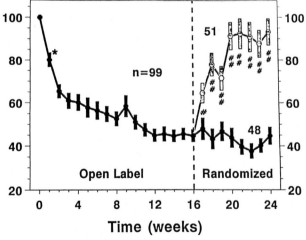

Plasma iPTH (% of Baseline)

FIG. 92-28. Changes in plasma parathyroid hormone during treatment with intermittent oral doxercalciferol in patients on dialysis. All patients received doxercalciferol during the open label (0 to 16 weeks) and were then randomized to either placebo *(shaded)* or continued doxercalciferol. [From Frazao JM, et al. Intermittent doxercalciferol (1α-hydroxyvitamin D$_2$) therapy for secondary hyperparathyroidism. *Am J Kidney Dis* 2000;36:550, with permission.]

Dihydrotachysterol

Dihydrotachysterol (DHT) is a synthetic compound that, after undergoing hepatic hydroxylation, resembles calcitriol structurally. Early studies with DHT confirmed its effectiveness in causing an increase in intestinal calcium absorption (245) as well as a decrease in serum PTH and alkaline phosphatase (142). In a more recent study of patients on hemodialysis with osteitis fibrosa, Cordy and Mills demonstrated significant decreases in bone resorption and osteoid volume after a minimum of 12 months of treatment with DHT at a dosage of 0.25 to 1.00 mg/day (284). Unfortunately, tetracycline labeling was not performed to assess possible reductions in bone formation. It appears from limited bone histologic studies that DHT can cause healing of osteitis fibrosa. Whether similar effects in patients with pure osteomalacia also occur has not been determined. DHT has a potency approximately three times that of calciferol. It takes approximately 1 to 2 weeks to correct hypercalcemia after cessation of therapy.

In summary, treatment of osteitis fibrosa with vitamin D metabolites is best begun early in the disease process. Although oral calcifediol therapy seems sufficient in some patients, a favorable response is not universal. A prolonged half-life renders it less useful than the 1-hydroxylated vitamin D metabolites. DHT is inexpensive and effective at doses of 0.5 to 1.0 mg/day for the treatment of osteitis fibrosa, but also has the hazard of a long half-life. Oral calcitriol in doses of 0.25 to 1.00 μg/day or alfacalcidol in doses of 1.0 to 2.0 μg/day is effective in healing osteitis fibrosa. However, patients with severe hyperparathyroidism or pure osteomalacia are at an increased risk for development of hypercalcemia. In patients where hypercalcemia limits the dosing of calcitriol, pulse intermittent therapy with doxercalciferol or paricalcitol may prove to be more effective. Rarely have these metabolites been helpful in the treatment of pure osteomalacia.

TREATMENT OF ADVANCED DISEASE

Osteitis Fibrosa (Hyperparathyroid Bone Disease)

With severe hyperparathyroid bone disease, a sequential approach is useful. First, all of the preventive measures discussed previously should be introduced: phosphate control, calcium supplementation, and oral calcitriol or 1α-hydroxyvitamin D$_3$ therapy. Phosphate levels below 6 mg/dL and calcium levels between 10.0 and 10.5 mg/dL are desirable. If these measures fail, intravenous infusions of calcitriol or paricalcitol may be tried.

The intravenous form of calcitriol has proven effective in the treatment of severe hyperparathyroidism refractory to oral calcitriol. In the initial studies, Slatopolsky et al. demonstrated that the infusion of calcitriol in doses of 1.75 to 4.00 μg thrice weekly at the end of each dialysis resulted in a decline of serum PTH by 35% over 3 weeks (54). Although serum calcium eventually rose in all patients, the decline in serum PTH was noted before increases in serum calcium were evident. Subsequent studies evaluating bone histologic

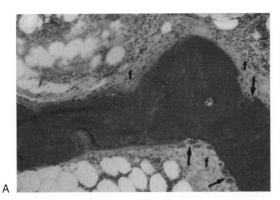
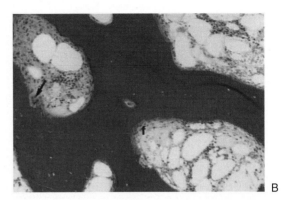

FIG. 92-29. A: Osteitis fibrosa in a patient on dialysis refractory to treatment with oral calcitriol. **B:** Histologic section from the same patient after treatment with intravenous calcitriol. Amount of fibrosis *(f)* and number of osteoclasts *(arrows)* are decreased after treatment. (**A** and **B,** Goldner's stain, magnification ×115.) (See Color Fig. 92-29 following page 2624.)

changes indicated that long-term treatment with intravenous calcitriol ameliorates the osteitis fibrosa lesion in patients who are refractory to oral calcitriol (286) (Fig. 92-29). In patients on dialysis who had previously failed daily oral calcitriol treatment, intravenous calcitriol given thrice weekly effectively lowered serum PTH levels, significantly improved marrow fibrosis, and lowered bone turnover to more normal levels (Figs. 92-30 and 92-31). It was noted that transient episodes of asymptomatic hypercalcemia were quickly reversed by temporarily halting treatment or by decreasing the dosage (286). Since then, a number of reports have documented that intravenous calcitriol effectively lowers PTH levels (285,287). Unfortunately, because of the exclusive use of calcium salts for phosphate binding, a higher frequency of hypercalcemia also has been reported (288).

Because hypercalcemia frequently limits the use of higher calcitriol doses, newer vitamin D compounds have been developed to counteract this effect. Intravenous paricalcitol (19-nor-1,25-dihydroxyvitamin D_2) was shown in normal rats to be less calcemic than calcitriol and to suppress PTH in uremic rats without increasing ionized serum calcium (289). Martin et al. demonstrated that intravenous paricalcitol decreased PTH levels in patients on dialysis by approximately 60% over the 12-week treatment period, with few episodes of hypercalcemia (290) (Fig. 92-32). Although anecdotal evidence suggests that there may be less hypercalcemia with this product compared with calcitriol, prospective studies that actually show this possibility are lacking. Bone histologic data also are lacking in paricalcitol-treated patients, although in uremic rats, intravenous paricalcitol appears to be approximately ten times less active than calcitriol in mobilizing calcium and phosphorus from bone (291). Another new vitamin D compound, 22-oxacalcitriol, also appears to be less calcemic in rats while effectively suppressing PTH levels (292), but it has not yet been approved for use in patients on dialysis.

A promising new form of PTH suppression involves activating the calcium-sensing receptors in parathyroid tissue (293). A phase I trial of one such calcium receptor agonist,

NPS-R568, showed that it was very effective in acutely suppressing serum PTH in patients on dialysis (66) (Fig. 92-3). Declines in PTH usually were noticeable within 1 to 2 hours after oral ingestion of the drug, with peak effects occurring

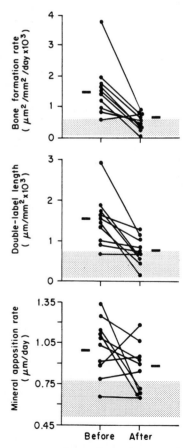

FIG. 92-30. Response of bone formation rate, double tetracycline label length, and mineral apposition rate to intravenous calcitriol in ten patients on dialysis previously refractory to oral calcitriol. *Shaded areas* represent normal range for values. (From Andress DL, et al. Intravenous calcitriol in the treatment of refractory osteitis fibrosa of chronic renal failure. *N Engl J Med* 1989;321:274, with permission.)

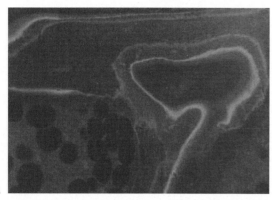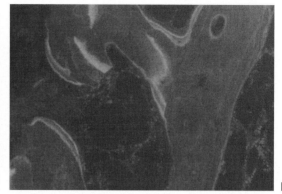

FIG. 92-31. A: Tetracycline labels in a patient on dialysis with osteitis fibrosa and high bone formation. **B:** Tetracycline labels in the same patient after treatment with intravenous calcitriol. The reductions in the interlabel distance and the length of double labels after treatment indicate a decrease in bone formation to normal. (**A** and **B,** Unstained fluorescent micrographs, magnification ×115.) (See Color Fig. 92-31 following page 2624.)

4 to 6 hours later (66). Newer calcium receptor analogs are being tested.

Parathyroidectomy is reserved for patients on dialysis who have severe osteitis fibrosa unresponsive to vitamin D therapy. Other indications for parathyroidectomy have included persistent hypercalcemia, intractable pruritus, progressive extraskeletal calcifications, and calciphylaxis (110). In general, removal of hyperplastic parathyroid glands is effective in relieving symptoms (294–297), although a minority of patients require repeated neck explorations for displaced or supernumerary parathyroid glands that result in persistent elevations of PTH (294,296). In a small number of patients, it has been shown that parathyroidectomy results in bone demineralization and osteomalacia (92,161,219,220). Because the decline in bone formation that follows parathyroidectomy is associated with accelerated bone surface aluminum

accumulation (91), it is suggested that all potential candidates for parathyroidectomy be evaluated for aluminum excess before surgery. This would be particularly important in those undergoing total parathyroidectomy because this procedure results in markedly reduced rates of bone formation (298). It is possible that intravenous calcitriol or paricalcitol therapy will replace the need for surgical parathyroidectomy in many patients. Failure to respond to treatment with any vitamin D analog may indicate irreversible reductions in vitamin D receptor density, which is characteristic of nodular parathyroid hyperplasia (299).

Aluminum-Associated Osteodystrophy

Treatment of aluminum bone disease involves taking preventive measures with respect to parenteral and oral aluminum intake as well as initiating chelation therapy once aluminum toxicity is diagnosed (Table 92-6). Water treatment with deionization or reverse osmosis is essential in maintaining dialysate aluminum concentrations below 10 μg/L

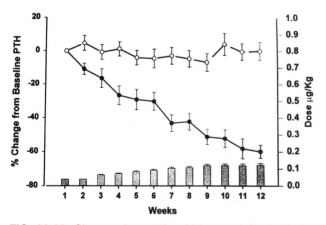

FIG. 92-32. Changes in parathyroid hormone levels during treatment with intermittent intravenous paricalcitol in patients on dialysis. Patients were randomized to placebo *(open circles)* or paricalcitol *(closed circles)*. Bars depict the doses of paricalcitol that increased according to the protocol. [From Martin KJ, et al. 19-nor-1α-25-dihydroxyvitamin D$_2$ (paricalcitol) safely and effectively reduces the levels of parathyroid hormone in patients on hemodialysis. *J Am Soc Nephrol* 1998;9:1427, with permission.]

TABLE 92-6. *Treatment of aluminum overload*

I. Asymptomatic or minimal symptoms—eliminate all sources of aluminum
  A. Check and correct dialysate
  B. Check and eliminate all medication sources
  C. Use calcium carbonate or calcium acetate as phosphate binder
  D. Add or substitute sevelamer as the phosphate binder

II. Moderate to marked symptoms
  A. Eliminate all sources of aluminum
  B. Initiate deferoxamine therapy at 5–10 mg/kg intravenously during the last 2 hr of dialysis once a week for 3 months
  C. Monitor closely for fungus infection
  D. Discontinue deferoxamine when symptoms abate

III. Symptoms worsen with chelation
  A. Administer half the dose of deferoxamine 4–6 hr before dialysis once a week
  B. After 1–2 mo, gradually increase the dose

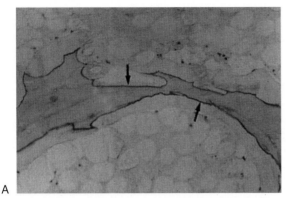 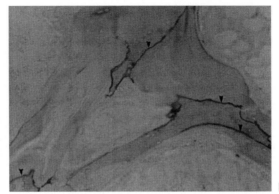

A   B

FIG. 92-33. A: Aluminum-associated bone disease in a patient on dialysis. Aluminum deposits *(arrows)* cover the mineralized bone surface. **B:** Aluminum stain in the same patient after treatment with intravenous deferoxamine. Most of the aluminum is now within the mineralized bone *(arrowheads),* indicating that new bone formation occurred despite the presence of aluminum at the mineralization front. (**A** and **B,** Aurin-tricarboxylic acid stain, magnification ×115.) (See Color Fig. 92-33 following page 2624.)

(300,301). Restricting the oral intake of aluminum now seems warranted owing to the association of aluminum bone disease with a high intake of aluminum-containing phosphate binders (172). Studies suggest that both calcium carbonate (223,302) and calcium acetate (232,303) are effective in binding intestinal phosphate when taken with meals.

Long-term aluminum chelation with deferoxamine is effective in the treatment of aluminum bone disease (160,304–308). Aluminum removal from the bone surface (Fig. 92-33) is accompanied by improvements in bone formation (Fig. 92-34) and bone symptoms. Some patients with a prior parathyroidectomy appear not to respond as readily to deferoxamine (305), suggesting that increased PTH secretion may be important in the healing of aluminum-related low-turnover bone disease. Because this poor response is related in part to the extent of bone surface aluminum, it is suggested that patients with a prior parathyroidectomy have a quantitative assessment of bone surface aluminum to determine whether more prolonged treatment with deferoxamine may be needed.

Only approximately 30% of the total circulating deferoxamine–aluminum chelate is removed by hemodialysis using cuprophane membranes (309). Until recently, there had been few improvements in the removal efficiency of deferoxamine–aluminum complexes using the different membranes (310). Polysulfone dialysis, however, appears to provide more efficient removal than dialysis with the cuprophane membrane, a result that is due only partly to the larger surface area (311). Charcoal hemoperfusion also may accelerate removal (312,313).

Although aluminum chelation with deferoxamine appears promising in the treatment of aluminum bone disease, a major side effect, the fungal infection mucormycosis, markedly limits its use (314–317). Almost always fatal, this complication may occur in 10% of treated patients on dialysis. Cataracts and retinal changes (318,319) and thrombocytopenia (320) also have been reported as complications of chronic deferoxamine therapy. The development of dialysis dementia with the initiation of deferoxamine treatment has been reported in a few patients (321). Avoidance of aluminum is

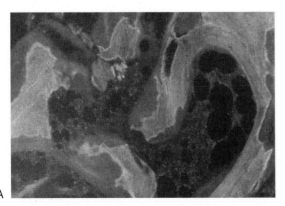 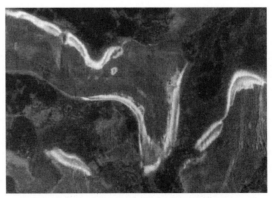

A   B

FIG. 92-34. A: Absence of tetracycline labels in a patient on dialysis with aluminum-associated osteomalacia. **B:** Tetracycline labels in the same patient after treatment with intravenous deferoxamine. The calculated bone formation rate is normal. (**A** and **B,** Unstained fluorescent micrographs, magnification ×115.) (See Color Fig. 92-34 following page 2624.)

preferable and chelation therapy is recommended only in critically toxic patients. Because of these concerns, it often is necessary to document aluminum toxicity by bone biopsy. When necessary, deferoxamine should be given at low doses (5 to 10 mg/kg/week), by either intravenous, intramuscular (322), or intraperitoneal routes (323) for no more than 3 months at a time.

Renal Transplantation

Renal transplantation, in most instances, corrects the abnormal calcium and phosphorus metabolism of uremia. Improvements in bone pathology, however, can be delayed depending on the severity of the underlying lesion (324). For example, patients who have had renal failure for a short duration may have essentially normal skeletons at the time of transplantation. In contrast, those who have had renal disease for a long duration plus a prolonged course of dialysis are likely to have significant bone disease at the time of transplantation. Transplant recipients in the latter group usually have more long-term problems with bone disease.

Renal synthesis of calcitriol resumes normally after transplantation (325). Resolution of hyperparathyroidism is seen in most patients within the first 4 months after transplantation (326). Those who continue to have persistent elevations of PTH often are hypercalcemic (327). In some, however, enhanced PTH secretion is present despite normal calcium levels (328). Hypophosphatemia or phosphate depletion can also elevate serum calcium levels (326). The prevalence of hypophosphatemia and hypercalcemia in transplant recipients is approximately 25% (327,328). The cause of the hypophosphatemia probably is multifactorial. Possible mechanisms include renal tubular phosphate leak (329), decreased phosphorus absorption secondary to corticosteroid therapy (330), and persistent hyperparathyroidism (331). Usually the hypercalcemia and hypophosphatemia are mild and can be controlled with oral phosphate supplements. Occasionally the hypophosphatemia results in osteomalacia, although more often it is not associated with significant bone histologic abnormalities (332).

Although several factors may be involved in decreasing bone mineral content during the early posttransplantation period, the deleterious effects of corticosteroids are the predominant concern (333). The debilitation of osteonecrosis in renal transplant recipients has been well described (252,334–337). Total hip replacement sometimes is indicated. Although osteonecrosis has occurred in patients on dialysis who have not received corticosteroids (338), the prevalence and severity of the disease in transplant recipients appear to be related to the cumulative steroid intake (339,340). Fortunately, early detection of osteonecrosis during the asymptomatic stage may be possible using MRI (340).

Glucocorticoids affect bone by decreasing bone formation and increasing bone resorption (339,341). Osteoblast function is thought to be decreased by steroids because the synthesis of bone cell protein (342) and collagen (343) is

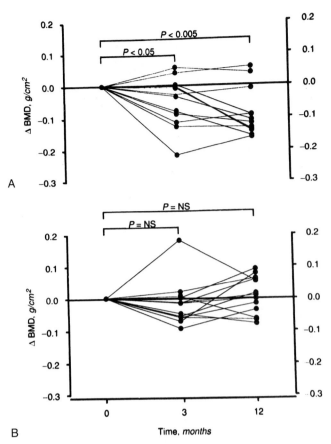

FIG. 92-35. Effect of pamidronate on femoral neck bone mineral density in renal transplant recipients. **A:** Control patients. **B:** Pamidronate-treated patients. (From Fan SS, et al. Pamidronate therapy as prevention of bone loss following renal transplantation. *Kidney Int* 2000;57:684, with permission.)

inhibited and because osteoblasts are induced to undergo apoptosis (programed cell death) (344). The increased osteoclast activity and bone resorption probably are secondary to the enhanced PTH secretion (339,345,346) because parathyroidectomy in glucocorticoid-treated animals abolishes the response (347).

In addition to increased PTH levels, intestinal calcium absorption is decreased and serum levels of 25-hydroxyvitamin D$_3$ are normal (339,348,349) or low (350) in renal transplant recipients. Even though serum levels of 25-hydroxyvitamin D$_3$ were normal in one group of patients studied by Hahn et al. who were receiving an average of 17.5 mg/day of prednisone or an equivalent, they noted that intestinal calcium absorption increased and serum PTH levels decreased after treatment with calcifediol (339). In a study by Rickers et al., there was no significant difference in bone mineral content among steroid-treated transplant recipients receiving sodium fluoride, vitamin D$_2$, and calcium phosphate compared with the control group that received prednisone alone (351). Certainly, more controlled trials are necessary before specific recommendations about treatment of steroid bone disease can be given. However, correction of abnormally low serum levels of calcium, phosphorus, or 25-hydroxyvitamin D$_3$ is certainly indicated.

The bisphosphonates, described as beneficial in postmenopausal osteoporosis (352,353) and in glucocorticoid-induced osteoporosis (354), may have potential in preventing osteoporosis in transplant recipients. Fan et al. demonstrated that two doses of intravenous pamidronate, given at the time of transplantation and 1 month later, effectively prevented the rapid bone loss that characterized the first year posttransplantation (355) (Fig. 92-35).

In summary, the bone disease seen in patients with renal disease has a complicated pathogenesis and therapy. Increased understanding of the factors involved has provided a rationale for management. A knowledgeable physician and compliant patient should be able to avoid most of the difficulties described in this chapter.

REFERENCES

1. Garner A, Ball J. Quantitative observations on mineralized and unmineralized bone in chronic renal azotaemia and intestinal malabsorption syndrome. *J Pathol Bacteriol* 1966;91:545.
2. Avioli LV. Collagen metabolism, uremia and bone. *Kidney Int* 1973; 4:105.
3. Price PA, Nishimoto SK. Radioimmunoassay for the vitamin K-dependent proteins of bone and its discovery in plasma. *Proc Natl Acad Sci USA* 1980;77:2234.
4. Baylink D, et al. Formation, mineralization and resorption of bone in vitamin D-deficient rats. *J Clin Invest* 1970;49:1122.
5. Parfitt AM. Plasma calcium control at quiescent bone surfaces: a new approach to the homeostatic function of bone lining cells. *Bone* 1989;10:87.
6. Frame B, Parfitt AM. Osteomalacia: current concepts. *Ann Intern Med* 1978;89:966.
7. Manologas SC. Birth and death of bone cells: basic regulatory mechanisms and implications for the pathogenesis and treatment of osteoporosis. *Endocrine Rev* 2000;21:115.
8. Canalis E, McCarthy T, Centrella M. Isolation of growth factors from adult bovine bone. *Calcif Tissue Int* 1988;43:346.
9. Centrella M, McCarthy T, Canalis E. Transforming growth factor β is a bifunctional regulator of replication and collagen synthesis in osteoblast enriched cell cultures from fetal rat bone. *J Biol Chem* 1987; 262:2869.
10. Hauschka PV, et al. Growth factors in bone matrix: isolation of multiple types by affinity chromatography on heparin Sepharose. *J Biol Chem* 1986;261:12665.
11. Robey PG, et al. Osteoblasts synthesize and respond to TGF-beta in vitro. *J Cell Biol* 1987;105:457.
12. Rosen V, Cox K, Hattersley G. Bone morphogenetic proteins. In: Bilezikian JP, Raisz LG, Rodan GA, eds. *Principles of bone biology.* San Diego, CA: Academic Press, 1996:661.
13. McCarthy TL, Centrella M, Canalis E. Regulatory effects of insulin-like growth factors I and II on bone collagen synthesis in rat calvarial cultures. *Endocrinology* 1989;124:301.
14. Mohan S, et al. Development of valid methods to measure insulin-like growth factors I and II in bone cell-conditioned medium. *Endocrinology* 1990;126:2534.
15. Andress DL. Heparin modulates the binding of insulin-like growth factor (IGF) binding protein-5 to a membrane protein in osteoblastic cells. *J Biol Chem* 1995;270:28289.
16. Andress DL, et al. Carboxy-truncated insulin-like growth factor binding protein-5 stimulates mitogenesis in osteoblast-like cells. *Biochem Biophys Res Commun* 1993;195:25.
17. Hruska KA, Teitelbaum S. Renal osteodystrophy. *N Engl J Med* 1995; 333:166.
18. Gonzalez EA, Martin KJ. Bone cell response in uremia. *Semin Dial* 1996;9:339.
19. MacDonald BR, Gallagher JA, Russell RGG. Parathyroid hormone stimulates the proliferation of cells derived from human bone. *Endocrinology* 1986;118:2445.
20. Oursler MJ, et al. Modulation of transforming growth factor-β production in normal human osteoblast-like cells by 17 β-estradiol and parathyroid hormone. *Endocrinology* 1991;129:3313.
21. Greenfield EM, et al. Aenyl cyclase and interleukin 6 are downstream effectors of parathyroid hormone resulting in stimulation of bone resorption. *J Clin Invest* 1995;96:1238.
22. Canalis E, et al. Insulin-like growth factor-I mediates selective anabolic effects of parathyroid hormone in bone cultures. *J Clin Invest* 1989;83:60.
23. Torring O, et al. Parathyroid hormone and parathyroid hormone-related peptide stimulate insulin-like growth factor-binding protein secretion by rat osteoblast-like cells through an adenosine 3′,5′-monophosphate-dependent mechanism. *Endocrinology* 1991;128:1006.
24. Herbelin A, et al. Elevated circulating levels of interleukin-6 in patients with chronic renal failure. *Kidney Int* 1992;39:954.
25. Herbelin A, et al. Influence of uremia and hemodialysis on circulating interleukin-1 and tumor necrosis factor alpha. *Kidney Int* 1990;37: 116.
26. Andress DL, et al. Plasma insulin-like growth factors and bone formation in uremic hyperparathyroidism. *Kidney Int* 1989;36:471.
27. Burger EH, Van Der Meer JW, Nijweide PJ. Osteoclast formation from mononuclear phagocytes: role of bone forming cells. *J Cell Biol* 1984;99:1901.
28. Parfitt AM. The coupling of bone formation to bone resorption: a critical analysis of the concept and its relevance to the pathogenesis of osteoporosis. *Metab Bone Dis Rel Res* 1982;4:1.
29. Parfitt AM. The actions of parathyroid hormone on bone: relation to bone remodeling and turnover, calcium homeostasis, and metabolic bone disease. *Metabolism* 1976;25:809.
30. Deftos LJ. The thyroid gland in skeletal and calcium metabolism. In: Avioli LV, Krane SM, eds. *Metabolic bone disease.* New York: Academic Press, 1978.
31. Green J, Kleeman CR. Role of bone in regulation of systemic acid-base balance. *Kidney Int* 1991;39:3.
32. Bushinsky DA. The contribution of acidosis to renal osteodystrophy. *Kidney Int* 1995;47:1816.
33. Phillips LS, et al. Somatomedin inhibitor in uremia. *J Clin Endocrinol Metab* 1984;59:764.
34. Russell JE, Termine JD, Avioli LV. Abnormal bone mineral maturation in the chronic uremic state. *J Clin Invest* 1973;52:2848.
35. Andress DL, Howard GA, Birnbaum RS. Identification of a low molecular weight inhibitor of osteoblast mitogenesis in uremic plasma. *Kidney Int* 1991;39:942.
36. Massry SG, Coburn JW, Kleeman CR. Evidence for suppression of parathyroid gland activity by hypermagnesemia. *J Clin Invest* 1970; 49:1619.
37. Mennes P, et al. Hypomagnesemia and impaired parathyroid hormone secretion in chronic renal disease. *Ann Intern Med* 1978;88:206.
38. Burnell JM, et al. Bone crystal maturation in renal osteodystrophy in humans. *J Clin Invest* 1974;53:52.
39. Sackler JP, Liu L. Heparin induced osteoporosis. *Br J Radiol* 1973;46: 548.
40. Llach F, et al. Skeletal resistance to endogenous parathyroid hormone in patients with early renal failure: a possible cause for secondary hyperparathyroidism. *J Clin Endocrinol Metab* 1975;41:339.
41. Bricker N. On the pathogenesis of the uremic state: an exposition of the "trade-off" hypothesis. *N Engl J Med* 1972;286:1093.
42. Slatopolsky E, et al. On the prevention of secondary hyperparathyroidism in experimental chronic renal disease using proportional reduction of dietary phosphorus intake. *Kidney Int* 1972;2:147.
43. Slatopolsky EA, et al. On the pathogenesis of hyperparathyroidism in chronic experimental renal insufficiency in the dog. *J Clin Invest* 1971;50:492.
44. Brown EM, et al. Abnormal regulation of parathyroid hormone release by calcium in secondary hyperparathyroidism due to chronic renal failure. *J Clin Endocrinol Metab* 1982;54:172.
45. Shen FH, et al. Serum immunoreactive parathyroid hormone and 25-hydroxy-vitamin D in patients with uremic bone disease. *J Clin Endocrinol Metab* 1975;40:1009.
46. Lopez-Hilker S, et al. Hypocalcemia may not be essential for the development of secondary hyperparathyroidism in chronic renal failure. *J Clin Invest* 1986;78:1097.
47. Wilson L, et al. Altered divalent ion metabolism in early renal failure: Role of 1,25(OH)$_2$ D. *Kidney Int* 1985;27:565.

48. Chertow BD, et al. Decrease in serum immunoreactive parathyroid hormone in rats and in parathyroid hormone secretion in vitro by 1,25-dihydroxycholecalciferol. *J Clin Invest* 1975;56:668.

49. Portale AA, et al. Effect of dietary phosphorus on circulating levels of $1,25(OH)_2$ D and immunoreactive parathyroid hormone in children with moderate renal insufficiency. *J Clin Invest* 1984;73:1580.

50. Silver J, Russell J, Sherwood LM. Regulation by vitamin D metabolites of messenger RNA for pre-pro-parathyroid hormone in isolated bovine parathyroid cells. *Proc Natl Acad Sci USA* 1985;82:4270.

51. Pitts TO, et al. Hyperparathyroidism and 1,25-dihydroxyvitamin D deficiency in mild, moderate, and severe renal failure. *J Clin Endocrinol Metab* 1988;67:876.

52. Delmez JA, et al. Parathyroid hormone suppression by intravenous 1,25-dihydroxyvitamin D: a role for increased sensitivity to calcium. *J Clin Invest* 1989;83:1349.

53. Dunlay R, et al. Direct inhibitory effect of calcitriol on parathyroid function (sigmoidal curve) in dialysis. *Kidney Int* 1989;36:1093.

54. Slatopolsky E, et al. Marked suppression of secondary hyperparathyroidism by intravenous administration of 1,25-dihydroxycholecalciferol in uremic patients. *J Clin Invest* 1984;74:2136.

55. Korkor AB. Reduced binding of [^{3}H]-1,25-dihydroxyvitamin D_3 in the parathyroid glands of patients with renal failure. *N Engl J Med* 1987;316:1573.

56. Freitag J, et al. Impaired parathyroid hormone metabolism in patients with chronic and renal failure. *N Engl J Med* 1978;298:29.

57. Brown EM. Physiology and pathophysiology of the extracellular calcium-sensing receptor. *Am J Med* 1999;106:238.

58. Lopez-Hilker S, et al. Phosphorus restriction reverses hyperparathyroidism in uremia independent of changes in calcium and calcitriol. *Am J Physiol* 1990;259:F432.

59. Slatopolsky E, et al. Phosphate restriction prevents parathyroid cell growth in uremic rats: high phosphate directly stimulates PTH secretion in vitro. *J Clin Invest* 1996;97:2534.

60. Almaden Y, et al. Direct effect of phosphorus on parathyroid hormone secretion from whole rat parathyroid glands in vitro. *J Bone Miner Res* 1996;11:970.

61. Canalejo A, et al. The effect of a high phosphorus diet on the parathyroid cell cycle. *Nephrol Dial Transplant* 1998;13[Suppl 3]:19.

62. Kates DM, Sherrard DJ, Andress DL. Evidence that serum phosphate is independently associated with serum PTH in patients with chronic renal failure. *Am J Kidney Dis* 1997;30:809.

63. Brown AJ, et al. Decreased calcium-sensing receptor expression in hyperplastic parathyroid glands of uremic rats: role of dietary phosphate. *Kidney Int* 1999;55:1284.

64. Kifor O, et al. Reduced immunostaining for the extracellular calcium-sensing receptor in primary and uremic secondary hyperparathyroidism. *J Clin Endocrinol Metab* 1996;81:1598.

65. Gogusev J, et al. Depressed expression of calcium receptor in parathyroid gland tissue of patients with hyperparathyroidism. *Kidney Int* 1997;51:328.

66. Antonsen JE, Sherrard DJ, Andress DL. A calcimimetic agent acutely suppresses parathyroid hormone levels in patients with chronic renal failure. *Kidney Int* 1998;53:223.

67. Wada M, et al. Calcimimetic NPS R-568 prevents parathyroid hyperplasia in rats with severe secondary hyperparathyroidism. *Kidney Int* 2000;57:50.

68. Parkinson IS, et al. Fracturing dialysis osteodystrophy and dialysis encephalopathy. *Lancet* 1979;1:406.

69. Alfrey AC, Hegg A, Craswell P. Metabolism and toxicity of aluminum in renal failure. *Am J Clin Nutr* 1980;33:1509.

70. Ittel TH, et al. Enhanced gastrointestinal absorption of aluminum in uremic rats. *Kidney Int* 1987;32:821.

71. Salusky IB, et al. Role of aluminum hydroxide in raising serum aluminum levels in children undergoing continuous ambulatory peritoneal dialysis. *J Pediatr* 1984;105:717.

72. Berlyne GM, et al. Hyperaluminemia from aluminum resins in renal failure. *Lancet* 1970;2:494.

73. Felsenfeld AJ, et al. Osteomalacia in chronic renal failure: a syndrome previously reported only with maintenance dialysis. *Am J Nephrol* 1982;2:147.

74. Altmann P, et al. Residual renal function in hemodialysis patients may protect against hyperaluminemia. *Kidney Int* 1987;32:710.

75. Buchanan MRC, Ihle BU, Dunn CM. Hemodialysis related osteo-malacia: a staining method to demonstrate aluminum. *J Clin Pathol* 1981;34:1352.

76. Cournot-Witmer G, et al. Aluminum localization in bone from hemodialyzed patients: relationship to matrix mineralization. *Kidney Int* 1981;20:375.

77. Maloney NA, et al. Histological quantitation of aluminum in iliac bone from patients with renal failure. *J Lab Clin Med* 1982;99:206.

78. De Vernejoul MC, et al. Effects of iron overload on bone remodelling in pigs. *Am J Pathol* 1984;116:377.

79. Pierce-Myli M, Pierides A. Iron and aluminum osteomalacia during hemodialysis: a new syndrome. *Kidney Int* 1984;25:151A.

80. Van de Vyver FL, et al. Iron overload and bone disease in chronic dialysis patients. *Contrib Nephrol* 1988;64:134.

81. D'Haes PC, et al. Increased bone strontium levels in hemodialysis patients with osteomalacia. *Kidney Int* 2000;57:1107.

82. Andreoli SP, Cohen M. Intraperitoneal deferoxamine therapy for iron overload in children undergoing CAPD. *Kidney Int* 1989;35:1330.

83. Schrooten I, et al. Strontium induced osteomalacia: a new disease entity in patients with end-stage renal failure in dialysis. An epidemiological survey. *Kidney Int* 1999;56:1886.

84. Romberg RW, et al. Inhibition of hydroxyapatite crystal growth by bone specific and other calcium-binding proteins. *Biochemistry* 1986;25:1176.

85. Schrooten I, et al. Strontium causes osteomalacia in chronic renal failure rats. *Kidney Int* 1998;54:448.

86. Hercz G, et al. Aplastic osteodystrophy without aluminum: the role of "suppressed" parathyroid function. *Kidney Int* 1993;44:860.

87. Andress DL, et al. Bone histomorphometry of renal osteodystrophy in diabetic patients. *J Bone Miner Res* 1987;2:525.

88. Vincenti F, et al. Parathyroid and bone response of the diabetic patient to uremia. *Kidney Int* 1984;25:677.

89. Sugimoto T, et al. Effects of high concentrations of glucose on PTH secretion in parathyroid cells. *Kidney Int* 1990;37:1522.

90. Goodman WG, Ramirez JA, Belin TR, et al. Development of adynamic bone in patients with secondary hyperparathyroidism after intermittent calcitriol therapy. *Kindney Int* 1994;46:1160.

91. Andress DL, et al. Effect of parathyroidectomy on bone aluminum accumulation in chronic renal failure. *N Engl J Med* 1985;312:468.

92. Charon SA, et al. Effects of parathyroidectomy on bone formation and mineralization in hemodialyzed patients. *Kidney Int* 1985;27:426.

93. De Vernejoul MC, et al. Increased bone aluminum deposition after subtotal parathyroidectomy in dialyzed patients. *Kidney Int* 1985;27:785.

94. Cann CE, Prussin SG, Gordon GS. Aluminum uptake by the parathyroid glands. *J Clin Endocrinol Metab* 1979;49:543.

95. Morrissey J, et al. Suppression of parathyroid hormone secretion by aluminum. *Kidney Int* 1983;23:699.

96. Plachot JJ, et al. Bone ultrastructure and x-ray microanalysis of aluminum-intoxicated hemodialyzed patients. *Kidney Int* 1984;25:796.

97. Blumenthal NC, Posner AS. In vitro model of aluminum-induced osteomalacia: Inhibition of hydroxy-apatite formation and growth. *Calcif Tissue Int* 1984;36:439.

98. Zhu JM, Huffer W, Alfrey AC. Effect of aluminum on bone matrix inductive properties. *Kidney Int* 1990;38:1141.

99. Costin G, et al. Endocrine abnormalities in thalassemia major. *Am J Dis Child* 1979;133:497.

100. Sherman LA, Pfeferbaum A, Brown EB. Hypoparathyroidism in a patient with long standing iron storage disease. *Ann Intern Med* 1970;73:259.

101. Sherrard DJ, Ott SM, Andress DL. Pseudo-hyperparathyroidism: a syndrome associated with aluminum intoxication in chronic renal failure. *Am J Med* 1985;79:127.

102. Richards P, Chamberlain MJ, Wrong OM. Treatment of osteomalacia of renal tubular acidosis by sodium bicarbonate alone. *Lancet* 1972;2:994.

103. Andreoli SP, Bergstein JM, Sherrard DJ. Aluminum intoxication from aluminum-containing phosphate binders in children with azotemia not undergoing dialysis. *N Engl J Med* 1984;310:1079.

104. Mitch WE, et al. The effect of a keto acid-amino acid supplement to a restricted diet on the progression of chronic failure. *N Engl J Med* 1984;311:623.

105. Massry SG, Goldstein DA. Role of parathyroid hormone in uremic toxicity. *Kidney Int* 1978;13:S39.

106. Denney JD, et al. Total body calcium and long-term calcium balance in chronic renal disease. *J Lab Clin Med* 1973;82:226.

107. Massry SG, et al. Skeletal resistance to parathyroid hormone in renal failure. *Ann Intern Med* 1973;78:357.

108. Alfrey AC, et al. Extraosseous calcification: evidence for abnormal pyrophosphate metabolism in uremia. *J Clin Invest* 1976;57:692.

109. Conger JD, et al. Pulmonary calcification in chronic dialysis patients. *Ann Intern Med* 1975;83:330.

110. Block GA, et al. Association of serum phosphorus and calcium × phosphate product with mortality risk in chronic hemodialysis patients: a national study. *Am J Kidney Dis* 1998;31:607.

111. Goodman WG, et al. Coronary-artery calcification in young adults with end-stage renal disease who are undergoing dialysis. *N Engl J Med* 2000;342:1478.

112. Massry SG, et al. Skeletal resistance to the calcemic action of parathyroid hormone in uremia. *Kidney Int* 1976;9:467.

113. Alfrey AC, Solomons CC. Bone pyrophosphate in uremia and its association with extraosseous calcification. *J Clin Invest* 1976;57:700.

114. Hodsman AB, et al. Vitamin-D-resistant osteomalacia in hemodialysis patients lacking secondary hyperparathyroidism. *Ann Intern Med* 1981;94:629.

115. Sherrard DJ, et al. Renal osteodystrophy: classification, cause and treatment. In: Frame B, Potts JT Jr, eds. *Clinical disorders of bone and mineral metabolism.* Amsterdam: Excerpta Medica, 1983:254.

116. Escobedo EM, et al. Magnetic resonance imaging of dialysis-related amyloidosis of the shoulder and hip. *Skeletal Radiol* 1996;25:41.

117. Mottet JJ, et al. Evidence for preservation of cortical bone mineral density in patients on continuous ambulatory peritoneal dialysis. *J Bone Miner Res* 1996;11:96.

118. Stein MS, et al. Prevalence and risk factors for osteopenia in dialysis patients. *Am J Kidney Dis* 1996;28:515.

119. Stehman-Breen CO, et al. Risk factors for hip fracture among patients with end-stage renal disease. *Kidney Int* 2000;58:2200.

120. Rix M, et al. Bone mineral density and biochemical markers of bone turnover in patients with predialysis chronic renal failure. *Kidney Int* 1999;56:1084.

121. Brickman AS, et al. Clinical effects of 1,25-dihydroxyvitamin D_3 in uremic patients with overt osteodystrophy. *Contrib Nephrol* 1980;18:29.

122. Charon SA, et al. Serum bone gla-protein in renal osteodystrophy: comparison with bone histomorphometry. *J Clin Endocrinol Metab* 1986;63:892.

123. Urena P, et al. Short-term effects of parathyroidectomy on plasma biochemistry in chronic uremia. *Kidney Int* 1989;36:120.

124. Malluche HH, et al. Plasma levels of bone Gla-protein reflect bone formation in patients on chronic maintenance dialysis. *Kidney Int* 1984;26:869.

125. Hruska KA, et al. Metabolism of immunoreactive parathyroid hormone in the dog: the role of the kidney and the effects of chronic renal disease. *J Clin Invest* 1975;56:39.

126. Andress DL, et al. Comparison of parathyroid hormone assays with bone histomorphometry in renal osteodystrophy. *J Clin Endocrinol Metab* 1986;63:1163.

127. Quarles LD, Lobaugh B, Murphy G. Intact parathyroid hormone overestimates the presence and severity of parathyroid-mediated osseous abnormalities in uremia. *J Clin Endocrinol Metab* 1992;75:145.

128. Andress DL, et al. Parathyroid hormone in aluminum bone disease: a comparison of parathyroid hormone assays. *Kidney Int Suppl* 1986;18:87.

129. McCarthy JT, et al. Serum bioactive parathyroid hormone in hemodialysis patients. *J Clin Endocrinol Metab* 1989;68:340.

130. Andress D, et al. Parathyroid hormone responsiveness to hypocalcemia in hemodialysis patients with osteomalacia. *Kidney Int* 1983;24:364.

131. Savory J, Wills MR. Analytical methods for aluminum measurement. *Kidney Int Suppl* 1986;18:24.

132. Nebeker HG, et al. Indirect methods for the diagnosis of aluminum bone disease: plasma aluminum, the deferoxamine infusion test and serum parathyroid hormone. *Kidney Int Suppl* 1986;18:96.

133. Pei Y, et al. Non-invasive prediction of aluminum bone disease in hemo- and peritoneal dialysis patients. *Kidney Int* 1992;41:1374.

134. Gejyo F, et al. Serum levels of B_2-microglobulin as a new form of amyloid protein in patients undergoing long-term hemodialysis. *N Engl J Med* 1986;314:585.

135. Zaoul PM, Stone WJ, Hakim RM. Effects of dialysis membranes on beta 2-microglobulin production and cellular expression. *Kidney Int* 1990;38:962.

136. Floege J, et al. Imaging of dialysis-related amyloid (AB-amyloid) deposits with ^{131}I-β_2-microglobulin. *Kidney Int* 1990;38:1169.

137. Sherrard DJ, Maloney NA. Single-dose tetracycline labeling for bone histomorphometry. *Am J Clin Pathol* 1989;91:682.

138. Albright F, Drake TG, Sulkowitch HW. Renal osteitis fibrosa cystica: report of case with discussion of metabolic aspects. *Bull Johns Hopkins Hosp* 1937;60:377.

139. Sherrard DJ, et al. The spectrum of bone disease in end-stage renal failure: an evolving disorder. *Kidney Int* 1993;43:436.

140. Bishop MC, et al. Effects of hemodialysis on bone in chronic renal failure. *BMJ* 1972;3:644.

141. Delmez JA, et al. Continuous peritoneal dialysis and bone. *Kidney Int* 1986;30:379.

142. Dent CE, Harper CM, Philpot GR. Treatment of renal-glomerular osteodystrophy. *QJM* 1961;30:1.

143. Dunstan CR, et al. Secondary hyperparathyroidism in chronic haemodialysis patients: a clinico-pathologic study. *Proc Eur Dial Transplant Assoc* 1983;20:731.

144. Duursma SA, Visser WJ, Njio LA quantitative histological study of bone in 30 patients with renal insufficiency. *Calcif Tissue Res* 1972;9:216.

145. Follis RH Jr, Jackson DA. Renal osteomalacia and osteitis fibrosa in adults. *Bull Johns Hopkins Hosp* 1943;72:232.

146. Ingham JP, Stewart JH, Posen S. Quantitative skeletal histology in untreated end-stage renal failure. *BMJ* 1973;2:745.

147. Stanbury SW. Azotemic renal osteodystrophy. *Br Med Bull* 1957;13:57.

148. Stanbury SW, Lumb GA. Parathyroid function in chronic renal failure. *QJM* 1966;35:1.

149. Sherrard DJ, et al. Quantitative histological studies on the pathogenesis of uremic bone disease. *J Clin Endocrinol Metab* 1974;39:119.

150. Teitelbaum SL, et al. Do parathyroid hormone and 1,25-dihydroxyvitamin D modulate bone formation in uremia? *J Clin Endocrinol Metab* 1980;51:247.

151. McGuire JL, Marks SC Jr. The effects of parathyroid hormone on cell structure and function. *Clin Orthop* 1974;100:392.

152. Teitelbaum SL, et al. Tetracycline fluorescence in uremic and primary hyperparathyroid bone. *Kidney Int* 1977;12:366.

153. Tam CS, Wilson DR, Harrison JE. Effect of parathyroid extract on bone apposition and the interaction between parathyroid hormone and vitamin D. *Miner Electrolyte Metab* 1980;3:74.

154. Malluche HH, et al. Bone histology in incipient and advanced renal failure. *Kidney Int* 1976;9:355.

155. Kopp JB, et al. Bone aluminum accumulation in hemodialysis patients: a longitudinal perspective. *Am J Kidney Dis* 1988;12:214.

156. Kaye M, et al. Osteoclast enlargement in end-stage renal disease. *Kidney Int* 1985;27:574.

157. Hitt O, et al. Tissue-level bone formation rates in chronic renal failure, measured by means of tetracycline bone labeling. *Can J Physiol Pharmacol* 1970;48:824.

158. Campos C, Arata RO, Mautalen CA. Parathyroid hormone and vertebral osteosclerosis in uremic patients. *Metabolism* 1976;25:495.

159. Ellis HA, Peart KM. Azotaemic renal osteodystrophy: a quantitative study on iliac bone. *J Clin Pathol* 1973;26:83.

160. Malluche HH, et al. The use of deferoxamine in the management of aluminum accumulation in bone in patients with renal failure. *N Engl J Med* 1984;311:140.

161. Teitelbaum SL, et al. Calcifediol in chronic renal insufficiency: skeletal response. *JAMA* 1976;235:164.

162. Voigts A, et al. Parathyroid hormone and bone histology: response to hypocalcemia in osteitis fibrosa. *Kidney Int* 1984;25:445.

163. Andress DL, et al. Plasma insulin-like growth factors and bone formation in uremic hyperparathyroidism. *Kidney Int* 1989;36:471.

164. Jehle PM, et al. Insulin-like growth factor system components in hyperparathyroidism and renal osteodystrophy. *Kidney Int* 2000;57:423.

165. Andress DL. Insulin-like growth factor-binding protein-5 (IGFBP-5) stimulates phosphorylation of the IGFBP-5 receptor. *Am J Physiol* 1998;274:E744.

166. Richman C, et al. Recombinant human insulin-like growth factor-binding protein-5 stimulates bone formation parameters in vitro and in vivo. *Endocrinology* 1999;140:4699.

167. Teitelbaum SL. Pathological manifestations of osteomalacia and rickets. *Clin Endocrinol Metab* 1980;9:43.

168. Ott SM, et al. The prevalence of bone aluminum deposition in renal osteodystrophy and its relation to the response to calcitriol therapy. *N Engl J Med* 1982;307:709.

169. Ward MK, et al. Osteomalacic dialysis osteodystrophy: evidence for a water-borne aetiological agent, probably aluminum. *Lancet* 1978;1:841.

170. Faugere MC, Malluche HH. Stainable aluminum and not aluminum content reflects histologic changes in bone of dialyzed patients. *Kidney Int* 1986;30:717.

171. Hodsman AB, et al. Do serum aluminum levels reflect underlying skeletal aluminum accumulation and bone histology before or after chelation by deferoxamine? *J Lab Clin Med* 1985;106:674.

172. Andress DL, et al. Aluminum-associated bone disease in chronic renal failure: high prevalence in a long-term dialysis population. *J Bone Miner Res* 1986;1:391.

173. Llach F, et al. Prevalence of various types of bone disease in dialysis patients. In: Robinson RR, ed. *Proceedings of the Ninth International Congress of Nephrology*. Berlin: Springer-Verlag, 1984.

174. Smith AJ, et al. Aluminum-related bone disease in mild and advanced renal failure: evidence for high prevalence and morbidity and studies on etiology and diagnosis. *Am J Nephrol* 1986;6:275.

175. Andress DL, et al. Osteomalacia and aplastic bone disease in aluminum-related osteodystrophy. *J Clin Endocrinol Metab* 1987;65:11.

176. Andress DL, et al. Early deposition of aluminum in bone in diabetic patients on hemodialysis. *N Engl J Med* 1987;316:292.

177. Bourdeau AM, et al. Parathyroid response to aluminum in vitro: ultrastructural changes and PTH release. *Kidney Int* 1987;31:15.

178. O'Hare JA, Murnaghan DJ. Evidence of increased parathyroid activity on discontinuation of high-aluminum dialysate in patients undergoing hemodialysis. *Am J Med* 1984;77:229.

179. Chan YL, et al. Effect of aluminum on normal and uremic rats: tissue distribution, vitamin D metabolites, and quantitative bone histology. *Calcif Tissue Int* 1983;35:344.

180. Ellis HA, McCarthy JH, Herrington J. Bone aluminum in hemodialyzed patients and in rats injected with aluminum chloride: relationship to impaired bone mineralization. *J Clin Pathol* 1979;32:832.

181. Goodman WG, Gilligan J, Horst R. Short-term aluminum administration in the rat. *J Clin Invest* 1984;73:171.

182. Lewis-Finch J, et al. The effects of discontinuation of aluminum exposure (with or without deferoxamine) on aluminum-induced osteomalacia in the uremic rat. *Kidney Int* 1986;30:318.

183. Ott SM, et al. Development and reversibility of aluminum-induced bone lesion in the rat. *J Lab Clin Med* 1987;109:40.

184. Robertson JA, et al. Animal model of aluminum-induced osteomalacia: role of chronic renal failure. *Kidney Int* 1983;23:327.

185. Goodman WG, et al. Parenteral aluminum administration in the dog: II. induction of osteomalacia and effect on vitamin D metabolism. *Kidney Int* 1984;25:370.

186. Goodman WG. Thyroparathyroidectomy modifies the skeletal response to aluminum loading in the rat. *Kidney Int* 1987;31:923.

187. Felsenfeld AJ, et al. The effect of high parathyroid hormone levels on the development of aluminum-induced osteomalacia in the rat. *J Am Soc Nephrol* 1991;1:970.

188. Quarles LD, et al. Aluminum deposition in bone: an epiphenomenon of the osteomalacic state. *J Clin Invest* 1985;75:1441.

189. Mayor GH, et al. Aluminum absorption and distribution: effect of parathyroid hormone. *Science* 1977;197:1187.

190. Hodsman AB, et al. Bone aluminum and histomorphometric features of renal osteodystrophy. *J Clin Endocrinol Metab* 1982;54:539.

191. Lieberherr M, et al. In vitro effects of aluminum on bone phosphatases: a possible interaction with bPTH and vitamin D_3 metabolites. *Calcif Tissue Int* 1982;34:280.

192. Blair HC, et al. Micromolar aluminum levels reduce ^{3}H-thymidine incorporation by cell line UMR 106-01. *Kidney Int* 1989;35:1119.

193. Howard GA. Chick kidney and calvaria cells: in vitro aluminum effects on DNA synthesis and vitamin D metabolism. *Calcif Tissue Int* 1984;36:13A.

194. De Vernejoul MC, et al. Histomorphometric evidence of deleterious effects of aluminum on osteoblasts. *Bone* 1985;6:15.

195. Andress DL, et al. Human bone cell metabolism of 25(OH)D in chronic renal failure: effect of surface bone aluminum. In: Norman AW, et al., eds. *Vitamin D, chemical, biochemical and clinical endocrinology of calcium metabolism*. New York: de Gruyter, 1985:960.

196. Pun KK, Ho PWM, Lau P. Effects of aluminum on the parathyroid hormone receptors of bone and kidney. *Kidney Int* 1990;37:72.

197. Faugere MC, et al. Loss of bone resulting from accumulation of aluminum in bone of patients undergoing dialysis. *J Lab Clin Med* 1986;107:481.

198. Ritz E, et al. Skeletal abnormalities in chronic renal insufficiency before and during maintenance hemodialysis. *Kidney Int* 1973;4:116.

199. DiRaimondo CR, et al. Pathologic fractures associated with idiopathic amyloidosis of bone in chronic hemodialysis patients. *Nephron* 1986;43:22.

200. Gorevic PA, et al. β_2-Microglobulin is an amyloidogenic protein in man. *J Clin Invest* 1985;76:2425.

201. Connors LH, et al. In vitro formation of amyloid fibrils from intact β_2-microglobulin. *Biochem Biophys Res Commun* 1985;131:1063.

202. Casey TT, et al. Tumoral amyloidosis of bone of beta-2-microglobulin origin in association with long-term hemodialysis: a new type of amyloid disease. *Hum Pathol* 1986;17:731.

203. Onishi S, et al. Beta-2 microglobulin deposition in bone in chronic renal failure. *Kidney Int* 1991;39:990.

204. Kataoka H, et al. Inhibitory effects of β_2-microglobulin on in vitro calcification of osteoblastic cells. *Biochem Biophys Res Commun* 1986;141:360.

205. Moe SM, et al. Role of IL-1β and prostaglandins in β_2-microglobulin induced bone mineral dissolution. *Kidney Int* 1995;47:587.

206. Chesney RW, et al. Influence of long-term oral 1,25-dihydroxyvitamin D in childhood renal osteodystrophy. *Contrib Nephrol* 1980;18:55.

207. Hodson EM, et al. Quantitative bone histology in children with chronic renal failure. *Kidney Int* 1982;21:833.

208. Milliner DS, et al. Soft tissue calcification in pediatric patients with end-stage renal disease. *Kidney Int* 1990;38:931.

209. Salusky IB, et al. Bone disease in pediatric patients undergoing dialysis with CAPD or CCPD. *Kidney Int* 1988;33:975.

210. Salusky IB, et al. "High dose" calcitriol for control of renal osteodystrophy in children on CAPD. *Kidney Int* 1987;32:89.

211. Trachman H, Bauthier B. Parenteral calcitriol for treatment of severe renal osteodystrophy in children with chronic renal insufficiency. *J Pediatr* 1987;110:966.

212. Blum WF, et al. Growth hormone resistance and inhibition of somatomedin activity by excess of insulin-like growth factor binding protein in uremia. *Pediatr Nephrol* 1991;5:539.

213. Hokken ACS, et al. Placebo-controlled, double-blind, cross-over trial of growth hormone treatment in prepubertal children with chronic renal failure. *Lancet* 1991;338:585.

214. Powell DR, et al. Modulation of growth factors by growth hormone in children with chronic renal failure. *Kidney Int* 1997;51:1970.

215. Powell DR, et al. Effects of chronic renal failure and growth hormone on serum levels of insulin-like growth factor-binding protein-4 (IGFBP-4) and IGFBP-5 in children: a report of the Southwest Pediatric Nephrology Study Group. *J Clin Endocrinol Metab* 1999;84:596.

216. Sedman AB, et al. Aluminum loading in children with chronic renal failure. *Kidney Int* 1984;26:210.

217. Griswold WR, et al. Accumulation of aluminum in a non-dialyzed uremic child receiving aluminum hydroxide. *Pediatrics* 1983;71:56.

218. Salusky IB, et al. Aluminum accumulation during treatment with aluminum hydroxide and dialysis in children and young adults with chronic renal disease. *N Engl J Med* 1991;324:527.

219. Slatopolsky E, et al. Long-term effects of calcium carbonate and 2.5 mEq/liter calcium dialysate on mineral metabolism. *Kidney Int* 1989;36:897.

220. Weinstein RS. Decreased mineralization in hemodialysis patients after subtotal parathyroidectomy. *Calcif Tissue Int* 1982;34:16.

221. Stewart AF, et al. Calcium homeostasis in immobilization: an example of resorptive hypercalciuria. *N Engl J Med* 1982;30:1136.

222. Coburn JW, Hartenbower DL, Massry SG. Intestinal absorption of calcium and the effect of renal insufficiency. *Kidney Int* 1973;4:96.

223. Slatopolsky EA, et al. The control of phosphate excretion in uremia. *J Clin Invest* 1966;45:672.

224. Tanaka Y, DeLuca HF. The control of 25(OH) vitamin D by inorganic phosphorus. *Arch Biochem Biophys* 1973;154:566.

225. Portale AA, et al. Reduced plasma concentration of 1,25-dihydroxyvitamin D in children with moderate renal insufficiency. *Kidney Int* 1982;21:627.

226. Combe C, Aparicio M. Phosphorus and protein restriction and parathyroid function in chronic renal failure. *Kidney Int* 1994;46:1381.

227. Llach F, Massry SG. On the mechanism of secondary hyperparathyroidism in moderate renal insufficiency. *J Clin Endocrinol Metab* 1985;61:601.

228. Hercz G, et al. Reversal of aluminum-related bone disease after substituting calcium carbonate for aluminum hydroxide. *Am J Kidney Dis* 1988;11:70.

229. Clarkson EM, McDonald SJ, De Wardener AE. The effect of a high intake of calcium carbonate in normal subjects and patients with chronic renal failure. *Clin Sci* 1966;30:425.

230. Makoff DL, et al. Chronic calcium carbonate therapy in uremia. *Arch Intern Med* 1969;123:15.

231. Slatopolsky E, et al. Calcium carbonate as a phosphate-binder in patients with chronic renal failure undergoing dialysis. *N Engl J Med* 1986;315:157.

232. Mai ML, et al. Calcium acetate, an effective phosphorus binder in patients with renal failure. *Kidney Int* 1989;36:690.

233. Froment DP, et al. Site and mechanism of enhanced gastrointestinal absorption of aluminum by citrate. *Kidney Int* 1989;36:978.

234. Molitoris BA, et al. Citrate: a major factor in the toxicity of orally administered aluminum compounds. *Kidney Int* 1989;36:949.

235. Nolan CR, Califano JR, Butzin CA. Influence of calcium acetate or calcium citrate on intestinal aluminum absorption. *Kidney Int* 1990; 38:937.

236. Partridge NA, et al. Influence of dietary constituents on intestinal absorption of aluminum. *Kidney Int* 1989;35:1413.

237. O'Donovan R, et al. Substitution of aluminum salts by magnesium salts in control of dialysis hyperphosphataemia. *Lancet* 1986;1:880.

238. Delmez JA, et al. Magnesium carbonate as a phosphorus binder: a prospective, controlled, crossover study. *Kidney Int* 1996;49:163.

239. Slatopolsky EA, et al. RenaGel, a nonabsorbed calcium- and aluminum-free phosphate binder, lowers serum phosphorus and parathyroid hormone. *Kidney Int* 1999;55:299.

240. Brickman AS, Coburn JW, Norman AW. Action of 1,25-dihydroxycholecalciferol, a potent, kidney-produced metabolite of vitamin D₃, in uremic man. *N Engl J Med* 1972;287:891.

241. Meyrier A, Marsac J, Richet G. The influence of a high calcium carbonate intake on bone disease in patients undergoing hemodialysis. *Kidney Int* 1973;4:146.

242. Indridason OS, Quarles LD. Comparison of treatments for mild secondary hyperparathyroidism in hemodialysis patients. *Kidney Int* 2000;57:282.

243. Bouillon R, Verberckmoes R, Moor PD. Influence of dialysate calcium concentration and vitamin D on serum parathyroid hormone during repetitive dialysis. *Kidney Int* 1975;7:422.

244. Goldsmith RS, Johnson WJ. Role of phosphate depletion and high dialysate calcium in controlling dialytic renal osteodystrophy. *Kidney Int* 1973;4:154.

245. Liu SH, Chu HI. Studies of calcium and phosphorus metabolism with special reference to pathogenesis and effects of dihydrotachysterol (ATIO) and iron. *Medicine (Baltimore)* 1943;22:103.

246. Eastwood JB, et al. The contrasting effects on bone histology of vitamin D and of calcium carbonate in the osteomalacia of chronic renal failure. *Clin Sci* 1974;47:23.

247. Potter DE, Wilson CJ, Ozonoff MB. Hyperparathyroid bone disease in children undergoing long-term hemodialysis: treatment with vitamin D. *J Pediatr* 1974;85:60.

248. Stanbury SW, Lumb GA. Metabolic studies of renal osteodystrophy: I. calcium, phosphorus and nitrogen metabolism in rickets, osteomalacia and hyperparathyroidism complicating chronic uremia and in the osteomalacia of adult Fanconi syndrome. *Medicine (Baltimore)* 1962; 41:1.

249. Smith JE, Goodman DS. The turnover and transport of vitamin D and a polar metabolite with the properties of 25-hydroxycholecalciferol in human plasma. *J Clin Invest* 1971;50:2159.

250. Recker R, et al. The efficacy of calcifidiol in renal osteodystrophy. *Arch Intern Med* 1978;138:857.

251. Bordier P, Marie JP, Arnaud CD. Evolution of renal osteodystrophy: correlation of bone histomorphometry and serum mineral and immunoreactive parathyroid hormone values before and after treatment with calcium carbonate or 25-hydroxycholecalciferol. *Kidney Int Suppl* 1975;2:102.

252. Potter DE, Genant HK, Salvatierra O. Avascular necrosis of bone after renal transplantation. *Am J Dis Child* 1978;132:125.

253. Frost HM, et al. Histomorphometric changes in trabecular bone of

254. Fraser DR, Kodicek E. Unique biosynthesis by kidney of a biologically active vitamin D metabolite. *Nature* 1970;228:764.

255. Berl T, et al. 1,25-Dihydroxycholecalciferol effects in chronic dialysis. *Ann Intern Med* 1978;88:774.

256. Delling G, et al. The actions of 1,25(OH)₂ D₃ on turnover kinetic, remodeling surfaces and structure of trabecular bone in chronic renal failure. *Contrib Nephrol* 1980;18:105.

257. Malluche HH, Goldstein DA, Massry SG. Effects of 6 months therapy with 1,25(OH)₂D₃ on bone disease of dialysis patients. *Contrib Nephrol* 1980;18:98.

258. Sherrard DJ, et al. Skeletal response to treatment with 1,25-dihydroxyvitamin D in renal failure. *Contrib Nephrol* 1980;18:92.

259. Brickman AS, et al. 1,25-Dihydroxyvitamin D₃ in normal man and patients with renal failure. *Ann Intern Med* 1974;80:161.

260. Brickman AS, et al. 1,25-Dihydroxycholecalciferol: effect on skeletal lesions and plasma parathyroid hormone levels in uremic osteodystrophy. *Arch Intern Med* 1974;134:883.

261. Quarles LD, et al. Oral calcitriol and calcium: efficient therapy for uremic hyperparathyroidism. *Kidney Int* 1988;34:840.

262. Kanis JA, Russell RGG. Rate of reversal of hypercalcemia and hypercalciuria induced by vitamin D and its 1α-hydroxylated derivatives. *BMJ* 1977;1:78.

263. Brickman AS, et al. Comparison of effects of 1α-hydroxyvitamin D₃ and 1-25-dihydroxyvitamin D₃ in man. *J Clin Invest* 1976;57:1540.

264. Pierides AM, et al. 1α-Hydroxycholecalciferol in hemodialysis renal osteodystrophy: adverse effects of anti-convulsant therapy. *Clin Nephrol* 1976;5:189.

265. Kanis JA, et al. An evaluation of 1α-hydroxy- and 1,25-dihydroxyvitamin D₃ in the treatment of renal bone disease. *Contrib Nephrol* 1980;18:12.

266. Bordier P, et al. The effect of 1α(OH)O₃ and 1α,25(OH)₂D₃ on the bone in patients with renal osteodystrophy. *Am J Med* 1978;64:101.

267. Kanis JA, et al. Treatment of renal bone disease with 1α-hydroxylated derivatives of vitamin D₃: clinical, biochemical, radiographic and histological responses. *QJM* 1979;48:289.

268. Peacock M, et al. Bone disease and hyperparathyroidism in chronic renal failure: the effect of 1α-hydroxyvitamin D. *Clin Endocrinol* 1977; 7:73.

269. Prior JC, et al. Experience with 1,25-dihydroxycholecalciferol therapy in patients undergoing hemodialysis with progressive vitamin D₂-treated osteodystrophy. *Am J Med* 1979;67:583.

270. Lefebvre A, et al. Optimal correction of acidosis changes progression of dialysis osteodystrophy. *Kidney Int* 1989;36:1112.

271. Davie MW. J, et al. 1-Alphahydroxycholecalciferol in chronic renal failure: studies of the effect of oral doses. *Ann Intern Med* 1976;84: 281.

272. Healy MD, et al. Effects of long-term therapy with calcitriol in patients with moderate renal failure. *Arch Intern Med* 1980;140:1030.

273. Melsen F, Nielsen HE, Romer FK. The Effect of 1α-OH D₃ on bone changes in nondialyzed patients with chronic renal insufficiency. In: Norman AW, et al., eds. *Vitamin D basic research and its clinical application.* Berlin: de Gruyter, 1979.

274. Massry GR, et al. Use of 1,25(OH)₂ D₃ in the treatment of renal osteodystrophy in patients with moderate renal failure. In Frame B, Potts TJ Jr, eds. *Clinical disorders of bone and mineral metabolism.* Amsterdam: Excerpta Medica, 1983:260.

275. Baker LR. I, et al. 1,25(OH)₂D₃ administration in moderate renal failure: a prospective double-blind trial. *Kidney Int* 1988;35:661.

276. Nordal KP, Dahl E. Low dose calcitriol versus placebo in patients with predialysis chronic renal failure. *J Clin Endocrinol Metab* 1988;67:929.

277. Christiansen C, et al. Deterioration of renal function during treatment of chronic renal failure with 1,25-dihydroxycholecalciferol. *Lancet* 1978;2:700.

278. Tougaard L, et al. Controlled trial of 1α-hydroxycholecalciferol in chronic renal failure. *Lancet* 1976;1:1044.

279. Farrington K, Varghese F, Moorhead JE. Vitamin D analogues and renal function. *Lancet* 1978;2:150.

280. Naik RB, et al. Effects of vitamin D metabolites and analogues on renal function. *Nephron* 1981;28:17.

281. Sjoden G, Lindgren JU, DeLuca HF. Antirachitic activity of 1α-hydroxyergocalciferol and 1a-hydroxycholecalciferol in rats. *J Nutr* 1984;114:2043.

renal failure patients treated with calcifediol. *Metab Bone Dis Rel Res* 1981;2:285.

282. Sjoden G, et al. 1α-Hydroxyvitamin D_2 is less toxic than 1α-hydroxyvitamin D_3 in the rat. *Proc Soc Exp Biol* 1985;178:432.

283. Frazao JM, et al. Intermittent doxercalciferol (1α-hydroxyvitamin D_2) therapy for secondary hyperparathyroidism. *Am J Kidney Dis* 2000; 36:550.

284. Cordy PE, Mills DM. The early detection and treatment of renal osteodystrophy. *Miner Electrolyte Metab* 1981;5:311.

285. Quarles LD, et al. Prospective trial of pulse oral versus intravenous calcitriol treatment of hyperparathyroidism in ESRD. *Kidney Int* 1994;45:1710.

286. Andress DL, et al. Intravenous calcitriol in the treatment of refractory osteitis fibrosa of chronic renal failure. *N Engl J Med* 1989;321:274.

287. Llach F, Hervas J, Cerezo S. The importance of dosing intravenous calcitriol in dialysis patients with severe hyperparathyroidism. *Am J Kidney Dis* 1995;26:845.

288. Ginsburg DS, Kaplan EL, Katz AI. Hypercalcemia after oral calcium-carbonate therapy in patients on chronic hemodialysis. *Lancet* 1973; 1:1271.

289. Slatopolsky E, et al. A new analog of calcitriol, 19-nor-$1,25(OH)_2D_2$, suppresses parathyroid hormone secretion in uremic rats in the absence of hypercalcemia. *Am J Kidney Dis* 1995;28:852.

290. Martin KJ, et al. 19-Nor-1α,25-dihydroxyvitamin D_2 (paricalcitol) safely and effectively reduces the levels of intact parathyroid hormone in patients on hemodialysis. *J Am Soc Nephrol* 1998;9:1427.

291. Finch JL, Brown AJ, Slatopolsky E. Differential effects of 1,25-dihydroxyvitamin D_3 and 19-nor 1,25-dihydroxyvitamin D_2 (paricalcitol) on calcium and phosphorus resorption in bone. *J Am Soc Nephrol* 1999;10:980.

292. Brown AJ, et al. The noncalcemic analogue of vitamin D, 22-oxacalcitriol, suppresses parathyroid hormone synthesis and secretion. *J Clin Invest* 1989;84:728.

293. Wada M, et al. The calcimimetic compound NPS R-568 suppresses parathyroid cell proliferation in rats with renal insufficiency: control of parathyroid cell growth via a calcium receptor. *J Clin Invest* 1997;100:2977.

294. Dawborn JK, et al. Parathyroidectomy in chronic renal failure. *Nephron* 1983;33:100.

295. Johnson WJ, et al. Results of subtotal parathyroidectomy in hemodialysis patients. *Am J Med* 1988;84:23.

296. Memmos DE, et al. The role of parathyroidectomy in the management of hyperparathyroidism in patients on maintenance hemodialysis and after renal transplantation. *Nephron* 1982;30:143.

297. Mozes MF, et al. Total parathyroidectomy and autotransplantation in secondary hyperparathyroidism. *Arch Surg* 1980;115:378.

298. Kaye M, D'Amour P, Henderson J. Elective total parathyroidectomy without autotransplant in end-stage renal disease. *Kidney Int* 1989;35:1390.

299. Fukuda N, et al. Decreased 1,25-dihydroxyvitamin D_3 receptor density is associated with a more severe form of parathyroid hyperplasia in chronic uremic patients. *J Clin Invest* 1993;92:1436.

300. Graf H, et al. Aluminum removal by hemodialysis. *Kidney Int* 1981; 19:587.

301. Hodge KC, et al. Critical concentrations of aluminum in water used for dialysis. *Lancet* 1981;1:802.

302. Moriniere P, et al. Substitution of aluminum hydroxide by high doses of chronic hemodialysis: disappearance of hyperaluminemia and equal control of hyperparathyroidism. *Proc Eur Dial Transplant Assoc* 1982; 19:784.

303. Schiller LR, et al. Effect of the time of administration of calcium acetate on phosphorus binding. *N Engl J Med* 1989;320:1110.

304. Ackrill P, et al. Treatment of fracturing renal osteodystrophy by desferrioxamine. *Proc Eur Dial Transplant Assoc* 1982;19:203.

305. Andress DL, et al. Bone histologic response to long-term deferoxamine therapy for aluminum bone disease. *Kidney Int* 1987;31:1344.

306. Brown DJ, et al. Treatment of dialysis osteomalacia with desferrioxamine. *Lancet* 1982;2:343.

307. Charon SA, et al. Deferoxamine-induced bone changes in hemodialysis patients: a histomorphometric study. *Clin Sci* 1987;73:227.

308. Felsenfeld AJ, et al. Desferrioxamine therapy in hemodialysis patients with aluminum-associated bone disease. *Kidney Int* 1989;35:1371.

309. Kaehny WD, et al. Aluminum transfer during hemodialysis. *Kidney Int* 1977;12:361.

310. Muirhead N, et al. Removal of aluminum during hemodialysis: effect of different dialyzer membranes. *Am J Kidney Dis* 1986;8:51.

311. Molitoris BA, et al. Rapid removal of DFO-chelated aluminum during hemodialysis using polysulfone dialyzers. *Kidney Int* 1988;34:98.

312. Delmez J, et al. Accelerated removal of deferoxamine mesylate-chelated aluminum by charcoal hemoperfusion in hemodialysis patients. *Am J Kidney Dis* 1989;13:308.

313. McCarthy JT, et al. Deferoxamine and coated charcoal hemoperfusion to remove aluminum in dialysis patients. *Kidney Int* 1988;34:804.

314. Boelaert JR, et al. The role of desferrioxamine in dialysis-associated mucormycosis: report of three cases and review of the literature. *Clin Nephrol* 1988;29:261.

315. Daly AL, et al. Mucormycosis: association with deferoxamine therapy. *Am J Med* 1989;87:468.

316. Van Cutsem J, Boelaert JR. Effects of deferoxamine, feroxamine and iron on experimental mucormycosis (zygomycosis). *Kidney Int* 1989;36:1061.

317. Windus DW, et al. Fatal *Rhizopus* infections in hemodialysis patients receiving deferoxamine. *Ann Intern Med* 1987;107:678.

318. Davies SC, et al. Ocular toxicity of high-dose intravenous deferoxamine. *Lancet* 1983;2:181.

319. Olivieri NF, et al. Visual and auditory neurotoxicity in patients receiving subcutaneous deferoxamine infusions. *N Engl J Med* 1986;314:869.

320. Walker JA, Sherman RA, Eisinger RP. Thrombocytopenia associated with intravenous deferoxamine. *Am J Kidney Dis* 1985;6:254.

321. Sherrard DJ, Walker JV, Boykin JL. Precipitation of dialysis dementia by deferoxamine treatment of aluminum-related bone disease. *Am J Kidney Dis* 1988;12:126.

322. Molitoris BA, et al. Efficacy of intramuscular and intraperitoneal deferoxamine for aluminum chelation. *Kidney Int* 1987;31:986.

323. Hercz G, et al. Aluminum removal by peritoneal dialysis: intravenous vs. intraperitoneal deferoxamine. *Kidney Int* 1986;30:944.

324. Pierides AM, et al. Assessment of renal osteodystrophy following renal transplantation. *Proc Eur Dial Transplant Assoc* 1974;11:481.

325. Piel CF, Roof BS, Avioli LV. Metabolism of tritiated 25-hydroxycholecalciferol in chronically uremic children before and after successful renal transplantation. *J Clin Endocrinol Metab* 1973;37:944.

326. Alfrey AC, et al. Resolution of hyperparathyroidism, renal osteodystrophy and metastatic calcification after renal homotransplantation. *N Engl J Med* 1968;279:1349.

327. David DS, et al. Hypercalcemia after renal transplantation: long-term follow-up data. *N Engl J Med* 1973;289:398.

328. Mitlak BH, et al. Parathyroid function in normocalcemic renal transplant recipients: evaluation by calcium infusion. *J Clin Endocrinol Metab* 1991;72:350.

329. Rosenbaum RW, et al. Decreased phosphate reabsorption after renal transplantation: evidence for a mechanism independent of calcium and parathyroid hormone. *Kidney Int* 1981;19:568.

330. Walker GS, et al. Factors influencing the intestinal absorption of calcium and phosphorus following renal transplantation. *Nephron* 1980;26:225.

331. Kleerekoper M, et al. Hyperparathyroidism after renal transplantation. *BMJ* 1975;3:680.

332. Felsenfeld A, et al. Hypophosphatemia in long-term renal transplant recipients: effects on bone histology and $1,25(OH)_2D$ levels. *Kidney Int* 1984;25:342.

333. Gottlieb MN, et al. A longitudinal study of bone disease after successful renal transplantation. *Nephron* 1978;22:239.

334. Fisher DE, Bickel WH. Corticosteroid induced avascular necrosis. *J Bone Joint Surg Am* 1971;53:849.

335. Gustafson LA, Meyers MH, Berne TV. Total hip replacement in renal transplant recipients with aseptic necrosis of the femoral head. *Lancet* 1976;2:606.

336. Haberman ET, Cristofaro RL. Avascular necrosis of bone as a complication of renal transplantation. *Semin Arthritis Rheum* 1976;6:189.

337. Murray WR. Hip problems associated with organ transplants. *Clin Orthop* 1973;90:57.

338. Bailey GL, et al. Avascular necrosis of the femoral head in patients on chronic hemodialysis. *Trans Am Soc Artif Intern Organs* 1972;18:401.

339. Hahn TJ, et al. Altered mineral metabolism in glucocorticoid-induced osteopenia. *J Clin Invest* 1979;64:655.

340. Kopp JB, et al. Prospective evaluation of renal transplant bone disease. *Kidney Int* 1989;35:518(abstr).

341. Frost HM, Villanueva AR. Human osteoblastic activity. Part III: the effect of cortisone on lamellar osteoblastic activity. *Henry Ford Hosp Med J* 1961;9:97.

342. Peck WA, Brandt J, Miller I. Hydrocortisone-induced inhibition of protein synthesis and uridine incorporation in isolated bone cells in vitro. *Proc Natl Acad Sci USA* 1967;57:1599.

343. Thompson JS, Urist MR. Effects of cortisone on bone metabolism in intact and thyroidectomized rabbits. *Calcif Tissue Res.* 13:197,1973.

344. Weinstein RS, et al. Inhibition of osteoblastogenesis and promotion of apoptosis of osteoblasts and osteocytes by glucocorticoids. *J Clin Invest* 1998;102:274.

345. Fucik RF, et al. Effect of glucocorticoids on function of the parathyroid glands in man. *J Clin Endocrinol Metab* 1975;40:152.

346. Lukert BP, Adams JS. Calcium and phosphorus homeostasis in man: effect of corticosteroids. *Arch Intern Med* 1976;136:1249.

347. Aloia JF, et al. Skeletal metabolism and body composition in Cushing's syndrome. *J Clin Endocrinol Metab* 1974;39:981.

348. Hahn TJ. Drug-induced disorders of vitamin D and mineral metabolism. *Clin Endocrinol Metab* 1980;9:107.

349. Hahn TJ, Halstead LR, Haddad JG Jr. Serum 25-hydroxyvitamin D concentrations in patients receiving chronic corticosteroid therapy. *J Lab Clin Med* 1977;90:399.

350. Klein RG, et al. Intestinal calcium absorption in exogenous hypercortisolism: role of 25-hydroxyvitamin D and corticosteroid dose. *J Clin Invest* 1977;60:253.

351. Rickers H, et al. Corticosteroid-induced osteopenia and vitamin D metabolism: effect of vitamin D_2, calcium phosphate and sodium fluoride administration. *Clin Endocrinol* 1982;16:409.

352. Storm T, et al. Effect of intermittent cyclical etidronate therapy on bone mass and fracture rate in women with postmenopausal osteoporosis. *N Engl J Med* 1990;322:1265.

353. Black DM, et al. Randomized trial of effect of alendronate on risk of fracture in women with existing vertebral fractures: fracture intervention trial research group. *Lancet* 1996;348:1535.

354. Saag KG, et al. Alendronate for the prevention and treatment of glucocorticoid-induced osteoporosis. *N Engl J Med* 1998;339:292.

355. Fan SS, et al. Pamidronate therapy as prevention of bone loss following renal transplantation. *Kidney Int* 2000;57:684.

CHAPTER 93

Nervous System Manifestations of Renal Failure

Cosmo L. Fraser and Allen I. Arieff

Advancements in dialysis therapy, renal transplantation, and their medical management have resulted in improvement of both the duration and quality of life in patients with end-stage renal disease (ESRD). However, patients with renal failure continue to manifest a variety of neurologic disorders. Those with chronic renal failure who have not yet received dialysis therapy may develop a symptom complex progressing from mild sensorial clouding tremor to delirium and coma. Even after the institution of otherwise adequate maintenance dialysis therapy, patients may continue to manifest more subtle nervous system dysfunction such as impaired mentation, generalized weakness, and peripheral neuropathy. The central nervous system (CSN) disorders of untreated renal failure and those persisting despite dialysis are referred to as uremic encephalopathy. The treatment of end-stage renal disease with dialysis has itself been associated with the emergence of at least four distinct disorders of the CNS: dialysis dysequilibrium, dialysis dementia, stroke, and sexual dysfunction. The dialysis disequilibrium syndrome (DDS) is a consequence of the initiation of dialysis therapy in a minority of patients. Dialysis dementia is a progressive, generally fatal encephalopathy that can affect patients on chronic hemodialysis as well as children with chronic renal failure who have not been treated with dialysis. Cardiovascular disorders are the major cause of death in hemodialysis patients, accounting for 40% of deaths (1). These include myocardial infarction, cardiomyopathy, ischemic heart disease, and stroke (2). The factors associated with uremia that lead to an increased incidence and mortality from stroke are not well known, but are beginning to be elucidated (1–3).

In addition to the preceding manifestations of neurologic dysfunction, which are specifically related to uremia, dialysis, or both, a number of other neurologic disorders occur with increased frequency in patients who have end-stage

renal disease and are being treated with chronic hemodialysis. Subdural hematoma, acute stroke, certain electrolyte disorders (hyponatremia, hypernatremia, phosphate depletion, hypercalcemia), vitamin deficiencies, Wernicke's encephalopathy, drug intoxication, hypertensive encephalopathy, and acute trace element intoxication must be considered in patients with chronic renal failure who manifest an altered mental state. In the recent past renal transplantation was associated with a variety of nervous system infections and neoplasms, such as reticulum cell sarcoma and lymphoma, which were probably a direct result of immunosuppressive therapy. This may be altered with the widespread use of cyclosporin for renal transplantation (4).

Patients with renal failure are also at risk of developing organic brain disease and metabolic encephalopathy, which can afflict the general population. Therefore, a thorough and complete evaluation is necessary when a patient with end-stage kidney disease presents with altered mental status.

UREMIC ENCEPHALOPATHY

Uremic encephalopathy is an acute or subacute organic brain syndrome that regularly occurs in patients with acute or chronic renal failure when the glomerular filtration rate declines below 10% of normal. As with other organic brain syndromes, these patients display variable disorders of consciousness, psychomotor behavior, thinking, memory, speech, perception, and emotion (5–7). The term *uremic encephalopathy* is used to describe the early appearance and dialysis responsiveness of the nonspecific neurologic symptoms of uremia. Other systemic abnormalities observed in patients with chronic renal failure are separable from uremic encephalopathy on the grounds that they tend to appear late in the progressive clinical course, infrequently produce symptoms, are detected in tissues and organs rather than as integrated whole organism phenomena, and respond sluggishly and irregularly to dialysis procedures. The symptoms may include sluggishness and easy fatigue; daytime drowsiness and

C. L. Fraser and A. I. Arieff: Department of Medicine, University of California School of Medicine, San Francisco, California

insomnia with a tendency toward sleep inversion; itching; inability to focus or sustain attention or to perform mental (cognitive) tasks and manipulation; inability to manage ideas and abstractions; slurring of speech; anorexia, nausea, and vomiting probably of central origin; restlessness; imprecise memory; diminished sexual interest and performance; volatile emotionality and withdrawal; myoclonus and "restless legs"; "burning feet"; asterixis; hiccoughs; paranoid thought content; disorientation and confusion with bizarre behavior; hallucinosis, muttering, and mumbling; meningeal signs, nystagmus; vertigo and ataxia; transient pareses and aphasic episodes; coma; and convulsions.

Certain salient characteristics of the symptoms of uremic encephalopathy are especially noteworthy: They are caused by dysfunction of the nervous system and are manifested as cognitive, neuromuscular, somatosensory, and autonomic impairments; their severity and overall rates of progression vary directly with the rate at which renal function develops. Uremic symptoms are generally more severe and progress more rapidly in patients with acute renal failure than in those with chronic renal failure. In slowly progressive renal failure the number and severity of symptoms also typically vary cyclically, with intervals of acceptable well being in an otherwise inexorable downhill course toward increasing disability. The symptoms are readily ameliorated by dialysis procedures and suppressed by maintenance dialysis regimens. They are also usually relieved entirely following restoration of renal function (e.g., after successful renal transplantation). Thus, the encephalopathy of renal failure is important to recognize precisely because it is promptly and decisively treatable by clinical methods that are generally available. The causes of uremic encephalopathy doubtless are multiple and complex. Recent studies demonstrate that brain oxygen utilization is diminished in patients with end-stage renal disease (8). Most such individuals had anemia, and partial correction of the anemia did not improve the impaired brain oxygen utilization (8). However, since the widespread introduction of recombinant human erythropoietin (EPO) as a therapeutic agent in patients with end-stage renal disease (ESRD) treated with hemodialysis (9), it is now clear that brain function and quality of life are improved by correction of the anemia associated in ESRD with EPO (10–12).

Diagnosis

The diagnosis of uremic encephalopathy in most patients is suspected if there is a constellation of clinical signs and symptoms that indicate renal or urologic disease or injury. However, the presenting symptoms of uremia, as mentioned earlier, are similar to many other encephalopathic states; thus, there is a risk of misdiagnosis and mistreatment. The differential diagnosis is even more complex, because patients with renal failure are subjected to other intercurrent illnesses that may also induce additional encephalopathic effects. Moreover, if a drug or its metabolites with potential CNS

toxicity is excreted or significantly metabolized by the kidney, the ensuing encephalopathic symptoms may not be entirely attributable to "uremia" but to the drug that has reached toxic levels at ordinary dose rates. When levels of azotemia are discovered that are sometimes associated with uremic encephalopathy in the absence of associated illness, differentiation of the effects of drug versus renal failure may be very difficult. One or more dialysis treatments may both restore more normal body fluid composition and also reduce drug levels, so that the question remains moot while the patient recovers. Despite the possibilities that such multiple causes of encephalopathy might occur simultaneously, uremic encephalopathy may be successfully differentiated in most instances by means of the usual clinical methods.

In patients who have other medical problems, such as advanced liver disease with hepatic insufficiency, it is often difficult to differentiate whether the cause of encephalopathy is owing to either hepatic or renal causes. Under normal conditions, protein and amino acids in the gastrointestinal tract are metabolized by colonic bacteria and mucosal enzymes to form ammonia (13). Ammonia then enters the liver through the portal circulation where it participates in the urea cycle to form urea. Over 90% of the urea produced is excreted in the urine and the remainder enters the colon via hepatoportal recirculation. However, in patients with renal failure, the major route for elimination of urea is not available; thus, there is an increase in blood urea. The amount of urea that enters the colon is increased because of the elevated plasma urea. Urea is then acted on by colonic bacteria and mucosal enzymes in a similar manner to protein and amino acids. This leads to increased ammonia production in uremic subjects that may either increase plasma ammonia levels or lead to misinterpretation of this test.

If the patient with kidney failure also has cirrhosis or some other form of liver failure, this additional ammonia load may present a stress that cannot be adequately handled by the diseased liver. The result may be increased blood and CNS ammonia levels with development of encephalopathy (13). Thus, patients with cirrhosis and end-stage kidney disease are at particular risk for developing encephalopathy because both conditions act synergistically to increase both blood and CNS ammonia. Consequently, it would be prudent to institute early dialysis in patients with end-stage liver and kidney diseases in order to reduce the plasma urea and thus the production of ammonia from urea in the gut. Ammonia also can be removed from the blood by hemodialysis. It should be noted that plasma urea and serum creatinine do not always adequately reflect renal function in patients with severe liver disease. Recent studies suggest that many patients who have cirrhosis, ascites, and normal plasma urea and creatinine may in fact have severe renal functional impairment (14–16). Differentiation of hepatic from uremic encephalopathy on clinical grounds can be very difficult in such individuals.

ACUTE RENAL FAILURE

The clinical manifestations of acute renal failure have been studied in several large patient series (7,17,18). Abnormalities of mental status have been noted as early and sensitive indices of a neurologic disorder, which progressed rapidly into disorientation and confusion (19,20). Fixed attitudes, torpor, and other signs of toxic psychosis were common. When uremia is untreated and allowed to progress, coma often supervenes. Cranial nerve signs such as nystagmus and mild facial asymmetries are common, although usually transient. There can be visual field defects and papilledema of the optic fundi. About half the patients have dysarthria, and many have diffuse weakness and fasciculations. Marked variation of deep tendon reflexes is noted in most patients, often in an asymmetric pattern. Progression of hyperreflexia, with sustained clonus at the patella or ankle, is common (21).

Electroencephalograms (EEG) in patients with acute renal failure (18) generally have been grossly abnormal when the diagnosis of renal failure is first established (Fig. 93-1). In most instances, the percentage of EEG power less than 5 and 7 Hz, which are standard measurements of the percentage of EEG power devoted to abnormal (delta) slow wave activity, are over 20 times the normal value. The percentage of EEG frequencies above 9 Hz and below 5 Hz are not affected by dialysis for 6 to 8 weeks, but return to normal with recovery of renal function. Similar findings have been shown in experimental animals with renal failure (22). The EEG may worsen both during and for several hours after hemodialysis and up to 6 months after initiation of dialytic therapy (23,24). In patients with acute renal failure, the EEG is abnormal within 48 hours of the onset of renal failure (18) and is generally not affected by dialysis within the first 3 weeks

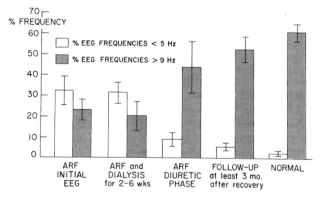

FIG. 93-1. Percentage of EEG frequencies below 5 Hz and above 9 Hz. Normal values are on the right. Patients with acute renal failure (ARF) have significant changes in both frequencies above 9 Hz and below 5 Hz. These changes are unaffected by dialysis but become normal with return of renal function. Data from 16 patients with ARF are illustrated. Data are mean ± SE. (From: Cooper JD, Lazarowitz VC, Arieff AI. Neurodiagnostic abnormalities in patients with acute renal failure: evidence for neurotoxicity of parathyroid hormone. *J Clin Invest* 1978;61:1448, with permission.)

(Fig. 93-1). During this interval, patients with acute renal failure have been shown to have elevated levels of parathyroid hormone (PTH) in plasma (18,25). Several months after return of renal function, plasma PTH levels also return to normal. Although there are doubtless many factors that contribute to uremic encephalopathy, many investigators have shown no correlation between encephalopathy and any of the commonly measured indicators of renal failure (e.g., blood urea nitrogen [BUN], creatinine, bicarbonate, arterial pH, and potassium) (18,20,25). For this and other reasons, parathyroid hormone has been postulated to be a major CNS "uremic toxin" (25,26).

CHRONIC RENAL FAILURE

The incidence of ESRD in the United States is 180 cases per million population (27). Among patients with ESRD treated with chronic hemodialysis, the mortality in the United States is 21% per year (28). The most frequent causes of ESRD in the United States are diabetes, hypertension, and glomerulonephritis (29). The neurologic manifestations reported with chronic renal failure (CRF) are numerous (20,30). The EEG findings in patients with CRF are usually less severe than those observed in patients with acute renal failure (5). Several investigations have shown a good correlation between the percentage of EEG frequencies and power below 7 Hz and the decline of renal function as estimated by serum creatinine (6,7). After the initiation of dialysis, there may be an initial period of clinical stabilization during which time the EEG deteriorates (up to 6 months) but it then approaches normal values (24); however, still more improvement is seen after renal transplantation (6,31). Cognitive functions also have been shown to be impaired in uremia. These include sustained attention, selective attention, speed of decision making, short-term memory, and mental manipulation of symbols (5).

The causes of the EEG abnormalities observed in uremic patients are probably multifactorial but there is evidence that a very important element may be an effect of parathyroid hormone (PTH) on brain. In experimental animals with either acute or chronic renal failure, many of the EEG abnormalities can be shown to be related to a direct effect of PTH on brain, which leads to an elevated brain content of calcium Ca^{2+} (22). Studies in patients with either acute renal failure or chronic renal failure suggest a similar pathogenesis (32,33).

Psychological Testing

Several different types of psychological tests have been applied to subjects with chronic renal failure. These have been designed to measure the effects of either dialysis, renal transplantation, or parathyroidectomy (6,25,30).

The Trailmaking Test has been administered to a number of uremic subjects. In general, their performance was less effective than that of normal; improvement with practice limits repeated use of this test. The Continuous Memory Test correlates quite well with the degree of renal failure, as does the Choice Reaction Time (CRT). Scores in both tests improve with treatment by dialysis or renal transplantation. Similar but less impressive results are obtained with the Continuous Performance Test. Of all these tests, it appears that the CRT is best correlated with renal function and improvement in the patient's condition as a result of dialysis or transplantation (5,34).

Patients who had chronic renal failure who were maintained on dialysis have been evaluated as to the possible effects of PTH on psychological function (25). After establishment of baseline values, patients with chronic renal failure underwent parathyroidectomy for other medical reasons (e.g., bone disease, soft tissue calcification, and persistent hypercalcemia, all of which were unresponsive to medical management). In these patients, parathyroidectomy resulted in a significant improvement in several areas of psychological testing. They showed significant improvement in Raven's Progressive Matrices percentile scores and visual motor index (VMI) raw and percentage scores. These are tests of general cognitive function, nonverbal problem solving and visual motor or visual spatial skills (5,34).

In addition, they manifested significantly fewer errors on the Trailmaking Test as well as significantly lower raw and T-score values on the Profile of Mood States Fatigue Scale postoperatively, in which they reported feeling significantly less fatigue, weariness, and inertia after undergoing surgery. Control subjects who underwent neck surgery for other reasons showed significant postoperative improvement in the Trailmaking Test but showed no change in any of the other tests (25). Other studies have shown that there is intellectual impairment in most patients with chronic renal failure who are being treated with dialysis (35–37). In these studies the procedures included the full Wechsler Adult Intelligence Scale (WAIS), the Walton-Black Modified Word Learning Test (MWLT), and the Block Design Learning Test (BDLT).

The overall intellectual level, as measured by the WAIS full-scale IQ, did not differ significantly from normal. The patients' performance was owing mainly to the digit symbol, block design, and picture arrangement subtests, all of which produced scores significantly below normal. The impairment of intellectual level as represented by the Wechsler deterioration quotient also was outside the normal range. The data on verbal learning obtained with the MWLT and performance learning obtained with the BDLT did not indicate any gross learning abnormality. Cognitive data were compared with other information, such as age, sex, length of dialysis, and biochemical variables by a multiple regression technique. The analysis suggested that of the cognitive data, those obtained with the BDLT bore the strongest relation to duration of dialysis. Other studies have suggested that the WAIS full-scale IQ in dialysis patients is below that of the general population (5). There appears to be a consensus, based on psychological testing, that chronic renal failure results in organiclike losses of intellectual function, particularly information-processing capacities (35–37).

BIOCHEMICAL BRAIN CHANGES

To determine the possible causes of the EEG abnormalities and clinical manifestations observed in patients with either acute or chronic renal failure, *in vivo* biochemical studies have been carried out in brain of both patients and laboratory animals. Measurements have included brain intracellular pH and concentrations of Na^+, K^+, Cl^-, Al^{3+}, Ca^{2+}, Mg^{2+}, urea, adenine nucleotides (creatine phosphate, ATP, ADP, AMP), lactate, and $(Na^+ + K^+)$-activated adenosine triphosphatase (ATPase) enzyme activity (18,20,38–44). In patients with acute renal failure, the brain content of water, K^+ and Mg^{2+} is normal, whereas Na^+ is modestly decreased and Al^{3+} is slightly elevated (18). However, cerebral cortex Ca^{2+} content is almost twice the normal value (18,25,32). Similar findings have been observed in dogs with acute renal failure (22,42). Permeability of uremic rat brain to inert molecules (e.g., insulin and sucrose) is increased. The permeability of brain to weak acids, such as sulfate, penicillin, and dimethadione, is normal to low (43–45).

Alterations of cerebral metabolism that might be related to the changes in permeability mentioned in the preceding also have been studied in animals (39,46–48). There are at least four studies that have attempted to evaluate the effects of uremia on the CNS using subcellular analysis. The first two studies evaluated Na-K-ATPase enzyme activity in crude microsomal fractions obtained from brains of acutely uremic rats (38,40). There was a significantly decreased Na-K-ATPase enzyme activity in their preparation and they suggested that the depressed enzyme activity was not owing to acidosis but the uremic state itself (38). On the other hand, an earlier study by Van den Noort and associates (40) found no significant difference in cationic ATPase activity in normal and uremic rat brains. In the brain of rats with acute renal failure, creatine phosphate, ATP, and glucose were increased, but there were corresponding decreases in AMP, ADP, and lactate. Total brain adenine nucleotide content and $(Na^+ - K^+)$-activated ATPase were normal to low. The uremic brain utilized less ATP and thus failed to produce ADP, AMP, and lactate at normal rates. The brain energy charge was normal, as was the redox state, and these findings were not altered by hypoxia (39). There was a corresponding decrease in brain metabolic rate, along with elevated glucose and low lactate levels (39). Other studies of uremic brain have shown a decrease in cerebral oxygen consumption (8), but such findings were not apparently related to the presence of anemia. Patients with chronic renal insufficiency (glomerular filtration rate below 20 mL/min) have decreased brain uptake of glutamine and increased ammonia uptake. The relevance of these findings, in terms of neurotransmitters or other brain function, is unknown (46).

Studies have been carried out in neurons and glia of uremic rat brain (49). Two different cytoskeletal proteins, both early indicators of brain injury, were examined. These included glial fibrillary acidic protein (GFAP), which is specific to astrocytes, and microtubule-associated protein-2 (MAP-2), which localizes to neuronal cell bodies and dendrites. Its loss

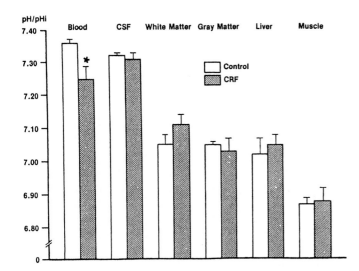

FIG. 93-2. The effects of 4 months of chronic renal failure (CRF) on the intracellular pH (pHi). In dogs with CRF, the arterial pH is significantly below control values. However, pHi is normal in brain white and gray matter, the liver, and skeletal muscle (*$P < 0.01$). *CSF,* cerebrospinal fluid. (From: Mahoney CA, Arieff AI. Central and PNS effects of chronic renal failure. *Kidney Int* 1983;24:170, with permission.)

provides one of the earliest indications of neuronal degeneration. In uremic brain (12 hours of acute renal failure), there was a diffuse increase in GFAP in cerebral cortex. Changes in MAP-2 immunoreactivity were observed in all regions of the cerebral cortex. These data suggest that there may be profound degenerative changes in neurons even with only moderate azotemia. These studies suggest subcellular anatomic changes in brain of animals with acute renal failure, but do not elucidate any metabolic abnormalities.

In animals with either acute or chronic renal failure, both urea concentration and osmolality are similar in brain, cerebrospinal fluid, and plasma. The solute content of brain in animals with acute renal failure is such that essentially all of the increase in brain osmolality is owing to an increase of brain urea concentration. However, in animals with chronic renal failure, about half of the increase in brain osmolality is owing to the presence of undetermined solute (idiogenic osmoles) with the other half owing to an increase of urea concentration (41,48).

In dogs with chronic renal failure, brain content of Na^+, K^+, Cl^- and water are not different from control values. Similarly, the extracellular space was not different from control (48). Calcium content was measured in eight parts of the brain in dogs who had chronic renal failure for 4 months. Calcium content was found to be normal in the subcortical white matter, pons, medulla, cerebellum, thalamus, and caudate nucleus. However, as shown in Fig. 93-2, calcium was about 60% above control values in both cortical gray matter and hypothalamus. Magnesium content was normal in all eight parts of the brain, as was water content (48). Other investigators also have found an elevated cerebral cortex calcium content in dogs with chronic renal failure (50). In animals who have acute renal failure and metabolic acidosis, the intracellular pH (pHi) of brain and skeletal muscle is normal (43) (Fig. 93-2). In dogs with chronic renal failure, intracellular pH is normal in brain, liver, and skeletal muscle (48). In patients with renal failure, intracellular pH has been reported to be normal in both skeletal muscle and leukocytes, as well as in the "whole body" (51–54) (Fig. 93-2). The pH of CSF

also has been shown to be normal in both patients and laboratory animals with renal failure (41,43,48). Thus, despite the presence of extracellular metabolic acidemia in patients or laboratory animals with either acute renal failure or chronic renal failure, the intracellular pH is normal in brain, white cells, liver, and skeletal muscle.

In general then, studies of brain tissue from both intact animal models of uremia and humans with renal failure have revealed many different biochemical abnormalities associated with the uremic state. However, such investigations have not yet revealed much about the fundamental mechanisms that might induce such abnormalities. Such studies probably will have to be done in isolated cell systems or subcellular systems from the brain. These systems have the advantage of permitting one to study isolated manifestations of the uremic state while removing the numerous potential confounding influences present in an *in vivo* model.

UREMIC NEUROTOXINS

Central Nervous System

Uremic neurotoxins would imply retention of solutes that have detrimental effects on nervous system function, whether peripheral nervous system (PNS) or CNS (55).

There are at least three different types of uremic solutes that can be characterized (56). These include: (a) small water-soluble compounds, such as urea and creatinine (57); (b) middle molecules; and (c) protein-bound compounds. Most of the small water-soluble compounds, such as urea and creatinine, are not particularly toxic and are easily removed with dialysis. Guanidine compounds have been postulated to be "uremic toxins" for many years (58), based on possible detrimental effects on the CNS.

This is based in part on the effects of guanidine compounds on mitochondrial function (59,60). Guanidino compounds were measured in 28 different regions in brain of uremic patients (61). Guanidinosuccinic acid was elevated by up to 100-fold in uremic brain versus control brain, and levels increased with increasing levels of uremia. The brain levels of guanidinosuccinic acid were similar to those observed in animal brain following injection to blood levels that cause convulsions (61). Guanidines inhibit neutrophil superoxide production, can induce seizures, and suppress natural killer cell response to interleukin-2 (62). Other guanidines, which are arginine analogs, are competitive inhibitors of nitric oxide (NO) synthetase, and can lead to vasoconstriction, hypertension, ischemic glomerular injury, immune dysfunction, and neurologic changes (62).

Middle molecules are large molecular weight compounds (300 to 12,000 daltons) that have been felt to be responsible for many of the manifestations of uremia. Despite the fact that at one time dialysis membranes were designed with the specific intent of removing more middle molecules, evidence of their toxicity generally is lacking (63–66). Recently, there has been a renewed interest in these molecules (64,67), but evidence of their toxicity is still conjectural (62). Advanced glycosylation end products (AGEs) can modify tissues, enzymes, and proteins and may play a role in the pathogenesis of dialysis-associated amyloidosis (56). Advanced glycosylation end products also may play a role in the pathogenesis of diabetic nephropathy (68). Advanced glycosylation end products are markedly elevated in plasma of patients with ESRD (69). The AGEs react with vascular cells to inactivate endothelial nitric oxide and may increase the propensity of patients with ESRD to develop hypertension. Current dialysis therapy is relatively ineffective in removal of AGEs, so that there is accumulation of AGEs in patients with ESRD, particularly those with diabetes mellitus (69). The AGEs are "middle molecules" and have the potential to cause tissue damage and lead to hypertension. Thus, at least some "middle molecules" actually may be deleterious in patients with ESRD, and they are poorly removed with conventional dialysis (69). Parathyroid hormone (PTH) is a high-molecular-weight compound and may be an important CNS uremic toxin (18,22,25,26). Protein-bound compounds (toxins) are not substantially removed by dialysis, and almost all are lipophilic. Such compounds include polyamines such as spermine. Spermine is postulated to be a uremic toxin and appears to react with the N-methyl-D-aspartate (NMDA) receptor, which affects calcium and sodium permeability in brain cells (70). Stimulation of the NMDA receptor in brain is the final common pathway for brain cell death in a number of pathologic pathways (71,72). The uremic state is associated with increased oxidative stress, resulting in protein oxidation products in plasma and cell membranes. There is eventual alteration of proteins with formation of oxidized amino acids, including glutamine and glutamate (56). Such reactions eventually may lead to stimulation of the NMDA receptor in brain, with brain cell damage or death (3). In recent reviews, there are no new candidates for uremic toxins that impair the CNS (73). The anemia of renal failure had been suggested as a contributor to uremic toxicity (74), but this has been largely eliminated by the widespread use of erythropoietin (9,11,75).

Peripheral Nervous System

There are a number of solutes that are purported to impair peripheral nerve function. Several possible uremic toxins have been identified that appear to be correlated with depression of MNCV in laboratory animals (58,76,77). However, these studies do not take into account the facts that: (a) depressed MNCV is cyclical, with abnormal low values one day and normal values the next (17); (b) there is a day-to-day variation in MNCV that approaches 20% (78); and (c) the finding of depressed MNCV in laboratory animals associated with high plasma levels of potential uremic neurotoxins generally has not been confirmed in human subjects with renal failure (65,79–81). Although it is possible to relate impairment in MNCV with levels in blood of various substances, the best correlation was obtained between reduced MNCV versus a reduction in glomerular filtration rate.

Among the potential peripheral nerve uremic neurotoxins is parathyroid hormone (PTH) based on a correlation between plasma PTH levels and MNCV in patients with chronic renal failure (79). Parathyroid hormone is of high molecular weight, and if neurotoxic, could thus qualify as a high molecular weight uremic toxin (82). Some earlier studies suggested a possible effect of PTH on MNCV in the dog (77) but these impressions have not been confirmed (48). In patients who have hyperparathyroidism without uremia, PTH has no observable effect on peripheral nerve function (83). In both patients and laboratory animals with acute renal failure, the MNCV has been found to be normal (18,84,85). In all studies of both patients and laboratory animals with chronic renal failure, the MNCV had not been shown to be affected by PTH (48). Thus, in both patients and laboratory animals with either acute or chronic renal failure, or primary or secondary hyperparathyroidism, no effect of PTH on nerve function can be demonstrated. In patients with chronic renal failure, there is no change in MNCV as a result of either recovery of renal function or chronic hemodialysis; there was also no effect of parathyroidectomy (84). In addition, when patients begin dialysis therapy, MNCV either stabilizes or improves (86). However, virtually all of these patients have elevated plasma PTH levels (87).

Animal studies suggest that in either acute or chronic renal failure, changes in MNCV take longer than 6 months to develop and are probably not related to an effect of PTH. Mahoney and associates studied dogs who had renal failure for periods of 3.5 days to 6 months (39). There was no change in the MNCV after any of the aforementioned intervals of renal failure, and the MNCV was normal even after 6 months with glomerular filtration rate below 22% of control.

SUBCELLULAR STUDIES

One system that appears to lend itself particularly well to studies of metabolic abnormalities in uremia is the synaptosome. When brain tissue is homogenized in isoosmotic media, the presynaptic nerve terminals are seared off and resealed to form intact membrane vesicles called synaptosomes. Like the intact nerve endings, synaptosomes contain mitochondria and synaptic vesicles and are metabolically active (88,89). The synaptosome can be studied as an intact system or hypotonically lysed into its constituents and ghost synaptic plasma membrane (90,91). Although the synaptic junction was first isolated at the turn of the 19th century and first described histologically by Cajal, (92,93), it was not until the late 1950s that the synaptosome was finally isolated (94,95). Isolation of synaptosomes subsequently proved to be an important step in understanding the response of the brain to numerous metabolic insults. Synaptosomes have been used in the investigation of neurotransmitter substances, ion transport, drug actions, and effects of nervous system toxins on numerous metabolic processes (47,90). Synaptosomes are that portion of the nerve cell where neurotransmitter substances are synthesized, stored, and released. Thus, any abnormalities present in the uremic state might be expected to affect synaptosomal function and information transfer in the CNS. There are at least two ways by which information transfer occurs between neurons in the CNS, and both of which may be abnormal in the uremic state. Communication between cells is either by chemical or electrical transmission at the synaptic junction. Because both of these methods of communication cross the synaptic space, the nerve cells are able to communicate quite rapidly with each other over great distances. Conduction via the axon and transmission at the synaptic junction make possible this rapid and precise communication. Transmission at most synapses is by chemical means, although some synapses operate purely by electrical conduction. The type of transmission utilized at the synapses appears to be dependent on the type of synaptic junction in question. Transmission through the gap junction is primarily electrical, whereas transmission through the unabridged, larger synaptic junction, is felt to be strictly a chemical phenomenon (96). Because of these intricate interrelationships at the synapses in the CNS, it is not surprising that dysfunction in information transfer at the synapses does occur in uremia (97).

Physiology of Neurotransmission

The neuron is the vehicle of communication and the center for the processing of information in the CNS. The neuron consists of three major portions: the axon, the dendrites, and the soma (cell body). Each neuron is contacted by hundreds of axons from other neurons that may either inhibit or excite the receptor area of the cell (98).

The synaptosome is usually about 0.6 to 1.2 μ in diameter. The two most important internal organelles in the synaptosomes are synaptic vesicles and mitochondria. The synaptic vesicles contain neurotransmitter substances that, when released into the synaptic space, either inhibit or excite the postsynaptic receptor area. Mitochondria provide the energy for the metabolic processes in the neuron. They are the source of ATP, which is required to synthesize transmitter substances

and maintain ionic equilibrium at the nerve terminals. When an action potential reaches the presynaptic terminal of a neuron, the plasma membrane depolarizes, causing a rapid influx of calcium into the terminal. The accumulated calcium serves to aggregate the synaptic vesicles to teach other and to the surface of contact with the opposing neuron. This facilitates the release of neurotransmitter substances from the synaptic vesicles into the synaptic space by exocytosis. The neurotransmitter substance acts on the postsynaptic terminal in such a way as to change the membrane permeability of the postsynaptic neuron. The affecter neuron is then either excited or inhibited, depending on the type or receptor present on the affected cell.

Del Castillo and Datz first suggested that a relationship existed between extracellular calcium concentration and quantal release of acetylcholine from the synaptic vesicles (99). They showed that calcium concentration did not affect the number of acetylcholine molecules packaged into each quantum but that calcium concentration did affect the number of acetylcholine molecule packaged into each quantum and that calcium concentration increased the probability that a given quantum of acetylcholine will be released. In subsequent work, Katz and Miledi (100–102) proposed that the influx of calcium into nerve terminals by action potential causes calcium to interact with synaptic vesicles to cause neurotransmitter release. After emptying their content into the synaptic space, the vesicles separate from the plasma membrane and are used repeatedly for storage and release of transmitter substances. After these vesicles and mitochondria are used repeatedly for synthesis, storage, and release of neurotransmitter substances, they eventually degenerate. Fortunately, new organelles are continually made in the cell soma and are transported to the nerve terminal where they serve to replace the degenerated organelles in the nerve terminals. This process provides a constant supply of the machinery required for information processing by the CNS.

Studies by Fraser, Sarnacki, and Arieff (90,91) in rat brain synaptosomes demonstrated abnormalities of both sodium and calcium transport and decreased Na-K-ATPase pump activity in the brains of rats with uremia (Figs. 93-3 and 93-4). They suggested that these findings may affect neurotransmitter release in the uremic state (90,91). This defect did not appear to be owing to the uremic environment at the time of study, because synaptosomes were washed several times and frozen before uptake studies were carried out. The defect observed in uremia appeared to be due to a physical alteration of the synaptosomal membrane in acute uremia. These workers also demonstrated alterations of calcium transport in uremic rat brain (103) (Fig. 93-4). Based on the relationship between extracellular calcium and the release of neurotransmitter substances in nerve terminals, they concluded that this defect may affect neurotransmitter release and information processing in the uremic state.

In subsequent studies, the increase in calcium transport in uremia appeared to be PTH dependent (90,103). When calcium transport by both the Na-Ca exchanger and the

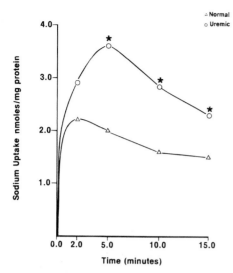

FIG. 93-3. The difference between the veratridine-stimulated Na+ uptake and the control uptake (without addition of neurotoxins) in both groups of synaptosomes is plotted in this graph. The top curve shows the veratridine-stimulated sodium uptake in uremic synaptosomes, whereas the uptake in normal synaptosomes is represented by the lower curve. The increased veratridine-stimulated sodium uptake in uremic rats is significantly less than in normal rats (*P < 0.001) at 5, 10, and 15 minutes. (From: Fraser CL, Sarnacki P, Arieff AI. Abnormal sodium transport in synaptosomes from brain of uremic rats. *J Clin Invest* 1985;75:2014, with permission.)

ATP-dependent calcium pump was carried out in brain of parathyroidectomized uremic rats, calcium accumulation into these vesicles returned to normal values. Additionally, parathyroidectomized uremic rats that were injected with parathyroid extract showed abnormalities of calcium transport similar to those described in uremia (104). These findings suggested that in uremic animals, PTH may be responsible for some of the alterations in synaptosomal calcium transport (103). It was also interesting to note that clinically, the

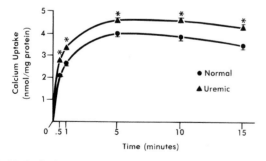

FIG. 93-4. Sodium–calcium exchange in normal versus uremic synaptosomes. The top curve shows calcium uptake in uremic synaptosomes. The lower curve shows uptake in normal synaptosomes. This graph is a mean of eight experiments, and each time point was done in triplicate. The result is expressed as mean +SE. The points indicated by the asterisks represent differences that are significant to P < 0.005. (From: Fraser CL, Sarnacki P, Arieff AI. Abnormal sodium transport in synaptosomes from brain of uremic rats. *J Clin Invest* 1985;76:1789, with permission.)

uremic parathyroidectomized rats tolerated uremia better than control uremic rats and uremic parathyroidectomized rats treated with PTH. Thus, there appear to be both clinical and physiologic changes in the uremic brain that may be PTH dependent.

Regulation of cytosolic Ca^{2+} by inositol triphosphate (1,4, 5-IP3) is owing primarily to release of Ca^{2+} from intracellular stores (105). It also was found that 1,4,5-IP3 may increase cytosolic Ca^{2+} by the transport of Ca^{2+} from the extracellular to the intracellular space, through other mechanisms (106,107). Injections of 1,4,5-IP3 into cells produce a rise in intracellular Ca^{2+}. This is owing to both an immediate Ca^{2+} release from intracellular pool and a more prolonged phase attributed to calcium influx from extracellular space (108–110). Injections of 1,4,5-IP3 into cells also was shown to increase permeability of plasma membrane vesicles to Ca^{2+} and to increase Ca^{2+} current through lymphocyte membranes (111).

More recently, Fraser and associates (90,112) evaluated the effects of acute uremia on sodium and calcium transport in uremic rat brain. They demonstrated decreased Na-K-ATPase pump activity in uremia (112). There appeared to be to a physical alteration of the synaptosomal membrane in uremic rat brain. These contentions were based on the observation that veratridine-stimulated sodium uptake was markedly greater in synaptosomes from uremic rats than from normal rats (112) (Fig. 93-3).

Fraser and associates also demonstrated alterations of calcium transport in uremic rat brain synaptosomes (90) (Fig. 93-4). The increase in calcium transport observed in uremia may be PTH dependent (104). When calcium transport was studied in synaptosomes from parathyroidectomized uremic rats, calcium accumulation into these vesicles returned to normal control values. Additionally, parathyroidectomized uremic rats that were injected with intact bovine parathyroid extract showed abnormalities of calcium transport similar to those previously described in uremia (104). Thus, in the presence of a uremic environment, PTH may be responsible for the alterations in calcium transport observed in uremic brain (104).

As mentioned, when a neuron in the CNS is stimulated, an action potential is generated which results in a change in the membrane permeability to calcium of the synaptic nerve terminal. This results in calcium influx from the extracellular space to the cytosol of the nerve terminal (113). The mechanisms by which calcium enters cells include sodium channels, calcium channels, and the Na-Ca exchanger (114). As opposed to nonexcitable cells where the Na-Ca exchanger participates only in calcium efflux (114), in excitable cells such as neurons and myocardium the exchanger participates in both calcium influx and efflux (115,116). In order to maintain calcium balance, calcium that enters the cell from the extracellular space has to be pumped out, and this is achieved by the Na-Ca exchanger and the Ca-ATPase pump. These two mechanisms comprise the primary exporter of calcium from either excitable or nonexcitable tissues (115,117,118). The overall effect of these transporters is to maintain a calcium gradient of 10,000:1 (outside-inside cells) and in the study state they maintain a net calcium flux across the plasma membrane of zero. The Na^+-Ca^{2+} exchanger which operates electrically (exchanging three Na^+ for one Ca^{2+}) is a high-capacity, low-affinity system, whereas the Ca^{2+}-ATPase is a low-capacity, high-affinity system that continuously pumps calcium out of cells. Thus, in cellular regulation of calcium, the Ca^{2+}-ATPase pump modulates subtle changes in cytosolic calcium, whereas the Na^+-Ca^{2+} exchanger is important in regulating major changes in calcium flux (119).

Prior investigations established the importance of both the Na^+-Ca^{2+} exchanger and the Ca^{2+}-ATPase pump in regulating calcium movement across neuronal membranes, and led to the suggestion that PTH-mediated calcium uptake in uremia was independent of cAMP (103). These led to investigations as to whether inositol phosphates were possible intracellular messengers for PTH action in brain (120). The regulation of cytosolic Ca^{2+} by inositol 1,4,5-IP3 is known to be primarily owing to the release of Ca^{2+} from intracellular stores (105,121). However, recent evidence indicates that 1,4,5-IP3 may also increase cytosolic Ca^{2+} by mobilizing Ca^{2+} from the extracellular to the intracellular space (107).

To determine whether 1,4,5-IP3 may regulate cell cytosolic Ca^{2+} by acting on the plasma membrane-bound Na^+-Ca^{2+} exchanger, Fraser and associates investigated Ca^{2+} transport by this method (120). In the presence of either an inhibitor of voltage-gated Na^+ channels (tetrodotoxin) or the K^+ ionophore (valinomycin), Ca^{2+} uptake was significantly inhibited by 1,4,5-IP3 in a concentration-dependent manner. Similarly, Ca^{2+} efflux from synaptosomes by the exchanger was also significantly inhibited by 1,4,5-IP3. The inhibitory effect of 1,4,5-IP3 on the Na^+-Ca^{2+} exchanger was observed in the presence of Ca^{2+} channel blockers, and in vesicles pretreated with caffeine to deplete the 1,4,5-IP3-sensitive stores of Ca^{2+}. Taken together, these results suggest that during signal transduction in brain, 1,4,5-IP3 may increase cytosolic (Ca^{2+}) in part by inhibiting the Na^+-Ca^{2+} exchanger and thus, Ca^{2+} efflux from cell (120).

Although calcium transport in synaptosomes in uremia appears to be influenced by PTH, not all transport processes are affected in this manner. Verkman and Fraser evaluated water and urea transport in synaptosomes by stopped-flow light scattering technique and found no differences in either water or urea permeabilities in normal rats compared to those with uremia, or uremic animals subjected to parathyroidectomy (47). From these studies they were also able to show that synaptosomal water and urea transport occurred by a lipid diffusive pathway and was not affected by uremia (47).

CENTRAL NERVOUS SYSTEM PATHOLOGY WITH UREMIA

Pathologic studies of brain have been reported in over 400 patients dying with chronic renal failure (51,122). It has been shown that there is some necrosis of the granular layer of the cerebral cortex. Small intracerebral hemorrhages and necrotic foci are seen in about 10% of uremic patients and focal glial proliferation is seen in about 2%. In general, changes in the brain of patients who died with chronic renal failure are probably nonspecific and related more to any of a number of concomitant underlying disease states (123). Subdural hemorrhage, once a common finding in autopsied uremic patients, is now quite unusual (23). Cerebral edema has not been observed in the brains of humans and laboratory animals with either acute or chronic renal failure (18,25,124).

The recent use of advanced neuroimaging techniques has led to substantial in vivo study of uremic brain in humans (125). Acute and subacute movement disorders have been observed in patients with ESRD (126). These have been associated with bilateral basal ganglia and internal capsule lesions (126,127). Cerebral atrophy has been observed in chronic hemodialysis patients (128), and it tends to worsen as dialysis therapy continues (129,130). Cerebral atrophy had previously been thought to be associated with dialysis dementia, but this is apparently not the case (131). End-stage renal disease has also been reported to lead to deterioration of vision (132). Some cases are associated with uremic pseudotumor cerebri, and in these elected cases, surgical optic nerve fenestration may improve visual loss (133).

Pathophysiology

Although many factors contribute to uremic encephalopathy, most investigators have shown no correlation between encephalopathy and any of the commonly measured indicators of renal failure. In recent years, there has been considerable discussion of the possible role of PTH as a uremic toxin. There is a substantial amount of evidence to suggest that PTH may exert an adverse effect on the CNS (18,22,25,48).

Role of Parathyroid Hormone

In patients dying with acute or chronic renal failure, the calcium content in brain cerebral cortex is significantly elevated (18,22,25) (Fig. 93-5). Dogs with acute or chronic renal failure show increases of brain gray matter calcium and EEG changes similar to those seen in humans with acute renal failure (39,42,48). In dogs, both the EEG and brain calcium abnormalities can be prevented by parathyroidectomy. Conversely, these abnormalities can be reproduced by administration of PTH to normal animals while maintaining serum calcium and phosphate in the normal range. Thus, PTH is essential to produce some of the CNS manifestations in the canine model of uremia (22,50).

Parathyroid hormone is known to have CNS effects in humans even in the absence of impaired renal function. Neuropsychiatric symptoms are reported to be among the most common manifestations of primary hyperparathyroidism (134–139). Patients with primary hyperparathyroidism also have EEG changes similar to those observed in patients with acute renal failure (18,140). The common denominator appears to be elevated plasma levels of PTH (18,22,25,42). In

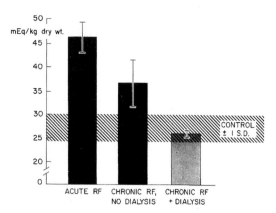

FIG. 93-5. The brain (cerebral cortex) content of calcium (Ca^{2+}) in patients who had acute renal failure, those with chronic renal failure treated with dialysis, or patients with end-stage chronic renal failure treated for at least 2 years with hemodialysis. Brain Ca^{2+} content is significantly greater than control values in patients who had acute renal failure ($P < 0.001$) or chronic renal failure not treated with dialysis ($P < 0.03$). However, in patients treated with dialysis, brain Ca^{2+} content is normal. Data are mean +SE. *RF,* renal failure. (From: Arieff AI. Neurological complications of uremia. In: Brenner BM, Rector FC Jr, eds. *The kidney.* Philadelphia: WB Saunders, 1986, with permission.)

patients with acute renal failure the EEG is abnormal within 18 hours of the onset of renal failure and is generally not affected by dialysis for periods of up to 8 weeks (18). In patients with either primary or secondary hyperparathyroidism, parathyroidectomy results in an improvement of both EEG and psychological testing, suggesting a direct effect of PTH on the CNS. Similarly, dialysis results in a decrement of brain (cerebral cortex) calcium toward normal in both patients and laboratory animals with renal failure concomitant with improvement of the EEG (18,22,25,42). In uremic patients, both EEG changes and psychological abnormalities are improved by parathyroidectomy or medical suppression of PTH (25). Parathyroid hormone, a high brain calcium content, or both are probably responsible, at least in part, for many of the encephalopathic manifestations of renal failure.

The mechanisms by which PTH might impair CNS function are only partially understood. The increased calcium content in such diverse tissues as skin, cornea, blood vessels, brain, and heart in patients with hyperparathyroidism suggests that PTH may somehow facilitate the entry of Ca^{2+} into such tissues. The finding of increased calcium in the brains of both dogs and humans with either acute or chronic renal disease and secondary hyperparathyroidism is consistent with the concept that part of the CNS dysfunction and EEG abnormalities found in acute renal failure or chronic renal failure may be owing in part to a PTH-mediated increase in brain calcium (Fig. 93-5). Calcium is essential for the function of neurotransmission in the CNS and for a large number of intracellular enzyme systems. Thus, an increased brain calcium content could disrupt cerebral function by interfering with either of these processes (32,141). It is also possible that PTH itself may have a detrimental effect on the CNS.

NEUROLOGIC COMPLICATIONS OF END-STAGE RENAL DISEASE AND ITS THERAPY

Dialysis Disequilibrium Syndrome

In patients with ESRD, there are several CNS disorders that may occur as a consequence of dialytic therapy. Dialysis disequilibrium syndrome is a clinical condition that occurs in patients being treated with hemodialysis. The syndrome was first described in 1962 (142) and may include symptoms such as headache, nausea, emesis, blurring of vision, muscular twitching, disorientation, hypertension, tremors, and seizures (143,144). The syndrome of DDS has been expanded to include milder symptoms, such as muscle cramps, anorexia, restlessness, and dizziness (144–147). Although DDS has been reported among all age groups, it is more common among younger patients, particularly the pediatric age group (148). The syndrome most often is associated with rapid hemodialysis of patients with acute renal failure, but it also has occasionally been reported following maintenance hemodialysis of patients with chronic renal failure (149–152). The pathogenesis of DDS has been extensively investigated and the findings are summarized elsewhere (41,144,153,154). The symptoms are usually self-limited but recovery may take several days. It appears that present methods of dialysis have altered the clinical picture of DDS. Most reports of seizures, coma, and death were reported prior to 1970. The symptoms of DDS as reported in the last 25 years (1975 to 2000) generally have been mild, consisting of nausea, weakness, headache, fatigue, and muscle cramps. Almost all cases have occurred in patients undergoing their initial four hemodialyses. It is also unclear whether any patient ever actually died from DDS or in fact from other neurologic complications associated with dialysis, such as acute stroke, subdural hematoma, subarachnoid hemorrhage, or hyponatremia (144). A differential diagnosis of patients presenting with these symptoms are shown in Table 93-1. Recently, the diagnosis of DDS has become a "wastebasket" for a number of disorders that can occur in

TABLE 93-1. *Differential diagnosis of dialysis dysequilibrium syndrome*

Copper intoxication
Subdural hematoma
Uremia, per se
Nonketotic hyperosmolar coma with hyperglycemia
Cerebral embolus secondary to shunt clotting
Acute cerebrovascular accident
Dialysis dementia
Cardiac arrhythmia
Depletion syndrome
Malfunction of fluid-proportioning system
Excessive ultrafiltration
Hypoglycemia
Wernicke's encephalopathy
Hyperparathyroidism with hypercalcemia
  (serum Ca > 14 mg/dl)
Malignant hypertension
Hyponatremia (serum Na$^+$ < 125 mEq/liter)
Nickel intoxication

patients with renal failure and may affect the CNS (144). It is important to recognize that the diagnosis of DDS should be one of exclusion.

Dialysis disequilibrium syndrome has been treated either by addition of osmotically active solute (glucose, glycerol, albumin, urea, fructose, NaCl, mannitol) to the dialysate, or by intravenous infusion of mannitol or glycerol. With the technique of *pure ultrafiltration* the patient is subjected to ultrafiltration without dialysis. The net result is loss of fluid without the patient undergoing dialysis. The role of ultrafiltration followed by dialysis in prevention of DDS is currently being evaluated (155,156). Additionally, DDS can be prevented by decreasing the time on dialysis and increasing the frequency of dialysis at the initiation of hemodialysis in patients. Mannitol infusion accompanying the initial three hemodialyses has been successful in prevention of DDS (146). Administration of 50 mL of 50% mannitol both at the initiation of dialysis and after 2 hours of dialysis generally has been successful in preventing symptoms of DDS. The same effects can be obtained by addition of glycerol to the dialysate, but technical considerations render this option less popular (147,157).

Chronic peritoneal dialysis is currently in use worldwide. Different types of peritoneal dialysis are carried out either in-center, at home, or combinations of ambulatory plus home. Patients undergo continuous low-volume peritoneal dialysis for as long as 24 hours per day (158) (159). Symptoms of dialysis disequilibrium syndrome presently have not been reported in patients utilizing this mode of dialysis.

Dialysis Dementia

Dialysis dementia (also called dialysis encephalopathy) is a progressive, frequently fatal neurologic disease that was initially described in several reports from 1970 to 1973 (160–162). Existence of the syndrome was then independently confirmed worldwide by several different groups in the early to mid-1970s (131,163–173). In adults, the disease is seen almost exclusively in patients being treated with chronic hemodialysis. The early literature focused on the distinctive neurologic findings (123,161,162,164–166). However, more recent reports from both Europe and the United States suggest that some forms of dialysis dementia may be a part of a multisystem disease, which may include encephalopathy, osteomalacic bone disease, proximal myopathy, and anemia (20,123,174–176).

The etiology of this syndrome remains controversial (177). Although an increase in brain aluminum content has been strongly implicated in some cases of dialysis dementia, the evidence is far less convincing in others. At this stage of our knowledge it seems useful to subdivide dialysis dementia into three categories (Table 93-2): (a) an epidemic form related to contamination of the dialysate, often with aluminum; (b) sporadic cases in which aluminum intoxication is less likely to be a contributory factor; and (c) dementia associated with congenital or early childhood renal disease. This entity has

TABLE 93-2. *Subgroups of dialysis dementia*

Sporadic endemic
  No clear relation to aluminum
  Worldwide distribution
  No known therapy
Epidemic
  Geographic clusters
  Often related to aluminum in dialysis water
  Epidemic usually stops with treatment of water supply
  Probably often related to other trace elements in water
    such as Sn, Mn, Co, Mg, Fe
Childhood
  May be owing to a nonspecific effect of uremia on
    immature brain
  No clear association with aluminum

been reported in several children who were never dialyzed or exposed to aluminum compounds. These early childhood cases may represent developmental neurologic defects resulting from exposure of the growing brain to a uremic environment (37).

The initial reports of dialysis dementia in the 1970s were soon followed by reports throughout the world (178). These patients all had the endemic form and usually had been on chronic hemodialysis for over 2 years before the onset of symptoms. Early manifestations consisted of a mixed dysarthria-apraxia of speech with slurring, stuttering, and hesitancy. Personality changes, including psychoses, led to dementia, myoclonus, and seizures. Symptoms initially were intermittent and were often worse during dialysis, but generally became constant. In most cases, the disease progressed to death within 6 months. Speech disturbances were found in 90% of patients, affective disorders culminating in dementia in 80%, motor disturbances in 75%, and convulsions in 60% to 90%. In contrast to this fairly distinct clinical picture, brain histology generally has been normal or nonspecific.

Early in the disease, the EEG shows multifocal bursts of high amplitude delta activity with spikes and sharp waves, intermixed with runs of more normal appearing background activity. These EEG abnormalities may precede overt clinical symptoms by 6 months. As the disease progresses, the normal background activity also deteriorates to slow frequencies (148). The EEG has been said to be pathognomic, but a similar pattern also may be seen in other metabolic encephalopathies. The diagnosis depends on the presence of the typical clinical picture and is confirmed by the characteristic EEG pattern (166). Magnetoencephalography (MEG) only recently has been used in the evaluation of uremic patients (179). Magnetoencephalography has not yet been used in the evaluation of patients with dialysis dementia.

Aluminum intoxication was first implicated in this disorder by Alfrey and associates (169). Aluminum content of brain gray matter was elevated to eleven times the normal value in patients with dialysis dementia, versus an increase of three times normal in patients on chronic hemodialysis without dialysis dementia. Aluminum content was also increased in bone and other soft tissue. Oral phosphate binders containing aluminum [Al(OH)$_3$ and Al$_2$(CO$_3$)$_2$] were originally suspected as the source of the aluminum.

Most of the aluminum in blood is bound to transferrin, so that there is very little free aluminum in the blood (180). The brain contains few transferrin receptors, so that normally, aluminum uptake into brain is negligible. Any free aluminum in blood, usually in the form of aluminum-citrate, can readily enter the CNS. Normally, there is an excess of gallium-binding sites in plasma, so that even in situations where blood aluminum is increased, there is still almost no free aluminum in blood. Aluminum binding can be studied with the aluminum analog gallium (181). In studies of gallium-transferrin binding in blood of patients having either Alzheimer's disease, Down's syndrome, or renal failure treated with chronic hemodialysis, gallium binding to transferrin was significantly reduced in patients with either Down's syndrome or Alzheimer's disease (180). However, gallium binding to transferrin was normal in patients with chronic renal failure treated with hemodialysis. In such patients, there was accumulation of aluminum in those brain regions with high densities of transferrin receptors (102).

The aforementioned findings involve studies in only nine patients with dialysis dementia (180,182) and five with chronic renal failure treated with hemodialysis. More such studies are needed before it can be conclusively stated that the distribution of aluminum in brain of patients with dialysis dementia is not similar to that in patients with Alzheimer's disease. Neurofibrillary changes are not present in patients with chronic renal failure without dialysis dementia (102,103).

Recent studies have further added to our knowledge of the possible effects of aluminum on the CNS in patients with chronic renal failure. A possible pathophysiologic basis for detrimental effects of aluminum on the CNS has been described by Altmann and associates (183). Dihydropteridine reductase is an important enzyme in the synthesis of several important neurotransmitters, such as tyrosine and acetylcholine. They found that erythrocyte levels of dihydropteridine reductase activity were less than predicted values, and correlated with plasma aluminum levels (183). Red cell dihydropteridine reductase activity levels doubled after treatment with desferrioxamine. Although brain levels of dihydropteridine reductase activity were not evaluated, it was suggested that high brain aluminum levels might lead to decreased availability of dihydropteridine reductase in the brain. It has been suggested that the mere presence of an increased body aluminum burden has an adverse effect on overall mortality (184). More specifically, an increased body aluminum burden (estimated by the desferrioxamine infusion test) has been associated with memory impairment and increased severity of myoclonus with decreased motor strength (185).

Altmann and associates evaluated patients with chronic renal failure and apparently normal cerebral function (183,186). They found that when compared to a control group with similar IQ, the patients with chronic renal failure had abnormalities in six tests of psychomotor function. Plasma aluminum levels were only mildly elevated (59 ± 9 μm/L). Anemia improved and the erythrocyte activity of dihydropteridine reductase rose significantly when 15 of these patients were treated for 3 months with desferrioxamine. Changes in erythrocyte dihydropteridine reductase activity correlated significantly with changes in psychomotor performance (183,186). Even at high blood Al levels, most Al is bound to transferrin (180) and thus cannot bind to the cerebral transferrin receptors. It may be that patients who develop dialysis dementia have less transferrin binding capacity, less transferrin, or a greater density of transferrin receptors in the brain. These issues have not been studied to date.

Thus, aluminum may be toxic in patients with chronic renal failure, possibly leading to both dialysis dementia and osteomalacia (167,168,174–176). Most nephrologists would agree that the potential hazards of poor control of plasma phosphate are worse than the potential toxicity of aluminum accumulation from oral aluminum-containing antacids. However, recent studies suggest that calcium carbonate (or acetate) may be more effective for the control of hyperphosphatemia than is aluminum hydroxide (187–189). More recently, sevelamer (Renagel), a polymeric phosphate binder, has come into wide usage for control of phosphate in chronic dialysis patients (190). Sevelamer has been found to be more effective than calcium carbonate, calcium acetate, or aluminum hydroxide for the treatment of hyperphosphatemia in dialysis patients (190,191), and it does not introduce aluminum into the body.

Nevertheless, aluminum is still the second most prevalent element in the earth's crust, and a substantial quantity will enter the body, even without administration of aluminum-containing antacids (192–194).

Deionization of the water used to prepare dialysate recently has been employed as a preventive measure (195), although deionization may be beneficial by removing any number of other agents. Other trace elements may be present in water that can result in CNS toxicity. Such elements include cadmium, mercury, lead, manganese, copper, nickel, thallium, boron, and tin (Fig. 93-5A). Among these potentially neurotoxic elements no one has measured brain content of cadmium, mercury, nickel, thallium, vanadium, or boron. Manganese has been found to be increased in cortical white matter in the eight encephalopathic patients in whom it was measured (173). These patients also had elevated aluminum levels in gray matter.

Most of the controversy over the etiology of dialysis dementia has involved those cases that occur sporadically. As noted, dialysate aluminum levels are not always elevated. The use of aluminum-containing antacids is no different in patients with dialysis dementia than in unaffected patients, and brain aluminum levels in patients with dialysis dementia may overlap with those of unaffected patients (177). The largest group of "sporadic cases" has been reported from

Nashville, Tennessee (174). The reported incidence of dialysis dementia in the area is 5%, despite the use of deionized water for dialysate with aluminum levels below 5 μg/L. Osteomalacic bone disease was not clinically apparent in this group. Serum aluminum levels in the encephalopathic group were three to four times higher than other dialyzed patients, despite equivalent prescribed doses of aluminum-containing phosphate binders. These results suggest greater absorption and/or retention of aluminum or other trace metal contamination in this group of encephalopathic patients. No other metals were measured in the Nashville study.

The evidence available thus far indicates that aluminum is elevated in the brain (cortical gray matter) of patients with dialysis dementia; however, the actual contribution of aluminum to the encephalopathy remains unclear. Aluminum content has been reported to be elevated in the brain of patients with other disorders, including senile dementia and Alzheimer's syndrome, and might actually be a nonspecific finding associated with dementia. Aluminum also is elevated in the brains of patients who have other disorders associated with altered blood-brain barrier. Such disorders include renal failure, hepatic encephalopathy, and metastatic cancer (Fig. 93-5B). Other evidence suggests that brain aluminum content may also increase as a function of the aging process. Thus, blood-brain barrier abnormalities can result in increased brain aluminum content (196).

Despite these unresolved questions, most outbreaks of the epidemic form of dialysis dementia have been associated with high levels of aluminum in the dialysate (167,197,198). Lowering the dialysate aluminum to below 20 μg/L, usually by deionization, appears to prevent the onset of the disease in patients who are beginning dialysis. New cases may continue to appear in those patients who were previously exposed to the high aluminum dialysate, although the course is milder and mortality is somewhat decreased. Eliminating the source of aluminum has resulted in improvement in some but not all patients with overt disease. Renal transplantation has generally not been helpful in patients with established dialysis dementia. Diazepam or clonazepam are useful in controlling seizure activity associated with the disease, but become ineffective later on and do not alter the final outcome (165).

Treatment of sporadic cases, in which the etiology is not clear, is more difficult. Every effort should be made to identify a treatable cause. Dialysis dementia must be differentiated from other metabolic encephalopathies, such as hypercalcemia and hypophosphatemia, hyperparathyroidism, acute heavy metal intoxications, and structural neurologic lesions, such as subdural hematoma (199) (Table 93-3). Because of the low incidence, the uncertain etiology, and the poor correlation of plasma with tissue aluminum levels, screening tests generally have not been employed.

The source of excess Al^{3+} in brain is not entirely clear. Some Al^{3+} apparently is absorbed after oral administration of aluminum-containing antacids (37,141). Significant absorption of oral aluminum can occur in patients with chronic

TABLE 93-3. *Differential diagnosis of dialysis dementia*

Metabolic encephalopathies
  Hypercalcemia
  Hypophosphatemia
  Hypoglycemia
  Hyperosmolarity
  Hyponatremia
  Overt uremia
  Drug intoxications
  Trace element intoxications: manganese, mercury,
    lead, nickel, thallium, boron, vanadium, chromium,
    tin, cadmium
  Hyperparathyroidism
Hypertensive encephalopathy
Dialysis dysequilibrium
Structural lesions
  Subdural hematoma
  Normal pressure hydrocephalus
  Stroke

renal failure but the weight of evidence is against oral aluminum as the major source. The retention of Al^{3+} after oral administration of Al^{3+} salts is greater in patients with renal failure than in normal subjects (200,201). The typical daily dietary Al^{3+} intake is 10 to 100 mg (194), although absorption is normally minimal. This quantity of dietary Al^{3+} is more than enough to account for the entire increase of brain Al^{3+} observed in patients with dialysis dementia. Among 22 such patients, the mean brain Al^{3+} content (116) was 22 mg/kg dry weight. The normal human brain weighs about 1,500 gm and is about 80% water, or 300 gm dry weight. Thus, the total increase in Al^{3+} content for the whole brain is less than 7 mg in patients with dialysis dementia. Therefore, the entire increase of brain Al^{3+} in such patients can theoretically be accounted for by dietary aluminum. The increase in body aluminum stores may also be, in part, the result of Al^{3+} contamination from other sources, such as Al^{3+} in dialysate water, dialysis system aluminum pipes, or aluminum leaked from anodes (113,115).

There are a large number of children who have renal insufficiency and also require hospitalization with intravenous therapy. Such children may receive large quantities of intravenous aluminum (Al^{3+}) from contamination of intravenous solutions with aluminum salts (202–207). Thus, even in the absence of hemodialysis therapy, children with chronic renal failure may receive large quantities of intravenous aluminum, which may explain the development of dialysis dementia even in the absence of dialysis (207). The location of the aluminum in brain of patients with dialysis dementia has not been well established. In Alzheimer's disease, it initially appeared that the aluminum was localized only to the nuclear regions of neurofibrillary tangles (208). More recent investigations reveal that aluminum accumulates in at least four different sites in Alzheimer's disease: DNA-containing structures of the nucleus; protein moieties of neurofibrillary tangles; amyloid cores of senile plaques; and cerebral ferritin (209—211).

Senile plaques and neurofibrillary tangles of course are diagnostic features of Alzheimer's disease (212). It is not generally appreciated that the brain also contains senile plaques and neurofibrillary tangles in the majority of cases of dialysis dementia (182); however, in dialysis dementia, aluminum was not located in the neurons but rather in glial cells and the walls of blood vessels (195). The aforementioned findings involve studies in small numbers of patients (chronic renal failure treated with hemodialysis = 5; dialysis dementia = 9) (189,182). More such studies are needed before it can be stated conclusively that the distribution of aluminum in brain of patients with dialysis dementia is not similar to that in patients with Alzheimer's disease.

Deionization of the water used to prepare dialysate recently has been employed as a preventive measure (195). However, deionization may be beneficial by removing any number of other agents. Other trace elements may be present in water that can result in CNS toxicity. Such elements include cadmium, mercury, lead, manganese, copper, nickel, thallium, boron, and tin (Fig. 93-5A). Among these potentially neurotoxic elements no one has measured brain content of cadmium, mercury, nickel, thallium, vanadium, or boron. Manganese was found to be increased in cortical white matter in the eight encephalopathic patients in whom it was measured (173). These patients also had elevated aluminum levels in gray matter.

Treatment of sporadic cases in which the etiology is not clear is more difficult. Every effort should be made to identify a treatable cause. Dialysis dementia must be differentiated from other metabolic encephalopathies, such as hypercalcemia and hypophosphatemia, hyperparathyroidism, acute heavy metal intoxications, and structural neurologic lesions, such as subdural hematoma (199) (Table 93-3). Screening tests generally have not been employed because of the low incidence, uncertain etiology, and poor correlation of plasma with tissue aluminum levels.

The source of the increased Al^{3+} in brain of patients with dialysis encephalopathy theoretically can be accounted for on the basis of increased Al^{3+} intake. However, it is unclear as to how the Al^{3+} enters brain in increased quantities. It may be that the increased body aluminum burdens present in uremic subjects may contribute to increased Al^{3+} content in brain of such individual. To clarify the role of oral ingestion of aluminum salts in the causation of increased brain Al^{3+} content, it would be instructive to examine brain tissue from patients without renal failure who had ingested large quantities of Al(OH)3 (e.g., patients with chronic peptic ulcer disease). However, because such material is not likely to be available, studies in laboratory animals given large quantities of aluminum salts should provide similar information. In both rats and dogs receiving oral aluminum salts, there is a significant increment in brain Al^{3+} content (172,213,214). Administration of parathyroid hormone to rats receiving aluminum salts results in an additional increment of brain Al^{3+} content (200,214,215). Thus, in laboratory animals, both a chronic increase in oral Al^{3+} ingestion, or

parathyroid hormone excess, can lead to an increase of cerebral cortex Al^{3+}, even in the absence of renal failure.

Alternative Etiologies

Many other possible causes of dialysis dementia have been proposed. These include other trace element contaminants, (162,177,214) normal pressure hydrocephalus (177), slow virus infection of the CNS (63), and regional alterations in cerebral blood flow (214a). Some patients with dialysis dementia may have altered cerebrospinal fluid dynamics, which are at least suggestive of normal pressure hydrocephalus (216). Six patients with dialysis dementia were found to have normal cerebrospinal fluid dynamics, but only mild dilatation of the cerebral ventricles (216). In this study, however, control subjects (uremic patients treated with hemodialysis but not having dialysis dementia) were not evaluated, and results of recent studies suggest that many patients who have end-stage renal disease without dialysis encephalopathy also may have ventricular dilatation with cerebral atrophy (129). Furthermore, there is a generally poor correlation between ventricular dilatation, cerebral atrophy, and the presence of dementia (217).

Slow virus infection of the nervous system is a possible etiology for dialysis dementia. The clinical manifestations resemble those of other slow virus infections, such as Kuru or Creutzfeldt-Jakob disease (218,219). In at least once instance, a slow virus (foamy virus) has been isolated from the brain of patients who died with dialysis encephalopathy (218).

In summary, dialysis dementia probably represents an endpoint in a disease of multiple etiology. There are at least three subgroups and in two of them the etiology of dialysis encephalopathy must be regarded as unknown. The possible role of aluminum or other trace element abnormalities is unclear. At this time, there is no known satisfactory treatment for patients with dialysis encephalopathy. Most patients reported in the literature thus far have not survived, usually dying within 18 months of diagnosis. The syndrome is not alleviated by increased frequency of dialysis, and usually not by renal transplantation (123,220). Definitive therapy must await a better understanding of the pathogenesis of this disorder. The use of deferoxamine to chelate aluminum or other trace elements is experimental and currently under extensive investigation. There have been several reports of improvement in patients with dialysis dementia treated with deferoxamine (216).

OTHER CENTRAL NERVOUS SYSTEM COMPLICATIONS OF DIALYSIS

In addition to dialysis dementia and dialysis disequilibrium syndrome, there are several other neurologic disorders that have been reported in patients being treated with dialysis. In most instances, patients have initially presented with headache, nausea, emesis, or hypotension, whereas some have had seizures. Most such patients have initially been diagnosed as having DDS, whereas others, particularly those with chronic subdural hematoma, have been suspected of having dialysis dementia. The disorders include: copper intoxications, subdural hematoma, muscle cramps, nonketotic hyperosmolar coma with hyperglycemia, cerebral embolus secondary to shunt declotting, acute cerebrovascular accident, depletion syndrome, malfunction of fluid proportioning system, excessive ultrafiltration with hypotension and seizures, hypoglycemia, and Wernicke's encephalopathy (34,48). Subdural hematoma is not an infrequent cause of death in patients maintained with chronic hemodialysis (23,221). This condition initially may present with headache, drowsiness, nausea, and vomiting. If the patient loses consciousness or develops signs of increased intracranial pressure, a diagnosis of subarachnoid bleeding should be considered. Such episodes in uremic patients are usually fatal unless operated on. If the preceding symptoms persist between hemodialysis, or progressively worsen, subdural hematoma is likely, particularly if the patient is taking anticoagulants. On physical examination, there is often evidence of localized neurologic disease; there may be signs of meningeal irritation, and somnolence and focal seizures may be observed. The diagnosis usually can be made by modern neuroimaging techniques such as computed axial tomography (CAT scan) or magnetic resonance imaging (MRI) (125,222). Subarachnoid bleeding in hemodialysis patients is probably often related to anticoagulant excess (223). The initial symptom when intracranial hemorrhage occurs is usually depression of sensorium: convulsions may follow, and the patients may lapse into coma.

Improper proportioning of dialysate, owing to either human or mechanical error, is still an important cause of neurologic abnormality in dialysis patients (224). The usual effect of such dialysate abnormalities is the production of either hyponatremia or hypernatremia. Both of these abnormalities of body fluid osmolality can lead to seizures and coma, although different mechanisms are involved. In acute hypernatremia, there will be excessive thirst, lethargy, irritability, seizures, and coma, with spasticity and muscle rigidity. In acute hyponatremia there is weakness, fatigue, and dulled sensorium, which may also progress to seizures and coma, respiratory arrest, and death. Such symptoms developing soon after initiation of hemodialysis should alert the physician to the possibility of such an error. A check of the dialysate osmolality or sodium concentration is the most rapid means of detecting this problem. Death has been reported as a consequence of either hypernatremia or hyponatremia (225,226).

About one liter of fluid per hour can be removed by ultrafiltration hemodialysis, and about 300 mL/hour by peritoneal dialysis using hypertonic dialysate. Such a rate of fluid removal from the intravascular space may be faster than the rate at which fluid can be replaced from the interstitial compartment, and hypotension may develop. Symptoms of hypotension may include seizures that, although actually owing to cerebrovascular insufficiency, may be mistaken for DDS, particularly in diabetic subjects.

Most of the neurologic complications of renal transplantation relate to secondary afflictions, such as infection and neoplasia (23). As already discussed, most of the neurologic complications of the uremic state tend to improve following renal transplantation. These include the neuropathy, encephalopathy, and EEG changes (23,227,228).

STROKE IN PATIENTS TREATED WITH CHRONIC HEMODIALYSIS

Cerebrovascular disease is a common cause of death in chronic hemodialysis patients (229), and stroke represents the second most frequent cause of death (229,230) (the three most frequent are heart attack, stroke, and infection) (27,231). In the United States and western Europe (including Israel), cardiovascular disease is far more common in dialysis patients than the rest of the population (2,232). Part of the reason may be that the major cause of end-stage renal disease in the United States is diabetes mellitus (27%), far more than in Europe (19%) and Japan (10%) (233,234). Among the factors that undoubtedly contribute to the high incidence of stroke in patients with ESRD treated with hemodialysis are the high incidence of hypertension, the large number of such patients who have diabetes mellitus, and the accelerated arteriosclerosis in such patients (23,235). In addition, uremic patients tend to have high cholesterol levels and a high incidence of obesity, and they tend to smoke cigarettes (236,237). There is a high incidence of chronic infection in dialysis patients, which leads to elevated blood levels of atherogenic risk factors, such as cytokines, which appear to contribute to the increased incidence of stroke in such patients (238,239). The elevated cytokines are largely owing to the high incidence of chronic inflammatory conditions in chronic hemodialysis patients (239).

There is substantial recent evidence that chronic inflammation plays a role in the pathogenesis of cardiovascular disease (240). Cytokines released from involved tissues stimulate the liver to synthesize acute phase proteins, including C-reactive protein (CRP). Elevated levels of CRP and other cytokines constitute an independent risk factor for cardiovascular disease (241). Advanced glycosylation end products (AGEs) can modify tissues, enzymes, and proteins and may play a role in the pathogenesis of dialysis-associated amyloidosis (56,242). Advanced glycosylation end products are markedly elevated in plasma of patients with ESRD (69), particularly if they also have diabetes mellitus (68,234). These AGEs react with vascular cells to inactivate endothelial nitric oxide and may increase the propensity of ESRD patients to develop arteriosclerosis and hypertension (69). There is evidence for increased cytokine production secondary to blood interaction with bioincompatible dialysis components. In particular, blood–dialyzer interaction can activate mononuclear cells, leading to production of inflammatory cytokines (243). Synthetic high-flux dialyzer membranes are permeable to the proinflammatory cytokines, and are capable of removing interleukin-1B (IL-1B), tumor necrosis factor α (TNFα), and

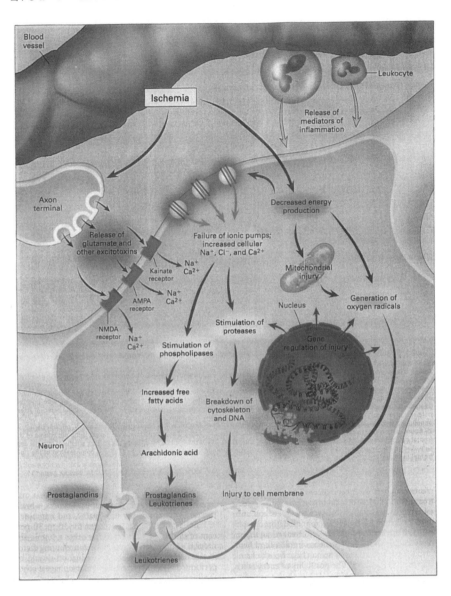

FIG. 93-6. The molecular events initiated in brain tissue by acute cerebral ischemia. Interruption of cerebral blood flow results in decreased energy production, which in turn causes failure of ionic pumps, mitochondrial injury, activation of leukocytes (with release of mediators of inflammation), generation of oxygen radicals, and release of excitotoxins. Increased cellular levels of sodium, chloride and calcium ions result in stimulation of phospholipases and proteases, followed by generation and release of prostaglandins and leukotrienes, breakdown of DNA and the cytoskeleton, and ultimately, breakdown of the cell membrane. Alteration of genetic components regulates elements of the cascade to alter the degree of injury. AMPA denotes α-amino-3-hydroxy-5-methyl-4-isoxazole propionic acid and N-methyl-D-aspartate. (From: Brott T, Bogousslavsky J. Treatment of acute ischemic stroke. *N Engl J Med* 2000;343:710, with permission.) (See Color Fig. 93-6 following page 2624.)

interleukin-6 (IL-6), thus offering a potential therapeutic approach (244). It is unclear whether cytokine removal by continuous renal replacement therapy will decrease the incidence of stroke (245). The use of sorbents with continuous plasma filtration offers another possibility for a novel therapeutic approach (246,247). Some of the cytokines, such as IL-1B, TNFα, and IL-6, may induce an inflammatory state, and are believed to play an important role in dialysis-related mortality (239,243). Recent prospective studies have demonstrated that patients with ESRD and higher blood levels of certain cytokines have a greater mortality and have a larger number of cardiovascular events (248). Contaminated dialysate water can result in pyogenic substances of bacterial origin being absorbed into the dialysis membrane (249). The consequence could be induction of an inflammatory response in certain dialysis patients. Substances of bacterial origin activate circulating mononuclear cells to produce proinflammatory cytokines. The cytokines include IL-1B, TNFα, and IL-6, and they mediate the acute phase response resulting in elevated

levels of acute phase proteins, including CRP (249). The effects of dialysis reuse on cytokine production has not been evaluated, but may be important, as reuse could theoretically lead to more contamination of dialysate (249,250). Reactive carbonyl compounds and AGEs, which tend to modify proteins in a deleterious manner (56), can be decreased by use of a peritoneal dialysate containing icodextrin and amino acids instead of glucose (251).

The cardiovascular disease and cerebrovascular disease can lead to cerebral ischemia. Cerebral ischemia initiates a number of processes that can lead to progressive brain damage (Fig. 93-6) (252). Cerebral ischemia can lead to activation in brain of free radicals, NMDA, and apoptosis, all potential mechanisms of brain damage in patients with hypoperfusion or stroke (253–255) (Fig. 93-6). Anoxic injury to brain endothelial cells can increase production of nitric oxide, which can lead to free radical formation (256,257). Apoptosis, or programed cell death, is another mode of destruction of brain cells in stroke (255). Glutamate activates the NMDA receptor complex and also can lead to later activation of apoptosis (258). In general, the ischemic event of a stroke only serves to initiate the biochemical events that may lead to brain damage. Interventions that counter these biochemical events may decrease the brain damage associated with acute stroke (259,260).

Recent knowledge of the pathogenesis of stroke has led to a major expansion in the opportunities for prevention of stroke. High-grade carotid stenosis can lead to stroke, although the exact numbers of patients who will suffer stroke when they have carotid stenosis is not known (261). Screening patients who have renal failure for the presence of carotid stenosis will diagnose a substantial number of such patients, although at considerable cost. However, because of noninvasive diagnostic techniques such as duplex Doppler ultrasonography, screening for carotid stenosis involves essentially no morbidity (262). Studies of the aortic arch for the presence of large atherosclerotic plaques (more than 4 mm thick) is an important predictor for the possibility of stroke in the future (23,263), as is the presence of atrial fibrillation (263). Other common preventive measures include treatment of hypertension, cessation of smoking, lowering of plasma cholesterol, control of plasma glucose (in diabetic patients), weight loss, increased exercise, and decreased alcohol consumption (237). Other possible preventive measures include dietary antioxidants, low-dose aspirin, and a decrease of intake of saturated fatty acids (237). The last word is far from in, but substantial evidence suggests that administration of hormone replacement therapy in postmenopausal women is associated with a reduced risk of stroke (237,264–266). Such therapy may include other compounds that have estrogenlike effects (267). Although treatment of hypertension is known to decrease the incidence of stroke, not all antihypertensive agents are of equal efficacy. In general, only ß-blockers, thiazide diuretics, and angiotensin-converting enzyme (ACE) inhibitors have been shown to reduce the incidence of stroke, whereas α-adrenergic blocking agents and calcium channel blockers may not (268–271).

Given that the aforementioned are likely mechanisms of brain damage in stroke, a whole new field is opened as far as potential therapeutic agents for decreasing brain damage associated with stroke. Such agents include calcium channel blockers (272,273), inhibitors of NMDA receptors (274), and agents that scavenge free radicals (275). It is now clear that in many cases acute stroke often can be successfully treated, but only if physicians realize that stroke should now be considered a medical emergency where timely therapy can make the difference in functional survival of the brain (276). Therapies for acute stroke that are now being administered in teaching hospitals in the United States start with acute neuroimaging in the emergency room. An initial CT scan will usually reveal acute stroke and if present, serves to differentiate occlusive from hemorrhagic stroke. If a nonhemorrhagic stroke is present, treatment prospects can be examined with magnetic resonance angiography (MRA), which is noninvasive. Contrast should not be administered to patients with impaired renal function, but can be given to dialysis patients (277). When acute stroke is diagnosed within the appropriate time window (within 3 hours of the onset of symptoms) current therapies may include intravenous thrombolytic therapy (278), intraarterial thrombolytic therapy, antithrombotic and antiplatelet drugs, defibrinogenation agents, and neuroprotective drugs (252,279–281). Administration of the defibrinogenation agent ancrod to patients with acute ischemic stroke resulted in a better functional status after 3 months follow-up (281). Nizofenone can scavenge free radicals and inhibit glutamate release, and may prove useful as a cerebroprotective agent (282).

Some cases of acute stroke are caused by dissection of the carotid or vertebral artery systems. These patients have lesions that are not amenable to dissolution of clot, as the obstructing lesions is in fact a hemorrhage in the arterial wall (283–285). Dissection of the carotid or vertebral artery system can be initiated by chiropractic manipulation of the cervical spine, so that such maneuvers should probably be avoided in dialysis patients (283). In addition, some cases of apparent acute stroke in dialysis patients are caused by subdural hematoma, which always must be considered in the differential diagnosis of stroke in dialysis patients (23).

SEXUAL DYSFUNCTION IN UREMIA

Disturbances in sexual function are a common complication of chronic renal failure (286,287). These complications include erectile dysfunction, decreased libido, and decreased frequency of intercourse (288). Studies in uremic rats showed that erectile impairment was associated with a disturbance in nitric oxide synthetase gene expression (289). Sexual dysfunction in men with ESRD treated with maintenance hemodialysis is common, and previously, impotence was observed in at least 50% of such patients (290). A number of abnormalities associated with renal failure appear to be important in the genesis of impotence. There are abnormalities in autonomic nervous system function (288), impairment in arterial and venous systems of the penis (along with vascular pathology in other vascular beds), hypertension (many drugs used to treat hypertension cause secondary impotence) and other associated endocrine abnormalities (291). There are also the associated effects of aging, with impotence observed in over 50% of men over 60 years old who do not have renal failure (292). There are a variety of approaches to the evaluation of impotence in men with uremia (293). Patients with ESRD have a high incidence of cardiovascular disease (1), which impairs penile vessels along with those of the rest of the body (232). The incidence of hypertension is also higher in ESRD patients than the rest of the population, and hypertension is a major contributor to vascular disease (1,294). Many drugs used to treat hypertension can lead to impotence (calcium channel blockers, thiazides, and guanethidine). The incidence of depression is high in patients with ESRD, and many drugs used to treat depression can lead to impotence (phenothiazines, tricyclics, fluoxetine). Although appreciation of the aforementioned abnormalities may increase our understanding, until very recently there was little that could be done other than to discontinue certain drugs used to treat hypertension or depression (290). There are now a number of drugs that can successfully treat impotence (295). Alprostadil was successful but had to be delivered transurethrally (296). In particular, sildenafil can be administered orally and is highly effective, even in men who have cardiovascular disease (297) or uremia (298). Other treatments for impotence among men with ESRD include penile prostheses, direct injection of α blocking agents or other vasodilators (papaverine, phentolamine, alprostadil) into the penis, and vacuum constrictive devices (286,295).

UREMIC NEUROPATHY

Clinical Manifestations

Peripheral neuropathy in patients with renal failure has been recognized for over 100 years (299). This disorder, however, was not fully appreciated until the early 1960s (86). Prior to the institution of chronic dialysis therapy, approximately 65% of patients with end-stage renal disease probably did not live long enough to develop clinically apparent neuropathy. Although existing data are difficult to evaluate, neuropathy is probably present in about 65% of patients with end-stage renal disease at the time of the institution of dialysis (300).

Many patients with chronic renal failure who are neurologically asymptomatic may exhibit abnormalities on physical examination. They also may have evidence of autonomic neuropathy such as impotence and postural hypotension. Moreover, abnormal nerve conduction may be present in the absence of symptoms or abnormal findings on physical examination in patients who have renal insufficiency. Additionally, alternations in nerve conduction do no necessarily indicate structural changes in the peripheral nerves.

The motor nerve conduction velocity (MNCV) is a test that is frequently used to assess peripheral neuropathy. The test, however, is somewhat unreliable because there is a large normal variation in MNCV (up to 20% on a day-to-day basis) (78) and the test has very limited utility in detecting moderate impairment of peripheral nerve function. Sensory nerve conduction velocity (SNCV) is more sensitive than MNCV, but the test is quite painful and most patients do not permit repeated tests.

In general, there are two broad categories of peripheral neuropathy. These are described in terms of the pattern of involvement of the PNS. First, there are processes that result in a bilaterally symmetric disturbance of function that can be designated as polyneuropathies. Polyneuropathy tends to be associated with agents such as toxic substances, metabolic disorders (uremia, diabetes, deficiency states), and certain examples of immune reaction that act diffusely on the PNS. The second category comprises isolated lesions of peripheral nerves (mononeuropathy) or multiple isolated lesions (multiple mononeuropathy). In severe symmetric polyneuropathies, a generalized loss of peripheral nerve function may occur, and

the impairment is usually maximal distally in the limbs. A mixed motor and sensory polyneuropathy with a distal distribution results in weakness and wasting most frequently observed peripherally in the arms and legs. There are also distal sensory changes of "glove and stocking" distribution. In those neuropathies that involve "dying back" of the axons from the periphery (299), it is possible that the neurons that have the longest axons to maintain appear to be the first to suffer.

Uremic neuropathy is a distal, symmetric, mixed polyneuropathy. Motor and sensory modalities are both generally affected and lower extremities are more severely involved than are the upper extremities. Clinically, uremic polyneuropathy cannot be distinguished from the neuropathies associated with certain other metabolic disorders such as diabetes mellitus, chronic alcoholism, and various deficiency states. The occurrence of neuropathy bears no relationship to the type of underlying disease process (e.g., glomerulonephritis or pyelonephritis). However, certain diseases that can lead to renal failure may simultaneously affect peripheral nerve function in a manner separate from the manifestations of uremia. Such diseases include amyloidosis, multiple myeloma, systemic lupus erythematosus, polyarteritis nodosa, diabetes mellitus, and hepatic failure (86). The clinical manifestations of uremic neuropathy are characterized by several different stages. It appears that when glomerular filtration rate exceeds 12 mL/minute, clinical evidence of neuropathy generally is absent (7,122,225).

Peripheral Nerves

The restless leg syndrome is a common early manifestation of chronic renal failure. Clinically, patients experience sensations in lower extremities such as crawling, prickling, and pruritus. The sensations are worse distally than proximally and generally are more prominent in the evening. The restless leg syndrome may initially be present in up to 40% of patients with chronic renal failure (301). Another symptom experienced by patients with early uremic neuropathy is the burning foot syndrome, which is present in less than 10% of patients with chronic renal failure (302). Rather than "burning," the actual symptoms consist of swelling sensations, constriction, and tenderness of the distal lower extremities.

The physical signs of peripheral nerve dysfunction often begin with loss of deep tendon reflexes, particularly knee and ankle jerks (225,226). Impaired vibratory sensation also is an early sign of uremic neuropathy. Loss of sensation in the lower leg is common and often takes the form of "stocking-glove" anesthesia of the lower leg. The sensory loss includes pain, light touch, vibration, and pressure.

Metabolic Neuropathy

Uremic neuropathy is one of a group of central–peripheral axonopathies, also known as dying-back polyneuropathies, which have been described by Spencer and Schaumberg (303). The causes of such central–peripheral axonopathies include many types of toxic compounds. These include neuropathies associated with diabetes, multiple myeloma, certain hereditary polyneuropathies, and uremia (303). The causes of such central–peripheral axonopathies include many types of toxic compounds (303). These include neuropathies associated with diabetes, multiple myeloma, amyloidosis, certain hereditary polyneuropathies, and uremia (303). There is also an associated degeneration of the spinal cord, particularly involving posterior columns, as well as other portions of the CNS. Such findings are usually attributed either to local CNS disease or to damage of spinal ganglion cells secondary to ascending PNS damage. It is likely, however, that the CNS components of distal axonopathies. The clinical characteristics of such distal axonopathies as described by Schaumberg and Spencer include the following (303):

1. *Insidious onset.* In most human toxic neuropathies, there is a steady low-level exposure. Because only the distal portion of selected, scattered fibers are affected, the patient may still function well despite the axonal degeneration.
2. *Onset in legs.* Large and long axons are affected early, and fibers of the sciatic nerve are especially vulnerable.
3. *Stocking-glove sensory loss.* Degeneration in the distal axon proceeds toward the cell body, resulting in clinical signs in the feet and hands initially.
4. *Early loss of Achilles reflex.* Fibers to the calf muscles are of large diameter and among the first affected by many toxins, even when longer, smaller-diameter axons in the feet are spared.
5. *Moderate slowing of motor nerve conduction.* In demyelinating neuropathies, motor nerves or roots are diffusely affected; in axonal neuropathies, scattered motor fibers often are intact and motor nerve conduction velocity may appear normal or only slightly slow despite severe paresis.
6. *Normal cerebrospinal fluid protein content.* Pathologic changes usually are distal and nerve roots are spared.
7. *Slow recovery.* Axonal regeneration (in contrast to remyelination) is slow—about 1 mm/day. Thus, after institution of dialysis or renal transplantation, recovery of nerve function may take months or years.
8. *Residual disability.* Most toxic axonopathies are characterized by tract degeneration of long, large-diameter fibers in the CNS concomitant with changes in the PNS. Signs of lesions in the corticospinal and spinocerebellar pathways may not be clinically apparent if there is severe peripheral neuropathy. However, on recovery from the neuropathy, there may be spasticity or ataxia.

It can be recognized readily that the preceding features are similar to many descriptions of uremic neuropathy (86, 299,304). The cellular basis for distal axonopathies, however, remains unclear. Spencer and associates (305) emphasized that a number of chemically unrelated neurotoxic compounds and several types of metabolic abnormalities can cause strikingly similar patterns of distal symmetric polyneuropathy in humans and animals.

These authors suggest a possible common metabolic basis for many distal axonopathies. Neurotoxic compounds may deplete energy supplies in the axon by inhibiting nerve fiber enzymes required for the maintenance of energy synthesis. Resupply of enzymes from the neuronal soma may fail to meet the increased demand for enzyme replacement in the axon, causing the concentration of enzymes to decrease in distal regions. This could lead to a local blockade of energy-dependent axonal transport, which could then produce a series of pathologic changes culminating in distal nerve fiber degeneration.

Uremic Toxins and Nerve Conduction

Several possible uremic toxins have been identified that appear to be correlated with depression of MNCV in laboratory animals (58,76,77); however, these studies do not take into account the facts that: (a) depressed MNCV is cyclical, with abnormal low values one day and normal values the next; (b) there is a day-to-day variation in MNCV that approaches 20% (78); and (c) the finding of depressed MNCV in laboratory animals associated with high plasma levels of potential uremic neurotoxins generally has not been confirmed in human subjects with renal failure (20). Although it is possible to relate impairment in MNCV with levels in blood of various substances, the best correlation was obtained between reduced MNCV versus a reduction in glomerular filtration rate (Table 93-4).

Parathyroid Hormone

Among the potential uremic neurotoxins is PTH (306), based on a possible correlation between plasma PTH levels and MNCV in patients with chronic renal failure (79). Some earlier studies suggested a possible effect of PTH on MNCV in the dog (77), but these impressions have not been confirmed (48,84). In patients who have hyperparathyroidism without uremia, PTH has no observable effect on peripheral nerve function (48,83,84). In both patients and laboratory animals with acute renal failure, the MNCV has been found to be normal (18,20,65,85) (Fig. 93-7). In all studies of both patients and laboratory animals with chronic renal failure, the MNCV had not been shown to be affected by PTH (20) (Fig. 93-7). Thus, in both patients and laboratory animals with either acute renal failure or chronic renal failure, or primary or secondary hyperparathyroidism, no effect of PTH on nerve function can be demonstrated. In patients with chronic renal failure, there is no change in MNCV as a result of either recovery of renal function or chronic hemodialysis; there was also no effect of parathyroidectomy (84). In addition, when patients begin dialysis therapy, MNCV either stabilizes or improves (86). However, virtually all of these patients have elevated plasma PTH levels (307).

Animal studies suggest that in either acute or chronic renal failure, changes in MNCV take longer than 6 months to develop and are probably not related to an effect of PTH (Fig. 93-7). Mahoney and associates studied dogs who had renal failure for periods of 3.5 days to 6 months (39). There was no change in the MNCV after any of the aforementioned

TABLE 93-4. *Relation between nerve function and various "uremic neurotoxins"*

Reference	Putative uremic neurotoxin	Correlation coefficient with MNCV	Other
Giulio SD, et al. Parathormone as a nerve poison in uremia. *N Engl J Med* 1978;299:1134.	Parathyroid hormone	0.09	No effect of PTH on motor nerve function
Avram MM, et al. Search for the uremic toxin. *N Engl J Med* 1978;298:1000.	Parathyroid hormone	0.45	
Nielsen VK. The peripheral nerve function in chronic renal failure: VI. *Acta Med Scand* 1973; 194:455.	Urea Creatinine Glomerular filtration rate	0.41 0.51 0.68–0.84	
Blagg CR, et al. Nerve conduction in relationship to the severity of renal disease. *Nephron* 1968;5:290.	Urea Creatinine	0.51 0.57	
Blumberg A, et al. Myoinositol-uremic neurotoxin? *Nephron* 1978;21:186.	Myoinositol	0.03	
Reznek RH, et al. Plasma myoinositol concentrations in uraemic neuropathy. *Lancet* 1977;1:675.	Myoinositol	0.67	
Clements RSJ, et al. Raised plasma-myoinositol levels in uraemia and experimental neuropathy. *Lancet* 1973;1:1137.	Myoinositol	NA	Detrimental effect of myoinositol on nerve function
Man NK, et al. An approach to "middle molecules" identification in artificial kidney dialysate, with reference to neuropathy prevention. *TASAIO* 1973;19:320.	Middle molecules	NA	No *in vivo* evidence of MNCV impairment with renal failure
Scribner BH, and Babb AL. Evidence for toxins of "middle" molecular weight. *Kidney Int* 1975;7:S349.	Middle molecules	NA	As above
Kjellstrand CM, et al. Considerations of the middle molecule hypothesis II. *TASAIO* 1973;19:325.	Middle molecules	NA	As above
Giovannetti S, et al. Methylguanidine in uremia. *Arch Intern Med* 1973;131:709.	Methylguanidine	NA	Chronic injection; depressed MNCV in patients
Lonergan ET, et al. Erythrocyte transketolase activity in dialyzed patients. *N Engl J Med* 1971;284:1399.	Transketolase deficiency	NA	Deficiency related to impaired MNCV in patients
Mahoney CA, et al. Central and peripheral nervous system effects of chronic renal failure. *Kidney Int* 1983;24:170.	Parathyroid hormone	0.05	No effect of PTH on motor nerve function
Kanda F, et al. Somatosensory evoked potentials in acute renal failure. *Kidney Int* 1990;38:1085.	Parathyroid hormone	NA	No effect of PTH on sensory nerve function

MNCV = motor nerve conduction velocity.

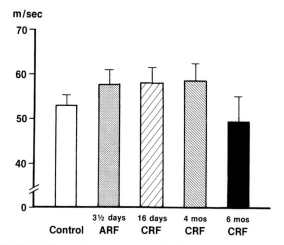

FIG. 93-7. The motor nerve conduction velocity (MNCV) in the peroneal nerve in control dogs (N = 12) and in dogs who had renal failure for the following periods: acute renal failure (ARF) 3.5 days (N = 10); chronic renal failure (CRF) 16 days (N = 11); CRF 4 months (N = 10); and CRF 6 months (N = 5). None of the values of MNCV in dogs with renal failure is significantly different from the control value. (From: Mahoney CA, Arieff AI. Central and peripheral nervous system effects of chronic renal failure. *Kidney Int* 1983;24:170, with permission.)

intervals of renal failure, and the MNCV was normal even after 6 months with glomerular filtration rate below 22% of control.

It also has been suggested that either PTH or acute renal failure somehow resulted in an increase of nerve calcium content and that this might be related to impaired MNCV (77). However, in dogs with renal failure for periods of 3.5 days to 4 months, there were no observed increases in nerve calcium content (39) (Fig. 93-8). Nerve calcium values in dogs with

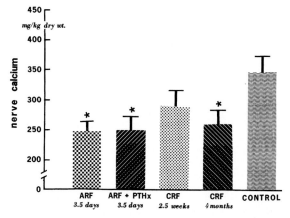

FIG. 93-8. Nerve calcium content in peripheral (sciatic) nerve of dogs with renal failure for intervals indicated. Renal failure for all intervals shown caused significant decrement in nerve calcium content compared to control values. *ARF,* acute renal failure; *CRF,* chronic renal failure; *PTHx,* parathyroidectomy. (Data from: Mahoney CA, Arieff AI. Central and peripheral nervous system effects of chronic renal failure. *Kidney Int* 1983;24:170, with permission.)

acute renal failure with or without parathyroidectomy also were not different and in fact actually fell significantly (versus control) in dogs with chronic renal failure (Fig. 93-8).

REFERENCES

1. Meeus F, Kourilsky O, Guerin AP, et al. Pathophysiology of cardiovascular disease in hemodialysis patients. *Kidney Int* 2000;58:S140.
2. Parfrey PS. Cardiac and cerebrovascular disease in chronic uremia. *Am J Kidney Dis* 1993;21:77.
3. Wratten ML, Tetta C, Ursini F, et al. Oxidant stress in hemodialysis: prevention and treatment strategies. *Kidney Int* 2000;58: S126.
4. Slomowitz LA, Wilkinson A, Hawkins R, et al. Evaluation of kidney function in renal transplant patients receiving long-term cyclosporine. *Am J Kidney Dis* 1990;15:530.
5. Teschan PE, Arieff AI. Uremic and dialysis encephalopathies. In: McCandless DW, ed. *Cerebral energy metabolism and metabolic encephalopathy.* New York: Plenum Press, 1985:263.
6. Teschan PE, Bourne JR, Reed RB. Electrophysiological and neurobehavioral responses to therapy: The National Cooperative Dialysis Study. *Kidney Int* 1983;23:558.
7. Teschan PE, Ginn HE, Bourne JR, et al. Quantitative indices of clinical uremia. *Kidney Int* 1979;15:676.
8. Hirakata H, Yao H, Osato S, et al. CBF and oxygen metabolism in hemodialysis patients: effects of anemia correction with recombinant human EPO. *Am J Physiol* 1992;262:F737.
9. Ifudu O, Feldman J, Friedman EA. The intensity of hemodialysis and the response to erythropoietin in patients with end-stage renal disease. *N Engl J Med* 1996;334:420.
10. Nissenson AR. Epoetin and cognitive function. *Am J Kidney Dis* 1992; 20:21.
11. Grimm G, Stockenhuber F, Schneeweiss B, et al. Improvement of brain function in hemodialysis patients treated with erythropoietin. *Kidney Int* 1990;38:480.
12. Moreno F, Sanz-Guajardo D, Lopez-Gomez J, et al. Increasing the hematocrit has a beneficial effect on quality of life and is safe in selected hemodialysis patients. *J Am Soc Nephrol* 2000;11:335.
13. Fraser CL, Arieff AI. Hepatic encephalopathy. *N Engl J Med* 1985; 313:865.
14. Takabatake T, Ohta H, Ishida Y, et al. Low serum creatinine levels in severe hepatic disease. *Arch Intern Med* 1988;148:1313.
15. Papadakis MA, Arieff AI. Unpredictability of clinical evaluation of renal function in cirrhosis. *Am J Med* 1987;82:945.
16. Gines P, Arroyo V. Hepatorenal syndrome. *J Am Soc Nephrol* 1999; 10:1833.
17. Locke SJ, Merrill JP, Tyler HR. Neurological complications of acute uremia. *Arch Intern Med* 1961;108:519.
18. Cooper JD, Lazarowitz VC, Arieff AI. Neurodiagnostic abnormalities in patients with acute renal failure. Evidence for neurotoxicity of parathyroid hormone. *J Clin Invest* 1978;61:1448.
19. Fraser CL, Arieff AI. Neurological problems with acute renal failure. In: Ronco C, Bellomo R, eds. *Critical care nephrology.* Hingham, MA: Kluwer Academic Publishers, 1997:819.
20. Fraser CL, Arieff AI. Nervous system complications in uremia. *Ann Intern Med* 1988;109:143.
21. Moe SM, Sprague SM. Uremic encephalopathy. *Clin Nephrol* 1994; 42:251.
22. Guisado R, Arieff AI, Massry SG, et al. Changes in the electroencephalogram in acute uremia. Effects of parathyroid hormone and brain electrolytes. *J Clin Invest* 1975;55:738.
23. Reese GN, Appel SH. Neurologic complications of renal failure. *Semin Nephrol* 1981;1:137.
24. Kiley JE, et al. Evaluation of encephalopathy by EEG frequency analysis in chronic dialysis patients. *Clin Nephrol* 1976;5:245.
25. Cogan MG, Covey C, Arieff AI, et al. CNS manifestations of hyperparathyroidism. *Am J Med* 1978;65:963.
26. Slatopolsky E, Martin K, Hruska K. Parathyroid hormone metabolism and its potential as a uremic toxin. *Am J Physiol* 1980;239:F1.
27. Agodoa LY, Eggers PW. Renal replacement therapy in the United States: data from the United States renal data system. *Am J Kidney Dis* 1995;25:119.

28. Garg PP, Frick KD, Diener-West M, et al. Effect of the ownership of dialysis facilities on patient's survival and referral for transplantation. *N Engl J Med* 1999;341:1653.

29. Beddhu S, Bruns FJ, Saul M, et al. A simple comorbidity scale predicts clinical outcomes and costs in dialysis patients. *Am J Med* 2000;108:609.

30. Fraser CL, Arieff AI. Neuropsychiatric complications of uremia. In: Brady HR, Wilcox CS, eds. *Therapy in nephrology and hypertension.* Philadelphia: WB Saunders, 1999:488.

31. Bowling PS, Bourn JR. Discriminant analysis of electroencephalograms recorded from renal patients. *IEEE Trans Biomed Eng* 1978; 25:12.

32. Mahoney CA, Arieff AI. Uremic encephalopathies: clinical, biochemical and experimental features. *Am J Kidney Dis* 1982;2:324.

33. Fraser CL, Arieff AI. Metabolic encephalopathy as a complication of acid base, and electrolyte disorders. In: Arieff AI, DeFronzo RA, eds. *Fluid, electrolyte and acid-base disorders,* 2nd ed. New York: Churchill Livingstone, 1995:685.

34. Fraser CL, Arieff AI. Metabolic encephalopathy as a complication of renal failure: mechanisms and mediators. In: Matuschak GM, ed. *New horizons: the science and practice of acute medicine,* 5th ed, vol 2. Baltimore: Williams & Wilkins, 1994:518.

35. Osberg JW, Meares GJ, McKee DC, et al. Intellectual functioning in renal failure and chronic dialysis. *J Chronic Dis* 1982;35:445.

36. English A, Savage RD, Britton PG, et al. Intellectual impairment in chronic renal failure. *Br Med J* 1978;1:888.

37. Greenberg MD. Brain damage in hemodialysis patients. *Dial Transplant* 1978;7:238.

38. Minkoff L, Gaertner M, Darah C, et al. Inhibition of brain sodium-potassium ATPase in uremic rats. *J Lab Clin Med* 1972;80:71.

39. Mahoney CA, Sarnacki P, Arieff AI. Uremic encephalopathy: role of brain energy metabolism. *Am J Physiol* 1984;247:F527.

40. Van den Noort S, Eckel RE, Brine K, et al. Brain metabolism in uremic and adenosine-infused rats. *J Clin Invest* 1968;47:2133.

41. Arieff AI, Massry SG, Barrientos A, et al. Brain water and electrolyte metabolism in uremia: effects of slow and rapid hemodialysis. *Kidney Int* 1973;4:177.

42. Arieff AI, Massry SG. Calcium metabolism of brain in acute renal failure. Effects of uremia, hemodialysis, and parathyroid hormone. *J Clin Invest* 1974;53:387.

43. Arieff AI, Guisado R, Massry SG. Central nervous system pH in uremia and the effects of hemodialysis. *J Clin Invest* 1977;58:306.

44. Perry TL, Yong VW, Kish SJ, et al. Neurochemical abnormalities in brain of renal failure patients treated by repeated hemodialysis. *J Neurochem* 1985;45:1043.

45. Fishman RA. Permeability changes in experimental uremic encephalopathy. *Arch Int Med* 1970;126:835.

46. Deferrari G. Brain metabolism of amino acids and ammonia in patients with chronic renal insufficiency. *Kidney Int* 1981;20:505.

47. Verkman AS, Fraser CL. Water and non-electrolyte permeability in brain synaptosomes isolated from normal and uremic rats. *Am J Physiol* 1986;250:R306.

48. Mahoney CA, Arieff AI, Leach WJ, et al. Central and peripheral nervous system effects of chronic renal failure. *Kidney Int* 1983; 24:170.

49. Sadowski RH, Hayne BD, He J. Acute renal failure induces rapid glial and neuronal changes in the rat cerebral cortex. *Kidney Int* 2001, in press.

50. Akmal M, Goldstein DA, Multani S, et al. Role of uremia, brain calcium and parathyroid hormone on changes in electroencephalogram in chronic renal failure. *Am J Physiol* 1984;246:F575.

51. Arieff AI. Neurological manifestations of uremia. In: Brenner BM, Rector FC Jr, eds. *The kidney,* 3rd ed, vol II. Philadelphia: WB Saunders, 1986:1731.

52. Levin GE, Baron DN. Leucocyte intracellular pH in patients with metabolic acidosis or renal failure. *Clin Sci* 1977;52:325.

53. Maschio G, Bazzato G, Bertaglia E, et al. Intracellular pH and electrolyte content of skeletal muscle in patients with chronic renal acidosis. *Nephron* 1970;7:481.

54. Tizianello A, Deferrari G, Gurreri G, et al. Effects of metabolic alkalosis, metabolic acidosis and uraemia on whole-body intracellular pH in man. *Clin Sci Mol Med* 1977;52:125.

55. Vanholder R. Pathogenesis of uremic toxicity. In: Ronco C, Bellomo R, eds. *Critical care nephrology.* Hingham, MA: Kluwer, 1998:845.

56. Miyata T, Kurokawa K, van Ypersele de Strihou C. Relevance of oxidative and carbonyl stress to long-term uremic complications. *Kidney Int* 2000;58:S120.

57. Vanholder R. Low molecular weight uremic toxins. In: Ronco C, Bellomo R, eds. *Critical care nephrology.* Hingham, MA: Kluwer, 1998:855.

58. Giovannetti S, Balestri PL, Barsotti G. Methylguanidine in uremia. *Arch Intern Med* 1973;131:709.

59. Davidoff F. Effects of guanidine derivatives on mitochondrial function I. *J Clin Invest* 1968;47:2331.

60. Davidoff F. Guanidine derivatives in medicine. *N Engl J Med* 1973; 289:141.

61. De Deyn P, Marescau B, D'Hodge R, et al. Guanidino compound levels in brain regions of non-dialyzed uremic patients. *Neurochem Int* 1995;27:227.

62. Dhondt A, Vanholder R, van Beisen W, et al. The removal of uremic toxins. *Kidney Int* 2000;58:S47.

63. Man NK. An approach to "middle molecules" identification in artificial kidney dialysate, with reference neuropathy prevention. *Trans Am Soc Artif Intern Organs* 1973;19:320.

64. Kjellstrand CM. The clinical significance of middle molecules. *Dialysis Trans* 1979:860.

65. Scribner BH, Farrell PC, Milutinovic J. Evolution of the middle molecular hypothesis. *Proc 5th Int Congr Nephrol (Mexico)* 1972;5:190.

66. Scribner BH, Babb AL. Evidence for toxins of "middle" molecular weight. *Kidney Int* 1975;7:S349.

67. Vanholder R, DeSmet R, Hsu C, et al. Uremic toxins: the middle molecule hypothesis revisited. *Semin Nephrol* 1994;14:205.

68. Makita Z, Radoff S, Rayfield EJ, et al. Advanced glycosylation end products in patients with diabetic nephropathy. *N Engl J Med* 1991; 325:836.

69. Haag-Weber M. AGE-modified proteins in renal failure. In: Ronco C, Bellomo R, eds. *Critical care nephrology.* Hingham, MA: Kluwer, 1998:878.

70. Koenig H, Goldstone AD, Lu CY, et al. Polyamines: transducers of osmotic signals at the blood-brain barrier. *Proc Amer Soc Neurochem* 1988;19:79.

71. Beal MF. Mechanisms of excitotoxicity in neurologic disease. *FASEB J* 1992;6:3338.

72. Lipton SA, Rosenberg PA. Excitatory amino acids as a final common pathway for neurologic disorders. *N Engl J Med* 1994;330:613.

73. Ringoir S. An update on uremic toxins. *Kidney Int* 1997;62:S2.

74. Kokot FWA. Evidence that the anemia of renal failure participates in overall uremic toxicity. *Kidney Int* 1997;52:S83.

75. Evans RW, Rader B, Manninen DL. The quality of life of hemodialysis recipients treated with recombinant human erythropoietin. *JAMA* 1990;263:825.

76. Clements RSJ, DeJesus PVJ, Winegrad AI. Raised plasma-myoinositol levels in uraemia and experimental neuropathy. *Lancet* 1973;1:1137.

77. Goldstein DA, Chui LA, Massry SG. Effect of parathyroid hormone and uremia on peripheral nerve calcium and motor nerve conduction velocity. *J Clin Invest* 1978;62:88.

78. McQuillen MP, Gorin FJ. Serial ulnar nerve conduction velocity measurements in normal subjects. *J Neurol Neurosurg Psychiatry* 1969;32:144.

79. Avram MM, Feingold DA, Huatuco AH. Search for the uremic toxin: decreased motor nerve conduction velocity and elevated parathyroid hormone in uremia. *N Engl J Med* 1978;298:1000.

80. Lonergan ET, Semar M, Sterzel RB, et al. Erythrocyte transketolase activity in dialyzed patients. *N Engl J Med* 1971;284:1399.

81. Reznek RH, Salway JG, Thomas PK. Plasma myoinositol concentrations in uraemic neuropathy. *Lancet* 1977;1:675.

82. Horl WH. High molecular weight uremic toxins. In: Ronco C, Bellomo R, eds. *Critical care nephrology.* Hingham, MA: Kluwer, 1998:867.

83. Mallette LE, Pattern BM, Engle WK. Neuromuscular disease in secondary hyperparathyroidism. *Ann Intern Med* 1975;82:474.

84. Giulio SD, Chkoff N, Lhoste F, et al. Parathormone as a nerve poison in uremia. *N Engl J Med* 1978;299:1134.

85. Aurbach GD. Neuromuscular disease in primary hyperparathyroidism. *Ann Intern Med* 1974;80:182.

86. Asbury AK. In: Dyck PJ, Thomas PK, Lambert EH, eds. *Uremic neuropathy,* vol. 2. Philadelphia: WB Saunders, 1975.

87. Arnaud CD. Hyperparathyroidism and renal failure. *Kidney Int* 1973; 4:89.

88. Deutch C, Drown C, Rafalowska U, et al. Synaptosomes from rat brain: morphology, compartmentation, and transmembrane pH and electrical gradients. *J Neurochem* 1981;36:2062.

89. Whittaker VP. The synaptosome. In: Lajtha A, ed. *Handbook of neurochemistry,* vol II. New York: Plenum Press, 1978:327.

90. Fraser CL, Sarnacki P, Arieff AI. Calcium transport abnormality in uremic rat brain synaptosomes. *J Clin Invest* 1985;76:1789.

91. Fraser CL, Arieff AI. Abnormalities of transport in synaptosomes from uremic rat brain: role of parathyroid hormone. *J Gen Physiol* 1986;88:24.

92. Cajal SR. La fine structure des centres nerveux. *Proc R Soc (Lond)* 1984;55:444.

93. Sherrington CS. The central nervous system. In: Fosters M, ed. *A textbook of physiology,* 7th ed. London: Macmillan, 1987.

94. De Robertis E. Ultrastructure and cytochemistry of the synaptic region. *Science* 1967;156:907.

95. De Robertis E, Arwee G, Salganicoff L, et al. Isolation of synaptic vesicles and structural organization of the acetylcholine system within brain nerve endings. *J Neurochem* 1963;10:255.

96. Makowski L, Casper DLD, Phillips NC, et al. Gap junction structures. II. Analysis of the x-ray diffraction data. *J Cell Biol* 1977;74:629.

97. Bennett WVL. Electrical transmission: a functional analysis and comparison to chemical transmission. In: Kendal ER, ed. *Handbook of physiology.* Bethesda, MD: American Physiological Society, 1977:357.

98. Gray EG, Whittaker VP. The isolation of nerve endings from brain: an electron-microscopic study of cell fragments derived by homogenization and centrifugation. *J Anat (Lond)* 1962;96:79.

99. Del Castillo J, Datz B. The effect of magnesium on the activity of motor nerve endings. *J Physiol (Lond)* 1954;124:553.

100. Katz B, Miledi R. The release of acetylcholine from nerve endings by graded electric pulses. *Proc R Soc Lond (Biol)* 1967;167:23.

101. Katz B, Miledi R. A study of synaptic transmission in the absence of nerve impulses. *J Physiol (Lond)* 1967;192:407.

102. Katz B, Miledi R. The timing of calcium action during neuromuscular transmission. *J Physiol (Lond)* 1967;189:535.

103. Fraser CL, Sarnacki P, Budayr A. Evidence that parathyroid hormone-mediated calcium transport in rat brain synaptosomes is independent of cyclic adenosine monophosphate. *J Clin Invest* 1988;81:982.

104. Fraser CL, Sarnacki P. Parathyroid hormone mediates changes in calcium transport in uremic rat brain synaptosomes. *Am J Physiol* 1988; 254:F837.

105. Berridge MJ. Inositol triphosphate and diacylglycerol: two interacting second messengers. *Ann Rev Biochem* 1987;56:159.

106. Putney JW Jr. A model for receptor-regulated calcium entry. *Cell Calcium* 1986;7:1.

107. Putney JW Jr, Takemura H, Hughes AR, et al. How do inositol phosphates regulate calcium signaling? *FASEB J* 1989;3:1899.

108. Irvine RF, Letcher AJ, Lander DJ, et al. Inositol triphosphates in carbachol-stimulated rat parotid glands. *Biochem J* 1984;223:237.

109. Irvine RF, Moor RM. Micro-injection of 1,3,4,5-tetrakisphosphate activates sea urchin eggs by a mechanism dependent on external calcium. *Biochem J* 1986;240:917.

110. Irvine RF, Moor RM. Inositol (1,3,4,5) tetrakis phosphate-induced activation of sea urchin eggs requires the presence of inositol triphosphate. *Biochem Biophys Res Commun* 1987;146:184.

111. Kuno M, Gardner P. Ion channels activated by inositol 1,4,5-triphosphate in plasma membrane of human T-lymphocytes. *Nature (Lond)* 1987;326:301.

112. Fraser CL, Sarnacki P, Arieff AI. Abnormal sodium transport in synaptosomes from brain of uremic rats. *J Clin Invest* 1985;75:2014.

113. Requena J, Mullins LJ. Calcium movement in nerve fibres. *Quart Rev Biophys* 1979;12:371.

114. Barritt GJ. Calcium movement across the cell membrane. The role of calcium in biological systems. Boca Raton, FL: CRC Press, 1982:17.

115. Blaustein MP, Nelson M. Na^+-Ca^{2+} exchange: its role in the regulation of cell calcium. In: Carafoli E, ed. *Membrane transport of calcium.* New York: Academic, 1982:217.

116. Kalix P. Uptake and release of calcium in rabbit vagus nerve. *Pflugers Arch Physiol* 1971;326:1.

117. Philipson KD, Nishimoto AY. Stimulation of Na^+-Ca^{2+} exchange in cardiac sarcolemmal vesicles by proteinase pretreatment. *Am J Physiol* 1982;243:C191.

118. Varecka L, Carafoli E. Vanadate movement of Ca^{2+} and K^+ in human red blood cells. *J Biol Chem* 1982;257:7414.

119. Carafoli E. Intracellular calcium homeostasis. *Ann Rev Biochem* 1987;56:395.

120. Fraser CL, Sarnacki P. Inositol 1,4,5 tris-phosphate may regulate systolic Ca^{2+} in rat brain synaptosomes. *J Clin Invest* 1990;86:2169.

121. Berridge MJ. Inositol phosphates as second messengers. In: Putney JW Jr, ed. *Phosphoinositides and receptor mechanisms.* New York: Alan R. Liss, 1986:25.

122. Rotter W, Roettger P. Comparative pathologic-anatomic study of cases of chronic global renal insufficiency with and without hemodialysis. *Clin Nephrol* 1974;1:257.

123. Burks JS, Alfrey AC, Huddlestone J, et al. A fatal encephalopathy in chronic haemodialysis patients. *Lancet* 1976;1:764.

124. Arieff AI, Guisado R, Massry SG. Uremic encephalopathy: studies on biochemical alterations in the brain. *Kidney Int* 1975;7:S194.

125. Arieff AI, Fraser CL, Rowley H, et al. Metabolic encephalopathy. In: Kucharczyk J, Moseley M, Barkovich AJ, eds. *Magnetic resonance neuroimaging,* 1st ed, vol 1. Boca Raton, FL: CRC Press, 1994:319.

126. Okada J, Yoshikawa K, Matsuo H, et al. Reversible MRI and CT findings in uremic encephalopathy. *Neuroradiology* 1991;33:524.

127. Wang HC, Brown P, Lees AJ. Acute movement disorders with bilateral basal ganglia lesions in uremia. *Mov Dis* 1998;13:952.

128. Savazzi GM. Pathogenesis of cerebral atrophy in uraemia. *Nephron* 1988;49:94.

129. Passer JA. Cerebral atrophy in end-stage uremia. *Proc Clin Dialy Trans Forum* 1977;7:91.

130. Savazzi GM, Cusamo F, Vinci S, et al. Progression of cerebral atrophy in patients on regular hemodialysis treatment: long-term follow-up with cerebral computed tomography. *Nephron* 1995;69:29.

131. Mahurkar SD, Myers L, Cohen J, et al. Electroencephalographic and radionucleotide studies in dialysis dementia. *Kidney Int* 1978;13:306.

132. Korzets Z, Zeltzer E, Rathaus M, et al. Uremic optic neuropathy. A uremic manifestation mandating dialysis. *Am J Nephrol* 1998;18:240.

133. Guy J, Johnston P, Corbett J, et al. Treatment of visual loss in pseudotumor cerebri associated with uremia. *Neurology* 1990;40:28.

134. Crammer JL. Calcium metabolism and mental disorder. *Psychol Med* 1977;7:557.

135. Gatewood JW, Organ CH, Mead BT. Mental changes associated with hyperparathyroidism. *Psychiatry* 1975;123:129.

136. Heath H, Hodgson SF, Kennedy MA. Primary hyperparathyroidism: incidence, morbidity, and potential impact in a community hospital. *N Engl J Med* 1980;302:189.

137. Peterson P. Psychiatric disorders in primary hyperparathyroidism. *J Clin Endocrinol Metab* 1968;28:1491.

138. Luxenberg J, Feigenbaum LZ, Aron JM. Reversible long-standing dementia with normocalcemic hyperparathyroidism. *J Am Geriat Soc* 1984;32:546.

139. Silverberg SJ, Shane E, Jacobs TP. A 10-year prospective study of primary hyperparathyroidism with or without parathyroid surgery. *N Engl J Med* 1999;341:1249.

140. Goldstein DA, et al. The relationship between the abnormalities in EEG and blood levels of parathyroid hormone in dialysis patients. *J Clin Endocrinol Metab* 1980;51:130.

141. Rasmussen H, Goodman DBP. Relationships between calcium and cyclic nucleotides in cell activation: cellular calcium metabolism and calcium-mediated cellular processes. *Physiol Rev* 1977;57:428.

142. Kennedy AC, Linton AL, Eaton JC. Urea levels in cerebrospinal fluid after hemodialysis. *Lancet* 1962;1:410.

143. Arieff AI. Dialysis disequilibrium syndrome: current concepts on pathogenesis. In: Schreiner GE, Winchester JF, eds. *Controversies in nephrology,* vol 4. Washington, DC: George Washington University Press, 1982:376.

144. Arieff AI. Dialysis disequilibrium syndrome: current concepts on pathogenesis and prevention. *Kidney Int* 1994;45:629.

145. Pagel MD, Ahmad S, Vizzo JE, et al. Acetate and bicarbonate fluctuations and acetate intolerance during dialysis. *Kidney Int* 1982;21:513.

146. Rodrigo F, Shideman J, McHugh R, et al. Osmolality changes during hemodialysis: natural history, clinical correlations, and influence of dialysate glucose and intravenous mannitol. *Ann Intern Med* 1977;86:554.

147. Van Stone JC, Carey J, Meyer R, et al. Hemodialysis with glycerol containing dialysate. *ASAIO J* 1979;2:119.
148. Grushkin CM, Korsch B, Fine RN. Hemodialysis in small children. *JAMA* 1972;221:869.
149. de Peterson H, Swanson AG. Acute encephalopathy occurring during hemodialysis. *Arch Intern Med* 1964;113:877.
150. Fukusige M, Tado O, Matsuki S, et al. Hemodialysis with kill-type artificial kidney: clinical study on disequilibrium syndrome. *Acta Urol (Jap)* 1971;17:89.
151. Mawdsley C. Neurological complications of hemodialysis. *Proc R Soc Med* 1972;65:871.
152. Porte FK, Johnson WJ, Klass DW. Prevention of dialysis disequilibrium syndrome by use of high sodium concentration in the dialysate. *Kidney Int* 1973;3:327.
153. Arieff AI, Leach W, Park R, et al. Systemic effects of NaHCO3 in experimental lactic acidosis in dogs. *Am J Physiol* 1982;242:F586.
154. Greca G, Dettori P, Biasoli S. Brain density studies in dialysis. *Lancet* 1980;2:582.
155. Kliger AS. Complications of dialysis: hemodialysis, peritoneal dialysis and CAPD. In: Arieff AI, DeFronzo RA, eds. *Fluid, electrolyte and acid-base disorders.* New York: Churchill Livingstone, 1985:777.
156. Rouby JJ, Rottenbourg J, Durande JP. Hemodynamic changes induced by regular hemodialysis and sequential ultrafiltration hemodialysis: a comparative study. *Kidney Int* 1980;17:801.
157. Arieff AI, Lazarowitz VC, Guisado R. Experimental dialysis disequilibrium syndrome: prevention with glycerol. *Kidney Int* 1978;14:270.
158. Burkart J. Adequacy of peritoneal dialysis. In: Henrich WL, ed. *Principles and practice of dialysis.* Baltimore: Williams & Wilkins, 1994:111.
159. Gutman RA, Blumenkrantz MJ, Chan YK. Controlled comparison of hemodialysis and peritoneal dialysis: Veterans Administration multicenter study. *Kidney Int* 1984;26:459.
160. Siddiqui JY, Fitz AE, Lawton RL. Causes of death in patients receiving long-term hemodialysis. *JAMA* 1970;212:1350.
161. Mahurkar SD, Dkar SK, Salta R, et al. Dialysis dementia. *Lancet* 1973;1:1412.
162. Alfrey AC, Mishell J, Burks SR, et al. Syndrome of dyspraxia and multifocal seizures associated with chronic hemodialysis. *Trans Amer Soc Artif Intern. Organs* 1972;18:257.
163. Barratt LJ, Lawrence JR. Dialysis-associated dementia. *Aust NZ J Med* 1975;5:62.
164. Chokroverty S, Bruetman ME, Berger V, et al. Progressive dialytic encephalopathy. *J Neurol Neurosurg Psychiatry* 1976;39:411.
165. Nadel AM, Wilson WP. Dialysis encephalopathy: a possible seizure disorder. *Neurology* 1976;26:1130.
166. Noriega-Sanchez A, Martinez-Maldonado M, Haiffe RM. Clinical and electroencephalographic changes in progressive uremic encephalopathy. *Neurology* 1978;28:667.
167. Dunea G, Mahurkar SD, Mamdami B. Role of aluminum in dialysis dementia. *Ann Intern Med* 1978;88:502.
168. Flendrig JA, et al. Aluminum and dialysis dementia. *Lancet* 1976;1:235.
169. Alfrey AC, LeGendre GR, Kaehny WD. The dialysis encephalopathy syndrome: possible aluminum intoxication. *N Engl J Med* 1976;294:184.
170. McDermott JR, Smith AI, Ward MK, et al. Brain aluminum concentration in dialysis encephalopathy. *Lancet* 1978;1:901.
171. Parkinson ID, et al. Fracturing dialysis osteodystrophy and dialysis encephalopathy. *Lancet* 1979;1:406.
172. Arieff AI, Cooper JD, Armstrong D, et al. Dementia, renal failure and brain aluminium. *Ann Intern Med* 1979;90:741.
173. Cartier F, Allain P, Gary J, et al. Encephalopathie myoclonique progressive des dialyses: role de l'eau utilisee pour l'hemodialyse. *Nouv Presse Med* 1978;7:97.
174. Ward MK, et al. Osteomalacia dialysis osteodystrophy: evidence for a water-borne aetiological agent, probably aluminum. *Lancet* 1978;1:841.
175. Pierides AM. Hemodialysis encephalopathy with osteomalacic fractures and muscle weakness. *Kidney Int* 1980;18:115.
176. Prior JC. Dialysis encephalopathy and osteomalacic bone disease. *Am J Med* 1982;72:33.
177. Arieff AI. Aluminum and the pathogenesis of dialysis dementia. *Environ Geochem Health* 1990;12:89.
178. Fraser CL, Arieff AI. Nervous system manifestations of renal failure. In: Schrier RW, Gottschalk CW, eds. *Diseases of the kidney,* 5th ed, vol III. Boston: Little, Brown, 1993:2789.
179. Thodis E, Anninos PA, Pasadakis P. Evaluation of CNS function in CAPD patients using magnetoencephalography (MEG). *Adv Periton Dial* 1992;8:181.
180. Farrar G, Altmann P, Welch S, et al. Defective gallium-transferrin binding in Alzheimer disease and Down syndrome: possible mechanism for accumulation of aluminum in brain. *Lancet* 1990;335:747.
181. Farrar G, Morton AP, Blair JA. The intestinal speciation of gallium: possible models to describe the bioavailability of aluminum. In: Bratter P, Schramel P, eds. *Trace element analytical chemistry in medicine and biology,* vol 5. Berlin: Walter de Gruyter, 1988:343.
182. Brun A, Dictor M. Senile plaques and tangles in dialysis dementia. *Acta Pathol Microbiol Scand* 1981;89:193.
183. Altmann P, Al-Salihi F, Butter K, et al. Serum aluminum levels and erythrocyte dihydropteridine reductase activity in patients on hemodialysis. *N Engl J Med* 1987;317:80.
184. Chazan JA, Blonsky SL, Abuelo JG, et al. Increased body aluminum: an independent risk factor in patients undergoing long-term hemodialysis? *Arch Intern Med* 1988;148:1817.
185. Sprague SM, Corwin HL, Tanner CM, et al. Relationship of aluminum to neurocognitive dysfunction in chronic dialysis patients. *Arch Intern Med* 1988;148:2169.
186. Altmann P, Hamon C, Blair J, et al. Disturbance of cerebral function by aluminum in haemodialysis patients without overt aluminum toxicity. *Lancet* 1989;ii:7.
187. Slatopolsky E, Weerts C, Lopez-Hilker S. Calcium carbonate as a phosphate binder in patients with chronic renal failure undergoing dialysis. *N Engl J Med* 1986;315:157.
188. Emmett M, Sirmon MD, Kirkpatrick WG, et al. Calcium acetate control of serum phosphorus in hemodialysis patients. *Am J Kidney Dis* 1991;17:544.
189. Mai ML, Emmett M, Sheikh MS, et al. Calcium acetate, an effective phosphorus binder in patients with renal failure. *Kidney Int* 1989;36:690.
190. Slatopolsky EA: Renagel, a nonabsorbed calcium- and aluminum-free phosphate binder, lowers serum phosphorus and parathyroid hormone. *Kidney Int* 1999;55:299.
191. Bleyer AJ, Burke SK, Dillon M. A comparison of the calcium-free phosphate binder sevelamer hydrochloride with calcium acetate in the treatment of hyperphosphatemia in hemodialysis patients. *Am J Kidney Dis* 1999;33:694.
192. Perl DP, Good PF. Uptake of aluminum into CNS along nasal-olfactory pathways. *Lancet* 1987;329:1028.
193. Rifat SL, Eastwood MR, McLachlan DRC, et al. Effect of exposure of miners to aluminum powder. *Lancet* 1990;336:1162.
194. Campbell IR, Cass JF, Cholak J. Aluminum in the environment of man. *AMA Arch Indust Health* 1957;15:359.
195. Good PF, Perl DP. A laser microprobe mass analysis study of aluminum distribution in the cerebral cortex of dialysis encephalopathy. *J Neuropathol Exp Neurol* 1988;47:321.
196. Banks WA, Kastin AJ. Aluminium increases permeability of the blood-brain barrier to labelled DSIP and b-endorphin: possible implications for senile and dialysis dementia. *Lancet* 1983;2:1227.
197. Wing AJ. Dialysis dementia in Europe: report from the registration committee of the EDTA. *Lancet* 1980;1:190.
198. Berkseth RO, Shapiro FL. An epidemic of dialysis encephalopathy and exposure to high aluminum dialysate. In: Schriener GE, Winchester JF, eds. *Controversies in nephrology.* Georgetown, MD: Georgetown University Press, 1980:42.
199. Arieff AI. Effects of water, acid base, and electrolyte disorders on the central nervous system. In: Arieff AI, DeFronzo RA, eds. *Fluid, electrolyte and acid-base disorders,* vol 2. New York: Churchill Livingstone, 1985:969.
200. Graf H, Stummvoll HK, Messinger V. Aluminum removal by hemodialysis. *Kidney Int* 1981;19:587.
201. Kaehny WD, Hegg AP, Alfrey AC. Gastrointestinal absorption of aluminum from aluminum-containing antacids. *N Engl J Med* 1977;296:1389.
202. Sedman AB, Wilkening GN, Warady BA. Encephalopathy in childhood secondary to aluminum intoxication. *J Pediatr* 1984;105:836.

203. Sedman AB, Klein GL, Merritt RJ, et al. Evidence of aluminum loading in infants receiving intravenous therapy. *N Engl J Med* 1985;312:1337.

204. Santos F, Massie MD, Chan JCM. Risk factors in aluminum toxicity in children with chronic renal failure. *Nephron* 1986;42:189.

205. Salusky IB, Foley J, Nelson P, et al. Aluminum accumulation during treatment with aluminum hydroxide and dialysis in children and young adults with chronic renal disease. *N Engl J Med* 1991;324:527.

206. Polinsky MS, Gruskin AB. Aluminum toxicity in childhood secondary to aluminum toxicity. *J Pediatr* 1984;105:758.

207. Andreoli SP, Bergstein JM, Sherrard DJ. Aluminum intoxication from aluminum-containing phosphate binders in children with azotemia not undergoing dialysis. *N Engl J Med* 1984;310:1079.

208. Perl DP, Brody AR. Alzheimer's disease: x-ray spectrometric evidence of aluminum accumulation in neurofibrillary tangle-bearing neurons. *Science* 1980;208:297.

209. Kogeorgos J, Scholtz C. Neurofibrillary tangles in aluminum encephalopathy: a new finding. *Neuropathol Appl Neurobiol* 1982;8:246.

210. Garruto RM, Fukatsu R, Yanagihara R, et al. Imaging of calcium and aluminum in neurofibrillary tangle-bearing neurons in parkinsonism-dementia of Guam. *Proc Natl Acad Sci USA* 1983;81:1875.

211. Candy JM, McArthur FK, Oakley AE, et al. Aluminum accumulation in relation to senile plaque and neurofibrillary tangle formation in the brains of patients with renal failure. *J Neurol Sci* 1992;107:210.

212. Katzman R. Alzheimer's disease. *N Engl J Med* 1986;314:964.

213. Berlyne GM, Ben-Ari J, Pest D. Hyperalbuminemia from aluminum resins in renal failure. *Lancet* 1970;2:494.

214. Mayor GH, Sprague SM, Hourani MR, et al. Parathyroid hormone-mediated aluminum deposition and egress in the rat. *Kidney Int* 1980;17:40.

214a. Mathew RJ, Rabin P, Stone WJ, et al. Regional cerebral blood flow in dialysis encephalopathy and primary degenerative dementia. *Kidney Int* 1985;28:64.

215. Cantin M, Genest J. The heart and the atrial natriuretic factor. *Endocrinol Rev* 1985;6:107.

216. Malluche HH, Smith AJ, Abreo K. The use of deferoxamine in the management of aluminum accumulation in bone in patients with renal failure. *N Engl J Med* 1984;311:140.

217. Smith JS. The investigation of dementia: results in 200 consecutive admissions. *Lancet* 1981;1:824.

218. Gajdusek DC. Hypothesis: interference with axonal transport of neurofilament as a common pathogenetic mechanism in certain diseases of the central nervous system. *N Engl J Med* 1985;312:714.

219. Selkoe DJ. Cerebral aging and dementia. In: Tyler HR, Dawson DM, eds. *Current neurology,* vol 1. Boston: Houghton Mifflin, 1978:360.

220. Arieff AI, Mahoney CA. Pathogenesis of dialysis encephalopathy. *Neurobehav Toxicol Teratol* 1983;5:641.

221. Farley PC, Kam-Yung L, Suba S. Severe hypernatremia in a patient with psychiatric illness. *Arch Intern Med* 1986;146:1214.

222. Kucharczyk W, Brant-Zawadzki M, Norman D. Magnetic resonance imaging of the central nervous system. An update. *West J Med* 1985;142:54.

223. Weber DL, Reagan T, Leeds M. Intracerebral hemorrhage during hemodialysis. *NY State J Med* 1972;72:1853.

224. Bleumle LW. Current status of chronic hemodialysis. *Am J Med* 1968;44:749.

225. Smith RJ, Block MR, Arieff AI, et al. Hypernatremic, hyperosmolar coma complicating chronic peritoneal dialysis. *Proc Clin Dialysis Trans Forum* 1974;4:96.

226. Arieff AI. CNS manifestations of disordered sodium metabolism. In: Morgan DB, ed. *Clinics in endocrinology and metabolism: electrolyte disorders,* vol 13. Philadelphia: WB Saunders, 1984:269.

227. Bolton CF. Electrophysiologic changes in uremic neuropathy after successful renal transplantation. *N Engl J Med* 1976;284:1170.

228. Anderson RJ, Schafer LA, Olin DB. Infectious risk factors in the immunosuppressed host. *Am J Med* 1973;54:453.

229. Iseki K, Kinjo K, Kimura Y, et al. Evidence for a high risk of cerebral hemorrhage in chronic dialysis patients. *Kidney Int* 1993;44:1086.

230. Iseki K, Fukiyama K. Predictors of stroke in patients receiving chronic hemodialysis. *Kidney Int* 1996;50:1672.

231. Mazzuchi N, Carbonell E, Fernandez-Caen J. Importance of blood pressure control in hemodialysis patient survival. *Kidney Int* 2000;50:2147.

232. Rostand SG, Branzell JD, Cannon RO, et al. Cardiovascular complications in renal failure. *J Am Soc Nephrol* 1991;2:1053.

233. Held P, Brunner F, Okada M, et al. Five year survival for end-stage renal disease patients in the USA, Europe and Japan, 1982–1987. *J Am Soc Nephrol* 1990;15:451.

234. Breyer JA. Medical management of nephropathy in type I diabetes mellitus. *J Am Soc Nephrol* 1995;6:1523.

235. Foley RN, Harnett JD, Parfrey PS. Cardiovascular complications of end-stage renal disease. In: Schrier RW, Gottschalk CW, eds. *Diseases of the kidney,* 6th ed, vol III. Boston: Little, Brown, 1997:2647.

236. Orth SR, Stockman A, Conradt C, et al. Smoking as a risk factor for end-stage renal failure in men with primary renal disease. *Kidney Int* 1998;54:926.

237. Bronner LL, Kanter DS, Manson JE. Primary prevention of stroke. *N Engl J Med* 1995;333:1392.

238. Ayus JC, Sheikh-Hamad D. Silent infection in clotted hemodialysis access grafts. *J Am Soc Nephrol* 1998;9:1314.

239. Zimmerman J, Herringer S, Pruy A. Inflammation enhances cardiovascular risk and mortality in hemodialysis patients. *Kidney Int* 1999;55:648.

240. Panichi V, Migliori M, dePietro S, et al. The link of biocompatibility to cytokine production. *Kidney Int* 2000;58:S96.

241. Ballou SP, Kushner I. C-reactive protein and the acute phase response. *Adv Intern Med* 1992;37:313.

242. Miyata T, Inagi R, Iida Y, et al. Involvement of B2-microglobulin modified with advanced glycation end products in the pathogenesis of hemodialysis-associated amyloidosis. *J Clin Invest* 1994;93:521.

243. Pertosa G, Grandaliano G, Gesualdo L, et al. Clinical relevance of cytokine production in hemodialysis. *Kidney Int* 2000;58:S104.

244. Lonnemann G, Linnenweber S, Burg M, et al. Transfer of endogenous pyrogens across artificial membranes? *Kidney Int* 1998;53:S43.

245. Sieberth HG, Kierdorf HP. Is cytokine removal by continuous hemofiltration feasible. *Kidney Int* 1999;56:S79.

246. Tetta C, Cavaillon JM, Camussi G, et al. Continuous plasma filtration coupled with sorbents. *Kidney Int* 1998;53:S186.

247. Ronco C, Brendolan A, Dan N. Adsorption in sepsis. *Kidney Int* 2000;58:S148.

248. Balakrishnan VSCHS, Jaber BL, Natov SN, et al. Interleukin-1 receptor antagonist synthesis by peripheral blood mononuclear cells: a novel predictor of morbidity among hemodialysis patients. *J Am Soc Nephrol* 2000;11:2114.

249. Lonnemann G. The quality of dialysate. *Kidney Int* 2000;58:S112.

250. Ayus JC, Arieff AI. The effect of dialysis dosage and reuse on mortality in hemodialysis patients. *J Am Soc Nephrol* 2000;11:225A.

251. Ueda Y, Goffin E, Yoshino A, et al. Effect of dwell time on carbonyl stress using icodextrin and amino acid peritoneal dialysis fluids. *Kidney Int* 2000;58:2518.

252. Brott T, Bogousslavsky J. Treatment of acute ischemic stroke. *N Engl J Med* 2000;343:710.

253. Coyle JT, Puttfarcken P. Oxidative stress, glutamate and neurodegenerative disorders. *Science* 1993;262:689.

254. Bonfoco E, Krainc M, Ankarcrona M, et al. Apoptosis and necrosis. *Proc Natl Acad Sci USA* 1995;92:7162.

255. Vexler ZS, Roberts TPL, Bollen AW, et al. Transient cerebral ischemia: association of apoptosis induction with hypoperfusion. *J Clin Invest* 1997;99:1453.

256. Kumar M, Liu GJ, Floyd RA, et al. Anoxic injury of endothelial cells increases production of nitric oxide and hydroxyl radicals. *Biochem Biophys Res Commun* 1996;219:497.

257. Kurose I, Wolf R, Grisham MH, et al. Microvascular responses to inhibition of nitric oxide production: role of active oxidants. *Circ Res* 1995;76:30.

258. Ankarcrona M, Dypbukt JM, Bonfoco E. Glutamate-induced neuronal death. *Neuron* 1995;15:961.

259. Collins RC, Dobkin BH, Choi DW. Selective vulnerability of the brain: new insights into the pathophysiology of stroke. *Ann Intern Med* 1989;110:992.

260. Lee JM, Grabb MC, Zipfel GJ, et al. Brain tissue responses to ischemia. *J Clin Invest* 2000;106:723.

261. ECACAS. Surgery was superior in asymptomatic patients with high-grade carotid stenosis. *JAMA* 1996;273:1421.

262. Lee TT, Solomon NA, Heidenreich PA, et al. Cost-effectiveness of screening for carotid stenosis in asymptomatic persons. *Ann Intern Med* 1997;126:337.

263. Amarenco P, Heinzlef O, Lucas C. Atherosclerotic disease of the aortic arch as a risk factor for recurrent ischemic stroke. *N Engl J Med* 1996;334:1216.

264. Nabulsi AA, Folsom AR, White A, et al. Association of hormone-replacement therapy with various cardiovascular risk factors in postmenopausal women. *N Engl J Med* 1993;328:1069.

265. Lieberman EH, Gerhard MD, Uehata A, et al. Estrogen improves endothelium-dependent, flow-mediated vasodilation in postmenopausal women. *Ann Intern Med* 1994;121:936.

266. Mendelsohn ME, Karas RH. The protective effects of estrogen on the cardiovascular system. *N Engl J Med* 1999;340:1801.

267. Sato M, Rippy MK, Bryant HU. Raloxifene, tamoxifen, nafoxidine, or estrogen effects on reproductive and nonreproductive tissues in ovariectomized rats. *FASEB J* 1996;10:905.

268. Parmley WW. Evolution of angiotensin-converting enzyme inhibition in hypertension, heart failure, and vascular protection. *Am J Med* 1998;105:27S.

269. ALLHAT. Major cardiovascular events in hypertensive patients randomized to doxazosin vs chlorthalidone. *JAMA* 2000;283:1967.

270. Yusuf S, Sleight P, Pogue J. Effects of an angiotensin-converting enzyme inhibitor, Ramipril, on cardiovascular events in high-risk patients. *N Engl J Med* 2000;342:145.

271. Gueyffier F, Boutitie F, Boissel JP, et al. Effect of antihypertensive drug treatment on cardiovascular outcomes in women and men. *Ann Intern Med* 1997;126:761.

272. Kucharczyk J, Mintorovitch J, Moseley ME, et al. Ischemic brain edema is reduced by a novel calcium and sodium channel entry blocker. *Radiology* 1991;179:221.

273. Kucharczyk J, Chew W, Derugin N, et al. Nicardipine reduces ischemic brain injury. An in vivo magnetic resonance imaging/spectroscopy study in cats. *Stroke* 1989;20:268.

274. Albers GW, Atkinson RP, Kelley RE, et al. Safety, tolerability and pharmacokinetics of the NMDA antagonist dextrorphan in patients with acute stroke. *Stroke* 1995;26:254.

275. Gress DR. Stroke: revolution in therapy. *Western J Med* 1994;161:288.

276. Alberts MJ, Lyden PD, Zivin JA, et al. Emergency brain resuscitation. *Ann Intern Med* 1995;122:622.

277. Parfrey PS, Griffiths SM, Barrett BJ, et al. Contrast material-induced renal failure in patients with diabetes mellitus, renal insufficiency, or both. A prospective controlled study. *N Engl J Med* 1989;320:143.

278. Study Group E. Thrombolytic therapy with streptokinase in acute ischemic stroke. *N Engl J Med* 1996;335:145.

279. Tissue plasminogen activator for acute ischemic stroke. The National Institute of Neurological Disorders and Stroke rt-PA Stroke Study Group. *N Engl J Med* 1995;333:1581.

280. del Zoppo GJ. Acute stroke-on the threshold of a therapy. *N Engl J Med* 1995;333:1632.

281. Sherman DG, Atkinson RP, Chippendale T. Intravenous ancrod for treatment of acute ischemic stroke. *JAMA* 2000;283:2395.

282. Yasuda H, Nakajima A. Brain protection against ischemic injury by nizofenone. *Cerebrovasc Brain Metabol Rev* 1993;5:264.

283. Frisoni GB, Anzola GP. Vertebrobasilar ischemia after neck motion. *Stroke* 1991;11:1452.

284. Schievink WI, Mokri B, O'Fallon WM. Recurrent spontaneous cervical-artery dissection. *N Engl J Med* 1994;330:393.

285. Mitiguy J. Ischemic stroke in young adults. *Headlines* 1993; July/Aug:2.

286. Droller MJ, Anderson JR, Beck JC. Impotence. *JAMA* 1993;270:83.

287. Palmer BF. Sexual dysfunction in uremia. *J Am Soc Nephrol* 1999;10:1381.

288. Campese VM, Romoff MS, Levitan D. Mechanisms of autonomic nervous system dysfunction in uremia. *Kidney Int* 1981;20:246.

289. Abdel-Gawad M, Huynh H, Brock GB. Experimental chronic renal failure-associated erectile dysfunction: molecular alterations in nitric oxide synthetase pathway and IGF-I system. *Mol Urol* 1999;3:117.

290. Massry SG, Smogorzewski MJ, Klahr S. Metabolic and endocrine dysfunctions in uremia. In: Schrier RW, Gottschalk CW, eds. *Diseases of the kidney,* 6th ed, vol III. Boston: Little, Brown, 1997:2661.

291. Massry SG, Bellinghieri G. Metabolic and endocrine disturbances in uremia: sexual dysfunction. In: Massry SG, Glassock RJ, eds. *Textbook of nephrology,* 3rd ed, vol 2. Baltimore: Williams & Wilkins, 1995:1416.

292. Lamberts SWJ, van den Beld AW, van der Lely A. The endocrinology of aging. *Science* 1997;278:419.

293. Campese VM, Liu CL. Sexual dysfunction in uremia. *Contrib Nephrol* 1990;77:1.

294. Rostand SG, Brown G, Kirk KA, et al. Renal insufficiency in treated hypertension. *N Engl J Med* 1989;320:684.

295. Leland J. A pill for impotence? *Newsweek* 1997;Nov 17:62.

296. Nathan HP, Hellstrom WJG, Kaiser FE. Treatment of men with erectile dysfunction with transurethral alprostadil. *N Engl J Med* 1997;336:1.

297. Herrmann HC, Chang G, Klugherz BD, et al. Hemodynamic effects of sildenafil in men with severe coronary artery disease. *N Engl J Med* 2000;342:1622.

298. Utiger RD. A pill for impotence. *N Engl J Med* 1998;338:1458.

299. Nielsen VK. The peripheral nerve function in chronic renal failure. VI. *Acta Med Scand* 1973;194:455.

300. Raskin NH, Fishman RA. Neurologic disorders in renal failure. *N Engl J Med* 1976;294:143.

301. Fernandez JP, McGinn JT, Hoffman RS. Cerebral edema from blood-brain glucose differences complicating peritoneal dialysis second membrane syndrome. *NY State J Med* 1968;68:677.

302. Schneck SA. Neuropathological features of human organ transplantation 1. *J Neuropathol Exp Neurol* 1965;24:415.

303. Spencer PS, Schaumberg HH. Central peripheral distal axonopathy. The pathology of "dying-back" polyneuropathies. *Prog Neuropathol* 1977;3:255.

304. Thomas PK, Hollinrake K, Lascelles RG. The polyneuropathy of chronic renal failure. *Brain* 1971;94:761.

305. Spencer PS, Sabri MI, Schaumberg HH. Does a defect of energy metabolism in the nerve fiber underlie axonal degeneration in polyneuropathies? *Ann Neurol* 1979;5:501.

306. Massry SG. Is parathyroid hormone a uremic toxin? *Nephrology* 1977;19:125.

307. Andress DL, Sherrard DJ. The osteodystrophy of chronic renal failure. In: Schrier RW, Gottschalk CW, eds. *Diseases of the kidney,* 6th ed, vol III. Boston: Little, Brown, 1997:2597.

CHAPTER 94

Cardiac Disease in Chronic Renal Disease

Sean W. Murphy, Claudio Rigatto, and Patrick S. Parfrey

End-stage renal disease (ESRD) and cardiovascular disease have been inextricably linked since the earliest days of chronic dialysis. Clyde Shields, the first patient on long-term dialysis, died of myocardial infarction (MI) in 1970, aged 50 years, 11 years after starting hemodialysis (1). Several statistics accrued since that time attest to the impact of cardiovascular disease in renal patients. Approximately one-half of all deaths in patients with ESRD are attributable to cardiovascular disease, a proportion that is remarkably similar throughout the world (2–10). The annual incidence of MI or angina requiring hospitalization among patients on hemodialysis is 8%, and that of heart failure requiring hospitalization or treatment with ultrafiltration is 10% (11). Among patients starting maintenance dialysis, approximately 80% exhibit left ventricular hypertrophy (LVH) or systolic dysfunction disorders that are predictive of congestive heart failure (CHF), ischemic heart disease (IHD) and death (12). This high prevalence of LV abnormalities pertains to patients receiving renal transplants as well (13). Furthermore, this rate of cardiovascular death in patients on dialysis is substantially higher than that of the general population at all age groups, particularly in the younger group (Fig. 94-1).

Several factors are thought to contribute to this high burden of cardiac disease in chronic renal disease. First, the prevalence of many traditional risk factors for cardiovascular disease and death, such as diabetes and hypertension, is higher among patients with renal disease than in the general population. Second, several metabolic and hemodynamic disturbances that occur and progress in relation to declining renal function may modify cardiovascular risk. There is growing evidence that these uremia-related risk factors (e.g., anemia, hyperhomocysteinemia, hypoalbuminemia, divalent ion abnormalities, oxidative stress) contribute to the excess

burden of cardiovascular disease in renal patients. Finally, it has become clear that cardiovascular disorders arise early in chronic renal insufficiency (CRI), progress during dialysis, and may partially regress subsequent to transplantation, only to progress again as the allograft fails. The burden and relative importance of traditional and uremia-related cardiac risk factors likely evolve parallel to these phases of renal disease as well.

In this chapter, we discuss the pathogenesis, risk factors, and treatment of IHD and disorders of LV geometry and function. As demonstrated in Fig. 94-2, IHD may result from critical coronary artery disease (CAD) or nonatherosclerotic disease and is associated with cardiomyopathy; heart failure (the major manifestation of pump dysfunction) results from ischemic disease or cardiomyopathy, and cardiomyopathy may be the result of concentric LVH, LV dilation, or systolic dysfunction. Emphasis is placed where possible on direct evidence obtained in epidemiologic studies of clinically relevant populations. Where the data permit, differences in clinical profile, risk factors, and treatment during CRI, dialysis, and transplantation are highlighted. The topic of cardiovascular disease in renal failure is in ferment and many questions, particularly those regarding treatment, cannot be answered definitively because adequate studies are lacking. Where reasonable, these gaps are filled by extrapolation from nonrenal populations.

ISCHEMIC HEART DISEASE

Pathogenesis

Symptomatic myocardial ischemia usually results from flow-limiting critical coronary atherosclerotic disease, but may be present in the absence of significant angiographic CAD in approximately 25% of patients (14–16) (Fig. 94-3). In the latter case, small vessel disease or a decrease in myocardial capillary density consequent to LVH or fibrosis may be the culprits (17–20). LVH itself may predispose to ischemia.

In nonrenal failure populations, the initiating event of atherosclerosis appears to be endothelial injury caused by

S. W. Murphy and P. S. Parfrey: Departments of Medicine, Memorial University of Newfoundland and The Health Sciences Centre, St. John's, Newfoundland, Canada

C. Rigatto: Faculty of Medicine, University of Manitoba; and Section of Nephrology, St. Boniface General Hospital, Winnipeg, Manitoba, Canada

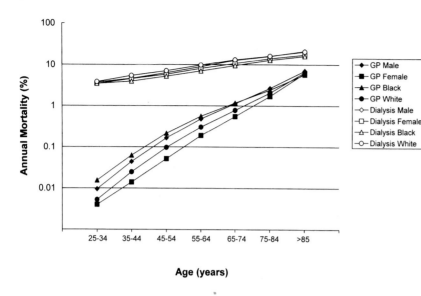

FIG. 94-1. Annual cardiovascular mortality by age group in the general population and in patients on dialysis. (From Foley RN, Parfrey PS, Sarnak MJ. Epidemiology of cardiovascular disease in chronic renal disease. *J Am Soc Nephrol* 1998;9:S16, with permission.)

mechanical stress (e.g., hypertension) or endothelial toxins (nicotine, oxidative stress, hyperlipidemia, and inflammation) that alter the endothelial phenotype to a more permeable, procoagulant state (21). Endothelial denudation or, more commonly, alterations in cell surface receptor expression permit access of lipoproteins and macrophages into the subintimal space (21,22). Oxidative modification of lipoproteins, particularly low-density lipoprotein (ox-LDL), is chemotactic for macrophages and facilitates uptake of oxidized lipids by macrophages, resulting in formation of foam cells (23). Ox-LDL stimulates elaboration of growth factors that are mitogenic for smooth muscle and profibrotic (24). These processes result in the accumulation of oxidatively modified lipids and inflammatory cells at the center of a fibrous "cap" of variable thickness. This cap may rupture, causing subocclusive thromboses that may be minimally symptomatic or associated with acute coronary syndromes (e.g., unstable angina, MI). These thrombi eventually become organized in the wall of the vessel. Calcific

deposits may develop. The mature atheroma thus may contain, in addition to lipids, inflammatory cells, collagen, organized thrombus, and calcium (25). The propensity for rupture varies with the composition of the atheroma. Lipid- and inflammatory cell–rich atheromas with thin fibrous caps are thought to be more unstable than those with a greater degree of fibrosis and less lipid (26). The presence of calcium by electron beam tomography correlates with advanced atherosclerosis and appears to be more prevalent in patients with ESRD (27,28).

Theoretically, renal failure can modify this process at multiple levels. Hypertension and flow overload may increase stresses on the vascular wall. In many patients on dialysis, a prooxidant and chronic inflammatory state pertains, and both may contribute to endothelial dysfunction (29). Hyperhomocysteinemia may promote endothelial activation and thrombosis by mechanisms that are yet unclear (30,31).

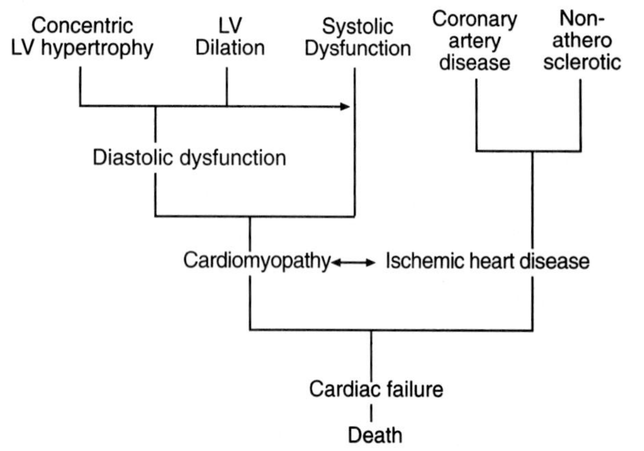

FIG. 94-2. Cardiomyopathy and ischemic heart disease in chronic uremia.

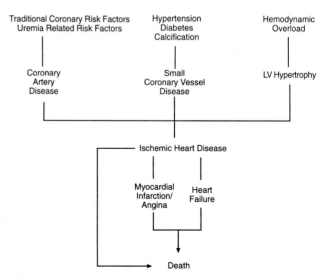

FIG. 94-3. The etiology of ischemic heart disease in chronic uremia.

Hyperparathyroidism may promote vascular calcification and medial hypertrophy (29).

In the absence of flow-limiting CAD, ischemic symptoms may result from a reduction in coronary vasodilator reserve and altered myocardial oxygen delivery. Intracoronary ultrasonography has shown that angiographically normal vessel segments may contain areas of nonencroaching atheroma. Endothelial function is impaired in these vessels and may reduce coronary vasodilator reserve (i.e., the ability of the vessel to dilate above baseline) in response to increased myocardial oxygen demand (32). Vasodilator reserve is clearly impaired in vessels with lumen-encroaching disease (33). The resulting mismatch of supply and demand may give rise to symptomatic ischemia.

Small vessel disease may occur in LVH and diabetes, and because of uremia *per se*. In LVH, small vessel smooth muscle hypertrophy and endothelial abnormalities can diminish coronary reserve. Diabetes may be associated with microvascular disease characterized by endothelial proliferation, subendothelial fibrosis, and exudative deposits of hyaline in the intima (34). In uremic rats, LVH is associated with a severe reduction in myocardial capillary density compared with hypertensive rats matched for weight and blood pressure (19). Small vessel calcification may impair coronary reserve; an association between elevated $Ca \times PO_4$ product and CAD has been reported (35).

Dysregulation of energy metabolism in the myocyte may increase cellular susceptibility to ischemia. A reduced myocardial phosphocreatine–adenosine triphosphate ratio under stress has been observed in uremic animals (36). Hyperparathyroidism may play a critical role in the dysregulation of cellular energetics, and may thus exacerbate ischemic damage to the myocardium (37).

Diagnosis

Symptoms of myocardial ischemia in patients with CRI are in general similar to those in the nonuremic population. However, the prevalence of silent myocardial ischemia in this group of patients is very high (38,39). This has been best demonstrated in diabetic patients with ESRD because they often are subjected to screening coronary angiography before renal transplantation. In one series of 100 diabetic patients with ESRD, for example, 75% of the patients with angiographically demonstrated CAD had no typical angina symptoms (40). The prevalence of asymptomatic CAD in nondiabetic patients with ESRD is not as well studied. Patients with CRI and symptomatic IHD should be investigated in a manner similar to patients with normal renal function, provided that revascularization be undertaken should critical CAD be identified. In the general population, there is some suggestion that silent ischemia might lead to an increased mortality rate (41). There is no evidence, however, that revascularization of such patients prolongs their survival. Routine screening for CAD in asymptomatic patients with CRI therefore is not recommended (42). Several organizations have issued clinical practice guidelines for screening patients before noncardiac surgery (43,44), and it is appropriate to apply these to the CRI population as well. These groups recommend screening before surgery when the combination of risk factors and the nature of the operation put the patient at moderate or higher risk of a cardiovascular event. Patients being evaluated for renal transplantation are an exception to the aforementioned recommendations. The adverse prognostic implications of CAD, the desire to avoid allograft injury from posttransplantation invasive cardiac testing, and the need to ration transplantable organs are justification for screening all but the lowest-risk patients. The American Society of Transplant Physicians has published guidelines for the evaluation of renal transplantation candidates that include recommendations for the investigation of CAD (45).

Noninvasive Testing for Coronary Artery Disease

Exercise electrocardiography has been the traditional method of noninvasive diagnosis of CAD. The sensitivity of this test is only 50% to 60% for single-vessel disease but is greater than 85% for triple-vessel CAD in the general population (46). These figures are based on the assumption that the patient reaches an adequate exercise level (i.e., 85% of the age-adjusted predicted maximal heart rate). A large proportion of patients with ESRD are unable to achieve this target because of poor exercise tolerance or the use of cardiac medications. One study of 85 diabetic uremic patients showed that only 6 achieved an adequate exercise level (47). In another study, only 12 of 60 diabetic patients with ESRD achieved target heart rates (48). Pharmacologic agents therefore often are used for noninvasive testing for CAD in these patients. The sensitivity of dipyridamole-thallium testing in patients with ESRD ranges from 37% to 86%, with a specificity of approximately 75% (49–51). Dobutamine stress echocardiography may be the method of choice where it is available because the reported sensitivity in patients with CRF is relatively high at 69% to 95%, with a specificity of approximately 95% (52–54).

Coronary Angiography

Cardiac catheterization and coronary angiography remain the gold standard for the diagnosis of CAD. A major disadvantage associated with this mode of investigation is the potential for renal toxicity from radiocontrast agents. CRI, especially in diabetic patients, is a major risk factor for contrast-induced acute renal failure (55). The risk of clinical nephrotoxicity is related to the severity of prior renal impairment. Administration of contrast during coronary angiography may precipitate ESRD in patients with severe impairment in renal function at baseline. The risk of contrast nephropathy in high-risk patients may be reduced by using nonionic contrast media and by saline infusion (55).

Burden of Disease

The prevalence and incidence of IHD and cardiovascular death among patients with mild to moderate renal failure are not well studied but may approach those seen in ESRD (56). In a small prospective study in France, age-adjusted annual incidence of MI or ischemic stroke was three times that in the general population (57). In the Modification of Diet in Renal Disease (MDRD) Study of nondiabetic CRI, the annual incidence of first hospitalizations for cardiovascular disease was 3% (58). In a study of the effect of the angiotensin-converting enzyme (ACE) inhibitor benazepril on the progression of renal disease, the combined annual incidence of sudden cardiac death or fatal or nonfatal MI was 1% (59). Because these data are drawn from clinical trial inductees, they likely represent conservative estimates of the true event rates (60).

In Canada, by the time patients reach ESRD, the prevalence of CAD approaches 40%; approximately 22% have angina pectoris, whereas 18% have had a prior MI (4). The annual incidence of angina or MI among Canadian patients on hemodialysis is 10% (11). MI is the cause of death in approximately 14% of patients on dialysis in the United States (2).

Among renal transplant recipients (RTR), the overall prevalence of CAD is approximately 15% (61). The annual incidence of MI, revascularization, or death from MI among RTR is 1.5% (62).

Risk Factors

Although experimental studies in animal models and cross-sectional or case-control studies in small groups of patients can lend insight into the mechanisms of IHD in renal failure, only large, rigorous, prospective studies in relevant clinical populations can identify widely generalizeable risk factors for cardiovascular disease. The Framingham Study (63) is the archetypal population-based cohort study in the field of cardiovascular disease, and the risk factors identified by it have been widely vindicated in subsequent intervention trials on blood pressure control and cholesterol reduction (64–66). Unfortunately, few large, adequately designed prospective cohort studies on cardiovascular outcomes have been performed in renal failure populations (67). An analysis of risk factors for cardiovascular disease in renal failure must of necessity include data from retrospective cohorts, national registries, and cross-sectional and case-control studies that, in declining order of reliability, provide less conclusive information.

Nonmodifiable Risk Factors

Age

Advancing age is associated with an increased risk of IHD in the general population (63,68). Older age has been independently associated with arteriographic CAD (16), *de novo*

occurrence of angina pectoris, MI, or coronary revascularization in patients on dialysis [relative risk (RR) 1.6 per decade] (67), and increased risk of death among patients on dialysis (4). Little is known about the impact of age in the CRI population, but because this group is intermediate between the general population and the ESRD population in terms of renal function, age is likely a risk factor as well.

Among RTR, age is an independent risk factor for MI or coronary revascularization or death from MI (RR 1.5 per decade) (62), and for all-cause death (RR 1.5 per decade) (69).

Diabetes Mellitus

Diabetes is an independent risk factor (RR 1.5 to 2.2) for the development of CAD in the general population (70–74). The link with IHD events in the CRI population has not been explicitly studied but is probably intermediate between the general population and patients on dialysis. Among patients on dialysis, diabetes is independently associated with the development of *de novo* IHD and death (adjusted RR 3.98 and 3.86, respectively) (67–69). Among RTR, diabetes is strongly associated with multiple cardiovascular outcomes (RR of 2.09 for MI, revascularization, or death from MI; RR of 2.98 for ischemic stroke; and RR of 25.7 for development of peripheral vascular disease) (62).

The impact of diabetes in all renal populations may well be underestimated. Angiographic studies in asymptomatic diabetic patients on dialysis show that approximately one-third have at least one coronary artery stenosis of 50% or greater (38). Among asymptomatic diabetic patients referred for renal transplantation, 88% of those older than 45 years had significant coronary stenosis (75).

Modifiable Risk Factors

Hypertension

Hypertension is a long-established risk factor for IHD in the general population (76,77). Pharmacologic therapy of hypertension reduces the risk of MI by 14% to 16% for each 6 mm Hg reduction in diastolic blood pressure (78,79).

The prevalence of hypertension in patients with CRI is approximately 80% and varies with the cause of renal disease. In the MDRD Study, although 91% of patients were treated with antihypertensive agents, only 54% had blood pressures of 140/90 mm Hg or less (80). Unfortunately, no studies to date have directly assessed the role of hypertension in the evolution of IHD in CRI. Levin et al. have shown that hypertension is associated with the development and progression of LVH in patients with CRI (81). Because LVH is independently associated with IHD in the general population (RR 3.0 in men with LVH, 4.6 in women) (74) and in patients on dialysis (RR 5.9 for concentric, 5.35 for eccentric LVH) (67), by inference it also should be associated with cardiovascular events in CRI. This is indirect reasoning; observational and experimental studies of IHD in CRI are badly needed. The need is particularly acute when one considers that the high burden of IHD among patients with ESRD likely originated or progressed during the CRI phase.

The link between hypertension and IHD or mortality among patients on dialysis is complex. Studies have shown an inverse relationship between blood pressure and mortality, with hypertension predicting longer survival (67–82). However, the high prevalence of cardiac disease at the start of ESRD therapy is a confounding issue even for well executed, prospective cohort studies. Because cardiac dysfunction can cause low blood pressure (so-called reverse causality) and is independently associated with death, even prospective studies cannot exclude the possibility that low blood pressure is simply a surrogate marker for poor pump function, unless patients with cardiac abnormalities at baseline are excluded from analysis. This is difficult to do in practice because most (75% to 80%) patients have echocardiographic abnormalities at the start of maintenance dialysis. In one prospective cohort study of 433 patients on dialysis, high blood pressure was positively associated with the development if IHD and LVH but negatively associated with mortality (83). In this same cohort, LVH was predictive of CHF, which in turn was associated both with mortality and with a drop in mean arterial pressure. Lower mean arterial pressure after an episode of CHF was independently associated with mortality. These observations suggest, but do not prove, the following causal sequence:

$$\text{Hypertension} \rightarrow \text{IHD and LVH} \rightarrow$$

$$\text{pump failure} \rightarrow \text{hypotension and death}$$

Although definitive proof for this chain of events still is lacking, the authors believe that hypertension is deleterious in patients on dialysis, as it is in the general population.

The prevalence of hypertension among RTR is 70% to 80% (62). Elevated blood pressure has been associated with shortened graft and patient survival, as well as higher rates of CAD (2,84). However, retrospective analyses of large transplant cohorts have not found an association between hypertension and mortality after adjustment for age, diabetes, tobacco use, and time on dialysis before transplantation (62,85).

Clearly, further study is needed of the hypertension/IHD link, particularly in CRI and RTR populations, where the prevalence of IHD at baseline is lower and confounding by "reverse causality" less likely, and thus causal relationships more reliably discerned. In the interim, on the basis of strong biologic rationale, robust evidence in the general population, and strong evidence in renal disease populations for hypertension as a risk factor for LVH and IHD, hypertension should be considered a risk factor for IHD in patients with renal failure.

Smoking

Smoking is a powerful risk factor for IHD in the general population, approximately doubling the risk of cardiovascular events in the Framingham cohort (86). Smoking cessation can reduce the risk of IHD by 50% even in longtime heavy smokers (87).

The impact of smoking in patients with CRI has not been well studied. It has been associated with thrombotic stroke in one prospective study (57). In ESRD, approximately 30% to 40% of patients starting dialysis are smokers (11,67), and smoking has been associated with an excess mortality rate of 26% in incident patients on hemodialysis, even after extensive covariate adjustment (2).

Among RTR, 25% to 40% smoke at the time of transplant assessment and, despite admonitions to quit, most continue to smoke after transplantation (88–90). A smoking exposure of 10 to 25 pack-years has been independently associated with ischemic stroke (RR 1.2 to 1.6), peripheral vascular disease (RR 1.2 to 1.6), and death (RR 1.4 to 2.0) (62,88,89).

Dyslipidemia

Elevated total cholesterol (TC), LDL-C, lipoprotein(a) [Lp(a)], and triglycerides (TG) and low high-density lipoprotein (HDL-C) are associated with IHD in the general population, and the efficacy of targeted LDL-C lowering with HMG-CoA reductase inhibitors has been established by clinical trials (66,91–95). An atherogenic lipid profile is highly prevalent in patients with renal disease (Table 94-1), particularly in patients with nephrotic syndrome (96).

With respect to clinical outcomes, there are yet no data linking hypercholesterolemia to cardiovascular disease in CRI. Among patients on dialysis, the data are conflicting. The highest mortality risk appears to be associated with low, not high cholesterol (97). However, low TC is strongly correlated with poor nutritional status and low albumin levels, both of which are associated with increased mortality risk. It therefore is unclear whether low TC is causally related to death, or is a marker for malnutrition, hypoalbuminemia, or other, yet unknown factors associated with death. Although definitive data are lacking, it is biologically plausible that high TC and LDL-C are risk factors in adequately nourished patients on dialysis, as they are in the general population.

Lipoprotein(a) deserves special consideration because it is elevated in patients on dialysis and, unlike TC and LDL-C, has been prospectively and independently associated with IHD and death (98,99). However, in both renal and nonrenal disease populations, total experience with Lp(a) as a risk stratification tool is still limited and clinical intervention trials with IHD endpoints are nonexistent. Ongoing studies may address these concerns (100).

In RTR, hypercholesterolemia (61,101) and low HDL (62) have been linked to ischemic events.

TABLE 94-1. *Estimated prevalence (%) of lipoprotein abnormalities in renal disease*

Category	TC >240 mg/dL	LDL-C >130	HDL-C <35	TG >200	Lp(a) >30
General population	20	40	15	15	15
Dialysis					
Hemodialysis	20	30	50	45	30
Peritoneal dialysis	25	45	20	50	50
Chronic renal insufficiency					
Nephrotic	90	85	50	60	60
Nonnephrotic	30	10	35	40	45
Renal transplant recipients	60	60	15	35	25

TC, total cholesterol; *LDL-C,* low-density lipoprotein; *HDL-C,* high-density lipoprotein; *TG,* triglycerides; *Lp(a),* lipoprotein (a). Adapted from Kasiske B. Hyperlipidemia in patients with chronic renal disease. *Am J Kidney Dis* 1998;32:S142.

Homocysteine

Homocysteine (Hcy) is a byproduct of methionine metabolism, a sulfhydryl-containing essential amino acid, and lies at the junction of two metabolic pathways, trans-sulfuration and remethylation. The rate of Hcy elimination by both pathways depends on an adequate supply of B vitamin cofactors, particularly B_{12} and folate. An association between Hcy and cardiovascular disease was first suggested by observations that patients with homocysteinuria, a rare genetic disorder, have marked elevations in serum Hcy and markedly accelerated rates of atherosclerosis. More recently, several large observational studies have shown that variations in Hcy levels in the general population are independently associated with cardiovascular disease (102–104). Although the epidemiologic link is strong, there is yet no clinical trial evidence that reducing Hcy levels will reduce cardiovascular event rates in the general population.

Progressive renal failure is associated with increasing Hcy levels: 83% of patients have Hcy levels above the 90th percentile for the general population by the time they reach ESRD (105). Cross-sectional studies of the association between Hcy and cardiovascular disease in patients on dialysis have yielded conflicting results (105). Two small, prospective studies have found an association between Hcy and combined cardiovascular endpoints (106,107). Total numbers were small, limiting the generalizability of these results. Moreover, extensive multivariate adjustment was not possible, so the independence of the Hcy effect from other cardiovascular risk factors in patients on dialysis remains to be established. Limited prospective data in RTR and CRI suggest that Hcy may be an independent risk factor in these populations as well (108,109).

High-dose folate supplementation (15 mg/day) reduces Hcy levels in ESRD by 25% to 30%, but cannot normalize levels in most patients. In RTR, combination therapy with vitamins B_6 and B_{12} and folate normalized Hcy in most patients in one small study (110). Data in CRI are lacking. As yet, no clinical trials in renal patients have been performed to assess whether high-dose folate therapy, with or without vitamin B_6 or B_{12}, reduces cardiovascular events.

Other Risk Factors

Hypocalcemia has been associated independently with excess mortality in cross-sectional analyses of patients on dialysis (97) and with *de novo* development of IHD in an inception cohort of Canadian patients on dialysis (111). The pathogenetic mechanism is unclear but may relate to an association with hyperparathyroidism, which itself is associated with lipid disturbances, LVH, myocardial fibrosis, and impaired cellular bioenergetics, all of which may cause or exacerbate ischemia or cardiomyocyte death (37,112,113). Chronic endothelial activation or injury, activation of prothrombotic factors, oxidative stress, chronic inflammation, and advanced glycosylation end products all may contribute to cardiovascular risk (29,114–116).

Outcome

Registry and retrospective cohort data show that presence of IHD in patients starting dialysis is associated with excess short- and long-term mortality rates (2,6). In a Canadian prospective cohort study, patients with clinical IHD at the start of dialysis were more likely to have an admission for CHF (RR 1.7) or to die (RR 1.5) than patients free of IHD at baseline, after adjustment for age and diabetes (67). In these patients, most of the excess mortality associated with IHD seemed to be through the development of CHF. In diabetic RTR, presence of IHD is associated with a fourfold risk of future events and death (75).

LEFT VENTRICULAR HYPERTROPHY AND SYSTOLIC DYSFUNCTION

Diagnosis

Because echocardiography is widely available, simple, and reproducible, it has become the method of choice for assessment of LVH (117–119). Systolic dysfunction is defined as an ejection fraction of less than 40%, indicating impaired myocardial contractility. It often is associated with LV dilatation (LV end-diastolic diameter $\geq$ 5.6 cm), defined echocardiographically as LV cavity volume index greater than

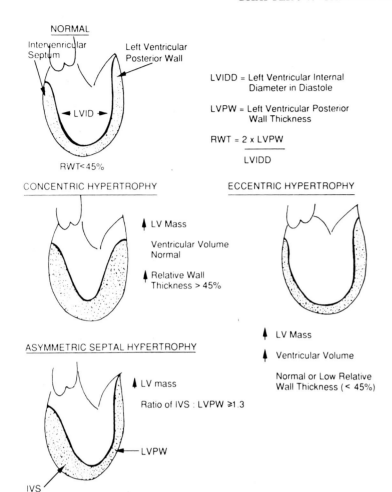

LVIDD = Left Ventricular Internal
Diameter in Diastole

LVPW = Left Ventricular Posterior
Wall Thickness

$$RWT = \frac{2 \times LVPW}{LVIDD}$$

FIG. 94-4. Patterns of left ventricular hypertrophy on echocardiography.

90 mL/m² (117). Concentric LVH is characterized by a thickened LV wall (≥1.2 cm during diastole) with normal cavity volume. LV mass index is a calculated parameter that reflects the degree of muscular hypertrophy in the LV. Epidemiologic studies in nonrenal patients have established that the upper limits of LV mass index are 130 g/m² for adult men and 102 g/m² for adult women (120). Values above these limits indicate hypertrophy. The patterns of LVH on echocardiography are shown in Fig. 94-4.

The calculation of LV mass and volume are not independent of volume status. As a result, the patient should be as close as possible to a "dry weight." In patients on hemodialysis, it is important to standardize the time and conditions of the study in relation to the dialysis session. Echocardiograms in these patients probably should be obtained the day after the dialysis session, with the patient at dry weight or at most 1 kg above it.

Pathogenesis

Ventricular growth occurs in response to mechanical stresses, primarily volume or pressure overload (121) (Fig. 94-5). Volume overload results in addition of new sarcomeres in series, leading to increased cavity diameter (122). A larger diameter results in increased wall tension, a direct consequence of Laplace's law, which states that wall tension (T) is proportional to the product of intraventricular pressure (P) times the ventricular diameter (D): in symbols, T = PD/4. An increase in wall tension secondarily stimulates the addition of new sarcomeres in parallel. This remodeling thickens the ventricular wall, distributing the tension over a larger cross-sectional area of muscle and returning the tension in each individual fiber back to normal, alleviating the stimulus to further hypertrophy. This combination of cavity enlargement and wall thickening is called *eccentric hypertrophy*. Pressure overload increases wall tension by increasing intraventricular pressure, resulting directly in the parallel addition of new sarcomeres and its functional consequences as described. Because sarcomeres are not added in series, isolated pressure overload does not lead to cavity enlargement (concentric hypertrophy).

Both eccentric and concentric hypertrophies are initially beneficial. Dilatation permits an increase in stroke volume without an increase in the inotropic state of the myocardium and as such is an efficient adaptation to volume overload (123). It also permits the maintenance of a normal stroke volume and cardiac output in the presence of *decreased* contractility. Muscular hypertrophy returns the tension per unit muscle fibre back to normal, decreasing ventricular stress.

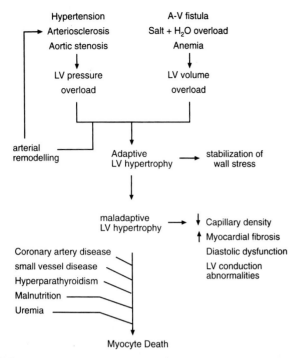

FIG. 94-5. The etiology of myocyte death in chronic uremia.

Ultimately, however, LVH becomes maladaptive. Muscular hypertrophy is associated with several progressive, deleterious changes in cell function and tissue architecture. Early in the evolution of LVH, slow reuptake of calcium by the sarcoplasmic reticulum leads to abnormal ventricular relaxation. Combined with decreased passive compliance of a thickened ventricular wall, these changes may precipitate diastolic dysfunction (124). More advanced sarcoplasmic reticulum dysfunction is associated with calcium overload and cell death. Decreased capillary density, impaired coronary reserve, and abnormal relaxation may decrease subendocardial perfusion, promoting ischemia (125). Frequent coexistence of CAD may exacerbate ischemia and myocyte attrition (121). Fibrosis of the cardiac interstitium also occurs (126) and appears to be more marked in pressure than volume overload. Myocyte apoptosis, ischemia, and neurohormonal activation (e.g., increased catecholamines, angiotensin II, aldosterone) are thought to contribute to myocardial dysfunction (123,127,128). In the late phases of chronic and sustained overload, oxidative stress is prominent and contributes to cellular dysfunction and demise (129). Together, these various processes lead to progressive cellular attrition, fibrosis, pump failure, and, ultimately, death.

The uremic milieu of chronic renal disease can potentiate many of these processes. Anemia, salt and water excess, and arteriovenous fistulae in patients on dialysis are prevalent causes of volume overload, whereas hypertension is a major cause of pressure overload. These disturbances are probably the primary stimuli to ventricular remodeling in uremia. These same stimuli promote arterial remodeling in the large and resistance arteries, characterized by diffuse arterial thick-

ening and stiffening (arteriosclerosis), which can increase the effective load on the left ventricle independently of mean arterial pressure (129,130). Secondary hyperparathyroidism may be associated with aortic valve calcification and in some cases stenosis, a less frequent cause of pressure overload (131).

The attrition of myocytes in chronic uremia may be exacerbated by several factors. Underlying CAD promotes ischemia and infarction. Hyperparathyroidim increases susceptibility to ischemia through dysregulation of cellular energy metabolism (37), and appears to promote myocardial fibrosis directly (132). Clinical studies have shown that the extent of myocardial fibrosis in patients with ESRD is more marked than in patients with diabetes mellitus or essential hypertension with similar LV mass (133). Malnutrition, oxidative stress, and inadequate dialysis may all additionally promote myocyte death (29,121,134). Such cell death in the presence of LVH and continuing pressure and volume overload may be catastrophic, leading to a severe "overload cardiomyopathy" and, ultimately, death (135).

Burden of Disease

Disorders of LV geometry begin well before the initiation of dialysis. In a cross-sectional study conducted by Greaves and coworkers, patients with CRI (serum creatinine >3.4 mg/dL) had a mean LV mass index of 120 g/m², which was intermediate between that of sex- and age-matched control subjects (79 g/m²) and patients on dialysis (136 g/m²) (136). An abnormal echocardiogram, primarily LVH, was observed in 63% of patients with CRI, versus 72% of patients on dialysis, suggesting a relationship between LV morphology and worsening renal function. Levin et al. have reported a prevalence of LVH of 26.7% in patients with a creatinine clearance rate greater than 50 mL/minute, 30.8% in those with clearances of 25 to 49 mL/minute, and 45.2% in those with clearances less than 25 mL/minute (137). In the prospective arm of this study, an association between rising LV mass index and falling glomerular filtration rate was observed. Another cross-sectional study has yielded comparable results (138). The overall prevalence of LVH among patients beginning dialysis is 75% (139–142). In a large prospective cohort study, only 16% had normal echocardiograms at inception. Fifteen percent (15%) had systolic dysfunction, 28% had dilatation with preserved contractility, and 41% had concentric LVH (134). In a subset of patients on dialysis who underwent yearly consecutive echocardiograms, LV mass index and LV cavity volume progressively increased, the biggest increase occurring between baseline and 1 year (143).

In patients about to undergo transplantation, the distribution of echocardiographic abnormalities is similar to those in patients on dialysis: normal 17%, concentric LVH 41%, dilatation 32%, and systolic dysfunction 12% (144). In one longitudinal study, the proportion of patients with normal studies doubled (36%) and systolic function normalized in all patients with fractional shortening of less than 25% 1 year posttransplantation (144).

Risk Factors

Nonmodifiable Risk Factors

Age

As with IHD, age is an important clinical marker of risk for LVH in the general, CRI, ESRD, and transplant populations (120,137,145,146).

Sex

The role of sex as a risk factor for LVH and systolic dysfunction is less clear. In a registry-based study, women were found to be more likely to have radiographic cardiomegaly or a history of CHF and less likely to exhibit electrocardiographic or echocardiographic evidence of LVH than men (147). In contrast to this result, a large prospective cohort study of patients beginning dialysis found no relationship between sex and development of heart failure. Moreover, female sex was associated with concentric LVH, whereas male sex was predictive of LV dilatation and CHF (148). These contradictory findings may relate to differences in sample size, design, and criteria for LV geometry.

Diabetes Mellitus

There is evidence for a specific diabetic cardiomyopathy in diabetic patients without ESRD (149,150). LVH is a more frequent finding in hypertensive diabetic patients than in hypertensive nondiabetic patients, as is cardiac fibrosis (150,151). Diabetes has been identified as a predictor of hypertrophy in patients on dialysis (134,136).

Modifiable Risk Factors

Hypertension

The prevalence of hypertension in the various renal populations has already been discussed. Hypertension is associated with increased risk of progression of CRI and earlier onset of dialysis. A lower-than-usual target blood pressure (<125/75 mm Hg) appears more effective in delaying renal decline than the usual goal (<140/90) in patients with proteinuria (>1 g/day), suggesting a lower threshold for hypertensive damage among proteinuric renal patients. Hypertension has been shown to promote LV growth in a large cohort of patients with CRI (81).

In patients on dialysis, each 10 mm Hg increment in blood pressure is associated with a 48% higher risk for development of LVH (83). Paradoxically, *low* blood pressure has been linked with increased mortality rates in cross-sectional and longitudinal studies (82,97). As was discussed earlier, the resolution of this paradox may lie in the observation that low blood pressure is more likely the result, not the cause, of pump failure, which is known to predispose to death.

In RTR, elevated blood pressure has been associated with shortened graft and patient survival, as well as higher rates of CAD (2,84). However, a recent retrospective study of a large transplant cohort did not find an association between hypertension and death after adjustment for age, diabetes, tobacco use, and time on dialysis before transplantation (152). Only one study has examined the natural history of cardiomyopathy after transplantation (146). In this analysis, hypertension was associated with progression to LVH in patients with normal hearts at transplantation.

Anemia

Anemia has been associated with LV dilatation and LVH in CRI and in patients on dialysis (RR for LVH progression, per 10 g/L drop, is 1.74 in CRI and 1.48 in dialysis) (81,134,143,153–155). Anemia also is a risk factor for the development of *de novo* cardiac failure and death in dialysis (156). Partial correction of anemia is associated with regression of hypertrophy in cohort studies (157,158).

Two trials have studied the impact of full correction of hemoglobin on cardiovascular endpoints in dialysis. A large American trial compared normalization of hemoglobin versus partial correction in patients on hemodialysis *with* preexisting IHD or cardiac failure (159). The primary outcome was death or MI. The trial was stopped early because an interim analysis precluded the possibility of demonstrating survival benefit in the normalization group by the end of the trial. Increased mortality and increased dialysis access loss were observed among patients randomized to normalization. In a Canadian trial, patients on hemodialysis without symptomatic cardiac disease were allocated to normalization of hemoglobin with erythropoietin or to partial correction of anemia (160). Normalization of hemoglobin seemed to prevent progressive LV dilatation in those with normal cardiac volumes at baseline. These two studies suggest that full correction of anemia is not beneficial in patients with established cardiac disease, but may prevent development of cardiomyopathy in those without it. Whether hemoglobin normalization at an earlier stage of renal disease (e.g., in CRI) may be beneficial is unresolved.

The impact of anemia on the heart of RTR has not been studied. A retrospective cohort study currently underway in two Canadian centers will try to illuminate this question (C. Rigatto et al., personal communication).

Ischemic Heart Disease

The risk factors and outcome for IHD are discussed elsewhere in this chapter. It is worth repeating that CAD is an important cause of systolic and diastolic dysfunction in the general population and in patients on dialysis (134,161).

Mode and Quantity of End-Stage Renal Disease Therapy

Declining function of native kidneys has been associated with LV growth in patients with CRI (81). Once patients are on dialysis, the impact of the dialysis dose on LVH is not definitively known. One randomized, crossover trial has suggested that more intensive dialysis tends to ameliorate echocardiographic abnormalities (162). Analyses of data from multiple large, prospective studies have shown that a dialysis dose threshold exists below which mortality rates increase sharply (163,164). These inflection points have been used to formulate targets for Kt/V$_{urea}$ for both peritoneal dialysis (weekly Kt/V>2.0) and hemodialysis (per treatment Kt/V>1.2). Whether higher dosing targets will result in improvements in cardiac outcomes or mortality rates is not known. The HEMO study underway in the United States may shed light on this question.

Whether one modality (peritoneal dialysis vs. hemodialysis) is less "cardiotoxic" than the other remains the subject of debate. Observational data suggest that the relative risk of death and hospitalization may be less for patients on peritoneal dialysis in the first 2 years (RR 0.6 to 0.8), but this benefit disappears later on (RR 1.00). More study is needed because results are highly sensitive to the mode of analysis and to inclusion criteria (incident vs. prevalent patients) (165–167).

Renal transplantation appears to induce normalization of systolic dysfunction and regression of concentric LVH and LV dilatation, at least in patients without clinically evident IHD (144). This effect seems to persist for at least 3 years posttransplantation (146). It is not known which adverse risk factors characteristic of the uremic state have been corrected to produce the improvement in LV contractility, but blood pressure control may play a role (144,146).

Hypoalbuminemia

Several studies have shown that hypoalbuminemia is a powerful predictor of poor outcome in patients with ESRD. Hypoalbuminemia has been associated with LV dilatation and predisposes to *de novo* cardiac failure and IHD (168). The mechanisms underlying this association are unknown. Hypoalbuminemia is associated with a hypercoagulable state and therefore may predispose to MI and ischemic cardiomyopathy. Alternatively, it may be a marker for malnutrition, inadequate dialysis, vitamin deficiency, or a chronic inflammatory state, all of which hypothetically could accelerate myocyte death and the development of cardiomyopathy, as discussed earlier. The cardiovascular impact of hypoalbuminemia among patients with CRI and RTR is unknown.

Aortic Stenosis

Acquired aortic stenosis may occur in a minority of patients (131) and may induce concentric LVH. Calcification of the aortic valve has been observed in 28% to 55% of patients on dialysis in various series, whereas hemodynamically important stenosis has been reported in 3% to 13%. Progression at times may be extremely rapid. The major factors predisposing to aortic valve calcification appear to be hyperparathy-roidism, duration of dialysis, and degree of elevation of the calcium × phosphate product.

Salt and Water Overload

Salt and water overload is a persistent problem in patients on dialysis and is problematic to a lesser extent in patients with CRI and in RTR. Blood volume correlates directly with LV diameter in patients on hemodialysis (169), as does the magnitude of interdialytic weight changes (170). LV diameter decreases with volume contraction during hemodialysis (119). Keeping the patient's dry weight optimal can minimize the degree of enlargement of the LV (153). Despite these associations, it is difficult clearly to discern cause and effect. Salt and water overload is by definition blood volume overload and hence probably plays a causal role in the development of LVH. However, it is possible that salt and water retention is induced by preexisting systolic or diastolic dysfunction in some patients.

Outcome

The presence of concentric LVH, LV dilatation with normal contractility, and systolic dysfunction at baseline has been associated with progressively worse survival, independent of age, sex, diabetes, and IHD (140) (Fig. 94-6). All three abnormalities also were associated with increased risk for the development of CHF. Excessive hypertrophy in concentric LVH (high LV mass to volume ratio) and inadequate hypertrophy in LV dilatation (low LV mass to volume ratio) were independently associated with late mortality in a Canadian dialysis cohort (12).

CONGESTIVE HEART FAILURE

Pathogenesis

Congestive heart failure may result from systolic dysfunction or diastolic dysfunction, the latter occurring because of concentric or eccentric hypertrophy (Fig. 94-2). IHD is an additional independent predictor (148).

Among patients with diastolic dysfunction, CHF results from impaired ventricular relaxation; this leads to an exaggerated increase in LV end-diastolic pressure for a given increase in end-diastolic volume. As a result, a small excess of salt and water can rapidly lead to a large increase in LV end-diastolic pressure, culminating in pulmonary edema.

In dilated cardiomyopathy, cardiac output is maintained at the expense of an increase in both end-diastolic fiber length and end-diastolic volume (i.e., through the Frank-Starling mechanism). As ventricular volume increases, failure to achieve adequate hypertrophy leads to an increase in wall stress and an increase in end-diastolic pressure, leading ultimately to pulmonary edema.

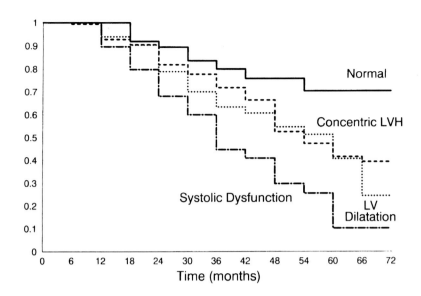

FIG. 94-6. The cumulative survival of patients starting dialysis with a normal echocardiogram *(solid line),* concentric left ventricular (LV) hypertrophy *(dotted line),* LV dilatation *(short-dashed line),* and systolic dysfunction *(long-dashed line).* (From Parfrey PS, Foley RN, Harnett JD, et al. The outcome and risk factors for left ventricular disorders in chronic uremia. *Nephrol Dial Transplant* 1996;11:1277, with permission.)

Diagnosis

The development of CHF, even in the presence of salt and water overload, suggests an underlying cardiac abnormality. Because the management of diastolic dysfunction differs from that of systolic dysfunction, an echocardiogram of the left ventricle is useful in planning management.

Burden of Disease

On starting dialysis, 37% of patients have had a previous episode of CHF (6). A baseline history of CHF carries a twofold risk of death independent of age, diabetes, and heart disease (6,140,171). The risk for development of pulmonary edema requiring hospitalization or ultrafiltration after starting maintenance hemodialysis is 10% annually (11). Among patients free of CHF at initiation of dialysis, *de novo* CHF developed in 25% over 41 months of observation. In contrast to the explicit data available for patients with ESRD, the incidence of CHF with or without need for hospitalization has not been described in patients with CRI or in RTR.

Risk Factors

In a group of patients with ESRD followed prospectively from initiation of dialysis, two groups were identified: one without a previous history of CHF, and one with a history of CHF at initiation. The independent predictors of CHF at initiation were age, diabetes, IHD, systolic dysfunction on echocardiogram, and low serum albumin. In patients free of baseline CHF, the significant predictors of the *de novo* development of CHF, independent of age, diabetes, and systolic dysfunction at baseline, were hypertension, anemia, low albumin, and hypocalcemia (11,148). It appears that factors that predispose to volume or flow overload (e.g., anemia), pressure overload (e.g., hypertension), and cell death

(e.g., malnutrition, hypocalcemia/hyperparathyroidism, IHD) are associated with CHF in dialysis.

In patients with CRI or in RTR, studies linking risk factors with clinical CHF are lacking. The risk factors for LVH in CRI have been discussed and include anemia and hypertension. Because LVH is a risk factor for CHF in the general and ESRD populations, it is likely that anemia and hypertension predispose to CHF in CRI.

Outcome

Data are available only for patients with ESRD. In the cohort discussed in the previous section, the median survival of patients who had heart failure at or before initiation of ESRD therapy was 36 months, compared with 62 months in subjects without baseline CHF. This adverse prognosis was independent of age, diabetes, and IHD. Among patients who had heart failure at baseline, recurrent heart failure developed in 56% and 44% remained failure-free during follow-up. Median survival in those with recurrent CHF was 29 months, significantly less than in those without recurrence (45 months) (148).

MANAGEMENT

The goals of treatment of cardiac disease are to alleviate symptoms, minimize hospitalization, and improve mortality rates. Because relatively few trials have been conducted in the CRF and ESRD population, many of the following recommendations are based on data from patients without renal impairment.

Ischemic Heart Disease

The treatment of both the acute (unstable angina and acute MI) and the nonacute presentations of CAD (stable angina and CHF) are in general the same as in the nonuremic population (42,172). Control of extracellular fluid volume by ultrafiltration and partial correction of anemia is an important therapeutic adjunct specific to CRF and patients on dialysis.

Medical Management

As in the general population, patients with CRI and stable angina pectoris who have not had an MI should be treated with antianginal agents for relief of symptoms. Coronary arteriography is recommended for patients with symptoms at rest or after minimal exertion, LV dysfunction, or signs of severe ischemia at low level of exercise during a stress test. For patients who have an MI, β-adrenergic blockade is recommended indefinitely, as is an ACE inhibitor for patients with LV dysfunction (173). In the general population, aspirin therapy is of proven benefit in the treatment of acute MI and after acute MI, as well as for long-term use in patients with a wide range of prior manifestations of cardiovascular disease (174). Although there is no evidence for the efficacy of aspirin in the CRI population, the improvement in cardiovascular disease outcomes in nonuremic patients with preexisting cardiovascular disease is significant enough that the benefits are likely to outweigh the harm. Consequently, patients with CRI or ESRD with acute presentations of CAD or established CAD should be treated with aspirin in a manner similar to patients with normal renal function. However, given that the complications from aspirin probably are more frequent in patients with CRI, the universal use of aspirin for the primary prevention of CAD in these patients is not recommended (42). Individual patient risks and benefits must be considered before beginning such therapy.

Dyslipidemia

There is no strong evidence linking dyslipidemia to CAD in patients with CRI or ESRD, and no trials of lipid-lowering therapy have been completed. Despite this, the clear benefit observed in the general population makes it reasonable to treat uremic patients in a similar manner. The National Kidney Foundation's (NKF) Task Force on Cardiovascular disease recommends using the National Cholesterol Education Program (NCEP) Adult Treatment Panel (ATP II) guidelines for classification and treatment in patients with renal disease (175). Patients with CRI should be considered the highest-risk group, and thus LDL cholesterol levels of 100 mg/dL (2.56 mmol/L) or more and 130 mg/dL (3.33 mmol/L) or more are treatment thresholds for diet and drug therapy, respectively. The target LDL level is 100 mg/dL (2.56 mmol/L) or less. A cholesterol-lowering diet should be part of the treatment program, but most patients require pharmacologic therapy. HMG-CoA reductase inhibitors are safe and effective in uremic patients, but screening for myositis should be undertaken. Fibrates also are effective, but dose reduction appropriate to the level of renal failure is important. The combination of an HMG-CoA reductase inhibitor and a fibrate is

associated with a high risk of muscle toxicity and in general should be avoided. Until further information becomes available, elevated triglycerides and low HDL-C without elevated LDL-C should be treated with diet and exercise but not drug therapy.

Revascularization

The potential risks and benefits of coronary revascularization procedures in patients with CRI or ESRD are different from those in the general population. The reported perioperative mortality rate of coronary artery bypass graft (CABG) surgery in patients on dialysis has ranged from 0% to 20%, significantly higher than in the general population, but the studies on which these figures are based are mostly small and retrospective, and do not make adjustment for comorbid factors (176–187). When the results of these studies are combined, the perioperative mortality rate is approximately 8% to 9%, roughly three times the expected rate for patients without ESRD. The perioperative morbidity rate of CABG surgery also is greater both in patients on dialysis and non–dialysis-dependent patients with CRI than in matched control patients (179,183,188,189). Unadjusted 2-year survival rates for patients on dialysis undergoing CABG have been reported to range from 45% to 92% (178,181,183,184,187). The few studies that have been long enough to determine the 5-year cumulative survival rate of patients on dialysis after CABG indicate that it is approximately 50% (176,184,185). These survival rates are comparable with those seen in the overall ESRD population (2), but are considerably lower then the overall 5-year survival rate of 85% after CABG observed in the Coronary Artery Surgery Study (190). There are few data as to the outcome of revascularization procedures in patients who have had renal transplantation. However, case reports and small series of patients suggest that transplanted patients with near-normal renal function have a perioperative mortality rate and long- term survival rate close to those observed in the non-ESRD population (177,191–195).

There have been no randomized trials of CABG versus medical management in patients with CRI and symptomatic CAD, but one retrospective study has suggested that patients with severe CAD do benefit from the procedure (178). The only randomized trial of revascularization versus medical therapy in patients with ESRD to date enrolled 26 asymptomatic diabetic patients who were found to have CAD on screening coronary angiography before renal transplantation (196). Ten of 13 medically managed and 2 of 13 revascularized patients had a cardiovascular endpoint (unstable angina, MI, or cardiac death) and the trial was stopped early by an external review committee. This provides some evidence that revascularization may improve the prognosis of asymptomatic CAD in this select population, but medical therapy in this instance consisted only of a calcium channel blocking drug and aspirin. Regardless of any survival benefit, CABG usually offers good relief from angina pain (176,177,181,183).

There has been some recent debate over the role of percutaneous transluminal angioplasty (PTCA) in patients with CRI or ESRD. Despite a high rate of initial technical success in patients with ESRD, PTCA seems to be associated with frequent recurrence of symptoms, usually resulting from restenosis (184,185,197–200). Early results from studies using PTCA with stenting of dilated vessels in the dialysis population suggest a lower recurrence rate with this procedure (201,202).

To date, there have been no studies comparing PTCA with medical management of patients with ESRD or CRI and CAD. Most retrospective and uncontrolled comparisons of patients on dialysis who underwent PTCA and patients who had CABG have demonstrated no overall survival difference in the two groups. Patients treated with PTCA do, however, have a significantly higher long-term risk of MI or recurrence of ischemic symptoms (184,185).

In summary, the indications for coronary revascularization in patients with CRI or ESRD are in general the same as those in the nonuremic population. Revascularization appears to be beneficial in high-risk patients and those with persistent symptoms of myocardial ischemia despite maximal medical therapy, provided that their life expectancy is otherwise reasonable. Based on the existing evidence, CABG appears to be the revascularization procedure of choice. PTCA with stenting seems to be a reasonable alternative in single-vessel disease or multiple-vessel disease with culprit lesions.

Congestive Heart Failure

For all patients with symptoms of heart failure, potentially reversible precipitating and aggravating factors (e.g., ischemia, tachycardia, arrhythmias, or hypertension) should be sought and appropriately managed. The treatment of heart failure differs for those with systolic and diastolic dysfunction (Fig. 94-7).

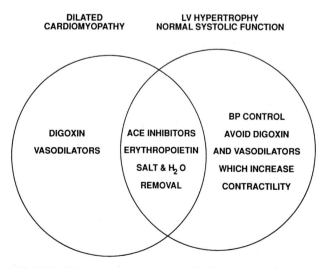

FIG. 94-7. The management of cardiac failure in chronic uremia. See text for discussion of β-adrenergic receptor blockers.

Angiotensin-Converting Enzyme Inhibitors

The utility of this class of drugs for the management of heart failure has been well demonstrated in the general population. ACE inhibitors have been found to improve symptoms, reduce morbidity, and improve survival (203,204), making them an important component of CHF therapy. Although trials in the CRI or ESRD population have not been conducted, the high degree of benefit shown in other patients makes it very reasonable to treat these patients in a similar manner. ACE inhibitor therapy therefore is recommended for patients with symptomatic heart failure, post-MI patients with an LV ejection fraction less than 40%, and asymptomatic patients with an LV ejection fraction less than 35% (203).

Digoxin

The benefit of digoxin in the setting of symptomatic LV systolic dysfunction and atrial fibrillation is widely accepted. The use of digoxin in similar patients with normal sinus rhythm has been more controversial, but a substantial body of evidence supporting its use does exist (205–208). Nonuremic patients with symptomatic LV systolic dysfunction have less morbidity and improved exercise tolerance when given digoxin in conjunction with standard therapy (i.e., diuretics and ACE inhibitors) (208), but digoxin does not appear to improve survival (205). Digoxin therefore should be considered for patients with CRI and systolic dysfunction, with a reduction in dose appropriate to their level of renal impairment. Digoxin should not be given to patients whose heart failure is due primarily to diastolic dysfunction because the increased contractility could worsen diastolic impairment.

β-Adrenergic Receptor Blockers

A large amount of data from recent, well designed trials supports the use of β-adrenergic receptor antagonists in the management of LV systolic dysfunction. Improvements in mortality or hospitalization rates have been shown in patients with mild to moderate symptomatic heart failure treated with carvedilol, bisoprolol, or controlled-release metoprolol (209–212). β Receptor antagonists with intrinsic sympathomimetic activity appear to be detrimental and should not be used in patients with heart failure. Current guidelines for the general population suggest the routine use of β receptor antagonists in clinically stable patients with an LV ejection fraction less than 40% and mild to moderate heart failure symptoms who are on standard therapy (i.e., diuretics, an ACE inhibitor, and digoxin) (213). Such therapy also should be considered for asymptomatic patients with an LV ejection fraction less than 40%, but the evidence supporting its use in this setting is not as strong. β Receptor antagonists are not currently recommended for patients with severe symptomatic heart failure (i.e., those with symptoms at rest). These guidelines are generally applicable to the CRI and ESRD population as well. As in the nonrenal population, however, the agents should be started in low doses with careful clinical reevaluation during the titration phase.

Other Drugs

Diuretics remain an essential component of the symptomatic treatment for heart failure in non–dialysis-dependent patients with CRI, although multiple agents at high doses may be required in patients with more advanced renal impairment. Long-acting nitrates may be useful in some patients, particularly those with diastolic dysfunction. Direct vasodilators are considered inadvisable in this setting (203).

Data regarding the use of angiotensin II type 1 (AT$_1$) receptor blockers in patients with heart failure are beginning to accumulate. Although a number of trials are underway, only the Evaluation of Losartan in the Elderly (ELITE) studies have been completed. Although ELITE I suggested a survival advantage in the losartan group, this was not confirmed in ELITE II (214,215). Although it is possible that the AT$_1$ receptor blockers will prove to have an efficacy in heart failure similar to that of ACE inhibitors, the latter remain the agents of choice for the treatment of LV dysfunction, with or without symptomatic heart failure (213).

Uremia-Related Interventions

Anemia

The optimal target hematocrit for improving outcomes in patients with CAD or LV dysfunction is not known. At least one trial has shown that maintaining a normal hematocrit, compared with the usual target level of 33% to 36%, in patients with established cardiac disease is not of benefit and may be detrimental (159) (Fig. 94-8). Partial correction of anemia consistently has been shown to induce some regression of LVH (216–220), and normalization of hemoglobin may prevent progressive LV dilatation in those with normal cardiac volumes at baseline (160). Until further data become available, however, it is reasonable to follow the current

NKF-Dialysis Outcomes Quality Initiative guidelines for treatment of anemia for all patients, including those with cardiac disease. These guidelines recommend a target hematocrit of 33% to 36%, based on improvement in quality of life and exercise tolerance (221).

Hypertension

As in the general population, there is evidence that treatment of hypertension leads to regression of LVH in patients with renal disease (222–224). It is not known whether the regression of LVH in patients with CRI leads to greater improvement in outcomes than control of hypertension alone. It is likely that a number of classes of antihypertensive agents lead to regression of LVH, although there is increasing evidence that ACE inhibitors are more effective than other classes of drugs (225). Despite this report, there is not enough evidence to support the superiority of one class of antihypertensive agents for this purpose. For the general population, the Joint National Committee recommendations for hypertension treatment do not differ for patients with and without LVH (76). It therefore is reasonable to use the recommendations developed for target blood pressure and antihypertensive agents of choice in patients with CRI independent of their cardiac disease status (226).

Mode and Quantity of Dialysis

The recommended target Kt/V$_{urea}$ is more than 2.0 per week for peritoneal dialysis and more than 1.2 per treatment for hemodialysis (163,164). Whether higher doses of dialysis may improve cardiac outcomes is not known. The establishment and maintenance of an accurate dry weight is extremely important. Symptoms of heart failure clearly can be worsened by salt and water retention. Myocardial ischemia may be aggravated by increased LV end-diastolic pressure associated with extracellular fluid volume overload and by the fluid shifts accompanying rapid ultrafiltration during hemodialysis.

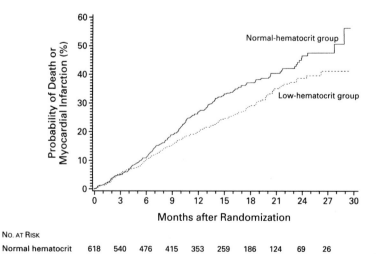

No. at Risk

Normal hematocrit	618	540	476	415	353	259	186	124	69	26
Low hematocrit	615	537	485	434	391	292	216	131	80	20

FIG. 94-8. Cumulative survival of patients on hemodialysis with preexisting cardiac disease, treated with erythropoietin, randomly allocated to partial correction of hematocrit or to normal hematocrit. (From Besarab A, Bolton WK, Brown JK, et al. The effects of normal as compared with low hematocrit values in patients with cardiac disease who are receiving hemodialysis and epoetin. *N Engl J Med* 1998;339:584, with permission.)

Some patients who are unable to tolerate the intradialytic volume expansion associated with intermittent hemodialysis may be more easily managed with peritoneal dialysis. There is no good evidence, however, that either modality is associated with improved outcomes for patients with cardiac disease.

CONCLUSIONS

The burden of cardiac disease in all phases of renal failure is high, and its clinical impact grave. The most frequent clinical manifestations are IHD and CHF. IHD may be atherosclerotic or nonatherosclerotic in origin. CHF results from IHD, cardiomyopathy, or both. The manifestations of uremic cardiomyopathy include concentric and eccentric LVH and systolic dysfunction. Risk factors for cardiac disease in uremia include age, diabetes, hypertension, anemia, volume overload, hyperparathyroidism, dyslipidemia, and perhaps uremia itself.

Although studies have traditionally focused on the dialysis population, it has become evident that risk factors for cardiovascular disease and their initial consequences to the heart already are present during the predialysis phase and persist despite significant amelioration in the transplantation phase. Even so, our knowledge of these risks and consequences remains far from definitive, particularly in the CRI and transplantation phases. The dearth of experimental evidence is particularly acute with regard to therapy. Although much data exist on the impact of risk factor modification and therapy of CHF for the general population, corresponding trials in the renal population have not been done. In the interim, it is useful to remember that many of the risks for cardiac dysfunction are common to both renal and nonrenal patients, that many of these risks are higher in the renal failure population, and that the absolute benefit of any intervention tends to increase with increasing risk. It is likely, therefore, that the validity of extrapolations from the general population will be vindicated in future trials. The most logical approach at present seems to be to treat according to recommendations for the nonrenal population unless there is a compelling contraindication, or there are convincing contrary data from studies in the renal failure population. Ultimately, this approach will have to be validated by clinical trials of adequate statistical power.

REFERENCES

1. Drukker W. Haemodialysis: a historical review. In: Maher JF, ed. *Replacement of renal function by dialysis.* 3rd ed. Boston: Kluwer Academic, 1989:20.
2. United States Renal Data System. *USRDS 1998 annual data report.* Bethesda, MD: U.S. Department of Health and Human Services, National Institutes of Health, National Institute of Diabetes and Digestive and Kidney Diseases, August 1998.
3. Raine AE, Margreiter R, Brunner FP, et al. Report on management of renal failure in Europe, XXII. *Nephrol Dial Transplant* 1992;7:S7.
4. Canadian Organ Replacement Register. *1999 Report, volume 1: dialysis and renal transplantation.* Ottawa, Ontario: Canadian Institute for Health Information, June 1999.
5. El-Reshaid K, Johny K, Sugathan T, et al. End-stage renal disease and renal replacement therapy in Kuwait: epidemiological profile over the last 4 1/2 years. *Nephrol Dial Transplant* 1994;9:532.
6. Foley RN, Parfrey P, Hefferton D, et al. Advance prediction of early death in patients starting maintenance dialysis. *Am J Kidney Dis* 1994;23:836.
7. Morduchowicz G, Winkler J, Derazne E, et al. Causes of death in patients with end-stage renal disease treated by dialysis in a center in Israel. *Isr J Med Sci* 1992;28:776.
8. Fernandez JM, Carbonell ME, Mazzucchi N, et al. Simultaneous analysis of morbidity and mortality factors in chronic hemodialysis patients. *Kidney Int* 1992;41:1029.
9. Mailloux LU, Bellucci A, Wilkes B, et al. Mortality in dialysis patients: analysis of the causes of death. *Am J Kidney Dis* 1991;18:326.
10. Viglino G, Cancarini G, Catizone L, et al. Ten years of continuous ambulatory peritoneal dialysis: analysis of patient and technique survival. *Perit Dial Int* 1993;13:S175.
11. Churchill D, Taylor D, Cook R, et al. Canadian Hemodialysis Morbidity Study. *Am J Kidney Dis* 1992;19:214.
12. Foley RN, Parfrey PS, Harnett JD, et al. The prognostic importance of left ventricular geometry in uremic cardiomyopathy. *J Am Soc Nephrol* 1995;5:2024.
13. Parfrey PS, Harnett JD, Foley RN, et al. Impact of renal transplantation on uremic cardiomyopathy. *Transplantation* 1995;60:908.
14. Roig E, Betriu A, Castaner A, et al. Disabling angina pectoris with normal coronary arteries in patients undergoing long term dialysis. *Am J Med* 1981;71:431.
15. Rostand SG, Kirk KA, Rutsky EA. Dialysis associated ischemic heart disease: insights from coronary angiography. *Kidney Int* 1984;25:653.
16. Rostand SG, Rutsky E. Ischemic heart disease in chronic renal failure: demography, epidemiology and pathogenesis. In: PS Parfrey, JD Harnett, eds. *Cardiac dysfunction in chronic uremia.* Boston: Kluwer Academic, 1992:53.
17. Mosseri M, Yarom R, Gotsman MS, et al. Histologic evidence for small vessel coronary artery disease in patients with angina pectoris and patent large coronary arteries. *Circulation* 1986;74:964.
18. James TN. Morphologic characteristics and functional significance of focal fibromuscular dysplasia of small coronary arteries. *Am J Cardiol* 1990;65:12G.
19. Amann K, Wiest G, Zimmer G, et al. Reduced capillary density in the myocardium of uremic rats: a stereological study. *Kidney Int* 1992;42:1079.
20. Rambusek M, Amann K, Mall G, et al. Structural causes of cardiac dysfunction in uremia. *Ren Fail* 1993;15:421.
21. Diaz M, Frei B, Vita J, et al. Antioxidants and atherosclerotic heart disease. *N Engl J Med* 1997;337:408.
22. Cominacini L, Garbin U, Pasini A, et al. Antioxidants inhibit the expression of ICAM-1 and VCAM-1 induced by oxidized LDL on human umbilical vein endothelial cells. *Free Radic Biol Med* 1997;22:117.
23. Westhuyzen J. The oxidation hypothesis of atherosclerosis: an update. *Ann Clin Lab Sci* 1997;27:1.
24. Ananyeva N, Tjurmin A, Berliner J, et al. Oxidized LDL mediates the release of FGF-1. *Arterioscler Thromb Vasc Biol* 1997;17:445.
25. Stary H. Composition and classification of human atherosclerotic lesions. *Virchows Arch A Pathol Anat* 1992;421:277.
26. Schwarz U, Buzello M, Stein G, et al. Morphology of coronary atherosclerotic lesions in patients with end-stage renal failure. *Nephrol Dial Transplant* 2000;15:218.
27. Achenbach S, Moshage W, Ropers D, et al. Value of electron beam computed tomography for the non-invasive detection of high grade coronary artery stenosis and occlusions. *N Engl J Med* 1998;339:1964.
28. Goodman W, Goldin J, Kuizon B, et al. Coronary-artery calcification in young adults with end-stage renal disease who are undergoing dialysis. *N Engl J Med* 2000;342:1478.
29. Rigatto C, Singal P. Oxidative stress in uremia: impact on cardiac disease in dialysis patients. *Semin Dial* 1999;12:91.
30. Hankey I, Eikelbloom J. Homocysteine and vascular disease. *Lancet* 1999;354:407.
31. Bostom A, Culleton B. Hyperhomocysteinemia in chronic renal disease. *J Am Soc Nephrol* 1999;10:891.
32. Erbel R, Ge J, Bockisch A, et al. Value of intracoronary ultrasound and Doppler in the differentiation of angiographically normal coronary arteries: a prospective study in patients with angina pectoris. *Eur Heart J* 1996;17:880.

33. Uren N, Melin J, De Bruyne B, et al. Relation between myocardial blood flow and the severity of coronary artery stenosis. *N Engl J Med* 1994;330:1782.

34. Zoneraich S. Unravelling the conundrums of the diabetic heart diagnosed in 1876: prelude to genetics. *Can J Cardiol* 1994;10:945.

35. Rostand SG, Kirk K, Rutsky EA. The epidemiology of coronary artery disease in patients on maintenance hemodialysis: implications for management. *Contrib Nephrol* 1986;52:34.

36. Raine A, Seymour A, Roberts A, et al. Impairment of cardiac function and energetics in experimental renal failure. *J Clin Invest* 1993; 92:2934.

37. Massry SG, Smogorzewski M. Mechanisms through which parathyroid hormone mediates its deleterious effects on organ function in uremia. *Semin Nephrol* 1994;14:219.

38. Weinrauch L, D'Elia JA, Healy RW, et al. Asymptomatic coronary artery disease: angiographic assessment of diabetics evaluated for renal transplantation. *Circulation* 1978;58:1184.

39. Lorber MI, Van Buren CT, Flechner SM, et al. Pre-transplant coronary arteriography for diabetic renal transplant recipients. *Transplant Proc* 1987;19:1539.

40. Braun WE, Philips DF, Vidt DG, et al. Coronary artery disease in 100 diabetics with end-stage renal failure. *Transplant Proc* 1984;16:603.

41. Cohn PF. Detection and prognosis of asymptomatic patients with silent myocardial ischemia. *Am J Cardiol* 1988;61[Suppl 3]:4B.

42. Murphy SW, Foley RN, Parfrey PS. Screening and treatment for cardiovascular disease in patients with chronic renal disease. *Am J Kidney Dis* 1998;32[5 Suppl 3]:S184.

43. Eagle KA, Brundage BH, Chaitman BR, et al. Guidelines for perioperative cardiovascular evaluation for non-cardiac surgery: report of the ACC/AHA Task Force on Practice Guidelines (Committee on Perioperative Cardiovascular Evaluation for Non-cardiac Surgery). *J Am Coll Cardiol* 1996;27:910.

44. American College of Physicians. ACP clinical guideline: guidelines for assessing and managing the perioperative risk from coronary artery disease associated with major non-cardiac surgery. *Ann Intern Med* 1997;127:309.

45. Kasiske BL, Ramos EL, Gaston RS, et al. The evaluation of renal transplant candidates: clinical practice guidelines. *J Am Soc Nephrol* 1995;6:1.

46. Coley CM, Eagle KA. Preoperative assessment and perioperative management of cardiac ischemic risk in non-cardiac surgery. *Curr Probl Cardiol* 1996;5:290.

47. Morrow CE, Schwartz JS, Sutherland DE, et al. Predictive value of thallium stress testing for coronary and cardiovascular events in uremic diabetic patients before renal transplantation. *Am J Med* 1983; 81:63.

48. Philipson JD, Carpenter BJ, Itzkoff J, et al. Evaluation of cardiovascular risk for renal transplantation in diabetic patients. *Am J Med* 1986; 81:630.

49. Dahan M, Lagallicier B, Himbert D, et al. Diagnostic value of myocardial thallium stress scintigraphy in the selection of coronary artery disease in patients undergoing chronic hemodialysis. *Arch Mal Coeur* 1995;88:1121.

50. Boudreau RJ, Strony JT, du Cret RP, et al. Perfusion thallium imaging of type I diabetes patients with end-stage renal disease: comparison of oral and intravenous dipyridamole administration. *Radiology* 1990;175:103.

51. Marwick TH, Steinmuller DR, Underwood DA, et al. Ineffectiveness of dipyridamole SPECT thallium imaging as a screening technique for coronary artery disease in patients with end stage renal failure. *Transplantation* 1990;49:100.

52. Resis G, Marcovitz PA, Leichtman AB, et al. Usefulness of dobutamine stress echocardiography in detecting coronary artery disease in end-stage renal disease. *Am J Cardiol* 1995;75:707.

53. Albanese J, Nally J, Marwick T, et al. Dobutamine echocardiography is effective in the non-invasive detection of prognostically important coronary artery disease in patients with end-stage renal disease. *J Am Soc Nephrol* 1994;5:322(abstr).

54. Bates JR, Sawada SG, Segar DS, et al. Evaluation using dobutamine stress echocardiography in patients with insulin dependent diabetes mellitus before kidney and/or pancreas transplant. *Am J Cardiol* 1996; 77:175.

55. Murphy SW, Barrett BJ, Parfrey PS. Contrast nephropathy. *J Am Soc Nephrol* 2000;11:177.

56. Foley RN, Parfrey PS, Sarnak MJ. Epidemiology of cardiovascular disease in chronic renal disease. *J Am Soc Nephrol* 1998;9:S16.

57. Jungers P, Massy ZA, Khoa TN, et al. Incidence and risk factors of atherosclerotic cardiovascular accidents in predialysis chronic renal failure patients: a prospective study. *Nephrol Dial Transplant* 1997; 12:2597.

58. Lazarus JM, Bourgoignie JJ, Buckalew VM, et al., for the Modification of Diet in Renal Disease Study Group. Achievement and safety of a low blood pressure goal in chronic renal disease. *Hypertension* 1997;29:641.

59. Maschio G, Alberti D, Janin G, et al. Effect of the angiotensin converting enzyme inhibitor benazepril on the progression of chronic renal insufficiency. *N Engl J Med* 1996;334:939.

60. Fletcher RH, Fletcher SW, Wagner EH. *Clinical epidemiology: the essentials.* 3rd ed. Baltimore: Williams & Wilkins, 1996.

61. Kasiske BL. Risk factors for accelerated atherosclerosis in renal transplant recipients. *Am J Med* 1988;84:985.

62. Kasiske BL, Guijarro C, Massy ZA, et al. Cardiovascular disease after renal transplantation. *J Am Soc Nephrol* 1996;7:158.

63. Kannel WB, Castelli W, McNamara P. The coronary profile: 12 year follow-up in the Framingham Study. *J Occup Med* 1967;9:611.

64. SHEP Cooperative Research Group. Prevention of stroke by antihypertensive drug treatment in older persons with isolated systolic hypertension: final results of the Systolic Hypertension in the Elderly Program. *JAMA* 1991;265:3255.

65. Gong L, Zhang W, Zhu Y, et al. Shanghai trial of nifedipine in the elderly (STONE). *J Hypertens* 1996;14:1237.

66. The Scandinavian Simvastatin Survival Study Group. Randomized trial of cholesterol lowering in 4444 patients with coronary disease: the Scandinavian Simvastatin Survival Study (4S). *Lancet* 1994;344: 1383.

67. Parfrey PS, Foley RN, Harnett JD, et al. Outcome and risk factors of ischemic heart disease in chronic uremia. *Kidney Int* 1996;49: 1428.

68. Castelli WP, Anderson KM. A population at risk. *Am J Cardiol* 1986; 80[Suppl 2]:S23.

69. Rabbat CG, Thorpe KE, Russell JD, et al. Comparison of mortality risk for dialysis patients and cadaveric first renal transplant recipients in Ontario, Canada. *J Am Soc Nephrol* 2000;11:917.

70. Kannel WB, Mcgee DL. Diabetes and glucose tolerance as risk factors for cardiovascular disease: the Framingham Study. *Diabetes Care* 1979;2:120.

71. Kannel WB, McGee DL. Diabetes and cardiovascular disease: the Framingham Study. *JAMA* 1979;241:2035.

72. Valsania P, Zarich S, Kowalchuk G, et al. Severity of coronary artery disease in young patients with insulin-dependent diabetes mellitus. *Am Heart J* 1991;122:695.

73. Singer DE, Nathan DM, Wilson PW, et al. Association of HbA1C with prevalent cardiovascular disease in the original cohort of the Framingham Heart Study. *Diabetes* 1992;41:202.

74. Culleton BF, Wilson PWF. Cardiovascular disease: risk factors, secular trends, and therapeutic guidelines. *J Am Soc Nephrol* 1998;9:S5.

75. Manske CL, Thomas L, Wang Y, et al. Screening diabetic transplant candidates for coronary artery disease: identification of a low risk subgroup. *Kidney Int* 1993;44:617.

76. Joint National Committee on Prevention, Detection, Evaluation and Treatment of High Blood Pressure. The sixth report of the Joint National Committee on Prevention, Detection, Evaluation and Treatment of High Blood Pressure. *Arch Intern Med* 1997;157:2413.

77. Kannel WB. Role of blood pressure in cardiovascular disease: the Framingham Study. *Angiology* 1975;26:1.

78. Collins R, Peto R, MacMahon S, et al. Blood pressure, stroke, and coronary heart disease. Part 2: Short term reductions in blood pressure: overview of randomized drug trials in their epidemiological context. *Lancet* 1990;335:827.

79. Hebert P, Moser M, Mayer J, et al. Recent evidence on drug therapy of mild to moderate hypertension and decreased risk of coronary heart disease. *Arch Intern Med* 1993;153:578.

80. Buckalew VM, Berg RL, Wang SR, et al. prevalence of hypertension in 1,795 subjects with chronic renal disease: the Modification of Diet in Renal Disease Study baseline cohort. *Am J Kidney Dis* 1996;28:811.

81. Levin A, Thompson CR, Ethier J, et al. Left ventricular mass index increase in early renal disease: impact of decline in hemoglobin. *Am J Kidney Dis* 1999;34:125.

82. Zager PG, Nikolic J, Brown RH, et al. "U" curve association of blood pressure and mortality in hemodialysis patients. *Kidney Int* 1998;54: 561.

83. Foley RN, Parfrey PS, Harnett JD, et al. Impact of hypertension on cardiomyopathy, morbidity and mortality in end-stage renal disease. *Kidney Int* 1996;49:1379.

84. Opelz G, Wujciak T, Ritz E, for the Collaborative Transplant Study. Association of chronic kidney graft failure with recipient blood pressure. *Kidney Int* 1998;53:217.

85. Cosio FG, Alamir A, Yim S, et al. Patient survival after renal transplant: 1. the impact of dialysis pre-transplant. *Kidney Int* 1998;53:762.

86. Kannel WB. Update on the role of cigarette smoking in chronic renal disease. *Am Heart J* 1981;101:319.

87. Gordon T, Kannel W, Mcgee D, et al. Death and coronary attacks in men after giving up cigarette smoking: a report from the Framingham Study. *Lancet* 1974;2:1345.

88. Cosio FG, Falkenhain ME, Pesavento ET, et al. Patient survival after renal transplantation: II. the impact of smoking. *Clin Transplantation* 1999;13:336.

89. Kasiske BL, Klinger D. Cigarette smoking in renal transplant recipients. *J Am Soc Nephrol* 2000;11:753.

90. Kasiske BL. Risk factors for cardiovascular disease after renal transplantation. *Miner Electrolyte Metab* 1993;19:186.

91. Criqui M, Heiss G, Cohn R, et al. Plasma triglyceride level and mortality from coronary artery disease. *N Engl J Med* 1993;328:1220.

92. Schaefer EJ, Lamon-Fava S, Jenner JL, et al. Lipoprotein(a) levels and risk of coronary artery disease in men: the Lipid Research Clinics coronary primary prevention trial. *JAMA* 1994;271:999.

93. Goldbourt U, Yaari S, Medalie J. Isolated low HDL cholesterol as a risk factor for coronary heart disease mortality: a 21-year follow-up of 8000 men. *Arterioscler Thromb Vasc Biol* 1997;17:107.

94. Castelli WP. Incidence of coronary artery disease and lipoprotein cholesterol levels: the Framingham Study. *JAMA* 1986;256:2835.

95. Kannel WB. Cholesterol and risk of coronary artery disease in men. *Clin Chem* 1988;34:B53.

96. Kasiske B. Hyperlipidemia in patients with chronic renal disease. *Am J Kidney Dis* 1998;32:S142.

97. Lowrie EG, Lew NL. Commonly measured laboratory values in hemodialysis patients: relationships among them and to death risk. *Semin Nephrol* 1992;12:276.

98. Cressman MD, Heyka RJ, Paganini EP, et al. Lp(a) is an independent risk factor for cardiovascular disease in hemodialysis patients. *Circulation* 1992;86:475.

99. Cressman MD, Abood D, O'Neill J, et al. Lp(a) and mortality during chronic hemodialysis treatment. *Chem Phys Lipids* 1994;67:419.

100. Coresh J, Longenecker JC, Miller ER, et al. Epidemiology of cardiovascular risk factors in chronic renal disease. *J Am Soc Nephrol* 1998;9:S24.

101. Aakhus S, Dahl K, Wideroe TE. Cardiovascular morbidity and risk factors in renal transplant patients. *Nephrol Dial Transplant* 1999;14:648.

102. Eikelboom J, Lonn E, Genest J, et al. Homocysteine and cardiovascular disease: a critical review of the epidemiological evidence. *Ann Intern Med* 1999;131:363.

103. Kark J, Selhub J, Adler B, et al. Nonfasting plasma homocysteine level and mortality in middle aged and elderly men and women in Jerusalem. *Ann Intern Med* 1999;131:321.

104. Bostom A, Rosenberg I, Silbershatz H, et al. Non-fasting plasma total homocysteine levels and stroke incidence in elderly persons: the Framingham Study. *Ann Intern Med* 1999;131:352.

105. Bostom A, Lathrop L. Hyperhomocysteinemia in end-stage renal disease: prevalence, etiology, and potential relationship to arteriosclerotic outcomes. *Kidney Int* 1997;52:10.

106. Bostom A, Shemin D, Verhoef P, et al. Elevated fasting total homocysteine levels and cardiovascular disease outcomes in maintenance dialysis patients: a prospective study. *Arterioscler Thromb Vasc Biol* 1997;17:2554.

107. Moustapha A, Naso A, Nahlawi M, et al. Prospective study of hyperhomocysteinemia as an adverse cardiovascular risk factor in end-stage renal disease. *Circulation* 1998;97:138.

108. Jungers P, Chauveau P, Bandin O, et al. Hyperhomocysteinemia is associated with atherosclerotic occlusive arterial accidents in predialysis chronic renal failure patients. *Miner Electrolyte Metab* 1997; 23:170.

109. Doucloux D, Motte G, Challier B, et al. Serum total homocysteine and cardiovascular disease occurrence in chronic stable renal transplant patients: a prospective study. *J Am Soc Nephrol* 2000;11: 134.

110. Bostom A, Gohh R, Beaulieu A, et al. Treatment of hyperhomocysteinemia in renal transplant patients: a randomized placebo controlled trial. *Ann Intern Med* 1997;127:1089.

111. Foley RN, Parfrey PS, Harnett J, et al. Chronic hypocalcemia: a major morbidity and mortality factor in ESRD patients. *J Am Soc Nephrol* 1994;5:446.

112. Lacour B, Basile C, Drueke T, et al. Parathyroid function and lipid metabolism in the rat. *Miner Electrolyte Metab* 1982;7:157.

113. London G, Parfrey P. Cardiac disease in chronic uremia: pathogenesis. *Adv Ren Replace Ther* 1997;4:194.

114. Gris J, Branger B, Vecina F, et al. Increased cardiovascular risk factors and features of endothelial activation and dysfunction in dialyzed uremic patients. *Kidney Int* 1994;46:807.

115. Korbet S, Makita Z, Firanek C, et al. Advanced glycosylation end products in continuous ambulatory peritoneal dialysis. *Am J Kidney Dis* 1993;22:588.

116. Makita Z, Bucala R, Rayfield E, et al. Reactive glycosylation end products in diabetic uremia and treatment of renal failure. *Lancet* 1994; 343:1519.

117. Pombo JF, Troy BL, Russell RO Jr. Left ventricular volumes and ejection fractions by echocardiography. *Circulation* 1971;43:480.

118. Devereux R, Roman M. Ultrasonic techniques for the evaluation of hypertension. *Curr Opin Nephrol Hypertens* 1994;3:644.

119. Harnett JD, Murphy B, Collingwood P, et al. The reliability and validity of echocardiographic measurement of left ventricular mass in hemodialysis patients. *Nephron* 1993;65:212.

120. Levy D, Savage DD, Garrison RJ, et al. Echocardiographic criteria for left ventricular hypertrophy: the Framingham Study. *Am J Cardiol* 1987;59:956.

121. London GM, Parfrey PS. Cardiac disease in chronic uremia: pathogenesis. *Adv Ren Replace Ther* 1997;4:194.

122. Grossman W, Jones D, Maclaurin L, et al. Wall stress and patterns of hypertrophy in the human left ventricle. *J Clin Invest* 1975;56:56.

123. Grossman W. Cardiac hypertrophy: useful adaptation or pathological process? *Am J Med* 1980;69:576.

124. Rozich JD, Smith B, Thomas JD, et al. Dialysis induced alterations in left ventricular filling: mechanisms and clinical significance. *Am J Kidney Dis* 1991;3:277.

125. Hofman JI. Transmural myocardial perfusion. *Prog Cardiovasc Dis* 1987;29:429.

126. Amann K, Ritz E. Cardiac disease in chronic uremia: pathophysiology. *Adv Ren Replace Ther* 1997;4:212.

127. Cheng W, Li B, Kajstura J, et al. Stretch induced programmed myocyte death. *J Clin Invest* 1995;96:2247.

128. Suzuki H, Schaefer L, Ling H, et al. Prevention of cardiac hypertrophy in experimental chronic renal failure by long term ACE inhibitor administration: potential role of lysosomal proteinases. *Am J Nephrol* 1995;15:129.

129. London GM, Guerin AP, Marchais SJ, et al. Cardiac and arterial interactions in end stage renal disease. *Kidney Int* 1996;50:600.

130. London GM, Drueke TB. Atherosclerosis and arteriosclerosis in chronic renal failure. *Kidney Int* 1997;51:1678.

131. Raine AEG. Acquired aortic stenosis in dialysis patients. *Nephron* 1994;68:159.

132. Amann K, Wiest G, Klaus G, et al. The role of parathyroid hormone in the genesis of interstitial cell activation in uremia. *J Am Soc Nephrol* 1994;4:1814.

133. Mall G, Huther W, Schneider J, et al. Diffuse intermyocardiocytic fibrosis in uremic patients. *Nephrol Dial Transplant* 1990;5:39.

134. Parfrey PS, Foley RN, Harnett JD, et al. The outcome and risk factors for left ventricular disorders in chronic uremia. *Nephrol Dial Transplant* 1996;11:1277.

135. Katz A. The cardiomyopathy of overload: an unnatural growth response in the hypertrophied heart. *Ann Intern Med* 1994;121:363.

136. Greaves S, Gamble G, Collins J, et al. Determinants of left-ventricular hypertrophy and systolic dysfunction in chronic renal failure. *Am J Kidney Dis* 1994;24:768.

137. Levin A, Singer J, Thompson CR, et al. Prevalent left ventricular hypertrophy in the predialysis population: opportunities for intervention. *Am J Kidney Dis* 1996;27:347.

138. Tucker B, Fabbian F, Giles M, et al. Left ventricular hypertrophy and ambulatory blood pressure monitoring in chronic renal failure. *Nephrol Dial Transplant* 1997;12:724.

139. Silberberg JS, Barre PE, Prichard SS, et al. Impact of left ventricular hypertrophy on survival in end-stage renal disease. *Kidney Int* 1989; 36:286.

140. Foley R, Parfrey P, Harnett J, et al. Clinical and echocardiographic disease in end- stage renal disease: prevalence, associations, and risk factors. *Kidney Int* 1995;47:186.

141. Covic A, Goldsmith DJ, Georgescu G, et al. Echocardiographic findings in long-term long hour hemodialysis patients. *Clin Nephrol* 1996; 45:104.

142. Dahan M, Siohan P, Viron B, et al. Relationship between left ventricular hypertrophy, myocardial contractility, and load conditions in hemodialysis patients: an echocardiographic study. *Am J Kidney Dis* 1997;30:780.

143. Foley RN, Parfrey PS, Kent GM, et al. The long term evolution of cardiomyopathy in dialysis patients. *Kidney Int* 1998;54:1720.

144. Parfrey PS, Harnett JD, Foley RN, et al. Impact of renal transplantation on uremic cardiomyopathy. *Transplantation* 1995;60:908.

145. Disney APS, ed. *Report 1996, Australia and New Zealand Dialysis and Transplant Registry.* Adelaide, South Australia: Australia and New Zealand Dialysis and Transplant Registry, 1996.

146. Rigatto C, Foley R, Kent G, et al. Long-term changes in left ventricular hypertrophy after renal transplantation. *Transplantation* 2000;70:570.

147. Bloembergen WE, Carroll C, Gillespie B, et al. Why do males with ESRD have higher mortality than females? *J Am Soc Nephrol* 1996; 7:1440.

148. Harnett JD, Foley RN, Kent GM, et al. Congestive heart failure in dialysis patients: prevalence, incidence, prognosis and risk factors. *Kidney Int* 1995;47:884.

149. Galdeisi M, Anderson K, Wilson P, et al. Echocardiographic evidence for a distinct diabetic cardiomyopathy (the Framingham Heart Study). *Am J Cardiol* 1991;68:85.

150. Grossman E, Messerli FH. Diabetic and hypertensive heart disease. *Ann Intern Med* 1996;125:304.

151. Van Hoeven K, Factor S. A comparison of the pathological spectrum of hypertensive, diabetic, and hypertensive-diabetic heart disease. *Circulation* 1990;82:848.

152. Cosio FG, Alamir A, Yim S, et al. Patient survival after renal transplant: 1. the impact of dialysis pre-transplant. *Kidney Int* 1998;53:762.

153. Huting J, Kramer W, Schutterle G, et al. Analysis of left ventricular changes associated with chronic hemodialysis: a non-invasive follow-up study. *Nephron* 1988;49:284.

154. Parfrey P, Foley R, Harnett J, et al. The clinical course of left ventricular hypertrophy in dialysis patients. *Nephron* 1990;55:114.

155. Foley RN, Parfrey PS, Harnett JD, et al. The impact of anemia on cardiomyopathy, morbidity and mortality in end stage renal disease. *Am J Kidney Dis* 1996;28:53.

156. Foley RN, Parfrey PS, Harnett JD, et al. The impact of anemia on cardiomyopathy, morbidity and mortality in end stage renal disease. *Am J Kidney Dis* 1996;28:53.

157. Martinez-Vea A, Bardaji A, Garcia C, et al. Long term myocardial effects of correction of anemia with recombinant human erythropoietin in aged dialysis patients. *Am J Kidney Dis* 1992;14:353.

158. Fellner S, Lang R, Neumann A, et al. Cardiovascular consequences of the correction of anemia of renal failure with erythropoietin. *Kidney Int* 1993;44:1309.

159. Besarab A, Bolton WK, Brown JK, et al. The effects of normal as compared with low hematocrit values in patients with cardiac disease who are receiving hemodialysis and epoetin. *N Engl J Med* 1998;339: 584.

160. Foley RN, Parfrey PS, Morgan J, et al. Effect of hemoglobin levels in hemodialysis patients with asymptomatic cardiomyopathy. *Kidney Int* 2000;58:1325.

161. Saxon L, Stevenson W, Middelkauff H, et al. Predicting death from progressive heart failure secondary to ischemic or idiopathic dilated cardiomyopathy. *Am J Cardiol* 1993;72:62.

162. Churchill D, Taylor D, Tomlinson C, et al. Effects of high flux hemodialysis on cardiac structure and function among patients with end-stage renal disease. *Nephron* 1993;65:573.

163. CANUSA (Canada-USA) Peritoneal Dialysis Study Group. Adequacy of dialysis and nutrition in continuous peritoneal dialysis: association with clinical outcomes. *J Am Soc Nephrol* 1996;7:198.

164. Gotch F, Levin N, Port F, et al. Clinical outcome relative to dose of dialysis is not what you think: the fallacy of the mean. *Am J Kidney Dis* 1997;30:1.

165. Fenton S, Schaubel D, Desmeules M, et al. Hemodialysis vs. peritoneal dialysis: a comparison of adjusted mortality rates. *Am J Kidney Dis* 1997;30:334.

166. Murphy SW, Foley R, Barrett B, et al. Comparative mortality of hemodialysis and peritoneal dialysis in Canada. *Kidney Int* 2000; 57:1720.

167. Collins A, Hao W, Xia H, et al. Mortality risks of peritoneal dialysis versus hemodialysis. *Am J Kidney Dis* 1999;34:1065.

168. Foley RN, Parfrey PS, Harnett JD, et al. Hypoalbuminemia, cardiac morbidity and mortality in end stage renal disease. *J Am Soc Nephrol* 1996;7:728.

169. Chaignon M, Chen WT, Tarazi RC, et al. Effect of hemodialysis on blood volume distribution and cardiac output. *Hypertension* 1981; 3:327.

170. London GM, Marchais SJ, Guerain AP, et al. Cardiovascular function in hemodialysis patients. *Adv Nephrol* 1991;20:249.

171. Hutchinson T, Thomas C, MacGibbon B. Predicting survival in adults with end stage renal failure: an age equivalence index. *Ann Intern Med* 1982;96:417.

172. Wizemann V. Coronary artery disease in dialysis patients. *Nephron* 1996;74:642.

173. Solomon AJ, Gersh BJ. Management of chronic stable angina: medical therapy, percutaneous transluminal coronary angioplasty, and coronary artery bypass graft surgery. *Ann Intern Med* 1998;128:216.

174. Hennekens CH, Dyken ML, Fuster V. Aspirin as a therapeutic agent in cardiovascular disease. *Circulation* 1997;96:2751.

175. Kasiske BL. Hyperlipidemia in patients with chronic renal disease. *Am J Kidney Dis* 1998;32[Suppl 3]:S142.

176. Marshall WG, Rossi NP, Meng RL, et al. Coronary artery bypass grafting in dialysis patients. *Ann Thorac Surg* 1986;42[Suppl 6]:S12.

177. Rostand SG, Kirk KA, Rutsky EA, et al. Results of coronary artery bypass grafting in end-stage renal disease. *Am J Kidney Dis* 1988;12:266.

178. Opsahl JA, Husebye DG, Helseth HK, et al. Coronary artery bypass surgery in patients on maintenance hemodialysis: long term survival. *Am J Kidney Dis* 1988;12:271.

179. Deutsch E, Berstein RC, Addonizio VP, et al. Coronary artery bypass surgery in patients on chronic hemodialysis: a case-control study. *Ann Intern Med* 1989;110:369.

180. Blakeman BP, Sullivan HJ, Foy BK, et al. Internal mammary artery revascularization in the patient on long term hemodialysis. *Ann Thorac Surg* 1990;50:776.

181. Batiuk TD, Kurtz SB, Oh JK, et al. Coronary artery bypass operation in dialysis patients. *Mayo Clin Proc* 1991;66:45.

182. Ko W, Krieger KH, Isom OW. Cardiopulmonary bypass procedures in dialysis patients. *Ann Thorac Surg* 1993;55:677.

183. Owen CH, Cummings RG, Sell TL, et al. Coronary artery bypass grafting in patients with dialysis-dependent renal failure. *Ann Thorac Surg* 1994;58:1729.

184. Rinehart AL, Herzog CA, Collins AJ, et al. A comparison of coronary angioplasty and coronary artery bypass grafting outcomes in chronic dialysis patients. *Am J Kidney Dis* 1995;25:281.

185. Koyanagi T, Nishida H, Kitamura M, et al. Comparison of clinical outcomes of coronary artery bypass grafting and percutaneous transluminal coronary angioplasty in renal dialysis patients. *Ann Thorac Surg* 1996;61:1793.

186. Samuels LE, Sharma S, Morris RJ, et al. Coronary artery bypass grafting in patients with chronic renal failure: a reappraisal. *J Card Surg* 1996;11:128.

187. Jahangiri M, Wright J, Edmondson S, et al. Coronary artery bypass graft surgery in dialysis patients. *Heart* 1997;78:343.

188. Zanardo G, Michielon P, Paccagnella A, et al. Acute renal failure in the patient undergoing cardiac operation. *J Thorac Cardiovasc Surg* 1993;107:1489.

189. Rao V, Weisel RD, Buth KJ, et al. Coronary artery bypass grafting in patients with non-dialysis dependent renal insufficiency. *Circulation* 1997;96[Suppl 2]:II-38.

190. CASS Principal Investigators and Their Associates. Coronary Artery Surgery Study (CASS): a randomized trial of coronary artery bypass surgery: survival data. *Circulation* 1983;68:939.

191. De Meyer M, Wyns W, Dion R, et al. Myocardial revascularization in patients on renal replacement therapy. *Clin Nephrol* 1991;36:147.

192. Christiansen S, Splittgerber FH, Marggraf G, et al. Results of cardiac operations in five kidney transplant patients. *Thorac Cardiovasc Surg* 1997;45:75.

193. Hueb WA, Oliveira SA, Bittencourt D, et al. Coronary artery bypass surgery for patients with renal transplantation. *Cardiology* 1986; 73:151.

194. Defraigne JO, Meurisse M, Limet R. Valvular and coronary surgery in renal transplant patients. *J Cardiovasc Surg* 1990;31:581.

195. Bolman RM, Anderson RW, Molina JE, et al. Cardiac operations in patients with functioning renal allografts. *J Thorac Cardiovasc Surg* 1984;88:537.

196. Manske CL, Wang Y, Rector T, et al. Coronary revascularization in insulin-dependent diabetic patients with chronic renal failure. *Lancet* 1992;340:998.

197. Kahn JK, Rutherford BD, McConahay DR, et al. Short and long term outcomes of percutaneous transluminal angioplasty in chronic dialysis patients. *Am Heart J* 1990;119:484.

198. Reusser LM, Osborn LA, White HJ, et al. Increased morbidity after coronary angioplasty in patients on chronic hemodialysis. *Am J Cardiol* 1994;73:965.

199. Ahmed WH, Shubrooks SJ, Gibson M, et al. Complications and long term outcome after percutaneous coronary angioplasty in chronic hemodialysis patients. *Am Heart J* 1994;128:252.

200. Schoebel FC, Gradaus F, Ivens K, et al. Restenosis after elective coronary balloon angioplasty in patients with endstage renal disease: a case-control study using quantitative coronary angiography. *Heart* 1997;78:337.

201. Toriyama T, Yokoya M, Matsuo S, et al. Effects of intervention with new devices on calcified coronary artery in hemodialysis (HD) patients. *J Am Soc Nephrol* 1997;8:255A(abstr).

202. Kishore KK, Silver M, Vatsavai SR, et al. Coronary stenting in ESRD patients. *J Am Soc Nephrol* 1997;8:140A(abstr).

203. Steering Committee and Membership of the Advisory Council to Improve Outcomes Nationwide in Heart Failure. Consensus recommendations for the management of chronic heart failure. *Am J Cardiol* 1999; 83:2A.

204. Garg RG, Yusuf S. Overview of randomized trials of angiotensin-converting enzyme inhibitors on mortality and morbidity in patients with heart failure. *JAMA* 1995;273:1450.

205. The Digitalis Investigation Group. The effect of digoxin on mortality and morbidity in patients with heart failure. *N Engl J Med* 1997;336: 525.

206. Uretsky BF, Young JB, Shahidi FE, et al. Randomized study assessing the effect of digoxin withdrawal in patients with mild to moderate chronic congestive heart failure: results of the PROVED trial. *J Am Coll Cardiol* 1993;22:955.

207. Packer M, Gheorghiade M, Young JB, et al. Withdrawal of digoxin from patients with chronic heart failure treated with angiotensin converting enzyme inhibitors. *N Engl J Med* 1993;329:1.

208. Young JB, Gheorghiade M, Uretsky BF, et al. Superiority of "triple" drug therapy in heart failure: insights from the PROVED and RADIANCE trials. *J Am Coll Cardiol* 1998;32:686.

209. Packer M, Bristow MR, Cohn JN, et al. The effect of carvedilol on morbidity and mortality in patients with chronic heart failure. *N Engl J Med* 1996;334:1349.

210. CIBIS Investigators and Committees. The Cardiac Insufficiency Bisoprolol Study II (CIBIS II): a randomized trial of beta-blockade in heart failure. *Lancet* 1999;353:9.

211. MERIT-HF Study Group. Effect of metoprolol CR/XL in chronic heart failure: Metoprolol CR/XL Randomized Intervention Trial in Congestive Heart Failure (MERIT-HF). *Lancet* 1999;353:2001.

212. MERIT-HF Study Group. Effects of controlled-release metoprolol on total mortality, hospitalizations, and well-being in patients with heart failure. *JAMA* 2000;283:1395.

213. Heart Failure Society of America. HFSA guidelines for management of patients with heart failure caused by left ventricular systolic dysfunction-pharmacological approaches. *Pharmacotherapy* 2000; 20:495.

214. Pitt B, Segal R, Martinez FA, et al. Randomized trial of losartan versus captopril in patients over 65 with heart failure (ELITE). *Lancet* 1997;349:747.

215. Pitt B, Poole-Wilson P, Segal R, et al. Effects of losartan versus captopril on mortality in patients with symptomatic heart failure: rationale, design, and baseline characteristics of the patients in the Losartan Heart Failure Survival Study (ELITE II). *J Card Fail* 1999;5:146.

216. Madore F, Lowrie EG, Brugnara C, et al. Anemia in hemodialysis patients: variables affecting this outcome predictor. *J Am Soc Nephrol* 1997;8:1921.

217. London GM, Zins B, Pannier B, et al. Vascular changes in hemodialysis patients in response to recombinant human erythropoietin. *Kidney Int* 1989;36:878.

218. Low I, Grutzmacher P, Bergmann M, et al. Echocardiographic findings in patients on maintenance hemodialysis substituted with recombinant human erythropoietin. *Clin Nephrol* 1989;31:26.

219. Silberberg J, Racine N, Barre PE, et al. Regression of left ventricular hypertrophy in dialysis patients following correction of anemia with recombinant human erythropoietin. *Can J Cardiol* 1990;6:1.

220. Pascual J, Teruel JL, Moya JL, et al. Regression of left ventricular hypertrophy after partial correction of anemia with erythropoietin in patients on hemodialysis: a prospective study. *Clin Nephrol* 1991;35: 280.

221. National Kidney Foundation-Dialysis Outcomes Quality Initiative. NKF-DOQI clinical practice guidelines for the treatment of anemia of chronic renal failure. *Am J Kidney Dis* 1997;30[4 Suppl 3]:S192.

222. Cannella G, Paoletti E, Delfineo R, et al. Regression of left ventricular hypertrophy in hypertensive dialyzed uremic patients on long-term antihypertensive therapy. *Kidney Int* 1993;44:881.

223. Dydadyk AI, Bagriy AE, Lebed IA, et al. ACE inhibitors captopril and enalapril induce regression of left ventricular hypertrophy in hypertensive patients with chronic renal failure. *Nephrol Dial Transplant* 1997;12:945.

224. London GM, Pannier B, Guerin AP, et al. Cardiac hypertrophy, aortic compliance, peripheral resistance, and wave reflection in end-stage renal disease: comparative effects of ACE inhibition and calcium channel blockade. *Circulation* 1994;90:2786.

225. Cruikshank JM, Lewis J, Moore V, et al. Reversibility of left ventricular hypertrophy by differing types of antihypertensive therapy. *J Hum Hypertens* 1992;6:85.

226. Mailloux LU, Levey AS. Hypertension in patients with chronic renal disease. *Am J Kidney Dis* 1998;32[Suppl 3]:S120.

CHAPTER 95

Metabolic and Endocrine Dysfunctions in Uremia

Shaul G. Massry, Miroslaw J. Smogorzewski, and Saulo Klahr

DISORDERS OF CARBOHYDRATE METABOLISM IN UREMIA

A multitude of abnormalities in carbohydrate metabolism are encountered in uremia (Table 95-1). Patients with chronic renal failure (CRF) and those treated with hemodialysis almost always display resistance to the peripheral action of insulin (1,2). The normal response of β cells to the presence of insulin resistance is to enhance their secretion of insulin. If for any reason, the β cells are unable to augment their secretion of insulin appropriately, an impaired glucose tolerance would ensue. The increase in the blood levels of insulin in response to hyperglycemia in uremic patients may be decreased, normal, or increased (3,4). These variations may reflect differences in insulin secretion and/or in its metabolic clearance.

Peripheral Resistance to Insulin Action

Usually, pancreatic β cells enhance their insulin secretion in the presence of insulin resistance (5,6), and therefore, glucose intolerance becomes apparent only when this adaptive response of β cells is impaired. Indeed, glucose intolerance is encountered in CRF patients who have both resistance to insulin action and impaired insulin secretion by β cells (1,7).

As early as 1962, Westervelt and Schreiner (8), using the forearm perfusion technique, showed that peripheral glucose uptake is reduced in uremic patients. This observation is consistent with the presence of resistance to the peripheral action of insulin. The introduction of the euglycemic insulin clamp technique provided the opportunity to measure the amount

S. G. Massry: Keck School of Medicine, University of Southern California School of Medicine, Los Angeles, California

M. J. Smogorzewski: Department of Medicine, Division of Nephrology, University of Southern California, Los Angeles, California

S. Klahr: Department of Medicine, Washington University School of Medicine; and Department of Science, Research and Science Affairs, Barnes-Jewish Hospital, St. Louis, Missouri

of glucose metabolized per unit of insulin (9) and confirmed the presence of decreased tissue sensitivity to insulin action (10). Castellino and colleagues (11) report that the peripheral resistance to insulin action occurs in patients with moderate renal failure and before the onset of signs and symptoms of the uremic syndrome.

The liver and skeletal muscles are the major sites for peripheral uptake of glucose. Therefore, resistance to insulin action in uremia may, theoretically, be present in both these organs and may result from (a) impaired uptake of glucose by these tissues and/or (b) increased production of glucose by the liver. However, the available data indicate that glucose metabolism by the liver is usually not impaired in uremia. Indeed hepatic glucose production (10,12,13) and its suppression by insulin (10,13) are not altered in CRF. Also glucose uptake by the liver is small and not affected by uremia (10). Thus, it is apparent that the skeletal muscles are the primary site for the decreased sensitivity to insulin action.

The insulin action on glucose transport by muscle is mediated through a complex process (14). First, insulin must bind to its receptor, which is made of two dimers (α and β) connected by a disulfide bond. The α subunit is located extracellularly and represents the ligand binding site. The β subunit is a transmembrane protein and contains an extracellular, transmembrane, and cytoplasmic domain; this β subunit has a tyrosine kinase activity. After insulin binding to the α-subunit, a signal is transmitted to the β subunit and results in autophosphorylation of the tyrosine residues causing a marked increase in tyrosine kinase activity. This is followed by tyrosine phosphorylation of insulin receptor substrate 1 (IRS1). The IRS1 is thought to operate as a multisite docking protein linked with insulin receptor and subsequently serves an important signaling role in the pathways for the various actions of insulin. One of these is the phosphatidylinositol 3-kinase pathway which is involved in the modulation of glucose transport.

The number of insulin receptors and their affinity to the hormone in erythrocytes (15), monocytes (10,13,16),

TABLE 95-1. *Characteristics of glucose and insulin metabolism in uremia*

Normal fasting blood glucose
Spontaneous hypoglycemia
Fasting hyperinsulinemia[a]
Normal, elevated, or decreased blood insulin levels in response to hyperglycemia induced by oral or intravenous glucose administration
Elevated blood levels of proinsulin and C peptide
Elevated blood levels of immunoreactive glucagon
Impaired insulin secretion by pancreatic islets[b]
Multiple derangements in metabolism and function of pancreatic islets
   Impaired glycolytic pathways
   Reduced basal and glucose-stimulated adenosine triphosphate content
   Elevated basal levels of cytosolic calcium
   Decreased V_{max} of Ca^{2+} ATPase and Na^+–K^+–ATPase
   Reduced calcium signal in response to glucose and potassium
Normal hepatic glucose production
Normal suppression of hepatic glucose production by insulin
Decreased peripheral sensitivity to insulin action
Impaired glucose tolerance[c]
Decreased requirement for insulin by diabetic patients with diabetic nephropathy and uremia

---

[a]Normal blood insulin levels may be encountered.
[b]This is observed only in the presence of established secondary hyperparathyroidism.
[c]This is present only when insulin secretion is impaired in the presence of the commonly encountered resistance to the peripheral action of insulin.

adipocytes (17–19), and hepatocytes (19) are normal. An increase in the number of insulin receptors was found in uremic patients compared to age- and sex-matched controls (20); also, insulin affinity to its receptors and insulin receptor kinase activity were unchanged (20). Similarly, insulin receptor kinase activity in skeletal muscles of chronic uremic rats is not different from control animals (21). All these data indicate that the insulin-resistant state in uremia is not due to abnormalities in the initial step (binding to receptor) of the cascade of the events that are involved in the peripheral action of insulin. It appears, therefore, that the cellular abnormality that underlies the reduced insulin sensitivity in CRF is a postreceptor defect. This notion implies that even very high levels of insulin may not correct the defect in glucose uptake by skeletal muscle. This postulate was confirmed by Smith and DeFronzo (12). The nature of this postreceptor defect is not as yet defined.

An insulin-regulated glucose transporter (GLUT-4), unique to muscle and adipose tissue, has been cloned and characterized (22,23). A decrease in the abundance of this transporter, in its translocation to cell surface, and/or in its intrinsic activity in uremia would provide an explanation for the reduced glucose uptake in response to insulin. Friedman and associates (24), however, report that the abundance of GLUT-4 in the muscle of a uremic patient is not different from that in normal subjects.

The peripheral resistance to insulin action occurs early in the course of renal failure and before the onset of signs and symptoms of the uremic syndrome become apparent. It is observed in the majority of patients with advanced renal failure and those treated with hemodialysis.

The resistance to the peripheral action of insulin is markedly improved after 10 weeks of hemodialysis (10,25) or following treatment of uremic patients with dietary protein restriction and supplementation with keto and amino acids for 6 months (26,27). Also, treatment with continuous ambulatory peritoneal dialysis (CAPD) is associated with improvement in peripheral insulin action (28). Further, glucose intolerance may even improve with CAPD therapy. These data suggest that a dialyzable uremic toxin, which may be a product of protein breakdown, is at least partly responsible for the derangement in insulin actions. Certain data have shown that uremic sera contain a compound that inhibits glucose metabolism by normal rat adipocytes (29). This compound has a molecular weight of 1,000 to 2,000 daltons, contains a protein component, and is specific for uremia because it is absent in the blood of patients with insulin-resistant state and without uremia. Others have found that hippurate, which accumulates in the blood of CRF patients, inhibits glucose utilization by rat diaphragm, brain, kidney cortex, and erythrocytes and may contribute to the insulin resistance in CRF (30).

Blood levels of glucagon (31,32) and growth hormone (33,34) are elevated in uremia. These hormones are antagonistic to insulin action and may contribute to the insulin-resistant state in CRF. However, the demonstration that dialysis therapy improves insulin sensitivity without an effect on the elevated blood levels of growth hormone and glucagon casts a doubt on their role in this phenomenon.

Sedentary lifestyle may be associated with insulin-resistant state (35). This phenomenon may contribute to the insulin-resistant state of uremic patients because they are weak, lead a sedentary lifestyle, and do not perform adequate exercise. Indeed, certain studies have shown that exercise training of uremic patients was followed by improvement in insulin sensitivity (36).

Insulin Secretion and Pancreatic Islet Metabolism

Changes in plasma insulin levels during glucose tolerance tests in uremic patients do not necessarily reflect insulin secretion because the metabolic clearance of insulin is impaired in uremia (37). The use of the hyperglycemic clamp technique has provided a better insight into the dynamics of insulin secretion in uremia. This technique evaluates both the initial (0 to 10 minutes) and late (10 to 20 minutes) responses in plasma insulin during sustained hyperglycemia. The results obtained with the hyperglycemic clamp in uremia are not uniform. Normal initial and exaggerated late responses (25), exaggerated initial and late responses (38), and decreased initial and late responses (13) have been reported. Since glucose utilization, even in the studies where insulin response

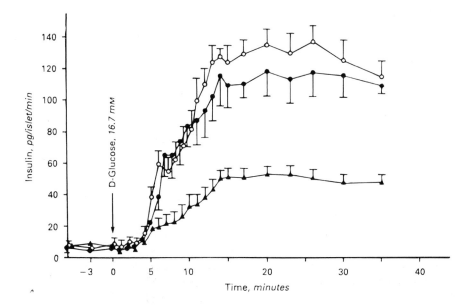

FIG. 95-1. Dynamic insulin release from perfused pancreatic islets of normal rats (○), animals with chronic renal failure (CRF)(▲), and normocalcemic parathyroidectomized rats with CRF (●). Each datum point represents the mean value, and brackets denote 1 SE. Note that both initial and late phases of glucose-induced insulin secretion are impaired. (From Fadda GZ, et al. Insulin release from pancreatic islets: effects of CRF and excess PTH. *Kidney Int* 1988;33:1066, with permission.)

was exaggerated, was not completely normalized (25,38), one may conclude that these data (13,25,38) indicate that insulin secretion in uremia is inappropriate relative to the state of insulin resistance. Direct evidence for impaired insulin secretion in CRF was provided by *in vitro* dynamic perfusion studies of pancreatic islets obtained from rats with CRF. Nakamuro and colleagues (39) and Fadda and others (40,41) reported impaired initial and late phase insulin secretion (Fig. 95-1).

Insulin secretion by β cells of the pancreatic islets is a complex process. The β cells are stimulated by nutrients (glucose, amino acids, or fatty acids) or nonnutrient agents such as hormones and neurotransmitter. The scope of this chapter does not permit a detailed presentation of this process. Although the mechanisms of recognition by the β cells of nutrient and nonnutrient stimuli may be different, the secretory process of insulin uses the same intracellular processes when the β cells are activated by nutrient or nonnutrient secretagogues.

In the case of glucose-induced insulin secretion, the process begins by the uptake of glucose by the β cells. Glucose is then metabolized to produce adenine triphosphate (ATP). The latter facilitates the closure of ATP-dependent potassium channels, followed by cell depolarization, and subsequent activation of voltage-sensitive calcium channels. As a consequence, calcium enters the islets causing an acute rise in cytosolic calcium concentration that triggers cellular events that lead to insulin secretion. Others propose that the ATP/adenosine diphosphate (ADP) ratio is an important factor in the sequence of events described above, and a rise in ATP/ADP ratio initiates the closure of the ATP-sensitive potassium channel and the depolarization of islets. Thus, a lower ATP content and/or a lower ATP/ADP ratio of islets in CRF, both in the resting state or after the stimulation with glucose, may contribute to the reduced insulin secretion.

Several studies indicate that the impairment of insulin secretion in uremia is mediated, in major part, by the state of secondary hyperparathyroidism that is commonly encountered in CRF. First, measurement of insulin secretion during hyperglycemic clamp studies before and after the medical suppression of the parathyroid gland or their surgical removal in children undergoing dialysis showed a significant improvement in insulin secretion after the normalization of the blood levels of parathyroid hormone (PTH) (42,43). Second, both initial and late plasma insulin responses during hyperglycemic clamp were reduced in dogs with CRF but normal in normocalcemic parathyroidectomized animals with CRF (13). Third, glucose-induced insulin secretion by pancreatic islets obtained from rats with CRF is reduced, but it is normal by islets from normocalcemic parathyroidectomized rats with CRF (40,41) (Fig. 95-1). Fourth, rats with normal renal function subjected to daily administration of PTH for 6 weeks displayed impaired glucose-induced insulin secretion by their islets (40,44) (Fig. 95-2). Thus, excess PTH inhibits insulin secretion in the presence or absence of uremia.

The severity of secondary hyperparathyroidism varies greatly among patients with CRF (45). It is possible that those with mild secondary hyperparathyroidism have appropriate response in insulin secretion during hyperglycemia as dictated by the insulin-resistant state and hence normal glucose metabolism. In contrast, impaired insulin secretion and glucose intolerance will be present in those with moderate to marked hyperparathyroidism. This postulate would provide an explanation for the variability in the presence of glucose intolerance among uremic patients.

Available data indicate that the chronic excess of PTH in the presence (41) or absence (44) of CRF causes a sustained rise in basal levels of cytosolic calcium ([Ca^{2+}]i) of pancreatic islets, and this abnormality plays an important role in the impaired insulin secretion (46). The processes involved in this elevation of [Ca^{2+}]i are complex. Both intact PTH

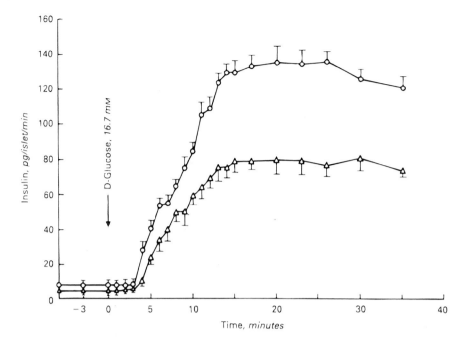

FIG. 95-2. Dynamic insulin release from perfused pancreatic islets of normal rats (○) and rats treated with parathyroid hormone (PTH) with normal renal function (△). Each datum point represents the mean value, and brackets denote 1 SE. Note the impaired insulin secretion in PTH-treated animals. (From Fadda GZ, et al. Insulin release from pancreatic islets: effects of CRF and excess PTH. *Kidney Int* 1988;33:1066, with permission.)

and its aminoterminal fragment enhance the entry of calcium into pancreatic islets (47,48). This action of PTH is receptor-mediated and is produced by generation of cyclic adenosine monophosphate (cAMP), stimulation of protein kinase C, and activation of voltage-dependent calcium channels through the stimulation of G proteins (48); further, verapamil, a calcium channel blocker, significantly inhibits the PTH-induced elevation in [Ca^{2+}]i of the islets (48). Several studies have shown that chronic and sustained entry of calcium into cells is associated with inhibition of mitochondrial oxidation with consequent reduction in ATP production (49–51). Indeed, the ATP content of pancreatic islets of rats with CRF is significantly lower than that of normal animals (41). Since the pumps that are directly (Ca^{+2}-ATPase) and indirectly (Na^+-K^+-ATPase) involved in calcium extrusion out of the islets require ATP, the lower ATP content of the islet in CRF would result in reduced activity of their Ca^{2+}-ATPase (41) and Na^+-K^+-ATPase (52) with consequent decrease in calcium efflux. Thus, it appears that the sustained rise in basal levels of [Ca^{2+}]i of pancreatic islets in CRF is due to both increased entry of calcium into and decreased exit of calcium out of the islets. This sequence of events is presented schematically in Fig. 95-3.

Several lines of evidence support the proposition that the elevated sustained elevation in the levels of [Ca^{2+}]i of the islets are responsible, in major part, for the impairment in their insulin secretion. First, rats with chronic excess of PTH in the presence or absence of CRF have elevated [Ca^{2+}]i and impaired insulin secretion (41,44). Second, normalization of [Ca^{2+}]i of pancreatic islets of rats with CRF by prior parathyroidectomy (40,41) or by their treatment with verapamil (53,54), which blocks the effect of PTH, prevents the impairment in insulin secretion. Finally, in the model of phosphate depletion, where the renal function is normal and

the parathyroid gland activity is inhibited, the basal levels of [Ca^{2+}]i of pancreatic islets are elevated and their insulin secretion is reduced (55).

The increased entry of calcium into islets in CRF and the elevation in basal levels of [Ca^{2+}]i may impair insulin secretion through an effect on ATP content of the islets. ATP is important in the process of insulin secretion because it facilitates the closure of the ATP-dependent potassium channels (56,57), which is followed by cell depolarization (57,58) and subsequent activation of voltage-sensitive calcium channels (57,59). As a consequence, calcium enters the islets, causing an acute rise in [Ca^{2+}]i (calcium signal), which triggers cellular events that lead to insulin secretion. Thus, a reduction in islet ATP content in CRF would be associated with a reduced glucose-induced calcium signal. This has been demonstrated by Fadda and Massry (60), who showed that the glucose-induced calcium signal in islets from rats with CRF was significantly smaller than that observed in islets from normal rats.

The sustained elevation in the basal levels of [Ca^{2+}]i and the reduction in the basal levels of ATP content of islets in CRF may affect glucose-induced insulin secretion through other metabolic pathways as well. For glucose-induced insulin secretion to occur, glucose must enter the islets and be appropriately metabolized. Fadda and coworkers (41) report that glucose uptake by islets from CRF animals is normal, but glucose metabolism by these islets is impaired.

After entry of glucose into the islets, it is phosphorylated to glucose-6-phosphate, converted by an isomerase to fructose-6-phosphate, and further phosphorylated by phosphofructokinase 1 (PFK-1) to fructose 1,6-biphosphate (61). These processes require an adequate amount of ATP and intact function of PFK-1. Thus, the low ATP content of islet in CRF and the finding that the V_{max} of PFK-1 is reduced in these islets (41)

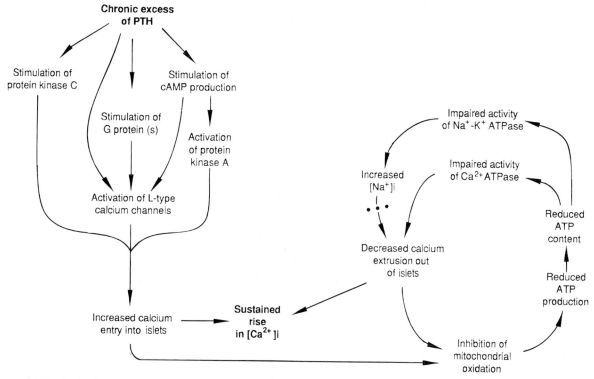

FIG. 95-3. A schematic presentation of the sequence of events that lead to a rise in the basal level of cytosolic calcium [Ca^{2+}]i in pancreatic islets from rats with chronic renal failure (CRF). *ATP*, adenosine triphosphate; *cAMP*, cyclic adenosine monophosphate; *PTH*, parathyroid hormone.

indicate that glucose metabolism is impaired at steps of the glycolytic pathways before the production of glyceraldehyde 3-phosphate. This notion is supported by the observation that glucose-induced ATP and lactic acid production by islets are impaired in CRF and that insulin secretion induced by glyceraldehyde, which enters the glycolytic pathways after the PFK-1 step (61), is normal in CRF (41). The disturbances in glucose metabolism of islets in CRF are induced mainly by the PTH-mediated sustained rise in [Ca^{2+}]i in islets of CRF. Indeed, glucose metabolism of islets is normal in normocalcemic parathyroidectomized rats with CRF (no elevation in blood levels of PTH and normal [Ca^{2+}]i of islets) (41) and in rats with CRF treated with verapamil (elevated blood levels of PTH but normal [Ca^{2+}]i of islets [54]).

Glucose is not the only nutrient that induces insulin secretion. Other stimuli include amino acids, the most potent of which is L-leucine (62), and potassium (63). CRF is associated with the impairment in both potassium-induced (64) and L-leucine-induced (65) insulin secretion. These abnormalities are also secondary to the PTH-mediated rise in basal levels of [Ca^{2+}]i of islets (64,65). Thus, a generalized failure of insulin secretion in response to a variety of secretagogues is present in CRF, and this defect is, in major part, due to chronic excess of PTH.

A number of studies point toward an interaction between 1,25-dihydroxyvitamin D$_3$ (1,25[OH]$_2$D$_3$) and insulin secretion. The endocrine pancreas of the chick contains a receptor protein for 1,25(OH)$_2$D$_3$ (66,67) and a Vitamin D-dependent calcium binding protein (68). The latter was found in the pancreas of other animals and is localized in the β cells of the islets (69, 70). Also labeled 1,25(OH)$_2$D$_3$ given to rats was found in the β cells of their pancreas (71). Finally, insulin secretion was inhibited in Vitamin D-deficient rats with normal renal function (72), and the defect was restored to normal after supplementation of Vitamin D to these animals (73).

Patients with CRF have low blood levels of 1,25(OH)$_2$D$_3$ and are usually Vitamin D-deficient (74). It is theoretically possible that the 1,25(OH)$_2$D$_3$ deficiency in these patients also plays a role in the impaired insulin secretion encountered in CRF. A study is available demonstrating that the acute intravenous administration of 1,25(OH)$_2$D$_3$ to dialysis patients was followed by a significant increment in early and late phases of insulin secretion as well as in correction of the glucose intolerance (75); these effects of 1,25(OH)$_2$D$_3$ occurred without changes in blood levels of PTH.

Insulin Clearance

The kidney plays an important role in insulin metabolism and clearance. Insulin is filtered by the glomeruli and reabsorbed by the proximal tubule (76). The renal clearance of insulin in normal subjects is about 200 mL/minute (77), a value greater than the glomerular filtration rate (GFR) indicating that peritubular uptake of insulin also occurs (78). It is estimated that 6 to 8 U of insulin are removed daily by the kidney, accounting for the clearance of 25% to 40% of insulin secreted by the pancreatic islets.

The decrease in metabolic clearance rate of insulin becomes apparent in patients with a GFR less than 40 mL/minute, but significant prolongation of the half-life of insulin is observed when GFR falls below 20 mL/minute (37). Treatment of uremic patients with dialysis is followed by marked improvement in insulin clearance presumably due to augmented removal of insulin by the liver and muscles. This observation is consistent with the notion that certain dialyzable uremic toxins are responsible for the decreased extrarenal clearance of insulin. The nature of these toxins is not known as yet.

In patients with CRF, impairment in both the renal (37) and the extrarenal (liver and muscles) (79) clearances of insulin is responsible for the fasting hyperinsulinemia, for the higher blood levels of insulin after glucose administration, for the decreased requirement of insulin in patients with diabetic nephropathy and uremia, and at least in part for the hypoglycemia that is occasionally encountered in nondiabetic patients with CRF.

Hypoglycemia

Both diabetic and nondiabetic patients with renal failure may develop spontaneous hypoglycemia. In the diabetic patients, decreased degradation of the administered insulin may result in higher blood levels of insulin than those expected and would therefore precipitate hypoglycemia; careful adjustment of the dosage of insulin therapy is needed in these patients.

Spontaneous hypoglycemia has been encountered in CRF (80–82). The mechanism of spontaneous hypoglycemia in nondiabetic uremic patients is not clear. In one such patient, a reduction in hepatic glucose output due to diminished alanine availability for gluconeogenesis was found (80). In another patient, spontaneous hypoglycemia occurred after parathyroidectomy, which was followed by a significant increase in insulin secretion (81). In a study of 21 nondiabetic hemodialysis patients treated with glucose-free dialysate, nine developed hypoglycemia (83). Poor nutritional status, diminished gluconeogenesis, impaired glycogenolysis, and impaired degradation in insulin may contribute to the spontaneous hypoglycemia (82).

Uremic diabetic patients treated with oral hypoglycemic agents, which are cleared by the kidney, may also require appropriate adjustment of the dosage of these drugs to avoid hypoglycemia. In these patients, it is also advisable to use short-acting oral hypoglycemic agents.

Clinical Consequences

Excess PTH in CRF may interfere with extrarenal disposal of potassium loads (84). It is possible that this abnormality is linked with the impairment in insulin secretion of CRF. Potassium stimulates insulin secretion (63,85), and insulin is an important regulator of extrarenal disposition of potas-

sium (86,87). Since potassium-induced insulin secretion by pancreatic islets obtained from rats with CRF is markedly reduced (64), one would expect that this abnormality would contribute to the impairment in the extrarenal disposal of potassium loads in CRF and may contribute to the appearance of hyperkalemia.

An increase in atherogenesis and other cardiac diseases is encountered in uremic patients (88). Several factors may be responsible for this phenomenon. The disturbances in glucose metabolism and insulin secretion and the secondary hyperparathyroidism may all contribute to the increased risk for atherogenesis in these patients. Postprandial hyperglycemia in the glucose-intolerant uremic patient may, by itself, be a risk factor for atherosclerotic cardiovascular disease. Hyperinsulinemia and insulin-resistant state may be associated with hypertension (89), which is a well-recognized risk factor for cardiac disease in uremia.

Insulin is also an important regulator of lipoprotein lipase activity, and insulin deficiency or resistance to its action is associated with reduced availability and hence activity of this enzyme (90). This enzyme plays a major role in triglyceride removal. Indeed postheparin lipolytic activity in patients with CRF is impaired, and this defect is the primary cause of hypertriglyceridemia in these patients (91). Further support for the role of insulin in this regard is provided by the observation that administration of insulin to rats with CRF corrected the defect in postheparin lipolytic activity as well as the hypertriglyceridemia (92).

Other studies have shown that excess PTH plays a significant role in the genesis of the reduced postheparin lipolytic activity and in the hypertriglyceridemia of CRF. Normocalcemic parathyroidectomized dogs (93) and rats (94) with CRF have normal postheparin lipolytic activity and normal blood levels of triglycerides. It is possible that the excess PTH exerts its effects by a direct action on the metabolism of both hepatic (95) and lipoprotein lipases (96) and/or through an indirect effect on insulin secretion. Indeed, the production, activity, secretion, and the molecular machinery of both hepatic and lipoprotein lipases are adversely affected by CRF.

It should also be mentioned that insulin is an anabolic hormone. It promotes amino acid uptake by skeletal muscle and inhibits protein degradation. Resistance to insulin action in patients with CRF may contribute to protein catabolism in these patients.

DISORDERS OF LIPID METABOLISM IN UREMIA

Lipids, Lipoproteins, and Lipid Transport and Metabolism

Altered lipid metabolism is common in patients with chronic renal insufficiency (97). Lipids circulate in plasma, incorporated into spheric, water-soluble particles (lipoproteins) that contain a core of nonpolar lipids (cholesterol, cholesterol esters, and triglycerides) surrounded by a monolayer composed of specific proteins (apoproteins), polar lipids, and esterified cholesterol and phospholipids (98,99). This monolayer permits the lipoprotein to remain miscible in plasma. Lipoproteins are an efficient vehicle for the transport of triglycerides and cholesterol in plasma.

Lipoproteins can be separated by electrophoresis and ultracentrifugation in salt solutions. The classification of lipoproteins is usually reported on the basis of their separation by ultracentrifugation. The density and hence the ultracentrifugation characteristics of lipoproteins differ widely and depend on the ratio between surface and core components (98,99). Based on their density, four classes of lipoproteins are present in plasma from fasting individuals: very-low-density lipoprotein (VLDL), intermediate-density lipoprotein (IDL), low-density lipoprotein (LDL), and high-density lipoprotein (HDL). Chylomicrons (large triglyceride-rich particles of intestinal origin) are the fifth class of lipoproteins, transiently present in plasma in the postprandial state. Each of these lipoproteins is heterogeneous in terms of size, lipid composition, and apoprotein content. Subfractions of the major lipoprotein classes can be isolated by electrophoresis, gradient ultracentrifugation, or affinity column chromatography. A sixth lipoprotein, Lp(a) lipoprotein, is present in plasma. This lipoprotein has a hydrated density between 1.06 and 1.08 g/mL. Lp(a) lipoprotein consists of an LDL particle to which an additional protein, apoprotein (a), is covalently bound (100,101).

The protein components of lipoproteins (apoproteins) are classified by letters of the alphabet and roman numeral suffixes (Table 95-2). Some of these apoproteins, such as apoprotein A-I in HDL, apoprotein B-100 in LDL, and apoprotein B-48 in chylomicrons, play a structural role. Some apolipoproteins are ligands for receptors such as apoprotein B-100 for the LDL receptor and apoprotein E for the chylomicron remnant receptor. The potential functions of some of these apoproteins are described in Table 95-2.

Three enzymes (98,99) play a pivotal role in lipid metabolism: lipoprotein lipase, hepatic triglyceride lipase (HTGL),

and lecithin-cholesterol acyltransferase (LCAT). In addition, a specific transfer protein, cholesteryl ester transfer protein (CETP), facilitates the exchange of cholesteryl esters and triglycerides between HDL and triglyceride-rich lipoproteins. The major physiologic action of lipoprotein lipase is to degrade triglyceride-rich particles in the postprandial state. The activity of the enzyme is dependent on the presence of a cofactor, apoprotein C-II. The enzyme apparently exerts its action at the level of the endothelial surface. It releases fatty acids that can be utilized to satisfy energy needs or can be stored in adipose tissue, depending on the metabolic conditions. As a consequence of this hydrolysis, triglyceride particles develop a reduced core size, lose a portion of the surface components such as phospholipids and proteins, and become smaller in size and denser. Hepatic lipase has two major actions: (a) hydrolysis of triglycerides and phospholipids on HDL_2, and (b) hydrolysis of triglycerides on VLDLs and IDLs. The enzyme LCAT, which is synthesized in the liver, catalyzes the formation of all cholesterol esters in the plasma by transferring a fatty acyl chain of phospholipids to the hydroxy group of unesterified cholesterol. This action, which occurs in the circulation, accounts for the balance between cholesterol on the surface and in the core of each lipoprotein particle.

Metabolism of Very-Low-Density Lipoproteins

The liver is the main site of VLDL synthesis. VLDL particles transport endogenous triglycerides from the liver to peripheral tissues (102,103). The intravascular hydrolysis of VLDL triglycerides depends on the activity of lipoprotein lipase (Fig. 95-4). Remnant particles that result from VLDL lipolysis are either taken up by the liver via apo E-mediated metabolism or subsequently converted to LDL (Fig. 95-4). LDL is the major product of VLDL metabolism in human plasma. Several factors, including diet, plasma concentrations of free fatty acids, and levels of insulin, glucagon, and

TABLE 95-2. *Metabolic functions of plasma apoproteins*

Apoprotein	Molecular weight	Metabolism role
A-I	28,000	Activates LCAT
A-II	17,500	Activates hepatic lipase; may inhibit LCAT
A-IV	46,000	Unknown, possibly involved in lipid transfer between lipoproteins
B-48	264,000	Transport of lipids from the gut as chylomicrons
B-100	512,000	Transport of lipids from the liver as VLDL and LDL; recognized by cellular LDL receptors
C-I	7,000	Activates LCAT
C-II	9,000	Activates lipoprotein lipase
C-III	9,000	May inhibit activation of lipoprotein lipase by apo C-II
D	22,000	May be involved in lipid transfer between lipoproteins
E	34,000	Recognized by hepatic apo E receptors and cellular LDL receptors; recognition facilitates hepatic uptake of chylomicron and VLDL remnants
Transfer proteins	Variable	Facilitate the transfer of triglycerides, phospholipids, and cholesteryl esters between lipoproteins

LCAT, lecithin–cholesterol acyltransferase; *LDL,* low-density lipoprotein; *VLDL,* very-low-density lipoprotein
(From Illingworth DR. Lipoprotein metabolism. *Am J Kidney Dis* 1993;22:90, with permission.)

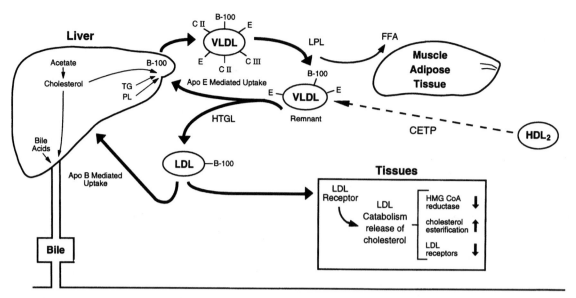

FIG. 95-4. Metabolic interconversions of very-low-density (VLDL) and low-density lipoproteins (LDL) in plasma and the intracellular effects of receptor-mediated uptake of LDL free fatty acids (FFA). *CETP,* cholesteryl ester transfer protein; *HDL$_2$,* HDL with a density between 1.063 and 1.125 g/mL; *HMG CoA,* 3-hydroxy-3-methylglutaryl coenzyme A; *HTGL,* hepatic triglyceride lipase; *LPL,* lipoprotein lipase; *PL,* phospholipid; *TG,* triglyceride. (From Illingworth DR. Lipoprotein metabolism. *Am J Kidney Dis* 1993;22:90, with permission.)

epinephrine in plasma, appear to modulate the secretion of hepatic VLDL, which in turn influences VLDL concentrations in plasma. In subjects with normal triglyceride levels, all the apo B that enters plasma as a component of VLDL is preserved, as the particle is metabolized to IDL and to LDL. In contrast, in patients with severe hypertriglyceridemia, most of the VLDL particles are removed prior to conversion to LDL, leading to low plasma concentrations of LDL. Moderate hypertriglyceridemia, plasma triglycerides of 300 to 800 mg/dL, usually reflects the accumulation of endogenous VLDL particles in plasma. Such an accumulation may result from enhanced rates of LDL synthesis, genetic or acquired defects in triglyceride hydrolysis, or combinations of both.

Metabolism of Low-Density Lipoproteins

LDL is the major cholesterol-carrying particle present in human plasma. Metabolically, LDL may be considered an end product of VLDL metabolism. The liver accounts for 70% of the catabolism of LDL, and peripheral tissues account for the remaining 30%. LDL catabolism is facilitated by both receptor-mediated and nonreceptor-mediated pathways. In normal subjects, receptor-mediated pathways account for about 75% of the clearance of plasma LDL. The uptake of LDL by receptor-mediated endocytosis results in the suppression of endogenous cholesterol biosynthesis, an enhanced rate of intracellular cholesterol esterification, and a reduction in the number of high-affinity LDL receptors expressed on the cell surface. Hypercholesterolemia, with increased plasma concentrations of LDL cholesterol, may be the consequence of a number of genetic and acquired

disorders. These may lead to an enhanced rate of VLDL and LDL apo-B synthesis from either genetic (104,105) or acquired defects in LDL catabolism (due to impaired expression of high-affinity LDL receptors), from disturbances in the receptor binding domain of LDL, which causes impaired LDL catabolism, or from combined defects resulting in enhanced synthesis and impaired catabolism.

Metabolism of High-Density Lipoproteins

HDL is generated in the liver and from the intravascular lipolysis of VLDL particles and chylomicrons. The newly synthesized HDL contains predominantly protein, free cholesterol, and phospholipids, but when exposed to LCAT it becomes rich in cholesterol esters (106). The apoprotein content of individual HDL particles differs, and it is apparent that some HDL particles contain apo A-I and apo A-II, whereas others may only contain apo A-I. The half-life of HDL is from 4 to 6 days and is influenced by both diet and a number of drugs. Diets rich in carbohydrates, which raise VLDL, reduce HDL concentrations and result in an enhanced rate of HDL turnover, whereas nicotinic acid, which depresses VLDL synthesis, raises the concentrations of HDL and prolongs the half-life of apo A-I in plasma. Epidemiologic studies show an inverse correlation between the plasma concentrations of HDL cholesterol and the risk of coronary artery disease. Factors that increase HDL concentrations include a moderate consumption of alcohol, sustained regular exercise, and correction of hypertriglyceridemia (107,108).

In summary, the transport and metabolism of lipoproteins in humans are relatively well understood. A number of factors, both genetic and acquired, may modify this transport system and result in abnormal concentrations of lipoproteins in plasma. Increased plasma concentrations of cholesterol-rich VLDL and chylomicron remnants of LDL and of Lp(a), all appear to be highly atherogenic, whereas on the basis of epidemiologic studies, increased concentrations of HDL cholesterol appear to afford protection from the premature development of atherosclerosis. Modifications in lipoproteins, particularly oxidation or glycosylation of LDL, may also affect the metabolism of these lipoproteins and result in enhanced rates of uptake by scavenger receptors present in tissue macrophages, with the resultant formation of foam cells (109,110).

Abnormalities of Lipoprotein Metabolism in Renal Disease

The mechanisms by which loss of renal function affects lipoprotein metabolism are not well understood (97,102). Although disorders of lipoprotein metabolism increase in frequency with advancing renal insufficiency, this is not always reflected in the degree of hyperlipidemia. Dyslipoproteinemias found in patients with renal disease may be secondary to their renal insufficiency (111–113) or may be due to genetic abnormalities. To rule out genetic abnormalities, important information can be obtained from examination of family members and from family histories and a careful analysis of the events preceding the onset of renal insufficiency. Early in renal disease, disturbances of apoprotein metabolism may be found without any changes in lipid levels. Significantly reduced levels of apo A-I or apo A-II may be detected in renal insufficiency and in patients with normal lipid levels (103). However, reduced levels of these two major HDL apoproteins are more marked in patients with advanced renal failure and in patients with hypertriglyceridemia (114,115). In some studies, no significant decreases of plasma apo A-I and apo A-II concentrations were found in patients with CRF (116,117). Male patients may have lower HDL cholesterol levels and apo A-I concentrations than female patients (115,118). Concentrations of apo B are usually normal in early renal insufficiency, and reduced, normal, or increased concentrations of apo B have been reported in patients with advanced renal insufficiency and in those on dialysis (103,114,115,119).

In CRF, a moderate elevation of triglyceride concentrations represents the characteristic plasma lipid abnormality (112), but a significant number of patients have normal triglyceride levels (103,114). The occurrence of hypertriglyceridemia varies considerably among reported patient populations. Among patients in dialysis, about 30% to 70% of the total patient population will demonstrate elevated triglyceride values. In contrast, plasma cholesterol levels are usually within the normal range. This lipid profile, which resembles lipoprotein phenotype IV, has been a consistent finding in most reports. In contrast with the numerous studies of plasma lipids in patients with advanced renal insufficiency, relatively

little information is available on the earlier asymptomatic stages of renal insufficiency. Plasma triglyceride levels may be normal when GFR exceeds 20 mL/minute in nondiabetic patients. Grützmacher and colleagues (120) have reported increased serum triglyceride levels when the GFR decreased below 30 mL/minute. Others have found elevated triglyceride concentrations in only 30% of patients with a GFR greater than 15 mL/minute in comparison with 62% of patients with more advanced renal failure and 76% of patients on hemodialysis (121). However, plasma cholesterol levels were increased in only 25% of patients with advanced renal insufficiency.

Platelet-activating factor (PAF) is a potent inflammatory mediator associated with several disorders, including renal disease. PAF is degraded to the inactive metabolic lyso-PAF by PAF-acetyl hydrolase (PAF-AH), which is considered a potent antiinflammatory and antiatherogenic associated with lipoproteins. Milionis and coworkers (122) report that plasma PAF-AH activity is increased in uremic patients. This elevation is greater in patients in CAPD. These patients also exhibit a more atherogenic lipid profile and more pronounced alterations in the specific activity and the kinetic constants of Lp(a)-associated PAF-AH.

Some of the lipid changes associated with renal disease include a decrease in cholesterol in HDL and an increase in cholesterol in VLDL and IDL. The LDL cholesterol is usually within normal limits. Thus, there is a redistribution of cholesterol from HDL to VLDL and IDL even when the plasma levels of cholesterol are within normal limits (123–125). As a consequence of this redistribution, the ratio of either total cholesterol or LDL cholesterol to HDL cholesterol is increased. The reduced levels of HDL are reflected in reductions in both HDL_2 and HDL_3 subfractions (126). Although patients with moderate renal insufficiency often have normal levels of plasma triglycerides and cholesterol, more subtle changes in the lipid distribution may be found, including an increase in the concentration of LDL triglyceride and a reduction in the concentration of HDL cholesterol (120,127). There are also changes in the concentrations of apoproteins. In advanced renal failure, there are decreased concentrations of apo A-I and A-II, normal or minimal elevations of apo B, and normal or, in male patients, decreased levels of apo E. In addition, there is a significantly greater concentration of apo C-III and less pronounced increases in the levels of apo C-I and C-II (115,120,128). Increased concentrations of apo C-III tend to correlate with triglyceride levels but may also be found in patients with normal levels of triglycerides. The ratios of apo A-I to C-III and apo A-I to B are reduced, and the ratio of apo C-III to apo E is increased (115,119,125). The changes in apo C-III ratios in patients with renal insufficiency are greater in patients with hypertriglyceridemia than in those who have normal lipid levels in plasma (115,121,128). Apoproteins may be an excellent marker of dyslipoproteinemia because other observations suggest that in the earliest stages of renal insufficiency it is possible to detect marked changes in apoprotein profiles and major lipoprotein density classes in plasma (115,121). In patients with GFR values greater than 15 mL/minute and normal plasma levels of lipids, there is a significant decrease in the concentrations of apo A-I and A-II and increased concentrations of apo C-III. The redistribution of apo B, C-III, and E characteristics of advanced renal insufficiency can also be found in patients with incipient to moderately advanced renal insufficiency (119).

Mechanisms of Altered Lipid Metabolism in Chronic Renal Insufficiency

The rates of production and catabolism of lipoproteins determine their plasma concentration. The mechanisms responsible for hypertriglyceridemia in chronic renal disease have not been fully clarified, but the major defect appears to be reduced lipolysis of triglyceride-rich lipoproteins (129–132). Several of the factors that may affect the metabolism of triglyceride-rich lipoproteins in renal failure are listed in Table 95-3. Substantial evidence suggests impaired transport and catabolism of triglyceride-rich lipoproteins in renal failure (130,132,133). This results in accumulation of lipoproteins at various stages of catabolism, as reflected in the increased concentrations of IDL and remnants of intestinal lipoproteins (chylomicron remnants) often found in patients with renal insufficiency (133,134). The catabolism of triglyceride-rich lipoprotein is mediated by lipoprotein lipase and by HTGL, possibly via the apo B and apo E receptors in the liver (135). In uremic patients, VLDL may be directly removed without being converted into LDL (136). Several studies have reported decreased activities of lipoprotein lipase in the plasma and adipose tissue of uremic patients (137–139).

Patients with GFR values less than 50 mL/minute may have reduced lipolytic activity after heparin administration without increases in plasma triglycerides (140). The factors responsible for the decrease in lipoprotein lipase activity are unknown. Insulin resistance or deficiency may have a role in this process (141). A nondialyzable inhibitor of lipoprotein lipase may also accumulate in uremia (137,142).

Apo C-II is a cofactor for lipoprotein lipase activity, whereas apo C-III inhibits this reaction. A decreased ratio of apo C-II to C-III as found in uremia may therefore affect the activity of lipoprotein lipase (143–145). Patients with chronic renal insufficiency also have a reduced activity of HTGL (146–148). Thus, a decreased activity of both lipases may account for the defective catabolism of triglyceride-rich lipoproteins in uremia. Reduced lipoprotein lipase activity could explain the decreased catabolism of newly secreted chylomicrons and VLDL, whereas reduced activity of HTGL may impair the clearance of partially metabolized lipoproteins and chylomicron remnants. Normal lipid metabolism also requires the removal by peripheral cells and adipose tissue of fatty acids generated during lipolysis. Uremic patients with hypertriglyceridemia exhibit a lower rate of fatty acid incorporation into adipose tissue than do uremic patients with normal levels of triglycerides (149). A reduced activity of LCAT in uremia (123,150,151) may also have a role in the decreased catabolism of triglyceride-rich lipoproteins. Alterations of LCAT may also lead to changes in HDL composition and impaired cholesterol transport.

An increase in triglyceride production may also contribute to the hypertriglyceridemia. Some patients, particularly those with elevated triglyceride levels, may have increased triglyceride synthesis compared to patients with normal triglyceride levels (136). Because of the decreased catabolism of triglycerides, even modest increases in triglyceride production may increase triglyceride levels substantially (152). Insulin resistance may also have a role in the hypertriglyceridemia observed in CRF, although this suggestion is conjectural at present (153,154).

TABLE 95-3. *Factors that may contribute to hypertriglyceridemia in patients with chronic renal insufficiency*

Decreased triglyceride catabolism and removal	Increased triglyceride production
Decreased activity of lipolytic enzymes	Increased ingestion of carbohydrates
Lipoprotein lipase	
Insulin deficiency or resistance	Uptake of glucose from dialysate in CAPD
Increased PTH	
Inhibitors in uremic plasma	
Reduced apo C-II/C-III ratio	Hyperinsulinemia (?)
Hepatic triglyceride lipase	
Lecithin–cholesterol acyltransferase (LCAT)	
Alterations of lipoprotein substrate	
Triglyceride-enriched LDL	
Altered apolipoprotein composition	
Increased apo C-III/E in IDL-LDL	
Modifications of lipoproteins	
Decreased receptor- and nonreceptor-mediated cellular uptake of lipoproteins	

CAPD, continuous ambulatory peritoneal dialysis; *IDL,* intermediate-density lipoprotein; *LDL,* low-density lipoprotein; *PTH,* parathyroid hormone
(Adapted from Attman PO, Alaupovic P. Lipid abnormalities in chronic renal insufficiency. *Kidney Int* 1991;31:S16, with permission.)

Lp(a) Lipoprotein in End-Stage Renal Disease

Lp(a) lipoprotein is a plasma lipoprotein, the protein component of which consists of apo B covalently bound to apoprotein (a), a glycoprotein that is structurally homologous to plasminogen (154,155). Several reports suggest that increased levels of Lp(a) in plasma represent an important and independent risk factor for coronary artery disease (155–157). A number of studies indicate that patients with end-stage renal disease (ESRD) have a two- to threefold increase in the concentration of Lp(a) in plasma before and after replacement therapy when compared to normal subjects (158,159). Both normal and increased levels of Lp(a) have been reported in patients after a kidney transplant (160,161). Although normal levels of Lp(a) have been reported in patients on CAPD (162), other reports indicate that the levels of Lp(a) are elevated in CAPD patients (159,163). Whether the conflicting findings are due to differences in analytic techniques, to genetic differences, or to some other factors remains to be established. The potential mechanisms by which ESRD leads to increased levels of Lp(a) are not presently known.

Treatment of Lipid Disorders in Patients with Renal Insufficiency

Several factors in addition to the lipid abnormalities, including hypertension, smoking, electrolyte imbalances, hemostatic abnormalities, and accumulation of uremic toxins, may contribute to the development of atherosclerosis in the patient with chronic renal insufficiency. The potential contribution of elevated levels of triglycerides to this increased risk for atherogenesis is unclear. Whether hypertriglyceridemia per se is a risk factor for coronary heart disease is questionable (164). Certainly triglycerides do not greatly contribute to the composition of the atherosclerotic plaques. However, high levels of triglycerides are known to raise the concentrations of other "atherogenic" lipoproteins that apparently do promote plaque formation. These include chylomicron remnants (165), VLDL remnants (166,167), and small, dense LDL (168,169). Moreover, elevated triglycerides are often associated with reduced levels of apoproteins that may "prevent" atherosclerosis, such as HDL (170,171). Thus, although elevated levels of triglycerides in plasma may not be atherogenic per se, they may increase the risk of coronary artery disease through secondary effects on lipoprotein metabolism. If this were the case, treatment of hypertriglyceridemia would be advisable. Unfortunately, safe and effective modalities of therapy for reducing triglyceride levels are not available. Dietary modifications including weight loss in obese patients and reduced intake of carbohydrates will minimize the overproduction of VLDL triglycerides by the liver and thereby lower plasma triglyceride levels (152,172,173). These dietary manipulations, however, do not affect the underlying defect, that is, the decreased lipolysis of VLDL triglycerides, and they would not be expected to eliminate elevated triglyceride levels in most patients. According to

some reports, restricting carbohydrates and cholesterol with no change in protein intake may significantly reduce fasting levels of serum triglycerides and triglyceride production (152). Low-protein diets supplemented with keto acids or essential amino acids may reduce triglycerides (mainly in male patients) and cholesterol (174,175). Such diets also may normalize high cholesterol levels even in diabetic patients with overt nephropathy and chronic renal insufficiency (176). Exercise apparently promotes catabolism of VLDL triglycerides. Goldberg and associates (177) describe a 23% decrease in plasma levels of triglycerides and a 30% decrease in the levels of VLDL triglycerides in hemodialysis patients who underwent 12 months of exercise training. In sedentary patients, by contrast, total triglyceride and VLDL triglyceride levels increased during the same period.

Several classes of drugs seem effective in the treatment of hypercholesterolemia. These include the fibric acids, probucol, nicotinic acid, inhibitors of the 3-hydroxy-3-methylglutaryl coenzyme A (HMG CoA) reductase, and bile acid sequestrants.

Fibric Acids

One group of lipid-lowering drugs most extensively used in patients with chronic renal insufficiency is the fibric acids. A major effect of fibric acids is to enhance the activity of lipoprotein lipase. Thus, they tend to correct the underlying cause of elevated triglycerides in patients with renal failure. Among the fibric acids studied clinically in renal failure patients are clofibrate (178–180), gemfibrozil (181), and bezafibrate (182). Most studies suggest that with these agents triglyceride levels decrease significantly and HDL levels often rise as well (178,179,181). Since fibric acids are excreted mainly by the kidneys, their dosage has to be adjusted to prevent toxicity. Toxicity usually is manifested by myopathy accompanied by high serum levels of serum creatine kinase. Although some patients with chronic renal insufficiency can tolerate fibric acids without developing myopathy, several investigators (180,181) suggest that the risk is sufficient to prevent the use of these drugs in the treatment of hypertriglyceridemia in patients with renal failure. Other lipid-lowering drugs have not been adequately tested in patients with chronic renal insufficiency. Omega-3 polyunsaturated fatty acids (found in fish oils) can lower triglyceride levels. However, they mainly decrease the secretion rate for VLDL triglycerides and do not modify the underlying lipolytic defect. In addition, they may increase the likelihood of bleeding by interfering with platelet function. Their use in uremic patients cannot be recommended at this time because they have not been adequately studied and information regarding their safety during long-term administration is not available.

Probucol

Probucol causes a modest reduction of LDL cholesterol levels. It also reduces the levels of HDL cholesterol. Its major benefit may be related to its antioxidant effects. This drug appears to be devoid of major side effects.

Nicotinic Acid

Nicotinic acid reduces LDL cholesterol, lowers VLDL triglyceride levels, and raises HDL cholesterol. This drug appears to inhibit the hepatic secretion of lipoproteins containing apo B. The drug has several side effects. It may cause flushing and itching of the skin, hyperglycemia, liver dysfunction, and hyperuricemia. Some of the side effects may be minimized by giving very low doses of the drug and increasing the dosage slowly.

3-Hydroxy-3-Methylglutaryl Coenzyme a Reductase Inhibitors

These drug "statins" inhibit a rate-limiting enzyme in cholesterol synthesis (183). They inhibit hepatic cholesterol synthesis and enhance LDL receptor formation. They lower the plasma levels of both LDL cholesterol and VLDL triglycerides. Studies both *in vivo* and *in vitro* have demonstrated that "statins" may affect the progressive course of renal disease by modifying monocyte infiltration, mesangial cell proliferation, mesangial matrix expansion and tubulointerstitial inflammation, and fibrosis. These effects may be related, at least in part, to inhibition of small G-protein isoprenylation involved in early gene products, transcription factors, and modulation of the cell-cycle regulatory proteins. Few side effects are encountered with these drugs. In some patients, they may cause elevated liver enzymes, gastrointestinal discomfort, and insomnia. A more serious complication is the development of myopathy. Factors predisposing to myopathy include the simultaneous use of cyclosporine, fibric acids, or nicotinic acid and the presence of hepatic disease.

Lipid abnormalities in renal disease are associated with progressive loss of renal function in experimental animals. Recently the "statins" have demonstrated a beneficial effect in different animal models of progressive renal failure. Lovastatin ameliorated the extent of glomerular disease in the model of renal ablation, in obese Zucker rats and in rats given puromycin aminonucleoside with the nephrotic syndrome.

Bile Acid Sequestrants

Bile acid sequestrants are nonabsorbable resins (cholestyramine, colestipol) that bind bile acids in the intestine. They cause increased conversion of cholesterol to bile acids and decrease the cholesterol content of the liver, thus promoting the synthesis of LDL receptors. The final result is a decrease in LDL cholesterol in plasma. At doses of 8 to 20 g/day, the levels of LDL cholesterol in plasma may decrease by 30 to 60 mg/dL. These drugs can cause constipation and may prevent the adequate absorption of certain drugs (digoxin, warfarin, thiazide diuretics, and β-blockers).

Prospective, randomized clinical trials designed to reduce lipid abnormalities using a combination of hypolipidemic drugs and angiotensin-converting enzyme (ACE) inhibitors, LDL apheresis, and supplemental vitamins are lacking. Such clinical trials would clarify the role of treating lipid abnormalities in the progression of renal disease and their role in cardiovascular complications (184).

DISORDERS OF PROTEIN AND AMINO ACID METABOLISM IN UREMIA

Nutrients can be divided into six general classes: proteins, lipids, carbohydrates, minerals, vitamins, and water. The first three classes are organic compounds that serve as sources of energy required for carrying out the biochemical and functional activities of organs and cells (185). In addition to being an energy source, proteins in the diet provide the amino acids that are used to synthesize body proteins. Proteins and their constituent amino acids are essential to life. They fulfill a variety of physiologic roles including effecting the growth and maintenance of new tissue and regulating many functions, such as enzymatic activity, growth, and ion and solute transport. They also serve as signaling molecules across cell membranes, as hormones, in immunity as antibodies, in differentiation, in gene expression, and so on.

The protein requirement of an individual is defined as the lowest level of dietary protein intake that will balance the losses of nitrogen from the body in persons maintaining energy balance at modest levels of physical activity. The need for dietary protein arises largely because turnover of tissue and organ proteins is accompanied by an inefficient capture of their constituent amino acids to form new body proteins. The amino acids are lost via oxidative metabolism. Most estimates of protein and amino acid requirements in humans have been obtained directly or indirectly from measurements of nitrogen balance. In the course of carrying out their functional roles, proteins and amino acids turn over, and part of their nitrogen and carbon is lost via excretory pathways, including carbon dioxide in expired air and urea and ammonium in urine. Thus, to maintain an adequate protein and amino acid balance, these losses must be replaced by an appropriate dietary supply of a usable source of nitrogen and by indispensable and conditionally indispensable amino acids to replace those that are lost during the course of their daily metabolic transactions or those that are deposited during growth and tissue replacement.

Traditionally, the 20 amino acids present in body proteins have been classified in two categories: essential or nonessential, depending on whether they are required in the diet for the maintenance of nitrogen balance in healthy adult subjects. The essential amino acids initially reported in 1954 were valine, leucine, isoleucine, threonine, methionine, phenylalanine, lysine, and tryptophan. The nonessential amino acids were glycine, alanine, serine, cystine, tyrosine, aspartic acid, glutamic acid, proline, hydroxyproline, histidine, citrulline, and arginine. Since the seminal work of Rose (186), additional information suggests that this is no longer a satisfactory classification. Thus, histidine has now been shown to be an essential (indispensable) amino acid, and the amino acids glycine, cystine, tyrosine, proline, and arginine, together with glutamine and taurine, are now more appropriately classified as being conditionally indispensable. This means there are either specific dietary or host conditions under which function is best maintained or improved when these amino acids are part of the nutrient intake.

Amino Acid Levels in Serum and Tissues of Patients with Renal Insufficiency

Changes in the levels of serum amino acids are observed in patients with chronic renal insufficiency prior to and after renal replacement therapy (187,188). In general, the serum levels of tryptophan, histidine, tyrosine, and the branched-chain amino acids, particularly valine, are low, whereas elevated concentrations of citrulline, of the conjugated amino acids, and of the sulfur-containing amino acids cystine and methionine are found. Low amino acid levels in uremic patients may be due to anorexia, a decrease in amino acid synthesis, an increase in catabolism, or impaired binding to serum albumin caused by substances that accumulate in the blood in uremia. Decreased utilization of amino acids by the kidney as renal mass is lost may contribute to the accumulation in plasma of certain amino acids such as citrulline. Decreased uptake in other organs may also account for decreased amino acid catabolism. However, the concentration of amino acids is much greater inside cells. Thus, plasma levels of amino acids are not as representative as intracellular levels. About 80% of the free amino acids are stored in muscle tissue. Changes in intracellular amino acid levels have also been described in uremia. The intracellular levels of valine are decreased, while normal concentrations of other branched-chain amino acids are found in humans (189,190). An inverse correlation between the levels of intracellular valine and plasma bicarbonate concentrations has been demonstrated in patients undergoing hemodialysis (191). This is in keeping with observations by Hara and associates (190) of increased catabolism of branched-chain amino acids as a consequence of metabolic acidosis in rats with experimental chronic renal disease. Low intracellular levels of taurine with normal or slightly elevated concentrations of this amino acid in plasma are also present in uremic subjects. Since the precursors of taurine such as cystine, methionine, and cystine sulfonic acid are elevated, a selective metabolic block at the level of cystine sulfonic acid decarboxylase has been proposed to explain the decrease in intracellular taurine (192). In addition, low intracellular levels of threonine and lysine and low ratios of essential to nonessential amino acids (valine–glycine, phenylalanine–tyrosine) have been reported in patients with ESRD. It has been suggested that the insulin resistance that develops in uremia may impair the uptake of amino acids by cells. In support of this hypothesis are studies in acutely uremic rats, in which a normal basal uptake but diminished insulin-stimulated uptake by muscle tissue was observed using β-aminoisobutyrate as a tracer (193). Some of the changes in plasma amino acids observed in uremia

may be the result of dietary manipulations, such as decreased ingestion of certain amino acids. Anorexia may also contribute to the altered pattern of amino acids. In one study, correction of the anemia of CRF by the administration of erythropoietin led to partial or complete normalization of decreased levels of serine, valine, and leucine and of elevated lysine, hydroxyproline, and ornithine levels. In addition, the tyrosine–phenylalanine ratio increased toward normal (194). All of these changes may be related to improved intake of nutrients as a consequence of the correction of the anemia.

Effects of Chronic Renal Insufficiency on Protein Metabolism

There is a high prevalence of protein malnutrition in patients with ESRD on maintenance dialysis therapy (195). The presence of hypoalbuminemia, decreased levels of prealbumin, and decreased levels of other markers indicative of protein malnutrition are potent predictors for morbidity and mortality in patients with ESRD (196). Although anorexia may be an important contributing factor, other evidence suggests that chronic renal insufficiency per se may cause abnormalities in protein metabolism. As mentioned previously, alterations in free amino acid concentrations occur both in plasma and intracellularly (in muscle) in individuals with ESRD. As also mentioned previously, essential amino acid concentrations are lower in the plasma of patients with chronic renal disease than in control subjects eating identical amounts of dietary protein (188,189). The decreased concentrations of essential amino acids in uremic patients have been attributed to poor absorption from the gastrointestinal tract or increased metabolism by either the small intestine or the liver (197). Individuals with ESRD have an accelerated metabolism of essential amino acids. Thus, patients with ESRD should not be expected to adapt normally to diets with limiting amounts of protein because one of the adaptations to a decrease in protein intake is a marked decrease in essential amino acid degradation (198). Nitrogen balance has been examined in small groups of patients with CRF and in control subjects receiving 0.6 g/kg body weight/day of high–biologic-value protein (199). After a prolonged lead-in period, both groups achieved neutral nitrogen balance without a discernible difference in their ability to adapt.

The rates of synthesis and degradation of proteins can be quantitated by the infusion of either radiolabeled or stable isotopes bearing amino acids. This allows the calculation of total body protein synthesis and total average proteolysis, as well as amino acid oxidation (200). Patients with stable CRF have been studied using this methodology when ingesting either of two different levels of dietary protein, 0.6 g/kg body weight or 1.0 g/kg body weight. Studies were performed both after overnight fasting and in the fed state (201). No differences were found in either the rate of protein turnover or amino acid oxidation compared to control subjects. Thus, the dynamics of amino acid metabolism are apparently normal at the whole body level in stable, nonacidotic patients with chronic renal insufficiency. However, the presence of malnutrition in patients with ESRD suggests that under certain circumstances uremia may be accompanied by increased protein catabolism. It is possible that patients with ESRD fail to adapt adequately to diets limiting protein intake due to an inadequate caloric intake. Caloric intakes in excess of 35 to 40 kcal/kg body weight may be needed for these patients to adapt to diets severely restricted in protein content (202). Evidence derived mainly from studies in experimental animals also indicates that metabolic acidosis may be a major catabolic factor in uremia. In addition, depressed insulin-stimulated synthesis of protein in muscle may contribute to abnormal protein metabolism.

Caloric Requirements of Uremic Patients

Although protein-calorie malnutrition is common in patients with ESRD, few studies have examined the caloric requirements of these patients. Inadequate caloric intake may be present when energy requirements are increased, caloric intake is decreased, or a combination of both. When protein intake is restricted, supplemental calories may improve nitrogen balance (202–204). If calorie intake is inadequate in patients eating a low-protein diet, the risk of catabolizing body protein is increased (202,204). Maroni (204) examined the caloric needs of patients on low-protein diets as well as the nutritional adequacy and mechanisms of adaptation to a very-low-protein diet containing 0.28 g/kg body weight and supplemented with either essential amino acids or a mixture of keto acids. He reports that when reduced intakes of protein are consumed, increasing caloric intake improves nitrogen balance.

Kopple and associates (202) examined the energy requirements of six patients with chronic renal disease prior to dialysis. They varied the caloric intake from 15 to 45 kcal/day, while the subjects ingested a constant protein intake of 0.55 to 0.6 g/kg body weight/day. They report that nitrogen balance became more positive as energy intake was increased and urea nitrogen appearance correlated inversely with caloric intake. Thus, an increase in caloric intake improves protein utilization and reduces net protein catabolism in patients with CRF. Monteon and coworkers (205) also report that the energy expenditure of patients with chronic renal disease measured during rest and exercise did not differ from that of control subjects. These investigators suggest that 35 kcal/kg body weight/day should be administered to patients with CRF consuming low-protein diets. Most studies of patients on dialysis indicate that these individuals are malnourished (206–209). One study found that wasting was already present at the initiation of dialysis, suggesting that malnutrition preceded the onset of hemodialysis therapy. Another recent report also described findings that indicate that patients with chronic renal disease receiving conservative treatment or hemodialysis had decreased calorie and protein intakes, and anthropometric measurements revealed the presence of

malnutrition (210). Resting energy expenditure was normal, indicating that wasting presumably was due to decreased food intake and not increased energy expenditure. The finding of a decreased respiratory quotient (despite normal resting energy expenditure) in patients with advanced chronic renal insufficiency suggested oxidation of endogenous fat, a pattern similar to that seen in patients with starvation (211).

Nutrition in Hemodialysis Patients

An extensive body of literature indicates that dialysis patients have protein-calorie malnutrition. It has been reported that hypoalbuminemia, negative nitrogen balance, loss of muscle mass, and wasting are commonly seen in long-term dialysis patients (212). Several indices of malnutrition have been utilized. These range from the well-known anthropometric measurements such as skinfold thickness and midarm muscle circumference to skin testing for anergy and other indices of immune deficiency (213–216). The most convincing link between malnutrition and mortality has been provided by measurements of serum albumin concentration. Even small decrements in albumin concentration (in the range of 3.5 to 4.0 g/dL) have been associated with increased mortality in hemodialysis patients; in addition, albumin appears to be a late index of malnutrition. Because of its relatively long half-life (21 days) and the vast capacity of the liver to synthesize albumin, a decrease in serum albumin concentration may follow the onset of malnutrition by several months (217). Prealbumin, with a half-life of 2 days, may be a more useful earlier indicator of malnutrition in normal individuals. Other indicators of malnutrition include serum cholesterol levels below 150 mg/dL, decreased concentration of transferrin, and a decrease in body weight to less than 80% of ideal body weight. Other indices of malnutrition in patients with ESRD undergoing renal replacement therapy are shown in Table 95-4. Several reports indicate a substantial

TABLE 95-4. *Indices of malnutrition in patients with end-stage renal disease*

Serum albumin < 4.0 g/dL
Prealbumin concentration < 29 mg/dL
Cholesterol concentration < 150 mg/dL
Transferrin concentration < 200 mg/dL
Body weight < 80% of ideal weight
Marked reduction in anthropometric measurements
Low serum creatinine and urea concentration in patients
  without residual renal function
Insulinlike growth factor I concentration < 300 μg/L
Protein catabolic rate < 0.8 g/kg/d
Continuous decline of estimated dry weight
Low predialysis serum potassium (and possibly serum
  phosphorus)

(Adapted from Hakim RM, Levin N. Malnutrition in hemodialysis patients. *Am J Kidney Dis* 1993;21:125, with permission.)

prevalence of protein-energy malnutrition in patients undergoing maintenance hemodialysis (209,218–223).

Factors that Affect Nutritional Status

As mentioned before, several factors in patients with ESRD prior to the initiation of replacement therapy contribute to the prevalence of protein-energy malnutrition in CRF. These factors include the development of anorexia, changes in the motility and function of the gastrointestinal tract including gastroparesis, malabsorption, and constipation, the prescription of long-term low-protein diets without adequate supplementation with keto acids or amino acids, and evidence of acidosis or low hematocrit, all of which may contribute to a patient feeling ill and presumably to anorexia. In addition, the initiation of dialysis increases catabolism, and adjustments in protein and caloric intake are necessary to maintain adequate protein balance. Factors that affect the nutritional status of dialysis patients prior to therapy and after therapy is initiated are summarized in Table 95-5.

Although protein-calorie malnutrition is the most commonly recognized nutritional deficiency in patients with ESRD, other nutritional deficits may occur if the patient does not receive supplemental nutrition. Deficiencies of 1,25-dihydroxycholecalciferol, Vitamin B_6, folic acid, iron, carnitine, and probably zinc are not uncommon in patients with ESRD if they are not provided with dietary supplements of these nutrients (224–230).

TABLE 95-5. *Factors that affect the nutritional status of dialysis patients*

Gastrointestinal disturbances
  Anorexia
  Gastroparesis
  Malabsorption
  Esophagitis, gastritis
  Constipation
  Patients on long-term, low-protein intake
Biochemical derangements
  Acidosis
  High parathyroid hormone levels (?)
  Anemia (?)
  Low insulinlike growth factor I
  Insulin resistance, increased gluconeogenesis, and
    decreased glycogen stores
Miscellaneous events
  Depression
  Low socioeconomic status
  Multiple medications, particularly sedatives
  Underlying illness
  Frequent hospitalizations
Dialysis factors
  Kt/V < 1.0
  Bioincompatible membranes
  Loss of amino acid and peptides in dialysate
  Use of acetate and high-calcium dialysate

(Adapted from Hakim RM, Levin N. Malnutrition in hemodialysis patients. *Am J Kidney Dis* 1993;21:125, with permission.)

Dietary and Energy Intake Recommended in Patients Undergoing Dialysis Replacement Therapy

The dietary protein requirements of patients on hemodialysis or peritoneal dialysis are greater than the recommended dietary allowances for normal adults (231–234). Energy requirements in dialysis patients appear to be similar to those of normal adults who have the same level of physical activity (234,235). Table 95-6 summarizes the recommended nutrient intake for patients undergoing maintenance hemodialysis or peritoneal dialysis (236).

If severe malnutrition develops, despite adequate dialysis and measures designed to ameliorate anorexia and increased catabolism, it may be necessary to initiate enteral or parenteral alimentation to supply adequate calories and nutrients. Severely malnourished patients may need to be hospitalized for such treatment. It is preferable to use enteral alimentation through a thin nasogastric tube rather than parenteral alimentation, which carries the risk of catheter-related infections and sepsis. Parenteral nutrition with amino acids has been used with some success to improve nutrition. A mixture of essential and nonessential amino acids should be used. Special amino acid solutions for use in patients with CRF are available and have been used with some success (237–239).

ENDOCRINE DISORDERS

Sexual Dysfunction and Abnormalities in the Hormones of the Hypothalamic–Pituitary–Gonadal Axis

Both female and male patients with CRF and those receiving dialysis therapy display a variety of derangements in their sexual function (Table 95-7) and in the hormones of the hypothalamic–pituitary–gonadal axis (Table 95-8).

Most of the studies on sexual dysfunction in CRF patients have focused on impotence. Impotence is defined as the inability to obtain or maintain erection satisfactorily for completing intercourse. Impotence is common in patients with CRF and is observed in excess of 50% of these patients (240–242). These data are based on results obtained from interviews with or by the completion of questionnaires by the patients and/or their spouses. Despite the limitations inherent in these techniques, the results are in agreement with other data obtained by objective criteria such as nocturnal penile tumescence (NPT). Indeed, Procci and colleagues (242) find that the values of NPT among a large population of uremic patients are significantly lower than normal. Several factors appear to participate in the genesis of impotence in CRF patients. These include abnormalities in the neurohormonal control system of erection hormones of the hypothalamic–pituitary–gonadal axis, secondary hyperparathyroidism (autonomic nervous system) and, dysfunction of the corporal smooth muscles of the penis or in their response to relaxing stimuli, and/or derangements in the arterial supply or the venous drainage of the penis (243,244).

TABLE 95-6. *Recommended dietary protein and energy intake for patients undergoing maintenance hemodialysis or peritoneal dialysis*

	Maintenance hemodialysis[a]	Continuous ambulatory or cyclic peritoneal dialysis[a]
Protein	1.0–1.2 g/kg/d ≥50% high-biologic-value protein 1.2 g/kg/d is prescribed unless patient has normal protein status with intakes of 1.0–1.1 g protein/kg/d	1.2–1.5 g/kg/d ≥50% high-biologic-value protein 1.2–1.3 g protein/kg/day is generally prescribed; for malnourished patients, up to 1.5 g/kg/d may be given
Energy[b]	≥35 kcal/kg/d unless the patient's relative body weight is >120% or the patient gains or is afraid of gaining unwanted weight; ≥30 kcal/kg/d for patients older than 60 years	
Fat (percent of total energy intake)[c]	30%–40%	30%–40%
Polyunsaturated–saturated fatty acid ratio	1.0:1.0	1.0:1.0
Carbohydrate[d]	Remaining nonprotein calories	Remaining nonprotein calories
Total fiber intake	20–25 g/d	20–25 g/d

[a]When recommended intake is expressed as kilogram body weight, this refers to the standard weight as determined from the NHANES data (233) or the adjusted body weight (ABW) for patients whose body weight differs by more than 15% to 20% from standard. ABW = actual weight + [(actual weight − standard weight) × 0.25].

[b]Total energy intake (diet plus dialysate).

[c]If serum triglyceride levels are very high, the percentage of fat in the diet may be increased to approximately 40% of total calories; otherwise, 30% of total calories is preferable.

[d]Should be primarily complex carbohydrates.

(Adapted from Kopple JD. Effect of nutrition on morbidity and mortality in maintenance dialysis patients. *Am J Kidney Dis* 1994;24:1002, with permission.)

The basal levels of serum prolactin are elevated in the majority of the male uremic patients, and the response to thyrotropin-releasing hormone (TRH) is reduced and delayed (245–248). Females with CRF also have elevated serum levels of prolactin (249). The mechanisms for the hyperprolactinemia in CRF are not well defined. Increased autonomous production rate of prolactin is a major mechanism for the hyperprolactinemia, but decreased metabolic clearance rate may also play a role (250). The demonstration of resistance to stimulation or suppression of prolactin in CRF is consistent with increased autonomous production (246,247,250,251). The state of secondary hyperparathyroid-

ism of CRF may contribute to the increased production rate of prolactin because PTH stimulates prolactin secretion (252). The treatment of CRF patients with erythropoietin was associated with a decrease in serum prolactin levels and improvement of sexual dysfunction (253) but did not normalize the response to TRH (254). These observations suggest that either anemia and/or deficiency of erythropoietin per se participates in the genesis of the hyperprolactinemia of CRF. It is of interest that in some patients correction of the hyperprolactinemia by bromocryptine is also associated with improvement of sexual dysfunction (255). Thus, it appears

TABLE 95-7. *Derangements in sexual function in uremic patients*

Male	Female
Delayed sexual maturation	Delayed sexual maturation
Decreased libido	Amenorrhea
Reduced frequency of intercourse	Menorrhagia
Partial or total impotence	Conception is rare
Reduced nocturnal penile tumescence	Spontaneous abortion is usual if conception occurs
Gynecomastia and galactorrhea	Decreased libido
Atrophic testes	Frigidity
Oligospermia or azoospermia	Galactorrhea
Unconcealed masturbation among dialysis patients	
Priapism	
Retrograde ejaculation	

TABLE 95-8. *Abnormalities in the hormones of hypothalamic–pituitary–gonadal axis in uremic patients*

	Male	Female
Basal prolactin	↑ majority	N or ↑
Prolactin response to TRH	↓ and prolonged	↓ and delayed
Prolactin suppression test	Impaired	Impaired
Basal FSH	↑ majority	N
FSH response to GnRH	N but delayed	N
Basal LH	↑ majority	N majority
LH response to GnRH	↓, N, ↑ and delayed	N
Testosterone	↓ majority	
Estradiol	N occasionally ↑	↓ majority
Progesterone		N, ↓

FSH, follicle-stimulating hormone; *GnRH,* gonadotropin-releasing hormone; *LH,* luteinizing hormone; *N,* normal; *TRH,* thyrotropin-releasing hormone

that the elevation of serum levels of prolactin plays a role in the impotence of the male uremic patient.

The basal levels of follicle-stimulating hormone (FSH) are usually elevated, but normal values are also encountered, and the response to gonadotropin-releasing hormone (GnRH) is normal but delayed (256–261). The mechanisms responsible for the derangements in FSH in uremia are not well elucidated. FSH is an important hormone for spermatogenesis. It stimulates testicular growth and increases the production of testosterone-binding protein by Sertoli's cells; this protein permits high local concentration of testosterone around the testicular tubules, which is necessary for the maturation of sperm (262). Basal levels of FSH are usually elevated in patients with testicular damage but without CRF (263). In patients with CRF, there is testicular damage and impaired spermatogenesis (259,264,265) despite elevated blood levels of FSH. This finding could be consistent with (a) a testicular damage being a primary process in CRF and the elevated blood levels of FSH representing a normal response of the hypothalamic–pituitary axis and/or (b) a resistance to the action of FSH on the testes, leading to testicular damage with a consequent rise in blood levels of FSH. In either case, the negative feedback between the testes and the hypothalamic–pituitary axis appears to be normal in CRF.

Inhibin, a factor secreted by the Sertoli's cells of the seminiferous tubules of the testes, inhibits FSH secretion, and it is probably an important mediator of the negative feedback interaction between the testes and the hypothalamic–pituitary axis (266). It is, therefore, possible that the production and/or the secretion of inhibin is impaired in CRF, and such an abnormality may lead to elevation of the blood levels of FSH. A study of prepubertal boys with CRF showed that the blood levels of both FSH and immunoreactive inhibin were elevated, and there was no correlation between them (267).

The basal blood levels of luteinizing hormone (LH) are elevated in the majority of patients with CRF, and the response to GnRH may be normal, subnormal, or exaggerated (257,258,261,268,269). The mechanisms for these abnormalities in LH are not completely understood. A decrease in the metabolic rate of LH is present in CRF (259,270), and the half-life of LH in CRF patients is two to four times higher than in normal subjects (271); these abnormalities certainly contribute to the elevations in the blood levels of prolactin and in the delayed response of prolactin to GnRH.

It should be mentioned that Veldhuis and associates (272), using highly sensitive and specific immunoradiometric assay of LH and utilizing deconvolution analysis, report that the response of LH to GnRH in patients with CRF is not different from normal. LH stimulates production of testosterone by the Leydig's cells of the testes, and testosterone exerts a negative feedback control on GnRH and consequently on LH. Thus, the low blood levels of testosterone in CRF (256–259,265,273) may also contribute to the elevation of the blood levels of LH. However, this process may not be of

paramount importance in the genesis of the elevated blood levels of LH because testosterone is not the only signal for GnRH release. Further Schaefer and colleagues (271) report that in uremic patients, there is a decrease in the amplitude of the secretory bursts of bioactive and immunoreactive LH without a change in the number of bursts, leading to a decrease in pulsatile secretion of LH. This phenomenon may be due to decreased pulsatile secretion of GnRH. On the other hand, the basal nonpulsatile immunoreactive LH was increased in these patients. Thus, it is apparent that in CRF there are disturbances in both LH secretion and in its metabolic clearance rate.

The majority of patients with CRF have low blood levels of testosterone (256–259,265,273). Testosterone production is reduced, but its metabolic clearance rate is normal except in dialysis patients with significant arteriovenous shunt; the latter patients may have accelerated metabolic clearance rate (273). The conversion of testosterone to dihydrotestosterone is reduced (274). The serum levels of estradiol are normal (275). Thus, the free testosterone to estradiol ratio is reduced. Administration of human gonadotropin for 4 days did not increase testosterone levels in uremic patients within 8 hours but produced a two- to threefold increase after 4 days (273). These observations suggest a sluggish Leydig's cell function in uremic patients.

The mechanisms responsible for the low blood levels of testosterone in uremia are not well defined. As mentioned, LH stimulates testosterone secretion; however, despite the large body of work on LH metabolism in CRF, it is still not clear as to how the derangements in LH metabolism are related to the reduced blood levels of testosterone. If the reduced amplitude of the pulsatile burst of LH secretion is more critical for testosterone secretion than the sustained elevation of blood levels of LH, testosterone production would be impaired and blood levels of testosterone would be reduced. It is also possible that the testosterone-producing cells are resistant to the action of LH, and therefore testosterone production and/or secretion is impaired. In this context, the elevated blood levels of prolactin may interfere with the action of LH on the testes and participate in the resistance to the action of LH (276). Secondary hyperparathyroidism in CRF may also participate in the genesis of the reduced testosterone levels in blood (277,278).

Disturbances in the normal profile of the hypothalamic–pituitary–gonadal axis also exist in female uremic patients as well. These disturbances are responsible for an anovulatory menstrual cycle. The blood levels of estradiol are normal or low (279,280), the midmenstrual cycle surge of FSH and LH is lacking (279), and the blood levels of progesterone are low in the second half of the menstrual cycle (280). The available data from these studies suggest that these derangements in females with CRF are due to hypothalamic defects (281).

A significant portion of uremic patients and those treated with hemodialysis display abnormalities in the function of the autonomic nervous system (282). Such derangements may participate in the genesis of the impotence in uremia. Indeed, a significant correlation exists between both NPT and frequency of intercourse and autonomic nerve function as evaluated by the Valsalva ratio (283).

Arterial penile insufficiency is associated with impotence. Indeed, obstructive vascular disease of the internal iliac arteries and/or pudendal arteries and pelvic arterial steal syndrome are associated with erectile dysfunction. Patients with ESRD have vascular calcifications, and such a derangement has been reported in the vessels of the penis. These patients also have hyperlipidemia and increased incidence of atherogenesis that could affect the penile arterial system. In addition, many of them have hypertension and are treated with medication that affect the vascular tone. All these factors may interfere with the arterial blood flow to the penis and, therefore, adversely affect the erectile process. Venous occlusion or disturbances in venous vascular tone may also impair erection.

The hypogastric–cavernous arterial bed and/or venoocclusive dysfunction of the corpora cavernosa was evaluated in 20 patients with ESRD and impotence using pharmacocavernosometry, pharmacocavernosography, and pharmacoarteriography (284). Almost all had vascular disease of the penis as evidenced by abnormal intracavernous pressure response to repeated intracavernous injections of vasoactive agents. Other findings included cavernous artery occlusive disease, atherosclerotic disease of the distal penile arteries, corporal venoocclusive dysfunction, diffuse pan-cavernous leakage involving the dorsal, cavernous, and crural veins, glans penis, and corpus spongiosum.

The function of the corporal musculature is controlled by adrenergic and cholinergic neurotransmitters. As mentioned earlier, dysfunction of the autonomic nervous system is common in uremia, and it is not surprising that the relaxation of the corporal muscles that is essential for erection may be defective. Also the response of these smooth muscles to local relaxant agonists may be impaired. Finally, the production of these relaxants may be reduced.

Structural alterations in the corporal smooth muscle cells may also occur in uremia. Fine-needle biopsy of the cavernous bodies demonstrated deposits of membrane debris, vacuoles, and granular material in the perinuclear region as compared to normal. More extensive changes include significant thickening of basal lamina and subplasmalemmal vesicles.

A state of zinc deficiency has been incriminated in the pathogenesis of impotence. This claim is based on two observations. First, the treatment of four impotent uremic patients for several months with dialysate-containing zinc was associated with hyperzincemia and improvement in their sexual function. This may not necessarily mean that zinc deficiency is responsible for impotence but rather that hyperzincemia improves sexual performance. Second, oral zinc administration to uremic patients was associated with normalization of serum levels of testosterone and a fall toward normal of the

serum levels of FSH and LH. It should be mentioned that neither of these observations have been confirmed by others. Also, the serum levels of zinc are not always reduced in patients with renal failure, and the majority of these patients have normal blood zinc levels. Thus, the potential role of a possible zinc-deficient state in uremia as the cause of impotence awaits further studies.

Most uremic patients also have hypertension, and one of the side effects of most of the medications for the treatment of the high blood pressure is impotence.

Therapy for sexual dysfunction in uremia has been difficult. Testosterone injections (100 to 200 mg per day) have provided inconsistent results (285,286). Bromocryptine (1.25 to 5.0 mg per day) or clomiphene (100 mg per day) have been reported to improve potency and sexual performance (255). Certain data suggest that the correction of the anemia of chronic renal failure with erythropoietin has been associated with improvement in potency (253). Others report that dialysis patients with similar hematocrits with or without treatment with erythropoietin did not differ in their sexual performance (287), although some patients claimed an increase in their libido. However, those with erythropoietin therapy had elevated blood level of testosterone and sex hormone-binding globulin but normal free testosterone.

A major advance in the treatment of impotence in general and in patients with renal failure as well is the introduction of intracavernosal pharmacotherapy. This requires the injection of relaxant agents into the corpora cavernosa of the penis. The best approach utilizes polytherapy, which includes the injections of several relaxants. In most patients two agents are adequate. The most widely used are prostaglandin E_1 (20 mg per mL) and phentolamine (1.25 mg per mL). This therapy is usually followed by a successful erection permitting a successful intercourse culminating in orgasm. In some patients, pharmacotherapy is needed before every intercourse, whereas in others several therapies may be followed by restoration of the erectile function and no further therapy is needed; this is especially true in those with psychogenic impotence. Failure of pharmacotherapy may then necessitate surgical treatment of impotence; this requires the implantation of penile prostheses.

The discovery of sildenafil (Viagra) constitutes a breakthrough in the medical treatment of impotence (288). This drug is a selective inhibitor of cyclic guanosine monophosphate (cGMP)-specific phosphodiesterase type 5, which is the predominant isoform in the corpus cavernosum. cGMP stimulates relaxation of the smooth muscles of the cavernous body. Therefore, sildenafil allows relaxation of corporal smooth muscle and facilitates erection after sexual stimulation. Its effect occurs within 1 to 2 hours after its administration. Dosage of 25, 50, or 100 mg may be effective. The use of sildenafil is contraindicated in patients taking nitrates. Medications that inhibit cytochrome 450 reduce the clearance of sildenafil and results in higher blood levels of the drug for any given dose. These medications include cimetidine, erythromycin, ketoconazole, and itroconazole. Cardiac arrhythmias, myocardial infarction, and death has been reported in elderly patients with the use of sildenafil. Significant improvement in erectile dysfunction occurred after the use of Viagra by patients with CRF treated with dialysis therapy (289).

Gynecomastia

Variable degrees of gynecomastia are often encountered in the male uremic patient treated with maintenance hemodialysis. Gynecomastia usually develops during the initial months of dialysis and regresses with prolonged time on dialysis. The gynecomastia is less common in uremic patients who are not receiving dialysis therapy. It may be transient or may last for periods of several months. The mechanism of the gynecomastia is not known. The etiology may be related to the improvement in the nutritional status of the uremic patients with dialysis therapy and, as such, is similar to the mechanism of refeeding gynecomastia. It must be emphasized that in almost all cases of gynecomastia, there is an alteration either in the ratio between the serum levels of androgen and estrogen, in favor of the latter, or in the ratio between the action of androgen and estrogen at the tissue level. Indeed, in patients with advanced chronic renal failure and those treated with hemodialysis, the ratio between the serum levels of free testosterone and estradiol is reduced because of a decrease in testosterone levels.

Growth Hormone and Somatomedins

Growth hormone (GH) is produced and secreted by the somatotrophs of the pituitary glands. The latter contains GH (22,000 daltons) and pre-GH (28,000 daltons), and both forms may be secreted into the blood. The secretion of GH is pulsatile and displays diurnal rhythmicity, with the secretion being high before the awakening hours and decreasing toward the end of the day. The secretion of GH is controlled by two hypothalamic factors: growth hormone-releasing hormone (GHRH), which stimulates GH secretion, and somatostatin, which inhibits GH secretion. Other hormones and metabolic parameters affect GH secretion as well. Hypoglycemia, amino acid infusion, and a protein meal stimulate GH secretion, while hyperglycemia inhibits GH secretion. The majority of GH in plasma is monomeric (22,000 daltons), but larger molecules (dimer or "big" GH and "big big" GH) are also found (290,291). About 95% of GH is cleared by the liver (292), but GH is also filtered by the glomeruli and subsequently absorbed and catabolized by the renal tubular cells (293). The normal half-life of GH is about 20 minutes (294).

GH promotes linear growth, and it mediates its action via somatomedins. The latter are polypeptides that are synthesized by the liver, kidney, and muscle, and their synthesis is stimulated by GH. There are three types of somatomedins: A (2,000 daltons), B (5,000 daltons), and C (8,000 daltons).

Their secretion is constant throughout the 24 hours, and they circulate in blood bound to a protein. Insulin growth factor-I (IGF-I), which has been cloned, is identical to somatomedin C (295,296) and is the main somatomedin through which GH mediates its action. IGF-I inhibits GH most likely through stimulation of somatostatin secretion by the hypothalamus (297).

Basal blood levels of GH are elevated in CRF (298,299). Since only a small portion of GH is cleared by the kidney, the half-life of GH is either normal or modestly increased in patients with CRF (294,300). It appears, therefore, that the major reason for the elevation in the basal levels of GH in CRF is dysregulation of GH production and/or secretion. Several lines of evidence support this notion. First, hyperglycemia produced by glucose infusion does not suppress GH secretion (301); second, exaggerated response in GH secretion is observed after the administration of GHRH (302) or L-dopa (301); third, paradoxical release of GH is noted after TRH administration (301); finally, blockade of opioid receptors by naloxone causes a greater suppression of GH secretion in normal subjects than in patients with CRF (34,303). It is of interest that correction of anemia of CRF by treatment with erythropoietin exerts a beneficial effect on the derangements of GH secretion. These patients display a decrease in basal blood levels of GH (254,304,305) without a change in the exaggerated response to GHRH (305) and amelioration of the exaggerated response in GH secretion to insulin-induced hypoglycemia and in the paradoxical response in GH release to TRH administration (254,304).

Despite the elevated basal levels of GH in CRF, growth failure is common in children with CRF (306), suggesting an impaired action of GH. Since the effect of GH on growth is mediated through IGF-I, attention has been focused on the metabolism of the latter in CRF. The basal levels of IGF-I are low (307) or increased (308) in CRF. Other studies show that there is an increase in IGF-I binding proteins (IGFBP 1, 2, and 6) in plasma of patients with CRF (309,310), and this increase in binding capacity of IGF-I results in a decrease in the concentrations of free IGF-I (311). Also, inhibitors of IGF-I are present in plasma of patients with CRF (312,313). Thus, there is reduced bioavailability of IGF-I in uremia and therefore decreased action. Further, Ding and colleagues (314) report a postreceptor defect to IGF-I action in the epitrochlearis muscle of rats with CRF as compared to sham-operated, pair-fed controls. Finally, Fouque and associates (315) demonstrate the presence of resistance to the metabolic effects of recombinant human IGF-I in patients with advanced renal failure.

The demonstration of the resistance to the action of GH and IGF-I in CRF provides the rationale for the use of GH in the treatment of children with CRF with retarded growth. A multicenter study in 17 pediatric nephrology departments in the United States demonstrated that administration of recombinant human GH to 125 prepubertal children with CRF for 2 years was associated with an increase in growth rate and in standardized height without undue advancement of bone age or significant side effects (316).

Adrenocorticotropin–Cortisol Axis

In patients with end-stage CRF, plasma adrenocorticotropin (ACTH) levels are normal or elevated (34,317–321). ACTH secretion following the administration of corticotropin-releasing hormone (CRH) is blunted in patients with CRF (320–322), while others report the response to be normal (323). In hemodialysis patients, the ACTH response to hypoglycemia is normal (34) or blunted (324).

Both in patients with CRF and in those treated with dialysis, the basal blood levels of cortisol are normal (320,324–328) or modestly elevated (34,321,322,329–333). No correlation between free cortisol levels and the degree of CRF (GFR 2 to 44 mL/minute/1.73 m^2) was found (334), and the circadian rhythmicity of cortisol secretion is not disturbed (324,329,335,336). The half-life of cortisol is prolonged in CRF (335), and this may contribute to the elevated basal levels of cortisol reported in some patients. An increase in plasma levels of cortisol has been observed in children and adults during hemofiltration or hemodialysis by some (337) but not by others (329). In hemodialysis patients, a normal (329) or blunted (338) response of cortisol secretion to stimulatory factors was found, while in patients undergoing CAPD treatment, a normal response of cortisol secretion to ACTH or insulin-induced hypoglycemia (319) was reported. Both normal and incomplete suppression of cortisol with dexamethasone have been observed in patients with CRF (326,329,336,338). These data indicate that the adrenocorticotropin–cortisol axis is either normal or mildly altered in CRF. The clinical significance of such alterations is not evident.

Vasopressin

Blood levels of vasopressin are elevated in children (339) and adults (340) with CRF, in hemodialysis patients (341,342), and in those receiving CAPD (343). The major cause of this abnormality is the decrease in the metabolic clearance rate of the hormone by the kidneys (344,345). Abnormal osmotic regulation of vasopressin secretion may also be present in CRF. Indeed, some studies show no direct correlation between plasma osmolality and vasopressin in CRF (346,347), while other investigators demonstrate that the osmotic regulation of vasopressin is intact (348). The vasopressin response to nonosmotic stimuli appears to be normal in CRF in that blood vasopressin levels increased during ultrafiltration (349) and plasma volume contraction (346,350) and decreased during central hypervolemia produced by water immersion (342). On the other hand, angiotensin II infusion did not stimulate vasopressin secretion in patients with CRF (351). The clinical significance of the elevated blood levels of vasopressin in CRF is not obvious, and it is not clear whether this abnormality plays a role in the genesis of hypertension in patients with CRF.

Thyroid Gland and Hormones

Abnormalities in the structure and function of the thyroid gland and in the metabolism and blood levels of thyroid hormones are common in patients with CRF (352–354). These derangements may be due to the uremic state, to other nonthyroid disorders, or to concomitant disorders of the thyroid gland, the pituitary, or the hypothalamus. Table 95-9 lists the various factors that may cause abnormalities in thyroid hormone metabolism, and Table 95-10 details the changes in the profiles of thyroid hormone indices and their mechanisms and compares them with those in other thyroid disorders. Blood levels of thyroid-stimulating hormone (TSH) are normal in CRF, but the TSH response to TRH is usually blunted (352,355–357). Also the nocturnal TSH surge is reduced in both children and adults with CRF (358,359). These abnormalities are observed when GFR is reduced by 50% (360).

Patients with CRF often have reduced serum total thyroxine (T$_4$) and free T$_4$ index, low serum total triiodothyronine (T$_3$) and free T$_3$ index, and normal total serum reverse triiodothyronine (rT$_3$) levels. These alterations in thyroid hormone indices do not indicate a state of hypothyroidism but rather reflect the state of chronic illness and/or malnutrition of CRF. These changes in thyroid hormone indices do not

TABLE 95-9. *Causes of altered thyroid hormone metabolism in chronic renal failure*

Primary diseases of the hypothalamic–pituitary–thyroid axis
  Hypothyroidism
    Thyroid gland failure
    Pituitary gland failure
    Hypothalamic defect
  Hyperthyroidism
    Thyroid gland hyperfunction
    Exogenous thyroid hormone administration
  Euthyroid goiter
Nonthyroidal disorders
  Chronic renal failure
  Nephrotic syndrome
  Secondary endocrine and metabolic derangements
  Malnutrition and catabolism
  Concurrent systemic illnesses
  Pharmaceutical agents
    Dilantin
    β-Blockers (high doses)
    Glucocorticoids
    Iodinated contrast agents
      Ipodate
      Iopanoic acid
      Iodine solutions
    Amiodarone
    Dialysis therapy

(From Kaptein EM, Massry SG. Thyroid hormone metabolism. In: Massry SG, Glassock RJ, eds. *Textbook of nephrology,* 2nd ed. Baltimore: Williams & Wilkins, 1989.)

TABLE 95-10. *Serum thyroid hormone levels in thyroidal and nonthyroidal disorders*

	TT_4	Free T_4	Free T_4^a	T_4-binding capacity	TT_3	Free T_3 index	TSH	TSH response to TRH	Etiology
High TT_4 state of illness including CRF	↑	↑	↑	N, ↓	N, ↓	N, ↓	N	N, ↓	Decreased T_4 clearance from serum
Hyperthyroidism	↑	↑	↑	N, ↓	↑	↑	↓	Absent	Thyroid hormone excess
Low TT_4 state of illness including CRF	↓	↓	N, ↓	↓	↓	↓	↓, N↓	N, ↓	Reduced T_4 binding in serum
Primary hypothyroidism	↓	↓	↓	↑	↓	↓	↑	↑	Decreased thyroid gland function

↑, increased; ↓, decreased; CRF, chronic renal failure; N, normal; TRH, thyrotropin-releasing hormone; TSH, thyroid-stimulating hormone; T_4, thyroxine; T_3, triiodothyronine; TT_4, total T_4; TT_3, total T_3

^{a}Free T_4 by equilibrium dialysis or clinical assay two-step method.

(Modified from Kaptein EM. Thyroid hormone metabolism. In: Massry SG, Glassock RJ, eds. *Massry and Glassock's Textbook of nephrology,* 3rd ed. Baltimore: Williams & Wilkins, 1995.)

require therapy. It has been reported that the expression of messenger RNA (mRNA) of α and β T_3 receptors on mononuclear cells are increased in CRF (361), and this phenomenon may maintain euthyroid state despite low T_3 levels. The low T_3 state of CRF is considered to be protective for protein conservation, and therefore, supplementation of T_3 to these patients may be harmful. Measurement of free T_4 with analog radioimmunoassay or with label antibody assay yields lower values than those determined with equilibrium dialysis assay. This is due to interference with assay by indoxyl sulfate and hippuric acid which are elevated in blood of uremic patients (362).

Available data indicate that the prevalence of goiter is increased in patients with CRF and in those treated with dialysis, although the reported incidence varies from 0% to 58% (352,353). Kaptein and colleagues (352) studied 306 patients with ESRD and compared them to 139 hospitalized patients without renal disease (control groups). Goiter was present in 40% of the patients with renal failure and in 43% of those treated with dialysis, compared to 6.5% in the control group. The frequency of goiter was higher in patients treated for more than 1 year with hemodialysis (50%) than in those treated for less than 1 year (39%). Since goiter in renal failure patients was noticed in all geographic areas, one may conclude that uremia or some of its consequences are responsible for the high prevalence of goiter in these patients. Several factors including iodine metabolism, elevated serum levels of TSH or PTH, and goitrogens in the water supply have been incriminated.

Primary hypothyroidism is two to three times more frequent in patients with CRF than in the general population (352,353); this thyroid disorder is noted usually in females whose renal failure is due to diabetic nephropathy (352). Hypothyroidism has been observed in children with CRF due to cystinosis (363); cystine crystals deposit in the thyroid gland, leading to structural change and hypothyroidism. It is very difficult to make the clinical diagnosis of hypothyroidism in patients with CRF because the signs and symptoms of hypothyroidism are also encountered in patients with renal

failure without hypothyroidism (364). The only reliable way to diagnose hypothyroidism in renal failure is the finding of elevated serum levels of TSH. There is no increased frequency of hyperthyroidism in patients with CRF.

Parathyroid Glands

Patients with ESRD almost always have hyperplasia of the parathyroid glands, but the volume and mass of the glands vary among patients and among the four glands in the same patients. The size of the gland may reach 10 to 50 times normal, but rarely, the glands may be of normal size (365–367). These enlarged glands display chief cell hyperplasia with or without oxyphil cell hyperplasia, and nodular or adenomatouslike masses (nodules) may also be encountered within the hyperplastic glands (365–367). These nodules are well circumscribed and are surrounded by fibrous capsules (368,369). The cells in the nodular hyperplasia have less Vitamin D receptors (VDRs) density (370) and calcium sensing receptors (CaR) (371) and higher proliferative potential than the cells of diffuse hyperplasia (372,373). The change in structure of the parathyroid glands begins as polyclonal diffuse hyperplasia. However, the cells with the lower density for VDRs and CaR start to proliferate monoclonally (early nodularity in diffuse hyperplasia) and form nodules. Several monoclonal nodules of different size may develop resulting in nodular hyperplasia. The cells of one nodule may proliferate faster and more vigorously giving rise to a very large nodule that almost occupies the entire gland (single nodular gland). Several studies have shown that there are abnormalities in chromosome 11 on which the suppressor gene MEN-1 is located, allelic loss of 11q 13 and losses of several gene markers located on chromosome 11p (375,376,379). These molecular changes are implicated in the tumorigenesis of the parathyroid gland in CRF. Arnold and colleagues (374) report that the majority of parathyroid cells in patients with CRF have a monoclonal origin.

Available data indicate that three factors including phosphate retention (378,379), skeletal resistance to the calcemic action of PTH (380–385), and altered Vitamin D metabolism (386,387) interact to cause hyperplasia of the parathyroid glands in CRF. It appears that phosphate retention, which may develop as renal insufficiency ensues, may interfere with the ability of patients to augment the renal production of $1,25(OH)_2D_3$ to meet their increased need.

This notion is supported by the studies of Llach and Massry in adults (386) and of Portale and coworkers (388) in children. These patients had dysfunction of organs that were targets for Vitamin D action such as impaired intestinal absorption of calcium and skeletal resistance to the calcemic action of PTH (386) despite normal blood levels of $1,25(OH)_2D_3$. Dietary phosphate restriction was followed by a significant increment in blood levels of $1,25(OH)_2D_3$ (386,388) and normalization of the abnormalities cited above (386). Thus, it appears that a state of relative $1,25(OH)_2D_3$ deficiency is present in early renal failure, leading to defective absorption of calcium and impaired calcemic response to PTH (386). These two abnormalities produce hypocalcemia and, subsequently, secondary hyperparathyroidism. Hypocalcemia stimulates PTH secretion (389) and causes parathyroid cell hypertrophy (390). Dietary phosphate restriction in these patients restored the blood levels of PTH to normal (386,388).

It should be mentioned that with more advanced renal failure when hyperphosphatemia develops, the elevated blood levels of phosphorus may suppress blood levels of calcium and contribute to the hypocalcemia of advanced renal failure. In addition, experimental evidence indicates that the very high blood levels of phosphorus may directly affect the function of the parathyroid glands (391); such high phosphorus may induce hyperplasia of the parathyroid glands independent of calcium or $1,25(OH)_2D_3$, and by posttranscriptional mechanism, increase PTH synthesis and secretion.

The relative deficiency of $1,25(OH)_2D_3$ in patients with early and moderate renal failure may, directly and independent of the hypocalcemia, affect parathyroid gland activity. Several lines of evidence indicate an interaction between $1,25(OH)_2D_3$ and parathyroid glands. First, the parathyroid cells have intracellular receptors for $1,25(OH)_2D_3$ and contain the mRNA for this receptor (392,393). Second, $1,25(OH)_2D_3$ inhibits prepro-PTH mRNA in a dose-dependent manner (394,395), and a deficiency of $1,25(OH)_2D_3$ is associated with an increase in prepro-PTH mRNA and in the weight of the parathyroid glands in experimental renal failure (390–398). Third, $1,25(OH)_2D_3$ inhibits PTH secretion (399) as well as parathyroid cell proliferation (400). Fourth, Oldham and associates (401) and Madsen and others (402) report that $1,25(OH)_2D_3$ renders the parathyroid glands more susceptible to the suppressive action of an increase in ionized calcium.

The relationship between blood levels of PTH and calcium is best described by a sigmoidal curve (403); and the value of set point for calcium, defined as the calcium concentration that produces half maximal inhibition of PTH, is the midpoint between the maximal and minimal PTH secretions (403). Alterations in set point for calcium with a shift to right (i.e., 50%

inhibition of PTH secretion occurs at higher calcium concentration) were observed in parathyroid glands of patients with primary (404) or secondary hyperparathyroidism (403,405).

The cells of the parathyroid glands possess CaR (406). This receptor protein is located in the membrane of these cells. The levels of serum calcium and $1,25(OH)_2D_3$ as well as dietary phosphate do not appear to regulate the synthesis of CaR. In renal failure, there is a reduction in density of CaR in the parathyroid gland cells (371).

The CaR interacts with calcium as well as with other divalent-, trivalent-, and polycations (407). This receptor protein plays an important role in the ability of parathyroid glands to recognize changes in the concentration of calcium ion in the blood; and as such, CaR mediates the effect of calcium on the secretion of PTH from the parathyroid glands. A decrease in the concentration of calcium ion in blood is recognized by a G protein-coupled CaR and subsequently leads to PTH release. An increase in the concentration of calcium in the blood activates the CaR, an event that leads to an increase in the concentration of cytosolic calcium secondary to mobilization of calcium from intracellular calcium stores. This rise in cytosolic calcium results in inhibition of PTH release from the parathyroid glands.

Change in intracellular content of cAMP affects PTH secretion. Any factor that increases cAMP content (hypocalcemia, β-adrenergic agonists, dopaminergic agents, secretin, prostaglandin E, and cholera toxin) enhances PTH secretion. On the other hand, factors that reduce intracellular cAMP (hypercalcemia, hypermagnesemia, α-adrenergic agonists, prostaglandins of the F series, and nitroprusside) inhibit PTH release. Calcium is the most important regulator of PTH secretion, and the effect is mediated by changes in intracellular concentration of calcium. An increase in the concentration of intracellular calcium influences PTH secretion through several mechanisms: (a) inhibition of cAMP accumulation, (b) inhibition of cAMP action, and (c) stimulation of intracellular degradation of performed PTH.

The available data strongly support the proposition that deficiency of $1,25(OH)_2D_3$ may initiate secondary hyperparathyroidism even in the absence of overt hypocalcemia; this has been demonstrated in dogs with a 70% decrease in GFR (408). Since patients with CRF have both hypocalcemia and deficiency of $1,25(OH)_2D_3$, they are in double jeopardy regarding the development of secondary hyperparathyroidism. They could develop very large glands due to hyperplasia or hypertrophy of the parathyroid cells.

The formulation for the pathogenesis of secondary hyperparathyroidism in CRF discussed previously has important clinical implications. It is evident that dietary phosphate restriction in proportion to the fall in GFR in patients with early renal failure is adequate to reverse and correct secondary hyperparathyroidism and other abnormalities in divalent ion metabolism. However, achieving the proper and adequate dietary phosphate restriction and successful patient compliance with the dietary regimen may prove difficult. Since the available data indicate that dietary phosphate restriction exerts its effect through the increased production of $1,25(OH)_2D_3$ and since this Vitamin D metabolite also exerts a direct effect on the parathyroid glands, an alternative therapeutic approach would be supplementation of $1,25(OH)_2D_3$. Indeed, treatment of patients with moderate renal failure with $1,25(OH)_2D_3$ for 6 to 12 months was associated with improvement or normalization of the disturbances in divalent ion metabolism, including secondary hyperparathyroidism and bone disease (409,410).

The hyperplasia of the parathyroid glands in CRF causes marked elevation in blood levels of PTH (45,366,411,412) which becomes evident early in the course of renal failure (411,412). There is marked variation in the serum concentrations of PTH in patients with advanced renal failure and in those treated with hemodialysis (45,366); the levels may be 2 to 200 times normal. Low or undetectable levels of PTH may be encountered in patients with advanced renal failure who are hypomagnesemic and magnesium deficient (413), those who have low turnover osteomalacia with (414) and without (415,416) increased body burden of aluminum, and those who have primary hypoparathyroidism. Patients with diabetes mellitus and renal failure may have lower levels of PTH than those with renal failure due to other causes (417). The serum levels of PTH in the patients on dialysis may be affected by the concentration of calcium in the dialysate; patients treated with high calcium dialysate may have lower serum levels of PTH than those treated with lower calcium dialysate.

The PTH in the serum of the renal failure patients is made up of many fragments but mostly of the midregion and C-terminal fragments. Therefore, assays using an antibody directed toward these moieties of PTH yield high values; in contrast, the use of an antibody to the N-terminal fragment may reveal modest elevation in the serum levels of PTH. A two-site immunoradiometric assay (IRMA), which measures intact PTH molecule, has been developed (418). It is precise and provides reliable values of the serum levels of intact PTH in patients with CRF (419).

A large body of evidence has accumulated indicating that the excess blood levels of PTH in patients with CRF are deleterious to the function of many organs (46). Excess PTH has been implicated in the pathogenesis of the abnormalities of the central (419–429), peripheral (430,431), and autonomic (282,432–434) nervous systems; myocardiopathy (435–439); skeletal myopathy (440,441); glucose intolerance and impaired insulin secretion (13,40–44,55); hyperlipidemia (93,94); disorders of red blood cells (442–446), polymorphonuclear leukocytes (447–452), and T-cell (453,454) and B-cell (455,456) function; and abnormalities of the immune system (457).

This widespread effect of PTH on so many cells indicates that these cells must have receptors for PTH. Both Urena and colleagues (458) and Tian and colleagues (459) have demonstrated that the mRNA for the PTH-parathyroid hormone-related protein (PTH-PTHrP) receptor is present in many cells including kidney, bone, heart, brain, liver, spleen, aorta,

ileum, skeletal muscle, lung, and testes. Thus, both pathophysiologic and molecular evidence exist supporting the notion that almost all body organs are targets for PTH actions, and therefore, it is not surprising that chronic excess of PTH in CRF may exert widespread deleterious effects on body function in uremia. Hence, PTH is being considered a major uremic toxin.

In CRF, the mRNA of the PTH-PTHrP receptor is downregulated in both the traditional (kidney) and nontraditional (liver and heart) cells for PTH action (460–462). The mechanism underlying this phenomenon is not fully elucidated. However, since PTH causes a rise in $[Ca^{2+}]i$ in many cells in CRF (46), and since the elevation in $[Ca^{2+}]i$ is a major contributor to cell dysfunction in CRF (46), it is plausible that the rise in $[Ca^{2+}]i$ provides a negative feedback control mechanism through which the mRNA of the PTH-PTHrP is downregulated so that the increment in $[Ca^{2+}]i$ of cells does not progress unabated as the blood levels of PTH continue to rise with progression of renal failure. Tian and associates (461) and Smogorzewski and associates (462) provide evidence supporting this notion. They report that normalization of the $[Ca^{2+}]i$ of the kidney and heart in animals with CRF, through their treatment with verapamil, prevents the downregulation of the mRNA of the PTH-PTHrP receptor despite significant elevation in the blood levels of PTH.

Vitamin D Metabolites

The parent Vitamin D is first hydroxylated in liver to 25-hydroxyvitamin D (25[OH]D) (463,464). The turnover of Vitamin D may be accelerated by infection or drugs stimulating microsomal liver enzymes, resulting in lower plasma levels of 25(OH)D (465). This Vitamin D metabolite binds to an α-globulin (Vitamin D binding protein [DBP]) (466). In patients with nephrotic syndrome, the DBP is lost in the urine and with it 25(OH)D (467). Therefore, these patients have low blood levels of 25(OH)D. Similarly, DBP and 25(OH)D are lost in the peritoneal fluid in patients treated with CAPD. These patients may also have low blood levels of 25(OH)D (468,469). The normal blood level of 25(OH)D in adults living in the United States is 15 to 30 ng/mL (470). These levels display seasonal fluctuation related to sun exposure; they are higher in the summer and lower in the winter (471). The half-life of 25(OH)D is about 12 days (472).

In uremic patients with normal function of the gastrointestinal tract and liver, plasma 25(OH)D levels are usually normal (473–475) but are increased (476) in patients treated with Vitamin D. Excessive proteinuria (467,474) and concomitant severe extrarenal diseases (474,477) are associated with low blood levels of 25(OH)D. In uremic patients treated by CAPD or hemofiltration (478), plasma levels of 25(OH)D are usually low normal, while they are normal in hemodialysis patients. Low plasma 25(OH)D levels in uremic patients are usually due to reduced exposure of the skin to ultraviolet light, reduced intake of Vitamin D, intestinal malabsorption, or impaired hepatic 25-hydroxylation.

The 25(OH)D is carried out to the kidneys for further hydroxylation, resulting in the production of the active metabolite $1,25(OH)_2D_3$ (479–481). This metabolite also binds to DBP, but its binding efficiency to DBP is less than that of 25(OH)D. $1,25(OH)_2D_3$ may also be produced by other cells such as normal alveolar (482) and peritoneal (483) macrophages, peripheral blood macrophages (484), and macrophages of granulomas (485).

The main factors that regulate the function of renal 1 α-hydroxylase enzyme and hence the production of $1,25(OH)_2D_3$ are PTH, calcium, and phosphorus (486,487). Plasma levels of $1,25(OH)_2D_3$ are dependent on several factors including biosynthesis of Vitamin D in the skin, intake of Vitamin D or its metabolites, absorption of Vitamin D by the intestinal tract, intensity of 25-hydroxylation in the liver and of 1 α-hydroxylation of 25(OH)D in the kidneys (488), and loss of Vitamin D metabolites in urine of patients with nephrotic syndrome (467) or in the dialysate of CAPD patients (468,469). The normal blood levels of $1,25(OH)_2D_3$ range between 25 and 33 pg/mL in adults and between 49 and 66 pg/mL in children (489). The half-life of $1,25(OH)_2D_3$ is about 20 hours (490), which is considerably shorter than that of 25(OH)D.

The blood levels of $1,25(OH)_2D_3$ are usually normal in patients with moderate renal failure (386,388). Despite these normal levels, these patients display abnormalities in the function of the target organs for Vitamin D action (386). These observations indicate that these patients have a Vitamin D-resistant state. As renal failure progresses, an absolute Vitamin D-deficient state develops, with the blood levels of $1,25(OH)_2D_3$ being reduced when GFR falls below 50 mL/minute in children (388,491) and below 30 mL/minute in adults (386,492). In anephric patients and in those treated with dialysis, the blood levels of $1,25(OH)_2D_3$ are usually very low or undetectable (493–495). The finding of low blood levels of $1,25(OH)_2D_3$ in anephric patients and especially in those receiving Vitamin D indicates that $1,25(OH)_2D_3$ is produced by extrarenal sites in these patients. Patients with CRF and granulomatous diseases such as sarcoidosis may have elevated blood levels of $1,25(OH)_2D_3$ (496) caused by the extrarenal production of this metabolite by the macrophages of the granulomatous tissue (485).

The metabolic clearance rate (MCR) of $1,25(OH)_2D_3$ in uremic dogs (497) and humans (498) is not different from normal values. In contrast, Hsu and colleagues (499,500) report that the MCR of $1,25(OH)_2D_3$ in rats with CRF is lower than in normal rats. These authors attribute this phenomenon to suppression of the activity of 24-hydroxylase activity (an enzyme that is involved in the degradation of $1,25(OH)_2D_3$) by an unidentified factor present in the uremic serum (501). In contrast, Taylor and associates (502) report that the MCR of $1,25(OH)_2D_3$ is normal in rats after unilateral nephrectomy.

The deficiency of $1,25(OH)_2D_3$ in CRF plays a paramount role in the genesis of many of the disturbances of divalent ions observed in patients with CRF. These abnormalities include secondary hyperparathyroidism, defective intestinal absorption of calcium, skeletal resistance to the calcemic action of PTH, defective mineralization of bone, growth retardation in children, and proximal myopathy.

$1,25(OH)_2D_3$ exerts its action by binding to an intracellular Vitamin D receptor (VDR), which is located predominantly in the nucleus (503). The hormone-receptor complex interacts with DNA-responsive elements in target genes with the synthesis of bioactive proteins (504), which in turn mediate the actions of $1,25(OH)_2D_3$. Patients with CRF display end-organ resistance to the action of $1,25(OH)_2D_3$. This phenomenon is due to impairment in the cascade of the cellular events culminating in the biologic actions of $1,25(OH)_2D_3$. First, there is a decrease in the concentration of $1,25(OH)_2D_3$ receptors in rats (505,506), dogs (507), and humans (508) with renal failure. Second, certain as yet unidentified uremic toxin inhibits the binding of the $1,25(OH)_2D_3$-receptor complex with DNA-responsive elements in the target gene (506). This defect would, therefore, interfere with the production of the bioactive protein required for the action of $1,25(OH)_2D_3$. In advanced renal failure, the number of VDRs is reduced (370,507) leading to Vitamin D resistance. Thus, in patients with chronic renal failure, there is Vitamin D deficiency and Vitamin D resistance as well.

The factors responsible for the decrease in the number of VDRs in uremia are not fully elucidated but may include:

1. Reduced levels of $1,25(OH)_2D_3$ since this metabolite affects the production of VDR (509); specifically, low levels of $1,25(OH)_2D_3$ downregulate the mRNA of VDR.
2. Hyperparathyroidism of renal failure may play a role since high levels of PTH interfere with the $1,25(OH)_2D_3$-induced upregulation of VDR (510).
3. Uremic toxins may decrease the stability of the mRNA of VDRs, resulting in transcriptional reduction of VDR protein (511).

Renin–Angiotensin–Aldosterone System

In patients with CRF, the basal values of plasma renin activity (PRA) vary, and low, normal, or elevated levels have been reported (512–516) despite a preserved structure of the juxtaglomerular apparatus. Therefore, these variations are most likely due to variable degrees of renal ischemia in different renal diseases or to disturbances in the negative feedback control system between body fluid volume and renin secretion. Indeed, Weidmann and Maxwell (517) report that the levels of PRA are highest in patients with nephrotic syndrome, elevated in those with a glomerulonephritis, and normal in patients with tubulointerstitial disease. Meltzer and coworkers (518) report that PRA is high in patients with nephrotic syndrome due to minimal change disease but low or normal in other forms of nephrotic syndrome. Further, in some patients with diabetic nephropathy, obstructive uropathy, or interstitial nephritis, PRA is low as part of hyporeninemic hypoaldosteronism (519–523). In another study, Weidmann and associates (513) show that for any given level of exchangeable

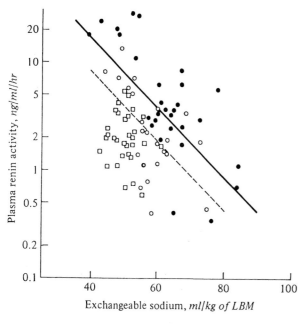

		N =	r =	P <
□	Normal subjects	31	−0.10	NS
	Hemodialysis patients			
○--	BP < 110 mm Hg	23	−0.75	0.0025
●—	BP ≥ 110 mm Hg	29	−0.74	0.001

FIG. 95-5. Relationship between exchangeable body sodium and plasma renin activity in normal subjects and patients being treated with hemodialysis with normal or elevated blood pressure. For any given body sodium, plasma renin activity is on average more than twice as high in hypertensive as in normotensive subjects. *BP*, mean blood pressure; *LBM*, lean body mass. (From Weidmann P, et al. Hypertension in terminal renal failure. *Kidney Int* 1976;9:294, with permission.)

body sodium, PRA is higher in hemodialysis patients, with or without hypertension, than in normal subjects (Fig. 95-5). These observations demonstrate reduced suppressibility of renin secretion by the state of volume and indicate the presence of impaired negative feedback between the state of body volume and renin secretion. It should also be mentioned that patients with CRF and those treated with hemodialysis have hypertension and are treated with medications that may affect renin secretion and as such contribute to the variability in PRA in these patients. After hemodialysis, PRA may increase (524,525). In CAPD patients, PRA is usually higher than in those treated with hemodialysis (328,343). Thus, the interpretation of the values of PRA in patients with CRF should take into consideration the type of renal disease, the state of body volume, and the therapeutic modalities given to the patients.

Normal (526,536), decreased (518–523,527,531,532), and elevated (527,531–534) basal levels of plasma aldosterone have been observed. This variability may be related to differences in the plasma concentrations of potassium and in PRA. Indeed, in patients with CRF with hyporeninemia and hyperkalemia, plasma aldosterone levels are low, and these patients have the syndrome of hyporeninemic hypoaldostero-

nism (519–523). In these patients, ACTH and angiotensin II administration fails to stimulate aldosterone secretion (520,521).

In patients with CRF with normal PRA and normokalemia, plasma aldosterone levels are normal (526,528–530) or increased (519–523,527–536). In these patients, the response of plasma aldosterone to ACTH or angiotensin II administration is intact (526,529,532,533). In a study in which plasma aldosterone levels were measured in patients with various degrees of renal insufficiency, the levels were normal in those with GFR greater than 50 mL/minute and increased progressively with the decline in GFR (534). Available data indicate that an adequate amount of aldosterone is critical for maintaining normokalemia in patients with CRF. Indeed, in those with hyporeninemic hypoaldosteronism, hyperkalemia is always present (519–523), and the administration of spironolactone to CRF patients is quickly followed by hyperkalemia (533,535,537).

The plasma concentrations of aldosterone in hemodialysis patients are variable (526,527,536), and they correlate well with the plasma concentrations of potassium and PRA. In these patients, plasma aldosterone increases with upright posture and after administration of ACTH (527,536). The changes in plasma aldosterone levels following the dialysis procedure are also dictated by the changes in body volume and in the concentrations of plasma potassium. Thus, during ultrafiltration without changes in plasma potassium, plasma aldosterone increases (538–541). A decline in plasma potassium during hemodialysis would blunt the rise in aldosterone levels induced by fluid removal (538–541). In anephric hemodialysis patients, plasma aldosterone levels are usually reduced (526,536–539,542–551), but normal levels may be encountered (341,342). These patients may have impaired responses to angiotensin II (526,544), ACTH (526,536,544), upright posture (526,542), or changes in volume status (526, 542,544).

In uremic patients treated with CAPD, plasma aldosterone concentrations may be normal or increased (343,448) and are responsive to weight loss (328) or administration of ACTH (318). Patients undergoing CAPD have higher plasma levels of aldosterone (343) and 18-hydroxycorticosterone (328) than those treated by hemodialysis (328,343).

Catecholamines

Plasma norepinephrine (NE) levels are usually normal in patients with mild renal insufficiency but are elevated in patients with advanced renal failure (282,549,551). In predialysis patients, the upright posture is associated with about a threefold increase in plasma NE levels, a change that is significantly greater than in normal subjects (282). In hemodialysis patients, the basal levels of NE are normal (282,552) or elevated (553,554). Campese and colleagues (282) and Zucchelli and coworkers (555) report that basal levels of NE did not change during the hemodialysis procedure, while Lake and associates (552) report an increase in the plasma levels of NE during dialysis. In contrast, plasma NE levels increase significantly during hemofiltration (556). This difference between hemodialysis and hemofiltration may partly explain the lower incidence of hypotensive episodes during hemofiltration compared with hemodialysis. In nondiabetic patients with CRF treated with CAPD, plasma levels of NE are elevated (554,557). Plasma levels of epinephrine are also elevated in patients with CRF (282,549).

The metabolism of NE is altered in CRF. The activity of tyrosine hydroxylase, the rate-limiting enzyme of NE synthesis, is reduced in myocardial homogenate (558) and in brain synaptosomes (428) of animals with CRF. Also the activity of dopamine β-hydroxylase, the enzyme that catalyzes the conversion of dopamine into NE, is reduced (559) or normal (560). Thus, it seems unlikely that increased production of NE is responsible for the elevation in the blood levels of NE in CRF. Further, the activities of the enzymes responsible for the degradation of NE are impaired in CRF. Atuk and coworkers (551) report that the activity of the red blood cells' catechol O-methyltransferase is reduced in patients with CRF, and the activity of monoamine oxidase is decreased in brain synaptosomes (428) and skeletal muscles and remnant kidney tissue (561) of rats with CRF. Thus, it appears that a decrease in the degradation of NE in CRF, at least partly, contributes to its elevated blood levels. A substantial part of plasma catecholamines is excreted by the kidney (562,563), and therefore reduction in renal function is associated with decreased renal clearance of these hormones, which in turn contributes to the elevation in their blood levels in CRF.

Depletion of catecholamine stores has also been observed in salivary glands of uremic patients (564) and in brain synaptosomes of rats with CRF (426) as well as reduced NE release and uptake by brain synaptosomes of rats with CRF (426) and by vesicles isolated from myocardium of uremic rats (558).

Atrial Natriuretic Peptide

In patients with CRF, the plasma levels of atrial natriuretic peptide (ANP) are elevated (565–569), and there is a significant correlation between these levels and those of plasma creatinine (569). In patients treated with dialysis, the plasma levels of ANP are also elevated (570–574). These elevated levels are most likely due to an increase in intravascular filling and to atrial distention and reflect fluid overload in these patients (571,575). Indeed, removal of fluid by ultrafiltration during dialysis therapy is associated with a decrease in the plasma levels of ANP (108,109,113). The latter are not influenced by the type of buffer (acetate or bicarbonate) of dialysate (573). Pruszczynski and associates (576) report that the basal levels of ANP are higher and the response of ANP to volume expansion is greater in patients with CRF with cardiac parasympathetic dysfunction than in those with intact parasympathetic function.

Endothelin

The plasma levels of immunoreactive (IR) endothelin are elevated in patients with CRF and in those treated with hemodialysis or CAPD (576–583). Although Warrens and colleagues (580) did not find a relationship between plasma levels of IR endothelin, a recent study by Stockenhuber and coworkers (581) claims a significant direct correlation between the plasma concentrations of IR endothelin and serum creatinine. Endothelin is detected in dialysate (579), indicating that it is dialyzable; however, there is no significant change in plasma levels of IR endothelin during the dialysis procedure (579,580). These observations suggest that either the amount removed by dialysis is small and/or endothelin production is increased during dialysis. IR endothelin is also detected in the peritoneal dialysate in patients treated with CAPD, but its clearance is significantly lower than that of creatinine (583).

Shichiri and colleagues (584) report that the plasma levels of IR endothelin are elevated in hypertensive but not in normotensive dialysis patients. In contrast, others report elevated plasma levels of IR endothelin in normotensive hemodialysis patients as well (578–580). After the correction of the anemia in hemodialysis patients with erythropoietin therapy, plasma levels of IR endothelin increased in those who developed hypertension but not in those whose blood pressure did not rise (582).

Several mechanisms may contribute to the elevation in plasma levels of IR endothelin. These include decreased renal excretion, increased production, and/or reduced metabolism of endothelin in CRF. The clinical significance of the high plasma levels of IR endothelin in patients with CRF is not fully understood. However, the high plasma endothelin levels may participate in the genesis of hypertension in patients with CRF. Also since endothelin has mitogenic activity (585,586), it may cause mitogenesis of vascular smooth muscle cells and contribute to atherogenesis in CRF.

Prostaglandins

In patients with advanced CRF (GFR less than 25 mL/minute), the urinary excretion of prostaglandins is usually reduced (587,588). Others report that the urinary excretion of prostaglandins A, E_2, and F_2 is normal or increased in CRF (589–593). It appears that the urinary excretion of prostaglandins is dependent on the residual renal mass (587) and/or the type of renal disease underlying the CRF (589,590). Indeed, in patients with CRF due to lupus erythematosus (590) or due to chronic renal ischemia (589), the urinary excretion or prostaglandin E_2 is markedly increased.

Administration of nonsteroidal antiinflammatory drugs to humans with CRF can cause acute deterioration of the residual excretory function of the kidney (588,594,595). As a result, it seems that increased production of endogenous prostaglandins per gram of remaining renal parenchyma may be necessary for the maintenance of the function of the residual nephrons by exerting a cytoprotective, diuretic, natriuretic, and/or vasodilatory effect (595).

In uremic patients not receiving dialysis, the plasma levels of thromboxane B_2 are in the normal range, showing a significant decline after acetaminophen administration (588). During hemodialysis, elevated plasma levels of prostaglandin E and 6-keto-prostaglandin $F_1\alpha$, which is a metabolite of prostacyclin (prostaglandin I_2), have been found (593). As the pulmonary endothelium is rich in prostaglandins (596) and lung damage occurs during hemodialysis (597), the potential participation of prostaglandin I_2 in the pathogenesis of circulatory disturbances during dialysis such as hypotension, headache, and nausea seems likely. This idea, however, does not seem to be supported by studies showing that administration of indomethacin, which is a nonspecific inhibitor of cyclooxygenase, does not influence hemodialysis-induced hypotension (596).

The urinary excretion of a stable prostacyclin metabolite is decreased in patients with hyporeninemic hypoaldosteronism and CRF (598); further, the urinary excretion of this prostacyclin metabolite could not be increased by norepinephrine or calcium infusion. These observations are consistent with these patients having prostacyclin deficiency as well as unresponsiveness of prostacyclin synthesis to stimuli.

Kallikrein–Kinin System

In patients with CRF, the absolute amount of urinary kallikrein, which is a marker of the renal kallikrein–kinin system, is moderately or markedly decreased, while kallikrein excretion calculated per unit of residual GFR is significantly increased (593). It is possible that the increased kallikrein secretion by the distal tubules of residual nephrons may be involved in the genesis of increased fractional sodium and water excretion in uremic patients.

Ouabainlike Factors

Endogenous inhibitors of the sodium pump have been implicated in the physiologic adaptation to CRF (599). Increased plasma levels of Na^+–K^+–ATPase inhibitors have been reported in renal failure (600–604). After long-term dialysis, normalization of Na^+–K^+–ATPase inhibitory activity was found (601). These reports are in contrast to findings in other studies in which low Na^+–K^+–ATPase inhibitory activity (605) or digoxinlike immunoreactive substances were found in only one-fourth of hemodialysis patients. These discrepancies seem to be related to the assay method and the type of antibody used for the assessment of digitalislike substances. It should be emphasized that in some studies a correlation has been shown between immunoreactive digitalislike substances and Na^+–K^+–ATPase inhibition (602,606), while in others a dissociation of these two parameters was reported (68). The chemical structure of the ouabainlike factors seems to be heterogeneous (601,602) and not well defined. It is not evident at the present time whether endogenous ouabainlike factors are involved in the pathogenesis of hypertension and the adaptive increase in urinary sodium excretion per nephron in uremic patients (600,607).

Gastrointestinal Hormones

Elevated plasma gastrin levels have been reported both in patients with CRF and in those treated with hemodialysis (608–612). Hypergastrinemia in CRF is due predominantly to "big" gastrin (G34); this molecule is biologically six to eight times less active than "little" gastrin (G17), levels of which are normal in CRF (611). This may explain a "normal" incidence of peptic ulcer in uremic patients (613). These findings are in contrast to those of other authors, who observed hyperchlorhydria and an increased incidence of peptic ulcer in patients with CRF (614).

Long-term hemodialysis treatment does not often affect the elevated plasma levels of gastrin (611,615), although in some studies a decline in gastrinemia was observed (612). Only trace amounts of gastrin could be detected in dialysate. A significant decline of gastrinemia after treatment with erythropoietin was found (616).

Since the kidney is the main site of gastrin biodegradation (617), hypergastrinemia in uremic patients is regarded as the consequence of reduced renal degradation of this hormone. Several other factors have also been incriminated in increased production of gastrin, including hypochlorhydria or achlorhydria (611), resistance of the gastric mucosa to gastrin (612), and gastrin cell density (618).

The plasma levels of other gastrointestinal hormones such as cholecystokinin (619,620), gastric inhibitory peptide (621), pancreatic polypeptide (610,616,622,623), secretin (619), and motilin (610) are elevated in patients with CRF. Both normal (610) and markedly elevated (624) plasma levels of vasoactive intestinal polypeptide were found in patients with CRF. The pathophysiologic importance of these findings remains to be elucidated.

Cytokines

Plasma levels of interleukin-1 (IL-1) in patients with CRF are not different from those in normal subjects (625,626), but they are markedly elevated in patients undergoing hemodialysis (627,628). During the dialysis session, the plasma concentration of IL-1 increases significantly in patients dialyzed with cellulose membranes (629). Plasma levels of IL-6 are normal in patients with CRF (630) but increased in patients undergoing dialysis (630,631). Plasma levels of tumor necrosis factor-α (TNF-α) are modestly elevated in patients with CRF (632) but significantly increased in patients undergoing hemodialysis (626). All of these observations are consistent with the notion that hemodialysis causes an increase in the production of these cytokines. Herbelin and associates

(626) report that the increase in plasma cytokine levels during dialysis was observed with both cellulose and synthetic (PAN-AN69) membranes.

In contrast, Pereira and Dinarello (633) studied a selected group of patients using specific radioimmunoassays and ELISA and report that the plasma levels of IL-1, TNF-α, and IL-1 receptors were elevated in patients with CRF, and those being treated with hemodialysis or CAPD. There were no significant differences in the levels of these cytokines among the three groups of patients. These authors further report that a significant correlation existed between the plasma concentrations of the cytokines and the degree of renal insufficiency. These data indicate that the elevation in the plasma concentrations of the cytokines are due to decreased clearance and not to increased production.

Finally, Powell and colleagues (634), using ELISA for the measurement of IL-1 and TNF-α, report that the plasma levels of these cytokines in patients with CRF, and those being treated with hemodialysis or CAPD are not different from those in normal subjects; further, these cytokines did increase during dialysis. These observations do not support decreased clearance or increased production of these cytokines in CRF.

Beta-Lipotropin and Opioid Peptides

Plasma β-lipotropin levels, like most of the other pituitary-derived polypeptide hormones, are moderately or markedly elevated in patients with ESRD (635–636), due to decreased renal clearance (636). Similarly elevated plasma levels of β-endorphin (637–641) and met-enkephalin (637,638) have been found in uremic patients. Plasma met-enkephalin levels were directly correlated with plasma creatinine and urea concentrations (642). In contrast, plasma leu-enkephalin levels are significantly lower in uremic patients than in healthy subjects (642). After treatment with a low-phosphorus, low-protein diet supplemented with essential amino acids and keto analogs, a significant decline of plasma α-endorphin levels was reported (640).

The elevated plasma levels of the opioid peptides suggest a state of hyperendorphinism, which may play a role in many of the endocrine abnormalities in CRF. Support for this notion is provided by studies by Kokot and others (303,643), who demonstrate that the administration of naloxone, which causes blockade of opioid receptors, is followed by amelioration of many of the endocrine derangements in CRF.

Leptin

Leptin is a 16-kd peptide (644) exclusively produced by adipocytes; therefore there is a strong relationship between body fat mass and serum leptin levels. Leptin is a regulator of appetite. High plasma levels of leptin reduce appetite. Leptin also increases metabolism. In obese subjects leptin circulates in the blood in the free form. It exerts its effect through a receptor that belongs to the class 1 cytokine receptor family.

The interaction of leptin with its receptor in the hypothalamus results in modulation of the activity neuromodulators that affect feeding behaviors; these neuromodulators include neuropeptide and melanocortin. The current basic and clinical aspects of leptin and its metabolism are provided in the excellent review of Sinha and Caro (645).

Patients with advanced renal failure and those treated with hemodialysis have elevated serum levels of leptin (646–648). However, certain patients with ESRD, especially males with low body mass index may have normal or even low levels of serum leptin. Several factors may underlie the hyperleptinemia in renal failure patients. These include impaired renal clearance, increased production, hyperinsulinemia, obesity, the chronic inflammatory state of renal failure, and therapy with glucocorticoids.

It is of interest that plasma leptin levels in patients treated with peritoneal dialysis are higher than in those managed with hemodialysis. Leptin levels in serum are not reduced by low-flux dialysis membranes, whereas high-flux dialysis membrane decreases leptin levels by 30% to 40%.

The significance of the hyperleptinemia in patients with ESRD is not adequately clarified, but certain data suggest that the hyperleptinemia may participate in the genesis of the anorexia of renal failure.

REFERENCES

1. De Fronzo RA, Andres R, Edgar P, et al. Carbohydrate metabolism in uremia: a review. *Medicine (Baltimore)* 1973;52:469.
2. De Fronzo RA, et al. Insulin resistance in uremia. *J Clin Invest* 1981;67:563.
3. Hampers CL, Soeldner JS, Doak PB, et al. Effect of chronic renal failure and hemodialysis on carbohydrate metabolism. *J Clin Invest* 1966;45:1719.
4. Lowrie EG, Soeldner JS, Hampers CL, et al. Glucose metabolism and insulin secretion in uremic, prediabetic, and normal subjects. *J Lab Clin Med* 1976;76:603.
5. Perley M, Kippnis DM. Plasma insulin responses to glucose and tolbutamide of normal weight and obese diabetic and non-diabetic subjects. *Diabetes* 1966;15:867.
6. Beck P, et al. Correlative studies of growth hormone and insulin plasma concentrations with metabolic abnormalities and acromegaly. *J Lab Clin Med* 1965;66:366.
7. De Fronzo RA. Pathogenesis of glucose intolerance in uremia. *Metab Clin Exp* 1978;27:1866.
8. Westervelt FB Jr, Schreiner GE. The carbohydrate intolerance of uremic patients. *Ann Intern Med* 1962;57:266.
9. De Fronzo RA, Tobin JD, Andrez R. Glucose clamp technique: a method for quantifying insulin secretion and resistance. *Am J Physiol* 1979;237:E241.
10. De Fronzo RA, Alverstrand A. Glucose intolerance in uremia: site and mechanism. *Am J Clin Nutr* 1980;33:1938.
11. Castellino P, et al. Glucose and amino acid metabolism in chronic renal failure: effect of insulin and amino acids. *Am J Physiol* 1992;262:F168.
12. Smith D, De Fronzo RA. Insulin resistance in uremia mediated by postbinding defects. *Kidney Int* 1982;22:54.
13. Akmal M, et al. Role of parathyroid hormone in glucose intolerance of chronic renal failure. *J Clin Invest* 1985;75:1037.
14. Jones M, Persaud SJ. Protein kinase, protein kinase, protein phosphorylation, and the regulation of insulin secretion from pancreatic islets. *Endocrine Rev* 1998;19:429.
15. Weisinger J, et al. Insulin binding and glycolytic activity in erythrocytes from dialyzed and non-dialyzed uremic patients. *Nephron* 1988;48:190.

16. Schmitz O, Alberti KGMM, Christensen NJ. Aspects of glucose home-ostasis in uremia as assessed by the hyperinsulinemic clamp technique. *Metabolism* 1985;34:465.

17. Taylor R, et al. Adipocyte insulin binding and insulin action in chronic renal failure before and during continuous ambulatory peritoneal dialysis. *Metabolism* 1986;35:430.

18. Pedersen O, et al. Postbinding defects of insulin action in human adipocytes from uremic patients. *Kidney Int* 1985;27:780.

19. Maloff, BL, McCaleb ML, Lockwood DH. Cellular basis of insulin resistance in chronic uremia. *Am J Physiol* 1983;245:E178.

20. Bak J, et al. Activity of insulin receptor kinase and glycogen synthase in skeletal muscle from patients with chronic renal failure. *Acta Endocrinol (Copenh)* 1989;121:744.

21. Cecchin F, et al. Insulin resistance in uremia: insulin receptor kinase activity in liver and muscle from chronic uremic rats. *Am J Physiol* 1988;254:E394.

22. James DE, Strube M, Mueckler M. Molecular cloning and characterization of an insulin-regulatable glucose transporter. *Nature (Lond)* 1989;338:83.

23. Mueckler M, et al. Sequence and structure of a human glucose transporter. *Science* 1985;229:941.

24. Friedman JE, et al. Muscle insulin resistance in uremic humans: glucose transport, glucose transporters, and insulin receptors. *Am J Physiol* 1991;261:E87.

25. De Fronzo RA, et al. Glucose intolerance in uremia: quantification of pancreatic beta cell sensitivity to glucose and tissue sensitivity to insulin. *J Clin Invest* 1978;62:425.

26. Gin H, et al. Low protein and low phosphorus diet in patients with chronic renal failure: influence on glucose tolerance and tissue insulin sensitivity. *Metabolism* 1987;36:1080.

27. Mak R, et al. The effect of a low protein diet with amino acid/keto acid supplements on glucose metabolism in children with uremia. *J Clin Endocrinol Metab* 1986;63:985.

28. Heaton A, et al. Hepatic and peripheral insulin action in chronic renal failure before and during continuous ambulatory peritoneal dialysis. *Clin Sci* 1989;77:383.

29. McCaleb ML, Wish JB, Lockwood DH. Insulin resistance in chronic renal failure. *Endocrinol Res* 1985;11:113.

30. Dzurik R, et al. The isolation of an inhibitor of glucose utilization from the serum of uraemic subjects. *Clin Chim Acta* 1983;46:77.

31. Kuku SF, et al. Heterogeneity of plasma glucagon-circulating components in normal subjects and patients with chronic renal failure. *J Clin Invest* 1976;58:742.

32. Emmanouel DS, et al. Pathogenesis and characterization of hyperglucagonemia in the uremic rat. *J Clin Invest* 1976;58:1266.

33. Lim VS, Kathpalia SC, Henriquez C. Endocrine abnormalities associated with chronic renal failure. *Med Clin North Am* 1978;62:1341.

34. Grzeszczak W, Kokot F, Dulawa J. Effects of naloxone administration on endocrine abnormalities in chronic renal failure. *Am J Nephrol* 1987;7:93.

35. Stuart CA, et al. Bed-rest-induced insulin resistance occurs primarily in muscle. *Metabolism* 1988;37:802.

36. Goldberg AP, et al. The metabolic and psychological effects of exercise training in hemodialysis patients. *Am J Clin Nutr* 1980;33:1620.

37. Rabkin R, Simon NM, Steiner S, et al. Effect of renal disease on renal uptake and excretion of insulin in man. *N Engl J Med* 1970;282:182.

38. Schmitz O. Effects of physiological and supraphysiologic hyperglycemia on early and late-phase insulin secretion in chronically dialyzed uremic patients. *Acta Endocrinol (Copenh)* 1989;121:251.

39. Nakamura Y, et al. Insulin release from column-perfused isolated islets of uremic rats. *Nephron* 1985;40:467.

40. Fadda GZ, et al. Insulin release from pancreatic islets: effects of CRF and excess PTH. *Kidney Int* 1988;33:1066.

41. Fadda GZ, et al. On the mechanism of impaired insulin secretion in chronic renal failure. *J Clin Invest* 1991;87:255.

42. Mak RH, et al. The influence of hyperparathyroidism on glucose metabolism in uremia. *J Clin Endocrinol Metab* 1985;60:229.

43. Mak RH, et al. Secondary hyperparathyroidism and glucose intolerance in children with uremia. *Kidney Int* 1983;24:S128.

44. Perna AF, Fadda GZ, Zhou X-J, et al. Mechanisms of impaired insulin secretion after chronic excess of parathyroid hormone. *Am J Physiol* 1990;259:F210.

45. Massry SG, Coburn JW, Peacock M, et al. Turnover of endogenous parathyroid hormone in uremic patients and those undergoing hemodialysis. *Trans Am Soc Artif Int Organs* 1972;18:416.

46. Massry SG, Smogorzewski M. Mechanisms through which parathyroid hormone mediates the deleterious effects on organ function in uremia. *Semin Nephrol* 1994;14:219.

47. Fadda GZ, Akmal M, Lipson LG, et al. Direct effect of parathyroid hormone on insulin secretion from pancreatic islets. *Am J Physiol* 1990;258:E975.

48. Fadda GZ, Thanakitcharu P, Smogorzewski M, et al. Parathyroid hormone raises cytosolic calcium in pancreatic islets: study on mechanisms. *Kidney Int* 1993;43:554.

49. Baczynski R, et al. Effect of parathyroid hormone on myocardial energy metabolism in the rat. *Kidney Int* 1985;27:618.

50. Denton RM, McCormack JG. Ca^{2+} transport by mammalian mitochondria and its role in hormone action. *Am J Physiol* 1985;299:E543.

51. Trump BE, Berezski IF. The role of ion deregulation in toxic cell injury. *Adv Modern Environ Tox* 1987;14:27.

52. Hajjar SM, et al. Reduced activity of Na^+-K^+ ATPase of pancreatic islets in chronic renal failure: role of secondary hyperparathyroidism. *J Am Soc Nephrol* 1992;2:1355.

53. Fadda GZ, et al. Correction of glucose intolerance and the impaired insulin release of chronic renal failure by verapamil. *Kidney Int* 1989;36:773.

54. Thanakitcharu P, Fadda GZ, Hajjar SM, et al. Verapamil prevents the metabolic and functional derangements in pancreatic islets of chronic renal failure in rats. *Endocrinology* 1991;129:1749.

55. Fadda GZ, Hajjar SM, Zhou X-J, et al. Verapamil corrects abnormal metabolism of pancreatic islets and insulin secretion in phosphate depletion. *Endocrinology* 1992;130:193.

56. Cook DL, Hales CN. Intracellular ATP directly blocks K^+ channels in pancreatic β-cells. *Nature (Lond)* 1984;311:271.

57. Prentki M, Matchinsky M. [Ca^{2+}]i, cAMP and phospholipid-derived messengers in coupling mechanisms of insulin secretion. *Physiol Rev* 1987;67:1185.

58. Henquin JC, Meissner HP. Significance of ionic fluxes and changes in membrane potential for stimulus secretion coupling in pancreatic β-cells. *Experientia (Basel)* 1984;40:1043.

59. Hedeskov CJ. Mechanisms of glucose-induced insulin secretion. *Physiol Rev* 1980;60:442.

60. Fadda GZ, Massry SG. Impaired glucose-induced calcium signal in pancreatic islets in chronic renal failure. *Am J Nephrol* 1991;11:475.

61. Stadtman ER. Allosteric regulation of enzyme activity. *Adv Enzymol Relat Areas Mol Biol* 1966;28:141.

62. Milner RDG. Stimulation of insulin secretion in vitro by essential amino acids. *Lancet* 1969;1:1075.

63. Oberwetter JM, Boyd AE II. High K^+ rapidly stimulates Ca^{2+}-dependent phosphorylation of three protein concomitant with insulin secretion from HIT cells. *Diabetes* 1984;36:864.

64. Fadda GZ, et al. Impaired potassium-induced insulin secretion in chronic renal failure. *Kidney Int* 1991;40:413.

65. Oh H-Y, et al. Abnormal leucine-induced insulin secretion in chronic renal failure. *Am J Physiol* 1994;267:F853.

66. Christakos S, Norman AW. Studies on the mode of action of calciferol XXXIX: biochemical characterization of 1,25-dihydroxyvitamin D_3 receptors in chick pancreas and kidney cytosol. *Endocrinology* 1981;108:140.

67. Pike JW. Receptors for 1,25-dihydroxyvitamin D_3 in chick pancreas: a partial physical and functional characterization. *J Steroid Biochem* 1981;16:385.

68. Roth J, Bonner-Weir S, Norman AW, et al. Immunocytochemistry of vitamin D-dependent calcium binding protein in chick pancreas: exclusive localization in β cells. *Endocrinology* 1982;110:2216.

69. Morrisey RL, Bucci TJ, Empson RN, et al. Calcium-binding proteins: its cellular localization in jejunum, kidney and pancreas. *Proc Soc Exp Biol Med* 1975;148:56.

70. Pochet R, Pipeleers DG, Malaisse WJ. Calbindin D-27 KDa preferential localization in non-β islet cells of the rat pancreas. *Biol Cell* 1987;61:155.

71. Narbaitz R Stumpf WE, Sar M. The role of autoradiographic and immunocytochemical techniques in the clarification of sites of metabolism and action of vitamin D. *J Histochem Cytochem* 1981;29:91.

72. Norman AW, Frankel BJ, Heldt AW, et al. Vitamin D₃ deficiency inhibits pancreatic secretion of insulin. *Science* 1980;209:823.

73. Cade C, Norman AW. Vitamin D₃ improves impaired glucose tolerance and insulin secretion in the vitamin D-deficient rat in vivo. *Endocrinology* 1986;119:84.

74. Mawer B, et al. Failure of formation of 1,25-dihydroxycholecalciferol in chronic renal failure. *Lancet* 1973;1:626.

75. Mak RHK. Intravenous 1,25-dihydroxycholecalciferol corrects glucose intolerance in hemodialysis patients. *Kidney Int* 1992;41:1049.

76. Rabkin R, Rubenstein AH, Colwell JA. Glomerular filtration and maximal tubular absorption of insulin [¹²⁵I]. *Am J Physiol* 1972;223:1093.

77. Rubenstein AH, Mako ME, Horwitz DL. Insulin and the kidney. *Nephron* 1975;15:306.

78. Rabkin R, Jones J, Kitabchi AE. Insulin extraction from the renal peritubular circulation in the chicken. *Endocrinology* 1977;101:1828.

79. Rabkin R, Unterhalter SA, Duckworth WC. Effect of prolonged uremia on insulin metabolism by isolated liver and muscle. *Kidney Int* 1979;16:433.

80. Garber AJ, Bier DM, Cryer PE, et al. Hypoglycemia in compensated chronic renal insufficiency: substrate limitations of gluconeogenesis. *Diabetes* 1974;23:982.

81. Nadkarni M, Berns JS, Rudnick MR, et al. Hypoglycemia with hyperinsulinemia in a chronic hemodialysis patient following parathyroidectomy. *Nephron* 1992;60:100.

82. Arem R. Hypoglycemia associated with renal failure. *Endocrinol Metab Clin North Am* 1989;18:103.

83. Jackson MA, et al. Occult hypoglycemia caused by hemodialysis. *Clin Nephrol* 1999;51:242.

84. Soliman AR, Akmal M, Massry SG. Parathyroid hormone interferes with extrarenal disposition of potassium in chronic renal failure. *Miner Electrolyte Metab* 1989;52:262.

85. Gomez M, Curry DL. Potassium stimulation of insulin release by the perfused rat pancreas. *Endocrinology* 1973;92:1126.

86. De Fronzo RA, Lee R, Jones A, et al. Effect of insulinopenia and adrenal hormone deficiency on acute potassium tolerance. *Kidney Int* 1980;17:586.

87. Bia M, De Fronzo RA. Extrarenal potassium homeostasis. *Am J Physiol* 1981;240:F257.

88. Linder A, Charra B, Sherrard DJ, et al. Accelerated atherogenesis of prolonged maintenance hemodialysis. *N Engl J Med* 1974;290:697.

89. Ferrannini E, et al. Insulin resistance in essential hypertension. *N Engl J Med* 1987;317:350.

90. Cryer A. Tissue lipoprotein lipase activity and its action in lipoprotein metabolism. *Int J Biochem* 1981;13:525.

91. Chan MK, Varghese Z, Moorhead JF. Lipid abnormalities in uremia, dialysis and transplantation. *Kidney Int* 1981;19:625.

92. Roullet JB, Lacour B, Drueke T. Partial correction of lipid disturbances by insulin in experimental renal failure. *Contrib Nephrol* 1986;50:203.

93. Akmal M, Kasim SE, Soliman AR, et al. Excess parathyroid hormone adversely affects lipid metabolism in chronic renal failure. *Kidney Int* 1990;37:854.

94. Akmal M, et al. Verapamil prevents CRF induced abnormalities in lipid metabolism. *Am J Kidney Dis* 1993;22:158.

95. Klin M, Smogorzewski M, Ni Z, et al. Abnormalities in hepatic lipase in chronic renal failure. *J Clin Invest* 1996;97:2167.

96. Wang Y, Smogorzewski M, Varuzhan G, et al. Abnormalities lipoprotein lipase (LPL) metabolism in chronic renal failure (CRF). *J Am Soc Nephrol* 9:625A, 1998.

97. Attman P-O, Alaupovic P. Lipid abnormalities in chronic renal insufficiency. *Kidney Int Suppl* 1991;31:S16.

98. Havel JR, Kane JP. Structure and metabolism of plasma lipoproteins. In: Scriver CR, et al, eds. *The metabolic basis of inherited disease*. New York: McGraw-Hill, 1989:1129.

99. Scanu AM. Physiopathology of plasma lipoprotein metabolism. *Kidney Int Suppl* 1991;31:S3,.

100. Alaupovic P. Apoproteins and lipoproteins. *Atherosclerosis* 1971;13:141.

101. Utermann G. The mysteries of lipoprotein (a). *Science* 1989;246:904.

102. Illingworth DR. Lipoprotein metabolism. *Am J Kidney Dis* 1993;22:90.

103. Attman PO, Samuelsson O, Alaupovic P. Lipoprotein metabolism and renal failure. *Am J Kidney Dis* 1993;21:573.

104. Russell DW, Esser V, Hobbs, HH. Molecular basis of familial hypercholesterolemia. *Arteriosclerosis* 1989;9[Suppl]:I8.

105. Hobbs HH, et al. The LDL receptor locus in familial hypercholesterolemia: mutational analysis of a membrane protein. *Annu Rev Genet* 1990;24:133.

106. Brewer HB Jr, Raider DJ. HDL: structure, function and metabolism. *Prog Lipid Res* 1991;30:139.

107. Krauss RM. Regulation of high density lipoprotein levels. *Med Clin North Am* 1982;66:403.

108. Williams PJ, et al. Association of diet and alcohol intake with high density lipoprotein subclasses. *Metabolism* 1985;34:524.

109. Steinberg D, et al. Beyond cholesterol: modifications of low density lipoprotein that increases its atherogenecity. *N Engl J Med* 1989;320:915.

110. Gaziano JM, Hennekens CH. Vitamin antioxidants and cardiovascular disease. *Curr Opin Lipidol* 1992;3:291.

111. Bagdade JD, Casaretto A, Albers J. Effects of chronic uremia, hemodialysis, and renal transplantation on plasma lipids and lipoproteins in man. *J Lab Clin Med* 1976;87:38.

112. Bagdade JD, Porte D, Bierman EL. Hypertriglyceridemia: a metabolic consequence of chronic renal failure. *N Engl J Med* 1968;279:181.

113. Huttunen JK, et al. Lipoprotein metabolism in patients with chronic uremia. *Acta Med Scand* 1978;204:211.

114. Alsayed N, Rebourcet R. Abnormal concentrations of CII, CIII and E apolipoproteins among apolipoprotein B-containing, B-free, and A-1-containing lipoprotein particles in hemodialysis patients. *Clin Chem* 1991;37:387.

115. Attman PO, Alaupovic P, Gustafson A. Serum apolipoprotein profile of patients with chronic renal failure. *Kidney Int* 1987;32:368.

116. Joven J, et al. Apoprotein A-I and high density lipoprotein subfractions in patients with chronic renal failure receiving hemodialysis. *Nephron* 1985;40:451.

117. Shoji T, et al. Impaired metabolism of high density lipoprotein in uremic patients. *Kidney Int* 1992;41:1653.

118. Goldberg AP, et al. Racial differences in plasma high-density lipoproteins in patients receiving hemodialysis: a possible mechanism for accelerated atherosclerosis in men. *N Engl J Med* 1983;308:1245.

119. Ohta T, Matsuda I. Apolipoprotein and lipid abnormalities in uremic children on hemodialysis. *Clin Chim* 1985;147:145.

120. Grützmacher P, et al. Lipoproteins and apolipoproteins during the progression of chronic renal disease. *Nephron* 1988;50:103.

121. Attman PO, Alaupovic P. Lipid and apolipoprotein profiles of uremic dyslipoproteinemia—relation to renal function and dialysis. *Nephron* 1991;57:401.

122. Milionis HJ, Elisaf MS, Tselepis A, et al. Plasma and Lp(a) associated PAD-acetylhydrolase activity in uremic patients undergoing different dialysis procedures. *Kidney Int* 1999;56:2276.

123. Dieplinger H, Schoenfeld PY, Fielding CJ. Plasma cholesterol metabolism in end-stage renal disease: difference between treatment by hemodialysis or peritoneal dialysis. *J Clin Invest* 1986;77:1071.

124. Ibels LS, et al. Studies on the nature and causes of hyperlipidemia in uraemia, maintenance dialysis and renal transplantation. *Q J Med* 1975;176:601.

125. Lacour B, et al. Comparison of several atherogenicity indices by the analysis of serum lipoprotein composition in patients with chronic renal failure with or without haemodialysis, and in renal transplant patients. *J Clin Chem Clin Biochem* 1985;23:805.

126. Rubiés-Prat J, et al. High-density lipoprotein cholesterol subfractions in chronic uremia. *Am J Kidney Dis* 1987;9:60.

127. Attman P-O, et al. The compositional abnormalities in lipoprotein density classes of patients with chronic renal failure (CRF). *Am J Kidney Dis* 1989;14:432(abst).

128. Parsy D, et al. Lipoprotein abnormalities in chronic hemodialysis patients. *Nephrol Dial Tranplant* 1988;3:51.

129. Cattran DC, et al. Defective triglyceride removal in lipemia associated with peritoneal dialysis and haemodialysis. *Ann Intern Med* 1976;85:29.

130. Cramp DG. Plasma lipid alterations in patients with chronic renal disease. *Crit Rev Clin Lab Sci* 1982;17:77.

131. Gregg R, et al. Effect of acute uremia on triglyceride kinetics in the rat. *Metabolism* 1976;25:1557.

132. Sanfelippo M, Grundy S, Henderson L. Transport of very low density lipoprotein triglyceride (VLDL-TG): comparison of hemodialysis (HD) and hemofiltration (HF). *Kidney Int* 1979;16:868,(abst).

133. Norbeck HE, Carlson LA. Increased frequency of late pre-beta-lipoproteins (LPbeta) in isolated serum very low-density lipoproteins in uraemia. *Eur J Clin Invest* 1980;10:423.

134. Ron D, et al. Accumulation of lipoprotein remnants in patients with chronic renal failure. *Atherosclerosis* 1983;46:67.

135. Demant T, et al. Lipoprotein metabolism in hepatic lipase deficiency: studies on the turnover of apolipoprotein B and on the effect of hepatic lipase on high density lipoprotein. *J Lipid Res* 1988;29:1603.

136. Chan PC, et al. Apolipoprotein B turnover in dialysis patients: its relationship to pathogenesis of hyperlipidemia. *Clin Nephrol* 1989;31:88.

137. Crawford GA, Mahony JF, Stewart JH. Impaired lipoprotein lipase activation by uraemic and post-transplant sera. *Clin Sci* 1981;60:73.

138. Goldberg A, Sherrard DJ, Brunzell JD. Adipose tissue lipoprotein lipase in chronic hemodialysis: role in plasma triglyceride metabolism. *J Clin Endocrinol Metab* 1978;47:1173.

139. Kraemer FB, Chen YD, Reaven GM. Hypertriglyceridemia and lipoprotein lipase activity in experimental uremia. *Nephron* 1982;30:274.

140. McCosh EJ, et al. Hypertriglyceridemia in patients with chronic renal insufficiency. *Am J Clin Nutr* 1975;28:1036.

141. Roullet JB, et al. Correction by insulin of disturbed TG-rich LP metabolism in rats with chronic renal failure. *Am J Physiol* 1986;250:E373.

142. Murase T, et al. Inhibition of lipoprotein lipase by uremic plasma, a possible cause of hypertriglyceridemia. *Metabolism* 1976;24:1279.

143. Atger V, et al. Presence of Apo B48, and relative Apo CII deficiency and Apo CIII enrichment in uremic very-low density lipoproteins. *Ann Biol Clin (Paris)* 1989;47:497.

144. Erkelens DW, Mocking JA. The CII/CIII ratio of transferable apolipoprotein in primary and secondary hypertriglyceridemia. *Clin Chim Acta* 1982;121:59.

145. Wakabayashi Y, et al. Decreased VLDL apoprotein C-II/apoprotein C-III ratio may be seen in both normotriglyceridemic and hypertriglyceridemic patients on chronic hemodialysis treatment. *Metabolism* 1987;36:815.

146. Applebaum-Bowdem D, et al. Postheparin plasma triglyceride lipases in chronic hemodialysis: evidence for a role for hepatic lipase in lipoprotein metabolism. *Metabolism* 1979;28:917.

147. Attman P-O, et al. Effect of protein-reduced diet on plasma lipids, apolipoproteins and lipolytic activities in patients with chronic renal failure. *Am J Nephrol* 1984;4:92.

148. Chan MK. Gemfibrozil improves abnormalities of lipid metabolism in patients on continuous ambulatory peritoneal dialysis: the role of postheparin lipases in the metabolism of high-density lipoprotein subfractions. *Metabolism* 1989;38:939.

149. Walldius G, Norbeck HE, Wahlberg G. Low fatty acid and glucose incorporation into adipose tissue in hypertriglyceridemia: a removal defect. In: Carlson LA, Pernow B, eds. *Metabolic risk factors in ischemic cardiovascular disease.* New York: Raven, 1982:225.

150. Guarnieri GF, et al. Lecithin-cholesterol acyltransferase (LCAT) activity in chronic uremia. *Kidney Int* 1978;13[Suppl 8]:S26.

151. McLeod R, Reeve CE, Frohlich J. Plasma lipoproteins and lecithin: cholesterol acyltransferase distribution in patients on dialysis. *Kidney Int* 1984;25:683.

152. Sanfelippo ML, Swenson RS, Reaven GM. Reduction of plasma triglycerides by diet in subjects with chronic renal failure. *Kidney Int* 1977;11:54.

153. Heuck CC, Ritz E. Hyperlipoproteinemia in renal insufficiency. *Nephron* 1980;25:1.

154. Berg K. A new serum type system in man: the Lp system. *Acta Pathol Microbiol Scand* 1963;59:369.

155. Scanu AM, Fless GM. Lipoprotein (a): heterogeneity and biological relevance. *J Clin Invest* 1990;85:1709.

156. Rader DJ, Brewer HB Jr. Lipoprotein (a): clinical approach to a unique atherogenic lipoprotein. *JAMA* 1992;267:1109.

157. Dahlen GH, Guyton JR, Attar M. Association of levels of lipoprotein (a), plasma lipids, and other lipoproteins with coronary artery disease documented by angiography. *Circulation* 1986;74:758.

158. Cressman MD, et al. Lipoprotein (a) is an independent risk factor for cardiovascular disease in hemodialysis patients. *Circulation* 1992;86:475.

159. Murphy BG, et al. Increased serum apolipoprotein (a) in patients with chronic renal failure treated with continuous ambulatory peritoneal dialysis. *Atherosclerosis* 1992;93:53.

160. Irish AB, et al. Lipoprotein (a) levels in chronic renal disease states, dialysis and transplantation. *Aust NZ J Med* 1992;22:243.

161. Black IW, Wilcken DEL. Decreases in apolipoprotein(a) after renal transplantation: implications for lipoprotein(a) metabolism. *Clin Chem* 1992;38:353.

162. Kandoussi A, et al. Plasma level of lipoprotein Lp(a) is high in pre-dialysis or hemodialysis, but not in CAPD. *Kidney Int* 1992;42:424.

163. Wanner C, et al. Effect of simvastatin on qualitative and quantitative changes of lipoprotein metabolism in CAPD patients. *Nephron* 1992;62:40.

164. Hulley SB, et al. Epidemiology as a guide to clinical decisions: the association between triglyceride and coronary heart disease. *N Engl J Med* 1980;302:1383.

165. Grundy SM, Mok HY. I. Chylomicron clearance in normal and hyperlipidemic man. *Metabolism* 1976;25:1225.

166. Reardon MF, et al. Lipoprotein predictors of the severity of coronary artery disease in men and women. *Circulation* 1985;71:881.

167. Tatami R, et al. Intermediate-density lipoprotein and cholesterol-rich very low density lipoprotein in angiographically determined coronary artery disease. *Circulation* 1981;64:1174.

168. Austin MA, et al. Low-density lipoprotein subclass patterns and risk of myocardial infarction. *JAMA* 1988;260:1917.

169. Richards EG, Grundy SM, Cooper K. Influence of plasma triglycerides on lipoprotein patterns in normal subjects and in patients with coronary artery disease. *Am J Cardiol* 1969;63:1214.

170. Castelli WP, et al. Incidence of coronary heart disease and lipoprotein cholesterol levels: the Framingham Study. *JAMA* 1986;256:2835.

171. Miller GJ, Miller NE. Plasma-high-density-lipoprotein concentration and development of ischaemic heart disease. *Lancet* 1975;1:16.

172. Cattran DC, et al. Dialysis hyperlipemia: response to dietary manipulations. *Clin Nephrol* 1980;13:177.

173. Sanfelippo ML, Swenson RS, Reaven GM. Response of plasma triglycerides to dietary change in patients on hemodialysis. *Kidney Int* 1978;14:180.

174. Aparicio M, et al. Effect of a low-protein diet on urinary albumin excretion in uremic patients. *Nephron* 1988;50:288.

175. Barsotti G, et al. Restoration of blood levels of testosterone in male uremics following a low protein diet supplemented with essential aminoacids and ketoanalogues. *Contrib Nephrol* 1985;49:63.

176. Barsotti G, et al. Effects of a vegetarian, supplemented diet on renal function, proteinuria, and glucose metabolism in patients with "overt" diabetic nephropathy and renal insufficiency. *Contrib Nephrol* 1988;65:87.

177. Goldberg PA, et al. Exercise training reduces coronary risk and effectively rehabilitates hemodialysis patients. *Nephron* 1986;42:311.

178. Goldberg AP, et al. Control of clofibrate toxicity in hypertriglyceridemia. *Clin Pharmacol* 1977;21:317.

179. Goldberg AP, et al. Increase in lipoprotein lipase during clofibrate treatment of hypertriglyceridemia in patients on hemodialysis. *N Engl J Med* 1979;301:1073.

180. Pierides AM, Alvarez-Ude F, Kerr DNS. Clofibrate-induced muscle damage in patients with chronic renal failure. *Lancet* 1975;2:1279.

181. Pasternack A, et al. Normalization of lipoprotein lipase and hepatic lipase by gemfibrozil results in correction of lipoprotein abnormalities in chronic renal failure. *Clin Nephrol* 1987;27:163.

182. Grützmacher P, et al. Lipid lowering treatment with bezafibrate in patients on chronic haemodialysis: pharmacokinetics and effects. *Klin Wochenschr* 1986;64:910.

183. Oda H, Keane WF. Recent advances in statins and the kidney. *Kidney Int Suppl* 1999;71:S2.

184. Yukawa S, et al. Ongoing clinical trials of lipid reduction therapy in patients with renal disease. *Kidney Int Suppl* 1999;71:S141.

185. Young VR. Nutritional requirements of normal adults. In: Mitch WE, Klahr S, eds. *Nutrition and the kidney,* 3rd ed. Philadelphia: Lippincott–Raven Publishers, 1998:253.

186. Rose WC. Amino acid requirements of man. *Fed Proc* 1979;8:546.

187. Kalliomäki JL, Markkanen TK, Sourander LB. Correlation between insulin requirement and renal retention in diabetic nephropathy. *Acta Med Scand* 1960;166:423.

188. Kopple JD. Abnormal amino acid and protein metabolism in uremia. *Kidney Int* 1978;14:340.

189. Bergström J, et al. Intracellular free amino acids in muscle tissue of patients with chronic uraemia: effect of peritoneal dialysis and infusion of essential amino acids. *Clin Sci Mol Med* 1978;54:51.

190. Hara Y, et al. Acidosis, not azotemia, stimulates branched-chain, amino acid catabolism in uremic rats. *Kidney Int* 1987;32:808.

191. Bergström J, Alvestrand A, Fürst P. Metabolic acidosis induces selective intracellular valine depletion in maintenance hemodialysis patients. Tokyo: *Proceedings of the Eleventh International Congress on Nephrology*, 1990:A 16A.

192. Fürst P. Amino acid metabolism in uremia. *J Am Coll Nutr* 1989;8:310.

193. Arnold WC, Holliday MA. Tissue resistance to insulin stimulation of amino acid uptake in acutely uremic rats. *Kidney Int* 1979;16:124.

194. Riedel E, et al. Correction of amino acid metabolism by recombinant human erythropoietin therapy in hemodialysis patients. *Kidney Int* 1989;36[Suppl 27]:S216.

195. Kopple JD. Causes of catabolism and wasting in acute or chronic renal failure. In: Robinson RR, ed. *Nephrology*. New York: Springer, 1984:1498.

196. Lowrie EG, Lew NL. Death risk in hemodialysis patients: the predictive value of commonly measured variables and an evaluation of death rate differences between facilities. *Am J Kidney Dis* 1990;15:458.

197. Deferrari G, et al. Splanchnic exchange of amino acids after amino acid ingestion in patients with chronic renal insufficiency. *Am J Clin Nutr* 1988;48:72.

198. Harper AE, Benjamin E. Relationship between intake and rate of oxidation of leucine and alpha-ketoisocaproate in vivo in the rat. *J Nutr* 1984;114:431.

199. Kopple JD, Coburn JW. Metabolic studies of low protein diets in uremia: nitrogen and potassium balances. *Medicine* 1973;52:583.

200. Bier DM. Intrinsically difficult problems: the kinetics of body proteins and amino acids in man. *Diabetes Metab Rev* 1989;5:111.

201. Goodship THJ, Mitch WE, Hoerr RA. Adaptation to low-protein diets in renal failure: Leucine turnover and nitrogen balance. *J Am Soc Nephrol* 1990;1:66.

202. Kopple JD, Monteon FJ, Shaib JK. Effect of energy intake on nitrogen metabolism in nondialyzed patients with chronic renal failure. *Kidney Int* 1986;29:734.

203. Food and Agriculture Organization/World Health Organization/United Nations University. *Energy and protein requirements.* Technical Report Series 724. Geneva: World Health Organization, 1985:1.

204. Maroni BJ. Caloric needs of patients on low protein diets. *Clin Appl Nutr* 1992;2:7.

205. Monteon FJ, et al. Energy expenditure in patients with chronic renal failure. *Kidney Int* 1986;30:741.

206. Ikizler TA, Hakim RM. Nutritional requirements of hemodialysis patients. In: Mitch WE, Klahr S, eds. *Handbook of nutrition and the kidney,* 3rd ed. Philadelphia, Lippincott–Raven Publishers, 1998:253.

207. Blumenkrantz MJ, Kopple JD, Gutman RA. Methods for assessing nutritional status of patients with renal failure. *Am J Clin Nutr* 1980;33:1567.

208. Kopple JD. Dietary considerations in patients with advanced chronic renal failure, acute renal failure and transplantation. In: Schrier RW, Gottschalk C, eds. *Diseases of the kidney,* 4th ed. Boston: Little, Brown and Company, 1988:3387.

209. Thunberg BJ, Swamy AP, Cestero RV. Cross-sectional and longitudinal nutritional measurements in maintenance hemodialysis patients. *Am J Clin Nutr* 1981;34:2005.

210. Schneeweiss B, et al. Energy metabolism in acute and chronic renal failure. *Am J Clin Nutr* 1990;52:596.

211. Cahill GF Jr. Starvation in man. *N Engl J Med* 1970;282:668.

212. Hakim RM, Levin N. Malnutrition in hemodialysis patients. *Am J Kidney Dis* 1993;21:125.

213. Nelson EE, et al. Anthropometric norms for the dialysis population. *Am J Kidney Dis* 1990;16:32.

214. Bansal VK, et al. Protein calorie malnutrition and cutaneous energy in hemodialysis maintained patients. *Am J Clin Nutr* 1980;33:1608.

215. Mattern WD, et al. Malnutrition, altered immune function and the risk of infection in maintenance hemodialysis patients. *Am J Kidney Dis* 1982;1:206.

216. Hak LJ, et al. Reversal of skin test anergy during maintenance hemodialysis by protein and calorie supplementation. *Am J Clin Nutr* 1982;36:1089.

217. Bischel M. Albumin turnover in chronically hemodialyzed patients. *Trans Am Soc Intern Organs* 1969;15:298.

218. Allman MA, et al. Body protein of patients undergoing haemodialysis. *Eur J Clin Nutr* 1990;44:123.

219. Bergström J, Alvestrand A, Fürst, P. Plasma and muscle free amino acids in maintenance hemodialysis patients without protein malnutrition. *Kidney Int* 1990;38:108.

220. Marckmann P. Nutritional status and mortality of patients in regular dialysis therapy. *J Intern Med* 1989;226:429.

221. Blagg CR. Importance of nutrition in dialysis patients. *Am J Kidney Dis* 1991;17:458.

222. Marckmann P. Nutritional status of patients on hemodialysis and peritoneal dialysis. *Clin Nephrol* 1988;29:75.

223. Piraino AJ, Firpo J, Powers DV. Prolonged hyperalimentation in catabolic chronic dialysis therapy patients. *J Parenter Enteral Nutr* 1981;5:463.

224. Bellinghieri G, et al. Correlation between increased serum and tissue L-carnitine levels and improved muscle symptoms in hemodialyzed patients. *Am J Clin Nutr* 1983;38:523.

225. Delano BG, Manis JG, Manis T. Iron absorption in experimental uremia. *Nephron* 1977;19:26.

226. Kopple JD, Swendseid ME. Vitamin nutrition in patients undergoing maintenance hemodialysis. *Kidney Int* 1975;7[Suppl 2]:S79.

227. Lawson DH, et al. Iron metabolism in patients with chronic renal failure on regular dialysis treatment. *Clin Sci* 1971;41:345.

228. Mackenzie JC, et al. Erythropoiesis in patients undergoing regular dialysis treatment (R.D.T.) without transfusion. *Proc Eur Dial Transplant Assoc* 1968;5:172.

229. Mahajan SK, et al. Improvement of uremic hypogeusia by zinc: a double-blind study. *Am J Clin Nutr* 1980;33:1517.

230. Sprenger KBG, et al. Improvement of uremic neuropathy and hypogeusia by dialysate zinc supplementation: a double-blind study. *Kidney Int* 1983;24[Suppl 16]:S315.

231. Kopple JD. Dietary considerations in patients with advanced chronic renal failure, acute renal failure, and transplantation. In: Schrier RW, Gottschalk CW, eds. *Diseases of the kidney,* 5th ed. Boston: Little, Brown and Company, 1992:3167.

232. Mitch W, Klahr S, eds. *Nutrition and the kidney,* 2nd ed. Boston: Little, Brown and Company, 1993.

233. Frisancho AR. New standards of weight and body composition by frame size and height for assessment of nutritional status of adults and the elderly. *Am J Clin Nutr* 1984;40:808.

234. *Recommended dietary allowances,* 10th ed. Washington, DC: National Academy Press, 1989.

235. Slomowitz LA, et al. Effect of energy intake on nutritional status in maintenance hemodialysis patients. *Kidney Int* 1989;35:704.

236. Kopple JD. Effect of nutrition on morbidity and mortality in maintenance dialysis patients. *Am J Kidney Dis* 1994;24:1002.

237. Cano N, et al. Perdialytic parenteral nutrition with lipids and amino acids in malnourished hemodialysis patients. *Am J Clin Nutr* 1990;52:726.

238. Piraino AJ, Firpo JJ, Powers, DV. Prolonged hyperalimentation in catabolic chronic dialysis therapy patients. *J Parenter Enteral Nutr* 1981;5:463.

239. Toigo G, et al. Effect of intravenous supplementation of a new essential amino acid formulation in hemodialysis patients. *Kidney Int Suppl* 1989;27:S278.

240. Levy NB. Sexual adjustment to maintenance hemodialysis and renal transplantation: national survey by questionnaire: preliminary report. *Trans Am Soc Artif Organs* 1973;19:138.

241. Abram HS, Hester LR, Epstein BA, et al. Sexual activity and renal failure. Mexico City 1972. *Proceedings of the Fifth International Congress on Nephrology* 1974:3:207.

242. Procci WR, Goldstein DA, Adelstein J, et al. Sexual dysfunction in the male patient with uremia: a reappraisal *Kidney Int* 1981;19:317.

243. Bennett AH, ed. *Impotence: diagnosis and management of erectile dysfunction.* Philadelphia: WB Saunders, 1994.

244. Massry SG, Bellinghieri G. Sexual dysfunction. In: Massry SG, Glassock RJ, eds. *Massry and Glassock's textbook of nephrology.* Baltimore: Williams & Wilkins, 1995:1416.

245. Hagen C, Olgaard K, McNeilly AS, et al. Prolactin and the pituitary–gonadal axis in male uraemic patients on regular dialysis. *Acta Endocrinol* 1976;82:29.

246. Ramirez G, O'Neil WM Jr, Bloomer HA, et al. Abnormalities in the regulation of prolactin in patients with chronic renal failure. *J Clin Endocrinol Metab* 1977;45:658.

247. Lim VS, Kathpalia SC, Frohman LA. Hyperprolactinemia and impaired pituitary response to suppression and stimulation in chronic

renal failure: reversal after transplantation. *J Clin Endocrinol Metab* 1979;48:101.

248. Gomez F, de la Cueva R, Wauters J-P, et al. Endocrine abnormalities in patients undergoing long-term hemodialysis. *Am J Med* 1980;68:522.

249. Ferraris JR, et al. Hormonal profile in pubertal females with chronic renal failure: before and under hemodialysis and after renal transplantation. *Acta Endocrinol* 1987;115:289.

250. Cowden EA, Ratcliffe WA, Ratcliffe JG, et al. Hypothalamic–pituitary function in uraemia. *Acta Endocrinol* 1981;98:488.

251. Peces R, et al. Prolactin in chronic renal failure, haemodialysis, and transplant patients. *Proc Eur Dial Transplant Assoc* 1979;16:700.

252. Isaac R, et al. Effect of parathyroid hormone on plasma prolactin in man. *J Clin Endocrinol Metab* 1978;47:18.

253. Schaefer RM, et al. Improved sexual function in hemodialysis patients on recombinant erythropoietin: a possible role of prolactin. *Clin Nephrol* 1989;31:1.

254. Ramirez G, O'Neil W, Jubiz W, et al. Thyroid dysfunction in uremia: evidence for thyroid and hypophyseal abnormalities. *Am Intern Med* 1976;84:672.

255. Ramirez G, et al. Bromocriptine and the hypothalamic hypophyseal function in patients with chronic renal failure on chronic hemodialysis. *Am J Kidney Dis* 1985;6:111.

256. Guevara A, et al. Serum gonadotropin and testosterone levels in uremic males undergoing intermittent dialysis. *Medicine* 1969;18:1062.

257. Chen JC, et al. Pituitary-Leydig cell function in uremic males. *J Clin Endocrinol Metab* 1970;31:14.

258. Lim VS, Fang S. Gonadal dysfunction in uremic men: a study of the hypothalamo–pituitary–testicular axis before and after renal transplantation. *Am J Med* 1975;58:655.

259. Holdsworth S, Atkins R, de Kretser D. The pituitary–testicular axis in men with chronic renal failure. *N Engl J Med* 1977;296:1245.

260. Czekalski S, et al. Serum concentration of pituitary thyroid and gonadal hormone in nondialyzed and dialyzed males with chronic renal failure. *Proc Eur Dial Transplant Assoc* 1978;15:599.

261. Semple CG, et al. The pituitary–testicular axis of uremic subjects on hemodialysis and continuous ambulatory peritoneal dialysis. *Acta Endocrinol* 1982;101:464.

262. Means AR, Vaitukatis J. Peptide hormone "receptors": specific binding of ^{3}H-FSF to testis. *Endocrinology* 1972;90:39.

263. de Kretser DM, Burger HG, Hudson B. The relationship between germinal cells and serum FSH in males with infertility. *J Clin Endocrinol Metab* 1974;38:787.

264. Phadke AG, MacKinnon KJ, Dossetor JB. Male fertility in uremia: restoration after renal allografts. *Can Med Assoc J* 1970;102:607.

265. de Kretser DM, Atkins RC, Hudson B, et al. Disordered spermatogenesis in patients with chronic renal failure and undergoing maintenance hemodialysis. *Aust NZ J Med* 1974;4:178.

266. de Jong FH. Inhibin. *Physiol Rev* 1988;68:555.

267. Mitchell R, et al. Elevated serum immunoreactive inhibin levels in peripubertal boys with chronic renal failure: Cooperative Study Group on Pubertal Development in Chronic Renal Failure. *Clin Endocrinol* 1993;39:27.

268. Distiller LA, et al. Pituitary-gonadal function in chronic renal failure: the effect of luteinizing hormone-releasing hormone and the influence of dialysis. *Metabolism* 1975;24:711.

269. Krolner B. Serum levels of testosterone and luteinizing hormone in patients with chronic renal disease. *Acta Med Scand* 1979;205:623.

270. de Kretser DM, Atkins RC, Paulsen CA. Role of the kidney in the metabolism of luteinizing hormone. *J Endocrinol* 1973;58:425.

271. Schaefer F, et al. Immunoreactive and bioactive luteinizing hormone in pubertal patients with chronic renal failure: Cooperative Study Group in Pubertal Development in Chronic Renal Failure. *Kidney Int* 1994;45:1465.

272. Veldhuis JD, et al. Evidence for attenuation of hypothalamic gonadotropin-releasing hormone (GnRH) impulse strength with preservation of GnRH pulse frequency in men with chronic renal failure. *J Clin Endocrinol Metab* 1993;76:648.

273. Stewart-Bently M, Gans D, Horton R. Regulation of gonadal function in uremia. *Metabolism* 1974;23:1065.

274. Oertel PJ, et al. The hypothalamo–pituitary–gonadal axis in prepubertal children with chronic renal failure (CRF). *Kidney Int* 1983;24:S34.

275. Sawin CT, Longcope C, Schmitt GW, et al. Blood levels of gonadotropins and gonadal hormones in gynecomastia associated with chronic hemodialysis. *J Clin Endocrinol Metab* 1973;36:988.

276. Carter JN, et al. Prolactin-secreting tumors and hypogonadism in 22 men. *N Engl J Med* 1978;299:847.

277. Massry SG, Goldstein DA, Procci WR, et al. Impotence in patients with uremia: a possible role for parathyroid hormone. *Nephron* 1977;19:305.

278. Akmal M, Goldstein DA, Kletzky OA, et al. Hyperparathyroidism and the hypotestosteronemia of acute renal failure. *Am J Nephrol* 1988;8:166.

279. Lim VS, Henriquez C, Sievertsen G, et al. Ovarian function in chronic renal failure: evidence suggesting hypothalamic anovulation. *Ann Intern Med* 1980;93:21.

280. Zingraff J, et al. Pituitary and ovarian dysfunctions in women on haemodialysis. *Nephron* 1982;30:149.

281. Ginsburg ES, Owen WF Jr. Reproductive endocrinology and pregnancy in woman on hemodialysis. *Semin Dial* 1993;6:105.

282. Campese VM, et al. Mechanisms of autonomic nervous system dysfunction in uremia. *Kidney Int* 1981;20:246.

283. Campese VM, et al. Autonomic nervous system dysfunction and impotence in uremia. *Am J Nephrol* 1982;2:140.

284. Kaufman JM, Hatzichristou DG, Mulhall JP, et al. Impotence of chronic renal failure. A study of the hemodynamic pathophysiology. *J Urol* 1994;151:612.

285. Barton CH, Mirahmadi MK. Administration on the pituitary testiculas axis and end stage renal failure. *Nephron* 1982;31:61.

286. Lawrence IG, et al. Correcting impotence in the male dialysis patient: experience with testosterone replacement and vacuum tumescence therapy. *Am J Kid Dis* 1998;31:313.

287. Lawrence IG, Price DE, Howlett TA, et al. Erythropoietin and sexual dysfunction. *Nephrol Dial Transplant* 1997;12:741.

288. Goldstein I, Lue TF, Padma-Nathan H, et al. Oral sildenafil in the treatment of erectile dysfunction. *N Engl J Med* 338:1397–1404, 1998.

289. Roses SE, et al. Preliminary observations of sildenfil treatment of erectile dysfunction in dialysis patients. *Am J Kidney Dis* 2001;37:134.

290. Stolar MW, Amburn K, Baumann G. Plasma "big" and "big big" growth hormone (GH) in man: an oligometric series composed of structurally diverse GH monomers. *J Clin Endocrinol Metab* 1984;59:212.

291. Leung DW, et al. Growth hormone receptor and serum binding protein: purification, cloning and expression. *Nature* 1987;330:537.

292. Taylor AL, Lipman RL, Salam A, et al. Hepatic clearance of human growth hormone. *J Clin Endocrinol Metab* 1972;34:395.

293. Johnson V, Mack T. Renal extraction filtration, absorption and catabolism of growth hormone. *Am J Physiol* 1977;233:F185.

294. Haffner D, et al. Metabolic clearance of recombinant human growth hormone in health and chronic renal failure. *J Clin Invest* 1993;93:1163.

295. Klapper DG, Svoboda ME, Van Wyk JJ. Sequence analysis of somatomedin-C: confirmation of identity with insulin-like growth factor I. *Endocrinology* 1983;112:2215.

296. Li CH, et al. Total synthesis of insulin-like growth factor I (somatomedin-C). *Proc Natl Acad Sci* 1983;80:2216.

297. Berelowitz M, et al. Somatomedin-C mediates growth hormone negative feedback by effects on both the hypothalamus and the pituitary. *Science* 1981;212:1279.

298. Samaan NA, Freeman RM. Growth hormone levels in severe renal failure. *Metabolism* 1970;19:102.

299. Wright AD, Lowy D, Fraser TR. Serum growth hormone and glucose intolerance in renal failure. *Lancet* 1968;2:798.

300. Pimpston BL, et al. Disappearance rates of plasma growth hormone after intravenous somatostatin in renal and liver disease. *J Clin Endocrinol Metab* 1975;41:392.

301. Ramirez G, O'Neill WA, Bloomer HA, et al. Abnormalities in the regulation of growth hormone in chronic renal failure. *Arch Intern Med* 1978;138:267.

302. Ramirez G, et al. Response to growth hormone-releasing hormone in adult renal failure patients on hemodialysis. *Metabolism* 1990;39:764.

303. Kokot F, Wiecek A, Grzeszczak W. Role of endogenous opioids in the pathogenesis of endocrine abnormalities in chronic renal failure. *Semin Dial* 1988;1:213.

304. Kokot F, Wiecek A, Grzeszczak W, et al. Influence of erythropoietin treatment on the function of the pituitary–adrenal axis and somatotropin secretion in hemodialysis patients. *Clin Nephrol* 1990;33: 241.

305. Ramirez G, et al. The effects of corticotropin and growth hormone releasing hormones on their respective secretory axis in chronic hemodialysis patients before and after correction of anemia with recombinant human erythropoietin. *J Clin Endocrinol Metab* 1994;78:63.

306. Schaefer F, et al. Pubertal growth in chronic renal failure. *Pediatr Res* 1990;28:5.

307. Goldberg AC, et al. Uremia reduces insulin-like growth factor I, increases insulin growth factor II and modifies their serum protein binding. *J Clin Endocrinol Metab* 1982;55:1040.

308. Euberg G, Hall K. Immunoreactive IGF-II in serum of healthy subjects and patients with growth hormone disturbance and uremia. *Acta Endocrinol* 1984;107:164.

309. Blum WF, et al. Growth hormone resistance and inhibition of somatomedin activity by excess of insulin-like growth factor binding protein in uremia. *Pediatr Nephrol* 1991;5:539.

310. Powell DR, et al. Insulin-like growth factor-binding protein-6 levels are elevated in serum of children with chronic renal failure. *J Clin Endocrinol Metab* 1997;82:2978.

311. Powell DR, et al. Serum concentrations of insulin-like growth factor (IGF)-1, IGF-2 and unsaturated somatomedin carrier proteins in children with chronic renal failure. *Am J Kidney Dis* 1987;4:287.

312. Phillips LS, et al. Somatomedin activity and inorganic sulfate in children undergoing hemodialysis. *J Clin Endocrinol Metab* 1978;46: 165.

313. Phillips LS, Kopple JD. Circulating somatomedin activity and sulfate levels in adults with normal and impaired kidney function. *Metabolism* 1981;30:1091.

314. Ding H, Gao X-L, Hirschberg R, et al. Impaired actions of insulin-like growth factor 1 on protein synthesis and degradation in skeletal muscle of rats with chronic renal failure: evidence for a postreceptor defect. *J Clin Invest* 1996;97:1064.

315. Fouque D, Peng SC, Kopple JD. Impaired metabolic response to recombinant insulin-like growth factor I in dialysis patients. *Kidney Int* 1995;47:876.

316. Fine RN, Kohaut EC, Brown D, et al. Growth after recombinant human growth hormone treatment in children with chronic renal failure: report of a multicenter randomized double-blind placebo-controlled study. *J Pediatr* 1994;124:374.

317. Wallace EZ, et al. Pituitary-adrenocortical function in chronic renal failure: studies of episodic secretion of cortisol and dexamethasone suppressibility. *J Clin Endocrinol Metab* 1980;50:46.

318. Zager PG, et al. Low dose adrenocorticotropin infusion in continuous ambulatory peritoneal dialysis patients. *J Clin Endocrinol Metab* 1985;61:1205.

319. Rodger RSC, et al. Anterior pituitary dysfunction in patients with chronic renal failure treated by hemodialysis or continuous ambulatory peritoneal dialysis. *Nephron* 1986;43:169.

320. Luger A, et al. Abnormalities in the hypothalamic–pituitary–adrenocortical axis in patients with chronic renal failure. *Am J Kidney Dis* 1987;9:51.

321. Siamopoulos KC, et al. Ovine corticotropin-releasing hormone stimulation test in patients with chronic renal failure: pharmacokinetic properties, and plasma adrenocorticotropic hormone, and serum cortisol responses. *Horm Res* 1988;30:17.

322. Siamopoulos KC, et al. Pituitary adrenal responsiveness to corticotropin releasing hormone in chronic uremic patients. *Peritoneal Dial Int* 1990;10:153.

323. Ramirez G. Abnormalities in the hypothalamic–hypophyseal axis in patients with chronic renal failure. *Semin Dial* 1994;7:138.

324. Ramirez G, Brueggemeyer C, Ganguly A. Counterregulatory hormonal response to insulin-induced hypoglycemia in patients on chronic hemodialysis. *Nephron* 1988;49:231.

325. Bacon GE, et al. Prolonged serum halflife of cortisol in renal failure. *Johns Hopkins Med J* 1973;132:127.

326. Barbour GL, Sevier BR. Adrenal responsiveness in chronic hemodialysis. *N Engl J Med* 1974;290:1258.

327. Ramirez G, Gomez-Sanchez C, Meikle WA, et al. Evaluation of the hypothalamic hypophyseal adrenal axis in patients receiving long-term hemodialysis. *Arch Intern Med* 1982;142:1449.

328. Zager PG, Fry HJ, Gredes BG. Plasma 18-hydroxycorticosterone during continuous ambulatory peritoneal dialysis. *J Lab Clin Med* 1983;102:604.

329. McDonald WJ, et al. Adrenocorticotropin–cortisol axis abnormalities in hemodialysis patients. *J Clin Endocrinol Metab* 1979;48:92.

330. Rosman PM, et al. Cortisol binding in uremic plasma I: absence of abnormal cortisol binding to corticosteroid-binding globulin. *Nephron* 1984;37:160.

331. Ivic MA, Stefanovic V. Does high cortisol in uremic patients influence their glucagon levels? *Exp Clin Endocrinol* 1988;91:362.

332. Carlstrom K, Posette A, Stege R, et al. Serum hormone levels in men with end-stage renal disease. *Scand J Urol Nephrol* 1990;24:75.

333. Ferraris JR, Ramirez JA, Goldberg V, et al. Glucocorticoids and adrenal androgens in children with end-stage renal disease. *Acta Endocrinol* 1991;124:245.

334. Betts PR, et al. Serum cortisol concentrations in children with chronic renal insufficiency. *Arch Dis Child* 1975;50:3.

335. Feldman HA, Singer I. Endocrinology and metabolism in uremia and dialysis: a clinical study. *Medicine* 1974;54:345.

336. Wallace EZ, et al. Pituitary-adrenocortical function in chronic renal failure: studies of episodic secretion of cortisol and dexamethasone suppressibility. *J Clin Endocrinol Metab* 1980;50:46.

337. Akmad M, Manzier AD. Simplified assessment of pituitary–adrenal axis in a stable group of chronic hemodialysis patients. *Trans Am Soc Artif Intern Organs* 1977;23:703.

338. Rosman PM, et al. Pituitary-adrenocortical function in chronic renal failure: blunted suppression and early escape of plasma cortisol levels after intravenous dexamethasone. *J Clin Endocrinol Metab* 1982;54:528.

339. Rauh W, et al. Vasoactive hormones in children with chronic renal failure. *Kidney Int* 1983;15:S27.

340. Ardaillou R, Pruszynski W, Benmansour M. Secretion and catabolism of antidiuretic hormone in renal failure. *Contrib Nephrol* 1986;50: 46.

341. Fasanella d'Amore T, et al. Response of plasma vasopressin to change in extracellular volume and/or plasma osmolality in patients on maintenance hemodialysis. *Clin Nephrol* 1985;23:299.

342. Kokot F, et al. Water immersion induced alterations of plasma atrial natriuretic peptide level and its relationship to the renin–angiotensin–aldosterone system and vasopressin secretion in acute and chronic renal failure. *Clin Nephrol* 1989;31:247.

343. Zabetakis PM, et al. Increased levels of plasma renin–aldosterone, catecholamines and vasopressin in chronic ambulatory peritoneal dialysis patients. *Clin Nephrol* 1987;28:147.

344. Benmansour M, et al. Metabolic clearance rate of immunoreactive vasopressin in man. *Eur J Clin Invest* 1982;12:475.

345. Argent NB, Wilkinson R, Baylis PH. Metabolic clearance rate of arginine vasopressin in severe chronic renal failure. *Clin Sci* 1992;83: 583.

346. Javadi MH, et al. Regulation of plasma arginine vasopressin in patients with chronic renal failure maintained on hemodialysis. *Am J Nephrol* 1986;6:175.

347. Shimamoto R, Watari J, Migahara M. A study of plasma vasopressin in patients undergoing chronic hemodialysis. *J Clin Endocrinol Metab* 1977;45:714.

348. Os I, Nordby G, Lyngdal PT, et al. Plasma vasopressin, catecholamines and atrial natriuretic factor during hemodialysis and sequential ultrafiltration. *Scand J Urol Nephrol* 1993;27:93.

349. Pruszczynski W, et al. Massive plasma arginine vasopressin (AVP) removal during hemofiltration stimulates AVP secretion in humans. *J Clin Endocrinol Metab* 1987;64:383.

350. Vaziri ND, Skousky R, Warner A. Effect of isoosmolar volume reduction during hemofiltration on plasma antidiuretic hormone in patients with chronic renal failure. *Int J Artif Organs* 1980;3:322.

351. Hammer M, Olgaard K, Madsen S. The inability of angiotensin II infusion to raise plasma vasopressin levels in haemodialysis patients. *Acta Endocrinol (Copenh)* 1980;95:422.

352. Kaptein EM, et al. The thyroid in end-stage renal disease. *Medicine* 1988;67:187.

353. Kaptein EM. Thyroid hormone metabolism. In: Massry SG, Glassock RJ, eds. *Massry and Glassock's textbook of nephrology*, 3rd ed. Baltimore: Williams & Wilkins, 1995:1406.

354. Silverberg DS, et al. Effects of chronic hemodialysis on thyroid function in chronic renal failure. *Can Med Assoc J* 1973;189:282.

355. Gonzalez-Barcens D, et al. Response to thyrotropin releasing hormone in patients with renal failure and after infusion in normal man. *J Clin Endocrinol Metab* 1973;36:117.

356. Ramirez G, et al. Thyroid abnormalities in renal failure. *Am Intern Med* 1973;79:500.

357. Ramirez G, O'Neil W, Jubiz W, et al. Thyroid dysfunction in uremia: evidence for thyroid and hypophyseal abnormalities. *Am Intern Med* 1976;84:672.

358. Bartalena L, et al. Lack of nocturnal serum thyrotropin (TSH) surge in patients with chronic renal failure undergoing regular maintenance hemofiltration: a case of central hypothyroidism. *Clin Nephrol* 1990;34:30.

359. Pasqualini T, et al. Evidence of hypothalamic-pituitary thyroid abnormalities in children with end-stage renal disease. *J Pediatr* 1991;118:873.

360. Giordano C, et al. Thyroid status and nephron loss—a study in patients with chronic renal failure, end-stage renal disease and/or on hemodialysis. *Int J Artif Organs* 1984;7:119.

361. Williams GR, Franklyn JA, Newberger JM, et al. Thyroid hormone receptor expression in the sick euthyroid syndrome. *Lancet* 1989;2:1477.

362. Makato I, et al. Serum substances that interfere with thyroid hormone assays in patients with chronic renal failure. *Clin Endocrinol* 1998;48:734.

363. Burke JR, et al. Hypothyroidism in children with cystinosis. *Arch Dis Child* 1978;53:947.

364. Tang WW, Kaptein EM, Massry SG. Diagnosis of hypothyroidism in patients with end-stage renal disease. *Am J Nephrol* 1987;7:192.

365. Roth SL, Marshal RB. Pathology and structure of the human parathyroid glands in chronic renal failure. *Arch Intern Med* 1969;124:397.

366. Katz AI, Hampers CL, Merrill JP. Secondary hyperparathyroidism and renal osteodystrophy in chronic renal failure. *Medicine* 1969;48:33.

367. Katz AD, Kaplan L. Parathyroidectomy for hyperplasia in renal disease. *Arch Surg* 1973;107:51.

368. Fukagawa M. Cell biology of parathyroid hyperplasia in uremia. *Am J Med. Sci* 1999;317:377.

369. Malmaeus J, Glimelius L, Johansson G, et al. Parathyroid pathology in hyperparathyroidism secondary to chronic renal failure. *Scand J Urol Nephrol* 1984;18:157.

370. Fukuda N, et al. Decreased 1,25-dihydroxyvitamin D_3 receptor density is associated with a more severe form of parathyroid hyperplasia in chronic uremic patients. *J Clin Invest* 1993;92:1436.

371. Kifor O, et al. Reduced immunostaining for the extracellular Ca^{2+}-sensing receptor in primary and uremic secondary hyperparathyroidism. *J Clin Endocrinol Metab* 1996;81:1596.

372. Tominaga Y, et al. DNA ploidy pattern of parathyroid parenchymal cells in renal secondary hyperparathyroidism with relapse. *Anal Cell Pathol* 1991;3:325.

373. Tominaga Y, et al. Recurrent renal hyperparathyroidism and DNA analysis of autografted parathyroid tissue. *World J Surg* 1992;16:595.

374. Arnold A, et al. Monoclonality of parathyroid tumors in chronic renal failure and in primary parathyroid hyperplasia. *J Clin Invest* 1995;95:2047.

375. Farnebo F, et al. Differential loss of heterozygosity in familial, sporadic, and uremic hyperparathyroidism. *Hum Genet* 1997;99:342.

376. Heppner C, et al. Somatic mutation of the MEN1 gene in parathyroid tumors. *Nat Genet* 1997;16:375.

377. Falchetti A, et al. Progression of uremic hyperparathyroidism involves allelic loss on chromosome 11. *J Clin Endocrinol Metab* 1993;76:139.

378. Bricker NS, et al. Calcium, phosphorus and bone in renal disease and transplantation. *Arch Intern Med* 1969;123:543.

379. Slatopolsky E, et al. On the prevention of secondary hyperparathyroidism in experimental chronic renal disease using "proportional reduction" of dietary phosphorus intake. *Kidney Int* 1972;2:147.

380. Llach F, et al. Skeletal resistance to endogenous parathyroid hormone in patients with early renal failure: a possible cause for secondary hyperparathyroidism. *J Clin Endocrinol Metab* 1975;41:339.

381. Massry SG, et al. Divalent ion metabolism in patients with acute renal failure: studies on mechanism of hypocalcemia. *Kidney Int* 1974;5:437.

382. Massry SG, et al. Skeletal resistance to parathyroid hormone in renal failure: study in 105 human subjects. *Ann Intern Med* 1973;78:357.

383. Massry SG, et al. Role of uremia in the skeletal resistance to the calcemic action of parathyroid hormone. *Miner Electrolyte Metab* 1978;1:172.

384. Massry SG, et al. Skeletal resistance to the calcemic action of PTH in uremia: role in 1,25(OH)$_2$D$_3$. *Kidney Int* 1976;9:467.

385. Massry SG, et al. Restoration of skeletal resistance to PTH in uremia by vitamin D metabolites: evidence for synergism between 1,25(OH)$_2$D$_3$ and 24,25(OH)$_2$D$_3$. *J Lab Clin Med* 1979;94:152.

386. Llach F, Massry SG. On the mechanism of secondary hyperparathyroidism in moderate renal insufficiency. *J Clin Endocrinol Metab* 1985;61:601.

387. Massry SG. Divalent ion metabolism and renal osteodystrophy. In: Massry SG, Glassock RJ, eds. *Massry and Glassock's textbook of nephrology*, 3rd ed. Baltimore: Williams & Wilkins, 1995:1441.

388. Portale AA, Booth BE, Halldran BP, et al. Effect of dietary phosphorus on circulating concentrations of 1,25-dihydroxyvitamin D and immunoreactive parathyroid hormone in children with moderate renal insufficiency. *J Clin Invest* 1984;73:1580.

389. Brent GA, et al. Relationship between the concentration and rate of change of calcium and serum intact parathyroid hormone levels in normal humans. *J Clin Endocrinol Metab* 1988;67:944.

390. Wernerson A, Widholm SM, Svensson O, et al. Parathyroid cell number and size in hypocalcemic young rats. *APMIS* 1991;99:1096.

391. Slatopolsky E, et al. Phosphorus prevents parathyroid gland growth. High phosphorus directly stimulates PTH secretion in vitro. *J Clin Invest* 1996;97:34.

392. Naveh-Many T, et al. Regulation of 1,25-dihydroxyvitamin D_3 receptor gene expression by 1,25-dihydroxyvitamin D_3 in the parathyroid in vivo. *J Clin Invest* 1990;86:1968.

393. DeMay MB, Kiernan MS, DeLuca HF, et al. Sequences in the human parathyroid hormone gene that bind the 1,25-dihydroxyvitamin D_3 receptor and mediate transcriptional repression in response to 1,25-dihydroxyvitamin D_3. *Proc Natl Acad Sci USA* 1992;89:8097.

394. Silver J, Russell J, Sherwood KM. Regulation by vitamin D metabolites of messenger ribonucleic acid for preproparathyroid hormone in isolated bovine parathyroid cells. *Proc Natl Acad Sci USA* 1985;82:4270.

395. Silver J, et al. Regulation by vitamin D metabolites of parathyroid hormone gene transcription in vivo in the rat. *J Clin Invest* 1986;78:1296.

396. Fukagawa M, et al. Regulation of parathyroid hormone synthesis in chronic renal failure in rats. *Kidney Int* 1991;39:874.

397. Shvil Y, Naveh-Many T, Barach P, et al. Regulation of parathyroid cell gene expression in experimental uremia. *J Am Soc Nephrol* 1990;1:99.

398. Reichel H, et al. Intermittent versus continuous administration of 1,25-dihydroxyvitamin D_3 in experimental renal hyperparathyroidism. *Kidney Int* 1993;44:1259.

399. Cantley LK, Russell J, Letteri D, et al. 1,25-dihydroxyvitamin D suppresses parathyroid hormone secretion from bovine parathyroid cells in tissue culture. *Endocrinology* 1985;117:2114.

400. Kramer R, Bolivar I, Goltzman D, et al. Influence of calcium and 1,25-dihydroxycholecalciferol on proliferation and proto-oncogene expression in primary cultures of bovine parathyroid cells. *Endocrinology* 1989;125:935.

401. Oldham SB, et al. The acute effects of 1,25-dihydroxycholecalciferol on serum immunoreactive parathyroid hormone in the dog. *Endocrinology* 1979;104:248.

402. Madsen S, Olgaard K, Ladefoged J. Suppressive effect of 1,25-dihydroxyvitamin D_3 on circulating parathyroid hormone in acute renal failure. *J Clin Endocrinol Metab* 1981;53:823.

403. Felsenfeld AJ, Llach F. Parathyroid gland function in chronic renal failure. *Kidney Int* 1993;43:771.

404. Brown EM, et al. Dispersed cells prepared from human parathyroid glands: distinct calcium sensitivity of adenomas vs. primary hyperplasia. *J Clin Endocrinol Metab* 1978;46:267.

405. Brown EM, et al. Abnormal regulation of parathyroid hormone release by calcium in secondary hyperparathyroidism due to chronic renal failure. *J Clin Endocrinol Metab* 1982;54:172.

406. Brown EM, et al. Cloning and characterization of an extracellular Ca2+-sensing receptor from bovine parathyroid. *Nature* 1993;366:575.

407. Coburn JW, et al. Calcium sensing and calcimimetic agents. *Kidney Int* 1999;56:S52.

408. Lopez-Hilker S, et al. Hypocalcemia may not be essential for the development of secondary hyperparathyroidism in chronic renal failure. *J Clin Invest* 1986;78:1097.

409. Healy M, et al. Effects of long-term therapy with 1,25(OH)$_2$D$_3$ in patients with moderate renal failure. *Arch Intern Med* 1980;140:1030.

410. Baker LRI, et al. 1,25(OH)$_2$D$_3$ administration in moderate renal failure: a prospective double blind trial. *Kidney Int* 1989;35:661.

411. Arnaud CD. Hyperparathyroidism and renal failure. *Kidney Int* 1973;4:89.

412. Berson SA, Yalow RS. Parathyroid hormone in plasma in adenomatous hyperparathyroidism, uremia and bronchogenic carcinoma. *Science* 1966;154:907.

413. Mennes P, Rosenbaum R, Martin K, et al. Hypomagnesemia and impaired parathyroid hormone secretion in chronic renal disease. *Ann Intern Med* 1978;88:206.

414. Coburn JW, Alfrey AC. Aluminum toxicity. In: Massry SG, Glassock RJ, eds. *Massry and Glassock's textbook of nephrology*, 3rd ed. Baltimore: Williams & Wilkins, 1995:1303.

415. Sherrard DJ, et al. The spectrum of bone disease in end-stage renal failure: an evolving disorder. *Kidney Int* 1993;43:436.

416. Hercz G, et al. Aplastic osteodystrophy without aluminum: the role of suppressed parathyroid function. *Kidney Int* 1993;44:860.

417. Andress DL, et al. Bone histomorphometry and renal osteodystrophy in diabetes mellitus. *J Bone Miner Res* 1987;2(6):525.

418. Nussbaum SR, et al. A highly sensitive two site immunoradiometric assay of parathyroid (PTH) and its clinical utility in evaluating patients with hypercalcemia. *Clin Chem* 1987;33:1364.

419. Kao PC, et al. Clinical performance of parathyroid hormone immunometric assays. *Mayo Clin Proc* 1992;67:637.

420. Akmal M, et al. Role of uremia, brain calcium and parathyroid hormone in changes in electroencephalogram in chronic renal failure. *Am J Physiol* 1984;246:F575.

421. Arieff AI, Massry SG. Calcium metabolism of brain in acute renal failure: effects of uremia, hemodialysis and parathyroid hormone. *J Clin Invest* 1974;53:387.

422. Goldstein DA, et al. The relationship between the abnormalities in electroencephalogram and blood levels of parathyroid hormone in dialysis patients. *J Clin Endocrinol Metab* 1980;51:130.

423. Goldstein DA, Massry SG. Effect of parathyroid hormone administration and its withdrawal on brain calcium and electroencephalogram. *Miner Electrolyte Metab* 1978;1:84.

424. Guisado R, Arieff AI, Massry SG. Changes in the electroencephalogram in acute uremia: effects of parathyroid hormone and brain electrolytes. *J Clin Invest* 1975;55:738.

425. Islam A, Smogorzewski M, Massry SG. Effect of chronic renal failure and parathyroid hormone on phospholipid content of brain synaptosomes. *Am J Physiol* 1989;256:F705.

426. Smogorzewski M, Campese VM, Massry SG. Abnormal norepinephrine uptake and release in brain synaptosomes in chronic renal failure. *Kidney Int* 1989;36:458.

427. Smogorzewski M, et al. Chronic parathyroid hormone excess in vivo increases resting levels of cytosolic calcium in brain synaptosomes: studies in presence and absence of chronic renal failure. *J Am Soc Nephrol* 1991;1:1162.

428. Islam A, Smogorzewski M, Zayed MA, et al. Effect of chronic renal failure with and without secondary hyperparathyroidism on the activities of synaptosomal tyrosine hydroxylase and monoamine oxidase. *Nephron* 1992;61:33.

429. Ni Z, Smogorzewski M, Massry SG. Derangements in acetylcholine metabolism in brain synaptosomes in chronic renal failure. *Kidney Int* 1993;44:630.

430. Akmal M, Massry SG. Role of PTH in the prolonged motor nerve conduction velocity of chronic renal failure. *Proc Exp Biol Med* 1990;195:202.

431. Goldstein DA, Chui LA, Massry SG. Effect of parathyroid hormone and uremia on peripheral nerve calcium and motor nerve conduction velocity. *J Clin Invest* 1978;62:88.

432. Collins J, Massry SG, Campese VM. Parathyroid hormone and the altered vascular response to norepinephrine in uremia. *Am J Nephrol* 1985;5:110.

433. Iseki K, Massry SG, Campese VM. Evidence for a role of PTH in the reduced pressor response to norepinephrine in chronic renal failure. *Kidney Int* 1985;28:11.

434. Saglikes Y, et al. Effect of PTH on blood pressure response to vasoconstrictor agonists. *Am J Physiol* 1985;248:F674.

435. Baczynski R, et al. Effect of parathyroid hormone on myocardial energy metabolism in the rat. *Kidney Int* 1985;27:718.

436. Bogin E, Massry SG, Harary I. Effect of parathyroid hormone on heart cells. *J Clin Invest* 1981;67:1215.

437. El-Belbessi S, et al. Effect of chronic renal failure on heart: role of secondary hyperparathyroidism. *Am J Nephrol* 1986;6:369.

438. Smogorzewski M, et al. Fatty acid oxidation in the myocardium: effect of parathyroid hormone and CRF. *Kidney Int* 1988;34:797.

439. Zhang Y-B, Smogorzewski M, Massry SG. Altered cytosolic calcium homeostasis in rat cardiac myocytes in CRF. *Kidney Int* 1994;45:1113.

440. Baczynski R, et al. Effect of parathyroid hormone on energy metabolism of skeletal muscle. *Kidney Int* 1985;28:722.

441. Perna AF, Smogorzewski M, Massry SG. Verapamil reverses PTH- or CRF-induced abnormal fatty acid oxidation in muscle. *Kidney Int* 1985;34:744.

442. Akmal M, et al. Erythrocyte survival in chronic renal failure: role of secondary hyperparathyroidism. *J Clin Invest* 1985;76:1969.

443. Bogin E, et al. Effects of parathyroid hormone on osmotic fragility of human erythrocytes. *J Clin Invest* 1982;69:1017.

444. Brautbar N, et al. Calcium, parathyroid hormone and phospholipid turnover of human red blood cells. *Miner Electrolyte Metab* 1985;11:111.

445. Meytes D, et al. Effect of parathyroid hormone on erythropoiesis. *J Clin Invest* 1981;67:1263.

446. Saltissi D, Carter GD. Association of secondary hyperparathyroidism with red cell survival in chronic hemodialysis patients. *Clin Sci* 1985;68:29.

447. Alexiewicz JM, et al. Impaired phagocytosis in dialysis patients: studies on mechanisms. *Am J Nephrol* 1991;11:102.

448. Doherty CC. Effect of parathyroid hormone on random migration of human polymorphonuclear leukocytes. *Am J Nephrol* 1988;8:212.

449. Chervu I, Kiersztejn M, Alexiewicz JM. Impaired phagocytosis in chronic renal failure is mediated by secondary hyperparathyroidism. *Kidney Int* 1992;41:1501.

450. Kiersztejn M, Smogorzewski M, Thanakitcharu P. Decreased O$_2$ consumption by polymorphonuclear leukocytes from humans and rats with CRF: role of secondary hyperparathyroidism. *Kidney Int* 1992;42:602.

451. Alexiewicz J, et al. Effect of treatment of hemodialysis patient with nifedipine on metabolism and function of polymorphonuclear leucocytes. *Am J Kidney Dis* 1995;25:440.

452. Hörl WH, Heray-Weker M, Mai B, et al. Verapamil reverses abnormal [Ca^{2+}]i and carbohydrate metabolism in PMNL of dialysis patients. *Kidney Int* 1995;47:1741.

453. Klinger M, et al. Effects of parathyroid hormone on human T cell activation. *Kidney Int* 1990;37:1543.

454. Alexiewicz JM, et al. Evidence for impaired T cell function in hemodialysis patients. A potential role for secondary hyperparathyroidism. *Am J Nephrol* 1990;10:495.

455. Alexiewicz JM, et al. Parathyroid hormone inhibits B cell proliferation: implications in chronic renal failure. *J Am Soc Nephrol* 1990;1:236.

456. Gaciong Z, et al. Inhibition of immunoglobulin production by parathyroid hormone: implications in chronic renal failure. *Kidney Int* 1991;40:96.

457. Massry SG, et al. Secondary hyperparathyroidism and the immune system in chronic renal failure. *Semin Nephrol* 1991;11:186.

458. Urena P, et al. Parathyroid hormone (PTH)/PTH-related peptide (PTHrP) receptor mRNA are widely distributed in rat tissues. *Endocrinology* 1993;133:617.

459. Tian J, Smogorzewski M, Kedes L, et al. Parathyroid hormone-related protein receptor messenger RNA is present in many tissues beside the kidney. *Am J Nephrol* 1993;13:210.

460. Urena P, et al. The renal PTH/PTHrP receptor is down-regulated in rats with chronic renal failure. *Kidney Int* 1994;45:605.

461. Tian J, Smogorzewski M, Kedes L, et al. PTH-PTHrP receptor mRNA is down-regulated in chronic renal failure. *Am J Nephrol* 1994;14:41.

462. Smogorzewski M, Tian J, et al. Down-regulation of PTH-PTHrP receptor of heart in CRF: role of [Ca^{2+}]i. *Kidney Int* 1995;47:1182.

463. Ponchon G, Kenna AL, DeLuca HF. Activation of vitamin D by the liver. *J Clin Invest* 1969;48:2032.

464. Horsting M, DeLuca HF. In vitro production of 25-hydroxy-cholecalciferol. *Biochem Biophys Res Commun* 1969;36:251.

465. Hahn TJ, Hendin BA, Scharp CR, et al. Effect of chronic anticonvulsant therapy on serum 25-hydroxycholecalciferol levels in adults. *N Engl J Med* 1972;287:900.

466. Imawari M, Kida K, Goodman DS. The transport of vitamin D and its 25-hydroxy metabolite in human plasma: isolation and partial characterization of vitamin D and 25-hydroxyvitamin D binding protein. *J Clin Invest* 1976;58:514.

467. Goldstein DA, Yoshitaka O, Kurokawa K, et al. Blood levels of 25-hydroxyvitamin D in hepatic syndrome: studies in 26 patients. *Ann Intern Med* 1972;87:664.

468. Delmez JA, et al. Mineral, vitamin D and parathyroid hormone in continuous ambulatory peritoneal dialysis. *Kidney Int* 1982;21:862.

469. Aloni Y, Shany S, Chaimovitz C. Losses of 25-dihydroxyvitamin D in peritoneal fluid: possible mechanism for bone disease in uremic patients treated with chronic ambulatory peritoneal dialysis. *Miner Electrolyte Metab* 1983;9:82.

470. Haddad JG Jr, Kyong JC. Competitive protein-binding radio-assay for 25-hydroxycholecalciferol. *J Clin Endocrinol Metab* 1971;22:992.

471. Arnaud SB, Matthusen M, Gilkinson JB, et al. Components of 25-hydroxyvitamin D in serum of young children in upper midwestern United States. *Am J Clin Nutr* 1977;30:1082.

472. Haddad JG Jr, Rojanasathit S. Acute administration of 25-hydroxycholecalciferol in man. *J Clin Endocrinol Metab* 1976;42:284.

473. Lucas PA, Woodhead JS, Brown RC. Vitamin D_3 metabolites in chronic renal failure and after renal transplantation. *Nephrol Dial Tranplant* 1988;3:70.

474. Pietrek J, Kokot F. Serum 25-dihydroxyvitamin D in patients with chronic renal disease. *Eur J Clin Invest* 1977;7:283.

475. Rickers H, et al. Serum concentrations of vitamin D metabolites in different degrees of impaired renal function. Estimation of renal and extrarenal secretion rate of 24,25-dihydroxyvitamin D. *Nephron* 1985;39:267.

476. Frohling PT, et al. Serum 25-hydroxyvitamin D in patients with chronic renal failure on long-term treatment with high doses of vitamin D_2. *Nephron* 1980;26:116.

477. Desai TK, Carlson RW, Geheb MA. Parathyroid-vitamin D axis in critically ill patients with unexplained hypocalcemia. *Kidney Int* 1987;22[Suppl]:S225.

478. Bettinelli AL, et al. Plasma 25(OH)D levels in children on long-term hemofiltration. *Nephron* 1987;46:327.

479. Fraser DR, Kodicek E. Unique biosynthesis by kidney of a biologically active vitamin D metabolite. *Nature* 1970;228:769.

480. Gray R, Boyle L, DeLuca HF. Vitamin D metabolism: the role of kidney tissue. *Science* 1971;172:1232.

481. Norman AW, Midgett RJ, Myrtle JF, et al. Studies on calciferol metabolism: I. production of vitamin D metabolite 4B from 25-OH-cholecalciferol by kidney homogenates. *Biochem Biophys Res Commun* 1971;42:1082.

482. Pryke AM, et al. Tumor necrosis factor-alpha induces vitamin D-1-hydroxylase activity in normal human alveolar macrophages. *J Cell Physiol* 1990;142:652.

483. Shany S, et al. Metabolism of 25-OH-vitamin D_3 by peritoneal macrophages from CAPD patients. *Kidney Int* 1991;39:1005.

484. Dusso A-S, et al. Extrarenal production of calcitriol in normal and uremic humans. *J Clin Endocrinol Metab* 1991;72:154.

485. Adams JS, Gacad MA. Characterization of 1α-hydroxylation of vitamin D_3 sterols by cultured macrophages from patients with sarcoidosis. *J Exp Med* 1985;121:755.

486. Holick F. Vitamin D and the kidney. *Kidney Int* 1987;32:912.

487. Portale AA, Halloran BP, Morris RC Jr. Physiologic regulation of the concentration of 1,25-dihydroxyvitamin D by phosphorus in normal men. *J Clin Invest* 1989;83:1494.

488. DeLuca MF. The physiology and biochemistry of vitamin D. In: Kumar R, ed. *Vitamin D* Boston: Martinus Nyhoff, 1984.

489. Eisman JA, et al. A sensitive, precise, and convenient method for determination of 1,25 hydroxyvitamin D in human plasma. *Anal Biochem Biophys* 1976;80:298.

490. Mawer EB, et al. Metabolic fate of administered 1,25 dihydroxycholecalciferol in controls and patients with hypoparathyroidism. *Lancet* 1976;1:1203.

491. Portale AA, Boothe BE, Tsai HC, et al. Reduced plasma concentration of 1,25-dihydroxy-vitamin D in children with moderate renal insufficiency. *Kidney Int* 1982;21:627.

492. Juttmann JR, et al. Serum concentrations of metabolites of vitamin D in patients with chronic renal failure (CRF): consequences for the treatment of 1-α-hydroxyderivatives. *Clin Endocrinol* 1981;14:225.

493. Jongen MJM, van der Vijgh WJF, Lips P, et al. Measurement of vitamin D metabolites in anephric subject. *Nephron* 1984;36:230.

494. Lund B, et al. 1,25-dihydroxycholecalciferol in anephric, haemodialyzed and kidney transplanted patients. *Nephron* 1980;25:30.

495. Lambert PW, et al. Evidence for extra renal production of 1α 25-dihydroxy vitamin D in man. *J Clin Invest* 1982;69:772.

496. Barbour SG, et al. Hypercalcemia in an anephric patient with sarcoidosis: evidence for extra renal generation of 1,25-dihydroxyvitamin D. *N Engl J Med* 1981;305:440.

497. Dusso A, et al. Metabolic clearance rate and production rate of calcitriol in uremia. *Kidney Int* 1989;35:860.

498. Salusky IB, et al. Plasma kinetics of intravenous calcitriol in normal and dialyzed subjects and acute effect on serum nPTH levels. In: Proceedings of the 7th Workshop of Vitamin D; April 24–29; 1988 Rancho Mirage, California. Abstract:186.

499. Hsu CH, Patel S, Young EW, et al. Production and degradation of calcitriol in renal failure rats. *Am J Physiol* 1987;253:F1015.

500. Hsu CH, Patel S, Young EW, et al. Production and metabolic clearance of calcitriol in acute renal failure. *Kidney Int* 1988;33:530.

501. Hsu CH, Patel SR, Young EW. Mechanism of decreased calcitriol degradation in renal failure. *Am J Physiol* 1992;262:F192.

502. Taylor CM, et al. Unilateral nephrectomy and 1,25-dihydroxyvitamin D_3. *Kidney Int* 1983;24:37.

503. Haussler MR, et al. Molecular biology of the vitamin D hormone. *Recent Prog Horm Res* 1988;49:263.

504. Pike JW. Emerging concepts on the biologic role and mechanism of action of 1,25-dihydroxyvitamin D_3. *Steroids* 1987;49:3.

505. Merke J, et al. Diminished parathyroid 1,25(OH)$_2$D$_3$ receptors in experimental uremia. *Kidney Int* 1987;32:350.

506. Hsu CH, Patel SR, Vanholder R. Mechanism of decreased intestinal calcitriol receptor concentration in renal failure. *Am J Physiol* 1993; 264:F662.

507. Brown AJ, et al. 1,25(OH)$_2$D receptors are decreased in parathyroid glands from chronically uremic dogs. *Kidney Int* 1989;35:19.

508. Korkor AB. Reduced binding of [H] 1,25-dihydroxyvitamin D_3 in the parathyroid glands of patients with renal failure. *N Engl J Med* 1987; 316:1573.

509. Naveh-Many T, et al. Regulation of 1,25-dihydroxyvitamin D_3 receptor gene expression by 1,25-dihydroxyvitamin D_3 in the parathyroid in vivo. *J Clin Invest* 1990;86:1968.

510. Reinhardt TA, Horst RL. Parathyroid hormone down-regulates 1,25(OH)$_2$D receptors (VDR) and VDR messenger ribonucleic acid in vitro and blocks hemologous up-regulation of VDR in vivo. *Endocrinology* 1990;127:942.

511. Patel SR, Ke HQ, Hsu CH. Regulation of calcitriol receptor and its mRNA in normal and renal failure rats. *Kidney Int* 1994;45:1020.

512. Kokot F, Kuska J. Plasma renin activity in patients with chronic renal insufficiency treated by hemodialysis. *Proc Eur Dial Transplant Assoc* 1971;8:542.

513. Weidmann P, et al. Hypertension in terminal renal failure. *Kidney Int* 1976;9:294.

514. Kuska J, Kokot F. Plasma renin activity and plasma aldosterone level in patients with chronic renal failure on maintenance haemodialysis. *Acta Med Pol* 1976;17:183.

515. Rauh W, et al. Vasoactive hormones in children with chronic renal failure. *Kidney Int* 1983;24:S27.

516. Saxuta T, et al. Renin, aldosterone and other mineralocorticoids in hyperkalemic patients with chronic renal failure showing mild azotemia. *Nephron* 1981;29:128.

517. Weidmann P, Maxwell MH. The renin-angiotensin system in terminal renal failure. *Kidney Int* 1975;8:S219.

518. Meltzer JI, et al. Nephrotic syndrome: vasoconstriction and hypervolemic types indicated by renin-sodium profiling. *Ann Intern Med* 1979;91:688.

519. Schambelan M, Sebastian A, Biglieri E. Prevalence pathogenesis, and functional significance of aldosterone deficiency in hyperkalemic patients with chronic renal insufficiency. *Kidney Int* 1980;17:89.

520. DeFronzo RA. Hyperkalemia and hyporeninemic hypoaldosteronism. *Kidney Int* 1980;17:118.

521. DeFronzo RA, Bia M, Smith D. Clinical disorders of hyperkalemia. *Annu Rev Med* 1982;33:521.

522. Phelps KR, Lieberman RL, Oh MS, et al. Pathophysiology of the syndrome of hyporeninemic hypoaldosteronism. *Metabolism* 1980; 29:186.

523. Battle DC. Hyperkalemic hyperchloremic metabolic acidosis associated with selective aldosterone deficiency and distal renal tubular acidosis. *Semin Nephrol* 1981;1:260.

524. Iitake K, et al. Effect of haemodialysis in plasma ADH levels, plasma renin activity and plasma aldosterone levels in patients with end-stage renal disease. *Acta Endocrinol (Copenh)* 1985;110:207.

525. Sasamura H, et al. Response of plasma immunoreactive active renin, inactive renin, plasma renin activity and aldosterone to hemodialysis in patients with diabetic nephrology. *Clin Nephrol* 1990;33:288.

526. Williams GH, et al. Studies on the metabolism of aldosterone in chronic renal failure and anephric man. *Kidney Int* 1973;4:280.

527. Weidmann P, Maxwell MH, Lupu AN. Plasma aldosterone in terminal renal failure. *Ann Intern Med* 1973;78:13.

528. Reubi FC, Weidmann P, Gluck Z. Interrelationships between sodium clearance, plasma aldosterone, plasma renin activity, renal hemodynamics and blood pressure in renal disease. *Klin Wochenschr* 1979; 57:1273.

529. Kahn T, et al. Potassium transport in chronic renal disease. *Clin Res* 1976;24:403A.

530. Brown JJ, Dusterdieck G, Fraser R. Hypertension and chronic renal failure. *Br Med Bull* 1971;27:128.

531. Saruta T, et al. Renin, aldosterone, and other mineralocorticoids in hyperkalemic patients with chronic renal failure showing mild azotemia. *Nephron* 1981;29:128.

532. Weidmann P, et al. Role of the renin–angiotensin–aldosterone system in the regulation of plasma potassium in chronic renal disease. *Nephron* 1975;15:35.

533. Berl T, et al. Role of aldosterone in the control of sodium excretion in patients with advanced chronic renal failure. *Kidney Int* 1978;14:228.

534. Hene RJ, Boer P, Koomans HA, et al. Plasma aldosterone concentrations in chronic renal disease. *Kidney Int* 1982;21:98.

535. Schrier RW, Regal EM. Influence of aldosterone on sodium, water, and potassium metabolism in chronic renal disease. *Kidney Int* 1972;1: 156.

536. Weidmann P, et al. Control of aldosterone responsiveness in terminal renal failure. *Kidney Int* 1975;7:351.

537. Kleeman CR, Okun R, Heller RJ. The renal regulation of sodium and potassium in patients with chronic renal failure (CRF) and the effects of diuretics in the excretion of these ions. *Ann NY Acad Sci* 1966;139: 520.

538. Henrich WL, Katz FH, Molinoff PB, et al. Competitive effects of hypokalemia and volume depletion on plasma renin activity, aldosterone and catecholamine concentrations in hemodialysis patients. *Kidney Int* 1977;12:279.

539. Olgaard K, Madsen S. Regulation of plasma aldosterone in anephric and non-nephrectomized patients during hemodialysis treatment. *Acta Med Scand* 1977;201:457.

540. Farinelli A, et al. Response of plasma aldosterone to sequential ultrafiltration, dialysis, and conventional hemodialysis. *Nephron* 1980; 26:274.

541. Zager PG, Frey HJ Gerdes BG, et al. Increased plasma levels of 18-hydroxycorticocosterone and 18-hydroxy, 11-deoxycorticosterone during continuous ambulatory peritoneal dialysis. *Kidney Int* 1982;12: 121.

542. Bayard F, et al. The regulation of aldosterone secretion in anephric man. *J Clin Invest* 1971;50:1585.

543. Walker GW, Cooke CR. Plasma aldosterone regulation in anephric man. *Kidney Int* 1973;3:1.

544. Weidmann P, et al. Dynamic studies of aldosterone in anephric man. *Kidney Int* 1973;4:289.

545. Sealey JE, et al. Studies of plasma aldosterone in anephric people: evidence for the fundamental role of the renin system in maintaining aldosterone secretion. *J Clin Endocrinol Metab* 1978;47:52.

546. Mitra S, Genuth SM, Berman LB, et al. Aldosterone secretion in anephric patients. *N Engl J Med* 1972;286:61.

547. McCaa RE, et al. Increased plasma aldosterone concentration in response to hemodialysis in nephrectomized man. *Circ Res* 1972;31:473.

548. Maher JF. Modifications of endocrine-metabolic abnormalities of uremia by continuous ambulatory peritoneal dialysis. *Am J Nephrol* 1990;10:1.

549. Ksiazek A. Dopamine-beta-hydroxylase activity and catecholamine levels in the plasma of patients with renal failure. *Nephron* 1979; 24:170.

550. Weidmann P, et al. Catecholamines and their possible role in hypertension associated with impaired renal function. *Contrib Nephrol* 1987;54:159.

551. Atuk NO, et al. Red blood cell catechol-o-methyl transferase, plasma catecholamines and renin in renal failure. *Trans Am Soc Artif Intern Organs* 1976;22:195.

552. Lake CR, Ziegler MG, Coleman MD, et al. Plasma levels of norepinephrine and dopamine-beta-hydroxylase in CRF patients treated with dialysis. *Cardiol Med* 1979;9:1099.

553. Brecht HM, Ernst W, Koch KM. Plasma noradrenaline levels in regular hemodialysis patients. *Proc Eur Dial Transplant Assoc* 1975;12: 281.

554. Henrich WL, Katz FH, Molinoff B, et al. Competitive effects of hypokalemia and volume depletion on plasma renin activity, aldosterone, and catecholamine concentrations in hemodialysis patients. *Kidney Int* 1977;12:279.

555. Zucchelli P, et al. Influence of ultrafiltration on plasma renin activity and adrenergic system. *Nephron* 1978;21:316.

556. Quellhorst E, Schuenemann B, Hildebrand V, et al. Hypertension and hemofiltration. *Contrib Nephrol* 1982;32:46.

557. Ratge D, Augustin R, Wisser H. Plasma catecholamines and alpha-and beta-adrenoreceptors in circulating blood cells in patients on continuous ambulatory peritoneal dialysis. *Clin Nephrol* 1987;28:15.

558. Hennemann H, Hevendehl G, Horler E, et al. Toxic sympathicopathy in uraemia. *Dial Transplant Nephrol* 1973;3:166.

559. Aoki K, Tazumi K, Takikawa K. Serum dopamine-beta hydroxylase activity in essential hypertension and in chronic renal failure. *Jpn Circ J* 1975;39:1111.

560. Lilley JJ, Golden J, Stone RA. Adrenergic regulation of blood pressure in chronic renal failure. *J Clin Invest* 1976;57:1190.

561. Wang M, Tam CF, Swendseid MD, et al. Monoamine and diamine oxidase activities in uremic rats. *Life Sci* 1975;17:653.

562. Baines AD, Craan A, Chan W, et al. Tubular secretion and metabolism of dopamine, norepinephrine, methoxytyramine and normetanephrine by the rat kidney. *J Pharmacol Exp Ther* 1979;208:144.

563. Willis LR, et al. Urinary excretion of radiolabelled norepinephrine after release from renal sympathetic nerves. *Life Sci* 1980;27:2541.

564. Winckler J, Hennemann H, Heidland A, et al. Katecholamingehalt adrenerger nerven in speicheldrusen mit gestorter elektrolytausscheidung bei uramie. *Klin Wochenschr* 1973;51:1115.

565. Rascher W, Tulassay T, Lang RE. Atrial natriuretic peptide in plasma of volume overloaded children with chronic renal failure. *Lancet* 1985;2: 303.

566. Anderson JV, et al. Effect of haemodialysis on plasma concentrations of atrial natriuretic peptide in adult patients with chronic renal failure. *J Endocrinol* 1986;110:193.

567. Ogawa K, et al. Plasma atrial natriuretic peptide concentrations and circulating forms in normal man and patients with chronic renal failure. *Clin Exp. Pharmacol* 1987;14:95.

568. Yamamoto Y, et al. Plasma concentrations of human atrial natriuretic polypeptide in patients with impaired renal function. *Clin Nephrol* 1987;27:84.

569. Predel HG, et al. Human atrial natriuretic peptide in non-dialyzed patients with chronic renal failure. *Clin Nephrol* 1989;31:150.

570. Marrissey EC, et al. Atrial natriuretic factor in renal failure and posthemodialytic postural hypotension. *Am J Kidney Dis* 1982;12: 510.

571. Cannella G, et al. Effects of changes in intravascular volume on atrial size and plasma levels of immunoreactive atrial natriuretic peptide in uremic man. *Clin Nephrol* 1988;30:187.

572. Deray G, et al. Plasma levels of atrial natriuretic peptide in chronically dialyzed patients. *Kidney Int* 1988;25 [Suppl]:S86.

573. Manno C, et al. Increased plasma levels of human atrial natriuretic factor in patients treated with acetate or bicarbonate hemodialysis. *Nephron* 1989;53:290.

574. Tikkanen I, et al. Plasma levels of atrial natriuretic peptide as an indicator of increased cardiac load in uremic patients. *Clin Nephrol* 1990;34:167.

575. Os I, Nordby G, Lyngdal PT, et al. Plasma vasopressin, catecholamines and atrial natriuretic factor during hemodialysis and sequential ultrafiltration. *Scand J Urol Nephrol* 1993;27:93.

576. Pruszczynski W, et al. Role of cardiac parasympathetic dysfunction in atrial natriuretic peptide response to volume changes in patients with chronic renal failure. *Miner Electrolyte Metab* 1987;13:333.

577. Webb DJ, Cockcroft JR. Plasma immunoreactive endothelin in uraemia. *Lancet* 1989;1:1211.

578. Koyama H, et al. Plasma endothelin levels in patients with uraemia. *Lancet* 1989;1:991.

579. Totsune K, et al. Detection of immunoreactive endothelin in plasma of hemodialysis patients. *FEBS Lett* 1989;249:239.

580. Warrens AN, et al. Endothelin in renal failure. *Nephrol Dial Transplant* 1990;5:418.

581. Stockenhuber F, et al. Plasma levels of endothelin in chronic renal failure and after renal transplantation: impact on hypertension and cyclosporin A-associated nephrotoxicity. *Clin Sci* 1992;82:255.

582. Takahashi K, Totsune K, Mouri T. Endothelin in chronic renal failure. *Nephron* 1994;66:373.

583. Lightfoot BO, Caruana RJ. Endothelin-1 in continuous ambulatory peritoneal dialysis and hemodialysis patients: a preliminary study. *Peritoneal Dial Int* 1993;13:55.

584. Shichiri M, et al. Plasma endothelin levels in hypertension and chronic renal failure. *Hypertension* 1990;15:493.

585. Komuro I, et al. Endothelin stimulates c-fos and c-myc expression and proliferation of vascular smooth muscle cells. *FEBS Lett* 1988;238:249.

586. Takuwa N, et al. A novel vasoactive peptide, endothelin, stimulates mitogenesis through inositol lipid turnover in Swiss 3T3 fibroblasts. *J Biol Chem* 1989;264:7856.

587. Lebel M, Grose JH. Abnormal renal prostaglandin production during the evolution of chronic nephropathy. *Am J Nephrol* 1986;6:96.

588. Berg KJ, et al. Acute effect of paracetamol on prostaglandin synthesis and renal function in normal man and in patients with renal failure. *Clin Nephrol* 1990;34:255.

589. McGiff JC, et al. Prostaglandin-like substances appearing in canine renal venous blood during renal ischemia. Their partial characterization by pharmacologic and chromatographic procedures. *Circ Res* 1970;27:765.

590. Kimberly RP, et al. Elevated urinary prostaglandins and the effects of aspirin on renal function in lupus erythematosus. *Ann Intern Med* 1978;89:336.

591. Blum M, et al. Urinary prostaglandin E in chronic renal disease. *Clin Nephrol* 1981;15:87.

592. Schneider M, et al. Urinary prostaglandins E_2 and $F_2\alpha$ in chronic renal failure. *Nephron* 1985;40:152.

593. Borges MF, Kjellstrand CM. The effect of prostaglandin inhibition on the clinical course of chronic hemodialysis. *Nephron* 1986;42:119.

594. Berg K. J. Acute effects of acetylsalicylic acid in patients with chronic renal insufficiency. *Eur J Clin Pharmacol* 1977;11:111.

595. Schlondorff D, Ardaillou R. Prostaglandins and other arachidonic acid metabolites in the kidney. *Kidney Int* 1986;29:108.

596. Gryglewski RJ, Korbut R, Ocetkiewcz A. Generation of prostacyclin by lungs in vivo and its release into the arterial circulation. *Nature* 1978;273:765.

597. Craddock PR, et al. Complement and leukocyte-mediated pulmonary dysfunction in hemodialysis. *N Engl J Med* 1977;296:769.

598. Nadler JL, Lee FO, Hsueh W, et al. Evidence of prostacyclin deficiency in the syndrome of hyporeninemic hypoaldosteronism. *N Engl J Med* 1986;314:1015.

599. DeWardener HE, Clarkson EM. Concept of natriuretic hormone. *Physiol Rev* 1985;65:658.

600. Kramer HJ, et al. Digoxin-like immunoreacting substance(s) in the serum of patients with chronic uremia. *Nephron* 1985;40:297.

601. Kelly RA, et al. Endogenous digitalis-like factors in hypertension and chronic renal insufficiency. *Kidney Int* 1986;30:723.

602. Vasdev S, et al. Plasma endogenous digitalis-like factors in healthy individuals and in dialysis dependent and kidney transplant patients. *Clin Nephrol* 1987;27:169.

603. Walker JA, et al. Digoxin-like immunoreactive substance in chronic hemodialysis patients: effect on digitoxin radioimmunoassay. *Am J Nephrol* 1987;7:300.

604. Bosch RJ, et al. Endogenous digoxin-like immunoreactivity and erythrocyte sodium transport in uremic patients undergoing dialysis. *Clin Sci* 1989;76:157.

605. Greenway DC, Nanji AA. Digoxin-like immunoreactive substance in renal failure: a reappraisal. *Nephron* 1986;44:108.

606. Seccombe DW, et al. Digoxin-like immunoreactivity, displacement of ouabain and inhibition of Na^+, K^+-ATPase by four steroids known to be increased in essential-hypertension. *Clin Biochem* 1989;22:17.

607. Graves SW, Brown B, Waldes R. An endogenous digoxin-like substance in patients with renal impairment. *Ann Intern Med* 1983;99:604.

608. Korman MG, Laver MC, Hansky J. Hypergastrinemia in chronic renal failure. *Br Med J* 1972;1:209.

609. Kokot F, et al. Äber die beziehung zwischen gastrin-und kalzitoninsekretion bei kranken mit akuter und chronischer niereninsuffizienz. *Dtsch Gesundh Wesen* 1981;36:429.

610. Sirinek KR, et al. Chronic renal failure: effect of hemodialysis on gastrointestinal hormones. *Am J Surg* 1984;148:732.

611. El Ghonaimy E, et al. Serum gastrin in chronic renal failure: morphological and physiological correlations. *Nephron* 1985;39:86.

612. Muto S, et al. Hypergastrinaemia and achlorhydria in chronic renal failure. *Nephron* 1985;40:143.

613. Gold CH, et al. Gastric acid secretion and serum gastrin levels in patients with chronic renal failure on regular hemodialysis. *Nephron* 1980;25:92.

614. Sullivan SN, Tustanoff E, Slaughter DN. Hypergastrinemia and gastric acid secretion in uremia. *Clin Nephrol* 1976;5:25.

615. Wesdorp RIC, et al. Gastrin and gastric acid secretion in renal failure. *Am J Surg* 1981;141:334.

616. Kokot F, et al. Influence of erythropoietin treatment on glucose tolerance, insulin, glucagon, gastrin and pancreatic polypeptide secretion in haemodialyzed patients with end-stage renal failure. *Contrib Nephrol* 1990;87:42.

617. Grace SG, Davidson WD, State D. Renal mechanism for removal of gastrin from the circulation. *Surg Forum* 1974;25:323.

618. Ala-Kaila K, Kekki M, Paronen I, et al. Serum gastrin in chronic renal failure: its relation to acid secretion, G-cell density, and upper gastrointestinal findings. *Scand J Gastroenterol* 1989;24:939.

619. Grekas DM, Raptis S, Tourkantonis AA, et al. Plasma secretin, pancreozymin and somatostatin-like hormone in chronic renal failure patients. *Uremia Invest* 1984;8:117.

620. Lauritzen JB, et al. Gastric inhibitory polypeptide (GIP) and insulin release in response to oral and intravenous glucose in uremic patients. *Metabolism* 1982;9:1096.

621. Owyang C, et al. Gastrointestinal hormone profile in renal insufficiency. *Mayo Clin Proc* 1979;63:769.

622. Bodgen G, et al. Human pancreatic polypeptide in chronic renal failure and cirrhosis of the liver: role of kidneys and liver in pancreatic polypeptide metabolism. *J Clin Endocrinol Metab* 1980;51:573.

623. Lugari R, et al. Human pancreatic polypeptide and somatostatin in chronic renal failure. *Proc Eur Dial Transplant Assoc–Eur Renal Assoc* 1984;21:614.

624. Henriksen JH, et al. Circulating endogenous vasoactive intestinal polypeptide (VIP) in patients with uraemia and liver cirrhosis. *Eur J Clin Invest* 1986;16:211.

625. Pereira BJ, et al. Plasma levels of IL-1 beta, TNF alpha and their specific inhibitor in undialyzed chronic renal failure CAPD and hemodialysis patients. *Kidney Int* 1994;45:890.

626. Herbelin A, et al. Influence of uremia and hemodialysis on circulating interleukin-1 and tumor necrosis factor. *Kidney Int* 1990;37:116.

627. Descamps-Latscha B, et al. Haemodialysis-membrane-induced phagocyte oxidative metabolism activation and interleukin-1 production. *Life Support Syst* 1986;4:349.

628. Lonneman G, et al. Plasma interleukin-1 activity in humans undergoing hemodialysis with regenerated cellulosic membranes. *Lymphokine Res* 1987;6:63.

629. Luger A, et al. Blood membrane interaction in hemodialysis leads to increased cytokine production. *Kidney Int* 1988;32:84.

630. Poignet JL, Fitting C, Delons S, et al. Circulating interleukin-6 in long term hemodialyzed patients. *J Am Soc Nephrol* 1990;1:372(abst).

631. Herbelin A, et al. Elevated circulating levels of interleukin-6 in patients with chronic renal failure. *Kidney Int* 1991;39:954.

632. Ghysen J, DePlaen JF, van Ypersele de Strihou C. The effect of membrane characteristic on tumor necrosis factor kinetics during haemodialysis. *Nephrol Dial Transplant* 1990;5:270.

633. Pereira BJG, Dinarello CA. Production of cytokines and cytokine inhibitory proteins in patients on dialysis. *Nephrol Dial Transplant* 1994;9[Suppl 2]:60.

634. Powell AC, et al. Lack of plasma interleukin-1 beta or tumor necrosis factor-alpha elevation during unfavorable hemodialysis conditions. *J Am Soc Nephrol* 1991;2:1007.

635. Gilkdes JJH, et al. Plasma immunoreactive melanotropic hormones in patients on maintenance hemodialysis. *Br. Med. J* 1975;1:656.

636. Aronin N, et al. Impaired clearance of beta-lipotropin in uremia. *J Clin Endocrinol Metab* 1981;53:797.

637. Hegbrant J, Thysell H, Ekman R. Elevated plasma levels of opioids peptides and delta sleep-inducing peptide but not of corticotropin-releasing hormone in patients receiving chronic hemodialysis. *Blood Purif* 1991;9:188.

638. Smith R, et al. Studies on circulating met-enkephalin and beta-endorphin in normal subjects and patients with renal and adrenal disease. *Clin Endocrinol* 1981;15:291.

639. Aronin N, Krieger DT. Plasma immunoreactive beta-endorphin is elevated in uraemia. *Clin Endocrinol* 1983;18:459.

640. Ciardella F, et al. Effects of a low-phosphorus, low-nitrogen diet supplemented with essential amino acids and ketoanalogues on serum beta-endorphin in chronic renal failure. *Nephron* 1989;53:129.

641. Thornton JR, Losowsky MS. Plasma beta endorphin in cirrhosis and renal failure. *Gut* 1991;32:306.

642. Zoccalli C, et al. Plasma met-enkephalin and leu-enkephalin in chronic renal failure. *Nephrol Dial Transplant* 1987;1:219.

643. Grzeszczak W, Kokot F, Dulawa J. Influence of naloxone on prolactin secretion in patients with acute and chronic renal failure. *Clin Nephrol* 1984;21:47.

644. Zhang Y, et al. Positional cloning of the mouse ob gene and its human homologue. *Nature* 1994;372:425.

645. Sinha MK, Caro JF. Clinical aspects of leptin. *Vitam Horm* 1998;54:1.

646. Heimburger O, et al. Serum immunoreactive leptin concentrations and its relation to body fat content in chronic renal failure. *J Am Soc Neprol* 1997;8:1423.

647. Iida M, et al. Hyperleptinemia in chronic renal failure. *Horm Metab Res* 1996;28:724.

648. Sharma K, et al. Plasma leptin is partly cleared by the kidney and is elevated in hemodialysis patients. *Kidney Int* 1997;51:1980.

SECTION XIII

Management of End-Stage Renal Disease

CHAPTER 96

Immunobiology and Immunopharmacology of Graft Rejection

Terry B. Strom and Manikkam Suthanthiran

There is broad consensus that renal transplantation is the treatment of choice for the majority of patients afflicted with end-stage renal disease (1). A better comprehension of the antiallograft response, improved and shorter periods of preservation of donor kidneys, judicious usage of new immunesuppressive drugs and antilymphocytic agents for the prevention and/or treatment of rejection, and the adaptation of infection prophylaxis protocols have all contributed to the steady improvement in the short-term as well as long-term rates of engraftment.

IMMUNOBIOLOGY OF RENAL TRANSPLANTATION

The Antiallograft Response

Allograft rejection is contingent on the coordinated activation of alloreactive T cells and antigen-presenting cells (APCs). Through the intermediacy of cytokines and cell-to-cell interactions, a heterogeneous contingent of lymphocytes, including CD4+ helper T cells, CD8+ cytotoxic T cells, antibody-forming B cells, and other proinflammatory leukocytes are recruited into the antiallograft response (Fig. 96-1 and Table 96-1).

T-Cell Activation and the Immunologic Synapse: Signal One

The immunologic synapse consisting of a multiplicity of T-cell surface protein forms and clusters, thereby creating a platform for antigen recognition and generation of various

T. B. Strom: Department of Medicine, Harvard School of Medicine; and Division of Immunology, Beth Israel Hospital, Boston, Massachusetts

M. Suthanthiran: Division of Nephrology, Departments of Medicine, Weill Medical College of Cornell University; and Department of Transplantation Medicine and Extracorporeal Therapy, New York-Presbyterian Hospital, New York, New York

crucial T-cell activation-related signals (2). The synapse begins to form when the initial adhesions between certain T-cell (e.g., CD2, LFA-1) and APC surface proteins (e.g., CD58, ICAM-1) are formed (Table 96-2). These adhesions create intimate contact between T cells and APCs and thereby provide an opportunity for T cells to recognize antigen. Antigendriven T-cell activation, a tightly regulated, preprogrammed process, begins when T cells recognize intracellularly processed fragments of foreign proteins (approximately 8 to 16 amino acids) embedded within the groove of the major histocompatibility complex (MHC) proteins expressed on the surface of APCs (3–5). Some recipient T cells directly recognize the allograft (i.e., donor antigen(s) presented on the surface of donor APCs), while other T cells recognize the donor antigen after it is processed and presented by self-APCs (6) (Fig. 96-1).

The T-cell antigen receptor (TCR)/CD3 complex is composed of clonally distinct TCR α and β peptide chains that recognize the antigenic peptide in the context of MHC proteins and clonally invariant CD3 chains that propagate intracellular signals originating from antigenic recognition (2,7,8) (Fig. 96-2). The TCR variable, diversity, junction, and constant region genes (i.e., genes for regions of the clone-specific antigen receptors) are spliced together in a cassettelike fashion during T-cell maturation (7). A small population of T cells express TCR γ and δ chains instead of the TCR α and β chains.

CD4 and CD8 proteins, expressed on reciprocal T-cell subsets, bind to nonpolymorphic domains of human leukocyte antigen (HLA) class II (DR, DP, DQ) and class I (A, B, C) molecules, respectively (2,7) (Fig. 96-1, Table 96-2). A threshold of TCR to MHC-peptide engagements is necessary to stabilize the immunologic synapse stimulating a redistribution of cell surface proteins and coclustering of the TCR/CD3 complex with the T-cell surface proteins (8–10). CD5 proteins (9,10) join the synapse. The TCR cluster already includes integrins (e.g., LFA-1) and nonintegrins, e.g., CD2 (2,8,9) that have created T-cell–APC adhesions. Hence,

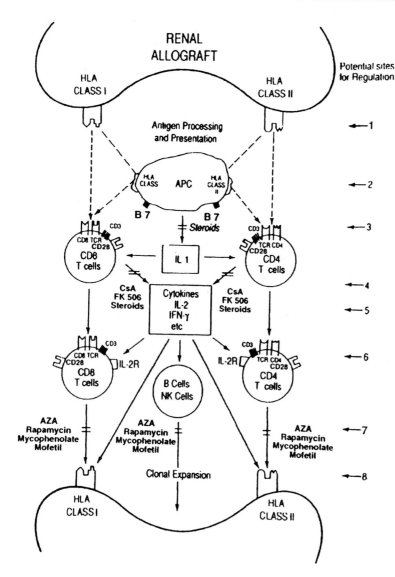

FIG. 96-1. The antiallograft response. Schematic representation of human leukocyte antigen (HLA), the primary stimulus for the initiation of the antiallograft response; cell surface proteins participating in antigenic recognition and signal transduction; contribution of the cytokines and multiple cell types to the immune response; and the potential sites for the regulation of the antiallograft response. **Site 1:** Minimizing histoincompatibility between the recipients and the donor (e.g., HLA matching). **Site 2:** Prevention of monokine production by antigen-presenting cells (APCs) (e.g., corticosteroids). **Site 3:** Blockade of antigen recognition (e.g., OKT3 mAbs). **Site 4:** Inhibition of T-cell cytokine production (e.g., cyclosporin A [CsA]). **Site 5:** Inhibition of cytokine activity (e.g., anti-interleukin-2 [IL-2] antibody). **Site 6:** Inhibition of cell cycle progression (e.g., anti-IL-2 receptor antibody). **Site 7:** Inhibition of clonal expansion (e.g., azathioprine [AZA]). **Site 8:** Prevention of allograft damage by masking target antigen molecules (e.g., antibodies directed at adhesion molecules). HLA class I: HLA-A, B, and C antigens; HLA class II: HLA-DR, DP, and DQ antigens. *IFN-γ*, interferon-γ; *NK cells,* natural killer cells.

antigen recognition stimulates a redistribution of cell-surface proteins and coclustering of the TCR/CD3 complex with the T-cell surface proteins (2,7–9) and signaling molecules. This multimeric complex functions as a unit in initiating T-cell activation.

Following activation by antigen, the TCR/CD3 complex and coclustered CD4 and CD8 proteins are physically associated with intracellular protein–tyrosine kinases (PTKs) of two different families, the src (including $p59^{fyn}$ and $p56^{lck}$) and ZAP 70 families (2). The CD45 protein, a tyrosine phosphatase, contributes to the activation process by dephosphorylating an autoinhibitory site on the $p56^{lck}$ PTK. Intracellular domains of several TCR/CD3 proteins contain activation motifs that are crucial for antigen-stimulated signaling. Certain tyrosine residues within these motifs serve as targets for the catalytic activity of src family PTKs. Subsequently, these phosphorylated tyrosines serve as docking stations for the SH2 domains (recognition structures for select phosphotyrosine-containing motifs) of the ZAP-70 PTK. Following antigenic engagement of the TCR/CD3 complex,

select serine residues of the TCR and CD3 chains are also phosphorylated (2,5).

The wave of tyrosine phosphorylation triggered by antigen recognition encompasses other intracellular proteins and is a cardinal event in initiating T-cell activation. Tyrosine phosphorylation of the phospholipase $C\gamma_1$ activates this coenzyme and triggers a cascade of events that lead to full expression of T-cell programs: hydrolysis of phosphatidylinositol 4,5-biphosphate (PIP_2) and generation of two intracellular messengers, inositol 1,4,5-triphosphate (IP_3) and diacylglycerol (11); (Fig. 96-2). IP_3, in turn, mobilizes ionized calcium from intracellular stores, while diacylglycerol, in the presence of increased cytosolic free Ca^{2+}, binds to and translocates protein kinase C (PKC)—a phospholipid/Ca^{2+}-sensitive protein serine/threonine kinase—to the membrane in its enzymatically active form (5,11). Sustained activation of PKC is dependent on diacylglycerol generation from hydrolysis of additional lipids such as phosphatidylcholine.

The increase in intracellular free Ca^{2+} and sustained PKC activation promote the expression of several nuclear

TABLE 96-1. *Cellular elements contributing to the antiallograft response*

Cell type	Functional attributes
T cells	The CD4+ T cells and the CD8+ T cells participate in the antiallograft response. CD4+ T cells recognize antigens presented by HLA-class II proteins, and CD8+ T cells recognize antigens presented by HLA-class I proteins. The CD3/TCR complex is responsible for recognition of antigen and generates and transduces the antigenic signal.
CD4+ T cells	CD4+ T cells function mostly as helper T cells and secrete cytokines such as IL-2, a T cell growth/death factor, and IFN-γ, a proinflammatory polypeptide that can upregulate the expression of HLA proteins as well as augment cytotoxic activity of T cells and NK cells. Recently, two main types of CD4+ T cells have been recognized: CD4+ TH1 and CD4+ TH2. IL-2 and IFN-γ are produced by CD4+ TH1 type cells, and IL-4 and IL-5 are secreted by CD4+ TH2 type cells. Each cell type regulates the secretion of the other, and the regulated secretion is important in the expression of host immunity.
CD8+ T cells	CD8+ T cells function mainly as cytotoxic T cells. A subset of CD8+ T cells expresses suppressor cell function. CD8+ T cells can secrete cytokines such as IL-2, IFN-γ, and can express molecules such as perforin, granzymes that function as effectors of cytotoxicity.
APCs	Monocytes/macrophages and dendritic cells function as potent APCs. Donor's APCs can process and present donor antigens to recipient's T cells (direct recognition) or recipient's APCs can process and present donor antigens to recipient's T cells (indirect recognition). The relative contribution of direct recognition and indirect recognition to the antiallograft response has not been resolved. Direct recognition and indirect recognition might also have differential susceptibility to inhibition by immunosuppressive drugs.
B cells	B cells require T cell help for the differentiation and production of antibodies directed at donor antigens. The alloantibodies can damage the graft by binding and activating complement components (complement-dependent cytotoxicity) and/or binding the Fc receptor of cells capable of mediating cytotoxicity (antibody-dependent, cell-mediated cytotoxicity).
NK cells	The precise role of NK cells in the antiallograft response is not known. Increased NK cell activity has been correlated with rejection. NK cell function might also be important in immune surveillance mechanisms pertinent to the prevention of infection and malignancy.

APCs, antigen presenting cells; *IFN,* interferon; *IL,* interleukin; *NK,* natural killer; *TCR,* T-cell antigen receptor

(Reproduced from Suthanthiran M, Morris RE, Strom TB. Transplantation immunobiology. In: Walsh PC, Retik AB, Vaughn ED Jr, et al., eds. *Campbell's urology,* 7th ed. Philadelphia: WB Saunders, 1997:491–504, with permission.)

TABLE 96-2. *Cell-surface proteins important for T cell activation*[a]

T cell surface	APC Surface	Functional response	Consequence of blockade
LFA-1 (CD11a, CD18)	ICAM (CD54)	Adhesion	Immunosuppression
ICAM1 (CD54)	LFA-1 (CD11a, CD18)		
CD8, TCR, CD3	MHCI	Antigen recognition	Immunosuppression
CD4, TCR, CD3	MHCII		
CD2	LFA3 (CD58)	Costimulation	Immunosuppression
CD40L (CD154)	CD40		
CD5	CD72		
CD28	B7-1 (CD80)	Costimulation	Anergy
CD28	B7-2 (CD86)		
CTLA4 (CD152)	B7-1 (CD80)	Inhibition	Immunostimulation
CTLA4 (CD152)	B7-2 (CD86)		

APC, antigen-presenting cell; *ICAM,* intercellular adhesion molecule; *LFA,* leukocyte function-associated; *MHC,* major histocompatibility complex

[a]Receptor/counter-receptor pairs that mediate interactions between T cells and APCs are shown in this table. Inhibition of each protein-to-protein interaction, except the CTLA4–B7.1/B7.2 interaction results in an abortive *in vitro* immune response. Initial contact between T cells and APCs requires an antigen-independent adhesive interaction. Next, the T cell antigen receptor complex engages processed antigen presented within the antigen-presenting groove of MHC molecules. Finally, costimulatory signals are required for full T cell activation. An especially important signal is generated by B7-mediated activation of CD28 on T cells. Activation of CD28 by B7.2 may provide a more potent signal than activation by B7.1. CTLA4, present on activated but not resting T cells, imparts a negative signal.

(Reproduced from Suthanthiran M, Morris RE, Strom TB. Transplantation immunobiology. In: Walsh PC, Retik AB, Vaughn ED Jr, et al., eds. *Campbell's urology,* 7th ed. Philadelphia: WB Saunders, 1997:491–504, with permission.)

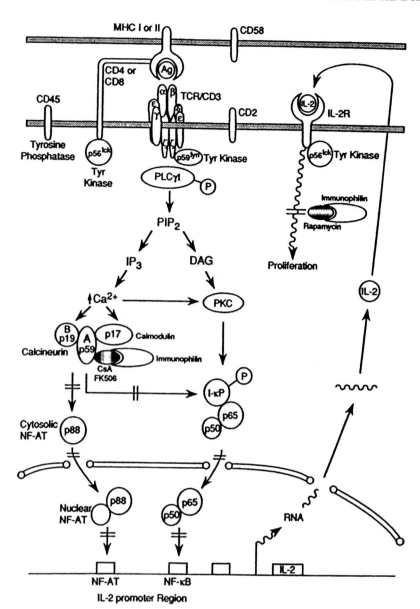

FIG. 96-2. Signal transduction in T cells and mechanisms of action of cyclosporin A (CsA), FK-506, or rapamycin. Signaling molecules and transmembrane signaling events participating in the transduction of antigenic signals from the plasma membrane of the T cells to the nucleus are schematically shown. The sites of action of the drug (CsA/FK-506/rapamycin)–immunophilin complex are also shown. *Ag,* antigen; *Ap59* and *Bp19,* subunits of calcineurin; *DAG,* diacylglycerol; *I-κB,* inhibitory factor kappa B; *IL-2,* interleukin-2; *immunophilin,* cyclophilin or FK binding protein; *IP₃,* inositol 1,4,5-triphosphate; *MHC,* major histocompatibility complex; *NF-AT,* nuclear factor of activated T cells; *NF-κB,* nuclear factor kappa B; *P,* phosphotyrosine; *PIP₂,* phosphatidylinositol 4,5-biphosphate; *PKC,* protein kinase C; *PLCγ1,* phospholipase C gamma-1; *Tyr kinase,* tyrosine kinase. (Adapted from Schreier MH, et al. *Transplant Proc* 1993;25:502.)

regulatory proteins (e.g., nuclear factor of activated T cells [NF-AT], nuclear factor kappa B [NF-κB], activator protein 1 [AP-1]) and the transcriptional activation and expression of genes central to T-cell growth (e.g., interleukin-2 [IL-2] and receptors for IL-2 and IL-15) (2,5,12).

Calcineurin, a Ca²⁺- and calmodulin-dependent serine/threonine phosphatase, is crucial to Ca²⁺-dependent, TCR-initiated signal transduction (13,14). Inhibition by cyclosporine and tacrolimus (FK-506) of the phosphatase activity of calcineurin is considered central to their immunosuppressive activity (15).

Costimulatory Signals: Signal Two

Signaling of T cells via the TCR/CD3 complex (signal one) is necessary, albeit insufficient, to induce T-cell proliferation; full activation is dependent on both the antigenic signals and

the costimulatory signals (signal two) engendered by the contactual interactions between cell surface proteins expressed on antigen-specific T cells and APCs (16,17) (Fig. 96-3, Table 96-2). Interaction of the CD2 protein on the T-cell surface with the CD58 (leukocyte function-associated antigen 3 [LFA-3]) protein on the APCs of the CD11a/CD18 (LFA-1) proteins with the CD54 (intercellular adhesion molecule 1 [ICAM-1]) (18) proteins, and/or the CD5 with the CD72 proteins (10) aids in imparting such a costimulatory signal.

Recognition of the B7-1 (CD80) and B7-2 (CD86) proteins expressed upon CD4+ T cells generates a very powerful T-cell costimulus (19). Monocytes and dendritic cells constitutively express CD86. Cytokines (e.g., granulocyte–macrophage colony-stimulating factor [GMCSF] or interferon-γ [IFN-γ]) stimulate expression of CD80 on monocytes, B cells, and dendritic cells (19). Many T cells express B7 binding proteins (i.e., CD28 proteins that are constitutively

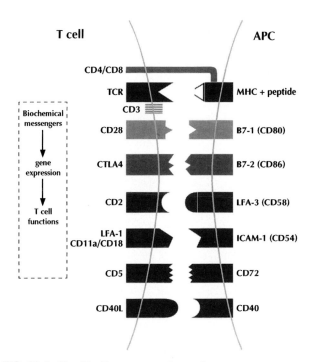

T cell   **APC**

CD4/CD8

TCR   MHC + peptide

CD3

CD28   B7-1 (CD80)

CTLA4   B7-2 (CD86)

CD2   LFA-3 (CD58)

LFA-1
CD11a/CD18   ICAM-1 (CD54)

CD5   CD72

CD40L   CD40

Biochemical
messengers

↓

gene
expression

↓

T cell
functions

FIG. 96-3. T-cell/antigen-presenting cell contact sites. In this schema of T-cell activation, the antigenic signal is initiated by the physical interaction between the clonally variant T-cell antigen receptor (TCR) α-, β-heterodimer and the antigenic peptide displayed by MHC on antigen-presenting cells (APCs). The antigenic signal is transduced into the cell by the CD3 proteins. The CD4 and the CD8 antigens function as associative recognition structures, and restrict TCR recognition to class II and class I antigens of MHC, respectively. Additional T-cell surface receptors generate the obligatory costimulatory signals by interacting with their counterreceptors expressed on the surface of the APCs. The simultaneous delivery to the T cells of the antigenic signal and the costimulatory signal results in the optimum generation of second messengers (such as calcium), expression of transcription factors (such as nuclear factor of activated T cells), and T-cell growth promoting genes (such as IL-2). The CD28 antigen as well as the CTLA4 antigen can interact with both the B7-1 and B7-2 antigens. The CD28 antigen generates a stimulatory signal, and the recent studies of CTLA4-deficient mice suggest that CTLA4, unlike CD28, generates a negative signal. *CD,* cluster designation; *ICAM-1,* intercellular adhesion molecule-1; *LFA-1,* leukocyte function-associated antigen-1; *MHC,* major histocompatibility complex. (From Suthanthiran M. Transplantation tolerance: fooling mother nature. *Proc Natl Acad Sci USA* 1996;93:12072.)

expressed on the surface of CD4+ T cells and CTLA-4 [CD152]), a protein whose ectodomain is closely related to that of CD28, and is expressed upon activated CD4+ and CD8+ T cells. CD28 binding of B7 molecules stimulates a Ca^{2+}-independent activation pathway that leads to stable transcription of the IL-2, IL-2 receptors, and other activation genes resulting in vigorous T-cell proliferation (19). For some time, the terms CD28 and the costimulatory receptor were considered synonymous by some, but the demonstration that robust T-cell activation occurs in CD28-deficient mice indicated that other receptor ligand systems contribute to

signal two (20). In particular the interaction between CD40 expressed upon APCs and CD40 ligand (CD154) expressed by antigen-activated CD4+ T cells has received great attention as a potent second signal (21). The delivery of the antigenic first signal and the costimulatory second signal leads to stable transcription of the IL-2, several T-cell growth factor receptors, and other pivotal T-cell activation genes (Table 96-2). The Ca^{2+}-independent costimulatory CD28 pathway is resistant to inhibition by cyclosporine or FK-506 as compared to the calcium-dependent pathway of T-cell activation. In contrast, recognition of B7 proteins by CTLA-4, a protein primarily expressed on activated T cells, stimulates a negative signal to T cells. This signal is a prerequisite for peripheral T-cell tolerance (22).

The formulation that full T-cell activation is dependent on the costimulatory signal as well as the antigenic signal is most significant, as T-cell molecules responsible for costimulation and their cognate receptors on the surface of APCs then represent target molecules for the regulation of the antiallograft response. Indeed, transplantation tolerance has been induced in experimental models by targeting a variety of cell-surface molecules that contribute to the generation of costimulatory signals.

Interleukin-2/Interleukin-15 Stimulated T-Cell Proliferation

Autocrine type of T-cell proliferation occurs as a consequence of the T-cell activation-dependent production of IL-2 and the expression of multimeric high affinity IL-2 receptors on T cells (Fig. 96-2) formed by the noncovalent association of three IL-2 binding peptides (α, β, γ) (12,23–25). IL-15 is a paracrine-type T-cell growth factor family member with very similar overall structural and identical T-cell stimulatory qualities to IL-2 (12). The IL-2 and IL-15 receptor complexes share β and γ chains which are expressed in low abundance upon resting T cells; expression of these genes is amplified in activated T cells. The α-chain receptor components of the IL-2 and IL-15 receptor complexes are distinct and expressed upon activated, but not resting, T cells. The intracytoplasmic domains of the IL-2 receptor β and γ chains are required for intracellular signal transduction. The ligand-activated, but not resting, IL-2/IL-15 receptors are associated with intracellular PTKs (12,26–28). Raf-1, a protein serine/threonine kinase that is prerequisite to IL-2/IL-15–triggered cell proliferation, associates with the intracellular domain of the shared β chain (29). Translocation of IL-2 receptor-bound Raf-1 serine/threonine kinase into the cytosol requires IL-2/IL-15–stimulated PTK activity. The ligand-activated common γ chain recruits a member of the Janus kinase family, Jak 3, to the receptor complex that leads to activation of a member of the STAT family. Activation of this particular Jak-STAT pathway is prerequisite for proliferation of antigen-activated T cells. The subsequent events leading to IL-2/IL-15–dependent proliferation are not fully resolved; however, IL-2/IL-15–stimulated expression of several DNA binding proteins including bcl-2, c-jun, c-fos, and c-myc contributes to cell-cycle progression (30,31). It is interesting and probably significant that IL-2, but not IL-15, triggers apoptosis of many antigen-activation T cells. In this way, IL-15–triggered events are more detrimental to the allograft response than IL-2. As IL-15 is not produced by T-cells, IL-15 expression is not regulated by cyclosporine or FK-506.

Immunobiology and Molecular Diagnosis of Rejection

The net consequence of cytokine production and acquisition of cell-surface receptors for these transcellular molecules is the emergence of antigen-specific and graft-destructive T cells (Fig. 96-1). Cytokines also facilitate the humoral arm of immunity by promoting the production of cytopathic antibodies. Moreover, IFN-γ and tumor necrosis factor-α (TNF-α) can amplify the ongoing immune response by upregulating the expression of HLA molecules as well as costimulatory molecules (e.g., B7) on graft parenchymal cells and APCs (Fig. 96-1). We and others have demonstrated the presence of antigen-specific cytotoxic T lymphocytes (CTL) and anti-HLA antibodies during or preceding a clinical rejection episode (32,33). We have detected messenger RNA (mRNA) encoding the CTL-selective serine protease (granzyme B) perforin, and Fas-ligand attack molecules and immunoregulatory cytokines, such as IL-10 and IL-15, in human renal allografts undergoing acute rejection (reviewed in reference 34). Indeed these gene-expression events can anticipate clinically apparent rejection. More recent efforts to develop a noninvasive method for the molecular diagnosis of rejection have proved rewarding. Using either peripheral blood (35) or urinary leukocytes (36) rejection-related, gene-expression events evident in renal biopsy specimens are also detected in peripheral blood or urinary sediment specimens. We suspect that a noninvasive, molecular diagnostic-approach rejection may prove pivotal toward detection of insidious, clinically silent rejection episodes that, although rarely detected through standard measures, are steroid-sensitive but usually lead to chronic rejection (37).

Immunopharmacology of Allograft Rejection

The Calcineurin Inhibitors: Cyclosporine and Tacrolimus (FK-506)

Cyclosporine, a small cyclic fungal peptide, and FK-506, a macrolide antibiotic, block the Ca^{2+}-dependent antigen triggered T-cell activation (signal one) (38) (Fig. 96-2). The immunosuppressive effects of cyclosporine and FK-506 are dependent on the formation of a heterodimeric complex that consists of the native compound (cyclosporine or FK-506) and its respective cytoplasmic receptor "immunophilin" proteins, cyclophilin and FK binding protein (FKBP). Cyclosporine–cyclophilin and FK-506/FKBP complexes bind to calcineurin and inhibit its phosphatase activity (Table 96-3).

TABLE 96-3. *Mechanisms of action of immunosuppressants*

Immunosuppressant	Subcellular site(s) of action
Azathioprine	Inhibits purine synthesis
Corticosteroids	Blocks cytokine gene expression
CsA/tacrolimus	Blocks Ca^{2+}-dependent T-cell activation pathway via binding to calcineurin
Mycophenolate mofetil	Inhibits inosine monophosphate dehydrogenase and prevents *de novo* guanosine and deoxyguanosine synthesis in lymphocytes
Sirolimus	Blocks IL-2 and other growth factor signal transduction; blocks CD28-mediated costimulatory signals

CsA, cyclosporin A; *IL*, interleukin

The inhibition of the enzymatic activity of calcineurin is central to the immunosuppressive effects of cyclosporine and FK-506.

Since the phosphorylation status of transcription factors may alter their intracellular localization, it is interesting that cyclosporine/FK-506 inhibition of phosphatase activity of calcineurin apparently interferes with the dephosphorylation of cytoplasmic NF-AT and its subsequent import into the nucleus. The phosphorylation status of transcription factors can also affect their DNA binding ability and interaction with the rest of the transcriptional machinery. For example, the DNA binding activities of c-jun increase on dephosphorylation. Also, cyclosporine inhibits the expression of not only NF-AT but other DNA binding proteins such as NF-κB and AP-1 (39).

Blockade of cytokine gene activation does not totally account for the antiproliferative effect of cyclosporine and FK-506. It is significant that cyclosporine, in striking contrast to its inhibitory activity on the induced expression of IL-2, enhances the expression of transforming growth factor-β (TGF-β) (40). Because TGF-β is a potent inhibitor of T-cell proliferation and generation of antigen-specific CTL (41), heightened expression of TGF-β must contribute to the antiproliferative/immunosuppressive activity of cyclosporine. This novel effect of cyclosporine also suggests a mechanism for some of the complications (e.g., renal fibrosis and tumor metastasis) of therapy with cyclosporine because TGF-β is a fibrogenic and proangiogenic cytokine.

Glucocorticosteroids

Glucocorticosteroids inhibit T-cell proliferation, T-cell–dependent immunity, and cytokine gene transcription (including IL-1, IL-2, IL-6, IFN-γ, and TNF-α genes) (42–44). While no single cytokine can reverse the inhibitory effects of corticosteroids on mitogen-stimulated T-cell proliferation, a combination of cytokines is effective (45). The glucocorticoid and glucocorticoid-receptor bimolecular complex block IL-2 gene transcription via impairment of the cooperative effect of several DNA binding proteins (46). Corticosteroids also inhibit formation of free NF-κB, a DNA binding protein required for cytokine and other T-cell activation gene expression events (47) (Fig. 96-1 and Table 96-3).

Azathioprine

A thioguanine derivative of 6-mercaptopurine (48), azathioprine is a purine analog that acts as a purine antagonist and functions as an effective antiproliferative agent (Fig. 96-1 and Table 96-3) (48,49).

Mycophenolate Mofetil

Mycophenolate mofetil (MMF) is a semisynthetic derivative of mycophenolic acid. It inhibits allograft rejection in rodents, diminishes proliferation of T and B lymphocytes, decreases generation of cytotoxic T cells, and suppresses antibody formation (50–52). MMF inhibits inosine monophosphate dehydrogenase (IMPDH), an enzyme in the *de novo* pathway of purine synthesis. Lymphocytes are dependent upon this biosynthetic pathway to satisfy their guanosine requirements (Table 96-3) (reviewed in reference 52). Early clinical trials have utilized MMF to replace azathioprine in the cyclosporine- and steroid-based immunosuppressive regimen. These controlled, prospective trials have shown a diminished incidence of early acute rejection episodes (52–54). Follow-up studies over a 3-year period have indicated an advantage for MMF over azathioprine (54).

Sirolimus (Rapamycin)

Rapamycin (55–57) is a macrocyclic lactone isolated from *Streptomyces hygroscopicus* that, like FK-506, binds to FKBP. However, rapamycin and FK-506 affect different and distinctive sites in the signal transduction pathway (Fig. 96-2 and Table 96-3). Whereas rapamycin blocks IL-2 and other growth factor-mediated signal transduction, FK-506 (or cyclosporine) has no such capacity. Also, the rapamycin/FKBP complex, unlike the FK-506/FKBP complex, does not bind calcineurin. The antiproliferative activity of the rapamycin/FKBP complex is linked to blockade of the activation of the 70-kd S6 protein kinases and blockade of expression of the bcl-2 proto-oncogene. Rapamycin also blocks the Ca^{2+}-independent CD28-induced costimulatory pathway. Substitution of rapamycin for azathioprine in a triple therapy regimen reduced the frequency and severity of acute rejection (58).

Immunosuppressive Regimens

The basic immunosuppressive protocol used in most transplant centers involves the use of at least two and often three drugs, each directed at a discrete site in the T-cell activation cascade (Fig. 96-1) and each with distinct side effects. While cyclosporin A (CsA) plus MMF plus glucocorticoids is the most widely used regimen, there are several popular variations of the basic calcineurin inhibitor-based triple drug protocol. A calcineurin free nonnephrotoxic regimen consisting of rapamycin, MMF, and glucocorticosteroids has also been developed and may have merit for use in recipients at high risk for delayed graft function (59).

Many centers employ a sequential immunosuppressive protocol. Monoclonal anti–T-cell (OKT3) or polyclonal antilymphocyte antibodies are used as induction therapy for 10 to 14 days in the immediate posttransplant period, thereby establishing an immunosuppressive umbrella that enables early engraftment without immediate use of cyclosporine during the early posttransplant period. During this critical period, the graft is particularly vulnerable to CsA/FK-506-induced nephrotoxic effects. The incidence of early rejection episodes is reduced by the prophylactic use of antilymphocyte antibodies. This protocol is particularly beneficial for patients at high risk for immunologic graft failure (e.g., broadly presensitized or retransplant patients). The efficacy of the polyclonal antilymphocyte antibody preparation (e.g., thymoglobulin) or mAbs (e.g., OKT3) in preventing rejection is impressive, but profound lymphopenia and an increase in the incidence of opportunistic infections and lymphoma results. Because of selective targeting of IL-2R+ T cells, anti-CD25 mAb treatment might be safer than treatment with thymoglobulin or anti–T-cell mAbs. Insofar as activated but not resting T cells express the IL-2 receptor α chain, anti-CD25 mAbs are employed as humanized (60,61) or chimeric (62,63) mAbs to selectively target and destroy alloreactive T cells. These efforts are based on successful exploration and application of IL-2–receptor targeted therapy in preclinical models (64). Human anti-IL-2–receptor α mAbs are being explored as replacements for OKT3 (which targets both resting and activated T cells) or polyclonal antilymphocyte antibodies in a sequential immunosuppressive protocol. Preliminary results with a low dose tacrolimus and sirolimus protocol (65) may prove to rival the current sequential immune therapy regimens for use in patients at high risk to reject an allograft.

Immunologic considerations, including antirejection therapy, are organized around a few general principles. The first consideration is careful patient preparation and, in the circumstance of living donor renal transplantation, selection of the best available ABO-compatible HLA match in the event that several potential living related donors are available for organ donation. Second is a multitiered approach to immunosuppressive therapy similar in principle to that used in chemotherapy; several agents are used simultaneously, each of which is directed at a different molecular target within the allograft response (Fig. 96-1 and Table 96-3). Additive/synergistic effects are achieved through application of each agent at a relatively low dose, thereby limiting the toxicity of each individual agent while increasing the total immunosuppressive effect. Third is the principle that higher immunosuppressive drug doses and/or more individual immunosuppressive drugs are required to gain early engraftment

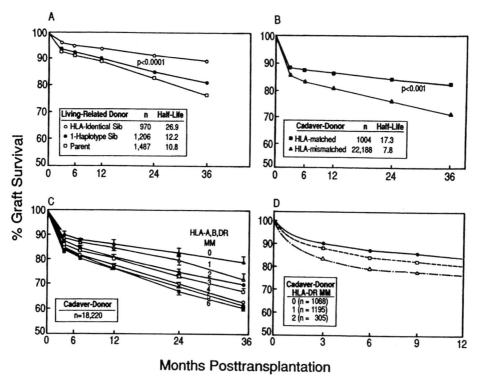

FIG. 96-4. Impact of human leukocyte antigen (HLA) matching on renal allograft survival rates. **A:** The effect of haplotype matching in living related renal transplantation (68). **B:** The superior results found with HLA-matched (A, B, and DR antigens) cadaveric renal grafts compared with HLA-mismatched cadaveric renal grafts (70). **C:** The impact of different levels of HLA-A, B, and DR mismatching on the survival of cadaveric grafts (72). **D:** The stepwise improvement in the survival of cadaveric grafts following matching for the HLA-DR antigens identified by DNA typing (number of DR mismatches: ●—●: 0;———: 1; ●—△—●: 2.) (75).

and to treat established rejection than are needed to maintain immunosuppression in the long term. Hence, intensive induction and lower dose maintenance drug protocols are used. Fourth is careful investigation of each episode of posttransplant graft dysfunction, with the realization that most of the common causes of graft dysfunction, including rejection, can (and often do) coexist. Successful therapy, therefore, often involves several simultaneous therapeutic maneuvers. Fifth is the appropriate reduction or withdrawal of an immunosuppressive drug when that drug's toxicity exceeds its therapeutic benefit.

HLA and Renal Transplantation

The genes that code for the HLA antigens are lodged within the short arm of chromosome 6 (66,67). The class I proteins, HLA-A, B, and C antigens, are composed of a 41-kd polymorphic chain linked noncovalently to a 12-kd β_2-microglobulin chain that is encoded in chromosome 15. The class I molecules are expressed by all nucleated cells and platelets. The class II molecules, HLA-DR, DP, and DQ, are composed of an α chain of 34 kd and a β chain of 29 kd. MHC class II molecules are constitutively expressed on the surface of B cells, monocytes/macrophages, and dendritic cells. Additional lymphoid cells such as T cells and many nonlymphoid

cells such as renal tubular epithelial cells express class II proteins only on stimulation with cytokines.

The clinical benefits of HLA matching are readily appreciable in the recipients of renal grafts from living related donors. An analysis of the United Network for Organ Sharing (UNOS) scientific renal transplant registry data has revealed that the 1-year graft survival rate is 94% in recipients of two haplotype-matched, HLA-identical kidneys. It is 89% and 90%, respectively, when a one haplotype-matched parent or sibling is the donor (68). (Fig. 96-4A). The Collaborative Transplant Study, an international study that draws on 305 transplant centers located in 47 countries for data, has also demonstrated that the survival rate of HLA-identical transplants is superior to that of one-haplotype-matched grafts, even in the cyclosporine era (69).

The advantage of HLA-matching is maintained beyond the first year of transplantation. UNOS registry data (68) show estimated half-lives (the time needed for 50% of the grafts functioning at 1 year post-transplantation to fail) of 26.9 years for HLA-identical grafts and 12.2 years and 10.8 years for one-haplotype-matched sibling grafts and parental grafts, respectively. Data from the Collaborative Transplant Study, comprising 22,414 living related grafts, have also revealed a substantial long-term benefit (69) of HLA matching in recipients of living related grafts.

The effect of matching for HLA in cadaveric graft recipients has been examined in a prospective U.S. study (70) in which kidneys were shared nationally on the basis of matching for HLA-A, B, and DR antigens. All transplantation centers in the United States participated in this study. The 1-year graft survival rate was 88% for HLA-matched kidneys and 79% for HLA-mismatched kidneys (Fig. 96-4B). Moreover, the benefit of HLA matching persisted beyond the first year posttransplantation; the estimated half-life of the HLA-matched renal graft was 17.3 years and that of HLA-mismatched renal allografts, 7.8 years.

Since the inception of the U.S. national kidney sharing program in 1987, more than 7,500 cadaveric kidneys have been distributed to transplantation centers located in 48 states, and a recent analysis confirmed and extended the observation that HLA-matched transplants have a superior outcome compared to HLA-mismatched transplants (71). The estimated 10-year rate of cadaveric graft survival was 52% for HLA-matched transplants and was 37% for HLA-mismatched transplants. Furthermore, the incidence of rejection was lower in HLA-matched transplants compared to mismatched ones. Interestingly, the mean duration of cold-ischemia time of nationally shared kidneys was not that different from locally transplanted kidneys; it was 23 hours compared to 22 hours for nonshared kidneys (71).

A stepwise increase in the survival rate of cadaveric renal allografts has also been documented with increasing levels of HLA-A, B, and DR antigen matching (Fig. 96-4C). The improvement in the graft survival rate following HLA matching is more apparent when matching is based on better resolved HLA antigens (HLA split antigens) than when based on broad HLA antigens; the improvement in the graft survival rate between the best-matched and the worst-matched grafts increases with time (72). In the UNOS registry data, the difference in the graft survival rate between the best-matched and worst-matched recipient was 10% at 1-year posttransplantation, and this difference increased to 18% by 3-years posttransplantation. The Collaborative Transplant Study of more than 67,000 primary cadaver grafts has also demonstrated a significant correlation between the number of HLA mismatches and graft loss (69).

A threshold level of HLA matching might exist: Allografts that are matched for four or more HLA antigens (or two or less HLA mismatches) have a superior short- as well as long-term outcome compared to less than four HLA antigen matches (or greater than two antigen mismatches) (72). It is noteworthy that the beneficial effect of different degrees of matching/mismatching for the HLA-A, B, and DR antigens (73), with the exception of phenotypically identical HLA transplants, is more evident in white recipients as compared to black recipients of cadaveric renal allografts (68,72).

The impact of each of the HLA loci, HLA-A locus, HLA-B locus, and HAL-DR locus, on renal allograft outcome has been investigated. Each locus impacts graft outcome. In the Collaborative Transplant Study, the influence of HLA-DR mismatches was greater than that of HLA-A or HLA-B mismatches in the first year following transplantation; with increased posttransplantation time, mismatches at any of the three loci impacted adversely on graft survival rates (69).

Molecular techniques for the finer resolution of the HLA system hold considerable promise (74). However, existing molecular methodologies have already helped resolve the discrepancies associated with the serologic identification of the HLA-DR antigens. The clinical advantage of molecular matching is suggested by the observation that the 1-year cadaveric renal graft survival rate is 87% in patients who receive kidneys that are HLA-DR identical not only by the serologic methods but also by molecular methods (DNA-RFLP method). This figure drops to 69% for patients who receive kidneys that are not HLA-DR identical by the molecular methodology (75). Application of molecular techniques for the identification of HLA-DR antigens has also resulted in the appreciation of a stepwise increase in the survival of cadaveric renal allografts matched for zero, one, or two HLA-DR antigens (Fig. 96-4D) (69,74). Molecular typing has also been used to detect mismatches at the HLA-A or HLA-B locus. Mismatches that were missed by conventional serologic techniques but identified by molecular techniques were found to adversely impact graft survival (69).

Current data suggest minimal impact of matching for HLA-C locus antigens. Matching for the HLA-DP antigen, on the other hand, appears to be important in repeat but not primary grafts (69).

Crossmatch

Crossmatches, testing of recipient's serum for antibodies reacting with the donor's HLA antigens, must be performed prior to renal transplantation. The standard crossmatch test consists of incubating the serum from the recipient with the donor's lymphocytes in the presence of rabbit serum as a source of complement.

The presence in the recipient's serum of cytotoxic antibodies directed at the donor's class I antigen (positive T-cell crossmatch) is an absolute contraindication to transplantation because 80% to 90% of transplants performed in the presence of a positive crossmatch are subject to hyperacute rejection (76). The sensitivity of the standard crossmatch test has been increased by the addition of sublytic concentrations of anti-human globulin (AHG) to the test system. The graft survival rate is about 5% lower in recipients with a positive AHG test compared to recipients with a negative AHG test (77).

The significance of antibodies reacting with the donor's class II antigens (positive B-cell crossmatch) is not fully resolved. A survival disadvantage, 7% in primary transplants and 15% in repeat transplants, however has been noted in recipients with a positive B-cell crossmatch (77).

A number of centers are currently evaluating the usefulness of flow cytometry-based methodology to detect donor-specific antibodies. Flow cytometry crossmatches permit detection of low, sublytic concentrations of complement fixing as well as noncomplement-fixing antibodies. The clinical impact of a positive flow cytometry crossmatch is currently being analyzed. In the UNOS kidney transplant registry data (78), a positive flow cytometry crossmatch was associated with an increased incidence of early graft dysfunction requiring dialytic support, primary nonfunction of the allograft, prolonged hospitalization, and a greater incidence of allograft rejection. The negative impact of a flow cytometry crossmatch was greater in repeat transplants compared to primary transplants. Whereas a positive flow crossmatch was associated with a 5% decrease in the 3-year survival rate of primary grafts, a 19% decrease was observed in the 3-year survival of repeat grafts. In primary transplants, a T+B+ flow cytometry crossmatch and a T−B+ crossmatch had a similar outcome (76% 3-year graft survival rate versus 74%), and in repeat transplants a T+B+ flow cytometry crossmatch has a much inferior outcome compared to a T−B+ crossmatch (60% 3-year graft survival rate versus 73%).

TRANSPLANTATION TOLERANCE

Transplantation tolerance can be defined as an inability of the organ graft recipient to express a graft destructive immune response. While this statement does not restrict either the mechanistic basis or the quantitative aspects of immune unresponsiveness of the host, true tolerance is antigen-specific, induced as a consequence of prior exposure to the specific antigen, and is not dependent on the continuous administration of exogenous nonspecific immunosuppressants.

A classification of tolerance on the basis of the mechanisms involved, site of induction, extent of tolerance, and the cell primarily tolerized is provided in Table 96-4. Induction strategies for the creation of peripheral tolerance are listed in Table 96-5.

Several hypotheses, not necessarily mutually exclusive and at times even complementary, have been proposed for the cellular basis of tolerance. Data from several laboratories support the following mechanistic possibilities for the

TABLE 96-4. *Classification of tolerance*

A. Based on the major mechanism involved
 1. Clonal deletion
 2. Clonal energy
 3. Suppression
B. Based on the period of induction
 1. Fetal
 2. Neonatal
 3. Adult
C. Based on the cell tolerized
 1. T cell
 2. B cell
D. Based on the extent of tolerance
 1. Complete
 2. Partial, including split
E. Based on the main site of induction
 1. Central
 2. Peripheral

TABLE 96-5. *Potential approaches for the creation of tolerance*

A. Cell depletion protocols
 1. Whole body irradiation
 2. Total lymphoid irradiation
 3. Panel of monoclonal antibodies
B. Reconstitution protocols
 1. Allogeneic bone marrow cells with or without T-cell depletion
 2. Syngeneic bone marrow cells
C. Combination of strategies A and B
D. Cell-surface molecule targeted therapy
 1. Anti-CD4 mAbs
 2. Anti-ICAM-1 + anti-LFA-1 mAbs
 3. Anti-CD3 mAbs
 4. Anti-CD2 mAbs
 5. Anti-IL-2 receptor α (CD25) mAbs
 6. CTLA4Ig fusion protein
 7. Anti-CD40L mAbs
E. Drugs
 1. Azathioprine
 2. Cyclosporine
 3. Rapamycin
F. Additional approaches
 1. Donor-specific blood transfusions with concomitant mAb or drug therapy
 2. Intrathymic inoculation of cells/antigens
 3. Oral administration of cells/antigens

creation of a tolerant state: clonal deletion, clonal anergy, and immunoregulation.

Clonal Deletion

Clonal deletion is a process by which self–antigen-reactive cells, especially those with high affinity for the self-antigens, are eliminated from the organism's immune repertoire. This process is called central tolerance. In the case of T cells, this process takes place in the thymus, and the death of immature T cells is considered to be the ultimate result of high-affinity interactions between a T cell with productively rearranged TCR and the thymic nonlymphoid cells, including dendritic cells that express the self-MHC antigen. This purging of the immune repertoire of self-reactive T cells is termed negative selection and is distinguished from the positive selection process responsible for the generation of the T-cell repertoire involved in the recognition of foreign antigens in the context of self-MHC molecules. Clonal deletion or at least marked depletion of mature T cells as a consequence of apoptosis can also occur in the periphery (reviewed in reference 79). The form of graft tolerance occurring as a consequence of mixed hematopoietic chimerism entails massive deletion of alloreactive clones (80). Tolerance to renal allografts has been achieved in patients that have accepted a bone marrow graft from the same donor (81,82). It is interesting that IL-2, the only T-cell growth factor that triggers T-cell proliferation as well as apoptosis, is an absolute prerequisite for the acquisition of organ graft tolerance through use of nonlymphoablative treatment regimens (83,84). Tolerance achieved under these circumstances also involves additional mechanisms, including clonal anergy and suppressor mechanisms (85–87).

Clonal Anergy

Clonal anergy refers to a process in which the antigen-reactive cells are functionally silenced. The cellular basis for the hyporesponsiveness resides in the anergic cell itself, and the current data suggest that the anergic T cells fail to express the T-cell growth factor, IL-2, and other crucial T-cell activation genes because of defects in the antigen-stimulated signaling pathway.

T-cell clonal anergy can result from suboptimal antigen-driven signaling of T cells, as mentioned earlier. The full activation of T cells requires at least two signals, one signal generated via the TCR/CD3 complex, and the second (costimulatory) signal initiated/delivered by the APCs. Stimulation of T cells via the TCR/CD3 complex alone—provision of signal 1 without signal 2 —can result in T-cell anergy/paralysis (Fig. 96-5 and Table 96-2).

B-cell activation, in a fashion analogous to T-cell activation, requires at least two signals. One signal is initiated via the B-cell antigen receptor immunoglobulin, and a costimulatory signal is provided by cytokines or cell surface proteins of T-cell origin. Thus, delivery of the antigenic signal alone to the B cells without the instructive cytokines or T-cell help can lead to B-cell anergy and tolerance.

Immunoregulatory (Suppressor) Mechanisms

Antigen-specific T or B cells are physically present and are functionally competent in tolerant states resulting from suppressor mechanisms. The cytopathic and antigen-specific cells are restrained by the suppressor cells or factors or express noncytopathic cellular programs. Each of the major subsets of T cells, the CD4 T cells and the CD8 T cells, has been implicated in mediating suppression. Indeed, a cascade involving MHC antigen-restricted T cells, MHC antigen-unrestricted T cells, and their secretory products have been reported to collaborate to mediate suppression. At least four distinct mechanisms have been advanced to explain the cellular basis for suppression:

1. An antiidiotypic regulatory mechanism in which the idiotype of the TCR of the original antigen-responsive T cells functions as an immunogen and elicits an antiidiotypic response. The elicited antiidiotypic regulatory cells, in turn, prevent the further responses of the idiotype-bearing cells to the original sensitizing stimulus.
2. The veto process by which recognition by alloreactive T cells of alloantigen-expressing veto cells results in the targeted killing (veto process) of the original alloreactive T cells by the veto cells.
3. Immune deviation, a shift in CD4+ T-cell programs away from Th1-type (IL-2, IFN-γ expressing) toward the Th2-type (IL-4, IL-10 expressing) program.
4. The production of suppressor factors or cytokines. For example, the production of TGF-β by myelin basic protein-specific CD8 T cells or other cytokines with antiproliferative properties. The process leading to full tolerance is infectious. Tolerant T cells recruit nontolerant T cells into the tolerant state (86). The tolerant state also establishes a condition in which foreign tissues housed in the same microenvironment as the specific antigen to which the host has been tolerized are protected from rejection (86). Tolerance is a multistep process (85–87).

Clearly more than one mechanism is operative in the induction of tolerance (Fig. 96-5). The tolerant state is not an all-or-nothing phenomenon but is one that has several gradations. Of the mechanisms proposed for tolerance, clonal deletion might be of greater importance in the creation of self-tolerance, and clonal anergy and immunoregulatory mechanisms might be more applicable to transplantation tolerance. More recent data suggest both clonal depletion and immunoregulatory mechanisms are needed to create and sustain central or peripheral tolerance. From a practical viewpoint, a nonimmunogenic allograft (e.g., located in an

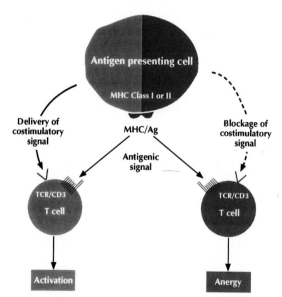

FIG. 96-5. T-cell activation/anergy decision points. Several potential sites for the regulation of T-cell signaling are shown. The antigenic peptide displayed by major histocompatibility complex (MHC) (**site 1**), costimulatory signals (**site 2**), T-cell antigen receptor (TCR) (**site 3**), and cytokine signaling (**site 4**) can influence the eventual outcome. Altered peptide ligands, blockade of costimulatory signals, downregulation of TCR, and interleukin (IL)-10 favor anergy induction, whereas fully immunogenic peptides, delivery of costimulatory signals, appropriate number of TCRs, and IL-12 prevent anergy induction and facilitate full activation of T cells. (From Suthanthiran M. Transplantation tolerance: fooling mother nature. *Proc Natl Acad Sci USA* 1996;93:12072.)

immunologically privileged site or physically isolated from the immune system) might also be "tolerated" by an immunocompetent organ-graft recipient.

Authentic tolerance has been difficult to identify in human renal allograft recipients. Nevertheless, the clinical examples, albeit infrequent, of grafts functioning without any exogenous immunosuppressive drugs (either due to noncompliance of the patient or due to discontinuation of drugs for other medical reasons) do suggest that some long-term recipients of allografts develop tolerance to the transplanted organ and accept the allografts. The recent progress in our understanding of the immunobiology of graft rejection and tolerance and the potential to apply molecular approaches to the bedside hold significant promise for the creation of a clinically relevant tolerant state and transplantation without exogenous immunosuppressants—the cherished goal of the clinician specializing in transplant procedures.

CONCLUSION

Successful renal transplantation represents the fruition of the dedicated efforts of basic scientists, clinicians, and allied personnel. An excellent paradigm for the effective application of knowledge gained by basic research to the alleviation of life-threatening illness, renal transplantation also affords marvelous opportunities for the investigation of the systemic basis for renal disease independent of organ-specific mechanisms. In the near future, one can anticipate clinical application of synergistic therapeutic protocols that target discrete steps in antigen recognition, signal transduction, and effector immunity. Finally, the ultimate prize of transplantation would be that the basic principles learned would facilitate the prevention of the disease that necessitated transplantation in the first place.

Acknowledgments

The authors are grateful to Ms. Frances Pechenick and Ms. Linda Stackhouse for their meticulous help in the preparation of this chapter.

REFERENCES

1. Suthanthiran M, Strom TB. Renal transplantation. N Engl J Med 1994; 334:365.
2. Dustin ML, Cooper JA. The immunological synapse and the actin cytoskeleton: molecular hardware for T cell signaling. Nature Immunol 2000;1:23.
3. Unanue ER, Cerottini JC. Antigen presentation. FASEB J 1989;3:2496.
4. Germain RN. MHC-dependent antigen processing and peptide presentation: providing ligands for T lymphocyte activation. Cell 1994;76:287.
5. Acuto O, Cantrell D. T cell activation and the cytoskeleton Annu Rev Immunol 2000;18:165.
6. Shoskes DA, Wood KJ. Indirect presentation of MHC antigens in transplantation. Immunol Today 1994;15:32.
7. Jorgensen JL, Reay PA, Ehrich EW, et al. Molecular components of T-cell recognition. Annu Rev Immunol 1992;10:835.
8. Suthanthiran M. A novel model for the antigen-dependent activation of normal human T cells: transmembrane signaling by crosslinkage of the CD3/T cell receptor-alpha/beta complex with the cluster determinant 2 antigen. J Exp Med 1990;171:1965.
9. Brown MH, et al. The CD2 antigen associates with the T-cell antigen receptor CD3 antigen complex on the surface of human T lymphocytes. Nature 1989;339:551.
10. Beyers AD, Spruyt LL, Williams AF. Molecular associations between the T-lymphocyte antigen receptor complex and the surface antigens CD2, CD4, or CD8 and CD5. Proc Natl Acad Sci USA 1992;89:2945.
11. Nishizuka Y. Intracellular signaling by hydrolysis of phospholipids and activation of protein kinase C. Science 1992;258:607.
12. Waldmann T, Tagaya Y, Bamford R. Interleukin-2, interleukin-15, and their receptors. Int Rev Immunol 1998;16:205.
13. O'Keefe SJ, et al. FK506- and CsA-sensitive activation of the IL-2 promoter by calcineurin. Nature 1992;357:692.
14. Clipstone NA, Crabtree GR. Identification of calcineurin as a key signalling enzyme in T-lymphocyte activation. Nature 1992;357:695.
15. Liu J, et al. Calcineurin is a common target of cyclophilin-cyclosporin A and FKBP-FK506 complexes. Cell 1991;66:807.
16. Schwartz RH. T cell anergy. Sci Am 1993;269:62.
17. Suthanthiran M. Signaling features of T cells: implication for the regulation of the anti-allograft response. Kidney Int Suppl 1993;43:S3.
18. Dustin ML, Springer TA. T-cell receptor cross-linking transiently stimulates adhesiveness through LFA-1. Nature 1989;341:619.
19. Lenschow DJ, Walunas TL, Bluestone JA. CD28/B7 system of T cell costimulation. Annu Rev Immunol 1996;14:233.
20. Shahinian A, Pfeffer K, Lee KP, et al. Differential T cell costimulatory requirements in CD28-deficient mice. Science 1993;261:609.
21. Noelle RJ. CD40 and its ligand in host defense. Immunity 1996;4:415.
22. Oosterwegel MA, Greenwald RJ, Mandelbrot DA, et al. CTLA-4 and T cell activation. Curr Opin Immunol 1999;11:294.
23. Smith KA. Interleukin-2: inception, impact, and implications. Science 1988;240:1169.
24. Waldman TA. The interleukin-2 receptor. J Biol Chem 1991;266:2681.
25. Takeshita T, Asao H, Ohtani K. Cloning of the gamma chain of the human IL-2 receptor. Science 1992;257:379.
26. Hatakeyama M, et al. Interaction of the IL-2 receptor with the src-family kinase p56^{lck}: identification of novel intermolecular association. Science 1991;252:1523.
27. Fung MR, et al. A tyrosine kinase physically associates with the alpha-subunit of the human IL-2 receptor. J Immunol 1991;147:1253.
28. Remillard B, et al. Interleukin-2 receptor regulates activation of phosphatidylinositol 3-kinase. J Biol Chem 1991;266:14167.
29. Maslinski W, Remillard B, Tsudo M, et al. Interleukin-2 (IL-2) induces tyrosine kinase-dependent translocation of active Raf-1 from the IL-2 receptor into the cytosol. J Biol Chem 1992;267:15281.
30. Shibuya H, et al. IL-2 and EGF receptors stimulate the hematopoietic cell cycle via different signaling pathways: demonstration of a novel role for c-myc. Cell 1992;70:57.
31. Taniguchi T. Cytokine signalling through non-receptor protein tyrosine kinases. Science 1995;260:251.
32. Strom TB, Tilney NL, Carpenter CB, et al. Identity and cytotoxic capacity of cells infiltrating renal allografts. N Engl J Med 1975;292:1257.
33. Suthanthiran M, Garovoy MR. Immunologic monitoring of the renal transplant recipient. Urol Clin North Am 1983;10:315.
34. Strom TB, Suthanthiran M. Prospects and applicability of molecular diagnosis of allograft rejection. Semin Nephrol 2000;20:103.
35. Vasconcellos LM, Schachter AD, Zheng XX, et al. Cytotoxic lymphocyte gene expression in peripheral blood leukocytes correlates with rejecting renal allografts. Transplantation 1998;66:562.
36. Li B, Hartono C, Ding R, et al. Noninvasive diagnosis of renal-allograft rejection by measurement of messenger RNA for perforin and granzyme B in urine. N Engl J Med 2001;344:947.
37. Rush D, Nickerson P, Gough J, et al. Beneficial effects of treatment of early subclinical rejection: a randomized study. J Am Soc Nephrol 1998;9:2129.
38. Schreiber SL. Immunophilin-sensitive protein phosphatase action in cell signaling pathways. Cell 1992;70:365.
39. Li B, Sehajpal PK, Khanna A, et al. Differential regulation of transforming growth factor beta and interleukin-2 genes in human T cells: demonstration by usage of novel competitor DNA constructs in the quantitative polymerase chain reaction. J Exp Med 1991;174:1259.
40. Sehajpal PK, Sharma VK, Ingulli E, et al. Synergism between the CD3 antigen- and CD2 antigen-derived signals: exploration at the level of

induction of DNA-binding proteins and characterization of the inhibitory activity of cyclosporine. *Transplantation* 1993;55:1118.

41. Kehrl JH, Wakefield LM, Roberts AB, et al. Production of transforming growth factor beta by human T lymphocytes and its potential role in the regulation of T cell growth. *J Exp Med* 1986;163:1037.

42. Knudsen PJ, Dinarello CA, Strom TB. Glucocorticoids inhibit transcriptional and post-transcriptional expression of interleukin-1 in U937 cells. *J Immunol* 1987;139:4129.

43. Zanker B, Walz G, Wieder KJ, et al. Evidence that glucocorticosteroids block expression of the human interleukin-6 gene by accessory cells. *Transplantation* 1990;49:183.

44. Arya SK, Won-Staal J, Gallo RC. Dexamethasone-mediated inhibition of human T cell growth factor and gamma-interferon messenger RNA. *J Immunol* 1984;133:273.

45. Almawi WY, et al. Abrogation of glucocorticosteroid-mediated inhibition of T cell proliferation by the synergistic action of IL-1, IL-6 and IFN-gamma. *J Immunol* 1991;146:3523.

46. Vacca A, et al. Glucocorticoid receptor-mediated suppression of the interleukin-2 gene expression through impairment of the cooperativity between nuclear factor of activated T cells and AP-1 enhancer elements. *J Exp Med* 1992;175:637.

47. Auphan N, DiDonato J, Rosette C, et al. Immunosuppression by glucocorticoids: inhibition of NF-κB activity through induction of IκB synthesis. *Science* 1995;270:286.

48. Elion GB. Biochemistry and pharmacology of purine analogues. *Fed Proc* 1967;26:898.

49. Bach JF, Strom TB. The Mode of action of immunosuppressive agents. In: Bach JF, Strom TB, eds. *Research monographs in immunology.* Amsterdam: Elsevier, 1986:105.

50. Morris RE, Wang J. Comparison of the immunosuppressive effects of mycophenolic acid and the morpholinoethyl ester of mycophenolic acid (RS-61433) in recipients of heart allografts. *Transplant Proc* 1999;23:493.

51. Sweeney MJ. Metabolism and biochemistry of mycophenolic acid. *Cancer Res* 1972;32:1803.

52. Lui SL, Halloran PF. Mycophenolate mofetil in kidney transplantation. *Curr Opin Nephrol Hypertens* 1996;5:508.

53. Sollinger HW and U.S. Renal Transplant Mycophenolate Mofetil Study Group. Mycophenolate mofetil for the prevention of acute rejection in primary cadaveric renal allograft recipients. *Transplantation* 1995; 60:225.

54. European Mycophenolate Mofetil Cooperative Study Group. Mycophenolate mofetil in renal transplantation: 3-year results from the placebo-controlled trial. *Transplantation* 1999;68:391.

55. Morris RE. Rapamycins: antifungal, antitumor, antiproliferative, and immunosuppressive macrolides. *Transplant Rev* 1992;6:39.

56. Chung J, Kuo CJ, Crabtree GR, et al. Rapamycin-FKBP specifically blocks growth-dependent activation of and signaling by the 70-kd 56 protein kinases. *Cell* 1992;69:1227.

57. Kuo CJ, et al. Rapamycin selectively inhibits interleukin-2 activation of p70 56 kinase. *Nature* 1992;358:70.

58. Kahan BD. Efficacy of sirolimus compared with azathioprine for reduction of acute allograft rejection: a randomized multicentre study. *Lancet* 2000;356:194.

59. Kreis H, Cisterne JM, Land W, et al. Sirolimus in association with mycophenolate mofetil induction for the prevention of acute graft rejection in renal allograft recipients. *Transplantation* 2000;69:1252.

60. Vincenti F, Kirkman R, Light S, et al. Interleukin-2 receptor blockade with daclizumab to prevent acute rejection in renal transplantation. Daclizumab Triple Therapy Study Group. *N Engl J Med* 1998;338:161.

61. Ekbergh H, Backman L, Tufveson G, et al. Daclizumab prevents acute rejection and improves patient survival post transplantation: 1 year pooled analysis. *Transplant Int* 2000;13:151.

62. Kahan BD, Rajagopalan PR, Hall M. Reduction of the occurrence of acute cellular rejection among renal allograft recipients treated with basiliximab, a chimeric anti-interleukin-2-receptor monoclonal antibody. United States Simulect Renal Study Group. *Transplantation* 1999; 67:276.

63. Hong JC, Kahan BD. Use of anti-CD25 monoclonal antibody in combination with rapamycin to eliminate cyclosporine treatment during the induction phase of immunosuppression. *Transplantation* 1999;68: 701.

64. Strom TB, et al. Interleukin-2 receptor-directed therapies: antibody- or cytokine-based targeting molecules. *Annu Rev Med* 1993;44:343.

65. McAlister VC, Gao Z, Peltekian K, et al. Sirolimus tacrolimus combination immunosuppression. *Lancet* 2000;355:376.

66. Klein J, Sato A. The HLA system. First of two parts. *N Engl J Med* 2000; 343:702.

67. Klein J, Sato A. The HLA system. Second of two parts. *N Engl J Med* 2000;343:782.

68. Cecka JM, Terasaki PI. The UNOS Scientific Renal Transplant Registry—1991. In: Terasaki PI, Cecka JM, eds. *Clinical transplants 1991.* Los Angeles: UCLA Tissue Typing Laboratory, 1992:1.

69. Opelz G, Wujciak T, Dohler B, et al. HLA compatibility and organ transplant survival. *Rev Immunogen* 1999;1:334.

70. Takemoto S, Terasaki PI, Cecka JM, et al. Survival of nationally shared, HLA-matched kidney transplants from cadaveric donors. *N Engl J Med* 1992;327:834.

71. Takemoto SK, Terasaki PI, Gjertson DW, et al. Twelve years' experience with national sharing of HLS-matched cadaveric kidneys for transplantation. *N Engl J Med* 2000;343:1078.

72. Cicciarelli J, Cho Y. HLA matching: univariate and multivariate analyses of UNOS Registry data. In: Terasaki PI, Cecka JM, eds. *Clinical transplants 1991.* Los Angeles: UCLA Tissue Typing Laboratory, 1992: 325.

73. Terasaki PI, et al. UCLA and UNOS Registries: overview. In: Terasaki PI, Cecka JM, eds. *Clinical transplants 1992.* Los Angeles: UCLA Tissue Typing Laboratory, 1992:409.

74. Opelz G, Wujciak T, Mytilineos J, et al. Revisiting HLA matching for kidney transplants. *Transplant Proc* 1993;25:173.

75. Opelz G, et al. Survival of DNA HLA-DR typed and matched cadaver kidney transplants. *Lancet* 1991;338:461.

76. Williams GM, et al. "Hyperacute" renal-homograft rejection in man. *N Engl J Med* 1968;279:611.

77. Ogura, K. Clinical transplants 1992. In: Terasaki PI, Cecka JM, eds. *Clinical transplants 1992.* Los Angeles: UCLA Tissue Typing Laboratory, 1993:357.

78. Cook DJ, El Fettouh, HIA, Gjertson DW, et al. Flow cytometry crossmatching (FXCM) in the UNOS kidney transplant registry. In: Terasaki PI, Cecka JM, eds. *Clinical transplants 1998.* Los Angeles: UCLA Tissue Typing Laboratory, 1999:413.

79. Van Parijs L, Abbas AK. Homeostasis and self-tolerance in the immune system: turning lymphocytes off. *Science* 1998;280:243.

80. Wekerle T, Sayegh MH, Hill J, et al. Extrathymic T cell deletion and allogeneic stem cell engraftment induced with costimulatory blockade is followed by central T cell tolerance. *J Exp Med* 1998;187:2037.

81. Sayegh MH, Fine NA, Smith JL, et al. Immunologic tolerance to renal allografts after bone marrow transplants from the same donors. *Ann Intern Med* 1991;114:954.

82. Spitzer TR, Delmonico F, Tolkoff-Rubin N, et al. Combined histocompatibility leukocyte antigen-matched donor bone marrow and renal transplantation for multiple myeloma with end stage renal disease: the induction of allograft tolerance through mixed lymphohematopoietic chimerism. *Transplantation* 1999;68:480.

83. Dai Z, Konieczny BT, Baddoura FK, et al. Impaired alloantigen-mediated T cell apoptosis and failure to induce long-term allograft survival in IL-2-deficient mice. *J Immunol* 1998;161:1659.

84. Li Y, Li XC, Zheng XX, et al. Blocking both signal 1 and signal 2 of T-cell activation prevents apoptosis of alloreactive T cells and induction of peripheral allograft tolerance. *Nature Med* 1999;5:1298.

85. Li SC, Wells AD, Strom TB, et al. The role of T cell apoptosis in transplantation tolerance. *Curr Opin Immunol* 2000;12:522.

86. Waldmann H. Transplantation tolerance—where do we stand? *Nature Med* 1999;5:1245.

87. Suthanthiran M. Transplantation tolerance: fooling mother nature. *Proc Natl Acad Sci USA* 1996;93:12072.

CHAPTER 97

Outcomes and Complications of Renal Transplantation

Laurence Chan, Wei Wang, and Igal Kam

Treatment options for patients with end-stage renal disease (ESRD) fall into three broad categories: hemodialysis, peritoneal dialysis, and transplantation. In most developed countries, there is a choice for each patient as to the modality of treatment that best suits the individual. The availability of these different methods of treatment has allowed flexibility in the management of each patient. Since the first successful renal transplantation more than 40 years ago (1), more than 400,000 patients with renal failure have had their lives prolonged with renal allografts (2–4). Renal transplantation has now become a preferred treatment modality for patients with ESRD. However, the number of patients with functioning grafts is still small when compared with the number of patients on maintenance dialysis (Fig. 97-1).

With improved transplantation outcomes, and widespread expectation that renal transplantation will be available, the growth in the number of patients wanting or waiting for a transplant has outpaced the supply of available organs (Fig. 97-2). The United Network for Organ Sharing (UNOS) reported that as of July 2000, 45,600 people on its national patient list were waiting for a kidney. Kidney transplantations are currently being performed in the United States at a rate of about 12,000 per year. The reported average waiting time for a cadaveric kidney transplant is approaching 3 years. More patients are now being considered for living donor kidney transplantation; 30% to 35% of all kidney transplantations performed in the United States are with living donors (Fig. 97-3).

In the United States, Medicare funding was meant to achieve equal access to transplantation and dialysis for all patients with ESRD in the Social Security System by removing the financial barrier to care. There is no doubt that access to dialysis care is reasonably equal; demographic distribution of dialysis reflects the population at large and also seems to match the population in need. However, there are relatively large racial and gender differences regarding kidney transplantation (Table 97-1). In a retrospective analysis of the effect of patient and dialysis unit characteristics on access to kidney transplantation, Held et al. (3) concluded that white, young, nondiabetic men with high incomes treated in a small dialysis unit are more likely to receive a cadaveric kidney than other patients. This is in agreement with a previous report by Kjellstrand (4).

The outcomes of renal transplantation are affected by many variables (Table 97-2). These factors include age, sex, and race of the recipient and the donor; tissue compatibility; prior sensitization to human leukocyte antigen (HLA); original renal disease, pretransplantation health status, and concomitant extrarenal disease of the recipient; compliance of the recipient; donor factors such as cold ischemia time and nephron dosing effect; and the experience of the transplantation center and the nature and extent of immunosuppressive therapy. Each of these factors contributes to some extent to the ultimate outcome of renal transplantation, as assessed by the survival of both the patient and the functioning graft. The short-term outcome has improved substantially in the past 15 years. One-year graft survival for cadaveric donor transplants now approaches 90% in experienced centers, but improvement in long-term graft survival has been more difficult to achieve. It has been empirically observed that after the first year, fractional graft survival over time is linear when plotted logarithmically. The half-lives can be a useful method of analyzing long-term survival. Despite significant improvement in 1-year graft survival between 1972 and 1990, the half-life has shown little improvement. However, in a recent analysis by Hariharan et al. (5) on graft survival for all 93,934 renal transplantations performed in the United States between 1988 and 1996, the 1-year survival rate for grafts from living donors increased from 88.8% to 93.9%, and the rate for cadaveric donor grafts increased from 75.7% to 87.7%. The half-life for grafts from living donors increased steadily from

L. Chan, W. Wang, and I. Kam: Department of Medicine, University of Colorado Health Sciences Center, Denver, Colorado

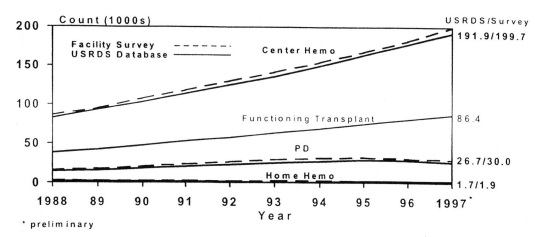

FIG. 97-1. Point prevalence counts of patients with end-stage renal disease by treatment modality, data source, and year, 1988–1997. Percentages include Puerto Rico and U.S. territories. (From United States Renal Data System. *USRDS 1999 annual data report.* Bethesda, MD: National Institutes of Health and National Institute of Diabetes and Digestive and Kidney Diseases, 1999, with permission.)

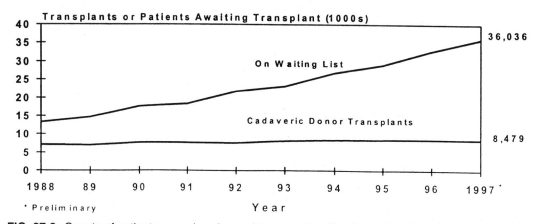

FIG. 97-2. Counts of patients on cadaveric renal transplant waiting list and counts of renal transplants from a cadaveric donor by year, 1989–1997. (United States Renal Data System. *USRDS 1999 annual data report.* Bethesda, MD: National Institutes of Health and National Institute of Diabetes and Digestive and Kidney Diseases, 1999, with permission.)

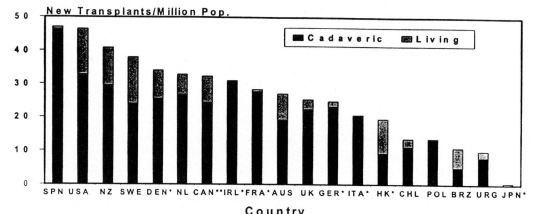

FIG. 97-3. Transplantation rates (count of new renal transplants per million total population) in Australia, New Zealand, Canada, selected European countries, Japan, Hong Kong, Chile, Brazil, Uruguay, and the United States during 1997, by donor type (cadaveric or living donor). (Data from Germany, Denmark, Ireland, France, Hong Kong, and Japan are from 1996.)

TABLE 97-1. *Patients with functioning grafts by sex and race, 1997*

Patient characteristic	No.	ESRD Modality (%) Functioning transplant	Dialysis
Total no. of patients	307,967	(100%)	72%
Male	167,478	(30.8%)	69.2%
Female	140,489	(24.8%)	75.2%
Native American	4,620	(20.7%)	79.3%
Asian/Pacific islander	11,076	(28.8%)	71.2%
Black	97,906	(15.6%)	84.4%
White	188,732	(34.7%)	65.3%
Other/unknown	5,633	(26.2%)	73.8%

Source: From US Renal Data System. *USRDS 1999 Annual data report.* Bethesda, MD: National Institutes of Health and National Institute of Diabetes and Digestive and Kidney Diseases, 1999, with permission.

12.7 to 21.6 years, and that for cadaveric grafts increased from 7.9 to 13.8 years. The improvement is not attributable to any of the newer immunosuppressive drugs, because it occurred in the era of treatment with cyclosporine, azathioprine, and prednisone. With the availability of better therapeutic protocols in the past 10 years, we may expect even better outcome in renal transplantation with better long-term graft and patient survival rates. In the subsequent sections of this chapter, we discuss each of the factors influencing outcome of renal transplantation, the recipient and donor evaluation before transplantation, immunosuppressive drugs, and posttransplantation management and complications.

PATIENT SELECTION AND PRETRANSPLANTATION EVALUATION

General Philosophy in Recipient Selection

Each transplantation center has its own criteria in selecting patients for transplantation. The decision to place a patient on the waiting list for a transplant should be made jointly by the nephrologist and the transplant surgeon. Most patients receive a transplant after undergoing maintenance hemodialysis or, to a lesser extent, peritoneal dialysis. However, many patients undergo transplantations before they require dialysis. Indeed, if the supply of kidneys were to increase, this shortcut would become an increasingly common practice. In general, patients with ESRD should be given the option to choose between

TABLE 97-2. *Factors influencing the outcome of cadaveric renal transplantation*

Immunologic	Nonimmunologic
Immunosuppressive protocol	Delayed graft function/ischemic time
Matching for human leukocyte antigen	Compliance
Sensitization	Cardiovascular disease
Rejection	Recipient age
	Center effect/clinical care
	Nephron dose/donor and recipient sex

TABLE 97-3. *Contraindications to transplantation*

Absolute	Relative
Active infection	Renal disease with high recurrence rate
Disseminated malignancy	Urologic abnormalities
Extensive vascular disease	Active systemic illness
High risk for perioperative mortality	Ongoing substance abuse
Persistent coagulation abnormality	Uncontrolled psychosis
	Refractory noncompliance
Informed patient refusal	

dialysis and transplantation. Patients who have expressed an interest in undergoing kidney transplantation should be fully evaluated by the transplant team as an outpatient during a clinic visit or on an inpatient basis in a few centers.

Criteria for acceptance were more stringent in the past. Today, there are few absolute contraindications to kidney transplantation (6,7), and many of the contraindications are relative (Table 97-3). Successful renal transplantation in Jehovah's Witnesses has also been reported (8). Several medical and immunologic factors of the recipient, however, have been identified with a higher risk of death and graft loss. These include older age, diabetes, and heart disease. These factors are also associated with a higher risk of death in the general population and in patients with ESRD treated by dialysis.

Age

The very young patient (younger than 5 years) and the older adult recipient do have a poorer patient and graft survival rates than patients of ages between these extremes (9–11). This is due to complications of immunosuppressive therapy leading to death or nontransplant-related complications, in particular cardiovascular disease in older adults, leading to death (12–13).

Until recently, patients older than 65 years generally were not considered for transplantation if significant cardiovascular disease was present (14–16). However, the ESRD population is rapidly "graying" (17). There has been a striking change over the past 10 years in the type of patient considered suitable for transplantation. The reluctance to accept transplantation in older patients was previously due to the belief that the perioperative and postoperative complication rates outweighed the advantages. However, with the improvements in perioperative management and immunosuppressive strategies, advanced age itself is no longer a contraindication to renal transplantation. Based on a retrospective analysis of patients from UNOS, it appears that older patients may have better immunologic survival, despite the higher mortality rate from cardiovascular disease (18,19). One explanation may be an age-related change in immunologic function that confers less alloreactivity with aging. For this reason, many centers advocate the use of lower immunosuppression in older adult patients (20).

Transplantation can now be safely and successfully performed in the older adult patient and will become much more widely practiced in this group of patients with end-stage renal failure (21–23).

Obesity

Obesity alone is rarely an absolute contraindication to transplantation, although it is a well-defined risk factor. Lower graft survival rates and more postoperative mortalities and complications have been demonstrated in patients with a body mass index (BMI; weight (kg)/[height (m)]^2) of more than 30 kg/m^2 (24). The large body size is also a risk factor for progression and subsequent premature failure due to the physiologic changes that have been linked to nephron hyperfiltration (25,26). Thus, weight reduction is important for obese patients on dialysis before proceeding to transplantation.

Prior Kidney Transplantation

Renal allograft failure is now one of the most common causes of ESRD, accounting for about 30% of patients awaiting renal transplantation. Graft survival of a second and third kidney transplant has been reported to be inferior to that of the first. Evaluation of a potential recipient for a second or third allograft requires careful attention to the reason for the graft failure (27–30). Factors such as noncompliance with immunosuppressive medications, loss of the graft in association with recurrent renal disease, or high alloreactivity with high panel reactive antibody titers. These patients may also manifest complications of prior immunosuppressive therapy, and as such, they should be screened for complications such as infection and malignancy associated with these medications. No controlled, prospective studies have been performed to determine the best method for tapering or withdrawing immunosuppression after renal allograft failure (31). Most centers have adopted a policy of immediate withdrawal of immunosuppression, combined with preemptive nephrectomy for patients with early allograft failure. However, this practice is less common for patients with late graft failure. A longer taper of immunosuppression may permit the maintenance of some residual renal function while the patient is on dialysis. Several small studies have noted that patients who have undergone transplant nephrectomy have higher panel reactive antibody titers than those undergoing

dialysis with the allograft still in place. An unresolved issue is whether there might be some benefit for retransplantation, compared with leaving the failed transplanted kidney in place (32). However, there appears to be no significant difference in outcome after retransplantation among those with or without nephrectomy. Further studies are needed to determine whether slower taper of calcineurin inhibitors or other immunosuppression can reduce the incidence of nephrectomy without untoward side effects in these patients while on dialysis.

Underlying Renal Diseases

It is most important to assess the cause of the potential recipient's renal failure. The primary pathologies leading to renal failure are expected to influence outcome, depending on the etiologic mechanisms, propensity for recurrence, and status of the immune system.

Diabetes Mellitus

Patients with diabetes mellitus are at increased risk with all forms of therapy for ESRD. The most dramatic change in patient selection has been the increase in diabetic patients with renal failure who are being offered transplantation as the treatment of choice (Fig. 97-4). For example, in the United States, diabetic patients now comprise more than 40% of all patients accepted for treatment on ESRD programs; 12% classified as type I and 28% as type II. This number is much lower than that for Europe but is steadily growing and is now around 20% overall. Although the diabetic patient is considered high risk for transplantation, it is now generally accepted that transplantation is the treatment of choice for many of these patients (33,34).

There is an increasing use of combined kidney and pancreas transplantation in selected patients with ESRD due to diabetes (35–38). Pancreas transplantation is performed mostly with a simultaneous kidney from the same donor. Benefits of pancreas transplantation include better glycemic control and improvement in some of the secondary complications

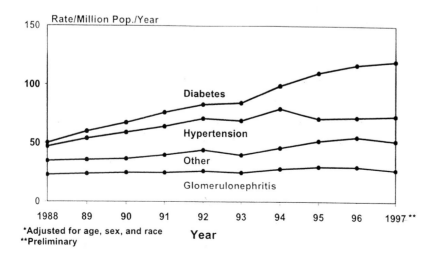

FIG. 97-4. End-stage renal disease incidence rates per year by primary diagnoses, 1988–1997. Rates by diagnoses adjusted for age, sex, and race. Rates do not include patients from Puerto Rico or the U.S. territories. (United States Renal Data System. *USRDS 1999 annual data report.* Bethesda, MD: National Institutes of Health and National Institute of Diabetes and Digestive and Kidney Diseases, 1999, with permission.)

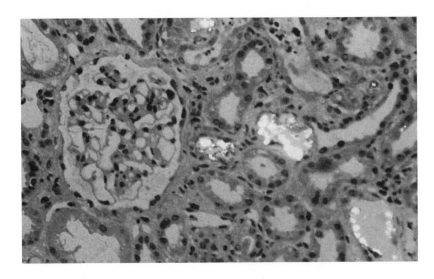

FIG. 97-5. Renal biopsy specimen from a transplanted kidney showing recurrence of oxalosis. (From Dr. William Hammond, Denver, CO, with permission.)

of diabetes. As of 1998, more than 11,000 pancreas transplantations were reported to the International Pancreas Transplant Registry. Patient survival and pancreas graft survival rates were 94% and 81%, respectively, at 1 year, 92% and 77% at 2 years, and 91% and 74% at 3 years (39).

Recurrence of the diabetic nephropathy in type I diabetic recipients is a late and slowly developing complication. In a detailed follow-up of 100 type I diabetic recipients who were alive with a functioning graft 10 years after transplantation, only two patients went on to lose the graft due to recurrence. No patient from the 265 diabetic recipients had graft loss due to recurrence in the first 10 years (40).

Examination of biopsy specimens early after transplantation indicates that there are few glomerular pathologic abnormalities other than frequent afferent and efferent arteriosclerosis. Glomerular basement immunoglobulin G (IgG) deposition is seen in less than 2 years after transplantation, but the onset and progression of glomerular basement membrane (GBM) thickening and mesangial expansion only occurs after 2 years. However, the typical nodular glomerular hyalinosis is rarely seen in these patients. Long-term follow-up has shown that recurrent nephropathy progresses to ESRD with the same time course as that of primary type I diabetic nephropathy. The mean time to recurrent ESRD is estimated to be 15 to 20 years. Therefore, recurrence of the lesion is not a barrier to long-term renal graft survival in diabetic recipients. The frequency and natural history of recurrence in type II diabetic recipients remain to be elucidated (41–44).

Metabolic and Congenital Disorders

Results of renal transplantation in patients with metabolic and congenital disorders causing end-stage renal failure such as Alport's syndrome, amyloidosis, cystinosis, familial nephritis, gout, and cystic disease are generally similar to those of the more common cause of end-stage renal failure, with the exception of oxalosis, sickle cell, and Fabry's disease (45,46).

Oxalosis. The early transplant experience was disappointing because of early graft failure due to recurrent urolithiasis (Fig. 97-5), nephrocalcinosis, renal failure, and systemic oxalate deposition (47). Earlier recommendations to consider primary oxalosis a contraindication to transplantation are being challenged by recent reports of successfully prolonged graft function despite persistent hyperoxalosis (48–50). Those grafts with good long-term function have usually passed urine promptly after the operation and have had little rejection. To reduce the chance of oxalate accumulation, dialysis treatment or kidney transplantation should be considered when the glomerular filtration rate (GFR) approaches 20 mL per minute. Aggressive dialysis schedules should be implemented before transplantation to deplete the oxalate metabolic pool. Medical therapy with pyridoxine, neutral phosphate, and magnesium should be started after transplantation to reduce oxalate deposition and recurrence. Combined renal and hepatic transplantation has also been recommended as a more definitive approach, and early results have been encouraging (51,52).

Unlike primary oxalosis, which is a congenital condition with enzymatic defects in oxalate metabolism, secondary oxalosis is due to excessive intake or absorption of oxalates from the diet. Secondary oxalosis is seen primarily in fat malabsorption, short-bowel syndromes after gastrointestinal (GI) surgery, and high-oxalate diets. For these patients, consideration should be given to reanastomosis of gastric bypass, hydration, and dietary restriction of oxalates.

Good allograft function can be achieved when attention is paid to reduce the oxalate excretion load (53).

Cystinosis. Cystine stones recur after transplantation but have little effect on graft function (54). Renal transplantation has been recommended as a preferred therapy in children with ESRD caused by cystinosis. However, the systemic effects of cystine accumulation, including corneal crystallization and retinal degeneration leading to blindness, progress after renal transplantation. Despite recurrence of the disease, long-term survival has been reported (55,56).

Sickle Cell Disease. The autosomal-recessive conditions of sickle cell disease and sickle cell trait may be complicated by various renal abnormalities that may eventually lead to

ESRD. Glomerular lesions are relatively rare and in some instances may be traced to an acquired chronic hepatitis B infection from multiple transfusions. There is little experience with renal transplantation in patients with sickle cell nephropathy (57). The overall results of the report by Barber et al. (57) from the University of Alabama were disappointing, with a 25% 1-year survival rate in eight patients. Others have claimed a more reasonable outcome (58). The importance of recurrence after transplantation is difficult to determine because of the relative nonspecific nature of sickle cell nephropathy. The North American Pediatric Renal Transplant Cooperative Study reports a more favorable outcome in pediatric patients, with a patient survival rate of 89%, and graft survival rates at 12 and 24 months posttransplantation of 89% and 71%, respectively (59).

Fabry's Disease. Fabry's disease is an X-linked disorder of glycosphingolipid metabolism due to a ceramide trihexosidase. Renal transplantation results have been disappointing with poor graft and patient survival. This poor outcome mostly has been due to continued morbidity from the underlying disease, which appears to be unaffected by successful restoration of normal renal function (60). However, European data concerning transplantation in patients with Fabry's disease disagree with what has been previously stated (61). Despite recurrence of the disease, long-term survival has recently been reported (62). Recently, it has been postulated that genetic correction of bone marrow cells derived from patients with Fabry's disease may have use for phenotypic correction of patients with this disorder (63,64).

Amyloidosis. Recurrent nephrotic syndrome and graft failure can occur in primary and secondary amyloidosis, but there is some indication that patients with amyloid-induced renal disease do better after renal transplantation than with dialysis as replacement therapy. The graft survival rate of patients with amyloid-induced ESRD who receive transplants now appears to be equal to the survival rate of patients with nonamyloid-induced ESRD who receive transplants (65). Familial Mediterranean fever, rheumatoid arthritis, and osteomyelitis are the most common causes of secondary amyloidosis. Familial Mediterranean fever is an autosomal-recessive disorder that occurs in Sephardic Jews, Armenians, Turks, Arabs of the Levant. In Israel, amyloidosis constitutes 6% of all patients on dialysis, compared with 0.6% in Europe. Although there has been a higher early mortality rate for patients who have received a transplant in the past, the incidence of rejection episodes is lower than that in patients without amyloidosis. Reduced immunosuppression has reduced postoperative mortality and morbidity rates. Colchicine at 1 to 2 mg per day dramatically relieves the symptoms and reduces the incidence of attacks in familial Mediterranean fever.

Alport's Syndrome. Dialysis and transplantation pose no particular problems for patients with Alport's syndrome. Recurrent disease has not been well documented. Improvement or stabilization of deafness after renal transplantation has occasionally been reported. There is a remote risk of developing *de novo* anti-GBM nephritis after transplantation (66–68).

Polycystic Kidney Disease. Autosomal-dominant polycystic kidney disease is responsible for approximately 4% to 12% of patients with ESRD in the United States and Europe. Early studies suggested that renal allograft and patient survival rates were better in those who had bilateral nephrectomy (69), but in more recent studies, the results of renal transplantation without bilateral nephrectomy are excellent (70). The polycystic kidneys will shrink considerably after successful transplantation. Thus, removal is only required if the kidneys are massive due to polycystic disease or there is associated persistent infection or severe hypertension. However, nephrectomy is indicated if cyst-related complications occur repeatedly (71). There is no increased risk of renal cell carcinoma in patients with autosomal-dominant polycystic kidney disease. Polycystic patients on dialysis should be followed for cardiac valve abnormalities and cerebral aneurysms (72).

Glomerulonephritis

Glomerulonephritis remains the second most common cause of ESRD. Because of the more frequent use of renal biopsy early in the course of most glomerular diseases, the pathologic diagnosis has often been well established for potential transplant recipients. Almost all types of glomerulonephritis have been reported to recur after transplantation. There is however much variation among the various types of glomerulonephritis with regard to the frequency of recurrence, the clinical course, and the prognosis (73–75). The overall incidence of recurrence is less than 10% to 20% and recurrent disease accounts for less than 2% to 4% of all graft failures.

Focal Segmental Glomerular Sclerosis. Recurrent focal sclerosis may be seen early after transplantation, presenting with nephrotic-range proteinuria and a rapid decline in renal function (76). Histologically, the features on light microscopy that permit categorization are focal and segmental sclerosis affecting a small number of glomeruli, often those in the deep juxtamedullary cortex. The development of foot process fusion can be immediate after transplantation and precede glomerular segmental sclerosis by weeks to months (Fig. 97-6). The frequency of recurrence is about 20% in adults and may be as high as 40% in children. It is likely that some of these patients had secondary focal segmental glomerular sclerosis (FSGS) due to nephron loss in reflux nephropathy, which would not be expected to recur in the transplant. Thus, the recurrence rate in primary FSGS may be substantially higher than the reported values. Patients presenting with rapid progression of renal disease from the time of diagnosis of nephrotic syndrome to ESRD have a higher risk for recurrence. If a patient who has undergone transplantation lost the graft because of recurrent FSGS, there is a 50% risk of subsequent allograft failure within 5 years of a second transplantation.

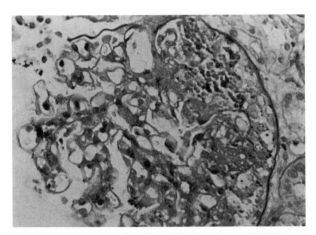

FIG. 97-6. Renal biopsy specimen of a transplanted kidney showing recurrence of focal segmental glomerulosclerosis. (periodic acid-Schiff stain, magnification ×250)

Treatment of recurrent FSGS remains disappointing. Heavy proteinuria and nephrotic syndrome are usually resistant to steroids (77). Cyclosporin A (CsA) has not proved effective in preventing recurrence. Because of the high risk of recurrence and rapid progression to ESRD, living donors generally are not used for the first allograft (78,79). Use of a cadaveric kidney, however, is not precluded, because the disease will not recur in all cases and not all patients with recurrence will lose the graft. Some centers have also suggested that if a first graft is lost to recurrent disease, a second transplantation should be delayed for 1 to 2 years.

The rapidity of recurrence strongly suggests the presence of a circulating factor in primary FSGS that is toxic to the capillary wall. It has been shown that serum from some patients with FSGS increases the permeability of isolated glomeruli to albumin. Testing of pretransplant sera with this approach can be used to predict recurrence after transplantation. Use of a regenerating protein adsorption column or plasma exchange can reduce protein excretion in patients with recurrent FSGS in the transplant. More prolonged remissions have been achieved using plasma exchange, which is initiated promptly after onset of proteinuria, or the combination of plasma exchange and cyclophosphamide. These prolonged beneficial results have also been reported in children treated with plasma exchange and cyclophosphamide (80–84).

Antiglomerular Basement Membrane Disease. Based on histology and fluorescence study results, anti-GBM disease is associated with a more than 50% recurrence rate in the allograft. However, only 25% of patients with biopsy-proven IgG staining along the capillary wall have evidence for clinical disease activity. Furthermore, graft failure due to recurrence disease is less common. Although engraftment during the presence of anti-GBM antibodies has been reported to be successful (85), many transplantation centers still prefer serologic quiescence of anti-GBM antibody production for 6 to 12 months before proceeding with transplantation to reduce the risk for recurrent anti-GBM disease. Despite delaying

transplantation to allow the anti-GBM antibody level to fall, recurrence has been reported (86,87).

Hemolytic-Uremic Syndrome. Hemolytic-uremic syndrome (HUS) has a recurrence rate of 20% to 50% (88,89). It has pathologic features common to the small vessel findings in acute vascular rejection, CsA toxicity, and malignant hypertension. The recurrence rate is higher in recipients of living-related transplants. Live kidney donation should proceed with caution in view of the possibility of a familial tendency to an abnormality of prostacyclin synthesis. A meta-analysis of 159 grafts in 126 patients by Ducloux et al. (90) in 1998 found that recurrent HUS was significantly associated with an older age at onset of HUS, a short duration between disease onset and ESRD or transplantation, the use of living related donors, and to a lesser degree, the administration of calcineurin inhibitors (CsA or tacrolimus). In high-risk patients with history of HUS, prevention by the administration of low-dose aspirin and dipyridamole should be used. Calcineurin inhibitors and antilymphocyte serum should be used with caution in these patients. A review of 114 patients with both recurrent and *de novo* HUS after organ transplantation found that two-thirds of patients had been treated with CsA. There is no successful treatment of recurrent HUS. Salicylates, dipyridamole, plasma infusion, and plasma exchange have been shown to be of limited benefit. Once established, HUS often does not remit in the allograft and typically results in rapid graft loss within days. CsA has been associated with altered coagulation mechanisms and the development of *de novo* HUS in renal transplant recipients (91). CsA should therefore be used with caution in patients whose original kidney disease was caused by HUS. If CsA has been associated with recurrent HUS in the first transplant, it should be avoided subsequently. Preliminary evidence suggests that patients with allograft loss due to recurrent HUS associated with CsA may successfully undergo retransplantation without the use of calcineurin inhibitors. An immunosuppressive protocol without calcineurin inhibitors consisting of mycophenolate mofetil (MMF), corticosteroids, and antilymphocyte antibody induction therapy was administered to six patients. No patient experienced disease recurrence, allograft loss, or episodes of acute rejection (92–95).

IgA Nephropathy/Henoch-Schönlein Purpura. In many parts of the world, immunoglobulin A (IgA) nephropathy is the most common type of glomerulonephritis. The true incidence of recurrence is best seen in Berger's series (96), in which all 32 patients had routine follow-up biopsies and 17 (50%) showed recurrent IgA nephropathy. However, there is a low incidence of allograft dysfunction that leads to allograft loss (97). IgA nephropathy with mesangial IgA deposit tends to disappear after transplanted to a patient with non-IgA nephropathy. Recent studies demonstrate that patients with IgA nephropathy had a highly significant survival rate compared with that of those with other diseases (98,99)

The closely related Henoch-Schönlein purpura (HSP) has been reported to recur with mesangial deposits of IgA,

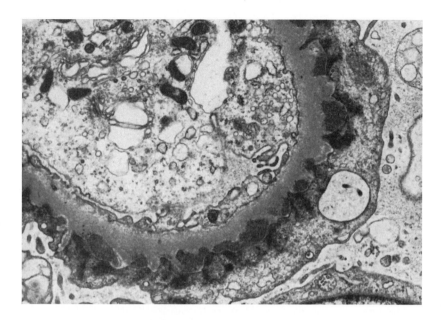

FIG. 97-7. Electron micrograph of *de novo* membranous glomerulonephritis. (From Dr. William Hammond, Denver, CO, with permission.)

occurring in 17 of 20 patients with minimal clinical manifestations in one series (96). Clinically, recurrent HSP can be severe with crescentic glomerulonephritis, nephrotic syndrome, graft failure, and variable recurrence of purpura (100). To reduce recurrence, one should delay engraftment for at least 6 to 12 months after the skin lesions of HSP have resolved (101,102).

Type I Membranoproliferative Glomerulonephritis. Type I membranoproliferative glomerulonephritis (MPGN) can resemble transplant rejection glomerulopathy on light microscopy (103). Crescents, C3 deposition in the capillary wall, and dense subendothelial deposits on electron microscopy are common to both. The early development of nephrotic syndrome and persistent microscopic hematuria from the time of transplantation are clinical markers suggesting recurrence rather than rejection. The frequency of recurrence was estimated to be 20% to 30%. Approximately 30% to 40% of patients with recurrent type I MPGN will lose their allograft (104). Graft rejection is often a confounding factor. Reduced C3 levels before transplantation usually return to within the normal range after transplantation and do not correlate with disease activity.

Type II MPGN (Dense-Deposit Disease). The recurrence rate is reported to be 50% to 100%, with graft failure in 20% to 50% of patients (105). Proteinuria with or without hematuria is the usual clinical presentation. A decrement in serum C3 levels and the appearance of C3 nephritic factor may be present in some cases. Recurrence is usually evident within the first year after engraftment. The unique ultrastructural appearance of extensive deposit within the basement membrane allows this diagnosis to be made with certainty before and after transplantation (106).

Membranous Nephropathy. An accurate rate of recurrence of membranous nephropathy is difficult to establish because of the relatively high frequency of primary *de novo* occurrence in allograft recipients (107). Recurrent membranous

nephropathy with nephrotic syndrome generally occurs earlier, at an average of 10 months, compared with *de novo* membranous nephropathy, which is usually seen about 18 to 20 months after transplantation (Fig. 97-7). It seems more likely to recur when the primary disease has been aggressive, but the overall incidence is only about 10%. *De novo* membranous nephropathy is not reported to lead to graft loss. Recurrent membranous nephropathy, however, can have early and heavy proteinuria and an increased chance of graft loss.

Systemic Lupus Erythematosus. Recurrence is relatively rare in patients with systemic lupus erythematosus (SLE). Similarly, reactivation of SLE after transplantation is extremely infrequent and is often controlled by immunosuppressive medications when it does occur (108,109). Recurrence is not predictable with serologic monitoring. However, there should be no systemic disease activity before transplantation (110,111). Recurrences can be successfully treated with steroids, MMF, or chlorambucil.

Wegener's Granulomatosis. There are few data on transplantation in patients with Wegener's granulomatosis. Recurrence is generally rare after transplantation (112–114). Recurrence can be treated successfully by adding cyclophosphamide and by increasing the steroid dose.

Progressive Systemic Sclerosis (Scleroderma). Recurrence of progressive systemic sclerosis in the graft can occur within the first few months after transplantation (115,116). Earlier reports have suggested that graft loss may be accelerated due to uncontrolled hypertension. Many of the reports on recurrence came from patients before the use of CsA and angiotensin-converting enzyme (ACE) inhibitors. Those patients with recurrence had malignant manifestations of scleroderma before transplantation, suggesting that it may be possible to clinically separate a subset of patients in whom early recurrence was more likely. The highest patient survival rate was noted in those individuals who have had bilateral native nephrectomies usually to control severe hypertension. The current recommendation for transplantation is that the patient should be clinically stable with absence of visceral progressive systemic sclerosis activity before transplantation. Patients with early diffuse scleroderma should be closely monitored for new onset of hypertension and be treated continuous with ACE inhibitors. Most patients with scleroderma will improve generally after transplantation with loss of Raynaud's syndrome and improvement of the skin condition. Therefore, transplantation is justified if the patient has not been severely debilitated by the systemic effects of scleroderma.

Interstitial Disease

Chronic Pyelonephritis. Chronic pyelonephritis is a diagnosis that has been frequently used for nonspecific interstitial nephritis not necessary caused by bacterial infection. The presence or history of significant urinary infection is important to identify. Because of the risk of residual foci of infection that may predispose to bacteremia or seed the urinary tract and transplanted kidney, pretransplant nephrectomy may be indicated in these patients.

Analgesic Nephropathy. Patients with analgesic nephropathy need to be identified because cessation of the use of nephrotoxic analgesics is essential for these patients. Kidney function may improve after cessation of the use of analgesics, and damage to the allograft is a significant risk if this use persists. There is an increase in the incidence of transitional cell carcinoma of the urinary tract in patients with analgesic nephropathy.

General Evaluation

This assessment should include not only a complete medical evaluation and determination where possible of the underlying disease causing renal failure, but also a careful surveillance for problems that might arise after transplantation (117) (Table 97-4).

A careful physical examination should be performed to identify coexisting cardiovascular, GI, or genitourinary (GU) disease. Additional examinations should assess pulmonary reserve, define potential sources of infection including dental caries, and assess the gynecologic risks for women.

The laboratory evaluation should include routine hematologic tests to detect leukopenia or thrombocytopenia, liver function tests to identify patients in whom the metabolism of cyclosporine may be abnormal, complete hepatitis and human immunodeficiency virus (HIV) profiles, viral titers, and throat and urine cultures.

Risk Factors

The major risk factors that have an impact on the recipient include age, the presence of diabetes mellitus, arteriosclerotic heart disease, chronic pulmonary disorders, and malignancy. Patient compliance has also been identified as an important

TABLE 97-4. *Pretransplantation recipient medical evaluation*

1. History and physical examination
2. Social and psychiatric evaluation
3. Determine primary kidney disease activity and residual kidney function
4. Dental evaluation
5. Laboratory studies:
   Complete blood cell count and blood chemistry
   Hepatitis B virus surface antigen
   Human immunodeficiency virus
   Antibodies to cytomegalovirus and Epstein-Barr virus
   Human leukocytes antigen typing and antibodies screening
   Urine analysis and urine culture
6. Chest radiograph
7. Electrocardiogram
8. Special procedures for selected patients:
   Abdominal ultrasound of gallbladder
   Upper gastrointestinal tract study or endoscopy
   Barium enema or colonoscopy
   PPD skin test
   Treadmill/exercise electrocardiogram
   Thallium scan
   Angiogram: coronary
   Cystoureterography
9. Consultation (optional):
   Psychiatric
   Gynecology evaluation and mammography (for women older than 40 yr)
   Urologic assessment (voiding cystoureterography, cystoscopy, or urodynamic studies in patients with vesicoureteric reflux, neurogenic bladder, bladder neck obstruction, or strictures)

cause of late graft failure (118). It is important to have social and psychiatric evaluation with a view to give support to these patients (119,120). Conditions excluding a patient from renal transplantation would probably be the presence of severe ischemic heart disease [although this might be approached by coronary artery bypass surgery, where appropriate, before transplantation (121)], older age (perhaps older than 70 years), although attitudes are still changing, and the presence of persistent infection or cancer. When a patient has had previous curative therapy for cancer, it is generally thought appropriate to wait at least 1 year, and possibly 2 years, with proven freedom from recurrence before going ahead with transplantation (122,123).

Cardiovascular Evaluation

Cardiovascular disease is a major cause of morbidity and mortality for the patient with ESRD, whether the patient remains on dialysis or chooses to have a kidney transplantation (124). It is therefore important to carefully screen the patient for any cardiovascular problems, especially in diabetic patients (125). Initial assessment of the severity of cardiovascular disease consists of careful clinical examination, an electrocardiogram, and radiograph of the chest and peripheral vessels for calcification. Evidence of moderate or severe myocardial ischemia is an indication for further investigation with thallium stress test or coronary angiography (126). Coronary artery bypass grafting should be considered before transplantation in the presence of severe angina or double- or triple-vessel disease. Any patient who has had a recent myocardial infarction should be reassessed for a transplant 6 months after the incident. Approximately 20% to 30% of diabetic transplant candidates have significant coronary artery disease, which may be asymptomatic. Noninvasive testing and, if indicated, cardiac catheterization should be performed before renal transplantation, because active intervention may improve patient outcome. For the nondiabetic, asymptomatic patient, extensive cardiac evaluation appears unnecessary, unless risk factors such as smoking, hypertension, hyperlipidemia, or family history of heart disease are present.

GI Evaluation

Although the incidence of peptic ulcer after renal transplantation is decreasing, complications of a peptic ulcer such as perforation or hemorrhage are associated with a high mortality rate in patients undergoing transplantation (127,128). For this reason, many centers actively screen patients for evidence of peptic ulceration before accepting them for transplantation and in the past have been quite aggressive about the management of these patients before transplantation. Similarly, in patients with symptomatic cholelithiasis or asymptomatic gall stones seen with ultrasonography, cholecystectomy should be performed to eliminate the risk of cholelithiasis and possible sepsis after transplantation. Patients with colonic disease, particularly those with diverticulitis, should be evaluated with barium enema and colonoscopy and if appropriate should be treated with surgical resection before transplantation.

GU Evaluation

Accurate evaluation of the lower urinary tract function before transplantation is important to minimize postoperative urologic complications. The original renal disease must be clearly defined. Any history of repeated urinary infections and current reports of urine cultures should be obtained. In the past, a voiding cystourethrogram has been performed on all patients to evaluate the urinary tract for evidence of outflow obstruction or vesicoureteral reflux. It is now considered necessary only if there is clinical evidence of a bladder or ureteric abnormality. Cystoscopy and urodynamic studies should be performed in patients with evidence of bladder dysfunction. Urologic operations are necessary either to correct or to improve obstructive lesions or sometimes to provide a conduit in the presence of a neurogenic bladder or a previous cystectomy.

HBsAg Screening

Successful renal transplantation in patients with positive hepatitis B virus surface antigen (HBsAg) has been reported (129). However, when patients positive for HBsAg are retrospectively compared with an age-matched group of patients on hemodialysis known to be surface antigen–positive, the transplant recipients have a higher frequency of chronic hepatitis and mortality due to hepatitis. The adverse effects are not apparent during the first 2 years after transplantation but become evident over the long term (130). Patients on hemodialysis have a high rate of surface antigen persistence but rarely develop chronic hepatitis, and the rate of seroconversion to surface antigen negativity is 15% to 20% per year. Because of this, some centers do not recommend renal transplantation in chronic HBsAg carriers. This decision however should be individualized. The better quality of life for the patient considered for transplantation should be weighed against the low but definite risk of development of chronic liver failure.

In a study by Pol et al. (131) from the Necker Hospital, patient and graft survival rates were similar between HBsAg-positive and HBsAg-negative kidney recipients. Their data suggest that renal transplantation may be appropriate for patients with chronic hepatitis regardless of their hepatitis virus status.

However, no patient should undergo transplantation when he or she has evidence of active hepatitis. Before transplantation, potential recipients should have stable liver enzymes, preferably less than two or three times the normal range for several months.

Hepatitis C Virus Screening

Transplant recipients are potentially at risk of developing hepatitis C virus (HCV) infection due to reactivation of pretransplantation HCV infection or to infection acquired from blood products or from HCV-infected organ donors (132). In potential recipients with serologic evidence of HCV, a liver biopsy should be performed to assess the histologic severity of the disease (133).

HIV Screening

The HIV antibody status of all potential donors and recipients should be determined before transplantation. Potential recipients who are highly sensitized may have false-positive enzyme-linked immunosorbent assay (ELISA) results because of a higher incidence of antibodies in their serum that react with HLA on the target cell used in the serologic assay (134). The Western blot technique, which detects viral envelope protein, may be more accurate in these situations. Polymerase chain reaction (PCR) analysis to detect small amounts of HIV viral DNA in serum may further improve accuracy, but the assay is not widely available for routine screening (135).

Preparation for Transplantation

Nephrectomy

Nephrectomy before transplantation is now an uncommon procedure and may be associated with a significant morbidity rate (136,137). Thus, bilateral nephrectomy is only performed in the presence of persistent urinary tract infection (usually associated with vesicoureteral reflux) or in the presence of renal cancer, nephrolithiasis, or medically intractable hypertension (138). There is some evidence that pretransplantation bilateral nephrectomy improves renal graft survival (139).

Unilateral nephrectomy may be necessary in patients with large polycystic kidneys to provide room for a subsequent transplant on that side (140).

Transfusion

Before the use of CsA, the beneficial effect of blood transfusions on cadaveric graft survival was reported to be 10% to 20% better than that of nontransfused recipients (141–143). Recently, however, the role of blood transfusion as an adjunct to transplantation has been a controversial topic. With the availability of recombinant erythropoietin (EPO), there is also less need for blood transfusion in patients with ESRD (144). The two main disadvantages of blood transfusions are the induction of cytotoxic antibodies (145,146) and the risk of infections (147). In 1983, Kahan (148) reported that patients who received CsA immunosuppression showed diminished beneficial effects of pretransplantation blood transfusion after cadaveric renal transplantation.

The Collaborative Transplant Study Data (149) demonstrated that the benefit of transfusion has diminished to a point at which the risks of infection and presensitization due to transfusion may outweigh any benefit on graft survival. The loss of transfusion effect is independent of the use of CsA and whether donor-specific or random transfusions were given. Iwaki et al. (150) reexamined the UCLA database in 1989 to determine whether a beneficial blood transfusion was present since the introduction of CsA. Their data showed an increase in the 1-year graft survival rate by 8% in first cadaveric kidney transplants when one HLA-DR mismatch was present (P < 0.01), by 10% when two HLA-DR mismatches were present (P < 0.01), and 0% when no HLA-DR mismatches were present. The transfusion effect was greater in Black than White recipients. Their analysis suggests two to three deliberate pretransplantation blood transfusions may still be helpful unless transplant candidates are to wait for a zero-mismatched HLA-DR cadaveric donor. Because the effect of transfusion is long lasting, it is not necessary to give deliberate additional blood if the patient has received two to three transfusions during a lifetime.

In the case of donor-specific transfusions, in which the recipient is given planned transfusions of blood from the potential donor before transplantation, there is a risk of a specific sensitization against the donor that could preclude subsequent transplantation from that donor (151). Sensitization occurs in approximately one-third of these patients. It is now customary to give either azathioprine or CsA with the donor-specific transfusions to lower the incidence of sensitization (152). This does appear to reduce the sensitization rate to about 5%. More recently, the concept of donor-specific transfusion

has been challenged, and evidence has been produced that random blood transfusions will result in equally good graft survival in this situation. After transplantation, patients who have received donor-specific transfusions often have a fairly characteristic course with an acute cellular rejection episode occurring within the first 4 days of transplantation, but in general, one that responds briskly to increased steroid therapy. Many transplantation units now feel that donor-specific transfusion is no longer necessary since the advent of CsA (153).

Immunologic Evaluation

In addition to determining HLA at the A, B, C, and DR loci, the potential recipient's serum should be screened regularly for HLA antibodies. Prophylactic measures are most important in the management of presensitization leading to hyperacute and accelerated rejection. The avoidance of both ABO incompatibility and positive T-cell crossmatches has eliminated the major cause of hyperacute rejection seen in the early days of transplantation. The presence of lymphocyte cytotoxic antibodies in the patient's serum is due to sensitization to HLA. It can occur after pregnancies, a blood transfusion, and a renal transplantation. Autoantibodies, on the other hand, often occur spontaneously and are not related to any obvious antigenic challenge (154). One method of defining the highly sensitized patient is to include subjects who at any time have developed lymphocytotoxic antibodies, which react with 90% or more of random panel cells. One approach to this is to remove the anti-HLA antibodies before transplantation (155,156). An alternative approach is to characterize the antibodies and to perform a crossmatch with different serologic techniques. Recently a technique using dithiothreitol (DTT) to eliminate immunoglobulin M (IgM) cytotoxic antibodies in the sera of sensitized recipients has allowed successful renal transplantation when the unmodified crossmatch test result is positive and the DTT-treated crossmatch result is negative (157), which indicates that the positive crossmatch is due to irrelevant IgM antibodies.

The resurgence of transplantation across ABO incompatibility has been brought on by the lack of availability of suitable (ABO-compatible) cadaveric donor kidneys for type O recipients, the blood group with the largest waiting list, as well as the inability to transplant HLA-identical but ABO-incompatible siblings (158). One approach is to transplant blood group A donors with A_2 subtype into O recipients. The A antigen has been found to be weakly immunogenic and does not elicit an isohemagglutinin response. Several centers have found this to be successful, with a 71% to 83% graft survival rate at around 1 year, providing a preformed anti-A_2 isohemagglutinin titer is absent. Another experimental approach is to perform pretransplantation splenectomy (159), plasmapheresis on recipients to deplete circulating anti-A and anti-B antibodies (160), or infusion of intravenous immunoglobulin (IVIG) (161).

Patients who have rejected their first graft acutely represent a very high-risk group of patients for subsequent transplant

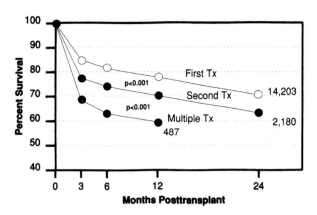

FIG. 97-8. Graft survival rates of cadaveric kidney transplants. Graft survival rates for 14,203 first cadaveric donor transplants (tx) were 78% and 70% at 1 and 2 years, respectively. Graft survival rates for those receiving their second transplant were 70% and 63% at 1 and 2 years, respectively. Data are from the United Network for Organ Sharing Scientific Renal Transplant Registry, 1990. (From Cecka J, Terasaki P, eds. *Clinical transplants 1990.* Los Angeles: UCLA Tissue Typing Laboratory, 1990:2, with permission.)

(162). On the other hand, patients in whom the graft has functioned for at least a year have survival rates for second grafts that are no different from that of the first graft. Matching for both HLA-A and HLA-B appears to exert a much greater influence on the survival of second grafts than in the case of first grafts (163,164), and although it does not appear necessary to avoid previous HLA-A and HLA-B incompatibilities with a second graft, it would appear logical to do so (164). In general, a second graft has a poorer graft survival rate than that of a first graft (Fig. 97-8), and this is particularly evident if the first graft was lost from irreversible rejection during the first few months after transplantation (165). In addition to a standard immunosuppressive regimen, the use of OKT-3 or polyclonal antibodies as part of an induction therapy may be indicated. With appropriate immunosuppression, it is possible to have successful transplantation of

highly sensitized patients without regards to HLA matching (166).

CADAVERIC VERSUS LIVING DONOR

Living related donor transplantations comprise about 30% of all transplantations performed in the United States (Fig. 97-9), although their proportion is much less (10% to 15%) in Europe and Australia (167). In addition, many programs will now accept living non–blood-related or distantly related donors (spouses, cousins, uncles, aunts, stepchildren, stepparents, or even close friends).

The ethical aspects of accepting kidneys from family are somewhat controversial (168,169). There has been concern for many years about the long-term outcome of a healthy donor. In particular, the concerns regarding the possibility of long-term renal dysfunction resulting from hyperfiltration in the solitary kidney have prompted transplantation centers to reevaluate their living related donor program. Several long-term follow-up studies have not revealed any adverse problems in living related donors with a single kidney (170,171). The donor mortality risk has been less than 0.1%. Life expectancy in the donor remains unaffected. Long-term study of more than 600 donors has shown no increased incidence of hypertension or impaired renal function (172). In one report, however, mild proteinuria and hypertension were found in male but not in female donors (173). Further studies and follow-up of kidney donors are necessary. In view of the shortage of cadaveric kidneys, transplantation of a graft from a histocompatible living related donor should be considered if there is a suitable donor. Excellent results were also observed in kidney transplants from spousal and living unrelated donors (174,175) On the other hand, the proposal that kidneys might be purchased from living unrelated donors should be condemned. It is with these issues in mind that the Transplantation Society has issued guidelines for the practice of transplantation that avoid exploitation and commercialization of organ donation (176). Similarly, the U.S.

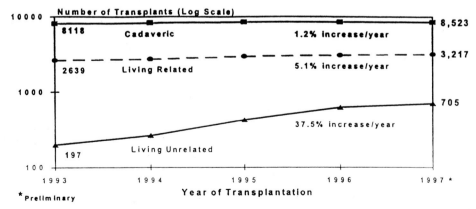

FIG. 97-9. Total number of renal transplants by donor source and year, 1993–1997. Number of transplants shown on log scale. (United States Renal Data System. *USRDS 1999 annual data report.* Bethesda, MD: National Institutes of Health and National Institute of Diabetes and Digestive and Kidney Diseases, 1999, with permission.)

Organ Transplantation Act of 1984 (House of Representatives 5580, title 2) makes it a federal crime to engage in organ sale and commerce. Hopefully, the new legislation will help strengthen the organ procurement program and increase the number of cadaveric kidneys available for transplantations (177). Globally, barriers to widen development of effective cadaveric programs of renal transplantation were not due to religious objections. The main factor seemed to be a lack of public concern about the need for cadaveric donor programs in patients with ESRD.

Living Donor Evaluation

Living donors are usually first-degree relatives who are one- or two-haplotype matched. However, there is good evidence that zero-haplotype–matched relatives can donate kidneys that provide an excellent chance of short- and long-term graft survival. Similarly, good results have been reported with emotionally related living donors. Most living unrelated donors are spouses or companions with long-standing emotional ties. This practice will likely become an important source of organs for transplantation. By 1995, about 10% of transplants were from living unrelated donors. This source of organs is expected to grow, particularly in light of the fact that a high graft survival rate has been associated with these donors. Initial screening should concentrate on related donors, and tissue typing should be used to help choose the best potential donor among ABO-compatible candidates. The attitude toward the use of unrelated living donors varies considerably among centers. In general, living donor transplantation is fraught with potential psychologic problems and it is important to ensure that the prospective donor has not been subjected to family pressure (178). A very careful psychologic evaluation will be needed to determine that the motivation to donate the kidney is indeed genuine (179). HLA genotyping should be used to decide on the most suitable donor if there are several family members who are all keen to give a kidney. The initial series of tests, which include ABO blood group and HLA tissue typing, can be completed at a brief outpatient visit. Possible living donor transplantation can then be considered with the individuals best matched to the recipient. The living donor not only needs a thorough medical evaluation with particular attention to renal function and the urinary tract, but also must undergo a renal angiography or magnetic resonance angiography to identify vascular or anatomic variation of the kidneys or the collecting systems. It is important to ascertain that both kidneys are of normal size and configuration, and that a donor kidney with a single renal artery can be obtained (Table 97-5).

Living Donor Nephrectomy

Standard Open Nephrectomy

The standard method for removing a kidney from a living donor is through a flank incision by open nephrectomy. The

TABLE 97-5. *Exclusion criteria for live, related donors*

Age <18 yr or >65–70 yr
Significant medical illness (e.g., cardiovascular/pulmonary diseases, recent malignancy)
History of recurrent kidney stones
History of thrombosis or thromboembolism
Strong family history of renal disease, diabetes, and hypertension
Psychiatric contraindications
Obesity (30% above ideal weight)
Hypertension (>140/90 mm Hg or necessity for medication)
Proteinuria (>250 mg/24 hr)
Microscopic hematuria
Abnormal glomerular filtration rate (<80 mL/min)
Diabetes (abnormal glucose tolerance test results or hemoglobin A_{Ic})
Urologic/vascular abnormalities in donor kidneys

approach to the kidney, which will usually be the left kidney because this has the longer renal vein, may be either below or through the bed of the twelfth rib using a retroperitoneal approach or rarely via an anterior transperitoneal approach using a midline incision. Care must be given to retraction of the kidney during its removal to avoid traction injury of the renal artery, and dissection in the hilum of the kidney, particularly between the ureter and the renal artery, should be avoided to prevent damage to the ureteric blood supply. Furthermore, in removing the ureter down to the brim of the pelvis, care should be taken to leave an adequate amount of periureteric tissue.

Laparoscopic Nephrectomy

Living donor nephrectomy for transplantation can also be performed by laparoscopic approach. The techniques of endoscopically assisted nephrectomy are now well established. Over the last few years, there has been an increased rate of donation with laparoscopic donor nephrectomy (180,181). This approach results in less postoperative surgical pain, a shorter hospital stay, and a quicker recovery than the standard open donor nephrectomy.

Cadaveric Donor Evaluation

The criteria for the diagnosis of brain death have been well defined in most Western countries, although the requirements vary little from country to country (182) (Table 97-6). In the United States, there are an estimated 20,000 brain-dead patients per year who would be acceptable donors, but fewer than 5,000 actually donate their organs for transplantation. The general acceptance of brain death (183) and improved preservation in recent years has led to the supply of better-quality kidneys and establishment of organ-sharing programs to match donor and recipient on the basis of ABO blood group compatibility and HLA matching (184,185).

Although there is a slight influence of donor age on renal function in transplant recipients (186,187), acceptable donors

TABLE 97-6. *Medical evaluation of the potential cadaver donor*

I. Diagnosis of brain death
  A. Preconditions
    1. Comatose patient, on ventilator
    2. Positive diagnosis of cause of coma (irremediable structural brain damage)
  B. Exclusions
    1. Primary hypothermia ($<33°C$)
    2. Drugs
    3. Severe metabolic or endocrine disturbances
  C. Tests
    1. Absent brainstem reflexes
    2. Apnea (strictly define)
II. No preexisting renal disease
III. No active infection
  Tests:
  A. HBsAg; antibodies to cytomegalovirus and hepatitis C virus
  B. HIV antibodies
  C. HIV antigen in high-risk patients

HBsAg, hepatitis B virus surface antigen; HIV, human immunodeficiency virus.

are between 3 and 65 years old, and in some centers, even younger and older donors are being considered. There should be no evidence of primary renal disease, and no generalized viral or bacterial infection. A major consideration is the risk of transmitting infection with the allograft to an immunosuppressed recipient (188). Because of the possibilities of HIV transmission, HIV screening should be performed (189). All donors who are confirmed positive for HIV antibody should be excluded from donation. Those donors at high risk for HIV infection generally should not be accepted for donation because there is a period of seronegativity in early HIV infection before antibodies appear. HIV antigen testing should be performed in such donors.

Cadaveric Donor Nephrectomy

Today most kidneys will be removed as part of a multiple-organ harvesting procedure in which not only the kidneys are removed, but also the liver and heart, and occasionally, the lungs and pancreas. This necessitates coordination and careful cooperation between the interested parties (190). With experience and care, a donor may provide all the previously mentioned organs, all of which can be satisfactorily transplanted (191). There are two basic approaches to cadaveric donor nephrectomy: The first is one in which each kidney is removed individually with a patch of aorta via an anterior approach, and the second, which is the more satisfactory technique, is one in which both kidneys are removed en bloc with the appropriate segment of aorta and vena cava. The dissection of the vessels and the kidneys can then be completed after hypothermic perfusion and storage. *In situ* perfusion may be performed in both cases before and during removal.

Renal Reservation

Effective preservation of the kidney is an integral part of a kidney transplantation program and has evolved on the basis of known principles of preservation because of a need for longer storage of kidneys (192–194). The ability to preserve kidneys provides time for tissue typing, cross-matching, and selecting the most appropriate recipients for a particular donor on the basis of matching, as well as the preparation of the patients selected, who often may need dialysis before transplantation, and finally the transport of the kidneys to a center where an appropriately matched recipient may be awaiting a transplant.

There are two methods of preservation: simple cold storage in ice after flushing with a hypothermic solution to give a renal core temperature of $0°C$ and a more complicated approach of continuous perfusion of the kidney with an oxygenated colloid solution (192). In general, preservation methods do not affect cadaveric renal allograft outcome (195). The simple cold-storage approach is now the most commonly used, because this provides adequate preservation for at least 24 hours, and even up to 48 hours with newer approaches to preservation.

The kidneys are initially flushed free of blood with a cold solution via the aorta and renal artery while the kidney is *in situ*. Many different flushing solutions have been used (e.g., Collins, citrate, and University of Wisconsin solution) and the search for the optimal solution continues (Table 97-7). Drugs, metabolites, and other agents have been used to enhance the effects of cold preservation. The aim of these maneuvers is to reduce the incidence of posttransplantation acute tubular necrosis (ATN). The University of Wisconsin solution has revolutionized the preservation of livers and pancreas, but whether it represents an improved method of preservation for kidneys has not yet been clearly established (192).

TABLE 97-7. *Composition of flushing solutions*

	Collins'	Citrate	University of Wisconsin
Sodium (mmol)	10	78	30
Potassium (mmol)	108	84	120
Magnesium (mmol)	—	40	5
Sulfate (mmol)	—	40	5
Bicarbonate (mmol)	10	—	—
Phosphate (mmol)	60	—	25
Citrate (mmol)	—	54	—
Glucose (mmol)	180	—	—
Mannitol (mmol)	—	120	—
Lactobionate (mmol)	—	—	100
Raffinose (mmol)	—	—	30
Adenosine (mmol)	—	—	5
Allopurinol (mmol)	—	—	1
Glutathione (mmol)	—	—	3
Insulin (U/L)	—	—	100
Dexamethasone (mg/L)	—	—	8
Hydroxyethyl starch (g/L)	—	—	50

In the absence of any warm ischemia, which is generally the case with a brain-dead donor on a ventilator, immediate function can be obtained in most kidneys with up to 24 hours of preservation and even after 48 hours of preservation in some patients. However, from 24 hours onward, most kidneys will have a significant period of delayed function, ranging from a week to several weeks, and there will be a significant incidence of permanent nonfunction (196). It has been suggested that for short-term outcome, local use of kidneys with poor HLA matching is as good as shared use with good matches (197).

Because 18 to 36 hours is an adequate time for most units and also allows time for transport of kidneys within a region or country, there has been widespread adoption of the simple cold-storage technique for preservation.

Unlike simple cold storage, machine preservation is more complex and expensive with limited benefits. With this system, a cold perfusate, either plasma protein fraction (PPF) or albumin (198), is used to perfuse the kidney at low pressures using either pulsatile or continuous perfusion, with the perfusate being oxygenated within the circuit. Both the temperature and the pressure of the perfusate are monitored and the flow is generally kept at 1 to 3 mL/g of kidney per minute. Progressively rising resistance with a fall in flow rates and a rise in pressure indicates inadequate preservation, but this is rarely seen within 3 days (192). However, normal perfusion characteristics are no guarantee of organ viability and function.

Prevention of Acute Tubular Necrosis

Despite the advances made, many centers continue to report up to a 50% incidence of acute renal failure in the first few weeks posttransplantation when cadaveric kidneys are used. The problem is more apparent with the use of CsA. The implication of this acute renal failure may not be limited to simple delay of allograft function but may affect eventual levels of function and probability of long-term graft survival (Fig. 97-10). A varying proportion of grafts never achieve satisfactory function after transplantation and are removed ("primary nonfunction"). Rejection is, of course, more difficult to diagnose in such circumstances than in a functioning kidney. Therefore, the benefits of immediate function after

transplantation, in terms of early recognition of rejection, are obvious. New approaches might be expected with better understanding of renal metabolism and its modification by hypothermia and other manipulations. Agents have been used to provide metabolic inhibition or substrate use for cellular energy requirements. Pretreatment with purine nucleotide precursors or addition of these precursors to the perfusate has given variable results (199). Recently, there have been abundant data that intracellular calcium accumulation plays a significant role in organ dysfunction after ischemic injury (200). The demonstration of cellular and organ protection in several models of ischemic acute renal failure using calcium channel blockers led to the introduction of verapamil or other calcium channel blockers as a component of preservation fluid.

THE TRANSPLANTATION OPERATION

The surgical technique of renal transplantation is standardized (201). The cadaveric transplant kidney must first be inspected to ensure that it is suitable for transplantation before undertaking the operation. This procedure should be performed in operating room on a sterile backtable. This procedure is to remove the unnecessary fatty tissue and to prepare the donor vessels. In small pediatric donors, both kidneys can be used en bloc for transplantation in adults.

The transplanted kidney is implanted in the retroperitoneal space in either the right or the left iliac fossa through an oblique incision extending from the suprapubic area to a point just above and medial to the anterior superior iliac crest. For transplantation after failed transplants in both iliac fossae, a lower midline intraperitoneal approach should be used.

The iliac vessels should be carefully dissected (202) and the lymphatics must be ligated to prevent lymphocele formation (203). The donor renal vein is end-to-side anastomosed to the external iliac vein. The renal artery is end-to-side anastomosed to the external or common iliac artery using an aortic cuff as a patch for the anastomosis, or it is end-to-end anastomosed to the internal iliac artery, which has been previously ligated and divided. The end-to-side anastomosis using an aortic cuff is the simpler anastomosis; it is the most appropriate one to use in cadaveric transplants when the renal artery is provided with an aortic cuff. The end-to-end anastomosis

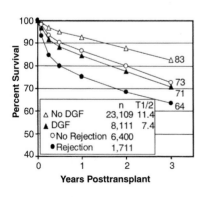

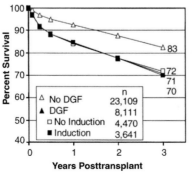

FIG. 97-10. Effects of delayed graft function (DGF), early rejections, and induction immunosuppression. Data are from the United Network for Organ Sharing Scientific Renal Transplant Registry, 1999. (From Cecka J, Terasaki P, eds. *Clinical transplants 1999.* Los Angeles: UCLA Tissue Typing Laboratory, 1999, with permission.)

to the internal iliac artery is technically more demanding and should only be used in living donor kidney transplants.

Implantation of the ureter in the bladder is performed in one of two ways (204). The first is to anastomose the spatulated end of the ureter mucosa to the dome of the bladder, drawing muscle over the anastomosis to provide a tunnel (205). The second technique is to bring the ureter through the lateral wall of the bladder and down through a 2- to 3-cm submucosal tunnel and out near the patient's own ureteric orifices at the trigone, where it is anastomosed mucosa to mucosa. The success rate of the first technique is greater than that of the second. Preventive antibiotics with appropriate broad-spectrum activity should be given with the premedication, particularly to protect against the possibility of infection being transmitted with the transplanted kidney.

General Postoperative Management and Follow-Up

Routine postoperative observations should include monitoring of vital signs, fluid intake, and urine output. Postoperative hematuria is usually transient. The Foley catheter is generally left in these patients for 3 to 4 days to prevent overdistention of the bladder, which might result from the high urine outflow rates that occur during this time. This is particularly important in diabetic patients who frequently have neurogenic bladders and can have extremely larger bladder volumes before they develop an urge to micturate. Catheters should also be carefully monitored for obstruction and irrigated under sterile conditions if occluded by a clot.

Immediate function of the transplanted kidney makes postoperative management of the patient in the first few days much simpler than if the kidney is not functioning. The patient, particularly in the case of a living related transplant, may have a massive diuresis in the first 48 hours, and for this reason, hourly monitoring of the urine output and a central venous line are essential to balance the fluid requirements appropriately. A very basic regimen, at least for the first few hours, is to replace fluid at the rate of the last hour's output plus 50 mL per hour of intravenous fluid. This can then be modified according to the kidney function and the central venous pressure.

Within 48 hours, particularly with a functioning kidney, the patient's restored sense of well being is quite remarkable, and most patients can get out of bed on the second postoperative day. Provided that no complications ensue and that any early rejection episode can be dealt with satisfactorily with appropriate treatment, these patients are ready to leave the hospital by the fifth or sixth postoperative day.

After discharge from hospital, the patient should continue to follow-up daily in the first week and the patient should then be seen two to three times a week in the first month after operation. Thereafter, the follow-up interval will depend on the patient's general condition and the development of additional problems. Routine biochemistry, hematology, and urine analysis test should be performed at each clinic visit (206).

IMMUNOSUPPRESSIVE THERAPY

Immunosuppressive options in kidney transplantation are rapidly expanding. Experience with newer immunosuppressive molecules is traditionally first obtained in kidney transplantation. Standard immunosuppressive therapy in renal transplant recipients consists of (a) baseline therapy to prevent rejection and (b) short courses of antirejection therapy using high-dose methylprednisolone, monoclonal antibodies, or polyclonal antisera such antilymphocyte globulin (ALG) and antithymocyte globulin (ATG). Most induction regimens incorporate elements of the maintenance immunosuppressive regimen. The basic approach involves the use of multiple drugs, each directed at a discrete site in the T-cell activities cascade and each with distinct side effects. The immunosuppressants can be classified, on the basis of their primary site of action, as inhibitors of transcription (CsA, tacrolimus), inhibitors of nucleotide synthesis (azathioprine, MMF), and inhibitors of growth factor signal transduction (sirolimus). The calcineurin inhibitor used will be either CsA or tacrolimus; an adjunctive agent will be chosen from MMF or sirolimus; and low-dose prednisone is used as a basic immunosuppressive drug for the induction and maintenance immunosuppressive therapy. Prednisone is started with a 200-mg dose, tapered by 40 mg per day until reaching 30 mg per day, then further tapered by 2.5 to 5 mg every 2 weeks to a maintenance dose of 5 to 10 mg per day. Most centers do not routinely discontinue or switch to alternate-day steroids unless the patient is having problems with side effects (including worsening glucose control, hypercholesterolemia, or difficulties in blood pressure control) and has had stable renal allograft function with no episodes of acute rejection within the preceding 6 to 12 months. Polyclonal or monoclonal antibodies directed at cell surface proteins are also being used in the clinical setting as induction therapy or antirejection treatment. In the absence of delayed graft function (DGF), CsA or tacrolimus can be started as a daily maintenance dose. The use of these immunosuppressive agents both to prevent and to treat rejection is associated with a number of side effects. The common medical problems in patients who have undergone transplantation are related to the use of these immunosuppressive agents. Overall, cumulative high-dose immunosuppression leads to increased infectious morbidity and mortality. The ideal of therapies in transplantation, therefore, is to reduce the level of immunosuppression that will prevent or suppress rejection while minimizing the risk of life-threatening infections and other problems related to the treatment (207,208).

Antibody Induction

Many centers use a prophylactic course of antilymphocyte agents for induction in the immediate posttransplantation period. This strategy establishes an immunosuppressive cover that enables early engraftment without the use of potential nephrotoxic drugs such as CsA and tacrolimus during the early posttransplantation period. These antibody protocols have reduced the incidence of early rejection and are particularly useful for high-risk patients such as presensitized patients with high panel reactive antibodies or patients undergoing retransplantation. Most clinical experience has been with the use of the pan-T monoclonal antibody, OKT-3, or a polyclonal antilymphocyte antibody such as Atgam at 15 mg/kg per day or Thymoglobulin at 1.5 mg/kg per day (or every other day) for 7 to 14 days (209–212). The need for antibody induction is still controversial. However, a recent meta-analysis of seven randomized, controlled trials of antibody induction therapy suggested a modest improvement in graft survival in those patients treated with antilymphocyte agents (213,214). In one recent study evaluating different induction therapies, acute rejection occurred in only 4% of those receiving Thymoglobulin compared with 25% of those receiving Atgam (211,212). Prophylactic OKT-3 appears to be most effective in high-risk cadaveric transplant recipients, including those who are sensitized or have two HLA-DR mismatches or a prolonged cold ischemia time (209,210). A report from the Collaborative Transplant Study clearly showed that sequential induction therapy with OKT-3 followed by cyclosporine resulted in better 3-year graft survival rates in first and subsequent transplants (215). These benefits were not seen with simultaneous OKT-3 and cyclosporine administration. Furthermore, the benefit of sequential therapy was greatest in high-risk patients with preformed panel reactive lymphocytotoxic antibodies of more than 50% and in Black and pediatric transplant recipients. In the highly presensitized patients, for example, 3-year graft survival rates were higher in both first transplants (80% versus 63% in those not treated with OKT-3) and in retransplants (73% versus 58%).

Anti–IL-2 receptor (CD25) monoclonal antibodies have been used for induction and can also reduce the incidence of early rejection episodes. Randomized prospective studies of two humanized antibodies against the alpha chain of the IL-2 receptor have recently shown a significant decrease in the incidence of acute rejection with few or no adverse events accompanying their use. In the first study, basiliximab (Simulect) was used in a double-blind trial in which 376 patients undergoing a primary cadaveric renal transplantation and receiving cyclosporine and corticosteroids were randomized to placebo or 20 mg of basiliximab administered on day zero and day four posttransplantation (216). There was no evidence of a cytokine release syndrome with basiliximab, and the incidence of infection and other adverse events was similar in the two groups. The benefits of this induction therapy include a lower incidence of biopsy-confirmed acute rejection at 6 months (30% versus 40%), a lower incidence of steroid-resistant first rejection episodes that required antibody therapy (10% versus 23%), and a lower mean daily dose of steroids at 2 and 4 weeks posttransplantation. Daclizumab (Zenapax) is another humanized anti–IL-2 receptor monoclonal antibody (217). Like basiliximab, daclizumab decreases the incidence of acute rejection. In one study of 153 renal transplant recipients receiving cyclosporine, azathioprine, and prednisone, the administration of daclizumab lowered the incidence of rejection (22% versus 35% with placebo). Both basiliximab and daclizumab have been approved by the Food and Drug Administration (FDA) for use in renal transplantation. No trials have yet directly compared the efficacy of these two agents, but they differ in cost and frequency of administration. A total of five doses is recommended for daclizumab, with each dose separated by 2 weeks; only two doses are recommended for basiliximab, with each separated by 4 days. The lower incidence of acute rejection and the apparent safety and lack of side effects associated with these antibodies suggest that these agents may eventually assume a significant role in induction immunosuppressive therapy in renal transplant recipients.

Treatment of Rejection

In the treatment of acute rejection, the most practical approach is probably to start a course of intravenous methylprednisolone, and if there is not an early regression of the symptoms associated with the rejection, one should perform a needle biopsy of the kidney to establish the diagnosis and consider giving OKT-3 or polyclonal anti–T-cell antibodies (see Table 97-14). The use of these potent therapies should be confined to acute rejections with acute components that are potentially reversible, for example, mononuclear interstitial cell infiltrate with tubulitis (see Fig. 97-16) or endovasculitis with acute inflammatory endothelial infiltrate (see Fig. 97-17).

Immunosuppressive Agents

Corticosteroids

Corticosteroids have been known for more than 40 years to have a suppressive effect on the immune system. Their first use in renal transplantation was in 1960 when cortisone was used to reverse a rejection episode in a living related donor transplant recipient who had been immunosuppressed by total body irradiation. Since then, steroids have been used for treatment of rejection episodes and as part of the standard immunosuppressive regimen for the prevention of rejection. The complications of steroid therapy are numerous and involve many organ systems. Acute side effects include fluid and salt retention, which may exacerbate hypertension, steroid-induced diabetes, which may result from impaired glucose tolerance, or preexisting diabetes, and rarely central nervous system (CNS) changes such as steroid psychosis or pseudotumor cerebri. These changes occur when high doses of prednisone or methylprednisolone are given during the initial posttransplantation period or in the treatment of a rejection episode. Generally, these short-term effects lessen or disappear when the doses of steroids are tapered. The long-term side effects are more insidious in onset and are associated with cushingoid changes, poor wound healing, and increased frequency of infections. Other side effects include cataracts, proximal myopathy, osteoporosis, and osteonecrosis.

In an effort to reduce the incidence of metabolic and infectious complications, the current trend is to use lower doses of steroids for maintenance (218–221) and intravenous pulses of methylprednisolone for treatment of rejection (222). Because of the growth-suppressive effects of corticosteroids, alternate-day steroid therapy was introduced for transplantation in children (223–224). However, this regimen has not been evaluated in randomized, controlled trials in adults and concerns have been expressed that conversion to alternate-day therapy has been associated with an increase in the incidence of rejection (225).

Steroid Withdrawal

Although steroid withdrawal after renal transplantation has definite advantages with a reduction in weight, hypertension, hypercholesterolemia, and improved appearance, there is concern that withdrawal of steroids from cyclosporine-based protocols will be associated with a deterioration in renal function (225,226). However, several institutes have reported successful withdrawal of steroids in kidney (227–231), pancreas (232), and liver transplantation (233–235). Data from uncontrolled studies of stable patients who have had no rejection episodes for at least 6 months have noted a successful outcome in 80% to 90% of cases maintained on cyclosporine and azathioprine. Cessation of steroid therapy is often associated with a fall in blood pressure and, in diabetic patients, better glycemic control; total cholesterol levels also fall, but there is an equivalent reduction in high-density lipoprotein (HDL) cholesterol and therefore an uncertain effect on cardiovascular risk. Prevention of osteopenia and aseptic necrosis of bone are other potential benefits; however, there are limited data to confirm this benefit. These beneficial metabolic effects must be balanced against the effect of steroid withdrawal on graft outcome. The Collaborative Transplant Study Registry data suggest that graft survival is superior in those patients in whom steroids are withdrawn. A similar analysis from the Australian and New Zealand Dialysis and Transplantation Registry also found the patients with a functioning graft at 1 year who were not on steroids had a better patient and graft survival thereafter, compared with patients who remained on steroids (236). However, these uncontrolled data have a possible defect in that patients may have remained on steroids because they had a more difficult early course, which might be associated with a poorer long-term graft survival course. Furthermore, a meta-analysis of prospective trials of steroid withdrawal in the first 3 months after transplantation suggested an increased incidence of acute rejection after withdrawal. Thus, early (within 3 months) cessation of steroids is associated with an increased incidence of acute rejection and a possible decrease in long-term graft survival. The effect of late withdrawal of steroids on graft function was examined in a randomized, prospective, controlled trial of patients on triple immunosuppressive therapy. One hundred patients in whom renal transplantation had been performed 1 to 6 years before the study entry were randomized to total prednisone withdrawal over 4 months or to continuation of triple therapy. Among the 49 patients randomized to steroid withdrawal, 42 (86%) were able to achieve complete cessation. Withdrawal of steroids was associated with decreases in blood pressure (although not completely sustained) and in total cholesterol levels (a decrease on average of 38 mg/dL). Although no defined episodes of acute reaction were observed among these patients, a significant decrease in renal function and a significant increase in the percentage of patients with proteinuria were found, compared with control patients. At 1 year, more steroid-withdrawal patients had a plasma creatinine concentration that was more than 25% more than the baseline value than control patients (53% versus 25%). Further increases were observed in the steroid-withdrawal patients at 2 and 3 years. After correction for differences in baseline creatinine values, the steroid-withdrawal patients had higher serum creatinine values at study exit and at 1 year than those of controls. This study confirmed the benefits of steroid withdrawal, namely an improvement in weight, hypertension, and hypercholesterolemia. However, there was an associated 10% decline in renal function, which appears to be stable at 3 years. Furthermore, the study was able to define a group of patients in whom steroids could be withdrawn without risk (237). Thus, an element of caution is required before recommending routine use of steroid withdrawal. However, the introduction of the newer immunosuppressive drugs such as tacrolimus, MMF, and sirolimus (rapamycin) may allow steroids to be withdrawn at an earlier stage after transplantation.

Azathioprine

Despite newer immunosuppressive regimens, azathioprine will continue to be used for patients with successful transplants who are already receiving azathioprine, for patients who are intolerant of other agents, and for some patients because of economic reasons. Azathioprine was first used as an immunosuppressive agent for kidney transplantation in 1962 (238), and shortly afterward, steroids were added for the prevention of rejection. For many years, azathioprine, at a dose of 1.75 to 2.5 mg/kg per day, was used with high-dose steroids, which were responsible for most of the significant complications accompanying renal transplantation. Then, in 1970, McGeown and colleagues reported excellent graft survival with azathioprine and low-dose steroids (239,240). Their patients were not typical in that nearly all had bilateral nephrectomies and all had many blood transfusions. For this reason, the Oxford group undertook a prospective, randomized, controlled trial of high-dose versus low-dose steroids in combination with azathioprine and showed not only that graft survival was identical but that the reduction in steroids-related complications was striking (218,219). These data were subsequently confirmed in other prospective trials, and low-dose steroids became the norm in combination with azathioprine (241). Before the 1980s, azathioprine and steroids were the mainstays of maintenance immunosuppression before the introduction of CsA (242–244). The side effects of azathioprine include bone marrow depression with granulocytopenia, hepatic dysfunction, pancreatitis, and an increased risk of infection and neoplasia. Macrocytic anemia with megaloblastic erythrocytosis (245), pure red cell aplasia (246), thrombocytopenia, and suppression of all marrow cell lines have been reported. Trimethoprim-sulfamethoxazole, when administered with azathioprine, may lead to neutropenia and thrombocytopenia (247), possibly because of the antibiotic's antifolate effect, resulting in enhanced 6-MP marrow toxicity.

Cyclosporin A

CsA is a fungal peptide with potent antilymphocyte properties. Cyclosporine was introduced to renal transplantation by Calne et al. (248) in 1978. The initial use of CsA in Europe was based on the early Cambridge experience of using CsA alone, whereas in North America, CsA was used with steroids. There were a number of studies evaluating cyclosporine protocols (249–252). The initial recommended dose of 14 to 18 mg/kg per day was used in most clinical trials. There is a trend of using a lower initial dose for renal transplantation, in the range of 8 to 12 mg/kg per day. This dosage was then adjusted to achieve specific plasma serum or whole blood levels. Although the need for steroids in patients treated with CsA remains unsolved (249,253), most patients are likely to need high-dose methylprednisolone for the treatment of rejection episodes. For this reason, most centers do use steroids with CsA from the time of transplantation. However, many patients can be managed without steroids or weaned off steroids during the first few months after transplantation. The Canadian Multicenter Study showed that steroids could be withdrawn successfully at 3 months, and the results were comparable with those of the control patients who were maintained on steroids (252). The Australian Multicenter Study (254) achieved 83% 1-year graft survival using CsA alone, and more than 60% of patients remained off maintenance steroids, which were only used for treatment of rejections. Salaman et al. (255) in a small study found no benefit of adding steroids, compared with CsA alone, but commented that a nephrotoxic side effect was more frequent in patients not on steroids. Other groups have successfully used a combination of azathioprine and CsA to avoid steroids (254,256,257).

Side Effects

A number of side effects have been observed in patients receiving CsA (248,258–261). Nephrotoxicity is the most worrying side effect of cyclosporine. Dose-related, reversible acute nephrotoxicity is observed in about 20% of patients (260,261). Nephrotoxic episodes tend to occur after 1 month. In addition to nephrotoxicity, other side effects include hypertrichosis, neurasthenia, convulsions, hepatic dysfunction, gingival hypertrophy, hyperkalemia, hypomagnesemia, hypertension, and fluid retention. CsA infrequently causes a microangiopathic hemolytic anemia in association with hemolytic-uremic syndrome. An autoimmune hemolytic anemia has also been reported in patients receiving CsA when ABO blood group O kidneys are engrafted into patients in blood group A or B. It is postulated that passenger B lymphocytes cause graft-verses-host disease by secreting hemolytic antibodies; an autoimmune neutropenia and thrombocytopenia have also been reported in this setting of ABO incompatibility (262–264).

Pharmacokinetics

Oral absorption of CsA is slow and incomplete, with peak blood concentrations occurring 2 to 4 hours after a dose. On average, 37% of an orally administered dose will be absorbed. It then undergoes some first-pass metabolism, yielding an absolute bioavailability of 27% in the blood. It is primarily eliminated from the body via hepatic metabolism. Cyclosporine is administered either as a single daily dose or as two 12-hourly doses. The starting oral dosage is 8 to 12 mg/kg per day. The dose is further tapered to a maintenance dosage of 3 to 6 mg/kg per day depending on the graft function and trough levels. The rationale for the twice-daily dose is based on the pharmacokinetics observed: that trough levels are reached between 12 and 16 hours after a single oral dose and on the assumption that nephrotoxicity might be related to peak levels, rather than trough levels (265,266).

Intravenous CsA, which may aggravate postoperative ATN, is to be avoided in the perioperative period. Patients with ileus or other GI dysfunction however may require intravenous coverage of CsA. The intravenous dose for CsA is 2 mg/kg or one-third of the oral dose and should be given in a slow infusion with 0.9% sodium chloride or 5% dextrose over 2 to 6 hours (267–269).

Drug Interactions

Cyclosporine is metabolized almost entirely in the liver, probably through the cytochrome P450 system. Most of the drug is excreted in the bile, and liver dysfunction causes it to accumulate and serum levels to rise. Thus, drugs that induce hepatic enzymes such as rifampicin, phenytoin, phenobarbitone, neflocin, and nafcillin will increase the rate of metabolism of cyclosporine and lower blood levels of the parent compound. Drugs that increase cyclosporine levels include calcium entry blockers such as diltiazem, verapamil, nicardipine, erythromycin, and ketoconazole. The well-known interactions are listed in Table 97-8. Impaired renal function does not affect plasma or whole blood levels because only about 0.1% of the native drug is detected in the urine and only 10% of the metabolites of the parent compound is excreted in the urine. A number of drugs are now known to enhance nephrotoxicity of CsA. These are aminoglycosides, ketoconazole, amphotericin B, trimethoprim, and cotrimoxazole (270–272).

TABLE 97-8. *Cyclosporine drug interactions*

Increase level	Decrease level	Additive nephrotoxicity
Erythromycin	Barbiturate	Aminoglycosides
Diltiazem	Carbamazepine	Amphotericin B
Ketoconazole	Isoniazid	Co-trimoxazole
Metoclopramide	Phenytoin	Trimethoprim
Oral contraceptives	Rifampicin	Acyclovir
Nicardipine		

Monitoring CsA Levels

Therapeutic monitoring of CsA levels is an important part of the management because of the variation in the interpatient and intrapatient metabolism. The trough level, rather than the peak level, is measured because its timing is more consistent and appears to correlate better with toxic complications. Measurements to calculate the area under the curve (AUC) will reflect the bioavailability of the drug and may allow more precise and individualized patient management (275,276). Plasma or whole blood levels of the drug can be measured either by radioimmunoassay (RIA) using polyclonal or monoclonal antibodies, which detect the parent drug and its metabolites, or high-pressure liquid chromatography (HPLC), which selectively measures parent compound. Recently, a number of nonisotopic immunoassays have also been commercially developed. One of the most successful method is the Abbot TDX System, which uses fluorescence polarization immunoassay to monitor the reaction between the drug and the antibody. The results are comparable to those using RIA (Table 97-9). Values obtained by RIA are approximately 1.3 times higher than those obtained by HPLC. Forty percent to 60% of the drug concentration in whole blood is bound to red cells, lymphocytes, and granulocytes. Because drug binding to red cells is temperature-dependent, plasma must be separated from the red cells at 37°C to obtain reproducible results. There is considerable disagreement as to whether plasma or blood levels correlate with either CsA toxicity or immunosuppression. Nevertheless, most physicians would feel that CsA trough levels, along with all clinical, biochemical, and histological parameters, are helpful to distinguish between nephrotoxicity and rejection (273–276).

TABLE 97-9. *Methods of determining cyclosporine levels*

Assay	Specific for parent compound	Recommended trough levels (ng/mL)
RIA (monoclonal)	+	Serum 50–125
		Blood 100–400
HPLC	+	Blood 100–400
RIA (polyclonal)	−	Serum 150–300
		Blood 200–800
FPIA (Abbott TDX system)	−	Blood 200–350

RIA, radioimmunoassay; HPLC, high-pressure liquid chromatography; FPIA, fluorescence polarization immunoassay.

Cyclosporine Nephrotoxicity

Nephrotoxicity is the most frequently encountered and most important side effect of CsA therapy. CsA nephrotoxicity can occur acutely within days or weeks after renal transplantation. The pathogenesis of acute nephrotoxicity is due to a decline in renal blood flow with a consequent fall in the GFR.

Acute CsA Nephrotoxicity. Acute cyclosporine toxicity tends to occur about 3 or 4 weeks after transplantation, rather than within the first 2 weeks when the typical rejection episode might occur and is not associated with swelling or tenderness of the graft or with fever. A small increment in the serum creatinine level occurs, which is frequently correlated with high serum CsA trough levels. The serum creatinine level returns to baseline within 24 hours of the reduction of the CsA dose (260,261).

Drugs that Cause Additive Nephrotoxicity. Along with CsA-induced nephrotoxicity, other drugs may cause renal dysfunction including antibiotics, diuretics, and H_2 receptor blockers. Trimethoprim-sulfamethoxazole, commonly used for infection prophylaxis, can cause an interstitial nephritis, or the trimethoprim moiety may interfere with tubule secretion of creatinine, leading to an elevation in the serum creatinine in the absence of a fall in GFR. Other antibiotics (aminoglycosides, amphotericin B) may be directly nephrotoxic. Diuretics may cause volume depletion or interstitial nephritis and should be avoided, if possible, in the early posttransplantation period. Cimetidine, an H_2-receptor antagonist, used for peptic ulcer disease prophylaxis, may compete with creatinine for tubule secretion and also cause a "false" increase in the serum creatinine; this was not seen with ranitidine. Concomitant administration of CsA and sirolimus increased absorption of CsA. Lower doses of CsA are required to maintain a therapeutic trough level (277–279).

Chronic CsA Nephrotoxicity. The debate about long-term nephrotoxicity of CsA remains unresolved. The pathogenesis of chronic CsA nephrotoxicity is currently unclear. Dose reduction does not reverse this form of chronic toxicity. There is evidence that renal prostaglandins and thromboxane production is stimulated in chronic CsA nephrotoxicity. Substitution of an oil-based fluid with fish oil leads to generation of vasodilatory arachidonate metabolites in the kidney. It has been suggested that CsA induces an arteriolar lesion in the kidney by reducing prostacyclin production secondary to decreased synthesis of prostacyclin stimulating factor. The prostacyclin stimulating factor may be a cytokine produced by helper T cells or interleukin 1 produced by macrophages. This may explain both immunosuppressive and nephrotoxic effects of CsA. Increased incidence of glomerular thrombosis in CsA treated renal and other organ transplant patients tend to support this hypothesis.

The stability of renal allograft function associated with long-term CsA therapy has been documented (256–258). In some cases, the deteriorating long-term renal function might be due to inadequate immunosuppression and chronic rejection rather then CsA nephrotoxicity. However, conversion from cyclosporine to azathioprine and prednisone is performed for documented nephrotoxicity or other worrying side effect of CsA. Several protocols have been proposed in the past (256,263,264). To avoid acute rejection after conversion, it was recommended that an overlap between discontinuation of CsA and the commencement of azathioprine and prednisone.

Differential Diagnosis of CsA Nephrotoxicity. In the early posttransplantation period, functional CsA nephrotoxicity has clinical features similar to those of acute renal allograft rejection. In the CsA treated patients, rejection may present with or without decline in urine output along with a rise in serum creatinine. Because CsA nephrotoxicity may present in a similar fashion, an allograft biopsy specimen should be obtained if the diagnosis is uncertain. Histologically, acute CsA nephrotoxicity can be distinguished from acute rejection chiefly by the absence of an extensive inflammatory infiltrate (280).

However, direct tubular toxicity has been described when CsA levels are elevated above 1000 ng/mL in whole blood. Whereas morphologic evidence of tubular injury was commonly seen in transplant biopsies obtained in the early years with CsA therapy, the incidence of this form of nephrotoxicity has fallen. The glomeruli may be small because of chronic ischemia; they may have wrinkled or thickened basement membranes or increased mesangial matrix; or they may be completely hyalinized or sclerosed. The vascular changes may include intimal proliferation with luminal obliteration most striking in the interlobular and arcuate arteries, and medial necrosis with degenerative changes of the internal elastic lamina. Tubular atrophy with luminal obliteration and interstitial fibrosis complete the picture (281,282). Needle biopsy evaluation of Class II MHC antigen expression has also been used for the differential diagnosis of CsA nephrotoxicity from kidney graft rejection (208). In the absence of the specimen, a clinical picture suggestive of CsA toxicity includes hypertension, tremor, elevated CsA trough levels, hyperkalemia, and a temporal relationship of improvement in allograft function after CsA dose reduction.

Neoral

The new microemulsion formulation of cyclosporine A is Neoral. The absorption of CsA from its classic formulation is slow and incomplete, and varies from day to day. The new microemulsion of CsA (Neoral) may overcome these shortcomings (271). Absorption is more rapid, complete, and consistent, and relatively independent of blood and bile flow. Maximum concentration is increased by 30 to 60%; mean time to reach maximum concentration is only 1.4 hours; and absorption, as measured by the area under the time-concentration curve, is 20 to 30% greater than with the classic CsA formulation. In addition, day-to-day variability is reduced by at least 50% for each of these parameters (273). Neoral has been approved by the Food and Drug Administration (FDA) in the United States. Initial trials have confirmed

that Neoral is equivalent to cyclosporine A for prevention of graft rejection and no differences have been shown in graft or patient survival. The dose of the microemulsion is 10% to 20% lower than standard cyclosporine; however, the exact conversion dose must be carefully undertaken.

Generic Formulations of Cyclosporine

A number of generic formulations of cyclosporine have been developed. These include the Gengraf capsule (Abbott Laboratories), the Cyclosporine USP capsule (Eon Labs), and the SangCya liquid have been approved for use in the United States. Other generic formulations are also available outside the United States. SangCya (Sang-35) is an oral liquid formulation of cyclosporine that has pharmacokinetic properties similar to those of Neoral. Like Neoral, it does not appear to be dependent on bile salts for absorption. Because of its bioequivalency, the impact of these generic formulations remains to be seen. Overall, these generic formulations are about 20% less expensive than Neoral. No adverse events have been reported regarding their use (283–289).

Tacrolimus

FK506, now called tacrolimus (Prograf), is a macrolide immunosuppressant and is similar to CsA in its mode of action (290,291). Both tacrolimus and CsA prevent the transcription of several T-cell growth promoting genes such as IL-2. Whereas CsA binds to cyclophilin, tacrolimus binds to an immunophilin, FK506 binding protein (FKBP). The drug's immunosuppressive action is mediated via blockade of calcineurin-mediated T-cell receptor signal transduction and inhibition of IL-2. By inhibiting cytokine gene transcription, tacrolimus suppresses T-cell and T-cell–dependent B-cell activation (292).

The initial experience with tacrolimus was mostly in liver transplantation because the drug was originally approved by the FDA for use in liver transplantation. The drug has now been used in kidney transplantation (293–295). Although recent trials have shown similar graft survival outcomes with tacrolimus when compared with Sandimmune CsA-based regimens in the setting of renal transplantation, the incidence of acute rejection and requirement for intensive immunosuppression may be less with tacrolimus. The multicenter FK506 Kidney Transplant Study Group trial (296) randomized 412 cadaveric renal transplant recipients to either tacrolimus or Sandimmune CsA-based immunosuppressive regimens. Both Sandimmune- and tacrolimus-based therapy resulted in similar graft survival rates at 1 year. However, tacrolimus was associated with a significantly decreased incidence of biopsy-proven acute rejection episodes (30.7% versus 46.4%) and requirement for antilymphocyte antibody therapy (10.7% versus 25.1%). The European Tacrolimus Multicenter Renal Study Group reported similar beneficial effects with tacrolimus in a 12-month follow-up (297) (Table 97-10). A meta-analysis of four studies involving more

TABLE 97-10. *Patient and graft survival and the incidence of acute rejection in two large randomized prospective multicenter trials of tacrolimus and cyclosporine in Europe and the United States*

	Tacrolimus (%)	Cyclosporine (%)	P
European trial (N = 448)			
One-yr patient survival	93.0	96.5	NS
One-yr graft survival	82.5	86.2	NS
Cumulative acute rejection	34.2	57.2	<0.001
Steroid-resistant rejection	11.3	21.6	<0.001
U.S. trial (N = 412)			
One-yr patient survival	95.6	96.6	NS
One-yr graft survival	91.2	87.9	NS
Cumulative acute rejection	30.7	46.4	<0.001
Steroid-resistant rejection	10.7	25.1	<0.001

NS, not significant.

than 1,000 patients also found that tacrolimus, compared with CsA, significantly reduced the incidence of acute rejection (298).

Tacrolimus may also be beneficial in renal transplantation as rescue therapy in patients with recurrent or resistant rejection episodes on CsA (299,300). Patients with biopsy-proven ongoing acute renal allograft rejection were switched from CsA to tacrolimus. The overall response rate was 74%. These beneficial results were confirmed in another trial that examined the use of tacrolimus among 73 patients in whom acute renal allograft rejection was refractory to therapy with corticosteroids (100%) and antilymphocyte antibodies (81%). The graft survival rate was 75% at 12 months after tacrolimus administration.

Tacrolimus has a toxicity profile slightly different from that of CsA. Both short- and long-term studies in liver and renal transplant recipients suggest that tacrolimus is at least as nephrotoxic as CsA (301,302). Tacrolimus can also cause hyperkalemia, hyperuricemia, and rarely hemolytic-uremic syndrome (303–306). However, there are differences in toxicity between tacrolimus and CsA. These include more prominent neurologic (307) and metabolic side effects; less frequent hirsutism, gingival hyperplasia, and hypertension; more frequent alopecia; and an increased proclivity for susceptibility to polyoma virus infection (308). Hypertrophic cardiomyopathy has also been reported in children treated with tacrolimus (309). The multicenter FK506 Renal Transplant Study (296–298) found an important difference in the toxicity profile between the two drugs: a relatively high incidence of insulin-dependent diabetes mellitus in tacrolimus-treated patients, compared with cyclosporine-treated individuals (19.9% versus 4.0%, respectively).

The recommended starting dosage for tacrolimus is 0.15 to 0.3 mg/kg per day administered in a split dose every 12 hours. Doses are adjusted to maintain tacrolimus drug levels at between 10 and 20 ng/dL during the first few posttransplantation months and between 5 to 15 ng/dL thereafter. African American patients were found to need a mean 37% higher dose than White patients to achieve comparable blood concentrations (310). Tacrolimus is absorbed primarily by small intestine and its oral bioavailability is about 25% with large interpatient and intrapatient variability. Like CsA, it is primarily metabolized by hepatic cytochrome P450. Therefore, the drug level will be influenced by concomitant administration of medications that affect cytochrome P450. Two commercial kits are available for tacrolimus-level determination. The microparticle immunoassay (Abbott Laboratories) is simpler and faster than ELISA (311–315).

Mycophenolate Mofetil

MMF (CellCept) is a new immunosuppressive agent that has been recently approved by the FDA for use in patients undergoing kidney transplantation. The drug is converted *in vivo* to mycophenolic acid (MPA), a noncompetitive and reversible inhibitor of inosine monophosphate (IMP) dehydrogenase (316). This enzyme is responsible for the conversion of IMP to guanosine monophosphate (GMP), which is required for the production of nucleic acids and other critical steps in cellular activation. Lymphocytes require the *de novo* synthesis of GMP, so MPA causes a profound inhibition of T- and B-cell function. Most other cells possess a salvage pathway that permits a resynthesis of guanine derivatives and are relatively resistant to MPA.

MMF has been used in renal transplant recipients in dual, triple, or sequential therapy in combination with CsA. In each protocol, the incidence and severity of acute rejection and the requirement for antirejection therapy were decreased significantly in the patients receiving MMF. The biopsy-proven rejection incidence rate fell overall by 45% to 55%, the number of patients treated for rejection declined by 35% to 50%, and the use of OKT-3 or ATG for refractory rejection fell by 40% to 66%, compared with patients administered azathioprine (317,318). In the study comparing mycophenolate (2 or 3 g per day) with placebo in 491 recipients of a cadaveric renal transplant treated with cyclosporine and prednisone, at 6 months, the biopsy-proven incidence of acute rejection was 14% to 17% with mycophenolate versus 46% with placebo. Placebo patients were also much more likely to require high doses of corticosteroids and antilymphocyte therapy to reverse the rejection episodes. Follow-up at 3 years revealed that the incidence of graft loss was significantly lower by 7.6% among those randomized to MMF. Another trial compared mycophenolate (2 to 3 g per day in divided doses) with azathioprine in 499 patients who were also treated with CsA, prednisone, and ATG. Although 6- and 12-month patient and graft survival rates were similar in the two groups, there were fewer first rejection episodes (18% to 20% versus 38% with azathioprine). The other trial is a randomized clinical report by the Tricontinental Mycophenolate Mofetil Renal Transplantation Study Group (319,320). It also compared the effectiveness of MMF at two doses, 3 g per day (164 patients) and 2 g per day (173 patients), with that of azathioprine, at 100 to 150 mg per day (166 patients). Patients were treated with equivalent doses of corticosteroids and CsA. Again, the MMF groups had a lower incidence of treatment failure at 6 months—35% and 38% versus 50% with azathioprine; a lower incidence of rejection—16% and 20% versus 36%; decreased use of antilymphocyte antibody for severe or steroid-resistant rejection episodes (4.9% and 8.8% versus 15.4%); and a nonsignificant trend toward improved graft survival at 1 year. At 3 years, both MMF groups continued to show a nonsignificant trend toward better graft survival and a lower rate of graft loss from rejection as compared with the azathioprine group (321,322). Despite the higher expense of mycophenolate, the lower incidence of rejection may make the use of this agent cost effective. Mycophenolate has also been successfully used as the third agent in tacrolimus-based regimens (323). In one randomized study of 208 patients comparing tacrolimus and prednisone versus tacrolimus, prednisone, and mycophenolate, the incidence of rejection 1 year posttransplantation was lower among the group given mycophenolate (27% versus 36%).

The major side effects of MMF include mild neutropenia and GI intolerance such as diarrhea, esophagitis, and gastritis at high doses. The toxicity profile was greater with a 3-g dose compared with 2 g of MMF. The reason for leukopenia in transplant recipients treated with MMF remains to be determined because leukopenia was not predicted based on the mechanism of action of MMF and was not noted in patients with psoriasis or rheumatoid arthritis who were treated with this drug. The incidence of infection is not increased overall, although there may be a slight increase in tissue invasive cytomegalovirus (CMV) infection of the GI tract and liver (324,325). The use of MMF was associated with an increase in HCV viremia (326).

A safe and effective dosage of MMF is 1 to 2 g per day. Therapeutic drug monitoring is still at a preliminary stage. HPLC methods have been established for the measurement of MMF, MPA, and mycophenolic acid glucuronide (MPAG), the principal metabolite that is pharmacologically inactive. Orally administered MMF is rapidly absorbed and hydrolyzed to MPA in the liver and is then glucuronidated to an inactive form MPAG. Bioavailability of MMF is 90% with a half-life of 12 hours. There is no accumulation of MPA in hepatic or renal impairment (327–329). However,

there are substantial intrapatient and interpatient variations in both adults and children. The maximum concentration of MPA and the AUC value determined immediately after transplantation were only 30% to 50% of those measured for patients 3 months after transplantation (326,330). In these patients, the free levels of MPA remained unchanged, suggesting that the increase in MPA levels was mainly due to increased levels of MPA bound to plasma proteins. Because the pharmacologic effects of MMF is thought to be correlated with free and not bound MPA levels, a reduction in plasma protein levels may increase the free levels of MPA without affecting whole blood concentrations (326). There is evidence of pharmacologic interaction between MMF and tacrolimus. MPA levels increase when MMF is used with tacrolimus (331,332). Monitoring the pharmacodynamic activity of MMF, by monitoring the activity of the enzyme IMP dehydrogenase, which is inhibited by MPA, has also been suggested as a potential method to monitor the efficacy of MMF and adjust its dose (333,334). The variability in MPA levels suggests that measurements of plasma MPA levels could be beneficial. There appears to be a good correlation between the drug exposure and the probability of rejection (335,336).

Sirolimus (Rapamycin)

Sirolimus, formerly designated *rapamycin,* is a macrolide antibiotic produced by the fungus, *Streptomyces hygroscopicus.* It was first isolated from soil samples that had been collected on Easter Island (or Rapa Nui) in 1969 (337,338). At that time, rapamycin was observed to arrest cell growth in *Candida* species and filamentous fungi. It was also shown to have tumoricidal activity, indicating that the antiproliferative effects seen in yeast could be extended to the mammalian system. Sirolimus activity in animal models of autoimmune disease was demonstrated in 1977 (339,340). The immunosuppressant activity of the drug was not documented in animal models until 1988 (341). Clinical trials were initiated 4 years later, and it was not until 1999 that FDA approval was granted for the use of sirolimus for the prophylaxis of organ rejection in patients receiving renal transplants.

The immunosuppressive function of sirolimus ultimately results from the dampening of cytokine and growth factor activity upon T, B, and nonimmune cells. Sirolimus binds to the immunophilins, a property shared with CsA and tacrolimus. Whereas tacrolimus and CsA both inhibit calcineurin-dependent T-cell receptor signal transduction, sirolimus inhibits a different pathway required for full T-cell activation, by blocking the phosphorylation of p70(s6) kinase and the eukaryotic initiation factor 4E binding protein, PHAS-1. Like tacrolimus, sirolimus binds to FKBP. Therefore sirolimus and tacrolimus compete for the same binding site on FKBP, but the resulting complexes, the functional unit for each, have different actions. The FKBP complex with tacrolimus blocks T-cell activation and the release of IL-2. The complex with sirolimus, on the other hand, blocks T-cell proliferation in response to IL-2. Furthermore, the sirolimus FKBP complex, unlike the tacrolimus FKBP complex, does not bind calcineurin. The cellular receptors for the sirolimus FKBP complex are being elucidated. Two proteins, designated as targets of rapamycin (TOR1 and TOR2), were identified as receptors for sirolimus. The antiproliferative activity of sirolimus appears to be a result in part of the sirolimus FKBP complex blocking the activation of the protein kinases that are involved in cell proliferation. *In vitro*, sirolimus and tacrolimus compete for the same binding protein and are antagonists pharmacologically. However, both drugs interact *in vivo* to produce immunosuppression that is additive or synergistic (342–345).

Sirolimus is currently being developed for combination maintenance immunosuppressive therapy with cyclosporine. Results of a phase I/II study suggest that combined therapy with CsA and sirolimus may permit the withdrawal of corticosteroids in most patients and reduce the incidence of acute rejection (346,347). In addition, another phase II trial found that among White recipients, a regimen consisting of rapamycin, corticosteroids, and CsA lowered the incidence of acute rejection and may be cyclosporine sparing.

The major side effects of sirolimus are dyslipidemia and thrombocytopenia. Although the drug is minimally nephrotoxic when used alone, the combination of sirolimus and CsA has caused synergistic toxicity in animals (348,349). In healthy volunteers, concomitant administration of sirolimus and the Neoral formulation of CsA increased the AUC for sirolimus by 230%, compared with administration of sirolimus alone, whereas administration 4 hours after the CsA dose increased the AUC by 80%. For this reason, it is recommended that sirolimus be administered 4 hours after the morning CsA dose. The pharmacologic interaction between sirolimus and tacrolimus has not been rigorously explored. Careful surveillance for drug interactions with sirolimus will be required. Sirolimus-based immunosuppression has a different adverse effect profile among renal transplant recipients, compared with a cyclosporine-based regimen. In this multicenter European trial, 83 patients were randomized to sirolimus or CsA, with all individuals receiving corticosteroids and azathioprine. At 12 months, no significant difference was observed in graft or patient survival rates or the incidence of biopsy-confirmed acute rejection. However, compared with cyclosporine, sirolimus was associated with a higher incidence of hypertriglyceridemia (51% versus 12%), hypercholesterolemia (44% versus 14%), thrombocytopenia (37% versus 0%), and leukopenia (39% versus 14%) (350–353).

Sirolimus is given at a dosage of 2 mg orally once daily 4 hours after the morning dose of either CsA or tacrolimus. A loading dose of 6 mg is given on the first day of treatment. African American patients may benefit from a maintenance dose of 5 mg per day. The drug is rapidly absorbed, reaching peak concentrations in 1 to 2 hours. It has a long half-life, averaging 62 hours. The recommended target trough levels vary between 5 and 15 ng/dL. Blood levels of sirolimus can be determined by HPLC with ultraviolet light detection or HPLC mass spectrometry. Drug levels of sirolimus exhibit considerable intrapatient and interpatient variability. Therapeutic drug monitoring by measuring trough blood levels could be expected to improve efficacy and reduce toxicity (354–356).

Overall, sirolimus is a new promising drug. Its potential role in slowing the progression of chronic transplant nephropathy has not yet been evaluated. In animal models, sirolimus has shown to attenuate or prevent chronic rejection. In a preliminary study, the switch from calcineurin-dependent drugs to sirolimus in patients with chronic rejection led to renal function improvement. However, these preliminary data need further randomized studies to clarify the role of sirolimus in chronic transplant nephropathy (357,358).

Polyclonal Antisera

ALG or ATG are polyclonal antisera derived from immunization of lymphocytes, lymphoblasts, or thymocytes into rabbits, goats, or horses and have been used prophylactically as induction therapy during the early posttransplantation period and for treatment of acute rejection (359–362).

The precise mechanism of action of the polyclonal antibodies is fully understood. The immunosuppressive product contains cytotoxic antibodies directed against various T-cell markers. After the administration, there is depletion of peripheral blood lymphocytes. The lymphocytes are either lysed or cleared by the reticuloendothelial system, and their surface antigen may be masked by the antibody.

Until recently, Atgam (Pharmacia & Upjohn, Kalamazoo, MI) was the only approved polyclonal agent available in the United States. Atgam is a purified γ-globulin solution obtained by immunization of horses with human thymocytes. It contains antibodies to a wide variety of human T-cell surface antigens, including the major histocompatibility complex (MHC) antigens. Thymoglobulin (SangStat Medical Corporation, Menlo Park, CA) is another polyclonal immunosuppressive agent derived from the rabbit (363,364). It recently gained approval for the treatment of rejection from the FDA. Like Atgam, Thymoglobulin contains antibodies to a wide variety of T-cell antigens and MHC antigens. Both Thymoglobulin and Atgam reverse acute rejection, thereby reducing the risks of developing chronic allograft nephropathy. Data suggest that Thymoglobulin may be superior to Atgam for the prevention or reversal of rejection. The ability of Thymoglobulin (1.5 mg/kg per day) and Atgam (15 mg/kg per day) to reverse rejection and prevent recurrent acute rejection was evaluated in one randomized study of 163 patients (365). Thymoglobulin was associated with a higher rejection reversal rate (88% versus 76%; P = 0.027) and a lower incidence of recurrent rejection 90 days after therapy (17% versus 36%). A third polyclonal preparation, the Minnesota ALG (MALG), is no longer available. Its efficacy, when compared with other immunosuppressive agents, has been extensively studied in multiple clinical trials (366–368).

Potential side effects of ALG include fever, chills, erythema, thrombocytopenia, local phlebitis, serum sickness, and anaphylaxis (369). The potential for development of host anti-ALG antibodies has not been a significant problem because of the use of less immunogenic preparations and probably because ALG suppresses the immune response to the foreign protein itself. To avoid allergic reactions, the patients receive intravenous medications consisting of methylprednisolone (30 mg) and diphenhydramine hydrochloride (50 mg) 30 minutes before injection. Acetaminophen should be given before and 4 hours after commencement of infusion for fever control. Thrombocytopenia and leukopenia may necessitate reduction or curtailment of the drug dose.

OKT3 Monoclonal Antibodies

OKT3 is a mouse monoclonal antibody directed against the CD3 molecule of the T lymphocyte. OKT3 has been used either from the time of transplantation to prevent rejection or to treat an acute rejection episode (370–377). It has been shown in a randomized clinical trial (371) to reverse 95% of primary rejection episodes, compared with 75% with high-dose steroids in patients who received azathioprine-prednisone immunosuppression. In patients receiving triple therapy (CsA azathioprine prednisone), 82% of primary rejection episodes were successfully reversed by OKT3 versus 63% with high-dose steroids. As with ALG, reduction of concomitant immunosuppression (discontinuation of CsA and reduction of azathioprine or mofetil dose) decreases the incidence of infectious complications. Side effects include fever, rigors, diarrhea, myalgia, arthralgia, aseptic meningitis, dyspnea, and wheezing, but these rarely persist after the second day of therapy. Release of tumor necrosis factor (TNF), IL-2, and interferon-γ (IFN-γ) in serum is found after OKT3 injection. The acute pulmonary compromise due to a capillary leak syndrome has rarely been seen because patients are brought to within 3% of dry weight before initiation of OKT3 treatment. Infectious complications, particularly infection with CMV, are increased after multiple courses of OKT3 (374–377). To avoid these potential complications during OKT3 treatment, one should follow a recommended protocol (Table 97-11).

The development of host anti–OKT3 antibodies is a potential problem for the use of this drug in patients previously treated with it. About 33% to 100% of patients develop antimouse antibodies after the first exposure to OKT3, depending on concomitant immunosuppression (376). Anti–OKT3 titers of 1 : 10,000 or more usually correlate with lack of clinical response. If anti–OKT3 antibodies are of low titer, retreatment with OKT3 is almost always successful. If retreatment is attempted with antimouse titers of 1 : 100 or more, certain laboratory parameters, including the peripheral lymphocyte count, CD3 T cells, and trough free circulating OKT3, should be monitored. If the absolute CD3 T-lymphocyte count is

TABLE 97-11. *Recommended protocol for OKT3 treatment*

I. Evaluation and treatment before administration
  A. Physical examination
  B. Laboratory tests including complete blood count
  C. Monitor intake and output, record weight changes
  D. Chest radiograph
  E. Hemodialysis or ultrafiltration for volume overload
  F. Premedication on day 0 and 1
    1. Methylprednisolone, 250–500 mg IV given 1 hr before the dose
    2. Methylprednisolone or hydrocortisone sodium succinate, 250–500 mg IV given 30 min after the dose
  G. Diphenhydramine, 50 mg IV 30 min before dose daily
  H. Acetaminophen, 650 mg PO 30 min before dose
  I. Discontinue or decrease dose of cyclosporin A or tacrolimus
II. Administer OKT3 (Orthclone), 5 mg/d IV, days 0–13
III. Monitor clinical course
  A. Check CD3 level on day 3
  B. Increase OKT3 dosage to 10 mg/d if either
    1. Anti-OKT3 antibody level is high
    2. OKT3 level is low
    3. CD3 level is not low
IV. CMV chemoprophylaxis

CMV, cisplatin, methotrexate, and vinblastine.

more than 10 per microliter or free circulating trough OKT3 level is not detected, it may be indicative of an inadequate dose of OKT3. The dose of OKT3 can be increased from 5 to 10 mg per day (375–377).

Intravenous Immunoglobulin

Infusion of IVIG may provide blocking or antiidiotypic antibodies that can reduce the production of anti-HLA antibodies in the pretransplantation period (378–381). There is also limited experience in the use of IVIG for the treatment of allograft rejection. Successful prevention and treatment of acute humoral rejections were reported in a series of living donor kidney transplants (381).

Plasma Exchange

The role of plasmapheresis in the therapy for acute rejection is to remove circulating lymphocytotoxic antibodies that may be mediating allograft destruction. Given the few controlled studies on the therapy for acute rejection, plasmapheresis has not been shown to offer any advantage over steroids or antibodies in the reversal of acute vascular rejection and has no long-term benefit on graft survival (382,383). Recently, a number of studies have reported favorable outcome of highly sensitized patients induced with pretransplant plasma exchange (384–386).

Total Lymphoid Irradiation

Several groups have used total lymphoid irradiation (TLI) in renal transplantation. Myburgh et al. (387) have reported 1- and 5-year graft survival rates of 86% and 60%, respectively.

Because of the complexity and troublesome side effects of TLI, it is unlikely that this method will be adopted for routine use (387–389).

New Immunosuppressive Agents

New agents such as deoxyspergualin, brequinar sodium, myriocin and its semisynthetic derivative FTY20, leflunomide, and prostaglandin E_1 (PGE$_1$) analog are currently under experimental and clinical studies for maintenance immunosuppression and for the treatment of acute rejection.

Experimental antibody therapies are now being designed to directly target the CD4 molecule, the CD3 molecule by a humanized form of monoclonal anti-CD3, and adhesion molecules such as intercellular adhesion molecule (ICAM-1) or leukocyte function-associated antigen-1 (LFA-1). A large multicenter study of induction with an anti-ICAM antibody failed to show any benefit in terms of the incidence of DGF. A multicenter trial with anti–LFA-1 antibody however showed a nonsignificant trend in the incidence of DGF in patients at risk (390–399).

FTY20 appears to be a very promising drug in experimental models. It reduces the number of T and B cells in the peripheral blood while increasing their numbers in lymph nodes and Peyer's patches. This redirected cell "homing" is thought to be due to modification by FTY20 of chemokine receptors on lymphocytes (400–405). The drug may potentiate the immunosuppressive effect of CsA. Phase II clinical trials are in progress. Phase III clinical trials studying FTY20-CsA combination will soon be started.

Modifications of available drugs such as MMF and sirolimus are currently under investigation. ERL080A is an enteric-coated form of MMF that may produce fewer GI side effects and perhaps permit a reduced dose. SDZ-RAD is a derivative of sirolimus. It has a hydroxyethyl chain that makes the drug more polar and improves its oral bioavailability. In this case, it may be administered simultaneously with CsA. The half-life of RAD is shorter than that of sirolimus. Phase II trials for both of these drugs are in progress (406–408). Both MMF and sirolimus have been shown to prevent chronic allograft rejection in experimental animals. Whether this important observation is reproducible in human remains to be determined by long-term study.

Optimal and sustained T-cell response after antigen recognition (signal 1) requires a costimulatory signal (signal 2) delivered through accessory T-cell surface molecules (409–412). Recently, the central role of the B7-CD28 and CD40-CD40L costimulatory pathway in acute allograft rejection has been well studied. Blocking the B7-CD28 pathway with the fusion protein CTLA4-Ig, blocking the CD40-CD40L pathway with anti-CD40L antibodies, or blocking both pathways simultaneously results in long-term allograft acceptance in rodents. This treatment with antibodies directed against molecules involved in the delivery of the second signal of the T cell is promising and may offer future prospects for tolerance induction. Clinical trials will begin soon for anti-CD40

TABLE 97-12. *Causes of acute renal failure associated with renal transplantation*

Prerenal	Hypovolemia
	Arterial stenosis or thrombosis
	Venous thrombosis
Renal	Acute tubular necrosis
	Hyperacute/accelerated rejection
	Acute rejection
	Nephrotoxicity
Postrenal	Ureteral obstruction
	Urinary leak
	Lymphocele
	Hematoma

ligand and CTLA4-Ig in renal transplant recipients. Because T-cell activation is a prerequisite for the induction of T-cell anergy, the concurrent use of conventional immunosuppressive drugs may interfere with the mechanisms of action and tolerance induction by these antibodies.

PROBLEMS RELATED TO THE TRANSPLANTED KIDNEY

Acute Renal Failure in the Transplanted Kidney

In the immediate posttransplantation period, there may be DGF or cessation of function after initial good function (413–418). The most likely cause of renal failure during this period is ischemic tubular damage, but a vascular accident, ureteric obstruction, a urine leak, or rejection are all possible causes (Table 97-12).

Acute Tubular Necrosis

The pathogenesis of ATN commonly begins with ischemic damage secondary to hypovolemia and hypotension in the donor (usually a cadaver) and prolonged warm ischemia and cold ischemia during preservation (419). Some evidence shows that a delay in onset of function of the transplanted kidney is harmful in terms of long-term impairment to renal function (420–422). This may even be more important with the use of calcineurin inhibitors such as CsA or tacrolimus, with which there is a good deal of evidence suggesting that kidneys with delayed function have a much poorer graft survival than kidneys with immediate function. It should also be remembered that a not uncommon presentation of ATN is reasonable urine output within the first 12 or 24 hours that gradually diminishes and is followed by oliguria. This pattern is seen more commonly with the use of calcineurin inhibitors and probably reflects some acute nephrotoxicity in an already damaged kidney.

Allograft Rejection

Rejection is the major cause of graft failure, and if the injury to the tubules and glomeruli is sufficiently severe, the kidney may not recover. It is therefore important to diagnose acute rejection as soon as possible to institute antirejection therapy promptly.

Hyperacute Rejection

Hyperacute rejection is very rare and is caused by antibodies against alloantigens that have appeared in response to previous exposure to antigens through prior transplantations, blood transfusions, or multiple pregnancies. The clinical manifestation of hyperacute rejection is a failure of the kidney to perfuse properly on release of the vascular clamps just after vascular anastomosis is completed. The kidney initially becomes firm and then rapidly becomes blue, spotted, and flabby. The presence of neutrophils in the glomeruli and peritubular capillaries in the kidney biopsy specimen confirms the diagnosis. It can be prevented by careful testing of recipients for the presence of the preformed cytotoxic antibodies (378,423).

Accelerated Rejection

An accelerated rejection that may start on the second or third day and that tends to occur in the previously sensitized patient in whom preformed anti-HLA antibodies are present. It occurs in patients who have had a previous graft, presents with a decrease in renal function, and has a similar clinical picture to that mentioned for hyperacute rejection (424,425).

Acute Rejection

Acute rejection episodes may occur as early as 5 to 7 days but are generally seen between 1 and 4 weeks after transplantation. The classic acute rejection episode of the earlier era in a patient treated with azathioprine-prednisone was accompanied by swelling and tenderness of the kidney and the onset of oliguria with an associated rise in the serum creatinine level; it was usually accompanied by a significant fever. However, in patients who have been treated with CsA, the clinical features of an acute rejection are really quite minimal in that there is perhaps some swelling of the kidney, usually no tenderness, and there may be a minimal to moderate degree of fever. Because such an acute rejection may occur at a time when there is a distinct possibility of acute CsA or tacrolimus toxicity, the differentiation between the two entities may be extremely difficult.

Differential Diagnosis

Acute renal failure after transplantation is a common and often treatable entity. The differential diagnosis of ATN, acute rejection, and CsA- or tacrolimus-induced nephrotoxicity may be difficult, particularly in the early posttransplantation period when more than one cause of dysfunction can occur together. Knowledge of the natural history of several clinical entities is extremely helpful in limiting the differential

TABLE 97-13. *Approach to the patient with acute renal failure after transplantation*

Immediate acute renal failure (48 hr)
Rule out catheter obstruction
Rule out hypovolemia
Radioisotope scan to rule out vascular catastrophe
Ultrasound to rule out urinary extravasation or obstruction
Radiocontrast studies (if indicated by above)
Early or late acute renal failure (after 48 hr)
History and physical examination to detect oliguria, tender swelling graft, fever
Urine sodium, FENa (especially if baseline available)
Cyclosporin A or tacrolimus levels
Radioisotope scan (to follow serially)
Ultrasound
Therapeutic trial of steroids/lowering cyclosporine dose
Renal biopsy

diagnosis. Many nonspecific tests are available to aid in the differential diagnosis (Table 97-13).

Noninvasive imaging of the transplanted kidney has been quite useful in differentiating the causes of acute allograft dysfunction in the early posttransplantation period. Local expertise however is a major factor in selection.

Radionuclide Imaging

Renal perfusion can be assessed by technetium diethylenetriamine pentaacetic acid or mercaptoacetyl-triglycine and tubular function by iodohippurate (Hippuran) ^{131}I uptake. A decline in initial renal blood flow and a decrease in tubular function often occur during acute rejection (Fig. 97-11). Occasionally, scans can help diagnose uncommon posttransplantation complications such as venous thrombosis or urine leak (426–428).

Ultrasound

Real-time and duplex Doppler sonography of the renal allograft are useful for evaluating recipients with surgical complications including perinephric fluid collections, hydronephrosis (Fig. 97-12), and vascular complications (429–431). The sonography reveals variable findings in acute rejection such as graft enlargement, enhanced echogenicity of the parenchyma, and increased resistive index (more than 70%) of the vessels. The studies will not confirm the diagnosis of rejection but will serve to exclude allograft thrombosis and urinary obstruction and indicate that a percutaneous transplant kidney biopsy with pathologic examination should be performed.

Renal Transplant Biopsy

A biopsy will help to confirm the diagnosis of ATN by the exclusion of a histologic picture of severe rejection. Needle biopsy of the cadaveric kidney just after implantation is helpful to detect renal disease or preservation injury that might confound interpretation of delayed renal allograft function.

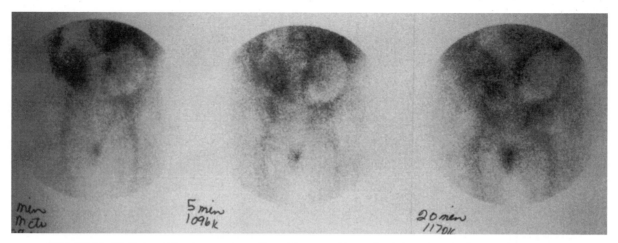

FIG. 97-11. Diethylenetriamine pentaacetic acid scan with marked decrease in flow possibly due to severe vascular rejection. Vascular catastrophe should be ruled out if there is no definite evidence of rejection.

However, a poor understanding of the natural history of transplant histology makes it an imperfect gold standard.

Technique of Renal Transplant Kidney Biopsy

The use of percutaneous biopsy of the transplanted kidney to diagnose rejection was first performed in 1967 (432). Since then, the technique has been well established as a useful tool in the differential diagnosis of allograft dysfunction (433–439). Transplant kidney biopsy can be more difficult than routine biopsy of a native kidney. The position and alignment of the transplanted kidney can vary from patient to patient (Fig. 97-13). In most instances, the transplanted kidney is palpable and the orientation kidney can be estimated by reviewing an isotope scan of the transplanted kidney (Fig. 97-14).

Biopsy can be obtained with a Vim-Silverman needle, a 14- to 16-G disposable Tru-Cut biopsy needle or an 18-G automatic Biopty or Monopty needle (Fig. 97-15A–C). It is best performed under sonographic guidance. Relative contraindications to biopsy include abnormal coagulation studies or a low platelet count, active urinary tract infection, and renal allograft hydronephrosis. Hydronephrosis indicative of

urinary tract obstruction should be further investigated. A small number of patients with urinary obstruction and rejection may coexist. It is interesting to note that significant macrophages infiltrate can occur with experimental urinary

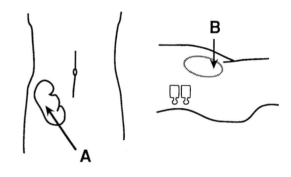

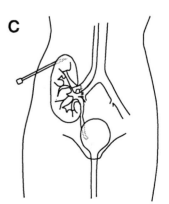

FIG. 97-13. Site of biopsy for the transplanted kidney. The orientation of the transplanted kidney is localized by palpation and review of the operative record and renal scan. The kidney is approached either tangentially or vertically, **(A)** in a plane tangential to the lateral curvature of the allograft or **(B)** in a plane perpendicular to the kidney directed to the lower pole. **C:** Tangential across the upper pole of the transplanted kidney.

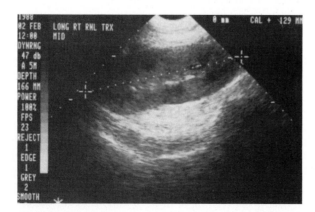

FIG. 97-12. Normal renal ultrasound of a transplanted kidney.

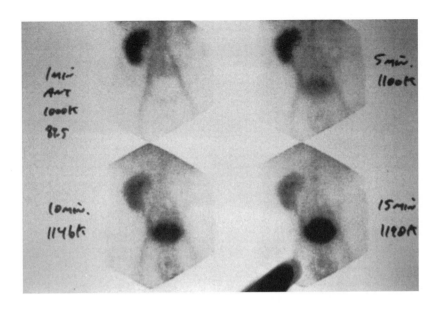

FIG. 97-14. Diethylenetriamine pentaacetic acid scan showing good renal perfusion in a transplanted kidney.

obstruction. In patients with a prolonged bleeding time due to uremia, intravenous l-desamino-8-D-arginine-vasopressin (0.3 μg/kg) can be used to correct the coagulation defect before the biopsy procedure. If the kidney has been transplanted via an intraabdominal approach or is difficult to localize, consideration should be given to the biopsy being performed using computed tomographic (CT) direction or occasionally via a limited open surgical approach in the operating room. The pathologic changes that occur with acute cellular rejection include interstitial infiltration with mononuclear cells and disruption of the tubular basement membranes (tubulitis) by the infiltrating cells (Fig. 97-16) (440). The presence of patchy mononuclear cell infiltrates without tubulitis is not uncommon in normal functioning renal allografts and is not sufficient to make the diagnosis of acute rejection. Vascular lesions are also common. The intrarenal arteries and arterioles show characteristic changes of intimal thickening and the presence of inflammatory cells within and adherent to the endothelium (Fig. 97-17). The glomerular changes are usually unremarkable in rejection. However, glomerular capillary and vascular intimal infiltrates can occur with acute vascular rejection (Fig. 97-18). Periodic examination of histologic features in the absence of changes in renal function may reveal silent allograft rejection (Tables 97-14 and 97-15). In a randomized, controlled trial, Rush et al. found that treatment of subclinical rejection detected by protocol biopsies lead to better graft function, compared with standard management without protocol biopsy (441,442). In addition to a conventional histopathologic approach, a technique using monoclonal antibodies has been used to identify the different types of cellular infiltrate (443). The infiltrate in grafts undergoing rejection comprises around 60% macrophages, 30% T lymphocytes, and less than 10% natural killer (NK) cells. This approach of identifying different T-cell subsets has been used for immunologic monitoring and treatment of rejection. HLA expression, which is increased on tubular cells during rejection, may be important in the rejection process. Immunohistologic evaluation of rejecting renal allografts shows an increased number of infiltrating MHC class II–positive and IL-2 receptor–positive mononuclear cells, when compared with controls.

Fine-Needle Aspiration Biopsy. An alternative approach to needle biopsy is to use fine-needle aspiration biopsy (FNAB) to sample parenchymal cells and infiltrating cells from the renal allograft. The technique allows serial sampling of cells for the determination of parenchymal cytology, nature of cellular infiltrate/T-cell subsets, and molecular markers (444–448). Good correlation with needle biopsy has been reported with respect to cellular infiltrate but not as good in showing vascular changes (449–451). Monoclonal antibody staining of the aspirate with antibodies to T-cell subsets, activation markers, and MHC antigen expression has advanced the usefulness of this technique.

New Techniques. Monitoring of other products of inflammation such as neopterin and lymphokines continues to be explored. It has been shown that acute rejection is associated with elevated plasma IL-1 in azathioprine-treated patients, and IL-2 in cyclosporine-treated patients (452). IL-6 is also increased in the serum and urine immediately after transplantation and during acute rejection episodes. The major problem however is that infection, particularly viral, can also elevate cytokine levels. PCR has also been used to detect messenger RNA for IL-2 in fine-needle aspirate of human transplant kidneys. Using this approach, IL-2 could be detected 2 days before rejection was apparent by histologic or clinical criteria. Similar PCR approaches can be used for quantitative analysis of intragraft gene expression such as granzyme B, perforin, transforming growth factor (TGFβ), IL-10, and IL-15 (453–456).

Urinary sediment cytology, coupled with immunologic and molecular techniques, should complement FNAB in the diagnosis and monitoring of rejection processes (456–459).

Magnetic resonance spectroscopy and imaging techniques (460–463) are being evaluated for the diagnosis of rejection. Magnetic resonance imaging (MRI) can demonstrate normal kidney architecture noninvasively without ionizing

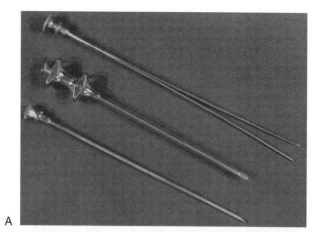

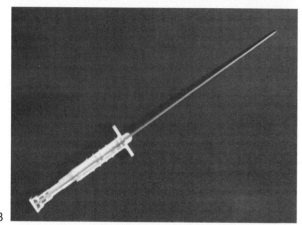

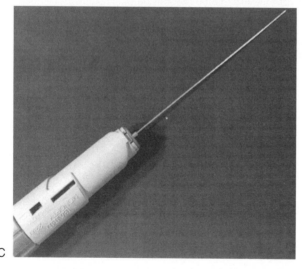

FIG. 97-15. Different types of biopsy needles. **A:** Vim-Silverman. **B:** Tru-Cut 14 G (disposable needle). **C:** Biopty gun 18 G (disposable needle).

radiation. It can evaluate corticomedullary demarcation, size of collecting system, presence of focal parenchymal changes, and shape of the kidney, and signal intensity of the sinus fat. Acute rejection can be diagnosed by the presence of a decreased or absent corticomedullary demarcation, with other signs of swelling, enlarged pyramids, and decreased signal intensity in the renal sinus fat (Fig. 97-19A,B). Changes for

ATN and nephrotoxicity are not specific. Therefore, it has not yet been established as a primary imaging modality in renal transplantation.

Chronic Rejection

Because chronic rejection is thought to be the end result of uncontrolled repetitive acute rejection episodes or a slowly progressive inflammatory process, its onset may be as early as the first few weeks after transplantation or any time thereafter. Progressive azotemia, proteinuria, and hypertension are the clinical hallmarks of chronic rejection (464–468). Immunologic and nonimmunologic mechanisms are thought to play a role in the pathogenesis of this entity including antibody-mediated tissue destruction possibly secondary to antibody-dependent cellular cytotoxicity leading to obliterative arteritis (Fig. 97-20), growth factors derived from macrophages, and platelets leading to fibrotic degeneration, and glomerular hypertension with hyperfiltration injury due to reduced nephron mass leading to progressive glomerular sclerosis.

Nonimmunologic causes can also contribute to the decline in renal function. Atheromatous renovascular disease of the transplanted kidney may also be responsible for a significant number of cases of progressive graft failure (Fig. 97-21). Although a smoldering subclinical inflammatory process may play a role in the pathogenesis of chronic rejection, the reduction in nephron mass (469,470) as a result of earlier immunologic injury most likely contributes to further decline in function. In patients with chronic rejection on azathioprine-prednisone immunosuppression, a switch from azathioprine to CsA (about 5 mg/kg) was shown in two studies to slow the decline in allograft function, compared with controls. On the other hand, adjustment of the CsA dosage to avoid nephrotoxicity, with the addition of azathioprine for immunosuppression, may preserve residual graft function.

Dietary protein restriction was also shown to reduce the rate of graft deterioration, compared with controls after 18 months of follow-up (471). Along with dietary protein restriction, aggressive control of hypertension may have a beneficial effect on hyperfiltration injury. Therefore, in the absence of a treatable rejection process or a surgically remediable cause, aggressive control of hypertension and dietary protein restriction may slow the inevitable decline in renal function. Clinical evidence suggests that control of hypertension with ACE inhibitor may preserve renal function in patients with (native) renal disease (472–476). Reduction of the urine protein excretion with ACE inhibitor or receptor antagonist may help to reduce lipid levels for patients with nephrotic-range proteinuria.

Patients with renal failure due to chronic allograft rejection should be evaluated early for initiation of dialysis treatment or retransplantation workup. Failed allografts, which were routinely removed in the past, usually are now left in place unless there are specific indications for surgery. Indications for transplant nephrectomy include infection; hemorrhage; signs of acute rejection with graft tenderness, swelling, and

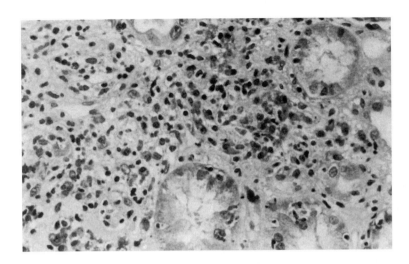

FIG. 97-16. Acute cellular rejection. Percutaneous renal transplant biopsy specimen showing tubulitis with tubular epithelial infiltrates of lymphocytes and plasma cells. (From Dr. Paul Shanley, Denver, CO, with permission.)

fever; and frank necrosis usually occurring on cessation of immunosuppressive drugs. For patients who are on the transplant waiting list, it is preferable to remove failed graft before or at the time of stopping immunosuppressive therapy in the hope of minimizing the production of HLA antibodies.

Glomerulonephritis in Allografts

Four main types of glomerulonephritis may occur in allografts: (a) The donor's kidney may be the seat of nephritis before grafting; (b) recurrent glomerulonephritis may develop due to the persistence of the original stimulus and recurrence of the original disease in the recipient; (c) transplant glomerulopathy may occur as a result of host response to the graft; and (d) *de novo* glomerulonephritis may arise in a healthy graft due to changes occurring in the recipient often as a result of immunosuppression (477–479).

Nephritis of Donor Origin

Cadaveric kidney donors may have unsuspected glomerulonephritis. It is therefore important to perform a graft biopsy during the transplantation. Kidneys from patients with early undetected IgA nephropathy and from patients with diabetes mellitus have been used for transplantation. IgA nephropathy in a transplant implanted into a non-IgA nephropathic recipient tends to disappear after the transplantation.

Recurrence of Primary Renal Disease

Essentially, all types of glomerulonephritis have been described to recur in renal allograft. However, there is much variation between the types of glomerulonephritis with regard to the frequency of recurrence, the clinical pattern, and the prognosis (290) (Table 97-16). The clinical manifestations of recurrent glomerulonephritis include microscopic hematuria and proteinuria, which may progress to nephrotic syndrome. Recurrent glomerulonephritis is the most common cause of nephrotic syndrome after transplantation. Proteinuria may also be a manifestation of *de novo* glomerular disease or chronic rejection. Although the documented overall incidence of graft failure from recurrent disease is less than 2%, this is an underestimate due to the difficulty in firmly establishing this diagnosis and in defining the cause of primary ESRD and graft dysfunction or loss occurred because of the same pathologic process (480–482).

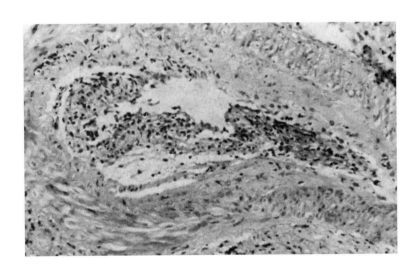

FIG. 97-17. Acute rejection. Renal transplant biopsy specimen showing marked endovasculitis and acute inflammatory endothelial infiltrates.

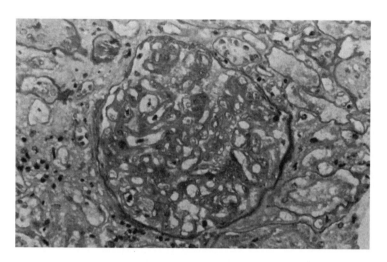

FIG. 97-18. Acute vascular rejection. Glomerular and vascular endothelial infiltrates and swelling.

Transplant Glomerulopathy

Transplant glomerulopathy is an entity that may be considered a special form of chronic rejection. It is believed to be related to the rejection process because the frequency of glomerular lesions was found to be inversely related to HLA compatibility. Histologically, it may resemble MPGN (type I) with mesangial proliferation and thickening or reduplication of the GBM. It is the most common cause of nephrotic syndrome in renal transplant recipients. Along with proteinuria, the clinical presentations include microscopic hematuria and progressive graft dysfunction.

CMV glomerulopathy is a controversial lesion (483). CMV infection of the allograft may produce a glomerulopathy,

TABLE 97-14. *Histopathology of renal allograft using needle biopsy*

Changes associated with rejection
Glomerular
  Swelling of endothelium
  Endothelial/mesangial proliferation
  Exudation of polymorphs, mononuclear cells
Interstitial
  Edema
  Infiltration of monocuclear cells
  Macrophages
  Eosinophils
Vascular
  Endothelial edema
  Mural infiltration
  Necrosis, hemorrhage
Severe vasculitis (especially interstitial hemorrhage)
  predicts eventual graft failure
Changes associated with cyclosporine
Tubular changes
  Giant mitochondria
  Vacuolization
  Microcalcification
Interstitium
  Mononuclear cell infiltration
Vascular changes
  Arteriolar necrosis

with impairment of function. It has been proposed that CMV infection, through elaboration of lymphokines and interferons, may cause upregulation of histocompatibility antigens on the allograft. This change results in induction of immune responses that lead histologically to glomerular endothelial changes and possibly vascular rejection and clinically to allograft dysfunction with decreased allograft survival (484).

De Novo *Glomerulopathy*

The development of glomerular lesions in patients with no history of glomerulonephritis suggests the presence of a *de novo* process in the allograft. *De novo* membranous nephropathy (Fig. 97-7) is reported to occur with an incidence of less than 1%. Nephrotic-range proteinuria occurred at a mean time of 1 to 2 years after transplantation. In contrast to the indolent course of idiopathic membranous glomerulonephritis in patients never receiving a transplant, *de novo* membranous nephropathy can lead to graft loss. This may be due to superimposed glomerular and interstitial lesions associated with chronic rejection.

FSGS is not uncommon among transplant recipients whose original disease was not FSGS (485). The mechanisms underlying *de novo* glomerulosclerosis are not clear. It may represent a nonspecific response to chronic rejection, glomerular ischemia, vesicoureteral reflux, or infections such as hepatitis B virus (HBV) and HIV. The use of heterologous ALG has been implicated in the development of *de novo* glomerulonephritis. Glomerulopathy may be related to antibodies cross-reacting with the GBM (486,487).

Circulating anti-GBM antibodies and anti-GBM disease can develop in some patients with Alport's disease after renal transplantation (66,68). Patients with Alport's disease lack a component of the GBM and do not bind anti-GBM antibodies isolated from patients with Goodpasture's syndrome. When the allograft that contains these GBM proteins is transplanted, the recipient may mount a humoral response against these proteins, which may lead to anti-GBM disease.

TABLE 97-15. *Banff 97 diagnostic categories for renal allograft biopsies*

1. Normal
   The presence of patchy mononuclear cell infiltrates without tubulitis is not uncommon in normally functioning renal allografts and when considered alone does not warrant the diagnosis of acute rejection

2. Antibody-mediated rejection
   Rejection demonstrated to be due, at least in part, to antidonor antibody
   A. Immediate (hyperacute)
   B. Delayed (accelerated acute)

3. Borderline changes: suggestive of acute rejection
   This category is used when no intimal arteritis is present, but there are foci of mild tubulitis (one to four mononuclear cells/tubular cross section)

4. Acute/active rejection

Type (Grade)	Histopathologic findings
IA	Cases with significant interstitial infiltration (>25% of parenchyma affected) and foci of moderate tubulitis (>4 mononuclear cells/tubular cross section or group of 10 tubular cells)
IB	Cases with significant interstitial infiltration (>25% of parenchyma affected) and foci of severe tubulitis (>10 mononuclear cells/tubular cross section or group of 10 tubular cells)
IIA	Cases with mild to moderate intimal arteritis
IIB	Cases with severe intimal arteritis comprising >25% of luminal area
III	Cases with "transmural" arteritis and/or arterial fibrinoid change and necrosis of medial smooth muscle cells

5. Chronic/sclerosing allograft nephropathy

Grade	Histopathological findings
I (mild)	Mild interstitial fibrosis and tubular atrophy
II (moderate)	Moderate interstitial fibrosis and tubular atrophy
III (severe)	Severe interstitial fibrosis and tubular atrophy

6. Other changes not considered to be due to rejection
   Posttransplant lymphoproliferative disorder
   Acute tubular necrosis
   Acute interstitial nephritis
   Cyclosporine or FK506-associated change

RESULTS OF KIDNEY TRANSPLANTATION

Patient Survival

In the 1960s and early 1970s, many patients received transplants when there were no supportive facilities if the graft failed. In those days, the high mortality rate was related to uncontrolled infection when excessive immunosuppression was used for rejection processes (2,5,488,489). With improvement in clinical care and the use of more specific immunosuppression, patient survival has improved both in the cadaveric and in the living related renal transplant recipient. Mortality rates at the end of the first year are currently less than 5% for living donors and less than 10% for cadaveric donors. Indeed, recent data indicate that patients currently receiving cadaveric donor transplants generally survive longer than patients treated by dialysis. Infectious complications of immunosuppressive therapy and cardiovascular diseases are the most important cause of death (490–497). Based on UNOS registry data, the major causes of death among cadaveric kidney transplant recipients were cardiovascular disease (26%) and infection (24%) during the first posttransplantation year. Between 1 and 3 years, the percentage of deaths due to infection fell to 15%, and malignancies accounted for 13% of patient death (498).

Graft Survival

Acute rejection is the most frequent cause of graft failure within the first year. Although patient survival rates have progressively improved, rates of graft survival after a cadaveric transplant have remained virtually unchanged in the 1970s and early 1980s (2,5,490,498). The failure to improve these results is due to the lack of more specific forms of immunosuppressive therapy. In the years immediately after 1983, there were dramatic gains in cadaveric graft survival, probably related to the introduction of cyclosporine (312). The overall cadaveric graft survival rate has increased from about 65% to about 80% to 85% at 1 year (Fig. 97-22A and B).

Based on data reported to the UNOS Scientific Renal Transplant Registry regarding transplantations performed between 1994 and 1998, the 1- and 3-year graft survival rates for 16,288 recipients of living donor kidneys were 93% and 86%, respectively, with a half-life of 17 years. The overall results of 35,289 cadaveric donor kidney transplantations were 87% and 76% graft survival at 1 and 3 years, respectively, with a half-life of 10 years (498). In addition to immunosuppressive agents, many other factors may influence graft survival (2,498,499). The recipient's race also influenced graft survival rates (Fig. 97-22C). Asian recipients of cadaveric

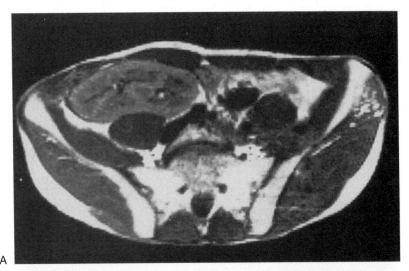

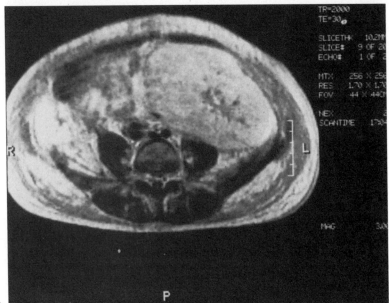

FIG. 97-19. Magnetic resonance imaging of transplanted kidney. **A:** Normal transplanted kidney. **B:** A transplanted kidney showing edema and loss of corticomedullary demarcation of the kidney during acute rejection.

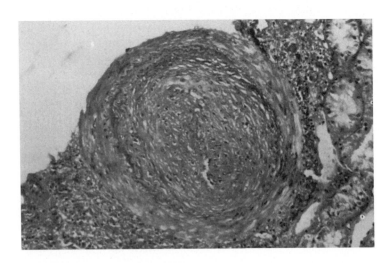

FIG. 97-20. Chronic rejection. Renal transplant biopsy specimen showing obliterative arteriopathy and fibrointimal vascular narrowing in chronic rejection.

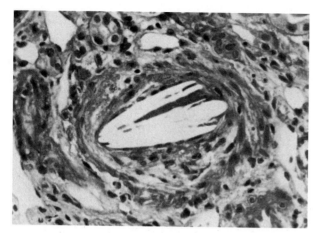

FIG. 97-21. Percutaneous needle biopsy of a kidney 20 years posttransplantation showing atheroembolus in a small artery. (trichrome stain, magnification ×400)

kidneys had the highest graft survival rates: 91% and 85% at 1 and 3 years, with a half-life of 18 years. The results of Whites and African Americans were significantly lower. The graft half-life was 12 years for Whites and 7 years for African Americans.

Living Related Transplantation

Monozygotic Twins

Provided there are no technical mishaps as a result of the operation itself, one should expect twin kidney transplants to survive indefinitely without the need for immunosuppression (500). However, there has been a significant incidence of

TABLE 97-16. *Recurrent disease in renal allografts*

Disease	Approximate recurrence rate (%)	Graft loss due to recurrence
Primary		
Glomerulonephritis		
FSGS	30–60	Common
HUS	20–50	Uncommon
Type I MPGN	20–30	Common
Type II MPGN	50–100	Uncommon
HSP	15–50	Uncommon
IgA nephrlopathy	50	Uncommon
Anti-GBM	25–50	Uncommon
Memembranous glomerulonephritis	10	Uncommon
Systemic disease		
Oxalosis	80–100	Common
Cystinosis	50–100	Common
Fabry's disease	Rare	Common
Sickle cell disease	Rare	Common
Diabetes type I	100	Uncommon
SLE	<1	Uncommon

FSGS, focal segmental glomerular sclerosis, hemolytic-uremic syndrome; MPGN, membranoproliferative glomerulo-nephritis; HSP, Henoch-Schönlein purpura; GBM, glomerular base membrane; SLE, systemic lupus erythematosus.

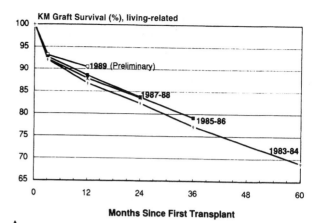

A

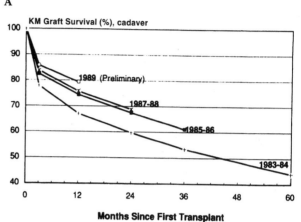

B

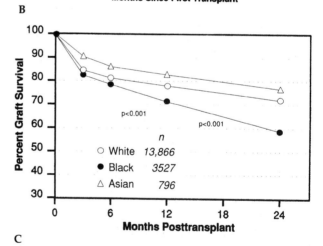

C

FIG. 97-22. Graft survival. **A:** Kaplan-Meier (KM) graft survival for living related donor *(LRD)* transplantations performed between 1983 and 1988. **B:** KM graft survival for cadaveric donor transplantations performed between 1983 and 1988. Graft survival rates for cadaveric grafts are improving over time. (From US Renal Data System. Annual data report, 1991. *Am J Kidney Dis* 1991;18[Suppl 2]:61, with permission.) **C:** Effect of race on graft survival. The race of the recipients was a significant factor in the outcome of the first cadaveric transplants. Asian patients had the highest graft survival rates—83% and 77% at 1 and 2 years, respectively—whereas Blacks had the poorest survival rates—71% and 59% at 1 and 2 years, respectively. (From Cecka J, Terasaki P, eds. *Clinical transplants 1990.* Los Angeles: UCLA Tissue Typing Laboratory, 1990:447, with permission.)

recurrent glomerulonephritis when this was the original disease in the recipient. In a series of 30 identical twin transplants followed for up to 27 years, 9 developed recurrent nephritis, one as late as 16 years after transplantation (501). Of 41 renal transplants between monozygotic twins recorded by the European Dialysis and Transplant Association, 36 were alive with functioning grafts from 1 to 14 years after transplantation (502). Two grafts failed from recurrent nephritis, two due to *de novo* glomerulonephritis, and one died in a traffic accident. This has been considered an indication for continuous low-grade immunosuppression in those patients in whom there is a risk of recurrent disease, but perhaps of greater importance is the withholding of transplantation until the original disease is completely quiescent.

HLA Identical Siblings

The HLA identical sibling transplant is ideal, and there have been recent reports of 3-year graft survival rates of 90% to 95% in such patients. Immunosuppression is still necessary because rejection does occur in a substantial number of patients and may even occasionally result in loss of a graft from rejection (503,504). These rejection episodes no doubt reflect recognition of, or sensitization to, minor histocompatibility antigens in the donor or to genetic recombination at the HLA-DR locus. Because excellent results are obtained with azathioprine and prednisone, this would seem to still be the immunosuppressive therapy of choice, in view of the nephrotoxicity associated with cyclosporine. However, some centers cover the recipient with cyclosporine for several months in case of unexpected rejection and then taper and discontinue the drug after 4 to 6 months. Steroids can usually be discontinued after 1 or 2 years if renal function is stable, although withdrawal of steroids should be done very cautiously over at least 6 months.

HLA Nonidentical Parent to Child or Siblings

A transplantation may be performed between a patient and a child who will differ for one HLA haplotype or between the two siblings who differ either for one or for both HLA haplotypes. The results of transplantation were related to the degree of HLA disparity, that is, two haplotype-disparate pairs were less successful than one haplotype-disparate pair and both were significantly worse than the results of transplantation between HLA identical siblings (505). However, CsA treatment and donor-specific blood transfusion have substantially improved the results of transplantation between HLA nonidentical family members. Actuarial graft survival is now very close to that achieved for transplantation between HLA identical siblings (506–509).

Living Unrelated Transplantation

A case can be made for the use of emotionally related donors such as a spouse or more distantly related members of the family such as cousins, and perhaps even between very close friends, now that the expectation of a successful transplant

is quite high (510–512). Despite greater histoincompatibility, the survival rates of these kidneys are greater than those of cadaveric kidneys. In a recent analysis by Terasaki et al. (511), the 3-year survival rates were 85% for kidneys from 368 spouses, 81% for kidneys from 129 living unrelated donors who were not married to the recipients, 82% for kidneys from 3,368 parents, and 70% for 43,341 cadaveric kidneys. The superior survival rate of grafts from unrelated donors could not be attributed to better HLA matching, White race, younger donor age, or shorter cold ischemia times but might be explained by damage due to shock before removal in 10% of the cadaveric kidneys. Living unrelated donors may thus become a major source of organs for kidney transplantation (513–515). However, living unrelated transplantation does give rise to a number of ethical and moral problems and should be considered only in exceptional circumstances, according to guidelines issued by The Transplantation Society (176,516–518).

Cadaveric Transplantation

Most kidneys used for transplantation have been from cadavers. Even though there may be variations from center to center (498), there has been a steady improvement in the results of cadaveric transplantation in terms of both patient and graft survival over the last 10 years. The patient survival rate is now around 96% at 1 year and the graft survival rate is approaching 80% (Fig. 97-22B); in selected groups of patients such as those who have received a transfusion and those who are receiving a first graft, the graft survival rate is more than 85% (498). This improvement in patient survival is due to the use of less immunosuppression and in particular the use of low-dose steroid protocols. Cardiovascular disease has replaced infectious complications as a major cause of morbidity and mortality.

The improved graft survival rate, which obviously is due partly to improved patient survival, can be attributed to the recognition of the transfusion effect, HLA matching (Fig. 97-23), and more recently to better immunosuppression. However, controversy still exists as to whether matching is of any relevance because of the better results achieved with better immunosuppression (498,519). Although this question has not been resolved, data are gradually accumulating suggesting that matching, and in particular matching for HLA-DR, does exert the same influence on graft survival in patients treated with CsA as with those on conventional immunosuppressive therapy (520). The 6-year half-life of kidney transplants from cadaveric donors has been unchanged since the early 1970s (521). This is in comparison with the 20- to 25-year half-life for the same period in HLA identical sibling transplants, emphasizing the effect of histocompatibility differences on graft survival (522).

With the improvement in patient and graft survival, renal transplantation has now become the treatment of choice by most patients with ESRD. However, there is a relatively lower percentage of Black patients with a functioning renal graft despite that the incidence rates of ESRD in the Black

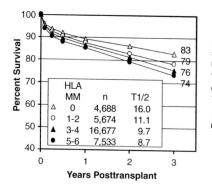
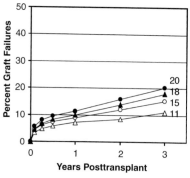

FIG. 97-23. Effects of human leukocyte antigen (HLA) mismatches on survival of first cadaveric transplants. Graft survival rates at 1 and 2 years posttransplantation declined as the number of HLA-A, HLA-B, and HLA-DR mismatches increased. The difference between the best- and the worst-matched grafts was 11% at 1 year and 14% at 2 years. (From Cecka J, Terasaki P, eds. *Clinical transplants 1990.* Los Angeles: UCLA Tissue Typing Laboratory, 1990:7, with permission.)

population in the United States are approximately three to four times as high as those in the White population. Although it has been suggested previously that Black recipients had significantly lower graft survival rates than White recipients in North America (Fig. 97-22C), more recent analysis has shown that factors other than race could explain the poorer survival of grafts in African American recipients and of African American kidneys in either race (498,523,524).

The results of cadaveric transplantation are now approaching a level at which, if there were an adequate supply of cadaveric kidneys, there probably would be little justification for continuing living related transplantations, except when high sensitization of the recipient makes cadaveric transplantation unlikely or impossible. Most patients who have rejected a first graft will be sensitized to histocompatibility antigens, and many of these patients are highly sensitized (525). This does make identification of a suitable donor much more difficult in that a negative crossmatch with the donor must be found; this in turn implies the need for a better matched graft. The patient who is highly sensitized and is awaiting a sequential graft provides one of the major reasons for the national and regional organ exchange network.

SURGICAL COMPLICATIONS OF RENAL TRANSPLANTATION

The surgical technique of renal transplantation is reasonably standardized, and overall direct surgical complication rates are low, accounting for only a small percentage of graft losses. Nevertheless, the transplant physician must be familiar with the diagnosis and treatment of surgically related complications to minimize recipient morbidity and mortality. The allograft is placed extraperitoneally into the iliac fossa in most cases. Thus, intraperitoneal bleeding, or bowel obstruction from adhesions or internal herniation, should not occur as a direct result of the surgery. In small children or in some recipients with a supravesical urinary diversion, the transplant is placed intraperitoneally and the potential surgical complications listed previously must be considered.

Wound Complications

The most important causes of wound infection stem from the operative complications of hematoma, urine leak, and lymphocele. Transplant recipients are vulnerable to wound infection because of postoperative immunosuppressive medications and poorly controlled uremia. Wound infections after transplantation are extremely bothersome because if they are deep-seated infections around the arterial anastomosis, secondary hemorrhage may occur. On presentation of a wound infection, adequate drainage should be provided immediately and appropriate antibiotic therapy introduced. However, prevention of contamination during donor nephrectomy and the use of preventive antibiotics before transplantation should ensure that the incidence of wound infection after transplantation is no more than 3% or 4%.

Patients with high fever but benign-appearing incision sites can harbor large purulent abscesses, emphasizing the effect of steroids on masking signs of inflammation. If unexplained fevers persist, ultrasonography or CT scanning of the wound may localize a fluid collection; needle aspiration of a fluid collection is indicated. Prophylaxis with the administration of intraoperative intravenous antibiotics has reduced both wound infection and sepsis.

Bleeding

Secondary hemorrhage after a renal transplantation fortunately is an unusual event and is always secondary to infection that usually has been introduced at the time of operation. During a fulminant rejection episode, acute swelling of the kidney may lead to rupture through its cortex, often originating at a previous biopsy site. Urgent surgical exploration is necessary in most cases of hemorrhage; the kidney and its surroundings should be examined, and the source of bleeding identified if possible and evacuated to eliminate a potential nidus of infection. If a small cortical rupture is present without venous obstruction, it may be repaired by packing with autologous muscle or microfibrillar collagen. If the rupture is large or venous compromise is present, transplant nephrectomy is almost invariably indicated.

Vascular Complications

Arterial Thrombosis

Thrombosis of the renal artery is a rare complication in the early days after transplantation, probably due both to the high flow through the kidney and to the associated anemia and coagulation defects present in most patients with end-stage renal failure (526). It occurs in less than 1% of renal transplantations. Factors that may predispose to thrombosis include preexisting hypercoagulable state, technical difficulties with the anastomosis, heavy arteriosclerotic involvement of recipient or donor vessels, kidneys with multiple renal arteries, and hypotension (527). Thrombosis may also occur because of CsA-associated arteriopathy or because of hyperacute humoral rejection. CsA has been associated with increased thromboembolic complications, possibly because of enhancement of platelet aggregation. Thrombosis due to an error in suture technique may occur in any case but would be extraordinarily rare in an end-to-side anastomosis performed between a patch of donor aorta to an arteriotomy in the common or external iliac artery. In the later weeks after transplantation, renal artery thrombosis may be seen secondary to arteriolar thrombosis in an acutely rejecting kidney, but the major vessel thrombosis is not the primary event. A renogram will quickly establish the presence of an arterial blood supply to the kidney if this is in doubt.

Sudden cessation of urine flow in the setting of a previously working allograft and a patent urinary catheter should suggest the possibility of renal artery thrombosis. An emergency renal ultrasound study or radionuclide renal scan will confirm the presence or absence of parenchymal blood flow. A digital subtraction angiogram is reserved for the very few cases with a "no flow" renal scan. Attempts to remove the thrombus are usually unsuccessful because of extensive intrarenal clotting beyond the main arterial branches (528).

Venous Thrombosis

Thrombosis of the renal vein as an acute event in the transplanted kidney is unusual and is usually due to a technical mishap at the time of operation. Thrombosis of the renal vein at some later period after transplantation is probably more common than is realized. It may occur secondary to thrombosis of the common iliac vein, or it may occur occasionally as the primary event. Venous thrombosis may be related to CsA use, but it may also occur after placement of the allograft into a tight scarred, retroperitoneal pocket after removal of a previous graft.

In the absence of the clinical features of thrombosis of the common iliac vein, thrombosis of the renal vein itself may present with proteinuria and a marked increase in the size of the kidney, but it may also occur without any notable features. Partial obstruction of the iliac vein by the pressure of the allograft can produce unilateral leg swelling on the side of the graft and rarely may lead to deep venous thrombosis. If the diagnosis of deep venous thrombosis is confirmed by Doppler plethysmography or venography, anticoagulation therapy should be initiated, unless there are absolute contraindications. Venography is the best test to confirm the diagnosis.

Treatment of well-localized thrombosis involves thrombectomy and revascularization. Alternatively, it can be treated with systemic anticoagulation. Treatment often is successful if the condition was due to a transient hypercoagulable state but rarely succeeds if the process was one manifestation of severe rejection and high renal vascular resistance with low flow. In practical terms, however, by the time the diagnosis is confirmed by angiography or radionuclide scanning, salvage of the kidney is unlikely and transplant nephrectomy is the usual outcome. Deep venous thrombosis occurs with a frequency of around 10% of transplant recipients. Anticoagulation of these patients for several months is required because pulmonary embolism is not an uncommon cause of death in renal transplant recipients.

Other Vascular Problems

In kidneys with multiple renal arteries, thrombosis of a polar branch can lead to ureteral necrosis or segmental parenchymal infarction with potential development of a caliceal cutaneous fistula. Careful attention to these tenuous, small caliber polar branches has decreased the incidence of these complications. In cadaveric kidneys harvested *en bloc,* a small aortic cuff (Carrel patch) can be made surrounding the orifices of the renal arteries. The cuff can then be end-to-side anastomosed to the external iliac artery, preventing any possibility of anastomotic compromise. If no cuff is available, the polar branches can be end-to-side anastomosed to the main renal artery, followed by anastomosis of the main artery to the recipient.

Many men with ESRD have erectile dysfunction because of decreased penile arterial flow, neuropathy, or both. Second transplant recipients should have an end-to-side renoiliac arterial anastomosis if the contralateral hypogastric artery was used in the first transplant.

Urologic Complications

Accurate evaluation of lower urinary tract function before transplantation is important to minimize postoperative urologic complications. There are many approaches to the correction of these urologic complications, but as a general rule, the approach should be early and aggressive, rather than conservative (529). Many of the complications are preventable with careful attention to the technique of donor nephrectomy.

Urine Leak

Urine leak is an infrequent but serious problem and occurs in approximately 2% of renal transplant recipients. It is seen early after transplantation and is usually secondary to necrosis of the entire or distal portion of the ureter or to infarction of the renal pelvis. This usually is due to the interruption or thrombosis of the ureteral artery, the main arterial supply to the donor ureter.

The source of the leak may be from the ureter, calices, or the bladder. Upper urinary tract leakage is due to ischemia resulting from the loss of vascular supply during organ procurement. Preservation of hilar vessels and periureteral fat and adventitia is the key to prevention of this problem. Bladder urine leak may occur at the site of the ureteral reimplant or along the cystotomy closure.

The clinical presentation of a urine leak may be subtle unless a wound drain is in place. Leakage of urine from the lower end of the ureter is not usually evident until at least 1 week after transplantation and often much later. It will be associated with a decrease in urine output, fever, local tenderness, and swelling due to the localized collection of urine, known as a *urinoma*. Other clinical signs include unexplained fever and edema of the scrotum, labia, or thigh ipsilateral to the graft.

Ultrasonography is the preferred study for diagnosis of a suspected urine leak. Aspiration of the fluid mass and comparison of the fluid creatinine or urea content to serum values confirms the diagnosis of urine leak. The dynamic phase of a renal scan also may demonstrate urinary extravasation. Cystography with oblique and drainage films will confirm whether the leak is from the bladder. Confirmation of upper urinary tract leakage is more difficult, because attempts at retrograde pyelography in the early postoperative period often are unsuccessful.

Urine is a strong chemical irritant to tissues and predisposes to infection of the fresh vascular anastomoses. Prolonged catheter drainage may be adequate treatment of a small bladder leak. Insertion of a percutaneous nephrostomy or ureteral stent can also be used to provide initial urinary drainage and to stabilize the patient. After function returns to baseline, surgical reexploration and repair is usually attempted. If the distal ureter is necrotic or stenotic, the necrotic portion can be removed and the vascularized proximal ureter can be reimplanted into the bladder. If the ureter is too short or the renal pelvis necrotic, the ipsilateral native ureter can be detached from the native kidney near the pelvis and connected to the renal transplant by means of a ureteropyeloplasty. The anastomosis is protected by a temporary nephrostomy and ureteral stent. If the native ureter is not available or adequate, the bladder can be mobilized and a Boari flap ureteronephrostomy constructed, or the bladder is anastomosed directly to the kidney pelvis, and a nephrostomy tube is left in place for several weeks (530).

Ureteral Obstruction

Acute ureteral obstruction in the early postoperative period may be due to distal ischemia, infarction, or rejection. Transient obstruction by clot in the ureter or bladder immediately postoperatively may cause erratic urine output and can usually be taken care of by bladder catheter irrigation. Technical error as an early cause of obstruction of the ureterovesical junction is rare. Oliguria or anuria in the immediate posttransplantation period should make one suspect the diagnosis. A cystogram is usually performed first to rule out a bladder leak. The diagnosis is confirmed by the presence of hydronephrosis by ultrasonography (Fig. 97-24) or by deceased

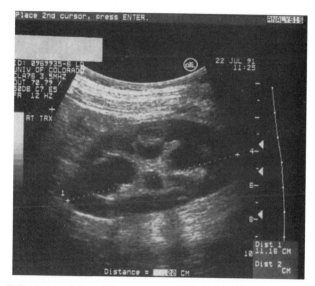

FIG. 97-24. Ultrasound scan of renal transplant showing hydronephrosis due to ureteric obstruction.

flow from ureter to bladder or evidence of extravasation on percutaneous nephrostogram (Fig. 97-25). The site of obstruction can be identified by an antegrade pyelogram. Occasionally, obstruction of the ureter may be secondary to a hydrocele or hematoma, which can occur after a percutaneous needle biopsy.

Obstruction of the ureter may occur at some time remote from transplantation, often due to the development of a stricture, presumably as a result of previous ischemia. Progressive stenosis of the distal transplant ureter secondary to fibrosis or chronic ischemia may present as progressive as azotemia over several months. Ultrasonography and an intravenous pyelogram or an antegrade pyelogram should confirm the diagnosis. Ureteric obstruction should always be considered in the patient with a gradual deterioration of renal function. Options for treatment include cystoscopic or percutaneous radiologic

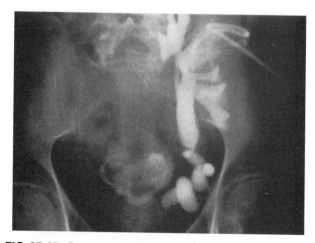

FIG. 97-25. Percutaneous nephrostogram of renal transplant. Nephrostomy tube placement with antegrade pyelogram to identify the site of obstruction.

placement of an indwelling double J ureteral stent, use of percutaneous nephrostomy, balloon dilation, and surgical repair (531,532).

Reflux

Vesicoureteral reflux into the transplanted ureter has a reported incidence of 4% to 65%, depending on the technique of ureteral anastomosis; the creation of a distinct submucosal tunnel through the bladder wall has resulted in a lower incidence. The presence of vesicoureteral reflux in the transplanted allograft has not been found to increase the rate of urinary tract infections, compared with nonrefluxing grafts (533). Mathew et al. (534) found an increased incidence of proteinuria, microhematuria, hypertension, and graft failure in the refluxing group, whereas Bootsma et al. (535) found no difference between refluxing and nonrefluxing groups with regard to proteinuria, graft function, and graft survival.

Lymphocele

The major complication associated with lymphatics is the occurrence of a lymphocele, which usually presents in the first 2 or 3 months after transplantation as a large cystic mass near the kidney (536,537). It is usually asymptomatic. Its presenting features are caused by pressure on surrounding structures; it may cause a deterioration in renal function due to pressure on the ureter, swelling of the leg due to pressure on the iliac vein, urgency due to pressure on the bladder, and diarrhea and tenesmus due to pressure on the rectum. Ultrasonography can confirm the presence of a perinephric (lymph) collection. Studies with radiolabeled lymph reveal that the major source of fluid in lymphoceles is from the lymphatics along the recipient iliac vessels and not from the renal hilum. Therefore, meticulous ligation of the lymphatics during exposure of the vessels is the best prevention. Aspiration of the mass and measurement of fluid creatinine and potassium levels, compared with the values in serum, help establish the diagnosis of lymphocele and exclude urine leak, hematoma, or abscess. Sometimes, the lymphocele will not recur after two or three aspirations. However, if the lymphocele continues to recur, it should be marsupialized into the peritoneal cavity, after checking the aspirate for urine products and bacterial growth.

SYSTEMIC COMPLICATIONS

Infection

The occurrence of infection is due primarily to the interplay between two factors: the degree of immunosuppression in the patient and the epidemiologic exposures that the patient encounters (538,539). Although the incidence of serious infection and the mortality rate from infection after transplantation have decreased dramatically during the last decade, infection

TABLE 97-17. *The diagnostic approach to the patient with an unexplained fever who underwent transplantation*

Possible sites of infection
  Chest: pulmonary infection, pericarditis, endocarditis
  Mouth: *Candida*
  Lower limb: deep venous thrombosis
  Soft tissues: skin (e.g., fungi, *Nocardia*, mycobacteria), joints
  Transplant wound: rejection, abscess, urine leak, hematoma
  Peritoneal cavity: pancreas, colon, dialysis catheter
  Urinary tract: bladder, prostate, native kidneys
  Central nervous system (CNS): *Listeria, Cryptococcus,* aspergilli, tuberculosis, *Nocardia*
  Systemic: viral infection, tuberculosis
Investigations
  Chest radiographs
  Ultrasound of transplanted kidney
  Cultures: mouth, sputum, urine, blood, stool, access sites
  Serology: viral antibodies, especially cytomegalovirus
  Lumbar puncture and computed tomography of head if CNS infection is suspected

remains a major hazard for the transplant recipient, particularly in the early months after the procedure (540,541). The fall in the incidence of infection is due to a number of factors, the main ones being the use of lower doses of immunosuppressive drugs and the general adoption of low-dose steroid protocols. The most common presentation of an infection in a transplant recipient is fever, and some guidelines to the approach to the patient with fever are given in Table 97-17. Some awareness of the times after transplantation when particular infections may occur is helpful in the diagnostic approach to a patient with a possible infection. During the first posttransplantation month, opportunistic infections are rare, and the major infectious disease hazards are similar to those for patients undergoing major urologic surgery. The period between 1 and 6 months after transplantation is when most serious infections occur. This is because of the maximal effect of the immunosuppressive drugs on the host's defense system, as well as its coinciding with the period when attempts are made to reverse rejection episodes with potent antirejection therapy. As in other states of immune deficiencies, opportunistic infections derived from endogenous flora including *Cryptococcus, Candida, Aspergillus, Pneumocystis carinii,* CMV, and herpes zoster are seen after transplantation. *Candida albicans,* a normal inhabitant of the oropharynx, intestine, and vagina in healthy individuals, may cause severe pharyngitis, esophagitis, vaginitis, and systemic infections in immunosuppressed patients (542). Wound infections and urinary infections are commonly due to bacterial infections. Septicemia is not uncommon after transplantation and is usually due to a Gram-negative organism with the primary focus in the urinary tract. However, *Staphylococcus aureus, Listeria,* and *Candida* may also cause septicemia. While awaiting the results of blood culture, one should commence appropriate broad-spectrum antimicrobial treatment.

A vigorous search for the focus of infection must be made and dealt with as appropriate.

Viral Infections

Cytomegalovirus

CMV is the most important viral infection occurring in transplant recipients. The incidence and severity of CMV infection depend on the presence of latent infection in the donor, the immune status of the recipient, and the amount of immunosuppressants used (542–544). CMV infection also causes considerable morbidity and may be associated with decreased allograft survival rates. CMV infection takes two forms, namely that of a primary infection of a secondary or reactivated infection. The primary infection is of most concern and occurs in patients who are seronegative at the time of transplantation and who received a kidney from a seropositive donor (545–547). Transfusions may also cause a primary infection in the seronegative patient, but this is far less common than the transmission of infection in the transplanted kidney (547).

The typical primary CMV infection commences as a fever that may be spiking or constant and usually occurs between 4 and 10 weeks after transplantation (548). It may be associated with neutropenia, and atypical lymphocytes may be identified in the blood smear. The leukopenia causes problems, particularly in patients receiving azathioprine in whom the dose will have to be reduced or often discontinued. The primary infection may lead to a CMV lung infection and less commonly to hepatitis, arthralgia, splenomegaly, myalgia, and GI ulceration (549). A deterioration in function of the renal transplant may also be seen during the early stages of the infection (550), and a frank glomerulopathy may occur (551). In rare instances, chorioretinitis can occur 4 to 6 months after transplantation, occasionally without prior evidence of CMV activity. CMV encephalitis, transverse myelitis (552), and cutaneous vasculitis (553) also have been reported.

Patients with secondary infection or reactivation of latent CMV often are not symptomatic, whereas those with superinfection of a new viral strain have the acute symptoms of active CMV (554–560). Most patients have antibodies against CMV at the time of transplantation. After transplantation, essentially all of these seropositive individuals shed the virus in saliva, urine, and blood, partly as a result of reactivation of endogenous latent virus. Recipients who shed CMV after transplantation do so between the first and sixth months, whereas the peak incidence of clinical illness due to CMV occurs 2 to 3 months after grafting (560). The appearance of CMV-specific IgM or IgG in the primary infection, or a rise in titer in the secondary infection, can be used in determining infectivity. Use of DNA restriction enzyme analytic methods to detect different CMV serotypes indicates that many of the clinical CMV infections in individuals seropositive for CMV before transplantation are due to superinfection with the donor virus strain (554,561,562).

During an active infection, CMV persists in the blood for several weeks. The presence of virus in the urine is only indicative of virus excretion. In the case of CMV pneumonia, virus can be isolated from bronchial lavage. A positive culture of the throat, urine, or blood (buffy coat) is generally sufficient evidence for the presence of active infection. Newer methods for determining the presence of viral infection include molecular hybridization using labeled viral DNA probes (563). They have been used successfully for the detection of viral DNA in blood during viremia, in urine, and in tissue biopsy specimens. PCR technique of urine and blood samples has also been used for more rapid and sensitive diagnosis of CMV. This technique can detect much smaller amounts of virus than other methods and can be potentially done in 7 hours (542).

Prior vaccination with live, attenuated CMV vaccine did not reduce the incidence of CMV infection and disease after renal transplantation. However, there was evidence that the vaccine reduced the severity of CMV disease, especially among seronegative recipients of grafts from seropositive donors (564,565). Primary infection can be prevented by avoiding transplantation of a kidney from a seropositive patient into a patient who is seronegative (566). CMV immune globulin given after transplantation has been shown to reduce the incidence of CMV syndromes. Prophylactic administration of oral acyclovir to renal allograft recipients for 12 weeks after transplantation has been shown to reduce symptomatic active CMV infection (567). Other agents such as ganciclovir and valacyclovir have been studied. Treating all transplant recipients with CMV prophylaxis is costly and may not be necessary. Chemoprophylaxis for CMV, however, should be used according to the risk of the patient for CMV (559).

The initial step in the treatment of overt CMV disease is to decrease the amount of immunosuppressive therapy being administered (568). Because of the association between CMV and *P. carinii* infection, trimethoprim-sulfamethoxazole prophylaxis is commonly given to the patients with clinical CMV disease (568). Specific treatment of CMV infection is indicated for those patients with life-threatening CMV pneumonitis or sight-threatening CMV chorioretinitis (544,569). Antiserum against CMV has been evaluated in the treatment of CMV pneumonia (570–572), both alone and in combination with ganciclovir, 9-(1,3-dihydroxy-2 propoxymethyl) guanine (DHPG), an antiviral agent that inhibits herpesvirus replication (573–575). When used as single-agent treatment, CMV immunoglobulin did not provide optimal therapy for CMV pneumonia in transplant recipients. The efficacy of ganciclovir has been shown in the treatment of pneumonia in bone marrow recipients. CMV pneumonitis and retinitis in renal transplants can also be ameliorated by ganciclovir. The major side effects of ganciclovir are bone marrow suppression, sterility, and potential nephrotoxicity (573–575). Dose adjustment is necessary for patients with renal impairment (Table 97-18).

TABLE 97-18. *Dosage adjustment for IV ganciclovir in the treatment of cytomegalovirus infection*

Serum creatinine (mg/dL)	Ganciclovir (IV)
<1.5	5 mg/kg q12h
1.5–2.5	2.5 mg/kg q12h
2.6–4.5	2.5 mg/kg q24h
>4.5; No dialysis	1.25 mg/kg q48h
Dialysis	1.25 mg/kg q24h

Herpes Simplex Virus

Reactivation of latent herpes simplex virus (HSV) infections is extremely common in transplant recipients. The most common lesion is the orolabial HSV type 1 infection. Occasionally, anogenital lesion due to HSV type 2 infection may occur. Rarely, Kaposi's varicelliform eruption due to disseminated HSV infection in the skin may develop in transplant recipients. Therapy for acute HSV infection with acyclovir will lead to clinical improvement (576,577).

Varicella Zoster

Varicella zoster is seen frequently in transplant recipients occurring at any time after transplantation. It is commonly presented as localized zoster due to reactivation of latent virus present in dorsal root ganglion since childhood chickenpox. Intravenous acyclovir is the treatment of choice. Chickenpox is a rare but often extremely virulent infection. Should a patient without humoral immunity to varicella zoster be exposed to chickenpox, varicella zoster immune globulin should be given within 72 hours of the exposure. If chickenpox develops, intravenous acyclovir needs to be instituted without delays (578).

Epstein-Barr Virus

The Epstein-Barr virus (EBV) is not in general a major problem in transplant recipients, although occasionally EBV may be the cause of a glandular feverlike illness. There has been some concern that patients immunosuppressed with CsA may be particularly prone to EBV infections because of the suppression of the generation of cytotoxic T cells against EBV-infected B lymphocytes. This in turn may cause an acute lymphoproliferative syndrome or even a polyclonal lymphoma (579,580). Using DNA hybridization technique, EBV has been identified in lymphoma and lymphoproliferative lesions of renal transplant recipients (581).

Human Immunodeficiency Virus

The impact of HIV infection and acquired immunodeficiency syndrome (AIDS) on recipients of organ transplants has not yet been fully realized. Immunosuppression may be associated with progression of the infection (582). As the population of asymptomatic HIV-seropositive individuals increases, it is of concern whether renal transplants in these individuals with concomitant chemical immunosuppression hastens the course of HIV infection (583,584). Surprisingly few cases of HIV infections or AIDS in transplant recipients have been reported. In general, the same clinical spectrum of disease is seen as that in the normal population (585,586). The transmission of HIV by blood transfusion and by the allograft itself has been well documented. In a case report of four individuals who received kidneys from donors with histories of intravenous drug use, HIV antibodies appeared 2 months after transplantation in two patients and were present in all four at 8 months. It is still unclear how patients who are HIV antibody–positive, either before or after transplantation should optimally be managed. A retrospective survey of 1,043 transplant recipients (all organs) at the University of Pittsburgh noted a 0.7% incidence of HIV-seropositivity in recipients before transplantation. Of 860 individuals who were seronegative at transplantation, 11 converted at a mean time of 96 days after transplantation. Half of the seropositive patients died within 6 months after surgery, and the other half were alive a mean of 43 months after transplantation (587). Hence, the Pittsburgh experience contributed to the enigma as to whether HIV antibody–positive patients should be excluded as transplant candidates. This report serves to emphasize that a large and more complete database is essential before it will be possible to design optimal policies and clinical practices for managing transplant candidates who are HIV antibody–positive, and for treating transplant recipients who either are HIV antibody–positive or have AIDS.

Polyomavirus

Both the BK virus (*Polyomavirus hominis*) and the JC virus (*Polyomavirus hominis*) belong to the human papovavirus family. They are nonenveloped, double-stranded DNA viruses. Both viruses have been cultured from the urine of transplant recipients. The excretion of the BK virus is associated with ureteral stricture and interstitial nephritis and that of the JC virus with progressive multifocal leukoencephalopathy. About 60% to 80% of adults are seropositive for the BK virus. In immunocompetent individuals, the virus has no great clinical significance. The virus resides in a latent state in the kidney in healthy individuals and can be activated without functional impairment or ill effects. Morphologic evidence of viral activation is the presence of polyomavirus-infected cells in the urine. In immunocompromised patients, polyomavirus can cause a morphologically manifested renal infection with cytopathic signs and functional impairment. In native and transplanted kidneys, the BK virus is found in areas of interstitial nephritis. In addition, renal allograft recipients were reported to have the virus associated with ureteral stenosis, and bone marrow transplant recipients from hemorrhagic cystitis. BK virus infection in renal transplant recipients has recently become more frequently recognized. It presents clinically as an acute rejection that appears unresponsive to treatment (588–592). The biopsy specimens have changes of severe tubulointerstitial nephritis (593–595). The presence of polyomavirus infection is suggested by the finding of large basophilic intranuclear viral inclusion bodies in tubular epithelial cells along the entire nephron and also the transitional cell layer. The affected tubular cells were enlarged and often necrotic. Confirmation of the diagnosis can be made by special staining with polyomavirus monoclonal antibody. Urine and blood samples from patients with persistent infection revealed positive PCR with abundant amplicons of BK virus. Urine microscopy showed decoy cells with ground glass–type intranuclear inclusions positive for BK virus by immunohistochemistry and electron microscopy. A major factor involved in the manifestation of BK virus disease is high-dose immunosuppression. No established therapeutic therapy for polyomavirus infection is available, and reduction of immunosuppression offers the best therapeutic option. Tacrolimus as a possible risk factor has been suggested in the past. Most infected patients have been taking tacrolimus, and alternative agents can be used if response is inadequate.

Hepatitis

Chronic liver function impairment is not rare after renal transplantation (596–598). Viral hepatitis and drug-related hepatitis are the most common causes. Despite the exclusion of patients with HBsAg from organ and blood donation, the incidence of chronic liver disease after transplantation has remained high, with abnormalities of liver function occurring in 7% to 24% of patients early in follow-up, and death due to liver failure in 8% to 28% of the long-term survivors of renal transplantation. It is also important to rule out other causes of hepatitis. Drugs that may cause hepatic dysfunction include CsA, azathioprine, antihypertensives, and lipid-lowering agents. CsA-induced liver enzyme elevation usually resolves after reducing the dosage. Azathioprine is also thought to be hepatotoxic (599). Reduction of the dose of azathioprine in patients with chronic hepatitis may be necessary (600). In patients with impaired liver function, cyclophosphamide at a dose of 1 mg/kg has been used in the past to replace azathioprine (601). In patients taking CsA or tacrolimus, azathioprine can be discontinued or substituted with MMF.

Hepatitis B Virus

HBV is a relatively uncommon viral infection after transplantation, but the main cause for concern is the outcome of transplantation in a patient who is a carrier of the hepatitis B antigen. Although graft survival in such hepatitis B–carrier patients is perhaps better than in other patients, reflecting some innate immunosuppressive defect in the patient, there is considerable concern about the possible progression of liver disease leading to liver failure. Furthermore, the incidence of hepatoma in those chronic carriers of hepatitis B is 15%, much higher than in the general population who contract hepatitis. It has been suggested that immunosuppression enables persistent viral replication, leading to a greater frequency of HBeAg, viral DNA, and viral DNA polymerase in the sera of individuals who have undergone transplantation.

The natural history of liver disease due to chronic hepatitis B differs from that in both the general population and patients on hemodialysis (602,603). Transplant recipients who have hepatitis B typically remain surface antigen–positive for longer than 6 months and do not revert to seronegativity. Most episodes of hepatitis in the early posttransplantation period are relatively mild, but an unusually high rate of transformation from chronic persistent to chronic active hepatitis occurs in this patient population. Patients who have persistent HBe-antigenemia or concomitant delta virus infection are at higher risk for chronic active hepatitis and more rapid deterioration.

Because of the poor conversion rate in patients with ESRD, hepatitis B vaccination of patients should be given early in the course of progressive renal failure. Previously vaccinated patients who are HBsAg-negative should be tested annually for anti-HBV antibodies and should receive booster vaccinations when the titer decreases to less than 10 mIU/mL. No known loss of graft function has occurred as a result of active vaccination with hepatitis B vaccine (604,605). HBsAg-positive transplant recipients should receive lamivudine starting at the time of transplantation and continuing for at least 18 to 24 months. Two small studies demonstrated good responses to treatment with lamivudine for renal allograft recipients, with clearance of HBV DNA and normalization of transaminase levels (606,607).

Hepatitis C Virus

Anti-HCV antibodies have been reported for 10% to 40% of renal transplant recipients. HCV is the major cause of non-A/non-B hepatitis. Patients with ESRD are at increased risk for HCV infection because of their continued exposure to blood and blood products, horizontal transmission within hemodialysis units (603,608–613).

A national collaborative study of 3,081 cadaveric organ donors from eight organ procurement organizations in the United States found that the mean prevalence of positive ELISA-1 for anti-HCV antibodies was 5% and the prevalence of circulating HCV RNA as detected by PCR was 2.4%. In comparison, the prevalence of anti-HCV among healthy blood donors in the United States is only 0.6%. The higher prevalence among cadaveric donors may reflect an increased incidence of risk factors associated with the spread of the viral infections. Stored sera from 716 consecutive cadaveric donors in the New England Organ Bank were screened for anti-HCV antibodies using ELISA-1 assay, and 13 anti–HVC-positive donors were identified. Twenty-nine recipients of organs from these anti-HCV donors were identified and studied. Fourteen (48%) of these recipients developed non-A and non-B hepatitis after transplantation; 12 had chronic liver disease. Posttransplantation sera tested positive for HCV RNA in all of the recipients from HCV RNA–positive donors, suggesting that almost all patients are at risk in this setting. However, standard clinical evaluation may not detect HCV infection, because 52% of the patients did not have any evidence of hepatic disease and seroconversion occurred in only 62%. Following antibody titer will underestimate both the transmission of HCV and the role of HCV in posttransplantation liver disease (614–616). An increased incidence of acute renal allograft dysfunction is associated with IFN-α treatment among kidney transplant recipients (617,618). This is because interferon can induce cytokine gene expression, increase cell surface expression of HLA, and enhance the function of NK cells, cytotoxic T cells, and monocytes. Hence, therapy with IFN-α carries the risk of inducing rejection in the allograft. Thus, the risk of rejection must be weighed against the potential benefits of slowing or preventing the progression of chronic liver disease (619). Therefore, a better strategy might be to screen and treat HCV with interferon (and possibly ribavirin) before, rather than after, transplantation (620).

Pulmonary Infection

The overall incidence of pneumonia in renal transplant recipients has decreased from 25% to 8% since 1980. The decrease in the incidence of pulmonary infections is related to the judicious use of immunosuppressive therapy and more aggressive treatment of infection (621). Nevertheless, infection of the lungs is still the most common form of life-threatening infections in renal transplant recipients.

Opportunistic infections occur less commonly many years after transplantation, especially in the patient who has good renal function and is on minimal immunosuppression. However, pneumococcal pneumonia can occur at any time and may have a very rapid progression, leading to death if not diagnosed and treated promptly. Finally, the definitive diagnosis can only be established by identification of a pathogen, and it is important that an aggressive approach be adopted for obtaining specimens for microbiologic examination.

CMV Pneumonia

Lung infection is a serious complication of CMV infection. In the patient who presents with a fever and radiologic pulmonary changes between 1 and 4 months after transplantation and who was seronegative at the time of transplantation and who had received a kidney from a seropositive donor, an initial diagnosis of CMV infection of the lung should be made once all other possible causes of the fever have been excluded. *P. carinii* may also occur as a superinfecting organism during active CMV infection (568). If significant leukopenia develops in association with the infection, immunosuppressive drugs may have to be reduced. Possible treatment should be withheld until a pathogen can be identified. If no indication of the diagnosis is available, bronchoscopy and bronchial alveolar lavage or open lung biopsy should be performed (Fig. 97-26).

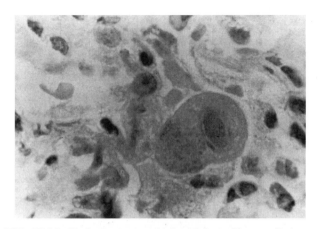

FIG. 97-26. Typical cytomegalovirus-infected lung cell showing cytomegaly, large intracellular inclusions with peripheral chromatin clumping, and abundant intracytoplasmic inclusions. (hematoxylin and eosin stain, magnification ×1,000)

Pneumocystis Carinii Pneumonia

This is a relatively common cause of pulmonary infection (622). The patient usually presents with a fever, often associated with some dyspnea, but with very few physical signs on examination. Chest radiograph shows diffuse shadowing that tends to be linear in distribution. Patients with suspected *P. carinii* pneumonia should have blood gas and vital signs closely monitored. Cotrimoxazole in high doses is the antimicrobial of choice. Prophylactic cotrimoxazole is commonly used during the first few months after transplantation because of the high incidence of this infection (623).

Legionella Pneumonia

Legionella pneumonia has become much more common in recent years; rather, it is probably being identified more commonly. The bacteria proliferates in stagnant water and so may be spread by way of air conditioning, plants, and showers (624). The chest radiograph in the early stages shows irregular, nodular shadows that progress, often quite rapidly, to a lobar or diffuse consolidation. Identification of the organism is difficult with conventional staining techniques but may be identified with direct immunofluorescent staining and may be grown from appropriate sputum or biopsy samples on specialized media. A high level of suspicion for this infection is needed, and erythromycin in high doses is the drug of choice.

Mycobacterial Infections

The incidence of tuberculosis in transplant recipients varies from region to region but certainly is more common in transplant recipients than in the general population (625). The symptoms are frequently nonspecific and the site of infection is often in organs other than the lungs. Treatment of the established case should be the routine antituberculous therapy (i.e., rifampicin and isoniazid), but it should be remembered that both these drugs are metabolized in the liver. Rifampicin induces hepatic enzymes; therefore, if the patient is being immunosuppressed with CsA or tacrolimus, the dose should be closely monitored. Chemoprophylaxis should be considered in patients with calcification on a chest roentgenogram and in the presence of a positive tuberculin skin test result. Six to 9 months of therapy with isoniazid should be given to patients who have never received adequate treatment and who are PPD-positive (626). Guidelines for targeted tuberculin testing and treatment of latent tuberculosis were recently developed jointly by the American Thoracic Society and the Centers for Disease Control and Prevention (627). The PPD (Mantoux) skin test involves an intradermal injection of 5 U of tuberculin PPD, with examination of the injection site 48 to 72 hours later. The minimal criterion for a positive skin test result is 5 mm diameter in duration for individuals at very high risk (including patients receiving immunosuppressive therapy).

Fungal Infections

Fungal infections are relatively common in transplant recipients and must always be considered as a possible cause of fever and pneumonia, especially in the presence of excessive immunosuppressive therapy (628). Pulmonary infiltrates due to fungal infection include *Aspergillus, Cryptococcus, Coccidiodes, Candida,* and *Histoplasmosis. Aspergillus* is a hyphal saprophytic fungus in which infection is by inhalation of spores and the lungs are therefore the primary site of infection. In the lung, *Aspergillus* causes a patchy infiltration followed by consolidation and abscess formation (Fig. 97-27).

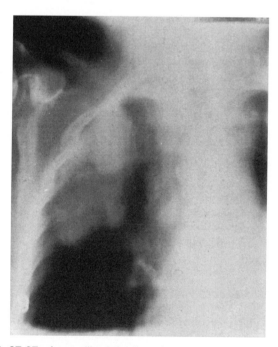

FIG. 97-27. *Aspergillus* infection of the lung in a patient who underwent renal transplantation after several courses of antirejection therapy with high-dose intravenous methylprednisolone. (From Morris PJ. *Kidney transplantation: principles and practice,* 2nd ed. New York: Grune & Stratton, 1984, with permission.)

Histoplasmosis is another fungal pneumonia that can occur in renal transplant recipients. This may also be acquired or result from reactivation and usually presents with fever, pulmonary infiltrates, and skin lesions at any time after transplantation. These infections require aggressive therapy with conventional amphotericin B, a lipid-based amphotericin B preparation (Abelcet, AmBisome, or Amphotec) (629), or an appropriate azole antifungal agent. Ketoconazole, fluconazole, and itraconazole are useful for treating mucocutaneous fungal infection and infection of the GU tract and GI system, lungs, and under specific conditions, CNS. All of the triazole antifungals impair calcineurin inhibitor metabolism and increase blood levels of CsA and tacrolimus. CsA or tacrolimus dose reduction may be necessary while patients are on triazole treatment (630).

Central Nervous System Infection

Infections of the CNS after renal transplantation typically present between 1 and 12 months posttransplantation and are characterized by a subacute onset and the frequent lack of systemic signs. Organisms commonly associated with CNS infection in renal transplant recipients include *Listeria, Cryptococcus, Mycobacterium, Nocardia, Aspergillus,* mucormycosis, *Toxoplasma, Candida,* and *Strongyloides. Listeria* may cause an acute or focal brain infection. *Cryptococcus* and, less often, *Mycobacterium* and *Coccidioides* are important causes of subacute meningitis. Focal lesions are most common with *Aspergillus, Toxoplasma,* and *Nocardia.* HIV can cause a variety of CNS syndromes, most predominantly a global dementing illness. JC virus infection can also cause dementia with progressive multifocal leukoencephalopathy (631).

In acute meningoencephalitis, nuchal rigidity may be absent. The development of fever and mild headache should be sufficient to alert the physician to the possibility of CNS infection. The aseptic meningitis that occurs during OKT-3 administration is self limited but if severe or persistent, may require diagnostic workup to rule out infection. Focal findings on neurologic examination are not common, except with well-developed focal brain infections. Because the early findings in these infections are often nonspecific, lumbar puncture and cranial CT scanning or MRI should not be delayed.

Aspergillus

Aspergillus may cause pneumonia in the immunocompromised host and may disseminate to the brain, skin, kidney, and gut. *Aspergillus,* which infiltrates the vasculature, is not found free in the cerebrospinal fluid (CSF) and is often impossible to diagnose before death. The organism may be suspected in patients with clinical evidence for meningitis and CSF cytology and chemistry determinations consistent with meningitis, especially in the absence of a positive culture, inflammatory foci, and culture or serologic findings consistent with cryptococcal infection. The treatment of choice is amphotericin B.

Cryptococcus

Although rare, *Cryptococcus* is another cause of meningitis in the transplant recipient. It tends to be seen relatively late in the transplantation course and has a rather nonspecific presentation; hence, the diagnosis is often delayed. Lung involvement is also common when this infection is present. Amphotericin B is again the indicated treatment.

Coccidioides

This is quite rare in Europe but does occur commonly in parts of the United States. It may cause destructive lesions of the lungs, liver, brain, and spleen and is sometimes due to reactivation of an existing latent infection. Amphotericin B is the appropriate treatment.

Listeria Monocytogenes

Listeria monocytogenes may present as meningitis, brain abscess, or meningoencephalitis. It may occur at any time after transplantation but is usually associated with increased or excessive immunosuppressive therapy for rejection. *Listeria* should be the primary suspect in a patient with meningoencephalitis because other causes of meningitis are rare in transplant recipients. CSF findings may not be striking. Treatment with ampicillin should be commenced as soon as CSF and other specimens for culture have been taken.

Nocardia

Nocardia usually presents as respiratory illness with an unproductive cough, fever, malaise, and a nodular infiltrate on the chest radiograph. Occasionally, the infection may spread to the brain presenting as a space-occupying lesion but may also be seen as skin abscesses or joint infections. The treatment of choice is probably sulfonamide, which is given for at least 2 months, although some would advocate treatment for 12 months.

Urinary Tract Infection

Urinary tract infection is the most common bacterial infection after transplantation. The incidence however has improved in recent years, most likely due to increased attention to urologic techniques and to the use of antibiotic prophylaxis after transplantation (632,633). Urinary tract infections appearing within the first 3 or 4 months after transplantation are often associated with transplant pyelonephritis, septicemia, and relapse after standard antibiotic therapy. Patients with anatomic abnormality requiring urinary diversion or stent placement and those with pyelonephritis should receive chronic suppressive antibiotics in addition to the 4 to 6 weeks of primary treatment. Uncomplicated urinary tract infections that occur later after transplantation can be treated with a standard 1- or 2-week course of oral antibiotics.

Cancer in Transplant Recipients

The incidence of cancer in transplant recipients varies considerably from region to region, ranging from a low incidence of 1.6% of patients developing cancer after transplantation in Europe to as high as 24% of patients in Australia (634–636). Much of this variation is due to the high incidence of skin cancer in those areas at risk for these cancers. In regions with limited exposure to the risk, there is a fourfold to sevenfold increase, but in areas with copious sunshine, there is an almost 29-fold increase in incidence, compared with the control population. There is also a well-recognized and highly significant increase in the risk of developing a malignant (non-Hodgkin's) lymphoma. Even with skin cancers and malignant lymphomas excluded from the analysis, there is an increased incidence in all forms of cancer in patients after transplantation (637–639) (Table 97-19). Careful physical examination to detect the common malignancies is essential in the long-term follow-up of renal transplant recipients. The increased incidence of cervical cancer in women after transplantation implies that all women who have received a transplant should have an annual cervical smear.

A number of factors contribute to the increased risk of cancers in immunosuppressed recipients of a kidney transplant. These include depression of immune surveillance, chronic antigenic stimulation in the presence of immunosuppression, a directly neoplastic action of the immunosuppressive drugs themselves, and increased susceptibility to oncogenic viral infection. Alterations in the immune surveillance due to immunosuppressive therapy may allow potentially malignant cell mutants to become established in the host, because they cannot be detected and killed in the usual fashion. The

TABLE 97-19. *Common malignancies encountered in renal transplant receipts*

Cancers of skin and lips
  Squamous cell carcinomas
  Basal cell carcinomas
  Malignant melanoma
Malignant lymphomas
  Non-Hodgkin's lymphoma
  Reticulum cell sarcoma
  B-cell lymphoproliferative syndrome (Epstein-Barr virus)
Kaposi's sarcoma
  Cutaneous form
  Visceral and cutaneous form
Genitourinary cancer
  Carcinoma of native kidney (acquired cystic disease)
  Carcinoma of transplanted kidney (hypernephroma)
  Carcinoma of the urinary bladder (cyclophosphamide associated)
  Uroepithelial tumors (associated with analgesic nephropathy)
Gynecologic cancer
  Carcinoma of cervix
  Ovarian cancer

allograft with its foreign HLA may also stimulate the host lymphoreticular system, resulting in the development of lymphoid malignancies. It has been suggested that ALG or ATG may have an etiologic role in the production of neoplasia. These agents produce immunosuppression by eliminating certain types of lymphocytes involved in immune reactions. Recently, the incidence of lymphoma has increased with the use of monoclonal antibodies OKT-3 for immunosuppression (640,641). Finally, latent oncogenic viruses may be activated in immunosuppressed hosts who are simultaneously experiencing stimulation immunologically by antigen. An association exists between papilloma virus and the development of squamous skin cancer, as well as condyloma acuminatum with cervical carcinoma. EBV has also been implicated in polyclonal B-cell lymphoproliferative disease. In addition to primary cancer developed *de novo* in patients after transplantation, cancer may be transferred in the transplanted kidney from a donor with cancer undetected at the time of donor nephrectomy.

Skin cancer is the most common neoplasia in transplant recipients, with an incidence 4 to 21 times the population average (642–644). Squamous cell carcinoma predominates over basal cell skin cancer (645). Patients who live in warm climates should be carefully advised after transplantation to use sun-blocking creams and to wear appropriate clothing while in the sun. The appearance of neoplasia can be atypical, and early biopsy of any suspicious lesion is indicated. The prognosis after resection of skin cancer is excellent, provided strict avoidance of sun exposure is followed. Reduction in immunosuppression may be considered if the malignancy is extensive or rapidly progressive.

Lymphoma occurs earlier than other tumors and accounts for 20% to 30% of posttransplantation neoplasms. The incidence of this neoplasm is relatively higher in the last decade probably related to the use of monoclonal or polyclonal globulin and other immunosuppression. Two types of lymphoproliferative disease are seen in patients after transplantation. The first presents with an infectious mononucleosis-like illness within the first year of transplantation with fever, sore throat, and lymphadenopathy. The clinical course is often short and can be fatal. Cessation of the immunosuppression will lead to regression in some patients. This type of lymphoproliferative disease is due to infection with EBV. With acyclovir treatment, remission can be achieved without cessation of immunosuppression. The second group of lymphoproliferative diseases presents as localized solid tumor masses and is confined to the CNS in a high percentage of patients. Lymphoma therefore should be considered in the differential diagnosis of any CNS abnormality (646). These lymphomas are often more rapidly progressive than those seen in the normal population, and although responding to conventional therapy for non-Hodgkin's lymphoma, remission tends to be short. In addition to standard, established treatment of each malignancy, consideration must be given to reduction or cessation of immunosuppressive medications (647). Azathioprine usually is discontinued during chemotherapy because many of the therapeutic agents are cytotoxic and additive suppression of the bone marrow can occur. In most cases, regression does not appear to occur with cessation of immunosuppression and the patients do not respond to acyclovir (648–652).

The incidence of Kaposi's sarcoma is 300 to 400 times that of the normal population and accounts for 5% to 10% of posttransplantation neoplasms. Those with Kaposi's sarcoma involving only the skin do better than those with visceral disease, with complete remission in 50% compared with 14%, respectively, after chemotherapy or cessation of immunosuppression. One-third of the remissions in Kaposi's sarcoma confined to the skin occurred with discontinuation of immunosuppression as the sole therapy (653,654).

GI Complications

GI complications include peptic ulceration, esophagitis, intestinal or colonic perforation and hemorrhage, pseudomembranous colitis, necrotizing enterocolitis, and diverticulitis.

Complications of a peptic ulcer, either hemorrhage or perforation, are associated with a high mortality rate in the transplant recipients. About 4% of the deaths after transplantation were reported to be caused by GI hemorrhage. Of these deaths, hematemesis or melena is seen in 75% of patients on presentation, whereas pain is the presenting symptom in 20%, and gastroduodenal perforation in about 10%. The most significant risk factor is a history of peptic ulcer disease (655,656). Whereas about 8% of patients with negative peptic ulcer histories before engraftment later develop gastroduodenal complications, 19% of those with previous episodes of uremic gastritis develop further complications after transplantation. For this reason, many centers actively screen patients for evidence of peptic ulceration before accepting for transplantation and in the past have been quite aggressive about the management of these patients, many being treated surgically before transplantation. Although this would still be the treatment of choice for active ulceration not responding to treatment or recurrent ulceration after treatment, most patients would now be given histamine antagonists prophylactically during the first few months after transplantation in the presence of a past history of ulceration but with no evidence of active ulceration at the time of transplantation. Both hemorrhage and perforation from a peptic ulcer after transplantation should be treated promptly and aggressively by surgery.

Infection of the GI tract presents commonly as *Candida* stomatitis or esophagitis. This is particularly common in transplant recipients who are debilitated from other complications or infections or in the presence of leukopenia or excess immunosuppressive therapy. Esophageal candidiasis is probably the most severe form of local infection due to this pathogen, but occasionally a septicemia may ensue. The esophagitis responds to local nystatin, but more severe infections should be treated with amphotericin B or fluconazole. Classic enteric pathogens are not notably common after transplantation.

Spontaneous perforation of the small intestine is rare, and the etiology is often not understood, although CMV infection, obstruction, intestinal ischemia, and the use of steroids have been implicated (657). Hemorrhage of the large bowel with ulceration and perforation occurs in 0.9% of such patients. Possible causes include uremia, the effects of immunosuppressive therapy, use of antibiotics, atherosclerosis, and the sequelae of irradiation. Administration of sodium polystyrene resin in sorbitol to treat patients with hyperkalemia can also be complicated by colonic perforation (658).

Pseudomembranous colitis is an antibiotic-associated diarrhea and thus may occur in transplant recipients who are receiving broad-spectrum antibiotic therapy for a concomitant bacterial infection. However, it may also occur in transplantation units where *Clostridium difficile* infection is endemic (659). This condition is highly infectious and should be treated as such to avoid spread within a transplantation unit. Occasionally, a necrotizing enterocolitis with gangrene of part or all of the colon, and even occasionally involving only the small bowel, is seen. This is inevitably fatal and the cause is uncertain, although it has been associated with CMV infection. Solitary ulcers, which may bleed or perforate, may also be encountered, especially in the cecum. Colonoscopy is a useful diagnostic tool in some of these colonic complications.

Diverticulitis is no more common in the transplant recipient than in the normal population, except perhaps in patients with polycystic kidneys, but complicated diverticulitis does again present a very serious problem with a high mortality rate. For this reason, some surgeons believe that the presence of diverticulosis in patients before transplantation is an indication for colectomy to avoid complications arising after transplantation.

Pancreatitis

Although mild hyperamylasemia without pancreatitis is common in patients with poor graft function due to decreased clearance of the enzyme, high serum amylase and lipase levels suggest active pancreatitis (660). Acute pancreatitis has been reported to occur in 2% to 12% of transplant recipients. Several causes have been considered. Inflammatory changes, possibly due to secondary hyperparathyroidism, may be seen in the glands of uremic patients. Microscopic examination occasionally has revealed changes consistent with the presence of CMV, but the role of this organism is unknown. Corticosteroids may produce pancreatitis both experimentally and clinically. Azathioprine is a rare cause of pancreatitis (661). Recently, there are case reports of pancreatic insufficiency and pancreatitis in a small fraction of patients on CsA (662). The pancreatic abnormalities due to CsA may be dose-related because the abnormality improved with reduction of the CsA dose. Acute pancreatitis in renal transplant recipients often follows a fulminating course with an acute abdomen, electrolyte disturbances, tetany, jaundice, and hypotension (662,663).

Cardiovascular Complications

Cardiovascular Disease

Cardiovascular disease is a major cause of morbidity and death after renal transplantation. With increasing transplantation in older adults and diabetic patients and the longer survival of grafts, cardiovascular disease will take an increasingly prominent place in the problems of patients with successful renal transplants (664,665). Much of this risk is determined by the cause of the underlying disease for renal failure, and certainly patients with a primary diagnosis of hypertension or diabetes mellitus fare significantly worse in this respect than others. The cardiovascular disease can be attributed to the high prevalence of vascular pathology that is characteristic of both these diseases and is independent of their end-stage renal failure. Nevertheless, once the patient has undergone transplantation, it is essential that rigorous advice be given to a correction of any risk factors that would increase the risks of cardiovascular disease, namely, hyperlipidemia, hypertension, cigarette smoking, obesity, and carbohydrate intolerance.

Hyperlipidemia

It has been known for some time that uremic patients frequently have type IV hyperlipidemia with marked hypertriglyceridemia. Total cholesterol level is usually within the normal range or low. In particular, HDL levels are abnormally low (666–668). After transplantation, the hypertriglyceridemia of uremia shifts toward hypercholesterolemia. Very-low-density lipoprotein and low-density lipoprotein (LDL) cholesterol levels are elevated in transplant recipients. Hypertriglyceridemia may persist, but triglyceride levels often decrease. Overall, the incidence of hyperlipidemia after transplantation is about 50% (669–674).

High-dose prednisone may contribute to the development of hypercholesterolemia. Normalization of serum lipids, however, including HDL cholesterol, occurs after reduction of the initial steroid dose. HDL levels increase and return to within the normal range, with normal proportions of HDL3 and HDL2 (671). Studies imply that prompt tapering of prednisone dose after transplantation facilitates a return to normal lipid concentrations.

Dietary therapy should be initiated during the first 6 months after transplantation, when hypercholesterolemia is most often marked. Patients should be advised to avoid high-calorie, high-carbohydrate, and high-fat diets (672). Supplementation of the diet with ω-3 fatty acids may reduce triglyceride and cholesterol levels, and increase HDL levels. If hypercholesterolemia persists beyond 6 months on diet therapy and on maintenance steroid dose, drug therapy should be considered.

Potential pharmacologic agents include niacin, bile binding resins, gemfibrozil, and lovastatin. Niacin lowers triglyceride and cholesterol levels. A slow-release preparation of niacin may reduce the side effects of flushing and GI distress. Bile binding resins can also be used but may interfere with immunosuppressive drug absorption. Gemfibrozil primarily reduces triglyceride levels; but it can lower cholesterol when triglyceride levels are within the normal range. Lovastatin inhibits 3-hydroxy-3-methylglutaryl coenzyme A (HMG CoA) reductase, the rate-limiting enzyme in cholesterol biosynthesis, and is effective in reducing cholesterol levels. Liver enzymes should be monitored in all patients receiving niacin, gemfibrozil, and lovastatin because hepatitis is a major adverse effect. Reports have been made of myositis and myalgia occurring at a low frequency, secondary to gemfibrozil and lovastatin. An increased risk of myositis has been described in those patients receiving CsA who also were treated with lovastatin (673–677).

Hyperhomocystinemia

The association between fasting plasma total homocysteine levels and cardiovascular disease has been demonstrated by retrospective and prospective studies in the general population (678). A case-control study demonstrated that renal transplant recipients with cardiovascular disease exhibited higher fasting total homocysteine levels (more than 10 μmol/L) compared with renal transplant recipients without cardiovascular disease. Cross-sectional studies of renal transplant recipients also confirmed a similar association between total fasting homocysteine levels and cardiovascular disease. Because renal transplantation recipients typically have fasting total homocysteine levels that are twofold higher than those of age- and gender-matched control subjects, the incidence is high enough to warrant screening (679,680). Hyperhomocystinemia can be safely and effectively reduced by folate, Vitamin B_6 and Vitamin B_{12}. However, the lack of well-designed interventional trials makes it difficult to recommend routine screening (681,682).

Hypertension

Hypertension is extremely common after renal transplantation. It is more common in recipients of cadaveric grafts than those receiving living related grafts, suggesting that rejection is a significant factor in this high incidence of hypertension after transplantation (683–685). Hypertension before and after engraftment probably contributes to the accelerated vascular disease seen in patients with ESRD and is associated with reduced graft function (686).

Hypertension in the transplant recipient may be due to the patient's diseased native kidney, rejection of the transplanted kidney, renal artery stenosis in the transplanted kidney, corticosteroids, and CsA therapy (687,688).

The relationship between hypertension and activity of the renin–angiotensin system in patients with a renal transplant is confusing (689,690). It is apparent that the patient's native kidneys may contribute to hyperreninemia, but conflicting reports exist concerning the role of the renin–angiotensin system in the transplanted kidney as a cause of hypertension. Native kidney disease and chronic rejection are the two most common causes of hypertension in the transplant population, whereas hemodynamically significant renal artery stenosis accounts for about 5%.

Steroid therapy certainly contributes to hypertension, although this is less likely now that low-dose steroid protocols are used by most centers. It is now apparent that the incidence of hypertension in patients being treated with CsA, either with or without steroids, is greater than that seen in patients treated with prednisone and azathioprine (691). The degree to which CsA might increase blood pressure is dose-dependent, as demonstrated by the fact that there is a general decrease in blood pressure after the reduction of the CsA dose to maintenance therapy levels of 4 mg/kg per day.

Initial management of hypertension in patients with stable graft function includes salt restriction, weight reduction, elimination or reduction of medications that may contribute to hypertension, and the use of antihypertensive agents.

Most standard therapies have been demonstrated to be safe and effective after renal transplantation. There are however a number of management issues that are unique to transplant recipients. Transplant recipients may be more prone to decreased renal function resulting from diuretic use than hypertensive patients in the general population. Patients may occasionally develop decreased renal function after ACE inhibitor therapy, especially if the patient exhibits renal artery stenosis or chronic allograft nephropathy. Anemia and hyperkalemia may also be associated with the use of ACE inhibitors and angiotensin II receptor antagonists. Several studies however have shown that these drugs are generally safe, effective, and well tolerated. They may reduce proteinuria and stabilize the deterioration in renal function in chronic allograft failure, possibly by reducing TGF-β. They may also have additional benefit in reducing the incidence of cardiovascular events in high-risk patients.

ACE inhibitors such as captopril or enalapril are useful in treating posttransplantation hypertension in patients who do not have transplant artery stenosis. Calcium channel blockers are being used more frequently in the treatment of hypertension. The hemodynamic effects of CsA include decreased effective renal plasma flow and increased renovascular resistance. Calcium channel blockers such as verapamil have been shown to affect GFR and PGE_2 production (692). It has been suggested that the use of calcium channel blockers may have additional cytoprotective effect against ischemic and nephrotoxic injury in the transplanted kidney. Because calcium and its carrier protein, calmodulin, may be involved in various T-cell functions, calcium channel blockers and CsA may be directly additive with regards to the calcium cellular immune mechanism (693,694). If the native kidneys are believed to be the source of hypertension, nephrectomy (695–697) should be considered. Overall, nephrectomy has been shown to substantially reduce blood pressure in these patients.

If the hypertension persists, patients with hypertension associated with renal dysfunction should be evaluated to determine the cause of the dysfunction. Possibilities include chronic rejection, CsA nephrotoxicity, or a recurrence of the original disease. A renal biopsy may be appropriate to rule out rejection. If hypertension is severe or associated with worsening renal function, with no evidence for rejection, transplant artery stenosis may be pursued by arteriography.

Renal Artery Stenosis

When hypertension cannot be controlled, particularly if attempts to reduce blood pressure result in decreased renal function, the possibility of renal allograft artery stenosis should be considered. Transplant renal artery stenosis currently is diagnosed in approximately 2% of cases. In earlier reports, the incidence ranged from 1% to 25%. In the past, most stenoses had been described with the end-to-end anastomosis between the renal artery and the recipient hypogastric artery, presumably because of the discrepancy in size and quality of the two vessels, although rejection injury may be a predisposing factor (698,699). Occasionally, renal artery stenosis may occur in the early months after transplantation; at this time, it is always due to a technical defect at the anastomotic site. Because the use of end-to-side anastomosis of an aortic patch containing the renal artery origin onto the recipient external iliac artery, the incidence rate has become much lower (700,701). Today, renal artery stenosis presents one to several years after transplantation with poorly controlled hypertension and deterioration of renal function. Other causes of arterial stenosis include arteriosclerosis, development of a fibrous plaque in the artery at the anastomotic site or constriction beyond it, technical narrowing of the anastomosis, perfusion injury, kinking of the vessels, and chronic microvascular rejection. Sudden occurrence or increase in the severity of hypertension, the presence of a new bruit over the allograft, or a decline in renal function in the absence of rejection all suggest the possibility of renal artery stenosis. A rise in the serum creatinine level after treatment with an ACE inhibitor for hypertension is very suggestive of renal allograft arterial stenosis (1). On occasion, renal vein and peripheral renin levels may be of value. Renal artery stenosis is relatively common in the transplanted kidney, as demonstrated angiographically, but this does not necessarily mean that it is the cause of hypertension. Along with immunologic rejection (702), abnormal hemodynamics and flow turbulence at or just distal to the anastomotic site have been suggested as possible causes of arterial stenosis. An acute angle or kinking between donor and recipient arteries, or the excessive length of the hypogastric renal artery system, may contribute to the flow turbulence.

The diagnosis of a functional renal artery stenosis is difficult, but in the presence of poorly controlled hypertension and deteriorating renal function, magnetic resonance angiography of the kidney or renal arteriography, as well as renal biopsy, should be considered. If the biopsy shows evidence of moderate-to-severe chronic rejection with intimal fibrosis of the arteries and arterioles, correction of the renal artery stenosis is unlikely to be very successful. Another more diagnostic sign of a functional stenosis is a loss of renal function after treatment with an ACE inhibitor such as captopril or enalapril. This does imply a prominent role for the renin–angiotensin system in the etiology of the hypertension. Radionuclide scan may show a delay and decrease in allograft blood flow but is a relatively insensitive tool for diagnosis of renal artery stenosis. Doppler ultrasonography is a moderately sensitive and noninvasive means of establishing the diagnosis, however, many false-negative results occur. The technique is easy to perform and interpret in cases with only one artery and an end-to-end anastomosis. Other screening tests include magnetic resonance angiography (703) and spiral CT (704). Angiography is however the most sensitive test for the diagnosis of renal artery stenosis in a transplanted kidney and is essential in therapy. However, establishing that a renal artery stenosis demonstrated angiographically is the cause of the hypertension, renal dysfunction, or both is extremely difficult, because both may be due to the associated vascular changes of chronic rejection. A renal biopsy may be helpful in making the diagnosis if it excludes significant chronic rejection. The results of surgical correction of the stenosis are good (705,706), but because of the difficulty of the surgery, there has been considerable interest in percutaneous transluminal angioplasty of renal artery stenoses (707–710).

Polycythemia

An increased erythrocyte mass has been demonstrated in some 17% of graft recipients (711). Erythrocytosis, defined as a hematocrit value of more than 52%, most often occurs within the first year after transplantation and may be associated with good allograft function, chronic rejection, transplant renal artery stenosis (712), hydronephrosis, native kidney and hepatic EPO production, and the use of androgenic steroids. In patients with good allograft function, it is postulated that correction of the uremic milieu allows overzealous red blood cell production because of a reset marrow response to EPO (713,714). In patients with chronic rejection, renal artery stenosis, and hydronephrosis, intrarenal hypoxemia may stimulate EPO production (715). In most cases, the precise etiology is uncertain, but studies on EPO levels after transplantation indicate that graft function restores the hematopoietic response to normal. The phenomenon usually is self limited, lasting 3 to 12 months. Low doses of an ACE inhibitor (beginning with 2.5 mg of enalapril per day or 12.5 mg of captopril twice a day) reduce the hematocrit to normal or near-normal levels. The effect begins within 6 weeks and is complete in 3 to 6 months. An association between the ACE inhibitor–induced reduction in hematocrit and a fall in plasma EPO levels has been demonstrated in some studies. Also compatible with an EPO-independent mechanism is the observation that withdrawal of the ACE inhibitor results in a gradual rise in hematocrit without a concurrent elevation in EPO levels. ACE inhibitors can also induce anemia in some renal transplant recipients without erythrocytosis. The mechanism of action is unclear.

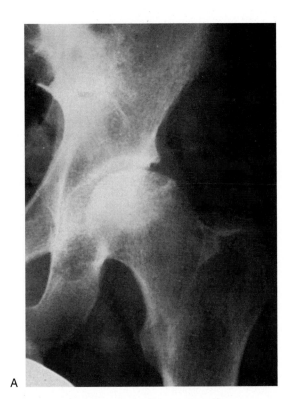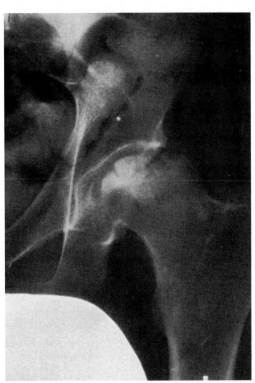

FIG. 97-28. Avascular necrosis of the head of the femur after transplantation. **A:** Normal radiograph of the hip 10 months after transplantation, at which time, the patient was complaining of pain. **B:** The same hip 8 months later. This patient had received azathioprine and high-dose steroids and subsequently had a successful hip replacement. (From Morris PJ. *Kidney transplantation: principles and practice,* 2nd ed. New York: Grune & Stratton, 1984, with permission.)

An alternative to ACE inhibition is theophylline. Theophylline appears to act as an adenosine antagonist in this setting, suggesting that adenosine facilitates both the release and perhaps the bone marrow response to EPO (716–719). In severe cases (hematocrit, more than 52%), phlebotomy is indicated to prevent thromboembolic complications, which may occur in as many as 20% of patients with erythrocytosis.

Bone Complications

The main types of renal osteodystrophy are secondary hyperparathyroidism and osteomalacia. After successful transplantation, the metabolic milieu of bone changes with correction of acidosis, cessation of aluminum hydroxide gel therapy, and improved Vitamin D metabolism (720). This leads to varying degrees of resolution of preexisting renal osteodystrophy and osteomalacia. A progressive resolution of the radiographic changes of hyperparathyroidism occurs as early as 3 months after transplantation, but abnormalities may persist for more than 12 months in some patients. However, many patients have sustained hyperparathyroidism. Indications for parathyroidectomy include progressive elevation of parathyroid hormone (PTH) and alkaline phosphatase levels, progressive or new metabolic bone disease, osteonecrosis, metastatic calcification, and severe symptoms of pruritus and proximal myopathy. Osteoporosis is related to steroid

therapy. It is much less of a problem now that low-dose steroid protocols are used, but the postmenopausal woman, even on low-dose steroid therapy, is likely to develop significant osteoporosis.

The main bone disorder that can be directly attributed to transplantation is avascular necrosis or osteonecrosis, which most commonly affects the hips (Fig. 97-28) and tends be bilateral but may affect other joints, including the wrists, elbows, knees, ankles, and shoulders. Pain may be severe and is the most common presenting symptom, usually occurring between 1 and 3 years after transplantation. The mean time to onset was 12 months after transplantation (range, 6 to 21 months). The incidence of avascular necrosis has been as high as 15% after transplantation, but this was due almost entirely to high-dose steroid therapy used in conjunction with azathioprine. Because of the general adoption of low-dose steroid protocols, the incidence of avascular necrosis has dropped dramatically to about 2% (721,722). Patients with preexisting secondary hyperparathyroidism at the time of transplantation may be at a higher risk for developing avascular necrosis of bone. Pain usually precedes any radiologic changes by several months. In well-established cases, the diagnosis can be made on plain radiographs, whereas CT scanning, MRI, and nuclear bone scanning may detect earlier changes. Percutaneous needle manometry of intramedullary pressures may demonstrate elevated pressures and venous outflow obstruction, which precede structural bone necrosis. If performed early, core decompression to relieve the intramedullary venous outflow obstruction can prevent osteonecrosis. With more severe disease, prosthetic total hip replacement has been used with excellent functional recovery. In general, surgery should be performed early to facilitate rehabilitation.

Prospective studies have demonstrated that bone loss occurs early and rapidly after renal transplantation (723–725). These patients lost 6.8% of their initial bone mass during the first 6 months after transplantation and developed a low-turnover bone disorder resembling that induced by glucocorticoids. By 18 months, bone loss had decreased 9% from baseline. The development of osteopenia places the patient at increased risk for pathologic fractures. The prevalence of atraumatic fractures in the renal transplant recipient may be as high as 22%; these fractures occur primarily at sites of high cancellous bone, such as the vertebrae and ribs. Posttransplantation bone loss involves both preexisting risk factors, such as hyperparathyroidism, and the adverse effects of immunosuppressive therapy. Glucocorticoid suppression of bone formation is the most important factor in the genesis of early bone loss. Steroids are directly toxic to osteoblasts and lead to increased osteoclast activity. They also have other effects that promote calcium loss and the development of osteopenia. These include decreased calcium absorption, reduced gonadal hormone production, diminished insulin-like growth factor-1 production, and decreased sensitivity to PTH. Cyclosporine, which induces a high-turnover osteopenia in rodents, also may contribute to bone loss, especially in long-term survivors and in subjects treated only with cyclosporine. It is important to monitor bone mineral density in the renal transplant recipient using dual-energy x-ray absorptiometry. It is recommended that lumbar spine and hip bone mineral densities be measured at the time of transplant, after 6 months, and then every 12 months if results are abnormal. Those subjects displaying rapid bone loss and/or a low initial bone density should be considered for treatment. Calcium supplementation (1 g per day) should be considered in nonhypercalcemic patients. The administration of Vitamin D analogs (such as calcitriol) can further improve calcium absorption. If bone loss is severe or rapid, consideration should be given to the administration of calcitonin or other antiresorptive agents such as the bisphosphonates (such as pamidronate) (726,727).

Renal Electrolyte and Tubular Disorders

Proximal bicarbonate wasting occurs most often in the early transplantation course and resolves gradually. Proximal renal tubular acidosis may be related to ischemic preservation injury, secondary hyperparathyroidism, malnutrition, ATN, and acute rejection (728–730). Distal renal tubular acidosis sometimes occurs either as a consequence of acute rejection or as a result of the interstitial nephropathy caused by chronic rejection. Hyperkalemia is common in patients on CsA and

is readily reversible with lowering of the dose. The mechanism is unclear, but the decreased potassium excretion may be due to diminished serum aldosterone levels or to a primary tubular defect.

Hypercalcemia

Acute hypercalcemia usually occurs in the setting of severe secondary hyperparathyroidism. Because of the improved management of secondary hyperparathyroidism preoperatively, this is less frequently seen with oral phosphate binders, calcium supplementation, and Vitamin D administration. Still, 10% to 20% of patients may develop hypercalcemia within the first 1 to 2 years after transplantation (731). Most hypercalcemic patients have transient elevations in serum calcium levels, in the range of 11 to 12 mg/dL. The treatment of hypercalcemia includes dietary reduction of calcium and cessation of thiazide diuretics and Vitamin D supplements, which may exacerbate hypercalcemia. Persistent mild hypercalcemia is generally managed conservatively with serial serum calcium determinations, unless there are indications for more aggressive intervention with parathyroidectomy. Serum intact PTH should be measured at 6 and 12 months and then annually posttransplantation (732–734).

There are two major indications for parathyroidectomy in these patients: severe symptomatic hypercalcemia, usually occurring in the early posttransplantation period; and persistent, marked hypercalcemia. Approximately 4% to 10% of patients remain hypercalcemic after 1 year. Elective parathyroidectomy should be considered if the plasma calcium concentration remains at more than 12.5 mg/dL (3.1 mmol/L) for more than 1 year, particularly if associated with radiologic evidence of increased bone resorption.

Hypophosphatemia

Hypophosphatemia (serum phosphorus levels of less than 2.6 mg/dL) is very common in the early weeks after transplantation. Newly transplanted kidneys may waste phosphate under the influence of a raised PTH level (735,736). Some transplanted kidneys continue to lose excessive phosphate despite resolution of the secondary hyperparathyroidism (737). Hypophosphatemia is usually not symptomatic and typically resolves over 6 to 12 months. Hypophosphatemia is observed in 60% to 70% of patients within 1 year after transplantation. Hypophosphatemia may persist for more than 1 year in 20% to 25% even in the absence of hyperparathyroidism. The most common cause is due to a renal phosphate–wasting syndrome in the absence of other evidence of proximal tubule dysfunction (738). The decrease in serum phosphorus levels is less among transplant recipients who receive corticosteroid-free immunosuppressive therapy. Plasma phosphate levels of less than 1.0 to 1.5 mg/dL (0.32 to 0.48 mmol/L) can cause muscle weakness. Severe and prolonged hypophosphatemia can lead to osteomalacia and fractures. Oral phosphate replacements are required if hypophosphatemia persists. One important exception is the patient with significant persistent hyperparathyroidism, as detected by elevated plasma intact PTH levels. In this setting, the administration of phosphate can exacerbate the hyperparathyroidism in part by complexing with calcium and lowering intestinal calcium absorption.

Hypomagnesemia

Hypomagnesemia (serum total magnesium levels of less than 1.5 mg/dL) is common in the early weeks after transplantation. It can result from CsA- or tacrolimus-induced renal magnesium leaks. The use of thiazide diuretics is another common cause of renal magnesium loss. Up to 25% of long-term CsA-treated patients manifest hypomagnesemia (739–741). The prevalence decreases with time after transplantation, possibly because of decreasing CsA blood levels. The prevalence of CsA-induced hypomagnesemia may be higher among diabetic patients. Muscle weakness, hypokalemia, hypocalcemia, and rarely seizures may result from severe hypomagnesemia. Low magnesium levels may be associated with hypertension in CsA-treated patients. Low magnesium levels have been linked to hyperlipidemia in renal transplant recipients and magnesium replacement was demonstrated to reduce elevated total and LDL cholesterol levels in a small uncontrolled trial by Gupta et al. (742).

Hyperuricemia

Renal handling of uric acid is affected by the use of CsA leading to higher serum urate levels in CsA-treated patients (743–745). Asymptomatic hyperuricemia occurs in 55% of patients receiving CsA and in 25% of those taking azathioprine. There is no report of graft failure due to urate nephropathy in the transplanted kidney. Crystal-induced erosive arthritis can occur in these patients. Nonsteroidal antiinflammatory agents should also be avoided because of potential negative influence on renal hemodynamics and the development of interstitial nephritis. Colchicine is the preferred treatment if symptoms persist. Allopurinol, a xanthine oxidase inhibitor, should be avoided in patients taking azathioprine. Concomitant administration of allopurinol and azathioprine results in marrow suppression and a fourfold increase in immunosuppression.

Hyperglycemia

Glycosuria occurs in about 60% of patients in the first 6 months after transplantation. Both tacrolimus and CsA may cause pancreatic toxicity, with hyperglycemia occurring when drug levels are high and in conjunction with prednisone administration (746–748). In large prospective and retrospective studies, the incidence varied from 4% to 18%. The incidence was reported to be higher among patients treated with CsA and prednisone, compared with those treated with azathioprine and prednisone. Tacrolimus has also been linked to a higher incidence of posttransplantation diabetes mellitus. Older individuals and African American or Hispanic patients are most susceptible. Glucose intolerance resolves with reduction of the steroid dose in most of these patients (749).

Cataracts

Posterior lenticular cataracts appear in up to 10% of transplant recipients receiving high-dose steroids. Usually the cataracts are small and do not present a severe handicap to the patient, although in some instances, cataracts are large and require removal of the lens.

Obesity

Many studies report the prevalence of obesity at the time of transplantation but few report its prevalence after transplantation. However, approximately 40% of renal transplant recipients are obese 1 year after transplantation. Obesity is defined as a BMI of more than 30% kg/m^2, or more than 130% ideal body weight (750,751). Increased caloric intake may occur after transplantation primarily because of enhanced appetite associated with corticosteroid use. If obesity ensues, it may contribute to the development or exacerbation of hypertension, hyperlipidemia, cardiovascular disease, and steroid-induced diabetes. A consistent correlation between obesity and graft survival has not been found, although patient survival may be reduced, largely because of cardiac death. Weight loss is recommended to improve lipid profile, lower blood pressure, and improve glycemic control for patients with type II diabetes mellitus. In addition to limitation of caloric intake, management of posttransplantation obesity includes behavior modification, an exercise program, and early nutritional counseling (752).

Malnutrition

Up to 70% of the patients on dialysis have some element of malnutrition, and low serum albumin level is a predictor of mortality risk for patients with ESRD on dialysis. Approximately 10% of patients exhibit hypoalbuminemia at 1 year and 20% at 10 years after transplantation. Low serum albumin levels may be the result of decreased production and/or increased catabolism (753,754). Increased urinary protein excretion, especially in patients with chronic transplant nephropathy, may also result in low serum albumin levels. Chronic allograft nephropathy with hypoalbuminemia is associated with a decrease in muscle mass, which is reflected in decreases in urinary creatinine excretion. Corticosteroids accelerate the protein catabolic rate and frequently create negative nitrogen balance. Studies by Hoy et al. have documented significant increases in the protein catabolic rate, accompanied by decreases in serum albumin levels, in the immediate posttransplantation period (755). Even maintenance low-dose corticosteroid therapy increases protein catabolism and muscle wasting. Severe protein catabolism contributes to poor wound healing and an increased susceptibility to infection (756). Early nutritional support is indicated in high-risk patients. Assessment of nutritional status by a renal dietitian should be incorporated into the clinic visit. Serum albumin levels should be monitored annually. Serum prealbumin levels should be measured if albumin levels are low or if clinical findings suggest possible malnutrition. The degree of protein catabolism can be assessed by the measurement of urea nitrogen appearance. A daily protein intake ranging from 0.55 to 1.0 g/kg has been recommended for stable posttransplantation patients.

Growth in Children

Children with end-stage renal failure will have retarded growth, and after transplantation, one of the major problems of the use of steroids in immunosuppressive protocols is the continuing retardation of growth. Although the rate of growth usually improves after transplantation, catch-up growth is less common. Growth rate is related to the age of the child, the presence of near-normal renal function, and the use of alternate-day steroids (757–759). The use of cyclosporine, especially if used without steroids, in children appears to allow normal growth and indeed there is now some evidence that catch-up growth may occur in these patients (760–762).

Parenthood After Renal Transplantation

Chronic renal failure is usually associated with a loss of libido, amenorrhea in women, and impotence in men. After successful transplantation, menstruation returns in young women, and men usually redevelop their libido and potency. Women have had successful pregnancies and men have fathered children. Of the first 697 transplant recipients at the University of Colorado (763), 50 male recipients were responsible for 67 pregnancies. There were 60 live births, 2 abortions, and 5 successful current pregnancies. Thirty-seven female recipients had 56 pregnancies resulting in 44 live births, 8 abortions, and 3 current pregnancies. Toxemia occurred in 27% of pregnancies, approximately four times the expected incidence in a nontransplant population. Further renal deterioration with preexisting renal impairment was considered a possible indication for termination of pregnancy. Irreversible deterioration of renal function attributable to pregnancy occurred in 7%. Forty-five percent of deliveries were premature and 30% of newborns had one or more complications. The occurrence of congenital anomalies was small. Since then, significant experience has accumulated enabling the physician to provide sound advice to women of childbearing age who have undergone transplantation (764). Before conception, immunosuppressive therapy should be stable and at low maintenance levels. Some recommend attempting conception between 2 and 5 years after transplantation when renal function is both normal and stable. Individuals with serum creatinine values of less than 2 mg/dL tend to do well with no decline in function. Proteinuria occurs in 40% of pregnant women with a kidney transplant, but it is usually insignificant and resolves after delivery. The rate of rejection is 9%

TABLE 97-20. *Criteria for renal transplantation recipient desiring pregnancy*

1. At least 1.5–2 yr after transplantation
2. Stable graft function with minimal immunosuppression, serum creatinine, <2.5 mg/dL
3. No evidence of graft rejection
4. No significant proteinuria
5. Good blood pressure control
6. No evidence of pelvicaliceal distortion

late in pregnancy, not significantly different compared with nonpregnant transplant recipients (Table 97-20).

Although the incidence of spontaneous abortion may be higher, there is no evidence of an increased incidence of congenital abnormalities in pregnancies successfully carried through to term (765–767). Some 45% to 60% of the deliveries are preterm, and low fetal birth weight for gestational age is present in about 20% of pregnancies. The pelvic location of the renal allograft is not a contraindication to vaginal delivery. Cesarean section, performed in about one-fourth of the deliveries, should be reserved for obstetric indications only. Delivery should be performed with aseptic technique and prophylactic antibiotics administered for any surgical procedures. The steroid dose should be increased if there are signs of adrenal insufficiency.

There are no reported adverse effects of CsA or tacrolimus on human fetuses. Although rare, steroids may cause adrenal insufficiency in the neonate. Steroids and low concentrations of azathioprine and CsA are found in breast milk. Because there are few data on the effects of continued exposure to low doses of immunosuppressive agents perinatally, breastfeeding is not recommended (768). Few data are available concerning the safety of pregnancy for patients receiving the newer immunosuppressive agents. Animal studies have raised the possibility of an increased risk of malformations in the newborns of women treated with MMF during pregnancy. It is recommended that MMF be discontinued 6 weeks before conception is attempted. However, outcomes of pregnancies among women exposed to MMF at conception or during pregnancy have been reported; no structural malformations have been noted among offspring exposed to MMF but exposure is limited (5 mothers, 29 fathers) (769).

CURRENT SUCCESS AND FUTURE CHALLENGE

Dramatic improvements have occurred in the outcome of renal transplantation over the past 40 years. Immunosuppressive drug regimens have become more sophisticated with better graft survival rates with less morbidity and mortality. Currently the 1-year graft and patient survival rates are 85% to 90% and more than 95% in most transplantation centers despite the fact that an increasing number of high risk patients are undergoing transplantation as a replacement therapy for ESRD (2,5,498). The long-term issues confronting the patient and physician are both the relentless decline in allograft function resulting in poor graft survival beyond 5 years for cadaveric transplants (464,674) and the medical complications, particularly those resulting from the use of chronic immunosuppression (206,770). Renal allograft failure is now one of the most common causes of ESRD, accounting for 20% to 30% of patients awaiting a renal transplant. Efforts must also be directed to increase supply of donor organs. The limited availability of kidneys for transplantation raises ethical questions such as patient selection and allocation of kidneys for transplantation (771).

REFERENCES

1. Hume DM, et al. Experiences with renal homotransplantation in the human: report of nine cases. *J Clin Invest* 1955;34:327.
2. United States Renal Data System. *USRDS 1999 annual data report.* Bethesda, MD: National Institutes of Health and National Institute of Diabetes and Digestive and Kidney Diseases, 1999.
3. Held PJ, et al. Access to kidney transplantation. Has the United States eliminated income and racial differences? *Arch Intern Med* 1988; 148:2594.
4. Kjellstrand CM. Age, sex, and race inequality in renal transplantation. *Arch Intern Med* 1988;148:1305.
5. Hariharan S, et al. Improved graft survival after renal transplantation in the United States, 1988 to 1996. *N Engl J Med* 2000;342:605.
6. Chan L, Schrier RW. New therapeutic protocols in kidney transplantation. *Semin Nephrol* 1985;6:168.
7. Ramos ER, et al. The evaluation of candidates for renal transplantation. *Transplantation* 1994;57:490.
8. Kaufman DB, et al. A single-center experience of renal transplantation in thirteen Jehovah's Witnesses. *Transplantation* 1988;45:1045.
9. Clark AGB, et al. Renal transplantation in children. *Transplant Rev (Orlando)* 1987;1:101.
10. Fine RN. In depth review: renal transplantation of the infant and young child and the use of pediatric cadaver kidneys for transplantation in pediatric and adult recipients. *Am J Kidney Dis* 1988;12:1.
11. Fine RN. The adolescent with end-stage renal disease. *Am J Kidney Dis* 1985;6:81.
12. Lauffer G, et al. Renal transplantation in patients over 55 years old. *Br J Surg* 1988;75:984.
13. Lee POC, Terasaki PI. Effect of age on kidney transplants. In: Terasaki PI, ed. *Clinical kidney transplants.* Los Angeles: UCLA Tissue Typing Laboratory, 1985;123.
14. Pirsch JD, et al. Cadaveric renal transplantation with cyclosporine in patients more than 60 years of age. *Transplantation* 1989;47: 259.
15. Shah B, et al. Current experience with renal transplantation in older patients. *Am J Kidney Dis* 1988;12:516.
16. Roza AM, et al. Renal transplantation in patients more than 65 years old. *Transplantation* 1989;48:189.
17. Eggers PW. Health care policies: economics of the geriatric renal population. *Am J Kidney Dis* 1990;16:384.
18. Chertow GM, et al. Antigen-independent determinants of graft survival in living-related kidney transplantation. *Kidney Int* 1997; 63[Suppl]:S84.
19. Chertow GM, et al. Antigen-independent determinants of cadaveric kidney transplant failure. *JAMA* 1996;276:1732.
20. Miller RA. The aging immune system: primer and prospectus. *Science* 1996;273:70.
21. Basar H, et al. Renal transplantation in recipients over the age of 60: the impact of donor age. *Transplantation* 1999;67:1191.
22. Roodnat JI, et al. The vanishing importance of age in renal transplantation. *Transplantation* 1999;67:576.
23. Wolfe RA, et al. Comparison of mortality in all patients on dialysis, patients on dialysis awaiting transplantation, and recipients of a first cadaveric transplant. *N Engl J Med* 1999;341:1725.
24. Gill IS, et al. Impact of obesity on renal transplantation. *Transplantation Proc* 1993;25:1047.
25. Brenner BM, Milford EL. Nephron underdosing: a programmed cause of chronic renal allograft failure. *Am J Kidney Dis* 1993;21:66.
26. Remuzzi G, et al. Early experience with dual kidney transplantation in adults using expanded donor criteria. Double Kidney Transplant Group (DKG). *J Am Soc Nephrol* 1999;10:2591.
27. Bersztel, et al. Is kidney transplantation in sensitized recipients justified? *Transplant Int* 1996;9:S49.
28. Heise ER, Thacker LR, MacQueen JM, et al. Repeated HLA mismatches and second renal graft survival in centers of the South-Eastern Organ Procurement Foundation. *Clin Transplantation* 1996;10:579.
29. Mahoney RJ, et al. Identification of high- and low-risk second kidney grafts. *Transplantation* 1996;61:1349.
30. Thorogood J, et al. Prognostic indices to predict survival of first and second renal allografts. *Transplantation* 1991;52:831.
31. Kiberd BA, Belitsky P. The fate of the failed renal transplant. *Transplantation* 1995;59:645.
32. Vanrenterghem Y, Khamis S. The management of the failed renal allograft [Editorial]. *Nephrol Dial Transplantation* 1996;11:955.
33. Friedman EA, et al. Post-transplant diabetes in kidney transplant recipients. *Am J Nephrol* 1985;5:196.
34. Najarian JS, et al. Ten year experience with renal transplantation in juvenile onset diabetics. *Ann Surg* 1979;190:487.
35. Najarian JS, Canafax DM, Sutherl DE. Renal transplantation in diabetic patients is confirmed therapy while pancreas transplantation should be performed only in an investigational setting. *J Diabetic Complications* 1988;2:158.
36. Rosen CB, et al. Morbidity of pancreas transplantation during cadaveric renal transplantation. *Transplantation* 1991;51:123.
37. Cheung AH, et al. Simultaneous pancreas-kidney transplant versus kidney transplant alone in diabetic patients. *Kidney Int* 1992;41:924.
38. Remuzzi G, Gugeneti P, Mauer SM. Pancreas and kidney/pancreas transplants: experimental medicine or real improvement? *Lancet* 1994; 343:27.
39. Gruessner A, Sutherl DER. Pancreas transplant results in the United Network for Organ Sharing (UNOS) Registry compared with Non-USA data in the International Registry. In: Terasaki PI, Cecka JM, eds. *Clinical transplants.* Los Angeles: UCLA, 1994:47.
40. Bohman SO, et al. Recurrent diabetic nephropathy in renal allografts placed in diabetic patients and protective effect of simultaneous pancreatic transplantation. *Transplantation Proc* 1987;19:2290.
41. Fioretto P, et al. Reversal of lesions of diabetic nephropathy after pancreas transplantation. *N Engl J Med* 1998;339:69.
42. Luzi L. Pancreas transplantation and diabetic complications. *N Engl J Med* 1998;339:115.
43. Smets YF, et al. Effect of simultaneous pancreas-kidney transplantation on mortality of patients with type-1 diabetes mellitus and end-stage renal failure. *Lancet* 1999;353:1915.
44. Sollinger HW, et al. Experience with 500 simultaneous pancreas-kidney transplants. *Ann Surg* 1998;228:284.
45. Groth CG, Ringden O. Transplantation in relation to the treatment of inherited disease. *Transplantation* 1984;38:319.
46. Renal transplantation in congenital and metabolic disease: a report from the ASC/NIH Renal Transplant Registry. *JAMA* 1975;232:148.
47. Vanrenterghem Y, et al. Severe vascular complications in oxalosis after successful cadaveric kidney transplantation. *Transplantation* 1984; 38:93.
48. Scheinman J, Najarian JS, Mauer SM. Successful strategies for renal transplantation in primary oxalosis. *Kidney Int* 1984;25:804.
49. Watts RWE, et al. Timing of renal transplantation in the management of pyridoxine resistant type I primary hyperoxaluria. *Transplantation* 1988;45:1143.
50. Whelchel JD, et al. Successful renal transplantation in hyperkaluria. *Transplantation* 1983;35:161.
51. McDonald JC, et al. Reversal by liver transplantation of the complications of primary hyperoxalemia as well as the metabolic defect. *N Engl J Med* 321:1100 1989.
52. Ruder H, et al. Combined renal and hepatic transplantation for correction of hyperoxalouria type I. *Eur J Pediatrics* 1990;150:56.
53. Roberts RA, et al. Renal transplantation in secondary oxalosis. *Transplantation* 1988;45:985.
54. Wilson RE. Transplantation in patients with unusual causes of renal failure. *Clin Nephrol* 1976;5:51.
55. Almond PS, et al. Renal transplantation for infantile cystinosis: long-term follow-up. *J Pediatr Surg* 1993;28:232.
56. Ehrich JH, et al. Renal transplantation in 22 children with nephropathic cystinosis. *Pediatr Nephrol* 1991;5:708.

57. Barber WH, et al. Renal transplantation in sickle cell anemia and sickle disease. *Clin Transplantation* 1987;1:169.

58. Chatterjee SN. National study on natural history of renal allografts in sickle cell disease or tract. *Nephron* 1980;25:199201.

59. Warady BA, Sullivan EK. Renal transplantation in children with sickle cell disease: a report of the North American Pediatric Renal Transplant Cooperative Study (NAPRTCS). *Pediatr Transplantation* 1998;2:130.

60. Maizel SE, et al. Ten years experience in renal transplantation in Fabry's disease. *Transplant Proc* 1981;13:57.

61. Donati D, Novario R, Gastaldi L. Natural history and treatment of uremia secondary to Fabry's disease. *Nephron* 1987;46:353.

62. Mosnier JF, et al. Recurrence of Fabry's disease in a renal allograft eleven years after successful transplantation. *Transplantation* 1991;51:759.

63. Ojo A, et al. Excellent outcome of renal transplantation in patients with Fabry's disease. *Transplantation* 2000;69:2337.

64. Takenaka T, et al. Long-term enzyme correction and lipid reduction in multiple organs of primary and secondary transplanted Fabry mice receiving transduced bone marrow cells. *Proc Natl Acad Sci USA* 2000;97:7515.

65. Pasternack A, Ahonen J, Kuhlback B. Renal transplantation in 45 patients with amyloidosis. *Transplantation* 1986;42:598.

66. Milliner DS, Pierides AM, Holley KE. Renal transplantation in Alport's syndrome: anti–glomerular basement membrane glomerulonephritis in the allograft. *Mayo Clin Proc* 1982;57:35.

67. Mazzarella V, et al. Renal transplantation in patients with hereditary kidney disease: our experience. *Contrib Nephrol* 1997;122:203.

68. Scolari F, et al. Kidney transplantation in Alport's syndrome. *Contrib Nephrol* 1997;122:140.

69. Advisory Committee to the Renal Transplant Registry: the 13th report of the Human Renal Transplant Registry. *Transplantation Proc* 1977;9:9.

70. Sanfillippo FP, et al. Transplantation for polycystic kidney disease. *Transplantation* 1983;36:54.

71. Brazda E, et al. The effect of nephrectomy on the outcome of renal transplantation in patients with polycystic kidney disease. *Ann Transplantation* 1996;1:15.

72. Jeyarajah DR, et al. Liver and kidney transplantation for polycystic disease. *Transplantation* 1998;66:529.

73. Cameron JS. Glomerulonephritis in renal transplants. *Transplantation* 1982;34:237.

74. Mathew TH, et al. Glomerular lesions after renal transplantation. *Am J Med* 1975;59:177.

75. Mathew TH. Recurrence of disease following renal transplantation. *Am J Kidney Dis* 1988;12:85.

76. Vincenti F, et al. Inability of cyclosporine to completely prevent the recurrence of focal glomerulosclerosis after kidney transplantation. *Transplantation* 1989;47:595.

77. Tejani A, Stablein DH. Recurrence of focal segmental glomerulosclerosis posttransplantation: a special report of the North American Pediatric Renal Transplant Cooperative Study. *J Am Soc Nephrol* 1992;2:S256.

78. Striegel JE, et al. Recurrence of focal segmental sclerosis in children with steroid resistant nephrotic syndrome following renal transplantation. *Kidney Int* 1986;30:544.

79. Artero M, et al. Recurrent focal segmental glomerulosclerosis: natural history and response to therapy. *Am J Med* 1992;92:375.

80. Briggs JD, Jones E. Recurrence of glomerulonephritis following renal transplantation. Scientific Advisory Board of the ERA-EDTA Registry. European Renal Association-European Dialysis and Transplant Association. *Nephrol Dial Transplantation* 1999;14:564.

81. Dall'Amico R, et al. Prediction and treatment of recurrent focal segmental glomerulosclerosis after renal transplantation in children. *Am J Kidney Dis* 1999;34:1048.

82. Dantal J, et al. Effect of plasma protein adsorption on protein excretion in kidney-transplant recipients with recurrent nephrotic syndrome [Comments]. *N Engl J Med* 1994;330:7.

83. Savin VJ, et al. Circulating factor associated with increased glomerular permeability to albumin in recurrent focal segmental glomerulosclerosis [Comments]. *N Engl J Med* 1996;334:878.

84. Toth CM, et al. Recurrent collapsing glomerulopathy [Letter; comment]. *Transplantation* 1998;65:1009.

85. Couser WG, et al. Successful renal transplantation in patients with anti-GBM antibody to glomerular basement membrane. *Clin Nephrol* 1973;1:381.

86. Netzer KO, Merkel F, Weber M. Goodpasture syndrome and end-stage renal failure—to transplant or not to transplant [Editorial]? *Nephrol Dial Transplantation* 1998;13:1346.

87. Trpkov KF, et al. Recurrence of anti-GBM antibody disease twelve years after transplantation associated with de novo IgA nephropathy. *Clin Nephrol* 1998;49:124.

88. Hebert D, Sibley RK, Mauer S. Recurrence of hemolytic uremic syndrome in renal transplant recipients. *Kidney Int* 1986;30:51.

89. Doutrelepont JM, et al. Early recurrence of hemolytic uremic syndrome in a renal transplant recipient during prophylactic OKT3 therapy. *Transplantation* 1992;53:1378.

90. Ducloux D, et al. Recurrence of hemolytic-uremic syndrome in renal transplant recipients: a meta-analysis. *Transplantation* 1998;65:1405.

91. Berden JHM, et al. Hemolytic-uremic syndrome during cyclosporine immunosuppression in renal allograft recipients. *Clin Transplantation* 1987;1:246.

92. Agarwal A, et al. Recurrent hemolytic uremic syndrome in an adult renal allograft recipient: current concepts and management. *J Am Soc Nephrol* 1995;6:1160.

93. Holman MJ, et al. FK506-associated thrombotic thrombocytopenic purpura. *Transplantation* 1993;55:205.

94. Nashan B, Vincenti F. Successful transplantation without recurrence in hemolytic uremic syndrome omitting calcineurin inhibitors for immunosuppression [Abstract]. *Transplantation* 1998;65:S92.

95. Trimarchi HM, et al. FK506-associated thrombotic microangiopathy: report of two cases and review of the literature. *Transplantation* 1999;67:539.

96. Berger J. Recurrence of IgA nephropathy in renal allografts. *Am J Kidney Dis* 1988;12:371.

97. Odum J, et al. Recurrent mesangial IgA nephritis following renal transplantation. *Nephrol Dialysis Transplantation* 1994;9:309.

98. Bachman U, et al. The clinical course of IgA-nephropathy and Henoch-Schönlein purpura following renal transplantation. *Transplantation* 1986;42:511.

99. Kessler M, et al. Recurrence of immunoglobulin A nephropathy after renal transplantation in the cyclosporine era. *Am J Kidney Dis* 1996;28:99.

100. Brensilver JM, et al. Recurrent IgA nephropathy in living-related donor transplantation: recurrence or transmission of a familial disease? *Am J Kidney Dis* 1988;12:147.

101. Nast CC, et al. Recurrent Henoch-Schönlein purpura following renal transplantation. *Am J Kidney Dis* 1987;9:39.

102. Ramos EL. Recurrent diseases in the renal allograft. *J Am Soc Nephrol* 1991;2:109.

103. Brunt EM, et al. Transmission and resolution of type I membranoproliferative glomerulonephritis in recipients of cadaveric renal allografts. *Transplantation* 1988;46:595.

104. Curtis JJ, et al. Renal transplantation for patients with type I and type II membranoproliferative glomerulonephritis: serial complement and nephritic factor measurements and the problem of recurrent disease. *Am J Med* 1979;66:216.

105. Eddy A, et al. Renal allograft failure due to recurrent dense intramembranous deposit disease. *Clin Nephrol* 1984;21:305.

106. Turner DR, et al. Transplantation in mesangiocapillary glomerulonephritis with intramembranous dense "deposits." Recurrence of disease. *Kidney Int* 1976;9:439.

107. Berger BE, et al. De novo and recurrent membranous glomerulopathy following kidney transplantation. *Transplantation* 1983;35:315.

108. Bumgardner GL, et al. Single center 1–15 year results of renal transplantation in patients with systemic lupus erythematosus. *Transplantation* 1988;46:703.

109. Yakub UM, Freeman RB, Pabico RC. Renal transplantation in patients with systemic lupus erythematosus. *Arch Intern Med* 1983;143:2089.

110. Goss JA, Cole BR, Jendrisak MD, et al. Renal transplantation for systemic lupus erythematosus and recurrent lupus nephritis. *Transplantation* 1991;52:805.

111. Grimbert P, et al. Long-term outcome of kidney transplantation in patients with systemic lupus erythematosus: a multicenter study. Groupe Cooperatif de Transplantation d'ile de France. *Transplantation* 1998;66:1000.

112. Aunsholt NA, Ahlbom G. Recurrence of Wegener's granulomatosis after kidney transplantation involving the kidney graft. *Clin Transplantation* 1989;3:159.

113. Steinman TI, et al. Recurrence of Wegener's granulomatosis after kidney transplantation: successful induction of remission with cyclophosphamide. *Am J Med* 1980;68:458.

114. Schmitt WH, et al. Renal transplantation in Wegner's granulomatosis. *Lancet* 1993;342:860.

115. Merino GE, et al. Renal transplantation for progressive systemic sclerosis with renal failure: case report and review of previous experience. *Am J Surg* 1977;133:745.

116. Richardson JA. Hemodialysis and kidney transplantation for renal failure from scleroderma. *Arthritis Rheum* 1973;16:265.

117. Kasiske BL, et al. The evaluation of renal transplant candidates: clinical practice guidelines. *J Am Soc Nephrol* 1995;6:1.

118. Didlake RH, et al. Patient noncompliance: a major cause of late graft failure in cyclosporine-treated renal transplants. *Transplant Proc* 1988;20[Suppl 3]:63.

119. Rovelli M, et al. Noncompliance in organ transplant recipients. *Transplant Proc* 1989;21[Pt 1]:833.

120. Stewart RS. Psychiatric issues in renal dialysis and transplantation. *Hosp Community Psychiatry* 1983;34:623.

121. Batuik JD, Kurtz SB, Orszulak TA. Coronary artery bypass operation in dialysis patients. *Mayo Clin Proc* 1991;66:45.

122. Matas AJ, et al. Successful renal transplantation in patients with prior history of malignancy. *Am J Med* 1975;59:791.

123. Penn I. The effect of immunosuppression on pre-existing cancers. *Transplantation* 1993;55:742.

124. Braun WE, et al. The course of coronary disease in diabetics with and without renal allografts. *Transplant Proc* 1981;13:57.

125. Rimmer JM, et al. Renal transplantation in diabetes mellitus: influence of preexisting vascular disease on outcome. *Nephron* 1986;4:304.

126. Morrow CE, et al. Predictive value of thallium stress testing for coronary and cardiovascular events in uremic diabetic patients before renal transplantation. *Am J Surg* 1983;146:331.

127. Feduska NJ, et al. Peptic ulcer disease in renal transplant recipients. *Am J Surg* 1984;148:51.

128. Kestens PJ, Alexandre GPJ. Gastroduodenal complications after transplantation. *Clin Transplantation* 1988;2:221.

129. Chatterjee SN, et al. Successful renal transplantation in patients positive for hepatitis B antigen. *N Engl J Med* 1974;291:62.

130. Pirson Y, Alexandre GPJ, de Strihou CVY. Long-term effect of HBs antigenemia on patient survival after renal transplantation. *N Engl J Med* 1977;296:194.

131. Pol S, et al. Chronic hepatitis in kidney allograft recipients. *Lancet* 1990;335:878.

132. Pereira BJ, Wright TL, Schmid C, et al. A controlled study of hepatitis C transmission by organ transplantation. *Lancet* 1995;345:484.

133. Pereira BJ, et al. Prevalence of HCV RNA in hepatitis C antibody positive cadaver donor and their recipients. *N Engl J Med* 1992;327:910.

134. Wittwer CT, et al. False-positive antibody tests for human immunodeficiency virus in transplant patients with antilymphocyte antibodies. *Transplantation* 1987;44:843.

135. Schwartz A, et al. The effect of cyclosporine on the progression of HIV type 1 infection transmitted by transplantation—data on four cases and review of the literature. *Transplantation* 1993;55:95.

136. Matas AJ, et al. Lethal complications of bilateral nephrectomy and splenectomy in hemodialyzed patients. *Am J Surg* 1975;129:6216.

137. Yarimizu SN, et al. Mortality and morbidity in pretransplant bilateral nephrectomy: analysis of 305 cases. *Urology* 1978;12:55.

138. Sheinfeld J, et al. Selective pretransplant nephrectomy: indications and perioperative management. *J Urol* 1985;133:379.

139. Sanfilippo FP, Vaughn WK, Spees EK. The association of pretransplant native nephrectomy with decreased renal allograft rejection. *Transplantation* 1984;37:256.

140. Sanfilippo FP, et al. Transplantation for polycystic kidney disease. *Transplantation* 1983;36:54.

141. Morris PJ, Ting A, Stocker JW. Leukocyte antigens in renal transplantation: the paradox of blood transfusion in renal transplantation. *Med J Aust* 1968;2:1088.

142. Opelz G, et al. Effect of blood transfusions on subsequent kidney transplants. *Transplant Proc* 1973;5:253.

143. Ahmed Z, Terasaki PI. Effect of transfusion. In: Terasaki PI, ed. *Clinical transplants.* Los Angeles: UCLA Tissue Typing Laboratory, 1991.

144. Eschbach JW. Nephrology forum: the anemia of chronic renal failure: pathophysiology and the effects of recombinant erythropoietin. *Kidney Int* 1989;35:134.

145. Burlingham WJ, et al. Risk factors for sensitization by blood transfusions. *Transplantation* 1989;47:140.

146. Pfaff WW, et al. Incidental and purposeful random donor blood transfusion—sensitization and transplantation. *Transplantation* 1989;47:130.

147. Alter HJ, et al. Detection of antibody to hepatitis C virus in prospectively followed transfusion recipients with acute and chronic non-A, non-B hepatitis. *N Engl J Med* 1989;321:1494.

148. Kahan BD. Donor-specific transfusions—a balanced view. In: Morris PJ, Tilney NL, eds. *Progress in transplantation I.* Edinburgh: Churchill Livingstone, 1984:115.

149. Opelz G. The Collaborative Transplant Study Data. *Transplantation Rev* 1988;2:77.

150. Iwaki Y, Cecka JM, Terasaki PI. The transfusion effect in cadaver kidney transplants-yes or no. *Transplantation* 1990;49:56.

151. Cochrum KC, et al. Donor-specific blood transfusions in HLA-D disparate one-haplotype related allografts. *Transplant Proc* 1979;11:1903.

152. Burlingham WJ, et al. Improved renal allograft survival following donor-specific transfusions—III. Kinetics of mixed lymphocyte responses before and after transplantation. *Transplantation* 1988;45:127.

153. Kahan BD. Cyclosporine. *N Engl J Med* 1989;321:1725.

154. Evans PR, et al. Detection of kidney-reactive antibodies at crossmatch in renal transplant recipients. Transplantation 1988;46:844.

155. Palmer A, et al. Removal of anti-HLA antibodies by extracorporeal immunoadsorption to enable transplantation. *Lancet* 1989;1:10.

156. Taube D, et al. Removal of anti-HLA antibodies prior to transplantation: an effective and successful strategy of highly sensitized renal allograft recipients. *Transplant Proc* 1989;21:694.

157. McCalman R, et al. Successful kidney transplant in the presence of IgM antibodies. *Clin Nephrol* 1991;5:255.

158. Alexandere GPJ, et al. ABO-incompatible related and unrelated living donor renal allograft. *Transplant Proc* 1986;18:452.

159. Sutherland DER, et al. The long-term effect of splenectomy versus no splenectomy on renal allograft survival: reanalysis of a randomised prospective study. *Transplant Proc* 1985;17:136.

160. Taube D. Immunoadsorption in the sensitized renal transplant recipients. *Kidney Int* 1990;38:350.

161. Tyan DB, Li VA, Czer L. Intravenous immunoglobulin suppression of HLA alloantibody in highly sensitized transplant candidates and transplantation with a histoincompatible organ. *Transplantation* 1994;57:553.

162. Gifford RR, et al. Duration of first renal allograft survival as indicator of second allograft outcome. *Surgery* 1980;88:611.

163. Ting A, Morris PJ. Successful transplantation with a positive T and B cell crossmatch due to autoreactive antibodies. *Tissue Antigens* 1983;21:219.

164. Hunsicker LG. Renal transplantation for the nephrologist: HLA matching and cadaveric kidney allocation [Editorial]. *Am J Kidney Dis* 1989;13:438.

165. Opelz G. Influence of HLA matching on survival of second kidney transplants in cyclosporine-treated recipients. *Transplantation* 1989;47:823.

166. Matas AJ, et al. Successful transplantation of highly sensitized patients without regard to HLA matching. *Transplantation* 1988;45:338.

167. European Dialysis and Transplantation Association (EDTA). Combined report on regular dialysis and transplantation in Europe. *Proceedings of the annual meeting of the European Dialysis and Transplantation Association, 1994.*

168. Donnelly PK, Clayton DG, Simpson AR. Transplants from living donors in the United Kingdom and Ireland: a centre survey. *Br Med J (Clin Res)* 1989;298:490.

169. Simmons RG. Long term reactions of renal recipients and donors. In: Levy NB, ed. *Psychonephrology 2: psychological problems in kidney failure and their treatment.* Plenum Publishing, 1983:275.

170. Anderson CF, et al. The risks of unilateral nephrectomy: status of kidney donors 10 to 20 years postoperatively. *Mayo Clin Proc* 1985;60:367.

171. Williams S, Oler J, Jorkasky DK. Long term renal function in kidney donors: a comparison of donors and their siblings. *Ann Intern Med* 1986;105:1.

172. Miller IJ, et al. Impact of renal donation: long-term clinical and biochemical follow-up of living donors in a single center. *Am J Med* 1985;79:201.

173. Hakim RM, Goldszer RC, Brenner BM. Hypertension and proteinuria: long-term sequelae of uninephrectomy in humans. *Kidney Int* 1984; 25:930.

174. Terasaki PI, et al. High survival rates of kidney transplants from spousal and living unrelated donors. *N Engl J Med* 1995;333:333.

175. Geffner SR, et al. Living unrelated renal donor transplantation: the UNOS experience, 1987–1991. In: Terasaki PI, Cecka JM, eds. *Clinical transplants 1994.* Los Angeles: UCLA Tissue Typing Laboratory, 1995:197.

176. Commercialisation in transplantation: the problems and some guidelines for practice. The Council of the Transplantation Society. *Lancet* 2:715 1985.

177. Salvatierra O. Optimal use of organs for transplantation. *N Engl J Med* 318:1329 1988.

178. Bay WH, Hebert LA. The living donor in kidney transplantation. *Ann Intern Med* 106:719 1987.

179. Simmons RG, Anderson CR. Social and psychological problems in living donor transplantation. *Transplant Proc* 17:1577 1985.

180. Jacobs SC, et al. Laparoscopic live donor nephrectomy: the University of Maryland 3-year experience. *J Urol* 2000;164:1494.

181. Schweitzer EJ, et al. Increased rates of donation with laparoscopic donor nephrectomy. *Ann Surg* 2000;232:392.

182. Office of Organ Transplantation, Task Force on Organ Transplantation. *Organ transplantation, issues and recommendation.* US Health Resources and Services; 1986.

183. Black PM. Brain death. *N Engl J Med* 1978;299:388.

184. Opelz G. The benefit of exchanging donor kidneys among transplant centers. *N Engl J Med* 1988;318:1289.

185. Takiff H, et al. The benefit and underutilization of sharing kidneys for better histocompatibility. *Transplantation* 1989;47:102.

186. Kasiske BL. The influence of donor age on renal function in transplant recipients. *Am J Kidney Dis* 1988;11:248.

187. Smith AY, et al. Short-term and long-term function of cadaveric kidneys from pediatric donors in recipients treated with cyclosporine. *Transplantation* 1988;45:360.

188. Kumar P, et al. Transmission of human immunodeficiency virus by transplantation of a renal allograft, with development of the acquired immunodeficiency syndrome. *Ann Intern Med* 1987;106: 244.

189. Bowen PA II, et al. Transmission of human immunodeficiency virus (HIV) by transplantation: clinical aspects and time course analysis of viral antigenemia and antibody production. *Ann Intern Med* 1988; 108:46.

190. Soifer BE, Gelb AW. The multiple organ donor: Identification and management. *Ann Intern Med* 1989;110:814.

191. Cosimi AB. The donor and donor nephrectomy. In: Morris PJ, ed. *Kidney transplantation: principles and practice,* 4th ed. Philadelphia: W.B. Saunders, 1994:56.

192. Belzer FO, Southard JH. Principles of solid-organ preservation by cold storage. *Transplantation* 1988;45:673.

193. Chan L, Bore PJ, Ross BD. Possible new approaches to organ preservation. *Int Urol* 1984;11:323.

194. Marshall VC, Jablonski P, Scott DF. Renal preservation. In Morris PJ, ed. *Kidney transplantation: principles and practice,* 4th ed. Philadelphia: W.B. Saunders, 1994:86.

195. Spees EK, et al. Preservation methods do not affect cadaver renal allograft outcome: the SEOPF Prospective Study 1977–1982. *Transplant Proc* 1984;16:177.

196. Novick AC, et al. Detrimental effect of cyclosporine on initial function of cadaver renal allografts following extended preservation. *Transplantation* 1986;42:154.

197. Alexander JW, Vaughn WK, Pfaff WW. Local use of kidneys with poor HLA matches is as good as shared use with good matches in the cyclosporine era: an analysis at one and two years. *Transplant Proc* 1987;19:672.

198. Hoffmann RM, et al. Combined cold storage–perfusion preservation with a new synthetic perfusate. *Transplantation* 1989;47:32.

199. Chan L, Bore PJ, Ross BD. Possible new approaches to organ preservation. *Int Urol* 1984;11:323.

200. Chan L, Schrier RW. Effects of calcium channel blockers on renal function. *Annu Rev Med* 1990;41:289.

201. Murray JE, Harrison JH. Surgical management of fifty patients with kidney transplants including eighteen pairs of twins. *Am J Surg* 1963; 105:205.

202. Gorey TF, et al. Iliac artery ligation: the relative paucity of ischemic sequelae in renal transplant patients. *Ann Surg* 1979;190:753.

203. Griffiths AB, Fletcher EW, Morris PJ. Lymphocele after renal transplantation. *Aust N Z J Surg* 1979;49:626.

204. Weil R III, et al. Prevention of urological complications after kidney transplantation. *Ann Surg* 1971:154.

205. Thrasher JB, Temple DR, Spees EK. Extravesical versus Leadbetter-Politano ureteroneocystostomy: a comparison of urological complications in 320 renal transplants. *J Urol* 1990;144:1150.

206. Kasiske BL, et al. Recommendations for the outpatient surveillance of renal transplant recipients. American Society of Transplantation. *J Am Soc Nephrol* 2000;11[Suppl 15]:S1.

207. Hong JC, Kahan BD. Immunosuppressive agents in organ transplantation: past, present, and future. *Semin Nephrol* 2000;20:108.

208. Suthanthiran M, Strom TB. Renal transplantation. *N Engl J Med* 1994; 331:365.

209. Norman DJ, et al. A randomized clinical trial of induction therapy with OKT3 in kidney transplantation. *Transplantation* 1993;55:44.

210. Hanto DW, et al. Induction immunosuppression with antilymphocyte globulin or OKT3 in cadaver kidney transplantation: results of a single institution prospective randomized trial. *Transplantation* 1994;57: 377.

211. Brennan DC, et al. A randomized, double-blinded comparison of Thymoglobulin versus Atgam for induction immunosuppressive therapy in adult renal transplant recipients. *Transplantation* 1999;67: 1011.

212. Brennan DC, et al. A pharmacoeconomic comparison of antithymocyte globulin and muromonab CD3 induction therapy in renal transplant recipients. *Pharmacoeconomics* 1997;11:237.

213. Szczech LA, et al. Effect of anti-lymphocyte induction therapy on renal allograft survival: a meta-analysis. *J Am Soc Nephrol* 1997;8:1771.

214. Szczech LA, Berlin JA, Feldman HI. The effect of antilymphocyte induction therapy on renal allograft survival. A meta-analysis of individual patient-level data. Anti-Lymphocyte Antibody Induction Therapy Study Group. *Ann Intern Med* 1998;128:817.

215. Opelz G. Efficacy of rejection prophylaxis with OKT3 in renal transplantation. Collaborative Transplant Study. *Transplantation* 1995;60: 1220.

216. Nashan B, et al. Randomised trial of basiliximab versus placebo for control of acute cellular rejection in renal allograft recipients. CHIB 201 International Study Group. *Lancet* 1997;350:1193.

217. Vincenti F, et al. Interleukin-2-receptor blockade with daclizumab to prevent acute rejection in renal transplantation. Daclizumab Triple Therapy Study Group. *N Engl J Med* 1998;338:161.

218. Chan L, et al. Prospective trial of high-dose versus low-dose prednisone in renal transplantation. *Transplant Proc* 1980;12:323.

219. Chan L, et al. High and low dose prednisone. *Transplant Proc* 1981; 13:336.

220. d'Apice AJF, et al. A prospective randomized trial of low-dose versus high-dose steroids in cadaveric renal transplantation. *Transplantation* 1984;37:373.

221. Morris PJ, et al. Low dose oral prednisolone in renal transplantation. *Lancet* 1982;2:525.

222. Gray D, et al. Oral versus intravenous high dose steroid treatment of renal allograft rejection. *Lancet* 1978;1:117.

223. DeVecchi A, et al. Long-term comparison between single-morning daily and alternate-day steroid treatment in cadaver kidney recipients. Transplant Proc 1980;12:327.

224. Dumler F, et al. Long-term alternate day steroid therapy in renal transplantation. *Transplantation* 1982;34:78.

225. Hricik DE, Almawi WY, Strom TB. Trends in the use of glucocorticoids in renal transplantation. *Transplantation* 1994;57:979.

226. Veenstra DL, et al. Incidence and long-term cost of steroid-related side effects after renal transplantation. *Am J Kidney Dis* 1999;33:829.

227. Kupin W, et al. Complete replacement of methylprednisolone by azathioprine in cyclosporine-treated primary cadaveric renal recipients. *Transplantation* 1988;45:53.

228. O'Connell PJ, et al. Results of steroid withdrawal in renal allograft recipients on low-dose cyclosporine A, azathioprine and prednisolone. *Clin Transplantation* 1988;2:102.

229. Stratta RJ, et al. Withdrawal of steroid immunosuppression in renal transplant recipients. *Transplantation* 1988;45:323.

230. Matl I, et al. Withdrawal of steroids from triple-drug therapy in kidney transplant patients. *Nephrol Dial Transplantation* 2000;15:1041.

231. Hollander AA, et al. Late prednisone withdrawal in cyclosporine-treated kidney transplant patients: a randomized study. *J Am Soc Nephrol* 1997;8:294.

232. Humar A, et al. Steroid withdrawal in pancreas transplant recipients. *Clin Transplantation* 2000;14:75.

233. Stegall MD, et al. Prednisone withdrawal 14 days after liver transplantation with mycophenolate: a prospective trial of cyclosporine and tacrolimus. *Transplantation* 1997;64:1755.

234. Stegall MD, et al. Prednisone withdrawal late after adult liver transplantation reduces diabetes, hypertension, and hypercholesterolemia without causing graft loss. *Hepatology* 1997;25:173.

235. Trouillot TE, et al. Successful withdrawal of prednisone after adult liver transplantation for autoimmune hepatitis. *Liver Transplant Surg* 1999;5:375.

236. Disney APS, Russ GR, Walker R, et al, eds. *Australian and New Zealand Dialysis and Transplant Registry report.* 1997:119.

237. Ratcliffe PJ, et al. Randomised controlled trial of steroid withdrawal in renal transplant recipients receiving triple immunosuppression. *Lancet* 1996;348:643.

238. Hitchings GH, Elion GB. Chemical immunosuppression of the immune response. *Pharmacol Rev* 1963;15:365.

239. McGeown MS, et al. One hundred kidney transplants in the Belfast City Hospital. *Lancet* 2:648, 1977.

240. McGeown MG, et al. Ten-year results of renal transplantation with azathioprine and prednisolone as only immunosuppression. *Lancet* 1988;1:983.

241. Salaman JR, Griffin PJA, Price K. A controlled clinical trial of low-dose prednisolone in renal transplantation. *Transplant Proc* 1982;14:103.

242. Murray JE, et al. Prolonged survival of human-kidney homografts by immunosuppressive drug therapy. *N Engl J Med* 1963;268:1315.

243. Salvatierra O, et al. The impact of one thousand renal transplants at one center. *Ann Surg* 1977;186:424.

244. Morris PJ, et al. Low dose oral prednisolone in renal transplantation. *Lancet* 1982;2:525.

245. McGrath BP, et al. Macrocytosis and selective marrow hypoplasias. *Q J Med* 1975;44:57.

246. Hogge DE, et al. Reversible azathioprine-induced erythrocyte aplasia in a renal transplant recipient. *Can Med Assoc J* 1972;126:512.

247. Bradley PP, et al. Neutropenia and thrombocytopenia in renal allograft recipients treated with trimethoprim-sulfamethoxazole. *Ann Intern Med* 1980;93:560.

248. Calne RY, et al. Cyclosporin A in patients receiving renal allografts from cadaver donors. *Lancet* 1978;2:1323.

249. Calne RY. Cyclosporine in cadaveric renal transplantation: 5-year follow up of a multicentre trial. *Lancet* 1987;2:506.

250. Starzl TE, et al. The use of cyclosporin A and prednisone in cadaver kidney transplantation. *Surg Gynecol Obstet* 1980;151:17.

251. Canadian Multicenter Transplant Study Group. A randomized clinical trial of cyclosporine in cadaveric renal transplantation. *N Engl J Med* 1983;309:809.

252. Canadian Multicentre Transplant Study Group. A randomized clinical trial of cyclosporine in cadaveric renal transplantation: analysis at three years. *N Engl J Med* 1986;314:1219.

253. Opelz G. Effect of the maintenance immunosuppressive drug regimen on kidney transplant outcome. *Transplantation* 1994;58:443.

254. Hall BM, et al. Comparison of three immunosuppressive regimens in cadaver renal transplantation: long-term cyclosporine, short-term cyclosporine followed by azathioprine and prednisolone, and azathioprine and prednisolone without cyclosporine. *N Engl J Med* 1988;318:1499.

255. Salaman JR, et al. Renal transplantation without steroids. *J Pediatr* 1987;111:1026.

256. Chapman JR, Morris PJ. Cyclosporine conversion. *Transplantation Rev (Orlando)* 1987;1:197.

257. Burke JF Jr, et al. Long term efficacy and safety of cyclosporine. *N Engl J Med* 1994;331.

258. Kahan BD, et al. Complications of cyclosporine-prednisone immunosuppression in 402 renal allograft recipients exclusively followed at a single center from one to five years. *Transplantation* 1987;43:197.

259. Sommer BG, et al. Serum cyclosporine kinetic profile—failure to correlate with nephrotoxicity or rejection episodes following sequential immunotherapy for renal transplantation. *Transplantation* 1988;45:86.

260. Myers BD. Cyclosporine nephrotoxicity. *Kidney Int* 1986;30:964.

261. Myers BD, et al. The long-term course of cyclosporine-associated chronic nephropathy. *Kidney Int* 1988;33:590.

262. Lewis RM, et al. Stability of renal allograft function associated with long-term cyclosporine immunosuppressive therapy—Five-year follow-up. *Transplantation* 1989;47:266.

263. Gonwa TA, et al. Results of conversion from cyclosporine to azathioprine in cadaveric renal transplantation. *Transplantation* 1987;43:225.

264. Kasiske BL, Heim-Duthoy JZ. Elective cyclosporine withdrawal after renal transplantation: a meta-analysis. *JAMA* 1993;269:395.

265. Sallas WM. Development of limited sampling strategies for characteristics of a pharmacokinetic profile. *J Pharmacokinet Biopharm* 1995;23:515.

266. Sallas WM, et al. A nonlinear mixed-effects pharmacokinetic model comparing two formulations of cyclosporine in stable renal transplant patients. *J Pharmacokinet Biopharm* 1995;23:495.

267. Actis GC, et al. Continuously infused cyclosporine at low dose is sufficient to avoid emergency colectomy in acute attacks of ulcerative colitis without the need for high-dose steroids. *J Clin Gastroenterol* 1993;17:10.

268. McGuire TR, et al. Influence of infusion duration on the efficacy and toxicity of intravenous cyclosporine in bone marrow transplant patients. *Transplant Proc* 1988;20:501.

269. Merion RM, et al. Bile refeeding after liver transplantation and avoidance of intravenous cyclosporine. *Surgery* 1989;106:604.

270. Awni WM, et al. Long-term cyclosporine pharmacokinetic changes in renal transplant recipients: effects of binding and metabolism. *Clin Pharmacol Ther* 1989;45:41.

271. Mueller EA, et al. Pharmacokinetics and tolerability of a microemulsion formulation of cyclosporine in renal allograft recipients. A concentration-controlled comparison with the commercial formulation. *Transplantation* 1994;57:1178.

272. Kovarik JM, et al. Cyclosporine pharmacokinetics and variability from a microemulsion formulation. A multicenter investigation in kidney transplant patients. *Transplantation* 1994;58:658.

273. Niese D. A double-blind randomized study of Sandimmune Neoral versus Sandimmune in new renal transplant recipients: results after 12 months. The International Sandimmune Neoral Study Group. *Transplant Proc* 1995;27:1849.

274. Mahalati K, et al. A 3-hour postdose cyclosporine level during the first week after kidney transplantation predicts acute rejection and cyclosporine nephrotoxicity more accurately than trough levels. *Transplant Proc* 2000;32:786.

275. Mahalati K, et al. Neoral monitoring by simplified sparse sampling area under the concentration-time curve: its relationship to acute rejection and cyclosporine nephrotoxicity early after kidney transplantation. *Transplantation* 1999;68:55.

276. Lipkowitz GS, et al. Long-term maintenance of therapeutic cyclosporine levels leads to optimal graft survival without evidence of chronic nephrotoxicity. *Transplant Int* 1999;12:202.

277. Bennett WM. The nephrotoxicity of new and old immunosuppressive drugs. *Renal Fail* 1998;20:687.

278. Andoh TF, et al. Comparison of acute rapamycin nephrotoxicity with cyclosporine and FK506. *Kidney Int* 1996;50:1110.

279. Andoh TF, et al. Synergistic effects of cyclosporine and rapamycin in a chronic nephrotoxicity model. *Transplantation* 1996;62:311.

280. Solez K, et al. International standardization of nomenclature for the histologic diagnosis of renal allograft rejection: the Banff working classification of kidney pathology. *Kidney Int* 1993;44:411.

281. Ruiz P, et al. Associations between cyclosporine therapy and interstitial fibrosis in renal allograft biopsies. *Transplantation* 1988;45:91.

282. Barrett M, et al. Needle biopsy evaluation of class II major histocompatibility complex antigen expression for the differential diagnosis of cyclosporine nephrotoxicity from kidney graft rejection. *Transplantation* 1987;44:223.

283. Christians U, First MR, Benet LZ. Recommendations for bioequivalence testing of cyclosporine generics revisited. *Ther Drug Monit* 2000;22:330.

284. Haug M 3rd, Wimberley SL. Problems with the automatic switching of generic cyclosporine oral solution for the innovator product. *Am J Health Syst Pharm* 2000;57:1349.

285. Bartucci MR. Issues in cyclosporine drug substitution: implications for patient management. *J Transplant Coord* 1999;9:137.

286. Guidelines for the use of cyclosporine formulations. Proceedings of a roundtable satellite meeting of the Transplantation Society; Montreal, Canada, 13 July 1998. *Transplant Proc* 1999;31:1631.

287. Johnston A, Holt DW. Bioequivalence criteria for cyclosporine. *Transplant Proc* 1999;31:1649.

288. Kahan BD. Recommendations concerning the introduction of generic formulations of cyclosporine. *Transplant Proc* 1999;31:1634.

289. Christians U. Generic immunosuppressants: the European perspective. *Transplant Proc* 1999;31:19S.

290. Ho S, Clipstone N, Timmermann L, et al. The mechanism of action of cyclosporin A and FK506. *Clin Immunol Immunopathol* 1996;80: S40.

291. Dumont FJ. FK506, an immunosuppressant targeting calcineurin function. *Curr Med Chem* 2000;7:731.

292. Peterson LB, et al. A tacrolimus-related immunosuppressant with biochemical properties distinct from those of tacrolimus. *Transplantation* 1998;65:10.

293. Klintmalm G. A review of FK506: a new immunosuppressant agent for the prevention and rescue of graft rejection. *Transplantation Rev* 1994;8:53.

294. Jordan ML, et al. FK506 "rescue" for resistant rejection of renal allografts under primary cyclosporine immunosuppression. *Transplantation* 1994;57:860.

295. Textor SC, et al. Systemic and renal hemodynamic differences between FK506 and cyclosporine in liver transplant recipients. *Transplantation* 1993;55:1332.

296. Pirsch JD, et al. A comparison of tacrolimus (FK506) and cyclosporine for immunosuppression after cadaveric renal transplantation. FK506 Kidney Transplant Study Group. *Transplantation* 1997;63:977.

297. Mayer AD, et al. Multicenter randomized trial comparing tacrolimus (FK506) and cyclosporine in the prevention of renal allograft rejection: a report of the European Tacrolimus Multicenter Renal Study Group. *Transplantation* 1997;64:436.

298. Knoll GA, Bell RC. Tacrolimus versus cyclosporin for immunosuppression in renal transplantation: meta-analysis of randomised trials. *BMJ* 1999;318:1104.

299. Woodle ES, et al. Meta-analysis of FK506 and mycophenolate mofetil refractory rejection trials in renal transplantation. Refractory Rejection Meta-Analysis Study Group. *Transplant Proc* 1998;30:1297.

300. Woodle ES, et al. A multicenter trial of FK506 (tacrolimus) therapy in refractory acute renal allograft rejection. A report of the Tacrolimus Kidney Transplantation Rescue Study Group. *Transplantation* 1996;62:594.

301. Finn WF. FK506 nephrotoxicity. *Renal Fail* 1999;21:319.

302. Andoh TF, et al. Comparison of acute rapamycin nephrotoxicity with cyclosporine and FK506. *Kidney Int* 1996;50:1110.

303. Rerolle JP, et al. Tacrolimus-induced hemolytic uremic syndrome and end-stage renal failure after liver transplantation. *Clin Transplantation* 2000;14:262.

304. Mihatsch MJ, et al. The side-effects of cyclosporine-A and tacrolimus. *Clin Nephrol* 1998;49:356.

305. Grupp C, Schmidt F, Braun F, et al. Haemolytic uraemic syndrome (HUS) during treatment with cyclosporin A after renal transplantation—is tacrolimus the answer [Editorial]? *Nephrol Dial Transplantation* 1998;13:1629.

306. Pham PT, et al. Cyclosporine and tacrolimus-associated thrombotic microangiopathy. *Am J Kidney Dis* 2000;36:844.

307. Mueller AR, et al. Neurotoxicity after orthotopic liver transplantation. A comparison between cyclosporine and FK506. *Transplantation* 1994;58:155.

308. Binet I, et al. Polyomavirus disease under new immunosuppressive drugs: a cause of renal graft dysfunction and graft loss. *Transplantation* 1999;67:918.

309. Nakata Y, et al. Tacrolimus and myocardial hypertrophy. *Transplantation* 2000;69:1960.

310. Neylan JF. Racial differences in renal transplantation after immunosuppression with tacrolimus versus cyclosporine. FK506 Kidney Transplant Study Group. *Transplantation* 1998;65:515.

311. Wong KM, et al. Abbreviated tacrolimus area-under-the-curve monitoring for renal transplant recipients. *Am J Kidney Dis* 2000;35:660.

312. van Hooff, et al. Dosing and management guidelines for tacrolimus in renal transplant patients. *Transplant Proc* 1999;31:54S.

313. Capone D, et al. Therapeutic monitoring of tacrolimus in pediatric and adult transplanted patients. *J Chemother* 1998;10:176.

314. Braun F, et al. Pitfalls in monitoring tacrolimus (FK 506). *Ther Drug Monit* 1997;19:628.

315. Ihara H, et al. Intra- and interindividual variation in the pharmacokinetics of tacrolimus (FK506) in kidney transplant recipients—importance of trough level as a practical indicator. *Int J Urol* 1995;2:151.

316. Allison AC, Eugui EM, Sollinger HW. Mycophenolate mofetil (RS-61443): mechanisms of action and effects in transplantation. *Transplantation Rev* 1993;7:129.

317. European Mycophenolate Mofetil Cooperative Study Group. Placebo-controlled study of mycophenolate mofetil combined with cyclosporin and corticosteroids for prevention of acute rejection. *Lancet* 1995; 345:1321.

318. Sollinger HW, for the US Renal Transplant Mycophenolate Mofetil Study Group: mycophenolate mofetil for the prevention of acute rejection in primary cadaveric renal allograft recipients. *Transplantation* 1995;60:225.

319. A blinded, randomized clinical trial of mycophenolate mofetil for the prevention of acute rejection in cadaveric renal transplantation. The Tricontinental Mycophenolate Mofetil Renal Transplantation Study Group. *Transplantation* 1996;61:1029.

320. Mathew TH. A blinded, long-term, randomized multicenter study of mycophenolate mofetil in cadaveric renal transplantation: results at three years. Tricontinental Mycophenolate Mofetil Renal Transplantation Study Group. *Transplantation* 1998;65:1450.

321. Mycophenolate mofetil in cadaveric renal transplantation. US Renal Transplant Mycophenolate Mofetil Study Group. *Am J Kidney Dis* 1999;34:296.

322. Danovitch GM. Mycophenolate mofetil in renal transplantation: results from the U.S. randomized trials. *Kidney Int* 1995;52[Suppl]:S93.

323. Mendez R. FK 506 and mycophenolate mofetil in renal transplant recipients: six-month results of a multicenter, randomized dose ranging trial. FK 506 MMF Dose-Ranging Kidney Transplant Study Group. *Transplant Proc* 1998;30:1287.

324. Halloran P, et al. Mycophenolate mofetil in renal allograft recipients: a pooled efficacy analysis of three randomized, double-blind, clinical studies in prevention of rejection. The International Mycophenolate Mofetil Renal Transplant Study Groups. *Transplantation* 1997;63: 39.

325. Sarmiento JM, et al. Mycophenolate mofetil increases cytomegalovirus invasive organ disease in renal transplant patients. *Clin Transplantation* 2000;14:136.

326. Rostaing L, et al. Changes in hepatitis C virus RNA viremia concentrations in long-term renal transplant patients after introduction of mycophenolate mofetil. *Transplantation* 2000;69:991.

327. Langman, L. J, LeGatt, D. F, Yatscoff, R. W. Blood distribution of mycophenolic acid. *Ther Drug Monit* 1994;16:602.

328. Shaw LM, Nowak I. Mycophenolic acid: measurement and relationship to pharmacologic effects. *Ther Drug Monit* 1995;17:685.

329. Yeung J, Wang W, Chan L. Determination of mycophenolic acid (MPA) level: comparison of high performance liquid chromatography (HPLC) with homogenous enzyme-immunoassay (EMIT). *Transplant Proc* 1999;31:1214.

330. Bullingham RE, Nicholls AJ, Kamm BR. Clinical pharmacokinetics of mycophenolate mofetil. *Clin Pharmacokinet* 1998;34:429.

331. Hubner GI, Eismann R, Sziegoleit W. Drug interaction between mycophenolate mofetil and tacrolimus detectable within therapeutic mycophenolic acid monitoring in renal transplant patients. *Ther Drug Monit* 1999;21:536.

332. Filler G, Zimmering M, Mai I. Pharmacokinetics of mycophenolate mofetil are influenced by concomitant immunosuppression. *Pediatr Nephrol* 2000;14:100.

333. Langman LJ, et al. Pharmacodynamic assessment of mycophenolic acid-induced immunosuppression in renal transplant recipients. *Transplantation* 1996;62:666.

334. Wang W, Yeung J, Chan L. Pharmacodynamic assessment of mycophenolic acid induced immunosuppression by measuring IMPDH activity. *J Am Soc Nephrol* 1999;10:716A.

335. Weber LT, et al. Therapeutic drug monitoring of total and free mycophenolic acid (MPA) and limited sampling strategy for determination of MPA-AUC in paediatric renal transplant recipients. The German Study Group on Mycophenolate Mofetil (MMF) Therapy. *Nephrol Dial Transplantation* 1999;14:34.

336. van Gelder T, et al. A randomized double-blind, multicenter plasma concentration controlled study of the safety and efficacy of oral

mycophenolate mofetil for the prevention of acute rejection after kidney transplantation. *Transplantation* 1999;68:261.

337. Vezina C, Kudelski A, Sehgal SN. Rapamycin (AY-22,989), a new antifungal antibiotic. I. Taxonomy of the producing streptomycete and isolation of the active principle. *J Antibiot (Tokyo)* 1975;28:721.

338. Sehgal SN, Baker H, Vezina C. Rapamycin (AY-22,989), a new antifungal antibiotic. II. Fermentation, isolation and characterization. *J Antibiot (Tokyo)* 1975;28:727.

339. Douros J, Suffness M. New antitumor substances of natural origin. *Cancer Treat Rev* 1981;8:63.

340. Eng CP, Sehgal SN, Vezina C. Activity of rapamycin (AY-22, 989) against transplanted tumors. *J Antibiot (Tokyo)* 1984;37:1231.

341. Calne RY, et al. Rapamycin for immunosuppression in organ allografting. *Lancet* 1989;2:227.

342. Morris RE, et al. Use of rapamycin for the suppression of alloimmune reactions in vivo: schedule dependence, tolerance induction, synergy with cyclosporine and FK 506, and effect on host-versus-graft and graft-versus-host reactions. *Transplant Proc* 1991;23:521.

343. Vu MD, et al. Tacrolimus (FK506) and sirolimus (rapamycin) in combination are not antagonistic but produce extended graft survival in cardiac transplantation in the rat. *Transplantation* 1997;64:1853.

344. Wiederrecht GJ, et al. Mechanism of action of rapamycin: new insights into the regulation of G_1-phase progression in eukaryotic cells. *Prog Cell Cycle Res* 1995;1:53.

345. Sehgal SN. Rapamune (RAPA, rapamycin, sirolimus): mechanism of action immunosuppressive effect results from blockade of signal transduction and inhibition of cell cycle progression. *Clin Biochem* 1998;31:335.

346. Murgia MG, Jordan S, Kahan BD. The side effect profile of sirolimus: a phase I study in quiescent cyclosporine-prednisone–treated renal transplant patients. *Kidney Int* 1996;49:209.

347. Kahan BD, Julian BA, Pescovitz MD, et al. Sirolimus reduces the incidence of acute rejection episodes despite lower cyclosporine doses in Caucasian recipients of mismatched primary renal allografts: a phase II trial. Rapamune Study Group. *Transplantation* 1999;68:1526.

348. Andoh TF, Burdmann EA, Fransechini N, et al. Comparison of acute rapamycin nephrotoxicity with cyclosporine and FK506. *Kidney Int* 1996;50:1110.

349. Serkova N, et al. Evaluation of individual and combined neurotoxicity of the immunosuppressants cyclosporine and sirolimus by in vitro multinuclear NMR spectroscopy. *J Pharmacol Exp Ther* 1999;289:800.

350. Groth CG, et al. Sirolimus (rapamycin)-based therapy in human renal transplantation: similar efficacy and different toxicity compared with cyclosporine. Sirolimus European Renal Transplant Study Group. *Transplantation* 1999;67:1036.

351. Kahan BD. Efficacy of sirolimus compared with azathioprine for reduction of acute renal allograft rejection: a randomised multicentre study. The Rapamune US Study Group. *Lancet* 2000;356:194.

352. McAlister VC, et al. Sirolimus-tacrolimus combination immunosuppression. *Lancet* 2000;355:376.

353. Sacks SH. Rapamycin on trial. *Nephrol Dial Transplantation* 1999;14:2087.

354. Holt DW, Lee T, Johnston A. Measurement of sirolimus in whole blood using high-performance liquid chromatography with ultraviolet detection. *Clin Ther* 2000;22:B38.

355. Kahan BD, et al. Therapeutic drug monitoring of sirolimus: correlations with efficacy and toxicity. *Clin Transplantation* 2000;14:97.

356. Svensson JO, Brattstrom C, Sawe J. Determination of rapamycin in whole blood by HPLC. *Ther Drug Monit* 1997;19:112.

357. Viklicky O, et al. SDZ-RAD prevents manifestation of chronic rejection in rat renal allografts. *Transplantation* 2000;69:497.

358. Ikonen TS, et al. Sirolimus (rapamycin) halts and reverses progression of allograft vascular disease in non-human primates. *Transplantation* 2000;70:969.

359. Hardy MA. Use of ATG in treatment of steroid-resistant rejection. *Transplantation* 1980;29:162.

360. Steinmuller DR, et al. Comparison of OKT3 with ALG for prophylaxis for patients with acute renal failure after renal transplantation. *Transplantation* 1991;52:67.

361. Frey DJ, Matas AJ, Gillingham KJ, et al. A prospective randomized trial of MALG versus OKT3 for prophylactic immunosuppression in cadaver renal allograft recipients. *Transplantation* 1992;54:50.

362. Hanto DW, Jendrisak MD, So SK, et al. Induction immunosuppression with antilymphocyte globulin or OKT3 in cadaver kidney transplantation: results of a single institution prospective randomized trial. *Transplantation* 1994;57:377.

363. Zaltzman JS, Paul LC. Single center experience with Thymoglobulin in renal transplantation. *Transplant Proc* 1997;29:27S.

364. Tesi RJ, et al. Thymoglobulin reverses acute renal allograft rejection better than Atgam—a double-blinded randomized clinical trial. *Transplant Proc* 1997;29:21S.

365. Gaber AO, et al. Results of the double-blind, randomized, multicenter, phase III clinical trial of Thymoglobulin versus Atgam in the treatment of acute graft rejection episodes after renal transplantation. *Transplantation* 1998;66:29.

366. Frey DJ, et al. MALG vs OKT3 following renal transplantation: a randomized prospective trial. *Transplant Proc* 1991;23:1048.

367. Frey DJ, et al. Sequential therapy—a prospective randomized trial of MALG versus OKT3 for prophylactic immunosuppression in cadaver renal allograft recipients. *Transplantation* 1992;54:50.

368. Wilson LG. The crime of saving lives. The FDA, John Najarian, and Minnesota ALG. *Arch Surg* 1995;130:1035.

369. Debets JM, et al. Evidence of involvement of tumor necrosis factor in adverse reactions during treatment of kidney allograft rejection with antithymocyte globulin. *Transplantation* 1989;47:487.

370. Schroeder TJ, First MR. Monoclonal antibodies in organ transplantation. *Am J Kidney Dis* 1994;23:138.

371. Ortho Multicenter Transplant Study Group. A randomized trial of OKT3 monoclonal antibody for acute rejection of cadaveric renal transplants. *N Engl J Med* 1985;313:337.

372. Norman DJ, et al. The use of OKT3 in cadaveric renal transplantation for rejection that is unresponsive to conventional anti-rejection therapy. *Am J Kidney Dis* 1988;11:90.

373. Norman DJ, et al. A randomized clinical trial of induction therapy with OKT3 in kidney transplantation. *Transplantation* 1993;55:44.

374. Norman DJ, et al. Effectiveness of a second course of OKT3 monoclonal anti-T cell antibody for treatment of renal allograft rejection. *Transplantation* 1988;46:523.

375. Mayes JT, et al. Reexposure to OKT3 in renal allograft recipients. *Transplantation* 1988;45:349.

376. Carey G, Lisi PJ, Schroeder TJ. The incidence of antibody formation to OKT3 consequent to its use in organ transplantation. *Transplantation* 1995;60:151.

377. Hirsch R, et al. Suppression of the humoral response to anti-CD3 monoclonal antibody. *Transplantation* 1989;47:853.

378. Montgomery RA, et al. Plasmapheresis and intravenous immune globulin provides effective rescue therapy for refractory humoral rejection and allows kidneys to be successfully transplanted into cross-match-positive recipients *Transplantation* 2000;70:887.

379. Jordan SC, et al. Posttransplant therapy using high-dose human immunoglobulin (intravenous gamma-globulin) to control acute humoral rejection in renal and cardiac allograft recipients and potential mechanism of action. *Transplantation* 1998;66:800.

380. Peraldi MN, et al. Long-term benefit of intravenous immunoglobulins in cadaveric kidney retransplantation. *Transplantation* 1996;62:1670.

381. Casadei D, et al. Immunoglobulin i.v. high dose (IVIgHD): new therapy as a rescue treatment of grafted kidneys. *Transplant Proc* 1996;28:3290.

382. Cardella CJ, et al. Effect of intensive plasma exchange on renal transplant rejection and serum cytotoxic antibody. *Transplant Proc* 1978;10:617.

383. Allen NH, et al. Plasma exchange in acute renal allograft rejection. *Transplantation* 1983;35:425.

384. Reisaeter AV, et al. Pretransplant plasma exchange or immunoadsorption facilitates renal transplantation in immunized patients. *Transplantation* 1995;60:242.

385. Torretta L, et al. Usefulness of plasma exchange in recurrent nephrotic syndrome following renal transplant. *Artif Organs* 1995;19:96.

386. Reisaeter AV, et al. Plasma exchange in highly sensitized patients as induction therapy after renal transplantation. *Transplant Proc* 1994;26:1758.

387. Myburgh JA, et al. Total lymphoid irradiation in clinical renal transplantation—results in 73 patients. *Transplant Proc* 1991;23:2033.

388. Saper V, et al. Clinical and immunological studies of cadaveric renal transplant recipients given total-lymphoid irradiation and maintained on low-dose prednisone. *Transplantation* 1988;45:540.

389. Strober S, et al. Acquired immune tolerance to cadaveric renal allografts. *N Engl J Med* 1989;321:28.

390. Morris RE. New small molecule immunosuppressants for transplantation: review of essential concepts. *J Heart Lung Transplantation* 1993;12:S275.

391. Katz SM, Hong JC, Kahan BD. New immunosuppressive agents. *Transplant Proc* 2000;32:620.

392. Moran M, et al. Prevention of acute graft rejection by the prostaglandin E₁ analogue misoprostol in renal-transplant recipients treated with cyclosporine and prednisone. *N Engl J Med* 1990;322:1183.

393. Soulillou JP, et al. Randomized controlled trial of a monoclonal antibody against the interleukin-2 receptor (33B3.1) as compared with rabbit antithymocyte globulin for prophylaxis against rejection of renal allografts. *N Engl J Med* 1990;322:1175.

394. Cantarovich D, et al. Anti-interleukin 2 receptor monoclonal antibody in the treatment of ongoing acute rejection episodes in human kidney graft—a pilot study. *Transplantation* 1989;47:454.

395. Carpenter CB, et al. Prophylactic use of monoclonal anti–IL-2 receptor antibody in cadaveric renal transplantation. *Am J Kidney Dis* 1989;14[Suppl 2]:54.

396. Powelson JA, et al. CRR-grafted OKT4A monoclonal antibody in cynomolgus renal allograft recipients. *Transplantation* 57:788 1994.

397. Haug CE, et al. A phase I trial of immunosuppression with anti–ICAM-1 (CD54) mAB in renal allograft recipients. *Transplantation* 1993;55:766.

398. Okubo M, et al. 15-Deoxyspergualin rescue therapy for methylprednisone resistant rejection of renal transplants as compared with OKT3. *Transplantation* 1993;55:505.

399. Cramer DV, Chapman FA, Makowka L. Use of brequinar sodium for transplantation. *Ann N Y Acad Sci* 1993;696:216.

400. Nagahara Y, et al. Evidence that FTY720 induces T cell apoptosis in vivo. *Immunopharmacology* 2000;48:75.

401. Furukawa H, et al. Prolongation of canine liver allograft survival by a novel immunosuppressant, FTY720: effect of monotherapy and combined treatment with conventional drugs. *Transplantation* 2000;69:235.

402. Tamura A, et al. Immunosuppressive therapy using FTY720 combined with tacrolimus in rat liver transplantation. *Surgery* 2000;127:47.

403. Kita Y, et al. Prolonged graft survival induced by CTLA4IG-gene transfection combined with FTY720 administration in rat heart grafting. *Transplant Proc* 1999;31:2787.

404. Suzuki S. FTY720: mechanisms of action and its effect on organ transplantation. *Transplant Proc* 1999;31:2779.

405. Suzuki S. FTY720: mechanisms of action and its effect on organ transplantation. *Transplant Proc* 1999;31:2779.

406. Hausen B, et al. Combined immunosuppression with cyclosporine (Neoral) and SDZ RAD in non-human primate lung transplantation: systematic pharmacokinetic-based trials to improve efficacy and tolerability. *Transplantation* 2000;69:76.

407. Neumayer HH, et al. Entry-into-human study with the novel immunosuppressant SDZ RAD in stable renal transplant recipients. *Br J Clin Pharmacol* 1999;48:694.

408. Kirchner GI, et al. Pharmacokinetics of SDZ RAD and cyclosporin including their metabolites in seven kidney graft patients after the first dose of SDZ RAD. *Br J Clin Pharmacol* 2000;50:449.

409. Kishimoto K, et al. The role of CD154-CD40 versus CD28-B7 costimulatory pathways in regulating allogeneic T_h1 and T_h2 responses in vivo. *J Clin Invest* 2000;106:63.

410. Abrams JR, et al. Blockade of T lymphocyte costimulation with cytotoxic T lymphocyte–associated antigen 4-immunoglobulin (CTLA4Ig) reverses the cellular pathology of psoriatic plaques, including the activation of keratinocytes, dendritic cells, and endothelial cells. *J Exp Med* 2000;192:681.

411. Li Y, et al. Blocking both signal 1 and signal 2 of T-cell activation prevents apoptosis of alloreactive T cells and induction of peripheral allograft tolerance. *Nat Med* 1999;5:1298.

412. Gudmundsdottir H, Turka LA. T cell costimulatory blockade: new therapies for transplant rejection. *J Am Soc Nephrol* 1999;10:1356.

413. Cecka JM. The UNOS Scientific Renal Transplant Registry. *Clin Transplantation* 1998:1.

414. Geddes CC, et al. Factors influencing long-term primary cadaveric kidney transplantation—importance of functional renal mass versus avoidance of acute rejections—the Toronto Hospital experience 1985–1997. *Clin Transplantation* 1998:195.

415. Land W. Delayed graft function and renal allograft outcome. *Transplantation* 1999;68:452.

416. Matas AJ, et al. Immunologic and nonimmunologic factors: different risks for cadaver and living donor transplantation [see comments]. *Transplantation* 2000;69:54.

417. Rowinski W, et al. Delayed kidney function risk score: donor factors versus ischemia/reperfusion injury. *Transplant Proc* 1999;31:2077.

418. Tejani AH, et al. Predictive factors for delayed graft function (DGF) and its impact on renal graft survival in children: a report of the North American Pediatric Renal Transplant Cooperative Study (NAPRTCS). *Pediatr Transplantation* 1999;3:293.

419. Ontario Renal Transplant Research Group. Factors influencing early renal function in cadaveric kidney transplants—a case control study. *Transplantation* 1988;45:122.

420. Halloran PF, et al. Early function as the principal correlate of graft survival—a multivariate analysis of 200 cadaveric renal transplants treated with a protocol incorporating antilymphocyte globulin and cyclosporine. *Transplantation* 1988;46:223.

421. Davison JM, Uldall PR, Taylor RM. Relation of immediate posttransplant renal function to long-term function in cadaver kidney recipients. *Transplantation* 1977;23:310.

422. Hall BM, et al. Post-transplant acute renal failure in cadaver renal recipients treated with cyclosporine. *Kidney Int* 1985;28:178.

423. Rodriguez PC, Arroyave IH, Mejia G, et al. Detection of alloantibodies against non-HLA antigens in kidney transplantation by flow cytometry. *Clin Transplantation* 2000;14:472.

424. Pratschke J, et al. Accelerated rejection of renal allografts from braindead donors. *Ann Surg* 2000;232:263.

425. Madan AK, et al. Treatment of antibody-mediated accelerated rejection using plasmapheresis. *J Clin Apheresis* 2000;15:180.

426. Akahira H, et al. Dynamic SPECT evaluation of renal plasma flow using technetium-99m MAG3 in kidney transplant patients. *J Nucl Med Technol* 1999;27:32.

427. Dunn EK. Radioisotopic evaluation of renal transplants. *Urol Radiol* 1992;14:115.

428. Dubovsky EV, et al. Report of the Radionuclides in Nephrourology Committee for evaluation of transplanted kidney (review of techniques). *Semin Nucl Med* 1999;29:175.

429. Allen KS, et al. Renal allografts: prospective analysis of Doppler sonography. *Radiology* 1988;169:371.

430. Hall JT, et al. Correlation of radionuclide and ultrasound studies with biopsy findings for the diagnosis of renal transplant rejection. *Urology* 1988;32:172.

431. Gankins SM, Sanfilippo FP, Carroll RA. Duplex Doppler sonography of renal transplants: lack of sensitivity and specificity in established pathologic diagnosis. *AJR Am J Roentgenol* 1989;152:535.

432. Mathew TH, et al. Percutaneous needle biopsy of renal homografts. *Med J Aust* 1968;1:6.

433. Chandraker A. Diagnostic techniques in the work-up of renal allograft dysfunction—an update. *Curr Opin Nephrol Hypertens* 1999;8:723.

434. Cosio FG, Pelletier RP, Sedmak DD. Predictive value of histopathology and function on outcome of renal allografts after acute rejection. *Transplant Proc* 1999;31:261.

435. Dean DE, et al. A blinded retrospective analysis of renal allograft pathology using the Banff schema: implications for clinical management. *Transplantation* 1999;68:642.

436. Oda A, Morozumi K, Uchida K. Histological factors of 1-h biopsy influencing the delayed renal function and outcome in cadaveric renal allografts. *Clin Transplantation* 1999;13:6.

437. Pascual M, et al. The clinical usefulness of the renal allograft biopsy in the cyclosporine era: a prospective study. *Transplantation* 1999;67:737.

438. Solez K, Vincenti F, Filo RS. Histopathologic findings from 2-year protocol biopsies from a U.S. multicenter kidney transplant trial comparing tacrolimus versus cyclosporine: a report of the FK506 Kidney Transplant Study Group. *Transplantation* 1998;66:1736.

439. Veronese FV, et al. Interpretation of surveillance kidney allograft biopsies according to the Banff criteria. *Transplant Proc* 1999;31:3019.

440. Racusen LC, et al. The Banff 97 working classification of renal allograft pathology. *Kidney Int* 1999;55:713.

441. Rush DN, et al. Protocol biopsies in renal transplantation: research tool or clinically useful? *Curr Opin Nephrol Hypertens* 1998;7:691.

442. Rush D, et al. Beneficial effects of treatment of early subclinical rejection: a randomized study. *J Am Soc Nephrol* 1998;9:2129.

443. Bishop GA, et al. Immunopathology of renal allograft rejection analyzed with monoclonal antibodies to mononuclear markers. *Kidney Int* 1986;29:708.

444. Pascoe MD, et al. Increased accuracy of renal allograft rejection diagnosis using combined perforin, granzyme B, and Fas ligand fine-needle aspiration immunocytology. *Transplantation* 2000;69:2547.

445. Chandraker A. Diagnostic techniques in the work-up of renal allograft dysfunction—an update. *Curr Opin Nephrol Hypertens* 1999;8:723.

446. Ribeiro-David DS, et al. Contribution of the expression of ICAM-1, HLA-DR and IL-2R to the diagnosis of acute rejection in renal allograft aspirative cytology. *Transplant Int* 1998;11:S19.

447. Oliveira G, et al. Cytokine analysis of human renal allograft aspiration biopsy cultures supernatants predicts acute rejection. *Nephrol Dial Transplantation* 1998;13:417.

448. Nast CC. Renal transplant fine needle aspiration and cytokine gene expression. *Pediatr Nephrol* 1995;9:S56.

449. Bishop GA, et al. Diagnosis of renal allograft rejection by analysis of fine-needle aspiration biopsy specimens with immunostains and simple cytology. *Lancet* 1986;2:645.

450. Helderman JH, et al. Confirmation of the utility of fine needle aspiration biopsy of the renal allograft. *Kidney Int* 1988;34:376.

451. Seron D, et al. Diagnosis of rejection in renal allograft biopsies using the presence of activated and proliferating cells. *Transplantation* 1989;47:811.

452. Forsythe JLR, et al. Plasma interleukin 2 receptor levels in renal allograft dysfunction. *Transplantation* 1989;48:155.

453. Strom TB, Suthanthiran M. Prospects and applicability of molecular diagnosis of allograft rejection. *Semin Nephrol* 2000;20:103.

454. Suthanthiran M. Clinical application of molecular biology: a study of allograft rejection with polymerase chain reaction. *Am J Med Sci* 1997;313:264.

455. Suthanthiran M. Molecular analyses of human renal allografts: differential intragraft gene expression during rejection. *Kidney Int* 1997;58[Suppl]:S15.

456. Wang W, Chan L, Reilly RF. Quantitative RT-PCR of TGF-β_1 in urinary cells is a diagnostic tool for chronic renal allograft rejection. *J Am Soc Nephrol* 2000;11:675A.

457. Segasothy M, et al. Urine cytologic profile in renal allograft recipients determined by monoclonal antibodies. *Transplantation* 1989;47:482.

458. Simpson MA, et al. Sequential determinations of urinary cytology and plasma and urinary lymphokines in the management of renal allograft recipients. *Transplantation* 1989;47:218.

459. Dooper PMM, et al. Immunocytology of urinary sediments in renal transplant patients with deteriorating graft function. *Transplant Proc* 1989;21:3596.

460. Chan L, et al. NMR and biochemical studies of the synergistic detrimental effects of ischemia and cyclosporine nephrotoxicity. *Transplant Proc* 1991;23:711.

461. Chan L, Shapiro JI. Magnetic resonance study of renal transplantation. *Renal Physiol Biochem* 1989;12:181.

462. Dunbar KR, et al. Loss of corticomedullary demarcation on magnetic resonance imaging: an index of biopsy-proven acute renal transplant dysfunction. *Am J Kidney Dis* 1988;12:200.

463. Feduska NJ, Terrier F, Vincenti F. Evaluation of acute renal allograft rejection and cyclosporine nephrotoxicity by magnetic resonance imaging. *Transplant Proc* 1985;17:2597.

464. Shaikewitz ST, Chan L. Chronic renal transplant rejection. *Am J Kidney Dis* 1994;23:884.

465. Almond PS, et al. Risk factors for chronic rejection in renal allograft recipients. *Transplantation* 1993;55:752.

466. Matas AJ, et al. The impact of an acute rejection episode on long-term renal allograft survival (t1/2). *Transplantation* 1994;57:857.

467. Paul LC. Chronic allograft nephropathy: an update. *Kidney Int* 1999;56:783.

468. Jindal RM, Hariharan S. Chronic rejection in kidney transplants. An in-depth review. *Nephron* 1999;83:13.

469. Brenner BM, Cohen RA, Milford EL. In renal transplantation, one size may not fit all. *J Am Soc Nephrol* 1992;3:162.

470. Terasaki PI, et al. The hyperfiltration hypothesis in human renal transplantation. *Transplantation* 1994;57:1450.

471. Salahudeen AK, et al. Effects of dietary protein in patients with chronic renal transplant rejection. *Kidney Int* 1992;41:183.

472. Bochicchio T, et al. Fosinopril prevents hyperfiltration and decreases proteinuria in post-transplant hypertensives. *Kidney Int* 1990;38:873.

473. Traindl O, et al. The effects of lisinopril on renal function in proteinuric renal transplant recipients. *Transplantation* 1993;55:1309.

474. Szabo A, et al. Effect of angiotensin-converting enzyme inhibition on growth factor mRNA in chronic renal allograft rejection in the rat. *Kidney Int* 2000;57:982.

475. Hausberg M, et al. ACE inhibitor versus beta-blocker for the treatment of hypertension in renal allograft recipients. *Hypertension* 1999;33:862.

476. Lufft V, et al. Antiproteinuric efficacy of fosinopril after renal transplantation is determined by the extent of vascular and tubulointerstitial damage. *Clin Transplantation* 1998;12:409.

477. Berger BE, et al. De novo and recurrent membranous glomerulopathy following kidney transplantation. *Transplantation* 1983;35:315.

478. Mathew TH. Recurrence of disease following renal transplantation. *Am J Kidney Dis* 1988;12:85.

479. Kim EM, et al. Recurrence of steroid-resistant nephrotic syndrome in kidney transplants is associated with increased acute renal failure and acute rejection. *Kidney Int* 1994;45:1440.

480. Cheigh JS, et al. Kidney transplant nephrotic syndrome: relationship between allograft histopathology and natural course. *Kidney Int* 1980;18:358.

481. Korbet SM, Schwartz MM, Lewis EJ. Recurrent nephrotic syndrome in renal allografts. *Am J Kidney Dis* 1988;11:270.

482. Morzycka M, et al. Evaluation of recurrent glomerulonephritis in kidney allografts. *Am J Med* 1982;72:588.

483. Herrera GA, et al. Cytomegalovirus glomerulopathy: a controversial lesion. *Kidney Int* 1986;29:725.

484. Dittmer R, et al. CMV infection and vascular rejection in renal transplant patients. *Transplant Proc* 1989;21:3600.

485. Cheigh JS, et al. Focal segmental glomerulosclerosis in renal transplants. *Am J Kidney Dis* 1983;2:449.

486. Schwartz A, et al. Impact of de novo membranous glomerulonephritis on the clinical course after kidney transplantation. *Transplantation* 1994;58:650.

487. Cameron JS. Glomerulonephritis in renal transplants. *Transplantation* 1982;34:237.

488. Vollmer WM, Wahl PW, Blagg CR. Survival with dialysis and transplantation in patients with end-stage renal disease. *N Engl J Med* 1983;308:1553.

489. Port FK, et al. Comparison of survival probabilities for dialysis patients vs cadaver renal transplant recipients. *JAMA* 1993;270:1339.

490. Suthanthiran M, Strom TB. Renal transplantation. *N Engl J Med* 1994;331:365.

491. Held PJ, et al. Trends in mortality rates among dialysis and transplant patients in the US. *Kidney Int* 1990;37:239.

492. Khauli RB, et al. A critical look at survival of diabetics with end-stage renal disease: transplantation versus dialysis. *Transplantation* 1986;41:598.

493. Grenfell A, et al. Renal replacement for diabetic patients: experience at King's College Hospital 1980–1989. *Q J Med* 1992;85:861.

494. Tilney NL, Chang A, Milford EL, et al. Ten-year experience with cyclosporine as primary immunosuppression in recipients of renal allografts. *Ann Surg* 1991;214:42.

495. Lim EC, Terasaki PI. Outcome of kidney transplantation in different diseases. In: Terasaki PI, ed. *Clinical transplants*. Los Angeles: UCLA Tissue Typing Laboratory, 1990:461.

496. Wolfe RA, et al. Comparison of mortality in all patients on dialysis, patients on dialysis awaiting transplantation, and recipients of a first cadaveric transplant. *N Engl J Med* 1999;341:1725.

497. Wolfe RA, et al. A critical examination of trends in outcomes over the last decade. *Am J Kidney Dis* 1998;32:S9.

498. Cecka JM. The UNOS Scientific Renal Transplant Registry. In Cecka J, Terasaki PI, ed. *Clinical transplants 1999*. Los Angeles: UCLA Tissue Typing Laboratory, 1999:1.

499. Opelz G, Mickey MR, Terasaki PI. Calculations on long term graft and patient survival in human kidney transplantation. *Transplant Proc* 1977;9:27.

500. Murray JE, Harrison JH. Surgical management of fifty patients with kidney transplants including eighteen pairs of twins. *Am J Surg* 1963;105:205.

501. Tilney NL. Renal transplantation between identical twins: a review. *World J Surg* 1986;10:381.

502. Brunner FP, Broyer M, Brynger H. Combined report on regular dialysis and transplantation in Europe. *Proc 15th Dial Transplant Assoc Meeting 1984.* 1985;22:5.

503. d'Apice AJF, et al. Possible rejection of an HLA-identical sibling renal allograft. *Med J Aust* 1976;1:195.

504. Salaman JR, et al. Rejection of HLA identical related kidney transplants. *Tissue Antigens* 1976;8:233.

505. Sutherland DER, et al. Renal allograft functional survival rates are similar for kidneys from sibling donors mismatched for one versus two haplotypes with the recipient. *Transplant Proc* 1985;17:110.

506. Fletchner SM, et al. The use of cyclosporine and prednisone for high MLC haploidentical living related renal transplants. *Transplant Proc* 1983;15:442.

507. Glass NR, et al. Can the results of live donor kidney transplantation be improved? *Surgery* 1983;94:636.

508. Kaufman DB, et al. Renal transplantation between living-related sibling pairs matched for zero-HLA haplotypes. *Transplantation* 1989;47:113.

509. Simmons RL, et al. One hundred sibling transplants followed 2–7 years—a multifactorial analysis. *Ann Surg* 1977;185:196.

510. Pirsch JD, et al. Cadaveric renal transplantation with cyclosporine in patients more than 60 years of age. *Transplantation* 1989;47:259.

511. Terasaki PI, et al. High survival rates of kidney transplants from spousal and living unrelated donors. *N Engl J Med* 1995;333:333.

512. Geffner SR, et al. Living unrelated renal donor transplantation: the UNOS experience, 1987–1991. In: Terasaki PI, Cecka JM, eds. *Clinical transplants 1994.* Los Angeles: UCLA Tissue Typing Laboratory, 1995:197.

513. Khajehdehi P. Living non-related versus related renal transplantation—its relationship to the social status, age and gender of recipients and donors. *Nephrol Dial Transplantation* 1999;14:2621.

514. Toronyi E, et al. Attitudes of donors towards organ transplantation in living related kidney transplantations. *Transplant Int* 1998;11:S481.

515. Marshall PA, Daar AS. Cultural and psychological dimensions of human organ transplantation. *Ann Transplantation* 1998;3:7.

516. Kaplan BS, Polise K. In defense of altruistic kidney donation by strangers. *Pediatr Nephrol* 2000;14:518.

517. Cunningham MA, et al. Kidney transplantation from living non-related donors. *Med J Aust* 1996;165:172.

518. Commercially motivated renal transplantation: results in 540 patients transplanted in India. The Living Non-Related Renal Transplant Study Group. *Clin Transplantation* 1997;11:536.

519. Opelz G. Influence of HLA matching on survival of second kidney transplants in cyclosporine-treated recipients. *Transplantation* 1989;47:823.

520. Morris PJ, Ting A, Muller G. Factors influencing, survival of sequential grafts and their influence on the selection of a donor and recipient for a sequential graft. In: *Transplantation and clinical immunology,* 13th ed. Amsterdam: Excerpta Medica,1981:89.

521. Mahony JF, Sheil AGR. Long-term complications of cadaver renal transplantation. *Transplantation Rev (Orlando)* 1987;1:47.

522. Wynn JJ, et al. Late results of renal transplantation. *Transplantation* 1988;45:329.

523. Galton J. Racial effect on kidney transplantation. In: Terasaki PI, ed. *Clinical kidney transplants 1985.* Los Angeles: UCLA Tissue Typing Laboratory, 1985:153.

524. Perdue ST, Terasaki PI. Analysis of interracial variation in kidney transplant and patient survival. *Transplantation* 1982;34:75.

525. Claas FH, Van Rood JJ. Transplantation in hyperimmunized patients. *Adv Nephrol* 1989;18:317.

526. Rijksen JFWB, Koolen MI, Wavaszewski JE. Vascular complications in 400 consecutive renal allotransplants. *J Cardiovasc Surg* 1982;23:91.

527. Goldman MH, et al. A twenty-year survey of arterial complications of renal transplantation. *Surg Gynecol Obstet* 1975;141:758.

528. Jones RM, et al. Renal vascular thrombosis of cadaveric renal allografts in patients receiving cyclosporine, azathioprine and prednisone triple therapy. *Clin Transplantation* 1988;2:122.

529. Loughlin KR, Tilney NL, Richie JP. Urologic complications in 718 renal transplant patients. *Surgery* 1984;95:297.

530. Thrasher JB, Temple DR, Spees EK. Extravesical versus Leadbetter-Politano ureteroneocystostomy: a comparison of urological complications in 320 renal transplants. *J Urol* 1990;144:1150.

531. Erlichman RJ, et al. The use of percutaneous nephrostomy in renal transplant patients with ureteric obstruction. *Surg Gynecol Obstet* 1986;162:121.

532. Nicholson ML, et al. Urological complications of renal transplantation: the impact of double J ureteric stent. *Ann R Coll Surg Engl* 1991;73:316.

533. Yadav RVS, et al. Vesico-ureteric reflux following renal transplantation. *Br J Surg* 1972;59:33.

534. Mathew TH, Kincaid-Smith P, Vikraman P. Risks of vesicoureteric reflux in the transplanted kidney. *N Engl J Med* 1977;297:414.

535. Bootsma M, et al. The clinical significance of vesico-ureteral reflux in transplanted kidneys. *Clin Transplantation* 1987;1:311.

536. Griffiths AB, Fletcher EW, Morris PJ. Lymphocele after renal transplantation. *Aust N Z J Surg* 1979;49:626.

537. Schweizer RT, et al. Lymphoceles following renal transplantation. *Arch Surg* 1977;104:42.

538. Rubin RH. Infectious disease complications of renal transplantation *Kidney Int* 1993;44:221.

539. Murphy J, et al. Factors influencing the frequency of infection in renal transplant recipients. *Arch Intern Med* 1976;136:670.

540. Peterson PK, et al. Infectious diseases in hospitalized renal transplant recipients: a prospective study of a complex and evolving problem. *Medicine* 1982;61:360.

541. Tanphaichitr NT, Brennan DC. Infectious complications in renal transplant recipients. *Adv Renal Replacement Ther* 2000;7:131.

542. Tong CY, Cuevas LE, Williams H, et al. Prediction and diagnosis of cytomegalovirus disease in renal transplant recipients using qualitative and quantitative polymerase chain reaction. *Transplantation* 2000;69:985.

543. Aquino VH, Figueiredo LT. High prevalence of renal transplant recipients infected with more than one cytomegalovirus glycoprotein B genotype. *J Med Virol* 2000;61:138.

544. Brennan DC, et al. Control of cytomegalovirus-associated morbidity in renal transplant patients using intensive monitoring and either preemptive or deferred therapy. *J Am Soc Nephrol* 1997;8:118.

545. Ho M, et al. The transplanted kidney as a source of cytomegalovirus infection. *N Engl J Med* 1975;293:1109.

546. Johnson PC, et al. The impact of cytomegalovirus infection on seronegative recipients of seropositive donor kidneys versus seropositive recipients treated with cyclosporine-prednisone immunosuppression. *Transplantation* 1988;45:116.

547. Betts RF, et al. Transmission of cytomegalovirus infection with renal allografts. *Kidney Int* 1975;8:385.

548. Betts RF, et al. Clinical manifestations of renal allograft derived primary cytomegalovirus infection. *Am J Dis Child* 1977;131:759.

549. Patel NP, Carey RJ. Cytomegalovirus as a cause of cecal ulcer with massive hemorrhage in a renal transplant recipient. *Ann Surg* 1980;46:260.

550. Pouteil-Noble C, et al. Cytomegalovirus infection: an etiological factor for rejection? A prospective study in 242 renal transplant recipients. *Transplantation* 1993;55:851.

551. Boyce NW, et al. Cytomegalovirus infection complicating renal transplantation and its relationship to acute transplant glomerulopathy. *Transplantation* 1988;45:706.

552. Spitzer PG, Tarsy O, Eliapoulos GM. Acute transverse myelitis during disseminated cytomegalovirus infection in a renal transplant recipient. *Transplantation* 1987;44:151.

553. Minars N, et al. Fatal cytomegalovirus inclusion disease associated skin manifestations in a renal transplant patient. *Arch Dermatol* 1977;113:1569.

554. Chou S. Acquisition of donor strains of cytomegalovirus by renal transplant recipients. *N Engl J Med* 1986;314:1418.

555. Snydman DR, Rubin RH, Werner BG. New developments in cytomegalovirus prevention and management. *Am J Kidney Dis* 1993;21:217.

556. Rubin RH. Preemptive therapy in immunosuppressed hosts. *N Engl J Med* 1991;324:1057.

557. Lewis RM, et al. The adverse impact of cytomegalovirus infection on clinical outcome in cyclosporine-prednisone treated renal allograft recipients. *Transplantation* 1988;45:353.

558. Hibberd PL, et al. Symptomatic cytomegalovirus disease in the cytomegalovirus antibody seropositive renal transplant recipient treated with OKT3. *Transplantation* 1992;53:68.

559. Jassal SV, et al. Clinical practice guidelines: prevention of cytomegalovirus disease after renal transplantation. *J Am Soc Nephrol* 1998;9:1697.

560. Peterson PK, et al. Cytomegalovirus disease in real allograft recipients: a prospective study of clinical features, risk factors and impact on renal transplantation. *Medicine* 1980;59:283.

561. Rubin RH, et al. Multicenter seroepidemiologic study of the impact of cytomegalovirus infection on renal transplantation. *Transplantation* 1985;40:243.

562. Grundy JE, et al. Symptomatic cytomegalovirus infection in seropositive kidney recipients: reinfection with donor virus rather than reactivation of recipient virus. *Lancet* 1988;2:132.

563. Kemnitz J, et al. Rapid identification of viral infections in liver, heart, and kidney allograft biopsies by in situ hybridization [Letter]. *Am J Surg Pathol* 1989;13:80.

564. Balfour HH, Welo PK, Sachs GW. Cytomegalovirus vaccine trial in 400 renal transplant candidates. *Transplant Proc* 1985;17:81.

565. Brayman KL, et al. Prophylaxis of serious cytomegalovirus infection in renal transplant candidates using live human cytomegalovirus vaccine—interim results of a randomized trial. *Arch Surg* 1988;123:1502.

566. Metselaar HJ, et al. Prevention of CMV infection by screening for CMV antibodies in renal allograft recipients and the blood and kidney donors. *Scand J Infect Dis* 1988;20:135.

567. Balfour HH, et al. A randomized placebo-controlled trial of oral acyclovir for the prevention of cytomegalovirus disease in recipients of renal allografts. *N Engl J Med* 1989;320:1381.

568. Higgins RM, et al. The risks and benefits of low-dose cotrimoxazole prophylaxis for Pneumocystis pneumonia in renal transplantation. *Transplantation* 1989;47:558.

569. Aulitzky WE, et al. Ganciclovir and hyperimmunoglobulin for treating cytomegalovirus infection in bone marrow transplant recipients. *J Infect Dis* 1988;158:488.

570. Snydman DR, et al. Use of cytomegalovirus immune globulin to prevent cytomegalovirus disease in renal-transplant recipients. *N Engl J Med* 1987;317:1049.

571. Syndman DR. Ganciclovir therapy for cytomegalovirus disease associated with renal transplants. *Rev Infect Dis* 1988;10[Suppl 3]:554.

572. Harbison MA, et al. Ganciclovir therapy of severe cytomegalovirus infections in solid-organ transplant recipients. *Transplantation* 1988;46:82.

573. Dunn DL, et al. Treatment of invasive CMV disease in solid organ transplant patients with ganciclovir. *Transplantation* 1991;51:98.

574. Turgeon N, et al. Effect of oral acyclovir or ganciclovir therapy after preemptive intravenous ganciclovir therapy to prevent cytomegalovirus disease in cytomegalovirus seropositive renal and liver transplant recipients receiving antilymphocyte antibody therapy. *Transplantation* 1998;66:1780.

575. Nichols WG, Boeckh M. Recent advances in the therapy and prevention of CMV infections. *J Clin Virol* 2000;16:25.

576. Goodman JL. Possible transmission of herpes simplex virus by organ transplantation. *Transplantation* 1989;47:609.

577. Griffin PJA, et al. Oral acyclovir prophylaxis of herpes infections in renal transplant recipients. *Transplant Proc* 1985;17:84.

578. Warrel MJ, et al. The effects of viral infection on renal transplants. *Q J Med* 1980;49:219.

579. Hanto, D. W, et al. Epstein-Barr virus, immunodeficiency and B-cell lymphoproliferation. *Transplantation* 1985;39:461.

580. Ho M, et al. The frequency of Epstein-Barr virus infection and associated lymphoproliferative syndrome after transplantation and its manifestations in children. *Transplantation* 1985;45:719.

581. Ho M, et al. Epstein-Barr virus infections and DNA hybridization studies in posttransplantation lymphoma and lymphoproliferative lesions: the role of primary infection. *J Infect Dis* 1985;152:876.

582. Oliveira DB, et al. Brief communications: severe immunosuppression in a renal transplant recipient with HTLV-III antibodies. *Transplantation* 1986;41:260.

583. Carbone LG, et al. Determination of acquired immunodeficiency syndrome (AIDS) after renal transplantation. *Am J Kidney Dis* 1988;11:387.

584. L'Age-Stehr J, et al. HTLV III infection in kidney transplant recipients. *Lancet* 1985;2:1361.

585. Rubin RH, et al. The acquired immunodeficiency syndrome and transplantation. *Transplantation* 1987;44:1.

586. Rubin H, Tolkoff-Rubin NE. The problem of human immunodeficiency virus (HIV) infection and transplantation. *Transplant Int* 1988;1:36.

587. Dummer JS, et al. Infection with human immunodeficiency virus in the Pittsburgh transplant population—a study of 583 donors and 1043 recipients, 1981. *Transplantation* 1989;47:134.

588. Gardner SD, et al. Prospective study of the human polyomaviruses BK and JC and cytomegalovirus in renal transplant recipients. *J Clin Pathol* 1984;37:578.

589. Hogan TF, et al. Rapid detection and identification of JC virus and BK virus in human urine by using immunofluorescence microscopy. *J Clin Microbiol* 1980;11:178.

590. Heritage J, Chesters PM, McCance DJ. The persistence of papovavirus BK DNA sequences in normal human renal tissue. *J Med Virol* 1981;8:143.

591. Nickeleit V, et al. Polyomavirus infection of renal allograft recipients: from latent infection to manifest disease. *J Am Soc Nephrol* 1999;10:1080.

592. Andrews CA, et al. A serological investigation of BK virus and JC virus infections in recipients of renal allografts. *J Infect Dis* 1988;158:176.

593. Drachenberg CB, et al. Human polyoma virus in renal allograft biopsies: morphological findings and correlation with urine cytology. *Hum Pathol* 1999;30:970.

594. Howell DN, et al. Diagnosis and management of BK polyomavirus interstitial nephritis in renal transplant recipients. *Transplantation* 1999;68:1279.

595. Mathur VS, et al. Polyomavirus-induced interstitial nephritis in two renal transplant recipients: case reports and review of the literature. *Am J Kidney Dis* 1997;29:754.

596. Sopko J, Anuras S. Liver disease in renal transplant recipients. *Am J Med* 1978;64:139.

597. Ware AJ, et al. Etiology of liver diseases in renal transplant patients. *Ann Intern Med* 1979;91:364.

598. Weir MR, et al. Chronic liver disease in recipients of long-term renal allografts: analysis of morbidity and mortality. *Kidney Int* 1985;28:839.

599. Ramalho JH, et al. Hepatotoxicity of azathioprine in renal transplant recipients. *Transplant Proc* 1989;21:1716.

600. Farge D, et al. Reduction of azathioprine in renal transplant patients with chronic hepatitis. *Transplantation* 1986;41:55.

601. Yadav RVS, et al. Cyclophosphamide in renal transplantation. *Transplantation* 1988;45:421.

602. Parfrey PS, et al. The clinical and pathological course of hepatitis B liver disease in renal transplant recipients. *Transplantation* 1984;37:461.

603. Chan L, Mo S, Wang W. Hepatitis and the renal patient. In: Massry SG, Glassock RJ, eds. *Textbook of nephrology,* 4th ed. Philadelphia: Lippincott Williams & Wilkins, 2001:1333.

604. Feuerhake A, et al. HBV-vaccination recipients of kidney allografts. *Vaccine* 1984;2:255.

605. Stevens DE, et al. Hepatitis B vaccine in patients receiving hemodialysis: immunogenicity and efficacy. *N Engl J Med* 1984;311:496.

606. Rostaing L, et al. Efficacy and safety of lamivudine on replication of recurrent hepatitis B after cadaveric renal transplantation. *Transplantation* 1997;64:1624.

607. Goffin E, et al. Lamivudine inhibits hepatitis B virus replication in kidney graft recipients. *Transplantation* 1998;66:407.

608. Morales JM, Campistol JM. Transplantation in the patient with hepatitis C. *J Am Soc Nephrol* 2000;11:1343.

609. Boyce NW, et al. Non-hepatitis B-related liver disease in a renal transplant population. *Am J Kidney Dis* 1988;11:307.

610. Atler HJ, et al. Detection of antibody to hepatitis C virus in prospectively followed transfusion recipients with acute and chronic non-A, non-B hepatitis. *N Engl J Med* 1989;321:1494.

611. Nampoory MR, et al. Organ-transmitted HCV infection in kidney transplant recipients from an anti-HCV negative donor. *Transplant Proc* 1999;31:3207.

612. Mahmoud IM, et al. A prospective study of hepatitis C viremia in renal allograft recipients. *Am J Nephrol* 1999;19:576.

613. Pereira BJ, et al. Transmission of hepatitis C virus by organ transplantation. *N Engl J Med* 1991;325:454.

614. Pereira BJ, et al. Screening and confirmatory testing of cadaver donors for hepatitis C virus infection: a U.S. National Collaborative Study. *Kidney Int* 1994;46:886.

615. Pereira BJ, et al. A controlled study of hepatitis C transmission by organ transplantation. *Lancet* 1995;345:484.

616. Morales JM, et al. Transplantation of kidneys from donors with hepatitis C antibody into recipients with pre-transplantation anti-HCV. *Kidney Int* 1995;47:236.

617. Rostaing L, et al. Treatment of chronic hepatitis C with recombinant interferon alpha in kidney transplant recipients. *Transplantation* 1995;59:1426.

618. Rostaing L, et al. Acute renal failure in kidney transplant patients treated with interferon alpha 2b for chronic hepatitis C. *Nephron* 1996;74:512.

619. Kovarik J, et al. Adverse effect of low-dose prophylactic human recombinant leukocyte interferon-alpha treatment in renal transplant recipients. *Transplantation* 1988;45:402.

620. Duarte R, et al. Interferon-alpha facilitates renal transplantation in hemodialysis patients with chronic viral hepatitis. *Am J Kidney Dis* 1995;25:40.

621. Moore FD Jr, et al. The declining mortality from pneumonia in renal transplant patients. *Infect Surg* 1983;2:13.

622. Talseth T, et al. Increasing incidence of Pneumocystis carinii pneumonia in renal transplant patients. *Transplant Proc* 1988;20:400.

623. Higgins RM, et al. The risks and benefits of low-dose cotrimoxazole prophylaxis for Pneumocystis pneumonia in renal transplantation. *Transplantation* 1989;47:558.

624. Tobin JO, et al. Legionnaires' disease in a transplant unit: isolation of the causative agent from shower baths. *Lancet* 1980;2:118.

625. Sayiner A, et al. Tuberculosis in renal transplant recipients. *Transplantation* 1999;68:1268.

626. John GT, et al. A double-blind randomized controlled trial of primary isoniazid prophylaxis in dialysis and transplant patients. *Transplantation* 1994;57:1683.

627. American Thoracic Society and Centers for Disease Control and Prevention: targeted tuberculin testing and treatment of latent tuberculosis infection. *MMWR Morb Mortal Wkly Rep* 2000;49(RR-6):1.

628. Bach MC, et al. Influence of rejection therapy on fungal and nocardial infections in renal transplant recipients. *Lancet* 1973;1:180.

629. Linden P, Williams P, Chan KM. Efficacy and safety of amphotericin B lipid complex injection (ABLC) in solid-organ transplant recipients with invasive fungal infections. *Clin Transplantation* 2000;14:329.

630. Tolkoff-Rubin NE, Rubin RH. Opportunistic fungal and bacterial infection in the renal transplant recipient. *J Am Soc Nephrol* 1992;2:S264.

631. ZuRhein GM, Varakis J. Progressive multifocal leukoencephalopathy in a renal allograft recipient. *N Engl J Med* 1974;291:798.

632. Tolkoff-Rubin NE, et al. A controlled study of trimethoprim-sulfamethoxazole prophylaxis of urinary tract infection in renal transplant recipients. *Rev Infect Dis* 1974;4:614.

633. Franz M, Horl WH. Common errors in diagnosis and management of urinary tract infection. II: Clinical management. *Nephrol Dial Transplantation* 1999;14:2754.

634. Penn I. Cancers complicating organ transplantation. *N Engl J Med* 1990;323:1767.

635. Sheil AG. Cancer after transplantation. *World J Surg* 1986;10:389.

636. Sheil AGR, et al. Cancer incidence in renal transplant patients treated with azathioprine or cyclosporine. *Transplant Proc* 1987;19:2214.

637. Penn I. Cancers following cyclosporine therapy. *Transplant Proc* 1987;29:2211.

638. Penn I. Neoplastic complications of transplantation. *Semin Respir Infect* 1993;8:233.

639. Opelz G, Henderson R, for the Collaborative Transplant Study. Incidence of non-Hodgkin lymphoma in kidney and heart transplant recipients. *Lancet* 1993;342:1514.

640. Swinnen JL, et al. Increased incidence of lymphoproliferative disorders after immunosuppression with the monoclonal antibody OKT3 in cardiac transplant recipients. *N Engl J Med* 1990;323:1723.

641. Wilkinson AH, et al. Increased frequency of posttransplant lymphomas in patients treated with cyclosporine, azathioprine and prednisone. *Transplantation* 1989;47:293.

642. Sheil AG. Cancer after transplantation. *World J Surg* 1986;10:389.

643. Sheil AGR, et al. Cancer incidence in renal transplant patients treated with azathioprine or cyclosporin. *Transplant Proc* 1987;19:2214.

644. Penn I. The changing patterns of posttransplant malignancies. *Transplant Proc* 1991;23:1101.

645. McLelland J, Chu AC. Skin tumours in renal allograft recipients. *J R Soc Med* 1989;92:110.

646. Nalesnik MA, et al. The pathology of posttransplant lymphoproliferative disorders occurring in the setting of cyclosporine A-prednisone immunosuppression. *Am J Pathol* 1988;133:173.

647. Starzl TE, et al. Reversibility of lymphomas and lymphoproliferative lesions developing under cyclosporine-steroid therapy. *Lancet* 1984;1:583.

648. Cockfield SM, et al. Post-transplant lymphoproliferative disorder in renal allograft recipients. Clinical experience and risk factor analysis in a single center. *Transplantation* 1993;56:88.

649. Patton DF, et al. Epstein-Barr virus–determined clonality in posttransplant lymphoproliferative disease. *Transplantation* 1990;49:1080.

650. Hanto DW, Frizzera G, Gajl-Peczalska KJ. Epstein-Barr-virus induced B-cell lymphoma after renal transplantation: acyclovir therapy and transition from polyclonal to monoclonal B cell proliferation. *N Engl J Med* 1982;306:913.

651. Randhawa PS, et al. Expression of Epstein-Barr virus-encoded small RNA (by the EBER-1 gene) in liver specimens from transplant recipients with post-transplantation lymphoproliferative disease. *N Engl J Med* 1992;327:1710.

652. Mosialos G, et al. The Epstein-Barr virus transforming protein LMP1 engages signaling proteins from the tumor necrosis factor receptor family. *Cell* 1995;80:389.

653. Harwood AR, et al. Kaposi's sarcoma in recipients of renal transplants. *Am J Med* 1979;67:759.

654. Ecder ST, et al. Kaposi's sarcoma after renal transplantation in Turkey. *Clin Transplantation* 1998;12:472.

655. Hadjuyannakis EJ, et al. Gastrointestinal complications after renal transplantation. *Lancet* 1971;2:781.

656. Kestens PJ, Alexandre GPJ. Gastroduodenal complications after transplantation. *Clin Transplantation* 1988;2:221.

657. Demling RH, et al. Intestinal necrosis and perforation after renal transplantation. *Arch Surg* 1975;110:251.

658. Misre MK, et al. Major colonic diseases complicating a renal transplantation. *Surgery* 1973;73:942.

659. Ritchie DB, et al. Clostridium difficile-associated colitis: cross infection in predisposed patients with renal failure. *N Z Med J* 1982;95:265.

660. Fernandez JA, Rosenberg JC. Post-transplantation pancreatitis. *Surg Gynecol Obstet* 1986;143:795.

661. Kawanishi H, Rudolph E, Bull F. Azathioprine-induced acute pancreatitis. *N Engl J Med* 1973;289:357.

662. Lorber M, et al. Hepatobiliary and pancreatic complications of cyclosporine therapy in 466 renal transplant recipients. *Transplantation* 1987;43:35.

663. Tilney NL, Collins JJ Jr, Wilson RE. Hemorrhagic pancreatitis: a fatal complication of renal transplantation. *N Engl J Med* 1966;274:1051.

664. Kasiske BL, et al. Cardiovascular disease after renal transplantation. *J Am Soc Nephrol* 1996;7:158.

665. Aakhus S, Dahl K, Wideroe TE. Cardiovascular morbidity and risk factors in renal transplant patients. *Nephrol Dial Transplantation* 1999;14:648.

666. Bagdade JD, Albers JJ. Plasma high-density lipoprotein concentrations in chronic hemodialysis and renal transplant patients. *N Engl J Med* 1977;296:1435.

667. Ibels LS, et al. Studies on the nature and causes of hyperlipidemia in uremia, maintenance dialysis and renal transplantation. *Q J Med* 1975;44:601.

668. Kasiske BL, Umen AJ. Persistent hyperlipidemia in renal transplant patients. *Medicine* 1987;66:309.

669. Cattran DC, et al. Hyperlipidemia after renal transplantation: natural history and pathophysiology. *Ann Intern Med* 1979;91:554.

670. Curtis JJ, et al. Effects of renal transplantation of hyperlipidemia and high-density lipoprotein cholesterol (HDL). *Transplantation* 1978;26:364.

671. Jung K, et al. Changed composition of high-density lipoprotein subclasses HDL2 and HDL3 after renal transplantation. *Transplantation* 1988;46:407.

672. Moore RA, et al. The effects of the American Heart Association step one diet on hyperlipidemia following renal transplantation. *Transplantation* 1990;49:60.

673. Roodnat JI, et al. Cholesterol as an independent predictor of outcome after renal transplantation. *Transplantation* 2000;69:1704.

674. Massy ZA, Kasiske BL. Post-transplant hyperlipidemia: mechanisms and management. *J Am Soc Nephrol* 1996;7:971.

675. Corpier CL, et al. Rhabdomyolysis and renal injury with lovastatin use. Report of two cases in cardiac transplant recipients. *JAMA* 1988;260:239.

676. Cheung AK, et al. A prospective study on treatment of hypercholesterolemia with lovastatin in renal transplant recipients receiving cyclosporine. *J Am Soc Nephrol* 1993;3:1884.

677. Lal SM, et al. Effects of nicotinic acid and lovastatin in renal transplant patients: a prospective, randomized, open-labeled study. *Am J Kidney Dis* 1995;25:616.

678. Welch GN, Loscalzo J. Homocysteine and atherothrombosis [Comments]. *N Engl J Med* 1998;338:1042.

679. Dimeny E, et al. Serum total homocysteine concentration does not predict outcome in renal transplant recipients. *Clin Transplantation* 1998;12:563.

680. Arnadottir M, et al. Serum total homocysteine concentration before and after renal transplantation. *Kidney Int* 1998;54:1380.

681. Ducloux D, et al. Serum total homocysteine and cardiovascular disease occurrence in chronic, stable renal transplant recipients: a prospective study. *J Am Soc Nephrol* 2000;11:134.

682. Bostom AG, et al. Treatment of hyperhomocystinemia in renal transplant recipients. A randomized, placebo-controlled trial. *Ann Intern Med* 1997;127:1089.

683. Luke RG. Nephrology forum: hypertension in renal transplant recipients. *Kidney Int* 1987;31:1024.

684. Bennett WM, et al. Post-transplant hypertension: studies of cortical blood flow and the renal pressor system. *Kidney Int* 1976;6:99.

685. Curtis JJ. Hypertension in the renal transplant patient. *Transplantation Rev (Orlando)* 1988;2:17.

686. Cheigh JS, et al. Hypertension in kidney transplant recipients—effect on long-term renal allograft survival. *Am J Hypertens* 1989;2[Pt 1]:341.

687. Curtis JJ, et al. Cyclosporin in therapeutic doses increases renal allograft vascular resistance. *Lancet* 1986;2:477.

688. Luke RG, et al. Mechanisms of posttransplant hypertension. *Am J Kidney Dis* 1985;A79.

689. Curtis JJ, et al. Inhibition of angiotensin converting enzyme in renal transplant recipients with hypertension. *N Engl J Med* 1983;308:377.

690. Linas SL, et al. Role of the renin-angiotensin system in posttransplantation hypertension in patients with multiple kidneys. *N Engl J Med* 1978;298:1440.

691. Chapman JR, et al. Hypertension after renal transplantation—a comparison of cyclosporine and conventional immunosuppression. *Transplantation* 1987;43:860.

692. Burke M, Wilder L. Effect of verapamil on glomerular filtration rate and glomerular prostaglandin production during cyclosporine administration. *Transplantation* 1988;46:919.

693. Birx DL, Berger M, Fleischer TA. The interference of T cell activation by calcium channel blocking agents. *J Immunol* 1984;133:904.

694. Weir MR, et al. Additive effect of cyclosporine and verapamil on the inhibition of activation and function of human peripheral blood mononuclear cells. *Transplant Proc* 1988;20[Suppl 2]:240.

695. Curtis JJ, et al. Surgical therapy for persistent hypertension after renal transplantation. *Transplantation* 1981;31:125.

696. Curtis JJ, et al. Benefits of removal of native kidneys in hypertension after renal transplantation. *Lancet* 1985;2:739.

697. Thompson JF, et al. Control of hypertension after renal transplantation by embolisation of host kidneys. *Lancet* 1984;2:424.

698. Morris PJ, et al. Renal artery stenosis in renal transplantation. *Med J Aust* 1971;1:1255.

699. Tilney NL, et al. Renal artery stenosis in transplant patients. *Ann Surg* 1984;199:454.

700. Lacombe M. Arterial stenosis complicating renal allotransplantation in man: a study of 38 cases. *Ann Surg* 1975;181:283.

701. Roberts JP, et al. Transplant renal artery stenosis. *Transplantation* 1989;48:580.

702. Simmons RL, et al. Renal allograft rejection simulated by arterial stenosis. *Surgery* 1970;68:800.

703. Loubeyre P, et al. Transplanted renal artery: detection of stenosis with color Doppler US. *Radiology* 1997;203:661.

704. Alfrey EJ, Rubin GD, Kuo PC, et al. The use of spiral computed tomography in the evaluation of living donors for kidney transplantation. *Transplantation* 1995;59:643.

705. Dickerman RM, et al. Surgical correction of posttransplant renovascular hypertension. *Ann Surg* 1980;192:639.

706. Miller AR, et al. Treatment of transplant renal artery stenosis: experience and reassessment of therapeutic options. *Clin Transplantation* 1989;3:101.

707. De Meyer M, et al. Treatment of renal graft artery stenosis. *Transplantation* 1989;47:784.

708. Greenstein SM, et al. Percutaneous transluminal angioplasty. *Transplantation* 1987;43:29.

709. Grossman RA, et al. Percutaneous transluminal angioplasty treatment of renal transplant artery stenosis. *Transplantation* 1982;34:339.

710. Sniderman KW, et al. Percutaneous transluminal dilation in renal transplant arterial stenosis. *Transplantation* 1980;30:440.

711. Wickre CG, et al. Postrenal transplant erythrocytosis: a review of 53 patients. *Kidney Int* 1983;23:731.

712. Besarab A, et al. Dynamics of erythropoiesis following renal transplantation. *Kidney Int* 1987;32:526.

713. Sun CH, et al. Serum erythropoietin levels after renal transplantation. *N Engl J Med* 1989;321:151.

714. Gaston RS, Julian BA, Curtis JJ. Posttransplant erythrocytosis: an enigma revisited. *Am J Kidney Dis* 1994;24:1.

715. Aeberhard JM, et al. Multiple site estimates of erythropoietin and renin in polycythemic kidney transplant patients. *Transplantation* 1990;50:613.

716. Ilan Y, et al. Erythrocytosis after renal transplantation. The response to theophylline treatment. *Transplantation* 1994;57:661.

717. Torregrosa JV, et al. Efficacy of captopril on posttransplant erythrocytosis. *Transplantation* 1994;58:311.

718. Rell K, et al. Correction of posttransplant erythrocytosis with enalapril. *Transplantation* 1994;57:1059.

719. Julian BA, et al. Erythropoiesis after withdrawal of enalapril in posttransplant erythrocytosis. *Kidney Int* 1994;46:1397.

720. Cundy T, et al. Calcium metabolism and hyperparathyroidism after renal transplantation. *Q J Med* 1983;205:67.

721. Chan L, et al. Prospective trial of high-dose versus low dose prednisone in renal transplantation. *Transplant Proc* 1980;12:323.

722. Parfrey PS, et al. The decreased incidence of aseptic necrosis in renal transplant recipients: a case control study. *Transplantation* 1986;41:182.

723. Julian BA, et al. Rapid loss of vertebral mineral density after renal transplantation. *N Engl J Med* 1991;325:544.

724. Julian BA, Quarles LD, Niemann KM. Musculoskeletal complications after renal transplantation: pathogenesis and treatment. *Am J Kidney Dis* 1992;19:99.

725. Gauthier VJ, Barbosa LM. Bone pain in transplant recipients responsive to calcium channel blockers. *Ann Intern Med* 1994;121:863.

726. Cueto-Manzano AM, et al. Effect of 1,25-dihydroxyvitamin D3 and calcium carbonate on bone loss associated with long-term renal transplantation. *Am J Kidney Dis* 2000;35:227.

727. Fan SL, et al. Pamidronate therapy as prevention of bone loss following renal transplantation. *Kidney Int* 2000;57:684.

728. Better OS, et al. Spontaneous remission of the defect in urinary acidification after cadaver kidney homotransplantation. *Lancet* 1970;1:110.

729. Gyory AZ, et al. Renal tubular acidosis, acidosis due to hyperkalemia, disordered citrate metabolism and other tubular dysfunctions following human renal transplantation. *Q J Med* 1969;38:321.

730. Wilson DR, Siddiqui AA. Renal tubular acidosis after kidney transplantation: natural history and significance. *Ann Intern Med* 1973;79:352.

731. Cundy T, et al. Calcium metabolism and hyperparathyroidism after renal transplantation. *Q J Med* 1983;52:67.

732. Messa P, et al. Persistent secondary hyperparathyroidism after renal transplantation. *Kidney Int* 1998;54:1704.

733. Mourad M, et al. Early posttransplant calcemia as a predictive indicator for parathyroidectomy in kidney allograft recipients with tertiary hyperparathyroidism. *Transplant Proc* 2000;32:437.

734. Garvin PJ, et al. Management of hypercalcemic hyperparathyroidism after renal transplantation. *Arch Surg* 1985;120:578.

735. Higgins RM, et al. Hypophosphataemia after renal transplantation: relationship to immunosuppressive drug therapy and effects on muscle detected by 31P nuclear magnetic resonance spectroscopy. *Nephrol Dial Transplantation* 1990;5:62.

736. Ambuhl PM, et al. Metabolic aspects of phosphate replacement therapy for hypophosphatemia after renal transplantation: impact on muscular phosphate content, mineral metabolism, and acid/base homeostasis. *Am J Kidney Dis* 1999;34:875.

737. Claesson K, et al. Prospective study of calcium homeostasis after renal transplantation. *World J Surg* 1998;22:635.

738. Rosenbaum RW, et al. Decreased phosphate reabsorption after renal transplantation: evidence for a mechanism independent of calcium and parathyroid hormone. *Kidney Int* 1981;19:568.

739. Ramos EL, et al. Hypomagnesemia in renal transplant patients: improvement over time and association with hypertension and cyclosporine levels. *Clin Transplantation* 1981;9:185.

740. Vannini SD, et al. Permanently reduced plasma ionized magnesium among renal transplant recipients on cyclosporine. *Transplant Int* 1999;12:244.

741. Cavdar C, et al. Hypomagnesemia and mild rhabdomyolysis in living related donor renal transplant recipient treated with cyclosporine A. *Scand J Urol Nephrol* 1998;32:415.

742. Gupta BK, Glicklich D, Tellis VA. Magnesium repletion therapy improved lipid metabolism in hypomagnesemic renal transplant recipients: a pilot study. *Transplantation* 1999;67:1485.

743. Lin HY, et al. Cyclosporine-induced hyperuricemia and gout. *N Engl J Med* 1989;321:287.

744. West C, Carpenter BJ, Hakala TR. The incidence of gout in renal transplant recipients. *Am J Kidney Dis* 1987;10:369.

745. Noordzij TC, Leunissen KM, Van Hooff JP. Renal handling of urate and the incidence of gouty arthritis during cyclosporine and diuretic use. *Transplantation* 1991;52:64.

746. Boudreaux JP, et al. The impact of cyclosporine and combination immunosuppression on the incidence of posttransplant diabetes in renal allograft recipients. *Transplantation* 1987;44:376.

747. Roth D, et al. Posttransplant hyperglycemia: increased incidence in cyclosporine-treated renal allograft recipients. *Transplantation* 1989;47:278.

748. Jindal RM. Posttransplant diabetes mellitus-a review. *Transplantation* 1994;58:1289.

749. Veenstra DL, et al. Incidence and long-term cost of steroid-related side effects after renal transplantation. *Am J Kidney Dis* 1999;33:829.

750. Meier-Kriesche HU, et al. The effect of body mass index on long-term renal allograft survival. *Transplantation* 1999;68:1294.

751. Holley JL, et al. Obesity as a risk factor following cadaveric renal transplantation. *Transplantation* 1990;49:387.

752. Patel MG. The effect of dietary intervention on weight gains after renal transplantation. *J Renal Nutr* 1998;8:137.

753. Guijarro C, et al. Serum albumin and mortality after renal transplantation. *Am J Kidney Dis* 1996;27:117.

754. Becker BN, et al. The impact of hypoalbuminemia in kidney-pancreas transplant recipients. *Transplantation* 1999;68:72.

755. Hoy WE, et al. The influence of glucocorticoid dose on protein catabolism after renal transplantation. *Am J Med Sci* 1986;291:241.

756. Seagraves A, et al. Net protein catabolic rate after kidney transplantation: impact of corticosteroid immunosuppression. *JPEN J Parenter Enteral Nutr* 1986;10:453.

757. DeVecchi A, et al. Long-term comparison between single-morning daily and alternate-day steroid treatment in cadaver kidney recipients. *Transplant Proc* 1980;12:327.

758. Diethelm AG, et al. Alternate-day prednisone therapy in recipients of renal allografts. *Arch Surg* 1976;111:867.

759. Dumler F, et al. Long-term alternate day steroid therapy in renal transplantation. *Transplantation* 1982;34:78.

760. Fletchner SM, et al. Impact of cyclosporine on renal function and growth in pediatric renal transplant recipients. *Transplant Proc* 1985;17:1284.

761. Rees L, Greene SA, Adlard P, et al. Growth and endocrine function after renal transplantation. *Arch Dis Child* 1988;63:1326.

762. Ghio L, et al. Advantages of cyclosporine as sole immunosuppressive agent in children with transplanted kidneys. *Transplantation* 1992;54:757.

763. Penn I, Makowski EI, Harris P. Parenthood following renal transplantation. *Kidney Int* 1981;18:221.

764. Registration Committee of the European Dialysis and Transplant Association. Successful pregnancies in women treated by dialysis and kidney transplantation. *Br J Obstet Gynaecol* 1980;87:839.

765. Davison JM. Renal transplantation and pregnancy. *Am J Kidney Dis* 1987;9:374.

766. Davison JM, Lindheimer MD. Pregnancy in women with renal allografts. *Semin Nephrol* 1981;4:240.

767. Davison JM, Uldall PR, Taylor RM. Relation of immediate posttransplant renal function to long-term function in cadaver kidney recipients. *Transplantation* 1977;23:310.

768. Armenti VT, et al. National transplantation pregnancy registry—outcome of 154 pregnancies in cyclosporine-treated female kidney transplant recipients. *Transplantation* 1995;57:502.

769. Armenti VT, et al. Report from the National Transplantation Pregnancy Registry (NTPR): outcomes of pregnancy after transplantation. In: Cecka JM, Teasaki PI, eds. *Clinical kidney transplants 1999.* Los Angeles: UCLA Tissue Typing Laboratory, 1999:111.

770. Halloran PF, et al. Strategies to improve the immunologic management of organ transplants. *Clin Transplantation* 1995;9:227.

771. US Department of Health and Human Services. 1999 Report to Congress on the Scientific and Clinical Status of Organ Transplantation. US House of Representatives and US Senate; September 1999.

CHAPTER 98

Peritoneal Dialysis

Thomas A. Golper, John M. Burkart, and Beth Piraino

Fifteen percent of the world's dialysis population utilizes peritoneal dialysis (PD). This fraction is growing at an increasing rate, particularly in developing countries. Peritoneal dialysis is used to treat almost 12% of the US dialysis population. When comparable populations are analyzed, patient survival rates by PD and hemodialysis (HD) are similar (1–7). The exception appears to be elderly diabetic patients treated by continuous ambulatory peritoneal dialysis (CAPD), who have a 1.26 relative risk of death compared to those treated by HD (8). Unmeasured comorbid factors may explain this difference, or there may be a selection bias undescribed by known comorbidities. Nonetheless, PD treatment affects thousands of patients and is growing in popularity. Furthermore, PD is receiving increasing industrial attention in the research and development of newer and superior technologies.

Space precludes us from describing an extensive physiologic basis for PD. This was done quite well in Chapter 106 of the fifth edition of this book. We discuss the current major issues of concern for PD in this chapter—the definition of "adequate" therapy and the control or management of therapy-related complications.

ADEQUACY OF PERITONEAL DIALYSIS AND ITS RELATION TO NUTRITION

Minimal Versus Optimal Dialysis

Adequate dialysis is a prerequisite for both technique and patient survival (9–11). The goals of renal replacement therapy (RRT) are listed in Table 98-1. In addition, nephrologists must provide enough RRT so that the amount of dialysis delivered is not the rate-limiting step that determines survival

T. A. Golper: Department of Medicine, Division of Nephrology and Hypertension, Vanderbilt University Medical Center, Nashville, Tennessee

J. M. Burkart: Department of Nephrology, Wake Forest University Medical Center, Winston-Salem, North Carolina

B. Piraino: Department of Medicine, University of Pittsburgh School of Medicine; and Peritoneal Dialysis Program, University of Pittsburgh Medical Center, Pittsburgh, Pennsylvania

(i.e., the concept of a "minimal" dialysis dose). "Optimal" dialysis prescriptions not only eliminate uremia as a potential variable that influences outcome but also facilitate blood pressure control, maximize protein intake, and optimize quality of life.

The National Cooperative Dialysis Study (NCDS) (12) was designed to compare morbidity and death in HD patient groups randomly assigned to two different target dialysis doses and treatment times. Lower morbidity was seen in patients with: (a) the lower time-averaged concentration of urea or higher dialysis dose, or (b) a total urea clearance over volume of distribution (Kt/V) of at least 0.8 per treatment and a protein catabolic rate of from 0.8 to 1.4 g/kg body weight/day (13). This study defined the minimally acceptable dose of dialysis, not optimal therapy. In the United States, the mean prescribed Kt/V is 1.02 (14). In contrast, Charra and colleagues (10) reported a 20-year follow-up for 445 unselected HD patients with a mean Kt/V of 1.67 (10). Outcome was not a function of Kt/V but correlated with blood pressure and age. The 20-year patient survival was 43%, approaching that for healthy individuals of the same age! This exemplifies an optimal dialysis prescription. Preliminary data for PD patients also suggest that the relative risk of death decreased as the dose of total solute clearance increased (11).

Impact of Nutritional Status and Dialysis Dose on Outcome

The present working hypothesis is that overall solute clearance is positively correlated with protein intake and patient outcome (15). This is based on the following arguments generated from cross-sectional studies: (a) that malnutrition correlates with an increased risk of adverse events such as hospitalizations and mortality; (b) that dietary protein intake (DPI) tends to correlate with nutritional parameters; (c) that DPI correlates with dialysis dose; and (d) that DPI increases as dialysis dose increases in the absence of comorbid conditions in an individual patient.

Unfortunately, the next link in the data (i.e., demonstration that dialysis dose correlates with serum albumin levels)

TABLE 98-1. *Goals of end-stage renal disease replacement therapy*

Prolong life
Reverse uremic symptoms
Optimize quality of life
Maintain positive nitrogen balance
Return to pre–end-stage renal disease functional status
Minimize patient inconvenience factors

remains to be proved. Additionally, if the leading cause of death in end-stage renal disease (ESRD) patients is cardiovascular (16), how does the presence of malnutrition translate into an increased risk of death from cardiovascular events? It is recognized that serum albumin levels are the net result of multiple processes. It is a negative acute phase reactant. Recent studies have linked serum C-reactive protein levels, an acute phase protein thought to be a marker of a chronic or acute inflammatory state, to survival and low serum albumin levels (17). A chronic inflammatory state has been associated with an increased risk of cardiovascular death. These data show that many factors influence serum albumin levels, only one of which is dialysis dose, and at the same time suggest that low serum albumin levels may be predictive of cardiovascular death.

Impact of Nutritional Status on Patient Outcome

Low serum albumin levels are known to be associated with an increased risk of death and morbidity in the general population (18). Lowrie and Lew (19) found that the relative risk of death increased as the serum albumin (a surrogate for visceral protein stores) decreased in HD patients. Interestingly, the relative risk of death also decreased as the serum creatinine (a surrogate for somatic protein stores) increased. Both of these values tend to be higher with better nutritional status. These findings were confirmed in Canadian HD patients (20). These observations were extended to PD patients, but with controversial results (21). Many, but not all publications have shown that low serum albumin levels are associated with an increased risk of death (11,22,23) and morbidity (11,22–25). In the preliminary report of the CANUSA study (26), serum albumin levels were the strongest independent predictor of outcome. Lean body mass, determined from creatinine kinetics, had an additive predictive value.

Other more specific measurements of nutritional status, such as global nutritional assessment, also have been shown to correlate with outcome (27). Furthermore, Pollock and coworkers (28) found that low total body nitrogen was associated with poor clinical outcome in CAPD.

Convincing as these data may be, however, the U.S. Renal Data System has reported that the relative risk of mortality for a subgroup of CAPD patients entering treatment in 1986 and 1987 did not increase unless the serum albumin level was less than 3.0 g/dL (29). Struijk and associates (30) similarly reported that the relative risk of death in CAPD patients did not increase until the serum albumin level was below approximately 3.1 g/dL.

The reasons for these different observations are complex. The determinants of serum albumin concentration include synthesis, catabolism, body distribution, body volume, extracorporeal losses, and acute or chronic inflammation. If dialysis dose is a major determinant of DPI, differences in dialysis dose in these studies could explain different outcomes (15). Additionally, differences in the presence of comorbid diseases also may affect both the synthesis and catabolism of albumin (27,31). The patient's volume and peritoneal membrane transport status also may be contributory. Rapid transporters on PD tend to have low serum albumin levels despite what is thought to be an adequate dose of dialysis (24,32–34). Perhaps this is owing to increased dialysate protein losses, subtle volume overload, or the need for hypertonic exchanges to maintain ultrafiltration (UF), which may be associated with excessive glucose absorption and appetite suppression (35).

Differences in the methods used to determine serum albumin concentration could be another reason for the varying results (36). The most commonly used method of serum albumin determination, the bromcresol green method, tends to markedly overestimate albumin levels when compared to nephelometry (37).

An international survey reported that 40% of CAPD patients manifested various degrees of malnutrition (38). This suggests that many PD patients are at an increased risk of death. If the working hypothesis is correct, perhaps this is a reflection of unrecognized underdialysis.

Measurements of Nutritional Status

Serum albumin levels are an easily obtainable surrogate marker for the patient's visceral protein stores and underlying nutritional status but do not single-handedly define malnutrition. In one study, low serum albumin levels correlated with evidence of malnutrition in women only (38). Furthermore, although increasing serum albumin levels correlated positively with changes in nitrogen balance (39) and serum albumin levels correlated positively with total body nitrogen (22), Heide and colleagues (40) found no correlation with the change in serum albumin and decreasing total body nitrogen; therefore, other surrogate markers for nutritional status have been evaluated. Estimates of DPI, such as the protein equivalent of nitrogen appearance (PNA), formerly called protein catabolic rate (PCR), tend to correlate with serum albumin levels and nutritional status in most (41,22,32) but not all studies (23,42,43). Keshaviah and Nolph (44) compared the many formulas available to calculate PNA from urea nitrogen appearance (UNA) in dialysate and urine, and the Randerson equation was recommended (45) (Table 98-2).

Actual DPI from food records correlates well with PNA calculations (46); however, the line of best fit is not the line of identity. At lower levels of DPI, presumably when a patient is catabolic, PNA tends to exceed DPI, and the

TABLE 98-2. *Commonly used formulas for protein nitrogen appearance*

PNA = 10.76 (G_{un} + 1.46) (Randerson)
PNA = 9.35 G_{un} + 0.294 V + protein losses
  (Modified Borah)
PNA = 6.25 (UN_{loss} + 1.81 + 0.031 × body weight)
  (Teehan)
PNA = 6.25 × N loss (Kjeldahl)
PNA (g/24 h) = 15.1 + (6.95 × urea nitrogen appearance in
  g/24 h) + dialysate and urine protein in g/24 h
  (Bergstrom)*
  In the absence of direct measurement of urinary and
    dialysate protein losses, this following less accurate
    formula may be used:
PNA (g/24 hours) = 20.1 + (7.50 × urea nitrogen
  appearance in g/24 h (Bergstrom)

PNA, protein nitrogen appearance; G_{un}, urea nitrogen generation rate; *V*, volume of urea distribution; UN_{loss}, urea nitrogen loss; *N*, nitrogen.

*Bergstrom J, Heimburger O, Lindholm B. Calculation of the protein equivalent of total nitrogen appearance from urea appearance, which formulas should be used? *Peritoneal Dial Int* 1998;18:467.

Modified from: Keshaviah P, Nolph K. Protein catabolic rate calculations in CAPD patients. *Trans Am Soc Artif Intern Org* 1991;37:M400.

estimation (PNA) may overestimate actual DPI. Conversely, when anabolic, PNA calculations may underestimate actual DPI. Davies and associates (47) have suggested that one can estimate net nitrogen balance by examining the ratio of DPI/PNA. If the patients were catabolic, one would expect to find a low DPI and a low DPI:PNA ratio. These patients may be uremic, and an increase in dialysis dose should be considered if no other cause for the catabolism is found.

Lean body mass (LBM) is an estimate of a patient's somatic protein stores. Nolph and coworkers (32) showed a correlation between LBM and serum albumin levels. The CANUSA study showed a correlation between increasing LBM and improvement in outcome (11). Wai-Kei Lo and colleagues (48) reviewed the multiple ways to assess LBM in PD patients, such as measurement of total body potassium, use of bioelectric impedance, near infrared interaction, and anthropometric measurements, and found that creatinine kinetics correlate well with other more standard methods of LBM determination. This calculation should not be influenced by the presence of subtle volume overload. Creatinine production can be determined from measurements of creatinine in 24-hour dialysate and urine collections (Table 98-3). Lean body mass is a sensitive index of nutritional status when normalized to a percentage of body weight or height (49).

Subjective nutritional assessment is another tool that can be used to assess a patient's nutritional status (38,50). This assessment tool uses 21 variables derived from history and physical examination and serum albumin levels. Although this tool is very predictive of nutritional status and outcome (11), it is labor intensive.

TABLE 98-3. *Creatinine kinetics*

Steady state, production (mg/d) = excretion (urinary and
  dialytic) + metabolic degradation
Excretion (mg/d) = $V_u C_u$ + $V_d C_d$
Metabolic degradation (mg/d) = 0.38 × S_{crt} (mg/dL) ×
  body weight (kg)
LBM (kg) = (0.029 × production) (mg/d) + 7.38

V_u, volume of urine (mL/24 h); V_d, volume of effluent dialysate (mL/24 h); C_u, creatinine concentration in urine (mg/mL); C_d, creatinine concentration in effluent dialysate (mg/mL); S_{crt}, serum creatinine (mg/dL); *LBM*, lean body mass.

Modified from: Keshaviah PR, et al. Lean body mass estimation by creatinine kinetics. *J Am Soc Nephrol* 1994;4: 1475.

Impact of Dialysis Dose on Protein Intake

Cross-sectional analysis of a PD population suggests that there is a positive linear correlation between dialysis dose and protein intake (15,32,51–53) (Fig. 98-1). If so, dialysis dose should positively correlate with biochemical estimates of nutritional status such as serum albumin levels; however, as noted in the previous discussion, only some studies have found such a correlation (43,54–56). Some reasons for their lack of correlation were discussed earlier.

Mathematical coupling between PNA and Kt/V has been proposed as another reason for the reported linear relationship (57). The same data (UNA) are used to calculate both. It needs to be proved for an individual patient that there is an increase in protein intake and nutritional parameters as dialysis dose increases. Several studies have shown this to be the case (53,58–61). Preliminary data correlating total energy intake and dietary protein intake from 9-day food records with dialysis dose show a positive correlation between PNA and Kt/V (59). These data suggest that this relationship truly is physiologic.

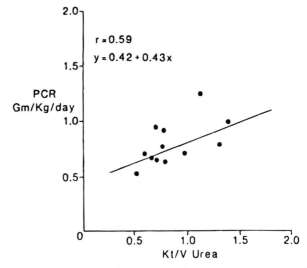

FIG. 98-1. Correlation between total urea clearance over volume of distribution (Kt/V) and protein catabolic rate (PCR).

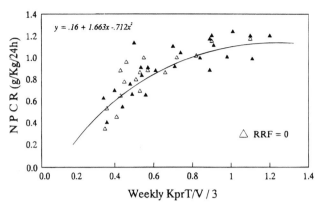

FIG. 98-2. Correlation between overall Kt/V (dialysate and renal) and protein catabolic rate appears to be curvilinear. *KprT/V/3*, total peritoneal and residual Kt/V divided by 3; *NPCR*, normalized protein catabolic rate; *RRF*, residual renal function. (From: Ronco C, et al. Assessment of adequacy in peritoneal dialysis. *Adv Renal Replacement Ther* 1994;1:15, with permission.)

Intuitively, one would postulate that this linear correlation could not continue indefinitely. Blake and colleagues (62) first suggested that the slope of the line relating Kt/V to PNA became less steep when Kt/V was greater than 1.7/week. Subsequently, Ronco and associates (63) reported that the best fit of the line correlating the two values in their CAPD patients was curvilinear, suggesting that once weekly Kt/V 2.3 further increases in dialysis dose resulted in only very small increases in DPI (Fig. 98-2). Preliminary data using 9-day food records to determine protein intake also suggest that this relationship does become curvilinear and eventually plateaus (59).

Based on these studies, the observed relationship between PNA and Kt/V is physiologic, and the point where the curve plateaus may define the "optimal" dose of dialysis for PD patients. The finding of a plateau in the correlation between Kt/V and DPI at a DPI of about 1.2 g/kg ideal weight per day for both HD and PD at different Kt/Vs (64) is consistent with the peak concentration hypothesis (65) and suggests that intermittent therapies for PD may need a higher weekly Kt/V than continuous therapies. Thus, minimal target doses of dialysis can be recommended (Table 98-4). However, to date, no studies in a large cohort of PD patients have shown conclusively that an increase in dialysis dose is associated with a corresponding increase in DPI.

TABLE 98-4. *Recommended target doses for peritoneal dialysis*

Continuous peritoneal dialysis (CAPD, CCPD)
Kt/V ≥ 2.0/wk
Creatinine clearance ≥60 L/wk/1.73 m², unless a low or low average transporter where the target is ≥50 L/wk/1.73 m²
Intermittent peritoneal dialysis
Kt/V ≥ 2.2/wk

Kt/V, total urea clearance over volume of distribution.

Residual Renal Function

Total solute clearance is the total of the net solute removed by both dialysis and residual renal function (RRF). Each 1 mL/minute of creatinine clearance owing to "glomerular filtration" adds 10 L/week of creatinine clearance. Similarly, for each 1 mL/minute of urea clearance, there is approximately 0.25 added to the total weekly Kt/V for a 70-kg man. A residual renal creatinine clearance of 6 mL/minute (possible glomerular filtration rate [GFR] of about 3 mL/minute) adds approximately 30 L/week of creatinine clearance to overall solute clearance. Considering that a total of 70 L/week of creatinine clearance is the minimal recommended for "adequate therapy," one can appreciate the magnitude of the RRF contribution to overall clearance. As RRF deteriorates, the patient may experience inadequate total clearance if the dialysis dose is not increased.

It is now well documented that RRF is better preserved with PD than HD (66,67). Unfortunately, RRF does deteriorate over time (43,46,51,61,68). Furthermore, patients with the most severe malnutrition tend to have the worst RRF (38).

At very low GFRs, much of the urine creatinine is owing to tubular secretion rather than glomerular filtration. Consequently, 24-hour collection measurements of creatinine clearance can significantly overestimate true GFR. Therefore, when attempting to determine the RRF clearance of small-molecular-weight substances, only the clearance owing to GFR is wanted. Small-solute clearance measured as Kt/V and creatinine clearance correlate best when adjusted for tubular secretion of creatinine (modified renal creatinine clearance). Keshaviah (61) recommends averaging the residual renal creatinine and urea clearances as an estimate of GFR when using creatinine kinetics. No adjustment is needed with urea kinetics.

Another clinical result of this difference in residual renal clearance of creatinine and urea is that the numerical value for creatinine clearance (in mL/minute, L/week, etc.) is relatively higher than that of urea. In contrast, as discussed in the following, the peritoneal clearance of urea is relatively more than that of creatinine. These differences become important when discussing target solute clearances goals in patients with varying amounts of residual renal and peritoneal clearances. Patients with significant amounts of residual renal clearance have relatively higher creatinine clearances than anuric patients who have the same urea clearance.

Dietary Protein Requirements in Peritoneal Dialysis

The precise DPI required to maintain nitrogen balance in PD patients is unclear. Blumenkrantz and associates (69) and Diamond and Henrich (70) suggested that a DPI of 1.2 g/kg per day was needed; however, cross-sectional studies suggest that patients who show no signs of malnutrition seem to eat less (0.88 to 0.99 g/kg per day) (52,71). In another study, during which nitrogen balance was measured in CAPD patients on a diet thought to correspond to their spontaneous daily energy

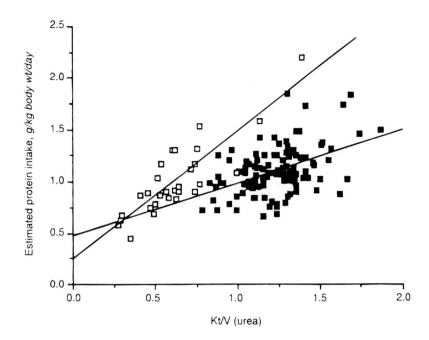

FIG. 98-3. The relationship via linear regression of protein catabolic rate to total urea clearance over volume of distribution in continuous ambulatory peritoneal dialysis *(hollow squares)* and hemodialysis *(solid squares)*. (From: Bergstrom J, Lindholm B. Nutrition and adequacy of dialysis: how do hemodialysis and CAPD compare? *Kidney Int* 1993;43:S39, with permission.)

intake, some patients with a protein intake as low as 0.7 g/kg per day were thought to be in nitrogen balance (72). These data were obtained using PNA and PCR to estimate DPI. Many reports have shown that DPI estimated from dietary recall is much higher than that estimated from urea generation rates using the Randerson equation (72–74); however, protein intake was still lower than the 1.2 g/kg per day recommended from balance studies. Nitrogen balance is related not only to protein intake but also to total energy intake (72), and this may explain some of these discrepancies.

If a DPI of 1.0 g/kg per day is considered adequate to maintain normal nutrition, then a "minimal" dose of PD needed to achieve this can be estimated from published data (Fig. 98-3). These data would suggest that for PD patients to achieve a PNA of approximately 1.0 g/kg per day, a HD equivalent dose of dialysis (Kt/V) of at least 0.6 is required, a dose similar to the minimal recommendations established from PD outcome studies (23,46,75). It is interesting to note that in the curvilinear relationships between Kt/V and DPI, the curve tends to plateau at a DPI of 1.0 to 1.2 g/kg per day in both HD and PD patients (Fig. 98-4).

STEPS IN PRESCRIPTION DIALYSIS

Determination of Peritoneal Transport Characteristics

There is interpatient variation in peritoneal membrane transport characteristics. Thus, peritoneal equilibration testing (PET) is the standard way to characterize these transport properties (76). After drainage of an overnight dwell, 2 L of 2.5% dextrose dialysate are instilled (time 0) and allowed to dwell for 4 hours. Dialysate urea, glucose, and creatinine are measured at time 0, and after 2 and 4 hours of dwell time, and compared to serum values obtained after 2 hours of dwell. Four-hour drain volume is also measured. For each

dwell time, dialysate to plasma ratios (D/P) of creatinine and urea are determined, as is the ratio of glucose at the drain time to the initial dialysate glucose concentration (D/D$_0$). These results are plotted against time and compared to known standard curves (Fig. 98-5). The patient's peritoneal membrane type can be characterized using the standard 2.5% dextrose PET, and the PD prescription is matched to the patient's transport characteristics (Table 98-5).

Dialytic solute clearance is composed of diffusively derived solute as well as solute derived convectively owing to ultrafiltration (UF). Patients with smaller drain volumes (i.e., less UF) tend to have lower dialytic clearances.

High (rapid) transporters of creatinine and urea also tend to be rapid absorbers of dialysate glucose. Therefore, although

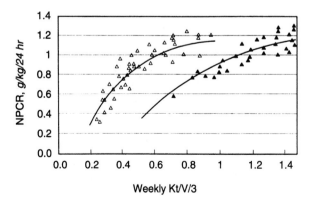

FIG. 98-4. Correlation between total urea clearance over volume of distribution (Kt/V) (weekly Kt/V divided by 3) and protein catabolic rate (NPCR) for hemodialysis (HD) patients *(solid triangles)* and continuous ambulatory peritoneal dialysis (CAPD) patients *(open triangles)*. In contrast to previous reports, the nonlinear correlation appears to be the stronger relationship. (From: Ronco C, et al. Adequacy of CAPD. *Kidney Int* 1994;46:S18, with permission.)

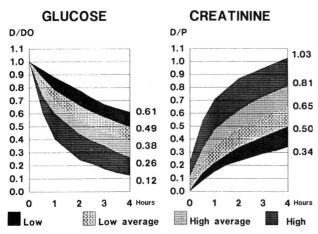

FIG. 98-5. Dialysate to plasma ratios (D/P) for creatinine and drain time to initial dialysis concentration (D/DO) ratios for glucose, generated from standard peritoneal equilibration testing. (From: Twardowski ZJ. Clinical value of standardized equilibration tests in CAPD patients. *Blood Purif* 1989;7:95, with permission.)

the D/P creatinine ratios for 4-hour dwell tend to be close to 1, drain volumes tend to be small. High transporters maximize their D/P ratios and intraperitoneal volumes early during the dwell. Once the osmotic gradient dissipates, UF ceases, followed thereafter by net fluid reabsorption caused by lymphatic reabsorption. With standard CAPD, these patients may have drain volumes that are actually less than instilled volumes. Short dwell times often are needed to optimize clearance (77) (Fig. 98-6).

In low (slow) transporters, peak UF occurs late during the dwell, and net UF can be obtained even after prolonged dwells because glucose absorption is slow. The D/P ratios for creatinine and urea increase almost linearly during the dwell. For these patients, dwell time is the crucial determinant of overall clearance. They do best with continuous therapies such as standard CAPD or continuous cycling PD (CCPD). Patients with very large body surface areas may need high doses of PD or possibly even adjunctive HD treatments.

Although the standard 2.5% dextrose PET is the most practical, there are alternative methods to classify membrane

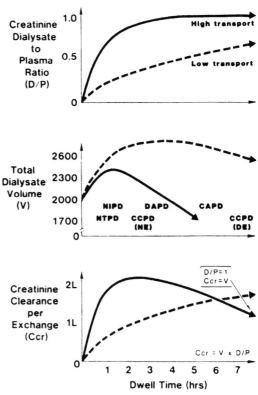

FIG. 98-6. Theoretical relationships between dwell time, dialysis to plasma (D/P) creatinine ratio, dialysate volume (V), and creatinine clearance (Ccr) per exchange compared for rapid or high transporters *(solid curves)* and slow or low transporters *(dashed curves)* during 2 L 2.5% dextrose exchanges. The lower panel curves are derived from the upper and middle panels. Nightly intermittent peritoneal dialysis (NIPD) and nightly tidal peritoneal dialysis (NTPD) use short dwell exchanges and are best suited for high or rapid transporters. In continuous ambulatory peritoneal dialysis (CAPD) and continuous cycling peritoneal dialysis (CCPD) with a diurnal (daytime) exchange (DE), there are longer dwells most suited for low or slow transporters. Daytime CAPD (DAPD) and the nocturnal exchanges (NE) of CCPD usually utilize dwell times of 2 to 4 hours and can be suitable for some fast transporters. The diurnal exchange of CCPD is not suitable for high transporters. (From: Twardowski ZJ. Nightly peritoneal dialysis (why? who? how? and when?). *Trans Am Soc Artif Intern Org* 1990;36:8, with permission.)

TABLE 98-5. *Predicted response to continuous ambulatory peritoneal dialysis: baseline peritoneal equilibration testing prognostic value*

Solute peritoneal transport	UF	Dialysis adequacy	Preferred dialysis modality
High	Poor	Yes	NDP, DAPD
High average	Adequate	Yes	Standard CAPD[a]
Low average	Good	Yes	Standard CAPD[a]
Low average	Good	No	High-flow PD[b]
Low	Excellent	No	High-flow PD[b]

UF, ultrafiltration; *NPD,* nightly peritoneal dialysis; *DAPD,* daytime ambulatory peritoneal dialysis; *CAPD,* continuous ambulatory peritoneal dialysis; *PD,* peritoneal dialysis.

[a]CAPD with 7.5 to 9.0 L/d, or continuous cycling peritoneal dialysis (CCPD) with dialysis solution inflow 6 to 8 L overnight and 2 L daytime.

[b]CAPD with >9.0 L/d, or CCPD with inflow >8 L overnight and/or 2 L daytime.

Modified from: Twardowski ZJ. Nightly peritoneal dialysis (why? who? how? and when?). *Trans Am Soc Artif Intern Org* 1990;36:8.

transport. Mass transfer area coefficients (MTAC) more succinctly define peritoneal transport by diffusion (78,79). These define transport independent of UF (convection-related solute removal) and consequently are not influenced by dwell volume or glucose concentration. The practical use of MTAC for modeling a peritoneal dialysis prescription requires additional laboratory measurements and computer models, but once these are obtained, MTAC can be used easily in the clinical setting (80). The PET is used specifically to characterize the patient's peritoneal membrane transport properties. It is not a measurement of dialysis dose. Although daily clearances can be estimated from PET studies, these estimates can significantly overestimate or underestimate actual daily clearances (81). Additionally, as more has become known about ultrafiltration and water transport across the peritoneal membrane, it has been recommended that a 4.25% dextrose PET be used to characterize transport and evaluate aquaporin-mediated water transport (82). The 4.25% PET has been compared to the 2.5% PET in a cohort of chronic PD patients and no clinically significant difference in D/P curves were found, although there was a significant difference in drain volume and decrease in dialysate sodium levels owing to aquaporin-mediated water transport as expected, suggesting that the 4.25% PET may be as clinically useful in prescription management as is the 2.5% PET (83).

Measurements to Monitor Dialysis Dose

There is no single documented "uremic toxin"; therefore, there is some controversy over which laboratory parameters should be used as an index for adequacy of dialysis. There are data to suggest that the outcome for PD patients is related to the dose of dialysis when measured in urea kinetics (23,51) and also when measured in creatinine kinetics (11,54,84,85). These studies support the use of clearance data to measure dialysis dose. Other studies have documented that serum albumin levels are inversely correlated with an increasing risk of death in PD patients and that DPI correlates with the dialysis dose.

Although a higher Kt/V is associated with a higher PCR, one should not monitor nutritional status only, such as monthly serum albumin levels. There are many diverse causes of low serum albumin levels, only one of which is inadequate dialysis. Both dose and protein intake should be monitored because the relationship among DPI, dose of dialysis, and uremic manifestations is different in each patient. As is clear from Table 98-6, small-solute clearance is substantially less for PD than HD. Yet outcome is no different for similar populations (86–88). It is also clear from Table 98-6 that solute clearances in CAPD exceed those of standard HD for all but the small-molecular-weight solutes. Is the reason that survival rates on CAPD and HD are similar because of comparable "middle-molecule" clearance? Should middle-molecule clearance be measured as the "PD yardstick?" It is a common clinical experience that when CAPD patients manifest uremic symptoms, they improve after increasing

TABLE 98-6. *Solute removal by dialysis and the natural kidney*

Solute clearance	Natural kidney	HD low flux	HD high flux	CAPD
Urea (L/wk)	750	130	130	70
Vitamin B$_{12}$ (L/wk)	1,200	30	60	40
Inulin (L/wk)	1,200	10	40	20
β_2-Microglobulin (mg/wk)	1,000	0	300	250

HD, hemodialysis; *CAPD,* continuous ambulatory peritoneal dialysis.
Modified from: Keshaviah P. Adequacy of CAPD: a quantitative approach. *Kidney Int* 1992;42:5160.

the volume or number of exchanges per day. Figure 98-7 demonstrates the theoretic influence of the number of CAPD exchanges on the weekly solute clearance for a wide range of molecular weights. It is clear that increasing the number of exchanges per day results in only a minimal increase in large- or middle-molecule clearance, but a marked increase in small-solute clearance. Therefore, based on Keshaviah's theoretic projections (61) and the available clinical experience, it seems that overall small-solute clearance, not middle- or large-molecular-weight clearance, is most closely related to uremic toxicity and urea or creatinine kinetics should be used for monitoring dialysis dose, with one caveat. This assumes that the middle molecule clearance is not decreased. It is important to note that clearances of middle molecular weight substances are markedly time-dependent (number of hours of dwell time). Maneuvers that increase small solute clearances while decreasing middle molecule clearance may be associated with an increase relative risk of an adverse outcome (89).

The choice between using urea kinetics or creatinine clearance as the measurement of dialysis dose is arbitrary. Current data in general suggest that there is no clinical advantage of one over the other. However, the CANUSA study proposes that creatinine kinetics are stronger predictors of outcome

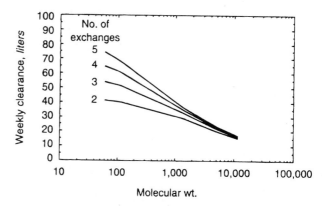

FIG. 98-7. The influence of the number of exchanges on the weekly solute clearance for a range of solute molecular weights derived from a computerized model of peritoneal transport. (From: Keshaviah P. Adequacy of CAPD: a quantitative approach. *Kidney Int* 1992;42:S160, with permission).

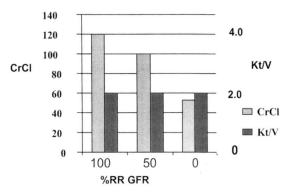

FIG. 98-8. Theoretical calculations of total solute clearance in terms of total urea clearance over volume of distribution (Kt/V) and creatinine clearance (CCr) in an average transporter of average weight with varying amounts of residual renal and peritoneal clearances (100% RR, 50% RR and 50% PD, 100% PD) assuming total Kt/V is 2.0/week in all cases. (From: Burkart J. Adequacy of peritoneal dialysis. *Advan Renal Replace Ther* 2000;7:310, with permission.)

than urea kinetics (11). This is probably because these were incident patients and their residual renal function was the component of their total solute clearance most likely to differ at baseline and change over time. As mentioned, patients who have a significant amount of residual renal function are likely to have relatively higher creatinine clearance than urea clearance because of the creatinine secretion by proximal tubules and urea reabsorption. In anuric patients the urea clearance in mL/minute or L/day is relatively higher than that of creatinine because of differences in diffusion rates for these solutes; consequently, the expected clearance of creatinine in L/week per 1.73 m^2 is different in a patient who is just starting PD with a residual renal Kt/V of 2.0/week than in an anuric patient with a peritoneal Kt/V urea of 2.0/week (Fig. 98-8). Thus, although both markers of solute clearance may be predictors of outcome, the target or goal for creatinine clearance may have to change over time as residual renal function decreases and is replaced by peritoneal clearance. On the other hand, it appears from outcome studies that the Kt/V target may not need change.

When changing from standard CAPD (long dwells) to cycler therapy (short dwells), it is important to remember the difference in transport rates of urea and creatinine. Transport of urea into the dialysate tends to occur faster than creatinine. For that reason, if dialysis dose is being monitored using urea kinetics, keeping Kt/V constant going from long to short dwells may decrease creatinine clearance. In contrast, if dialysis dose is measured using creatinine clearance, keeping creatinine clearance constant when changing from long to short dwells may keep Kt/V constant or even increase it. This concept has been termed "horizontal modeling" (90). This is clinically relevant. If one does switch from CAPD to intermittent PD (IPD) and at the same time there is a very slight increase in Kt/V, the weekly creatinine clearance is likely to decrease or stay the same. If creatinine kinetics were used and the prescription is modeled to keep the creatinine clearance

the same, then Kt/V will probably increase. These changes are amplified in high versus low transporters and become more apparent for creatinine as dwell times decrease (as with cycler therapies).

How to Monitor Dialysis Dose

It is recommended that monitoring should include both dialysis dose and nutritional parameters because outcomes correlate with both. Collections of dialysate and urine over 24 hours are relatively easy to obtain and can provide most of the clinically relevant data one needs to individualize a patient's prescription and monitor progress. These collections also can be used to calculate PNA, LBM, and other variables (Table 98-7). Mathematical estimations of daily clearance tend to correlate with the actual clearance measured from 24-hour collections, but there is a high degree of discordance (81). Peritoneal equilibration testing (PET) data are obtained to characterize and monitor the patient's peritoneal membrane transport characteristics. The two tests are complementary to each other and are routinely used together for developing a patient's dialysis prescription and problem solving.

It is common practice to obtain a PET periodically. In fact, the Health Care Finance Administration's ESRD Networks have mandated adequacy of PD testing twice per year. Peritoneal membrane transport tends to be stable over time (91). If there is a change over time, the D/P ratios are likely to increase slightly, and there may be a small decrease in UF.

TABLE 98-7. *Usefulness of 24-hour dialysate and urine collection*

Creatinine kinetics
Creatinine clearance[a]
Creatinine clearance[b]
Total creatinine clearance[a,b]
Creatinine production[a,b]
Lean body mass[a,b]
D/P creatinine[a]
Ratio of measure to predicted creatinine generation
Urea kinetics
Urea clearance[a]
Urea clearance[b]
Total urea clearance[a,b]
PNA[a,b]
Urea generation[a,b]
Creatinine and urea kinetics
Estimated glomerular filtration rate (modified creatinine clearance) 24-hour urine
Drain volume—ultrafiltration rates

D/P, dialysis to plasma ratio; *PNA,* protein equivalent of nitrogen appearance.
[a]Dialysis only.
[b]Urine only.
Modified from: Burkart JM, et al. 24-hour dialysate collection versus peritoneal equilibrium test for determining adequacy of peritoneal dialysis. *Peritoneal Dial Int* 1992;12:104.

Calculation of Dialysis Dose

To individualize dialysis dose and make comparisons of dose between patients, Twardowski and Nolph (92) recommend normalizing creatinine clearance to body surface area using 1.73 m² as the standard body surface area. If urea kinetics (Kt/V) are used, the sum of the daily dialysate and residual renal (RRUrCl/day) urea clearances (DialUrCl/day) are then divided by the volume of distribution (V), as with HD (93). The urea V can be estimated to be 60% (males) or 55% (females) of the patient's weight in kilograms. More accurate estimations of V can be obtained using standardized nomograms, such as Watson (94) or Hume and Weyers (95).

A controversial issue is what weight should one use when calculating V and body surface area (BSA) (96). Weight has a different effect on normalization (V or BSA) for male or female and for CCr versus Kt/V. The mathematical relationship between BSA and V is not fixed and is most disturbed by gender and obesity. These differences are most marked when a patient's weight differs significantly from the norm in patients with the same height and frame. The actual V is different in a patient with the same body weight if the increase in body weight from ideal is owing to overhydration or increase in adipose tissue. The same is true if loss of weight is due to malnutrition versus amputation. There are published recommendations for how to adjust for amputations when calculating V (97). Jones (98) noted that when actual body weight was used for normalization, there was no difference in total solute clearance (Kt/V or CCr) between nourished and malnourished patients. However, when calculated V and BSA were determined using desired body weight, there was a significant difference. The NKF-DOQI guidelines suggest that in malnourished patients one must adjust the total solute clearance goals for that patient to promote anabolism. The guidelines suggest that the minimal weekly total solute clearance goal should be adjusted by the ratio of desired:actual body weight. In those cases, the minimal solute clearance in terms of urea kinetics would be higher than 2.0 (i.e., 2.0 × desired:actual body weight). Further studies are needed to confirm the appropriateness of this recommendation.

Calculation of Dietary Protein Intake

Dietary protein intake (DPI) can be directly measured in metabolic wards, by dietary histories or food recall records. An advantage of using food records is that they also evaluate total energy intake. Energy intake and DPI often do not correlate. Unfortunately, food records are time consuming and difficult to obtain because they require trained dietitians. Therefore, most reports relating dialysis dose to DPI use estimations, based on UNA, total nitrogen appearance (TNA), or PNA (99–101). The most commonly used formulas to estimate PNA or PCR include: (a) the modified Borah equation (44), based on a linear correlation between urea generation

and DPI in HD patients with measured protein losses in the dialysate included; (b) the Randerson technique (102), based on a similar linear correlation between urea generation rates and DPI established in a CAPD population; (c) the Teehan technique (103), based on an estimate of total nitrogen losses by adding measured to averaged losses determined from a literature review, then multiplied by 6.25 (percent of protein that is nitrogen); and (d) the Kjeldahl technique (104), based on actual nitrogen losses in the effluent dialysate (Table 98-2).

The total PNA is then divided by the patient's body weight to determine the "normalized" PNA (nPNA), expressed in grams per kilogram of body weight per day. The target nPNA is at least 1.0 g/kg per day, corresponding to a DPI of about 1.0 g/kg per day. This term does not take into account differences in frame size and LBM. If a patient is markedly obese, the aforementioned calculations give a falsely low nPNA for the patient's actual LBM. Conversely, if a patient is malnourished and has a less than expected LBM, these equations give you a falsely elevated nPNA. Various attempts to avoid this problem are under investigation, but corrections have not been standardized. One modification uses actual measurements of V or data from nomograms that more accurately estimate V. This V is then "normalized" by dividing it by 0.58 kg/L to determine normalized body weight (NBW). The PCR is then divided by NBW to get nPNA. An extension of these principles is utilized to determine lean body mass from creatinine kinetics (105).

Compliance and Other Pitfalls in Prescribing Peritoneal Dialysis

For a variety of reasons, patients may be adherent to their prescribed regimen during the testing period, but not routinely, and consequently may be inadequately dialyzed on a daily basis. The ratio of measured to predicted creatinine generation might provide insight into a patient's overall compliance (106,107). If patients do their prescribed number of exchanges on the day that they collect their 24-hour collections after periods of underdialysis, a new steady state is created, and the measured creatinine production is higher than the predicted because of a "washout" effect. Additionally, because of the washout of creatinine and urea, the measured Kt/V, creatinine clearance, and PNA are all higher than those actually delivered. Further experience is needed with this approach. It appears likely that noncompliance is one possible cause for ratios above unity (108).

Some issues to consider in patients on standard CAPD are: (a) inappropriate dwell times (a rapid transporter would do better with short dwells); (b) failure to increase dialysis dose to compensate for loss of RRF; (c) inappropriate instilled volume (patient may only infuse 2 L of a 2.5-L bag); (d) multiple rapid exchanges and one very long dwell (patient may do three exchanges between 9 AM and 5 PM, and a long dwell from 5 PM to 9 AM, limiting overall clearances); and (e) inappropriate selection of dialysate glucose for long dwells that may not maximize UF and clearance.

TABLE 98-8. *Minimal total solute clearance goals for peritoneal dialysis: recommendations from various committees*

Continuous ambulatory peritoneal dialysis			
Committee		Kt/V	Creatinine clearance
NKF-DOQI (1997)		2.0	>60 L/wk/1.73 m²
Renal Association UK		1.7	>50 L/wk/1.73 m²
Canada[4] H and HA transporters		2.0	>60 L/wk/1.73 m²
L and LA transporters		2.0	>50 L/wk/1.73 m²
NKF-DOQI–II (revised 2000)		2.0	>60 L/wk/1.73 m²
H and HA transporters		2.0	>50 L/wk/1.73 m²
L and LA transporters			
Ad Hoc Committee			
Underdialysis	???Borderline	<1.7	<50
	???Acceptable	1.7–1.89	50–59
		1.9–2.09	60–69
	???Desirable	>2.09	>70
Continuous cycling peritoneal dialysis			
Committee		Kt/V	Creatinine clearance
NKF-DOQI (1997)		>2.1	>63 L/wk/1.73 m²
Canada		>2.0	>50 L/wk/1.73 m²
NKF-DOQI–II (2000)		>2.0	>63 L/wk/1.73 m²

Modified from: Burkart J. Adequacy of peritoneal dialysis. *Adv Renal Replace Ther* 2000;7:310.

Other problems are specific for those patients on cycler therapy. The drain time may be inappropriately long (more than 20 minutes). Inappropriately short dwell times may be such that clearances are not maximized. Failure to augment total dialysis dose with a daytime dwell ("wet" day versus "dry" day) could also result in underdialysis. Finally, inappropriate selection of dialysate glucose may not allow maximization of UF, resulting in less total clearance. One may be able to achieve weekly urea clearance targets but not creatinine or middle molecule clearance targets with short dwell and intermittent clearance—nightly intermittent peritoneal dialysis (NIPD). A shortened time with fluid in the peritoneum is accompanied by decreased middle molecule clearances and this may have an adverse effect on outcomes. There are no outcome data in patients on NIPD. It may be that when patients become anuric, they must maximize their "time" (most of day) on dialysis to maintain middle molecular weight clearances.

Minimal Total Solute Clearance Goals

Desirable targets for dialysis doses are outlined in Table 98-4. Original NKF-DOQI targets were developed based on outcome data and opinion available as of May 1997. Since then, more clinical experience with these targets and additional outcome data have become available. Hence, the NKF-DOQI committee has adjusted its recommendations and subsequent working groups have formulated slightly different targets. Reasons for these revised minimal total solute clearance goals have been reviewed elsewhere (109). These include issues such as new data on anuric patients (110), the observation that patients who are low and low-average solute transporters

have a lower relative risk of morbidity and or death than high and high-average transporters with the same solute clearances (111,112), and the known differences in solute transport of urea and creatinine by residual renal function and the peritoneum. The revised NKF-DOQI guidelines and subsequent guidelines from Canada (113) and the United Kingdom (114) reflect these observations. In general they are similar. Both the revised DOQI and the Canadian guidelines recommend a weekly Kt/V of 2.0 for CAPD patients with lower solute clearance goals in terms of CCr for low and low average transporters. The Canadian guidelines do not recommend adjusting targets for CCPD or NIPD. The guidelines from the UK recommend lower targets in general and as the Canadian guidelines, do not have different targets for CCPD or NIPD (Table 98-8).

Adjusting Dialysis Dose

When prescribing an individual patient's treatment program, one should aim for a dose in the optimal range. One must also monitor other indices of adequate dialysis such as quality of life, blood pressure, and DPI. If during routine monitoring or clinical evaluation the delivered dose of dialysis needs to be altered, this can be done in a scientific manner with knowledge of the PET, the present total clearance of urea or creatinine, and understanding the relationship among dialysis clearance, drain volume, and dwell time based on the measured D/P ratios. Increasing the instilled volume does not always result in an increase in clearance. For instance, in a low transporter in whom clearance is critically dependent on dwell time, changing from standard CAPD (infused volume of 8 L) to cycler therapy using 2-hour dwells and infused volumes of 10 to 14 L may not always result in an overall increase in clearance.

To adjust the dialysate prescription, one needs to know the D/P ratio at the anticipated dwell time and the patient's drain volume for that dwell time. By altering dwell time, one can change the D/P ratio and the drain volume. Altering instilled volume also affects total drain volume and convective clearance. In general, increasing the instilled volume without changing dwell time results in an increase in solute clearance.

PERITONEAL DIALYSIS MODALITY SELECTION

Technique variations for PD can be manual and/or automated and either continuous or intermittent. Peritoneal blood flow and dialysate flow are considerably less than that with typical HD. Therefore, clearance of small solutes such as urea or creatinine are less than that with HD. Weekly clearances approach those of HD because CAPD is performed in a continuous fashion. Urea and other small solutes readily diffuse from blood to dialysate, and equilibrium may even be reached during the dwell in high (rapid) transporters. There is continued removal of middle and larger molecules throughout the dwell. Smaller patients may be more comfortable with lower instilled volumes. Patients with respiratory disease may become symptomatic when supine. Thus, choosing a PD method is based on both medical and nonmedical factors (115).

Peritoneal Dialysis Techniques: Continuous Therapies

Continuous Ambulatory Peritoneal Dialysis

Continuous ambulatory peritoneal dialysis is the most commonly used form of PD. Since its original description, there have been few changes in the basic therapy, although there have been many changes in the connection devices or "connectology" used to make the exchange. The long dwells associated with CAPD achieve adequate daily small-solute clearances. Because of the long dwells and continuous nature of the therapy, most end-stage renal disease (ESRD) patients can achieve the minimal daily-recommended dialysis dose. Continuous ambulatory peritoneal dialysis is a manual therapy and usually uses less fluid than automated PD. The usual dialysis prescription for patients on this technique is four exchanges per day of 2.0- or 2.5-L dwells. Continuous ambulatory peritoneal dialysis must be individualized by increasing or decreasing dwell volume and by altering the number of exchanges per day.

Continuous Cycling Peritoneal Dialysis

Continuous cycling peritoneal dialysis uses an automated cycler to perform exchanges while the patient sleeps with a subsequent daytime dwell; therefore, this is a constant therapy. Weekly clearances for typical CCPD are similar to those of CAPD; however, CCPD adds the extra cost of the cycler and the need for fresh tubing on a daily basis. Modifications of this technique include altering the number of nightly exchanges, dwell time, instilled volume, and occasionally combining CAPD technology to augment clearances by having the patient do one or more manual exchanges during the day. Clearances with this technique can be augmented by longer times on the cycler, more rapid cycler exchanges, or by doing a daytime exchange.

Peritoneal Dialysis Techniques: Intermittent Therapies

Because intermittent therapies typically use multiple short dwells, they tend to be automated but can be done manually. For chronic therapy intermittent peritoneal dialysis (IPD) is best suited for patients who are found to be high transporters based on PET (76). It is estimated that 10% to 15% of patients on PD are high transporters who would do best on short dwell therapies. Patients who are average or low transporters typically cannot achieve adequate clearances with intermittent techniques unless they have a high level of residual renal function. These therapies also may be transiently indicated during peritonitis for some patients with UF failure (type I membrane failure).

Intermittent Peritoneal Dialysis

By definition, IPD implies that therapy periods alternate with times when the peritoneum has been drained ("dry abdomen"). Typically the patient uses multiple short dwell exchanges three or four times a week. Techniques include manual IPD, cycler IPD, reverse osmosis machine IPD, intermittent reciprocating dialysis with an extracorporeal reconstituting circuit, and others (116). Variations have led to the development of tidal peritoneal dialysis (TPD) (117). Based on presently recommended weekly minimal clearances, it is difficult to achieve these minimal targets in an anuric patient with three or four times a week therapy unless the patient has a prolonged treatment each time (classic IPD).

Nonetheless, classic IPD therapies continue to have their uses. A report from Mexico (where more than 90% of patients with ESRD are on a form of PD) suggested that cycler IPD may be more practical in countries where technical, social, and economic limitations restrict the use of CAPD (118). Other uses include treatment of refractory heart failure (119), as a transient therapy for immediately postoperative patients, or for those who are on CAPD and have developed hernias or leaks (see Hernias and Genital and Abdominal Wall Edema). Lowest intraabdominal pressures are achieved with low-volume supine dialysis.

Nightly Intermittent Peritoneal Dialysis

Nightly intermittent peritoneal dialysis (NIPD) with standard cycling techniques is best utilized by patients with high or high-average transport. Daytime ambulatory peritoneal dialysis (DAPD) is based on the same concept as NIPD, but DAPD is a manual technique, and the patient typically has a "dry time" during the night. Both NIPD and DAPD operate within an intermediate range of dwell times. In rapid transporters, 8 hours of nightly dialysis can yield creatinine clearances similar to or higher than those achieved with standard CAPD. The lower the peritoneal membrane transfer rates, the lower the 8-hour NIPD or DAPD clearances (120), and in some patients, time spent on NIPD or DAPD has to be prolonged by 10% to 40% to achieve minimal target clearances (121). Consequently, the efficiency of standard NIPD or DAPD must be improved to achieve adequate clearances in anuric patients with average or low-average transport characteristics without spending an excessive amount of time on the therapy.

Tidal Peritoneal Dialysis

Tidal peritoneal dialysis (TPD) consists of the repeated instillation of small tidal volumes of dialysis fluids with the use of an automated cycler. The procedure is usually performed nightly. It is assumed that by maintaining an intraperitoneal reservoir and not attempting a complete drain at each exchange, tidal dialysis may maintain more continuous contact of dialysate with the peritoneal membrane. Furthermore, the more rapid cycling of dialysis may increase mixing and prevent formation of stagnant intraperitoneal fluid layers. Although preliminary studies suggest that creatinine and urea clearances are augmented (122), many clinicians continue to reserve enthusiasm for this approach pending more outcome data. Variables to be chosen include reserve volume, tidal outflow volume, tidal replacement volume, flow rates, and frequency of the exchanges. Tidal peritoneal dialysis was developed in an attempt to increase the efficiency of NIPD techniques (123). Spencer and Farrell (124) have shown that MTACs increase as instilled volume is increased from 1 to 2 L, presumably because of an increase in dialysate–peritoneal surface area contact (124). However, an increase from 2 to 3 L does not always result in an increase in transport (125). Therefore, other mechanisms of increasing efficiency needed to be considered. A major disadvantage of TPD is the cost of the extra dialysate.

ULTRAFILTRATION

A certain minimal amount of daily UF is necessary to maintain water balance in patients with ESRD. This is achieved by an osmotic pressure gradient between blood and the dialysate using glucose as the effective osmotic force. During UF, retained solutes are swept along with the bulk solvent flow even in the absence of a concentration difference for diffusion. This contribution to net solute clearance has been termed solvent drag or convection; therefore, overall solute clearance is the sum of that owing to diffusion and convection.

Clinical Physiology

In addition to UF absorption of fluid from the peritoneal cavity, UF also occurs mainly via lymphatics (126). Intraperitoneal volume at any time is determined by the relative magnitudes of transcapillary UF and lymphatic reabsorption. Net UF at the end of any dwell is defined as the difference between drained volume and instilled volume. This definition assumes that the residual volume is constant, which is often not the case (127,128). This variation is insignificant for day-to-day clinical practice.

The driving force for UF decreases as the membrane becomes more permeable to solutes and the osmotic gradient diminishes. Ultrafiltration rates are highest at the beginning of the dwell. As glucose is absorbed, UF decreases as osmotic equilibrium is approached (129). Depending on the concentration of instilled glucose, osmotic equilibrium is reached at different times in the dwell cycle. For 2-L solutions containing 1.5% dextrose, osmotic equilibrium and maximal drain volume are reached after about 2 hours of dwell time in patients with average peritoneal membrane transport characteristics. For 4.25% dextrose solutions, peak intraperitoneal volumes are not likely to occur until after 3 or 4 hours (77). As osmotic equilibrium is approached, intraperitoneal volume and ultimate drain volume decrease owing to isosmotic absorption of fluids. In CAPD patients, this absorption rate ranges from 40 to 60 mL/hour and is attributable primarily to lymphatic drainage of the peritoneum (130).

Ultrafiltration Failure

Peritoneal UF is considered adequate when at least 5.5 mL of filtrate is generated per 1 g of absorbed glucose (92). Ultrafiltration failure can be defined as the failure of fluid removal by peritoneal dialysis to match the volume balance and blood pressure needs of the patient (i.e., there must be a balance of input and output). Ultrafiltration failure represents a failure to maintain volume homeostasis. This definition implies that clinically UF failure can result from inadequate fluid removal by PD or excessive salt and water intake. Furthermore, failure to remove adequate amounts of salt and water by the current PD prescription does not necessarily imply that there must be a pathologic alteration of the peritoneal membrane itself. Other possible causes include catheter malfunction, inadequate use of hypertonic fluids, inappropriately long dwell times, increased lymphatic reabsorption, fluid sequestration, and failure to match dwell time to peritoneal membrane transport status (132–134).

Ultrafiltration failure in CAPD may be defined as clinical evidence of fluid overload despite restriction of fluid intake and the use of three or more hypertonic (4.25% dextrose) exchanges per day (131). However, other definitions have been used in various publications; therefore, the exact incidence of UF failure is unknown. At one center, UF failure was observed in 6.2% of 227 CAPD patients over 10 years, and the

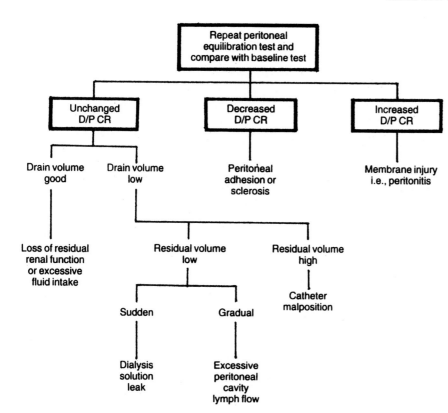

FIG. 98-9. Algorithm for loss of ultra-filtration in continuous ambulatory peritoneal dialysis (CAPD) patients. *D/P CR,* dialysis:plasma creatinine ratio. (From: Khanna R, Nolph KD, Oreopoulos DG, eds. *Essentials of peritoneal dialysis.* Dordrecht, The Netherlands: Kluwer Academic, 1993:98, with permission.)

risk increased with time on PD (135). The prevalence was 2.6% after 1 year on PD and 30.9% after 6 years. Others claim that UF failure is responsible for up to 15% of PD technique discontinuation (136,137). If one considers a more rigid definition such as one defined by the ability of a specified hypertonic dwell to remove a certain amount of fluid, the true incidence is rather low.

Clinical symptoms consistent with UF failure are not always caused by an actual loss of peritoneal UF capacity. Fluid overload, clinically mimicking UF failure, may occur when urine volume decreases and fluid intake is excessive or during noncompliance with the prescribed exchange regimen. Dialysate leaks from the intraabdominal cavity into extraabdominal tissue spaces may also result in loss of UF because of a decrease in dialysate contact with the peritoneal membrane. These causes are not associated with a change in peritoneal membrane transport characteristics. The first steps in the evaluation of a patient with suspected UF failure are to determine urine volume and to establish whether net effluent drain volume and/or peritoneal transport have changed. Apparent loss of UF is potentially reversible if caused by catheter malposition, dialysate leak, or recent peritonitis but usually is permanent if kinetic studies suggest a reduction in UF capacity of the membrane.

An ad hoc committee has recently reviewed UF issues in PD and recommended a specific clinical definition for membrane failure while outlining a rational approach to fluid management and blood pressure control (138). This is based in part on prior classifications based on transport findings and has been revised for patients with irreversible UF failure (133,134). This group recommends using a 4-hour dwell with 2.0 L of 4.25% dextrose dialysate to diagnose and work-up UF failure. Using this definition, less than 400 mL of net ultrafiltration after a 4-hour dwell is diagnostic of true peritoneal membrane failure. A rational approach to the patient with suspected UF failure is found in Fig. 98-9. If a patient presents with the clinical syndrome of volume overload, one first: (a) rules out dietary indiscretion; (b) assures that patient is on the appropriate prescription for his or her peritoneal membrane transport type; and (c) rules out mechanical problems. If these do not confirm the cause, then a 4.25% PET is done, UF volume and D/P creatinine ratios are noted. Further evaluation is based on D/P creatinine ratio.

Ultrafiltration Failure and High Solute Transport

Patients with loss of UF and current 4-hour PET ratios of D/D_0 glucose of less than 0.3 and D/P creatinine of greater than 0.81 are characterized as high solute transporters (Fig. 98-5). These patients tend to have rapid small-molecular-weight solute transport and poor UF owing to high (rapid) glucose absorption and resultant rapid dissipation of the osmotic gradient. These patients are the largest group with true UF failure. Some patients have these transport characteristics at baseline, and if their dwell times are mismatched for their membrane transport characteristics, they often appear to have UF failure as they lose residual renal function and no longer have urine flow to supplement dialysate daily fluid losses. In other patients, the loss of UF is owing to an increase in membrane transport. This increase is caused by either an acquired increase in transport (formerly called type I membrane failure) or membrane changes associated with a recent episode of peritonitis.

Recent Peritonitis

It is a common clinical experience for PD patients to experience fluid retention during peritonitis. Compared to baseline, during peritonitis PET reveals an increase in the D/P ratio for creatinine and a decrease in the D/D_0 ratio for glucose. There is also an increase in dialysate protein losses and a significant decrease in net UF (139). These changes associated with peritonitis are usually reversible after recovery. Microscopic findings in patients with acute peritonitis have revealed denudation of the mesothelial surface (140,141). However, in some patients, remesothelialization never occurs even after recovery from peritonitis (142). This leads to chronic UF loss and is referred to as type I membrane failure. Di Paolo and coworkers (143) have demonstrated that autoimplantation of labeled cultured mesothelial cells in rabbits and CAPD patients with peritonitis resulted in reimplantation, improvement in UF parameters, and normalization of dialysate phospholipid concentrations. Further studies are needed before widespread clinical use of this technique is advocated. These patients often need a temporary change in their standard dialysis prescription (shorter dwell times or increased tonicity) to maintain UF. If available, several studies have indicated that UF during an episode of peritonitis can be maintained with alternative osmotic agents such as icodextrin (144).

Acquired Increase in Membrane Transport

Patients who develop an increase in peritoneal transport over time on PD (formally called type I membrane failure) are the most common cause of chronic UF failure in CAPD. Peritoneal equilibration testing confirms high or high average transport rates with resultant rapid glucose absorption, loss of the osmotic gradient, and a decrease in net transcapillary UF. In contrast to the situation seen with peritonitis, where transport changes and protein losses usually are transient (145), small-solute transport changes and protein losses are more permanent with type I membrane failure (131). There also tends to be less of a decline in dialysate sodium owing to the sodium sieving with convective transport as seen in controls. These changes are thought to result from an increase in effective surface area of the peritoneal membrane.

These changes were originally described with acetate-containing dialysis solutions (146) but has also been seen in patients who have only used lactate-containing dialysis (131). Recurrent peritonitis and use of hypertonic dialysate have been implicated in some (147,148) but not all studies (131,149). The incidence of an increase in membrane transport seems to increase with time on PD, implicating repeated exposure of the peritoneum to dialysate as a possible cause.

Reported microscopic findings are similar to those seen with peritonitis.

Most cases can be managed by shortening dwell times. Because these patients have high (rapid) transport of small solutes, they have adequate urea and creatinine clearances even with short dwell exchanges. Occasionally resting the peritoneum for at least 4 weeks through temporary transfer to HD has been associated with an improvement (150,151). Di Paolo and coworkers (152) found low phosphatidylcholine levels in patients with various types of UF failure. Increases in UF were observed after intraperitoneal phosphatidylcholine administration in CAPD patients without UF failure (153,154). Possible explanations include direct membrane effects of phosphatidylcholine or decreased absorption via subdiaphragmatic lymphatics by: (a) an increase in cholinergic tone, causing contraction of subdiaphragmatic stomata (155); (b) neutralization of the anionic charges on the lymphatic endothelium by its cationic charge, which tends to keep stomas open; and (c) surface-acting properties of the molecule that tend to repel water and inhibit movement into the lymphatics. Despite these initial findings, routine use of intraperitoneal phosphatidylcholine cannot be recommended currently because of concerns about safety and the possibility of adhesion formation. The effects of oral phosphatidylcholine are conflicting (156–158).

Although it is often possible to achieve adequate small-solute clearance in these patients, they often require transfer to HD for volume and blood pressure control. There also is a concern that continued membrane damage may result in eventual progression to peritoneal sclerosis or type II membrane failure (159,160). If so, it would be important clinically to closely monitor patients with type I failure with PETs. If these patients continue on PD and their solute transport declines, it may be beneficial to temporarily switch them to HD to allow healing of the peritoneum (161).

Ultrafiltration Failure and No Change or Average Solute Transport

Loss of UF in patients with no change or average transport characteristics tends to result from catheter malfunction, fluid leaks, or excessive lymphatic reabsorption (formerly type III membrane failure) and aquaporin deficiency. If loss of UF is owing to catheter malfunction or fluid leaks, the patients do not have a functional change in their membrane and usually can be maintained on PD after the problem has been resolved.

Excessive Lymphatic Absorption

Excessive lymphatic absorption (historically called type III membrane failure) is a very uncommon cause of membrane failure caused by excessive rates of lymphatic absorption of fluid (131). Although these patients may not have a significant change in D/P values when compared to baseline, they do have drain volumes after 4 hours of dwell that are less than baseline values or what would be expected based on standard

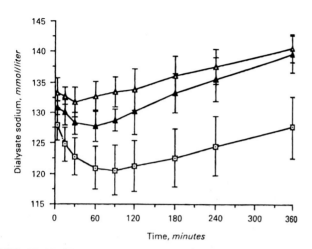

FIG. 98-10. Dialysate sodium concentrations as a function of time in patients using 4.25% dextrose exchanges over 6-hour dwells. Results are compared in patients with normal ultrafiltration kinetics *(hollow squares)*, those with high lymphatic absorption rates *(solid triangles)*, and those with high glucose absorption rates *(hollow triangles)*. (From: Heimburger O, et al. Peritoneal transport in CAPD patients with permanent loss of ultrafiltration capacity. *Kidney Int* 1990;38:495, with permission.)

therapy. A further diagnostic clue is that these patients tend to have higher dialysate sodium concentration during the dwell than controls (131,149) (Fig. 98-10).

Aquaporin Deficiency

This is a rare and only recently understood condition, which may become more prevalent as a more uniform diagnostic approach to UF failure is undertaken (162). Patients with suspected aquaporin deficiency have damage to, decreased number of, or no water channels or ultra-small pores that can lead to deficient crystalloid-induced UF (163). These patients are diagnosed clinically by finding less than 400 mL of UF with a 4.25% PET and lack of sodium sieving early in the dwell. However, one must be careful to exclude patients who are very rapid transporters whose sodium sieving does occur, but does so early in the dwell that if looked for after 60 to 90 minutes of dwell time may be masked. These patients should respond clinically to use of colloid osmotic agents (such as Icodextrin), which achieve ultrafiltration through a different mechanism and are not dependent on the water channels for UF.

Ultrafiltration Failure and Low Solute Transport

Patients with UF failure and low (slow) solute transport (D/D$_0$ glucose of more than 0.5 and a D/P creatinine of less than 0.5) tend also to have inadequate small-solute clearances. Poor UF occurs despite the maintenance of adequate osmotic gradients. These patients are found to have a loss of functional peritoneum and the differential would include: peritoneal sclerosis (formally called type II membrane failure)

or multiple peritoneal adhesions and at times patients with high lymphatic absorption rates. These patients often require transfer to HD.

Peritoneal Sclerosis

An uncommon cause of UF failure is sclerosing peritonitis (type II membrane failure). This is reported to affect less than 1% of PD patients. Patients present with both UF and small-solute transport failure but, because of the association with intestinal adhesions, may also present with intestinal obstruction (160). The etiology is uncertain. Peritoneal irritants, recurrent peritonitis, long-term use of PD, acetate-containing dialysis, chlorhexidine, ß-blockers, and endotoxins have all been implicated in the pathogenesis (160). These patients have low net UF, normal glucose absorption, and high lymphokines in the dialysate associated with low prostaglandin GE$_2$ levels when compared to individuals with normal or high peritoneal transport properties (164).

Tamoxifen, an antiestrogen agent that inhibits protein kinase C, has recently been used to stabilize the process of peritoneal sclerosis (165). It has also been used to treat retroperitoneal fibrosis, a process with pathologic findings similar to those of peritoneal sclerosis (166). A trial of tamoxifen may be reasonable in patients who are reluctant to switch to HD.

Peritoneal sclerosis should not be confused with the syndrome of sclerosing encapsulating peritonitis (SEP) (167). With SEP, patients present with a thick-walled membrane cocoon entrapping loops of bowel associated with anorexia, nausea, vomiting, malnutrition, and intestinal obstruction. This clinical picture is similar to a type II membrane failure pattern with a decrease in solute transport and UF (168). As opposed to patients with SEP, patients with simple type II membrane failure do not have the surgical findings of an encapsulating fibrosis but may have diffuse thickening and fibrosis of the parietal and visceral peritoneum.

Multiple Abdominal Adhesions

Extensive intraabdominal adhesions may result after recurrent or severe peritonitis and after catastrophic intraabdominal events. These processes can cause a decrease in the peritoneal membrane surface area in contact with dialysate. Although normal transport may occur in the membrane that is in contact with dialysate, overall transport and net UF decrease simply from loss of surface area. Surgical lysis of adhesions may result in improvement, and if an adequate increase in surface area can be achieved, PD could continue.

CATHETERS

Types of Peritoneal Catheters

The Tenckhoff catheter originally designed by Palmer and modified by Tenckhoff continues to be used in the majority of PD patients (169–172). A number of variations are available.

The straight or curved subcutaneous portion may have one or two cuffs. Double-cuffed catheters are used in the majority of patients (171). The intraabdominal portion of the catheter may be straight or curled. Curled catheters were designed to decrease outflow problems and infusion pain (173) but appear to have similar complication rates as straight Tenckhoff catheters (174,175).

The Toronto Western Hospital catheter has two silicone rubber disks 5 cm apart on the intraabdominal portion of the catheter (to prevent migration of the catheter tip) and a Dacron disk at the base of the second cuff (to decrease the risk of leaks) (176,177). The rates of complications are similar with the Toronto Western catheter and the Tenckhoff catheter (175), although Flanigan and colleagues (178) found catheter survival to be superior with the Tenckhoff catheter.

To decrease migration of the intraabdominal portion and exit site infections, Twardowski and associates (179) designed a catheter with a curved subcutaneous pathway in which both the internal and external exit sites are downward. Comparisons with the straight Tenckhoff catheter indicate similar 2-year catheter survival, peritonitis risk, and exit site infection (180,181), although catheter dislocation may be decreased with the Swan neck catheter (181). Hwang and colleagues (182) found superior 3-year catheter survival rates with the Swan neck catheter compared to the Tenckhoff catheter, which was attributed to lower rates of cuff extrusion and pericatheter leakage. Down-directed tunnels are associated with lower infection rates (183). A modification of the Swan neck catheter with a presternal exit site had excellent 2-year survival of 95%, in the hands of an experienced team (184).

The curled single-cuff Tenckhoff catheter is used in most children (185). Three lengths of catheters are available: neonatal (8 to 10 cm from cuff to tip), juvenile (16 cm cuff to tip), and adult, based on patient size (186).

Peritoneal Catheter Placement

The location of the exit site should be discussed with the patient prior to placement to avoid the waistline. Preoperative laxatives are indicated for constipation, commonly present in patients because of phosphate binders, and an important cause of catheter malfunction (187). The patient should void prior to the procedure; if the patient has a neurogenic bladder, then urethral catheterization is performed. In many patients, placement can be accomplished using local anesthesia with sedation, although general anesthesia is occasionally necessary (188). The patient usually does not require admission. Prophylactic antibiotics (generally a cephalosporin) for catheter placement (189,190) given before the skin incision decreases the risk of catheter related peritonitis (191).

Most peritoneal dialysis catheters are inserted by a surgeon using a dissection technique (171). A small paramedian incision is made overlying the rectus sheath down through the muscle to the peritoneum (192,193). The catheter is inserted so that the deep cuff is within the rectus muscle and the tip is in the pelvis. A purse string of nonresorbable suture (to decrease the risk of subsequent leaks) is placed where the catheter enters the peritoneum. Catheter function is assessed by infusing and draining fluid (194). The subcutaneous tunnel is formed such that the superficial cuff is 3 cm from the skin surface (187) and directed downward. A small exit site wound formed by a tapered tunneling device of the same diameter as the catheter is best for minimizing trauma and decreasing the risk of subsequent exit site infection and catheter-related peritonitis (195).

Placement via a peritoneoscope is used in a minority of catheters. This technique allows direct intraabdominal visualization (171,196,197). Adhesions can be avoided and the tip of the catheter placed to allow optimal catheter function. Outcomes were not different in a randomized comparison of laparoscopic versus conventional dialysis catheter insertion (both done by surgeons), except that the conventional placement was faster (14 versus 22 minutes, P < 0.0001) (198). The peritoneoscope is useful in patients with previous surgery or when placement by dissection results in a nonfunctioning catheter (199,200).

Blind percutaneous catheter placement may be used for placement of a catheter for acute renal failure to be used for a short time (186). Percutaneous blind catheter insertion is the least desirable technique, as it can be associated with organ perforation and drain failure (201–203). Percutaneous catheter placement using fluoroscopy is not widely performed (204).

To decrease the risk of peritonitis via the tunnel, Moncrief and coworkers (205) developed a new insertion technique. At insertion, the entire external portion of the catheter is buried in abdominal wall subcutaneous tissue. Three to 5 weeks later the catheter is externalized via a small incision, which becomes the exit site. Burying the external portion of the catheter for 6 weeks appears to lower the risk of S. aureus infections, but does not change technique survival (206).

Children require special consideration. In infants, the exit site is located above the diaper area to prevent contamination (207). Partial omentectomy is useful to prevent outflow problems. In boys, herniotomy and ligation of patent processus vaginalis at the time of catheter placement decrease the risk of subsequent inguinal hernia and hydrocele (207).

Perforation of the bladder or bowel or laceration of the spleen is an uncommon occurrence (208), but adhesions increase the risk (209). Perforation of a hollow viscus should be considered if the effluent is feculent or when watery diarrhea, polyuria, or watery vaginal discharge occurs with infusion of dialysate (209). Minor bleeding frequently occurs after catheter insertion but generally stops quickly and spontaneously. Flushing the catheter with heparinized (500 U/L) dialysate is useful to clear the catheter and prevent blockage by clots (210).

Postoperative Management and Exit Site Care

If possible, initiation of PD is postponed to allow healing and prevent leaks (189). Under these circumstances, the catheter should be flushed several times with 1 L of dialysate or saline until the effluent is clear and then capped until training begins (211). The use of 2-L exchange volumes may be used immediately with no increased risk of leaks if bed rest is prescribed for the first 3 days (212). Alternatively, the patient may be maintained on HD until healing occurs. The risk of catheter complications is the same for patients placed on IPD versus those on temporary HD during the healing phase (211); therefore, training on the cycler (with the abdomen empty when erect) can be initiated immediately after catheter placement.

Postoperative sterile dressing changes until healing takes place may help reduce infection risk (190,213). The surgical dressing may be left intact for several days unless there is bleeding. Povidone-iodine solution is commonly used for postoperative cleaning of the exit site (190).

Once healed, many centers advise washing the exit site with bactericidal soap and water during routine bathing (190). Cleaning with povidone-iodine and the use of nonocclusive dressing results in fewer exit site infections than use of non-bactericidal soap and water (214). The use of povidone-iodine ointment applied to sterile gauze used as a dressing to the exit site is effective to prevent early exit site infections (215). Once the exit site is well healed, swimming in chlorinated pools or the ocean is permitted, but swimming in creeks or ponds or the use of hot tubs should be avoided, because this may result in infection (190).

Mechanical Complications

Early inadequate outflow occurs after 7% of catheter insertions, requiring replacement in one-half of these patients (188,216). Constipation may lead to shifting of the catheter position, drainage failure, and catheter loss. Ideally, the catheter tip should be in a pelvic gutter, because this location results in maximum outflow rate (217). Tip migration to the epigastric or hypochondriac regions is generally associated with dysfunction (188,216,218). Poor drainage owing to catheter malposition in the upper quadrants may be corrected by manipulation with a laparoscope or Fogarty catheter, fluoroscopically using a guide wire, or surgically (180,219–225).

There are other causes of catheter dysfunction in addition to catheter malposition. One- or two-way obstruction may result from clots or fibrin within the lumen (194,209). Forcibly flushing with heparinized saline may resolve this problem, but fibrinolytic agents may be effective if this fails (226–228). Omental obstruction may necessitate omentectomy, especially in children (188,194,207–209,229). Partial omentectomy at catheter placement improves catheter survival, and is performed routinely in children (230).

Peritoneal dialysate leaks, which may occur at several different locations (192,231), develop in 5% to 10% of catheters in the immediate postoperative period (180,188,192,216) and in 2% to 4% (216) of catheters later in the course of CAPD. Dialysate leaking from the exit site presents as clear fluid that is strongly test-strip positive for glucose. Leaks at the internal cuff may present as abdominal wall edema, discussed in the following. These leaks may result from the use of resorbable suture material at the deep cuff, placement in a median rather than paramedian site, early initiation of CAPD, or hernia formation (177,194,209,232). Computed tomography scan peritoneography (using Omnipaque, 50 mL/L of dialysate) is the best way to evaluate leaks and hernias (233). A dialysate leak may resolve with PD in the supine position or temporary cessation of PD (using HD) (192,209). Dialysate leaks from the exit site often are associated with infection; thus prophylactic antibiotics should be given (234). If a leak occurring more than 1 month after catheter insertion does not resolve within 4 days of reduced dialysate volumes, or if it recurs after full volumes are resumed, surgical correction generally is required (235).

INFECTIONS

Definitions of Peritoneal Dialysis-Related Infections

Peritonitis is present when the effluent is cloudy with a white blood cell count 100 cells/L with more than 50% polymorphonuclear cells (236). The patient usually has abdominal pain but often does not have a fever (236–239). The effluent white blood cell concentration is a less sensitive indicator of peritonitis if the patient is already on antibiotics or if the patient is on automated PD with either a dry abdominal cavity or a short dwell time when presenting with peritonitis. In these circumstances, the percentage of neutrophils (more than 50%) is more useful than is total white blood cell concentration (236).

Approximately 6% of patients with culture-positive effluent present with abdominal pain and clear effluent (240). A delayed effluent cell reaction occurs in two-thirds of these patients, but one-third never develop an appropriate cellular response to infection. When not experiencing peritonitis such patients have a lower dialysate cell count (particularly macrophages and CD4 lymphocytes) and a delayed production of interleukin-6 and -8, compared to other patients. Any patient on PD who presents with abdominal pain should be considered to have peritonitis until proven otherwise.

An exit site infection is defined as erythema or purulent drainage or both at the catheter exit site (241,242). Induration and tenderness at the exit site are abnormal and may indicate infection. Erythema of the exit site (which is normally flesh colored) may result from either irritation or infection (243), but is seldom associated with catheter loss unless drainage also is present (244). Nonpurulent drainage and crusting of the exit site do not necessarily represent infection, nor does a positive culture of a normal-appearing exit site (245).

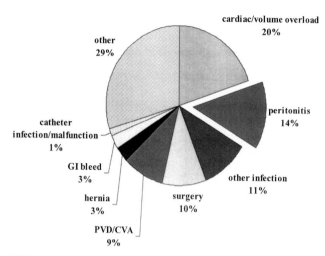

FIG. 98-11. Causes of 274 hospitalization for 126 peritoneal dialysis patients, as percentages. (From: Fried L, Abidi S, Bernardini J, et al. Hospitalization in peritoneal dialysis patients. *Am J Kidney Dis* 1999;33:927, with permission.)

An infection of the subcutaneous catheter (or "tunnel infection") is present when there is pain, tenderness, erythema, or induration over the subcutaneous pathway. Tunnel infections most often occur in the presence of an exit site infection (246,247). Tunnel infections often are clinically occult. This has been shown by numerous studies using sonography of the subcutaneous tunnel in patients with exit site infections (247–250). When peritonitis occurs in conjunction with an exit site infection owing to the same microorganism (particularly *S. aureus* or *P. aeruginosa*), the presumption should be that there is a tunnel infection (251).

Peritoneal dialysis-related infections remain a major problem. Such infections are responsible for the majority of catheters lost (191,252) and contribute to transfer of the patient to HD (22,246,253). Peritonitis is a major cause of hospitalization (11,22,254) (Fig. 98-11). Peritonitis occasionally results in death, either directly from sepsis or indirectly from ensuing complications (191,255–257).

Dialysate Solutions and Peritoneal Immune Function

Peritoneal host defenses are of great importance in preventing peritonitis. Bacteria are cleared from the peritoneum by the processes of opsonization, chemotaxis, phagocytosis, and intracellular killing (258). Thus, bacteria contamination of the peritoneal cavity does not always result in peritonitis if the peritoneal immune defenses are intact. Phagocytosis by peritoneal macrophages decreases in the majority of patients 1 to 2 days prior to the onset of clinical peritonitis, suggesting that not only entry of bacteria into the peritoneal cavity but also malfunction of peritoneal immune function contributes to peritoneal infection (259).

Peritonitis decreases peritoneal ultrafiltration (260,261). During peritonitis there is a sharp rise in the dialysate to plasma ratios for low, middle, and high molecular weight

TABLE 98-9. *Dialysate composition*

Dextrose, measured in g/dL (%) as the hydrous dextrose, available as 1.5%, 2.5%, and 4.25%
Sodium, measured as mEq/L, available at 132
Chloride, measured as mEq/L, available at 102, 96, and 95
Lactate, measured as mEq/L, available at 35 and 40
Calcium, measured as mEq/L, available at 2.5 and 3.5
Magnesium, measured as mEq/L, available at 0.5 and 1.5
Bag volumes, measured in L, available at 0.25, 0.5, 0.75, 1.0, 1.5, 2.0, 2.5, 3.0, 5.0, and 6

solutes, which returns to baseline by 2 weeks. However, ultrafiltration does not completely return to the baseline values, probably because of impairment of transcellular water transport (261). Effluent levels of interleukin-1 and -6, as well as transforming growth factor-ß and fibroblast growth factor (both of the latter being sclerogenic cytokines), remain elevated even 6 weeks after an episode of peritonitis (260), suggesting a mechanism for decreased ultrafiltration in some patients with increasing time on PD.

Dialysate interferes with peritoneal immune defenses. Dialysate contains sodium, chloride, lactate, calcium, magnesium, and dextrose (Table 98-9). The acidic pH, lactate content, and hypertonicity of dialysate are nonphysiologic and impair peritoneal immune function (262,263). The dilution effect of dialysate also increases peritonitis risk. The immunoglobulin and complement concentrations in dialysate are 1% to 2% of those in the peritoneal cavity of patients not on PD (258–264), and the concentration of the peritoneal macrophage, important in peritoneal defense against infection, is low (262).

Lactate is the commonly used alkali because dialysate containing both bicarbonate and glucose cannot undergo the routine heat sterilization procedures (265). Neutrophil function is better preserved with bicarbonate-containing dialysate compared to lactate-containing dialysate (266), although bicarbonate with a high glucose concentration remains cytotoxic (267). Lactate-containing dialysate with neutral pH is much less inhibitory of superoxide generation by neutrophils compared to standard lactate dialysate and almost similar to bicarbonate-containing dialysate (268). Bicarbonate-containing dialysate is feasible, in that the bicarbonate and dextrose can be kept in separate compartments and combined prior to infusion, but this process is expensive and not yet clinically available (265). Two-chambered bicarbonate lactate-buffered PD fluid confers better phagocytosis and is associated with lower glucose degradation products compared to standard dialysate (269). Whether bicarbonate-containing dialysate will result in lower peritonitis rates remains to be seen.

Polymers of glucose are an alternative to dextrose (270,271). Dextrose is rapidly absorbed during a dwell, thus decreasing the osmotic gradient and leading to considerable caloric load. Glucose polymers are isosmolar; UF is obtained through colloid osmosis. In a randomized multicenter study, icodextrin (a large-molecular-weight glucose polymer), used for the overnight exchange, was safe and provided effective UF, compared to 4.25 g/dL dextrose dialysate (271). The glucose polymer solution is less suppressive, compared to 2.5 g/dL and 4.25 g/dL dextrose dialysate, on bacterial phagocytosis; this effect is predominantly owing to the lower osmolality (272,273). Peritonitis results in increased degradation of icodextrin, an increase in dialysate osmolality, and therefore, increased ultrafiltration, in striking contrast to the changes seen with glucose dialysate in peritonitis (274). Icodextrin dialysate is available in Europe but not yet in the United States.

Amino acid-containing dialysate has been proposed as an alternative to glucose-containing dialysate. Polymorphonuclear cell function is not impaired by amino acid dialysate in contrast to dextrose-containing dialysate (275). Amino acid dialysate has similar small- and large-molecular-weight solute transport and UF to equimolar dextrose dialysate (276). The use of one exchange each day of a 1% amino acid dialysate for 6 months improved nitrogen balance but did not result in a rise in the serum albumin (277). Disadvantages of amino acid dialysate include a rise in the blood urea nitrogen level and a fall in the bicarbonate (277); therefore, close attention must be paid to urea nitrogen clearance to prevent uremia, and sodium bicarbonate orally often is necessary during use of amino acid dialysate.

Dialysate is available in 2.5 mEq/L and 3.5 mEq/L calcium. Dialysate with 3.5 mEq/L calcium places the patient in positive calcium balance (278). Parathyroid hormone is suppressed, which may contribute to the high prevalence of aplastic bone disease in PD patients (279,280). The use of 3.5 mEq/L calcium is associated with a higher risk of hypercalcemia (281). Dialysate with 2.5 mEq/L calcium results in negative calcium balance, allowing increased doses of calcium salts to be used for phosphate control (278,281); however, the use of 2.5 mEq/L calcium dialysate, especially without calcitriol, may lead to an exacerbation of hyperparathyroidism (281,282).

Connection Devices

New connection techniques have resulted in a dramatic lowering of peritonitis rates, particularly those owing to organisms such as coagulase negative Staphylococcus. For many years, the standard connection system was a straight line with an empty dialysate bag attached to the patient between dialysis exchanges (283). The exchange was performed manually. The straight-line system has been replaced with safer connection systems, such as the Y-set and double bag system. With the Y-set, the patient connects the catheter to a Y-set of tubing attached to a full dialysate bag and an empty bag. The patient sequentially flushes dialysate through the line into the drain bag to clear air, then drains the effluent from the peritoneum, infuses the fresh dialysate, and disconnects the Y tubing, either capping the catheter or snapping off the tubing. This strategy is known as "flush before fill" and was initially brought into practice by Buoncristiani (284). The double bag

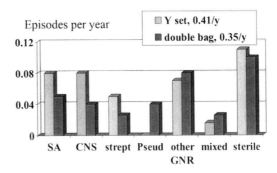

FIG. 98-12. Episodes of peritonitis per dialysis year at risk in patients randomly assigned to the Y set or the double bag system for continuous ambulatory peritoneal dialysis (CAPD). (Modified from: Li PKT, Szeto CC, Law MC, et al. Comparison of double bag and Y set disconnect systems in continuous ambulatory peritoneal dialysis: a randomized prospective multicenter study. *Am J Kidney Dis* 1999;33:535.)

system is a further improvement in technology, because both the drain and fill bags are already attached to the Y tubing; therefore, the only possible site of contamination is during the connection the patient makes to the exchange tubing attached to the catheter. Peritonitis rates are significantly lower with the double bag system compared to the Y-set in high-risk populations (285,286). The double bag system offers little advantage over the Y-set in centers with low peritonitis rates (287). However, a close analysis indicates lower rates of Gram-positive peritonitis with the double bag compared to the Y-set, suggesting that this method further reduces the risk of contamination (Fig. 98-12). Therefore, the best connection device is that with the preattached bags (the double bag system).

The data are conflicting on whether peritonitis rates are lower on the cycler compared to CAPD. De Fijter and coworkers (288,289) randomly assigned 82 patients beginning peritoneal dialysis to cycler PD (type not identified) or CAPD using a Y-set. Peritonitis rates were lower (0.51 versus 0.94 per dialysis year, respectively) on the cycler. Similar differences, although accompanied by overall lower rates, were seen in a larger, nonrandomized study from Spain (290). Because this center has a protocol treating *S. aureus* nasal carriage, the rates of *S. aureus* peritonitis were extremely low in both groups (0.03 episodes per year at risk in both). Lower rates of coagulase-negative Staphylococcus, streptococcus species, and Gram-negative bacteria reduced peritonitis in the cycler (Home Choice) group (Fig. 98-13). A strikingly high rate of Gram-negative peritonitis results from reuse of the cassettes (not recommended by the manufacturer) (291,292).

Catheter Infections

There is a marked variation in reported rates of exit site infections, in part because of differing definitions and because exit and tunnel infections are not always reported separately (293). The catheter infection rate is reported at about 0.6 per year in the National CAPD Registry and many single centers

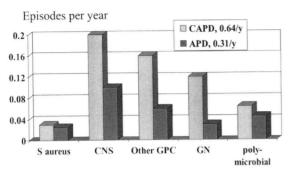

FIG. 98-13. Episodes of peritonitis per dialysis year at risk in patients on continuous ambulatory peritoneal dialysis (CAPD) versus ambulatory peritoneal dialysis (APD). The center uses prophylaxis for *S. aureus* nasal carriers; therefore, *S. aureus* peritonitis rates are very low in both groups. (Modified from: Rodriguez-Carmona A, Perez Fontan M, Garcia Falcon T, et al. A comparative analysis on the incidence of peritonitis and exit site infection in CAPD and automated peritoneal dialysis. *Perit Dial Int* 1999;19:253.)

(242,244,293–295). The rate of clinically obvious tunnel infection is 0.19 per year (22,296); however, when an exit site infection is present, fluid collections along the subcutaneous pathway can be demonstrated frequently by ultrasound examination. Tunnel involvement is common when an exit site infection is concurrent (247,297–300).

Microorganisms causing exit site infections are shown in Table 98-10. The most common organism causing exit site and tunnel infections is *Staphylococcus aureus,* which may be difficult to resolve and can lead to peritonitis and catheter loss (22,242,294,296,301–305). *P. aeruginosa* is the second most common cause of exit site and tunnel infections and frequently recurs or is refractory to antibiotic therapy and tunnel revision (306). Therefore, early catheter removal is appropriate if the patient does not respond to a course of antibiotics. *S. epidermidis* and culture-negative exit site infections are generally nonpurulent, and infrequently cause peritonitis (242).

The peritonitis rate in patients who have catheter infections is more than twice that of patients who do not (242,247). Involvement of the tunnel, especially the inner cuff as

TABLE 98-10. *Pathogens causing exit site infections*

Pathogens	Episodes per year
S. aureus	0.3–0.4[a]
S. epidermidis	0.1
Gram-negative	0.1–0.2
Culture-negative	0.03–0.1
Total	0.6–0.7

[a]Much lower in programs using *S. aureus* prophylaxis.
Modified from: Flanigan MJ, et al. Continuous ambulatory peritoneal dialysis catheter infections: diagnosis and management. *Peritoneal Dial Int* 1994;14:248; Holley JL, Bernardini J, Piraino B. Infecting organisms in continuous ambulatory peritoneal dialysis patients on the Y-set. *Am J Kidney Dis* 1994;23:569.

demonstrated by ultrasound, predicts subsequent peritonitis (247). Even in the absence of a clinical tunnel infection and with resolution of exit site infection with therapy, the deep cuff may harbor *S. aureus* or *P. aeruginosa,* resulting in recurrent peritonitis (307).

A number of studies have demonstrated the efficacy of local antibiotics applied to the exit site to prevent infections. Daily exit site mupirocin is highly effective in reducing *S. aureus* exit site infections (308,309). Ciprofloxacin otologic solution, 0.5 mL single dose vial applied daily as part of routine care, reduced both *S. aureus* and *P. aeruginosa* exit site infections compared to historical controls (310). The use of ciprofloxacin may be prohibitively expensive for many patients.

Peritonitis

Peritonitis rates with the disconnect systems generally are 0.4 to 0.6 per year (284,301,311,312). The organisms that cause peritonitis are listed in Table 98-11 (301,313,314). Many other organisms in addition to those listed have been identified in episodes of peritonitis, including those caused by fungi, protozoans, algae, viruses, and mycobacterium (315–317). The outcome of peritonitis is highly organism-specific (Fig. 98-14). Etiologies of peritonitis are shown in Fig. 98-15.

Contamination at the time of an exchange, usually but not invariably resulting in coagulase negative Staphylococcal peritonitis, remains a leading cause of peritonitis (301,318). *S. epidermidis* peritonitis is not usually caused by a catheter infection (246) or colonization of the skin, nose, or exit site (319,320); however, *S. epidermidis* can colonize the peritoneal catheter, producing a slime layer that can extend from the exit site through the cuff(s) into the peritoneal cavity (321). The rate of bacterial colonization of the catheter is related to the degree of bacterial contamination of the exit

TABLE 98-11. *Pathogens causing peritonitis using disconnect systems*

Pathogens	Episodes/year
S. epidermidis	0.1–0.2
S. aureus	0.15[a]
Other Gram-positive	0.1–0.2
Gram-negative	0.1
Polymicrobial	0.01
Fungi	0.01
Culture-negative	0.01–0.1
Total	0.4–0.6

[a]Approximately one-third this in programs using *S. aureus* prophylaxis.
Modified from: Holey JL, Bernardini J, Piraino B. Infecting organisms in continuous ambulatory peritoneal dialysis patients on the Y-set. *Am J Kidney Dis* 1994;23:569; Tofte-Jensen P, et al. PD-related infections of standard and different disconnect systems. *Adv Peritoneal Dial* 1994;10:214; Lupo A, et al. Long-term outcome in continuous ambulatory peritoneal dialysis: a 10 year survey by the Italian cooperative peritoneal dialysis study group. *Am J Kidney Dis* 1994;24:826.

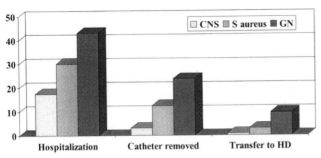

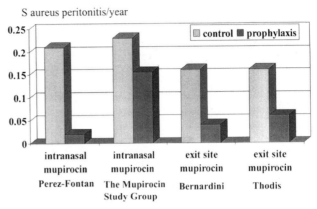

FIG. 98-14. Percentages of peritonitis episodes resulting in hospitalization, catheter removal and transfer to hemodialysis. (Modified from: Bunke CM, Brier ME, Golper TA, et al. Outcomes of single organism peritonitis in peritoneal dialysis: gram negatives versus gram positives in the Network 9 Peritonitis Study. *Kidney Int* 1997;52:524.)

FIG. 98-16. Rates of *S. aureus* peritonitis in episodes per dialysis year at risk, with and without mupirocin prophylaxis in four studies. (Modified from: Perez-Fontan M, et al. Treatment of *Staphylococcus aureus* nasal carriers in continuous ambulatory peritoneal dialysis with mupirocin: long-term results. *Am J Kidney Dis* 1993;22:708; Coles GA, The Mupirocin Study Group. Nasal mupirocin prevents *S. aureus* exit site infections during peritoneal dialysis. *J Am Soc Nephrol* 1996;7:2403; Mylotte JM, Kahler L, Jackson E. "Pulse" nasal mupirocin maintenance regimen in patients undergoing continuous ambulatory peritoneal dialysis. *Infect Control Hosp Epidemiol* 1999;20:741; Herwaldt LA. Reduction of *Staphylococcus aureus* nasal carriage and infection in dialysis patients. *J Hosp Infect* 1998;40:S13.)

site at the time of catheter insertion, but within 3 weeks of insertion most catheters are colonized (321,322). The relationship of biofilm to peritonitis is unclear. Recurrent or relapsing peritonitis (defined as a second episode owing to the same organism within 2 to 4 weeks of stopping antibiotics) is generally caused by staphylococcus (323,324) and may be caused by biofilm. Some recurrent *S. epidermidis* peritonitis episodes have the same plasmid profile as the organisms causing the first infection (325,326). The coagulase-negative staphylococci isolated from patients with peritonitis are more likely to be producers of biofilm than are isolates not associated with peritonitis (327,328); however, biofilm formation does not invariably lead to peritonitis (325,329). The keys to preventing peritonitis caused by coagulase negative Staphylococcal peritonitis are avoidance of connection techniques requiring spiking of bags and extensive training of the patient in aseptic technique. Miller and Findon have demonstrated that proper hand washing and drying prior to performance of an exchange sharply reduces bacterial numbers on the spike connection and in the peritoneal space after touch contamination (330).

S. aureus carriage and catheter infections are another source of peritonitis. *S. aureus* in the nares, at the exit site, or on the skin is strongly associated with *S. aureus* catheter infection and peritonitis (331–337). Several antibiotic protocols have been shown to decrease the risk of *S. aureus* infection in PD patients (308,309,336,338–342) (Fig. 98-16). These predominantly use intranasal mupirocin cream, bid for 5 days monthly for carriers, or daily at the exit site. These protocols are uniformly effective in reducing exit site infections. Exit site mupirocin is also effective in reducing *S. aureus* peritonitis (308,309). Use of exit site mupirocin for 1 year in a program did not lead to resistance (343). Prevention of *S. aureus* peritonitis is critical, because the outcome is worse compared to other staphylococci (344,345).

Gram-negative peritonitis, associated with considerable morbidity (344), is not well understood. The bowel may be a source, through translocation of bacteria across the bowel wall or secondary to organ pathology (346,347). Approximately one-third of peritonitis episodes owing to enteric organisms have underlying visceral injury (347). Peritonitis caused by intraabdominal pathology is associated with severe symptoms and commonly results in transfer of the patient to HD and death (255,256,346–350), especially if surgery is delayed. Causes of enteric peritonitis in PD patients include ischemic bowel, cholecystitis, appendicitis, perforated ulcers, colonic polypectomy, and diverticulae (347,350) (see section on intraabdominal catastrophes).

Procedures such as colonoscopy (351–353), endoscopy with sclerotherapy (354), dental manipulation, endometrial biopsy, liver biopsy, and laparoscopic cholecystectomy

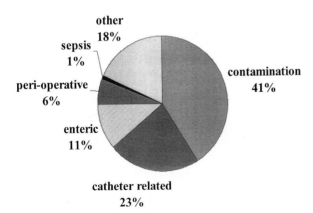

FIG. 98-15. Etiologies of peritonitis. (Modified from: Harwell CM, Newman LN, Cacho CP, et al. Abdominal catastrophe: visceral injury as a cause of peritonitis in patients treated by peritoneal dialysis. *Perit Dial Int* 1997;17:586.)

TABLE 98-12. *Fungal peritonitis without and with prophylaxis*

Reference	Prophylaxis	Incidence[a]
Zaruba (369)	Nystatin tid	0.20 vs 0.03
Robitaille (370)	Nystatin or ketoconazole	0.14 vs 0
Wadhwa (371)	Fluconazole qod	0.08 vs 0.01
Lo (372)	Nystatin qid	0.02 vs 0.01
Thodis (373)	Nystatin qid	0.02 vs 0.02
Williams (374)	Nystatin qid	0.01 vs 0.01

[a]Antibiotic associated fungal peritonitis, in episodes per year. Rate without prophylaxis given first.

(355–357) can result in peritonitis; thus, antibiotic prophylaxis is indicated. Other unusual causes of peritonitis are vaginal leak of dialysate (358,359) and the use of intrauterine devices (360).

Fungal peritonitis accounts for 2% to 3% of all peritonitis episodes (361) Abdominal pain may be severe and associated with fever (362). Patients may be acutely ill and appear to have a surgical abdomen; death may result (363), particularly if catheter removal is delayed (364,365). Mortality with fungal peritonitis is 14% to 27% (361,366,367). Prior antibiotic therapy and frequent bacterial peritonitis are predisposing causes (361,366–368). Prophylaxis, mainly using nystatin during antibiotic therapy, appears to be most effective in programs with high fungal peritonitis rates (Table 98-12) (369–374). Programs with a low fungal peritonitis rate do not appear to benefit from prophylaxis.

The culture is "sterile" in approximately 14% to 20% of episodes that meet the criteria for peritonitis based on cell count (301,375). A fastidious microorganism that has not grown in culture probably causes most of these episodes. When subsequently recultured, a microorganism is identified in one-third (375). Also recent antibiotic exposure can render dialysate "sterile," despite active peritonitis (376). Culturing dialysate by placing 10 mL in blood culture bottles enhances the yield of isolating the causative pathogen (377–379). The differential diagnosis for sterile cloudy fluid includes fibrin, effluent eosinophilia (380–382), hemoperitoneum, chyloperitoneum, and pancreatitis. Intraperitoneal generic vancomycin (383) and amphotericin cause chemical peritonitis (384). Mycobacteria always should be considered in peritonitis that is culture negative. Such patients have cloudy effluent, abdominal pain, and fever. Extraperitoneal TB is not necessarily present (385). Polymorphonuclear cells predominate in the effluent, and thus, do not distinguish *Mycobacterium* peritonitis from bacterial peritonitis. Acid-fast bacillus (AFB) smears of the effluent, even examining three concentrated specimens, are seldom positive; therefore, the diagnosis is generally made on culture, delaying treatment for weeks. Peritoneal tissue cultures are more optimal than culture of peritoneal fluid.

A number of demographic features are associated with an increased risk for peritonitis. White nondiabetic patients aged 20 to 59 years have the lowest risk of peritonitis (293). The reason for the increased risk seen in Blacks is not understood (386–388). Conflicting data exist on whether diabetic patients

have an increased risk of peritonitis (171,293,389,390). Age more than 60 years was a risk factor for peritonitis in the final report of the National CAPD Registry (293,391), but other studies indicate that elderly patients have similar peritonitis rates as younger patients (392–394). Peritonitis rates in children are higher than those of adults (185,395,396). Immunosuppressed patients are also at increased risk, especially for infections owing to *S. aureus* and fungi (397).

Other factors influencing peritonitis risk include connection technology; with the lowest rates occurring with the double bag system for CAPD and a cycler system that does not involve spiking (discussed in the preceding). Peritonitis risk is increased after an episode of peritonitis (171,318). Single-cuff catheters are associated with a higher risk of peritonitis than double-cuff catheters (171,191). Neither catheter design nor insertion technique is associated with higher or lower peritonitis rates (171,191); however, downward directed tunnels decrease the risk of catheter-associated peritonitis (191).

Treatment of Peritoneal Dialysis-Related Infections

Exit Site Infections

The initial antibiotic for an exit site infection must be active against staphylococci, with subsequent therapy dependent on the specific organism identified. Oral antibiotics are as effective as intraperitoneal antibiotics (244). Vancomycin should be reserved for methicillin-resistant organisms not sensitive to cotrimoxazole. Sonography of the tunnel is useful to determine length of therapy (Fig. 98-17). Those infections limited to the exit site require an average of 2 weeks of antibiotic therapy, whereas involvement of the superficial tunnel lengthens average therapy to 3 weeks or more. Involvement of the deep cuff requires 2 months or more of antibiotic therapy and may require removal of the catheter to prevent peritonitis (300). Local care of the exit site is generally intensified and in mild or equivocal exit site infection if the tunnel is not involved, this may be the only therapy (190). If prolonged antibiotic therapy fails to resolve the exit site infection, revision of the tunnel with removal of the external cuff (in two cuffed catheters) may help to prolong the life of the catheter (294,398) but often eventually results in peritonitis (294,399). An incision

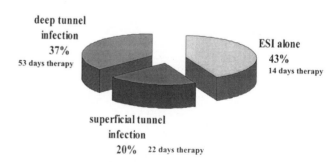

FIG. 98-17. Extent of *S. aureus* catheter infection (N = 49) using sonography with mean days of therapy also shown. (From: Vychytil A, Lilaj T, Lorenz M, et al. Ultrasonography of the catheter tunnel in peritoneal dialysis patients: what are the indications? *Am J Kidney Dis* 1999;33:722, with permission.)

TABLE 98-13. *Antibiotic doses for peritonitis*

Antibiotic	Dose intraperitoneally
Cefazolin or cephalothin	15–20[a] mg/kg once daily
Vancomycin	30 mg/kg once, then 15 mg/kg every 5 d
Ceftazidime	15–20[a] mg/kg once daily
Gentamicin, tobramycin, or netilmycin	0.6 mg/kg once daily

[a]Higher dose for patients with residual renal function.
Modified from: Keane WF, Bailie GR, Boeschoten E, et al. Adult peritoneal dialysis related peritonitis treatment recommendations. *Peritoneal Dial Int* 2000;20:396.

is made over the tunnel to expose the cuff, which is carefully shaved from the catheter. The area of granulation tissue and cellulitis may also be débrided (400). Cuff shaving and tunnel revision are never effective if catheter-related peritonitis is present (399). Pseudomonas exit site infections are particularly prone to recurrence and often lead to peritonitis, a devastating complication (401,402). Therefore, recurrent and refractory exit site infections might be best managed with catheter replacement. In such high-risk patients, to prevent recurrence in a new catheter, consideration should be given to using ciprofloxacin otic solution at the exit site as described.

Peritonitis

Empiric antibiotic therapy is begun once the diagnosis of peritonitis has been established based on the effluent cell count (403). Treatment should be given quickly because shock and death can ensue rapidly, especially with streptococcal peritonitis (404,405). Initial therapy should include coverage for both Gram-positive and -negative organisms (403,406).

A first-generation cephalosporin combined with ceftazidime provides appropriately broad coverage initially (Table 98-13). A single daily dose of cefazolin, 15 mg/kg, results in dialysate concentration levels above the minimum inhibitory concentration over 24 hours for sensitive organisms, allowing once a day dosing (for those without residual renal function) in CAPD patients (407). There are limited data on once daily dosing of cefazolin for CCPD patients. Therefore, these patients should be treated with continuous intraperitoneal cefazolin, until more data are available. An initial single dose of ceftazidime, 15 mg/kg IP, also results in serum and dialysate concentrations above the MIC (for susceptible organisms) for more than 24 hours because the serum elimination half-life is 22 hours (408). Aminoglycoside therapy should be avoided when possible to preserve residual renal function (409).

Vancomycin is necessary when the patient has a history of methicillin-resistant organisms or if the program has a high rate of methicillin resistance, as well as for the patient with a cephalosporin allergy (403,410). Onozato and coworkers reported a cure rate of only 56% using cefazolin and amikacin as empiric therapy, perhaps because only 67% of *S. aureus* and 20% of *S. epidermidis* in this program

were sensitive to cefazolin (411,412). For centers with a high rate of resistance to cephalosporins, van Biesen and associates recommended empiric therapy with a single initial dose of vancomycin, 15 mg/kg IP, combined with gentamicin, 1.5 mg/kg (for urine output of more than 500 mL/day) or 0.5 mg/kg (for urine output less than 500 mL/day), IP as a single dose (413). The authors recommend beginning ciprofloxacin, orally (500 mg twice daily) for those treated as outpatients, and 50 mg/exchange for those patients admitted on the second day. This protocol provides 96% coverage of the organisms causing peritonitis in their program.

Subsequent therapy after antibiotic loading depends on the organism isolated. *S. aureus, S. epidermidis,* and streptococcus can be treated with a first-generation cephalosporin alone, if methicillin-sensitive. Fifty percent or more of *S. epidermidis* causing peritonitis is resistant to cephalosporins (412,414). These patients should be switched to vancomycin as should patients with methicillin resistant *S. aureus* (MRSA) peritonitis (415). MRSA peritonitis has a failure rate of 60% when treated with vancomycin, and frequently results not only in catheter loss but also in peritoneal adhesions precluding further PD (416); therefore, rifampin should be added to vancomycin therapy. Peritonitis caused by vancomycin intermediate resistant *S. aureus* has been reported, and was successfully treated with rifampin and trimethoprim-sulfamethoxazole (417). Therapy for *S. aureus* peritonitis takes 3 weeks. Two weeks is generally sufficient for other Gram-positive cocci.

If a concomitant catheter infection is present, as is commonly the case for *S. aureus,* catheter removal is necessary (251). Although antibiotic therapy may lead to apparent resolution, persistent infection generally is present and eventually leads to catheter loss. Delayed catheter removal in such circumstances can lead to considerable morbidity as well as possible death (255).

Empiric cephalosporin is discontinued and ampicillin begun for peritonitis caused by enterococcus. Vancomycin-resistant enterococcus as a cause of peritonitis in PD patients is still rare, accounting for 0.4% to 4% of episodes (414,418). This is probably because colonization of PD patients with vancomycin-resistant enterococci is infrequent (419–421). Vancomycin-resistant enterococci should be treated with linezolid; catheter removal should be prompt if resolution does not occur within several days.

The subsequent therapy of Gram-negative organisms is dependent on the sensitivities. Aminoglycoside therapy should be reserved for those infections in which sensitivities dictate the use of these drugs because of the need to preserve residual renal function (409). Historically, aminoglycosides in PD patients have been given continuously in each PD exchange following a loading dose (422). However, continuous intraperitoneal dosing can lead to otovestibular toxicity if courses exceed 2 weeks (423). Once a day dosing of intraperitoneal aminoglycoside, shown to be effective, provides high local levels of the antibiotic while avoiding systemic toxicity (424,425). The index of suspicion should be high because one-third of peritonitis episodes with enteric organisms have underlying organ pathology (347). This possibility can be further evaluated with an abdominal CT scan.

P. aeruginosa peritonitis should be treated with two drugs for a minimum of 3 weeks. Peritonitis caused by *P. aeruginosa* is difficult to treat (303,304) and can sometimes result in the death of the patient (426,427). Aminoglycosides are often ineffective therapy for these infections (303,304), and long courses may result in vestibular toxicity (304,423). Antibiotic therapy is much more likely to be effective if a catheter infection is not present (304), although long courses of therapy may be required to prevent relapse (428). If a *Pseudomonas* catheter infection is present in conjunction with the peritonitis, it is wise to promptly remove the catheter.

Peritonitis owing to *Stenotrophomonas maltophilia* (formerly *Xanthomonas maltophilia*) is difficult to resolve. Despite treatment with multiple antibiotics, catheter removal may be necessary (429). Immunosuppression is a risk factor.

The growth of multiple Gram-negative or anaerobic organisms should lead to the strong suspicion of intraabdominal pathology. A surgical consult and an abdominal CT scan should be obtained, because delay in diagnosing an intraabdominal source can result in the patient's death. Metronidazole should be added to the therapy. Antibiotic therapy should be 21 days.

Antibiotic therapy of fungal peritonitis is not generally successful unless the catheter is removed. Amphotericin B has poor diffusion from blood into peritoneum (384), whereas intraperitoneal administration results in chemical peritonitis (384). Flucytosine, ketoconazole, and fluconazole diffuse readily from blood to peritoneum (384) and are more effective than amphotericin (362), although catheter removal still is often necessary (430–432). Fluconazole is particularly well tolerated when administered intraperitoneally. Chan and colleagues (367) found a cure rate of 9.5% using fluconazole therapy alone without catheter removal. Fluconazole plus catheter removal cured 67%, whereas 14% required amphotericin in addition. Most authorities feel that prompt catheter removal for fungal peritonitis is the most prudent approach in adults.

Fibrinolytic agents have been used in the treatment of patients with recurrent or refractory peritonitis (433–435) or in relieving catheter obstruction associated with peritonitis (228). Approximately two-thirds of episodes of refractory or relapsing peritonitis (predominantly *S. epidermidis*) resolved with intraperitoneal urokinase compared to only 8% of patients given only antibiotics (435). In another randomized trial (436), recurrent peritonitis (predominantly coagulase-negative staphylococcus) resolved in 59% of patients given urokinase, compared to 95% of patients whose catheters were replaced.

Temporary cessation of PD, which improves peritoneal immune function, has been successfully utilized to assist in resolving peritonitis, in conjunction with antibiotics (437–440). This approach has been useful in recurrent peritonitis episodes owing to coagulase-negative staphylococcus (441,442) but has also been helpful in resolving refractory

S. aureus (441). It is effective only if catheter infection is absent.

Catheter removal is necessary to resolve the infection in some cases. Peritonitis owing to *S. aureus, P. aeruginosa,* enteric peritonitis with an intraabdominal source, and fungus often requires catheter removal (255,443,444). Catheter-related peritonitis accounts for approximately one-third of the catheters removed (216,301), whereas the proportion and rate of catheter removal for isolated peritonitis have decreased with use of improved connection systems (301). Simultaneous catheter removal and replacement are quite successful for recurring peritonitis and tunnel infections (436,445–449). This eliminates an interim period on hemodialysis. This approach is best used when the effluent leukocyte cell count is under 100/μL. This approach is not recommended for fungal or *P. aeruginosa* peritonitis. These episodes require that the patient spend a period of time off PD (446,447).

OTHER COMPLICATIONS

Pancreatitis

Pancreatic abnormalities including pancreatitis occur with a higher frequency in uremic patients (450–454). The highest incidence of pancreatitis among ESRD patients is in transplant recipients, but within dialysis populations, it is not clear that PD patients have a higher incidence than do HD patients (453–456). Reports from the mid-1980s suggested a greater incidence in PD patients (453,456), prompting several etiologic hypotheses. Pancreatitis was thought to be related to higher uremic solute concentrations in PD patients or even to the potentially direct toxic effects of dialysate, which bathes a portion of the pancreas. The dialysate dextrose concentration, hypertonicity, hypercalcemia, foreign particulate debris, bacteria, or antibiotics may induce inflammation in the sensitive pancreas (453,456–458). That the direct toxicity of dialysate may be causative is supported by the recurrence of pancreatitis after reinstitution of PD after initial resolution (459). Hyperlipidemia is both a risk factor for and complication of pancreatitis. The hyperlipidemia seen more frequently in PD patients is low-density lipoprotein hypercholesterolemia, which is not particularly toxic to the pancreas. On the other hand, HD patients are more likely to suffer from hypertriglyceridemia, which is a predisposing factor for pancreatitis when severe enough to be associated with hyperchylomicronemia. The high intake of simple carbohydrates in PD patients may be a factor in inducing hyperlipidemia. This is a major difference between HD and PD patients.

Even though pancreatitis is an infrequent complication of PD, it carries a high mortality rate of 20% to 60% (453,455). The typical clinical presentation for acute pancreatitis in a PD patient is characterized by abdominal pain with normal bowel sounds, nausea, vomiting, absence of fever, hyperamylasemia (more than three times normal), elevated effluent dialysate amylase concentration (more than 100 U/L), and a variable appearance of effluent dialysate, including being clear, hemorrhagic, tea-colored, or even cloudy (453–456,460). Hyperlipidemia and/or hypercalcemia is frequently present and may be predisposing metabolic abnormalities (453,455,460). Pancreatitis should be strongly considered if appropriately treated "peritonitis" does not resolve because this presentation is quite similar to PD-associated microbial peritonitis. The effluent in pancreatitis is usually sterile, even if hemorrhagic cloudy or tea-colored. Burkart and associates (461) have suggested that dialysate effluent amylase concentration is low in bacterial peritonitis, even if slow to resolve, whereas it is more than 100 U/L with pancreatitis or other intraabdominal pathologies. If a diagnosis of pancreatitis is uncertain, computed tomography (CT) is the preferred imaging study over sonography because it is more sensitive (462). In addition to demonstration of an engorged pancreas, CT may be particularly useful to identify the ominous finding of a pseudocyst.

The principles of management do not differ from that in patients without ESRD. Offending agents should be discontinued, and if that includes dialysate, PD should be halted. However, peritoneal lavage can be helpful in removing inflammatory mediators, especially if the dialysate was not the culprit. There is no evidence to support a recommendation to halt PD in all patients with acute pancreatitis, and discontinuing PD probably does not alter the prognosis (455). Percutaneous pseudocyst drainage may be preferable to internal (jejunal) drainage, and this may preclude continuation of PD. Hyperlipidemia and hypercalcemia should be corrected. The role of lower concentrations of calcium in dialysate is unknown.

Chyloperitoneum

There have been a few scattered case reports of chylous fluid leaking into the peritoneum and draining with effluent dialysate (463–466). The dialysate is cloudy but on more careful examination looks milky, reflecting the lipid-rich content of chyle. The most common cause is trauma to intraperitoneal lymph vessels, either catheter-induced or from external trauma. Patients are usually asymptomatic. Treatment initially is conservative, to decrease abdominal lymph production by a low-fat, high-calorie diet supplemented with medium-chain triglycerides. The next step is discontinuation of PD, because the presence of dialysate may retard closure of the leak. If this is unsuccessful, a trial of total parenteral alimentation may be considered. Should these steps fail to resolve the leak, catheter removal is indicated. Lymphangiography may identify the source of the leak should other surgery be considered.

Hemoperitoneum

Just 1 mL of blood in 2 L of dialysate results in readily evident visual hemoperitoneum (467), and 7 mL results in effluent dialysate that looks like red fruit juice. Fortunately, this is an uncommon occurrence, but when it does occur,

TABLE 98-14. *Causes of hemoperitoneum in peritoneal dialysis patients*

Retrograde menstruation
Ovulation
Catheter-induced trauma (omental abrasion, repositioning, constipation)
Bowel disease (ischemic, inflammatory)
Peritonitis
Cysts (ovarian, polycystic kidney, acquired cystic kidney)
Abdominal trauma
Strenuous exercise (including sexual activity)
Systemic bleeding (thrombocytopenia, anticoagulants)
Hypertonic exchanges (hyperemia)
Pancreatitis
Vasculitis (systemic lupus erythematosus)
Sclerosing peritonitis
Adhesions
Granulosa cell tumor
Ectopic pregnancy
Cholecystitis
Colonoscopy
Dissection from adjacent sites (femoral hematoma, spleen, colon)
Previous hepatitis
Enema
Extracorporeal lithotripsy
Splenic infarction

it is very disturbing to the patient. It is also fortunate that hemoperitoneum is usually benign (468). Table 98-14 lists causes of hemoperitoneum in PD patients. When actually quantitated, hemoperitoneum occurs in a minimum of 10% of women undergoing PD and 4% of men (468). When it occurs in women of childbearing age, 64% of the causes are related to ovulation or menses. In one series, this population experienced an almost 90% incidence rate (469). There does not appear to be a connection with PD-associated peritonitis (468).

Menstrual and surgical histories are informative (Table 98-14). If the patient is asymptomatic and the bleeding stops spontaneously, no evaluation is absolutely necessary. In the absence of active menses, bloody dialysate should be evaluated by effluent cell count, differential, Gram stain and culture, and effluent fluid amylase concentration. An abdominal ultrasound may be informative. Obviously, symptoms referable to the abdomen prompt further evaluation, which ultimately could include a laparotomy. Treatment is directed at the specific cause. However, because patients often are asymptomatic, precluding an extensive evaluation, treatment generally is supportive. Heparin administered intraperitoneally may protect from subsequent catheter occlusion from clots but may prolong bleeding. Three rapid flushes with room temperature dialysate may induce peritoneal vasoconstriction and stop bleeding (467). Dialysate cooler than room temperature could precipitate cardiac dysrhythmias. Furthermore, cool dialysate should be avoided where mesenteric perfusion is compromised, because it could exacerbate ischemia of the bowel. This therapy is probably only effective in cases where the bleeding is secondary to a peritoneal membrane bleed. Gynecologic hormone therapy may be indicated in women who demonstrate hemoperitoneum during menses or ovulation (470).

Hernias and Genital and Abdominal Wall Edema

Intraabdominal pressure rises with increasing intraperitoneal volume, sitting, straining at stool, coughing, and strenuous physical activity. Combined with the extremes of age, debilitation of ESRD, and poor wound healing from uremia, it is no surprise that hernias are detected in 10% to 25% of PD patients (471,472). The most common sites are at the catheter insertion (inguinal ventral or umbilical), but other sites are not uncommon. Over 13% of the hernias present are strangulated. Half become clinically evident within the first year of PD (473,474), but many probably go undetected unless special scintigraphic studies are performed (475). Most of the scintigraphically diagnosed asymptomatic cases never progress to clinically appreciable disease. Many PD patients have hernias diagnosed prior to initiating PD, and herniorrhaphies are performed at the time of catheter insertion (476). Patients can perform PD immediately after repair about half the time, and by 3 weeks, all can perform some type of PD. Usually exchange volume is decreased and supine positioning for PD is recommended (i.e., some form of cycler PD) (474). Another alternative is to utilize prosthetic overlay mesh within the herniorrhaphy and not interrupt the PD (477).

There probably is no benefit from routine screening scintigraphy in adults because clinical manifestations alone dictate the need to repair (478). In children, some programs routinely perform intraoperative peritoneograms (and herniorrhaphies if positive) at the time of catheter placement. To ensure prompt strength postoperatively, especially for large hernias, supporting prosthetic overlay mesh is inserted at herniorrhaphy (477). Placement of catheters through the rectus muscle in a paramedian approach probably reduces the incidence of subsequent incisional or catheter site hernias. Postinsertion leakage increases the likelihood of subsequent hernias. The incidence of hernias is markedly lower in PD patients undergoing intermittent treatments rather than continuous (471), probably because of the lower intraabdominal pressures in the lying positions.

Abdominal wall edema or genital edema is caused by either dialysate leakage through acquired peritoneal defects such as the catheter insertion site, traumatic rents such as previous hernias or incisions, or congenital defects that go undetected until PD raises intraperitoneal PD pressures, opening them (patent processus vaginalis). Thus, the fluid could dissect between tissue layers or through natural pathways. Edema of the scrotum or perineal area is usually owing to a patent processus vaginalis (231,479). Scrotal edema develops in 10% of men on CAPD (231,480), whereas labial edema occurs in only 1.4% of women (480). This can be managed temporarily by supine PD, but surgical correction is generally required, certainly if a hernia is present (192). Postoperative management may include hemodialysis for 1 week or more (192). Vaginal

leakage of dialysate is rare but serious, because it can lead to recurrent peritonitis, often with fungus (358,359,481). This complication should be suspected in any woman with watery vaginal discharge that is positive for glucose. If the leak is through the fallopian tubes, then tubal ligation is corrective (482).

The site of a subcutaneous dialysate leak can be located with scintigraphy or contrast imaging (480,483–485). Contrast peritoneogram or scintigraphy is important to detect the leakage site or defect. Surgical closure is recommended, hence the precise identification of the leak site. Although watchful waiting is tempting, the collective PD experience suggests that elective operative intervention is the best approach to these complications related to increased abdominal pressure.

Hydrothorax

Fluid migrates from the peritoneal to pleural space in 2% to 5% of patients undergoing PD either via transdiaphragmatic lymphatics or defects in the tendinous portion of the diaphragm (486–488). There is an increased incidence in women, patients with polycystic kidney disease (489) or hernias, those prone to peritonitis, and children. Almost 90% of the cases are isolated to the right pleural space (488). The heart or pericardium probably protects the tendinous portion of the left hemidiaphragm. The hydrothorax can occur abruptly and painfully following exercise or trauma and can be immediately life threatening. A more common presentation is with gradual progression of orthopnea or dyspnea, usually without pain. Half of the cases present within the first month of PD, and only one-fifth present 1 year or more after initiation (488). Resolution (i.e., being able to continue PD) is more likely in those cases where the presentation is within 1 year of initiating PD.

The simultaneous measurement of the concentrations of albumin, glucose, and lactate dehydrogenase in peritoneal effluent, pleural fluid, and blood may be helpful diagnostically. Labeled albumin is a useful marker (490), but methylene blue should be avoided because of the pain it causes. Although helpful in localizing the defect, these diagnostic maneuvers probably do not alter management (491). If the origin of the hydrothorax is dialysate, therapy is indicated regardless of whether there is a distinct leak versus lymphatic transport.

Initial attempts should be made to decrease intraabdominal pressure by decreasing volumes (decrease fill, decrease UF), performing PD supine, and periods of an empty belly. Chemical pleurodesis with tetracycline, blood N-CWS (*Nocardia rubra* cell wall skeleton), triamcinolone, OK-432, pleurodesis with talc, or fibrin adhesive (492) has each been successful but can be painful with unpredictable results. Surgical treatment is recommended if pleurodesis fails. The operation involves a limited incision and a few sutures and is much less morbid than a full thoracotomy (493). Alternatively, transfer to HD is an option.

Hyperlipidemia

Compared to HD patients, PD patients demonstrate higher total cholesterol concentrations, apo A-I, and apo B and lower apo A-I:B ratios, serum albumin, and high-density lipoprotein (HDL) cholesterol concentrations (494,495). The cause of these abnormalities is multifactorial. Although total caloric intake is equal in PD and HD patients because of absorbed dextrose from peritoneal dialysate, oral caloric intake is actually less in PD patients (496,497). This absorbed simple carbohydrate may account for 25% of total caloric intake. The development of hypertriglyceridemia during the first year of PD has been correlated with glucose absorption (498). Patients who require frequent hypertonic exchanges do so because of increased fluid and/or food intake. Therefore, it is difficult to determine whether hyperlipidemia is secondary to diet or hypertonic dialysate. Furthermore, there is loss into effluent dialysate of oncotic proteins (e.g., albumin) and liporegulatory species (e.g., HDL cholesterol, apoproteins) (499,500). This sets the stage for hyperlipidemia and atherosclerosis.

By virtue of their uremic condition and hypertension, patients with chronic renal failure are also at increased risk for vascular disease. This risk is even greater in diabetic patients with chronic renal failure (16). Many of the vascular risk markers described in patients with diabetes are even more abnormal with the addition of renal failure and dialysis (501). In dialysis patients treated with subcutaneous insulin, type IV hyperlipidemia and hyperinsulinemia are considerably more frequent and severe than in nondiabetic dialysis patients. In addition to abnormally low levels of HDL cholesterol, dialysis patients also have significantly elevated levels of certain circulating markers of cardiovascular disease such as Lp(a) lipoprotein, factor VII coagulant activity, plasminogen activator inhibitor, and fibrinogen (501–503).

The treatment of hyperlipidemia in PD patients must include an attempt to decrease the use of hypertonic exchange. This should be done in conjunction with a dietary restriction of fluids, fats, and simple carbohydrates. Alternative osmotic agents such as amino acids and glucose polymer are undergoing long-term trials now. Preliminary results indicate only modest lipid-lowering effects of these agents (271,504). Lipid-lowering drugs of several classes have been utilized successfully. The major US experience with fibric acid derivatives is with gemfibrozil, which increases lipoprotein lipase activity, the catabolism of very-low-density lipoproteins (VLDL), and the concentration of HDL_2 and HDL_3 (505). The dose should be reduced by initiation with 300 mg once daily and titrated gradually upward. Gemfibrozil can cause myositis, which may be manifested by increased serum potassium and/or creatinine kinase concentrations. A less toxic but effective agent is clinofibrate (506). Hydroxymethylglutaryl-CoA reductase inhibitors, predominantly used to treat hypercholesterolemia, are safe and effective in PD patients (507–511). The role of omega-3 fatty acids (fish oils) is still to be determined because, although effective, they are poorly tolerated (512–514).

Intraabdominal Pathology in Peritoneal Dialysis Patients

Less than 6% of peritonitis episodes in PD patients are owing to intraabdominal pathology (IAP) (515). The culture isolation of multiple enteric pathogens, a single, unusual enteric pathogen, a peripheral leukocytosis, an increasing PD cell count on antibiotic therapy, and an expanding pneumoperitoneum are important clues to IAP (188,349,515). Obvious signs of IAP, such as fecal or biliary material in the dialysate or diarrhea containing dialysate, are not commonly observed. Risk factors for the development of IAP include diverticulosis, constipation and its treatment (516), and unrepaired hernia. Death with IAP is linked to bowel gangrene, malnutrition, and comorbidities such as liver failure, shock, bacteremia, pneumonia, and gastrointestinal or intracerebral hemorrhage, and delayed surgical intervention (517); therefore, by a broad consensus, early surgical intervention in suspected IAP is strongly recommended (347,518).

In general, slowly resolving peritonitis warrants close follow-up. Clear dialysate while on antibiotics is not an absolute sign of a benign process. Generalized abdominal peritonitis can mask localized signs and symptoms of IAP. Surgical consultation is urgently needed in the following conditions:

- Localized abdominal pain and tenderness
- Dilated loops of bowel on abdominal radiograph
- Progressive increase in intraperitoneal free air with continued peritonitis
- Mixed flora on dialysate gram stain or culture
- Refractory peritonitis
- Hemoperitoneum with measurable dialysate hematocrit

Those perioperative interventions that best allow continuation or quick return to PD postoperatively include:

1. Tight wound closure for prevention of dialysate leakage, possibly using nonresorbable sutures
2. Drain removal before resuming PD to allow adequate dialysis
3. Preoperative extensive PD to increase platelet function and allow a few days without PD postoperatively for healing
4. Elective repair of abdominal wall hernias (see Abdominal Hernias in Continuous Peritoneal Dialysis) both for patient comfort as well as prevention of bowel incarceration
5. Avoidance of constipation, because impacted stool often accompanies diverticulitis or perforated bowel
6. Optimization of nutrition to counter the marked protein loss through an inflamed peritoneum
7. Avoidance of PD with transfer to HD if extensive bowel wall repairs are made. A low threshold for transition to HD is generally a prudent decision.

8. Omentectomy at surgery if the omentum appears threatening to catheter flow function (519,520)

INTRAPERITONEAL INSULIN

Immediately after CAPD became a viable therapy, Flynn and Nanson (521) suggested that the intraperitoneal administration of insulin could act as an artificial pancreas. Shortly thereafter Madden and coworkers (522) showed that glycemic control was superior and peritonitis rates no worse with intraperitoneal insulin in CAPD patients. Subsequently, it was demonstrated that improved glycemic control is associated with better outcomes (523). Copley and Lindberg recently reviewed the use of insulin in PD patients (524).

The absorption of intraperitoneal insulin may be via diffusion and/or lymphatics. It is influenced by temperature, hormones, and dwell time, but less so by dextrose concentration, dialysate osmolality, and heparin (525–528). At 37°C, more insulin binds to dialysis-set plastics than at room temperature (526); therefore, once a routine regimen is established, it is prudent to adhere to it. The ultimate absorption from dialysate to circulation varies from 13% to 46% of the intraperitoneal dose (527,529,530). In CAPD, the total intraperitoneal dose is 2.5 to 3.5 times the previous subcutaneous dose, and in CCPD, 2 times the subcutaneous dose (522,531,532). The dose is larger in intraperitoneal administration because of loss of insulin in effluent dialysate, intraperitoneal degradation, hepatic metabolism, binding to dialysis-set plastics, and glucose absorption during dialysis.

The following protocols are our modifications of several previously described protocols, reviewed by Copley and Lindberg (524).

Conversion from Subcutaneous to Intraperitoneal Insulin in Continuous Ambulatory Peritoneal Dialysis Patients

1. Plan on four exchanges per day. Bag volume does not matter.
2. Total all of the subcutaneous insulin given the previous day (NPH, Lente, regular, or any other kind, plus multiple doses).
3. Hold all subcutaneous insulin after 8 PM the night before the conversion. No further subcutaneous insulin is administered.
4. Stop all IV insulin after 4 AM the day of the conversion. All further insulin is intraperitoneal regular insulin.
5. Perform autolets immediately before each exchange, and record.
6. To the first bag, add one-third of the total calculated in item 2, all as regular. This represents the basal dose. See item 10 for nighttime bag.
7. To item 6, for a 1.5% dextrose bag, add no more extra insulin (i.e., the usual basal dose); for a 2.5% dextrose bag, add 10% more units of regular insulin to basal dose;

and for a 4.25% dextrose bag, add 20% more units of regular insulin to the basal dose.

8. Suggested changes to basal dose of insulin:

Pre-Exchange Autolet Blood Sugar (Mg/dL) Amount of Insulin Change Per Whole Bag
<80 Decrease by 15%
81–160 No change
161–220 Add 10%
221–250 Add 15%
251–400 Add 20% to 25%
401–500 33%
>500 Consider hospitalization

9. Therefore, total insulin dose per bag is composed of three components: (a) basal dose as in item 6; (b) dextrose addition as in item 7; and (c) hyperglycemic addition as in item 8.
10. For nighttime bag do all the calculations in the preceding then reduce insulin dose for the bag by 50% because the patient will be asleep.

Conversion from Subcutaneous to Intraperitoneal Insulin in Continuous Cycling Peritoneal Dialysis Patients

1. Plan on a single 4.25% dextrose daytime exchange
2. Cycler exchanges to be determined individually
3. Total all of the previous daily subcutaneous insulin: (a) all types of insulin, plus (b) all doses.
4. Hold all subcutaneous insulin after 8 PM the night before. Hold all IV insulin by 4 AM the day of the conversion.
5. To the daytime 4.25% bag, add 120% of the previous day's total (see item 3) all as regular insulin. Most cycler patients who do not carry intraperitoneal fluid during the day, and thus do not have an intraperitoneal reservoir of insulin, require a subcutaneous injection in the morning of intermediate-acting insulin.
6. Eighty percent of the previous day's total subcutaneous dose is added to one bag hung on the cycler. Many patients ultimately need as much insulin at night on the cycler as they do during the day when they are eating. Starting the cycler dose at 80% of the diurnal dose is a cautious beginning range.
7. Perform autolet of blood sugar before meals and just before draining the daytime bag and q3h the first night on the cycler and at the end of the cycler run.

Conversion from Intraperitoneal Insulin in Continuous Ambulatory Peritoneal Dialysis to Continuous Cycling Peritoneal Dialysis

The mean total daily intraperitoneal insulin dose on CCPD is approximately 85% of that total intraperitoneal dose on

CAPD. About 40% of the total intraperitoneal dose in CCPD is required in the daytime exchange (533); therefore, when converting from CAPD to CCPD:

1. Total daily intraperitoneal dose on CAPD $\times$ 0.85 $\times$ 0.4 = daytime exchange dose.
2. Total daily intraperitoneal dose on CAPD $\times$ 0.85 $\times$ 0.6 = nighttime dose delivered steadily and equally throughout the night.

HYPERTENSION

The original reports of outcomes in patients receiving PD emphasized the control of hypertension and attributed this phenomenon to better volume control and/or the better removal of vasoconstrictor substances (534,535). Some of these originally described patients had been previously treated with HD and had higher blood pressure. Numerous studies now corroborate that during the early period of treatment by PD, hypertension is controlled at least as well as and often better than that achieved by HD (536–541). There is weak but suggestive evidence that this early improvement in hypertension is secondary to the correction of excess extracellular volume (540,542,543); however, there are data to suggest this is a gross oversimplification (541). It is conceivable that the presence of intraperitoneal fluid may alter hemodynamics; however, when measured, the instillation of dialysate into the peritoneal cavity essentially invokes only minor effects on splanchnic, central venous, and cardiac hemodynamics (544–550). Nonetheless, prolonged PD and presumably better blood pressure control have been associated with reduced left ventricular mass (539,551), which has not been demonstrated in HD patients (551–555). Volume control and sodium removal by PD are related to numerous factors, including dialysate composition (osmolality created by dextrose and sodium concentrations), peritoneal permeability and UF capacity, splanchnic circulation, and residual renal function (542,556).

After many months of PD, the antihypertensive effect of PD appears to be less likely secondary to volume control (540,557). At this time, weight may actually have risen, although this could reflect the increased caloric intake from the transperitoneal absorption of dextrose. Because the peritoneal membrane is associated with different transport properties than HD membranes, the more efficient removal of pressor substances by PD is speculated to play a role in this late hypertension control (540). These pressor compounds could include Na-K-ATPase inhibitors, norepinephrine, and endothelin. However, after a year or more of PD, hypertension is less effectively controlled than after PD initiation. This may be related to the development of peritoneal sclerosis (558), progressive obesity, dialysis prescription noncompliance (107), improved appetite and well being and dietary indiscretion, increased hematocrit, loss of residual renal function, or other as yet unidentified factors.

TRANSPLANTATION

Peritoneal dialysis patients may differ from their HD counterparts in several aspects that could influence transplant outcomes. Compared to HD patients, PD patients demonstrate a more normal immune response as characterized by T4:T8 lymphocyte ratios, T-cell counts, T-cell stimulation, cell-mediated immunity, and lymphocyte blastogenesis (559–563). Thus, it was not completely unexpected when two early small studies suggested that graft survival might be inferior in recipients previously treated by PD (559,564). It was speculated that the PD patients were more immunocompetent at the time of transplantation, thus decreasing graft tolerance. However, subsequent studies with larger population bases have shown that graft survival is essentially equal in recipients previously treated by HD or PD (565,566).

Another difference between PD and HD patients influencing transplantation is that the control of anemia, with or without erythropoietin, is easier with PD (567). Thus, PD patients are less likely to experience blood transfusions and subsequent enhanced graft tolerance. In fact, pretransplant blood transfusions appear to be of less benefit to PD patients (564). Furthermore, the decreased transfusion requirement of PD patients makes hepatitis less likely, which is important considering the adverse effects of viral hepatitis as graft survival (568).

Peritoneal dialysis patients when compared to HD patients have better blood pressure control and preserved residual renal function, which may affect care in the immediate posttransplant period. Patients receiving intraperitoneal insulin must be converted back to subcutaneous insulin as PD is terminated. Transperitoneal albumin losses with or without peritonitis contribute to protein malnourishment in PD patients. This may predispose them to wound infections or other steroid complications. Peritoneal dialysis patients are prone to develop higher plasma fibrinogen and Lp(a) lipoprotein concentrations (569–571), which could contribute to posttransplant steroid-exacerbated atherosclerosis. Murphy and coworkers (572) described an increased frequency of early graft thrombosis in PD patients from their center in Belfast as well as throughout the United Kingdom. This may be reflective of severe atherosclerosis present at the time of engraftment.

When specifically addressing wound, urinary tract, and respiratory infections, there is no difference in the frequency or types of non–peritonitis-related posttransplant infections in recipients having been dialyzed by PD or HD (565,566). Of graft recipients, 5% to 15% experience peritonitis in the posttransplant period (573–576), and 2.5% to 10% experience exit site infections (566,574). The course of posttransplant peritonitis generally is not different from that seen in PD patients who are not receiving immunosuppressive medications, and it requires essentially the same treatment with parenteral or intraperitoneal antibiotics, with the exception that allograft function may necessitate larger or more frequent doses. Posttransplant exit site or tunnel infections probably warrant catheter removal, especially if the flesh infection is in proximity to the graft incision.

Peritoneal dialysis catheters are sometimes removed at the time of engraftment because of the location of a pancreatic allograft in adults or the renal allograft in children, and because of the good expected immediate graft function in living related allografts. Leaving the catheters *in situ* for weeks to months has been shown to be safe, although frequent flushing is recommended to maintain patency and to avoid unlubricated or unbuffered bowel contact. Some transplant centers place prophylactic intraperitoneal antibiotics into flushing dialysate and cap off the system at the time of transplantation. Others simply cap off without antibiotics. If an exit site infection is present at the time of transplantation, most centers remove the catheter and proceed with the transplant. A tunnel infection or active peritonitis generally precludes transplantation at that time. A prudent policy is to observe the course of the peritonitis for at least 2 weeks following the discontinuation of antibiotics. If no relapse has occurred, the patient is then reactivated on the recipient list.

Posttransplant ascites can develop in PD patients, even with functioning grafts (577). This may require drainage, which can be done through the catheters into an empty dialysate bag. It is probably related to a hyperemic peritoneum whose mesothelium has been altered by the previous presence of dialysate. It may take weeks, but this does subside spontaneously. The ascites should be drained only when dictated by patient comfort because the protein content is generally high and negative protein balance may ensue.

REFERENCES

1. Nolph KD. Comparison of continuous ambulatory peritoneal dialysis and hemodialysis. *Kidney Int* 1988;33:S123.
2. Maiorca R, et al. Is CAPD competitive with hemodialysis for long-term treatment of uremic patients? *Nephrol Dial Transplant* 1989;4:244.
3. Vonesh EF, Lysaght MJ, Moran J, et al. Kinetic modeling as a prescription aid in peritoneal dialysis. *Blood Purif* 1991;9:246.
4. Disney APS, ed. *Thirteenth Report of the Australia and New Zealand Dialysis and Transplant Registry.* Woodville, South Australia: Queen Elizabeth Hospital, 1990.
5. Fenton SS, Schaubel DE, Desmeules M, et al. Hemodialysis versus peritoneal dialysis: a comparison of adjusted mortality rates. *Am J Kid Dis* 1997;30:334.
6. Golper TA, et al. Peritoneal dialysis results in the EDTA Registry. In: Nolph KD, ed. *Peritoneal dialysis,* 3rd ed. Boston: Kluwer Academic, 1988.
7. Collins AJ, Ma JZ, Umen A, et al. Urea index and other predictors of hemodialysis patient survival. *Am J Kidney Dis* 1994;23:272.
8. Held PJ, et al. Continuous ambulatory peritoneal dialysis and hemodialysis: comparison of patient mortality with adjustment for comorbid conditions. *Kidney Int* 1994;45:1163.
9. Nolph KD. Technique survival in continuous ambulatory peritoneal dialysis. *Perit Dial Int* 1994;14:322.
10. Charra B, et al. Survival as an index of adequacy of dialysis. *Kidney Int* 1992;41:1286.
11. Churchill DN, et al. Adequacy of peritoneal dialysis—Canada–USA study. *J Am Soc Nephrol* 1996;7:198.
12. Lowrie EG, et al. Effect of the hemodialysis prescription on patient morbidity: report from the National Cooperative Dialysis Study. *N Engl J Med* 1981;305:1176.
13. Gotch FA, Sargent JA. A mechanistic analysis of the National Cooperative Dialysis Study. *Kidney Int* 1985;28:526.
14. Delmez J, Windus D. Hemodialysis prescription and delivery in a metropolitan community. *Kidney Int* 1991;41:1023.
15. Lindsay RM, Spanner E. A hypothesis: the protein catabolic rate is dependent on the type and amount of treatment in dialyzed uremic patients. *Am J Kidney Dis* 1989;13:382.
16. United States Renal Data System. *USRDS 1993 Annual Report.* The National Institutes of Health, The National Institute of Diabetes and Digestive and Kidney Diseases, Bethesda, MD. March 1993.
17. Noh H, Lee SW, Kang SW, et al. Serum C-reactive protein: a predictor of mortality in continuos ambulatory peritoneal dialysis patients. *Perit Dial Int* 1998;18:387.
18. Herrman FR, et al. Serum albumin level on admission as a predictor of death, length of stay, and readmission. *Arch Intern Med* 1992;152:125.
19. Lowrie EG, Lew NL. Death risk in hemodialysis patients: the predictive value of commonly measured variables and an evaluation of death rate differences between facilities. *Am J Kidney Dis* 1990;15:458.
20. Churchill DN, et al. Canadian hemodialysis morbidity study. *Am J Kidney Dis* 1992;19:214.
21. Winchester J. The albumin dilemma. *Am J Kidney Dis* 1992;20:76.
22. Pollock CA, et al. Continuous ambulatory peritoneal dialysis: eight years of experience at a single center. *Medicine* 1989;68:293.
23. Teehan BP, et al. Urea kinetic analysis and clinical outcome on CAPD: a five-year longitudinal study. In: Khanna R, et al, eds. *Advances in peritoneal dialysis.* Toronto: Peritoneal Dialysis Bulletin, 1990:181.
24. Blake PG, et al. Serum albumin in patients on continuous ambulatory peritoneal dialysis—predictors and correlations with outcomes. *J Am Soc Nephrol* 1993;3:1501.
25. Young GA, et al. Nutrition and delayed hypersensitivity during continuous ambulatory peritoneal dialysis in relation to peritonitis. *Nephron* 1986;43:177.
26. Keshaviah P, et al. Impact of nutrition on CAPD mortality for the Canada–USA study of peritoneal dialysis adequacy. *J Am Soc Nephrol* 1994;5:494A.
27. Fenton SSA, et al. Nutritional assessment of continuous ambulatory peritoneal dialysis patients. *Trans Am Soc Artif Intern Organs* 1987;33:650.
28. Pollock CA, et al. Total body nitrogen by neutron activation in maintenance dialysis. *Am J Kidney Dis* 1990;16:38.
29. Fine A, Cox D. Modest reduction of serum albumin in continuous ambulatory peritoneal dialysis patients is common and of no apparent clinical consequence. *Am J Kidney Dis* 1992;20:50.
30. Struijk DG, et al. The effect of serum albumin at the start of continuous ambulatory peritoneal dialysis treatment on patient survival. *Perit Dial Int* 1994;14:212.
31. Acchiardo SR, et al. Evaluation of CAPD prescription. In: Khanna R, et al, eds. *Advances in peritoneal dialysis.* Toronto: Peritoneal Dialysis Bulletin, 1991:47.
32. Nolph KD, et al. Cross sectional assessment of weekly urea and creatinine clearances and indices of nutrition in continuous ambulatory peritoneal dialysis patients. *Perit Dial Int* 1993;13:178.
33. Kaysen GA, Schoenfeld PY. Albumin homeostasis in patients undergoing continuous ambulatory peritoneal dialysis. *Kidney Int* 1984;25:107.
34. Burkart JM, Jordan J, Rocco MV. Cross sectional analysis of D/P creatinine ratios versus serum albumin values in NIPD patients. *Perit Dial Int* 1994;14:S18.
35. Hylander B, Barkeling B, Rossner S. Eating behavior in continuous ambulatory peritoneal dialysis and hemodialysis patients. *Am J Kidney Dis* 1992;20:592.
36. Heimburger O, Bergstrom J, Lindholm B. Is serum albumin an index of nutritional status in continuous ambulatory peritoneal dialysis patients? *Perit Dial Int* 1994;14:108.
37. Koomen GCM, et al. Comparison between dye binding methods and nephelometry for the measurement of albumin in plasma of peritoneal dialysis. *Perit Dial Int* 1992;12:S133A.
38. Young GA, et al. Nutritional assessment of continuous ambulatory peritoneal dialysis patients: an international study. *Am J Kidney Dis* 1991;17:462.
39. Buchwald R, Pena JC. Evaluation of nutritional status in patients on continuous ambulatory peritoneal dialysis. *Perit Dial Int* 1989;9:295.
40. Heide B, et al. Nutritional status of patients undergoing continuous ambulatory peritoneal dialysis. *Perit Dial Bull* 1983;3:138.

41. Lindsay RM, Spanner E. The lower serum albumin does reflect nutritional status. *Semin Dial* 1992;5:215.
42. Cancarini G, et al. Nutritional status in long-term CAPD patients. In: Khanna R, et al, eds. *Advances in peritoneal dialysis.* Toronto: Peritoneal Dialysis Bulletin, 1992:84.
43. Blake PG, et al. Lack of correlation between urea kinetic indices and clinical outcome in CAPD patients. *Kidney Int* 1991;39:700.
44. Keshaviah P, Nolph K. Protein catabolic rate calculations in CAPD patients. *Trans Am Soc Artif Intern Organs* 1991;37:M400.
45. Randerson DH, Chapman GV, Farrell PC. Amino acid and dietary status in long-term CAPD patients. In: Atkins RC, Rarrell PC, Thomson N, eds. *Peritoneal dialysis.* Edinburgh: Churchill Livingstone, 1981:171.
46. Keshaviah P, Nolph KD, Prowant B. Defining adequacy of CAPD with urea kinetics. In: Khanna R, et al, eds. *Advances in peritoneal dialysis.* Toronto: Peritoneal Dialysis Bulletin, 1990:173.
47. Davies SJ, et al. A model of protein intake and urea kinetics that can predict catabolism/anabolism in CAPD patients. *Perit Dial Int* 1992;12:S18A.
48. Wai-Kei LO, et al. Comparison of different measurements of lean body mass in normal individuals and in chronic peritoneal dialysis patients. *Am J Kidney Dis* 1994;23:74.
49. Van Itallie TB, et al. Height-normalized indices of the body's fat free mass and fat mass: potentially useful indicators of nutritional status. *Am J Clin Nutr* 1990;52:953.
50. Detsky AJ, et al. What is subjective global assessment of nutritional status? *J Parenter Enteral Nutr* 1987;11:8.
51. Lameire NH, et al. A longitudinal, five-year study of urea kinetic parameters in CAPD patients. *Kidney Int* 1992;42:426.
52. Bergstrom J, Lindholm B. Nutrition and adequacy of dialysis: how do hemodialysis and CAPD compare? *Kidney Int* 1993;43:S39.
53. Lindsay RM, et al. Which comes first, Kt/V or PCR—chicken or egg? *Kidney Int* 1992;42:S32.
54. Blake PG, et al. Is total creatinine clearance a good predictor of clinical outcome? *Perit Dial Int* 1992;12:353.
55. Heimburger O, Bergstrom J, Lindholm B. Albumin and amino acid levels as markers of adequacy in CAPD. *Perit Dial Int* 1994;14:S123.
56. Brandes JC, et al. Clinical outcome of continuous ambulatory peritoneal dialysis predicted by urea and creatinine kinetics. *J Am Soc Nephrol* 1992;2:1430.
57. Harty JC, et al. Is the correlation between the normalized protein catabolic rate and Kt/V the result of mathematical coupling? *Am J Soc Nephrol* 1993;4:407.
58. Burkart JM, et al. Using a computer kinetic modeling program to prescribe PD. *Perit Dial Int* 1993;13:S77A.
59. Burkart JM, et al. Total energy and dietary protein intake from 9 day food records are related to dialysis dose in peritoneal dialysis and hemodialysis. *Perit Dial Int* 1995;15:S-37A.
60. Heimburger O, et al. The effect of increased PD on Kt/V, protein catabolic rate (PCR) and serum albumin. *Perit Dial Int* 1992;12:S19A.
61. Keshaviah P. Adequacy of CAPD: a quantitative approach. *Kidney Int* 199242:S160.
62. Blake P, et al. The relationship between Kt/V and normalized protein catabolic rate is not linear. *Perit Dial Int* 1993;13:S71A.
63. Ronco C, et al. Assessment of adequacy in peritoneal dialysis. *Adv Renal Replac Ther* 1994;1:15.
64. Nolph KD, et al. The relationship of net protein catabolic rate to weekly urea clearance in continuous ambulatory peritoneal dialysis: linear or curvilinear? *J Am Soc Nephrol* 1994;5:500A.
65. Keshaviah PR, Nolph KD, Stone JCV. The peak concentration hypothesis: a urea kinetic approach to comparing the adequacy of continuous ambulatory peritoneal dialysis and hemodialysis. *Perit Dial Int* 1989;9:257.
66. Rottembourg J, et al. Evolution of residual renal functions in patients undergoing maintenance hemodialysis or continuous ambulatory peritoneal dialysis. *Proc EDTA* 1983;19:397.
67. Cancarini GC, et al. Renal function recovery and maintenance of residual diuresis in CAPD and hemodialysis. *Perit Dial Bull* 1986;6:77.
68. Tattersall JE, et al. Maintaining adequacy of CAPD by individualizing dialysis prescription. *Nephrol Dial Transplant* 1995;9:749.
69. Blumenkrantz MJ, et al. Metabolic balance studies and dietary protein requirements in patients undergoing continuous ambulatory peritoneal dialysis. *Kidney Int* 1981;19:593.
70. Diamond SM, Henrich WL. Nutrition and peritoneal dialysis. In: Mitch WE, Klahr S, eds. *Nutrition and the kidney.* Boston: Little, Brown, 1988:198.
71. Nolph KD. What's new in peritoneal dialysis—an overview. *Kidney Int* 1992;42:S148.
72. Bergstrom J, et al. Protein and energy intake, nitrogen balance and nitrogen losses in patients treated with continuous ambulatory peritoneal dialysis. *Kidney Int* 1993;44:1048.
73. Harty JC, et al. The normalized protein catabolic rate is a flawed marker of nutrition in CAPD patients. *Kidney Int* 1994;45:103.
74. Lindholm B, et al. Urea kinetic modeling in peritoneal dialysis. In: Lopot F, ed. *Urea kinetic modeling.* Ruddervoorde: EDTNA-ERCA, 1990:134.
75. Blake PG, et al. Is total creatinine clearance a good predictor of clinical outcomes in continuous ambulatory peritoneal dialysis? *Perit Dial Int* 1992;12:353.
76. Twardowski ZJ. Clinical value of standardized equilibration tests in CAPD patients. *Blood Purif* 1989;7:95.
77. Twardowski ZJ. Nightly peritoneal dialysis (why? who? how? and when?). *Trans Am Soc Artif Intern Organs* 1990;36:8.
78. Garred LJ, et al. A simple kinetic model for assessing peritoneal mass transfer in chronic ambulatory peritoneal dialysis. *Trans Am Soc Artif Intern Organs* 1983;3:140.
79. Popovich RP, Moncrief SW. Transport kinetics. In: Nolph KD, ed. *Peritoneal dialysis,* 2nd ed. Boston: Martinus Nijhoff, 1985:115.
80. Vonesh EF, et al. Kinetic modeling as a prescription aid in peritoneal dialysis. *Blood Purif* 1991;9:246.
81. Burkart JM, Jordan JR, Rocco MV. Assessment of dialysis adequacy by measured clearance versus extrapolated PET data. *Perit Dial Int* 1993;13:184.
82. Pannakeet MM, Imholz ALT, Struijk DG, et al. The standard peritoneal permeability analysis: a tool for assessment of peritoneal permeability characteristics in CAPD patients. *Kidney Int* 1995;48:866.
83. Pride, Burkart, et al. Comparison of 2.5% PET with 4.25% PET. *Perit Dial Int* 2001, in press.
84. Brandes JC, Piering WF, Beres JA. A method to assess efficacy of CAPD: preliminary results. In: Khanna R, et al, eds. *Advances in peritoneal dialysis,* vol. 6. Nashville: Peritoneal Dialysis Bulletin, 1990:192.
85. Rocco MV, Jordan JR, Burkart JM. The efficacy number as a predictor of morbidity and mortality in peritoneal dialysis patients. *J Am Soc Nephrol* 1993;4:1184.
86. United States Renal Data System. *USRDS 1991 Annual Report.* The National Institutes of Health, The National Institute of Diabetes and Digestive and Kidney Diseases, Bethesda, MD. March 1991.
87. Posen GA, et al. Results from the Canadian Renal Failure Registry. *Am J Kidney Dis* 1990;15:397.
88. Maiorca R, et al. A six-year comparison of patient and technique survivals in CAPD and HD. *Kidney Int* 1988;34:518.
89. Brophy DF, Sowinski KM, Kraus MA, et al. Small and middle molecular weight solute clearance in nocturnal intermittent peritoneal dialysis. *Perit Dial Int* 1999;19:534.
90. Nolph KD, Twardowski ZJ, Keshaviah PR. Weekly clearances of urea and creatinine on CAPD and NIPD. *Perit Dial Int* 1992;12:298.
91. Blake PG, et al. Changes in peritoneal membrane transport rates in patients on long term CAPD. In: Khanna R, et al, eds. *Advances in peritoneal dialysis,* vol. 5. Toronto: Peritoneal Dialysis International, 1989:3.
92. Twardowski ZJ, Nolph KD. Peritoneal dialysis: how much is enough? *Semin Dial* 1988;1:75.
93. Gotch FA, Sargent JA. A mechanistic analysis of the National Cooperative Dialysis Study. *Kidney Int* 1985;28:526.
94. Watson PE, et al. Total body water volumes for adult males and females estimated from simple anthropometric measurements. *Am J Clin Nutr* 1980;33:27.
95. Hume R, Weyers E. Relationship between total body water and surface area in normal and obese subjects. *Clin Pathol* 1971;24:234.
96. Satko SG, Burkart JM. Frequency and causes of discrepancy between Kt/V and creatinine. *Perit Dial Int* 1998;19:31.
97. Tzamaloukas AH, Saddler MC, Murphy G, et al. Volume of distribution and fractional clearance of urea in amputees on continuous ambulatory peritoneal dialysis. *Perit Dial Int* 1994;14:356.

98. Jones MR. Etiology of severe malnutrition: results of an international cross-sectional study in continuous ambulatory peritoneal dialysis patients. *Am J Kidney Dis* 1994;23:412.

99. Borah MF, et al. Nitrogen balance during intermittent dialysis therapy of uremia. *Kidney Int* 1978;14:491.

100. Grodstein G, Kopple JD. Urea nitrogen appearance, a simple and practical indicator of total nitrogen output. *Kidney Int* 1979;16:953A.

101. Maroni BJ, Steinman TI, Mitch WE. A method for estimating nitrogen intake of patients with chronic renal failure. *Kidney Int* 1985;27:58.

102. Randerson DH, Chapman GV, Farrell PC. Amino acid and dietary status in CAPD patients. In: Atkins RC, Farrell PC, Thompson N, eds. *Peritoneal dialysis.* Edinburgh: Churchill Livingstone, 1981:179.

103. Teehan BP, Schleifer CR, Sigler MH, et al. A quantitative approach to the CAPD prescription. *Perit Dial Bull* 1985;5:152.

104. Kjeldahl J. Neue methode zur bestimmung des stickoffs nin organischen Korpern. *Zeit Anal Chem* 1983;22:366.

105. Keshaviah PR, et al. Lean body mass estimation by creatinine kinetics. *J Am Soc Nephrol* 1994;4:1475.

106. Keen M, Lipps B, Gotch F. The measured creatinine generation rate in CAPD suggests only 78% of prescribed dialysis is delivered. In: Khanna R, et al, eds. *Advances in peritoneal dialysis.* Toronto: Peritoneal Dialysis Publications, 1993:73.

107. Warren PJ, Brandes JC. Compliance with the peritoneal dialysis prescription is poor. *J Am Soc Nephrol* 1994;4:1627.

108. Burkart JM, Bleyer AJ, Jordan JR, et al. An elevated ratio of measured to predicted creatinine production in CAPD patients is not a sensitive predictor of noncompliance with the dialysis prescription. *Perit Dial Int* 1996;16:142.

109. Burkart JM. Adequacy of peritoneal dialysis. *Advan Renal Replac Ther* 2000;7:310.

110. Bhaskaran S, Schaubel DE, Jassal V, et al. The effect of small solute clearance on survival of anuric peritoneal dialysis patients. *Perit Dial Int* 2000;20:181.

111. Churchill DN, Thorpe KE, Nolph KD. Increased peritoneal transport is associated with poor patient and technique survival on continuous ambulatory peritoneal dialysis. *J Am Soc Nephrol* 1998;9:1285.

112. Davies SJ, Phillips L, Russell GI. Peritoneal solute transfer is an independent predictor of survival on CAPD. *J Am Soc Nephrol* 1996;7:1443.

113. Clinical Practice Guidelines of the Canadian Society of Nephrology for the Treatment of Patients with Chronic Renal Failure. *J Am Soc Nephrol* 1999;10:13.

114. The Renal Association and Royal College of Physicians of London. *Treatment of adult patients with renal failure. Recommended standards and audit measures.* London: Royal College of Physicians, 1997.

115. Nissenson AR, et al. Non-medical factors that impact on ESRD modality selection. *Kidney Int* 1993;43:S120.

116. Wegner G. Chirurgische bemerkungen uber die peritonealhohle, mit besonderer berucksichtigung der ovariotomie. *Arch Klin Chir* 1877;20:51.

117. Twardowski ZJ. New approaches to intermittent peritoneal dialysis therapies. In: Nolph KD, ed. *Peritoneal dialysis,* 3rd ed. Dordrecht: Kluwer Academic, 1989:133.

118. Trevino-Becerra A. Intermittent peritoneal dialysis with a cycler may be the answer. *Perit Dial Bull* 1984;4:112.

119. Shapira J, et al. Peritoneal dialysis in refractory congestive heart failure. Part I. Intermittent peritoneal dialysis. *Perit Dial Bull* 1983;3:130.

120. Nolph KD, Twardowski ZJ, Keshaviah PR. Weekly clearances of urea and creatinine on CAPD and NIPD. *Perit Dial Int* 1992;12:298.

121. Twardowski ZJ, et al. Daily clearances with continuous ambulatory peritoneal dialysis and nightly peritoneal dialysis. *Trans Am Soc Artif Intern Organs* 1986;32:575.

122. Twardowski ZJ, et al. Chronic nightly tidal peritoneal dialysis (NTDP). *Trans Am Soc Artif Intern Organs* 1990;36:M584.

123. Steinhauer HB, et al. Increased dialysis efficiency in tidal peritoneal dialysis compared to intermittent peritoneal dialysis. *Nephron* 1991;58:500.

124. Spencer PC, Farrell PC. Applications of kinetic monitoring in CAPD. In: Weimer W, Fieren MWJA, Diderich PPNN, eds. *Proc IV Benelux Symp* Rotterdam: November 24, 1984:9.

125. Twardowski ZJ, et al. Efficiency of high volume low frequency continuous ambulatory peritoneal dialysis (CAPD). *Trans Am Soc Artif Intern Organs* 1983;29:53.

126. Nolph KD, et al. The kinetics of ultrafiltration during peritoneal dialysis: the role of lymphatics. *Kidney Int* 1987;32:219.

127. Struijk DG, et al. Indirect measurement of lymphatic absorption in CAPD patients by the disappearance rate of dextran 70 is not influenced by trapping. *Kidney Int* 1992;41:1668.

128. Imholz ALT, et al. Residual volume measurements in CAPD patients with exogenous and endogenous solutes. In: Khanna R, et al, eds. *Advances in peritoneal dialysis.* Toronto: University of Toronto, 1992:33.

129. Popovich RP, Pyle WK. Kinetics of peritoneal transport. In: Nolph KD, ed. *Peritoneal dialysis.* The Hague: Martinus Nijhoff, 1981:79.

130. Koomen GC, et al. A fast reliable method for the measurement of intraperitoneal dextran 70, used to calculate lymphatic absorption. *Adv Perit Dial* 1991;7:10.

131. Heimburger O, et al. Peritoneal transport in CAPD patients with permanent loss of ultrafiltration capacity. *Kidney Int* 1990;38:495.

132. Ronco C, et al. Pathophysiology of ultrafiltration in peritoneal dialysis. *Perit Dial Int* 1990;10:119.

133. Mactier RA. Investigation and management of ultrafiltration failure in CAPD. In: Khanna R, et al, eds. *Advances in peritoneal dialysis.* Nashville: Peritoneal Dialysis Bulletin, 1991:57.

134. Verger C, Larpent L, Celicout B. Clinical significance of ultrafiltration failure on CAPD. In: La Greca G, et al, eds. *Peritoneal dialysis.* Milan: Wichtig Editore, 1986:91.

135. Heimburger O, et al. A quantitative description of solute and fluid transport during peritoneal dialysis. *Kidney Int* 1992;41:1320.

136. Faller B, Marichal JF. Loss of ultrafiltration in continuous ambulatory peritoneal dialysis: a role for acetate. *Perit Dial Bull* 1984;4:10.

137. Bazzato G, et al. Restoration of ultrafiltration capacity of peritoneal membrane in patients on CAPD. *Int J Artif Organs* 1984;7:93.

138. Mujais S, Nolph K, Gokal R, et al. Evaluation and management of ultrafiltration problems in peritoneal dialysis. *Perit Dial Int* 2000;20:S5.

139. Panasiuk E, et al. Characteristics of peritoneum after peritonitis in CAPD patients. *Adv Perit Dial* 1988;4:42.

140. Dobbie JW, Lloyd JK, Gall CA. Categorization of ultrastructural changes in peritoneal mesothelium, stroma, and blood vessels in uremia and CAPD patients. In: Nolph KD, ed. *Advances in peritoneal dialysis,* 3rd ed. Boston: Kluwer Academic, 1990:3.

141. Verger C, Luger A, Moore HL. Acute changes in peritoneal morphology and transport properties with infectious peritonitis and mechanical injury. *Kidney Int* 1983;23:823.

142. Dobbie J. Pathogenesis of peritoneal fibrosing syndromes (sclerosing peritonitis) in peritoneal dialysis. *Perit Dial Int* 1992;12:14.

143. Di Paolo N, Vanni L, Sacchi G. Autologous implant of peritoneal mesothelium in rabbits and man. *Clin Nephrol* 1990;34:179.

144. Posthuma N, ter Weel PM, Donnker AJM, et al. Icodextrin use in CCPD patients with peritonitis: ultrafiltration abd serum disaccharide concentrations. *Nephrol Dial Transplant* 1998;13:2341.

145. Krediet RT, et al. Alterations in the peritoneal transport of water and solutes during peritonitis in continuous ambulatory peritoneal dialysis patients. *Eur J Clin Invest* 1987;17:43.

146. Rottembourg J, et al. Role of acetate in loss of ultrafiltration during CAPD. *Contrib Nephrol* 1987;57:197.

147. Ota K, et al. Functional deterioration of the peritoneum: does it occur in the absence of peritonitis? *Nephrol Dial Transplant* 1987;2:30.

148. Shaldon S, et al. Pathogenesis of sclerosing peritonitis in CAPD. *Trans Am Soc Artif Intern Organs* 1984;30:193.

149. Pollack CA, et al. Loss of ultrafiltration in continuous ambulatory peritoneal dialysis (CAPD). *Perit Dial Int* 1989;9:107.

150. Verger C, Larpen L, Dumontet M. Prognostic values of peritoneal equilibration curves in CAPD patients. In: Maher JF, ed. *Frontiers in peritoneal dialysis.* New York: Field, Rich, 1986:88.

151. Miranda B, et al. Peritoneal resting and heparinization as an effective treatment for ultrafiltration failure in patients on CAPD. *Contrib Nephrol* 1991;89:199.

152. Di Paolo N, et al. Phosphatidylcholine and peritoneal transport during peritoneal dialysis. *Nephron* 1986;44:365.

153. Querques M, et al. Influence of phosphatidylcholine on ultrafiltration and solute transfer in CAPD patients. *Trans Am Soc Artif Intern Organs* 1990;36:M581.

154. Dombros N, et al. Phosphatidylcholine increases ultrafiltration in continuous ambulatory peritoneal dialysis patients. In: Avram MM, Giordano C, eds. *Ambulatory peritoneal dialysis.* New York: Plenum, 1990:39.

155. Mactier RA, et al. Pharmacological reduction of lymphatic absorption from the peritoneal cavity increases net ultrafiltration and solute clearances in peritoneal dialysis. *Nephron* 1988;50:229.

156. Di Paolo N, et al. Phosphatidylcholine: a physiological modulator of the peritoneal membrane. In: Avram MM, Giordano C, eds. *Ambulatory peritoneal dialysis.* New York: Plenum, 1990:44.

157. Chan H, Abraham G, Oreopoulos DG. Oral lecithin improves ultrafiltration in patients on peritoneal dialysis. *Perit Dial Int* 1989;9:203.

158. De Vecchi A, et al. Phosphatidylcholine administration in continuous ambulatory peritoneal dialysis (CAPD) patients with reduced ultrafiltration. *Perit Dial Int* 1989;9:207.

159. Huarte-Loza E, et al. Peritoneal membrane failure as a determinant of the CAPD future. *Contrib Nephrol* 1987;47:219.

160. Diaz-Buxo JA. Peritoneal sclerosis in a woman on continuous cyclic peritoneal dialysis. *Semin Dial* 1992;5:317.

161. Verger C, Celicout B. Peritoneal permeability and encapsulating peritonitis. *Lancet* 1985;1:986.

162. Monquil MC, Imholz AL, Struijk DJ, et al. Does impaired transcellular water transport contribute to net ultrafiltration failure during CAPD? *Perit Dial Int* 1995;15:42.

163. Goffin E, Combert S, Jamar F, et al. Expression of aquaporin (AQP1) in a long term peritoneal dialysis patient with impaired transcellular water transport. *Am J Kidney Dis* 1999;33:383.

164. Lamperi S, Carozzi S, Nasini MG. Lympho-monokine disorders and peritoneal fibroblast proliferation in CAPD. *Trans Am Soc Artif Intern Organs* 1986;32:35.

165. Turner MW, Holleman JH. Successful therapy of sclerosing peritonitis. *Semin Dial* 1992;5:316.

166. Clark CP, Vanderpool D, Preskitt JT. The response of retroperitoneal fibrosis to tamoxifen. *Surgery* 1991;109:502.

167. Bargman JM, Oreopoulos DG. Complications other than peritonitis or those related to the catheter and the fate of uremic organ dysfunction in patients receiving peritoneal dialysis. In: Nolph KD, ed. *Peritoneal dialysis,* 3rd ed. Dordrecht: Kluwer Academic, 1990:289.

168. Grefberg N, Nilsson P, Andreen T. Sclerosing obstructive peritonitis, beta blockers, and continuous ambulatory peritoneal dialysis. *Lancet* 1983;2:733.

169. Palmer RA, et al. Treatment of chronic renal failure by prolonged peritoneal dialysis. *N Engl J Med* 1966;274:248.

170. Tenckhoff H, Schechter H. A bacteriologically safe peritoneal access device. *Trans Am Soc Artif Intern Organs* 1968;14:181.

171. Port FK, et al. Risk of peritonitis and technique failure by CAPD connection technique: a national study. *Kidney Int* 1992;42:967.

172. Gokal R, Alexander S, et al. Peritoneal catheters and exit site practices toward optimum peritoneal access: 1998 update. *Perit Dial Int* 1998;18:11.

173. Rottembourg J, et al. Straight or curled Tenckhoff peritoneal catheter for continuous ambulatory peritoneal dialysis (CAPD). *Perit Dial Bull* 1981;1:123.

174. Akyol AM, Porteous C, Brown MW. A comparison of two types of catheters for continuous ambulatory peritoneal dialysis (CAPD). *Perit Dial Int* 1990;10:63.

175. Scott PD, et al. Peritoneal dialysis access: prospective randomized trial of 3 different peritoneal catheters—preliminary report. *Perit Dial Int* 1994;14:289.

176. Oreopoulos DG, et al. A prospective study of the effectiveness of three permanent peritoneal catheters. *Proc Clin Dial Transplant Forum* 1976;6:96.

177. Apostolidis NS, et al. The use of TWH catheters in CAPD patients: fourteen year experience in technique survival and complication rates *Perit Dial Int* 1998;18:424.

178. Flanigan MJ, et al. The use and complications of three peritoneal dialysis catheter designs: a retrospective analysis. *Trans Am Soc Artif Intern Organs* 1987;33:33.

179. Twardowski ZJ, et al. The need for a "swan neck" permanently bent, arcuate peritoneal dialysis catheter. *Perit Dial Bull* 1985;5:219.

180. Eklund BH, et al. Catheter configuration and outcome in patients on continuous ambulatory peritoneal dialysis: a prospective comparison of two catheters. *Perit Dial Int* 1994;14:70.

181. Nebel M, Marczewski K, Finke K. Three years of experience with the swan neck Tenckhoff catheter. *Adv Perit Dial* 1991;7:208.

182. Hwang TL, Huang CC. Comparison of swan neck catheter with Tenckhoff catheter for CAPD. *Adv Perit Dial* 1994;10:203.

183. Golper TA, et al. Catheters and peritonitis: the Network 9 peritonitis study. *J Am Soc Nephrol* 1993;4:405A.

184. Twardowski ZJ, Prowant BF, Nichols WK, et al. Six year experience with Swan neck presternal peritoneal dialysis catheter. *Perit Dial Int* 1998;18:598.

185. Alexander SR, et al. Maintenance dialysis in North American children and adolescents: a preliminary report. *Kidney Int* 1993;44:S104.

186. Lewis MA, Nycyk JA. Practical peritoneal dialysis—the Tenckhoff catheter in acute renal failure. *Pediatr Nephrol* 1992;6:470.

187. Gokal R, et al. Peritoneal catheters and exit-site practices: toward optimum peritoneal access. *Perit Dial Int* 1993;13:29.

188. Robison RJ, et al. Surgical considerations of continuous ambulatory peritoneal dialysis. *Surgery* 1984;96:723.

189. Khanna R. Acute management of the patient requiring a chronic peritoneal catheter. *Semin Dial* 1990;3:93.

190. Prowant BF, Warady BZ, Nolph KD. Peritoneal dialysis catheter exit site care: results of an international survey. *Perit Dial Int* 1993;13:149.

191. Golper TA, et al. Risk factors for peritonitis and catheter loss in patients on chronic peritoneal dialysis: the Network 9 peritonitis and catheter survival study. *Am J Kidney Dis* 1996;28:428.

192. Schleifer CR, et al. Management of hernias and Tenckhoff catheter complications in CAPD. *Perit Dial Bull* 1984;4:146.

193. Odor A, et al. Experience with 150 consecutive permanent peritoneal catheters in patients on CAPD. *Perit Dial Bull* 1985;5:226.

194. Lovinggood JP. Peritoneal catheter implantation for CAPD. *Perit Dial Bull* 1984;4:S106.

195. Crabtree JH, Fishman A, Siddiqi RA, et al. The risk of infection and peritoneal catheter loss from implant procedure exit site trauma. *Perit Dial Int* 1999;19:366.

196. Ash SR, Handt AE, Bloch R. Peritoneoscopic placement of the Tenckhoff catheter: further clinical experience. *Perit Dial Bull* 1983;3:8.

197. Nahman NS, et al. Modification of the percutaneous approach to peritoneal dialysis catheter placement under peritoneoscopic visualization: clinical results in 78 patients. *J Am Soc Nephrol* 1992;3:103.

198. Wright MJ, Bel'eed K, Johnson BF, et al. Randomized prospective comparison of laparoscopic and open peritoneal dialysis catheter insertion. *Perit Dial Int* 1999;19:372.

199. Kimmelstiel FM, et al. Laparoscopic management of peritoneal dialysis catheters. *Surg Gynecol Obstet* 1993;176:565.

200. Shyr YM. Complications of peritoneal catheters placed by a single surgeon. *Perit Dial Int* 1994;14:401.

201. Nielsen PK, et al. A consecutive study of 646 peritoneal dialysis catheters. *Perit Dial Int* 1994;14:170.

202. Bullmaster JR, et al. Surgical aspects of the Tenckhoff peritoneal dialysis catheter: a 7 year experience. *Am J Surg* 1985;149:339.

203. Mellotte GJ, et al. Peritoneal dialysis catheters: a comparison between percutaneous and conventional surgical placement techniques. *Nephrol Dial Transplant* 1993;8:626.

204. Jacobs IG, et al. Radiologic placement of peritoneal dialysis catheters: preliminary experience. *Radiology* 1992;182:251.

205. Moncrie JW, et al. The Moncrief-Popovich catheter: a new peritoneal access technique for patients on peritoneal dialysis. *ASAIO J* 1993;39:62.

206. Park MS, et al. Effect of prolonged subcutaneous implantation of peritoneal cathter on peritonitis rate during CAPD: a prospective randomized study. *Blood Purif* 1998;16:171.

207. Clark KR, et al. Surgical aspects of chronic peritoneal dialysis in the neonate and infant under 1 year of age. *J Pediatr Surg* 1992;27:780.

208. Sanderson MC, et al. Surgical complications of continuous ambulatory peritoneal dialysis. *Am J Surg* 1990;160:561.

209. Diaz-Buxo J. Mechanical complications of chronic peritoneal dialysis catheters. *Semin Dial* 1991;4:106.

210. Francis DMA, et al. Surgical aspects of continuous ambulatory peritoneal dialysis—3 years experience. *Br J Surg* 1984;71:225.

211. Lye WC, et al. Breaking-in after the insertion of Tenckhoff catheters: a comparison of two techniques. *Adv Peritoneal Dial* 1993;3:236.

212. Song JH, Kim GA, Lee SW, et al. Clinical outcomes of immediate full-volume exchange one year after peritoneal catheter implantation for CAPD *Perit Dial Int* 2000;20:194.

213. Copley JB. Prevention of peritoneal dialysis catheter-related infections. *Am J Kidney Dis* 1987;10:401.

214. Luzar MA, et al. Exit site care and exit site infection in continuous ambulatory peritoneal dialysis: results of a randomized multicenter trial. *Perit Dial Int* 1990;10:25.

215. Waite NM, Webser N, Laurel M, et al. The efficacy of exit site povidone iodine ointment in the prevention of early peritoneal dialysis-related infections. *Am J Kidney Dis* 1997;29:763.

216. Swartz R, et al. The curled catheter: dependable device for percutaneous peritoneal access. *Perit Dial Int* 1990;10:231.

217. Joffe P, Christensen AL, Jensen C. Peritoneal catheter tip location during non-complicated continuous ambulatory peritoneal dialysis. *Perit Dial Int* 1991;11:261.

218. Schleifer CR, et al. Migration of peritoneal catheters: personal experience and a survey of 72 other units. *Perit Dial Bull* 1987;7:189.

219. Moss JS, et al. Malpositioned peritoneal dialysis catheters: a critical reappraisal of correction by stiff-wire manipulation. *Am J Kidney Dis* 1990;15:305.

220. Smith DW, Rankin RA. Value of peritoneoscopy for nonfunctioning continuous ambulatory peritoneal dialysis catheters. *Gastrointest Endoscop* 1989;35:90.

221. Gibson DH, et al. Laparoscopic repositioning of blocked peritoneal dialysis catheters in patients on CAPD. *Clin Nephrol* 1990;33:208.

222. Wilson JAP, Swartz RD. Peritoneoscopy in the management of catheter malfunction during continuous ambulatory peritoneal dialysis. *Dig Dis Sci* 1985;30:465.

223. Gadallah MF, Arora N, Arumugam Moles K. Role of Fogarty catheter manipulation in management of migrated, nonfunctional peritoneal dialysis catheters. *Am J Kidney Dis* 2000;35:301.

224. Simons ME, Pron G, Voros M, et al. Fluoroscopically-guided manipulation of malfunctioning peritoneal dialysis catheters. *Perit Dial Int* 1999;19:544.

225. Dobrashian RD, Conway B, Hutchison A, et al. The repositioning of migrated Tenckhoff continuous amublatory peritoneal dialysis catheters under fluoroscopic control. *Br J Radiol* 1999;72:452.

226. Palacios M, Schley W, Daugherty JC. Use of streptokinase to clear peritoneal catheter. *Dial Transplant* 1982;11:172.

227. Benevent D, et al. Fungal peritonitis in patients on continuous ambulatory peritoneal dialysis. *Nephron* 1985;41:203.

228. Wiegmann TB, et al. Effective use of streptokinase for peritoneal catheter failure. *Am J Kidney Dis* 1985;6:119.

229. Allon M, Soucie JM, Macon EJ. Complications with permanent peritoneal dialysis catheters: experience with 154 percutaneously placed catheters. *Nephron* 1988;48:8.

230. Nicholson ML, Burton PR, Donnelly PK. The role of omentectomy in continuous ambulatory peritoneal dialysis. *Perit Dial Int* 1991;11:330.

231. Kopecky RT, Funk MM, Kreitzer PR. Localized genital edema in patients undergoing continuous ambulatory peritoneal dialysis. *J Urol* 1985;124:880.

232. Stegmayr BG, et al. Absence of leakage by insertion of peritoneal dialysis catheter through the rectus muscle. *Perit Dial Int* 1990;10:53.

233. Litherland J, Lupton EW, Ackrill PA, et al. Computed tomographic peritoneography: CT manifestations in the investigation of leaks and abnormal collections in patients on CAPD *Nephrol Dial Transplant* 1994;9:1449.

234. Holley JL, Bernardini J, Piraino B. Characteristics and outcome of peritoneal dialysate leaks and associated infections. *Adv Perit Dial* 1993;9:240.

235. Hirsch DJ, Jindal KK. Late leaks in peritoneal dialysis patients. *Nephrol Dial Transplant* 1990;5:670.

236. Flanigan M, Freeman RM, Lim VS. Cellular response to peritonitis among peritoneal dialysis patients. *Am J Kidney Dis* 1985;6:420.

237. Rubin J, et al. Peritonitis during continuous ambulatory peritoneal dialysis. *Ann Intern Med* 1980;92:7.

238. Fenton S, et al. Clinical aspects of peritonitis in patients on CAPD. *Perit Dial Bull* 1981;6:S4.

239. Gould IM, Casewell MW. The laboratory diagnosis of peritonitis during continuous ambulatory peritoneal dialysis. *J Hosp Infect* 1986;7:155.

240. Koopmans JG, Boeschoten EW, Pannekeet MM, et al. Impaired initial cell reaction in CAPD-related peritonitis. *Perit Dial Int* 1996;16:S362.

241. Pierratos A. Peritoneal dialysis glossary. *Perit Dial Bull* 1984;1:2.

242. Abraham G, et al. Natural history of exit-site infection in patients on continuous ambulatory peritoneal dialysis. *Perit Dial Bull* 1988;8:211.

243. Gonthier D, et al. Erythema: does it indicate infection in a peritoneal catheter exit site? *Adv Perit Dial* 1992;8:230.

244. Flanigan MJ, et al. Continuous ambulatory peritoneal dialysis catheter infections: diagnosis and management. *Perit Dial Int* 1994;14:248.

245. Luzar MA. Exit site infection in continuous ambulatory peritoneal dialysis: a review. *Perit Dial Int* 1991;11:333.

246. Piraino B, Bernardini J, Sorkin M. The influence of peritoneal catheter exit site infections on peritonitis, tunnel infections, and catheter loss in patients on continuous ambulatory peritoneal dialysis. *Am J Kidney Dis* 1986;8:436.

247. Plum J, Sudkamp S, Grabensee B. Results of ultrasound-assisted diagnosis of tunnel infections in continuous ambulatory peritoneal dialysis. *Am J Kidney Dis* 1994;23:99.

248. Korzets Z, Erdberg A, Golan E, et al. Frequent involvement of the internal cuff segment in CAPD peritonitis and exit-site infection—an ultrasound study. *Nephrol Dial Transplant* 1996;11:336.

249. Vychytil A, Lilaj T, Lorenz M, et al. Ultrasonography of the catheter tunnel in peritoneal dialysis patients: what are the indications? *Am J Kidney Dis* 1999;33:722.

250. Vychytil AS, Lorenz M, Schneider B, et al. New criteria for management of catheter infections in peritoneal dialysis patients using ultrasonography. *J Am Soc Nephrol* 1998;9:290.

251. Gupta B, Bernardini J, Piraino B. Peritonitis associated with exit site and tunnel infections. *Am J Kidney Dis* 1996;28:415.

252. Weber J, et al. Survival of 138 surgically placed straight double-cuff Tenckhoff catheters in patients on continuous ambulatory peritoneal dialysis. *Perit Dial Int* 1993;13:224.

253. Woodrow G, Turney JH, Brownjohn AM. Technique failure in peritoneal dialysis and its impact on patient survival. *Perit Dial Int* 1997;17:360.

254. Fried L, Abidi S, Bernardini J, et al. Hospitalization in peritoneal dialysis patients. *Am J Kidney Dis* 1999;33:927.

255. Tzamaloukas AH, Murata GH, Fox L. Peritoneal catheter loss and death in continuous ambulatory peritoneal dialysis peritonitis: correlation with clinical and biochemical parameters. *Perit Dial Int* 1993;13: S338.

256. Fenton SSA and the University of Toronto Collaborative Dialysis Group. Peritonitis related deaths among CAPD patients. *Perit Dial Bull* 1983;3:S9.

257. Fried LF, Bernardini J, Johnston JR, et al. Peritonitis influences mortality in peritoneal dialysis patients. *J Am Soc Nephrol* 1996;7:2176.

258. Holmes CJ. Peritoneal host defense mechanisms in peritoneal dialysis. *Kidney Int* 1994;46:S58.

259. Betjes MGH, et al. Analysis of the peritoneal cellular immune system during CAPD shortly before a clinical peritonitis. *Nephrol Dial Transplant* 1994;9:684.

260. Lai KN, Lai KB, Lam CWK, et al. Changes of cytokine profiles during peritonitis in patients on continuous ambulatory peritoneal dialysis. *Am J Kidney Dis* 2000;35:644.

261. Ates K, Koc R, Nergizoglu G, et al. The longitudinal effect of a single peritonitis episode on peritoneal membrane transport in CAPD patients. *Perit Dial Int* 2000;20:220.

262. Chaimovitz C. Peritoneal dialysis. *Kidney Int* 1994;45:1226.

263. Jorres A, et al. Impact of peritoneal dialysis solutions on peritoneal immune defense. *Perit Dial Int* 1993;13:S291.

264. Cairns HS. Continuous ambulatory peritoneal dialysis peritonitis: role and treatment of impaired host defenses. *Semin Dial* 1992;4:17.

265. Hutchison AJ, Gokal R. Peritoneal dialysis fluids for the future: do we have the solution? *Dial Transplant* 1992;21:57.

266. Dobos GJ, et al. Bicarbonate-based dialysis solution preserves granulocyte functions. *Perit Dial Int* 1994;14:366.

267. Pedersen FB. Biocompatibility studies with bicarbonate-based solutions. *Adv Perit Dial* 1994;10:245.

268. Yu AW, et al. Effects of euhydric peritoneal dialysis solutions containing a mixture of bicarbonate and lactate alone on neutrophilic superoxide production. *ASAIO J* 1994;40:M900.

269. Sundaram S, Cendoroglo M, Cooker LA, et al. Effect of two-chambered bicarbonate lactate-buffered peritoneal dialysis fluids on peripheral blood mononuclear cell land polymorphonuclear cell function in vitro. *Am J Kidney Dis* 1997;30:680.

270. Jorres A, Gahl GM, Frei U. Peritoneal dialysis fluid biocompatibility: does it really matter? *Kidney Int* 1994;46:S79.

271. Mistry C, Gokal R, Peers E, et al. A randomized multicenter clinical trial comparing isosmolar Icodextrin with hyperosmolar glucose solutions in CAPD. *Kidney Int* 1994;46:496.

272. de Fijter CWH, et al. Biocompatibility of a glucose-polymer-containing peritoneal dialysis fluid. *Am J Kidney Dis* 1993;21:411.

273. Posthuma N, Wee FM, Donker AJM, et al. Peritoneal defense using icodextrin or glucose for daytime dwell in CCPD patients. *Perit Dial Int* 1999;19:334.

274. Want T, Cheng H, Heimbruger O, et al. Effect of peritonitis on peritoneal transport characteristics: glucose solution versus polyglucose solution. *Kidney Int* 2000;57:1704.

275. Brulez HFH, et al. In vitro compatibility of a 1.1% amino acid containing peritoneal dialysis fluid with phagocyte function. *Adv Peritoneal Dial* 1994;10:241.

276. Park MS, et al. Peritoneal transport during dialysis with amino acid-based solutions. *Perit Dial Int* 1993;13:280.

277. Bruno M, et al. CAPD with an amino acid dialysis solution: a long-term cross-over study. *Kidney Int* 1989;35:1189.

278. Bender FH, Bernardini J, Piraino B. Calcium mass transfer with dialysate containing 1.25 and 1.75 mmol/L calcium in peritoneal dialysis patients. *Am J Kidney Dis* 1992;20:367.

279. Hercz G, et al. Aplastic osteodystrophy without aluminum: the role of "suppressed" parathyroid function. *Kidney Int* 1993;44:860.

280. Malluche HH, Monier-Faugere MC. Risk of adynamic bone disease in dialyzed patients. *Kidney Int* 1992;42:S62.

281. Piraino B, et al. The use of dialysate containing 2.5 mEq/L calcium in peritoneal dialysis patients. *Perit Dial Int* 1992;12:75.

282. Honkanen E, et al. CAPD with low calcium dialysate and calcium carbonate: results of a 24-week study. *Adv Perit Dial* 1992;8:356.

283. Oreopoulos DG, et al. A simple and safe technique for continuous ambulatory peritoneal dialysis (CAPD). *Trans Am Soc Artif Intern Organs* 1978;24:484.

284. Buoncristiani U. Continuous ambulatory peritoneal dialysis connection systems. *Perit Dial Int* 1993;13:S139.

285. Kiernan L, Kliger A, Gorban-Brennan N, et al. Comparison of continuous ambulatory peritoneal dialysis realted infections with different "Y-tubing" exchange systems. *J Am Soc Nephrol* 1995;5:1835.

286. Monteon F, Correa-Rotter R, Paniagua R, et al. Prevention of peritonitis with disconnect systems in CAPD: a randomized trial. *Kidney Int* 1998;54:2123.

287. Li PKT, Szeto CC, Law MC, et al. Comparison of double bag and Y set disconnect systems in continuous ambulatory peritoneal dialysis: a randomized prospective multicenter study. *Am J Kidney Dis* 1999;33:535.

288. de Fijter CWH, et al. Peritoneal defense in continuous ambulatory versus continuous cyclic peritoneal dialysis. *Kidney Int* 1992;42:947.

289. de Fijter CWH, Oe LP, Nauta J, et al. Clinical efficacy and morbidity associated with continuous cyclic compared with continuous ambulatory peritoneal dialysis *Ann Int Med* 1994;120:264.

290. Rodriguez-Carmona A, Perez Fontan M, Garcia Falcon T, et al. A comparative analysis on the incidence of peritonitis and exit site infection in CAPD and automated peritoneal dialysis. *Perit Dial Int* 1999;19:253.

291. Ponferrada LP, Prowant BF, Rackers JA, et al. A cluster of Gram negative peritonitis episodes associated with reuse of HomeChoice cycler cassettes and drain lines. *Perit Dial Int* 1996;16:636.

292. Chow J, Munro C, Wong M, et al. HomeChoice automated peritoneal dialysis machines: the impact of reuse of tubing and cassettes *Perit Dial Int* 2000;20:336.

293. Lindblad AS, Noval JW, Nolph KD, eds. *Continuous ambulatory peritoneal dialysis in the USA: final report of the National CAPD Registry 1981–1988.* Dordrecht: Kluwer Academic, 1989.

294. Scalamogna A, et al. Exit site and tunnel infections in continuous ambulatory peritoneal dialysis patients. *Am J Kidney Dis* 1991;18:674.

295. Rotellar C, et al. Ten years' experience with continuous ambulatory peritoneal dialysis. *Am J Kidney Dis* 1991;17:158.

296. Holley JL, Bernardini J, Piraino B. Risk factors for tunnel infections in continuous peritoneal dialysis. *Am J Kidney Dis* 1991;18:344.

297. Holley JL, et al. Ultrasound as a tool in the diagnosis and management of exit site infections in patients undergoing continuous ambulatory peritoneal dialysis. *Am J Kidney Dis* 1989;14:211.

298. Korzets Z, Erdberg A, Golan E, et al. Frequent involvement of the internal cuff segment in CAPD peritonitis and exit site infection—an ultrasound study. *Nephrol Dial Transplant* 1996;11:336.

299. Vychytil A, Lilaj T, Lorenz M, et al. Ultrasonography of the catheter tunnel in peritoneal dialysis patients: what are the indications? *Am J Kidney Dis* 1999;33:722.

300. Vychytil A, Lorenz M, Schneider B, et al. New criteria for management of catheter infections in peritoneal dialysis patients using ultrasonography. *J Am Soc Nephrol* 1998;9:290.

301. Holley JL, Bernardini J, Piraino B. Infecting organisms in continuous ambulatory peritoneal dialysis patients on the Y-set. *Am J Kidney Dis* 1994;23:569.

302. Bernardini J, et al. An analysis of ten-year trends in infections in adults on continuous ambulatory peritoneal dialysis (CAPD). *Clin Nephrol* 1991;36:29.

303. Krothapall R, et al. *Pseudomonas* peritonitis and continuous ambulatory peritoneal dialysis. *Arch Intern Med* 1982;142:1862.

304. Bernardini J, Piraino B, Sorkin M. Analysis of continuous ambulatory peritoneal dialysis related *Pseudomonas aeruginosa* infections. *Am J Med* 1987;83:829.

305. Gupta B, Bernardini J, Piraino B. Peritonitis associated with exit site and tunnel infections. *Am J Kidney Dis* 1996;28:415.

306. Lo CY, Chu WL, Wan KM, et al. Pseudomonas exit site infections in CAPD patients: evolution and outcome of treatment. *Perit Dial Int* 1998;18:637.

307. Bayston R, Andrews M, Rigg K, et al. Recurrent infection and catheter loss in patients on continuous ambulatory peritoneal dialysis. *Perit Dial Int* 1999;19:550.

308. Bernardini J, Piraino B, Holley J, et al. A randomized trial of *Staphylococcus aureus* prophylaxis in peritoneal dialysis patients: mupirocin calcium ointment 2% applied to the exit site versus cyclic oral rifampin. *Am J Kidney Dis* 1996;27:695.

309. Thodis E, Bhaskaran S, Pasadakis P, et al. Decrease in *Staphylococcus aureus* exit site infections and peritonitis in CAPD patients by local application of mupirocin ointment at the catheter exit site. *Perit Dial Int* 1998;18:261.

310. Montenegro J, Saracho R, Aguirre R, et al. Exit site care with ciprofloxacin otologic solution prevents polyurethane catheter infection in peritoneal dialysis patients. *Perit Dial Int* 2000;20:209.

311. Maiorca R, et al. Prospective controlled trial of a Y-connector and disinfectant to prevent peritonitis in continuous ambulatory peritoneal dialysis. *Lancet* 1983;2:642.

312. Burkart JM. Comparison of peritonitis rates using standard spike versus Y sets in CAPD. *Trans Am Soc Artif Intern Organs* 1988;34:433.

313. Tofte-Jensen P, et al. PD-related infections of standard and different disconnect systems. *Adv Peritoneal Dial* 1994;10:214.

314. Lupo A, et al. Long-term outcome in continuous ambulatory peritoneal dialysis: a 10 year survey by the Italian cooperative peritoneal dialysis study group. *Am J Kidney Dis* 1994;24:826.

315. Lunde NM, Messana JM, Swartz RD. Unusual causes of peritonitis in patients undergoing continuous peritoneal dialysis with emphasis on *Listeria monocytogenes*. *J Am Soc Nephrol* 1992;3:1092.

316. Saklayen MG. CAPD peritonitis incidence, pathogens, diagnosis, and management. *Med Clin North Am* 1990;74:997.

317. Cheng IKP, Chan PCK, Chan MK. Tuberculous peritonitis complicating long-term peritoneal dialysis. *Am J Nephrol* 1989;9:155.

318. Churchill DN, et al. Peritonitis in continuous ambulatory peritoneal dialysis (CAPD): a multi-centre randomized clinical trial comparing the Y connector disinfectant system to standard systems. *Perit Dial Int* 1989;9:159.

319. Brown AL, et al. Epidemiology of CAPD-associated peritonitis caused by coagulase negative *Staphylococci*: comparison of strains isolated from hands, abdominal Tenckhoff catheter exit site and peritoneal fluid. *Nephrol Dial Transplant* 1991;6:643.

320. Eisenberg ES, et al. Colonization of skin and development of peritonitis due to coagulase-negative *Staphylococci* in patients undergoing peritoneal dialysis. *J Infect Dis* 1987;156:478.

321. Read RR, et al. Peritonitis in peritoneal dialysis: bacterial colonization by biofilm spread along the catheter surface. *Kidney Int* 1989;35:614.

322. Gorman SP, et al. Confocal laser scanning microscopy of peritoneal catheter surfaces. *J Med Microbiol* 1993;38:411.

323. Bint AJ, et al. Diagnosis and management of peritonitis in continuous ambulatory peritoneal dialysis: report of a working party of the British Society for Antimicrobial Chemotherapy. *Lancet* 1987;1:845.

324. Golper TA, Hartstein AI. Analysis of the causative pathogens in uncomplicated CAPD-associated peritonitis: duration of therapy, relapses, and prognosis. *Am J Kidney Dis* 1986;7:141.

325. Horman GB, et al. Plasmid profile and slime analysis of coagulase-negative *Staphylococci* from CAPD patients with peritonitis. *Perit Dial Bull* 1986;6:195.

326. Al-Wali W, et al. Differing prognostic significance of reinfection and relapse in CAPD peritonitis. *Nephrol Dial Transplant* 1992;7:133.

327. Beaman M, et al. Peritonitis caused by slime-producing coagulase negative *Staphylococci* in continuous ambulatory peritoneal dialysis. *Lancet* 1987;1:42.

328. Dasgupta MK, Kowalewaska-Grochowska K, Costerton JW. Biofilm and peritonitis in peritoneal dialysis. *Perit Dial Int* 1993;13:S322.

329. Swartz R, et al. Biofilm formation on peritoneal catheters does not require the presence of infection. *Trans Am Soc Artif Intern Organs* 1991;37:626.

330. Miller TE, Findon G. Touch contamination of connection devices in peritoneal dialysis—a quantitative microbiologic analysis. *Perit Dial Int* 1997;17:560.

331. Sesso R, et al. *Staphylococcus aureus* skin carriage and development of peritonitis in patients on continuous ambulatory peritoneal dialysis. *Clin Nephrol* 1989;31:264.

332. Luzar MA, et al. *Staphylococcus aureus* nasal carriage and infection in patients on continuous ambulatory peritoneal dialysis. *N Engl J Med* 1990;322:505.

333. Lye WC, et al. *Staphylococcus aureus* CAPD-related infections are associated with nasal carriage. *Adv Perit Dial* 1994;10:163.

334. Sewell CM, et al. Staphylococcal nasal carriage and subsequent infection in peritoneal dialysis patients. *JAMA* 1982;248:1493.

335. Oxton LL, et al. Risk factors for peritoneal dialysis related infections. *Perit Dial Int* 1994;14:137.

336. Swartz R, et al. Preventing *Staphylococcus aureus* infection during chronic peritoneal dialysis. *J Am Soc Nephrol* 1991;2:1085.

337. Zimmerman SW, et al. *Staphylococcus aureus* peritoneal catheter related infections: a cause of catheter loss and peritonitis. *Perit Dial Bull* 1988;8:191.

338. Zimmerman SW, et al. Randomized controlled trial of prophylactic rifampin for peritoneal dialysis related infections. *Am J Kidney Dis* 1991;18:225.

339. Perez-Fontan M, et al. Treatment of *Staphylococcus aureus* nasal carriers in continuous ambulatory peritoneal dialysis with mupirocin: long-term results. *Am J Kidney Dis* 1993;22:708.

340. Coles GA, The Mupirocin Study Group. Nasal mupirocin prevents *S. aureus* exit site infections during peritoneal dialysis. *J Am Soc Nephrol* 1996;7:2403.

341. Mylotte JM, Kahler L, Jackson E. "Pulse" nasal mupirocin maintenance regimen in patients undergoing continuous ambulatory peritoneal dialysis. *Infect Control Hosp Epidemiol* 1999;20:741.

342. Herwaldt LA. Reduction of *Staphylococcus aureus* nasal carriage and infection in dialysis patients. *J Hosp Infect* 1998;40:S13.

343. Vas SI, Conly J, Bargman JM, et al. Resistance to mupirocin: no indication of it to date while using mupirocin ointment for prevention of *Staphylococcus aureus* exit site infections in peritoneal dialysis patients. *Perit Dial Intern* 1999;19:313.

344. Bunke CM, Brier ME, Golper TA, et al. Outcomes of single organism peritonitis in peritoneal dialysis: gram negatives versus gram positives in the Network 9 Peritonitis Study. *Kidney Int* 1997;52:524.

345. Peacock SJ, Howe PA, Day NP, et al. Outcome following staphylococcal peritonitis. *Perit Dial Int* 2000;20:215.

346. Van der Reijden HJ, et al. Fecal peritonitis in patients on continuous ambulatory peritoneal dialysis, an end-point in CAPD? *Adv Perit Dial* 1988;4:198.

347. Harwell CM, Newman LN, Cacho CP, et al. Abdominal catastrophe: visceral injury as a cause of peritonitis in patients treated by peritoneal dialysis. *Perit Dial Int* 1997;17:586.

348. Rubin J, et al. Management of peritonitis and bowel perforation during chronic peritoneal dialysis. *Nephron* 1976;16:220.

349. Wakeen MJ, Zimmerman SW, Bidwell D. Viscus perforation in peritoneal dialysis patients: diagnosis and outcome. *Perit Dial Int* 1994;14:371.

350. Bustos E, et al. Clinical aspects of bowel perforation in patients undergoing continuous ambulatory peritoneal dialysis. *Semin Dial* 1994;7:355.

351. Sprenger R, Neyer U. Enterococcus peritonitis after endoscopic polypectomy: need for prophylactic antibiotics. *Perit Dial Bull* 1987;7:263.

352. Holley J, Seibert D, Moss A. Peritonitis following colonoscopy and polypectomy: a need for prophylaxis? *Perit Dial Bull* 1987;7:105.

353. Verger C, Danne O, Vuillemin F. Colonoscopy and continuous ambulatory peritoneal dialysis. *Gastroint Endoscop* 1987;33:334.

354. Barnett JL, Elta G. Bacterial peritonitis following endoscopic variceal sclerotherapy. *Gastroint Endoscop* 1987;33:316.

355. Martinez E, Coll P, Donate T. Prevention of CAPD peritonitis. *Lancet* 1991;337:431.

356. Levy M, Balfe JW. Optimal approach to the prevention and treatment of peritonitis in children undergoing continuous ambulatory and continuous cycling peritoneal dialysis. *Semin Dial* 1994;7:442.

357. Fried L, Bernardini J, Piraino B. Iagrogenic peritonitis: the need for prophylaxis. *Perit Dial Int* 2000;20:343.

358. Swartz RD, et al. Recurrent polymicrobial peritonitis from a gynecologic source as a complication of CAPD. *Perit Dial Bull* 1983;3:32.

359. Coward RA, et al. Peritonitis associated with vaginal leakage of dialysis fluid in continuous ambulatory peritoneal dialysis. *Br Med J* 1982;284:1529.

360. Stuck A, Seiler A, Frey FJ. Peritonitis due to an intrauterine device in a patient on CAPD. *Perit Dial Bull* 1986;6:158.

361. Turkish Multicenter Peritoneal Dialysis Study Group. The rate, risk factors, and outcome of fungal peritonitis in CAPD patients: experience in Turkey. *Perit Dial Int* 2000;20:338.

362. Holdsworth SR, et al. Management of *Candida* peritonitis by prolonged peritoneal lavage containing 5-fluorocytosine. *Clin Nephrol* 1975;4:157.

363. Rault R. *Candida* peritonitis complicating chronic peritoneal dialysis: a report of five cases and review of the literature. *Am J Kidney Dis* 1983;2:544.

364. Kerr CM, et al. Fungal peritonitis in patients on continuous ambulatory peritoneal dialysis. *Ann Intern Med* 1983;99:334.

365. Goldie SJ, Kiernan-Troidle L, Torres C, et al. Fungal peritonitis in a large chronic peritoneal dialysis population: a report of 55 episodes. *Am J Kidney Dis* 1996;28:86.

366. Amici G, et al. Fungal peritonitis in peritoneal dialysis: critical review of 6 cases. *Adv Perit Dial* 1994;140:169.

367. Chan TM, et al. Treatment of fungal peritonitis complicating continuous ambulatory peritoneal dialysis with oral fluconazole: a series of 21 patients. *Nephrol Dial Transplant* 1994;9:539.

368. Johnson RJ, et al. Fungal peritonitis in patients on peritoneal dialysis: incidence, clinical features and prognosis. *Am J Nephrol* 1985;5:169.

369. Zaruba K, Peters J, Jungbluth H. Successful prophylaxis for fungal peritonitis in patients on continuous ambulatory peritoneal dialysis: six years' experience. *Am J Kidney Dis* 1991;17:43.

370. Robitaille P, Merouani A, Clermont M, et al. Successful antifungal prophylaxis in chronic peritoneal dialysis: a pediatric experience. *Perit Dial Int* 1995;15:77.

371. Wadhwa NK, Suh H, Cabralda T. Antifungal prophylaxis for secondary fungal peritonitis in peritoneal dialysis patients. *Adv Perit Dial* 1996;12:189.

372. Lo WK, Chan CY, Cheng SW, et al. A prospective randomized control study of oral nystatin prophylaxis for *Candida* peritonitis complicating continuous ambulatory peritoneal dialysis. *Am J Kidney Dis* 1996;28:549.

373. Thodis E, Vas SI, Bargman JM, et al. Nystatin prophylaxis: its inability to prevent fungal peritonitis in patietns on continuous ambulatory peritoneal dialysis. *Perit Dial Int* 1998;18:583.

374. Williams PF, Moncrieff N, Marriott J. No benefit in using nystatin prophylaxis against fungal peritonitis in peritoneal dialysis patients. *Perit Dial Int* 2000;20:352.

375. Bunke M, Brier ME, Golper TA. Culture-negative CAPD peritonitis: the Network 9 study. *Adv Perit Dial* 1994;10:174.

376. Sewell DL, et al. Comparison of large volume culture to other laboratory methods for isolation of microorganisms from peritoneal dialysate. *Perit Dial Int* 1990;10:49.

377. Luce E, et al. Improvement in the bacteriologic diagnosis of peritonitis with the use of blood culture media. *Trans Am Soc Artif Intern Organs* 1982;28:259.

378. Ryan S, Fessia S. Improved method for recovery of peritonitis-causing microorganisms from peritoneal dialysis. *J Clin Microbiol* 1987;25:383.

379. Lye WC, et al. Isolation of organisms in CAPD peritonitis: a comparison of two techniques. *Adv Perit Dial* 1994;10:166.

380. Chan MK, et al. Peritoneal eosinophilia in patients on continuous ambulatory peritoneal dialysis: a prospective study. *Am J Kidney Dis* 1988;11:180.

381. Humayun HM, et al. Peritoneal fluid eosinophilia in patients undergoing maintenance peritoneal dialysis. *Arch Intern Med* 1981;141:1172.

382. Gokal R, et al. "Eosinophilic" peritonitis in continuous ambulatory peritoneal dialysis. *Clin Nephrol* 1981;14:328.

383. Piraino B, et al. Chemical peritonitis due to intraperitoneal vancomycin (Vancoled). *Perit Dial Bull* 1987;7:156.

384. Fabris A, et al. Pharmacokinetics of antifungal agents. *Perit Dial Int* 1993;13:S380.
385. Lui SL, Lo CY, Choy BY, et al. Optimal treatment and long term outcome of tuberculous peritonitis complication continuous ambulatory peritoneal dialysis. *Am J Kidney Dis* 1996;28:747.
386. Holley JL, Bernardini J, Piraino B. A comparison of peritoneal dialysis related infections in black and white patients. *Perit Dial Int* 1993;13:45.
387. Korbet SM, Vonesh EF, Firanek CA. A retrospective assessment of risk factors for peritonitis among an urban CAPD population. *Perit Dial Int* 1993;13:126.
388. Farias MG, et al. Race and the risk of peritonitis: an analysis of factors associated with the initial episode. *Kidney Int* 1994;46:1392.
389. Lye WC, et al. A prospective study of peritoneal dialysis-related infections in CAPD patients with diabetes mellitus. *Adv Peritoneal Dial* 1993;9:195.
390. Viglino G, et al. Ten years experience of CAPD in diabetics: comparison of results with non-diabetics. *Nephrol Dial Transplant* 1994;9:1443.
391. Nolph KD, et al. Experiences with the elderly in the National CAPD Registry. *Adv Perit Dial* 1990;6:33.
392. Tranaeus A, Heimburger O, Lindholm B. Peritonitis during continuous ambulatory peritoneal dialysis (CAPD): risk factors, clinical severity, and pathogenetic aspects. *Perit Dial Int* 1988;8:253.
393. Holley JL, et al. A comparison of infection rates among older and younger patients on continuous ambulatory peritoneal dialysis. *Perit Dial Int* 1994;14:66.
394. Ismail N, et al. Renal replacement therapies in the elderly. Part 1. Hemodialysis and chronic peritoneal dialysis. *Am J Kidney Dis* 1993; 22:759.
395. Sieniawska M, et al. Continuous ambulatory peritoneal dialysis (CAPD) in children: a clinical report. *Perit Dial Int* 1988;8:159.
396. Yinnon AM, Gabay D, Raveh D, et al. Comparison of peritoneal fluid culture results from adults and children undergoing CAPD. *Perit Dial Int* 1999;19:51.
397. Andrews PA, Warr KJ, Hicks A, et al. Impaired outcome of continuous ambulatory peritoneal dialysis in immunosuppressed patients. *Nephrol Dial Transplant* 1996;11:1104.
398. Wadhwa NK, et al. Exit-site/tunnel infection and catheter outcome in peritoneal dialysis patients. *Adv Perit Dial* 1992;8:325.
399. Piraino B, et al. Failure of peritoneal catheter cuff shaving to eradicate infection. *Perit Dial Bull* 1987;7:179.
400. Nichols WK, Nolph KD. A technique for managing exit site and cuff infection in Tenckhoff catheters. *Perit Dial Bull* 1983;3:S4.
401. Szabo T, Siccion Z, Izatt S, et al. Outcome of *Pseudomonas aeruginosa* exit site and tunnel infections: a single center's experience. *Adv Perit Dial* 1999;15:209.
402. Lo CY, Chu WL, Wan KM, et al. Pseudomonas exit site infections in CAPD patients: evolution and outcome of treatment. *Perit Dial Int* 1998;18:637.
403. Keane WF, Bailie GR, Boeschoten E, et al. Adult peritoneal dialysis related peritonitis treatment recommendations. *Perit Dial Int* 2000;20:396.
404. Yinnon AM, Jain V, Magnussen CR. Group B streptococcus (Agalactiae) peritonitis and bacteremia associated with CAPD. *Perit Dial Int* 1993;13:241.
405. Winchester JF, Rakowski TA. Group A streptococcal peritonitis associated with continuous ambulatory peritoneal dialysis. *Am J Med* 1989;87:487.
406. Brier ME, Aronoff GR. Initial intraperitoneal therapy for CAPD peritonitis: the Network 9 peritonitis study. *Adv Perit Dial* 1994;10:141.
407. Manley HJ, Bailie GR, Asher RD, et al. Pharmacokinetics of intermittent intraperitoneal cefazolin in continuous ambulatory peritoneal dialysis patients. *Perit Dial Int* 1999;19:65.
408. Grabe DW, Bailie GR, Eisele G, et al. Pharmacokinetics of intermittent intraperitoneal ceftazidime. *Am J Kidney Dis* 1999;33:111.
409. Shemin D, Maaz D, Pierre D, et al. Effect of aminoglycoside use on residual renal function in peritoneal dialysis patients. *Am J Kidney Dis* 1999;34:14.
410. Mason NA, Zhang T, Messana JM. Methicillin resistance patterns associated with peritonitis in a University-Based Peritoneal Dialysis Center. *Perit Dial Int* 1999;19:483.
411. Onozato ML, Caramori JC, Barretti P. Initial treatment of CAPD peritonitis: poor response with association of cefazolin and amikacin. *Perit Dial Int* 1999;19:88.
412. Agraharkar M, Klevjer-Anderson P, Rubinsien E, et al. Use of cefazolin for peritonitis treatment in peritoneal dialysis patients. *Am J Nephrol* 1999;19:555.
413. van Biesen W, Vanholder R, Vogelaers D, et al. The need for a center tailored treatment protocol for peritonitis. *Perit Dial Int* 1998;18:274.
414. Ng R, Zabetakis P, Callahan C, et al. Vancomycin-resistant enterococcus infection is a rare complication in patients receiving PD on an outpatient basis. *Perit Dial Int* 1999;19:273.
415. Vas S, Bargman J, Oreopoulos DG. Treatment in PD patients of peritonitis caused by Gram positive organism with single daily dose of antibiotics. *Perit Dial Int* 1997;17:91.
416. Lye WC, Leong SO, Lee EJ. Methicillin resistant *Staphylococcus aureus* nasal carriage and infections in CAPD. *Kidney Int* 1993;43:1357.
417. Smith TL, Pearson ML, Wilcox KR, et al. *N Engl J Med* 1999;340:493.
418. Troidle L, Kliger AS, Gorban-Brennan N, et al. Nine episodes of CPD-associated peritonitis with vancomycin-resistant enterococci. *Kidney Int* 1996;50:1368.
419. Sandoe JAT, Gokal R, Struthers JK. Vancomycin-resistant enterococci and empirical vancomycin for CAPD peritonitis. *Perit Dial Int* 1997;17:617.
420. Low CL, Eisele G, Cerda J, et al. Low prevalence of vancomycin-resistant enterococcus in dialysis patients with a history of vancomycin use. *Perit Dial Int* 1996;16:651.
421. Brady JP, Snyder JW, Hasbargen JA. Vancomycin-resistant enterococcus in end stage renal disease. *Am J Kidney Dis* 1998;32:415.
422. Malacoff RF, Finkelstein FO, Andriole VT. Effect of peritoneal dialysis on serum levels of tobramycin and clindamycin. *Antimicrob Ag Chemother* 1975;8:574.
423. Chong TK, Piraino B, Bernardini U. Vestibular toxicity due to gentamicin in peritoneal dialysis patients. *Perit Dial Int* 1991;11:152.
424. Lye WC, van der Straaten JC, Leong SO, et al. Once-daily intraperitoneal gentamicin is effective therapy for Gram negative CAPD peritonitis. *Perit Dial Int* 1999;19:357.
425. Lau MN, Kao MT, Chen CC, et al. Intraperitoneal once daily dose of cefazolin and gentamicin for treating CAPD peritonitis. *Perit Dial Int* 1997;17:87.
426. Bunke M, Brier ME, Golper TA. *Pseudomonas* peritonitis in peritoneal dialysis patients: the Network 9 peritonitis study. *Am J Kidney Dis* 1995;25:769.
427. Tzamaloukas AH, Murata GH, Fox L. Death associated with *Pseudomonas* peritonitis in malnourished elderly diabetics on CAPD. *Perit Dial Int* 1993;13:241.
428. Pasadakis P, et al. Treatment and prevention of relapses of CAPD *Pseudomonas* peritonitis. *Adv Perit Dial* 1993;9:206.
429. Taylor G, McKenzie M, Buchanan-Chell M, et al. Peritonitis due to *Stenotrophomonas maltophilia* in patients undergoing chronic peritoneal dialysis. *Perit Dial Int* 1999;19:259.
430. Hoch BS, et al. The use of fluconazole in the management of *Candida* peritonitis in patients on peritoneal dialysis. *Perit Dial Int* 1993; 13:S357.
431. Levine J, et al. Fungal peritonitis complicating continuous ambulatory peritoneal dialysis: successful treatment with fluconazole, a new orally active antifungal agent. *Am J Med* 1989;86:825.
432. Eisenberg ES. Intraperitoneal flucytosine in the management of fungal peritonitis in patients on continuous ambulatory peritoneal dialysis. *Am J Kidney Dis* 1988;11:465.
433. Nankivell BJ, Lake N, Gillies A. Intracatheter streptokinase for recurrent peritonitis in CAPD. *Clin Nephrol* 1991;35:20.
434. Dasgupta MK. Use of streptokinase or urokinase in recurrent CAPD peritonitis. *Adv Perit Dial* 1991;7:169.
435. Innes A, et al. Treatment of resistant peritonitis in continuous ambulatory peritoneal dialysis with intraperitoneal urokinase: a double blind clinical trial. *Nephrol Dial Transplant* 1994;9:797.
436. Williams AJ, et al. Tenckhoff catheter replacement or intraperitoneal urokinase: a randomised trial in the management of recurrent continuous ambulatory peritoneal dialysis (CAPD) peritonitis. *Perit Dial Int* 1989;9:65.
437. Usberti M, et al. Treatment of acute peritonitis by temporary discontinuation of dialysis and low dose of oral ciprofloxacin in patients on CAPD. *Perit Dial Int* 1994;14:185.
438. Guiberteau R, et al. Treatment of peritoneal infection by the natural defenses of the peritoneal cavity. *Contrib Nephrol* 1987;57:92.
439. Pagniez DC, et al. Withdrawal of continuous ambulatory peritoneal dialysis to treat mild peritonitis. *Br Med J* 1988;297:1174.

440. Glancey GR, Cameron JS, Ogg CS. Peritoneal drainage: an important element in host defence against staphylococcal peritonitis in patients on CAPD. *Nephrol Dial Transplant* 1992;7:627.

441. Kant KS, et al. Relapsing peritonitis in continuous ambulatory peritoneal dialysis (CAPD): treatment by interruption of CAPD and prolonged antibiotic therapy. *Perit Dial Int* 1988;8:155.

442. Cairns HS, et al. Treatment of resistant CAPD peritonitis by temporary discontinuation of peritoneal dialysis. *Clin Nephrol* 1989;32:27.

443. Smith JL, Flanigan MJ. Peritoneal dialysis catheter sepsis: a medical and surgical dilemma. *Am J Surg* 1987;154:602.

444. Kim D, et al. *Staphylococcus aureus* peritonitis in patients on continuous ambulatory peritoneal dialysis. *Trans Am Soc Artif Intern Organs* 1984;30:494.

445. Paterson AD, et al. Removal and replacement of Tenckhoff catheter at a single operation: successful treatment of resistant peritonitis in continuous ambulatory peritoneal dialysis. *Lancet* 1986;2:1245.

446. Swartz R, et al. Simultaneous catheter replacement and removal in refractory peritoneal dialysis infections. *Kidney Int* 1991;40:1160.

447. Cancarini GC, et al. Simultaneous catheter replacement and removal during infectious complications in peritoneal dialysis. *Adv Perit Dial* 1994;10:210.

448. Goldraich I, et al. One-step peritoneal catheter replacement in children. *Adv Perit Dial* 1993;9:325.

449. Posthuma N, Borgstein PJ, Eijsbouts Q, et al. Simultaneous peritoneal dialysis catheter insertion and removal in catheter related infections without interruption of peritoneal dialysis. *Nephrol Dial Transplant* 1998;13:700.

450. Baggenenstoss AH. The pancreas in uremia: a histopathologic study. *Am J Pathol* 1948;24:1003.

451. Avram MM. High prevalence of pancreatic disease in chronic renal failure. *Nephron* 1977;18:68.

452. Robinson DO, et al. Pancreatitis and renal disease. *Scand J Gastroenterol* 1977;12:17.

453. Rutsky EA, et al. Acute pancreatitis in patients with end-stage renal disease without transplantation. *Arch Intern Med* 1986;146:1741.

454. Gupta A, et al. CAPD and pancreatitis: no connection. *Perit Dial Int* 1992;12:309.

455. Pannekeet MM, et al. Acute pancreatitis during CAPD in the Netherlands. *Nephrol Dial Transplant* 1993;8:1376.

456. Caruana RJ, et al. Pancreatitis: an important cause of abdominal symptoms in patients on peritoneal dialysis. *Am J Kidney Dis* 1986;7:135.

457. Singh S, Wadhwa N. Peritonitis, pancreatitis and infected pseudocyst in a continuous ambulatory peritoneal dialysis patient. *Am J Kidney Dis* 1987;9:84.

458. Evans DB, Slapak M. Pancreatitis in the hard water syndrome. *Br Med J* 1975;3:748.

459. Flynn CT, Chandran P, Shadur C. Recurrent pancreatitis in a patient on CAPD. *Perit Dial Bull* 1986;6:1060.

460. Donnelly S, Levy M, Prichard S. Acute pancreatitis in continuous ambulatory peritoneal dialysis (CAPD). *Perit Dial Int* 1988;8:187.

461. Burkart J, et al. Usefulness of peritoneal fluid amylase levels in the differential diagnosis of peritonitis in peritoneal dialysis patients. *J Am Soc Nephrol* 1991;1:1186.

462. Silverstein W, Isikoff MB, Hill MC. Diagnostic imaging of acute pancreatitis: prospective study using CT and sonography. *Am J Radiol* 1981;137:497.

463. Humayun H, et al. Chylous ascites in a patient treated with intermittent peritoneal dialysis. *Artif Organs* 1984;8:358.

464. Pomeranz A, et al. Chyloperitoneum: a rare complication of peritoneal dialysis. *Perit Dial Bull* 1984;4:35.

465. Roodhoft AM, Van Acker KJ, De Broe ME. Chylous peritonitis: an infrequent complication of peritoneal dialysis. *Perit Dial Bull* 1987;7:195.

466. Porter J, Wang WM, Oliveira DBG. Chylous ascites and continuous ambulatory peritoneal dialysis. *Nephrol Dial Transplant* 1991;6:659.

467. Goodkin DA, Benning MG. An outpatient maneuver to treat bloody effluent during continuous ambulatory peritoneal dialysis (CAPD). *Perit Dial Int* 1990;10:227.

468. Greenberg A, et al. Hemoperitoneum complicating chronic peritoneal dialysis: single-center experience and literature review. *Am J Kidney Dis* 1992;19:252.

469. Blumenkrantz MJ, et al. Retrograde menstruation in women undergoing chronic peritoneal dialysis. *Obstet Gynecol* 1981;57:667.

470. Harnett JD, et al. Recurrent hemoperitoneum in women receiving continuous ambulatory peritoneal dialysis. *Ann Intern Med* 1987;107:341.

471. Rocco MV, Stone WJ. Abdominal hernias in chronic peritoneal dialysis patients: a review. *Perit Dial Bull* 1985;July–September:171.

472. Bargman JM. Complications of peritoneal dialysis related to increased intraabdominal pressure. *Kidney Int* 1993;43:S75.

473. Digenis GE, et al. Abdominal hernias in patients undergoing continuous ambulatory peritoneal dialysis. *Perit Dial Bull* 1982;2:115.

474. Pauls DG, Basinger BB, Shield CF. Inguinal herniorrhaphy in the continuous ambulatory peritoneal dialysis. *Am J Kidney Dis* 1992;20:497.

475. Kopecky RT, et al. Complications of continuous ambulatory peritoneal dialysis: diagnostic value of peritoneal scintigraphy. *Am J Kidney Dis* 1987;10:123.

476. Nicholson ML, et al. Combined abdominal hernia repair and continuous ambulatory peritoneal dialysis (CAPD) catheter insertion. *Perit Dial Int* 1989;9:307.

477. Imvrios G, et al. Prosthetic mesh repair of multiple recurrent and large abdominal hernias in continuous ambulatory peritoneal dialysis. *Perit Dial Int* 1994;14:338.

478. Kopecky RT, et al. Prospective peritoneal scintigraphy in patients beginning continuous ambulatory peritoneal dialysis. *Am J Kidney Dis* 1990;15:228.

479. Orfei R, Seybold K, Blumberg A. Genital edema in patients undergoing continuous ambulatory peritoneal dialysis (CAPD). *Perit Dial Bull* 1984;14:251.

480. Tzamaloukas AH, et al. Scrotal edema in patients on CAPD: causes, differential diagnosis and management. *Dial Transplant* 1992;21:581.

481. Khanna R, et al. Fungal peritonitis in patients undergoing chronic intermittent or continuous peritoneal dialysis. *Proc Eur Dial Trans Assoc* 1980;17:291.

482. Caporale N, Perez D, Alegre S. Vaginal leak of peritoneal dialysis liquid. *Perit Dial Int* 1991;11:284.

483. Schultz SG, Harmon TM, Nachtnebel KL. Computerized tomographic scanning with intraperitoneal contrast enhancement in a CAPD patient with localized edema. *Perit Dial Bull* 1984;4:253.

484. Mandel P, Faegenburg D, Imbriano LF. The use of technetium-99m sulfur colloid in the detection of patent processus vaginalis in patients on continuous ambulatory peritoneal dialysis. *Clin Nucl Med* 1985;10:553.

485. Johnson BF, et al. A method for demonstrating subclinical inguinal herniae in patients undergoing peritoneal dialysis: the isotope "Peritoneoscrotogram." *Nephrol Dial Transplant* 1987;2:254.

486. Shemin D, Clark DD, Chazan JA. Unexplained pleural effusions in the peritoneal dialysis population. *Perit Dial Bull* 1989;9:143.

487. Benz RL, Schleifer CR. Hydrothorax in continuous ambulatory peritoneal dialysis: successful treatment with intrapleural tetracycline and a review of the literature. *Am J Kidney Dis* 1985;5:136.

488. Nomoto Y, et al. Acute hydrothorax in continuous ambulatory peritoneal dialysis: a collaborative study of 161 centers. *Am J Nephrol* 1989;9:363.

489. Fletcher S, Turney JH, Brownjohn AM. Increased incidence of hydrothorax complicating peritoneal dialysis in patients with adult polycystic kidney disease. *Nephrol Dial Transplant* 1994;9:832.

490. Spadaro JJ, Thakur V, Nolph KD. Technetium-99m-labeled macroaggregated albumin in demonstration of trans-diaphragmatic leakage of dialysate in peritoneal dialysis. *Am J Nephrol* 1982;2:36.

491. Green A, et al. The management of hydrothorax in continuous ambulatory peritoneal dialysis (CAPD). *Perit Dial Int* 1990;10:271.

492. Vlachojannis J, et al. A new treatment for unilateral recurrent hydrothorax during CAPD. *Perit Dial Bull* 1985;July–September:180.

493. Allen SM, Matthews HR. Surgical treatment of massive hydrothorax complicating continuous ambulatory peritoneal dialysis. *Clin Nephrol* 1991;36:299.

494. Avram MM, et al. The uremic dyslipidemia: a cross-sectional and longitudinal study. *Am J Kidney Dis* 1992;20:324.

495. Avram MM, et al. Cholesterol and lipid disturbances in renal disease: the natural history of uremic dyslipidemia and the impact of hemodialysis and continuous ambulatory peritoneal dialysis. *Am J Med* 1989;87:55N.

496. Gahl GM, et al. Outpatient evaluation of dietary intake and nitrogen removal in continuous ambulatory peritoneal dialysis. *Ann Intern Med* 1981;94:643.

497. Grodstein GP, et al. Glucose absorption during continuous ambulatory peritoneal dialysis. *Kidney Int* 1981;19:564.

498. Lamiere N, et al. Effects of long-term CAPD on carbohydrate and lipid metabolism. *Clin Nephrol* 1988;30:S53.

499. Kagan A, et al. Kinetics of peritoneal protein loss during CAPD. II. Lipoprotein leakage and its impact on plasma lipid levels. *Kidney Int* 1990;37:980.

500. Steele J, et al. Lipids, lipoproteins and apolipoproteins A-I and B and apolipoprotein losses in continuous ambulatory peritoneal dialysis. *Atherosclerosis* 1989;79:47.

501. Cressman MD, et al. Lipoprotein (a) is an independent risk factor for cardiovascular disease in hemodialysis patients. *Circulation* 1992;86:475.

502. Cavagna R, et al. Risk factors of ischemic cardiac disease in patients on continuous ambulatory peritoneal dialysis. *Perit Dial Int* 1993; 13:S402.

503. Valentine RJ, et al. Lp(a) lipoprotein is an independent, discriminating risk factor for premature peripheral atherosclerosis among white men. *Arch Intern Med* 1994;154:801.

504. Young GA, et al. The use of an amino-acid-based CAPD fluid over 12 weeks. *Nephrol Dial Transplant* 1989;4:285.

505. Chan MK. Gembribrozil improves abnormalities of lipid metabolism in patients on continuous ambulatory peritoneal dialysis: the role of postheparin lipases in the metabolism of high-density lipoprotein subfractions. *Metabolism* 1989;38:839.

506. Nishizawa Y, et al. Hypertriglyceridemia and lowered apolipoprotein C-II/C-II ratio in uremia: effect of a fibric acid, clinofibrate. *Kidney Int* 1993;44:1352.

507. Matthys E, et al. Effects of simvastatin treatment on the dyslipoproteinemia in CAPD patients. *Atherosclerosis* 1991;86:183.

508. Di Paolo B, et al. Therapeutic effects of simvastatin on hyperlipidemia in CAPD patients. *Trans Am Soc Artif Intern Organs* 1990;36:M578.

509. Marangoni R, et al. Dyslipidemia in patients undergoing continuous ambulatory peritoneal dialysis: pharmacological therapy (simvastatin) versus hemodialysis. *Perit Dial Int* 1993;13:S431.

510. Dimitriadis A, et al. The effect of simvastatin on dyslipidemia in continuous ambulatory peritoneal dialysis patients. *Perit Dial Int* 1993; 13:S434.

511. Li PKT, et al. Lovastatin treatment of dyslipoproteinemia in patients on continuous ambulatory peritoneal dialysis. *Perit Dial Int* 1993; 13:S428.

512. Van Acker BAC, et al. The effects of fish oil on lipid profile and viscosity of erythrocyte suspensions in CAPD patients. *Nephrol Dial Transplant* 1987;2:557.

513. Jones RG, et al. Effect of dietary fish oil on lipid abnormalities in patients on CAPD. *Perit Dial Int* 1988;8:203.

514. Lempert KD, Rogers JS, Albrinich MJ. Effects of dietary fish oil on serum lipids and blood coagulation in peritoneal dialysis patients. *Am J Kidney Dis* 1988;11:170.

515. Tzamaloukas AH, et al. Peritonitis associated with intraabdominal pathology in continuous ambulatory peritoneal dialysis patients. *Perit Dial Int* 1992;13:S335.

516. Singharetnam W, Holley J. Acute treatment of constipation may lead to transmural migration of bacteria resulting in gram-negative, polymicrobial, or fungal peritonitis. *Perit Dial Int* 1996;16:423.

517. Wellington JL, Rody K. Acute abdominal emergencies in patients on long-term peritoneal dialysis. *Can J Surg* 1993;36:522.

518. Spence PA, Mathews RE, Khanna R, et al. Indications for operation when peritonitis occurs in patients on chronic ambulatory peritoneal dialysis. *Surg Gyn Obstet* 1985;161:450.

519. Moffat FL, Deitel M, Thompson DA. Abdominal surgery in patients undergoing long-term peritoneal dialysis. *Surgery* 1982;92:598.

520. Fleisher AG, Kimmelstiel FM, Lattes CG, et al. Surgical complications of peritoneal dialysis catheters. *Am J Surg* 1985;149:726.

521. Flynn CT, Nanson JA. Intraperitoneal insulin with CAPD—an artificial pancreas. *Trans Am Soc Artif Intern Organs* 1979;25:114.

522. Madden MA, Zimmerman SW, Simpson DP. Continuous ambulatory peritoneal dialysis in diabetes mellitus. *Am J Nephrol* 1982;2:133.

523. Tzamaloukas AH, et al. Clinical associations of glycemic control in diabetics on CAPD. *Adv Peritoneal Dial* 1993;9:291.

524. Copley JB, Lindberg JS. Insulin: its use in patients on peritoneal dialysis. *Semin Dial* 1988;1:143.

525. Johnson CA, et al. Adsorption of insulin to the surface of peritoneal dialysis solution containers. *Am J Kidney Dis* 1983;3:224.

526. Twardowski ZJ. Insulin adsorption to peritoneal dialysis bags. *Perit Dial Bull* 1983;July–September:113.

527. Wideroe TE, et al. Intraperitoneal (^{125}I) insulin absorption during intermittent and continuous peritoneal dialysis. *Kidney Int* 1983;23:22.

528. Balducci A, et al. Intraperitoneal insulin in uraemic diabetics undergoing continuous ambulatory peritoneal dialysis. *Br Med J* 1981; 283:1021.

529. Schmitz O. Insulin-mediated glucose uptake in non-dialyzed and dialyzed uremic insulin-dependent diabetic subjects. *Diabetes* 1985; 34:1152.

530. Schade D, et al. The kinetics of peritoneal insulin absorption. *Metabolism* 1981;30:149.

531. Scarpioni L, et al. Insulin therapy in uremic diabetic patients on continuous ambulatory peritoneal dialysis: comparison of intraperitoneal and subcutaneous administration. *Perit Dial Int* 1993;14:127.

532. Diaz-Buxo JA, et al. Diabetic nephropathy: experience with various dialytic therapies. *Contemp Dial* 1983;4:9.

533. Aujla NS, Piraino B, Sorkin MI. An intraperitoneal insulin regimen for diabetics on continuous cyclic peritoneal dialysis. *Trans Am Soc Artif Intern Organs* 1990;36:119.

534. Oreopoulos DG, et al. Continuous ambulatory peritoneal dialysis: a new era in therapy of chronic renal failure. *Clin Nephrol* 1979;11:125.

535. Popovich RP, et al. Continuous ambulatory peritoneal dialysis. *Ann Intern Med* 1978;88:449.

536. Di Paolo BD, et al. Incidence and pathophysiology of hypertension in continuous ambulatory peritoneal dialysis. *Perit Dial Int* 1993;13:S396.

537. Ramos J, et al. CAPD: three years experience. *Q J Med* 1983;52:165.

538. Young MA, et al. Anti-hypertensive drug requirements in continuous ambulatory peritoneal dialysis. *Perit Dial Bull* 1984;4:85.

539. Alpert MA, et al. Comparative cardiac effects of hemodialysis and continuous ambulatory peritoneal dialysis. *Clin Cardiol* 1986;9:52.

540. Saldanha LF, Weiler EWJ, Gonick HC. Effect of continuous ambulatory peritoneal dialysis on blood pressure control. *Am J Kidney Dis* 1993;21:194.

541. Rodby RA, Vonesh EF, Korbet SM. Blood pressure in hemodialysis and peritoneal dialysis using ambulatory blood pressure monitoring. *Am J Kidney Dis* 1994;23:401.

542. DeVecchi AF. Adequacy of fluid/sodium balance and blood pressure control. *Perit Dial Int* 1994;14:S110.

543. Kurtz S, Wong V, Anderson C. Continuous ambulatory peritoneal dialysis: three years' experience at the Mayo Clinic. *Mayo Clin Proc* 1983;58:633.

544. Marquez-Julio A, et al. Hypotension in patients on continuous ambulatory peritoneal dialysis. In: Legrain M, ed. *Continuous ambulatory peritoneal dialysis.* Amsterdam: Excerpta Medica, 1980:263.

545. Schurig R, et al. Hemodynamic studies in long-term peritoneal dialysis patients. *Artif Organs* 1979;3:215.

546. Schurig R, et al. Central and peripheral hemodynamics in long term peritoneal dialysis patients. *Proc Eur Dial Transplant Assoc* 1979; 16:165.

547. Kong C, Raval U, Thompson F. Effect of 2 liters of intraperitoneal dialysate on the cardiovascular system. *Clin Nephrol* 1986;26:134.

548. Fleming S, et al. Influence of intraperitoneal dialysate on blood pressure during continuous ambulatory peritoneal dialysis. *Clin Nephrol* 1983;19:132.

549. Swartz C, et al. The acute hemodynamic and pulmonary perfusion effects of peritoneal dialysis. *Trans Am Soc Artif Intern Organs* 1978;15:367.

550. Acquatella H, et al. Left ventricular function in uremia: a hemodynamic and echocardiographic study. *Nephron* 1978;22:160.

551. Leenen F, et al. Changes in left ventricular hypertrophy and function in hypertensive patients started on continuous ambulatory peritoneal dialysis. *Am Heart J* 1985;110:102.

552. Maiorca R, et al. Morbidity and mortality of CAPD and hemodialysis. *Kidney Int* 1993;43:S4.

553. Timio M, et al. Evoluzione dell'pertrofia ventricolare sinistra negli uremici ipertesi dopo sei mesi emodialisi o di CAPD. *Ital Nefrol* 1988;5:257.

554. Silberberg JS, et al. Impact of left ventricular hypertrophy on survival in end-stage renal disease. *Kidney Int* 1989;36:286.

555. Parfrey PS, et al. The clinical course of left ventricular hypertrophy in dialysis patients. *Kidney Int* 1989;36:286.

556. Nolph KD, Sorkin MI, Moore H. Autoregulation of sodium and potassium removal during continuous ambulatory peritoneal dialysis. *Trans Am Soc Artif Intern Organs* 1980;26:334.

557. Stablein DM, et al. The effect of CAPD on hypertension control: a report of the National CAPD Registry. *Perit Dial Int* 1988;8:141.
558. Slingeneyer A, Canaud B, Mion C. Permanent loss of ultrafiltration capacity of the peritoneum in long-term peritoneal dialysis: an epidemiological study. *Nephron* 1983;33:133.
559. Gelfand M, et al. CAPD yields inferior transplant results compared to hemodialysis. *Perit Dial Bull* 1984;4:S26A.
560. Giangrande A, et al. Continuous ambulatory peritoneal dialysis and cellular immunity. *Proc Eur Dial Transplant Assoc* 1982;19:372.
561. Singh S, et al. Comparison of lymphocyte markers and lymphoblastic transformation studies of patients converted from hemodialysis to CAPD. In: Maher JF, Winchester JF, eds. *Frontiers in peritoneal dialysis.* New York: Field and Rich, 1986:591.
562. Giacchino F, et al. Improved cell-mediated immunity in CAPD patients as compared to those on hemodialysis. *Perit Dial Bull* 1984;4:209.
563. Langhoff E, Ladefoged J. Improved lymphocyte transformation in vitro in patients on continuous ambulatory peritoneal dialysis. *Proc Eur Dial Transplant Assoc* 1983;20:230.
564. Guillou PJ, et al. CAPD—a risk factor for renal transplantation? *Br J Surg* 1984;71:878.
565. Winchester JF, Rotellar C, Goggins M. Transplantation in peritoneal dialysis and hemodialysis. *Kidney Int* 1993;43:S101.
566. Maiorca R, et al. Kidney transplantation in peritoneal dialysis patients. *Perit Dial Int* 1994;14:S162.
567. Besarab A, Golper TA. Response of continuous peritoneal dialysis patients to subcutaneous recombinant human erythropoietin differs from that of hemodialysis patients. *Trans Am Soc Artif Intern Organs* 1991;37:M395.
568. First RM. Long-term complications after transplantation. *Am J Kidney Dis* 1993;22:477.
569. Murphy BG, et al. Plasma fibrinogen concentrations in renal replacement therapy. In: Ernst E, ed. *Fibrinogen—a new cardiovascular risk factor.* Vienna: Blackwell MZV, 1992.
570. Vaziri ND, et al. Coagulation cascade, fibrinolytic system, antithrombin III, protein C, and protein S in patients maintained on continuous ambulatory peritoneal dialysis. *Thrombos Res* 1989;53:173.
571. Murphy BG, et al. Increased serum apolipoprotein (a) in patients with chronic renal failure treated with continuous ambulatory peritoneal dialysis. *Atherosclerosis* 1992;93:53.
572. Murphy BG, et al. Increased renal allograft thrombosis in CAPD patients. *Nephrol Dial Transplant* 1994;9:1166.
573. Gokal R. Renal transplantation in patients on CAPD. In: La Greca G, et al, eds. *Peritoneal dialysis.* Milan: Wichtig Editore, 1986: 283.
574. O'Donoghue D, et al. Continuous ambulatory peritoneal dialysis and renal transplantation: a ten-year experience in one center. *Perit Dial Int* 1992;12:242.
575. Maher JF, Moore J Jr, Fernandez C. Renal transplantation after peritoneal dialysis in the United States. In: La Greca G, et al, eds. *Peritoneal dialysis.* Milan: Wichtig Editore, 1986:291.
576. O'Donoghue DJ, Dyer PA, Gokal R. Renal transplantation in patients treated with continuous ambulatory peritoneal dialysis. In: La Greca G, et al, eds. *Peritoneal dialysis.* Milan: Wichtig Editore, 1988: 259.
577. Dutton S. Transient post-transplant ascites in CAPD patients. *Perit Dial Bull* 1983;3:164.

CHAPTER 99

Center and Home Chronic Hemodialysis: Outcome and Complications

Anne Marie Miles and Eli A. Friedman

Maintenance hemodialysis is the only long-term form of mechanical organ replacement therapy currently available, and can prolong life for 20 or more years. In the years since the initial canine experiments in the laboratory of Abel and Rowntree at Johns Hopkins University in 1913 (1), and the first practical extension of life by repetitive hemodialysis in 1960 (2), hemodialytic therapy has burgeoned through the years. Presently, more than 1 million people around the world with end-stage renal disease (ESRD) are kept alive. Some of the seminal advances that have led to the current practice of chronic hemodialysis are listed in Table 99-1 (1,3–5); however, because less than 10% of normal kidney function is restored by dialytic therapy, complications of uremia still may occur and impact significantly on morbidity and mortality of hemodialysis patients. This chapter encompasses hemodialysis techniques and prescription, multisystem complications that may contribute to morbidity in maintenance hemodialysis patients, and factors contributing to death on hemodialysis.

EPIDEMIOLOGY

The 1999 United States Renal Data System (USRDS) report documents that in 1997, of 300,000 persons with end-stage renal disease (ESRD), 63% were treated with hemodialysis, 9% with peritoneal dialysis, and the rest with kidney transplantation (6). The cost of treating ESRD in America continues to rise and now stands at some $16 billion per year. A steady decline in utilization of home hemodialysis in the United States seen since 1983 may be explained by a combination of factors: noncompetitive reimbursement rates compared to center hemodialysis, the growing popularity of chronic ambulatory peritoneal dialysis (CAPD) in the 1980s, changing ESRD demographics (a more elderly population with

multisystem complications often related to diabetes mellitus, many unsuited for home dialysis), lack of adequate physician endorsement of the self-care "ideal," and physician bias (7). In some parts of the country, home hemodialysis is used predominantly for the elderly rich who are too debilitated to travel back and forth to an in-center dialysis unit, and who are willing to contribute copayments for each dialysis session.

Among center hemodialysis patients, the most common causes of renal failure are hypertension, diabetes, chronic glomerulonephritis, and polycystic kidney disease (Table 99-2) (6). A disproportionately high percentage of patients with polycystic kidney disease and chronic glomerulonephritis receive home hemodialysis, probably reflective of a younger and more self-reliant population, with medical disease usually confined to their renal problem.

Home Versus Center Hemodialysis

Home hemodialysis was initially instituted in response to inadequate funding and shortage of hospital staff and space for the fledgling hemodialysis programs of the early 1960s. The first home hemodialysis program in the United States was started in Seattle, Washington, where in 1970, over 90% of hemodialysis patients were treated at home (8). Washington State still has the largest home hemodialysis population in the United States, followed by New York, Mississippi, New Jersey, and Tennessee (6,9). In 1973, 42% of approximately 10,000 US ESRD patients were on home hemodialysis. Because of a combination of factors cited earlier, in 1997, there were only 1,848 patients on home hemodialysis in the United States (6). Any relatively stable patient who has a home and a partner, or who can afford a dialysis technician or nurse, is a candidate for home hemodialysis (Fig. 99-1), and this option of renal replacement therapy should be presented to almost all new patients with chronic renal insufficiency. Home hemodialysis may also allow for the new treatment regimens of slow nighttime or short daily

A.M. Miles and E.A. Friedman: Renal Disease Division, SUNY, Health Science Center at Brooklyn and University Hospital, Brooklyn, New York

TABLE 99-1. *The history of hemodialytic therapy*

1854	Scottish chemist Thomas Graham coins the term "dialysis" following work on solute movement across semipermeable membranes of ox bladder and vegetable parchment.
1913	John Jacob Abel, Leonard Rowntree, and BB Turner at Johns Hopkins University perform first dialysis on dogs using celloidin membranes and hirudin anticoagulation.
1942	George Haas in Germany performs first human hemodialysis, initially with hirudin, after 1928, with heparin.
1943	Willem Kolff in Holland constructs the rotating drum dialyzer using cellophane membranes from sausage casings.
1946	Nils Alwall in Sweden designs first ultrafiltration-controlled dialyzer.
1955	Twin coil dialyzer introduced by Watschinger and Kolff.
1960	Belding Scribner introduces the modified Kiil dialyzer, a low-volume, low-resistance, low-temperature continuous flow dialysis system, using a more permeable membrane, Cuprophane.
1960	Scribner, Quinton, and Dillard in Seattle, Washington introduce first means of chronic vascular access—the Teflon external shunt—and initiate the first patient on maintenance hemodialysis, Clyde Shields. He lives for 11 years.
1963	Albert Babb and others in Seattle design a central proportioning system for simultaneous supply of dialysis fluid to multiple patients.
1964	Home hemodialysis introduced in Boston, Seattle, and London.
1966	James Cimino and M. Brescia at the Bronx Veterans Administration Hospital, New York, construct the internal endogenous arteriovenous fistula.
1972	Medicare Act passed by Congress allowing the Federal Government to pay for the cost of dialysis.
1982	The National Cooperative Dialysis Study report affirms the importance of small molecular weight clearance as a measure of dialysis adequacy. Gotch and Sargent introduce the concept of urea kinetic modelling and Kt/V based on the results of the NCDS.
1989	Food and Drug Administration approves use of recombinant human erythropoietin in treatment of renal anemia.

TABLE 99-2. *Hemodialysis treatment, 1997 (USRDS, 1999)[a]*

	Percent utilizing	
Patient characteristic	Center hemodialysis	Home hemodialysis
All patients	62.3	0.6
Age		
0–19	17.3	0.4
20–24	41.5	0.4
45–64	58.4	0.6
65+	84.2	0.7
Male	60.1	0.6
Female	65.0	0.5
Native American	69.0	1.3
Asian/Pacific Islander	60.5	0.4
Black	76.8	0.5
White	54.7	0.6
Diabetes	72.2	0.5
Hypertension	74.9	0.5
Glomerulonephritis	44.8	0.6
Cystic kidney disease	39.8	0.7
All other	51.6	0.6

[a]By age, sex, race, and primary disease.

dialysis (which provide Kt/v values well over 2.0 and which are currently under intensive study) to become more widely accessible (10,11).

Contraindications to home hemodialysis include severe, uncompensated cardiovascular disease, uncontrolled or very brittle diabetes, and significant loss of mental acuity. There is no age cutoff. Successful home hemodialysis has been accomplished in the eighth decade of life, in diabetic patients with limb amputations or limited vision, and in patients with severe arthritis or lower limb paralysis.

A multidisciplinary team, including a physician, nurse, and social worker, best effects initial assessment of candidates for home hemodialysis. Patient motivation, psychosocial and vocational factors, intelligence, home environment, and level of social support are assessed. A paid dialysis helper may be employed if there is no family member to assist. Medicare does not reimburse these workers, but some insurance companies and state-funded renal agencies provide coverage for home dialysis assistants.

Training for home hemodialysis should take place in an area separate from the general hemodialysis treatment area. During initial training of 3 to 4 weeks, instruction in medical and dietary regimens, access cannulation, and operation of the dialysis machine are taught. Audiovisual aids, written material, and question-and-answer formats are useful. Subsequent training is usually completed in 3 to 6 weeks and includes problem solving, troubleshooting, and basic emergency intervention. Arrangements for installation of equipment (dialysis machine, deionizer, and reverse osmosis machine), delivery of disposable supplies, servicing, and repair, are made, permitting start of home hemodialysis usually within 3 to 4 months. A 24-hour on-call backup system involving a home hemodialysis nurse should be in place in case of emergencies. Monthly blood samples drawn at home are mailed or brought in to the affiliated center, and once yearly home follow-up visits by the training staff should be made.

Patient survival on home hemodialysis is equal to and often better than that on center hemodialysis (12); as with rehabilitation data, however, bias in assignment of healthier patients to home hemodialysis may be a factor. In some

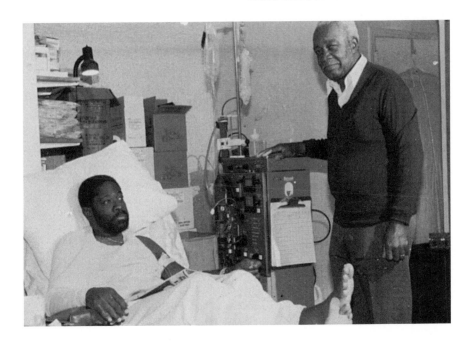

FIG. 99-1. A 47-year-old Brooklyn man on home hemodialysis for 17 years shown with his helper, his 67-year-old father. He worked as a teacher for over 15 years, when complications related to vascular access led to retirement. Note storage shelves and boxes of dialysis equipment in background.

locales, an overrepresentation of older, sicker patients in home hemodialysis programs may modify these statistics. At our institution, the actuarial survival at 10 years for home hemodialysis patients (mean age 39.3 years) was 77%, and strikingly, every one of our 20-year dialysis survivors is on home hemodialysis (13). Other advantages of home hemodialysis are listed in Table 99-3. Home hemodialysis is the means of uremia therapy advocated by the authors when a renal transplant is declined or not possible.

HEMODIALYSIS EQUIPMENT AND TECHNIQUE

Hemodialysis is performed using a dialyzer (Fig. 99-2), a hemodialysis machine (essentially a system of pumps and sensors), and blood tubing. These components form two major circuits: the blood circuit and the dialysate circuit (Fig. 99-3). The blood circuit consists of an input "arterial" needle (inserted about 3 cm from the arteriovenous anastomotic site and pointing toward the anastomosis) and line that carry blood from the patient's vascular access to the dialyzer under the negative pressure of a roller type positive-displacement blood pump. Blood passes through the dialyzer blood compartment and is returned to the patient

TABLE 99-3. *Advantages of home hemodialysis*

Flexibility in scheduling allows for vocational and lifestyle requirements
Self-care ideal leads to more informed, independent patient
Better rehabilitation
Cheaper than center dialysis or continuous ambulatory peritoneal dialysis
Fewer vascular access complications related to single, experienced venepuncturist
Allows for high-intensity dialysis regimens of short daily or slow nighttime dialysis

under positive pressure via an output "venous" blood tubing and needle, the latter placed at least 3 to 5 cm proximal to the arterial needle and pointing in the opposite direction, toward the heart. The dialysate circuit usually consists of a single-pass system in which concentrated dialysate is mixed with an appropriate amount of processed water (usually in a ratio of 1:34). The typical composition of dialysate is: sodium 135 to 145 mEq/L, potassium 1.0 to 3.0 mEq/L, calcium 6 to 7 mg/dL, magnesium 0.5 to 1.0 mEq/L, chloride 100 to 124 mEq/L, bicarbonate 35 to 40 mEq/L, and glucose 200 mg/dL. Dialysate is then pumped through the dialyzer at a flow rate of 500 to 800 mL/minute and discarded into a drain. Blood and dialysate flow counter current through the dialyzer, blood through the some 300,000 capillary tubes of the commonly used hollow fiber dialyzers, and dialysate between the capillary tubes. Plasma solutes including nitrogenous wastes in the blood diffuse across the dialyzer membrane down their concentration gradients. Convective loss or mass transfer of nitrogenous compounds occurs only at rates of high ultrafiltration. Most dialyzers used today are hollow fiber dialyzers developed in the mid-1970s. More than 70% of American dialysis centers (predominantly non–hospital-based, for-profit facilities) use dialyzers reprocessed with formaldehyde or peracetic acid (14). Parallel plate dialyzers are used infrequently and predominantly in patients with problems of anaphylactoid-type reactions thought to be related to the sterilizing agent ethylene oxide trapped within the potting compound in which the ends of the capillary tubes of hollow fiber dialyzers are embedded. Coil dialyzers and flat plate Kiil dialyzers are no longer in use in the United States. Membranes used to manufacture dialyzers and their ultrafiltration coefficients are shown in Table 99-4.

Hemodialytic techniques may be varied depending on the need for fluid versus solute removal and the dose of dialysis required:

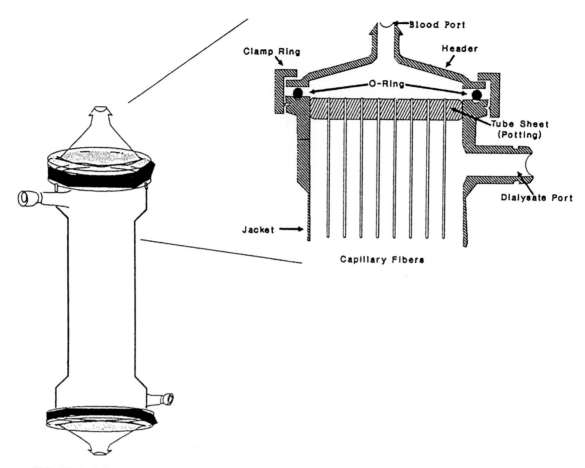

FIG. 99-2. Schematic diagram of a hollow fiber dialyzer. Enlargement depicts view of one end of the dialyzer. Number of capillary fibers (normally averaging 10,000) has been reduced for clarity. (From: Ahmad S, Blagg CR, Scribner BH. Center and home chronic hemodialysis. In: Schrier R, Gottschalk C, eds. *Diseases of the kidney*, 5th ed. Boston: Little, Brown, with permission).

1. Conventional Hemodialysis

Dialysis is performed using cellulosic membranes and blood flow rates of 200 to 350 mL/minute three times weekly for 3 to 4 hours at a time.

2. Isolated Ultrafiltration or Sequential Hemodialysis

Isolated ultrafiltration or sequential hemodialysis is performed in patients with predominant or severe fluid overload who are hemodynamically unstable or prone to precipitous decreases in blood pressure during usual combined dialysis and ultrafiltration. Isolated ultrafiltration is usually performed prior to dialysis. Typically, blood is circulated through the dialyzer at 150 to 300 mL/minute, under negative pressure in the dialysate compartment such that an ultrafiltrate of plasma (usually 2,000 to 3,000 mL) is formed and discarded. Dialysate solution is not circulated, and the solute composition of blood is unchanged by the convective transport that occurs in isolated ultrafiltration. By use of bicarbonate-based, slightly cooled dialysate with sodium concentrations of 135 to 140 mEq/L, and volumetric instead of pressure-controlled dialysis machines, combined dialysis and fluid removal is possible in most patients and is ideal. However, in a small subset of patients who are intolerant of aggressive fluid removal with conventional dialysis, benefit may be had from an initial period of isolated ultrafiltration, with removal of up to 30 mL/kg per hour of fluid.

3. Rapid Hemodialysis or High-Efficiency Hemodialysis

High-efficiency hemodialysis (HED) (15) is a reduced-time dialysis regimen in which solute and fluid removal is accomplished by: (a) increasing blood flow to more than 500 mL/minute; (b) increasing dialysate flow from 500 to 700 to 800 mL/minute; (c) use of dialyzers with a high mass transfer coefficient, low resistance to blood and dialysate flow, and a high ultrafiltration coefficient; (d) bicarbonate buffered dialysate because the capacity to metabolize acetate is exceeded at the high dialysate and blood flow rates; and (e) reliance on a mathematical model to calculate the length of each dialysis maintaining a midweek predialysis blood urea nitrogen (BUN) of about 80 ± 10 mg/dL for a patient with a protein catabolic rate of 0.8 to 1.4 g/kg per day and a Kt/V of 1.0 to 1.3 (vide infra). Treatment times are reduced to 2.5 to 3 hours.

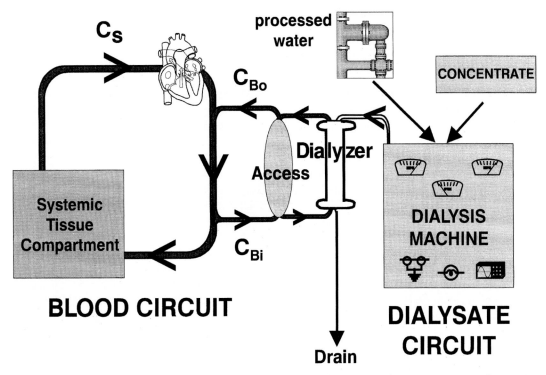

FIG. 99-3. Schematic diagram of the blood and dialysate circuits and their components. C_{Bo}, outlet (venous line) solute concentration; C_{Bi}, blood inlet (arterial line) solute concentration; C_S, systemic solute concentration.

4. High-Flux Dialysis

High-flux dialysis (HFD) is similar to HED in delivery of larger doses of dialysis and shorter treatment times, but the membranes employed and the dialyzer ultrafiltration coefficients are different. High-efficiency hemodialysis uses cellulosic membranes (ultrafiltration coefficient of 10 to 20 mL/hour per mm Hg), whereas HFD uses synthetic, "open" membranes, such as polysulfone (ultrafiltration coefficient of 20 to 60 mL/hour per mm Hg). High-efficiency hemodialysis involves the highly efficient removal of small molecules such as urea (molecular weight less than 300 daltons) with a prehemodialysis to posthemodialysis reduction in blood concentration of greater than or equal to 60%, whereas HFD efficiently removes larger, "middle" molecules (molecular weight 300 to 1,500 daltons) in addition.

5. Hemodialysis in Parallel

In large dialysis patients, who have inadequate dialysis by clinical or laboratory parameters despite use of large, synthetic dialyzers, high blood (greater than 500 mL/minute) and dialysate (greater than 800 mL/minute) flow rates, and dialysis times over 4 hours, use of two hemodialyzers in parallel

TABLE 99-4. *Types of dialyzer membranes*

Membrane material	Types	Tradename
Cellulose	Regenerated cellulose	
	Cuprammonium cellulose	Cuprophan
	Cuprammonium, Rayon	
	Saponified cellulose ester	SCE
Substituted cellulose	Cellulose acetate	Cellulate
	Cellulose triacetate	
Celluloso-synthetic (cellulose + tertiary ammonium compound)	Hemophan	
	Cellosyn	
Synthetic	Polyacrylonitrile	PAN
	PAN copolymerized with sodium methalyl sulfonate	AN69
	Polymethylmethacrylate	PMMA
	Polycarbamate	Gambrane
	Polyethylene vinyl alcohol	EVAL
	Polysulfone	

(HDP) can provide increased clearance at a cost of approximately $14 extra per dialysis session (16).

6. Slow Nighttime Dialysis and Short Daily Dialysis

These new modalities are under intensive study in the United States and abroad (10,11). They may be performed in-center or, more cheaply, in the patients home. Patients dialyze for 8 to 12 hours overnight three times per week or for 2 to 3 hours every day to provide increased urea and middle molecule clearance. Aksys Ltd. developed a modified dialysis machine (The Personal Hemodialysis System dialysis machine) to facilitate these new dialysis modalities that is currently under review by the US Food and Drug Administration. Preliminary reports from centers involved in small trials of these two new dialysis regimes indicate 30% to 50% reductions in erythropoietin doses and use of antihypertensives, improvement in nutritional indices, dramatic reduction in need for phosphate binders, reduced hospitalization costs, and improvement in well being and quality of life.

Assessing Adequacy of Dialysis: How Much is Enough?

The optimum dose of dialysis to deliver has been a pivotal question since the earliest days of maintenance dialysis. The difficulty in answering this question is related to the fact that the precise toxin(s) responsible for producing the uremic syndrome are still unidentified. Urea is a marker for products of protein catabolism, the source of most uremic toxins, and is the best surrogate marker for actual uremic toxins despite its large volume of distribution and dependence on liver function.

Optimum dialysis has been defined as "that dose of dialysis above which no further improvement in the morbidity and mortality associated with dialysis can be expected" (17). Objective parameters of dialysis adequacy include a midweek predialysis BUN level 75 to 85 mg/dL with consumption of a diet sufficient to generate a protein catabolic rate (PCR) greater than 0.8 g/kg per day; adequate muscle mass reflected in a creatinine generation rate of at least 125 micromol/kg per day; minimal or negligible acidosis, hyperkalemia, or hyperphosphatemia; hematocrit greater than 25%; minimal osteodystrophy; and no abnormalities on peripheral motor nerve conduction velocity studies or electroencephalography.

Attempts to quantitate dialysis originated in 1951, when Wolf (18) introduced the concept of dialysance and relative dialysance (the ratio of a substance's dialysance relative to that of urea) and described the effects of dialysance, blood flow, bath volume, and volume of distribution on dialysis kinetics. Dialysis prescription remained largely empiric, however, until Babb and Scribner propounded the "square meter per hour" hypothesis in 1971 (19). Solute transfer across the dialysis membrane was proposed to be a function of dialyzer surface area and permeability, duration of dialysis, and to a lesser degree, blood and dialysate flow rates. From this then completely new concept evolved the Dialysis Index Model (20). This simple calculation allowed for

residual glomerular filtration, and distinguished between small and middle molecule dialyzer clearance. The Dialysis Index relates a weekly creatinine clearance indexed to body size to a dialyzer surface area for a given amount of time. In two prospective studies (21,22) it was shown that a weekly B_{12} clearance of at least 30 L/week 1.73 m^2 was needed to prevent development of peripheral motor neuropathy in patients on hemodialysis. Based on the Dialysis Index, dialysis time was reduced to as little as 6 to 8 hours per week in patients with residual renal function, purportedly without ill effect (23), but the index was found to have limited correlative and predictive value overall. In 1974, Popovich and Moncrief (24) devised an expression: the maximum (predialysis) metabolite concentration ratio (PMCR), which in a dialysis patient relates the serum concentration of nitrogenous compounds to a "normalized" value for the same patient with normal kidney function. These workers concluded that "chronic uremics receiving adequate dialysis therapy ... have predicted middle molecule PMCRs greatly in excess of 15 (times the normal concentration)." They reasoned that tolerance of high middle molecule concentrations (a usual circumstance in most dialysis patients) meant that "either middle molecules are not important neurotoxins or that the assumptions implicit in the calculation of the PMCR are decidedly invalid."

The late 1970s then saw a shift from emphasis on middle molecules as the culprits in uremic toxicity to consideration of small molecules such as urea. Ginn and Teschan reduced the hours of dialysis based on total urea clearance (a combination of dialyzer clearance and residual glomerular filtration) and presence of neurologic abnormalities (25,26). A total urea clearance of 3,000 mL/week per liter body water was proposed to be adequate dialysis because survival without symptoms in patients with chronic renal insufficiency and glomerular filtration rates of as little as 10% of normal had been observed. Reduced dialysis time, however, caused impaired cognitive function (Choice Reaction Time and Continuous Memory Task), slowing of EEG frequency, and decreased "sense of well being." As was true for four other studies, urea level appeared to proffer a better marker for dialysis adequacy than did middle molecules. The potential value of serial EEG tracings as a guide to uremia therapy was inferred from these trials of reduced dialysis time (Figs. 99-4 and 99-5).

In 1981, the importance of urea as a marker of uremic toxicity was affirmed in the landmark National Cooperative Dialysis Study (NCDS) (27). This multicenter clinical trial prospectively examined the clinical outcomes (death or hospitalization) in 165 hemodialysis patients over a 6-month period. Patients were randomly assigned to four dialysis regimens (Table 99-5) differing on the basis of dialysis time and the time averaged clearance of urea (TAC$_{urea}$) in mg/dL.

$$TAC_{urea} = [Td(C1 + C2) + Id(C2 + C3)]/2(Td + Id)$$

where *Td* is dialysis time, *Id* is interdialytic interval, *C1* is predialysis BUN, *C2* is postdialysis BUN, and *C3* is BUN before the next dialysis.

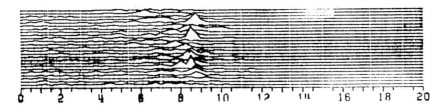

FIG. 99-4. Electroencephalogram (EEG) power-spectrum analysis displayed in compressed spectral arrays. This tracing was obtained from a uremic patient complaining of drowsiness, insomnia, lassitude, anorexia, and nausea. Quantifying the EEG yielded a discriminant score of +0.24. (Courtesy of PE Teschan.)

All study subjects received conventional dialysis three times per week with cellulose-based dialysis membranes. Analysis of the study results revealed that TAC$_{urea}$ (and not dialysis time) was the single most important factor determining outcome on dialysis. Later analysis and interpretation of the study data by Gotch and Sargent (28) led to the dissemination of urea kinetic modeling (UKM) that had been conceptualized a decade earlier (29). Reduced time dialysis (2.5 to 3 hours per session) was also widely adopted on the basis of the study results. Later, the importance of dialysis time in addition to urea levels in determining dialysis adequacy was reaffirmed (30), unfortunately not before thousands of hemodialysis patients on shortened treatment regimens had been subject to the effects of underdialysis (31). Urea kinetic modeling properly applied, however, is currently the best means of prescribing and assessing adequacy of dialysis. The urea product (Kt) (32) and the standardized Kt/v (eKt/v) are modifications that may have greater clinical accuracy and utility.

UREA KINETIC MODELING

Urea is assumed to be freely distributed throughout all tissues and circulating fluids in the body in a volume called the urea pool (or space). The urea pool is approximately equal to total body water (variable volume, single compartment model). During dialysis, the change in body urea content equals the difference between the urea generated and that removed.

change in body urea = urea generation − urea removal

$$d(V \times C)/dt = G - K \times C \qquad [1]$$

where V is volume of distribution of urea (L), C is urea concentration (mg/dL), t is dialysis time (minutes), G is urea generation rate (mg/minute), K is whole body urea clearance (mL/minute). Generation of urea during dialysis is assumed to negligible and solution of the differential equation [1] over time yields the formula:

$$K \times t/V = \log C_O/C \qquad [2]$$

where Kt/V is the normalized whole body urea clearance or dialysis dose, C_O is predialysis urea concentration, and C is postdialysis urea concentration. Values of K and V are calculated sequentially with the use of a computer or programmable calculator using the patient's height, weight, residual renal function, interdialytic weight gain, the dialyzer's expected urea clearance (manufacturer's data), calculated or nomogram-derived V (V is commonly taken to be 58% of total body weight, or read from standard nomograms using the patient's age, sex, weight, and height), and midweek predialysis and postdialysis BUN levels. The modeled value of K is obtained using the formula derived value of V, and the modeled value of V is obtained using the expected dialyzer clearance (manufacturer's data). The interdialytic urea generation rate, TAC$_{urea}$ (ideally 50 to 60 mg/dL), and normalized PCR in g/kg body weight per day (optimally greater than 0.8 g/kg per day) also can be derived (33). Protein catabolic rate is a measure of protein intake, muscle breakdown, and protein losses from the skin and gut. In stable dialysis patients in neutral nitrogen balance, PCR should equal daily protein intake and is defined by the following relationship.

$$PCR = 9.35 \times G + 0.29 \times V$$

where G is interdialytic urea generation rate in mg/minute, and V is volume of distribution of urea in liters. Proof of the long-held assumption that a well-dialyzed patient ingests more protein requires documentation of a direct correlation between PCR and Kt/V (34). The modeled value of K is compared to the expected value (manufacturer's data), and that of V to the formula- or nomogram-derived value in order to assess adequacy of delivered dialysis and detect blood-sampling errors (35). If the modeled value of V is much greater than the calculated value, errors in collection of postdialysis blood samples resulting in falsely low postdialysis BUN levels should be suspected. The Kt/V urea is calculated using modeled values of K, V, and dialysis time. The dialysis time needed to produce optimum values of PCR and K may also be calculated. TAC$_{urea}$, although not currently as popular as Kt/V as a measure of dialysis adequacy, is still favored by

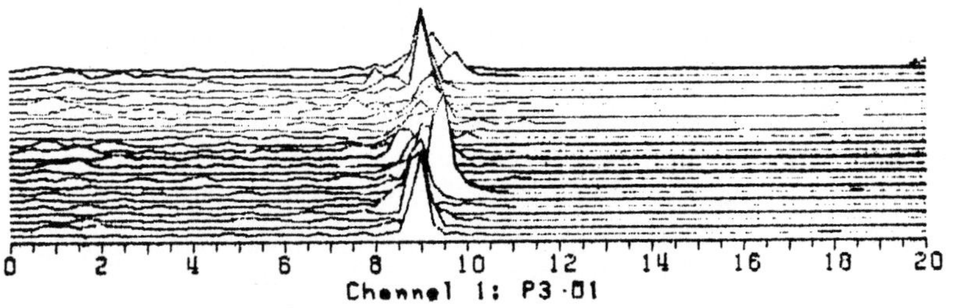

FIG. 99-5. Following the initial series of hemodialyses, the same patient shown in Fig. 99-4 improved clinically with disappearance of neurologic complaints. Normalized discriminant score corresponds to increased mean frequencies and power (amplitude) and decreased dispersion of wave frequencies. (Courtesy of PE Teschan.)

TABLE 99-5. *Four groups of the National Cooperative Dialysis Study*

Groups	Td (h)	Predialysis BUN (mg/dL)	TAC$_{urea}$ (mg/dL)	Patients (%)
Long Td, low BUN	4.5–5.0	60–80	50	86
Long Td, high BUN	4.5–5.0	110–130	100	46
Short Td, low BUN	2.5–3.5	60–80	50	69
Short Td, high BUN	2.5–3.5	110–130	100	31

Td, dialysis time; *BUN,* blood urea nitrogen; *TAC$_{urea}$,* time averaged concentration of BUN.

some and has the advantages of being unaffected by residual renal function, volume, and schedule changes, and errors inherent in urea modeling.

Controversy surrounds the optimum value of Kt/V urea. Initially thought to be 0.8 based on Gotch's discontinuous step function analysis of NCDS data (29), Keshaviah in a reanalysis of NCDS data has shown a continuous linear relationship between Kt/V and hospitalization or death, with the risk of adverse outcome being minimized at a Kt/V of approximately 1.3. This, in association with an increasing body of evidence confirming reduction in morbidity and mortality with Kt/V levels above 1.0 (36–40) has led to the current consensus of prescribing doses of dialysis of at least 1.3 with urea reduction ratio (URR) of 65%. A 15-year survival of 55% is reported in Tassin, France, with 24 hours of dialysis per week over the past 20 years in patients averaging 53 years of age and an average Kt/V of 1.67. Improved survival in this population is largely attributed to excellent blood pressure control without medication possible because of long, slow ultrafiltration (40). The Tassin population is younger and contains few diabetics compared to the US hemodialysis population, however, thereby avoiding groups at greater risk of death. A large multicenter trial under the aegis of the National Institutes of Health examining morbidity and mortality in hemodialysis patients and focusing on adequacy of dialysis, membrane type, and dialyzer reuse is currently underway, and should provide great insight into the vexing question of dialysis adequacy.

Pitfalls in Urea Kinetic Modeling

Many inaccuracies may arise during measurement of all three components of Kt/V, such as the following.

Clearance Measurements (K)

Use of Manufacturers' Urea Clearance Data for Dialyzers

Use of manufacturers' urea clearance data for dialyzers (measured with aqueous solutions of urea) can overestimate *in vivo* clearance by 15 to 20% (41,42). Conventional arteriovenous sampling for measurement of dialyzer clearance may also result in overestimation of up to 23% if corrections for hematocrit and access recirculation are not made (43). Direct dialysis quantification (DDQ) is the most accurate method of measuring urea clearance but is tedious and time consuming. In DDQ, the value of dialyzer clearance is not assumed. Paired measurements of predialysis and postdialysis urea blood levels, coupled with measurement of urea in spent dialysate permits direct assessment of solute transfer, which, together with residual glomerular filtration rate, allows for application of single pool kinetics. Comparative application of urea kinetic modeling and DDQ techniques to the same group of 40 hemodialysis patients showed that kinetic modeling overestimated V, PCR, and K (44).

Loss of Dialyzer Surface Area and Volume

Dialyzer fiber clotting may occur (particularly toward the end of dialysis) with reduction in clearance. Dialyzer reuse may also contribute to reductions in dialyzer clearance, and may go unrecognized if monitoring of residual fiber bundle volume of the reused dialyzer is not frequent and scrupulous.

Measurement of Volume of Distribution of Urea (V)

Inaccurate Urea Assumption

The first inaccuracy arises from the assumption that urea is equally and freely distributed throughout the body. In fact, urea distributes in only 93% of plasma volume and in 86% of red cell volume.

Presence of Recirculation

Presence of recirculation, intra-access and cardiopulmonary (vide infra), especially at high blood flow rates, resulting in falsely low postdialysis BUN levels.

Improper Collection of Blood Samples

The predialysis BUN sample should be drawn from the arterial line before the blood pump is started (serum BUN can fall significantly as soon as 1 minute after starting hemodialysis) and before administration of heparin or saline. The postdialysis BUN sample also should be drawn from the arterial line, at least 2 minutes after the blood pump is stopped in order to avoid recirculated blood being pumped through the access, and to reduce the effect of urea rebound. The arterial line is clamped or disconnected between the sampling port and the dialyzer, 5 to 30 cc of blood is withdrawn from the arterial needle (to flush venous blood that may have recirculated through the access), the sample for BUN is taken, and the 5 to 30 cc flush is returned to the patient.

TABLE 99-6. *Formulae for calculation of Kt/V*

$Kt/V = (4 \times URR) - 1.2$
$Kt/V = 1.18 \times -\ln(R)$
$Kt/V = 2.2 - 3.3 \times (R - 0.03 - UF/W)$
$Kt/V = -\ln(R - 0.03 - 0.75 \times OF/W)$
$Kt/V = -\ln(R - 0.03) + (4 - 3.5 \times R) \times UF/W$

URR, Pre-post BUN/pre BUN; *UF,* volume of fluid removed (L); *W,* postdialysis weight (kg); *R,* post/pre BUN ratio.

Accuracy of formulae increases from top to bottom.

From: Daugirdas JT. Chronic hemodialysis prescription: a urea kinetic approach. In: Daugirdas JT, Ing TD, eds. *Handbook of dialysis,* 2nd ed. Boston: Little, Brown, and Company, 1994:92; with permission.

Urea Rebound

Thirty minutes after termination of dialysis, urea levels often rise to 5 to 10 mg/dL above the level in samples drawn immediately after dialysis. This rebound of urea levels reflects equilibration of urea from the intracellular space, especially of relatively poorly perfused areas (skeletal muscle, bone, skin), and is most marked after short (2 to 2.5 hours) dialysis. Despite significant urea rebound within the first 30 minutes of dialysis termination, all clinical studies evaluating Kt/V have utilized values of postdialysis urea samples drawn 0 to 1 minutes after dialysis. Consequently, a Kt/V of 1.4, based on blood sampling 0 to 1 minute postdialysis often corresponds to Kt/V of only 1.1 to 1.2 if an equilibrated blood sample drawn 30 to 60 minutes after dialysis were drawn.

Shortened Dialysis Time (t)

Dialysis time may be lost owing to staff- or patient-related factors (Table 99-6).

Because of these problems, and the relative complexity of the calculations involved, alternative, simpler methods of assessing Kt/V have been formulated. The most popular is the URR percent reduction in urea (PRU) (45,46).

$$URR = (\text{predialysis BUN} - \text{postdialysis BUN})/$$
$$\text{predialysis BUN} \times 100$$

The URR is a measure of urea clearance during a single dialysis treatment and is a function of dialysis time, volume of distribution of urea, and dialyzer urea clearance. The URR has been graphically related to Kt/V (Fig. 99-6) and varies with the amount of ultrafiltrate removed. A URR of 55% corresponds to a KT/V of 1.0. The URR is also subject to drawbacks, however. Changes in K will not be detected because K is not directly assessed (falsely high value of K indicates either poor blood sampling technique or access recirculation); PCR values cannot be calculated; URR tends to underestimate Kt/V at high rates of ultrafiltration; and the URR is a less accurate measure of Kt/V at Kt/V values less than 0.8 or greater than 1.4.

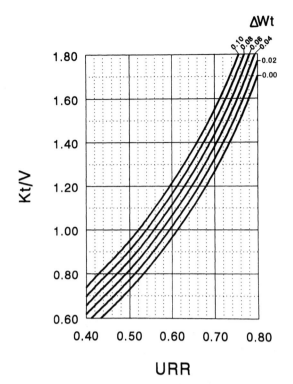

FIG. 99-6. Graphic estimation of Kt/V from the urea reduction ratio at varying levels of dialytic weight loss. Curves are derived from formal urea modeling assuming a 3-hour dialysis, no residual renal function, and a volume of distribution of urea 58% of body weight. The nonlinear relationship between Kt/V and urea reduction ratio for treatments with net ultrafiltration losses from 0% to 10% of final (dry) body weight is shown. (From: Depner TA. Special feature estimation of Kt/V from the urea reduction ratio for varying levels of dialytic weight loss: a bedside graphic aid. *Semin Dial* 1993;6:242. Reprinted by permission of Blackwell Scientific Publications.)

Several formulae computing Kt/V from predialysis and postdialysis BUN levels also are in use (Table 99-6). The use of on-line blood and dialysate-based urea sensors for clearance measurements will allow accurate computation of whole body Kt/V in the near future.

HEMODIALYSIS OUTCOME

The quality of life during the extra years offered by hemodialytic therapy varies in patients depending on several factors including age, renal diagnosis, comorbid conditions (diabetes, cardiovascular disease), nutritional status, presence of anemia, and dialysis dose (47). Some recipients of maintenance dialysis are fully or significantly rehabilitated, whereas others (unfortunately the majority) experience varying degrees of chronic debility that renders them unable to fulfill the early expectations of the Medicare Act of 1972, which ensured financial support for treatment of all patients found suitable for chronic hemodialysis. Erythropoietin (EPO) use has improved rehabilitation in many patients (48), but failure or resistance to the drug may blunt its potential beneficial effect of improving functional status in many patients.

TABLE 99-7. *Causes of death in end-stage renal disease patients (USRDS, 1994)*

Cause	Percent
Myocardial infarction	14.5
Other cardiac cause	29.9
Cerebrovascular disease	5.6
Septicemia	10.6
Withdrawal from dialysis	9.9
Malignancy	3.4
Pulmonary infection	2.4
Unknown cause	7.6
Other known cause	16.1

Crude mortality rates in US maintenance hemodialysis patients are higher than in other industrialized nations. Hemodialysis patients in the United States have a gross yearly mortality rate of 24% (6), and their life expectancy is worse than that of patients of the same age with prostate or colon cancer. A 49-year-old ESRD patient is estimated to have a life expectancy of 6.8 years and a 59-year-old ESRD patient, a life expectancy of 4.4 years. These values are 75% to 80% lower than those of the general population: an expected loss of life of 23 years for ESRD patients aged 49, and 17 years for those aged 59 years. Actuarial calculations reveal the average projected remaining lifetime of prevalently dialyzed patients with ESRD is one-fourth to one-sixth that of the general population through age 50. Mortality rates in American hemodialysis patients have improved over the past decade, however.

Higher ESRD mortality rates of 15% to 30% in the United States as compared to Europe and Japan (49–51) are explained by: (a) greater comorbidity in US patients because of advanced age and diabetes; (b) better death reporting in the United States; and (c) lower delivered dose of dialysis (related to shortened dialysis treatment times, use of smaller dialyzers ± widespread reuse of dialyzers) in US patients compared to other developed countries (53). Hence, the continuing trend toward higher dialysis dose in the United States and the intense interest in nocturnal and daily hemodialysis. Causes of death in hemodialysis patients are shown in Table 99-7.

COMPLICATIONS OF CHRONIC HEMODIALYSIS

Underdialysis

There has been a consistent increase in the delivered dose of dialysis from a URR of 63% and Kt/v of 1.21 in 1993 to 68% and 1.37 in 1996, respectively (6). Despite this increasing trend for more dialysis, URRs of less than or equal to 60% are not uncommon in many dialysis units and underdialysis remains one of the major contributors to dialysis morbidity and mortality. Causes of underdialysis are shown in Table 99-8. Recirculation of more than 15% to 20% of previously dialyzed venous blood into the arterial line is an important cause of underdialysis and may go unrecognized if not actively sought. This short-circuiting of blood (causing repeat dialysis of plasma) in an arteriovenous fistula or graft within an extremity, or in tubing leading to a single-needle (dependent on to and fro blood flow) dialysis circuit or a temporary double lumen catheter, reduces the efficiency of extracorporeal blood treatment. Although measured blood flow through the dialyzer may indicate attainment of a predetermined flow rate, dialysis of the same blood reduces effective solute extraction (clearance). Clues to the presence of blood recirculation during dialysis include the combination of an anticipated fall in BUN with a minimal decline in concentration of larger solutes (creatinine, Vitamin B_{12}), and signs of venous outflow stenosis or obstruction such as a swollen access limb, high venous pressures on dialysis, and a prominent, intermittent, tapping arterial inflow pulse. As a simple test for recirculation, simultaneous measurements of BUN levels in arterial blood entering the dialyzer, and systemic blood should not differ by more than 0 ± 2 mg/dL. To quantify the amount of recirculation, simultaneous measurements of the same solute (urea, creatinine) in samples drawn from arterial and venous bloodlines during dialysis are compared with the level of the same solute in a simultaneous venous blood sample from the contralateral extremity (the three-needle method) (Fig. 99-3).

$$\text{recirculation } (\%) = \frac{C_S - C_{Bi}}{C_S - C_{Bo}} \times 100$$

TABLE 99-8. *Causes of underdialysis*

Patient-related factors	Factors related to equipment malfunction or failure	Staff-related problems

Problems related to vascular access
  Venous outflow stenosis resulting in recirculation
  Poor access development or inflow stenosis resulting in low blood flow rates
Missed or shortened dialysis sessions (depression/psychosocial problems)
Cardiovascular disease with hemodynamic instability, need for repeated interruptions in dialysis, and reduced dialysis time
Unrecognized concurrent illness (malignancy, infection)
	Dialyzer deviation from manufacturer specifications
	Reduction in clearance of reused dialyzers
	Inadequate heparinization with dialyzer clotting and reduction in clearance
	Low blood flow rates secondary to improper blood pump calibration, collapse of pump line segment, or lack of total occlusion of blood pump
		Incorrect dialysis prescription (time × surface area × blood flow rate)
		Incorrect needle placement or reversal of blood lines with resultant recirculation
		Shortening or improper tallying of dialysis time (time during which the blood pump is turned off or blood flow rate significantly reduced should not be included)
		Improper collection of postdialysis blood samples for calculation of dialysis adequacy

where C_S is the systemic concentration, C_{Bi} is the blood inlet (arterial line) concentration, and C_{Bo} the outlet (venous line) concentration of an easily measured solute, such as urea, in mg/dL. It is important to distinguish the venous blood sample (C_{Bo}), also called a post-*dialyzer* blood sample from a post-*dialysis* blood sample that is drawn from the arterial line at least 2 minutes after termination of dialysis for purposes of calculating the URR. If significant recirculation (greater than 15% to 20%) is detected, contrast angiography of the access is indicated and a stenosis of the venous outflow tract of the access often is discovered.

A recent modification in the usual three-needle method of obtaining blood samples for the measurement of recirculation has been brought about by recognition of the presence of cardiopulmonary recirculation (CPR) (52,53). The BUN of dialyzed blood returning to the heart is reduced by admixture with blood volume returning to the heart from other areas of the body, such that during dialysis, arterial BUN is always lower than venous BUN by 3 to 4 mg/dL. This CPR (also called arteriovenous dysequilibrium) accounts for about 7% of recirculation, and becomes especially significant in patients with low cardiac outputs and therefore more time for dilution of dialyzed blood. CPR in patients with congestive heart failure may approach 11% to 12%. It is therefore incorrect to assume that the BUN level in a peripheral vein of the nonaccess arm is equal to that at the arterial inlet line of the dialyzer when recirculation is absent; the peripheral vein BUN is always lower because of CPR. To eliminate the effect of CPR, a two-needle method utilizing a stop-flow or low flow technique is used to collect the C_S (peripheral) blood sample: The blood pump is stopped or slowed to 50 mL/minute, and a blood sample drawn from the arterial line no more than 30 seconds later. Collection of this C_S blood sample at minimal or no blood flow prevents collection of recirculated blood. Collection of the sample within 30 seconds of stopping or slowing dialysis minimizes the effect of urea rebound. Samples for C_{Bo} and C_{Bi} are collected in the usual manner at the set blood flow rate. Cardiopulmonary recirculation does not occur with use of central venous catheters for dialysis access. If the standard three-needle technique is used for calculation of recirculation, samples should be drawn within the first 30 minutes of start of the hemodialysis treatment, as systemic blood venous BUN becomes lower than that of venous BUN in the nonaccess arm because of relatively poorer blood perfusion in the vasoconstricted extremity. The difference between nonaccess arm venous BUN and systemic venous BUN (veno-venous dysequilibrium) is most marked after 1 hour of initiation of hemodialysis, and can account for falsely high recirculation rates of up to 30%.

Underdialysis should be suspected in any patient who is deteriorating, without obvious cause, during maintenance hemodialysis. The integrity of the vascular access should be checked, the presence of blood recirculation excluded, and urea kinetic modeling performed and compared to previous analyses. To test the inference that underdialysis is responsible for the patient's worsening condition, the effect on clinical well being of an increase in effective dialysis should be determined. Substitution of a greater surface area dialyzer without change in dialysis time is an initial empiric step readily accepted by patient and staff. Should intradialytic hypotension, or prior selection of a large dialyzer preclude this approach, an extension of the duration of each dialysis is mandated as the next step. An increment of 1 hour per dialysis (for each dialysis), for 1 month, is usually sufficient to induce improvement in an underdialyzed patient. Improved work tolerance, and lessened pruritus, anorexia, and hiccoughs may be the first subjective indicators that the diagnosis of underdialysis was correct. A rising hematocrit and declining phosphorus and parathyroid hormones (PTH) levels over the ensuing 3 months afford further corroboration of the wisdom of having raised dialysis time. Changes in the amount of dialysis may require months to a year or longer to effect clinical well being.

Cardiovascular Disease

Hypertension

Hypertension is the second most serious threat (after diabetes) to longevity on maintenance hemodialysis (54). Hypertension requiring therapy is seen in 20% to 50% of dialysis patients on conventional hemodialysis. In Tassin, France where long, slow dialysis is practiced, fewer than 3% of patients need antihypertensive drugs, reflecting the better-tolerated and hence more adequate removal of fluid with slow dialysis (40). Normotensive hemodialysis patients live notably longer than their hypertensive unit-mates. Normotension appeared to be a "condition" for surviving through the tenth year of maintenance hemodialysis in Lundin and associates' series of 10-year patients (55).

By obtaining an ambulatory blood pressure (ABP) profile during 48 hours in 24 normotensive hemodialysis patients (4 hours, three times weekly), Battistella and coworkers provide insight into the response to worsening levels of uremia in the functionally anephric human (56). Ambulatory blood pressure is greater on the second postdialysis day (122/74 mm Hg) than on the day after dialysis (117/70 mm Hg); nocturnal decrease in blood pressure is less than 5%. Surprisingly, increases in ABP on the second day do not correlate with the degree of interdialytic weight gain. The *white coat syndrome* continues to impact on blood pressure even after initiation of maintenance hemodialysis. No matter when it is taken, blood pressure before hemodialysis is continually higher than the diurnal ABP (138/74 mm Hg versus 121/73 mm Hg), even if the ABP is analyzed 1 hour prior to hemodialysis (129/77 mm Hg). Hypertension in renal failure, although multifactorial, usually responds to contraction of plasma volume induced by dietary salt and water restriction and ultrafiltration on dialysis. Loop diuretics may be used to augment water excretion in patients with residual renal function and creatinine clearances greater than approximately 8 mL/minute.

The management goal in balancing interdialytic weight gain against intradialytic fluid extraction is to attain the patient's "dry weight"—the weight at which the patient is normotensive without use of antihypertensives and that permits interdialytic weight gain of 5 or more pounds without development of hypertension. At dry weight, protracted postdialysis hypotension or symptomatic circulatory insufficiency is unlikely. Very often, the limiting factor in fluid removal (ultrafiltration) during hemodialysis is a fall in blood pressure to hypotensive levels accompanied by leg and other muscle cramps. A vicious cycle of need for antihypertensive drug use, hypotension on dialysis with interruption of dialysis and need for saline replacement, weight gain, exacerbation of volume-sensitive hypertension, and increased dose of antihypertensive medications may afflict some patients and contribute to underdialysis as a result of shortened dialysis time.

Blood pressure lability during hemodialysis depends in part on the choice of dialysate buffer (acetate or bicarbonate) and the concentration of sodium in dialysate. Because sodium retention may aggravate underlying hypertension, the exact dialysis prescription seeks to minimize hypertension while protecting against intradialytic hypotension. Kramer and colleagues studied six ESRD patients with sequential bicarbonate and acetate dialysate at four different dialysate sodium concentrations (135, 140, 145, and 150 mmol/L) (57). During hemodialysis, bicarbonate buffer protected against hypotensive episodes, as did a sodium dialysate sodium concentration of 140 mmol/L. There was no advantage in raising dialysate sodium concentration above 140 mmol/L. Zuccala and associates explored the question of whether one class of antihypertensive drugs was superior to others in eight hemodialysis patients (58) with a high plasma renin activity (greater than 2 ng/mL per hour). Patients were given 50 mg of captopril, clonidine, and nifedipine in random order. All three drugs produced an equivalent fall in mean blood pressure from a pretest value of 121 ± 8 mm Hg to 111 to 112 ± 4 mm Hg.

Normalization of hypertensive blood pressure can be effected within 2 weeks of beginning maintenance hemodialysis without need for antihypertensive drugs in most patients. Low doses of a calcium blocker, angiotensin enzyme inhibitor or receptor blocker, or ß blocker may be added to the regimen of patients who remain hypertensive at their dry weight. Extraction of clonidine during hemodialysis, however, may precipitate hypertension, agitation, and headache—signs of withdrawal—in some patients. Persistent hypertension, continuing despite volume contraction and treatment with central or peripheral vasodilators has been responsive to a combination of ACE inhibitor plus calcium channel blocker in our hands. Only rarely have we needed to resort to minoxidil, which is highly effective but difficult to use. Minoxidil, in doses as high as 80 mg per day, has preempted the need for native binephrectomy, a previous last resort in difficult-to-control hypertensive patients. However, the side effects of minoxidil include hypertrichosis, tachycardia, and fluid retention in serous cavities. Concomitant prescription of a ß blocker to counteract reflex tachycardia and increased ultrafiltration should be performed with initiation of minoxidil therapy. Active participation by the patient in drug dose modification is aided by provision of an inexpensive and reliable blood pressure monitor. We employ a simple aneroid, blinking light, beeping device that is widely available, under a variety of brand names, in surgical supply stores for about $80 (DIGI+PLUS DSP-80, Ueda Electronic Works, Ltd., Japan).

About 80% of American ESRD patients on maintenance hemodialysis are now treated with erythropoietin, a recombinant hormone that was first thought to worsen hypertension. Our own experience, and that of others (59) indicates that about one-third of previously normotensive and hypertensive hemodialysis patients show an increase in blood pressure during erythropoietin treatment. There is no correlation between the rise in blood pressure and patient age, sex, duration of ESRD, and previous levels of blood pressure. Return to baseline (preerythropoietin) blood pressure generally is easily accomplished either by increasing ultrafiltration or antihypertensive drugs during hemodialysis.

Coronary Artery Disease

In a study of the earliest patients started on hemodialysis, Lindner and associates found that 85% had died by the thirteenth year of dialysis of presumed cardiovascular causes, probably because of accelerated atherosclerosis (60). The probability of myocardial infarction, angina, or pulmonary edema requiring hospitalization in hemodialysis patients is about 10% per year (61). The prevalence of congestive heart failure and complex ventricular ectopy are 10% and 18%, respectively (62,63). Cardiac dysfunction in the incident hemodialysis population is also common: Abnormalities of systolic function and/or left ventricular hypertrophy are found in over 70% of patients starting maintenance hemodialysis (72). Risk factors for atherosclerosis in dialysis patients include hypertension, cigarette smoking, diabetes mellitus, hyperlipidemia (30% to 50% of chronic dialysis patients are hypertriglyceridemic, with normal total cholesterol but unfavorable HDL:LDL ratios), abnormalities of calcium metabolism, hyperuricemia, and the presence in uremic serum of mitogenic factors that can stimulate smooth muscle proliferation, an early step in the genesis of atherosclerotic lesions. Investigators found that one such mitogenic substance, platelet-derived growth factor (PDGF), is increased in activity about threefold during dialysis with cuprophane membranes (64). Most of the dialysis prior to 1970 was performed with cuprophane membranes and they are still frequently used. An association between cuprophane and accelerated atherosclerosis is yet to be established, but the greater bioincompatibility of this material compared with newer membrane materials in use today mitigates against its continued widespread application in dialysis.

Cigarette smoking is a significant risk factor for coronary artery disease in dialysis patients. Of 20 patients who smoked cigarettes in Lundin and colleagues' retrospective study of dialysis patients begun on treatment between 1964 and 1968,

33% were dead by their seventh year of dialysis, and 75% by the eleventh year (55). Every patient who died of cardiovascular disease (5/5) was a cigarette smoker. By contrast, only 3/10 living patients were cigarette smokers. In dialysis patients assessed during transplantation for the presence and severity of atherosclerosis by Vincenti and associates (65), no correlation was found between preexisting "metabolic and lipid abnormalities, and duration of hemodialysis." Correlation was found, however, between degree of hypertension, age, and severity of atherosclerosis, which caused the authors to conclude that "atherosclerosis may not be accelerated by hemodialysis and may be prevented by more stringent control of hypertension in uremia."

The importance of calcium/phosphate balance in the genesis of obstructive coronary artery disease has been highlighted in recent studies utilizing magnetic resonance imaging or electron beam computed tomographic imaging of coronary artery plaque that documents increasing evidence of coronary plaque formation in hemodialysis patients with hyperphosphatemia or elevated calcium/phosphorus products (66,67). Metastatic or dystrophic deposits of calcium within coronary vessels and around cardiac valve rings can be significant contributors to cardiac mortality in dialysis patients.

Dialysis-Associated Pericarditis

Small asymptomatic pericardial effusions are common in dialysis patients who are volume overloaded. Fibrinous pericarditis with large effusions can produce cardiac tamponade, may occur in up to 8% to 10% of the chronic hemodialysis population, and is a reflection of underdialysis (68). Patients with dialysis-associated pericarditis may have chest pain, distended neck veins, a pericardial rub, or develop recurrent hypotension during the first 30 to 60 minutes of dialysis. Intensification of the dialysis regimen with daily heparin-free dialysis for 1 to 2 weeks brings about reduction in size of the effusion in 50% to 70% of patients. Surgical drainage of the pericardial space is indicated if the effusion is massive (greater than 250 mL), fails to respond to medical therapy, produces hemodynamic instability on dialysis, or if there are clinical or echocardiographic signs of early or imminent tamponade. Subxiphoid pericardiotomy is the procedure of choice; however, in emergent cases, needle aspiration of the pericardial space is necessary first.

Undernutrition

One-third of adult hemodialysis patients show evidence of moderate to severe protein calorie malnutrition (PCM). Factors contributing to PCM in hemodialysis patients include anorexia associated with uremia, advanced age, medications, or intercurrent illness; depression; economic constraints; and the catabolic stress of the hemodialytic technique itself. Causes of dialysis-induced catabolism include: membrane bioincompatibility (37) hypothesized to be caused by interleukin-1 (IL-1) and tumor necrosis factor; the loss of up to 8

to 12 gm of amino acids per week on dialysis; and metabolic acidosis (69,70). The importance of PCM in contributing to dialysis mortality has been emphasized by Lowrie and Lew (71), who documented that mortality risk in chronic dialysis patients correlated best with hypoalbuminemia, followed by increasing age and serum creatinine. Hemodialysis patients with serum albumin levels between 3.5 and 4.0 g/dL have a two times greater mortality risk compared to those with values above 4 g/dL. With serum albumins of 2.5 to 3.0 g/dL, mortality risk is increased 16-fold. Low serum BUN and cholesterol were also associated with increased mortality risk. Hypoalbuminemia in dialysis patients also correlates with the prevalence of infections, congestive heart failure, and pericarditis.

Routine dietary assessment is mandated in hemodialysis patients. Indices of nutritional status such as transferrin levels, lymphocyte counts, in addition to serum albumin levels should be monitored. Protein catabolic rate by kinetic modeling and anthropometric measurements also are useful adjuncts. In order to maintain neutral nitrogen balance it is recommended that patients on hemodialysis receive a total caloric intake of at least 35 kcal/kg per day, with high-biological-value protein intake of 1.2 g/kg per day. About 35% of nonprotein calories should be from carbohydrates and the rest from fat. Correcting comorbid illnesses and increasing dialysis dose (72) may also improve nutritional status. Early use of enteral or parenteral nutrition during acute illnesses in hemodialysis patients is advocated. The role of intradialytic parenteral nutrition (IDPN) providing 500 to 600 calories/day is currently under debate (73). For the present it is best limited to those patients who are unable to eat. Recombinant human growth hormone in doses of 5 to 10 mg subcutaneously three times weekly administered in conjunction with IDPN also has been shown to aid protein anabolism (74), but the cost of the hormone at $40/mg renders its widespread use prohibitive.

Vascular Access Complications

Problems related to vascular access account for one-fourth of all ESRD patient hospitalizations (75). A well-functioning vascular access is essential for delivery of dialysis and *adequate* dialysis. The economic and social cost of admissions for access declotting or repair is high, and morbidity is especially marked in the elderly. Long-term vascular access is best effected in the form either of an endogenous Brescia-Cimino radiocephalic fistula or a synthetic graft usually made of polytetrafluoroethylene (PTFE).

Thrombosis and Infection

Failure of vascular access because of thrombosis with or without associated infection occurs in PTFE grafts more frequently than in endogenous fistulae. Polytetrafluoroethylene grafts have an average duration of patency of 1 to 3 years (2-year patency rate of 70%), whereas a well-constructed

Brescia-Cimino fistula has a mean patency of 3 to 4 years or longer. The complication rate of PTFE grafts is four to five times that of fistulae. Access thrombosis usually is associated with an anatomic abnormality (venous stenosis, aneurysm formation, local scarring at a site of repeated needle puncture), extrinsic compression, or low flow state. Vascular accesses in diabetic patients have similar 1-year patency rates when compared to nondiabetic patients (76). In a large series from Boston (85), 324 arteriovenous accesses were created in 256 patients between June 1979 and October 1983. Thirty-four of the patients were diabetic and had 22 Cimino fistulae and 27 PTFE grafts placed. When compared to similar vascular accesses in nondiabetic patients, there was no difference in the patency rates at 1 year in diabetic and nondiabetic patients. Early failure of fistulae because of poor maturation or failure of maturation is more common in diabetic than nondiabetic patients, however.

The substrate for development of access thrombosis and occlusion is stenosis caused by myointimal hyperplasia and neovascularization of the outflow tract of the access just distal to the venous anastomosis where the jet of blood shunted across the access impinges (77,78). Impending thrombosis of the access related to venous outflow stenosis often can be detected by monitoring for high venous pressures (a venous pressure of greater than 150 mm Hg at a blood flow rate of 200 mL/minute is considered elevated); feeling a weakening access thrill; detecting an arterial pulse that is excessively prominent and tapping; and noting prolonged bleeding following removal of dialysis needles. Recirculation percentages also rise as a stenosis on the venous side of the access worsens, and recirculation rates therefore should be measured at least at 6-month intervals. In the presence of these warning signs, contrast angiography of the access (fistulogram) is indicated, and balloon angioplasty of the stenosed segment can be performed immediately to preempt access thrombosis (Fig. 99-7). Angioplasty is associated with at least a 50%

restenosis rate, however. Doppler ultrasonography may be unreliable in detecting early stenoses in many arteriovenous grafts because of complex, turbulent blood flow through the graft. A progressively weakening arterial pulse and low blood flow rates with collapse of the arterial line ("sucking") indicate inflow stenosis and also should prompt angiography of the access.

Early surgical thrombectomy utilizing a Fogarty catheter with repair or bypass of stenotic areas (if present) will restore graft patency if graft thrombosis does supervene. Thrombolysis using urokinase 60–500,000 U/hour can achieve graft patency in 60% to 90% of cases, but the risk of bleeding complications and rethrombosis is high (79). Use of composite grafts made partially of the usual expanded PTFE material along with the more resilient plasma PTFE, can allow early graft cannulation (within 24 hours) following construction or repair of a graft (80). Prospective trials using these composite grafts are underway.

Infection of arteriovenous grafts is more common than with fistulae, may occur in association with graft thrombosis, and may be present in the absence of obvious signs of local infection. Infection of a perigraft hematoma is a common initiating event. Strict attention to skin preparation before cannulation of the arteriovenous access is of great importance in reducing the incidence of graft infections.

Venous Hypertension

Another complication of placement of arteriovenous access is chronic swelling of the hand (Fig. 99-7), and especially the thumb ("sore thumb" syndrome), related to the presence of the distal segment of the vein used for creation of the access (81). Venous hypertension also may occur in association with venous stenosis of the access, or a more proximal stenosis at the level of the subclavian vein, which may have been previously catheterized for temporary vascular access. Ligature of the distal venous limb of the fistula or graft, or balloon dilatation of an area of stenosis usually corrects the problem.

Radial Steal Syndrome

The blood supply to the fingers may be compromised when the radial artery is used for construction of a side-to-side arteriovenous fistula with the cephalic vein. Radial arterial blood no longer supplies the fingers, whereas the fistula provides a low-pressure runoff system that short circuits the ulnar and interosseous arterial blood supply through the palmar arch, a system that may have been previously compromised because of medial arterial calcification, which is especially common in diabetics (82). Pain and numbness in the fingers may proceed to ischemia and gangrene (Figs. 99-8 and 99-9). A steal syndrome may be avoided or ameliorated by ligation of the distal radial artery segment to prevent retrograde flow of blood from the ulnar arterial system into the fistula, or by primary creation of an end-artery to side- or end-vein fistula.

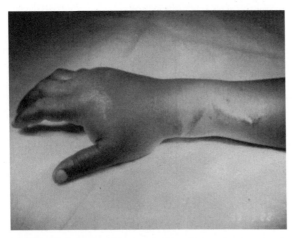

FIG. 99-7. Chronic swelling of the access hand and arm in a patient with proximal axillary vein stenosis. (Courtesy of JH Hong.)

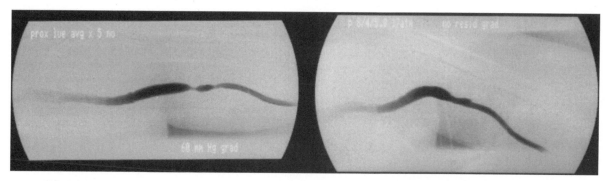

FIG. 99-8. Contrast angiography showing stenotic area of the axillary vein before and after percutaneous balloon angioplasty.

Ischemic Monomelic Neuropathy

Multiple distal mononeuropathies may occur in the upper limb following placement of a proximal arteriovenous access (83). The condition is particularly common in diabetic patients and is characterized by acute painful weakness of the forearm and hand muscles, which occurs within hours of the access creation and is related to ischemia of the peripheral nerves owing to sudden diversion of the blood supply by placement of a proximal brachiocephalic fistula. Early closure of the fistula or removal of the graft may result in reversal of the syndrome.

Hematologic Complications

Anemia

The introduction in 1980 of recombinant erythropoietin (EPO) for treatment of renal anemia was one of the most important advances in hemodialytic therapy. Doses of 50 to 100 U/kg of EPO three times weekly usually are required to keep Hct above 30%. The National Kidney Foundation's Dialysis Outcomes and Quality Initiatives study (DOQI) currently recommends a target hematocrit of 33% to 36% and hemoglobin 11 to 12 g/dL (84), but there is still active debate regarding the possible beneficial effect of higher target Hcts (85).

Iron deficiency should always be sought and treated first, even before initiation of EPO therapy because hemodialysis patients lose up to 1,000 mL/year of packed red blood cells equivalent to 1 g of iron. The transferrin saturation should be kept between 20% and 50% and serum ferritin 100 to 800 ng/mL during EPO therapy (86). Causes for failure of erythropoietin effect include iron deficiency, folate deficiency, infection or inflammation, malignancy, aluminum overload, red cell dyscrasia, and hyperparathyroidism with bone marrow fibrosis.

Bleeding Diathesis

Uremic platelets show abnormal aggregation and adhesion, and there is decreased activity of von Willebrand factor and decreased levels of platelet factor III, such that the bleeding time may be greatly prolonged. In association with frequent heparinization during dialysis, this results in a bleeding tendency that may produce spontaneous retroperitoneal bleeds or subdural hematomas. Improvement may be effected by intensive dialysis, correction of anemia by erythropoietin, and the use of cryoprecipitate (87), desmopressin (dDAVP) (88), or conjugated estrogens (89).

Sepsis

Bacterial infections occur commonly in hemodialysis patients, and may present insidiously yet progress rapidly. Staphylococcal and Gram-negative organisms (*Escherichia coli* in particular) usually are implicated. Opportunistic pathogens are uncommon. Septicemia was responsible for 10.6% of deaths in Medicare ESRD patients between 1989 and 1991 (6). Impaired neutrophil chemotaxis caused by reduced ability to bind C5A and variable derangements in macrophage Fc function and IL-1 production have been reported in dialysis patients, resulting in defective antigen internalization and processing (90). Iron overload (if present) contributes to defective neutrophil function. In addition, dialysis patients show reduced T- and B-cell response to various mitogens, as well as to viral vaccines (influenza, hepatitis B). Initiation of dialysis therapy leads to significant improvement in *in vitro* T-cell proliferation as measured by T-cell IL-6 and IL-10 production (91). Despite these defects in immunity, the high rate of bacterial infections in hemodialysis patients is probably most strongly related to frequent breaches in the skin during vascular access cannulation. Infected PTFE grafts may lack obvious signs of infection, so that the index of suspicion in a febrile dialysis patient with a prosthetic graft vascular access must be high, particularly if there is associated thrombosis of the graft. Bacterial infections in hemodialysis patients generally appear more severe and more likely to progress to septicemia with attendant risks of endocarditis and seeding of a prosthetic graft if this was not already the original site of infection.

The urinary tract may be a source of infection in patients with polycystic kidney disease (PKD) and diabetic patients

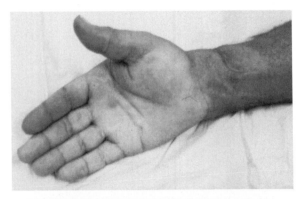

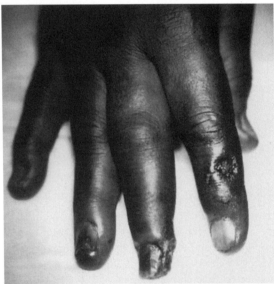

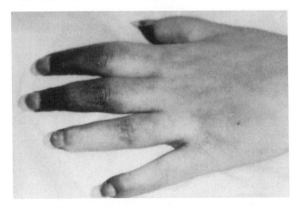

FIG. 99-9. Three cases of radial steal syndrome following placement of vascular access showing increasing degrees of severity of ischemia. The two most severe cases occurred in diabetics. (Courtesy of JH Hong.)

with neurogenic bladders. Lipid-soluble antibiotics such as ciprofloxacin or trimethoprim sulfamethoxazole that penetrate cyst walls well should be used to treat urinary infections in patients with PKD. The suspicion of diverticulitis in patients with PKD with abdominal symptoms and sepsis should also be high because of an association between colonic diverticula and PKD. Pneumonia is a significant cause of morbidity and mortality in dialysis patients and often presents

with atypical pulmonary infiltrates. Tuberculosis is 10 times as common in hemodialysis patients as in the general population, and disease often is extrapulmonary, miliary, and atypical. Infections with Yersinia, Mucor (vide infra), Listeria, and Salmonella also are reported to be more common and/or severe in hemodialysis patients.

Diseases of Bone and Soft Tissue

Renal Osteodystrophy

Three predominant types of renal osteodystrophy occur, but combinations and transitional forms sometimes related to therapy commonly are seen.

High Turnover Renal Bone Disease

This is due to secondary hyperparathyroidism and is characterized by increased osteoblastic and osteoclastic activity with varying degrees of bone marrow fibrosis, the presence of woven osteoid, and normal or accelerated mineralization of bone. Pathogenetic factors include hyperphosphatemia, hypocalcemia and low levels of 1,25-dihydroxycholecalciferol (92). The hypocalcemia may be absolute or merely relative, as a shift of the set point of calcium (the serum calcium level needed to reduce the maximal PTH level by 50%) to the right on the PTH/calcium curve occurs in uremia so that a higher serum calcium than normal is required to inhibit PTH secretion. Serum calcium levels in uremic patients should be kept between 9.5 and 11.5 mg/dL. Radiologic changes develop late in hyperparathyroidism. In established disease, subperiosteal resorption is best seen on the radial borders of the middle phalanges of the middle fingers, erosion of the terminal tufts of the fingers, and subperiosteal erosions and cysts involving the lateral one-third of the clavicles are characteristic (Fig. 99-10). Multiple bone cysts first observed in the outer one-third of the clavicles and middle phalanges but involving mainly long bones are noted in advanced disease (osteitis fibrosa cystica). Osteosclerosis involving the axial skeleton and giving rise to the characteristic "rugger jersey" spine appearance also is a feature of high turnover renal bone disease. Intact or N-terminal parathyroid hormone (PTH) levels measured by immunoradiometric assay (iPTH) are greater than 150 to 200 pg/mL in patients with clinically significant hyperparathyroidism. Some 90% of patients with iPTH levels less than 900 pg/mL respond to treatment with intravenous or oral calcitriol (medical parathyroidectomy) (93). A new Vitamin D analog, 19-nor-1α25-dihydoxyvitamin D2 (paricalcitol) with less calcemic effect, is rapidly gaining popularity in the United States. In patients with severe hyperparathyroidism and iPTH levels greater than 900 pg/mL, however, medical therapy may be ineffective in over 60% of cases owing to autonomy of the parathyroid glands (tertiary hyperparathyroidism). These patients often have associated hypercalcemia and hyperphosphatemia with pruritus and calciphylaxis and benefit from surgical parathyroidectomy. Tertiary

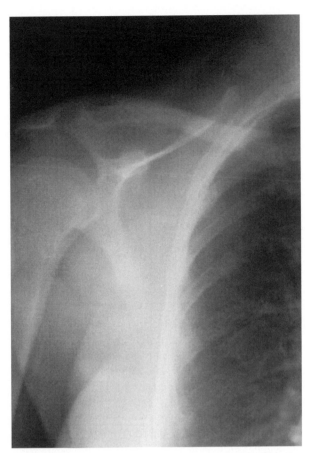

FIG. 99-10. Gross erosion of the distal one-third of the clavicle (Nathan's sign) in a hemodialysis patient with secondary hyperparathyroidism.

hyperparathyroidism may complicate renal transplantation, persisting after graft failure and resumption of maintenance hemodialysis.

Low Turnover Bone Disease

This multifactorial variant of renal osteodystrophy is characterized by low levels of parathyroid hormone (less than two times normal), a reduced number of osteoclasts and osteoblasts with low rates of bone turnover, and a tendency to develop hypercalcemia (particularly with treatment). Two types of low turnover bone disease are seen, aplastic bone disease and osteomalacia.

Aplastic Bone Disease. This disorder is characterized by decreased osteoclast and osteoblast activity, cessation of bone formation, and intact PTH levels less than 100 pg/mL. Etiologic factors include aluminum and iron overload, and the condition occurs more frequently in diabetic uremic patients, patients on CAPD, and uremic patients with previous parathyroidectomies. An increase in fractures and poor fracture healing may be features of aplastic bone disease. Aplastic bone disease accounted for 49% of bone lesions found in a population of 117 chronic hemodialysis patients and 142 CAPD

patients followed for a 1-year period in three Toronto hospitals; therefore, it is the most common form of renal bone disease currently seen (94). In this study, only osteomalacia was associated with increased stainable aluminum on bone biopsy.

Osteomalacia. This form of renal bone disease is characterized by underactivity of bone matrix and is marked by excess deposition of unmineralized osteoid in large osteoid seams. There may or may not be associated aluminum (Al) excess; however, in dialysis patients with osteomalacia, Al is the most common etiologic factor (97). Conditions that predispose to the development of Al bone disease include factors that enhance gastrointestinal absorption and those that favor deposition in the bone. Situations that enhance the gastrointestinal absorption of Al include ingestion of phosphate binders on an empty, acid-filled stomach; children, young adults (95), and diabetic patients (96) with renal disease; and citrate (97), lactate (98), and possibly other organic anions. Cases of Al intoxication occurring in predialytic uremic patients as a result of aluminum hydroxide therapy, especially if associated with concomitant ingestion of citrate-containing compounds such as Shohl's solution or effervescent analgesic tablets, have been described in children and adults (99,100). Low-turnover bone such as that following a parathyroidectomy (101) or after chronic treatment with intravenous calcitriol (102) can also permit Al deposition in the bone with its detrimental effects. In cases of aluminum bone disease, deposition of stainable aluminum over more than 25% to 30% of trabecular bone surface is seen. Bone pain, proximal myopathy, pathological fractures or pseudofractures of the bones of the axial skeleton (ribs, vertebrae, pelvis, hips), and long bone fractures (Fig. 99-11) are common features.

Although bone disease is a dominant feature of chronic aluminum excess, neurologic symptoms are seen most commonly with acute exposure to aluminum, and may occur as an epidemic within a dialysis unit where the water supply has become contaminated with aluminum. Alfrey and associates in Denver in 1972 first described the syndrome of dialysis encephalopathy related to Al intoxication (103). Scanning dysarthria, myoclonus, progressive dementia, mutism, and seizures are typical features. Diagnosis is supported by an electroencephalogram (EEG) showing generalized slowing, with multifocal bursts of delta activity and spikes most prominent in the frontal lobes (Fig. 99-12). Electroencephalogram abnormalities may precede clinical signs by 6 to 8 months. The source of aluminum may be oral aluminum hydroxide used as a phosphate binder (before or after start of hemodialytic therapy), or aluminum from surface water treated with alum (to produce flocculation and aid in production of potable water for communities), or passing through aluminum-containing soils.

Calcium and not aluminum, salts should be used as phosphate binders in dialysis patients *unless:* (a) The serum phosphate level is very high with a calcium phosphate product over 70 and risk of precipitating or worsening metastatic

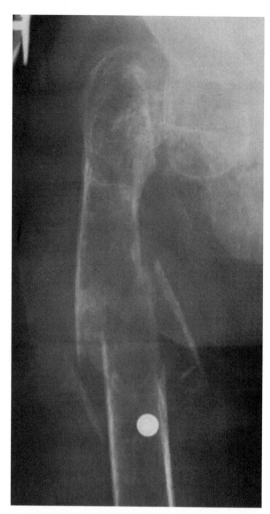

FIG. 99-11. Anteroposterior radiograph of the proximal femur in a 33-year-old man on home hemodialysis for over a decade, with severe renal osteomalacia. There is nonunion of a previous femoral neck fracture as well as an acute comminuted fracture of the femoral shaft. The bones are severely osteopenic, demonstrating a medullary density equivalent to the soft tissues of the thigh. (Courtesy of TA Einhorn.)

calcification if the serum calcium level is further raised by absorption of oral calcium. (b) Calcium salts have produced hypercalcemia. As many as one-third of hemodialysis patients (particularly those with aplastic bone disease) manifest hypercalcemia despite absorption of only 20% to 30% of ingested calcium carbonate. Before switching from calcium to an aluminum-based phosphate binder, however, dialysate calcium should be decreased to 2.0 to 2.5 mEq/L. Alternatively, the dose of 1,25-dihydroxycholecalciferol is reduced or the intravenous preparation used instead of the oral in an effort to reduce serum calcium level. In some patients, use of calcium acetate (2.3 g/day) instead of calcium carbonate may control hypercalcemia, as the acetate salt while binding twice as much phosphate as calcium carbonate is less well absorbed from the gut. (c) The serum phosphate remains high despite use of calcium in adequate doses taken with meals (3 to 12 grams per day calcium carbonate), such

that the largest dose of calcium is taken with the largest meal.

Aluminum intoxication in dialysis patients should be suspected in the setting of compatible clinical features (encephalopathy, fracturing osteomalacia, microcytic anemia), when serum aluminum levels are persistently over 50 to 100 μg/L, or a desferrioxamine (DFO) infusion test produces increments in serum aluminum levels of greater than 300 μg/L. If diagnostic tests are inconclusive or contradictory, bone biopsy following ingestion of aurine tetrahydrochloride demonstrates Al deposition on more than 25% to 30% of trabecular bone surfaces.

In mild Al intoxication, cessation of Al intake may suffice as therapy; in more severe cases, chelation therapy with intravenous DFO is used to mobilize Al from tissues and form stable diffusible complexes, which are dialyzable. Desferrioxamine is given in a dosage of 5 mg/kg once weekly (not exceeding 1 gm DFO per week) during the last hour of dialysis for 3 months. Serum Al increases and plateaus 12 to 24 hours after each dose of DFO. If levels rise above 350 to 400 μg/L, acute Al encephalopathy may be precipitated; therefore, the dose of DFO must be adjusted to keep serum Al below this level. Other side effects of DFO therapy include hypotension at infusion rates greater than 40 mg/kg per hour, anaphylaxis, skin rash, diarrhea, and visual and auditory abnormalities. Hyperparathyroidism may be unmasked and serum calcium levels fall as bone turnover and mineralization increases with therapy. Infections with certain species of fungi and bacteria (*Mucor* sp., *Yersinia* sp.) have been reported to be more common in patients treated with DFO; however, this risk has not been widely substantiated (104–106). Al removal at each dialysis session is between 15 and 20 mg per treatment, and clinical improvement is seen after several weeks.

Mixed Uremic Osteodystrophy

Here osteitis fibrosa is associated with evidence of defective bone mineralization.

Metastatic Calcification and Calciphylaxis

Deposition of calcium phosphate aggregates occurs when the product of calcium and phosphate in blood exceeds 70. Deposits are seen primarily in skin and subcutaneous tissues and may be massive. Elevated serum phosphate levels always should be treated with a short course of aluminum hydroxide before initiating therapy with calcium salts. These ectopic calcific deposits must be differentiated from calcified tophaceous gout, tumoral calcinosis, myositis ossificans, and calcified tumors.

Calciphylaxis is characterized by ischemic necrosis of the soft tissues of the extremities associated with extensive vascular calcification. Penetrating ulcers with eschar formation and secondary infection occur. The condition sometimes responds to parathyroidectomy.

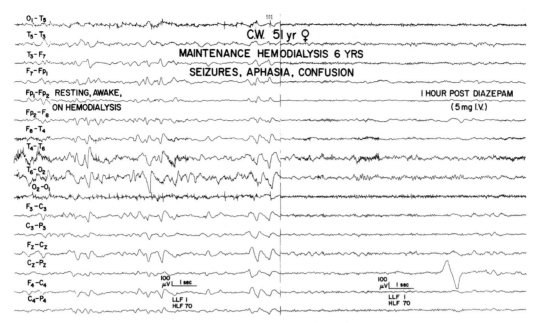

FIG. 99-12. Electroencephalogram in dialysis dementia. Tracing on left obtained from dying 51-year-old woman after 6 years of dialysis with progressive neurologic signs including dysarthria, seizures, and aphasia. Improvement by diazepam, shown on right, is characteristic, although not pathognomonic of dialysis dementia.

Amyloidosis

Amyloidosis was first recognized as the cause of the ubiquitous carpal tunnel syndrome of chronic hemodialysis patients in Tassin, France in 1980 when amyloid tissue was noted in the synovial membranes of uremic patients undergoing surgery for carpal tunnel release (107). Polymerized ß-2-microglobulin was then documented to be the constituent in deposits of amyloid found in the carpal tunnel and other musculoskeletal sites of long-term hemodialysis patients (108). ß-2-Microglobulin amyloidosis is noted in up to 80% of hemodialysis patients on treatment for more than 15 years, and has been described in CAPD patients and patients with chronic renal failure before initiation of dialysis (109,110). The pathogenesis of amyloid formation is incompletely understood but may result from abnormal processing of a precursor protein under the influence of local tissue factors such as protease inhibitors or glycosaminoglycans, or from an amyloid enhancing factor (111). Levels of serum ß-2-microglobulin in hemodialysis patients range between 30 and 50 mg/L, 15 to 20 times normal nonuremic levels, but levels in patients with and without amyloidosis do not differ. Part of the increased serum levels of ß-2-microglobulin in dialysis patients is owing to accumulation in plasma caused by loss of normal glomerular filtration. Cuprophane membranes can also increase production of ß-2-microglobulin (112). Although synthetic PAN membranes adsorb and filter ß-2-microglobulin by diffusion and convection, removing up to 300 mg of the substance in a 4-hour hemodialysis session, they have not been demonstrated to reduce the risk or severity of amyloidosis in dialysis patients. Deposition of amyloid occurs predominantly in articular and periarticular areas and produces a number of well-described syndromes.

Carpal Tunnel Syndrome

This is the most common manifestation of dialysis amyloidosis. A history of paraesthesia and pain on the palmar surfaces of the thumb, index, middle finger, and radial aspect of the fourth finger is elicited. Pain often is worse at night and during hemodialysis sessions. Later, weakened opposition and abduction of the thumb with atrophy of the thenar eminence is seen. Physical examination, including testing for Tinel's sign (paresthesia or pain in the fingers reproduced by percussion over the volar surface of the wrist) and Phalen's sign (paresthesia or pain in the fingers reproduced by full flexion of the wrist for over 1 min) often is negative. Diagnosis is best confirmed by use of motor and sensory nerve conduction studies. Prolonged remission of symptoms may be obtained by wrist splints, which prevent flexion and extension, particularly during sleeping hours. Relief also can be obtained with the injection of 0.75 mL of 1% Xylocaine mixed with 0.75 mL triamcinolone (40 mg/mL) into the carpal tunnel. Ultimately, surgery is needed to transect the transverse carpal ligament, especially if there is evidence of motor or sensory loss; however, the condition often recurs after surgery.

Chronic Synovitis

Chronic synovitis of the shoulders, knees, wrists, and hips—with or without associated effusion, crepitation, deformity, and decreased range of motion—are seen with increasing frequency in long-term dialysis patients (113); it involves almost 100% of those at risk by the twentieth year of treatment. Amyloid deposits are found in the fluid of affected joints, and in surrounding tissues. Shoulder ultrasonography is useful and may show thick rotator cuffs and echogenic pads of amyloid tissue between the muscle groups. Chronic tenosynovitis of the flexor tendons of the fingers also is seen and may produce flexion contractures sometimes associated with subcutaneous deposits of amyloid in the tendon sheaths of the palms. Tenosynovitis of the Achilles and quadriceps tendons may result in their spontaneous rupture.

Destructive Spondyloarthropathy

This variant of dialysis amyloidosis predilects for the intervertebral discs of the upper cervical area, producing paravertebral erosions and cystic radiolucencies within and around the bones (114). These radiolucencies consist of abundant amyloid deposits invading subchondral bone. A characteristic radiologic triad is described in destructive cervical spondyloarthropathy owing to amyloid: severe intervertebral disc space narrowing, erosion and geodes of the adjacent vertebral plates, and absence of osteophytosis. Localized neck pain may be the only symptom in early or mild cases, whereas vertebral collapse or subluxation may result in severe disease and can produce compressive myelopathy and even progress to paraplegia, particularly with neck manipulation (e.g., during induction of general anesthesia). Formation of periodontoid tumors of amyloid also may produce compressive myelopathy.

Pathologic Fractures of Long Bones

Juxtaarticular deposits of amyloid at sites of tendon insertions can produce large cystic lesions in the femoral heads, acetabula, humerus, and tibial plateaus that may fracture with minimal motion or injury. Total joint replacement may be required.

Systemic and visceral amyloid involvement is uncommon. Visceral amyloidosis in dialysis patients has been reported in a perivascular distribution in the gastrointestinal tract, heart, kidneys (with the formation of matrix stones) (115) and fatty tissue. Amyloidosis of the bowel wall may produce bleeding, intestinal obstruction, and deposits in the tongue odynophagia. Subcutaneous tumors in the buttocks, popliteal areas, elbows, and wrist also have been described.

There is no satisfactory treatment to prevent or arrest dialysis arthropathy. Renal transplantation is the only certain means of effecting improvement. Radiologic lesions take several years to heal following restoration of renal function by transplantation. Endoscopic resection of the coracoacromial joint may relieve shoulder pain (116). Prosthetic joint replacement of hip and knees may be necessary to preserve mobility, and spinal fusion with or without osteosynthetic grafts for cervical destructive arthropathy may prevent quadriplegia.

Muscle Cramps

Painful cramps involving the gastrocnemius, or small muscles of the feet, may occur in hemodialysis patients during dialysis or at night. Intradialytic or immediate postdialytic cramps probably reflect volume contraction and usually respond to fluid replacement with 0.9% saline, hypertonic saline, or hypertonic solutions of glucose or mannitol (117). Quinine sulfate 260 mg 2 hours before dialysis reduces the frequency of cramps from 17% to 6% of hemodialysis treatments (118). Carnitine supplementation (119) and Vitamin E 400 IU/day also are reported to be efficacious (120). Verapamil 120 mg at bedtime may help nocturnal cramps. Treatment is unsatisfactory in many patients, however, and patients learn to live with their annoying disability. Hypo- or hyperthyroidism, hypomagnesemia, hyponatremia, and hypocalcemia, as well as a variety of drugs also may produce muscle cramps; therefore, these factors should be ruled out as a cause of cramps in dialysis patients.

Machine- or Technique-Related Complications

Hemodialysis is extraordinarily safe despite the potential for mechanical failure and human error while processing blood and dialysate extracorporeally (121). Accidental death during hemodialysis is a rare event, occurring at a frequency of about 1 in 76,138 dialyses, whether performed by physicians, trained nurses and technicians, or the patient. Accidental injury to patients during hemodialysis results from overheated dialysate, contamination of dialysate with acid, sodium hypochlorite bleach (122) or formaldehyde (used to cleanse dialyzers for reuse), and chloramines used for water purification (123). An acute "new dialyzer" syndrome has been attributed to unidentified intoxicants leached from the dialyzer into the patient's blood (124). Disposable dialyzers and blood tubing are made of plastic, which may release organic intoxicants. Plasticizers such as diethylhexylphthalate, which are added to polyvinylchloride tubing to improve its low-temperature flexibility, may be leached out during hemodialysis. Plasticizers are highly toxic; exposure may cause necrotizing cutaneous vasculitis and a nonspecific, nonfatal, hepatitis. The risk of electrical shock during hemodialysis has been reduced to very little significance by attention to equipment design and periodic testing for current leakage (125). Rarely, when human intervention defeats (cancels) equipment safety monitors, fatal accidents have resulted from high or low dialysate temperatures, the exposure of blood to undiluted dialysate concentrate, high concentrations of chloramines, bleach, and formaldehyde or tap water lacking concentrate, all of which produce blood hemolysis. Air embolism should not occur if routine precautions are taken: ensuring tight tubing connections, intact tubing, proper clamping of the saline infusion port, and continuous arming of the air leak detector. In the event of this catastrophic and usually lethal complication the venous bloodline should be clamped immediately and the blood pump stopped. Then the patient should be placed in a reversed Trendelenburg position with the left side down, and cardiopulmonary support initiated.

Neurologic Complications

Clinical signs of uremic polyneuropathy do not occur in acute renal failure and appear late in the course of progressive chronic renal insufficiency. Uremic peripheral neuropathy has been categorized as sensory and motor. For unexplained reasons, motor neuropathy is more severe in men than women, but is not worse in elderly than young patients (126). Both motor and sensory conduction velocities are reduced, and distal latencies are prolonged to a similar degree (127). The main reason for faulty electrical conduction is axonal degeneration. In Bolton's view, repetitive measurements of motor nerve conduction velocity are of great value in assessing peripheral nerve integrity and as a sign of the course of renal failure (128). Numerous electrophysiologic tests were proposed as a means to monitor the quality of dialytic therapy under the premise that worsening neuropathy indicates failing dialysis, whereas stability or improvement suggests adequate dialysis; however, neuropathy reverses slowly with hemodialysis, and faster with use of highly permeable synthetic membranes that remove the implicated middle molecules more efficiently.

Peripheral motor neuropathy was noted in 29% of 17 randomly selected children undergoing dialysis (mean age 14.2 years) (129), and 87% of 30 uremic adults (18 receiving hemodialysis). The incidence and severity of uremic polyneuropathy have decreased significantly with refinement in the technique and amount of hemodialysis. Overt, severe neuropathy with foot drop and hand-muscle wasting now is only rarely observed. Motor neuropathy usually stabilizes or even improves during the course of hemodialysis in many patients, although controlled studies are lacking. In a careful study of 213 patients, Cadilhac and coworkers found that neuropathy stabilized during adequate dialysis, with few patients either worsening or improving (130). Routine practice no longer incorporates measurements of motor nerve conduction velocity because the information gained affords little benefit to direct patient care. Likewise, earlier employment of serial measurements of motor nerve conduction velocity (131) to define adequate dialysis (132) has been abandoned because of variability and imprecision in testing. Uremic neuropathy is best treated by increased dialysis dose, and use of tricyclic antidepressants such as amitriptyline, or the newer gabapentin. Mega doses of Vitamin B_6 and evening primrose oil supplements may ameliorate sensory symptoms of uremic peripheral neuropathy.

Acquired Cystic Renal Disease

The kidneys, although scarred and shrunken, do not completely cease function after the start of dialysis. Epithelial cells, mostly of proximal tubular, continue to proliferate, leading to the formation of cysts. The stimulus for this proliferation and function of the cysts, if any, is unknown. Grantham (133) proposed three possible causes for cyst formation in adult PKD that could be applicable to acquired cysts: (a) distal obstruction leading to high-pressure dilatation; (b) increased compliance of the tubular basement membrane with formation under normal pressure; or (c) proliferation of epithelial cells. The histologic nature of the proliferating cells points to the latter as the most likely cause. Stimuli for the development of cystic lesions lie within the uremic milieu. This is inferred from their regression after restoration of renal function following a successful renal transplant (134). Suggested factors include endogenous substances such as growth factors responsible for renal hypertrophy; retained toxins such as polyamines, which can cause cellular proliferation; or androgens. The latter has been implicated by the observation that cystic formation appears sooner in male dialysis patients (135) and that 20 of 24 renal malignancies were found in cystic kidneys in men.

In 1977, Dunnill and associates (136) noted a relationship of renal cysts in dialysis patients, found on postmortem, with spontaneous bleeding and tumors. Multiple renal cysts are discovered in 70% to 80% of patients on both hemodialysis and peritoneal dialysis for over 10 years. Cysts occur predominantly in the cortex; some arising in the corticomedullary junction. They can be few in number or can replace much of the renal parenchyma, to the point of resembling adult polycystic kidneys. The cysts range from microscopic to several centimeters in diameter; most are less than 0.5 cm. From histologic characteristics of tubular epithelium, Mickisch and coworkers (137) identified cysts as arising from proximal, distal, and collecting duct tubules. Ishikawa and associates (138), using lectins specific to proximal and distal tubular cells, however, found that 90% of the cysts had proximal tubular epithelium. Microscopically, the epithelium can range from simple cuboidal cells to papillary proliferation to a pattern of undifferentiated hyperplasia. The degree of cystic formation seems to correlate with the duration of renal disease, appearing even before the need for dialysis in some cases of long-standing azotemia. When studied by sonography, cysts were found in 22% of 120 nondialyzed azotemic patients with a mean serum creatinine level of 3 mg/dL; 35% of dialysis patients with a mean serum creatinine of 10 mg/dL; and 92% of patients on dialysis at least 8 years.

The feared complication of acquired cystic renal disease is the development of renal adenocarcinoma. On morphologic examination, up to 80% of contracted cyst-bearing kidneys in dialysis patients contain adenomas. Their malignant potential is unknown. The prevalence of renal cell carcinoma in long-term dialysis patients is reported to be 1% to 2%, 40 times that in the general population. Cancer can be heralded by hematuria, flank pain, renal mass, hypercalcemia with suppressed parathyroid hormone, or sudden reversal of anemia. Death has resulted from metastatic spread in a few cases. Because of this risk, some (139) have called for routine screening of dialysis patients with sonography or CT scanning, the latter being more sensitive. It is prudent to screen those on dialysis for more than 5 years because the cost is considerable and the yield low if every hemodialysis patient is studied in the absence of symptoms.

Neoplasia in Chronic Hemodialysis Patients

Several reports suggest an increased incidence of other malignancies as a result of persistent uremia in addition to malignant degeneration in cysts reported in long-term hemodialysis patients (vide supra) (140). Individual case reports by Oe and coworkers (141) of renal carcinoma development in hemodialyzed patients with polycystic kidneys, first suggested that cancer and dialysis are associated. De novo malignancy was noted in 15 patients on chronic hemodialysis (3% of the group at risk) and six kidney transplant recipients (4.9% of the risk group) leading Herr and associates to conclude that both uremia therapies impose a risk of neoplasia (142). Supporting this thesis is the finding in a nationwide survey of the Japanese dialysis population of an overall incidence of tumor death 2.3 times higher in males and 4.3 times higher in females than in the general population (143). Port and colleagues assessed the incidence of cancer in 4,161 ESRD patients on dialysis in Michigan compared to the calendar year-specific incidence rates of 4 million residents of the Detroit region (144). The tumor rate in dialysis patients "was significantly increased for all in situ tumors combined, as well as for invasive tumors of the kidney, the corpus uteri, and the prostate." A four to five times excess risk was observed for renal and endometrial cancers. Echoing the concern of Port and associates, DeSala and coworkers observed that 14 of 324 long-term dialysis patients in a Spanish unit developed malignant tumors, four of which were cancer of the bladder (145).

Despite these reports, the consensus is that recipients of maintenance hemodialysis are not at significantly increased risk of malignancy. Support for this view is afforded by Kantor's study of 28,049 Medicare ESRD patients whose cancer rates were compared to the National Cancer Institutes cancer incidence rates for the United States. No overall increase in cancer risk was found in the hemodialysis population, although patients with chronic glomerulonephritis had a small excess of non-Hodgkin's lymphoma and biliary tract cancers (146). Bush and Gabriel also assessed the course of 834 uremic patients, noting that only five who contracted malignant disease, an incidence of 0.6% that was no greater than the risk in the general age-matched population (147).

Gastrointestinal Complications

Liver Disease

Hepatic disease was recognized as a complication of long-term hemodialysis shortly after its inception as uremia therapy (148). Initial regimens for maintenance hemodialysis required repeated blood transfusions to sustain a hematocrit of 25% to 35%, fostering continuing hemolysis; hepatic hemosiderosis; and the transmission of hepatitis non-A, non-B, and hepatitis B (149). Alarm over the risk to staff of the

seemingly unavoidable risk of hepatitis B (as many as 20% of patients in some areas were hepatitis B antibody-positive) cast a pall over the growth of hemodialysis units during the early 1970s. Subsequently, elimination of pro forma transfusions and screening—exclusion of HBsAG-positive blood—reduced the prevalence of hepatitis in most dialysis units significantly, and after introduction of an effective hepatitis B vaccine (150), and institution of universal precautions, the incidence of new cases of hepatitis B within hemodialysis units has nearly disappeared. The prevalence of seropositivity for HBsAg in US hemodialysis patients varied between 2.7% to 7.8% in the 1970s (151,152), but fell to 1.2% in 1992 (153). Hepatitis C (formerly non-A, non-B) remains the most common cause of transfusion-acquired hepatitis, and also is transmitted through contact within dialysis units because time on dialysis is an independent risk factor for development of infection with the virus. The prevalence of antibodies to hepatitis C virus on ELISA II assay in US hemodialysis units varies between 25% and 36% (154,155). Problems with current antibody testing include the facts that 10% of HCV-infected dialysis patients never develop antibodies; that anti-HCV antibody may first be detectable as much as 6 to 12 months postinfection; and that a positive anti-HCV test may indicate recent and/or remote infection, but does not necessarily mean infectivity, because only 17% to 27% of anti-HCV ELISA-positive blood transmits HCV (156,157). Third-generation ELISA tests are more sensitive, but currently are not as widely used. Detection of HCV RNA using molecular hybridization studies therefore will prove to be the most reliable means of testing for the level of virus in serum and liver (103); however, its cost and technical difficulty will prevent widespread use. In the meantime, hand washing and changing gloves between patients are still some of the most important ways to prevent the spread of hepatitis within dialysis units. Dialysis patients with chronic hepatitis B infection should be isolated and dialyzed on dedicated dialysis machines. All dialysis patients and staff should receive hepatitis B vaccination. A hepatitis C vaccine is not available presently. It is not currently recommended to isolate patients with hepatitis C antibody positivity.

Parfrey and coworkers studied the impact of hepatitis B disease prospectively in hemodialysis and kidney transplant patients in Canada (158). Although immunosuppressed renal transplant recipients developed chronic active hepatitis or cirrhosis, resulting in death from liver disease at a rate of 5% per patient-year, a coincident group of 10 HBsAg-positive hemodialysis patients fared better. Persistent liver dysfunction occurred in only one dialysis patient; none died of liver disease. Confirmation of the relative benignity of HBsAG positivity in hemodialysis patients was reported by Marchesini and associates, who noted in a prospective study of 38 positive carriers followed for 6 to 66 months that none died of liver disease (159). Death owing to persistent hepatitis B antigenemia is rare; after a mean retrospective follow-up of 52 ± 5 months (some for 10 years), Harnett and coworkers noted that only one of 49 hemodialysis patients died of liver disease (160).

The wide variation in reported prevalence of liver disease in dialysis patients reflects differences in time of reporting and population studied; it is highest where transfusions are routine. Thus, in the review by Toussaint and colleagues, 33% of hemodialysis patients were found to have liver dysfunction (161). Granulomatous liver diseases including schistosomiasis and tuberculosis, and the late effects of viral infections such as cytomegalovirus should be considered, even in HbsAg-positive patients. Acquired immunodeficiency diseases syndrome (AIDS) in its agonal stages is frequently associated with multiple organ failure, including a hepatorenal syndrome.

Dialysis Ascites

Persistent ascitic fluid accumulation in a patient undergoing maintenance hemodialysis may be the consequence of disparate pathogenetic mechanisms, and the diagnosis of dialysis-associated ascites therefore is one of exclusion. Tuberculous peritonitis, whether miliary, or a direct extension of intraabdominal tuberculosis, has not been infrequent in our urban dialysis patients (162). Fungal peritonitis like bacterial and tuberculous peritonitis causes an exudative (protein content greater than 3 g/dL) ascitic fluid. In approximately half of our cases of proven tuberculosis, the diagnosis was made by peritoneal biopsy when staining for acid-fast organisms in ascitic fluid was negative. Advanced liver disease, usually associated with hypoalbuminemia, is an important cause of abdominal swelling owing to ascitic fluid. Gluck and Nolph reviewed 138 patients with ascites and ESRD reported through 1986 and cited contributing mechanisms as: fluid overload, hypoproteinemia, lymphatic drainage disturbances, and peritoneal membrane changes (163). A specific underlying cause was discovered in 15% of cases. When evaluating the etiology of ascites in a dialysis patient, the diagnosis of liver failure, like that of heart failure with anasarca, is not difficult. Having excluded specific causes of ascites, there remains a group of hemodialysis patients suffering ascites without explanation, leading to the term dialysis ascites (164). Dialysis ascites is a serious sign of failure of the hemodialysis regimen, often accompanied by muscle wasting, anorexia, and worsening neuropathy. Treatment involves restoration of positive nitrogen balance where hypoalbuminemia is linked to inadequate dialysis, and a clinical trial of increased dialysis time. Improvement is induced by intraperitoneal steroid instillation (165), albumin infusion, or intensive ultrafiltration during hemodialysis only rarely (166). Reinfusion of ascitic fluid (167) and resort to peritoneal dialysis (168) with gradual reduction in ascitic fluid volume are complex solutions to the therapeutic dilemma (169).

Reproductive Dysfunction

Illness mutes the sex drive. Hemodialysis patients remain azotemic, acidotic, and anemic with multiple endocrine abnormalities. Men on dialysis have low testosterone and high luteinizing hormone (LH) levels, which together with an elevated follicle stimulating hormone (FSH) level is associated with severe spermatogenic damage (170) and partial or complete impotence in 50% (171). Zinc deficiency is postulated to be one of 28 factors responsible for sexual malfunction in dialyzed men. A double-blind trial was conducted in hemodialyzed men given supplemental oral zinc using 50 mg of elemental zinc as zinc acetate (10 patients) with 10 control patients receiving placebo (172). Zinc treatment led to increased plasma zinc, serum testosterone, and sperm count, as well as an improvement in potency, libido, and frequency of intercourse. By contrast, Muir and associates (173) reported a negative study of the value of zinc treatment for impotence, leaving the issue unresolved at present. Muir and associates also conducted a double-blind crossover trial of bromocriptine for erectile impotence in dialyzed men, observing that 11 of 14 patients responded to bromocriptine with improved libido and/or quality of erections (174).

Fertility in women with renal insufficiency is reduced at serum creatinines as low as 1.5 mg/dL, and at a creatinine clearance of 10 to 15 mL/minute irregular menses develop and progress to amenorrhea and decreased libido as creatinine clearance falls below 4 mL/minute. Women on dialysis have low estrogen and high FSH and prolactin levels (175) that blunts sexual interest, causes anovulatory menstrual cycles and nearly always precludes successful pregnancy. A few successful pregnancies have been reported in women sustained by maintenance hemodialysis who were subjected to intensified dialysis (176), or who had some residual renal function. Almost 80% of the pregnancies that do occur end in spontaneous abortion (177).

In general, sexuality can be maximized by effective hemodialysis, proper nutrition, and awareness of the side effects (in men) of antihypertensive drugs that interfere with potency. Evaluation of the sexually incompetent man on dialysis requires assessment of historical performance (past ability to attain and maintain an erection), examination of a semen specimen, and, if all results are normal, sex hormone assay. Demonstration of nocturnal tumescence in impotent men desirous of intercourse indicates the patient's potential for development of an erection, while suggesting the possibility that sensitive counseling may improve sexual performance. Bromocriptine has been used in hyperprolactinemic men on dialysis, and some male dialysis patients report improved libido with testosterone supplements prescribed for therapy of anemia. Progesterone therapy may be warranted in some female dialysis patients who have irregular menstrual bleeding with anovulatory cycles and estrogen excess (178). Therapy with erythropoietin can reverse hyperprolactinemia and produce normal menses in some women on hemodialysis (179).

Psychosocial Problems

Maladjustment to the rigorous regimen of maintenance hemodialysis is a transient although common experience for nearly all dialysis patients. Depression, a sense of futility and hopelessness, and an unfavorably altered body image are common expressions of anxiety and fear over an uncertain future. Although gentle reassurance and repeated explanation may minimize patient stress, acceptance of the reality of life dependent on a machine is a persistent enervating and unbearable burden for some patients. According to Stewart (180), approximately one-fourth of dialysis patients are depressed at any time because of concern over compliance with diet, medication, and sexual dysfunction. From 1% to 6% of dialysis patients overtly commit suicide (181,182). The most recent report of the USRDS lists withdrawal from dialysis as the cause of death in 10% of patients who died between 1989 and 1991, the third most common cause of death in hemodialysis patients (6).

New and Kjellstrand reviewed a series of 1,766 ESRD patients in Minnesota and noted that 155 patients (9%) discontinued dialysis accounting for 22% of all deaths (183). Dialysis was stopped more often in older than younger nondiabetic patients, and more often in young diabetic patients than in young nondiabetic patients. Half of the patients were mentally competent when the decision to terminate dialysis was made. A derivative study of the same patients examined the course of 26 patients who withdrew from dialysis (4% of all deaths), although there was no evident medical or technical reason to do so (184). It was concluded that the competent patients who withdrew apparently die because they cannot stand the stress of the regimen. Approximately 10% of all deaths in a large Canadian dialysis program followed the elective decision to stop dialysis. Once dialysis was discontinued, patients lived a mean of 9.6 days and died for the most part without pain or prolonged suffering (185). In Brooklyn, very few of our predominantly Black patients elect to stop MD a reflection of the lower rate in Blacks than Whites observed nationally. To eliminate these *avoidable deaths,* the authors advocate better support, particularly from physicians, as well as careful patient selection to exclude those who elect not to have life prolongation.

Family support, optimal hemodialysis, and empathetic counseling usually are sufficient to overcome transient severe depression. Participation in patient group activities, such as programs sponsored by the American Association of Kidney Patients adds purpose and camaraderie to the dialysis patient's life. Beyond these generalizations, there are few data from which to extract specific measures to aid in coping with hemodialysis. For the growing number of Black and Hispanic patients in urban dialysis units, intractable poverty, shortages of social workers, and high unemployment rates frustrate implementation of usual social support mechanisms. Similarly, the increasing age of newly treated dialysis patients and the comorbid disorders of a geriatric population (stroke, heart attack, malignancy, and senility) stand in the way of joining groups and acting in their own interest.

REFERENCES

1. Abel JJ, Rowntree LG, Turner BB. On the removal of diffusible substances from the circulating blood of living animals by dialysis. *J Pharmacol Exp Ther* 1914;5:275.
2. Scribner BH, Caner JEZ, Buri R, et al. The technique of continuous hemodialysis. *Trans ASAIO* 1960;6:88.
3. Weisse AB. Turning bad luck into good: the alchemy of Willem Johan Kolff. *Semin Dial* 1993;6:52.
4. Scribner BH. A personalized history of chronic hemodialysis. *Am J Kidney Dis* 1990;16:511.
5. Drukker W. Hemodialysis: a historical review. In: Maher JF, ed. *Replacement of renal function by dialysis.* Dordrecht:Kluwer Academic, 1989:20.
6. United States Renal Data System, USRDS 1999 Annual Data Report, National Institutes of Health, National Institute of Diabetes and Digestive and Kidney Diseases, Bethesda, MD, 1999.
7. Nissenson AR, Prichard SS, Ignatius KP, et al. Non-medical factors that impact on ESRD treatment modality selection. *Kidney Int* 1993; 43:120.
8. Blagg CR. Home hemodialysis: a view from Seattle. *Nephrol News Issues* 1995;6:33.
9. Blagg CR. Home hemodialysis. *Semin Dial* 1994;7:293.
10. Buoncristiani U, et al. Rationale for daily dialysis. *Home Hemodial Int* 1995;1:21.
11. Pierratos R, et al. Two year experience with slow nocturnal hemodialysis (SNHD). *J Am Soc Nephrol* 1996;7:1417.
12. Capelli JP, Camiscioli TC, Vallorani RD, et al. Comparative analysis of survival on home hemodialysis, in-center hemodialysis and chronic peritoneal dialysis (CAPD-IPD) therapies. *Dial Transplant* 1985;14:38.
13. Delano BG, Lundin AP, Held PJ, et al. Imminent extinction of home hemodialysis. *JASN* 1991;2:320A.
14. Tokars JI, Alter MJ, Favero MS, et al. National surveillance of dialysis associated diseases in the United States, 1991. *Am Soc Artif Int Org J* 1993;39:966.
15. Keshaviah P. High efficiency hemodialysis. *Contrib Nephrol* 1989; 69:109.
16. Powers KM, et al. Improved urea reduction ratio and Kt/v in large hemodialysis patients using two dialyzers in parallel. *Am J Kidney Dis* 2000;35:266.
17. Hakim RM, Depner TA, Parker TF. Adequacy of hemodialysis. *Am J Kidney Dis* 1992;20:107.
18. Wolf RV, Remp DG, Kiley JE, et al. Artificial kidney function: kinetics of hemodialysis. *J Clin Invest* 1951;30:1062.
19. Babb AL, Popovich AP, Christopher TG, et al. The genesis of the square meter per hour hypothesis. *Trans ASAIO* 1971;17:81.
20. Babb AL, Strand MJ, Uvelli DA, et al. Quantitative description of dialysis treatment: a dialysis index. *Kidney Int* 1975;7:23.
21. Ahmad S, Babb AL, Multinovic J, et al. Effect of residual renal function on minimum dialysis requirements. *Proc Eur Dial Transplant Assoc* 1979;16:107.
22. Multinovic J, Babb AI, Eschbach JW, et al. Uremic neuropathy: evidence of middle molecule toxicity. *Artif Organs* 1978;2:45.
23. Multinovic J, Strand M, Casaretto A, et al. Clinical impact of residual glomerular filtration rate on dialysis time—a preliminary report. *Trans ASAIO* 1974;20:410.
24. Popovich RP, Moncrief JW. The prediction of metabolite accumulation concomitant with renal insufficiency: the middle molecule anomaly. *Trans ASAIO* 1974;20A:377.
25. Teschan PE, Ginn HE, Bourne JR, et al. Neurobehavioural probes for adequacy of dialysis. *Trans ASAIO* 1977;23:556.
26. Ginn HE, Teschan PE, Bourne JR, et al. Neurobehavioural and clinical responses to hemodialysis. *Trans ASAIO* 1978;24:376.
27. Lowrie EG, Laird NM, Parker TF, et al. Effect of the hemodialysis prescription on patient morbidity. Report from the National Cooperative Dialysis Study. *N Engl J Med* 1981;305:1176.
28. Gotch, FA, Sargent JA. A mechanistic analysis of the National Cooperative Dialysis Study (NCDS). *Kidney Int* 1985;28:526.
29. Sargent JA, Gotch FA. The analysis of concentration dependence of uremic lesions in clinical studies. *Kidney Int* 1975;7:35.
30. Held PJ, Levin NW, Bovberg RR, et al. Mortality and duration of hemodialysis treatment. *J Am Med Assoc* 1994;285:871.

31. Wizeman V, Kramer W. Short term dialyses, long term complications: ten years experience with short duration renal replacement therapy. *Blood Purif* 1987;5:193.

32. Zhensheng L, et al. Comparing urea reduction ratio and the urea product as outcome-based measures of hemodialysis dose. *Am J Kidney Dis* 2000;35:598.

33. Depner TA. Standards for dialysis adequacy. *Semin Dial* 1991;4:245.

34. Lindsay RM, Spanner E. A hypothesis. The protein catabolic rate is dependent upon the type and amount of treatment in dialyzed uremic patients. *Am J Kidney Dis* 1989;13:382.

35. Depner TA. *Prescribing hemodialysis: a guide to urea modeling.* Boston: Kluwer Academic, 1991.

36. Hakim R, Breyer J, Ismail N, et al. Effects of dose of dialysis on morbidity and mortality. *Am J Kidney Dis* 1994;23:661.

37. Hakim R, Lawrence P, Schulman G, et al. Increasing dose of dialysis improves mortality and nutritional parameters in hemodialysis patients. *J Am Soc Nephrol* 1992;3:367A.

38. Charra B, Calemard E, Ruffet M, et al. Survival as an index of adequacy of dialysis. *Kidney Int* 1992;41:1286.

39. Ahmad S, Cole JJ. Lower morbidity associated with higher Kt/V in stable hemodialysis patients. *J Am Soc Nephrol* 1990;1:346A.

40. Shen F-H, Hsu K-T. Lower mortality and morbidity associated with higher Kt/V in hemodialysis patients. *J Am Soc Nephrol* 1990;1:377A.

41. Collins A, Ilstrup K, Hanson G, et al. Rapid, high efficiency dialysis. *Artif Organs* 1986;10:185.

42. Ellis P, Malchesky P, Lankhorst B, et al. Evaluation of elevated blood urea nitrogen using direct dialysis quantification. *Co-Renal Nutrit* 1982;6:20.

43. Ellis PW, Malchesky PS, Magnusson MO, et al. Comparison of two methods of kinetic modeling. *Trans ASAIO* 1984;30:60.

44. Depner TA. Pitfalls in quantitating hemodialysis. *Semin Dial* 1993; 6:127.

45. Jindal KK, Manuel A, Goldstein MB. Percent reduction in blood urea concentration during hemodialysis (PRU): a simple and accurate method to estimate Kt/V urea. *Trans ASAIO* 1987;33:286.

46. Lowrie EG, Lew NL. The urea reduction ratio (URR): a simple method for evaluating hemodialysis treatment. *Contemp Dial Nephrol* 1991;12:11.

47. Keane WF, Collins AJ. Influence of comorbidity on mortality and morbidity in patients treated with hemodialysis. *Am J Kidney Dis* 1994;24:1010.

48. Evans RW, Rader B, Manninen DL, et al. The quality of life of hemodialysis recipients treated with recombinant human erythropoietin. *J Am Med Assoc* 1990;263:825.

49. Held PJ, Brunner FP, Odaka M, et al. Five year survival for end-stage renal disease patients in the United States, Europe and Japan, 1982–1987. *Am J Kidney Dis* 1990;15:451.

50. Held PJ, Blagg CR, Liska DW, et al. Adequacy of hemodialysis according to dialysis prescription in Europe and the United States. *Kidney Int* 1992;42:16.

51. Hull AR, Parker TF. Proceedings from the morbidity, mortality and prescription of dialysis symposium, Dallas, Texas, Sept 15–17,1989. *Am J Kidney Dis* 1990;15:375.

52. Schneditz D, Polaschegg HD, Levin NW, et al. Cardiopulmonary recirculation in dialysis: an underrecognized phenomenon. *ASAIO J* 1992;38:M194.

53. Sherman RA. The measurement of dialysis access recirculation. *Am J Kidney Dis* 1993;22:616.

54. Haire HM, Sherrard DJ, Scardapane D, et al. Smoking, hypertension and mortality in a maintenance dialysis population. *Cardiovasc Med* 1978;3:1163.

55. Lundin AP, Adler A, Feinroth MV, et al. Maintenance hemodialysis: survival beyond the first decade. *J Am Med Assoc* 1980;244:38.

56. Battistella P, de Cornelissen F, de Gaudemaris R, et al. Ambulatory blood pressure profiled during 48 hours in patients treated with chronic hemodialysis. *Arch Mal Coeur* 1990;83:1223.

57. Kramer BK, Ress KM, Ulshofer TM, et al. Hemodynamic and hormonal effects of low or high sodium dialysis. *Kidney Int* 1988; 34:192.

58. Zuccala A, Santoro A, Ferrari G, et al. Pathogenesis of hypertension in hemodialysis patients: a pharmacologic study. *Kidney Int* 1988;34:190.

59. Martins-Prat M, Teixera deSousa F, Barbas J, et al. Arterial hypertension in patients with chronic kidney insufficiency in hemodialysis with erythropoietin. *Rev Port Cardiol* 1990;9:119.

60. Lindner A, Farewell VT, Sherrard DJ. Accelerated atherosclerosis in prolonged maintenance hemodialysis. *N Engl J Med* 1981;290:697.

61. Churchill DN, Taylor DW, Cook RJ, et al. Canadian Hemodialysis Morbidity Study. *Am J Kidney Dis* 1992;19:214.

62. Parfrey PS, Harnett JD, Griffiths SM, et al. Congestive heart failure in dialysis patients. *Arch Int Med* 1992;148:1519.

63. Parfrey PS, Harnett JD, eds. *Cardiac dysfunction in chronic uremia.* Boston: Kluwer Academic, 1992.

64. Hemmendinger S, Neumann MR, Beretz A, et al. Mitogenic activity on human arterial smooth muscle cells in increased in the plasma of patients undergoing hemodialysis with cuprophane membranes. *Nephron* 1989;53:147.

65. Vincenti F, Amend WJ, Abele J, et al. The role of hypertension in hemodialysis-associated atherosclerosis. *Am J Med* 1980;68:363.

66. Goodman WG, et al. Coronary artery calcification in young adults with end-stage renal disease who are undergoing dialysis. *N Engl J Med* 2000;342:1478.

67. Block GA, et al. Re-evaluation of risks associated with hyperphosphatemia and hyperparathyroidism in dialysis patients: recommendations for a change in management. *Am J Kidney Dis* 2000;35:1226.

68. Rostand SG, Rutsky EA. Pericarditis in end stage renal disease. *Cardiol Clin* 1990;8:701.

69. Mitch WE, May RC, Maroni BJ, et al. Protein and amino acid metabolism in uremia: influence of metabolic acidosis. *Kidney Int* 1989;27:205.

70. Schulman D. How important is the problem of malnutrition in chronic dialysis patients? *Semin Dial* 1992;5:263.

71. Lowrie EG, Lew NL. Death risk in hemodialysis patients: the predictive value of commonly measured variables and evaluation of death rate differences between facilities. *Am J Kidney Dis* 1990;15:458.

72. Lindsay RM, Spanner E, Heidenheim RP, et al. Which comes first Kt/V or PCR—chicken or egg? *Kidney Int* 1992;38:S32.

73. Golgstein D, Strom J. Intradialytic parenteral nutrition: evolution and current concepts. *J Renal Nutr* 1991;1:9.

74. Schulman G, Wingard RL, Hutchinson R, et al. The influence of recombinant human growth hormone and intradialytic parenteral nutrition on malnutrition parameters of hemodialysis patients. *J Am Soc Nephrol* 1990;1:376A.

75. Carlson DM, Duncan DA, Naessens JM, et al. Hospitalization in dialysis patients. *Mayo Clin Proc* 1984;59:769.

76. Palder SB, Kirkman RL, Whittemore AD. Vascular access for hemodialysis. Patency rates and results of revision. *Ann Surg* 1985; 202:235.

77. Rekhter M, Nicholls S, Ferguson M, et al. Cell proliferation in human arteriovenous fistulas used for hemodialysis. *Arterioscler Thromb* 1993;13:609.

78. Swedberg SH, Brown BG, Sigley R, et al. Intimal fibromuscular hyperplasia at the venous anastomosis of PTFE grafts in hemodialysis patients: clinical, immunohistochemical, light and electron microscopic assessment. *Circulation* 1989;80:1726.

79. Schuman E, Quinn S, Blayne S, et al. Thrombolysis versus thrombectomy for occluded hemodialysis grafts. *Am J Surg* 1994;167:473.

80. Didlake R, Curry E, Bower J, et al. Composite dialysis access grafts. *J Am Coll Surg* 1994;178:24.

81. Butt KMH, Friedman EA, Kountz SL. Angioaccess. *Curr Probl Surg* 1976;12:9.

82. Tzamaloukas AH, Murata GH, Harford AM, et al. Hand gangrene in diabetic patients on chronic dialysis. *Trans ASAIO* 1991;37:638.

83. Riggs JE, Moss AH, Labosky DA, et al. Upper extremity ischemic monomelic neuropathy: a complication of vascular access procedures in uremic diabetic patients. *Neurology* 1989;39:997.

84. National Kidney Foundation-Dialysis Outcomes Quality Initiative (NKF-DOQI) Clinical Practice Guidelines for the treatment of anemia of chronic renal failure. *Am J Kidney Dis* 1997;30:S192.

85. Besarab A, Bolton WK, Browne JK, et al. The effects of normal as compared with low hematocrit values in patients with cardiac disease who are receiving hemodialysis and epoetin. *N Engl J Med* 1998;339:584.

86. Miles AM. Erythropoietin and iron therapy in patients with renal failure. In: Goodnough, LT. *Transfusion medicine and alternatives to blood transfusion.* Paris: R and J Editions Medicales, 2000:268.

87. Janson PA. Treatment of the bleeding tendency in uremia with cryoprecipitate. *N Engl J Med* 1980;303:1318.

88. Manucci PM, et al. Desamino-8-arginine vasopressin shortens the bleeding time in uremia. *N Engl J Med* 1983;308:8.

89. Livio M. Conjugated estrogens for management of bleeding associated with renal failure. *N Engl J Med* 1986;315:731.

90. Goldman M, Vanherweghem JL. Bacterial infections in chronic hemodialysis patients: epidemiologic and pathophysiologic aspects. *Adv Nephrol* 1990;19:315.

91. Kaul H, et al. Initiation of hemodialysis treatment leads to improvement of T-cell activation in patients with end stage renal disease. *Am J Kidney Dis* 2000;35:611.

92. Sherrard DJ. Control of renal bone disease. *Semin Dial* 1994;7:284.

93. Slatopoulsky E, Weerts C, Thielen J, et al. Marked suppression of secondary hyperparathyroidism by intravenous administration of 1,2 dihydroxycholecalciferol in uremic patients. *J Clin Invest* 1984;74:2136.

94. Sherrard DJ, Hercz G, Pei Y, et al. The spectrum of bone disease in end-stage renal failure: an evolving disorder. *Kidney Int* 1993;43:436.

95. Salusky IB, Foley J, Nelson P, et al. Aluminum accumulation during treatment with aluminum hydroxide and dialysis in children and young adults with chronic renal disease. *N Engl J Med* 1991;324:527.

96. Andress DL, Kopp JB, Maloney NA, et al. Early deposition of aluminum in bone in diabetic patients on hemodialysis. *N Engl J Med* 1987;316:292.

97. Slanina P, Frech W, Ekstrom L-G, et al. Dietary citric acid enhances absorption of aluminum in antacids. *Clin Chem* 1986;32:539.

98. Ittel TH, Griessner A, Sieberth HG. Effect of lactate on the absorption and retention of aluminum in the remnant kidney rat model. *Nephron* 1991;57:332.

99. Russo LS, Beale G, Sandroni S, et al. Aluminum intoxication in undialyzed adults with chronic renal failure. *J Neurol Neurosurg Psychiatry* 1992;55:697.

100. Main J, Ward MK. Potentiation of aluminum absorption by effervescent analgesic tablets in a hemodialysis patient. *Br Med J* 1992;304:1686.

101. Felsenfeld AJ, Harrelson JM, Gutman RA, et al. Osteomalacia after parathyroidectomy in patients with uremia. *Ann Int Med* 1982;96:34.

102. Andress DL, Norris KC, Coburn JW, et al. Intravenous calcitriol in refractory osteitis fibrosa of chronic renal failure. *N Engl J Med* 1989; 321:274.

103. Alfrey AC, Mishell JM, Burks J, et al. Syndrome of dyspraxia and multifocal seizures associated with chronic hemodialysis. *Trans ASAIO* 1972;18:251.

104. Windus DW, Stokes TJ, Julian BA, et al. Fatal rhizopus infections in hemodialysis patients receiving desferoxamine. *Ann Int Med* 1987; 107:678.

105. Segal R, Zoller KA, Sherrard DJ, et al. Mucormycosis: a life threatening infection in long term hemodialysis patients. *Kidney Int* 1988;33:238A.

106. Gallant T, Freedman MH, Vellend H, et al. Yersinia sepsis in patients with iron overload treated with DFO. *N Engl J Med* 1986;314:1643.

107. Assenat H, Calemard E, Charra B, et al. Syndrome du canal carpien et substance amyloide. *Nouv Press Med* 1980;24:1715.

108. Gorevic PD, Munoz PC, Casey TT, et al. Polymerization of intact beta₂-microglobulin in tissues causing amyloidosis in patients on chronic hemodialysis. *Proc Natl Acad Sci USA* 1986;83:7908.

109. Zingraff J, Noel LH, Bardin T, et al. Beta 2 microglobulin amyloidosis as a complication of chronic renal failure: a biopsy proven case. *N Engl J Med* 1990;323:1070.

110. Van Ypersele de Strihou C, Honhon B, Vandenbroucke Jm, et al. Dialysis amyloidosis. *Adv Nephrol* 1988;17:401.

111. Campistol JM, Skinner M. Beta 2 microglobulin amyloidosis—an overview. *Semin Dial* 1993;6:117.

112. Zaoui PM, Stone WJ, Hakim RM. Effects of dialysis membranes on beta₂ microglobulin production and cellular expression. *Kidney Int* 1990;38:962.

113. Goldstein S, Winston E, Chung TJ, et al. Chronic arthropathy in long-term hemodialysis. *Am J Med* 1985;78:82.

114. Cuffe MJ, Hadley MN, Herrera GA, et al. Dialysis-associated spondyloarthropathy. *J Neurosurg* 1994;80:694.

115. Linke RP, Bommer J, Ritz E, et al. Amyloid kidney stones of uremic patients consist of beta-2 microglobulin fragments. *Biochem Biophys Res Commun* 1986;136:665.

116. Okutsu I, Ninomiya S, Takatori Y, et al. Endoscopic management of shoulder pain in long term hemodialysis patients. *Nephrol Dial Transplant* 1990;6:117.

117. Canzanello VJ, Hylander-Rossner B, Sands RE, et al. Comparison of 50% dextrose water, 25% mannitol, and 23.5% saline for treatment of hemodialysis-associated muscle cramps. *ASAIO Trans* 1991;37: 649.

118. Kaji DM, Ackad A, Noltage WE, et al. Prevention of muscle cramps in hemodialysis patients by quinine sulfate. *Lancet* 1967;2:66.

119. Ahmad S. Multicenter trial of L-carnitine in maintenance hemodialysis patients. II. Clinical and biochemical effects. *Kidney Int* 1990;38:912.

120. Roca AO, Jarjoura D, Blend D, et al. Dialysis leg cramps: efficacy of quinine versus vitamin E. *ASAIO J* 1990;38:M481.

121. Friedman EA, Lundin AP. Environmental and iatrogenic obstacles to long life on hemodialysis. *N Engl J Med* 1982;306:167.

122. Hoy RH. Accidental systemic exposure to sodium hypochlorite (chlorox) during hemodialysis. *Am J Hosp Pharmacol* 1981;38:1512.

123. *Investigation of the risks and hazards associated with hemodialysis devices.* An FDA medical device standards publication, technical report. Washington, DC: Government Printing Office, 1980.

124. National Kidney Foundation revised standards for reuse of hemodialyzers. *Am J Kidney Dis* 1984;3:466.

125. Deller AG. Electrical safety in dialysis. *J Med Eng Technol* 1979; 3:186.

126. Nielsen VK. The peripheral nerve function in chronic renal failure. VI. The relationship between sensory and motor nerve conduction and kidney function, azotemia, age, sex and clinical neuropathy. *Acta Med Scand* 1973;94:455.

127. Nielsen VK. The peripheral nerve function in chronic renal failure. V. Sensory and motor conduction velocity. *Acta Med Scand* 1973; 194:445.

128. Bolton CF, Young GB. *Neurological complications of renal disease.* Boston: Butterworths, 1990.

129. Ackil AA, Shahani BT, Young RR. Sural nerve conduction studies and late responses in children undergoing hemodialysis. *Arch Phys Med Rehab* 1981;62:487.

130. Cadilhac J, Mion CH, Duday J, et al. Motor nerve conduction velocities as an index of the efficiency of maintenance dialysis in patients with end-stage renal failure. In: Canal N, Pozz G, eds. *Peripheral neuropathies.* New York: Elsevier/North-Holland, 1978:372.

131. Knoll O, Dierker E. Detection of uremic neuropathy by reflex response latency. *J Neurol Sci* 1980;47:305.

132. Ahmad S, Babb AL, Multinovic J et al. Effect of residual renal function on minimum dialysis requirements. *Proc Eur Dial Transplant Assoc* 1979;16:107.

133. Grantham JJ. Polycystic kidney disease: a predominance of giant nephrons. *Am J Physiol* 1983;244:F3.

134. Ishikawa I, Yuri T, Kitada H, et al. Regression of acquired cystic disease of the kidneys after successful renal transplantation. *Am J Nephrol* 1983;3:310.

135. Ishikawa I, Onouchi Z, Saito Y, et al. Sex differences in acquired cystic disease of the kidney on long-term dialysis. *Nephron* 1985;39:336.

136. Dunnill MS, Millard PR, Oliver D. Acquired cystic disease of the kidneys: a hazard of long-term intermittent maintenance hemodialysis. *J Clin Pathol* 1977;30:868.

137. Mickisch O, Bommer J, Bachmann S, et al. Multicystic transformation of kidneys in chronic renal failure. *Nephron* 1984;38:93.

138. Ishikawa I, Horiguchi T, Shikura N. Lectin peroxidase conjugate reactivity in acquired cystic disease of the kidney. *Nephron* 1989;51:211.

139. Gardner KD. Acquired renal cystic disease and renal adenocarcinoma in patients on long-term hemodialysis. *N Engl J Med* 1984;310:390.

140. Marple JT, MacDougall M. Development of malignancy in end-stage renal disease patient. *Sem Nephrol* 1993;13:306.

141. Oe PL, Tan KH, Donner R, et al. Development of renal carcinoma in a patient with polycystic kidneys undergoing chronic hemodialysis. *Eur Urol* 1980;6:316.

142. Herr HW, Engen DE, Hostetler J. Malignancy in uremia: dialysis versus transplantation. *J Urol* 1979;121:584.

143. Ota K, Yamashita N, Suzuki T, et al. Malignant tumors in dialysis patients: a nationwide survey. *Proc Eur Dial Transplant Assoc* 1981;18:724.

144. Port FK, Racheb NE, Schwartz AG, et al. Neoplasms in dialysis patients: a population based study. *Am J Kidney Dis* 1989;14:119.

145. DeSala O'Shea E, Morey Molina A, Ferrutxe Frau J, et al. Cancer of the bladder and hemodialysis. *Arch Esp Urol* 1990;43:359.

146. Kantor A, Hoover RN, Kinlen LJ, et al. Cancer in patients receiving long term dialysis. *Am J Epidemiol* 1987;126:370.

147. Bush A, Gabriel R. Cancer in uremic patients. *Clin Nephrol* 1984; 22:77.

148. Friedman EA, Thomson GE. Hepatitis complicating chronic hemodialysis. *Lancet* 1966;2:675.

149. Marmion BP, Burrell CJ, Tonkin RW, et al. Dialysis-associated hepatitis in Edinburgh; 1969–1978. *Rev Infect Dis* 1982;4:619.
150. Horak W, Leithner C, Kemenesi W, et al. Efficacy and tolerance of hepatitis B vaccination in medical personnel and hemodialysis patients. *Wien Klin Wochenschr* 1984;96:161.
151. Parfrey PS, Paradinas FJ, O'Driscoll JB, et al. Chronic liver disease in hemodialysis patients. *Proc Eur Dial Transplant Assoc* 1982;19:153.
152. Alter MJ, Favero MS. National surveillance of dialysis-associated diseases in the United States, 1989. *ASAIO Trans* 1991;37:97.
153. Tokars J, Alter M, Favero MS, et al. National surveillance of dialysis-associated diseases in the United States, 1992. *ASAIO J* 1994;40:1020.
154. Hardy NM, Sandroni S, Danielson S, et al. Antibody to hepatitis C virus increases with time on hemodialysis. *Clin Nephrol* 1992;38:44.
155. Kuhns M, De Medina M, McNamara A, et al. Detection of hepatitis C virus RNA in hemodialysis patients. *J Am Soc Nephrol* 1994;4:1491.
156. Van der Poel, Cuypers HTM, Reesink HW, et al. Confirmation of hepatitis C virus infection by new four-antigen recombinant immunoblot assay. *Lancet* 1991;337:317.
157. Garson JA, Tedder RS, Briggs M, et al. Detection of hepatitis C viral sequences in blood donations by "nested" polymerase chain reaction and prediction of infectivity. *Lancet* 1990;335:1419.
158. Parfrey PS, Forbes RD, Hutchinson TA, et al. The clinical and pathological course of hepatitis B disease in renal transplant recipients. *Transplantation* 1984;37:461.
159. Marchesini G, Zoli M, Angiolini A, et al. Relevance of HBe/anti-HBe system and DNA polymerase activity in chronic hepatitis-B virus carriers on hemodialysis. A prospective study. *Nephron* 1981;29:44.
160. Harnett JD, Parfrey PS, Kennedy M, et al. The long-term outcome of hepatitis B infection in hemodialysis patients. *Am J Kidney Dis* 1988;11:210.
161. Toussaint C, Dupont E, Vanherweghem JL, et al. Liver disease in patients undergoing hemodialysis and kidney transplantation. *Adv Nephrol* 1979;8:269.
162. Lundin AP, Adler AJ, Berlyne GM, et al. Tuberculosis in patients undergoing maintenance hemodialysis. *Am J Med* 1979;67:597.
163. Gluck Z, Nolph KD. Ascites associated with end-stage renal disease. *Am J Kidney Dis* 1987;10:9.
164. Popli A, Daugirdas JT, Ing TS. Dialysis ascites. *Int J Artif Organs* 1974;3:257.
165. Pascual JF, Melendez MT, Rivera-Viera JF. Local steroid therapy of refractory ascites associated with dialysis. *J Pediatr* 1979;94:319.
166. Bochler T, Dudley DA. Nephrogenous ascites. *Am J Gastroenterol* 1982;77:73.
167. Morgan AG, Sivapragasam S, Fletcher P, et al. Hemodynamic improvement after peritoneovenous shunting in nephrogenic ascites. *South Med J* 1982;75:373.
168. Bennett RR, Moore J Jr. Dialysis-induced ascites treated with peritoneal dialysis. *South Med J* 1987;80:379.
169. Ing TS, Daugirdas JT, Popli S, et al. Treatment of refractory hemodialysis ascites with maintenance peritoneal dialysis. *Clin Nephrol* 1981;15:198.
170. Holdsworth SR, de-Kretser DM, Atkins RC. A comparison of hemodialysis and transplantation in reversing the uremic disturbance of male reproductive function. *Clin Nephrol* 1978;10:146.
171. Procci WR. The study of sexual dysfunction in uremic males. Problems for patients and investigators. *Clin Exp Dial Apheresis* 1983;7:289.
172. Mahajan SK, Abbrasi AA, Prasad AS, et al. Effect of oral zinc therapy on gonadal function in hemodialysis patients. A double-blind study. *Ann Intern Med* 1982;97:357.
173. Rodger RS, Brook AC, Muirhead N, et al. Zinc metabolism does not influence sexual function in chronic renal insufficiency. *Contrib Nephrol* 1984;38:112.
174. Multinovic J, Strand M, Casaretto A, et al. Clinical impact of residual glomerular filtration rate (GFR) on dialysis time—a preliminary report. *Trans Am Soc Artif Intern Organs* 1974;20:410.
175. Hayslett JP. Interaction of renal disease and pregnancy. *Kidney Int* 1984;25:579.
176. Kobaykashi H, Maztsumoto Y, Otsubo O, et al. Successful pregnancy in a patient undergoing chronic dialysis. *Obstet Gynecol* 1981;57:382.
177. Registration Committee of the EDTA. Successful pregnancies in women treated by dialysis and kidney transplantation. *Br J Obstet Gynecol* 1980;87:839.
178. Ginsburg ES, Owen WF. Reproductive endocrinology and pregnancy in women on hemodialysis. *Semin Dial* 1993;6:105.
179. Schaefer RM, Kokot F, Wernze H, et al. Improved sexual function in hemodialysis patients on erythropoietin: a possible role for prolactin. *Clin Nephrol* 1989;31:1.
180. Stewart RS. Psychiatric issues in renal dialysis and transplantation. *Hosp Community Psychiatry* 1983;34:623.
181. Haenel T, Brunner F, Battegay R. Renal dialysis and suicide: occurrence in Switzerland and in Europe. *Compr Psychiatry* 1980;21:140.
182. Levy NB. Psychological problems of the patient on hemodialysis and their treatment. *Psychother Psychosom* 1979;31:260.
183. Neu S, Kjellstrand CM. Stopping long-term dialysis. An empirical study of withdrawal of life-supporting treatment. *N Engl J Med* 1986;314:14.
184. Roberts JC, Kjellstrand CM. Choosing death. Withdrawal from chronic dialysis without medical reason. *Acta Med Scand* 1988;233:181.
185. Cohen LM, McGue JD, Germain M, et al. Dialysis discontinuation. A good death. *Arch Intern Med* 1995;155:42.

CHAPTER 100

Ethical and Legal Considerations in End-Stage Renal Disease

Nancy B. Cummings

End-stage renal disease (ESRD) treatments have focused attention on biomedical ethical issues since the treatment modalities of dialysis and renal transplantation became actual modalities for patient care in the final four decades of the 20th century. The remarkable developments in genetics, molecular biology, and biomedical technology at the advent of the 21st century have increased the number of potential therapies, but this has been accompanied by diverse ethical dilemmas.

The quandary posed by the allocation of scarce resources for chronic renal failure raised a series of troubling issues for the medical profession in the 1960s. The treatment modalities of chronic hemodialysis and kidney transplantation had become available, but their overwhelming cost and the limited availability of donor kidneys put these treatments out of reach for most patients. The ethical dilemmas posed for patients with ESRD captured the attention of philosophers and theologians, as well as of medical professionals, and were a major factor in the development of the nascent field of biomedical ethics.

The selection of patients for chronic hemodialysis against the background of limited financial means, and issues surrounding the use of living related kidney donors, raised thorny ethical and moral dilemmas. There also were difficult moral issues when it became necessary to decide which patients would be selected to receive cadaver kidneys, always in limited supply.

The passage in 1972 of the amendment to the Social Security Act, Public Law (PL) 92-603, which called for the Medicare program through the Social Security system to pay for 80% of the health care costs of chronic renal failure for all entitled patients, eased some of the financial and allocation problems. However, new dilemmas arose: decisions about whom to treat, when to start treatment, and when to

discontinue treatment; the distribution of cadaver kidneys in the midst of scarcity; possible new sources for harvesting kidneys such as from the elderly and kidneys with slightly diminished function; the use of advance directives for health care; and the economic burden of high-technology treatments—of which dialysis and transplantation are prototypic.

Burgeoning health care costs in the United States capture newspaper headlines almost daily. The budgets of local, state, and federal governments are sorely stressed in their efforts to meet their many obligations, of which provision of health care is one of the weightiest. The inordinate escalation of health care costs, many of which are for "high technologies," not only has challenged health care providers, but government, business, industry, professional associations, voluntary health associations, and a spectrum of academic disciplines such as political science, economics, and health policy. All of these groups are trying to find solutions to the problem of providing affordable health care for the entire U.S. population. The magnitude of the fiscal situation underscores the scope of this challenge. The United States spent $204 billion (1989 dollars) on health care in 1970, and increased its spending on health care to $604 billion, or 9.2% of the country's gross domestic product (GDP), in 1980, and costs are projected to reach 16.2% ($2.2 trillion) of GDP by 2008 (1) by the Office of the Actuary, Health Care Financing Administration (HCFA). For comparison, in 1989 Canada spent 8.8%, West Germany, 8.1%, Japan, 6.8%, and the United Kingdom, 6.1%, according to the U.S. Congressional Budget Office (CBO) (2).

Public concern about issues often is reflected in what politicians are willing to address publicly and what is acceptable politically. Concerns over life-sustaining technologies (LSTs) in general and dialysis and transplantation specifically have been evident both in requests for studies and in legislation. In 1984, the U.S. Congress requested an Office of Technology Assessment (OTA) study, *Life-Sustaining Technologies and the Elderly* (3), which included dialysis; and in 1987, the Congress asked for an Institute of Medicine (IOM)

N. B. Cummings: Division of Nutrition Research Coordination, National Institute of Diabetes and Digestive and Kidney Diseases at the National Institutes of Health, Bethesda, Maryland; Center for Clinical Bioethics, Georgetown, University School of Medicine, Washington DC

study, *Kidney Failure and the Federal Government* (4). The fact that the U.S. Congress requested these studies is evidence that there is political concern about both the costs and the appropriate utilization of these expensive modalities of life-prolonging health care because senators and congressmen are not apt to deviate far from the interests of the electorate.

Because ESRD is the only catastrophic illness for which the federal government provides almost universal coverage, its costs are documented and more prominently highlighted than are those of other chronic, catastrophic illnesses. Medicare expenditures for the ESRD program were $7.7 billion (5) in 1993 and $12.3 billion in 1998 (Parts A and B, Medicare), approximately 89% of the costs of ESRD care (6). For comparative purposes, selected 2000 "personal consumption expenditures" (7) are presented: alcohol consumed "off premise" (not consumed in public establishments)—$6.9 billion; tobacco (for personal use)—$6.6 billion; casino gambling—$25.6 billion; and potato chips and similar products—$9,491 million (1991), projected for 2000—$12,359 million (8).

What are the significant ethical issues for clinical nephrologists (9)? Six leading issues have been salient for several decades; with advances in molecular biology/genetics, and the identification of the autosomal-dominant adult polycystic kidney disease (APKD) gene, a seventh issue needs to be addressed; and two more issues have arisen more recently: Access to renal transplantation has added one of the latter (10,11).

1. Questions surround the *allocation of resources,* scarce either because of limited funding or because of the absolute scarcity of a resource, such as kidneys for transplantation. These issues have troubled nephrologists since the advent of chronic hemodialysis and of immunosuppressive therapies, which made kidney transplantation a reality for most patients with chronic renal failure. Steps taken to increase recruitment of donor kidneys raise new issues: elderly donors or patients; transplantation of two kidneys; xenotransplantation; and the potential of cloning or assisted reproduction technology techniques such as *in vitro* fertilization to provide solid organs.
2. ESRD treatment is a prototype for the whole range of *LSTs,* all of which raise very difficult questions about the initiation, withholding, and withdrawal of dialysis (termination of care).
3. The *selection of the appropriate treatment* for patients with chronic renal failure, including the decision not to treat, was a uniquely difficult issue during the 1960s before the passage of PL 92-603 by the U.S. Congress in 1972. This law allowed physicians to select the proper treatment modality for patients: living related or cadaveric donor transplantation, peritoneal dialysis, or hemodialysis. For the latter two forms of treatment, it also allowed the physician to select the location of the treatment, either in-center or at home.

4. Under Medicare, 92% to 95% of patients with ESRD in the United States are eligible to be treated. Thus, as Belding Scribner pointed out, the prime sociomedical issue for chronic dialysis in the 1980s and 1990s is *"negative selection"*—deciding not to treat some patients definitively because they could not benefit from treatment (12).
5. *Patients' right of autonomy* to participate in their own health care decisions is recognized. The fact that this sometimes is in conflict with carefully considered recommendations of patients' physicians and of other health professionals has been troubling, especially when the patient elects to forego or terminate treatment.
6. Problems surround the issue of *dealing with "noncompliant" patients,* whose behavior not only jeopardizes their own health but frequently interferes with the health care team's ability to treat other patients in the dialysis unit.
7. Progress in molecular biology has led to improved understanding and technology concerning the genetics of renal disease. Already with identification of the APKD gene, nephrologists must be knowledgeable and experienced in prenatal diagnosis and gene therapy. However, the ethical dilemmas of privacy and confidentiality (13), as well as of testing minors and their right to know or not to know the diagnosis of a disease when there is no treatment, loom large for all genetic diagnoses. Presymptomatic APKD and Huntington's disease are two examples of genetic disease, knowledge of which may be threatening when there is no means for prevention or treatment.
8. *Patients whose behavior deviates from societal norms* raise especially troubling issues, particularly for those groups in society who try to change the behavior of others. Examples of such patients are homosexuals and those who use intravenous or injection drugs with resultant high rates of human immunodeficiency virus (HIV) infection. Should it become necessary to limit the availability of ESRD treatment, major ethical concerns will arise if some Americans advocate limiting the availability of treatment of patients with "lifestyle"-associated diseases.
9. *Disparities in access to renal transplantation* occur in the elderly, and in racial and ethnic groups compared with access for whites. Efforts to improve access to renal transplantation and conduct research into the reasons for the differential availability of renal transplantation for these underserved groups have been undertaken recently (10).

Ethical dilemmas related to ESRD thus cover a broad range of issues—from those of economics and macroallocation to those involved with individual physician–patient relationships and "bedside microallocation." Ethical issues include the costs of health care, the allocation of scarce resources, health disparities, the dilemmas surrounding starting and stopping life-sustaining treatment, and related quality-of-life issues, as well as those arising from advances in molecular biology.

ALLOCATION OF SCARCE RESOURCES

To understand how limited resources can be allocated fairly, as well as to understand the dilemma that presents itself when there are insufficient resources, it is helpful to consider two matters: (a) the American experience before the ESRD amendment to the Social Security Act passed, and (b) the distribution of health resources throughout the world. The first is well known to most nephrologists. It is dramatically evident when one looks at the problems the Seattle Admissions and Policy Committee faced in the early days of chronic hemodialysis. Heart-rending, difficult decisions had to be made about which patients would be treated because resources and funds were severely limited (14). After medical recommendations were made that chronic dialysis was indicated, patients to be considered were evaluated by this "faceless" Seattle committee, frequently known as the "God Committee." The committee reviewed patients' social and economic "worth," with weight given to factors such as income, number of children to be supported, use of alcohol or drugs, and contribution to the community and other similar considerations. At the time of the 25th anniversary meetings on chronic dialysis held in Seattle in April 1985, some of the members of the committee expressed their severe discomfort with the role they had to play in these life-and-death decisions. The committee members did not like to make these decisions about who should live and who should die, and they felt that deciding about access to treatment according to social worth was unjust.

Until the passage of the ESRD amendment (Section 2991) to PL 92-603, provision of ESRD treatment was restricted to those with sufficient personal funds or adequate private insurance coverage, or to those patients selected for the relatively limited number of clinical studies of ESRD modalities. The cost estimates, epidemiologic data, and the extent of insurance coverage provided when the law was enacted, as well as estimates of the potential for rehabilitation of patients with the anticipated concomitant economic benefits, proved to be quite inaccurate and overly optimistic (15).

Concerned about the mounting costs of the ESRD program and about criticisms of the effects of budgetary limitations on the quality of care, the U.S. Congress (Omnibus Reconciliation Act of 1987) requested that the IOM conduct a study, *Kidney Failure and the Federal Government* (4). This study was to address the major epidemiologic and demographic changes in the ESRD population that affect access to treatment, the quality of care, and the requirements for special resources by the program. The IOM committee examined (a) access to treatment by persons with chronic renal failure (both those eligible and those ineligible for Medicare benefits); (b) the quality of care provided to ESRD beneficiaries, as measured by clinical indicators and the functional status of patients, and patient satisfaction; (c) the effect of levels of reimbursement on quality of care; and (d) the adequacy of existing data systems to monitor these matters. The

IOM committee also examined patient perspectives, ethical issues, structure of the provider community, and ESRD research needs.

A U.S. CBO publication, *Rising Health Care Costs: Causes, Implications, and Strategies* (16), concluded that the factors responsible for the escalating health care costs per capita were (a) the aging population, (b) the availability of more effective and costly technologies, and (c) the failure of the normal discipline of the marketplace to limit the quantity of services supplied. Between 1970 and 1989, real health care spending per capita in the United States rose from $950 to $2,354 (in 1989 dollars)—an average annual real growth of 4.9% over this 19-year period. Another CBO paper (2) commented, "this growth rate reflects increases in quantity of services per capita, changes in quality, and increases in the price of medical services above general inflation in the economy."

It is helpful to look at comparable U.S. expenditures for other purposes, also given by the CBO: "During the 1980–1988 period, the consumer price index for all urban consumers increased 36 percent for food, 44 percent for entertainment, and 57 percent for shelter, compared with 85 percent for health care." This CBO policy paper stated that the disadvantages of the high and growing health care spending include (a) less income, both public and private, being available to spend on other goods and services; and (b) more difficulties in addressing problems of the underinsured population.

The American Medical Association (AMA) estimated that $11.7 billion per year was added to the cost of physicians' services by the practice of "defensive" medicine in the year 1985 (17). The CBO paper (2) reported that in 1988, the average malpractice insurance premium paid per year by employed physicians was $15,900, with the premiums varying by specialty ($35,300 for obstetricians/gynecologists to $4,400 for psychiatrists). Health care providers put a portion of their malpractice premiums and other overhead expenses into their charges for medical care. They also may change their patterns of practice in an effort to avoid lawsuits and to collect documentation for defense against potential suits. The AMA estimates that between 1982 and 1988, malpractice premiums for self-employed physicians rose at an average annual rate of 18.3% and that $5 billion was spent on medical malpractice premiums by all types of U.S. health care providers in 1988. Contrast this with the following year, 1989, when all U.S. public funds for medical research totaled only $10.2 billion.

World Health Resources

Those who live in the developed/high-income/industrialized countries have come to consider access to health care as a right. Hence for those fortunate Americans who have adequate insurance coverage for health care, it is difficult to realize that health care could be limited, albeit the United States has a tacit form of rationing by ability to pay. Although

TABLE 100-1. *Ranking of countries, health indicators (160 countries, 1994 or latest year available)*

Region	GNP per capita		Public expenditures per capita		Population per physician		Infant mortality		Life expectancy		Health (average rank)
	Rank	U.S. $	Rank	U.S. $	Rank	No.	Rank	Rate	Rank	Years	
World		4,580		231		899		56		65	
Industrial		24,180		1,376		428		6		77	
Transition		1,960		75		265		13		69	
Developing		1,100		22		1,622		60		63	
America											
North America		24,750		1,493		432		7		76	
United States	8	525,510		1,504	30	430	13	7	14	76	
Canada	12	1717,960		1,395	43	457	5	6	7	77	
Latin America		3,400		74		771		42		68	
Europe											
NATO Europe		17,060		1,012		427		18		75	
All NATO		20,240		1,211		429		13		75	
Eastern Europe		2,170		75		418		15		71	
Ex-USSR		1,870		74		230		18		69	
Other Europe		24,210		1,444		376		6		77	
Asia											
Middle East		2,340		55		1,435		42		65	
Israel	29	2314,170		240	40	439	25	8	14	76	
South Asia		320		4		2,711		83		59	
Far East		3,440		139		1,226		30		68	
Japan	4	337,100		1,767	51	590	1	5	1	79	
Oceania		14,270		748		559		19		73	
Africa		600		16		6,018		89		53	

From: R.L. Sivard, *World military and social expenditures 1996,* Washington, DC World Priorities, 1996.

92% to 95% of the citizens of the United States are entitled to Medicare coverage for ESRD treatment, it is estimated that 42.1 million individuals younger than 65 years of age in the United States in 1999 were uninsured and thus lacked means to cover even basic primary health care (18). Concomitant with the American emphasis on high-technology medicine (for those who can afford it) is a failure to provide elements of essential health care for pregnant women, infants, and children, which is reflected in high neonatal and infant mortality rates, serious nutritional deficiencies, and a failure to thrive among these groups. There are nine essential elements of primary health care: (a) adequate food and housing, with protection of houses against insects and rodents; (b) water adequate to permit cleanliness and safe drinking; (c) suitable waste disposal; (d) services for the provision of antenatal and postnatal care, including family planning; (e) infant and childhood care, including nutritional support; (f) immunization against the major infectious diseases of childhood; (g) prevention and control of locally endemic diseases; (h) elementary medical care of all age groups for injury and disease; and (i) easy access to sound and useful information on prevailing health problems, and on the methods to prevent and control them (19).

A look at the status of health care in the 160 countries throughout the world for which data are available underscores the limited funds that are available for even the most minimal of primary health coverage in situations of scarcity. The richest fifth of the world's population has 50 times the income of the poorest fifth (20). In 1994, public expenditure per capita for health in developing countries was $22 (Africa, $16; South Asia, $4), whereas that for the entire world was $231, and for industrial countries, $1,376 (Table 100-1). Thus, tertiary health care, which includes the high-technology, life-sustaining modalities such as hemodialysis and transplantation, which high-income countries take for granted, is far out of reach for most people living in low-income countries. There is a linear correlation between gross national product (GNP) per capita and public expenditures on health per capita. In addition to the fact that industrial countries have a larger GNP per capita, they spend a greater percentage of their GNP on health—approximately 6.18% (1993)—whereas "transition countries" spend 3.1%, and developing countries spend 2.0% of their GNP on health (Table 100-2).

When the United Nations was founded in 1945, it was agreed that "everyone had the right to a standard of living adequate for the health and well-being of himself and his family, including food, clothing, housing, and medical care and necessary social services ...." (21). The ethical dilemma that presents itself in attempting to satisfy this World Health Organization guideline is the question of how we can provide adequate medical care when resources are limited.

Even in the United States, with its greater economic resources, there are inadequate numbers of kidneys harvested for transplantation. Transplant physicians and surgeons, organ procurement agencies, voluntary health agencies

TABLE 100-2. *Comparative resources (160 countries, 1960 and 1994 or latest year available)*

Region	Gross national product (million 1987 U.S. dollars)		Population (thousand)		Physicians (thousand)		Million 1987 U.S. dollars for health care	
	1960	1994	1960	1994	1960	1993	1960	1993
World	5,740,482	18,686,317	3,007,578	5,585,674	1,587.8	6,092.9	143,235	978,140
Industrial	4,740,923	14,946,205		823,158		1,911.3		884,942
Transition	285,961	654,911		415,598		1,563.2		23,825
Developing	713,568	3,0085,201		4,346,921		2,617.3		69,372
America								
North America	2,100,745	289,650	198,580	289,650	279.1	663.0	28,238	350,803
United States	1,974,289	260,529	180,671	260,529	259.4	600.5	25,232	318,022
Canada	126,456	29,121	17,909	29,121	19.7	63.0	3,006	32,781
Latin America	233,317	468,862	213,520	468,882	113.3	597.5	2,885	19,806
Europe								
NATO Europe	1,865,322	5,3303,423		410,300	[a]	956.1	[a]	323,877
All NATO	3,968,067	11,080,149		699,950	[a]	1,619.1	[a]	674,680
Eastern Europe	104,116	218,318		122,673	[a]	293	[a]	6,909
Ex-U.S.S.R.	181,875	436,593		292,925	[a]	1,269.9	[a]	16,917
Other Europe	250,755	625,354		32,766	[a]	86.6	[a]	39,567
Asia								
Middle East	90,582	484,662	74,266	209,773	25.7	142.6	692	10,245
Israel	7,369	53,483	2,114	5,420	5.2	11.9	72	915
South Asia	108,080	443,415	573,788	1,216,035	102.6	439.9	496	5,089
Far East	587,959	3,865,851	1,012,152	1,877,272	208.3	1,494.3	8,886	179,277
Japan	446,698	3,000,848	94,096	124,782	96.0	211.0	7,810	155,113
Oceania	89,454	291,231	15,001	26,349	14.9	46.4	2,054	16,396
Africa	128,277	379,241	253,636	639,051	18.9	103.2	945	9,254

[a]Because of change in Eastern Europe and former U.S.S.R. data are not comparable for 1960.
From Sivard RL. *World military and social expenditures 1996.* Washington, DC: World Priorities, 1996.

involved with transplantation, and policy makers hope to find ways to increase the supply of kidneys for transplantation. Innovative sources such as transplantation of two "marginal" kidneys and use of kidneys from older donors are being evaluated. The importation of living unrelated kidney donors from less affluent countries of the world has allowed those wealthy enough to purchase a kidney to receive a transplant, whereas the impoverished donor potentially can live comfortably for a while with the payment received for a kidney (22). Transplant physicians and surgeons, ethicists, policy makers, clergy, and the public in industrialized countries have major ethical concerns about the purchase of body parts from living donors, and many countries, including the United States, have passed legislation forbidding the practice. Many physicians and surgeons from low-income countries, such as India, have countered in strong fashion and have provided a rationalization for the practice (23–27) (see later). A frequent defense of commercialism in organ procurement is that the "donor for hire" is able to improve the circumstances of his or her impoverished family.

Decisions About Allocation of Resources

The generic problems of resource allocation warrant the consideration of two factors. First, scarcity is inherent in the human condition. Resources rarely are adequate, and demands often increase faster than resources. Second, medical care is not the only determinant or even the chief determinant of health. The resources that are made available for medical care compete with the need for other public expenditures, some of which provide for health and safety, such as sanitation, pollution control, police and fire protection, as well as for other societal needs. Political, social, and economic decisions are made about needs such as education, defense, and the costs of operating the government. Decisions about expenditures for health care also compete with private funds that individuals spend according to their resources and their priorities, for food, clothing, shelter, and transportation, as well as for medical care.

In the allocation of resources, many questions must be asked:

1. Who chooses those who are to make allocation decisions?
2. Do those who are selected act as individuals, within *ad hoc* groups, or within institutionalized structures?
3. What are the requisite qualifications for the decision makers (e.g., medical competence, equitable representation of society, philosophical or economic or political representation)?
4. Should social worth of competing patients be weighted? And if so, how? (These were the sorts of issues facing the Seattle Admissions and Policy Committee in the 1960s.)
5. The selection process is so complex that many biomedical ethicists and philosophers espouse the use of a lottery, which adheres to the ethical principle of justice. Others, particularly those in the "Health Decisions Movement,"

believe that the public must set priorities for health care needs and benefits.

6. Demographic and medical criteria are overtly or covertly involved in treatment decisions. Race, sex, and age may affect decisions that should not be biased by other than objective medical considerations, such as comorbid conditions.

Accurate data are needed to substantiate how decisions are made and the criteria used. Numbers of articles and even books have been written about the United Kingdom's "rationing by age." However, this is not actually a government policy, as has been pointed out in a number of studies. In 1991, 31% of patients on renal dialysis in the United Kingdom were 65 years of age or older (28).

STARTING AND STOPPING TREATMENT: ADVANCED DIRECTIVES

The remarkable advances in medical science and technology require physicians to make weighty decisions about when to use "high technologies," and for how long. Issues arise in the decisions to use respirators, cardiopulmonary resuscitation, chemotherapy, enteral and parenteral nutrition, even antibiotics in special situations, and, of course, dialysis and transplantation. In the past several decades, society has moved from a state of awe at medical "miracles" to one of concern that these technologies may simply prolong the dying process and may even increase suffering. Ethicists, the media, policy makers, and the public increasingly are raising doubts about prolonging life for patients who are irreversibly unconscious (in a persistent vegetative state) or who are suffering inordinately. Thus, the foremost issue raised by the possible overuse of high-technology treatments is that of withholding or withdrawing care. On August 19, 1991, evidence of this societal concern was provided by *The New York Times* "Week in Review" lead article about patients' rights to reject aggressive care (29). The article discussed the public concern reflected in the rapid rise of Derek Humphry's book, *Final Exit,* published by the Hemlock Society, to the top of *The New York Times* "How To" Best Seller List—25% ahead of the next book on the list. The initial printing of 160,000 copies sold out within a week, nationwide.

End-stage renal disease treatment is a prototype of these high technologies. Most patients with ESRD have the advantage that they are conscious and able to discuss whether they wish to be treated and by what technique, and the eventualities that would make them wish to stop treatment. Patients and families increasingly make their views known about the quality of life they desire. Interestingly, health care professionals, patients, and families often have markedly different views about what is an acceptable quality of life. In the United States, whose demographic changes in patients with ESRD are representative of trends in other countries with ESRD programs, more than 40% of new patients were 65 years of age or older in 1990. Almost a third of the new patients were

diabetic. The current trend toward older and sicker patients starting dialysis has implications for the quality of life of patients with ESRD.

Considerations of quality of life are subjective. Nephrologists and other health professionals involved with patients on dialysis may have views of what constitutes a "good," "bearable," or "unbearable" quality of life that vastly differ from the views of the patients themselves (30–32).

Because it is difficult to obtain objective data about quality of life, there is a paucity of research in this area. Most quality-of-life studies have been done by nurses, social workers, sociologists, and psychiatrists, occasionally with input from nephrologists. In a prospective study, the Battelle National Kidney Dialysis and Kidney Transplantation Study (33), Evans and colleagues observed that "based on established standards of quality of life for the normal population, ESRD patients, despite their illness, appear to have adjusted reasonably well, even though they assess their quality of life to be somewhat lower than that of the general population."

The Battelle Study included 859 patients, of whom 347 were on in-center dialysis and 81 were on peritoneal dialysis. They found that in-center patients averaged 1.55 comorbid conditions per patient, whereas the overall average for all patients on dialysis was 1.1 comorbid conditions. The "total sickness impact profile score" and percentage distributions of comorbid conditions for patients on dialysis younger than 65 years of age and those 65 years of age and older were within one to two percentage points. Using the Karnovsky Index (34) to assess well-being and functional status, it was determined that the patients 65 years of age and older had greater satisfaction with the life parameters measured—feelings, satisfaction with marriages, family life, investments and savings, and standard of living—and with life in general than did those younger than 65 years. The older group did recognize that their health was less good than that of people of a comparable age without ESRD. They also realized that they had greater functional difficulties and a lesser ability to work or to be employed than did those without chronic renal failure.

There are obvious stresses in the lives of those dependent for their survival on a machine or on immunosuppressive therapy necessary to prevent rejection of a kidney transplant, because many patients experience side effects of the medications. The psychological and psychosocial effects of ESRD treatment on these patients cover a broad spectrum and cause substantial stresses on their families as well. A Canadian group (35) studied patients with ESRD, both on dialysis and after transplantation, and found a strong correlation between increased feelings of helplessness and depression on the one hand and low degrees of perceived control on the other. Changes in lifestyle caused by the loss of the patient's ability to participate in usual activities at work, at school, in the household, and at leisure because of ESRD treatment added to the stresses of the treatment itself. These changes also contributed to the depression related to loss of self-esteem, and to the loss of the usual quality of life with its accompanying satisfactions that are experienced by vigorous, healthy people.

The incidence of suicide is uncertain, and data about voluntary withdrawal from dialysis treatment are imprecise. Withdrawal from dialysis is no longer called "suicide," and the patient's death often is attributed to the primary renal disease. HCFA data on voluntary withdrawal from treatment indicate higher withdrawal rates in those 65 years of age and older. A survey of the literature (30) concerning quality of life includes these issues of support systems, adjustment, and rehabilitation. It also touches on special problems related to home dialysis and confirms many of the observations made about chronic and catastrophic diseases. Some patients cope remarkably well, whereas others cannot deal with the stresses. In addition to the stresses for patients and their families, there are major stresses for the deliverers of ESRD care. The impact of constantly caring for patients with irreversible disease causes "burnout" for many health professionals, especially nurses and dialysis technicians. Health professionals as well as patients have a need for support systems.

DEMOGRAPHICS

How do nephrologists make the difficult decisions about whom to treat and whom not to treat? It is helpful to study the demography of patients with ESRD over time to understand some factors affecting these decisions. Renee Fox (36) argued that "it appears that physicians have suspended all biomedical, as well as psychological and social, criteria of judgement concerning who should be dialyzed and who should not." To evaluate this contention, it may be helpful to look at some of the available data about withdrawal from dialysis treatment. Unlike the situation with some other LSTs, there are data that provide evidence about how patients feel about the stressful nature of dialysis treatment because patients on dialysis usually are alert and competent to make medical decisions.

Both the HCFA and the U.S. Renal Data System (USRDS), as well as the European Dialysis and Transplant Association (EDTA), the Australian and New Zealand Dialysis and Transplant Registry, and the Japanese Registry, provide demographic and modest medical data. Table 100-3 provides prevalence counts and rates for treated patients with ESRD in 18 selected countries that have a wide range in numbers of patients per million population (as well as in their GNP per capita). Figure 100-1 shows the treated ESRD incidence rate for seven countries from 1983 to 1992. The increasing age of patients entering ESRD treatment affects patterns of treatment, of withdrawal from treatment, and of complications because there are increasing numbers of comorbid conditions with increasing age.

The HCFA and the USRDS have demographic data that show the pattern of patients on the ESRD program in the United States. Germane to this discussion are the data about "withdrawal from dialysis." These numbers undoubtedly

TABLE 100-3. *Treated end-stage renal disease prevalence counts and rates (per million population) for selected countries, 1989*

Country	Prevalence	
	N	Rate (per million population)
United States	163,069	654
Japan[a]	83,489	726
West Germany[b]	31,512	516
France[b]	20,422	366
Italy[b]	19,203	334
Brazil[c]	16,045	104
Spain[b]	13,416	344
Canada	11,265	430
United Kingdom[b]	9,451	165
Netherlands	6,001	407
Australia	5,786	344
Yugoslavia	5,588	237
People's Republic of China	5,083	253

[a]Data for 1988.

[b]Incomplete counts according to the European Dialysis and Transplant Association.

[c]Excludes transplants.

represent underreporting because patients on dialysis usually are well informed about the hazards of excessive fluid intake and of potassium. Hence, deaths secondary to these causes may be masked and attributed to cardiovascular causes, rather than reported as instances of "voluntary" withdrawal from dialysis. HCFA no longer lists "withdrawal from dialysis" as a cause of death. Hence, the tables and figures from the USRDS 1991 report are presented. Eggers (6) considers that data designated as "failure to thrive" are similar to the earlier data for withdrawal as a cause of death (Tables 100-4, 100-5).

For the period 1987 to 1989, the USRDS (37) found that 8.51% of deaths were caused by withdrawal from dialysis, a percentage representing an average of 1,604 deaths per year. The distribution as percentage of deaths in specific

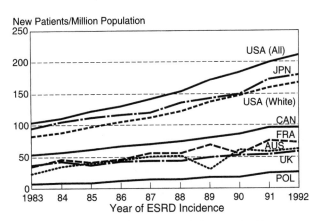

FIG. 100-1. Treated end-stage renal disease incidence rate for selected countries, 1983 to 1992. (From U.S. Renal Data System. *USRDS 1995 annual report.* Bethesda, MD: National Institutes of Health, National Institute of Diabetes and Digestive and Kidney Diseases, 1995.)

TABLE 100-4. *Medicare end-stage renal disease deaths 1997 through 1999: causes of death for stopping dialysis and possible withdrawal from dialysis (numbers of persons)*

Cause of death[a]	All deaths (N)	Dialysis not stopped	Dialysis stopped	Chronic failure to thrive
Total	177,784	152,906	24,878	12,964
[29] Cardiac arrest	36,269	32,772	3,497	2,064
[98] Other	11,942	8,300	3,642	2,187
[99] Unknown	12,405	10,873	1,532	994
[24] Hyperkalemia	2,734	1,325	1,408	930
[27] Cardiomyopathy	7,163	5,758	1,405	
[81] Cachexia	1,795	985	810	694
[26] Atherosclerotic heart disease	6,179	5,109	1,070	685
[28] Cardiac arrhythmia	9,288	8,315	973	522
[83] Malignancy, no immunosuppressives	4,203	3,189	1,014	485
[51] Septicemia, gangrene	4,442	3,381	1,061	440
[52] Septicemia, other	10,430	9,200	1,230	416
[84] Dementia	767	308	459	384
[36] Cerebral vascular accident, intracranial hemorrhage	8,026	6,277	1,749	381
[31] Pulmonary edema, exogenous fluid	1,575	1,098	477	307

[a]Medicare diagnostic numbers given in brackets.

groups was as follows: male—7.8%; female—9.35%; black—4.48%; white—10.41%. There also was an increasing percentage with increasing age, from 3.5% for those younger than 20 years to 11.45% for those 65 years of age and older. USRDS also reported withdrawal from dialysis as 11.2 per 1,000 patient years at risk, with those younger than age 20 years having only 0.6 death per 1,000 patient years, whereas those 65 years of age and older had 31.5 deaths per 1,000 patient years (Table 100-6). Figure 100-2 shows the latest available data on withdrawal from dialysis by age and race (1991 to 1992) from the HCFA (USRDS). In the three age groups, white patients on dialysis withdrew from dialysis over twice as frequently as did black patients on dialysis. Diabetic patients withdrew from dialysis three times more frequently than did patients whose primary renal disease was hypertension or glomerulonephritis (Table 100-7). Furthermore, considering the race and age of patients on hemodialysis, diabetic patients withdrew from dialysis more frequently in every category analyzed (Table 100-8). The mortality rates in the first 90 days listed as due to withdrawal from dialysis also are markedly higher for those between 65 and 74 years

of age and for those 75 years of age and older than for those between 45 and 64 years of age (Table 100-9).

Eggers studied voluntary withdrawal from dialysis (38) by evaluating the 20,028 deaths (Table 100-10) in 1987 that were linked with Medicare hospital stay records. (These records were drawn from the total of 22,670 deaths of patients with ESRD in 1987; 2,642 patients who died were covered by other forms of insurance.) Fifty-five percent of all deaths were in patients 65 years of age and older. In 1987 and 1986, 71,201 hospitalizations with an admission date within 365 days of the date of death were selected for analysis. HCFA death notification forms (No. 2746) were analyzed in two categories of death: voluntary withdrawal from dialysis, or death from another cause. Voluntary withdrawal was found to be directly related to age. No deaths in the youngest group (≤14 years) were reported as voluntary withdrawal, whereas the 15- to 24-year age group had less than 5% of deaths classified as voluntary withdrawal. In the 75 years and older group, more than 12% of the deaths were listed as voluntary.

In April 1996, Dr. Paul W. Eggers, of the Division of Health, Information and Outcomes, HCFA, reported that in

TABLE 100-5. *Medicare end-stage renal disease cardiac-related deaths 1997 through 1999: cause of death by reason for stopping dialysis (numbers of persons)*

Cardiac diagnosis[a]	All deaths	Dialysis not stopped	Dialysis stopped	Chronic failure to thrive
[23] Acute myocardial infarction	15,272	14,564	708	216
[28] Cardiac arrhythmia	9,288	8,315	973	522
[27] Cardiomyopathy	7,163	5,758	1,405	912
[26] Atherosclerotic heart disease	6,179	5,109	1,070	685
[30] Valvular heart disease	1,015	876	139	70
[25] Pericarditis	205	184	21	15
[29] Cardiac arrest	32,269	32,772	3,497	2,064
[31] Pulmonary edema	1,575	1,098	477	307

[a]Medicare diagnostic numbers given in brackets.

TABLE 100-6. *Mortality rates by cause of death*[a]

Cause of death	Total	Sex		Race		Age (yr)			
		Male	Female	Black	White	<20	20–44	45–64	65+
Pericarditis	1.0	1.1	0.8	1.1	0.9	0.3	0.5	1.0	1.8
Myocardial infarction	18.8	20.2	17.1	17.3	19.6	0.5	5.7	21.1	37.8
Cardiac	37.9	38.3	37.6	36.8	38.8	3.8	12.8	37.1	82.3
Cerebrovascular	8.5	7.2	10.1	9.8	8.0	1.1	3.0	8.5	17.9
Embolism, pulmonary	0.7	0.6	0.8	0.7	0.7	<0.1	0.4	0.8	1.0
Gastrointestinal hemorrhage	2.1	2.1	2.1	2.3	2.0	0.2	0.6	2.0	4.7
Hemorrhage, other	1.1	1.0	1.2	1.3	1.0	0.6	0.6	1.2	1.7
Pulmonary infection	4.4	4.8	3.9	3.5	4.7	0.9	1.7	3.6	10.1
Septicemia	13.5	11.8	15.6	16.0	12.6	2.5	5.6	14.3	26.1
Infection, other	2.2	2.1	2.3	2.2	2.2	0.8	1.2	2.3	3.7
Hyperkalemia	1.8	1.9	1.8	1.9	1.8	0.7	1.9	1.7	2.2
Malignancy	4.0	4.5	3.3	4.3	4.0	0.3	0.8	4.4	8.7
Withdrawal from dialysis	31.5	11.2	10.2	12.4	5.8	13.9	0.6	2.1	7.9
Unknown cause	10.4	10.4	10.3	13.1	9.1	1.9	5.4	10.8	18.5
Other	13.7	13.9	13.5	14.7	13.6	3.2	6.6	13.5	26.3
Missing data	25.6	27.0	23.9	25.0	26.2	4.7	11.8	26.9	47.8
Total patient years at risk	358,534	195,731	162,803	104,580	237,314	11,042	131,902	128,125	86,458

[a]Deaths of patients with end-stage renal disease (ESRD) per 1,000 patient years at risk, for all patients with ESRD, by cause of death, and by sex, race, and age, 1987–1989.
From U.S. Renal Data System. *USRDS 1991 annual data report.* Bethesda, MD: National Institutes of Health, National Institute of Diabetes and Digestive and Kidney Diseases, 1991.

the period from 1991 to 1994, there were 126,156 ESRD deaths, of which 17.8% (22,456) were listed as discontinuation of therapy or voluntary withdrawal (6). These data confirm those of earlier years noted previously: the percentage of deaths with voluntary withdrawal increased with age from 12.7% for people younger than 65 years of age to 18.3% for people 65 to 74 years, 23.6% for people 75 to 84 years, and 27.0% for people 85 years of age and older. Of all cardiac deaths, 12.7% were due to voluntary withdrawal. This number varied from 4.0% for acute myocardial infarction to 52.3% for hyperkalemia. Of the 8% of deaths due to vascular causes, 20.3% were due to voluntary withdrawal. Among the causes with particularly high rates of voluntary withdrawal are dementia (65.7%), cachexia (43.7%), malignancy and no history of immunosuppressive therapy (33.9%).

Those withdrawing were less likely (5.9%) to have had no hospitalizations (Table 100-11) than were other decedents (9.8%). They were slightly more likely to have been hospitalized for neoplasm (12.7% vs. 9.7%), but not more likely than other decedents to have been hospitalized for diabetes, hypertension, heart disease, congestive heart failure, or pneumonia. The greatest difference was noted in those with hospitalizations for mental disorders, who had 20.5% of deaths due to voluntary withdrawals and at least one hospital stay, compared with 12% among other decedents without mental illness. The length of stay per hospital episode was longer for those voluntarily withdrawing from dialysis than for the other decedents. In addition, the hospital expenditures were approximately $1,200 higher for those voluntarily withdrawing from dialysis.

Neu and Kjellstrand's earlier retrospective study (39) reported that diabetic patients stopped dialysis three to five times more frequently than did other patients, except in the oldest group. Withdrawal from dialysis was equally distributed among their patients who were and who were not mentally competent to make decisions about the termination of dialysis. They found that 22% of deaths were due to voluntary withdrawal.

In an evaluation of the cause of death among all Michigan patients on dialysis, from 1980 through 1985, Port (40) noted that the discontinuation of dialysis may be underreported and that there was a "markedly higher withdrawal rate in older, white, and diabetic patient groups, and that during

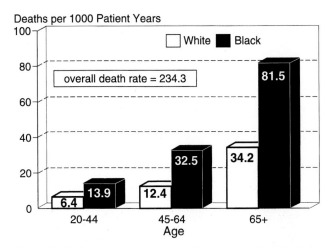

FIG. 100-2. Death rates due to withdrawal from dialysis by age and race, 1991 to 1992. (From U.S. Renal Data System. *USRDS 1995 annual report.* Bethesda, MD: National Institutes of Health, National Institute of Diabetes and Digestive and Kidney Diseases, 1995.)

TABLE 100-7. *Mortality rates by cause of death, by diagnosis[a]*

Cause of death	Diabetes	Hypertension	Glomerulonephritis
Pericarditis	1.9	1.1	0.7
Myocardial infarction	43.9	20.1	13.3
Cardiac	67.1	37.9	26.5
Cerebrovascular	16.5	8.1	5.3
Embolism, pulmonary	1.5	0.5	0.6
Gastrointestinal hemorrhage	2.2	2.5	2
Hemorrhage, other	1.3	1.4	0.7
Pulmonary infection	4	3.7	3.7
Septicemia	25	11.8	10.7
Infection, other	4.4	1.5	2
Hyperkalemia	3.1	1.8	1.2
Malignancy	2.7	4.5	3.7
Withdrawal from dialysis	17.4	5.6	5
Unknown cause	20.7	10.4	5.6
Other	18.3	14.5	10
Missing data	39.4	22.7	18.5
Total patient years at risk	26,282	27,451	22,574

[a]Deaths of patients with end-stage renal disease (ESRD) per 1,000 patient years at risk, for all patients with ESRD, by cause of death, for three major diagnoses, age 45–64 yr, 1987–1989.

From U.S. Renal Data System. *USRDS 1991 annual data report.* Bethesda, MD: National Institutes of Health, National Institute of Diabetes and Digestive and Kidney Diseases, 1991.

recent years, there has been a striking increase in withdrawal rates even when adjusted for other factors." Of 5,208 patients starting ESRD treatment in Michigan during 1980 to 1985, 282 died and 9.4% of these deaths were due to voluntarily stopping dialysis. This group included 11% of the women, 8% of the men, and 12% of the white patients (compared with 4% of the black patients). Between 1980 and 1986, this Michigan group had an increase in death rates due to stopping dialysis of approximately 60%. In the group younger than 49 years of age, 0.1% to 3.4% of deaths were from voluntarily stopping dialysis, whereas in those older than 80 years, 56% of deaths were from voluntary withdrawal. Port speculated that religious and cultural attitudes might affect the difference in withdrawal percentages between white and black patients on dialysis. Another explanation is possible differences in reporting (41).

TABLE 100-8. *Mortality rates by cause of death, by diabetic status, race, and age—hemodialysis[a]* *(deaths per 1,000 patient years at risk for all ESRD patients receiving hemodialysis [never transplanted] by cause of death, by diabetic status, race, and age, 1987–1989)*

Cause of death	Diabetic				Nondiabetic			
	Black	White	20–44 yr	45–64 yr	Black	White	20–44 yr	45–64 yr
Pericarditis	2.0	2.4	2.2	2.2	1.2	1.4	0.7	1.2
Myocardial infarction	34.2	55.6	29.5	46.6	18.5	26.6	5.1	19.4
Other cardiac	62.8	102.2	62.3	75.6	42.2	60.5	18.4	39.2
Cerebrovascular	17.4	22.2	15.9	18.1	11.0	11.1	4.0	8.8
Embolism, pulmonary	1.2	1.5	0.8	1.4	0.6	0.7	0.3	0.7
Gastrointestinal hemorrhage	2.7	3.8	2.5	2.5	3.1	3.7	0.9	2.7
Hemorrhage, other	0.8	1.0	<0.1	1.2	1.3	1.4	0.7	1.4
Pulmonary infection	4.0	7.7	4.9	4.2	4.3	8.1	2.3	4.2
Septicemia	27.5	31.3	20.8	26.9	16.3	17.2	7.7	13.5
Infection, other	4.3	4.6	4.0	4.3	2.0	2.2	1.6	1.6
Hyperkalemia	2.3	6.6	10.1	3.7	2.6	2.5	3.8	2.1
Malignancy	3.7	3.9	1.0	3.3	6.4	8.3	1.9	6.9
Withdrawal from dialysis	12.0	36.5	14.8	18.1	7.0	23.2	1.8	7.7
Unknown cause	21.2	26.3	24.3	23.1	14.7	12.1	7.6	11.0
Other	17.6	24.3	19.9	17.7	15.6	18.5	7.5	13.7
Missing data	34.2	49.9	29.2	37.8	24.2	32.4	12.1	21.6
Total patient years at risk	15,459	20,224	5,906	18,433	46,507	73,959	26,357	45,615

[a]Deaths per 1,000 patient years at risk for all patients with end-stage renal disease receiving hemodialysis (never transplanted), by cause of death, by diabetic status, race, and age, 1987–1989.

From U.S. Renal Data System. *USRDS 1991 annual data report.* Bethesda, MD: National Institutes of Health, National Institute of Diabetes and Digestive and Kidney Diseases, 1991.

TABLE 100-9. *Mortality rates in the first 90 days by cause of death and age[a]*

Cause of death	Age (yr) 45–64	65–74	75+
Pericarditis	0.1	0.7	0.9
Myocardial infarction	4.3	14.3	18.3
Other cardiac	8.8	32.9	49.1
Cerebrovascular	1.1	5.0	7.0
Embolism, air	<0.1	<0.1	<0.1
Embolism, pulmonary	0.1	0.5	0.4
Gastrointestinal hemorrhage	0.1	1.2	1.4
Vascular access	<0.1	<0.1	<0.01
Hemorrhage, other	0.2	0.5	0.8
Pulmonary infection	0.6	2.5	4.9
Septicemia	2.0	8.3	11.7
Viral hepatitis	<0.1	<0.1	0.1
Infection, other	0.2	0.6	1.2
Hyperkalemia	0.1	0.6	0.9
Pancreatitis	<0.1	0.1	0.1
Malignancy	0.9	2.9	3.2
Withdrawal from dialysis	1.6	9.6	19.4
Suicide	<0.1	0.4	0.2
Accidental, treatment related	<0.1	0.1	0.1
Accidental, not treatment related	0.1	0.1	<0.1
Unknown cause	2.0	6.7	10.4
Other	1.8	7.1	10.6
Missing data	8.6	19.3	32.2
Total patient years at risk	39,620	27,038	14,145

[a]Mortality rates during the first 90 days of end-stage renal disease (ESRD), by cause of death and age, all patients with ESRD, 1987–1989.

From U.S. Renal Data System. *USRDS 1991 annual data report.* Bethesda, MD: National Institutes of Health, National Institute of Diabetes and Digestive and Kidney Diseases, 1991.

SELECTION OF PATIENTS AND TREATMENT

In this era of broad entitlement for ESRD treatment, hard decisions about who can be treated do not have to be made in the way they were made before 1972. Nevertheless, many dialysis and transplantation centers have committees that consider treatment options for each patient with ESRD. Committee membership may include health professionals, lawyers, clergy, and laypeople. The patient with ESRD and his or her family may be invited to participate in the discussion. Recommendations are made about what sort of treatment would be advisable, including "no treatment." Frequently, a trial of therapy is suggested if there is doubt about its efficacy, or if the patient expresses a preference not to be treated.

Although overtly there is no committee such as the Seattle Admissions and Policy Committee, the "God Committee," there continue to be tacit and often outspoken societal judgments about patients' lifestyles. These frequently are expressed in the media and in protests about behavior. HIV-infected patients and those with acquired immunodeficiency syndrome (AIDS) are judged unfavorably because of either their sexual preferences or their substance abuse. Substance abuse often is involved in situations in which patients are disruptive in dialysis units, at times making the provision of treatment difficult for all patients. The issue of whether to isolate patients who are positive for either hepatitis B virus (HBV) or HIV raises the specter of violation of confidentiality for HIV-infected patients. Both ethical and legal issues (30,42) (cases discussed later) must be addressed in these situations.

An elusive issue related to the selection of a treatment modality is that of "sequestration" of patients. Although there is an absolute shortage of donor kidneys, some surgeons have questioned whether potential transplant recipients are not being offered the choice of transplantation as a treatment option. Aligned with this question is that of whether patients are not being put on and kept on dialysis for financial reasons. No objective data are available to substantiate these hypotheses. However, from 1982 to 1990, there was a 14% increase in the proportion of patients on dialysis treated in free-standing, for-profit dialysis units (Fig. 100-3). The for-profit chains have been able to benefit from economies of scale.

How are decisions actually made and how would they be affected if resources were limited? Such information often is anecdotal and has been more limited since entitlement for ESRD became so broad. Kilner (43) conducted a survey of decision making by the medical directors of dialysis facilities and kidney transplant centers in the United States. The

TABLE 100-10. *Distribution of patient deaths, by age at time of death and cause of death, by voluntary withdrawal from dialysis or other (1987)*

Age at time of death (yr)	No. of deaths Total	Other	Voluntary	Percent voluntary	Percent total
0–14	42	42	0	0%	0%
15–24	144	138	6	4%	1%
25–34	814	788	26	3%	4%
35–44	1,525	1,462	63	4%	8%
45–54	2,233	2,156	77	3%	11%
55–64	4,452	4,201	251	6%	22%
65–74	6,536	6,035	501	8%	33%
75–84	3,780	3,345	435	12%	19%
85+	502	430	72	14%	3%
All	20,028	18,597	1,431	7%	100%

From Health Care Financing Agency (HCFA), death notification forms.

TABLE 100-11. *Hospitalizations by specific diagnostic categories by cause of death, by voluntary withdrawal from dialysis or other*

Diagnostic category	Voluntary withdrawal from dialysis		Hospitalization		Chi-square P
	No (no.)	Yes (no.)	No	Yes	
Neoplasms	1,800	182	9.7%	12.7%	0.000
Diabetes	6,283	508	33.8%	35.5%	0.187
Hypertension	7,566	604	40.7%	42.2%	0.258
Acute myocardial infarction	1,906	91	10.2%	6.4%	0.000
Ischemic heart disease	1,420	107	7.6%	7.5%	0.828
Heart failure	6,344	520	34.1%	36.3%	0.087
Pneumonia	2,835	219	15.2%	15.3%	0.952
Malignant hypertension	578	39	3.1%	2.7%	0.420
Mental	2,238	293	12.0%	20.5%	0.000
Amputation	1,358	129	7.3%	9.0%	0.017
No stays	1,819	85	9.8%	5.9%	—
All persons	18,597	1,431	100.0%	100.0%	—

Modified from Health Care Financing Agency (HCFA), death notification forms.

response rates to the questionnaires were 40% and 50%, respectively. Sixteen selection criteria were evaluated. Both the dialysis and the transplant center directors agreed on the "very important criteria" for selection, which are listed in descending order of priority: medical benefit of treatment, likelihood of benefit, quality of benefit, willingness to cooperate with the treatment regimen, and the length of the benefit. The other 11 criteria were of lesser significance, at least in circumstances of plenty. These include psychological status, age, special responsibilities, required resources, support systems, social value, and scientific progress.

The impact of scarcity on dialysis selection criteria is striking. The percentage of center directors who would consider length of benefit as a selection criterion increased from 71% if resources were unlimited, to 96% if resources were limited. Likewise, the percentage for quality of benefit as a criterion went from 44% to 97%; for ability to pay, from

4% to 45%; and for medical benefit, from 62% to 95%. The most dramatic shift in consideration of a criterion was for age, which went from 10% to 85% of center directors who would consider age a criterion if resources shifted from being unlimited to limited. The ability to pay, in financially constricted circumstances, was considered relevant by 43% of the directors.

Eggers (44) studied the effects of comorbid conditions in patients who already were Medicare entitled before renal failure developed. With expansion of the apparent criteria for acceptance into dialysis, particularly the acceptance of increasingly older patients, Eggers found that more than 40% of patients with ESRD in the United States had Medicare entitlement before renal failure, representing a significant percentage of the eligible population, particularly of the elderly.

Although the mortality rate for all patients starting dialysis therapy was 21% to 22% in the first year after renal failure,

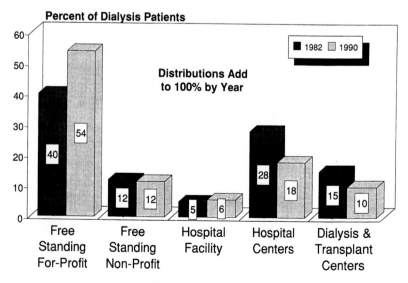

FIG. 100-3. Patients on dialysis by type of unit: distribution of patients by type of end-stage renal disease unit, 1982 to 1990. (From U.S. Renal Data System. *USRDS 1991 annual report.* Bethesda, MD: National Institutes of Health, National Institute of Diabetes and Digestive and Kidney Diseases, 1991.)

it was over 30% for patients who were older than 65 years of age at the onset of renal failure. Whereas questions are raised about the higher mortality rate for U.S. patients with ESRD than for patients with ESRD in other industrialized countries, many factors have been considered but none has proved to be the definitive answer. Shorter dialysis time, case mix, access to transplantation, patient compliance, and new dialysis techniques have produced variations. In 1981, 28% of new Medicare patients with ESRD were older than 65 years and 19% were diabetic, but in 1988, 39% were older than 65 years and 31% were diabetic. Eggers noted that "all of the risk categories had relative risks greater than 1.0 suggesting that these do represent meaningful added comorbid risks to renal failure." He reported that approximately one-third of patients older than 65 years of age at the time renal failure reached end stage die within 1 year of starting dialysis. The prerenal failure hospitalization rate is sufficiently high that this measure of comorbidity can be considered at the outset for most elderly patients who are Medicare entitled.

ETHICAL ISSUES AND PRINCIPLES

The remarkable scientific and technologic advances in medicine of the past 50 to 75 years resulted both in an unanticipated ability to prolong lives and in the need to consider ethical and moral problems never envisioned in the time of Hippocrates or even in the 19th century. The early success of renal transplantation, in which a healthy identical twin's kidney was transplanted in the twin with chronic renal failure, raised ethical issues in the 1950s about the use of living related donors. The development of dialysis and its empiric application for the treatment of acute renal failure during World War II, and the subsequent development of biocompatible Silastic cannulae to be used as indwelling arteriovenous shunts, which made chronic dialysis possible for individual patients, had a dramatic impact on medical practice. Both developments heightened awareness of the issues related to the allocation of limited resources, personnel, and funding available for chronic dialysis therapy in the 1960s.

These ethical issues, along with many others in the fields of medicine, biomedical research, and genetics, were seminal in the development of the field of biomedical ethics more than two decades ago. Ethical issues in the treatment of kidney disease continue to receive increasing attention, especially in the decade of 1990s continuing into the next decade. Although the precepts of medical ethics go back before the time of Hippocrates, the formal field of biomedical ethics that developed in the face of increasingly complex medical technologies is less than three decades old.

Foremost among the ethical dilemmas in high technology and especially in ESRD treatment are those involved in starting and stopping treatment. One of the prescient recommendations of the 1991 IOM report (4) acknowledged the import of biomedical ethics for nephrology: "ESRD clinicians should be encouraged to participate in continuing education in medical ethics and health law. Some specialists in [the] medical ethics of renal disease should be available to educate clinicians, to train members of ethics committees, and to do research on ethical issues in dialysis and transplantation." This recommendation accepts the fact that there are "no easy answers" to the ethical dilemmas facing nephrologists, who must be aware of all the nuances involved in making decisions to initiate and terminate treatment.

The development of and increased utilization of ethics consultations and ethics committees has provided a valuable resource for nephrologists facing difficult dilemmas. From 1971, when the first ethics committee was formed, to 1992, 66% to 75% of hospitals in the United States have established ethics committees. In addition, since 1995, the Joint Commission on Accreditation of Health Care Organizations (JCAHO) has required a "mechanism" to deal with ethical issues. Ethics committees have provided patients and health care professionals with a spectrum of support in coping with moral issues, facilitated communication, and enhanced education of all parties concerned as well as assisting with in conflict resolution. Cases brought to ethics committees often involve complex moral questions such as "patient autonomy, informed consent, competence, rights of conscience, medical futility, resource allocation, confidentiality, and surrogate decision making" (45).

In 1982, O'Brien (46), reported that patients on dialysis with a religious commitment survived longer than did those with no religious involvement. More recently, increased attention has been paid to the effect of religious faith on health, and medical schools have instituted programs in spirituality. Although objective reasons to explain the power of faith and spirituality in patient healing and well-being have not been elucidated, there have been a spate of articles about the effects of religion on patients' health (47). A meta-analysis assessed over 350 articles about religious involvement and health and concluded that religious involvement is a widespread practice that predicts successful coping with physical illness (49–51).

Principles and Models

How does one select patients fairly? What ethical principles are applied in fair selection? How are such principles helpful in decision making? The four ethical principles primarily used in biomedical considerations (51a) are (a) autonomy, (b) beneficence, (c) nonmaleficence, and (d) justice. These principles provide a useful framework for the assessment of patients' treatment. The shift in medical practice from paternalism to an emphasis on autonomy and informed consent is marked. In 1961, the *Journal of the American Medical Association (JAMA)* (52) reported that 88% of physicians did not tell their patients that they had cancer. Eighteen years later, a similar *JAMA* report (53) noted that 90% of physicians did tell their patients that they had cancer.

How do we use these four ethical principles in treating patients with ESRD? Autonomy, the independence to make one's own choices, includes the choices of never starting and of stopping treatment. Beneficence (doing good) is paternalistic if the decisions are made by the physician and not shared with the patient. Nonmaleficence is the familiar caveat: *Primum non nocere* ("First, do not harm"). Justice is a fairness principle. Justice requires fair consideration of access to medical benefits and an equitable distribution of these benefits. Consciously or unconsciously, those making decisions about treatment also may consider one or more of a number of similar principles to be ethically binding. These include integrity (truth telling), fidelity (the keeping of promises), confidentiality, privacy, liberty, charity, compassion, respect for persons and for the sanctity of life, and adherence to the "Golden Rule."

There also are five alternatives to the "principles approach" to bioethics. These constitute a "family of approaches" and include (a) phenomenology, (b) medical hermeneutics, (c) narrative, (d) the "new casuistry," and (e) virtue. Phenomenology (54) applies to descriptive accounts of clinical situations and their implications for solicitous care within clinically based ethics. A hermeneutic approach (55,56) to bioethics would use interpretation of moral experience as it occurs in relation to health care delivery, particularly the interactions of patients and health care professionals. (The term *hermeneutics* comes from the Greek *hermeneia*, which is translated as "interpretation.") The narrative approach (57) emphasizes the patient's "story." The casuistic mode of moral reasoning (58) emphasizes paradigm cases, a broad consensus of considered opinion, and probable certitude. Casuistry can be applied to the method of analysis and resolution of instances of moral perplexity by interpreting general moral rules in light of specific circumstances or cases. The virtue approach (59–61) focuses on both individuals' and communities' qualities of character. Virtue theories consider that judgments of character or of agents play a central role in good or appropriate performance.

In the decision-making process, several models that may influence treatment decisions by the physician have been identified. These include the warrior model, the parent model, and the contractual and covenantal models (62). These models, respectively, take approaches that consider medical treatment as a battle against death; the physician as playing a parental role of knowing what is best for the patient; the therapeutic interaction as two people entering an explicit contract in which the health professional is the giver and the patient is the recipient of services; and, last, medical care arrangements as a covenant in which there are mutual commitments. It is of great importance to the therapeutic relationship for the patient and his or her caregiver to have a similar view of and goals for the treatment process. This is achieved most felicitously with the covenantal model, in which both patient and caregiver are involved in the decision making (63).

For patients, one of the major health care issues, if not the most important issue, facing them today is how to maintain responsibility for their own medical destinies. Because patients and health professionals often have widely differing assessments of the quality of life a patient considers acceptable, it is essential that patients have a means to express their wishes and to exercise autonomy in their health care decisions. Concerns about this need for autonomy are evident in the spate of articles in the popular press, as well as in the increased use of advance directives by many people.

The advantage for physicians, other health professionals, and ethicists in considering relevant concerns of patients with ESRD is the fact that most patients on dialysis are alert at the initiation of dialysis or after a trial period, and thus are able to state their views about treatment. Although the issues involved are frequently discussed by nephrologists, no specific formal national guidelines have been delineated. Some centers have listed criteria for selection and for continuation of chronic dialysis. The Section on Renal Disease of the Health Sciences Center of the University of Arizona formalized their criteria in January, 1984 (30) (Table 100-12). Three objectives that the IOM study (4) recommends are (a) guaranteed access to ESRD treatment for all patients for whom it is medically appropriate, (b) the provision of high-quality care yielding desirable health outcomes consistent with both the patient's health status and current professional knowledge,

TABLE 100-12. *Criteria for selection for and continuation of chronic dialysis*

1. All patients shall be provided chronic dialysis therapy who:
   a. Grant fully informed consent; and
   b. Have chronic, irreversible end-stage renal disease; and
   c. Have a reasonable expectation of a quality of life acceptable to themselves; and
   d. Desire and can cooperate with such therapy; and
   e. Are legal residents of, or can establish legal residence in, the State of Arizona.
2. Patients will not be provided chronic dialysis therapy who suffer from a simultaneously present invariably rapidly fatal disease.
3. No patient shall be denied therapy on the basis of psychological, economic, or social factors, or on the basis of age, sex, ethnic origin or disability if criteria #1–5 above are otherwise met.
4. Patients shall have the right, and be informed of the right, to continue chronic dialysis, once initiated, if they so desire. Chronic dialysis may not be terminated against a patient's stated will.
5. Patients shall have the right, and be informed of the right, to discontinue chronic dialysis at any time they so desire by simply failing to appear for their scheduled treatments.
6. Chronic dialysis may be terminated in the event a patient is unable to state his will and cannot be reasonably expected to regain the ability to state his will, upon recommendation of the patient's physician with the consent of the legal next-of-kin, or, upon recommendation of the patient's physician and the consent of his legal guardian.

From Section on Renal Disease, Health Sciences Center, University of Arizona, January 2, 1984.

and (c) the development of policies that will facilitate continual improvement in both patient well-being and outcomes. The third recommendation, encouraging treatment centers to develop policies, is especially important because the discussions involved in the development of these policies will facilitate consideration of the weighty issues that often are hard to face. A major concern in decision making is adequate communication between patients/surrogates, families, significant others, and health care professional (64). Advance care planning should be a component of ongoing end-of-life discussions, which should be a routine, structured part of health care.

INITIATION AND WITHDRAWAL OF DIALYSIS

The ethical issues raised by the use of dialysis are prototypical of those raised by the use of many of the dramatic LSTs developed in the last half of the 20th century. Certainly the ethical issue of starting and stopping dialysis has been a central, often troubling one for physicians, other health professionals, patients, and families. This remarkable life-saving treatment can become a burden. Dependency on a machine for one's survival requires not only medical but also emotional support. The specific issues may vary according to the country involved. The success of dialysis in extending lives has been excellent. With the increased use of dialysis, a wider spectrum of patients with more complex diseases, multisystem complications, and serious comorbid conditions are entering ESRD therapy. Many patients with ESRD also are older. For these and other reasons, therefore, this LST is burdensome for many patients, and the question of whether to withdraw dialysis therapy has been one of the most difficult problems for the kidney health care team (65). Edmund Pellegrino has noted, "Quality of life is a valid criterion for discontinuance of treatment only if it is expressed as such by the patients or his valid surrogates.... Unilateral quality-of-life decisions by health professionals are invalid because of the possibilities of bias such as devaluation of the very young, very old, or disabled, or the growing pressure to contain expenditures at almost any cause" (66).

Professionals have developed guidelines for initiation and withdrawal of dialysis. The *International Yearbook of Nephrology* requested a chapter on termination of dialysis (67). Beginning in 1984, at least eight different medical groups have developed ethical and moral guidelines related to initiation, continuation, and withdrawal of intensive care (68–73).

The IOM committee that studied ESRD (4) identified three major ethical issues: (a) acceptance of patients for treatment, (b) termination of treatment, and (c) ethical questions arising for caregivers who deal with problem patients. The report (4) stated strongly that "the committee, recognizing this concern [an increasing number of patients with limited survival possibilities and relatively poor quality of life], believes that patient acceptance criteria should be medical, not economic,

and based on concern for the best interest of individual patients." The use of age was rejected explicitly as a criterion for accepting patients for ESRD treatment because it is not a predictor of the potential benefit of ESRD treatment for an individual patient. It was acknowledged that comorbidities, at whatever age of occurrence, tend to be "the primary determinants of quality of life and of survival."

The IOM report (4) further stated, "Decision-making about the initiation of treatment should result from informed discussion among the patient, the family, the physician, and other care-givers. Patients with ESRD usually rate their quality-of-life higher than do 'objective' observers." Patient preferences must be respected in decisions about their care. Clinical judgment along with patient or family preferences often may indicate that (compassionate) palliative terminal care is more appropriate than life-extending care. The options provided should not be treatment or abandonment, but rather a choice among different goals of treatment. "Three types of patients raise different ethical problems for clinicians today: 1. [the] non-compliant, self-destructive dialysis patient; 2. [the] hostile, abusive dialysis patient; and 3. [the] self-destructive transplant patient. [The] self-destructive transplant patient whose behavior threatens survival of [the] transplanted kidney may disqualify himself as a candidate for a subsequent transplant if the current organ fails."

The committee recommended that patients, clinicians in adult and pediatric nephrology, and bioethicists should develop guidelines for evaluating patients for whom the burdens of renal replacement therapy may substantially outweigh the benefits. The committee suggested that these guidelines should be flexible and encourage the physician to use discretion in assessing an individual patient. Nephrologists and other clinicians should discuss with all patients with ESRD their wishes about dialysis, cardiopulmonary resuscitation, and other life-sustaining treatments and encourage documented advance directives. Both the American Society of Nephrology and the Renal Physicians Association (74), and the Patient Services Committee of the National Kidney Foundation (75) (Table 100-13) developed guidelines about initiation and withdrawal of dialysis that were responsive to the 1991 IOM study (4).

There has been limited information on how decisions about the withdrawal of dialysis are made. A report prepared for the OTA by a University of Rochester dialysis group (76) reviewed their decision making and available objective data, along with a consideration of social, legal, and ethical tenets. The renal group sought agreement among three qualified physicians and the patient, or the patient's legal next of kin if the patient was not competent to make medical decisions. Autonomy was allowed for the competent patient, and documentation about what the incompetent patient would have wished were he or she competent to decide was required before therapy could be stopped. The Rochester group stated that if there was the slightest concern about litigation if ESRD therapy were to be terminated, the patient would be

TABLE 100-13. *National Kidney Foundation recommendations for initiation and withdrawal of dialysis treatment (75)*

1. Decisions patient specific and culturally, religiously, ethically sensitive decisions. Informed basis by individual patient/surrogate after consultation with care team and others.
2. Unethical to use mandatory standards, including patient's age, life expectancy, quality of life, intellectual or physical limitation, socioeconomic status (SES) or psychological condition to determine initiation or withdrawal.
3. Patient's values preferences goals are major factors in decision-making. Physician has right to refuse to provide treatment, which he/she regards as medically useless, futile or unwarranted (e.g., PVS, severe irreversible dementia).
4. Patient who has capacity to make own decisions has absolute right to make decision not to initiate or withdraw. His/her decision should be controlling.
5. Quality of life, mental functioning used to justify decision (if patient has capacity to make decision) and only patient's perception of his/her quality of life or level of functioning should be utilized.
6. Treatment not legally or ethically required if no substantive benefits.
7. When patient being evaluated for initiation, dialysis should be withheld if: (a) PVS; (b) irreversible, severe mental disorder so patient unable to react or to interact with environment.
8. Benefits, burdens unclear, recommend trial of about 30 days dialysis.
9. Reassessment of all patients after about 90 days.
10. When recommendation to withdraw: (a) adequate diagnosis of PVS; (b) irreversible mental disorder to patient; (c) cannot react or interact with environment
11. When patient or surrogate considers or desires withdrawal and health care team believes intervention measures could reverse decision, appropriate to recommend 30-day trial period or necessary time for assessment of interventions.
12. No federal or state laws or judicial decisions permit health care team and dialysis facilities to unilaterally withdraw therapy from patient who is abusive, persistently disruptive or "nonadherent" to his/her dialysis regimen.
13. Medical personnel treating patient have continuing responsibilities to patient/others after decision is made not to initiate/withdraw dialysis therapy.

treated vigorously, even if the personal or collective wisdom of the medical professionals was that treatment was inappropriate.

An issue of critical concern to patients is their quality of life. Patients, their physicians, and other health care professionals often differ in their view of quality of life. Patients may feel satisfied with a quality of life viewed as marginal by their physicians. Obversely, patients may feel that what their physicians view as a reasonable quality of life is intolerable. Judge Benjamin Cardozo, at the time a member of the New York State Supreme Court, affirmed the broader right to privacy in a statement interpreted by many courts to include

the right to make health care decisions for oneself. In a 1914 case, Justice Cardozo declared that "every human being of adult years and sound mind has a right to determine what shall be done with his own body and cannot be subjected to medical treatment without his consent" (77). This ruling is of special significance because in the second decade of the 20th century, paternalism and beneficence, as they are termed by biomedical ethicists now, were the rule in medical practice. The frequently discussed ethical principle of autonomy requires that the patient be allowed to decide if he or she wishes to make a commitment to such a long-term treatment as chronic dialysis and whether the commitment is worth the trade-off.

Studies of people's perceptions of quality of life, as seen by the health care team and as evaluated by the patient, often show a marked difference in the two viewpoints. Because it is difficult for a patient to comprehend what dialysis therapy may entail, patients frequently may be encouraged to undergo a trial period on dialysis—both to see if it will be beneficial and to allow the patient the opportunity to adapt to the therapy or even to decide that he or she does not wish to endure such demanding therapy.

The Ann Arbor Veterans Administration (VA) Medical Center, Michigan, has an ESRD committee that assesses patients' desires to stop dialysis therapy. Port (40) noted that health professionals have a responsibility not only to aid patients in their rehabilitation, but to provide support for patients and their families should withdrawal from dialysis be desired by or recommended for their patients. Port (40) added, "I believe that very rigid criteria for acceptance to chronic dialysis care may be more harmful by excluding patients who might benefit from therapy than an open acceptance policy that includes the willingness to discontinue dialysis according to a patient's request when there is no hope for reversibility."

A Canadian nephrologist (78) stated that "when patients have decided to start treatment, we should provide every guarantee that if things do not go well, they can discontinue it." This Canadian group believed it should provide appropriate support to deal with the consequences of whatever decision is made. If the treatment is to be withdrawn, the patient and family should have the reassurance that appropriate care and comfort will be provided, and that there is "hope even if it is for those who survive," including help with costs and insurance.

Allocation decisions other than those based purely on medical grounds are made, albeit subtly, in some situations and only in certain countries. Most analyses of ethical issues about ESRD treatment are considered against the background of Western culture and of high-income countries that can afford the high costs and that tend to place great weight on the individual and his or her rights of self-determination or autonomy.

Kidney teams make a major effort to inform patients of all aspects of this complex technology so that they are genuinely informed. The option of withdrawing from treatment, if it becomes too burdensome, usually is given. It is a fact that dialysis can sustain life in patients with kidney failure, but it is not without its drawbacks. Holden (79) stated:

> Even if an individual patient prefers death to a prolonged illness, the decision might be denied by the medical team which does not consider death an option and who fear legal entanglements. Dialysis patients who exercise their right to die must do so with many subtle harassments. For a great majority of patients on dialysis, a meaningful life is an increasingly reachable goal. Each person should be able to choose and should be assisted in making an independent choice by having adequate information and demonstration of emotional support. The presence of alternatives may tend to reinforce an individual's feeling that life, even with difficulty, is worth living as long as one is in control of the human decision-making process.

Because of the limited budget provided in Great Britain to that country's provinces, the ESRD experience in the United Kingdom has differed from that of most other industrialized nations. This is both because Britain has a more stringent budget for health expenditures in general and because funds available for ESRD are especially limited. A prospective study (80) of patients with ESRD in Northern Ireland was conducted during a 3-year period. McGeown and her colleagues followed these patients "until [the] patients' death, acceptance for regular dialysis, or the end of the survey period, and assessed them for their suitability for treatment" at the end of this time. Those patients who were not accepted for ESRD therapy in a situation of limited funding included 37% considered unsuitable because of mental disease, low IQ, or the designation "uncooperative patient," and also patients excluded for medical reasons such as malignancy and diabetes mellitus.

Decision making has evolved from the more paternalistic authoritarian pattern of earlier decades to a situation that provides a greater degree of autonomy for the patient. With this has come a great emphasis on the importance of "informed consent," accompanied by substantive discussions about how informed a patient can be, and what methods can be used to ensure a genuinely well informed patient who is able to make a reasonable decision about his or her care on the basis of available options. Informed consent must involve a presentation of the medical situation in terms the patient can comprehend. In this context, it is helpful for the physician to ask the patient to relate back his or her understanding of the information presented, and then for the physician to correct any misunderstandings.

Because of both the stress of the medical environment and the awe in which physicians often are held, patients may not "hear" the facts even when they are stated clearly. Treatment often is continued because of the perceived threat of a costly malpractice suit. Concerns about possible litigation and medical liability have resulted in major efforts by physicians and other members of the delivery team to prescribe or to continue expensive, sometimes futile treatment to avoid litigation, regardless of the cost of that treatment. Frequently, this is the situation even when the physician recognizes that cost containment should be a part of his or her responsibility.

KIDNEY TRANSPLANTATION

Numerous ethical issues arise in the field of organ transplantation. One of the most prominent issues, which matches in complexity the difficulties faced by the Seattle Policy and Admissions Committee for the field of dialysis in the 1960s, is how to allocate some very scarce resources, donor kidneys. There is a marked shortage of both living related organ donors and of cadaver donors. The latter source is problematic, because the availability of cadaver kidneys means that someone has to have died, and that someone usually is a young, healthy person injured or killed violently. Sir Roy Calne, the British transplantation surgeon, has said, "Most transplants are performed with organs taken from recently dead patients; there is therefore in every case an associated tragedy to permit life for the recipient. . . . I think the necessary tragedy to rescue a dying patient is a distressing concept for all transplant surgeons" (81). With stringent seat belt laws, efforts to diminish the incidence of drunken driving, and, until November 1995, lower highway speed limits, there has been a leveling off in the number of cadaver organs available for transplantation, even though aggressive public education programs stress the need for organ donation

The recruitment of organ donors is inadequate to provide the kidneys needed for the increasing numbers of patients on transplant waiting lists. Because of the limited number of donor organs, the ethical principle of justice looms large in the allocation of this scarce resource. Waiting lists have been the prominent means for assigning priorities in the United States. Ethicists periodically suggest using a lottery as a means to disperse scarce resources such as donor kidneys. The original means for allocating the scarce resource of hemodialysis by the Seattle Admissions and Policy Committee was troubling to many philosophers and theologians. As a result, it contributed significantly to the dialogues that gave rise to the field of biomedical ethics.

The suggestion that health care ethics committees (82) identify factors that could affect the success or failure of transplanting donor organs recalls the discomfort that decisions by the Seattle committee generated for its members. Attempts to judge the lifestyle choices that put people at increased risk for disease have resulted in efforts to charge the costs of these risks to the risk taker. Plato wrote that individuals have a responsibility to live in a manner that prevents illness. Recent suggestions have been made that "any strategy to allocate medical resources must take into account the choices of individuals that put them at heightened risk for diseases or conditions which necessitate costly medical intervention" (83). The potential use of xenotransplantation to produce solid organs for transplantation has been discussed for over a decade and recently cloning has been considered also (84).

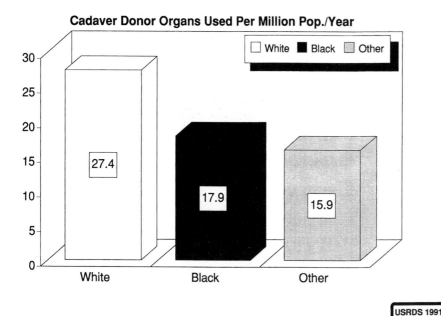

Cadaver Donor Organs Used Per Million Pop./Year

FIG. 100-4. Cadaveric donation by race: donor organs per U.S. population by race, 1989. (From U.S. Renal Data System. *USRDS 1991 annual report.* Bethesda, MD: National Institutes of Health, National Institute of Diabetes and Digestive and Kidney Diseases, 1991.)

Efforts to increase the number of cadaver donors have had limited success. Even when potential donor families understand the need for organ donation, they often have emotional reservations that prevent them from donating organs of their relative. Although blacks have a higher incidence of ESRD, they do not donate organs proportionally (Fig. 100-4). Because of the high incidence of ESRD among members of minority groups, but the relatively low number of minority kidney donors (United Network for Organ Sharing figure of approximately 9% black cadaver kidneys donated), there has been an attempt to increase donations by educational programs in churches and on radio and television. Although, in the past, kidney donors older than age 55 years had not been considered acceptable, the shortage of donor organs has led numerous transplantation surgeons and physicians to consider compromises in accepting older donors (85–88).

Among minorities, and especially those with low incomes, there exists the fear that their severely ill relative may not be given adequate care because of the possibility of an organ donation (83). A pilot project conducted by Callender and colleagues (89) indicated that the three reasons given by African American respondents for not donating kidneys (and for not filling out donor cards) were (a) religion or superstition, (b) a lack of trust in health care providers along with the suspicion that the potential donor might not receive adequate care in the hospital, and (c) the potential donor's being reminded of death. Negative connotations also were associated with cross-sex and cross-race kidney transplantations. Similar beliefs were reported as the reasons why two Hispanic adolescents with ESRD initially rejected the option of receiving a kidney transplant (89). The 17-year-old Ecuadorian woman and 17-year-old Argentinean man each were given psychiatric counseling in an effort to change their fears and accept a kidney transplant.

The shortage of donor kidneys is of such concern that new types of donors and new means of acquiring kidneys have been suggested: expanding the age limits for donors, loosening other criteria for kidney harvesting, and having states enact presumed consent laws. Presumed consent assumes that every person who dies would be presumed to consent to donate his or her organs unless the person or his or her family have indicated an unwillingness to donate. Walter Land (90) of Germany reported that although several European countries have presumed consent laws, they are not enforced, except in Austria. In addition, he believes the new European Community will not keep presumed consent. It also has been suggested in discussions by numerous nephrologists that a stipend be provided to donor families after organ donation. This suggestion has raised an ethical controversy, because many consider organ donation to be an altruistic act, and payment for organ donation could be coercive, especially for those who have a limited income.

The use of age as a criterion for selecting transplant recipients is a subject of controversy, as it is for other types of medical treatment (91,92). The 1984 Massachusetts Task Force report (93) suggested that transplantation should be made available to those who would benefit the most, especially in terms of posttransplantation longevity and the potential for rehabilitation. On the other hand, the Federal Age Discrimination Act of 1975 [codified at 42 USCA 6101 (1985)] prohibits "discrimination on the basis of age in programs or activities receiving federal assistance."

In Norway, unlike in the United States, transplantation is the treatment of choice for elderly patients. Fauchald and coworkers (94) reported that not only were the elderly recipients of kidney transplants in Norway, but that elderly donor kidneys were used for transplantation. Were the Norwegian approach to be applied in the United States, not only might there be an increase in the supply of donor kidneys, there might be an increase in the length of the transplantation waiting list as elderly recipients are entered.

Because of the shortage of cadaver kidneys, the transplantation community, including organizations such as the American Society of Transplant Surgeons, has agreed that not more than 5% of patients receiving cadaver kidneys should be foreign nationals. Foreign kidney transplant candidates who arrive in the United States with a bona fide living related donor usually will be accepted. However, ethical dilemmas arise when foreign patients arrive with a stated living unrelated donor or when there is a suspicion that the living related donor is not an actual blood relative. The debate about the treatment of foreign nationals may easily become chauvinistic, and one might ask whether justice is defined by national borders.

Living Donor Renal Transplantation

Living organ donation usually makes us think of voluntary and altruistic donation of a kidney to a close relative. The dilemmas raised by donation of an organ by a living relative, however, pose troublesome moral, ethical, and religious questions for society. These questions are even more troubling with regard to living unrelated organ donation. Renal transplantation using living donors who are not blood relatives has been considered as a possible solution to the shortage of kidneys available for transplantation. There are issues generic for both living related and for living unrelated donors: informed consent, donor autonomy, the absence of coercion, the decision to give or not to give a kidney, health risks, follow-up care for the donor, mechanisms for dealing with the donor's expenses and their reimbursement, and the impact of donation on the donor and on the donor's family.

Reports of the use of living unrelated donors, especially when tainted with commercialism, raise further issues: (a) the relationship of the donor to the recipient—emotionally related such as a spouse, a close friend, or a distant relative; (b) altruism; (c) conflict of interest; and (d) financial exploitation. Spital and Spital (95) polled a diverse group of health care professionals to determine their views about kidney donation from a variety of people, both living related and living unrelated potential donors. This poll showed that a very high percentage of those who care for patients with ESRD would consider the use of living unrelated donors.

In 1983, a Virginia physician formed an organization, the International Kidney Exchange, for the purchase of kidneys from living donors, primarily poor people, many from low-income countries (96,97). His plan was to sell these kidneys to patients needing transplants. The Virginia physician (whose license to practice medicine had been revoked in 1979 after a Medicare/Medicaid fraud conviction) said that a "monetary incentive system" might improve the shortage of transplantable organs. Moral outrage for both ethical and medical reasons was expressed by the National Kidney Foundation. To outlaw the sale of organs, Congressman Albert Gore, Jr.

(Democrat, Tennessee), introduced a bill (HR 4080) into the U.S. House of Representatives. Within the next year, Senator Edward M. Kennedy introduced a U.S. Senate bill to establish a study group to look into the potential for a national organ procurement system. The concept of the poor (notably the poor of developing countries) selling a kidney to the highest bidder sent shock waves through the transplant community and through the governments of high-income, developed countries. This has resulted in the development of guidelines and regulations, legislation, and means of discipline, as well as a spate of publications and conferences. Professional societies, both national and international, have made strong statements against financial exploitation of the poor "potential" donor. Other ethical issues in this sphere include the use of organ donors not competent to provide an autonomous decision: anencephalic infants (98), the mentally retarded (99,100), prisoners who are considered to be unavoidably coerced, and patients who are in a persistent vegetative state.

An innovative approach to another major issue related to the escalating costs of health care has been taken in the Oregon Senate. This plan for Medicaid recipients was applied to 100% of Oregon residents with incomes below the poverty line. The Oregon Senate and the Oregon Health Service Commission are set priorities for health care among a list of 709 treatment categories (101). Under the proposed plan, although a larger number of residents would be covered for health care, a smaller number of treatment categories are covered, a number projected to be 587. The effect of this experiment on expensive LSTs such as ESRD treatment, as contrasted to the impact on primary health care, is of great interest for nephrology. Earlier, the Oregon legislature decided not to fund solid organ transplantations other than kidney transplantation so that there would be funds available for prenatal and well-baby care (102).

There are considerable differences in the moral, ethical, and religious views of citizens from different nations of the world, differences between the views of those from high-income countries and those from low-income countries, as well as differences in resources, especially financial resources. These are reflected in the GDP per capita and in health expenditures per capita, the latter frequently reflecting national priorities. There are questions to be raised about the role of organizations in responding to these ethical dilemmas: professional societies, health professionals, organ procurement organizations, the media, organized religion, and academics from the disciplines of medicine, ethics, and philosophy.

These topics will never be ones for which there are simple, ready solutions. One must learn toleration for the disparate views of people from varied cultures and subcultures with vastly different bases of religion, ethics, and moral decision making. A review of some approaches to living unrelated donors can provide not only an understanding of how different cultures view these issues, but insight into the types of issues that may be faced in times of shortage, even by high-income countries. Five categories of living organ donation are

(a) living related, (b) emotionally related, (c) altruistic, (d) "rewarded" gifting, and (e) rampant commercialism (103). The first and occasionally the second form have been acceptable in the Western industrialized milieu. To varying degrees, the latter three are considered repugnant and unethical in Western terms. Dossetor (104) noted that living unrelated organ donation can be considered morally unacceptable. Living unrelated organ donation as a form of "rewarded giving" for countries whose economies do not allow other options may present the only possibility for a patient with ESRD to receive a kidney transplant. Further, living unrelated organ donation is an expression of toleration of marketplace commercialism for organ brokering to gain profit.

India: A Case Study of Living Unrelated Organ Donation

The two sides of a debate that has occurred in India are prototypical of the discussions aroused by the concept of living unrelated organ donation. India spent the equivalent of U.S. $3 of public funds per capita on health in 1987 (20). Yadav (27) listed Indian health priorities in descending order as follows: (a) family welfare and population control; (b) communicable diseases; (c) maternal and child health; (d) nutrition; (e) noncommunicable diseases; and (6) high-technology areas, which include transplantation and dialysis. In 1988 to 1989, the Indian health sector allocated approximately 542 crores, equivalent to approximately U.S. $374 million (1 crore = 10,000 rupees; 1988 exchange rate: 14.48 rupees/ 1 U.S. dollar), to the two centrally governed institutions that fund transplant programs, which funded five viable renal transplant programs. Nearly all transplantations are confined to the private sector, state-aided long-term hemodialysis is unavailable, and indigent patients without donors are sent home to die. Although India has no renal failure registry, it is estimated that there are approximately 80,000 new ESRD cases a year. A market survey by Parry and Company (105), conducted in 1988, concluded that with the 613 dialysis machines imported since 1971, 1,500 dialyses could be performed per day if all machines were working. This would allow biweekly dialysis for 3 months on average for a maximum number of 18,000 patients a year—approximately 22.5% of Indian patients with ESRD. Approximately 2,000 transplantations—approximately 2.5% of new ESRD cases—are performed annually. This market survey estimated that the cost of treating new patients in a fashion similar to Western treatment patterns would be approximately $20 billion a year.

Reddy and colleagues (25) commented, "ESRD patients will not accept the answer that occidental ethics and morals prevent us from performing paid donor transplantation. What about our conscience and ethics? Do we buy or let die?" They further argued that it is necessary to strike a balance among ethical, social, commercial, and scientific values, and render justice to all parties. They stated that "every system has merits as well as scope for corruption . . . people are at fault, not the system."

Yadav (27) noted that the Indian Kidney Foundation is working to eliminate the commercial procurement of kidneys and that India has many more pressing health problems to undertake before the nation can assign priority to sophisticated modalities such as transplantation. Reddy and coauthors (25) noted that "money often changes hands between related donors in India. . . . if commercial transplant [takes place] between relatives, what's wrong with unrelated?" They noted that there are frequent advertisements in the national press, both from patients requiring kidneys and from people willing to give kidneys—all for financial regard.

Others take a different view, however. Professor Abouna, in a letter to the *Journal of the Association of Physicians of India* quoted by Dr. M. K. Mani (23), wrote that living unrelated organ donation is a practice abhorrent to the conscience of civilized society; it causes patient care to be relegated to laws of the marketplace; unscrupulous brokers and methods are reminiscent of the slave trade; the welfare of donors and their families is not safeguarded; transplantation results are inferior; and the practice is a disincentive to cadaver and to living related kidney donation.

In 1993, both Houses of the Indian Parliament (106) cleared a Transplantation of Human Organs (THO) bill, which aimed to curb the burgeoning trade in human organs. The bill was enacted into law in 1994, thus banning the commercial trading of organs:

1. The law prohibits any commercial trading in human organs.
2. The law allows removal of organs for therapeutic purposes only (2 to 7 years' imprisonment and a fine of R10,000 to 20,000 are imposed for any individual involved in the supply of human organs for payment).
3. The law, for the first time, recognizes brainstem death as a criterion for removal of human organs for treatment; recognizes and defines a brainstem-dead person; and permits organ removal only when death has been certified by a four-member board of medical experts.
4. The law does not allow living organ donation for transplantation into a recipient unless the living donor is a "near" relative (e.g., spouse, sibling, parent, offspring).
5. The law requires special approval by an authorization committee appointed by the state or central government for donations based on affection, attachment, or other special reasons. Kumar (106) notes that for India, there is "a serious stumbling block facing cadaver transplant [because of] religious taboos and beliefs that relatives hold, [since] removal of body organs is often viewed as body mutilation."

This brief description of India's problems gives a sense of the dilemmas faced in that country. Different authors (107) provided differing rationalizations, suggested programs to limit abuse, and gave suggestions about how to benefit both the recipient and the donor who is paid the "solatium." Thiagarajan and colleagues (107) concluded that "as a transplant team, we sincerely believe that the values gained greatly overshadow the values lost."

In addition to the ethical dilemma related to the use of living unrelated organ donation is the difficult issue of commercialism. Abhorrent in Western societies, this practice in (108) reported on the status of 130 patients from the United Arab Emirates and Oman who elected to go to Bombay between June 1984 and May 1988 to buy kidneys from living unrelated donors for U.S. $2,600 to $3,300. The ethical principles of autonomy and informed consent need to be considered in such instances where patients were "not properly instructed about their treatment." In addition, inadequate information was provided to the original renal team of the transplant recipient when the patient returned to his own country. Furthermore, appropriate criteria for transplantation were not strictly followed, and patients were exposed to severe infections—the most common cause of the 25 deaths among these patients.

Other Views on Organ Donation

International and in Polls

When the commercialization of organ donations appeared to be on the rise and Western governments were enacting laws prohibiting the selling of organs, Kuwait enacted a Transplantation Law (No. 55) in 1987. This law allowed and defined procedures for the removal of organs from brain-dead subjects, and in its Article 7, considered the buying and selling of organs by any means, or for any material consideration, as a criminal offense. Kuwait became the first country in the Middle East to enact such a far-reaching and timely law. Abouna and colleagues (109) commented as follows: The "current practice of trading in human organs, using the poor and needy as victim donors, is medically, morally, and ethically objectionable." The practice has been condemned by the Transplantation Society, the American Society of Transplant Surgeons, and the European, British, and Canadian transplantation societies. In addition, as has been noted, it has been declared illegal in Kuwait. However, in the Middle East, especially in Egypt and Iraq, and in India and the Philippines, the practice of wealthy patients buying human kidneys from the poor has produced a lucrative market for brokers, middlemen, medical practitioners, and private hospitals. In 1987, the Islamic Organization for Medical Sciences, Kuwait (109), declared that "buying and selling of human organs was not allowed in Islam." The organization added, "It is clear to us that trading in human organs as a marketable commodity from the poor to the rich has no merit in a civilized and just society."

Spital (110) conducted a survey of U.S. transplantation centers concerning views on organ donation. There was a 59% response rate from the 169 centers to which questionnaires were mailed. Of the types of living donors that the responding centers would consider using, spouses were listed by 76% of centers; adult friends, by 48%; monozygotic twin minors, by 64%; and closely related nontwin minors, by 43%. The minimum donor age rated acceptable was 16, plus or minus 3 years. Many centers expressed reservations about donor sources such as minors and unrelated friends, and indicated that such donors seldom were used.

These concepts are controversial and must be addressed not only by physicians but by society, so that a code of behavior acceptable to physicians, potential donors, and patients can be developed. The possible increase in transplantation rates if living unrelated donor organs were used would not become apparent until this option was both widely available and adequately publicized. There is a concern that if living unrelated donors were used, there would be a drop in the altruistic donation of both cadaver kidneys and living related kidneys.

A broad view of medical policy suggests that it would be more beneficial, as well as more cost effective, if the emphasis of health care was placed increasingly on health maintenance and disease prevention, in addition to treatment. The ideal would be to arrest the progression of renal disease, or to prevent it, thereby eliminating ESRD and the need for donor kidneys. Thus, there is a moral imperative to support research to prevent or arrest kidney diseases that progress to ESRD. Stricter highway and road regulations affecting drinking and driving and more stringent speed limits have decreased deaths from automobile accidents, with a resultant decrease in the number of cadaver donors. In the United States, the Congress has just removed the federal speed limits, which were lowered in early 1970s, and returned speed limit regulation to the states. D'Apice and Walker (111) at Royal Melbourne Hospital, Australia, stated that "in spite of considerable efforts to increase the retrieval of these organs, the success of campaigns to lower the road toll has been reflected in a falling cadaveric transplantation rate and an increasing waiting list." Furthermore, most potential recipients have either no living relative or no suitable living related donor. The results of limitations on the number of transplants are a progressive overburdening of dialysis services and an increased waiting time for a kidney transplant.

Religious Views

Religious convictions may affect a person's willingness to donate organs or accept transplantation as a therapy. Although the United States is becoming increasing secular, it continues to have a great diversity of religions and religious sects. The symposium "Ethics, Justice, and Commerce in Transplantation: A Global View" (22), held in Canada in 1988, addressed ethical issues of unrelated organ donation. This conference also surveyed representatives of the major religions of the world about their religion's views of organ donation.

The following are some of the brief comments presented at the Canadian symposium by representatives of the major world religions. Islamic transplantation ethics, presented by Sahin (112), include the Koran's view that life is sacred, a gift from God, to be respected and preserved. Islam emphasizes the promotion of good health and disease prevention and considers that the "donor has to consent to the procedure by his own free will and . . . no fee is allowed to the donor."

According to Namihira (113), the gravity that the Japanese attribute to injuring a dead body is such that it still is difficult to obtain consent from bereaved families for organ donation (or for dissection for pathology or anatomy). The reason for refusal is fear of injuring the dead person's *itai* ("remains") by his or her own will. The Hindu (26), in considering cadaver organ donation, adhere to the basic theme of the Hindu religion: to help others who are suffering. Hindu mythology accepts the use of parts of the human body for the benefit of other humans. The Christian view, as expressed by Father Scorsone of the Roman Catholic Diocese of Toronto (114), is that giving organs for transplantation is both legitimate and a last act of generosity and love that the "person gone before us can offer someone still in the world."

The Jewish perspective on organ transplantation was presented by Rabbi Bilka (115) of Ottawa, who noted that the story of Adam and Eve suggests that surgical intervention is sanctioned and prescribed only if there is no other alternative. By extrapolation, he noted that transplantation procedures are not to be undertaken unless there is no other alternative. There is no obligation for an individual to take the risk of donating an organ to save someone else. "As long as in saving one life we do not destroy another life and the life-saving works within the context of moral and ethical responsibility, there is no concern that this is a denial of God's will." Sugunasiri, President of the Buddhist Council of Canada, delineated the Buddhist view of the dead body (116). Buddhism views transplantation of any part of the body as merely an act of technology and the rejection of an organ as a reflection of mental as well as material incompatibility.

LEGAL ISSUES

Background

The first successful kidney transplantations used a kidney from a healthy identical twin that was donated to the twin with chronic renal failure, and questions of "assault and battery" in the performance of surgery on the healthy twin were raised. The physicians and administrators of the Peter Bent Brigham Hospital (now the Brigham and Women's Hospital) in Boston obtained legal counsel and judicial opinions before operating on the healthy twin. At the same time, incidentally, ethical concerns that preceded the nascent field of biomedical ethics by a decade were expressed. Even today, legal issues intertwined with ethical issues continue to capture the concern of nephrologists and transplantation surgeons, as well as of politicians, lawyers, and health policy experts.

Concerns about potential liability suits have resulted in either the practice of very "defensive" medicine or in physicians dropping out of practice in high-risk fields, often the ones that have the highest malpractice insurance premiums. Taylor (117), President of Louis Harris and Associates, noted, "Nowhere else is the cost of malpractice insurance and the additional costs of unnecessary defensive medicine aimed

at frustrating lawsuits, nearly as high as here [in the United States]" (117). As Reiser (118) declared, "The current legal climate, rather than creating a helpful prudence toward others that makes doctors mindful of their responsibility toward patients (which law at its best induces), has instead become intimidating and encourages a damaging and self-protective response by physicians."

Legal instruments, often called *advance directives*, which include living wills and durable powers of attorney for health care, have attracted particular attention in the United States, especially since the passage of the Patient Self-Determination Act (PSDA) (119,120) sponsored by Senators John C. Danforth (Republican, Missouri) and Patrick Moynihan (Democrat, New York) and Congressman Sander Levin (Democrat, Mississippi). The PSDA became a provision of the Omnibus Budget Reconciliation Act of 1990 (121). Under the provisions of this act, by December 1, 1991, the HCFA was required to release regulations for all Medicare/Medicaid–eligible facilities such as nursing homes and hospitals. These regulations were to indicate how patients are to be made aware of the state laws and statutes about advance directives at the time of their admission to the health facility. Section 4751(a) of the PSDA requires (121) "that the State, acting through a State agency, association, or other private nonprofit entity, develop a written description of the law of the State (whether statutory or as recognized by the courts of the State) concerning advance directives that would be distributed by providers or organizations under the requirements of the [the Act]."

The five requirements for all Medicare- and Medicaid-funded facilities that must be met according to the regulations are that (a) written information be provided at the time of admission about "an individual's right under State law" to make decisions about his or her own medical care; (b) written policies and procedures about advance directives be maintained; (c) documentation shall be included in the person's medical record about whether an advance directive has been executed; (d) compliance with state law requirements shall be ensured; and (e) education about advance directives is to be provided for staff members and the community (122). Both before and after the PSDA was enacted into law, there have been numbers of publications about advance directives from professional and voluntary associations, such as the American Hospital Association (123), the American Bar Association (122), the Catholic Health Association of the United States, and the Society for the Right to Die, and from states, such as the publication from the Research Division of the Maryland Department of Legislative Reference (124).

Apart from the PSDA, the usefulness of a living will and durable power of attorney has been emphasized in the public arena by many legal cases in which evidence of patients' wishes about the use of LSTs has affected the continuation of high-technology treatment. Cases such as that of Nancy Cruzan (125,126), whose parents wanted to have her gastrostomy tube removed after she had remained in a persistent vegetative state for more than 7 years, and of Karen Ann Quinlan (127), whose parents obtained a court order for her respirator to be removed after she had been unconscious for more than 13 months, have focused public attention on the need for advance directives. After Karen Ann Quinlan's respirator was removed, she lived on for more than 9 years because, contrary to the expectations of her physicians, she was not ventilator dependent.

In the field of dialysis, questions have emerged about who should be treated and when treatment can be withdrawn—a reflection of the concerns of patients who desire to maintain autonomy in health care decisions and who may wish to determine their "right to die." Because of the litigious nature of contemporary American society, and the fact that LSTs are available to high percentages of patients in high-income, developed countries, some of the decisions about treatment have come before judges and into the courts. The United States has the highest number of patients with ESRD on dialysis therapy, and significant numbers of nephrologists are concerned about the possible legal implications of withdrawing dialysis therapy.

American nephrologists are wary about possible lawsuits, albeit the only three dialysis-related cases that reached higher courts were right-to-die cases. To understand the concerns of American physicians with the legal situation, it is helpful to understand that (17,128) the potential for lawsuits is raised more frequently in the United States, which has more lawyers than any other country in the world. The American Bar Association (129) estimates there were over a million (1,000,440) practicing lawyers as of June 30, 2000 (129a), an 18% increase since December 1993.* These numbers, as well as the greater use of the law for a myriad of transactions by Americans, highlight the reasons why the American system exercises its litigational capabilities.

In the field of transplantation, laws and regulations have been passed in the United States both to facilitate the procurement of organs for transplantation and to regulate conditions surrounding procurement and distribution. The Uniform Anatomical Gift Act, Uniform Determination of Death Act, and National Organ Transplantation Act of 1984 set regulations and criteria relevant to organ procurement at the

state and federal levels. In the United States, provisions of the Civil Rights Act of 1964 about equitable access are considered applicable to scarce organs. The shortage of organs for transplantation requires innovative means for the acquisition of increased numbers of kidneys. The suggestion that kidneys be harvested from living unrelated donors and the placement of advertisements offering kidneys for sale, primarily in the newspapers of low-income countries, shocked the high-income countries. After evidence of the use of living unrelated donor organs became available, many countries passed laws forbidding it or providing penalties if living unrelated donor organs are used. Nevertheless, there are still countries that allow the sale of kidneys by unrelated donors.

In the American legal system, three cases involving patients with ESRD reached state supreme courts, and the cases of two patients with ESRD were heard in lower courts. The former cases applied to patients' rights to withdraw from treatment or their right to die, and the latter cases pertained to the right to be treated—even when the health professionals determined that the patients' disruptive behavior interfered with proper functioning of the dialysis unit. The latter two cases and the British cases (see later) show the problems that develop when patients are unable to comply with the rigorous requirements of ESRD treatment, both on the renal units and in adhering to a therapeutic regimen, such as immunosuppressive therapy for transplant recipients.

Termination of Dialysis: Three State Supreme Court Cases

One of the ethical issues addressed earlier is the right of a patient to determine his or her own treatment, including the right to forgo treatment. This right also allows a patient to designate a surrogate decision maker, should the patient no longer be able to make medical decisions. The issue of termination of dialysis, either in comatose patients at the request of families or in the case of a blind diabetic patient who found existence too painful to continue, is addressed in three state supreme court cases.

The cases emphasize the anguish suffered by families when they must resort to the legal system to obtain what they consider compassionate care for their relative. The dichotomy between allowing a "good death" to occur versus prolongation of the dying process is poignantly evident in such ethical dilemmas. They show the legal and ethical issues to be faced when termination of dialysis treatment is determined to be medically appropriate. As with many aspects of ESRD treatment, the decisions to terminate dialysis are prototypical for other LSTs, especially in situations where patients have lost the mental capacity to make their own treatment decisions.

"To what extent should aggressive medical treatment be administered to preserve life after life itself, for reasons beyond anyone's control, has become irreversibly burdensome?" This question was asked by Judge Christopher Armstrong of the

---

*There is no single comprehensive source of current information about the number of lawyers in the world or in individual countries. Legal practitioners in different parts of the world have different responsibilities and different titles. To obtain a sense of the distribution throughout the world, an analysis was made of the 1978 reference Law and Judicial Systems of Nations (3rd ed.) (128). Practitioners of the law profession in different countries have markedly different responsibilities and titles. Of the 141 countries listed, according to the limited data available, 6 had no equivalent of lawyers, 65 had numbers listed, and 70 countries had no numbers listed. Thus, in this 1978 publication, there were approximately 754,691 lawyers, or equivalents, reported, of which the United States had 424,980 (December 1976), or 56%. The next largest groups of legal practitioners, in descending order of numbers and ranging from 40,000 to 16,000, were in the United Kingdom, Italy, Hungary, Philippines, Mexico, Argentina, and Egypt. (Canada and France did not report numbers.) The World Jurist Association (formerly the World Peace Through Law Center), Washington, D.C., reported in April 1996 that the fourth edition of their reference should go to the printer in late 1996.

Massachusetts Appellate Court, who heard the case of Earle Spring (130). Massachusetts requires that a judge approve the withdrawal of any life support system once it has been started. After judicial approval to stop dialysis was given, "right to lifers" protested the decision on Spring's return to the nursing home. Spring's wife of 55 years and his only son had requested that dialysis be discontinued because the 77-year-old man suffered from advanced senility in addition to ESRD. It took more than 15 months of hearings, appeals, reversals, and stays before the Massachusetts Supreme Judicial Court issued its opinion, upholding a probate court judgment that the temporary guardian not authorize further life-prolonging treatments. During this extended period, and before the final opinion was handed down, Earle Spring died.

Judge Armstrong of the Massachusetts Court made note of the "fearful strain" placed on Mr. Spring's family by the lengthy judicial process, and emphasized the need for "expediting such cases." The decision also noted that even a court order cannot guarantee total immunity to health professionals, because even when a physician makes a valid decision that a given treatment is not appropriate, there remains the hazard "that in subsequent litigation the omission will be found to have been negligent" (131). Earle Spring's nephrologist opined, "The way I practice medicine is very much determined by what the courts tell me to do."

The case of Peter Cinque, heard in the New York Supreme Court (132), illustrates the major efforts that patients or their families may have to exert when they wish to end treatment. Cinque, a 41-year-old, blind, diabetic amputee undergoing thrice-weekly dialysis, had numerous complications and pain that required medication. While still conscious, Cinque requested that dialysis be stopped and that he be allowed to return home to die. After his nephrologist and hospital authorities agreed with his request that he be allowed to stop dialysis, his treatment was continued. Reversing the terms of their agreement to withdraw dialysis, the hospital obtained a court order compelling that Cinque continue dialysis. Cinque then had respiratory arrest, became comatose, and was put on a respirator. His guardian *ad litem* recommended that his request to end treatment be granted, and the trial court ruled that the hospital should discontinue treatment.

The legal guardian of James Robert Smith (133), a comatose patient on hemodialysis, petitioned on Smith's behalf that dialysis be discontinued after the family, his physician, the hospital staff, and the court-appointed religious visitor unanimously agreed that Smith would have chosen this course had he been conscious and able to make his own decision. The New Mexico Right-to-Die Act of 1977 provided that a physician would be immune from legal liability if he or she honored a patient's written instructions directing that "maintenance medical treatment" not be used, if the patient had been certified terminally ill in compliance with the act. After the lower court ruled that dialysis could be discontinued, the Supreme Court of New Mexico reversed the ruling in an opinion stating that New Mexico had no statute

empowering a guardian to request or authorize ending dialysis of an incompetent person. Subsequently, the New Mexico legislature amended the Right-to-Die Act to allow a physician to remove life-sustaining medical treatment from an incompetent patient certified as terminally ill, or in an irreversible coma, if all family members who could be reached after reasonable effort agree that the patient, if competent, would have chosen such a course.

Noncompliant Patients

Adaptations to the chronicity of treatments such as dialysis are difficult because such patients suddenly have lost control of their lives. In different ways, patients try to maintain some degree of control within the stringent requirements of limitations on diet and fluid intake along with devoting a significant amount of time to dialysis treatment. Renal caregivers frequently attribute lapses from the tight controls imposed by dialysis schedules to "noncompliance." Haney has opined, "all noncompliance, resistance or aggressiveness can be perceived as an attempt on the part of the patient to either maintain or regain some semblance of control over her (his) life" (134–137). A group of experts (138) in patient behavior and compliance who have studied these issues for decades note that "the attitude of a patient towards himself and the illness often predicts behavior; in fact one of the best predictors of compliance is the patient's performance during a previous or concurrent illness." Haynes et al. (138) have provided a generic list of recommendations for improvement of compliance in an ambulatory setting: (a) be alert to possibility of noncompliance; (b) try to enlist family support; (c) take a sociobehavioral patient inventory; (d) try to contract with the patient for a therapeutic partnership; (e) educate, motivate, strengthen the patient; (f) keep medical regimen ritualized and simple; and (g) tailor appointments to the patient's needs.

Chronic dialysis teams occasionally have found that continued treatment of a disruptive patient interferes with the ability of the team to provide care to other patients on the dialysis unit. Two American cases illustrate legal actions for such problem patients and the outcomes. The first case, *Payton v. Weaver* (139), was instituted by Brenda Marie Payton, who alleged that her physician and the hospital had wrongfully refused to provide her with regular hemodialysis treatment. Payton, in addition to a confessed addiction to heroin and barbiturates for more than 15 years, had alcohol, weight, and emotional problems. In her lucid moments, she was noted to be marvelously sympathetic and articulate, but her behavior at other times made it extremely difficult to provide the medical care she needed.

Dr. Weaver, who had treated her since 1975, sent her a letter stating that he would no longer permit her to be treated in the outpatient dialysis unit because of her persistent uncooperative and antisocial behavior for more than 3 years, her persistent refusal to adhere to reasonable constraints of hemodialysis, the dietary schedules, and medical prescriptions, her use of barbiturates and other illicit drugs, and because all this resulted in disruption of the program.

After the County Superior Court denied her writ of mandate, the patient appealed. The Court of Appeal held that (a) no legal obligation to provide dialysis treatment arose from the physician's decision to abandon the patient only after due notice and ample opportunity had been afforded to secure the presence of other medical attendants; and (b) although ESRD is an extremely serious and dangerous disease, which can create imminent danger of loss of life if not properly treated, the need for continued treatment is not a condition qualifying for mandatory emergency services.

The court held that because "a hospital contains a unique, or scarce, medical resource needed to preserve life, it is arguably in the nature of a public service enterprise" and should not be permitted to withhold its services arbitrarily or without reasonable cause. The court recognized that a patient's disruptive conduct may constitute good cause for an individual hospital to refuse continued treatment and that it would be unfair to impose serious inconvenience on a hospital simply because such a patient selected it. However, the court recognized that there exists a collective responsibility on the part of providers of scarce health resources in a community, enforceable through equity, to share the burden of difficult patients over time, through an appropriately devised contingency plan. The trial court found that Brenda's disruptive conduct was, at least to some extent, in her power to control or modify, and, by implication at least, that absent such control or modification, her conduct was of such a nature as to justify respondent hospitals refusing her access to their facilities. Various types of conservatorships were discussed and the appeals court suggested that the trial court's order requiring Dr. Weaver to provide dialysis treatment to Brenda, pending appeal, remain in effect until the court's decision became final. The local networks' dialysis units informally arranged to provide dialysis care for Brenda in rotation so that the burden would not fall unduly on a single unit. (Within a month of the time this arrangement was made, Brenda Payton was hit by a bus and killed, in September 1982.)

The responsibility of a patient to participate in his or her own care was the issue raised in the suit, *Brown v. Bower* (140). Michael Brown was a noncompliant patient who was treated at the University of Mississippi Medical Center until he voluntarily left Jackson to be treated at Pascagoula, Mississippi. This 28-year-old patient's dialysis treatment had started when he was 18 years of age. From the beginning of his treatment, he was unable to adapt to the constraints imposed by his condition. He failed to cooperate with his treatment regimen, and he abused both drugs and alcohol. His two renal transplants failed because he did not take his immunosuppressive medications. He was given an opportunity to try peritoneal dialysis, but this too was unsuccessful because of his failure to follow necessary instructions. Brown persistently failed to comply with the prescribed dietary and fluid restrictions, thus

contributing to numerous medical crises. His behavior in the dialysis unit was abusive and threatening, compromising the delivery of care to other patients.

When Brown sought treatment at the University of Mississippi Medical Center on his return to Jackson, Dr. Bower refused, and Brown was returned to Pascagoula by ambulance for each dialysis session. The Fifth Circuit Court order mandated that Brown's right to treatment was conditional on his improved cooperation with treatment, that he be accompanied by some member of his family during the entire time he was receiving treatment, that he should not engage in abusive speech or conduct while receiving treatment, and that he should conform to the reasonable regimen for self-treatment and diet prescribed by the treating physician.

The aspect of Brown's defense that stood firm was his entitlement to treatment at the University of Mississippi under the Hill-Burton Act (42 USC S291 et seq), requiring that services be made available to all persons residing in the area of hospitals that had accepted federal grants. The Court concluded that Brown had not established a right to treatment against Dr. Bower, but that the University of Mississippi Medical Center was obligated to provide dialysis treatment under the Community Assurance required by the Hill-Burton Act. Brown, like Payton, met a violent death—in an automobile accident.

There have been marked limitations to the provision of dialysis therapy in the United Kingdom, but there have been very few instances of court cases such as those tried in the United States. In early 1984, under pressure from the social services and hostel staff, the Churchill Hospital, Oxford, offered dialysis to a high-risk patient, a 42-year-old man with a history of psychiatric illness and severe mental impairment, as well as advanced renal disease, after having cared for him for approximately a year (141). His behavior was increasingly disruptive, and he required sedation while being dialyzed to prevent him from removing the bloodlines from his arm. By degrees the staff of the renal unit came to the view that treatment by dialysis was a failure and would ultimately have to be discontinued. The dialysis sessions were proving a torment to both patient and medical staff, and the unit's capacity to deal with other patients was being affected.

The renal unit took the ultimate decision to discontinue treatment—a decision that appears to be in line with an earlier British court decision. In 1980, the Court of Appeal had taken the position that it could not be supposed that the Secretary of State for Social Services had to provide all the kidney machines asked for or all the new developments for every patient who would benefit from them. "The Court held that the limitation of health resources had to be determined in the light of current Government economic policy." It was stated that "though limitation of resources was not a dominant factor in this case, fair and sensible allocation of the unit's resources had to be taken into account, if justice was to be done to other patients, and treatment given to those most likely to benefit from it." The Court further noted that "as with any incurable and progressive condition, treatment to the bitter end may not be in the patient's best interest."

Advance Health Care Directives: Living Will and Durable Power of Attorney

The three state supreme court cases discussed illustrate the difficulties that arise when there is no advance written communication by patients indicating their wishes about treatment options should they become unable to make decisions because of physical or mental incapacity. Family members, caregivers, judges, and legal representatives are the people usually given the responsibility for making treatment decisions when adults are incapacitated. Without prior discussion with the patient, decision makers may have difficulty in determining what the patient might have wanted. They also may not agree about what the patient's wishes would be. Gradually into this morass, in the United States, have come options for two general types of written directives that can be used to avoid such difficulties. These directives allow the patient (a) to provide specific instructions about how he or she wishes to be treated or not treated in specific situations (both in the living will and in the durable power of attorney), and (b) to appoint an agent to make health care decisions should the patient become mentally incapacitated. (The patient's agent can be designated in the durable power of attorney for health care.)

These two types of advance directives for health care are recognized legally in most jurisdictions in the United States. By August 1991 (142), all but seven of the American states had enacted laws recognizing living wills, often referred to as declarations or directives, created in accordance with the State's Natural Death Act. These directives document a patient's wishes about health care should he or she have a terminal illness and be unable to provide further instructions. The seven states that do not have living will statutes have legislation pending that addresses the issues of artificial nourishment and hydration, a topic highlighted by the Cruzan case.

A durable power of attorney allows the power of attorney to endure even if the person making it is no longer competent to make medical decisions. Some form of durable powers of attorney are recognized throughout the United States and the District of Columbia. However, the field is changing rapidly. (Because of the rapid changes of statutes about living wills and durable powers of attorney, the most up-to-date information can be obtained from the Society for the Right to Die at 212-246-6962.) The durable power of attorney can be used to designate whether treatments are to be continued or discontinued in specified circumstances. As of July 1991, 27 states and the District of Columbia had specific forms to be used for durable powers of attorney for health care, an additional 11 states refer to health care decisions in their general durable powers of attorney statute, and Maryland (122) had a special durable powers of attorney form because of its differing views about artificial nutrition. In New Jersey, a court case is looking at durable powers of attorney, whereas Oklahoma does not allow these powers to be used for withdrawal of

nutrition or hydration. Coming from the state of Missouri where Nancy Cruzan's case raised these issues to prominence, Senator John Danforth studied all aspects of the need for advance directives and initiated the legislative efforts that resulted in the PSDA.

A 1982 Harris survey (143) revealed that only approximately one of every three persons in the U.S. adult population had given instructions to anyone about their treatment wishes should they become incompetent. Of these, only approximately one of every four had provided written instructions. Later studies showed that physicians often have not discussed these matters with their patients. Members of the groups who could counsel patients about such procedures (e.g., nurses, social workers, clergy) often are not as knowledgeable about the options as they should be. In addition, a diffidence about, or distaste for, discussions centered on death and dying unfortunately is common in the United States, even among physicians and clergy, the two groups who confront death most frequently. It is hoped that the PSDA of 1990 will encourage patients, physicians, and clergy to discuss advance directives and relevant treatment issues with all patients periodically—well ahead of the time when the directives might be necessary.

Physicians and other health care providers cannot treat a patient without his or her consent except in an emergency, when the law permits implied consent. Not only does a patient have the right of autonomy or self-determination, in regard to his or her choices, but the physician can refuse to treat a patient if the patient's choice conflicts with the physician's personal beliefs or values. In general, the capacity for wise health care decision making usually requires that the patient be able to understand the nature of his or her illness and the benefits and risks of the treatment options that are available. The patient also needs to be able to make and communicate a reasoned choice, and to appreciate the implications of various alternatives.

There have been relatively few studies of the use of advance directives among patients with ESRD. Two common concerns that patients may have about the execution of advance directives are the element of coercion that may arise when a health care professional addresses the issue of an advance directive with the patient, and the emotional impact that a decision about death and dying can have when the person recognizes that he or she has a life-threatening illness.

Preliminary data (144) from a questionnaire study of 321 residents living independently in a continuing care residential community indicate that discussion of advance directives in many different ways appears to be more effective in encouraging patients to execute advance directives. The response rate to this five-page questionnaire was 99.6% (319/321), and 80% of the respondents had both living wills and durable powers of attorney for health care. In addition, 10% each had either a living will or a durable power of attorney—for a total of 100% who had at least one type of advance directive. All of the respondents at this residential care community listed many different factors that influenced their decisions to executive advance directives. These included workshops, speakers, and discussions with family, friends, clergy, social workers, physicians, and other residents. It would seem that addressing this difficult subject in a less threatening way (e.g., through group discussions and free-wheeling conversations) while avoiding the element of coercion is preferable.

The next dilemma, of course, is adherence of the health care professional to the patient's expressed desires. Because of the element of uncertainty, it is preferable for the person to have a surrogate who is well informed about the patient's values and wishes and who is ready to defend the patient's preferences. This is especially important because no one can anticipate what future medical problems may arise when the person is not competent to make medical decisions.

In line with the views expressed by the life care community residents is the conclusion of a study (145) about advance directives (AD) in patients on dialysis: "Addressing AD before a medical crisis ensues may increase the likelihood of a 'good death' when complications bring the course of chronic dialysis to termination." This retrospective study of advance directives associated with "good deaths" in patients on chronic dialysis is based on a review (145) of consecutive deaths over more than 6 years in an academic health center. The study covered all adult patients older than 16 years of age who died from 1986 to early 1992. Of 182 patients who died in the period under review, 74 (41%) had advanced directives stated either verbally or in writing. The findings of this study included the following:

1. The prevalence of advance directives was highest among patients with age-related or chronically debilitating diseases.
2. Advance directives were significantly more prevalent among patients who withdrew from treatment in a reconciled fashion than among patients (a) who died suddenly or unexpectedly or (b) who died without having made a reconciled decision to forgo life-sustaining intervention.
3. Patients with an "internal" locus of decision making, rather than relying on an "external" locus (relatives or other agents), were more apt to have prior advance directives assessing their wishes about withdrawing from treatment on the basis of their own medical decisions.
4. Patients who had a definite spouse or spouse-equivalent relationship were more likely to have advance directives.
5. Patients with prior advance directives and situations in which patients withdrew from treatment were associated more frequently with an outcome favoring their wishes for care.

The authors concluded that when the renal team interacted with the patient and family closely on an ongoing basis, the medical treatment and outcome were more apt to be those that the patient requested. In addition, the authors did not believe that a government agency or a hospital committee is in a position to facilitate the most congenial interactive process about advance wishes for medical care. They (145) recommended:

"In managing patients with complicated chronic illness, sensitive attention to death as a possible outcome, even before the onset of preterminal complications is worthwhile. Death is inevitable, but recognizing patient concerns and fears engenders ongoing rapport and communication, favorably influencing the patient's decision making and the possibility of a good death."

The AIDS epidemic has raised widespread fears out of proportion to the risks for the general population because of the virtually universal fatal outcome for those afflicted. Public censure of those groups most likely to be infected with HIV (e.g., homosexuals and drug abusers) has been excessively vocal because of repugnance for their lifestyle. The media, always on the lookout for newsworthy and dramatic issues, usually do not analyze risks statistically, nor do they necessarily provide a balanced view of all the relevant issues. Thus, the stigma associated with HIV/AIDS has given rise to a number of ethical issues: patient privacy and confidentiality about the diagnosis, mandatory HIV/AIDS testing, the right of a person to know about potential exposure, health care professionals' right to know patients' HIV/AIDS status, and the responsibility of health care professionals to care for patients with HIV/AIDS.

Because of discrimination against patients with HIV/AIDS, the concerns about privacy (13) not only have received special attention in the media and in state legislation (146), but have resulted in lawsuits when there has been a breach of the right to privacy. The California Court of Appeals (147) ruled in 1991 that "a health care provider could be liable for invasion of the right to privacy . . . for improper disclosure of HIV-related information." In another case, the Superior Court of New Jersey, Law Division ruled that "an institutional provider (must) take affirmative steps to thwart the potentially damaging effects of the hospital 'grapevine'" in a situation of "hospital gossip" about a patient diagnosed with AIDS (148).

Because isolation of HIV-positive patients on a dialysis unit would identify them, neither infection-free dialysis areas nor isolation of those infected is acceptable. The exposures to blood that can occur with the treatment of patients with ESRD and the association of the AIDS epidemic with renal disease and dialysis therapy raise special ethical problems inherent in the practice of nephrology. Rao and colleagues (149) delineated some of these ethical problems for nephrologists: (a) resistance and even refusal by health care professionals to provide care for HIV-infected patients, (b) limitation or restriction of services, (c) controversy over routine or mandatory HIV testing of all patients with ESRD, (d) the initiation and termination of dialysis, and (e) transplantation for HIV-infected patients.

Resistance to Caring for Human Immunodeficiency Virus–Infected Patients

Incomplete knowledge about HIV and its transmission, coupled with the fatal outcome of AIDS, caused widespread fear that HIV (AIDS) would be transmitted in the dialysis setting. In addition, it became apparent that health care workers' moral values and deep-rooted psychological attitudes about sexual lifestyles and substance abuse were influencing health care decisions (150). Although there is a risk of seroconversion for health care workers, in combined data from ten prospective studies, the risk of HIV transmission was shown to be 0.37% for a single parenteral exposure (151,152). Risk is affected by the quantity of blood exposed and can be minimized by wearing gloves (151–153).

Health care professionals have an obligation to treat all patients in need, including those with AIDS. This precept has been less readily accepted as the AIDS epidemic has grown and spread throughout medical practice. The moral obligation of physicians to care for any and all illnesses that fall within their area of competence has been replaced in many physicians' thinking by the obligation to ensure that the patient receives treatment by medical professionals, but not necessarily by them individually. The professional obligations of physicians, nurses, dentists, and other health care workers are being scrutinized more intensely because of the Centers for Disease Control's (CDC) (153–155) recommendations that there be mandatory HIV screening of all providers and potential restrictions placed on HIV-positive individuals. Protection of those professionals found to be HIV infected under the Americans with Disabilities Act (ADA) would create moral as well as economic dilemmas for the institutions that employ them. Mandatory or coerced voluntary testing would create an atmosphere of intense caution among the specialists at greatest occupational risk for acquiring HIV (e.g., orthopedic surgeons and others who perform invasive procedures and who might be loath to treat HIV-positive patients). This might have a devastating effect on the availability of health care for HIV-infected patients.

Initially, some facilities considered that patients with ESRD infected with HIV should be treated by those few centers with the most experience treating AIDS and consequent greater expertise. Because the treatment of HIV-infected patients is underreimbursed, with resultant economic hardships, and because the necessary support systems might not be available, many patients were referred to other institutions.

During the 1970s, a precedent was set that it was not only acceptable, but even praiseworthy for dialysis facilities to exclude patients with infectious viruses (e.g., HBV infection) from treatment. The epidemic nature of HBV transmission in some dialysis centers before the development of HBV antigen testing and control of the blood supply caused many dialysis facilities to exclude HBV-infected patients. *Pari passu*, dialysis centers excluded HIV-infected patients as a threat to both staff members and other patients on dialysis, albeit the risk of HIV transmission was orders of magnitude less than that of HBV (151). The universal precautions established to control HBV infection in dialysis centers markedly reduced the transmission of the HBV virus (156). The CDC judged that these HBV universal precautions also would protect staff members and other patients on dialysis from HIV transmission (157). With the gradual spread of HIV infection throughout the United States and to most health care facilities, dialysis programs have had to accept responsibility for the care of HIV-infected patients, thus abandoning the concept of an "infection-free dialysis center."

Limitation or Restriction of Dialysis Services

The prognosis for patients with AIDS treated by dialysis was dismal initially. Most of these early patients on dialysis with HIV infection had advanced clinical AIDS and survived only a few months (158,159). The ethical question of whether it was even appropriate to start these patients on dialysis was raised. As HIV-infected patients in earlier stages of infection who had renal disease were dialyzed, longer survival times were noted, and treating HIV-infected patients with ESRD became more routine (158,160).

Various treatment limitations for HIV-infected patients on dialysis have been considered, and each raises ethical questions. Peritoneal dialysis has advantages from the perspectives of medical care and reduction of risks for the staff. Ethical dilemmas in limiting dialysis to the home setting for HIV-infected patients with ESRD arise because patients may not be motivated or may be too ill to perform self-care, or because they have an inadequate or no home support system. Limiting the type of dialysis for infection control is ethically questionable if that modality is not the most appropriate for a given HIV-infected patient. Vascular surgeons often are unwilling to put cannulae or fistulae in place for chronic dialysis in patients who are intravenous drug abusers because of the risk of HIV infection for surgeons and operating room personnel. Isolation of HIV-positive patients from other patients on dialysis in a fashion similar to that for HBV-positive patients would violate confidentiality by identifying these patients as infected—a major issue because the identification of HIV infection can have devastating social and ethical consequences owing to the stigma associated with AIDS/AIDS-related complex.

Human Immunodeficiency Virus Testing

Early in the AIDS epidemic, the stigmatization and serious socioeconomic repercussions of a positive HIV test result created major problems for HIV-positive patients on dialysis when the hope of medical benefit was minimal and health care professionals were wary of exposure to this dreaded disease. Initially, patients often were unable to obtain even transient dialysis, were isolated physically, and had virtually no hope for transplantation.

The development of a few effective means of treatment has moved the benefits of the HIV screening test beyond usefulness for mere prediction of outcome to diagnosis. Early in the AIDS epidemic, many physicians wanted to test all patients with ESRD to achieve infection control by restriction of therapy or by differential treatment of HIV-positive patients.

Development and wider availability of effective antiviral therapy and other effective means of infection prophylaxis (e.g., for *Pneumocystis carinii*) and tumor chemotherapy (e.g., for Kaposi's sarcoma) made early diagnosis of AIDS increasingly important for all patients at risk. As treatments to prevent the complication of blindness were developed, another benefit of early diagnosis was added. The emphasis has shifted from HIV screening for infection control or therapy restriction to identification of patients at risk so that more aggressive therapy may be used to prolong the lives of infected patients on dialysis and reduce the occurrence of serious complications.

The primary concerns in HIV testing are (a) accuracy; (b) need for informed consent, including adequate counseling both before and after test results are known; (c) the assessment of risks and benefits of the individuals involved; and (d) the use of required testing only when there is a clear benefit for patients and others. The use of Western blot and other, more specific tests virtually eliminated the initial difficulty with false-positive results, which occurred in 4% to 5% of patients tested (161–163).

Different countries may view HIV testing in different ways. In one study (164), 128 British and Irish nephrologists were questioned about their policy for HIV testing of patients with ESRD who were being considered for renal replacement therapy. Testing only with the patient's knowledge and consent was the policy of two-thirds of the nephrologists, with only 24 of 88 obtaining a signature. Of 101 (79%) who responded, one-third tested only those patients on dialysis whom they considered at risk for HIV. Potential transplant recipients would be tested by 68 of 100. A positive HIV test result was considered reason for exclusion from transplantation by 63 of 86, whereas 24 of 88 would use HIV positivity as a reason for excluding patients from hemodialysis, and 7 of 87 would use it as a reason to exclude patients from peritoneal dialysis. A consensus about the practice of HIV testing of patients with ESRD is needed. In Great Britain, the Royal College of Nurses Dialysis and Transplant Nurses Forum (165) developed guidelines for HIV testing after sending a questionnaire about current practices to 61 renal units. The responses indicated a diversity of practices: a lack of awareness of the ethical issues surrounding HIV testing, a practice that used HIV testing routinely only in the preparation of patients for a renal transplantation, and the conviction that hepatitis precautions were adequate for HIV. There was a concern that known HIV-positive patients might be alienated because of lack of awareness about the infectivity and means of transmission of HIV with consequent attendant prejudices. It was considered important to educate and inform patients before taking a blood sample for HIV testing.

An American nursing report (166) suggested that when caretakers are aware of a patient's HIV-positive status, they can offer available support systems and medications that provide an improved quality of life over an extended period. Even if a patient tests negative but is a member of a high-risk group, education can prove beneficial.

Al-Sulaiman and coauthors (167) noted that in the Riyadh Armed Forces Hospital, Saudi Arabia, all potential kidney donors and recipients, as well as patients with ESRD, are tested for HIV before commencing dialysis and at regular intervals. They observed that patients are at increased risk of acquiring HIV through blood transfusions or renal transplantation. Their routine testing showed that there were 8 HIV-positive patients among 830 potential kidney donors and recipients. HIV-positive patients are treated in a separate unit and precautions similar to those for HBV-positive patients are used. They recommended that staff members should have the option to be tested and that HIV carriers should be offered dialysis, and noted that dialysis for patients with AIDS and renal failure as part of the syndrome is "debatable."

Initiation and Termination of Dialysis

Initiation and termination of dialysis must be considered carefully for all patients with advanced disease who are not expected to live more than a few weeks or months. Each patient with HIV infection or AIDS must be evaluated in detail because of differences in people's perceptions of quality of life and of tolerable invasive treatments, and "trade-offs" between patients and health care professionals. With increasing numbers of AIDS complications, dialysis becomes more difficult technically and increasing demands are placed on the time and resources of the renal service. Against this background, guidelines for considering stopping dialysis are necessary, and the factors involved may include the following: (a) a competent patient's decision to withdraw from dialysis; (b) the use of advance directives, such as a living will or a durable power of attorney for health care; (c) progressive AIDS-associated dementia precluding the patient's ability to participate in dialysis care, especially if there is no available outside support system; and (d) the severity of AIDS complications, possibly making survival unlikely and dialysis not beneficial medically.

These considerations serve only as guidelines and the final decision often rests with the patient and his or her family or friends, assisted by health care professionals. Patients with AIDS who are intravenous drug abusers and are not compliant with their dialysis treatment, who refuse treatment for HIV complications, and who have neither advance directives nor a social support system make these decisions especially difficult. The major physical and emotional demands on the dialysis staff, the health risks to other patients on dialysis and staff members because of the transmission of diseases such as tuberculosis, and the ultimate necessity for institutional care raise ethical dilemmas about the continuation of dialysis.

Transplantation in Human Immunodeficiency Virus–Infected Patients

Fears about possible HIV-infected donor kidneys and ethical concerns over the exclusion of HIV-infected patients from organ transplant donation or receipt have been present since the early 1980s, when transmission of HIV infection by living related and cadaver organs was documented (168–170). Routine testing of prospective donors and recipients along with rejection of potential donors at high risk for HIV infection have settled many of the safety issues. Nevertheless, a modest and finite risk remains—in the use of blood products and in organ and tissue transplantation especially, and because of the window between HIV infection and seroconversion (171). The ethical principle of justice assumes central importance when the refusal of kidney transplantation to all HIV-infected patients with ESRD is contemplated. Data about the outcome of transplantation in HIV-infected patients are limited. The Pittsburgh center (172) reported the results of transplantation in 25 HIV-positive patients, of whom 13 (52%) were still alive. Their mean survival time after transplantation was 4.5 years for liver, 3.4 years for kidney, and 4.4 years for heart transplant recipients. The center did not observe a significant difference in survival time for patients who were HIV positive before transplantation surgery compared with those who tested positive only after transplantation. The Massachusetts General Hospital maintains an International Registry for the Study of AIDS in Transplantation under the joint sponsorship of the United Network for Organ Sharing, CDC, EDTA, Eurotransplant, and the journal *Transplantation* (173), and data are made available on a continuing basis. Although transplantation is medically feasible in asymptomatic HIV-positive patients, the scarcity of organs for transplantation raises the question of justice in allocating this scarce resource to patients who have a limited life expectancy. Medical benefit, potential length of survival, and presence of comorbid conditions must be considered. Center directors responding to Kilner's questionnaires (43) place great weight on these factors. All of the principles of medical ethics outlined in this chapter apply to the care of patients with ESRD with HIV infection or AIDS. These very difficult issues require careful and thoughtful analysis.

SUBSTANCE ABUSE AND END-STAGE RENAL DISEASE

Renal failure has been associated with the abuse of drugs, both illicit drugs and analgesics sold over the counter, for decades (174–177). Since the identification of the nephropathy caused by over-the-counter analgesics, both the medical community's awareness of the risk and the reformulation of analgesic combinations by pharmaceutical companies have diminished the risk of analgesic abuse, although analgesic-associated nephropathy remains a public health problem in many countries. The renal disease resulting in ESRD that is caused by addiction to "street drugs" and other illicit substances continues to be a problem of significant proportions in the United States, especially in larger American cities (178), as well as worldwide. The incidence of HIV infection is rising in the intravenous drug abuse population (179,180), and this group, especially black men, has an unusually high

incidence of renal disease (181–183). Glue sniffing (184,185), the putative toxin usually being toluene, is another type of drug abuse that has been associated with acute renal failure and distal renal tubular acidosis.

Analgesic nephropathy continues to be a renal disease of high prevalence in many European countries. A study by Noels and associates (186) provided the rationale for action by nephrologists to reduce the availability of hazards such as analgesics. This report showed a substantially lower prevalence of analgesic nephropathy when there was legislation that restricted the over-the-counter availability of most analgesic compounds, especially those containing two analgesics. The authors concluded that legislation prohibiting the availability of analgesic mixtures with at least one potentially addictive substance needs to be enacted to reduce access to these abusive compounds. Legislative restriction of analgesic sales in Australia (187) resulted in a decreased prevalence of analgesic abuse and of ESRD failure resulting from analgesic-associated nephropathy.

A further concern with an abusive drug that often is not viewed as a drug—alcohol—arises because of the concomitant alcohol intake of illicit drug abusers. A study (188) of 30 patients with postinfectious glomerulonephritis reported that 17 (57%) of the patients were alcoholics as determined by history and chemistry, and that chronic renal failure developed in 16 (53%) of the alcoholic but none of the nonalcoholic patients. The Klinikum Steglitz in Berlin (189) reported analgesic nephropathy as the most frequent diagnosis (30%) in patients on hemodialysis and the second most frequent diagnosis in their transplant recipients (17%), and that urothelial carcinoma was significantly more frequent in renal patients with analgesic nephropathy. Patients with analgesic nephropathy also comprised the oldest group of either patients on hemodialysis or transplant recipients.

Driesens and associates (190) recommended a more global approach to the analgesic abuse problem. They noted that "man experiences considerable difficulty adapting to sweeping social, technological and ideological changes of recent decades, and this transition contributes . . . to the analgesic problem. It should be a priority of government to find remedies for this state of affairs."

With the extraordinary expense of health care and the scarcity of resources for many treatment modalities, serious concerns have been expressed in many sectors of society about the wisdom and fairness of treating patients who are substance abusers. The frightening aspect of treatment decisions made by evaluation of social worth (i.e., a judgment that substance abusers cause their own difficulties) raises major ethical concerns, especially because there are other addictions or behaviors such as overeating, smoking, or drinking alcohol that society condones. Punishment for behaviors deemed unacceptable is inconsistent with many of the ethical principles and values that modern society accepts as important. Issues often discussed in reaching treatment decisions for substance abusers include the deferral or avoidance of health care for a long time, noncompliance, sociopathic behavior, limited potential for rehabilitation, recidivism, increased medical costs associated with excessive morbidity, a poor prognosis for a "normal" longevity, and the problem of allocating scarce resources such as kidneys for transplantation.

A sense of moral righteousness and society's disapproval of those who indulge in substance abuse are significant factors in the refusal of both physicians and dialysis centers to accept intravenous drug abusers as patients. In addition, these patients put unusual, often excessive and unreasonable, demands on the dialysis staff and service. Chronic drug addicts frequently are unreliable, and the potential for their rehabilitation to a more functional lifestyle is low. They do not adhere to treatment schedules and fail to take prescribed medications. Refusal to treat patients who are intravenous drug abuse or placing limitations on care for them often is justified by their increased morbidity with its related increased need for hospitalization. It also sometimes is justified by their decreased long-term survival time (191).

Because of their low socioeconomic status and limited Medicaid reimbursement for their health care, substance abusers receive marginal health care at best. Certainly, compassionate concern for fellow human beings and their misfortunes warrants special attention to the more specific clinical situations of this vulnerable group. Realistically, this is difficult to accomplish because physicians as well as society at large tend to make moral judgments about those whose lifestyle is unacceptable or even abhorrent.

The verbally and occasionally physically abusive behavior of substance abusers not only is disruptive in the dialysis unit, but makes patients and staff fear for their own safety. Handling such situations may require the use of security guards as well as other punitive means to control sociopathic behavior. Behavior that borders on the criminal can cause physicians, other health professionals, and hospital administrators to adopt a contractual model of the physician–and health professional–patient relationship rather than to provide treatment within the more desirable covenantal model. The attempted use of contracts and their legality are discussed both in the Payton and the Brown cases, examples of two noncompliant drug abusers whose cases came to court, as discussed earlier in this chapter.

There is great resistance among members of the transplantation community even to consider accepting patients who are or have been drug abusers (183). This resistance springs from the moral judgments mentioned, the experience that some patients who are drug abusers do not take immunosuppressive medications, and the limited number of kidneys available for transplantation. Again, contracts sometimes are considered. These may require (a) a reasonable degree of compliance with dialysis and other medical treatments, and (b) the completion of a recovery program with a documented drug-free period of at least 6 months before such a patient is placed on a waiting list.

In his analysis of noncompliant patients, Orentlicher (42) discussed the legal questions that are so unsettling for health care professionals. He implied that patients who are substance abusers may not be responsible for their actions because of their addiction and its resultant mental state. Health care staff members frequently are overextended and stressed in their efforts to care for patients with ESRD who depend on dialysis machines for survival. As a result, health care professionals often resent and are frustrated with any patient who makes no effort to care for herself or himself, much less a substance abuser who does not take responsibility for his or her own care. Many health professionals (e.g., surgeons and radiologists) have refused to use their skills in associated ESRD care and procedures for substance-abusing patients. Although it is essential for nephrologists and the dialysis staff who must care for these patients to recognize the importance of ethical issues and humane caring for substance abusers, the abusers usually require discipline and stringent actions. Participation of substance abusers in support groups, along with participation of professionals who are expert in recovery programs, often has been effective in achieving cooperation with the prescribed treatment regimen. Contracts between the health professionals and substance abusers also can limit the latter's manipulative actions.

GENETICS AND RENAL DISEASE

The burgeoning field of molecular genetics and its relevance to medical genetics have raised many new ethical issues. Patients' and health care professionals' continuing concerns about maintenance of the privacy and confidentiality of medical records are accompanied by an equally weighty concern about the use and protection of newly acquired knowledge about patients' genes identified for specific diseases by DNA testing. This concern has emerged as one of the major ethical issues accompanying the advances in the identification of genes and the potential for genetic diagnosis accompanying the Human Genome Project. Except for APKDs, the DNA polymorphisms causing progressive renal failure in people with the usual kidney diseases have not been identified (192). However, great progress has been made in the molecular genetics of a number of inherited renal diseases (193). The von Hippel-Lindau gene, which apparently acts as a tumor suppressor gene, has been implicated in both the sporadic and familial forms of renal cell carcinoma (194,195). The ethical issues involved with the genetics of renal disease and the intertwined factors of prenatal diagnosis and gene therapy achieved prominence earlier; they persist along with the issues of privacy and confidentiality.

The potential for genetic selection raises broad ethical issues for medicine in general, but also has implications for organ transplantation. In 1989, a California couple conceived a third child, at a time when preimplantation genetic diagnosis was not possible, in hopes that this infant might be a bone marrow donor for their 16-year-old daughter who had leukemia. At that time, there was a one in four chance that the child would be a match for their leukemic daughter. Ten years later, *in vitro* fertilization and embryo screening were used to select the appropriate embryo and produce a "test tube baby" that would have compatible cells for a transplant into his 6-year-old sister who had Fanconi's anemia. One month after the birth of this infant, whose umbilical cord cells had been collected, the sister received a transfusion of his umbilical cord cells (196). Ethical questions about the potential for "designer babies" have been raised since *in vitro* fertilization and embryo selection became reality. After what is believed to be the first instance of implanting an embryo with desired characteristics (i.e., compatible umbilical cord/bone marrow cells) into the uterus of the mother, the question of similar embryo selection for novel treatments for incurable diseases and for producing needed solid organs has been raised.

Rapid progress in the field of molecular genetics has widened the possibilities for prenatal diagnosis and has brought gene therapy into the realm of reality. As identifiable gene loci are found for more and more hereditary diseases, the ethical issues involved in prenatal diagnosis, genetic counseling, and gene therapy, as well as issues of presymptomatic testing, will need to be discussed openly and faced candidly.

The major concerns (143) about confidentiality of medical information and records, and about who other than the physician and patient has access to such data, reflect the use and abuse of such information. Siegler (197) scanned the medical chart of a patient who expressed concern about the confidentiality of his hospital record and enumerated "at least 25 and possibly as many as 100 health professionals and administrative personnel . . . [who] had access to the patient's record," all of whom had legitimate reasons to examine the chart.

The federal government has recognized the need to develop policies that address the restriction of medical information to patients and their physicians. A U.S. Public Health task force has been studying this issue for several years, and currently a bill addressing this topic is before the U.S. Congress.

Although broaching difficult ethical issues with patients is not easy, it is essential that nephrologists provide the available facts about familial and hereditary diseases to patients. Education about genetic diagnostic techniques such as amniocentesis, chorionic villus sampling, and selective abortion, with concomitant genetic counseling about the risk and occurrence of these genetic diseases, allow people to make informed choices when considering pregnancy.

Fletcher and Wertz (198) identified five factors that influence a given society's approach to prenatal diagnosis: scientific and medical resources, cultural traditions about the role of women and the family, abortion laws, the impact of religious groups and leaders on public policy, and the health care system in general. The ethical principles of autonomy, beneficence, nonmaleficence, and justice certainly are applicable when considering hereditary kidney diseases. Respect for the right of parents to make decisions autonomously requires that the available facts be presented to them in a fashion that they can comprehend and process before making a decision. The principle of justice requires that appropriate access to diagnostic techniques be ensured, and that adequate

genetic counseling about the meaning of the test results and the examinations be provided without coercion.

White and Caskey (199) analyzed the options in the diagnosis of APKDs that raise concerns about presymptomatic DNA testing. Presymptomatic diagnosis does not necessarily presage development of a disease and *a priori* does not mean that there is a preexisting condition. Patients with APKD and their families need to understand the pros and cons of the knowledge gained by DNA testing. The option concerning presymptomatic testing should be their autonomous choice. The options are:

1. No genetic testing, or
2. Proceed with genetic testing for APKD, in which case:
   a. Maintain confidentiality (provide information about test results only to the patient and physician), or
   b. Permit disclosure
      (i) Share positive or negative information with the patient's insurance company and Medicare
      (ii) Share positive or negative information with the patient's employer
      (iii) Share positive or negative information with the patient's family

These authors identified several consequences of testing:

1. The insurance carrier may believe that DNA testing for presymptomatic diseases is similar to testing for other known hereditary diseases, such as diabetes mellitus, and may use any positive results to rate the risk category for coverage as "normal" or "high."
2. An employer, concerned about the insurance pool risk or wanting predictions about the potential long-term impact of genetic disease on job performance, could require DNA studies to clarify genetic risk.
3. A spouse might request genetic information because reproductive decisions should be made jointly.

Genetic tests of asymptomatic family members would involve a type of family linkage study. Such tests require cooperation of at-risk family members, but this cooperation should not be assumed because of the potential risks of the knowledge.

The potential of gene therapy already is being studied, and an application of these principles has been used in a clinical trial at the U.S. National Institutes of Health. The adenosine deaminase gene (200) was introduced into T cells to treat a 4-year-old child with deficiency of this enzyme. A late 1991 Medlines search for articles about kidney disease and genetics produced more than 400 citations, and a 1995 search added more than 200 further references. These included numerous papers about APKD, Alport's syndrome, and Wilms' tumor, as well as references to other genetic kidney disorders.

The "testing [of] children at risk of genetic disorders has been a recognized part of both pediatrics and medical genetics for many years" (201,202) and sensitive radiographic imaging techniques were used in the diagnosis of APKD. Also now available is an international database (203) that is a subset of the International Studies of Genetic Renal Diseases, called *kidbase,* on the Internet (204). This database makes information on genetics broadly available, and measures must be enforced to maintain patient confidentiality. Abuse of genetic information can affect a patient's insurance, education, and employment.

Since the advent of DNA-based testing, there has been an ethical debate about testing for late-onset disorders such as Huntington's disease. Although APKD is primarily "adult," it may manifest in childhood. Harper and Clarke (201) noted, "The question (about presymptomatic tests in childhood) has not so far been adequately addressed, nor have the motives underlying childhood testing been clearly analyzed." When the onset is in childhood, there is good reason for early diagnosis. However,

> where there is only [a] remote chance of childhood onset, definitive testing for [a] gene should be deferred until the age of consent is reached or when there are suspicious clinical features. There is a strong argument for deferring testing until later childhood when the child can be actively involved in both medical decisions and possible career-related decisions. The availability of treatment would, of course, be a powerful argument for early testing.

The possible benefits of early APKD testing include the exclusion of APKD for a child who is not at risk. Such a child would be spared frequent assessments of his or her renal function and structure and frequent blood pressure measurements, all of which can cause anxiety. The child free of APKD and her family can benefit by avoiding the inconvenience of multiple testing, saving resources, and removing anxiety. On the other hand, there is a potential problem should a child be inappropriately assigned to a low-risk group and have necessary screening measures discontinued. The United Kingdom working group of the Institute of Medical Ethics (160) considered that testing of children for APKD is a research activity and should meet special research requirements.

Kielstein and Sass (204) stressed the ambiguity between a "right not to know" and a "duty to know," which they discussed in relation to parental decision making in prenatal screening for APKD. There are pros or cons to be weighed in considering selective abortion after prenatal screening for APKD. In Germany (205), there is a related public policy issue because preimplantation diagnosis is not available; selective abortion is allowed before the end of the first trimester only for certain medical or social indications.

Breuning and colleagues (206) recommended that before chorionic villus sampling is attempted, polymorphic DNA markers should be used for presymptomatic and prenatal diagnosis of an autosomal form of PKD, and the linkage phase of DNA markers should be established by determining haplotypes of the index family.

Background knowledge, experience, and perspectives on APKD as an example of hereditary disease have been provided by three studies. Together, these three studies constitute an analysis of the ethical issues associated with prenatal diagnosis and the related clinical situation. In the first study (207), information from interviews and a questionnaire of 190 subjects from 100 APKD families on the North Western

Regional Genetic Register was studied. The researchers sought to determine the potential interest of their respondents in prenatal diagnosis, and their understanding and experience of the clinical, therapeutic, and genetic aspects of APKD. The subjects understood the major aspects of the disease and its therapy. This cohort had had genetic counseling, and most knew the risk to their children. Although a high percentage of this group had had presymptomatic ultrasound studies, only a minority changed their reproductive behavior. Moreover, although most favored the availability of a prenatal test, only 23% of those at high risk of transmitting the disease who were contemplating having children expressed an interest in prenatal diagnosis.

The second study (208), of 45 patients with APKD in Israel, assessed the patients' knowledge about the familial nature of the disease and their attitudes. Most patients knew the name and prognosis of APKD, but only 9% knew their children were at risk. Thirty-eight percent of the patients wanted to know if they had APKD before they had children, but only 18% said they would not have had children if they had known the diagnosis beforehand. In spite of their disease, 45% of the patients on dialysis and 78% of patients not on dialysis would have had children.

The third study (209) looked at the prevalence and types of underlying hereditary renal diseases in Ireland among the dialysis population and in all patients who received a transplant at the national unit. Of 178 patients on dialysis, 28 (15.7%) had hereditary renal disease, as did 89 (10.3%) of 842 transplant recipients. APKD was the most common, affecting 68% of patients on dialysis and 64% of transplant recipients with hereditary renal disease. Alport's syndrome was the next most common disease (21.4% and 16.9%, respectively), whereas nephronophthisis ranked third, with an incidence of just over 10% in each group.

Although hereditary diseases resulting in ESRD account for approximately 10% of the ESRD population, it is unclear how those affected would react to prenatal diagnosis and genetic counseling. The recommendations of nephrologists about genetic counseling need to include a discussion of the risks and patterns of diseases as well as explanations of heredity.

SUMMARY

The remarkable success of kidney transplantation and chronic dialysis in the treatment of ESRD has been life saving for patients with chronic renal failure. At the same time, it has produced major new ethical dilemmas. These ethical issues are complex, troubling, and often elusive. There is a great temptation to avoid facing them because they are subjective and difficult to categorize. For those in the medical profession who feel more comfortable with precise, objective topics, dealing with these issues can be unsettling. However, moral and ethical concerns always have been part of the practice of medicine. With the remarkable advances in medicine and medical technology, the nature of the problems to be considered has outpaced the gradual development of codes of ethics devised to cope with innovative treatments and reinterpreted over the millennia since the development of the Hippocratic Oath.

There are no easy answers to the issues raised by LSTs. It is essential that a careful, thoughtful process be used in the analysis of these issues. This process calls for cooperative deliberations by a multidisciplinary group of health professionals, clergy, ethicists, lawyers, and laypeople, along with patients and their families. The mechanics of this deliberative process may vary according to the problem being addressed. Frequently, an ethics committee with broad representation of those with expertise as well as those concerned about the issues is convened. However, it is essential that physicians themselves continue to think deeply and in a disciplined fashion about the issues, rather than delegating difficult problems to a committee.

The major and most common issue confronting those treating patients with ESRD, an issue that is prototypical for all physicians and other health professionals treating patients with LSTs, is that of starting and stopping these treatments for critically ill patients. In the dialysis situation, most patients are alert and competent to make medical decisions for themselves about the initiation and termination of ESRD treatment. Variables that can affect the decisions made by both patients and nephrologists include age, comorbid conditions, and personal values and beliefs. Since the advent of the ESRD program, nephrologists in the United States rarely need to make hard decisions about whom to treat based on stringent financial considerations. In fact, nephrologists often are tempted to treat patients when medical judgment might suggest ESRD therapy is inappropriate. Other high-income countries, however, have had to limit provision of medical services, including dialysis, often tacitly. Low-income countries either can provide dialysis only for a privileged few or cannot provide this costly treatment.

The HCFA data show that the patients voluntarily requesting that dialysis be stopped account for at least 10% to 15% of deaths of patients on dialysis, with higher percentages reported for the elderly. Patients who withdraw voluntarily from dialysis or patients who are not compliant with the prescribed regimen, especially the fluid and potassium limitations for patients on dialysis and immunosuppressive therapy for transplant recipients, may have overtly or tacitly made the decision that they are not satisfied with their quality of life. Conversely, physicians caring for patients whose lifestyles and behavior are dissonant with that which health professionals expect must make an effort to understand, to be tolerant, and to find a means to achieve a *modus operandi* that includes appropriate care for the noncompliant patients, while not jeopardizing the care of other patients.

Appraisals of quality of life by patients and by health care professionals can be drastically different. It is essential for those treating patients to accept the desires and needs of patients to exercise autonomy in health care decision making, even when it may be at odds with considered medical judgment. The paternalistic fashion in which medicine was

practiced in the past often led physicians, including nephrologists, to rejoice in their ability to save lives, but sometimes to ignore the marginal nature of the life that was saved. The four ethical principles of autonomy, beneficence, nonmaleficence, and justice, as well as the developing approaches that encompass phenomenology, hermeneutics, casuistry, and the narrative and virtue approaches, provide a useful framework for assessing ethical issues. These are especially helpful when there is apparent disagreement among health professionals, patients, and families.

The occasional failure to listen to patients' sincere concerns about their treatment wishes are reflected in three right-to-die cases of patients on dialysis that reached higher courts. Against the background of the remarkable progress in medicine, the public has expressed its priorities about the kind of life and the manner of dying it prefers. Responses to these expressions have been codified in laws providing for advance directives, both living wills and durable powers of attorney for health care, as well as in the passage of the PSDA.

The allocation of scarce resources must be addressed by nephrologists, primarily in the sphere of kidney transplantation because of the shortage of cadaver kidneys for transplantation. Creative means to increase cadaver kidney donation need to be developed. Even more important, research efforts to find ways to prevent the diseases resulting in ESRD or to arrest their progression must be continued and increased. The macroallocation decisions about funding for medical care, both primary and tertiary, for the population are the responsibility of society as exercised by appropriate governmental bodies. The physicians' responsibility is to provide the best, most appropriate care for each individual patient. British nephrologists, with their stringent ESRD funding, have commented that although they may have no funds for a new transplant candidate whom they cannot accept, should that patient appear in the hospital, they would feel an immediate commitment to take care of him or her.

Included in considerations about the provision of care involving significant discomfort or pain must be a recognition of the fact that treatment that merely prolongs the dying process can be cruel. Helping the patient to experience a "good death" may be the kindest treatment when the medical situation is either futile or unbearable. Ideally, physicians should retain the responsibility that is graphically portrayed in many 19th-century paintings of the family physician seated by the bedside and supporting both patient and family during their travail when the course of disease cannot be reversed.

Special issues that occur with increasing frequency are associated with the specter of adverse societal judgment of what may be deemed deviant behavior. Often, these issues are associated with homosexuality and illicit drug use. These problems still must be confronted, and include dilemmas related to the treatment of patients with AIDS/HIV infection and of patients who have been substance abusers. The concern over risks of exposure to infection, along with the question of whether HIV-infected patients should be dialyzed in isolation, as are HBV-positive patients, is in conflict with the desire of patients with AIDS/HIV infection that their diagnosis be kept confidential. The criterion of "social worth," which was one of the most troubling for the Seattle "God Committee," may be tacitly or openly raised when patients with ESRD whose social behavior is deemed unacceptable are considered for dialysis and transplantation. Such criteria are in conflict with the obligation of physicians to care for the sick.

The high cost of health care in the United States effectively has resulted in rationing by ability to pay. Because there are so many persons who are not able to receive adequate health care, serious consideration is being given by politicians, insurance companies, corporations, economists, and the general population to the question of how to improve access to appropriate, affordable health care for all American people. Discussion of these issues is a fertile field for ethicists as well, and the criteria for inclusion in or exclusion from treatment have been considered, although exclusion from available treatment for any group of patients makes physicians extraordinarily uncomfortable. The costs of ESRD treatment are more visible than the costs of most treatments because of federal funding. This also has led to data gathering and analysis of ESRD at the federal level, along with a search for means to save money. Although the thought of rationing health care is abhorrent to most Americans, the efforts of the Oregon Senate and its Health Service Commission are being carefully observed by those who believe that priorities for medical treatments must be set.

Nephrologists already must face issues related to prenatal diagnosis and genetic counseling, whereas the potential for gene therapy may soon be realized. It is certain that the continuing progress in medical research will be accompanied by new ethical dilemmas. As nephrologists approach each new development and its application to patient care, they will need to learn how to make ethical decisions, often in the face of uncertainty, while recognizing that there are no simple formulas or universal answers to the complex issues raised. Although ready solutions to difficult situations will not be found, it is essential that considered and thoughtful approaches be used.

ACKNOWLEDGMENTS

The author thanks Dr. Paul Eggers for generous sharing of expertise in his specialty areas.

REFERENCES

1. Health Care Financing Administration. http://www.hcfa.gov/stats/NHE-Proj/proj1998/default.htm.
2. Congressional Budget Office. *Trends in health spending by Medicare and the nation.* Washington, DC: Congress of the United States, January 1991.
3. Office of Technology Assessment, U.S. Congress. *Life-sustaining technologies and the elderly.* OTA-BA-306, Washington, DC: U.S. Government Printing Office, July 1987.
4. Rettig RA, Levinsky NG, eds. *Kidney failure and the federal government: report of a study by a committee of the Institute of Medicine.* Washington, DC: National Academy, 1991.
5. Health Care Financing Administration Medicare Automated Data Retrieval System (MADRS). Baltimore, July 1991.
6. Eggers PW. Personal communication, 2000 (Division of Health, Information and Outcomes, Health Care Financing Administration, Washington, DC).
7. Department of Commerce, U.S. Government. NIWD/Bureau of Economic Analysis. July 27, 2000, Tables 2.6U and 2.4 PCE (http://www.esa.doc.gov).
8. McCully C. Personal communication, 2000 (U.S. Department of Commerce, Economic and Statistics Branch, Bureau of Economic Analysis, Washington, DC).
9. Cummings NB. Ethics and access to care: an overview. Presented at the annual meeting of the Renal Physicians Association, Phoenix, AZ, February 22, 1991 [condensation, *Nephrol News Issues* 1991;5:27, 30, 35].
10. Epstein AM, Ayanian JZ, Keogh JH, et al. Racial disparities in access to renal transplantation. *N Engl J Med* 2000;343:1537.
11. Young CJ, Gaston RS. Renal transplantation in black Americans. *N Engl J Med* 2000;343:1545.
12. Fox RC. The medical profession's changing outlook on hemodialysis (1950–1976). In: *Essays in medical sociology.* New York: John Wiley & Sons, 1979:122.
13. Cummings NB. Patient confidentiality. In: On the bioethics front. *Second Opin* 1993;19:112.
14. Alexander S. They decide who lives, who dies. *Life Magazine* November 9, 1962:102.
15. Rettig RA. Origins of the Medicare kidney disease entitlement: the Social Security Amendments of 1972. In: Hanna KE, ed. *Biomedical politics.* Washington, DC: National Academy, 1991:177.
16. Congressional Budget Office. *Rising health care costs: causes, implications, and strategies.* Washington, DC: Congress of the United States, 1991.
17. Hatlie MJ. Professional liability: the case for federal reform. *JAMA* 1990;263:585.
18. Silverman C, et al. *EBRI databook on employee benefits, 2000.* Washington, DC: Employee Benefit Research Institute, 2000:236, 257 (Table 8.8).
19. Cummings NB. Uremia therapy: the resource allocation dilemma from a global perspective. *Kidney Int Suppl* 1984;17:S133.
20. Sivard RL. *World military and social expenditures.* Washington, DC: World Priorities, 1991.
21. United Nations. Article 25, Universal Declaration of Human Rights.
22. First International Congress on Ethics, Justice and Commerce in Transplantation: A Global View. Ottawa, Canada, August 20–24, 1989. *Transplant Proc* 1990;22:891.
23. Mani MK. Letter to the editor. *N Engl J Med* 1986;315:716.
24. Panjwani DD, Kumar MS, White AG, et al. The ethical practice of medicine in India. *J Assoc Physicians India* 1986;34:895.
25. Reddy KC, et al. Unconventional renal transplantation in India. *Transplant Proc* 1990;22:910. (Sasruta Agencies Market Survey, 1988, quoted.)
26. Trivedi HL. Hindu religious view in context of transplantation of organs from cadavers. *Transplant Proc* 1990;22:942.
27. Yadav RVS. Transplantation as a health priority in India. *Transplant Proc* 1990;22:908.
28. Nicholson RH. Truth lies somewhere, if we knew but where. *Hastings Cent Rep* 1993;23:5.
29. Rosenthal E. In matters of life and death, the dying take control. *The New York Times,* August, 18, 1991: Section 4:1.
30. Cummings NB. Social, ethical and legal issues involved in chronic maintenance dialysis. In: Maher JF, ed. *Replacement of renal function by dialysis,* 3rd ed. Boston: Kluwer Academic Publishers, 1989:1141.
31. Johnson JP, McCauley CR, Copley JB. The quality of life of hemodialysis and transplant patients. *Kidney Int* 1982;22:286.
32. Kaplan-deNour A, Shanan J. Quality of life of hemodialysis and transplant patients. *Nephron* 1980;25:117.
33. Evans RW, Manninen DL, Garrison LP, et al. *The treatment of end-stage renal disease in the U.S.: selected findings from the National Kidney Dialysis and Kidney Transplantation Study.* Seattle, WA: Battelle Human Affairs Research Centers, 1985.
34. Karnofsky DA, Burchenal JHK. The clinical evaluation of chemotherapeutic agents in cancer. In: MacLeod CM, ed. *Evaluation of chemotherapeutic agents.* New York: Columbia University, 1949:191.

35. Devins GM., et al. Helplessness and depression in end-stage renal disease. *J Abnorm Psychol* 1981;90:531.

36. Fox RC, moderator. Exclusion from dialysis: a sociologic and legal perspective [Nephrology Forum]. *Kidney Int* 1981;19:739.

37. U.S. Renal Data System. *USRDS 1991 annual data report.* Bethesda, MD: National Institutes of Health, National Institute of Diabetes and Digestive and Kidney Diseases, 1991.

38. Eggers P. Voluntary withdrawal [draft manuscript]. Division of Health, Information and Outcomes, Health Care Financing Administration, Washington, DC.

39. Neu S, Kjellstrand CM. Stopping long-term dialysis: an empirical study of withdrawal of life-supporting treatment. *N Engl J Med* 1986; 314:14.

40. Port FK. Mortality and causes of death in patients with end-stage renal failure. *Am J Kidney Dis* 1990;15:215.

41. Port FK, Wolfe RA, Hawthorne VM, et al. Discontinuation of dialysis therapy as a cause of death. *Am J Nephrol* 1989;9:145.

42. Orentlicher D. Denying treatment to the noncompliant patient. *JAMA* 1991;265:1579.

43. Kilner JF. *Who lives? Who dies? Ethical criteria in patient selection.* New Haven, CT: Yale University, 1990:19–20.

44. Eggers P. The effect of comorbid conditions on mortality in Medicare's end stage renal disease population [draft manuscript]. Division of Health, Information and Outcomes, Health Care Financing Administration, Washington, DC.

45. Aulisio MP, Arnold RM, Younger SJ, for the Society for Health and Human Values–Society for Bioethics Consultation Task Force on Standards for Bioethics Consultation. Health care ethics consultation: nature, goals, and competencies, a position paper from the Society for Health and Human Values–Society for Bioethics Consultation Task Force on Standards for Bioethics Consultation. *Ann Intern Med* 2000;133:59.

46. O'Brien ME. Religious faith and adjustment to long-term dialysis. *J Relig Health* 1982;21:68.

47. Koenig HG, George L, Peterson B. Religiosity and remission from depression in medically ill older patients. *Am J Psychiatry* 1998;155:536.

48. Koenig HG, Hays J, Larson D, et al. Does religious attendance prolong survival? *J Gerontol A Biol Med Sci* 1999;54:M370..

49. Koenig HG, McCullough M, Larson D. *Handbook of religion and health.* New York: Oxford University Press, 2000:7–14.

50. Koenig HG. Religion, spirituality, and medicine: application to clinical practice. *JAMA* 2000;284:1708.

51. Hummer R, Rogers R, Nam C, et al. Religious involvement and US adult mortality. *Demography* 1999;36:273.

51a. Beauchamp T, Childress J. *Principles of biomedical ethics,* 3rd ed. New York: Oxford University Press, 1989.

52. Oken J. What to tell cancer patients. *JAMA* 1961;175:1120.

53. Novack DH, et al. Changes in physician attitudes towards the cancer patient. *JAMA* 1979;241:897.

54. Zaner RM. *Ethics and the clinical encounter.* Englewood Cliffs, NJ: Prentice Hall, 1988.

55. Daniel SL. The patient as text: a model of clinical hermeneutics. *Theor Med* 1986;7:195.

56. Graber GC, Thomasma DC. *Theory and practice in medical ethics.* New York: Continuum, 1989.

57. Brody H. *Stories of sickness.* New Haven, CT: Yale University Press, 1987.

58. Jonsen A, Toulmin S. *The abuse of casuistry: a history of moral reasoning.* Berkeley, CA: University of California Press, 1988.

59. Pellegrino E. Character, virtue, and self-interest in the ethics of the professions. *J Contemp Health Law Policy* 1989;5:53.

60. Pellegrino E, Thomasma DC. *For the patients' good: the restoration of beneficence in health care.* New York: Oxford University Press, 1988.

61. Shelp EE, ed. *Virtue and medicine.* Dordrecht, The Netherlands: D. Reidel, 1985.

62. May WF. *The physician's covenant.* Philadelphia: Westminster, 1983.

63. Kilner JF. Ethical issues and the ESRD patient. *Am J Kidney Dis* 1990; 15:218.

64. Larson DG, Tobin DR. End-of-life conversations: evolving practice and theory. *JAMA* 2000;284:1573.

65. Kaye M, Lella JW. Discontinuation of dialysis therapy in the demented patient. *Am J Nephrol* 1986;6:75.

66. Pellegrino ED. Decisions to withdraw life-sustaining treatment: a moral algorithm. *JAMA* 2000;283:1065.

67. Cummings NB. Termination of dialysis. In: Andreucci VE, Fine LG, eds. *International yearbook of nephrology.* Oxford: Oxford University Press, 1997:121.

68. Canadian Nurses Association, Canadian Medical Association, Canadian Hospital Association. Joint statement on terminal illness. *CMAJ* 1984;130:1357.

69. Stanley JM. The Appleton consensus: suggested international guidelines for decisions to forgo medical treatment. *J Med Ethics* 1989; 15:129.

70. Bone RC, Rackow EC, Weg JG, and members of AACP/SCCM. Consensus panel: ethical and moral guidelines for the initiation, continuation, and withdrawal of intensive care. *Chest* 1990;97:949.

71. Luce JM, Raffin TA. Withholding and withdrawal of life support from critically ill patients. *Chest* 1988;94:621.

72. American Medical Association, Council on Scientific Affairs. Good care of the dying patient. *JAMA* 1996;275:474.

73. Haverkate I, van der Wal G. Policies on medical decisions concerning the end of life in Dutch health care institutions. *JAMA* 1996;275: 435.

74. Renal Physicians Association and American Society of Nephrology. *Shared decision-making in the appropriate initiation and withdrawal from dialysis.* Clinical practice guideline. Washington, DC, and Rockville, MD: Renal Physicians Association and American Society of Nephrology, February 2000.

75. National Kidney Foundation. Initiation or withdrawal of dialysis in end stage renal disease. In: *Guidelines for the health care team.* New York: National Kidney Foundation. 1996.

76. Freeman RB. *Renal dialysis decision-making.* Prepared by contract to the University of Rochester for the Office of Technology Assessment, U.S. Congress. Washington, DC, March 1986.

77. *Schloendorff v New York Hospital,* 211 NY 125, 105, NE 92, 93 (1914) [New York State Supreme Court Decision].

78. Oreopoulos DG. Should we let them die? The moral dilemmas of economic restraints on life-support treatments [Editorial]. *CMAJ* 1982;126:745.

79. Holden MO. Dialysis or death: the ethical alternatives. *Health Soc Work* 1980;5:18.

80. McGeown MG. Chronic renal failure in Northern Ireland, 1968–1970. *Lancet* 1972;1:307.

81. Calne R. The gift of life. *Lancet* 1991;338:180.

82. Lawry K. Grappling with ethical issues in solid organ transplantation cases. *HEC Forum* 1994;6:47.

83. Blank RH. Lifestyle choices and medical technology: allocating organ transplants. *J Health Hum Resources* 1991;13:260.

84. Butcher J. Scientists propose two ways to clone a pig. *Lancet* 2000; 356:657.

85. Alexander JW, Vaughn WK. the use of "marginal" donors for organ transplantation. *Transplantation* 1991;51:135.

86. Kuo PC, Johnson LB, Schweitzer EJ, et al. Utilization of the older donor for renal transplantation. *Am J Surg* 1993;172:551.

87. Cofan F, Oppenheimer F, Campistol JM, et al. Advanced age donors in the evolution of renal transplantation. *Transplant Proc* 1995;27: 2248.

88. Lu AD, Carter JT, Weinstein RJ, et al. Outcome in recipients of dual kidney transplants. *Transplantation* 2000;69:281.

89. Callender CO, Bayton JA, Yeager C, et al. Attitudes among blacks towards donating kidneys for transplantation: a pilot project. *J Natl Med Assoc* 1982;74:6.

90. Land W, Dossetor JB. *Organ replacement therapy: ethics, justice, commerce.* New York: Springer-Verlag, 1991.

91. Delmar-McClure N. When organs match and health beliefs don't. *J Adolesc Health Care* 1985;6:233.

92. Cummings NB. Ethical issues in geriatric nephrology: overview. *Am J Kidney Dis* 1990;26:367.

93. Massachusetts Task Force on Organ Transplantation. *Report of the Massachusetts Task Force on Organ Transplantation.* Boston: Department of Public Health, Commonwealth of Massachusetts, 81, 1984.

94. Fauchald P, et al. Renal replacement therapy in elderly patients. *Transplant Int* 1988;1:131.

95. Spital A, Spital M. Living kidney donation: attitudes outside the transplant center. *Arch Intern Med* 1988;148:1077.

96. Sullivan W. Buying of kidneys of poor attacked. *The New York Times,* September 24, 1983: Section 1:9.

97. Gunby P. Bill introduced to thwart kidney brokerage. *JAMA* 1983; 250:2263.

98. Holzgreve W, et al. Renal transplantation from anencephalic donors. *N Engl J Med* 1987;316:1069.

99. Nelson JB. Organ transplants: their human dimensions. In: Nelson JB, ed. *Human medicine: ethical perspectives on new medical issues.* Minneapolis: Augsburg Publishers, 1973:149.

100. In re: *Guardianship of Richard Pescinski, Incompetent,* 67 Wisc 2d 4 [Supreme Court of Wisconsin, March 4, 1975].

101. Rich S. Advocates for the poor hit Oregon health plan: governor vows to prevent inadequate care. *The Washington Post,* September, 17, 1991:A3.

102. Welch HG, Larson EB. Dealing with limited resources: the Oregon decision to curtail funding for organ transplantation. *N Engl J Med* 1988;319:171.

103. Daar AS, Salahudeen AK, Pingle A, et al. Ethics and commerce in live donor renal transplantation: classification of the issues. *Transplant Proc* 1990;22:922.

104. Dossetor J, et al. Discussion. *Transplant Proc* 1990;19:933.

105. Parry and Co. Market survey, 1988 [Quoted in Reddy KC, et al. Unconventional renal transplantation in India. *Transplant Proc* 1990;22:910].

106. Kumar S. Curbing trade in human organs in India. *Lancet* 1994;344: 48.

107. Thiagarajan CM, et al. The practice of unconventional renal transplantation (UCRT) at a single centre in India. *Transplant Proc* 1990;22: 912.

108. Salahudeen AK. High mortality among recipients of bought living-unrelated donor kidneys. *Lancet* 1990;336:725.

109. Abouna GEM, et al. Commercialization in human organs: a Middle Eastern perspective. *Transplant Proc* 1990;22:918.

110. Spital A. Unconventional living kidney donors: attitudes and use among transplant centers. *Transplantation* 1989;48:243.

111. D'Apice AJF, Walker RG. Renal transplantation from living donors. *Med J Aust* 1988;148:427.

112. Sahin AF. Islamic transplantation ethics. *Transplant Proc* 1990;22: 939.

113. Namihira E. Shinto concept concerning the dead human body. *Transplant Proc* 1990;22:940.

114. Scorsone S. Christianity and the significance of the human body. *Transplant Proc* 1990;22:943.

115. Bilka RP. Jewish perspective on organ transplantation. *Transplant Proc* 1990;22:945.

116. Sugunasiri SHJ. The Buddhist view concerning the dead body. *Transplant Proc* 1990;22:947.

117. Taylor H. U.S. health care: built for waste. *The New York Times,* April 17, 1990:A15.

118. Reiser SJ. Malpractice, patient safety, and the ethical and scientific foundations of medicine. In: Huber PW, Litan RE, eds. *The liability maze: the impact of liability law on safety and innovation.* Washington, DC: The Brookings Institute, 1991.

119. LaPuma J, Orentlicher D, Moss RJ. Advance directives on admission: clinical implications and analysis of the Patient Self-Determination Act of 1990. *JAMA* 1991;266:402.

120. McCloskey EL. The Patient Self-Determination Act. *Kennedy Inst Ethics J* 1991;1:163.

121. Omnibus Budget Reconciliation Act of 1990. P. L. 101-508, Sections 4206, 4751.

122. Sabatino CP. *Patient Self-Determination Act: state law guide.* Washington, DC: American Bar Association, Commission of Legal Problems of the Elderly, 1991.

123. American Hospital Association (AHA). *Put it in writing: a guide to promoting advance directives.* Chicago: AHA Division of Public Relations, 1991.

124. McLean BG, Townsend P. The right to die. *Legislative Report Series,* vol. 8, no. 2. Annapolis, MD: Research Division, Department of Legislative Reference, 1990.

125. *Cruzan v Director,* Missouri Department of Health, 110 S. Ct. 2841, 2855–56 (1990).

126. *Cruzan v Director,* Missouri Department of Health, 760 S.W. 408 (1988).

127. In re: *Quinlan,* 137 N.J. Super. 227, 348A.2d 801; (Ch. Div. 1975),

modified, 70 N.J. 10, 355 A.2d 647 (cert. denied), 429 U.S. 922 (1976).

128. Rhyned CS. *Law and judicial systems of nations,* 3rd ed. Washington, DC: The World Peace Through Law Center, 1978.

129. American Bar Association Internal Report, February 1991.

129a. American Bar Association, *personal communication,* November, 2000.

130. In re: *Spring,* 380 Mass. 629, 405 NE 2d 115 (1980).

131. Society for the Right to Die, Inc. *Right-to-die court decisions.* New York: Society for the Right to Die, Inc., 1987.

132. In re: *Lydia E. Hall Hospital,* 116 Misc. 22d 477, 455 NYS 2d 706, Supreme Court, Nassau County (1982).

133. New Mexico ex rel *Smith v Fort,* No. 14, 768 (1983).

134. Haney SD. On being a problem patient. *AAKP Bull* 1993(Spring):3.

135. Johnson CC, Moss AH, Clarke SAD, et al. Working with noncompliant and abusive dialysis patients: practical strategies based on ethics and the law. *Adv Ren Replace Ther* 1996;3:77.

136. Bower JD. The issue: the role of the professional in management of noncompliant or problem dialysis patients. *Dial Transplant* 1995;24: 173.

137. Kottler J. *Compassionate therapy: working with difficult clients.* San Francisco: Jossey Bass.

138. Haynes BR, Taylor DW, Sackett DL. *Compliance in health care.* Baltimore: Johns Hopkins University Press, 1979:46–62.

139. *Payton v Weaver,* 131 Cal. App. 3d 38, App. 182 Cal. Report 225,1982.

140. *Brown v Bower,* U.S. District Court, Southern District of Mississippi, Jackson Division, Civil Action No. J86-8759 (B) (filed December 21, 1987).

141. Brahams D. When is discontinuation of dialysis justified? *Lancet* 1985;1:176.

142. Society for Right to Die. *Newsletter* 1991[Summer]:4.

143. President's Commission for the Study of Ethical Problems in Medicine and Biomedical and Behavioral Research. *Making health care decisions.* Vol. 2, appendix B. Washington, DC: U.S. Government Printing Office, 1982.

144. Cummings NB, Stocking C, Kohn G. Autonomy and advance directives for chronically ill patients. In: Kielstein R, ed. *Ethics and nephrology.* Bochum, Germany: Bochum Center for Medical Ethics, 1995.

145. Swartz RD, Perry E. Advance directives are associated with "good deaths" in chronic dialysis patients. *J Am Soc Nephrol* 1993;3:1623.

146. Smith RE. *Compilation of state and federal privacy laws.* Providence, RI: Privacy Journal, 1992.

147. *Estate of Urbaniak v Newton,* 277 Cal. Rptr. 354, 226, Cal. App. 3d 1128 Ct. App. 1st Dist. (1991).

148. *Behringer v Medical Center of Princeton,* Westlaw 690321 N.J. Super. Law Division, 25 April (1991).

149. Rao TKS, et al. Associated focal and segmental glomerulosclerosis in the acquired immunodeficiency syndrome. *N Engl J Med* 1984; 310:669.

150. Cooke M. Health-care workers and AIDS: an ethical overview. In: Cohen PT, Sande MA, Volberding PA, eds. *The AIDS knowledge base.* Waltham, MA: Medical Publishing Group, Division of Massachusetts Medical Society, 1990:1.

151. Gerberding JL, et al. Risk of transmitting the human immunodeficiency virus, cytomegalovirus, and hepatitis B virus to health care workers exposed to patients with AIDS and AIDS-related conditions. *J Infect Dis* 1987;156:1.

152. Henderson DK, Gerberding JL. Prophylactic zidovudine after occupational exposure to human immunodeficiency virus: an interim analysis. *J Infect Dis* 1989;160:321.

153. Centers for Disease Control. Recommendations for providing dialysis treatment to patients infected with human T-lymphotropic virus type III/lymphadenopathy-associated virus. *MMWR Morb Mortal Wkly Rep* 1986;35:376.

154. Centers for Disease Control. Recommendations for prevention of HIV transmission in health-care settings. *MMWR Morb Mortal Wkly Rep* 1987;36[Suppl 2S]:3S.

155. Centers for Disease Control. Update: human immunodeficiency virus infections in health-care workers exposed to blood of infected patients. *MMWR Morb Mortal Wkly Rep* 1987;36:285.

156. Alter MJ, Favero MS, Moyer LA, et al. National surveillance of dialysis-associated diseases in the United States, 1989. *Trans Am Soc Artif Intern Organs* 1991;37:97.

157. Favero MS. Precautions for dialyzing human immunodeficiency virus-infected patients. In: Monkhouse PM, ed. *Aspects of renal care 3.* London: Bailliére Tindall, 1989.

158. Carbone L, D'Agati V, Cheng J-T, et al. Course and prognosis of human immunodeficiency virus-associated nephropathy. *Am J Med* 1989;87:389.

159. Rao TKS, Friedman EA, Nicastri AD. The types of renal disease in acquired immunodeficiency syndrome. *N Engl J Med* 1987;316: 1062.

160. Ortiz C, et al. Outcome of patients with human immunodeficiency virus on maintenance hemodialysis. *Kidney Int* 1988;34:248.

161. Fassbinder W, Fursch A, Kuhnl P, et al. Human immunodeficiency virus antibody screening in patients on renal replacement therapy: prevalence of false-positive results. *Nephrol Dial Transplant* 1987;2: 248.

162. Monos DS, et al. Delineation of false-positive HIV antibody response in patients with renal failure and history of multiple transfusions. *Transfusion* 1989;29:119.

163. Peterman TA, et al. HTLV-III/LAV infection in hemodialysis patients. *JAMA* 1986;255:2324.

164. Stevens S, et al. HIV testing in patients with end stage renal disease. *BMJ* 1990;300:447.

165. Royal College of Nursing. *Royal College of Nursing guidelines for testing of renal patients for HIV and guidelines for dialysing HIV antibody positive patients.* London: Royal College of Nursing, 1991.

166. Collins D. HIV testing of great value to ESRD patient. *ANNA J* 1993; 20:114.

167. Al-Sulaiman M, Al-Khnader AA, Al-Hasani MK, et al. Impact of HIV infection on dialysis and renal transplantation. *Transplant Proc* 1989;21:1970.

168. Bowen PA, et al. Transmission of human immunodeficiency virus (HIV) by transplantation: clinical aspects and time course analysis of viral antigenemia and antibody production. *Ann Intern Med* 1988; 108:46.

169. Feduska NJ. Human immunodeficiency virus, AIDS, and organ transplantation. *Transplant Rev* 1990;4:93.

170. Kumar P, et al. Transmission of human immunodeficiency virus by transplantation of a renal allograft, with development of the acquired immunodeficiency syndrome. *Ann Intern Med* 1987;106:244.

171. Ward JW, et al. Transmission of human immunodeficiency virus (HIV) by blood transfusions screened as negative for HIV antibody. *N Engl J Med* 1988;318:473.

172. Tzakis AG, et al. Transplantation in HIV+ patients. *Transplantation* 1990;49:354.

173. Rubin RH, Tolkoff-Rubin NE. The problem of human immunodeficiency virus (HIV) infection and transplantation. *Transplantation* 1985;44:1.

174. Cunningham EE, et al. Heroin nephropathy: a clinicopathologic and epidemiologic study. *Am J Med* 1980;68:47.

175. Eknoyan G, et al. Renal involvement in drug abuse. *Arch Intern Med* 1973;132:801.

176. Rao TKS, Nicastri AD, Friedman EA. Natural history of heroin associated nephropathy. *N Engl J Med* 1974;290:19.

177. Stein MD. Medical complications of intravenous drug use. *J Gen Intern Med* 1990;5:249.

178. Cunningham EE, Ziclezny MA, Venuto RC. Heroin-associated nephropathy: a nationwide problem. *JAMA* 1983;250:2955.

179. Des Jarlais DC, Friedman EA. HIV infection among persons who inject illicit drugs: problems and prospects. *J AIDS* 1988;1:267.

180. Hahn RA, Onorato IM, Jones S, et al. Prevalence of HIV infection among intravenous drug users in the United States. *JAMA* 1989; 261:2677.

181. Friedman EA, Rao TKS. Why does uremia in heroin abusers occur predominately among blacks? *JAMA* 1983;250:2965.

182. Schoenfeld P, Feduska NJ. Acquired immunodeficiency syndrome and renal disease: report of the National Kidney Foundation-National Institutes of Health Task Force on AIDS and Kidney Disease. *Am J Kidney Dis* 1990;16:14.

183. Ross G, Weinstein S, Dutton S, et al. Renal transplantation in the end stage renal disease of drug abuse. *J Urol* 1983;129:14.

184. Gupta RK, van der Meulen J, Johny KV. Oliguric acute renal failure due to glue-sniffing: a case report scan. *J Urol Nephrol* 1991;25: 247.

185. Carlisle EJ, et al. Glue-sniffing and distal renal tubular acidosis: sticking to the facts. *J Am Soc Nephrol* 1991;1:1019.

186. Noels LM, Elseviers MM, de Broe ME. Impact of legislative measures on the sales of analgesics and the subsequent prevalence of analgesic nephropathy: a comparative study in France, Sweden, and Belgium. *Nephrol Dial Transplant* 1995;10:167.

187. Nanra RS. Analgesic nephropathy in the 1990s: an Australian perspective. *Kidney Int Suppl* 1993;42:S86.

188. Keller CK, Andrassy K, Waldherr R, et al. Postinfectious glomerulonephritis: is there a link to alcoholism? *QJM* 1994;87:97.

189. Schwarz A, Offerman G, Keller F. Analgesic nephropathy and renal transplantation. *Nephrol Dial Transplant* 1992;7:427.

190. Driesens F, Awouters F, Goossens T, et al. Analgesics abuse: theoretical and practical considerations. *Med Hypotheses* 1993;40:66.

191. Qiu C, Schoenfeld P, Burnell M, et al. Impact of the cocaine epidemic on end stage renal disease (ESRD) at San Francisco General Hospital. *J Am Soc Nephrol* 1990;1:373A.

192. Freedman BI, Bowden DW. The role of genetic factors in the development of end-stage renal disease. *Curr Opin Nephrol Hypertens* 1995;4:230.

193. Parfrey PS. Hereditary renal disease. *Curr Opin Nephrol Hypertens* 1993;2:192.

194. Jennings SB, Gnarra JR, Walther MM, et al. Renal cell carcinoma: molecular genetics and clinical implications. *Surg Oncol Clin North Am* 1995;4:219.

195. Linehan WM, Lerman MI, Zbar B. Identification of the von Hippel-Lindau (VHL) gene: its role in renal cancer. *JAMA* 1995;273:564.

196. Weiss R. Test tube baby born to save ill sister. *The Washington Post* 2000 Oct. 3:A1.

197. Siegler M. Confidentiality in medicine: a decrepit concept. *N Engl J Med* 1982;307:1518.

198. Fletcher JC, Wertz DC. Ethics and prenatal diagnosis: problems, positions, and proposed guidelines. In: Milunsky A, ed. *Genetic disorders and the fetus: diagnosis, prevention, and treatment,* 3rd ed. Baltimore: Johns Hopkins University Press, 1992:823.

199. White R, Caskey CT. Genetic predisposition and the Human Genome Project: case illustrations of clinical problems. In: Annas GJ, Elias S, eds. *Gene mapping: using law and ethics as guides.* New York: Oxford University Press, 1992:173.

200. Kohn DB, et al. Establishment and characterization of adenosine deaminase deficient human T-cell lines. *J Immunol* 1989;142: 3971.

201. Harper PS, Clarke A. Should we test children for "adult" genetic diseases? *Lancet* 1990;335:1205.

202. Hildebrandt F. Genetic diseases in children. *Curr Opin Pediatr* 1995;7:182.

203. Nicholson RH, ed. *Medical research with children: ethics, law and practice.* Oxford: Oxford University Press, 1986.

204. Kielstein R, Sass H-M. Right not to know or duty to know? Prenatal screening for polycystic kidney renal disease. *J Med Philos* 1992;17:395.

205. Embryo Protection Law Under Penal Code. Bundesrepublik, 1990. Paragraph 2,1; 2,2; 8,1.

206. Breuning MH, et al. Two step procedure for early diagnosis of polycystic kidney disease with polymorphic DNA markers on both sides of the gene. *J Med Genet* 1990;27:614.

207. Hodgkinson KA, Kerzin-Storrar L, Watters EA, et al. Adult polycystic kidney disease: knowledge, experience, and attitudes to prenatal diagnosis. *J Med Genet* 1990;27:552.

208. Lifshitz A, et al. Genetic counseling in adult polycystic kidney disease in Israel. *Nephron* 1990;55:386.

209. Green A, et al. Prevalence of hereditary renal disease. *Ir Med J* 1990;83:11.

SECTION **XIV**

Nutrition, Drugs, and the Kidney

CHAPTER 101

Protein Intake and Prevention of Chronic Renal Disease

Thomas H. Hostetter and William E. Mitch

NATURAL HISTORY OF CHRONIC RENAL FAILURE

In many normal adults, there is a decline in glomerular filtration rate (GFR) with age, but this should not be mistaken for the progressive loss of renal function that occurs with or after kidney damage because these subjects rarely require therapy for end-stage renal disease (ESRD). Specifically, approximately two-thirds of normal adults older than 40 years of age experience a decrease in GFR even if they have no obvious kidney disease (1), but in the remaining third, GFR remains stable (2). The proportions of those with a declining GFR can vary, however, because Fliser et al. noted that two-thirds of elderly subjects have values within the range of younger adults (3). The cause of the loss of GFR with normal aging is obscure but may be linked to the decline in dietary protein that occurs in most elderly subjects (4). Variation in dietary protein also accounts in part for the day-to-day variability in GFR (5). These data emphasize that the diet must be taken into account when evaluating a single value of GFR or changes in GFR with time (i.e., those with progression).

In contrast to normal aging, patients who experience kidney damage from different diseases and acquire manifestations of chronic renal failure (CRF) continue to lose function (i.e., experience "progression"), even when the disease that initially damaged the kidneys is no longer active [e.g., obstructive uropathy (6) or cortical necrosis after obstetric accidents (7)]. There are patients, however, including those with diabetic nephropathy, who do not exhibit progressive loss of GFR over periods of observation as long as 3 years despite kidney damage (8,9). In these reports, the investigators concentrated on controlling blood sugar and blood pressure, respectively, so it is likely that treating these abnormalities accounts at least in part for the lack of progression. There also are other, unidentified reasons for the lack of progression in patients with CRF, and in the largest published series of rates of loss of GFR [the Modification of Diet in Renal Disease (MDRD) Study (10)], less than 15% of patients had no progression over the average of 2.2 years of study even in the group with initially more advanced renal insufficiency (GFR, 13 to 23 mL/minute/1.73 m^2). The reason for the stability of renal function in these patients was not identified, but there were five factors that could be associated with faster rates of progression: (a) more proteinuria, (b) higher mean arterial pressure, (c) lower serum high-density lipoprotein cholesterol, (d) lower serum transferrin, and (e) polycystic kidney disease. This list does not include dietary protein, and this inconsistency is puzzling based on the foregoing discussion and the following review of published data.

By what methods can progression be assessed? Answering this question involves addressing two issues: knowing the accuracy of the method used to measure the remaining kidney function, and how accurately the method quantifies changes in renal function. These are distinct tasks because the former assesses GFR at one point in time, whereas the latter examines how rapidly renal function is being lost.

In earlier editions of this book, we evaluated how accurately creatinine clearance and serum creatinine estimate GFR and how well these methods approximate changes in GFR with time in patients with chronic renal insufficiency. This discussion will not be repeated except for a brief summary that includes new developments in measuring or estimating GFR.

Assessment of Glomerular Filtration Rate

The standard measure of GFR, the renal clearance of inulin, requires precise regulation of an intravenous infusion of inulin to achieve a steady-state plasma inulin concentration and at least three accurately timed urine collections with complete emptying of the bladder (11). To minimize the

T. H. Hostetter: National Institutes of Health, National Institute of Diabetes and Digestive and Kidney Diseases, Bethesda, Maryland

W. E. Mitch: Department of Medicine and Renal Division, Emory University School of Medicine, Atlanta, Georgia

influence of changes in posture, the patient should remain supine or be seated quietly, standing only to void (12,13). Patients usually are given a water load to improve the accuracy of collecting all the urine made during a collection period, and inulin is measured by chemical methods (14). Despite these precautions, the coefficient of variation of inulin clearance is at least 10% in patients with nearly "normal" GFR values and is higher in patients with CRF (11). To reduce the analytic error in measuring inulin, radiolabeled compounds cleared predominantly by glomerular filtration have been used; gamma-emitters usually are infused to avoid the error caused by the variable quenching when beta-emitting compounds (e.g., ^{14}C-inulin) are used. In individual subjects, there is a close concordance between the clearances of inulin and ^{125}I-iothalamate (or other labeled compounds) over a wide range of GFRs (12,15). As with inulin, measuring the renal clearance of ^{125}I-iothalamate or other radiolabeled markers requires considerable supervision to ensure an adequate urine flow and accurately timed blood and urine collections (15,16).

To avoid water loading and the timing of urine collections, methods based on calculating the total plasma disappearance of an injected radiolabeled compound have been devised (based on the demonstration that the renal clearance is insignificantly lower than the plasma clearance—any new method must be tested for the validity of this assumption). To calculate GFR from plasma clearance, at least three additional assumptions are made: (a) the extrarenal clearance of the radiolabeled compound is negligible; (b) the plasma clearance is constant during the period of sampling (with the prolonged infusion that is required for patients with advanced renal insufficiency, this assumption may not be valid); and (c) sampling includes the period that represents the monoexponential extrapolation of changes in radioactivity with time to infinity. If these prerequisites are missing, the plasma clearance calculation will be invalid. Satisfying these assumptions is most important when assessing the GFR of patients with severe CRF because there may be a small extrarenal clearance that is not detectable during short collection periods, and the time required to reach the monoexponential phase of removal can be many hours (16). For these reasons, most agree that the plasma clearance technique is not as accurate as the renal clearance, but the reproducibility of a ^{51}Cr-ethylenediaminetetraacetic acid (EDTA) plasma clearance is reportedly 4% to 5% in subjects with only mild impairment of renal function and approximately 12% for subjects with more advanced CRF [similar values were reported when the plasma clearance of nonradioactive iodinated compounds was measured (17)]. These values are similar to the variability of the renal clearance of inulin.

Some investigators have advocated a method of approximating the entire plasma disappearance curve based on a single plasma sample obtained several hours after an injection of a radiolabeled compound, but this leads to inaccuracies compared with multiple sampling techniques (16–21).

Nonradioactive markers (e.g., iothalamate, iohexol, iodixanol) have been shown to be acceptable for measuring GFR provided the dose is low so there is no risk of nephrotoxicity (17,22–25).

Creatinine Clearance

The 24-hour endogenous creatinine clearance usually exceeds inulin clearance because of tubular secretion, but the values of creatinine clearance and GFR become numerically close in patients with advanced CRF even though the percentage difference rises (11,26–28). Regardless, there are other reasons for avoiding creatinine clearance as a method of estimating GFR. These include the inconvenience to the patient of a 24-hour urine collection and the uncertainty of a complete urine collection. In addition, 24-hour creatinine clearances have a high coefficient of variation: in one study of 119 healthy ambulatory subjects, the coefficient of variation was 26%, and other reports indicate it varies from 6% to 22% (26,29,30). A major cause of this variability is the day-to-day differences in creatinine excretion (30–33); among hospitalized patients, creatinine excretion varies by at least 10% (34–36). Consequently, it is not surprising that the slope of sequential changes in creatinine clearance is poorly correlated with the slope of GFR (37,38). In fact, the relationship is so poor that many investigators recommend abandoning the 24-hour creatinine clearance (39,40). The same caveats apply to calculating the average of the 24-hour creatinine and urea clearances to estimate GFR, even though with proper collections, this value corresponds closely to inulin clearance (27).

A relatively recent strategy is to give cimetidine as an inhibitor of creatinine secretion to obtain a more accurate estimate of GFR. Regarding cimetidine dosage, 1.2 g usually achieves complete suppression of creatinine secretion, whereas 0.4 g often is insufficient (41). With water loading and carefully timed urine collections of 30 to 50 minutes, the cimetidine creatinine clearance procedure can give clearance values with a coefficient of variation of approximately 8% in patients with GFR values from 12 to 150 mL/minute (42). This eliminates the need to deal with radioactive material or purchase equipment, but still requires trained personnel.

Frustration with the variability in 24-hour creatinine clearances has led to the widespread practice of estimating creatinine clearance from serum creatinine and an estimated daily rate of creatinine excretion based on the age, weight, and sex of the patient (34,43). However, the widely used Cockcroft Gault formula (34) is derived from data of "normal, hospitalized" patients, but creatinine excretion declines in patients with CRF (43). This decrease in creatinine excretion in patients with CRF can be attributed to creatinine degradation, which, in turn, can be approximated by an average extrarenal creatinine clearance of 0.04 L/kg/day. This value for extrarenal clearance should be integrated with other factors affecting creatinine production when the creatinine clearance of patients with CRF is estimated from formulas. For example, the daily rate of creatinine production in milligrams per kilograms per day can be calculated as $28 - 0.2$ A for male and $23.8 - 0.17$ A for female subjects, where A is the age of the subject in years (34,43). Combining these formulas with the average extrarenal creatinine clearance yields a predicted creatinine clearance (C_{Cr}) in liters per kilogram per day: $C_{Cr} = (28 - 0.2 \text{ A}) S^{-1} - 0.04$ L/kg/day in men, and $C_{Cr} = (23.8 - 0.17 \text{ A}) S^{-1} - 0.04$ L/kg/day in women, where S^{-1} is the reciprocal of the serum creatinine in milligrams per liter. Using these formulas, the measured 24-hour creatinine clearances of 95% of uremic adults with stable serum creatinine values greater than 8 mg/dL were estimated to within 1.5 mL/minute (43). Obviously, this type of estimate incorporates several assumptions, and by relying on changes in serum creatinine alone, there is some reduction in the variability of estimated changes in GFR.

Serum Creatinine

Although rates of creatinine production are not constant but depend on lean body mass, the amount of meat in the diet and creatinine secretion by the kidney contributes a variable amount to total creatinine clearance (26,29,31,44). There have been attempts to estimate the GFR from serum creatinine: these methods seem to be satisfactory as long as the patient is in the steady state and has a near normal body habitus (34).

ASSESSMENT OF THE RATE OF PROGRESSION OF RENAL INSUFFICIENCY

Early studies suggested that the course of CRF was unpredictable, so prognosis was assessed by estimating the average time before ESRD occurred and dialysis became necessary, or a predetermined degree of renal insufficiency was reached (46–48) (Fig. 101-1). The field has advanced, however, and it now is recognized that most patients experience a loss of renal function that is not chaotic but rather constant and predictable when the decline in GFR with time is examined. Unfortunately, there have been very few examinations of the frequency of a linear decline in GFR with time in a large number of patients with kidney disease, but on average, a linear decline was observed in patients in the MDRD who were assigned to a high-protein diet, and there are several studies showing that the reciprocal of serum creatinine $(S^{-1};$ see later) declines linearly with time (26,49,50). As expected from any investigation of patients, a linear decline in kidney function is not uniformly observed. Shah and Levey reported that 32% of 77 patients had a "break-point" in the S^{-1} plot, suggesting that in those patients, the loss of renal function was not constant (51). Conversely, Coresh et al. found significant breakpoints in only 19% of a series of 67 patients followed until ESRD was reached (52). In addition, it remains unclear why the rate of loss of renal function is so variable even when

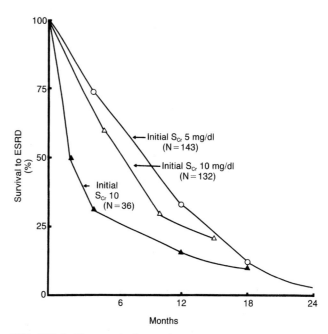

FIG. 101-1. The survival to end-stage renal disease (ESRD) of patients with chronic renal failure. Three reports are examined: data of 143 patients with an initial serum creatinine (S_{Cr}) of 5 mg/dL (47); of 132 patients with an initial S_{Cr} of 10 mg/dL (48); and of 36 patients with an initial S_{Cr} of 10 mg/dL (46). The criteria for diagnosing ESRD were not given in these reports, but the wide variability in survival of different populations is apparent.

each patient has a constant rate of progression and the same underlying kidney disease (53).

The optimal method for assessing the rate of progression is to measure sequential changes in GFR. Usually, this requires at least four measurements over 2 or more years (54,55). Like any measurement of a physiologic function, standardized methods must be strictly followed to achieve accuracy. Unfortunately, measuring GFR is costly because skilled personnel are required and reagents and measurements must be purchased. To be balanced against this problem is the fact that other methods (e.g., the time for a specified increase in serum creatinine to occur or repetitive measurements of creatinine clearance) provide less convincing evidence that the rate of progression has changed. Thus, the nephrologist is faced with deciding between organizing personnel plus purchasing the supplies required to establish a reliable method for measuring GFR (or at least investigating the accuracy of the method used by others, such as Nuclear Medicine colleagues), and relying on a less accurate method of estimating the loss of renal function.

For clinical purposes, the S^{-1} plot is the principal alternative to repetitive GFR measurements for assessing changes in GFR. There are two reasons for choosing this method to estimate the rate of loss of renal function. First, creatinine is simple to measure and reproducible [the day-to-day coefficient of variation in patients with renal disease is only 6.5% (57)], and usually there are preexisting values for the assessment of changes in renal function. Second, S^{-1} declines linearly with time in most patients with progressive renal insufficiency (26,50,52). Recognition that the decline in S^{-1} with time is linear in an individual patient led to the hypothesis that renal function is lost at a constant rate (58), and this seems to be true for most patients (26). For example, 80% of the patients reported by Rutherford et al. (59) and Coresh et al. (52) had linear slopes for their S^{-1} plots. An important issue is whether there is spontaneous slowing of the rate of loss of renal function when GFR falls to low levels. Based on data from patients with different causes of CRF, Gretz et al. (60) estimated that changes in the decline of S^{-1} are more likely to accelerate than to slow spontaneously, and Oksa et al. (61) attributed this to improved control of hypertension. Approximately half of patients with two slopes of S^{-1} (i.e., only five patients) in the study by Rutherford et al. (59) had spontaneous slowing of progression, indicating that this is an unusual occurrence. On the other hand, Walser et al. (38) reported there are important differences in the rates of progression measured as changes in S^{-1} compared with changes in the renal clearance of ^{99m}Tc-dithethylenetriamine pentaacetic acid (DTPA; i.e., GFR). They studied 17 patients eating a ketoacid-based, very-low-protein diet and corrected values of S^{-1} using average values of creatinine excretion to compare GFR with this "estimated" creatinine clearance. In four patients, they found a progressive loss of renal function based on the estimated creatinine clearances, even though the GFR values were stable. However, two patients had to begin dialysis, and changes in the GFR of the final patient suggested improvement in renal function while the estimated creatinine clearance remained stable. When they examined progression during different periods of these patients, there were 9 of 22 periods that exhibited a statistical difference between the slopes of estimated creatinine clearance and GFR: in two periods, GFR was stable but changes in the S^{-1} clearance suggested progression. In two other periods, both methods were consistent with progression, but the S^{-1} clearance method suggested faster progression, and in two other periods, GFR improved or worsened whereas the S^{-1} clearance method was stable. These last two instances are the most worrisome in terms of the S^{-1} method giving misleading information. Overall, however, it appears that in only 4 of 22 periods did the S^{-1} method yield an inappropriate conclusion regarding the direction of the change in renal function.

Although these differences are not great, there are other reasons why the S^{-1} method may not yield an accurate estimate of the loss of residual renal function. It is well known that creatinine secretion accounts for differences between creatinine clearance and GFR and that the S^{-1} method does not correct for it (28,45,62). Another problem is that creatinine production cannot be equated to creatinine elimination because of extrarenal elimination of creatinine [presumably degraded by gastrointestinal bacteria (63)]. As explained, this problem can be overcome by assuming a constant value of extrarenal clearance of 0.04 L/kg/day and, using this modi-

fication, it can be shown that the linear decline in creatinine clearance of patients with CRF is compatible with a linear decline in the S^{-1} (26,64). Unfortunately, it is not known whether extrarenal creatinine clearance does, indeed, remain constant throughout the course of CRF. Finally, there is the serious problem of dietary factors, especially variations in the amount of meat eaten. Meat, like other muscle, contains creatine, and varying meat in the diet varies the size of the creatine pool. In addition, cooking meat converts a portion of the creatine to creatinine, which increases the amount of creatinine that is excreted; contrariwise, an abrupt reduction in meat intake decreases the creatine and creatinine pools, leading to a lower serum creatinine (if creatinine clearance is constant). If, however, the protein (e.g., meat) content of the diet is relatively constant, the change induced by dietary creatinine is short lived; changes in creatine intake do last longer but they have a smaller effect on creatinine excretion (32,65,66). This is due to the slow rate of conversion of creatine in muscle (and other cells) to creatinine: the turnover of the endogenous creatine pool averages only 1.7% per day (67), which means that a new steady state of creatinine production after a sustained change in meat intake (i.e., the intake of creatine and preformed creatinine) occurs in approximately 4 months (26,43). The other problem with varying protein intake is that raising dietary protein increases GFR and, hence, creatinine clearance (68). In summary, changes in serum creatinine alone as a means of estimating the degree of renal damage should be discarded, but changes in the slope of S^{-1} can be used for screening to detect which patients are progressing or whether there has been a change in clinical status. If a specific therapy for progressive renal insufficiency is being investigated, changes in GFR are preferred.

Finally, it is important to determine the rate of progression of each patient individually because it is well known that variation of rates of progression among patients is high: Jones et al. (53) reported that patients with diabetic nephropathy had rates varying as much as 20-fold and Walser (54) found that changes in ^{99m}Tc-DTPA clearance in 34 patients with different causes of CRF varied from -0.96 to $+0.64$ mL/minute/month. The latter results led to the conclusion that 15% of patients may not show any progression (at least during the period of observation), a conclusion supported by results from the MDRD Study (66). These results not only emphasize the importance of evaluating progression rates in individual patients but point out why clinical trials in which there has been no screening to identify patients exhibiting progression are at risk of studying an inadequate number of patients to detect a benefit from any intervention.

PROGRESSION OF EXPERIMENTAL RENAL DAMAGE AND DIETARY PROTEIN

Dietary protein restriction reduces renal injury in virtually all models of experimental renal injury. This beneficial effect of

TABLE 101-1. *Experimental renal diseases improved by dietary protein restriction*

Remnant kidney
Nephrotoxic serum nephritis
Doxorubicin nephrosis
DOCA salt hypertension
Spontaneous hypertension with reduced renal mass
Salt-sensitive hypertension with glomerulonephritis
Diabetes mellitus
Spontaneous glomerular sclerosis of aging
Anti-tubular basement membrane nephritis

dietary protein has been recognized for more than 50 years (69) (Table 101-1), but the mechanisms whereby dietary protein restriction influences the progression of experimental renal diseases are unsettled. Both renal effects and systemic factors have been proposed to explain the beneficial effects of dietary manipulation. Dissection of the mechanisms would be useful not only for an understanding of how protein intake affects the kidney but for its contribution toward suggesting more specific therapies to improve renal preservation. Finally, it is clear that most of the proposed mechanisms are not mutually exclusive; restriction of dietary protein may well have several favorable effects on kidney damage.

Hemodynamic Mechanisms of Progression

Systemic Hypertension

Arterial hypertension arises in the course of most cases of chronic renal insufficiency and may contribute to renal damage. Clinical studies suggest that blood pressure control can reduce the rate of loss of renal function (70,71). Few studies have systematically explored the influence of dietary protein on systemic arterial pressure in experimental models of hypertension, and even fewer are available on humans with hypertension. Reduced dietary protein has been effective in lowering systemic arterial pressure in mineralocorticoid-induced hypertension in rats, so-called deoxycorticosterone salt hypertension (72). The mechanism of this antihypertensive effect is uncertain, but it may relate to changes in the interaction between calcium and contractile proteins in the vascular smooth muscle. However, in other forms of experimental hypertension, dietary protein restriction has not reduced systemic pressure. Notably, the systemic hypertension that develops in rats after subtotal nephrectomy persists even with severe dietary protein restriction. In addition, hypertension in the two-kidney, one-clip renovascular hypertension model is uninfluenced by reduced protein intake (73,74). Taken together, these experimental studies suggest no consistent effect of dietary protein on arterial pressure. Most important, in several models in which protein restriction diminishes renal injury, there has been no concomitant diminution in hypertension, indicating that the beneficial side effects of protein restriction do not necessarily depend on an antihypertensive action.

The effect of protein intake on arterial pressure in essential hypertension is unknown. In patients with hypertension related to chronic renal disease, systemic blood pressure has not been consistently reduced by restriction of dietary protein intake, similar to the results found in rats with subtotal nephrectomy (75,76). Although studies of protein restriction in patients with well characterized disorders such as mineralocorticoid-dependent or renovascular hypertension are not available, it remains possible that as in the animal models, dietary protein may influence the level of blood pressure in certain disorders, but additional studies are needed to test this possibility systematically. However, published controlled studies of protein restriction in patients with renal insufficiency did not note a consistent effect on arterial pressure (75–79).

Intrarenal Hemodynamics

Although systemic arterial pressure is not consistently influenced by dietary protein, intrarenal hemodynamics are regularly affected by the level of dietary protein. In this regard, dietary protein restriction appears almost unique in altering renal hemodynamics and protecting against experimental renal injury; other measures that successfully protect against progressive renal injury, including angiotensin-converting enzyme (ACE) inhibitors, heparin, antiplatelet agents, and thromboxane synthetase inhibitors, simultaneously reduce elevated systemic arterial pressure. However, the lack of effect of dietary protein on systemic arterial pressure does not preclude an important effect on intrarenal hemodynamics.

Consequent to loss of functional renal mass, animals ingesting a normal diet with unrestricted protein demonstrate functional and structural enlargement of residual renal tissue. Single-nephron GFR of the remaining nephrons rises substantially and in direct proportion to the nephron mass lost (i.e., the greater the loss, the greater the compensatory increase in filtration by the remnant units). Simultaneously, morphometric and biochemical indices of renal growth increase rapidly after reduction in renal mass. For example, renal RNA content begins to increase within 12 hours after unilateral nephrectomy, and incorporation of radiolabeled choline into renal membranes occurs in the first minutes after unilateral nephrectomy. The neurohumoral and cell biologic mechanisms underlying this remarkable increase in function and structure are disputed, but a number of studies identified forces and flows responsible for the augmentation of single-nephron GFR after loss of renal mass (80,81). The studies demonstrated that elevations in glomerular capillary pressure and plasma flow due to reduced renal vascular resistance cause the compensatory increase in single-nephron filtration rate in the remaining glomeruli.

One of the primary determinants of the degree of stimulated functional and structural growth in remnant nephrons is protein intake. Numerous studies in experimental animals demonstrated that a high protein intake augments the weight of the kidney and produces cellular evidence of enhanced growth. On the other hand, lowering dietary protein below standard levels reduces kidney size, even in animals with intact kidneys. Besides altered growth, functional changes can be produced in experimental animals and humans with intact kidneys by altering dietary protein intake. For example, GFR and renal blood flow both increase with either acute or chronic protein loading. Finally, the institution of a low-protein diet when renal mass is reduced markedly changes the functional and morphologic evidence of renal enlargement that normally occurs in residual nephrons after loss of renal mass.

The finding of blunted functional and structural changes induced by low-protein diets after nephron mass reduction and the observation that dietary protein restriction diminishes renal injury have led to the hypothesis that the deleterious effects of normal or increased dietary protein in the setting of renal damage are due to the adaptive increases in blood pressure and flow in the kidney. In this regard, studies in the remnant kidney rat model demonstrated that a low-protein diet diminishes both intrarenal pressures and evidence of renal injury, including proteinuria, abnormal glomerular permselectivity, and histologic damage, especially glomerular sclerosis (73,80). The same relation between glomerular capillary hypertension and glomerular injury and the reversal of this cycle by dietary protein restriction has been obtained in other models of renal injury, including mineralocorticoid hypertension, spontaneously hypertensive rats, and experimental diabetic nephropathy. With only a modest reduction in renal mass (uninephrectomy), dietary protein still influences glomerular injury (82,83). However, in this setting, no effect of the diet on glomerular capillary pressure was seen in one study (83). Finally, by imposing protein restriction after establishing that compensatory renal hypertrophy and hyperfunction have occurred and by studying several nondietary manipulations of renal diseases, it has been possible to incriminate increased glomerular capillary pressure as the injurious force. Based on these correlations, the hypothesis that protein restriction diminishes progressive renal injury by reducing intraglomerular pressure has been championed.

The neurohumoral basis for the hemodynamic effects of dietary protein on the normal and diseased nephron is uncertain. Somatostatin blocks the acute renal vasodilatation associated with intravenous amino acid infusion (84–86). However, somatostatin influences the secretion of so many hormones that this finding only suggests several candidates. Most attention has been focused on glucagon. Specifically, plasma glucagon levels rise with either oral protein feeding or intravenous amino acids (84,87,88), and intravenous infusion of exogenous glucagon at levels similar to those observed after an amino acid infusion provokes a rise in GFR and renal blood flow in humans (88). However, this action of glucagon appears to depend at least in part on prostaglandin (PG) synthesis because the simultaneous administration of a cyclooxy-

genase inhibitor with either amino acid or glucagon blunts the rises in GFR and blood flow (88). The exact cyclooxygenase-dependent product inducing the renal vasodilatation is uncertain because urinary excretions of PGE and the prostacyclin metabolite $PGF_{1\alpha}$ have been variably reported after protein loads (88). Attention also has been given to another local renal vasodilator system, the endothelium-derived relaxing factor, nitric oxide. Blockade of the synthesis of nitric oxide causes renal vasoconstriction in the rat (89). However, the renal vasodilatation after amino acid infusion appears to be particularly susceptible to this blockade, suggesting that nitric oxide also may be at work in the renal hemodynamic response to dietary protein. Furthermore, chronic increases in dietary protein intake in the normal rat not only provoked increases in GFR but augmented the renal excretion of metabolites of nitric oxide (90). Both of these phenomena are blunted by the competitive inhibitor of nitric oxide synthase, L-nitro-arginine methyl ester (L-NAME), suggesting a role of nitric oxide in dietary protein–induced alterations in renal hemodynamics. The more proximate stimulus to nitric oxide production is uncertain but could, to some degree, be arginine, the substrate for nitric acid production. However, other signals likely contribute to the hemodynamic effect because other amino acids also are capable of evoking renal vasodilatation (91).

Although the predominant action of increased dietary protein is to increase GFR largely by augmenting renal blood flow in normal kidneys, lesser effects on GFR and renal blood flow usually have been noted in diseased kidneys (76). However, alterations in glomerular capillary pressure due to shifts in efferent versus afferent vascular resistance have been noted rather regularly with protein feeding in the disease model. The shift toward greater efferent resistance in the setting of increased dietary protein with renal disease may be due to the increased renin secretion and intrarenal ACE activity. Associated higher levels of intrarenal angiotensin II with its predilection for efferent vasoconstriction might derive from the protein-induced stimulation of these two elements of the renin–angiotensin system (76,92–97). In addition, heightened dietary protein stimulates ACE activity along the proximal tubule (96). However, a tonic effect of angiotensin on the efferent arteriole seems to be an insufficient explanation for the heightened glomerular pressures of various disease models. Rather, some more chronic and long-acting effector seems more likely to be at fault because acute pharmacologic blockade of the production or action of angiotensin II does not alter the efferent vascular resistance or glomerular pressure in the remnant model, whereas chronic blockade with various drugs does effect these changes (98,99). Such chronically acting agents might include augmented levels of circulating aldosterone, which occur with higher protein intakes, or an angiotensin II–induced stimulus to yet another local intrarenal actor such as endothelin (76,100,101).

Indeed, aldosterone may enhance injury both through its hypertensive actions as well as direct fibrotic and tissue remodeling effects (100). Even though angiotensin II is capable of stimulating renal cell growth *in vitro,* protein-induced renal hypertrophy *in vivo* does not appear to depend on activity of the renin–angiotensin system because pharmacologic blockade of angiotensin does not attenuate renal growth on a high-protein diet (102). However, the enhanced renal growth associated with higher levels of protein intake may interact adversely with the renal hemodynamic actions of dietary protein. Several lines of evidence suggest that glomerular enlargement may be a forerunner of glomerular sclerosis (81,103–105). With increases in either glomerular capillary pressure or the diameter of glomerular capillaries, the wall tension of the capillaries would be predicted to rise; with coincident increases in both parameters, wall tension would rise still more. Such a mechanical load might further damage the glomerulus and cause or predispose to sclerosis. Yet, other nonhemodynamic liabilities could accrue to protein-induced renal growth—for example, heightened proteinuria due to associated defects in glomerular epithelial cell structure or altered mesangial clearance of macromolecules (106,107).

Inflammatory and Scarring Factors

An increasing number of cytokines and growth factors are being incriminated in the glomerulosclerosis and interstitial scarring characteristic of progressive renal disease (108,109). Dietary protein intake may influence the expression of some of these shaping and scarring factors and through this action determine progression of renal injury. Among these factors, transforming growth factor β (TGFβ) has received considerable attention and has been accorded substantial support for its role in progressive renal disease. The excess accumulation of TGFβ may produce glomerulosclerosis and perhaps chronic tubular interstitial disease in various models of progressive injury (110). The sources of the TGFβ may include both resident renal parenchymal cells, because all appear to have the capacity to produce this cytokine, and infiltrating cells, particularly monocytes. Furthermore, increased protein intake, angiotensin II, and aldosterone are capable of stimulating its renal accumulation; perhaps protein intake does so through the mediation of heightened angiotensin II or aldosterone levels (111,113,114,115). Also, not only may renal synthesis of nitric oxide under the stimulus of a high-protein diet evoke hemodynamic changes, as noted already, but toxic metabolites of nitric oxide such as peroxynitrite may be generated, leading to damaging free radical species (116). Increased insulin-like growth factor activity has been noted in tubular epithelium after high-protein diets (117). However, the effect of this phenomenon on progressive disease is uncertain. Whether dietary protein promotes chronic renal injury through the agency of other cytokines, such as interleukin-1 or platelet-derived growth factor, has been less examined, although an association with the latter has been noted (112). In view of the increasing evidence that these and other predominantly locally acting factors may participate in chronic

injury to the kidney, the effects of dietary protein may depend on several such mediators.

Opinion has emphasized the functional importance of the tubulointerstitial infiltrate seen in most chronic renal diseases. Studies by Agus et al. (118) of a model of interstitial nephritis induced by anti-tubular basement membrane antibody demonstrated that the course of this disease can be modified by restricting dietary protein. These investigators demonstrated that this immune-mediated interstitial injury was diminished despite continued high titers of the tubular basement membrane antibody. They hypothesized that the beneficial effect was due to the suppressive effect of relatively severe dietary protein restriction on effector T-cell immunity. Although the level of dietary protein restriction used in these studies was relatively severe, the authors nevertheless suggested that the beneficial effects of dietary protein restriction can be consequent on influences on the cellular immune system.

Deposition of complement component C3 and the terminal complement complex C5b-9 occurs around the renal tubules in most chronic progressive renal diseases, including those that do not have a primary immune etiology. The same pattern of deposition can be demonstrated in experimental models of renal injury, including the rat remnant kidney model (119). The mechanism whereby these complement components are deposited and the pathophysiologic significance of this deposition have been uncertain because immunoglobulins are not localized in the same peritubular areas. Although this deposition may represent a secondary effect of primary damage to renal cells, evidence supports a more primary role (119).

As with adaptive increases in renal hemodynamics to the loss of nephron mass, adaptive increases in tubular function, particularly ammonia production, also occur. Increased intrarenal ammonia could trigger the alternative complement pathway by a nucleophilic interaction of the free-base ammonia with the thiolester of complement component C3 to form an amidated C3 (119). Amidated C3 in turn could function as a convertase to generate chemotactic and membrane attack complexes and could interact with the leukocyte C3b receptor to stimulate an inflammatory response. Supporting this hypothetical mechanism are studies demonstrating that suppression of the enhanced ammonia production of remnant nephrons by chronic sodium bicarbonate loading reduces renal injury and peritubular deposition of complement components (119). Torres et al. (120) also produced evidence for renal ammoniagenesis as a process promoting cyst formation as well as interstitial inflammation in models of renal cystic disease. Thus, dietary protein restriction may be advantageous, at least in part, because it lowers the dietary acid load, thereby reducing ammonia production of the remnant nephron. A reduction in intrarenal ammonia could diminish activation of the complement system and its inflammatory, cystogenic, and cytotoxic consequences.

Proteinuria has long been recognized as a quantitative predictor of progressive renal disease. However, proteinuria may itself contribute to injury (121,122). Because increases in dietary protein in the setting of renal disease usually have been associated with higher rates of proteinuria, the deleterious effects of protein ingestion may be attributed in part to enhancement of proteinuria (76,123). Among the potentially deleterious effects of this enhanced trafficking of protein into the tubular lumen is the deposition of iron from circulating iron-containing proteins such as transferrin, thus potentially increasing oxidant damage. In addition, liberation of the chemoattractant substances attached to protein may fuel local inflammatory responses. Several biochemical cascades associated with inflammatory and oxidant injury have been identified as consequences of enhanced protein presentation to proximal tubular cells. Finally, inspissation of protein in the distal tubule may contribute to local, intrarenal obstruction (124).

Although higher dietary protein has, in general, been associated with worsening of the pathologic process of progressive renal disease, the exact contributions of increased fibrotic material as against the decreased degradation of these substances are unknown. Heightened levels of messages for various collagens and other matrix proteins have been identified with higher-protein diets in the puromycin aminonucleoside model (113). However, in this model, no change in message for several proteinases could be identified. On the other hand, a study of the remnant kidney model noted increases in several proteinases with lower-protein diets, thereby suggesting that low-protein diets may speed the degradation of fibrotic matrix (125).

Lipid and Mineral Metabolism

Although dietary protein restriction necessitates no change in dietary lipid intake, in practice, there often are alterations in the nature and quantity of lipid ingested when dietary protein is restricted. Hyperlipidemia accompanies ESRD. Although this abnormality probably contributes to large-vessel damage, its role in progressive glomerular capillary obliteration was suggested by Guijarro and Keane (126). Using the remnant kidney rat model, they demonstrated that clofibrate-induced reduction of the serum cholesterol level of rats ingesting a Standard diet lessened proteinuria and the prevalence of sclerotic glomeruli. The effects were achieved without altering the degree of hypertension or serum triglyceride levels. The role of protein intake *per se* in the hyperlipidemia of CRF is unknown, as are the detailed mechanisms whereby hypercholesterolemia contributes to glomerular disease. However, it seems reasonable to speculate that mechanisms analogous to those causing large-vessel disease, including direct endothelial injury and insinuation of cholesterol, its protein carrier, and other inflammatory agents into the capillary wall and mesangium, might contribute to progressive renal insufficiency.

A reduction in protein ingestion usually entails a reduction in phosphorus intake. Because dietary phosphate restriction

mitigates the progressive renal disease seen after subtotal nephrectomy or experimental glomerulonephritis in the rat, the possibility arises that the therapeutic benefits of protein restriction might derive from concomitant phosphorus restriction (127,128). However, studies in which dietary protein but not phosphorus has been varied indicated that dietary protein restriction without coincident phosphate restriction can be beneficial (82,129). On the other hand, phosphate restriction without simultaneous protein restriction also is capable of reducing progressive experimental renal disease (127,130). Thus, each of these dietary manipulations seems capable of independently diminishing progressive renal damage. The mechanism whereby phosphate restriction reduces renal injury remains uncertain (131). Four principal possibilities exist. First, phosphate restriction, at least in certain circumstances, has been associated with a reduction in GFR; hence, those advantages relating to diminution of hyperperfusion in residual nephrons may be achieved by phosphate restriction. This possibility has not yet been tested. Second, with severe phosphate restriction, defects in the inflammatory response due to dysfunction of leukocytes might be expected. Although the latter effect might contribute to the beneficial influence of phosphate restriction, it seems unlikely to be of clinical applicability, because severe phosphate depletion is required to achieve this antiinflammatory action. Third, it has been suggested that suppression of the intrarenal deposition of calcium phosphate crystals, which can be demonstrated histologically, may be an important mechanism whereby phosphate restriction slows the progression of chronic renal disease. Fourth, an effect of phosphate restriction to minimize nephron hypermetabolism in GFR also has been suggested (132). These mechanisms are not mutually exclusive and may all contribute to the beneficial effects of phosphate restriction.

Metabolic Effects

The augmented oxygen consumption of the remnant nephron has been emphasized as a potential mechanism of its ultimate injury. The increased single-nephron filtration rate in remnant nephrons is associated with an increased absolute sodium reabsorption per nephron. The mechanisms whereby enhanced sodium reabsorption occurs are multiple and include adjustment of peritubular capillary forces, augmentation of apical membrane ion transporters, and increased Na-K-adenosine triphosphatase (ATPase) activity. Whatever the mechanisms, the well documented influence of the sodium reabsorption rate on oxygen consumption by the normal kidney implies an increased oxygen consumption for residual nephrons. Furthermore, because hypertrophy as well as hyperplasia contribute to the compensatory growth of residual nephrons, oxygen consumption per cell almost certainly is enhanced in the remnant nephron. Increased oxygen consumption may give rise to damaging effects of its own because aerobically respiring cells such as those of renal cortical epithelium sequentially reduce oxygen to water in reactions that normally generate small amounts of potentially toxic oxygen free radicals. These reactive species, if unchecked, can cause biologic damage by several mechanisms, including peroxidation of membrane fatty acids, depolarization of hyaluronic acid, sulfhydryl oxidation and cross-linking, and nucleic acid damage. Evidence has been obtained in experimental acute renal failure that these free radicals cause several of these biochemical consequences, with resultant reduced renal function. Using the isolated perfused kidney technique, Harris et al. (132) found increased rates of oxygen consumption by remnant nephrons in the subtotally ablated rat kidney and suggested that heightened metabolic rates are damaging. Generally complementary results were obtained by Nath et al. (133) using the same model with *in vivo* measurements. Furthermore, the latter studies suggested that lipid peroxidation as well as oxygen consumption were augmented in the diseased kidneys when animals were ingesting a higher-protein diet (133). Phosphate restriction also may diminish renal injury by attenuation of the metabolic rate (134). Thus, elevated filtration rates impose potentially toxic metabolic demands on the tubular epithelium. Thus, dietary protein restriction appears to reduce renal oxygen demands and the production of toxic metabolites.

A wide range of potentially toxic materials accumulates with progressive renal disease. The study of these compounds usually has focused on their systemic toxicity and the "uremic syndrome." To date, no clear "uremic toxin" has been identified (135,136). However, a number of specific compounds and general classes have been examined, including advanced glycosylation end products, small nitrogenous wastes such as alka aminos, and other small organic compounds, including P-creosol and indoxyl sulfate. In the case of the last compound, evidence has been put forth linking it to ongoing renal injury in experimental models (137). Whether this or other substances contributing to the systemic debility of uremia also promote ongoing renal tissue damage is still unknown.

THE INFLUENCE OF DIETARY THERAPY ON PROGRESSION OF RENAL FAILURE

It is well known that dietary counseling improves uremic symptoms, and there is evidence that dietary protein restriction can change the course of renal insufficiency at least in some patients (138,139). There is, however, a concern—namely, that dietary protein restriction will increase the risk for development of malnutrition and, hence, compromise the patient's prognosis after dialysis therapy is initiated. This concern led some to conclude that dialysis therapy should be initiated "early" (e.g., creatinine clearance >20 mL/minute) to avoid the development of malnutrition (140,141). Before examining results from clinical trials of low-protein diets and progression, this issue must be addressed.

When properly administered, protein-restricted diets not only maintain nutritional status of patients with CRF but can reduce the metabolic consequences of renal insufficiency (142). Early studies (143–147) demonstrated that neutral nitrogen balance was achieved during long-term therapy with low-protein diets and maintenance of normal values of serum albumin. In fact, the use of supplemental essential amino acids (EAA) and ketoacids is associated with an increase in the level of serum albumin in patients with CRF who have low values (148). There also is evidence that restriction of dietary protein is safe for patients with the nephrotic syndrome (149,150). This raises the important issue of identifying factors that cause loss of lean body mass and low values of serum proteins in patients with CRF.

Abnormalities in Protein Turnover in Uremia

Concerns about the safety of low-protein diets arise in part because of the abundant evidence from cross-sectional analyses of patients on dialysis indicating that their nutritional state is abnormal; body weight is low and there is loss of muscle mass based on anthropometric evaluation, and serum proteins values are low (151–153). Evidence for nutritional abnormalities in patients with CRF who are not being treated by dialysis is less clear, in part because it is more difficult to categorize these patients into uniformly treated groups with similar degrees of renal insufficiency. Coles (154) did report results of a cross-sectional evaluation of patients with advanced renal insufficiency; there was evidence of decreased body weight, reduced muscle mass, and decreased serum proteins. The diet of these patients was unregulated, however. More recently, the biochemical status of 911 patients who also had had minimal attention to dietary factors for up to 7 years was reported (155). Patients with a serum creatinine greater than 5 mg/dL commonly had acidosis (one-third had a serum bicarbonate that was <15 mmol/L), hyperphosphatemia (one-third had values >7 mg/dL), and azotemia [one-third had blood urea nitrogen (BUN) values >120 mg/dL]. Such findings, however, are rare even in patients with advanced CRF when attention is given to instructing a patient on how to follow a low-protein diet and to eat sufficient calories, while regularly assessing the impact of the diet on nutritional status (146,147,156–161).

Are dietary factors responsible for nutritional abnormalities found in patients with CRF? In patients on dialysis, mechanisms causing loss of lean body mass are poorly defined; an inadequate diet and a catabolic response to inflammation arising from unknown stimuli have been implicated (153). In the treatment of patients with CRF, it has been known for over 100 years that excessive dietary protein aggravates the symptoms of CRF, leading to the constellation of findings termed *uremia* (138). The adverse effects of a high-protein diet were confirmed in rats with experimental CRF when they were fed a high-protein diet; both linear growth and weight gain were stunted and there were very high levels of BUN (162). In contrast, feeding lower amounts of protein led to improved protein utilization for growth and the lowest BUN values. Although no single factor causing these changes was identified, excess dietary protein commonly is associated with acidosis, and studies of rats as well as patients with CRF have demonstrated that metabolic acidosis stimulates the catabolism of protein and amino acids (163–166). These reports led Bergstrom to conclude that acidosis is the only factor demonstrated to be a uremic toxin (152). Another factor that might play a role in causing loss of lean body mass is stimulation of catabolism by inflammatory cytokines because uremia is associated with evidence of inflammation. First, high levels of acute-phase reactant proteins are linked to subnormal levels of serum albumin in patients on hemodialysis (167,168). Second, there are high circulating levels of tumor necrosis factor and interleukins in patients on hemodialysis and those with CRF (169,170). Third, high levels of these factors are associated with loss of lean body mass because of excessive protein catabolism (171–174).

If metabolic acidosis or inflammatory cytokines are stimuli causing loss of lean body mass, what catabolic mechanisms do they activate? The answer to this question requires understanding at least two metabolic principles: (a) the daily turnover rate of protein is quite large, and (b) there are robust metabolic responses that act to maintain protein balance in the face of nutritional stresses. Protein turnover in a 70-kg adult in neutral protein balance while eating 1 g protein/kg/day amounts to the synthesis and degradation of approximately 280 g of protein each day (i.e., four times the protein intake) (175,176). Consequently, even a small but sustained decrease in protein synthesis or increase in degradation has a major impact on lean body mass. The robust metabolic mechanisms acting to maintain lean body mass involve the ability of the patient to adjust metabolic rates of amino acids and protein in response to changes in the diet (e.g., if dietary protein falls because of anorexia, or is restricted to treat uremic symptoms) or possibly the occurrence of catabolic stimuli. The major metabolic response activated when dietary protein falls is suppression of the degradation of EAA. This response ensures that an adequate supply is available for protein synthesis. The ability to decrease EAA degradation is limited, however, and reaches a minimum level when dietary protein is at the lowest amount needed to achieve nitrogen balance. When dietary protein decreases below this amount, a second level of adaptive responses becomes more active, suppression of protein degradation (there also can be an increase in protein synthesis, although this response has been found less consistently). These responses were first identified in normal adults, but they are intact in patients with uncomplicated CRF (147,159,177). They are active even in patients with the nephrotic syndrome, but in this case, the response is even more remarkable. When net protein intake falls (i.e., the difference between dietary protein and protein lost in the urine), EAA degradation is suppressed accordingly (149). The importance of identifying these responses is not only that they act to maintain lean body mass, but that metabolic acidosis and cytokines activate catabolic mechanisms that

degrade amino acids and protein, resulting in an inability of the patient with CRF to respond to dietary protein restriction (178).

There is abundant evidence that metabolic acidosis causes amino acid and protein catabolism in infants, normal adults, and patients with CRF (147,159,177,179,180). For example, subnormal values of the essential branched-chain amino acids (BCAA) are common in patients with CRF (154), and correction of acidosis raises plasma BCAA levels (181,182). Hara et al. (183) found that plasma levels of valine, leucine, and isoleucine and the valine concentration in muscle water were lower in rats with CRF and metabolic acidosis compared with values in pair-fed, sham-operated rats. These abnormalities were corrected by feeding sodium bicarbonate. The underlying mechanism for this abnormality involves stimulation of the activity of branched-chain ketoacid dehydrogenase (BCKAD), the rate-limiting enzyme in the irreversible oxidation of BCAA. In fact, May et al. (184) reported that the V_{max} activity of BCKAD was increased in the muscle of rats with experimentally induced metabolic acidosis. England et al. identified the biochemical mechanisms accounting for increased BCKAD activity in the muscle of acidotic rats by showing that there is an increase in the fraction of the enzyme in the dephosphorylated, activated form; in addition, the levels of messenger RNA (mRNA) for the E1a, E1b, and E2 subunits of the enzyme are increased (193). These responses depend on both acidification and glucocorticoids (185) and are responsible for the increased degradation of BCAA in vivo and the lower levels of BCAA in plasma and muscle cells (163). In humans as well, metabolic acidosis stimulates the degradation of BCAA. When normal adults were fed NH_4Cl to induce acidosis, leucine oxidation was increased by 25% (180). When patients with CRF were given sodium bicarbonate to raise their serum bicarbonate from 16 to 21 mmol/L, the measured rate of leucine oxidation was suppressed by 29% (164). Lofberg et al. (182) reported that the free levels of BCAA measured in the intracellular pool of a muscle biopsy specimen taken from patients just before a dialysis treatment were corrected by adding sodium bicarbonate to the regimen to eliminate metabolic acidosis. Finally, Mochizuki (181) reported that low levels of BCAA and branched-chain ketoacids in plasma of acidotic patients with CRF were substantially increased when acidosis was treated. Besides acidosis, there are other metabolic abnormalities induced by renal failure that stimulate BCAA catabolism, at least in a model of acute renal failure in rats (186). How these factors induce BCAA catabolism has not been defined.

Metabolic acidosis also stimulates protein degradation in muscle, a catabolic response that blocks the second level of adaptation to stresses and results in loss of lean body mass. May et al. (187) studied rats with CRF complicated by acidosis and found a 22% higher rate of nitrogen excretion compared with that of sham-operated, pair-fed rats. The mechanism underlying this abnormality was linked to a 90% increase in the rate of protein degradation in muscle, but this was eliminated when acidosis in the rats was corrected by adding sodium bicarbonate to their diet. To identify mechanisms that could stimulate protein degradation, England et al. (188) studied protein turnover in BC$_3$H-1 myocytes. When the incubation media was acidified by reducing the concentration of sodium bicarbonate, cellular protein degradation increased and could not be corrected by adding insulin. Isozaki et al. (189) extended these studies to show that acidification-induced protein catabolism in BC$_3$H-1 myocytes requires glucocorticoids; they found no increase in protein degradation on acidification of the media unless glucocorticoids were present, and showed that stimulation by glucocorticoids could be blocked by adding RU 486, the steroid receptor antagonist.

Acidification of muscle cells activates the ATP-ubiquitin-proteasome–dependent pathway (176). This pathway uses energy to conjugate ubiquitin to proteins that are destined for degradation and to degrade protein. Ubiquitin is a member of the heat-shock protein family and its conjugation permits recognition of the protein by the 26S proteasome, which rapidly degrades the substrate protein to peptides in an energy-requiring reaction. Bailey and colleagues proved that the acidosis of CRF stimulates muscle protein catabolism in the ubiquitin-proteasome pathway (190). Stimulation of the ATP-ubiquitin-proteasome–dependent pathway in muscle not only accelerates muscle protein breakdown but increases the levels of mRNA for ubiquitin and for subunits of the proteasome. The latter response is due to transcription of the genes that encode ubiquitin and the proteasome subunits; a similar response occurs in rats with acute diabetes (191,192). This increase in mRNA in muscle is reminiscent of the increase in mRNA encoding subunits of BCKAD that occurs in muscle of rats with metabolic acidosis (193).

The mechanisms that activate the ATP-ubiquitin-proteasome–dependent proteolytic pathway are being hotly pursued because this pathway is involved in the degradation of so many types of proteins, including transcription factors, regulatory proteins, foreign molecules that become antigenic peptides in antigen-presenting cells, and the structural proteins of muscle (176). Moreover, activation of the pathway explains the excessive muscle protein degradation that occurs with diabetes, starvation, denervation, burns, sepsis, and cancer as well as metabolic acidosis; its involvement in these catabolic conditions suggests that its activation is part of a catabolic program (176). It also is relevant to understanding the poor nutritional condition of patients with CRF because inflammatory conditions stimulate it, and there is evidence that inflammation is common in uremia (see earlier discussion). Recent reports indicate that the interactions between inflammatory mediators and activation of the ATP-ubiquitin-proteasome pathway are complex. For example, it was found that NF-kB, the transcription factor activated by inflammatory cytokines, acts as a suppressor of transcription of proteasome subunit genes in muscle cells, and that glucocorticoids block NF-kB from suppressing transcription of proteasome subunit genes (194). Clearly, there is much to learn about the

regulation of mechanisms causing loss of lean body mass in uremia.

Several types of evidence indicate that acidosis is an important factor causing malnutrition in uremia. Papadoyannakis et al. (195) showed that treating patients with CRF with sodium bicarbonate led to an improvement in nitrogen balance. Williams and colleagues (196) studied acidotic patients with CRF who were eating a high-protein diet and reported that the rate of protein degradation did not decrease appropriately when the patients were switched to a low-protein diet. The normal suppression of protein degradation was restored, however, when the same patients with CRF were given sodium bicarbonate to raise their average serum bicarbonate level from 18 to 24 mmol/L. Using a similar strategy, Reaich et al. (164) found that the rate of protein degradation in acidotic patients with CRF is high. When they corrected the acidosis of CRF by feeding sodium bicarbonate, the rate of protein degradation decreased by 28%; it increased again when the patients were given an equimolar amount of sodium chloride and acidosis returned. This group (197) also reported that stimulation of proteolysis by acidosis in patients with CRF cannot be inhibited by insulin, but other reports confirm a key role for glucocorticoids in stimulating protein degradation (163,198). Garibotto et al. (199) measured the rate of protein degradation in the forearm muscle of patients with CRF and found that it was indirectly correlated with the serum bicarbonate value and directly correlated with the serum cortisol level. Ballmer and coworkers (200) reported that induction of metabolic acidosis in normal adults by feeding NH$_4$Cl not only caused a negative nitrogen balance but reduced the rate of albumin synthesis, whereas Movilli et al. reported that correcting the metabolic acidosis of patients on hemodialysis led to an increase in serum albumin concentration (201). The metabolic changes induced by acidosis also extend to hormones. Krapf and colleagues reported that induction of metabolic acidosis in normal adults impairs the function of growth hormone and thyroid hormone and the conversion of vitamin D to its most active form, 1,25(OH)$_2$ cholecalciferol (202–204).

Despite all these reports documenting the catabolic effects of metabolic acidosis, there are cross-sectional studies suggesting there is no relationship between the degree of acidosis and malnutrition in patients on dialysis (205). This conclusion should be ignored for two reasons: first, a single serum bicarbonate is not sufficient to define the presence of acidosis; and second, there is a major technical problem in measuring serum bicarbonate. The blood chemistry values for patients in many dialysis units are performed in laboratories at some distance from the unit and the delay in measuring the bicarbonate concentration creates unpredictable changes in plasma bicarbonate (206).

In summary, metabolic acidosis not only blocks the adaptive metabolic responses that maintain lean body mass, but activates specific catabolic responses, including the irreversible degradation of BCAA and the breakdown of protein. Consequently, metabolic acidosis should be corrected in all patients, especially those being treated with low-protein diets. However, when attention is given to ensuring an adequate intake of nutrients and avoiding metabolic abnormalities, an improved nutritional state in patients with CRF can be expected (142).

Assessment of Dietary Compliance

The classic report of Folin (207) pointed out that urea excretion is the principal change in urinary nitrogen after a change in dietary protein. This has been repeatedly confirmed and is the basis for assessing compliance with low-protein diets (143,144,208,209). The rate of urea production exceeds the steady-state rate of urea excretion in both normal and uremic subjects because there is an extrarenal clearance of urea due to its degradation by bacterial ureases present in the gastrointestinal tract (210–213). At one time, it was believed that urea degradation leading to an increase in ammonia nitrogen in the liver contributes substantially to amino acid synthesis and acts to improve the nutritional status of uremic patients (214). This is incorrect: the ammonia nitrogen simply is used to synthesize more urea (212,213). Stated more precisely, the rate of net urea production closely parallels dietary nitrogen (144,208,209) and is easily calculated because the concentration of urea is equal throughout body water (212,215). Because water represents 60% of body weight in nonedematous patients, changes in the urea nitrogen pool can be calculated by multiplying 60% of body weight (in kilograms) by the serum urea nitrogen concentration (in grams per liter). To calculate the net production of urea, termed the *urea appearance rate* (UNA), the change in the urea nitrogen pool (positive or negative) is added to urinary urea nitrogen excretion. If serum urea nitrogen and weight are stable, UNA equals the excretion rate.

Nonurea Nitrogen

Unlike urea nitrogen, nonurea nitrogen excretion (i.e., the nitrogen excreted in feces and in urinary uric acid, creatinine, and unmeasured nitrogenous products) varies minimally over a large range of dietary protein (208). Maroni et al. (208) found that nonurea nitrogen averages 0.031 g of nitrogen per kilogram per day (Fig. 101-2). This average value was derived from patients excreting less than 5 g protein per day, and if proteinuria exceeds this value, an additional amount of nitrogen equivalent to the urinary loss of protein nitrogen should be added to nonurea nitrogen excretion. More recently, nonurea nitrogen was reexamined by Kopple et al., who reported that fecal nitrogen of patients with CRF varies with dietary protein (209). We examined results of over 70 nitrogen balance measurements and could find no significant correlation between dietary nitrogen and fecal nitrogen or nonurea nitrogen excretion (Masud and Mitch, unpublished data). This is important because if nonurea nitrogen excretion is independent of dietary protein, it can be used in

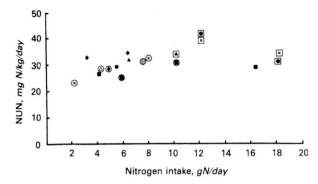

FIG. 101-2. Calculated values of total nonurea nitrogen excretion *(NUN)* in normal subjects *(solid symbols)* and patients with chronic renal failure. The average value for patients not being treated by dialysis is 0.031 g of nitrogen per kilogram per day. (From Maroni BJ, Steinman T, Mitch WE. A method for estimating nitrogen intake of patients with chronic renal failure. *Kidney Int* 1985;27:58, with permission.)

a relatively simple assessment of compliance with protein-restricted diets. Compliance is assessed by converting the prescribed value of protein intake to nitrogen by multiplying by 0.16, (protein is 16% nitrogen). If nitrogen balance is assumed to be zero, then nitrogen intake is equal to the sum of UNA (calculated as described) plus 0.031 g of nitrogen per kilogram per day (208). Clearly, this formulation does not apply to patients receiving total parenteral nutrition or eating completely digestible foods such as those eaten by astronauts. If the difference between the prescribed protein intake and the calculated total waste nitrogen excretion is found to exceed 20%, then reasons for noncompliance or reasons for the nitrogen balance to be negative should be investigated (139). Another use of the calculated dietary protein is to evaluate calorie intake. A patient's dietary history is used to estimate the ratio of protein to calories in his or her diet. Because the amount of dietary protein is determined from nitrogen excretion, calorie intake can be easily checked.

Other methods of assessing protein intake, including dietary histories, were exhaustively reviewed by Bingham (216): interview methods are less accurate and their reliability during repeated interviews is questionable because patients quickly learn the appropriate responses to questions about dietary habits. Thus, dietary compliance should be assessed from the measured urea nitrogen and estimated nonurea nitrogen excretion rates.

Dietary Protein Restriction and Progression of Renal Insufficiency

Beneficial effects of dietary restriction on progression were reported in the late 1970s, but these and subsequent reports have been criticized because they relied on changes in the serum creatinine or creatinine clearance to assess progression, and there were problems with achieving compliance with low-protein diets plus difficulties in study design (including the lack of randomization and retrospective analyses). Moreover, the largest trial of dietary protein restriction and progression led to the conclusion that there was no benefit of protein-restricted diets on progression when changes in GFR were evaluated by an intention-to-treat analysis. Thus, the role of dietary manipulation in treating patients with CRF to slow progression of renal insufficiency is controversial.

Three types of low-protein dietary regimens have been used in attempts to delay the progression of CRF: a diet providing the minimum daily requirement (0.6 g of protein/kg/day of predominantly high-quality protein that is rich in EAA); a diet providing approximately 0.3 g protein/kg/day but supplemented with a mixture of EAA; and the same diet supplemented with ketoacids. One of the first trials was reported by Maschio et al., who compared rates of progression in three groups of patients by assessing changes in serum creatinine and its reciprocal (217). The initial serum creatinine concentrations of patients in group I (25 patients) and group II (20 patients) were 1.5 to 2.7 and 2.9 to 5.4 mg/dL, respectively; both groups were prescribed a diet containing approximately 0.6 g of predominantly high-quality protein/kg/day, a phosphorus intake of less than 750 mg/day, and supplemental calcium to raise intake to 1.0 to 1.5 g/day. Thirty patients in group III served as a control group while eating an unrestricted diet (their initial serum creatinine values were between 1.6 and 4.7 mg/dL). The average intakes of protein, phosphorus, and calcium of the control group were 70 g, 900 mg, and 800 mg, respectively. It was reported that patients eating the restricted diets (i.e., groups I to II) lost renal function far more slowly than did the control group. The presence of proteinuria and hypertension diminished the beneficial effects of dietary therapy in all groups. However, the groups were not randomized, and the control group deteriorated more rapidly than did untreated patients in other reported series, so conclusions must be considered tenuous. No adverse effects of the restricted diet were noted and protein nutrition was well maintained.

In 1989, the Verona group reported results from 390 patients treated with a low-protein diet for an average of 54 months: 57% of the patients maintained stable serum creatinine values, 11% had slower deterioration (defined as a decrease in S^{-1} between -0.02 and -0.04 mg/dL/month), whereas 32% had rapid deterioration (i.e., > -0.04 mg/dL/month) compared with values obtained before changing the diet (218). Patients with interstitial nephritis fared better than those with chronic glomerulonephritis or polycystic kidney disease. Independent factors related to a poorer prognosis included a higher initial serum creatinine, more proteinuria, or higher systolic and diastolic blood pressures on presentation. No adverse effects of dietary therapy were reported and indices of protein nutrition were well maintained. Later, however, these investigators reported significant loss of muscle protein and a decrease in serum albumin and transferrin concentrations (despite stable anthropometric measurements) in a subgroup of eight patients who continued

the protein-restricted diet for an additional 5 years (219). Unfortunately, the energy intake of these eight patients was lower than prescribed (26 to 29 kcal/kg/day), so it is not clear that protein restriction alone caused loss of muscle.

In a prospective analysis of low-protein diets over at least 18 months, Rosman et al. studied 149 patients with creatinine clearances of less than 60 mL/minute/1.73 m² (220). The subjects were stratified according to age, sex, and renal function and then randomly assigned to a diet containing 0.4 to 0.6 g of protein per kilogram per day (predominantly high–biologic-value protein) or an unrestricted diet. All patients received a multivitamin supplement including vitamin D, and compliance was monitored by measuring the 24-hour urea nitrogen excretion every 3 months. Based on an analysis of changes in serum creatinine and its reciprocal, the authors concluded that the diet reduced the average rate of progression by a factor of approximately three. In contrast to the results of Maschio et al. (217), it appeared that older patients and those with chronic glomerulonephritis had a better response than did those with interstitial nephritis or polycystic kidney disease.

After 4 years of follow-up, Rosman et al. examined responses in 153 of the 248 patients initially entering the study (220). There was a smaller but significant benefit of dietary protein restriction on progression; it was most apparent in the group with more advanced renal insufficiency. Men but not women continued to show slowing of progression. However, the benefit was less than the response initially reported. Body weight and serum proteins were stable over 36 months of dietary therapy, indicating that the regimen preserved nutritional status. However, compliance with the diet [based on information given and the relationships described by Maroni et al. (208)] was not great; it can be estimated that on average, the diet contained more than 0.7 g protein/kg/day. Parenthetically, the prescribed intake of 0.4 g protein/kg/day for patients with advanced CRF would be below the minimum daily requirement of 0.6 g protein/kg/day, and hence cannot be recommended. The authors concluded that the most benefit accrued to patients with glomerulonephritis and that progression in patients with polycystic kidney disease appeared to be related entirely to blood pressure control. In the other diagnostic groups, blood pressure was not correlated with preservation of renal function.

In these reports as well as others, there is a recurring theme of a diminished response of patients with polycystic disease, whereas with other types of renal disease, hypertension or proteinuria is closely linked to progression (49,221,222). The mechanisms causing loss of renal function in polycystic kidney disease are unknown and the basis for the association between the severity of hypertension or proteinuria and progression is speculative. However, a low-protein diet reduces the degree of proteinuria and even augments the influence of ACE inhibitors on suppressing proteinuria (and, possibly, progression) (150,223,224).

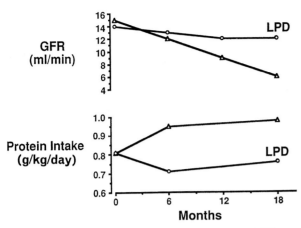

FIG. 101-3. Changes in glomerular filtration rate (GFR) measured as the plasma clearance of ^{51}Cr-EDTA in patients prescribed a protein-restricted diet *(open circles)* or an unrestricted diet *(open triangles)*. The calculated level of dietary protein based on urea excretion (210) also is shown. The low-protein regimen significantly reduced the decline in GFR. *LPD,* low-protein diet. [Figure drawn from the results of Ihle, et al. (77) and is reproduced with permission from Mitch WE, Klahr S. *Nutrition and the kidney,* 2nd ed. Boston: Little, Brown, 1993:254.]

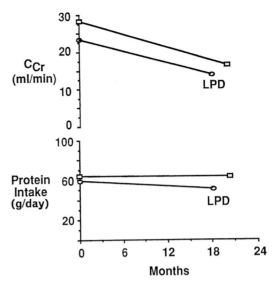

FIG. 101-4. Changes in creatinine clearance (C_{Cr}) during therapy with a low-protein *(LPD; open circles)* and control diet *(open squares)* in the trial conducted by Williams et al. (227). Protein intake was calculated from urea excretion (210). There was no effect on the progression of renal failure. (From Mitch WE. Dietary protein restriction in chronic renal failure. *J Am Soc Nephrol* 1991;2:823. © by American Society of Nephrology.)

In Australia, Ihle et al. conducted a prospective, randomized trial over an average of 18 months in 64 patients by comparing diets containing 0.4 g protein/kg/day or an unrestricted amount of protein (77). The groups initially were well matched for blood pressure, serum creatinine (range, 4.0 to 11.0 mg/dL), serum calcium, and phosphorus concentrations. Changes in GFR were determined from measurements of the plasma disappearance of ^{51}Cr-EDTA (Fig. 101-3). ESRD developed in 9 (27%) of 33 patients who followed the unrestricted diets, compared with only 2 (6%) of 31 who were believed to be compliant with the protein-restricted diet (P < 0.05). GFR decreased on average from approximately 15 to 6 mL/minute in the group eating an unrestricted diet but did not change significantly in the protein-restricted group (e.g., the average change was approximately 2 mL/minute). This was not an intention-to-treat design because the outcome of patients who did not comply with the restricted diet was not detailed. Based on urea excretion values, the average protein intake of the protein-restricted group was more than 0.7 g/kg/day (208). On average, serum albumin and anthropometric measurements remained stable over the 18 months of follow-up, but weight, serum transferrin, and total lymphocyte count decreased significantly. Because the phosphorus content of the protein-restricted diet was approximately 30% to 40% less than that of the unrestricted diet, the relative importance of dietary protein versus phosphorus restriction on progression cannot be determined. The decline in some, but not all, nutritional indices raises concern about prescribing less than the minimum daily requirement of protein to patients with CRF.

In contrast to these reports indicating a beneficial effect of dietary protein restriction on progression, other investigators

found no change in the loss of renal function. Williams et al. randomly assigned 95 patients with CRF to diets containing 0.6 g protein/kg/day or more than 0.8 g protein/kg/day; a third group was assigned to a diet with 0.8 g protein/kg/day plus a "low phosphorus intake" of 1 g/day (225). After a control period of 6 months during which all patients were assigned to 0.8 g protein/kg/day, the test diets were begun and patients were followed for an average of 19 ± 3 months while changes in creatinine clearance were measured. The decline in creatinine clearance of patients assigned to the 0.8-g protein diet was not different from that of the 0.6 g protein/kg/day group (Fig. 101-4). However, there was scarcely any difference in protein intake; the calculated average difference was only 8 g protein/day (208). As expected from the lack of a difference in protein intake (see earlier), creatinine excretion did not differ between the groups, nor did body weight change significantly (on average, there was a 1- to 2-kg decrease in weight in groups fed either the low-protein or the low-phosphorus diets). Because serum transferrin and immunoglobulins were normal, there was no evidence that prescribing the restricted diets adversely affected nutritional status.

A similar negative outcome was reported after the Northern Italian multicenter study (226). In that trial, 456 patients were evaluated and 311 satisfied the criteria for enrollment (165 in the low-protein group and 146 in the control group). The rate of loss of renal function was evaluated by analyzing the time to dialysis or to doubling of the serum creatinine level ("renal survival"). The outcome in terms of reaching end points was slightly, but not statistically better in patients prescribed the low-protein diet (27 vs. 42 in the control group).

Assuming the patients weighed an average of 70 kg, the urea excretion values indicate that the protein intake was approximately 0.9 g/kg/day by the unrestricted diet and 0.78 g protein/kg/day by the low-protein diet group [overall, the difference in protein intake was only approximately 9.5 g /day (208)]. Clearly, simply assigning patients to a low-protein diet will not affect progression if the patients do not eat the prescribed low-protein diet. Regarding changes in nutritional status, only weights were recorded and, on average, they did not change.

Meta-Analyses of Low-Protein Diets and Progression

Besides poor compliance, it is not clear why the outcomes in these studies were so different. One factor could be that the number of patients was too small. To address this problem, several groups have analyzed published data about low-protein diets and progression using the meta-analysis technique (227–230). The meta-analysis technique is a method for pooling results from several studies to determine if there is a difference in the frequency of a unique event that can be associated with the intervention. In three meta-analyses, it was concluded that a low-protein diet exerted a beneficial effect on progression of renal failure (227–229). In each, as well as the meta-analysis that pointed to only a minimal beneficial effect (230), the results were based on an intention-to-treat design. In an intention-to-treat design, there must be randomized assignment to the intervention (i.e., diet level), and a unique outcome (e.g., progression to dialysis, experiencing a rise in serum creatinine) must be discernible in each publication. However, in the intention-to-treat analysis, compliance with the diet is not considered, so this design tests for efficacy and practicality of the intervention but does not examine whether progression is slowed in patients who do comply with the dietary restriction. Fouque et al. analyzed results from six studies of randomly assigned patients who were followed until they required dialysis or died, and concluded that in five of the six trials there was a reduction in the number of renal "deaths" (61 in low-protein diet groups vs. 95 in control groups). The authors calculated an odds ratio to estimate the likelihood of progressing to ESRD and determined that dietary restriction significantly preserves renal function (P < 0.002). Pedrini et al. examined results of 1,413 patients participating in trials in which they were randomly assigned to a low-protein or control diet (228). They concluded that assignment to a low-protein diet reduces the risk of renal failure or death in nondiabetic patients by 33% (P < 0.001) and reduces the risk of a decrease in GFR or creatinine clearance or an increase in proteinuria by 46% in diabetic patients (P < 0.01). Fouque et al. reexamined the issue in an analysis of 7 trials and 1,494 patients (229). Again, it was concluded that assignment to a low-protein diet was associated with slowing of the loss of kidney function. In contrast, Kasiske et al. used many of the same data in a meta-analysis and concluded that the effect of dietary protein restriction was small (230).

Another factor that must be considered in assessing why there are contradictory conclusions about the influence of low-protein diets on progression is compliance. This is important because the hypothesis is that adherence to a low-protein diet will be associated with slowing of progression of renal insufficiency. Consequently, analysis of changes in renal function without taking compliance into account does not test this hypothesis. For example, secondary analyses of the MDRD trial indicate that patients who adhered to the diet did experience slowing of the rate of loss of GFR (see later).

Progression of Diabetic Renal Disease

Some, but not all patients with insulin-dependent diabetes experience renal failure, usually after 15 to 20 years of diabetes. Fortunately, the fraction of patients in whom kidney failure develops seems to be decreasing, but it is not known why only some patients are at risk. Factors that are associated with more rapid progression include hypertension and proteinuria, and means of treating these problems with ACE inhibitors have been reviewed (231). Dietary protein restriction could exert an additional beneficial effect because short-term restriction of dietary protein reduces urinary protein in diabetic patients with microalbuminuria (232–235). This is relevant because of the close association between proteinuria and the development of progression (236).

There are only a few publications examining whether a low-protein diet slows progression in diabetic nephropathy. In a 6-month evaluation of a diet set at 0.6 g protein/kg/day, Raal et al. found that there was a decrease in proteinuria and slower loss of GFR compared with results in patients eating an unrestricted diet (237). The degree of compliance was not detailed and the short period of observation makes it unclear whether these responses can be assigned to beneficial effects of the diet. Using a different design, Walker et al. changed the dietary protein of 19 insulin-dependent, proteinuric diabetic patients from an unrestricted protein intake (average, 1.13 g protein/kg/day) to a diet averaging 0.67 g protein/kg/day (232). They observed a significantly slower loss of GFR (from 0.61 to 0.14 mL/minute/month) that was independent of differences in blood pressure, energy intake, and glycosylated hemoglobin level. Zeller et al. compared results achieved by a diet containing 0.6 g protein/kg/day with those measured in patients eating an unrestricted diet (238). Changes in renal function were evaluated from albuminuria, serum creatinine, and the renal clearances of creatinine and ^{125}I-iothalamate (i.e., GFR). Based on urea excretion values (208), the patients assigned to the low-protein diet ate an average of approximately 0.7 g protein/kg/day; no signs of malnutrition developed and the average decline in GFR and creatinine clearance was slowed by the protein-restricted diet. Some of the patients given the unrestricted diet, however, did not exhibit progressive loss of GFR, emphasizing why it is important to ensure that patients in such trials have evidence of progression before beginning the trial (see earlier). The beneficial effects of the dietary regimen in the report by Zeller et al. could not be attributed to differences in blood pressure or glycemic control or to the frequency of examinations, leading to the conclusion that dietary restriction was the major factor. This conclusion is reinforced by meta-analyses of the influence of low-protein diets on progression (228,229).

Low-Protein Diets Supplemented with Essential Amino Acids or Ketoacids

The results just discussed were derived from patients eating natural foods to meet the requirements for protein, calories, and other nutrients. Dietary protein cannot be reduced safely below 0.6 g protein/kg/day unless energy intake is sufficient and a supplement of EAA or a mixture of EAA and their nitrogen-free analogs (ketoacids) are provided. In the United States, ketoacids are not commercially available, although EAA can be purchased as Aminess from Nestle Homelink or Calwood Nutritionals; both EAA and ketoacids are available in some other countries. During the 1980s, several reports provided evidence that a diet containing approximately 0.3 g protein/kg/day plus a supplement and sufficient calories was nutritionally sound in patients with advanced CRF because they promoted neutral nitrogen balance and maintained normal nutritional indices (e.g., serum proteins) during long-term therapy (142,145–147,159). Regarding the influence of these regimens on progression of CRF, Alvestrand et al. studied 17 patients with well defined rates of decline in S^{-1} despite treatment with a standard, low-protein diet. They prescribed an EAA-based regimen (0.3 g protein/kg/day plus an EAA supplement) and observed slowing of the decline in S^{-1} in 14 of 17 patients (239). Subsequently, this group conducted a prospective, randomized trial and concluded that the diet was not a major factor in achieving a slower rate of progression (240). Instead, they concluded that slowing of progression was more closely linked to a small (-2 mm Hg) reduction in diastolic blood pressure and, possibly, more frequent visits to the clinic. Examination of their data, however, reveals problems: first, 10 (18%) of the 57 enrolled patients did not exhibit any loss of renal function during the baseline period while they were eating an "unrestricted" diet; and second, there was poor compliance with the dietary regimen (the average difference in protein intake between the groups, 0.65 vs. 0.86 g/kg/day, was small).

There is evidence that the very-low-protein diet–ketoacid regimen can slow progression of CRF. Barsotti et al. (64) measured the decline in creatinine clearance in 31 patients who were eating the standard low-protein diet. They found that the loss of creatinine clearance was constant (i.e., linear) in patients with nondiabetic kidney diseases and the decline was interrupted in 11 of 12 patients who were switched to a regimen containing approximately 0.2 g protein/kg/day plus a supplement of the calcium salts of ketoacids. In a subsequent report, Barsotti et al. reported that 27 of 48 patients appeared to be compliant with the ketoacid-based regimen and in this subgroup, the average loss of creatinine

clearance was reversed from -0.65 to $+0.15$ mL/minute/ month (P < 0.005) (241). Other investigators used basic amino acid (i.e., ornithine and lysine) salts of ketoacids rather than the calcium salts to test whether progression is slowed. This formulation, used as a supplement to a diet containing 0.3 g protein/kg/day, seemed to slow the loss of renal function. In the initial study of 17 patients with well defined rates of decline in S^{-1}, 10 (59%) had a significantly slower rise in serum creatinine (or a decline in creatinine clearance) during an average of 20 months of therapy. Patients with advanced CRF (serum creatinine >8 mg/dL) did not experience slowing of progression (242). Subsequently, Walser et al. studied patients with advanced CRF (the initial GFR averaged 13 mL/minute) and compared this ketoacid-based regimen with an EAA-based regimen using a crossover design (158). The ketoacid regimen appeared to slow progression (measured as changes in GFR) more effectively than the EAA regimen, but only 12 patients were studied. As expected from earlier reports about metabolic effects of this regimen, there was no weight loss and serum albumin remained normal (146,242).

The efficacy of a ketoacid-based regimen has been compared with the standard low-protein regimen containing 0.6g protein/kg/day but no supplement. Di Landro et al. measured changes in the reciprocal of serum creatinine over 3 years in 44 patients assigned to the standard low-protein regimen, compared with 46 patients given the ketoacid regimen (243). Progression was significantly slower and parathyroid hormone and serum cholesterol both decreased in patients given the ketoacid regimen. These studies suffer because of the relatively small number of patients and the inclusion of results from some patients who had no evidence of progression.

The Modification of Diet in Renal Disease Study

The problem of small numbers of patients in these and other studies prompted the National Institutes of Health to undertake a multicenter study, the MDRD trial. Initially, there was a feasibility trial in which 96 patients participated to test acceptance of the regimens; progression was not formally evaluated (244). Subsequently, two groups of patients were studied in the full-scale trial: Study A patients had GFR values of 25 to 55 mL/minute/1.73 m². Subsequently, two groups of patients were studied in the full-scale trial: Study A patients had GFR values between 13 and 24 mL/minute/1.73 m². Patients in Study A were randomly assigned to one of two diets: at least 1 g protein/kg/day, or 0.6 g protein/kg/day; and to a mean blood pressure goal of either 105 or 92 mm Hg (49). Patients in Study B were randomly assigned to the 0.6 g protein/kg/day diet or to a regimen containing 0.3 g protein/kg/day plus a ketoacid supplement and the same two blood pressure goals (in Study B, there was no control group assigned to a high-protein or self-selected diet because such a diet could cause uremic symptoms). Average values of protein intake [estimated from urea appearance (208)] differed significantly among the groups in both Studies A and B; differences in blood pressure were less impressive. The impact on progression was analyzed by measuring changes in

^{125}I-iothalamate renal clearance over an average follow-up period of 2.2 years.

During the first 4 months, GFR declined more rapidly in Study A patients assigned to the low-protein diet and low-blood-pressure groups (P = 0.004 and P < 0.01, respectively). Thereafter, the rate of decline in GFR was 28% slower in patients assigned to the low-protein diet (P = 0.009) and 29% slower in the low-blood-pressure group (P = 0.006). In contrast, the loss of GFR of patients eating the unrestricted diet was remarkably linear with time. Using an intention-to-treat analysis, however, neither prescribing the low-protein diet nor assigning patients to the lower-blood-pressure goal was associated with slowing of the loss of GFR (Fig. 101-5).

In analyzing results from patients with more advanced CRF (Study B), the loss of GFR was 19% slower in the very-low-protein–ketoacid group compared with patients assigned to the standard low-protein diet (P = 0.065). However, there was no statistical difference in the cumulative incidence of ESRD or death of patients. In fact, the sole positive effect of the MDRD Study in this report was that a lower blood pressure goal was associated with slowing of progression in patients who had more than 1 g proteinuria/day. Patients with polycystic kidney disease did not benefit from either the diet or blood pressure control, and African American patients seemed to progress more rapidly than did other patients, but with a small number of subjects, the difference was not statistically significant.

Do the MDRD results settle whether a low-protein diet can slow progression? There are several reasons why this report does not settle the question (49,139,245). First, the sample size was based on the assumption that GFR would decline at a rate of 6 mL/minute/year in the control group (i.e., those prescribed an unrestricted diet and their usual blood pressure). However, progression was approximately 30% slower than expected overall, and approximately 15% of patients in the Study A control group did not progress. Obviously, it is impossible to determine if there is a beneficial influence of a low-protein diet on progression in these patients. Thus, the sample size may have been inadequate, and in support of this concern, the meta-analysis results lead to the conclusion that low-protein diets do slow the loss of renal function (see earlier). Second, there was a disproportionate number (~20%) of patients with polycystic disease, and progression in these patients appears to be unaffected by dietary manipulation or control of hypertension (246); inclusion of these patients could have obscured a benefit of a low-protein diet on progression in patients with other kidney diseases. Third, MDRD patients were give ACE inhibitors in an unregulated fashion, and use of this drug might have obscured the outcome (231). Fourth, the initial rapid decline in GFR in patients assigned the low-protein diet and low-blood-pressure groups was unexpected and could have obscured a beneficial effect on progression occurring in a more prolonged trial. Regarding the short duration of the study (2.2. years), the evaluation of another metabolic intervention on kidney function (i.e., the Diabetes Control and Complications Trial) (247) revealed no benefit of strict glycemic control for the initial 4 years, after which the suppressing of proteinuria became obvious. Finally, there are problems with accepting a lack of benefit in patients with more advanced CRF (Study B) because there was no control group eating an unrestricted diet. Moreover, the mixture of ketoacids was changed from the mixture that had shown a benefit in smaller trials conducted earlier (158,242,248). In fact, when changes in GFR of patients participating in the MDRD Feasibility Trial were analyzed, it was found that the loss of GFR was significantly slower (P < 0.03) compared with patients eating the standard low-protein diet.

These factors cast doubt on the conclusion that the MDRD Study (49) proved that low-protein diets do not slow the loss of renal function. In addition, the study was designed to evaluate the practicality of prescribing low-protein diets rather than rigorously test whether eating a low-protein diet slows the progression of CRF. In fact, when MDRD results were analyzed according to the amount of protein actually consumed, a benefit of dietary protein restriction in Study B patients was

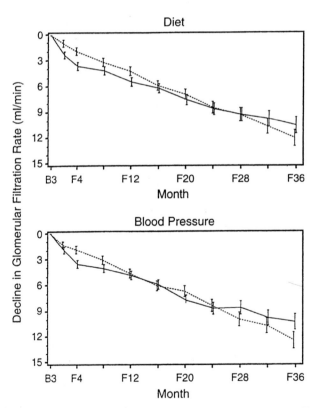

FIG. 101-5. The decline in the mean (±SEM) glomerular filtration rate from baseline values (B3) to the estimated value at 36 months (F36). In the **upper panel,** the results from those assigned to an unrestricted diet (approximately 1.3 g protein/kg/day, *dashed line*) and a low-protein diet (approximately 0.6 g protein/kg/day, *solid line*) are compared. In the **lower panel,** results from those assigned to a "usual" blood pressure (mean arterial pressure <107 mm Hg, *dashed line*) and a "low" blood pressure (mean arterial pressure <92 mm Hg, *solid line*) are compared. (Reproduced with permission from Klahr S, et al. The effects of dietary protein restriction and blood-pressure control on the progression of chronic renal disease. *N Engl J Med* 1994;330:882.)

obvious: each 0.2 g/kg/day reduction in protein intake was associated with a 29% slower rate of loss of GFR and a 51% prolongation in the time to dialysis (P < 0.01) (66,249). No independent influence of the ketoacid regimen was detected in this secondary analysis, but, as noted earlier, the ketoacid mixture used in the MDRD Study differed from the mixture showing positive results in earlier studies (248).

CONCLUSIONS

Results summarized in this and Chapter 103 show that dietary therapy reduces signs and symptoms of CRF and is nutritionally safe as long as there is no complicating factor such as acidosis or infection. Thus, dietary manipulation in a treatment program that includes monitoring protein and calorie intake in consultation with a dietitian (208,250) should be a mainstay of therapy for all patients. The observation that protein intake voluntarily decreases as renal insufficiency progresses is not a signal to urge an increase in dietary protein because this simply increases the degree of uremia but does not improve serum proteins (142,162,251). On the contrary, a well designed protein-restricted diet leads to an increase in serum albumin (251). Finally, a low-protein diet could delay the need for dialysis by ameliorating uremic symptoms while maintaining nutritional status. Two recent publications provide strong evidence for the long-term safety of this approach (160,161). Patients in these studies were followed for an average of 1.5 to 2 years after GFR had decreased to 10 to 13 mL/minute, and nutritional status was well maintained while they ate protein-restricted diets (Table 101-2). Clearly,

TABLE 101-2. *Nutritional therapy and delayed initiation of dialysis*

Study 1 (N = 56 patients)	
GFR (mL/min) on dialysis	6.6
Median survival (days) to dialysis	346
Nutritional status	
BUN	62 mg/dL
Serum CO_2	22 mM
Serum albumin	4.1 g/dL
Body weight (initial–final)	69.6–71.5 kg
Study 2 (N = 165 patients)	
GFR (mL/min) on dialysis	5.8
Median survival (months) to dialysis	29.8
Nutritional status	
BUN	47 mg/dL
Serum CO_2	22 mM
Serum albumin	3.9 g/dL
Body weight	64.2–64.6 kg

BUN, blood urea nitrogen; *GFR,* glomerular filtration rate.
In Study 1 (160) and Study 2 (161), patients were given a low-protein diet supplemented with essential amino acids or ketoacids and observed during the decline in renal function from GFR 10 mL/min (15 mL/min in diabetic patients) to a final value of 6.6 mL/min or 5.8 mL/min, respectively (the decision to initiate dialysis was made by physicians not monitoring the dietary therapy in Study 1 and by the investigators in Study 2). Measured indices of nutritional status demonstrate the absence of malnutrition at the end of each study.

successful implementation of dietary therapy requires the motivation of both the patient and the physician. The principal, if not the only disadvantage of such therapy (assuming that it is successful in eliminating uremic symptoms), is the dietary restriction it entails, but it is reasonable to expect that the time before dialysis therapy is required will be significantly prolonged.

ACKNOWLEDGMENTS

This work was made possible by grants DK37175 and AM 31437 from the National Institutes of Health and Clinical Research Center grant RR00039 of Emory University School of Medicine.

REFERENCES

1. Lindeman RD, Tobin J, Shock NW. Longitudinal studies on the rate of decline in renal function with age. *J Am Geriatr Soc* 1985;33:278.
2. Lindeman RD. Overview: renal physiology and pathophysiology of aging. *Am J Kidney Dis* 1990;16:275.
3. Fliser D, Feranek E, Joest M, et al. Renal function in the elderly: impact of hypertension and cardiac function. *Kidney Int* 1997;51:1196.
4. Kimmel PL, Lew SQ, Bosch JB. Nutrition, ageing and GFR: is age-associated decline inevitable? *Nephrol Dial Transplant* 11[Suppl 9]:85.
5. Levey AS, Adler S, Caggiula AW, et al. Effects of dietary protein restriction on the progression of moderate renal disease in the Modification of Diet in Renal Disease Study. *J Am Soc Nephrol* 1996;7:2616.
6. Torres VE, Velosa JA, Holley KE, et al. The progression of reflux nephropathy. *Ann Intern Med* 1980;92:776.
7. Kleinknecht D, Grunfeld JP, Gomez PC, et al. Diagnostic procedures and long-term prognosis in bilateral renal cortical necrosis. *Kidney Int* 1973;4:390.
8. Sawicki PT. Stabilization of glomerular filtration rate over 2 years in patients with diabetic nephropathy under intensified therapy regimens. *Nephrol Dial Transplant* 1997;12:1890.
9. Toto RD, Mitchell HC, Smith RD, et al. "Strict" blood pressure control and progression of renal disease in hypertensive nephrosclerosis. *Kidney Int* 1995;48:851.
10. Hunsicker LG, Adler S, Caggiula A, et al. Predictors of the progression of renal disease in the Modification of Diet in Renal Disease Study. *Kidney Int* 1997;51:1908.
11. Bauer JH, Brooks CS, Burch RN. Clinical appraisal of creatinine clearance as a measurement of glomerular filtration rate. *Am J Kidney Dis* 1982;2:337.
12. Rehling M, Moller ML, Thamdrup B, et al. Simultaneous measurement of renal clearance and plasma clearance of ^{99m}Tc-labelled diethylenetriaminepenta-acetate, ^{51}Cr-labelled ethylenediaminetetra-acetate and inulin in man. *Clin Sci* 1984;66:613.
13. Myers BD, Nelson RG, Williams GW, et al. Glomerular function in Pima Indians with noninsulin-dependent diabetes mellitus of recent onset. *J Clin Invest* 1991;88:524.
14. Nelson RG, Bennett PH, Beck GJ, et al. Development and progression of renal disease in Pima Indians with non-insulin-dependent diabetes mellitus. *N Engl J Med* 1996;335:1636.
15. Perrone RD, Steinman TI, Beck GJ, et al. Utility of radioisotopic filtration markers in chronic renal insufficiency: simultaneous comparison of ^{125}I-iothalamate, ^{169}Yb-DPTA, ^{99m}Tc-DTPA and inulin. *Am J Kidney Dis* 1990;16:224.
16. Gaspari F, Guerini E, Perico N, et al. Glomerular filtration rate determined from a single plasma sample after intravenous iohexol injection: is it reliable? *J Am Soc Nephrol* 1996;7:2689.
17. Gaspari F, Perico N, Matalone M, et al. Precision of plasma clearance of iohexol for estimation of GFR in patients with renal disease. *J Am Soc Nephrol* 1998;9:310.
18. Frennby B, Sterner G, Almen T, et al. The use of iohexol clearance to determine GFR in patients with severe chronic renal failure: a comparison between different clearance techniques. *Clin Nephrol* 1995;43:35.

19. Li Y, Lee HB, Blaufox MD. Single-sample methods to measure GFR with technetium-99M-DTPA. *J Nucl Med* 1997;38:1290.
20. Sambataro M, Thomaseth K, Pacini G, et al. Plasma clearance of 51Cr-EDTA provides a precise and convenient technique for measurement of glomerular filtration rate in diabetic humans. *J Am Soc Nephrol* 1996; 7:118.
21. Gaspari F, Perico N, Remuzzi G. Measurement of glomerular filtration rate. *Kidney Int Suppl* 1997;63:S151.
22. Isaka Y, Fujiwara Y, Yamamoto S, et al. Modified plasma clearance technique using nonradioactive iothalamate for measuring GFR. *Kidney Int* 1992;42:1006.
23. Gaspari F, Mosconi L, Vigano G, et al. Measurement of GFR with a single intravenous injection of nonradioactive iothalamate. *Kidney Int* 1992;41:1081.
24. Gaspari F, Perico N, Ruggenenti P, et al. Plasma clearance of nonradioactive iohexol as a measure of glomerular filtration rate. *J Am Soc Nephrol* 1995;6:257.
25. Kjaersgaard P, Jakobsen JA, Nossen JO, et al. Determination of glomerular filtration rate with Visipaque in patients with severely reduced renal function. *Eur Radiol* 1996;6:865.
26. Mitch WE. Measuring the rate of progression of renal insufficiency. In: Mitch WE, ed. *The progressive nature of renal disease.* New York: Churchill Livingstone, 1992:203.
27. Lubowitz H, Slatopolsky E, Shankel S, et al. Glomerular filtration rate: determination in patients with chronic renal disease. *JAMA* 1967; 199:252.
28. Shemesh O, Golbetz H, Kriss JP, et al. Limitations of creatinine as a filtration marker in glomerulopathic patients. *Kidney Int* 1985;28: 830.
29. Edwards OM, Bayliss RIS, Millen S. Urinary creatinine excretion as an index of the completeness of 24-hour urine collections. *Lancet* 1969;2:1165.
30. Doolan PD, Alpen EL, Theil GB. A clinical appraisal of the plasma concentration and endogenous clearance of creatinine. *Am J Med* 1962; 32:56.
31. Morgan DB, Dillon S, Payne RB. The assessment of glomerular function: creatinine clearance or plasma creatinine? *Postgrad Med J* 1978;54:302.
32. Bleiler RE, Schedle HP. Creatinine excretion: variability and relationships to diet and body size. *J Lab Clin Med* 1962;59:945.
33. Kelly RA, Mitch WE. Creatinine, uric acid and other nitrogenous waste products: clinical implication of the imbalance between their production and elimination in uremia. *Semin Nephrol* 1983;3:286.
34. Cockcroft DW, Gault MH. Prediction of creatinine clearance from serum creatinine. *Nephron* 1975;16:31.
35. Forbes GB, Bruining GS. Urinary creatinine excretion and lean body mass. *Am J Clin Nutr* 1978;29:1359.
36. Heymsfield SB, Arteaga C, McManus C, et al. Measurement of muscle mass in humans: validity of the 24-hour urinary creatinine method. *Am J Clin Nutr* 1983;37:478.
37. Levey AS, Gassman JJ, Hall PM, et al. Assessing the progression of renal disease in clinical studies: effects of duration of follow-up and regression to the mean. *J Am Soc Nephrol* 1991;1:1087.
38. Walser M, Drew HH, LaFrance ND. Creatinine measurements often yield false estimates of progression in chronic renal failure. *Kidney Int* 1988;34:412.
39. Adam W. All that is excreted does not glitter: or why do we keep on collecting urine to measure creatinine clearance [Editorial]? *Aust N Z J Med* 1993;23:638.
40. Payne RB. Creatinine clearance: a redundant clinical investigation. *Ann Clin Biochem* 1986;23:243.
41. van Acker BAC, Koomen GCM, Koopman MG, et al. Limitations of creatinine during cimetidine as a filtration marker in renal disease. *J Am Soc Nephrol* 1992;3:322.
42. Hellerstein S, Berenbom M, Alon US, et al. Creatinine clearance following cimetidine for estimation of glomerular filtration rate. *Pediatr Nephrol* 1998;12:49.
43. Mitch WE, Walser M. A proposed mechanism for reduced creatinine excretion in severe chronic renal failure. *Nephron* 1978;21:248.
44. Tripathy K, Klahr S, Lotero H. Utilization of exogenous urea nitrogen in malnourished adults. *Metabolism* 1970;19:253.
45. Walser M. Assessing renal function from creatinine measurements in adults with chronic renal failure. *Am J Kidney Dis* 1998;32:23.
46. Maher JF, Nolph KD, Bryan CW. Prognosis of advanced chronic renal failure: I. unpredictability of survival and reversibility. *Ann Intern Med* 1974;81:43.
47. Ahlmen J. Incidence of chronic renal insufficiency: a study of the incidence and pattern of renal insufficiency in adults during 1966–1971 in Gothenburg. *Acta Med Scand Suppl* 1975;582:3.
48. Johnson WJ, O'Kane HO, Elveback LR. Survival of patients with end-stage renal disease. *Mayo Clin Proc* 1973;48:18.
49. Klahr S, Levey AS, Beck GJ, et al. The effects of dietary protein restriction and blood-pressure control on the progression of chronic renal failure. *N Engl J Med* 1994;330:878.
50. Mitch WE, Buffington GA, Lemann J, et al. A simple method of estimating progression of chronic renal failure. *Lancet* 1976;2:1326.
51. Shah BV, Levey AS. Spontaneous changes in the rate of decline in reciprocal serum creatinine: errors in predicting the progression of renal disease from extrapolation of the slope. *J Am Soc Nephrol* 1992;2: 1186.
52. Coresh J, Walser M, Hill S. Survival on dialysis among chronic renal failure patients treated with a supplemented low-protein diet before dialysis. *J Am Soc Nephrol* 1995;6:1379.
53. Jones RH, Hayakawa H, MacKay JD, et al. The progression of diabetic nephropathy. *Lancet* 1979;1:1105.
54. Walser M. Progression of chronic renal failure in man. *Kidney Int* 1990; 37:1195.
55. Ruggenenti P, Perna A, Benini R, et al. In chronic nephropathies prolonged ACE inhibition can induce remission: dynamics of time-dependent changes in GFR. *J Am Soc Nephrol* 1999;10:997.
56. Austin SM, Lieberman JS, Newton LD, et al. Slope of serial GFR and the progression of diabetic glomerular disease. *J Am Soc Nephrol* 1993;3:1358.
57. Fraser CG, Williams P. Short-term biological variation of plasma analytes in renal disease. *Clin Chem* 1983;29:508.
58. Mitch WE. The influence of the diet on the progression of renal failure. *Annu Rev Med* 1984;35:249.
59. Rutherford WE, Blondin J, Miller JP, et al. Chronic progressive renal disease. *Kidney Int* 1977;11:62.
60. Gretz N, Manz F, Strauch M. Predictability of the progression of chronic renal failure. *Kidney Int Suppl* 1983;15:2.
61. Oksa H, Pasternack A, Luomala M, et al. Progression of chronic renal failure. *Nephron* 1983;35:31.
62. Gault MH, Longerich LL, Harnett JD, et al. Predicting glomerular function from adjusted serum creatinine. *Nephron* 1992;62:249.
63. Jones JD, Burnett PC. Creatinine metabolism in humans with decreased renal function: creatinine deficit. *Clin Chem* 1974;20:1204.
64. Barsotti G, Guiducci A, Ciardella F, et al. Effects on renal function of a low-nitrogen diet supplemented with essential amino acids and ketoanalogues and of hemodialysis and free protein supply in patients with chronic renal failure. *Nephron* 1981;27:113.
65. Levey AS, Beck GJ, Bosch JP, et al. Short-term effects of protein intake, blood pressure and antihypertensive therapy on glomerular filtration rate in the Modification of Diet in Renal Disease Study. *J Am Soc Nephrol* 1996;7:2097.
66. Levey AS, Greene T, Beck GJ, et al. Dietary protein restriction and the progression of chronic renal disease: what have all the results of the MDRD Study shown? *J Am Soc Nephrol* 1999;10:2426.
67. Crim MC, Calloway DH, Margen S. Creatinine metabolism in men: creatine pool size and turnover in relation to creatine intake. *J Nutr* 1976;106:371.
68. Lew SQ, Bosch JP. Effect of diet on creatinine clearance and excretion in young and elderly healthy subjects and in patients with renal disease. *J Am Soc Nephrol* 1991;2:856.
69. Mitch E. Measuring progression of renal insufficiency. In Mitch WE, ed. *The progressive nature of renal disease.* New York: Churchill Livingstone, 1986:167.
70. Parving HH, et al. Effective antihypertensive treatment postpones renal insufficiency in diabetic nephropathy. *Am J Kidney Dis* 1993;22:188.
71. Maschio G, et al. Effect of the angiotensin-converting-enzyme inhibitor benazepril on the progression of chronic renal insufficiency. *N Engl J Med* 1996;334:939.
72. Dworkin LD, et al. Hemodynamic basis for glomerular injury in rats with desoxycorticosterone salt hypertension. *J Clin Invest* 1984;73: 1448.
73. Nath KA, et al. Dietary protein restriction in established renal injury in the rat: selective role of glomerular capillary pressure in progressive glomerular dysfunction. *J Clin Invest* 1986;78:1197.

74. Schnermann J, et al. Tubuloglomerular feedback and glomerular morphology in Goldblatt hypertensive rats on varying protein diets. *Kidney Int* 1986;29:520.

75. Klahr S, et al. The effects of dietary protein restriction and blood-pressure control on the progression of chronic renal disease. *N Engl J Med* 1994;330:877.

76. Rosenberg ME, et al. Glomerular and hormonal responses to dietary protein intake in human renal disease. *Am J Physiol* 1987;253:F1083.

77. Ihle BU, et al. The effect of protein restriction on the progression of renal insufficiency. *N Engl J Med* 1989;321:1773.

78. Rosman JB, et al. Prospective randomised trial of early dietary protein restriction in chronic renal failure. *Lancet* 1984;2:1291.

79. Zeller K, et al. Effect of restricting dietary protein on the progression of renal failure in patients with insulin-dependent diabetes mellitus. *N Engl J Med* 1991;324:78.

80. Hostetter TH, et al. Hyperfiltration in remnant nephrons: A potentially adverse response to renal ablation. *Am J Physiol* 1981;241:F85.

81. Lafferty HM, Brenner BM. Are glomerular hypertension and "hypertrophy" independent risk factors for progression of renal disease? *Semin Nephrol* 1990;10:294.

82. Hostetter TH, et al. Chronic effects of dietary protein in the rat with intact and reduced renal mass. *Kidney Int* 1986;30:509.

83. O'Donnell MP, et al. High protein intake accelerates glomerulosclerosis independent of effects on glomerular hemodynamics. *Kidney Int* 1990;37:1263.

84. Castellino P, Coda B, De Fronzo RA. Effects of amino acid infusion on renal hemodynamics in humans. *Am J Physiol* 1986;251:F132.

85. Meyer TW, et al. The renal hemodynamic response to amino acid infusion in the rat. *Trans Assoc Am Physicians* 1983;156:76.

86. Premen AJ, Hall JE, Smith MJ. Postprandial regulation of renal hemodynamics: role of pancreatic glucagon. *Am J Physiol* 1985;248:F656.

87. Daniels BS, Hostetter TH. Effects of dietary protein intake on vasoactive hormones. *Am J Physiol* 1990;258:R1095.

88. Hirschberg RR, et al. Glucagon and prostaglandins are mediators of amino acid-induced rise in renal hemodynamics. *Kidney Int* 1988;33:1147.

89. Tolins JP, et al. Role of EDRF in the amino acid induced increase in GFR and renal blood flow. *Hypertension* 1991;17:1045.

90. Tolins JP, et al. Renal hemodynamic effects of dietary protein in the rat: role of nitric oxide. *J Lab Clin Med* 1995;125:228.

91. Lee KE, Summerill RA. Glomerular filtration rate following administration of individual amino acids in conscious dogs. *Q J Exp Physiol* 1982;67:459.

92. Fernandez-Repollet E, Tapia E, Martinez-Maldonado M. Effects of angiotensin-converting enzyme inhibition on altered renal hemodynamics induced by low protein diet in the rat. *J Clin Invest* 1987;80:1045.

93. Paller MS, Hostetter TH. Dietary protein increases plasma renin activity and reduces pressor reactivity to angiotensin II. *Am J Physiol* 1986;251:F34.

94. Rosenberg ME, Chmielewski D, Hostetter TH. Effect of dietary protein on rat renin and angiotensinogen gene expression. *J Clin Invest* 1990;85:1144.

95. Rosenberg ME, Kren SM, Hostetter TH. Effect of dietary protein on the renin-angiotensin system in subtotally nephrectomized rats. *Kidney Int* 1990;38:240.

96. Michel B, Grima M, Conquard C, et al. Effects of dietary protein and uninephrectomy on renal angiotensin converting enzyme activity in the rat. *Kidney Int* 1994;45:1587.

97. Inman SR, Stowe NT, Nally JV Jr, et al. Dietary protein does not alter intrinsic reactivity of renal microcirculation to angiotensin II in rodents. *Am J Physiol* 1995;282:F302.

98. Baboolal K, et al. The effect of acute angiotensin II blockade on renal function in rats with reduced renal mass. *Kidney Int* 1994;46:980.

99. Lafayette RA, et al. Angiotensin II receptor blockade limits glomerular injury in rats with reduced renal mass. *J Clin Invest* 1992;90:766.

100. Ibrahim HN, Rosenberg ME, Greene EL, et al. Aldosterone is a major factor in the progression of renal diseases. *Kidney Int* 1997;63:S115.

101. Fukui M, Nakamura T, Ebihara I. Effects of enalapril on endothelin-1 and growth factor gene expression in diabetic rat glomeruli. *J Lab Clin Med* 1994;123:763.

102. Smith LJ, Rosenberg ME, Hostetter TH. Effect of angiotensin II blockade on dietary protein-induced renal growth. *Am J Kidney Dis* 1993;22:120.

103. Daniels BS, Hostetter TH. Adverse effects of growth in the glomerular microcirculation. *Am J Physiol* 1990;258:F1409.

104. Fogo A, et al. Glomerular hypertrophy in minimal change disease predicts subsequent progression to focal glomerular sclerosis. *Kidney Int* 1990;38:115.

105. Yoshida Y, et al. Effects of antihypertensive drugs on glomerular morphology. *Kidney Int* 1989;26:626.

106. Fries JU, et al. Glomerular hypertrophy and epithelial cell injury modulate progressive glomerulosclerosis in the rat. *Lab Invest* 1989;60:205.

107. Grond J, et al. Analysis of renal structural and functional features in two rat strains with a different susceptibility to glomerular sclerosis. *Lab Invest* 1986;54:77.

108. Kettler M, Border WA, Noble NA. Cytokines and L-arginine in renal injury and repair. *Am J Physiol* 1994;267:F197.

109. Floege J, et al. Factors involved in the regulation of mesangial cell proliferation in vitro and in vivo. *Kidney Int* 1993;43:547.

110. Yoskioka K, et al. Transforming growth factor-b protein and mRNA in glomeruli in normal and diseased human kidneys. *Lab Invest* 1993;68:154.

111. Fukui M, et al. Low-protein diet attenuates increased gene expression of platelet-derived growth factor and transforming growth factor-b in experimental glomerular sclerosis. *J Lab Clin Med* 1993;121:224.

112. Kagami S, et al. Angiotensin II stimulates extracellular matrix protein synthesis through induction of transforming growth factor-β expression in rat glomerular mesangial cells. *J Clin Invest* 1994;93:2431.

113. Eddy AA. Protein restriction reduces transforming growth factor-beta and interstitial fibrosis in nephrotic syndrome. *Am J Physiol* 1994;266:F884.

114. Hostetter TH, Rosenberg ME, Kren S, et al. Aldosterone (Aldo) induces glomerular sclerosis in the remnant kidney. *J Am Soc Nephrol* 1995;6:1016.

115. Juknevicius I, Segal Y, Kren S, Hostetter TH. Aldosterone causes TGF-β expression. *J Am Soc Nephrol* (abstr) 2000;11:622A.

116. Snyder SH. Nitric oxide: more jobs for that molecule. *Nature* 1994;372:504.

117. Chin E, Bondy CA. Dietary protein-induced renal growth: correlation between renal IGF-I synthesis and hyperplasia. *Am J Physiol* 1994;266:C1037.

118. Agus D, et al. Inhibitory role of dietary protein restriction on the development and expression of immune-mediated antitubular basement membrane-induced tubulointerstitial nephritis in rats. *J Clin Invest* 1985;76:930.

119. Nath KA, Hostetter MK, Hostetter TH. Increased ammoniagenesis as a determinant of progressive renal injury. *Am J Kidney Dis* 1991;17:654.

120. Torres VE, et al. Renal cystic disease and ammoniagenesis in Han:SPRD rats. *J Am Soc Nephrol* 1994;5:1193.

121. Keane WF. Proteinuria: its clinical importance and role in progressive renal disease. *Am J Kidney Dis* 2000;35:S97.

122. Remuzzi G. Nephropathic nature of proteinuria. *Curr Opin Nephrol Hypertens* 1999;8:655.

123. Fitzgibbon WR, Webster SK, Imamura A, et al. Effect of dietary protein and enalapril on proximal tubular delivery and absorption of albumin in nephrotic rats. *Am J Physiol* 1996;270:F986.

124. Nath KA. Tubulointerstitial changes as a major determinant in the progression of renal damage. *Am J Kidney Dis* 1992;20:1.

125. Schaefer L, Meier K, Hafner C, et al. Protein restriction influences glomerular matrix turnover and tubular hypertrophy by modulation of renal proteinase activities. *Miner Electrolyte Metab* 1996;22:162.

126. Guijarro C, Keane WF. Lipid abnormalities and changes in plasma proteins in glomerular diseases and chronic renal failure. *Curr Opin Nephrol Hypertens* 1993;2:372.

127. Sanai T, et al. Advantage of early initiation of aluminum hydroxide administration for the prevention of experimental progressive renal disease. *Nephrol Dial Transplant* 1991;6:330.

128. Ibles LS, et al. Preservation of function in experimental renal disease by dietary restriction of phosphate. *N Engl J Med* 1978;298:122.

129. Kenner CH, et al. Effect of protein intake on renal function and structure in partially nephrectomized rats. *Kidney Int* 1985;27:739.

130. Lumlertgul D, et al. Phosphate depletion arrests progression of chronic renal failure independent of protein intake. *Kidney Int* 1986;29:658.

131. Lau K. Phosphate excess and progressive renal failure: the precipitation-calcification hypothesis. *Kidney Int* 1989;36:918.

132. Harris DCH, Chan L, Schrier RW. Remnant kidney hypermetabolism and progression of chronic renal failure. *Am J Physiol* 1988;254:F267.

133. Nath KA, Croatt AJ, Hostetter TH. Oxygen consumption and oxidant stress in surviving nephrons. *Am J Physiol* 1990;258:F1354.

134. Shapiro JI, et al. Attenuation of hypermetabolism in the remnant kidney by dietary phosphate restriction in the rat. *Am J Physiol* 1990;258: F183.

135. Bergstrom J. Uremic toxicity. In: Kopple JD, Massny SG, eds. *Nutritional management of renal disease*. Baltimore: Williams & Wilkins,1996:99.

136. Miyata T, van Ypersele de Strihou C, Kurokawa K, et al. Alterations in nonenzymatic biochemistry in uremia: origin and significance of "carbonyl stress" in long-term uremic complications. *Kidney Int* 1999;55:389.

137. Aoyama I, Miyazaki T, Niwa T. Preventive effects of an oral sorbent on nephropathy in rats. *Miner Electrolyte Metab* 1999;25:365.

138. Beale LS. *Kidney diseases, urinary deposits and calculous disorders: their nature and treatment*, 3rd ed. Philadelphia: Lindsay and Blakiston, 1869.

139. Maroni BJ, Mitch WE. Role of nutrition in prevention of the progression of renal disease. *Annu Rev Nutr* 1997;17:435.

140. Hakim RM, Lazarus JM. Initiation of dialysis. *J Am Soc Nephrol* 1995; 6:1319.

141. Anonymous. Clinical practice guidelines for peritoneal dialysis adequacy. *Am J Kidney Dis* 1997;30[Suppl 2]:S70.

142. Walser M, Mitch WE, Maroni BJ, et al. Should protein be restricted in predialysis patients? *Kidney Int* 1999;55:771.

143. Kopple JD, Coburn JW. Metabolic studies of low protein diets in uremia: I. nitrogen and potassium. *Medicine (Baltimore)* 1973;52: 583.

144. Cottini EP, Gallina DL, Dominguez JM. Urea excretion in adult humans with varying degrees of kidney malfunction fed milk, egg or an amino acid mixture: assessment of nitrogen balance. *J Nutr* 1973;103:11.

145. Alvestrand A, Ahlberg M, Furst P, et al. Clinical results of long-term treatment with a low protein diet and a new amino acid preparation in patients with chronic uremia. *Clin Nephrol* 1983;19:67.

146. Mitch WE, Abras E, Walser M. Long-term effects of a new ketoacid-amino acid supplement in patients with chronic renal failure. *Kidney Int* 1982;22:48.

147. Tom K, Young VR, Chapman T, et al. Long-term adaptive responses to dietary protein restriction in chronic renal failure. *Am J Physiol* 1995;268:E668.

148. Walser M. Does prolonged protein restriction preceding dialysis lead to protein malnutrition at the onset of dialysis? *Kidney Int* 1993;44: 1139.

149. Maroni BJ, Staffeld C, Young VR, et al. Mechanisms permitting nephrotic patients to achieve nitrogen equilibrium with a protein-restricted diet. *J Clin Invest* 1997;99:2479.

150. Walser M, Hill S, Tomalis EA. Treatment of nephrotic adults with a supplemented, very-low-protein diet. *Am J Kidney Dis* 1996;28:354.

151. Lim VS, Kopple JD. Protein metabolism in patients with chronic renal failure: role of uremia and dialysis. *Kidney Int* 2000;58:1.

152. Bergstrom J. Why are dialysis patients malnourished? *Am J Kidney Dis* 1995;26:229.

153. Qureshi AR, Alvestrand A, Danielsson A, et al. Factors predicting malnutrition in hemodialysis patients: a cross-sectional study. *Kidney Int* 1998;53:773.

154. Coles GA. Body composition in chronic renal failure. *QJM* 1972;41:25.

155. Hakim RM, Lazarus JM. Biochemical parameters in chronic renal failure. *Am J Kidney Dis* 1988;9:238.

156. Kopple JD, Sorensen MK, Coburn JW, et al. Controlled comparison of 20-g and 40-g protein diets in the treatment of chronic uremia. *Am J Clin Nutr* 1968;21:553.

157. Walser M, Hill S, Ward L. Progression of chronic renal failure on substituting a ketoacid supplement for an amino acid supplement. *J Am Soc Nephrol* 1992;2:1178.

158. Walser M, Hill SB, Ward L, et al. A crossover comparison of progression of chronic renal failure: ketoacids versus amino acids. *Kidney Int* 1993;43:933.

159. Masud T, Young VR, Chapman T, et al. Adaptive responses to very low protein diets: the first comparison of ketoacids to essential amino acids. *Kidney Int* 1994;45:1182.

160. Walser M, Hill S. Can renal replacement be deferred by a supplemented very-low protein diet? *J Am Soc Nephrol* 1999;10:110.

161. Aparicio M, Chauveau P, dePrecigout V, et al. Nutrition and outcome on renal replacement therapy of patients with chronic renal failure treated by a supplemented very low protein diet. *J Am Soc Nephrol* 2000; 11:708.

162. Meireles CL, Price SR, Pererira AML, et al. Nutrition and chronic renal failure in rats: what is an optimal dietary protein? *J Am Soc Nephrol* 1999;10:2367.

163. May RC, Bailey JL, Mitch WE, et al. Glucocorticoids and acidosis stimulate protein and amino acid catabolism in vivo. *Kidney Int* 1996; 49:679.

164. Reaich D, Channon SM, Scrimgeour CM, et al. Correction of acidosis in humans with CRF decreases protein degradation and amino acid oxidation. *Am J Physiol* 1993;265:E230.

165. Graham KA, Reaich D, Channon SM, et al. Correction of acidosis in CAPD decreases whole body protein degradation. *Kidney Int* 1996; 49:1396.

166. Graham KA, Reaich D, Channon SM, et al. Correction of acidosis in hemodialysis decreases whole-body protein degradation. *J Am Soc Nephrol* 1997;8:632.

167. Kaysen GA, Rathore V, Shearer GC, et al. Mechanisms of hypoalbuminemia in hemodialysis patients. *Kidney Int* 1995;48:510.

168. Kaysen GA. Biological basis of hypoalbuminemia in ESRD. *J Am Soc Nephrol* 1998;9:2368.

169. Nakanishi I, Moutabarrik A, Okada N, et al. Interleukin-8 in chronic renal failure and dialysis patients. *Nephrol Dial Transplant* 1994;9: 1435.

170. Herbelin A, Nguyen AT, Zingraff J, et al. Influence of uremia and hemodialysis on circulating interleukin-1 and tumor necrosis factor a. *Kidney Int* 1990;37:116.

171. Breuille D, Farge MC, Rose F, et al. Pentoxifylline decreases body weight loss and muscle protein wasting characteristics of sepsis. *Am J Physiol* 1993;265:E660.

172. Costelli P, Carbo N, Tessitore L, et al. Tumor necrosis factor-a mediates changes in tissue protein turnover in a rat cancer cachexia model. *J Clin Invest* 1993;92:2783.

173. Goodman MN. Interleukin-6 induces skeletal muscle protein breakdown in rats. *Proc Soc Exp Biol Med* 1994;205:182.

174. Hoshino E, Pichard C, Greenwood CE, et al. Body composition and metabolic rate in rat during continuous infusion of cachetin. *Am J Physiol* 1991;260:E27.

175. Motil KJ, Matthews DE, Bier DM, et al. Whole-body leucine and lysine metabolism: response to dietary protein intake in young men. *Am J Physiol* 1981;240:E712.

176. Mitch WE, Goldberg AL. Mechanisms of muscle wasting: the role of the ubiquitin-proteasome system. *N Engl J Med* 1996;335:1897.

177. Goodship THJ, Mitch WE, Hoerr RA, et al. Adaptation to low-protein diets in renal failure: leucine turnover and nitrogen balance. *J Am Soc Nephrol* 1990;1:66.

178. Price SR, Mitch WE. Metabolic acidosis and uremic toxicity: protein and amino acid metabolism. *Semin Nephrol* 1994;14:232.

179. Boirie Y, Broyer M, Gagnadoux MF, et al. Alterations of protein metabolism by metabolic acidosis in children with chronic renal failure. *Kidney Int* 2000;58:236.

180. Reaich D, Channon SM, Scrimgeour CM, et al. Ammonium chloride-induced acidosis increases protein breakdown and amino acid oxidation in humans. *Am J Physiol* 1992;263:E735.

181. Mochizuki T. The effect of metabolic acidosis on amino and keto acid metabolism in chronic renal failure. *Jpn J Nephrol* 1991;33: 213.

182. Lofberg E, Wernerman J, Anderstam B, et al. Correction of metabolic acidosis in dialysis patients increases branched-chain and total essential amino acid levels in muscle. *Clin Nephrol* 1997;48:230.

183. Hara Y, May RC, Kelly RA, et al. Acidosis, not azotemia, stimulates branched-chain amino acid catabolism in uremic rats. *Kidney Int* 1987;32:808.

184. May RC, Hara Y, Kelly RA, et al. Branched-chain amino acid metabolism in rat muscle: abnormal regulation in acidosis. *Am J Physiol* 1987;252:E712.

185. Wang X, Jurkovitz C, Price SR. Regulation of branched-chain ketoacid dehydrogenase flux by extracellular pH and glucocorticoids. *Am J Physiol* 1997;272:C2031.

186. Price SR, Reaich D, Marinovic AC, et al. Mechanisms contributing to muscle wasting in acute uremia: activation of amino acid catabolism. *J Am Soc Nephrol* 1998;9:439.

187. May RC, Kelly RA, Mitch WE. Mechanisms for defects in muscle protein metabolism in rats with chronic uremia: the influence of metabolic acidosis. *J Clin Invest* 1987;79:1099.

188. England BK, Chastain J, Mitch WE. Extracellular acidification changes protein synthesis and degradation in BC3H-1 myocytes. *Am J Physiol* 1991;260:C277.

189. Isozaki Y, Mitch WE, England BK, et al. Interaction between glucocorticoids and acidification results in stimulation of proteolysis and mRNAs of proteins encoding the ubiquitin-proteasome pathway in BC3H-1 myocytes. *Proc Natl Acad Sci USA* 1996;93:1967.

190. Bailey JL, Wang X, England BK, et al. The acidosis of chronic renal failure activates muscle proteolysis in rats by augmenting transcription of genes encoding proteins of the ATP-dependent, ubiquitin-proteasome pathway. *J Clin Invest* 1996;97:1447.

191. Price SR, Bailey JL, Wang X, et al. Muscle wasting in insulinopenic rats results from activation of the ATP-dependent, ubiquitin-proteasome pathway by a mechanism including gene transcription. *J Clin Invest* 1996;98:1703.

192. Mitch WE, Bailey JL, Wang X, et al. Evaluation of signals activating ubiquitin-proteasome proteolysis in a model of muscle wasting. *Am J Physiol* 1999;276:C1132.

193. England BK, Greiber S, Mitch WE, et al. Rat muscle branched-chain ketoacid dehydrogenase activity and mRNAs increase with extracellular acidemia. *Am J Physiol* 1995;268:C1395.

194. Du J, Mitch WE, Wang X, et al. Glucocorticoids induce proteasome C3 subunit expression in L6 muscle cells by opposing the suppression of its transcription by NF-kB. *J Biol Chem* 2000;275:19661.

195. Papadoyannakis NJ, Stefanides CJ, McGeown M. The effect of the correction of metabolic acidosis on nitrogen and protein balance of patients with chronic renal failure. *Am J Clin Nutr* 1984;40:623.

196. Williams B, Hattersley J, Layward E, et al. Metabolic acidosis and skeletal muscle adaptation to low protein diets in chronic uremia. *Kidney Int* 1991;40:779.

197. Reaich D, Graham KA, Channon SM, et al. Insulin mediated changes in protein degradation and glucose utilization following correction of acidosis in humans with CRF. *Am J Physiol* 1995;268:E121.

198. May RC, Kelly RA, Mitch WE. Metabolic acidosis stimulates protein degradation in rat muscle by a glucocorticoid-dependent mechanism. *J Clin Invest* 1986;77:614.

199. Garibotto G, Russo R, Sofia A, et al. Skeletal muscle protein synthesis and degradation in patients with chronic renal failure. *Kidney Int* 1994;45:1432.

200. Ballmer PE, McNurlan MA, Hulter HN, et al. Chronic metabolic acidosis decreases albumin synthesis and induces negative nitrogen balance in humans. *J Clin Invest* 1995;95:39.

201. Movilli E, Zani R, Carli O, et al. Correction of metabolic acidosis increases serum albumin concentration and decreases kinetically evaluated protein intake in hemodialysis patients: a prospective study. *Nephrol Dial Transplant* 1998;13:1719.

202. Brungger M, Hulter HN, Krapf R. Effect of chronic metabolic acidosis on the growth hormone/IGF-1 endocrine axis: new cause of growth hormone insensitivity in humans. *Kidney Int* 1997;51:216.

203. Brungger M, Hulter HN, Krapf R. Effect of chronic metabolic acidosis on thyroid hormone homeostasis in humans. *Am J Physiol* 1997;272:F648.

204. Krapf R, Vetsch R, Vetsch W, et al. Chronic metabolic acidosis increases the serum concentration of 1,25-dihydroxyvitamin D in humans by stimulating its production rate. *J Clin Invest* 1992;90:2456.

205. Uribarri J, Levin NW, Delmez J, et al. Association of acidosis and nutritional parameters in hemodialysis patients. *Am J Kidney Dis* 1999;34:493.

206. Kirschbaum B. Spurious metabolic acidosis in hemodialysis patients. *Am J Kidney Dis* 2000;35:1068.

207. Folin O. Laws governing the clinical composition of urine. *Am J Physiol* 1905;13:67.

208. Maroni BJ, Steinman T, Mitch WE. A method for estimating nitrogen intake of patients with chronic renal failure. *Kidney Int* 1985;27:58.

209. Kopple JD, Gao X-L, Oing P-Y. Diet protein and urea and total nitrogen appearance in chronic renal failure patients. *Kidney Int* 1997;52:486.

210. Gibson JA, Park NJ, Sladen GE, et al. The role of the colon in urea metabolism in man. *Clin Sci* 1976;50:51.

211. Jones EA, Smallwood RA, Craigie A, et al. The enterohepatic circulation of urea nitrogen. *Clin Sci* 1969;37:825.

212. Mitch WE, Lietman PS, Walser M. Effects of oral neomycin and kanamycin in chronic renal failure: I. urea metabolism. *Kidney Int* 1977;11:116.

213. Mitch WE, Walser M. Effects of oral neomycin and kanamycin in chronic uremic patients. II. nitrogen balance. *Kidney Int* 1977;11:123.

214. Giordano C. Use of exogenous and endogenous urea for protein synthesis in normal and uremic subjects. *J Lab Clin Med* 1963;62:231.

215. Mitch WE, Wilcox CS. Disorders of body fluids, sodium and potassium in chronic renal failure. *Am J Med* 1982;72:536.

216. Bingham SA. The dietary assessment of individuals: methods, accuracy, new techniques and recommendations. *Nutr Abstr Rev* 1987;57:705.

217. Maschio G, Oldrizzi L, Tessitore N, et al. Effects of dietary protein and phosphorus restriction on the progression of early renal failure. *Kidney Int* 1982;22:371.

218. Oldrizzi L, Rugiu C, Maschio G. The Verona experience on the effect of diet on progression of renal failure. *Kidney Int* 1989;36:S103.

219. Guarnieri GF, Toigo G, Situlin R, et al. Nutritional state in patients on long-term low-protein diet or with nephrotic syndrome. *Kidney Int* 1989;36:S195.

220. Rosman JB, Langer K, Brandl M, et al. Protein-restricted diets in chronic renal failure: a four year follow-up shows limited indications. *Kidney Int* 1989;36:S96.

221. The GISEN Group. Randomized placebo-controlled trial of effect of ramipril on decline in glomerular filtration rate and risk of terminal renal failure in proteinuric, non-diabetic nephropathy. *Lancet* 1997;349:1857.

222. Ruggenenti P, Perna A, Mosconi L, et al., GISEN. Urinary protein excretion rate is the best independent predictor of ESRF in non-diabetic proteinuric chronic nephropathies. *Kidney Int* 1998;53:1209.

223. Kaysen GA, Gambertoglio J, Jimenez I, et al. Effect of dietary protein intake on albumin homeostasis in nephrotic patients. *Kidney Int* 1986;29:572.

224. Gansevoort RT, De Zeeuw D, De Jong PE. Additive antiproteinuric effect of ACE inhibition and a low-protein diet in human renal disease. *Nephrol Dial Transplant* 1995;10:497.

225. Williams PS, Stevens ME, Fass G, et al. Failure of dietary protein and phosphate restriction to retard the rate of progression of CRF: a prospective, randomized, controlled trial. *QJM* 1991;81:837.

226. Locatelli F, Alberti D, Graziani G, et al. Prospective, randomised, multicentre trial of effect of protein restriction on progression of chronic renal insufficiency. *Lancet* 1991;337:1299.

227. Fouque D, Laville M, Boissel JP, et al. Controlled low protein diets in chronic renal insufficiency: meta-analysis. *BMJ* 1992;304:216.

228. Pedrini MT, Levey AS, Lau J, et al. The effect of dietary protein restriction on the progression of diabetic and nondiabetic renal diseases: a meta-analysis. *Ann Intern Med* 1996;124:627.

229. Fouque D, Wang P, Laville M, et al. Low protein diets delay end-stage renal disease in non diabetic adults with chronic renal failure. *Cochrane Database Syst Rev* 2000;2:CD001892.

230. Kasiske BL, Lakatua JDA, Ma JZ, et al. A meta-analysis of the effects of dietary protein restriction on the rate of decline in renal function. *Am J Kidney Dis* 1998;31:954.

231. Taal MW, Brenner BM. Renoprotective benefits of RAS inhibition: from ACEI to angiotensin II antagonists. *Kidney Int* 2000;57:1803.

232. Walker JD, Dodds RA, Murrells TJ, et al. Restriction of dietary protein and progression of renal failure in diabetic nephropathy. *Lancet* 1989;2:1411.

233. Yue DK, O'Dea J, Stewart P, et al. Proteinuria and renal function in diabetic patients fed a diet moderately restricted in protein. *Am J Clin Nutr* 1988;48:230.

234. Ciavarella A, DiMizio G, Stefoni S, et al. Reduced albuminuria after dietary protein restriction in insulin-dependent diabetic patients with clinical nephropathy. *Diabetes Care* 1987;10:407.

235. Evanoff GV, Thompson CS, Brown J, et al. The effect of dietary protein restriction on the progression of diabetic nephropathy: a 12-month follow-up. *Arch Intern Med* 1987;147:492.

236. Mogensen CE. Microalbuminuria as a predictor of clinical diabetic nephropathy. *Kidney Int* 1987;31:673.

237. Raal FJ, Kalk WJ, Lawson M, et al. Effect of moderate dietary protein restriction on the progression of overt diabetic nephropathy: a 6-mo prospective study. *Am J Clin Nutr* 1994;60:579.

238. Zeller KR, Whittaker E, Sullivan L, et al. Effect of restricting dietary protein on the progression of renal failure in patients with insulin-dependent diabetes mellitus. *N Engl J Med* 1991;324:78.

239. Alvestrand A, Bergstrom J. Amino-acid supplements and the course of chronic renal disease. In: Mitch WE, ed. *The progressive nature of renal disease.* New York: Churchill Livingstone, 1986:219.

240. Bergstrom J, Alvestrand A, Bucht H, et al. Progression of chronic renal failure in man is retarded with more frequent clinical follow-ups and better blood pressure control. *Clin Nephrol* 1986;25:1.

241. Barsotti G, Morelli E, Guiducci A. Three years' experience with a very low nitrogen diet supplemented with essential amino acids and keto-analogues in the treatment of chronic uremia. *Proc Eur Dial Transplant Assoc* 1982;19:773.

242. Mitch WE, Walser M, Steinman TL, et al. The effect of keto acid-amino acid supplement to a restricted diet on the progression of chronic renal failure. *N Engl J Med* 1984;311:623.

243. Di Landro D, Dattilo GA, Romagnoli GF. Comparative outcome of patients on a conventional low protein diet versus a supplemented diet in chronic renal failure. *Contrib Nephrol* 1990;81:201.

244. MDRD Study Group. The Modification of Diet in Renal Disease Study: design, methods and results from the feasibility study. *Am J Kidney Dis* 1992;20:18.

245. Mitch WE. Dietary therapy in uremia: the impact on nutrition and progressive renal failure. *Kidney Int* 2000;57:S38.

246. Klahr S, Breyer JA, Beck GJ, et al. Dietary protein restriction, blood pressure control, and the progression of polycystic kidney disease. *J Am Soc Nephrol* 1995;5:2037.

247. The Diabetes Control and Complications Trial Research Group. The effect of intensive treatment of diabetes on the development and progression of long-term complications in insulin-dependent diabetes mellitus. *N Engl J Med* 1993;329:977.

248. Teschan PE, Beck GJ, Dwyer JT, et al. Effect of a ketoacid-aminoacid-supplemented very low protein diet on the progression of advanced renal disease: a reanalysis of the MDRD Feasibility Study. *Clin Nephrol* 1998;50:273.

249. Levey AS, Adler S, Caggiula AW, et al. Effects of dietary protein restriction on the progression of advanced renal disease in the Modification of Diet in Renal Disease Study. *Am J Kidney Dis* 1996;27:652.

250. Rosman JB, Donker-Willenborg MA. Dietary compliance and its assessment in the Groningen trial on protein restriction in chronic renal failure. *Contrib Nephrol* 1990;81:95.

251. Yeh S-S, Schuster MW. Geriatric cachexia: the role of cytokines. *Am J Clin Nutr* 1999;70:183.

CHAPTER 102

Phosphate, Aluminum, and Other Elements in Chronic Renal Failure

Robert F. Reilly, Jr. and Allen C. Alfrey

In the attempt to define uremic toxins, a great deal of attention has been directed at organic compounds. However, at least two inorganic compounds, phosphate and aluminum, have been strongly implicated in the pathogenesis of a number of alterations that can occur in the uremic state. The metabolism and toxicity of phosphorus and aluminum in uremic patients and methods of preventing and treating disorders created by these two elements are reviewed in this chapter. Two other elements, magnesium and zinc, have also been implicated in the pathogenesis of some uremic symptomatology. However, the evidence of their involvement is much weaker than that for phosphorus and aluminum, and therefore these latter two elements are only briefly reviewed here. Finally, a variety of other disturbances in trace elements, both essential and nonessential, have also been recognized in uremic patients. Again, there is little evidence to date that any of these alterations are responsible for any clinical symptomatology.

PHOSPHORUS

An individual normally ingests 800 to 1,000 mg of phosphorus each day. The net absorption is approximately 60% of the ingested load, and this is readily excreted in the urine (1). In healthy persons, the serum phosphorus concentration is maintained in the normal range of 3.5 to 4.5 mg/dL. Even with renal failure, the serum phosphorus level is maintained within the normal range until the glomerular filtration rate falls below 25% of normal. This is accomplished initially by a reduction in renal tubular reabsorption of phosphorus and later by a combination of decreased renal tubular reabsorption of phosphorus and reduced gastrointestinal absorption of phosphorus. Renal tubular reabsorption of phosphorus is reduced as a consequence of increased secretion of parathyroid

R. F. Reilly: Department of Medicine, Yale University School of Medicine, New Haven, Connecticut

A. C. Alfrey: Department of Medicine, University of Colorado; and Department of Medicine, Veterans Administration Hospital, Denver, Colorado

hormone (PTH) (2), as well as a non–PTH-dependent mechanism that occurs as a result of a reduction in renal functional mass (3). The most apparent reason for a decrease in the gastrointestinal absorption of phosphorus is decreased 1,25-dihydroxyvitamin D_3 (1,25[OH]$_2$D$_3$) (calcitriol), which occurs with more advanced renal failure (4). However, as glomerular filtration falls below 25 mL/minute, these alterations in phosphorus metabolism are no longer sufficient to maintain normal serum phosphorus levels, and with further reductions in renal function there is a progressive rise in serum phosphorus levels (3,4). These interrelationships are shown in Fig. 102-1.

Consequences of Hyperphosphatemia

Hyperphosphatemia has been directly implicated in the pathogenesis of secondary hyperparathyroidism and its associated skeletal alterations (5) as well as metastatic calcifications (6), both of which occur with some frequency in uremic patients in whom phosphate control is not maintained. In addition, phosphate has been implicated as a factor that may in part be responsible for accelerating functional deterioration in a diseased or damaged kidney (7–9).

Secondary Hyperparathyroidism

Hyperphosphatemia has been strongly implicated in the pathogenesis of the secondary hyperparathyroidism that is commonly seen in uremic patients (5,10). The suggested mechanism by which hyperphosphatemia induces hyperparathyroidism is as follows: As glomerular filtration rate falls, there is a slight rise in serum phosphorus. This causes the serum calcium concentration to fall, which in turn stimulates the secretion of PTH. The increased PTH levels decrease renal tubular reabsorption of phosphorus, causing serum phosphorus levels to return to normal. As glomerular filtration rate progressively falls, increasing amounts of PTH are required to decrease tubular reabsorption of phosphorus

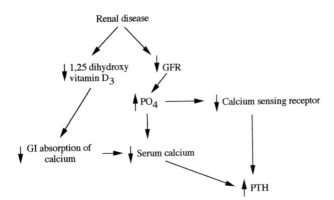

FIG. 102-1. Pathophysiologic mechanisms of secondary hyperparathyroidism. Renal disease results in a fall in glomerular filtration rate and a decrease in 1,25 dihydroxyvitamin D₃ levels. As a result of a decrease in gastrointestinal calcium reabsorption and an increase in serum phosphate there is a decrease in the serum calcium that leads to an increase in parathyroid hormone.

and maintain serum phosphorus in, or close to, the normal range. This process has been termed the trade-off hypothesis. It is suggested that to maintain normal phosphorus levels with progressive renal failure, the trade-off is the establishment of a hyperparathyroid state with its accompanying alterations.

Since it recently was shown that there are receptors on the parathyroid glands for 1,25(OH)$_2$D$_3$ and that this hormone can suppress PTH synthesis, it has been suggested that hypophosphatemia could suppress PTH levels by stimulating 1,25(OH)$_2$D$_3$ production (11). Although early during the course of renal failure, phosphorus depletion stimulates 1,25(OH)$_2$D$_3$ production (12), later in the course of renal failure, phosphorus has no effect on 1,25(OH)$_2$D$_3$ levels (13). In addition, phosphorus depletion suppresses PTH levels in the absence of any change in serum calcium or 1,25(OH)$_2$D$_3$ (13,14). Phosphate depletion also prevents the secondary hyperparathyroidism in Vitamin D deficiency (15). These studies suggest that phosphate per se has a direct effect on modulating PTH secretion.

Subsequent studies have verified this conclusion. Fresh rat parathyroid glands were incubated in media with increasing phosphate concentrations. A phosphorus concentration of 3 and 4 mm produced a 3- to 4-fold increase in PTH secretion compared to 1 mm phosphorus. These authors also report that incubation in high phosphorus medium suppressed the ability of increasing concentrations of calcium to inhibit PTH release (16). Nuclear transcript run-on experiments suggest that the effect of phosphorus is posttranscriptional (17). Recently, it has been shown that AUF1 binds to the 3'-UTR of the PTH transcript and stabilizes it (18). Perhaps this protein or others like it are regulated by phosphorus and or calcium in the parathyroid gland.

Dietary phosphate also plays a role in the expression of the calcium-sensing receptor. The calcium-sensing receptor is a G protein-coupled receptor expressed in parathyroid gland that couples to the production of inositol 1,4,5-triphosphate (IP$_3$). Calcium binds to the receptor and via IP$_3$ results in an inhibition of PTH release and transcription. In rats made uremic by 5/6 nephrectomy, the animals on a high phosphate diet (1.2% phosphate) showed a 55% decrease in calcium-sensing receptor mRNA levels and an increase in parathyroid gland weight (2.77 ± 0.95 μg/g body weight versus 0.77 ± 0.16 μg/g body weight in controls). Immunofluorescence studies indicated that the receptor was downregulated in areas of proliferation. Dietary phosphate restriction prevented both the decrease in calcium-sensing receptor transcript expression and parathyroid hyperplasia (19). This substantiates the view that the abnormal control of PTH secretion in uremia is due at least in part to the downregulation of the calcium-sensing receptor in hyperplastic parathyroid tissue. Although hyperphosphatemia appears to be important in the causation of secondary hyperparathyroidism, control of serum phosphorus alone has not been totally effective in the prevention of secondary hyperparathyroidism in uremia. In dogs, a reduction in dietary phosphorus intake that is proportional to the reduction in renal function initially prevents the expected rise in PTH levels (20). Eventually, however, PTH levels increase despite the dietary phosphorus restriction and the maintenance of phosphate levels within the normal range. In addition, although it has been routine practice for over a decade to attempt to control serum phosphorus levels in uremic patients, increased PTH levels and histologic evidence of hyperparathyroid bone disease, which may be symptomatic, are still commonly seen in uremic patients (21–23). This is additional evidence that phosphate restriction alone will not reverse the hyperparathyroid state.

Metastatic Calcification

Hyperphosphatemia has been strongly implicated in the pathogenesis of the extraosseous calcification that occurs in uremic patients (6,24). The various types of extraosseous calcium phosphate deposited in uremic patients are listed in Table 102-1. The best-documented types of extraosseous calcium phosphate deposits that result from hyperphosphatemia are tumoral, periarticular and articular, and conjunctival calcifications (25–28).

Tumoral calcification represents calcium phosphate deposits that are usually periarticular but do not involve the

TABLE 102-1. *Types of extraosseous calcifications*

Hyperphosphatemia-related
Conjunctival
Calcific periarthritis
Tumoral
Other etiologies
Vascular calcification
Visceral calcification
Heart
Lung
Kidney

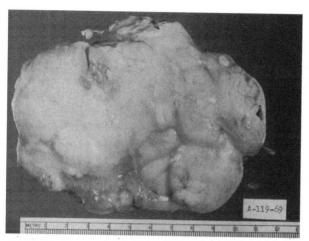

FIG. 102-2. Excised tumoral calcification demonstrating fibrous enclosure of the calcium phosphate deposit. (From LeGeros RZ, et al. Pathological calcification associated with uremia. Two types of calcium phosphate deposits. *Calcif Tissue Res* 1973;13:173, with permission.)

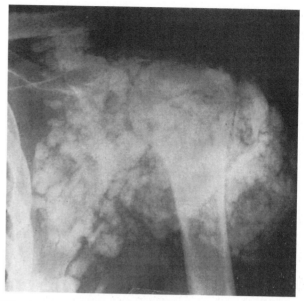

FIG. 102-3. Tumoral calcification around the left shoulder prior to renal transplantation.

joints or their capsules. These deposits are encapsulated with a thick fibrous wall and are multiloculated (29) (Fig. 102-2). Calcium phosphate deposits are present in a semisolid state as hydroxyapatite, and on examination the crystals are needle- and boat-shaped with a length of 30 to 40 nm and a width of 4.5 to 5.0 nm (24). In general, tumoral deposits cause little discomfort or other symptoms unless they are quite large, which may cause them to interfere with the range of motion of the joint.

Conjunctival calcifications are characterized by an unpleasant gritty sensation in the eyes that is associated with a marked redness or inflammation of the conjunctiva (25,30). As with tumoral calcification, the calcium phosphate deposit is hydroxyapatite.

Calcific periarthritis, like gout and pseudogout, is characterized by recurrent attacks of acute arthritis (26,31,32). However, in contrast to gout and pseudogout, the joint fluid contains neither uric acid nor calcium pyrophosphate crystals. Instead, there are extraarticular deposits of hydroxyapatite.

Tumoral, periarticular, and conjunctival calcifications share not only a similarity of the crystalline feature of the calcium phosphate deposits but also the fact that their occurrence is closely associated with overt hyperphosphatemia. Not only can the occurrence of these deposits be prevented, but also even when present they can be rapidly mobilized by lowering serum phosphorus levels (33). Additional evidence that hyperphosphatemia is responsible for the production of these deposits is a study of a patient with extensive tumoral deposits. Prior to renal transplantation and mobilization of these deposits, total body phosphorus was 969 g (normal 670 g), and calcium was 1,364 g (normal 1,185 g). Following transplantation, after the deposits had spontaneously mobilized (Figs. 102-3 and 102-4), total body phosphorus had fallen to 670 g and calcium to 1,282 g. This study showed that total body phosphorus was increased much more than total

body calcium, an increase that would be consistent with the fact that tumoral calcification is a condition of marked, total phosphorus excess.

In the two other major types of extraosseous calcifications, visceral and arterial, the role of hyperphosphatemia

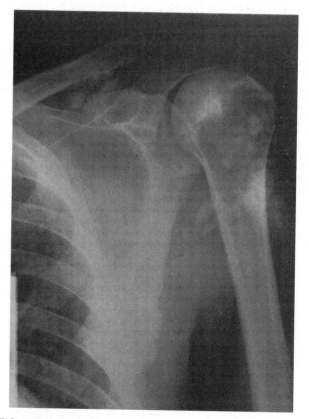

FIG. 102-4. Resolution of tumoral deposit about the left shoulder 3 months following successful renal transplantation.

in their pathogenesis is less clear. Visceral calcification occurs in a variety of tissues but exerts its major clinical consequences in the heart and lung, where it can cause pulmonary insufficiency, myocardial failure, or conduction disturbances (34,35). In older studies the reported incidence of visceral calcification was 40% to 45% in nondialyzed uremic patients and 75% in dialyzed uremic patients (36). Unfortunately, there are few recent studies reporting the frequency of visceral calcification in uremic patients. The available studies largely used indirect means of estimating visceral calcification (37–39). Because of the paucity of recent reports of this complication, it would appear that visceral calcification occurs much less often now than previously. The reason for this is unclear but it seems unlikely that phosphate control is responsible based on evidence suggesting that hyperphosphatemia is not important in the pathogenesis of these types of deposits. First, the presence of visceral calcification seems to bear no relationship to the presence or absence of tumoral, periarticular, or conjunctival calcifications, which are known to result from hyperphosphatemia. In addition, it is not known whether prevention or correction of hyperphosphatemia has any effect on the formation or mobilization of visceral calcification.

Finally, the calcium phosphate deposit in visceral calcification is markedly different from that in tumoral, periarticular, and conjunctival deposits. Unlike these latter deposits, which are hydroxyapatite, visceral calcification is an amorphous compound high in magnesium, aluminum, and pyrophosphate and has the thermochemical properties of whitlockite (29,35). These unique features of visceral calcification suggest that factors other than hyperphosphatemia are important in the pathogenesis of these deposits.

Although there is an impression that control of hyperphosphatemia may ultimately reduce the incidence of visceral calcification, there is no conclusive evidence supporting this supposition. In addition, other changes in dialytic techniques, such as more frequent dialysis, improved efficiency of dialysis, and water treatment for the preparation of the dialysate, were instituted about the time phosphate control was initiated, thus further confusing the issue of whether hyperphosphatemia is a major factor in the etiology of these deposits.

It seems equally as unlikely that hyperphosphatemia is important in the pathogenesis of vascular calcification (40–43). Vascular calcification is extremely common in uremic patients, being present in approximately 100% of uremic patients over 50 years old (40–42). Its presence does not correlate well with hyperphosphatemia, and there is little evidence that correction of the hyperphosphatemia causes its resolution (33,40–42). It has been suggested that the calcification represents an accelerated aging of the vascular tree. This causes calcium to be deposited locally and the calcification would appear not to be the result of hyperphosphatemia or some other alteration in the milieu (43).

Recently, a matrix gamma-carboxyglutamic acid (Gla) protein knockout mouse was generated (44). The mouse exhibited extensive and lethal calcification of the media of all elastic arteries. Matrix Gla protein (MGP) is an inhibitor of calcification in the vessel wall and its activity is dependent on

Vitamin K-dependent gamma carboxylation. MGP mRNA is constitutively expressed by normal vascular smooth muscle cells and is upregulated in cells adjacent to medial and intimal calcification (45). Several Gla-containing proteins are expressed in human vasculature. Dysregulation of these proteins by the uremic state may play a role in the vascular calcification observed in end-stage renal disease.

A final type of extraosseous calcification has been reported under the term *calciphylaxis* (46–49). It is a relatively rare condition in which the patient presents with a painful violaceous, mottled lesion of the extremities or trunk that progresses to skin and subcutaneous tissue necrosis, nonhealing ulcers, and gangrene. It is unclear what role, if any, hyperphosphatemia and secondary hyperparathyroidism play in the pathogenesis of this condition. Therapy has largely consisted of parathyroidectomy and phosphate-binding agents to normalize serum phosphorus levels. Results of such interventions have been inconsistent. More recently hyperbaric oxygen therapy has been employed with apparent success in one patient (50).

ALUMINUM

Normal Aluminum Metabolism

Aluminum is the fifth most common element in the earth's crust, but because of its insoluble nature only trace amounts of this element are actually ingested. Recent studies suggested that 2 to 8 mg of aluminum are ingested daily as a result of contamination in food (51,52). Because aluminum is used as a filler in some foods such as cheese and pickles and is a constituent of baking powder, eating habits can also affect the amount of aluminum ingested. An additional source of aluminum is municipal water supplies. Aluminum is commonly used to flocculate and remove turbidity from water sources. This can leave aluminum residues as high as 4 mg/L (53).

Most evidence suggests that the gastrointestinal tract represents a formidable barrier to aluminum absorption and little of the ingested aluminum is absorbed. This is based on the fact that total body aluminum is quite low, 35 to 40 mg, and does not increase with aging. In addition, urinary aluminum, which is believed to be the major pathway for the elimination of any systemic aluminum and reflects gastrointestinal absorption of aluminum, is approximately 10 μg/day (54).

The majority of studies show that aluminum is absorbed passively by the gastrointestinal tract. This appears to occur largely, if not entirely, through the paracellular pathway (55–57). Presently, only four factors have been clearly shown to modulate aluminum absorption. These are the amount of aluminum compound ingested (58), the solubility of the aluminum compound (59), the integrity of the tight junctions of the small intestine (55–57), and the uremic state (60). By increasing aluminum intake from milligram quantities to gram quantities, aluminum absorption can be increased by 20 to 50 times normal to as high as 500 μg/day (58). More soluble aluminum compounds such as aluminum lactate, as compared to aluminum hydroxide, are also more readily absorbed (59). The factor that has the largest effect on aluminum absorption is the opening of the tight junction between intestinal cells. This is exemplified by giving aluminum compounds with citrate (55). Not only is aluminum citrate relatively soluble as compared to other aluminum compounds, but also citrate, probably as a result of chelating the calcium necessary for the maintenance of tight junctions, opens the paracellular pathways (55,56). This results in a very rapid and markedly enhanced aluminum absorption (55,56). Recent studies further showed that normal individuals chronically ingesting calcium citrate, given as a calcium supplement, also have enhanced aluminum absorption from normal dietary sources (61).

Although it has been suggested that both Vitamin D (62) and PTH (63) may enhance aluminum absorption from the gastrointestinal tract, this has not been firmly established. In addition, the status of the body iron stores has been proposed to have an effect on aluminum absorption (64). Aluminum and iron metabolism may be closely interrelated, and there is a correlation between serum ferritin and plasma aluminum concentration in dialyzed uremic patients (64).

In the usual environmental exposure, the lungs represent major barriers to aluminum absorption. It seems that most inhaled aluminum is exhaled, and only a small amount of aluminum is retained in the pulmonary parenchyma. This supposition is based on the fact that pulmonary aluminum content increases with age but does not correlate with other tissue stores of this element (65,66). However, there is evidence that industrial workers exposed to aluminum fumes absorb some of the aluminum as manifested by an increase in urinary aluminum excretion (67).

The skin is largely impervious to aluminum; even with increased exposure, as can occur with antiperspirants, there is little evidence that any aluminum can be absorbed through the skin.

The kidney is the major avenue for the elimination of any absorbed aluminum. Although renal excretion of aluminum has not been fully evaluated, aluminum clearance seems to be 5% to 10% of the glomerular filtration rate (68,69). This is consistent with the finding that aluminum is approximately 90% to 95% protein bound in plasma (70). However, even the normal kidney has limited ability to excrete aluminum and when large parenteral loads of aluminum are administered, varying amounts of the administered aluminum are retained (69).

Normally, there is very little aluminum in bile, and even with acute aluminum loading, biliary excretion of aluminum increases only modestly (71). Thus, the biliary route of eliminating aluminum cannot replace that of the kidney, and loss of renal function markedly places the individual at risk of aluminum overload.

Effects Of Uremia On Aluminum Metabolism

There are several reasons why an increased body burden of aluminum would be expected in uremic patients. First, the uremic state in experimental animals is associated with

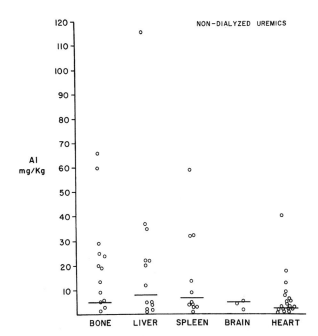

FIG. 102-5. Tissue aluminum levels in nondialyzed uremic patients. The upper limits of values found in nonuremic control subjects are shown by the horizontal line.

enhanced aluminum absorption from the gastrointestinal tract. The mechanism, however, has not been elucidated (60). The finding that tissue stores of aluminum were increased in over 85% of a group of nondialyzed uremic patients who were studied during a period when aluminum-containing, phosphate-binding gels were not routinely administered is in keeping with the finding of enhanced absorption of aluminum in the uremic state (65,66) (Fig. 102-5). In addition, uremic patients sometimes receive large oral loads of aluminum hydroxide, which is given to reduce dietary phosphate absorption.

In the dialyzed uremic patient the natural barriers to aluminum absorption—gastrointestinal tract, lungs, and skin—can be circumvented by the parenteral administration of aluminum. This can occur by dialyzing the patient with dialysate prepared with aluminum-contaminated water (72). Aluminum is bound in plasma largely to transferrin (70,73). Transferrin has been suggested as an ideal aluminum carrier in plasma because most of the iron sites are normally unoccupied. Transferrin-binding capacity would normally be around $600 \mu g$ of aluminum per liter of serum. Because of this binding capacity, any aluminum transferred from the dialysate to the patient is rapidly bound, maintaining a gradient from dialysate to patient and thus promoting additional aluminum uptake. Therefore, even a small amount of aluminum in the dialysate can result in the transfer of a large aluminum load to the patient during dialysis, appreciably enhancing the body burden of this element.

The compromised renal function prevents the elimination of most of the absorbed or administered aluminum, further enhancing the body burden of this element. In addition to enhanced gastrointestinal absorption and impaired urinary excretion of aluminum, uremic animals also tend to have an altered compartmentalization of aluminum in the body. In uremic animals, bone aluminum uptake is enhanced, whereas liver aluminum uptake seems to be slightly decreased (74).

Another tissue in which aluminum uptake may be enhanced in uremia is the brain (54). Although nonuremic-patient populations, such as individuals on chronic total parenteral nutrition (TPN) and premature infants receiving large amounts of albumin or TPN solutions, receive large intravenous loads of aluminum and have elevated bone and liver aluminum levels, aluminum neurotoxicity has not been observed with these conditions (69,75). Similarly, studies show that even animals given large parenteral loads of aluminum do not have nearly the high levels of aluminum in the brain as do uremic patients dying of aluminum neurotoxicity (76). This might suggest that the blood–brain barrier must be compromised for brain aluminum to be markedly increased. Such an abnormality in the blood–brain barrier may be found in advanced uremia (77).

Aluminum Toxicity

Neurotoxicity

Aluminum neurotoxicity was initially described in 1886 (78) and was rediscovered in 1937 (79). These studies showed that local administration or application of aluminum to the brain caused animals to develop a seizure disorder. Subsequently it was found that certain species of animals—cats and rabbits, in particular—also developed neurofibrillary tangles following the application (80–84) or parenteral administration of aluminum (85). The finding that aluminum could induce neurofibrillary tangles in animals prompted the suggestion that aluminum was a possible cause of Alzheimer's disease. However, this theory has been disputed because not all patients with Alzheimer's disease have high brain aluminum levels (84). Moreover, the neurofibrillary tangles and biochemical alterations in Alzheimer's disease and those of aluminum intoxication are different. Also, the senile plaques that are common in Alzheimer's disease are not seen in experimental aluminum toxicity (84).

In 1962 and 1975 two patients, one of whom had worked in an aluminum plant, developed a dementing neurologic disease in association with increased brain aluminum concentrations. These were the first reports to suggest that aluminum neurotoxicity could occur in humans (86,87).

In 1972, a new and distinct neurologic disease was first described in dialyzed uremic patients (88). The disease (dialysis encephalopathy or dialysis dementia) is characterized by an intermittent speech disturbance—a stuttering or stammering that is often first noted, and often intensified, during or immediately following the dialysis procedure. The speech disturbance is associated with personality changes, parietal lobe findings such as directional disorientation, seizures, myoclonus, and auditory and visual hallucinations. The findings are progressive, and over a 7- to 9-month period following the onset of symptoms the patients become totally mute and unable to perform purposeful movements. Death rapidly

ensues. Following the initial description of this disease, other dialysis patients from many different geographic areas were found to have a similar syndrome (88–96).

Initially the major considerations for the etiology of this disease were slow virus infection, communicating hydrocephalus, and an environmental toxin (97). Slow virus infection was excluded because of the lack of histologic changes in the brain and the failure to transmit the disease into primates by inoculating brain tissue from patients who had died of encephalopathy. Similarly, communicating hydrocephalus was excluded by computed tomography (CT) scans and lack of anatomic changes consistent with this condition. Based on the exclusion of these causes and the increasing awareness that dialysis encephalopathy was occurring in epidemic proportions in some dialysis units, but rarely, if ever, in other units, strongly suggested that an environmental toxin was responsible for the condition.

In 1976, one trace element, aluminum, was initially shown to be consistently higher in brain gray matter in patients dying of dialysis encephalopathy than in patients on dialysis dying of other causes and in nonuremic controls (98). This finding was confirmed by three other groups (90,92,94), and was followed by large epidemiologic studies in the United Kingdom which showed that in areas with a high incidence of dialysis encephalopathy aluminum was present in high concentrations in the water used to prepare the dialysate. In contrast, in areas where dialysis encephalopathy was rarely seen, aluminum content was low (99,100). This was subsequently supported by studies in France (90) and the United States (89,91,95,96,101), which also showed that centers with a high incidence of dialysis encephalopathy also had large amounts of aluminum in the dialysate. Further evidence incriminating aluminum as the toxin appeared when the number of cases of dialysis encephalopathy profoundly decreased when aluminum was removed from the water used to prepare the dialysate. Final evidence for the neurotoxicity of aluminum comes from reports showing that aluminum toxicity can be reversed with chelation (102,103).

In contrast to dialysis encephalopathy which results from a chronic exposure to aluminum from aluminum-contaminated dialysate or less commonly orally administered aluminum compounds, an acute form of aluminum neurotoxicity has been observed in uremic patients (104,105). This occurs under three different conditions: dialysis performed with dialysate highly contaminated with aluminum (106), the oral administration of citrate compounds in association with aluminum compounds (104,105), and marked elevation of plasma aluminum levels resulting from deferoxamine therapy (107). It would appear that virtually all nondialyzed children (108,109) and adults with uremia (104,105) who have developed aluminum neurotoxicity have done so from the ingestion of the combination of citrate and aluminum compounds. Although the patients may present with rather mild symptoms such as a speech disturbance similar to dialysis encephalopathy, more often there is an acute explosive onset of symptoms. In the adult patient, symptoms consist of agitation, confusion, myoclonic jerks, grand mal seizures, and obtundation, and can culminate in death within days of the onset of symptoms (104,105). In children, aluminum neurotoxicity tends to be somewhat different in that it is usually manifested by regression of verbal and motor skills (108,109). This is exemplified by the finding that children who have just started to walk and talk may lose these abilities.

If acute toxicity occurs as a consequence of high aluminum levels in the dialysate, it usually develops during the dialysis procedure (106). Symptoms resulting from deferoxamine therapy occur during or immediately following a dialysis for which deferoxamine was administered (107). Although symptoms of acute aluminum intoxication can occur after months of ingestion of the combination of citrate and aluminum compounds, it is not uncommon for symptoms to develop in a matter of weeks following the combined ingestion of these two compounds (104,105).

Standards for permissible levels of aluminum in water (less than 10 μg/L) used to prepare dialysate were established in 1981. By 1990 over 99% of dialysis units in the United States were treating water to remove aluminum. This was associated with a reduction in the number of dialysis patients developing dialysis encephalopathy from 229 cases (0.4%) in 61,450 dialysis patients in 1980 to 129 cases (less than 0.1%) in 140,555 dialysis patients in 1990 (110).

Recently, there have been two case reports of acute aluminum encephalopathy following alum bladder irrigation (111,112). Alum (aluminum ammonium sulfate) was introduced as a treatment for bladder hemorrhage in 1982 and is used as a second line agent if bleeding does not stop with saline irrigation. In general, alum does not cause symptoms in patients with normal renal function even though increases in serum aluminum levels do occur. Ten percent of alum by weight is aluminum; therefore, one liter of a 1% alum solution infused at a rate of a liter per hour exposes the bladder mucosa to 24 g of aluminum per day. Whether a damaged mucosa absorbs more aluminum than that of a normal bladder remains unclear. Acute encephalopathy has been reported at serum concentrations as low as 17 μg/L. There are at least 12 case reports in the literature and all but one have had some degree of renal insufficiency. Thus, alum should not be used as a bladder irrigant in patients with acute or chronic renal failure.

The diagnosis of aluminum neurotoxicity is largely based on a history of either oral or parenteral exposure to aluminum in uremic patients who demonstrate the classic clinical features and have had other neurologic disorders excluded by appropriate studies. The most useful laboratory test supporting the diagnosis of aluminum neurotoxicity is the electroencephalogram (EEG), where changes occur early and precede clinical symptoms (113). Unlike most metabolic encephalopathies, including uremic encephalopathy, which exhibit a generalized slowing on the EEG, in aluminum intoxication the background rhythm is relatively normal with multifocal bursts of slow or delta waves often accompanied by spike activity. The CT scan may appear normal or only

show mild cortical atrophy. There are no cerebrospinal fluid (CSF) abnormalities and aluminum levels in the CSF are not increased. The histologic changes that occur in the brains of patients dying of dialysis encephalopathy are nonspecific and similar to changes seen in patients on dialysis dying of other causes (97). Plasma aluminum levels in chronic intoxication are increased and often in the range of 100 to 200 μg/L. With acute aluminum intoxication plasma aluminum levels are usually in excess of 500 μg/L.

Because anatomic changes are minimal and the disease is reversible with treatment, aluminum appears to cause neurologic impairment by interfering with the brain's biochemistry. Although aluminum inhibits hexokinase activity (70,114,115) and affects brain calmodulin function (116), the specific mechanism by which aluminum interferes with neurologic function remains to be elucidated.

Skeletal Toxicity

Aluminum skeletal toxicity is characterized by Vitamin D-resistant osteomalacia, decreased or absent bone formation, low PTH levels, mildly elevated serum calcium levels, proximal myopathy, and failure to respond to Vitamin D therapy (117–119). Unlike virtually all other osteomalacic states, serum phosphorus levels are either normal or, more commonly, slightly elevated. The classic clinical feature of this disease is pathologic fractures (Fig. 102-6). Evidence for

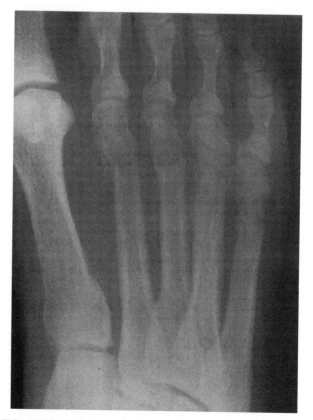

FIG. 102-6. Pathologic fractures of the metatarsals found in a patient with aluminum-associated osteomalacia.

the skeletal toxicity of aluminum seems to be as convincing as it is for the neurotoxicity of aluminum. The first evidence that aluminum caused bone disease in dialyzed uremic patients came from European epidemiologic studies, which showed that fracturing osteomalacia tends to occur in association with dialysis encephalopathy in dialyzed uremic patients in areas with high aluminum levels in the water used to prepare dialysate (99,100). As with encephalopathy, fracturing osteomalacia could be largely prevented or spontaneously healed by removing aluminum from the dialysate (95,100,120). However, this abnormality can also result from oral aluminum exposure. This was documented by two studies in which bone biopsies were randomly done in large populations of dialysis patients who only had oral aluminum exposure. These studies showed that 25% to 30% of these patients had aluminum-associated bone disease (21,22).

Besides the epidemiologic data, additional evidence for aluminum skeletal toxicity comes from the finding of markedly increased bone aluminum levels in this condition compared to levels found in other types of renal osteodystrophies (119). Experimentally, aluminum-induced osteomalacia in rats, dogs, and pigs provides even further data (76,121,122).

PTH seems to have a significant effect on the way aluminum manifests its skeletal toxicity. It was previously noted that patients with overt hyperparathyroid bone disease were protected from developing osteomalacia when they were dialyzed chronically with aluminum-contaminated dialysate (123). It has been found that patients with hyperparathyroid bone disease who have been treated by parathyroidectomy may subsequently develop aluminum-associated osteomalacia (124). Also, uremic, parathyroidectomized animals given parenteral aluminum subsequently develop more severe osteomalacia with less bone aluminum than do nonparathyroidectomized uremic animals given a comparable parenteral aluminum load (74). Conversely, it has been suggested that following chelation therapy for aluminum-induced osteomalacia, the patient may develop hyperparathyroid bone disease.

Diagnosis of aluminum-associated bone disease is based on the clinical features of bone pain; pathologic fractures, usually of the ribs and femoral neck; and proximal myopathy. Laboratory confirmation is based on bone biopsy specimens showing classic osteomalacia with aluminum, as determined by aluminum histochemical staining, present between the junction of calcified and noncalcified bone, and markedly increased quantitated bone aluminum levels (125). Plasma aluminum levels are characteristically elevated, documenting aluminum exposure. It would appear that uremia per se does not cause osteomalacia and the majority of cases of osteomalacia in uremic patients are a result of aluminum (126). Although it was initially believed that adynamic bone disease in uremic patients was also a result of aluminum intoxication (127), increasing evidence suggests that this is not the case (128).

Although the mechanism by which aluminum causes skeletal toxicity has not been elucidated, aluminum has several effects that could cause skeletal injury. Aluminum has been used in the tanning industry because of its ability to cross-link collagen fibrils (129). It was recently shown that aluminum cross-links collagen fibrils in bone matrix, destroying bone inductive properties (130). The presence of aluminum at the junction between calcified and noncalcified bone (125) could explain how it renders the osteoid noncalcifiable in spite of Vitamin D replacement and an increased calcium phosphate product. In addition, aluminum, especially in association with citrate, is a potent inhibitor of crystal formation, and this could affect bone formation (131). Aluminum also can inhibit bone phosphatases (132). Finally, aluminum is deposited in the mitochondria of osteoblasts (133), which could injure the osteoblasts and prevent bone formation.

Hematologic Toxicity

Aluminum also is toxic to the hematopoietic system. In humans it produces a microcytic hypochromic anemia in the setting of adequate iron stores (134–136). More recently, aluminum was shown to blunt or prevent the response to erythropoietin (137). Evidence that this effect is a result of aluminum is the finding that the anemia improves rapidly when aluminum exposure is eliminated or when aluminum is removed by chelation (135,136). Aluminum also can cause an anemia in rats and rabbits (138,139).

The specific mechanism responsible for aluminum-associated anemia has not been clearly identified. However, it appears that iron and aluminum metabolism are closely interrelated. As noted previously, like iron, aluminum is largely transported in plasma by transferrin. This suggests that the mechanism for the induction of aluminum-induced anemia is transferrin's deposition of aluminum at sites where iron is normally unloaded. However, aluminum also inhibits ferroxidase and ceruloplasmin activity, which could also affect iron metabolism (140).

Aluminum Speciation And Toxicity

The speciation of aluminum may determine aluminum toxicity for the various organ systems. Aluminum, because of its high formation constant with transferrin, citrate, phosphate, and hydroxides, cannot exist in plasma or the body in a free form. Formation constants are greater for aluminum with transferrin and citrate than with hydroxides (141). Therefore, in plasma, aluminum exists primarily in association with transferrin and secondarily with citrate. In view of the association between acute aluminum neurotoxicity and high levels of small molecular species of aluminum complexed to citrate and deferoxamine, it is suggested that these species most readily cross the blood–brain barrier and are responsible for neurotoxicity of this element. The aluminum effect on erythropoiesis and its interference with iron utilization has been studied *in vitro* (142). Whereas aluminum alone had no effect on human erythroid cultures, aluminum transferrin mixture caused a dose-dependent inhibition of erythroid colony growth. This is consistent with aluminum–transferrin complexes being responsible for the hematopoietic toxicity of aluminum noted *in vivo*. Evidence has been presented suggesting that aluminum forms coordinated complexes between carboxyl groups of collagen fibers in association with oxygen, cross-linking the collagen fibril and inhibiting bone induction properties (130). This type of aluminum complex in osteoid might explain the mechanism of aluminum-induced bone disease.

Management and Prevention of Hyperphosphatemia and Aluminum Intoxication

Because the treatment and prevention of hyperphosphatemia is now one of the major causes of aluminum excess and toxicity in uremic patients, it seems logical to discuss the two conditions together. For reasons cited already, it is essential to control serum phosphorus levels in uremic patients. Previously, the most widely used agent for this purpose was aluminum hydroxide. However, other types of oral phosphate binders are being increasingly used to reduce aluminum exposure. Calcium carbonate is a fairly effective phosphate binder and is now the most commonly used drug to control serum phosphorus in uremic patients (143). More recently, calcium acetate and calcium citrate have also been utilized (144,145). In fact, calcium acetate has been suggested to be a more effective phosphate binder than the other calcium compounds (145). Major side effects of the calcium compounds include hypercalcemia and constipation or diarrhea. The risk of hypercalcemia can be reduced by administering the calcium compounds at meal times. Because of its effect on enhancing aluminum absorption and promoting acute toxicity, calcium citrate is contraindicated in uremic patients.

Even when the calcium compounds are not adequate alone for control of serum phosphorus, they can reduce the amount of aluminum hydroxide supplemented to control serum phosphorus levels. To avoid toxicity, patients with advanced renal failure receiving aluminum compounds should have plasma aluminum levels measured serially and dosage modified if plasma aluminum levels exceed 20 to 30 μg/L.

Another possible means of phosphate control is more efficient removal of phosphorus during dialysis. This could possibly be accomplished by improved membranes or hemoperfusion of phosphate sorbents such as zirconium oxide.

However, until newer methods of control of serum phosphorus are available, the major method will continue to be the use of calcium compounds. At this time, it seems desirable to use calcium as a first line agent. If the phosphate remains high, then aluminum hydroxide can be used either alone or in combination with calcium, preferably for short periods of time. At no time should aluminum compounds be given in

dosages higher than 100 mg per kg per day. Such dosages can cause toxicity, especially in children (108,109,146). In fact, because of the risk of intoxication, aluminum compounds probably should not be used in uremic children.

Sevelamer hydrochloride is a calcium and aluminum free polymeric phosphate binder that has recently been approved for use in humans. Short- and long-term studies in patients with end-stage renal disease show that it reduces serum phosphate and low-density lipoprotein concentrations without raising serum calcium (147,148). Other noncalcium- and nonaluminum-containing compounds that have been shown to reduce intestinal phosphate absorption in laboratory animals include lanthanum chloride (149) and iron hydroxide complexes (150).

Ensuring that the water used to prepare dialysate is virtually free of aluminum (less than 10 μg/L) is obviously of major importance in the prevention of aluminum toxicity. A well-functioning reverse osmosis unit or a deionizer polisher will eliminate aluminum from the water used to prepare dialysate. In addition, aluminum tubing, pump headers, and other materials containing aluminum potentially leachable by treated water and dialysate should not be present in the dialysis system.

In dialyzed as well as nondialyzed uremic patients, plasma aluminum levels should be monitored two to three times yearly to document that the dialysate has been aluminum-free and that patients ingesting oral aluminum compounds are not in danger of developing aluminum intoxication. Generally, uremic patients ingesting aluminum compounds have plasma aluminum levels of about 50 μg/L. A small subset of 10% to 15% of patients have aluminum levels in excess of 100 μg/L. These patients are either aluminum intoxicated or in danger of becoming aluminum intoxicated. Dialysis patients receiving treatment with aluminum-contaminated dialysate will have plasma aluminum levels higher than 100 to 200 μg/L (151). Because aluminum levels vary considerably from day to day and season to season, merely one or two determinations in water may be misleading. Plasma aluminum levels remain high for weeks after patients are exposed to aluminum-contaminated dialysate and are therefore a good indicator of a previous exposure.

In general, water treatment to remove aluminum from the dialysate and substitution of calcium phosphate binders for aluminum binders have been very effective in preventing aluminum intoxication. As already stated, water treatment alone largely eliminates dialysis encephalopathy. With the combination of water treatment and use of calcium-containing phosphate binders, the incidence of aluminum bone disease in a large series decreased from 43% in 1985 to 8% in 1993 (152). A recent bone histomorphometric study also showed that aluminum-associated osteomalacia in both patients undergoing hemodialysis and peritoneal dialysis currently accounts for less than 8% of all bone disease (23).

For treatment of aluminum intoxication, all aluminum exposure should be removed. The dialysate should be routinely checked to ensure that it is aluminum-free, and calcium compounds should be substituted for the orally administered aluminum compounds. A number of patients with osteomalacia and far fewer with dialysis encephalopathy reportedly improved when they were no longer exposed to aluminum-contaminated dialysate (95,120). Moreover, a few patients with osteomalacia also improved following the discontinuation of oral aluminum compounds. However, the rate of improvement of osteomalacia can be markedly increased by chelation with deferoxamine (153,154). Dialysis encephalopathy is much less likely to improve spontaneously following discontinuation of aluminum exposure than is osteomalacia (155). Also, if chelation therapy is not given until late in the course of the disease, it may no longer be effective. Because of this observation, chelation seems to be indicated in all patients suspected of having dialysis encephalopathy.

A number of different approaches to chelation have been recommended. It appears that 2 g of deferoxamine is as effective as 4 g (156,157). In addition, symptomatic improvement of bone disease can occur as rapidly in patients given 0.5 g as in patients given 6 g weekly of deferoxamine (158). At this time, for the management of aluminum neurotoxicity it is unclear whether 1 to 2 g of deferoxamine should be given with each dialysis or only once weekly for maximum efficiency with the smallest dosage. At times, chelation therapy aggravates the symptoms in patients with aluminum neurotoxicity (107). If this occurs, it has been suggested that the deferoxamine dosage be reduced, possibly given intramuscularly the evening prior to dialysis, and maximally removed during the subsequent dialysis (158,159). Diazepam is effective in controlling deferoxamine-related seizures and myoclonic activity in the majority of patients.

The majority of patients with aluminum-associated bone disease experience improvement of clinical symptoms in 3 to 4 months, whereas patients with encephalopathy may require chelation for 10 to 12 months before there is any symptomatic improvement.

Therapy with deferoxamine is not without some risk. As already described, patients with marked aluminum overload may develop acute neurologic toxicity following deferoxamine therapy. Acute infections with *Yersinia* species and mucormycosis have been reported in patients receiving deferoxamine (160,161). It is believed that feroxamine is an iron supplier for these nonsiderophore-producing organisms, thus promoting their growth. Prior to treatment, therefore, the clinical diagnosis of aluminum intoxication should be reasonably well established and evidence of aluminum overload demonstrated either by a rise of plasma aluminum higher than 150 to 200 μg/L 24 to 48 hours following deferoxamine infusion (162) or increased bone aluminum levels in association with classic histologic findings of aluminum-associated bone disease.

Hydroxypyridones have undergone testing in rabbit and rat models of aluminum overload as alternatives to deferoxamine (163,164). These drugs significantly enhance excretion of aluminum in the urine and reduce aluminum levels in bone and brain. Advantages of these compounds over deferoxamine include lower cost and oral availability.

OTHER ELEMENTS

Magnesium

As renal function progressively falls, fractional magnesium clearance increases. As a result, even with advanced renal failure there is usually only a moderate rise in serum magnesium levels. Although severe hypermagnesemia can occur if patients with advanced renal failure are given large gastrointestinal loads of magnesium, it rarely, if ever, occurs with the usual exposure to magnesium.

Advanced uremia does represent a state of total magnesium excess. The two tissues consistently shown to have increased magnesium levels are serum and bone (165,166). Because magnesium is an inhibitor of crystal formation, it was once suggested that magnesium might be important in the deranged skeletal metabolism found in uremic patients (167). However, recent evidence that aluminum is intimately involved in this disturbance has cast some doubt on any important role for magnesium.

The possible role of magnesium in the pathogenesis of visceral calcification has not been clarified. In these deposits, magnesium is present in a constant molar ratio along with calcium and phosphorus. When incinerated, these deposits yield whitlockite $(CaMg)_3 (PO_4)_2$, again suggesting that magnesium is an integral component of these deposits (29). At this time, however, the role of magnesium in the formation of visceral calcium phosphate deposits remains to be defined.

Zinc

Another element that has received some attention is zinc. Because serum zinc levels have consistently been found to be subnormal in uremic patients, it has been suggested that a number of symptoms, including loss of appetite, an altered sense of taste and smell, and impotence, which are found in uremic patients, might result from zinc deficiency. Although some studies show that these symptoms could be improved with zinc supplementation, other investigations report no justification for zinc therapy (168–174). It should be noted that although serum zinc levels tend to be low, other tissue stores of zinc may be either unchanged or actually increased (175).

Minor Element Disturbances

The blood levels of a number of essential trace elements have been found to be decreased in both dialyzed and nondialyzed uremic patients. Blood selenium was found to be decreased in most but not all studies (176–183) as were serum manganese (184) and nickel (184–186). The level of copper in the blood of uremic patients has usually been reported as normal

(187,188). Blood vanadium levels largely have been reported to be increased (189–193). Two other essential trace elements have also been found to be increased in the blood of uremic patients, namely, chromium (188) and silicon (194–197). Of the nonessential elements, besides aluminum, blood levels of lithium (198) have been found to be increased, whereas blood rubidium and bromine levels have been found to be decreased (199).

Multiple tissue trace element profiles have been characterized in both dialyzed and nondialyzed uremic patients. As with blood, a number of trace elements in other tissues have been found to be abnormal in uremic patients. These can be divided into three groups. The first group represents a similar disturbance in multiple tissues documenting an alteration in the total body burden of these elements. Six elements belong to this group. Total body tin, zinc, and strontium, like aluminum, are increased, whereas total body rubidium is decreased in dialyzed and nondialyzed uremic patients. Total body bromine is decreased only in dialyzed uremic patients (175).

The second group of disturbances represents elements that may be increased or reduced in some tissues, whereas they are either normal or actually affected in the opposite direction in other tissues. Examples of this alteration are the increased copper concentration in lungs associated with a reduced copper concentration in heart of both dialyzed and nondialyzed uremic patients (175).

A third disturbance in trace elements is a translocation of an element from one organ to another. Two elements that fall into this group are cadmium and molybdenum, both of which are reduced in diseased kidneys and increased in the liver (175).

Of the remaining essential trace elements, selenium occurs in normal amounts in tissues from uremic patients (175). Silicon is increased in the spleen and liver in patients with chronic renal failure (200). Vanadium reportedly is increased in the bones of uremic patients (201). With regard to nonessential elements, tissue stores of lead (175,200,201) and mercury (175) appear to be normal in most uremic patients. Uranium may be increased in tissues from a limited number of dialysis patients. However, at this time, there is no evidence that any of these alterations, with the exception of aluminum, have any clinical consequences.

REFERENCES

1. Parfitt AM, Kleerekoper M. The divalent ion homeostatic system—physiology and metabolism of calcium, phosphorus, magnesium and bone. In: Maxwell MH, Kleeman CR, eds. *Clinical disorders of fluid and electrolyte metabolism*. New York: McGraw-Hill, 1980.
2. Slatopolsky E, et al. The control of phosphate excretion in uremia. *J Clin Invest* 1966;45:672.
3. Slatopolsky E, et al. Control of phosphate excretion in uremic man. *J Clin Invest* 1968;47:1865.
4. Slatopolsky E, et al. The pathogenesis of secondary hyperparathyroidism in early renal failure. In: Norman AW, ed. *Vitamin D basic research and its clinical application*. New York: deGruyer, 1979.
5. Bricker NS. On the pathogenesis of the uremic state: an exposition of the "trade-off hypothesis." *N Engl J Med* 1972;286:1093.
6. Katz AI, Hampers CH, Merrill JB. Secondary hyperparathyroidism and renal osteodystrophy in chronic renal failure: analysis of 195 patients with observations on the effects of chronic dialysis, kidney transplantation and subtotal parathyroidectomy. *Medicine* 1969;48:337.
7. Ibels LS, et al. Preservation of function in experimental renal disease by dietary restriction of phosphate. *N Engl J Med* 1978;298:122.
8. Karlinsky ML, et al. Preservation of renal function in experimental glomerulonephritis. *Kidney Int* 1980;17:293.
9. Lumlertgul D, et al. Phosphate depletion arrests progression of chronic renal failure independent of protein intake. *Kidney Int* 1986;29:658.
10. Slatopolsky E, et al. Non-suppressive secondary hyperparathyroidism in chronic progressive renal disease. *Kidney Int* 1972;1:38.
11. Korkor AB. Reduced binding of [^{3}H]1,25-dihydroxyvitamin D$_3$ in the parathyroid glands of patients with renal failure. *N Engl J Med* 1987;316:1573.
12. Portale AA, et al. Effect of dietary phosphorus on circulating concentrations of 1,25-dihydroxyvitamin D and immunoreactive parathyroid hormone in children with moderate renal insufficiency. *J Clin Invest* 1984;72:1580.
13. Lopez-Hilker S, et al. Phosphorus restriction reverses hyperparathyroidism in uremia independent of changes in calcium and calcitriol. *Am J Physiol* 1990;259:F432.
14. Lucas P A, et al. 1,25-dihydroxycholecalciferol and parathyroid hormone in advanced chronic renal failure: effects of simultaneous protein and phosphorus restriction. *Clin Nephrol* 1986;25:7.
15. Dabbagh S, et al. Aminoaciduria of vitamin D deficiency is independent of PTH levels and urinary cyclic AMP. *Miner Electrolyte Metab* 1989;15:221.
16. Almaden Y, et al. Direct effect of phosphorus on PTH secretion from whole rat parathyroid glands in vitro. *J Bone Miner Res* 1996;11: 970.
17. Kilav R, et al. Parathyroid hormone gene expression in hypophosphatemic rats. *J Clin Invest* 1995;96:327.
18. Sela-Brown A, et al. Identification of AUF1 as a parathyroid hormone mRNA 3′-untranslated region-binding protein that determines parathyroid hormone mRNA stability. *J Biol Chem* 2000;275:7424.
19. Brown AJ, et al. Decreased calcium-sensing receptor expression in hyperplastic parathyroid glands of uremic rats: role of dietary phosphate. *Kidney Int* 1999;55:1284.
20. Slatopolsky E, et al. On the prevention of secondary hyperparathyroidism in experimental chronic renal disease using "proportional reduction" of dietary phosphate intake. *Kidney Int* 1972;2:147.
21. Chan YL, et al. Dialysis osteodystrophy—a study involving 94 patients. *Medicine* 1985;64:296.
22. Llach F, et al. The natural course of dialysis osteomalacia. *Kidney Int* 1986;29[Suppl 18]:S74.
23. Sherrard DJ, et al. The spectrum of bone disease in end-stage renal failure—an evolving disorder. *Kidney Int* 1993;43:436.
24. Parfitt AM. Soft tissue calcification in uremia. *Arch Intern Med* 1969;124:544.
25. Berlyne GM. Microcrystalline conjunctival calcification in renal failure: a useful clinical sign. *Lancet* 1968;2:388.
26. Caner JEZ, Decker JL. Recurrent (gouty?) arthritis in chronic renal failure treated with periodic hemodialysis. *Am J Med* 1964;36:571.
27. Cassidy MJD, et al. Renal osteodystrophy and metastatic calcification in long-term continuous ambulatory peritoneal dialysis. *Q J Med* 1985;213:29.
28. De Francisco AM, et al. Parathyroidectomy in chronic renal failure. *Q J Med* 1985;218:289.
29. LeGeros RZ, Contiguglia SR, Alfrey AC. Pathological calcification associated with uremia: two types of calcium phosphate deposits. *Calcif Tissue Res* 1973;13:173.
30. Berlyne GM, Shaw AG. Red eyes in renal failure. *Lancet* 1962;1:4.
31. Mirahmadi KS, Coburn J, Bluestone R. Calcific periarthritis and hemodialysis. *JAMA* 1973;223:548.
32. Swannell AJ, Underwood FA, Dixon AS. Periarticular calcific deposits mimicking acute arthritis. *Ann Rheum Dis* 1970;29:380.
33. Alfrey AC, et al. Resolution of hyperparathyroidism, renal osteodystrophy and metastatic calcification after renal homotransplantation. *N Engl J Med* 1968;279:1349.
34. Conger JD, et al. Pulmonary calcification in chronic dialysis patients. *Ann Intern Med* 1975;83:330.
35. Terman DS, et al. Cardiac calcification in uremia: a clinical, biochemical and pathological study. *Am J Med* 1971;50:744.

36. Kuzela DC, et al. Soft tissue calcification in chronic dialysis patients. *Am J Pathol* 1977;86:403.

37. de Moraes CR. Calcification of the heart: a rare manifestation of chronic renal failure. *Pediatr Radiol* 1986;16:422.

38. Rostand SG, et al. Metastatic calcification and cardiac dysfunction in chronic renal failure. *Am J Med* 1988;85:651.

39. Sanders C, et al. Metastatic calcification of the heart and lungs in end-stage renal disease: detection and quantification by dual-energy digital chest radiography. *Am J Roentgenol* 1987;149:881.

40. Meema HE, Oreopoulos DG. Morphology, progression and regression of arterial and periarterial calcifications in patients with end-stage renal disease. *Radiology* 1986;158:671.

41. Meema HE, Oreopoulos DG, Rapoport A. Serum magnesium level and arterial calcification in end-stage renal disease. *Kidney Int* 1987;32:388.

42. Meema HE, Oreopoulos DG, de Veber GA. Arterial calcification in severe chronic renal disease and their relationship to dialysis treatment, renal transplant and parathyroidectomy. *Radiology* 1976;121:315.

43. Ibels LS, et al. Arterial calcification and pathology in uremic patients undergoing dialysis. *Am J Med* 1979;66:790.

44. Shanahan CM, et al. The role of Gla proteins in vascular calcification. *Crit Rev Eukaryot Gene Expr* 1998;8:357.

45. Shanahan CM, et al. High expression of genes for calcification regulating proteins in human atherosclerotic plaques. *J Clin Invest* 1994;93:2393.

46. Poche E, et al. Calciphylaxis in a hemodialysis patient: appearance after parathyroidectomy during a psoriatic flare. *Am J Kidney Dis* 1992;19:285.

47. Janigan DT, Morris J, Hirsch D. Acute skin and fat necrosis during sepsis in a patient with chronic renal failure. *Am J Kidney Dis* 1992;20:643.

48. Adroque HJ, et al. Systemic calciphylaxis revisited. *Am J Nephrol* 1981;1:177.

49. Roe SM, et al. Calciphylaxis: early recognition and management. *Am Surg* 1994;60:81.

50. Vassa N, Twardowski ZJ, Campbell J. Hyperbaric oxygen therapy in calciphylaxis-induced skin necrosis in a peritoneal dialysis patient. *Am J Kidney Dis* 1994;23:878.

51. Gorsky JE, et al. Metabolic balance of aluminum studied in six men. *Clin Chem* 1979;25:1739.

52. Greger JL, Baier MJ. Excretion and retention of low or moderate levels of aluminum by human subjects. *Fed Chem Toxicol* 1983;21:473.

53. Miller RG, et al. The occurrence of aluminum in drinking water. *Am Water Works Assoc* 1984;77:84.

54. Alfrey AC. Aluminum. *Adv Clin Chem* 1983;23:69.

55. Froment DH, et al. Site and mechanism of enhanced gastrointestinal absorption of aluminum by citrate. *Kidney Int* 1989;36:978.

56. Molitoris BA, et al. Citrate: a major factor in the toxicity of orally administered aluminum compounds. *Kidney Int* 1989;36:949.

57. Provan SD, Yokel RA. Aluminum uptake by the in situ rat gut preparation. *J Pharmacol Exp Ther* 1988;245:928.

58. Kaehny WD, Hegg AP, Alfrey AC. Gastrointestinal absorption of aluminum from aluminum-containing antacids. *N Engl J Med* 1977; 296:1389.

59. Froment DH, et al. Effect of solubility on the gastrointestinal absorption of aluminum from various aluminum compounds in the rat. *J Lab Clin Med* 1989;114:237.

60. Ittel TH, et al. Enhanced gastrointestinal absorption of aluminum in uremic rats. *Kidney Int* 1987;32:821.

61. Nolan CL, DeGoes JJ, Mantini SL, et al. Gastrointestinal absorption of aluminum and lead in women ingesting calcium citrate. *South Med J* 1994;87:894.

62. Adler AJ, Berlyne GM. Duodenal aluminum absorption in the rat: effect of vitamin D. *Am J Physiol* 1985;12:G209.

63. Mayor GH, et al. Parathyroid hormone-mediated aluminum deposition and egress in the rat. *Kidney Int* 1980;17:40.

64. Cannata JB, et al. Gastrointestinal aluminum absorption: Is it modulated by the iron-absorptive mechanism? *Proc EDTA-ERA* 1985; 21:354.

65. Alfrey AC. Aluminum metabolism in uremia. *Neurotoxicology* 1980; 1:43.

66. Alfrey AC, Hegg A, Craswell P. Metabolism and toxicity of aluminum in renal failure. *Am J Clin Nutr* 1980;33:1509.

67. Mussi I, et al. Behavior of plasma and urinary aluminum levels in occupationally exposed subjects. *Int Arch Occup Environ Health* 1984;54:155.

68. Burnatowska-Hledin MA, Mayor GH, Lau K. Renal handling of aluminum in the rat: clearance and micropuncture studies. *Am J Physiol* 1985;18:F192.

69. Klein GL, et al. Aluminum as a factor in the bone disease of long-term parenteral nutrition. *Trans Assoc Am Physicians* 1982;95:155.

70. Trapp GA. Plasma aluminum is bound to transferrin. *Life Sci* 1983; 33:311.

71. Kovalchik MT, et al. Aluminum kinetics during hemodialysis. *J Lab Clin Med* 1978;92:712.

72. Kaehny WD, et al. Aluminum transfer during hemodialysis. *Kidney Int* 1977;12:361.

73. Trapp GA. Studies of aluminum interaction with enzymes and proteins—the inhibition of hexokinase. *Neurotoxicology* 1980;1:89.

74. Alfrey AC, Sedman A, Chan YL. The compartmentalization and metabolism of aluminum in uremic rats. *J Lab Clin Med* 1985;2:227.

75. Sedman AB, et al. Evidence of aluminum loading in infants receiving intravenous therapy. *N Engl J Med* 1983;312:1337.

76. Chan Y, et al. The effect of aluminum on normal and uremic rats: tissue distribution, vitamin D metabolites and quantitative bone histology. *Calcif Tissue Int* 1983;35:344.

77. Jeppsson B, et al. Blood–brain barrier derangement in uremic encephalopathy. *Surgery* 1982;92:30.

78. Siem (1866). Quoted in Doeilken: Ober die wirkung des aluminum, unter besonder berucksichtigung der durch das aluminum versuracht-enlasionen im zentralnervensystem. *Naunyn Schmiedebergs Arch Exp Pathol Pharmak* 1897;40:98.

79. Scherp HW, Church CF. Neurotoxic action of aluminum salts. *Proc Soc Exp Biol Med* 1937;36:851.

80. Crapper DR, Kirshnan SS, Quittkat S. Aluminum, neurofibrillary degeneration and Alzheimer's disease. *Brain* 1976;99:67.

81. Klatzo L, Wisniewski H, Stretcher E. Experimental production of neurofibrillary degeneration: 1. Light microscopic observations. *J Neuropathol* 1965;24:187.

82. Petit TL, Biederman GB, McMullen PA. Neurofibrillary degeneration, dendritic dying back, and learning-memory deficits after aluminum administration: implications for brain aging. *Exp Neurol* 1980;67:152.

83. Terry RD, Pena C. Experimental production of neurofibrillary degeneration: 2. Electron microscopy, phosphatase histochemistry and electron probe analysis. *J Neuropathol* 1965;24:200.

84. Wisniewski HM, Sturman JA, Shek W. Aluminum chloride-induced neurofibrillary changes in the developing rabbit: a chronic animal model. *Ann Neurol* 1980;8:479.

85. De Boni U, et al. Neurofibrillary degeneration induced by systemic aluminum. *Acta Neuropathol (Berlin)* 1976;35:285.

86. Lipresle J, et al. A case of aluminum encephalopathy in man. *Comptes Rendus Seanes Societe Biologie* 1975;169:282.

87. McLaughlin AIG, et al. Pulmonary fibrosis and encephalopathy associated with the inhalation of aluminum dust. *Br J Ind Med* 1962;19:253.

88. Alfrey AC, et al. Syndrome of dyspraxia and multifocal seizures associated with chronic hemodialysis. *Trans Am Soc Artif Intern Organs* 1972;18:257.

89. Berkseth R, et al. Dialysis encephalopathy (DE): diagnostic criteria and epidemiology of 39 patients. *Am Soc Nephrol* 1978;11:36A.

90. Cartier F, et al. Encephalopathie myclonique progressive des dialyses: role de l'eau utilisee pour l'hemodialyse. *Nouv Presse Med* 1978;7: 97.

91. Dunea G, et al. Role of aluminum in dialysis dementia. *Ann Intern Med* 1978;88:502.

92. Flendrig JA, Kruis H, Das HA. Aluminum intoxication: the cause of dialysis dementia? *Proc Eur Dial Transplant Assoc* 1976;13:355. 87.

93. Galle P, et al. Encephalopathie myoclonique progressive des dialyses: presence d'aluminum et forte concentration dans les lysosomes des cellules cerebrates. *Nouv Presse Med* 1979;8:4091.

94. McDermott JR, et al. Brain-aluminum concentration in dialysis encephalopathy. *Lancet* 1978;1:901.

95. Pierides AM, et al. Hemodialysis encephalopathy with osteomalacic fractures and muscle weakness. *Kidney Int* 1980;18:115.

96. Rozas VV, Port KF, Rutt WM. Progressive dialysis encephalopathy from dialysate aluminum. *Arch Intern Med* 1978;138:1375.

97. Burks JS, et al. A fatal encephalopathy in chronic hemodialysis patients. *Lancet* 1976;1:764.

98. Alfrey AC, LeGendre GR, Kaehny WD. The dialysis encephalopathy syndrome: possible aluminum intoxication. *N Engl J Med* 1976; 294:184.

99. Parkinson IS, et al. Fracturing dialysis osteodystrophy and dialysis encephalopathy: an epidemiological survey. *Lancet* 1979;1:406.

100. Platts MM, Goode GC, Hislop JS. Composition of the domestic water supply and the incidence of fractures and encephalopathy in patients on home dialysis. *Br Med J* 1977;2:657.

101. Schreeder MT. Dialysis encephalopathy. *Arch Intern Med* 1979;139:510.

102. Ackrill P, et al. Successful removal of aluminum from patient with dialysis encephalopathy. *Lancet* 1980;2:692.

103. Ackrill P, Ralston AJ, Day JP. The role of desferrioxamine in the treatment of dialysis encephalopathy. *Kidney Int* 1986;18:S104.

104. Bakir AA, Hryhorczuk DO, Berman E, et al. Acute fatal hyperaluminemic encephalopathy in undialyzed and recently dialyzed uremic patients. *Trans Am Soc Artif Intern Organs* 1986;l32:171.

105. Kirschbaum GG, Schoolwerth AC. Acute aluminum toxicity associated with oral citrate and aluminum containing antacids. *Am J Med Sci* 1989;297:9.

106. FDA. Medical Alert. June 21, 1993:48.

107. Sherrard DJ, Walker JV, Boykin JL. Precipitation of dialysis dementia by deferoxamine treatment of aluminum-related bone disease. *Am J Kidney Dis* 1988;12:126.

108. Griswold WR, et al. Accumulation of aluminum in a nondialyzed uremic child receiving aluminum hydroxide. *Pediatrics* 1983;71:56.

109. Sedman AB, et al. Aluminum loading in children with chronic renal failure. *Kidney Int* 1984;26:201.

110. Tokars JI, et al. National surveillance of hemodialysis associated diseases in the United States, 1990. *ASAIO J* 1993;39:71.

111. Phelps KR, et al. Encephalopathy after bladder irrigation with alum: case report and literature review. *Am J Med Sci* 1999;318:181.

112. Nakamura H, et al. Acute encephalopathy due to aluminum toxicity successfully treated by combined intravenous deferoxamine and hemodialysis. *J Clin Pharmacol* 2000;40:296.

113. Alfrey AC. Dialysis encephalopathy syndrome. *Annu Rev Med* 1978;2:93.

114. Harrison WH, Codd E, Gray RM. Aluminum inhibition of hexokinase. *Lancet* 1972;2:277.

115. Viola RE, Morrison JF, Cleland WW. Interaction of metal (III)-adenosine 5′-triphosphate complexes with yeast hexokinase. *Biochemistry* 1980;19:3131.

116. Siegel N, Haug A. Aluminum interaction with calmodulin—evidence for altered structure and function from optical and enzymatic studies. *Biochim Biophys Acta* 1983;44:36.

117. Hodsman AB, et al. Bone aluminum and histomorphometric features of renal osteodystrophy. *Clin Endocrinol Metab* 1982;54:539.

118. Hodsman AB, et al. Vitamin D-resistant osteomalacia in hemodialysis patients lacking secondary hyperparathyroidism. *Ann Intern Med* 1981;94:629.

119. Ott SM, et al. The prevalence of bone aluminum deposition in renal osteodystrophy and its relation to the response to calcitriol therapy. *N Engl J Med* 1982;307:709.

120. Hudson GA, et al. Treatment of dialysis fracturing bone disease. *Kidney Int* 1980;18:532(abst).

121. Goodman WG. Parenteral aluminum administration in the dog: II. Induction of osteomalacia and effect on vitamin D metabolites. *Kidney Int* 1984;25:370.

122. Robertson JA, et al. Animal model of aluminum-induced osteomalacia: role of chronic renal failure. *Kidney Int* 1983;23:327.

123. Alfrey AC. Case against aluminum affecting parathyroid function. *Am J Kidney Dis* 1985;6:309.

124. Felsenfeld AJ, et al. Osteomalacia after parathyroidectomy in patients with uremia. *Ann Intern Med* 1982;96:34.

125. Maloney NA, et al. Histologic quantitation of aluminum in iliac bone from patients with renal failure. *J Lab Clin Med* 1982;99:206.

126. Dahl E, et al. Renal osteodystrophy in predialysis patients without stainable bone aluminum. *Acta Med Scand* 1988;224:157.

127. Andress DL, et al. Osteomalacia and aplastic bone disease in aluminum related osteodystrophy. *J Clin Endocrinol Metab* 1987;65:11.

128. Moriniere P, et al. Disappearance of aluminic bone disease in a long term asymptomatic dialysis population restricting Al(OH)$_3$ intake: emergence of an idiopathic adynamic bone disease not related to aluminum. *Nephron* 1989;53:93.

129. Heidemann E. The chemistry of tanning. In: Nimni ME, ed. *Collagen*, vol III, "Biotechnology." Boca Raton, FL: CRC, 1988.

130. Zhu JM, Huffer W, Alfrey AC. Effect of aluminum on bone matrix inductive properties. *Kidney Int* 1990;38:1141.

131. Thomas WC. Trace metal–citric acid complexes as inhibitors of calcification and crystal formation. *Proc Soc Exp Biol Med* 1982;170:321.

132. Lieberherr M, et al. In vitro effects of aluminum on bone phosphatases: a possible interaction with BPTH and vitamin D metabolites. *Calcif Tissue Int* 1982;34:280.

133. Cournot-Witmer G, et al. Effect of aluminum on bone and cell localization. *Kidney Int* 1986;18:S37.

134. O'Hare JA, Murnaghan DJ. Reversal of aluminum-induced hemodialysis anemia by low-aluminum dialysate. *N Engl J Med* 1982;306:654.

135. Short ALK, Winney RJ, Robsop JS. Reversible microcytic hypochromic anaemia in dialysis patients due to aluminum intoxication. *Proc Eur Dial Transplant Assoc* 1980;17:226.

136. Touam M, et al. Aluminum-induced, reversible microcytic anemia in chronic renal failure: clinical and experimental studies. *Clin Nephrol* 1983;19:295.

137. Casati S, et al. Aluminum interference in the treatment of haemodialysis patients with recombinant erythropoietin. *Nephrol Dial Transplant* 1990;5:441.

138. Kaiser L, et al. Microcytic anemia secondary to intraperitoneal aluminum in the rat. *Kidney Int* 1984;25:194(abst).

139. Seibert FB, Wells HG. The effect of aluminum on mammalian blood and tissue. *Arch Pathol* 1929;8:230.

140. Huber CT, Frieden E. The inhibition of feroxidase by trivalent and other metal ions. *Biol Chem* 1970;245:3979.

141. Martin RB. The chemistry of aluminum as related to biology and medicine. *Clin Chem* 1986;32:1797.

142. Mladenovic J. Aluminum inhibits erythropoiesis in vitro. *J Clin Invest* 1988;81:1661.

143. Fournier A, et al. Calcium carbonate, an aluminum-free agent for control of hyperphosphatemia, hypocalcemia and hyperparathyroidism in uremia. *Kidney Int* 1986;18:S114.

144. Mai ML, et al. Calcium acetate, an effective phosphorus binder in patients with renal failure. *Kidney Int* 1989;36:690.

145. Sheikh MS, et al. Reduction of dietary phosphorus absorption by phosphorus binders: a theoretical, in vitro and in vivo study. *J Clin Invest* 1989;83:66.

146. Andreoli SP, Bergstein JM, Sherrard DJ. Aluminum intoxication from aluminum containing phosphate binders in children with azotemia not undergoing hemodialysis. *N Engl J Med* 1984;310:1079.

147. Goldberg DI, et al. Effect of RenaGel, a non-absorbed, calcium- and aluminum-free phosphate binder, on serum phosphorus, calcium, and intact parathyroid hormone in end-stage renal disease patients. *Nephrol Dial Transplant* 1998;13:2303.

148. Chertow GM, et al. Long-term effects of sevelamer hydrochloride on the calcium x phosphate product and lipid profile of haemodialysis patients. *Nephrol Dial Transplant* 1999;14:2907.

149. Graff L, Burnel D. A possible non-aluminum oral phosphate binder? A comparative study on dietary phosphorus absorption. *Res Commun Mol Pathol Pharmacol* 1995;89:373.

150. Yamaguchi T, et al. Oral phosphate binders: phosphate binding capacity of iron (III) hydroxide complexes containing saccharides and their effect on the urinary excretion of calcium and phosphate in rats. *Ren Fail* 1999;21:453.

151. Winney RJ, Cowie JF, Robson JS. What is the value of plasma/serum aluminum in patients with chronic renal failure? *Clin Nephrol* 1985;24[Suppl 1]:S2.

152. Bonucci P, et al. Osteomalacia and aluminum intoxication: morphological aspects. In: Nicolini M, Zatta PF, Corain B, eds. *Aluminum in chemistry, biology and medicine*. Chur, Switzerland: Harwood Academic Publishers, 1994.

153. Brown DJ, et al. Treatment of dialysis osteomalacia with desferrioxamine. *Lancet* 1982;2:343.

154. Andress DL, et al. Bone histologic response to deferoxamine in aluminum related bone disease. *Kidney Int* 1987;31:1344.

155. Milne FJ, et al. The effect of low aluminum water and desferrioxamine on the outcome of dialysis encephalopathy. *Clin Nephrol* 1983;20:202.

156. Ciancioni C, et al. Plasma aluminum and iron kinetics in hemodialyzed patients after IV infusion of desferrioxamine. *Trans Am Soc Artif Intern Organs* 1984;30:479.

157. Ciancioni C, et al. Concomitant removal of aluminum and iron by haemodialysis and haemofiltration after desferrioxamine intravenous infusion. *Proc EDTA-ERA* 1984;21:469.

158. Kurokawa K, et al. Aluminum associated bone disease: considerations on the pathogenesis and the effects of deferoxamine treatment. *J Univ Occup Environ Health* 1987;9[Suppl]:133.

159. Molitoris BA, et al. Rapid removal of DFO-chelated aluminum during hemodialysis using polysulfone dialyzers. *Kidney Int* 1988;34:986.

160. Molitoris BA, et al. Efficacy of intramuscular and intraperitoneal deferoxamine for aluminum chelation. *Kidney Int* 1987;31:986.

161. Hoen B, et al. Septicemia due to *Yersinia enterocolitica* in a long-term hemodialysis patients after a single desferrioxamine administration. *Nephron* 1988;50:378.

162. Veis JH, et al. Mucormycosis in deferoxamine treated patients on dialysis. *Ann Intern Med* 1987;107:258.

163. Yokel RA, et al. The 3-hydroxypyridin-4-ones more effectively chelate aluminum in a rabbit model of aluminum intoxication than does desferrioxamine. *Drug Metab Dispos* 1996;24:105.

164. Gomez M, et al. Comparative aluminum mobilizing actions of deferoxamine and four 3-hydroxypyrid-4-ones in aluminum loaded rats. *Toxicology* 1998;130:175.

165. Milliner DS, et al. Use of the deferoxamine infusion test in the diagnosis of aluminum-related osteodystrophy. *Ann Intern Med* 1984;101:775.

166. Alfrey AC, Miller N, Butkus D. Evaluation of body magnesium stores. *J Lab Clin Med* 1974;84:153.

167. Alfrey AC. Disorders of magnesium metabolism. In: Seldin CW, Giebisch G, eds. *The kidney: physiology and pathophysiology*. New York: Raven, 1985.

168. Alfrey AC, Miller NL. Bone magnesium pools in uremia. *J Clin Invest* 1973;52:3019.

169. Antoniou LD, Shalhoub RJ. Zinc and sexual dysfunction. *Lancet* 1980;8:1034.

170. Antoniou LD, et al. Reversal of uraemic impotence by zinc. *Lancet* 1977;2:895.

171. Brook AC, et al. Absence of a therapeutic effect of zinc in the sexual dysfunction of haemodialyzed patients. *Lancet* 1980;2:618.

172. Mahaian SK, et al. Effect of oral zinc therapy on gonadal function in hemodialysis patients: a double blind study. *Ann Intern Med* 1982;97:357.

173. Mahajan SK, et al. Improvement of uremic hypogeusia by zinc: a double blind study. *Am J Clin Nutr* 1980;33:1517.

174. Vreman HJ, et al. Taste, smell and zinc metabolism in patients with chronic renal failure. *Nephron* 1980;26:163.

175. Zetin M, Stone RA. Effects of zinc in chronic hemodialysis. *Clin Nephrol* 1980;13:20.

176. Smythe WR, et al. Trace element abnormalities in chronic uremia. *Ann Intern Med* 1982;96:302.

177. Dworkin B, et al. Diminished blood selenium levels in renal failure patients on dialysis: correlations with nutritional status. *Am J Med Sci* 1987;293:6.

178. Turan B, et al. Serum selenium and glutathione-peroxidase activities and their interaction with toxic metals in dialysis and renal transplantation patients. *Biol Trace Elem Res* 1992;33:95.

179. Foote JW, Hinks LJ, Lloyd B. Reduced plasma and white blood cell selenium levels in haemodialysis patients. *Clin Chim Acta* 1987;164:323.

180. Girelli D, et al. Low platelet glutathione peroxidase activity and serum selenium concentration in patients with chronic renal failure: relations to dialysis treatments, diet and cardiovascular complications. *Clin Sci* 1993;84:611.

181. Kostakopoulos A, et al. Serum selenium levels in healthy adults and its changes in chronic renal failure. *Int Urol Nephrol* 1990;22:397.

182. Kallistratos G, et al. Selenium and haemodialysis: serum selenium levels in healthy persons, non-cancer and cancer patients with chronic renal failure. *Nephron* 1985;41:217.

183. Milly K, Wit L, Diskin C, et al. Selenium in renal failure patients. *Nephron* 1992;61:139.

184. Antos M, et al. Serum selenium levels in patients on hemodialysis. *Trace Elem Med* 1993;10:173.

185. Hosokawa S, Oyamaguchi A, Yoshida O. Trace elements and complications in patients undergoing chronic hemodialysis. *Nephron* 1990;55:375.

186. McNeely MD, et al. Abnormal concentrations of nickel in serum in case of myocardial infarction, stroke, burns, hepatic cirrhosis, and uremia. *Clin Chem* 1971;17:1123.

187. Hosokawa S, et al. Serum and corpuscular nickel and zinc in chronic hemodialysis patients. *Nephron* 1987;45:151.

188. Avasthi G, et al. Copper, zinc, calcium and magnesium in chronic renal failure. *J Assoc Physicians India* 1991;39:531.

189. Wallaeys B, et al. Trace elements in serum, packed cells and dialysate of CAPD patients. *Kidney Int* 1986;30:599.

190. Bello-Reuss EN, Grady TP, Mazumdar DC. Serum vanadium levels in chronic renal disease. *Ann Intern Med* 1979;91:743.

191. Tsukamoto Y, et al. Abnormal accumulation of vanadium in patients on chronic hemodialysis therapy. *Nephron* 1990;56:368.

192. Hosokawa S, Yoshida O. Serum vanadium levels in chronic hemodialysis patients. *Nephron* 1993;64:388.

193. Hosokawa S, Yoshida O. Vanadium in chronic hemodialysis patients. *Int J Artif Organs* 1990;13:197.

194. Hosokawa S, Yamaguchi O, Yoshida O. Vanadium transfer during haemodialysis. *Int Urol Nephrol* 1991;23:407.

195. Gitelman HJ, Alderman FR, Perry SJ. Silicon accumulation in dialysis patients. *Am J Kidney Dis* 1992;19:140.

196. Berlyne G, et al. Silicon metabolism: the basic facts in renal failure. *Kidney Int Suppl* 1985;17:S175.

197. Dobbie JW, Smith MJ. The silicon content of body fluids. *Scott Med J* 1982;27:17.

198. Mauras Y, et al. Increase in blood silicon concentration in patients with renal failure. *Biomedicine* 1980;33:228.

199. Durr JA, Miller NL, Alfrey AC. Lithium clearance derived from the natural trace blood and urine lithium levels. *Kidney Int Suppl* 1990;28:558.

200. Rudolph H, Alfrey AC, Smythe WR. Muscle and serum trace element profile in uremia. *Trans Am Soc Artif Intern Organs* 1973;19:456.

201. Indraprasit S, Alexander GV, Gonick HC. Tissue composition of major and trace elements in uremia and hypertension. *J Chron Dis* 1974;27:135.

CHAPTER 103

Dietary Considerations in Patients with Chronic Renal Failure, Acute Renal Failure, and Transplantation

Joel D. Kopple

IMPACT OF THE UREMIC SYNDROME ON NUTRITIONAL STATUS AND NUTRITIONAL REQUIREMENTS

In chronic renal failure (CRF), there are disorders in the intestinal absorption, urinary, intestinal, and dermal excretion or metabolism of a wide array of nutrients. These abnormalities may change the dietary requirements for many nutrients. The alterations include retention of products of protein, peptide, nucleic acid, and amino acid metabolism (1), as well as some products of carbohydrate metabolism (2–5); impaired urinary excretion of water, sodium, potassium, calcium, magnesium, phosphorus, trace elements, organic and inorganic acids, and other compounds (6–8); decreased intestinal absorption of calcium (9,10) and possibly iron (11,12), riboflavin (13), folate (14), Vitamin D_3 (15), and certain amino acids (intestinal dipeptide absorption appears to be normal [16]); possibly increased plasma clearance of pyridoxine hydrochloride; antagonism to the actions of several vitamins (due in part to medicines ingested and possibly to uremic factors); and a high risk of developing certain vitamin deficiencies, especially for folic acid, Vitamin B_6, Vitamin C, and the most potent metabolite of Vitamin D, 1,25-dihydroxycholecalciferol (17,18).

Patients with CRF also are prone to accumulate potential toxins that usually are eaten in small amounts and are readily excreted by the kidneys; notable among these are aluminum (19) and advanced glycosylation end products (20). There is mild carbohydrate intolerance that partly improves with hemodialysis therapy (2–4). In nondialyzed patients with CRF, patients on maintenance hemodialysis (MHD), and patients on chronic peritoneal dialysis (CPD), there is

a high incidence of type IV hyperlipoproteinemia with elevated serum triglyceride levels, a low serum high-density lipoprotein (HDL) cholesterol level, and elevated serum low-density lipoprotein (LDL) and intermediate-density lipoprotein levels (21–26). Plasma triglyceride, LDL cholesterol, and apolipoprotein B concentrations also tend to be higher in patients on CPD than in those undergoing MHD. Patients on CPD often have abnormally increased serum total cholesterol levels. Patients with CRF, including those on MHD, often display high serum concentrations of lipoprotein(a) (Lp[a]) (i.e., more than 30 mg/dL), which is associated with a high risk for coronary artery atherosclerosis, cerebrovascular arteriosclerosis, and stenosis of saphenous vein bypass grafts (25,26). In CRF, there are alterations in the concentrations or the composition of certain lipoproteins, with an abnormal proportion of individual lipids and apolipoproteins in the various lipoproteins (21–23,25,26). It has been suggested that this serum lipoprotein and apolipoprotein pattern is associated with an increased risk of atherosclerosis and coronary artery disease (25,26). Production of triglycerides generally is normal, but the metabolic clearance is impaired (27).

Potentially toxic oxidants (28,28a) and reactive carbonyl compounds (methylglyoxal, glyoxal [29], and 3-deoxyglucosone [30], which generate advanced glycosylation end products [31], and N^ϵ-carboxymethyllysine and pentosidine [32]) accumulate in plasma and tissues. Deficiencies of antioxidants (Vitamins C and E and possibly selenium) have been reported (18). This combination of alterations, which have been referred to as *oxidant and carbonyl stress,* may also cause endothelial injury and predispose to cardiovascular, cerebrovascular, and peripheral vascular disease.

Virtually every survey of the nutritional status of chronically uremic patients and patients undergoing MHD or CPD (i.e., continuous ambulatory peritoneal dialysis [CAPD] or automated peritoneal dialysis [APD]) indicates that they

---

J.D. Kopple: Department of Nephrology and Hypertension, Harbor-UCLA Medical Center, Torrance, California; and UCLA Schools of Medicine and Public Health, Los Angeles, California

TABLE 103-1. *Evidence for protein-energy malnutrition in advanced chronic renal failure*[a]

Anthropometry body composition	Biochemistry
Decreased	Decreased
Body weight	Serum
Height (children)	Total protein
Growth (children)	Albumin
Body fat (skinfold thickness)	Transferrin
Fat-free solid	Prealbumin
Intracellular water	Cholinesterase
Muscle mass (midarm muscle area, diameter, or circumference)	Pseudocholinesterase
Total body potassium (nondialyzed patients)	Plasma
Total body nitrogen (Patients on continuous ambulatory peritoneal dialysis)	Isoleucine
Total albumin mass, synthesis, and catabolism	Leucine
Valine pools (nondialyzed patients)	Total tryptophan
	Valine
	Valine : glycine ratio
	Essential : nonessential ratio
	Muscle
	Alkali soluble protein
	RNA : DNA ratio
	Valine
	Tyrosine
	Normal or increased
	Plasma
	Total nonessential amino acids
	Glycine

Note: This low body protein or muscle mass and/or total body fat mass have been determined by anthropometra, dual-energy x-ray absoptometry, bioelectrical impedance, and near-infrared interactance and total body nitrogen measurements.

[a]Nondialyzed patients with advanced chronic renal failure and patients on maintenance dialysis may have normal values for these parameters. However, statistical comparisons indicate that the levels are often abnormal in individual patients, and in group comparisons patients in chronic renal failure usually have significantly altered values.

frequently suffer from protein-energy malnutrition (33–58). The prevalence of protein-energy malnutrition is reported to vary from about 18% to 75% in various studies. In our experience, approximately one-third of these patients have mild to moderate malnutrition and 6% to 8% more have severe malnutrition. The evidence for protein-energy malnutrition, summarized in Table 103-1, includes decreased relative body weight (the individual's body weight divided by the weight of healthy people of the same age, height, sex, and frame size), skinfold thicknesses (an estimate of body fat), arm muscle diameter or cross-sectional area (a reflection of total muscle protein mass), total body nitrogen, increased total body water and extracellular water, decreased serum concentrations of many proteins (including albumin, prealbumin, transferrin, and certain complement proteins), low muscle alkali-soluble

protein, and low growth rates in children. The plasma amino acid pattern, which is unique to CRF, also shows many similarities to the amino acid pattern seen in protein-energy malnutrition (59). Total body potassium concentration is low in patients with CRF and within the normal range in individuals undergoing MHD. The above-mentioned findings are also not uncommonly observed in nondialyzed patients with advanced renal failure.

The problem of maintaining adequate protein nutrition is potentially more difficult for the patient on CPD, because the combined losses of proteins, amino acids, and peptides are greater than those in patients undergoing hemodialysis, particularly because the losses with CPD occur every day, whereas hemodialysis is generally performed only 3 times a week. Although patients on CPD may gain weight, the weight gain is generally of fat and water, even in the absence of visible edema; the mean serum total protein, albumin, and transferrin levels in patients on CPD tend to be lower than normal, although in most patients, the values do not decrease further during the course of treatment (41). One study reported extravascular albumin and total exchangeable albumin levels to be reduced in patients on CAPD (60); whereas in another study, body albumin pool levels were within the normal range (61). In a large series of patients on CPD, there was no change in arm muscle circumference during CPD therapy (62). Williams et al. (63) serially monitored total body potassium and nitrogen in patients undergoing CAPD; total body potassium did not change or increase, whereas total body nitrogen fell significantly. Other authors have reported a reduction in total body potassium in patients on CAPD who sustained multiple episodes of peritonitis (64).

Although the nutritional disorder most commonly associated with CRF is protein-energy malnutrition, other nutritional deficiencies also frequently occur if the patient does not receive supplemental nutrients. Particularly common in patients with CRF who do not take nutritional supplements are deficiencies for 1,25-dihydroxycholecalciferol, Vitamin B_6, folic acid, Vitamin C, iron, and possibly carnitine and zinc (11,12,17,18,66–70).

The following are causes of malnutrition in CRF.

1. Inadequate Nutrient Intake
   (i) Inadequate nutrient intake may be caused by anorexia due to uremic toxins, the debilitating effects of CRF and underlying illnesses (e.g., diabetes mellitus, lupus erythematosus), the impact of acute illness on the patient's ability to eat, and emotional disorders (40,41,71). Also, the fact that diets prescribed for patients with renal failure may be marginally adequate in protein and other nutrients, but less palatable to the patient and difficult to prepare may contribute to an inadequate intake.
   (ii) Serum leptin levels are elevated in uremia (72–74) and may induce anorexia. In rodents, leptin suppresses food intake via its actions on the hypothalamus and probably increases energy expenditure (75,76).

Whether leptin suppresses appetite in humans and specifically in patients with renal failure is less clear. Several studies describe an inverse relationship between serum leptin and dietary protein intake or a direct relation between serum leptin and weight loss in patients on MHD or CPD (73,74). Serum leptin levels are probably elevated in patients with CRF because of impaired degradation by the diseased kidney (77) and possibly because insulin stimulates leptin synthesis (78) and patients with CRF are often hyperinsulinemic. In addition, inflammation (see later discussion) and the acute-phase response increase serum leptin levels (79).

(iii) Inflammation, which is commonly present in patients on maintenance dialysis (80–83), is associated with increased levels of the cytokines, interleukin-1 (IL-1), IL-6, and tumor necrosis factor α (TNFα) (84,85). These cytokines may induce anorexia (86,87).

A cross-sectional study of the nutritional status of approximately 1,700 patients with chronic renal disease who were evaluated during the baseline period of the Modification of Diet in Renal Disease (MDRD) Study indicated that the dietary protein and energy intake and the nutritional status begin to decline when the glomerular filtration rate (GFR) (^{131}I-iothalamate clearance) is about 25 to 38 mL per minute per 1.73 m^2 (88). This decline was noted not only for protein and energy intake, but also for serum transferrin, body weight, midarm muscle circumference and percentage of body fat. The patients were not malnourished—indeed frank malnutrition was a criterion for exclusion from the study—but there were clearly statistically significant trends toward worsening nutritional status as the GFR decreased.

A decreased energy intake was also observed when the GFR was reduced to less than about 25 to 35 mL per minute per 1.73 m^2. This was noted in both the pilot study and the main clinical trial of the MDRD Study, even though these patients met with a trained nephrology research dietitian once monthly (89,90). These results may be particularly relevant because the patients in the MDRD Study were almost certainly a healthier subset of patients with chronic renal insufficiency because of the study's exclusionary criteria. Also in the pilot study for the HEMO Clinical Trial, the average dietary energy and protein intakes were observed to be less than the recommended levels (91). These results do not prove that a low protein or low energy intake is a common cause of the deterioration in nutritional status, but they are consistent with this possibility.

2. Increased Losses of Nutrients

(i) The dialysis procedure itself may promote wasting by removing nutrients. During routine hemodialysis with low-flux dialyzers, there are losses of about 6 to 8 g of free amino acids when patients are postabsorptive (fasting) and about 8 to 10 g when patients are postprandial (92–95). Approximately 2 to 3 g of peptides or bound amino acids is also removed.

Hemodialysis with high-flux membranes is reported to remove 8.0 ± 2.8 (SD) g of amino acids from patients postabsorptive and 9.3 ± 2.7 g of amino acids from patients postprandial (95,96). During the sixth reuse of high-flux polysulfone hemodialyzers with bleach and formaldehyde reprocessing, amino acid losses are reported to be 12.2 ± 4.4 g (95). About 2 to 3.5 g per day of free amino acids is removed during CAPD (97–99) (Table 103-2). In normoglycemic

TABLE 103-2. *Plasma amino acids and amino acid losses into dialysate in nine men undergoing CAPD*

	Plasma amino acids (μmol/L)		Dialysate amino acids (mg/24 hr)
	Patients on CAPD	Normal men	Patients on CAPD
No. of studies	14[a]	9	14[a]
Total essential[c]	963 ± 29[b]	$1,030 \pm 40$	$1,027 \pm 96$
Total nonessential[d]	$2,080 \pm 115$	$2,001 \pm 135$	$1,949 \pm 226$
Total[e]	$3,415 \pm 134$	$3,260 \pm 145$	$3,355 \pm 334$
Essential[c]:nonessential[d] ratio	0.48 ± 0.03	0.53 ± 0.03	0.59 ± 0.05

Note: CAPD, continuous ambulatory peritoneal dialysis.

[a]Fourteen studies were carried out in nine patients. Seven of these patients were studied twice in a clinical research center, once while ingesting a diet providing 1.0 g of protein per kilogram of body weight per day and once while eating a diet containing 1.4 g of protein per kilogram of body weight per day. There were no differences in plasma essential, nonessential, or total amino acid concentrations between the two diets. The other two patients were ingesting diets providing about 1.1–1.2 g of protein per kilogram of body weight per day.

[b]Mean $\pm$ standard error.

[c]Calculated as the sum of concentrations of histidine, isoleucine, leucine, lysine, methionine, phenylalanine, threonine, and valine.

[d]Calculated as the sum of the concentrations of alanine, arginine, asparagine, aspartate, glutamate, glutamine, glycine, ornithine, proline, and serine.

[e]Calculated as the sum of total essential amino acids, total nonessential amino acids, cystine, tyrosine, citrulline, and taurine.

Source: From Kopple JK, et al. Plasma amino acid levels and amino acid losses during continuous ambulatory peritoneal dialysis. *Am J Clin Nutr* 1982;36:395, with permission.

TABLE 103-3. *Serum proteins and dialysate protein losses in eight men undergoing continuous ambulatory peritoneal dialysis*

	Serum proteins[a]	Protein losses[b] per 24 hr
Total protein	6.6 ± 0.1[c] g/dL	8.8 ± 0.5 g
Albumin	3.5 ± 0.1 g/dL	5.7 ± 0.4 g
Transferrin	228 ± 11 mg/dL	333 ± 22 mg
IgG	1.41 ± 0.12 g/dL	1.25 ± 0.20 g
IgA	220 ± 18 mg/dL	173 ± 21 mg
IgM	234 ± 36 mg/dL	71 ± 18 mg
C3	107 ± 6 mg/dL	70 ± 7 mg
C4	32 ± 2 mg/dL	21 ± 2 mg

[a]Grand mean of values from 13 metabolic balance studies in eight men fed 1.0 or 1.4 g of protein per kilogram of body weight per day. Data were obtained periodically during the period of study with each diet.

[b]Losses of each protein into dialysate over 24 h were measured on 110 occasions in the eight patients.

[c]Mean ± standard error.

Source: From Blumenkrantz MJ, et al. Protein losses during peritoneal dialysis. *Kidney Int* 1981;19:593, with permission.

individuals, about 15 to 25 g of glucose may be removed when glucose-free dialysate is used (100). When the hemodialysate contains 200 mg/dL of glucose (180 mg/dL of anhydrous glucose), there is net absorption of approximately 10 to 12 g of glucose with each dialysis.

Usually, little protein is lost during hemodialysis. Formerly, when some hemodialyzers containing polysulfone membranes were reused with bleach and formaldehyde reprocessing procedures, the sieving coefficients of the membranes for large molecules increased dramatically (95,101). In one study, albumin losses were increased to 10.78 ± 7.87 (SD) g (range, 1.1 to 25.6 g) per hemodialysis as the number of reuses increased to more than 24 (95). Polysulfone membranes are now chemically modified, so this increase in permeability does not occur with multiple bleach and formaldehyde reprocessings.

In our experience, 8.8 ± 0.5 (SEM) g per day of total protein and 5.7 ± 0.4 g per day of albumin are lost into the dialysate with CAPD (Table 103-3) (102). Other investigators report similar results (102a,102b). During an acute peritoneal dialysis of about 36 hours' duration, about 22 g of total protein and 13 g of albumin are removed (102). Much of this loss is from the washout of ascitic fluid. With mild peritonitis, the quantity of protein removed increases to an average of 15.1 ± 3.6 g per day (102); protein losses can rise markedly with severe peritonitis, and we have observed peritoneal protein losses of as high as 100 g per day before initiating antibiotic therapy. Protein losses fall rapidly with antibiotic therapy but may remain elevated for many days to weeks (102).

Water-soluble vitamins and other bioactive compounds are removed by both hemodialysis and peritoneal dialysis (18,103–106). These vitamin losses can be easily replaced from the diet, but in patients with poor nutritional intake, such losses may enhance malnutrition.

(ii) Patients with renal failure often lose substantial quantities of blood secondary to occult gastrointestinal tract bleeding, frequent blood sampling for laboratory testing, and the sequestration of blood in the hemodialyzer (107,108). Because blood is rich in protein, these blood losses may contribute to protein wasting. For example, a person with a hemoglobin level of 12.0 g/dL and a serum total protein level of 7.0 g/dL will lose approximately 16.5 g of protein in each 100 mL of blood removed.

3. Increased Net Catabolism

(i) Patients with CRF frequently sustain superimposed illnesses (109–111). These comorbid conditions often induce a hypercatabolic state and may physically prevent ingestion, gastrointestinal absorption, or assimilation of foods (e.g., pancreatitis, gastrointestinal surgery).

(ii) There is now abundant evidence that even in the absence of overt clinical illness, patients with advanced CRF and patients on MHD may sustain inflammation with an acute-phase response and elevation of serum acute-phase proteins (APP) (e.g., C-reactive protein, [CRP], serum amyloid A, C3 complement, [SC]-acid glycoprotein, fibrinogen, haptoglobin, and [SC]-chymotrypsin) (80,83,112–114). A number of epidemiologic studies in patients on MHD have now shown that increased serum CRP is at least as strong a predictor of mortality as albumin (80,81,114,115). These elevations in serum APP levels are associated with an increase in inflammatory cytokines (IL-1, TNFα, and IL-6) (116,117). It has been argued that these elevated cytokines may promote protein-energy malnutrition in patients with CRF both by inducing anorexia (e.g., IL-1, IL-6, TNFα) (86,87) and by engendering protein catabolism (e.g., by activation of proteolytic enzymes released from granulocytes) or by suppressing protein synthesis (118,119). Indeed, evidence suggests that albumin synthesis is suppressed when the serum CRP level is elevated (119).

(iii) In this regard, it has been argued that hemodialyzers, particularly those composed of bioincompatible membranes, hemodialyzer tubing and filters, arteriovenous synthetic grafts and catheters, peritoneal dialysis catheters, and hemodialysate and possibly peritoneal dialysate solutions (presumably due to low levels of endotoxins), can stimulate this inflammatory response (120–123). Exposure to these artificial materials may activate monocytes or macrophages (124). These inflammatory cells then release the cytokines that stimulate the acute-phase response, IL-1, and TNFα. These cytokines, in turn, stimulate the release of IL-6, which further augments the acute-phase response with promotion of hepatic synthesis of the APP, as indicated earlier in this chapter (116,117).

In some *in vivo* studies in patients, hemodialysis with bioincompatible membranes increases the urea nitrogen appearance (UNA, or net urea generation) and hence enhances net protein breakdown and promotes negative nitrogen balance (125,126). There is a net release of amino acids from the leg, indicating enhanced net breakdown of skeletal muscle protein (126). Some research evidence indicates that more bioincompatible hemodialysis membranes, such as Cuprophan, are more likely to stimulate the release of interleukin and promote net protein degradation than are more biocompatible membranes (127,128). Several studies have provided evidence in support of the thesis that the artificial membranes, tubing, catheters, or dialysate used in the dialysis procedure can promote the acute-phase response (120–124, 129–133).

(iv) It would not be unexpected for the accumulation of endogenously formed uremic toxins to engender malnutrition. In renal failure, there are increased plasma or tissue concentrations of probably hundreds of metabolic products; more than 120 such compounds have already been identified (1,134,135). Some of these compounds are bioactive (1,134), and it is not unlikely that many have catabolic or antianabolic actions. Acidemia enhances decarboxylation of branched-chain amino acids and engenders protein catabolism in skeletal muscle (135a–138). Studies in humans suggest that metabolic acidemia causes protein catabolism and negative nitrogen balance (135a–138). Also, both oxidants and carbonyl compounds, as well as a deficiency of antioxidants, may cause tissue injury and inflammation and possibly a catabolic state.

(v) The endocrine disorders of uremia may also promote protein-energy malnutrition. Resistance to the actions of insulin (139,140) and insulin-like growth factor-1 (IGF-1) (141–143), as well as hyperglucagonemia (144) may promote protein wasting. Parathyroid hormone increases hepatic gluconeogenesis (145,146), and secondary hyperparathyroidism in renal failure therefore may cause protein wasting. The findings that 1,25-dihydroxycholecalciferol has pervasive effects on calcium metabolism, that Vitamin D deficiency may cause a proximal myopathy, and that 25-hydroxycholecalciferol stimulates muscle protein synthesis *in vitro* (147) suggest that deficiency of 1,25-dihydroxycholecalciferol may also cause muscle protein wasting. As indicated earlier in this chapter, serum leptin levels are elevated in renal failure and may contribute to anorexia (72–76).

(vi) Other possible but less well-established causes of wasting include exogenously derived uremic toxins, which may cause debility (e.g., aluminum) and possibly malnutrition.

(vii) Because the kidney synthesizes or degrades many biologically active compounds including certain amino acids, peptide hormones, other peptides, glucose, and fatty acids (148), it is possible that loss of these metabolic activities of the kidney in renal failure may disrupt the body's metabolism and promote malnutrition. In this regard, some possible mechanisms by which failure of renal metabolic activity might promote protein-energy malnutrition are described earlier in this chapter.

EFFECTS OF MALNUTRITION ON THE CLINICAL COURSE OF PATIENTS WITH CRF

Many studies indicate that in patients undergoing MHD or CPD, nutritional status is a powerful predictor of morbidity and mortality. Indeed, many epidemiologic studies indicate that the serum albumin level is one of the strongest predictors of mortality, following the age of the individual (52,149,150). Several reports have correlated morbidity or mortality rates in patients on MHD with low dietary protein intake (as indicated by protein nitrogen appearance (PNA), decreased body weight for a given height, and low serum albumin, urea, creatinine, cholesterol, and potassium levels (52,149–151). With the exception of albumin, the latter chemistries appear to correlate with mortality in a "J" curve relationship, in which both low and very high concentrations are negatively correlated with mortality (52). For patients on CPD, in whom retrospective analyses, in general, have been based on smaller sample sizes, morbidity or mortality has been correlated with serum albumin level and PNA in some (149,152,153) but not all studies (154). Body weight–for–height and anthropometric parameters of skeletal muscle mass or fat mass (e.g., skinfold thickness), a potential indicator of cumulative energy balance, also correlate with morbidity or mortality (155–157). No study has attempted to relate morbidity or mortality with dietary energy intake. The correlation between low serum cholesterol level and high mortality is consistent with such a relationship (52,149).

The epidemiologic association between nutritional status and morbidity or mortality does not prove that protein-energy malnutrition causes increased morbidity or mortality or that a greater protein and energy intake will reduce these adverse outcomes in such patients. Indeed, as indicated earlier in this chapter, comorbidity including conditions associated with inflammation may account for some of this relationship. Serum albumin level is negatively correlated with serum CRP in patients on MHD, and serum CRP level is at least as powerful a predictor of mortality as serum albumin (82,83,112,158,159). Some epidemiologic studies suggest that both protein-energy malnutrition and inflammation may each make independent contributions to the development of vascular disease in individuals with advanced CRF (160). Moreover, two retrospective analyses compared malnourished patients on MHD receiving intradialytic parenteral nutrition (IDPN) with malnourished patients on MHD not receiving this therapy (161,162). The data suggest that malnourished patients receiving IDPN had greater survival, compared with those who did not. In one study, when the serum albumin level was 3.3 g/dL or less, the patients who received IDPN had significantly greater survival rates than those who were not given IDPN (162).

DIETARY THERAPY FOR CHRONIC RENAL DISEASE AND CRF

General Approach to Dietary Management

The widespread nutritional and metabolic alterations, high incidence of malnutrition, and current evidence that dietary therapy may retard the rate of progression of CRF indicate that nutritional therapy is a critical aspect of the management of chronic renal disease. There are three goals for dietary treatment:

1. to maintain good nutritional status
2. to arrest or retard the progression of renal failure
3. to prevent or ameliorate uremic toxicity and the metabolic disorders of renal failure

Adherence to specialized diets is often a difficult and frustrating endeavor for patients and their families. Patients usually must make fundamental changes in their behavior and forsake some of their traditional sources of daily pleasure. Often, the patients must procure special foods, prepare special recipes, usually forgo or severely limit their intake of favorite foods, or eat foods that they may not desire. Demands are made on the patient's time and daily activities and on the emotional support system of the family or close associates. Therefore, it is incumbent on the physician not to prescribe radical changes in the patient's diet unless there is good reason to believe that these modifications may be beneficial. To ensure successful dietary therapy, patients with renal disease must undergo extensive training concerning the principles of nutritional therapy and the design and preparation of diets, and they need to be continuously encouraged to adhere to the prescribed diet. They usually require repeated training regarding their nutritional therapy. Without careful monitoring of nutritional intake, retraining, encouragement, and sensitivity to the cultural background, psychosocial condition, and lifestyle of the patients, they will be more likely to adhere poorly to their dietary prescription. They may eat too little rather than too much. (When the recommended nutrient intake is given in terms of body weight, it refers to standard body weight as determined from the National Health and Nutrition Evaluation Survey [NHANES] data [163,164].)

The recipes and meal plans should be designed specifically for the individual taste of the patient. A team approach—including the physician, dietitian, close family members, the nursing staff, and when available, social workers or psychiatrists—may improve adherence. Because the prescribed diet for patients with renal failure is complicated and obtaining an accurate diet history and maximizing dietary compliance for these individuals is a complex and subtle art, it is important for the physician to work with a dietitian who is knowledgeable and experienced in nephrology dietetics. It is often advantageous to organize the dietetic program in a medical center so the dietitians who treat nephropathic patients work exclusively in this specialty. Data indicate that a systematic, problem-oriented approach to dietary compliance can substantially improve compliance (165,166).

The physician should strongly support the dietitian's efforts to train and counsel the patient and to obtain dietary compliance. During each visit, the physician should assess the patient's dietary intake (see later discussion) and discuss the results with the patient. Generally, it is important for the spouse or other close relatives or friends to work closely with the patient to provide moral support and to assist, if needed, with the acquisition and preparation of foods. The entire medical team should assume an energetic, positive, and sympathetic approach to promote dietary adherence. A nurse, social worker, and psychiatrist can provide invaluable assistance by providing sympathetic counseling to the patient and informing other members of the team of problems that may impair the patient's adherence to the diet. The central issue is that if dietary therapy is prescribed to a patient, it requires a major commitment and effort by the patient and the medical staff to attain good results.

Because diets prescribed for renal insufficiency are often marginally low in some nutrients (e.g., protein) and high in others (e.g., calcium) and malnutrition is not infrequent, it is important to periodically evaluate the adequacy of the diet and the patient's nutritional status. The National Kidney Foundation Kidney Disease Outcomes Quality Initiative (NKF K/DOQI) Clinical Practice Guidelines for Nutrition in CRF has recommended that panels of nutritional measures should be used to assess protein-energy nutritional status in nondialyzed patients with CRF and patients on MHD (167,168). For nondialyzed patients with CRF with a GFR of less than 20 mL per minute, it is recommended that protein-energy nutritional status be evaluated by serial measurements of a panel of markers including at least one measure from each of the following clusters: (a) serum albumin; (b) edema-free actual body weight, percentage standard (NHANES II) body weight, or subjective global assessment; and (c) the normalized protein equivalent of total nitrogen appearance (TNA) or dietary interviews and diaries (167). The standard body weight for healthy individuals is obtained from the NHANES II (169). For patients on MHD or CPD, the recommended panel of measurements of protein-energy nutritional status is indicated in Table 103-4 and should routinely include predialysis or stabilized serum albumin, percentage of usual body weight, percentage of standard (NHANES II) body weight, subjective global assessment, dietary interviews and diaries, and normalized protein equivalent of TNA (168). (A predialysis serum measurement is obtained from an individual immediately before the initiation of a hemodialysis or intermittent peritoneal dialysis treatment. A stabilized serum

TABLE 103-4. *The National Kidney Foundation Kidney Disease Outcomes Quality Initiative recommendations for routine monitoring of nutritional status in patients on maintenance hemodialysis and chronic peritoneal dialysis*

Category	Measure	Minimum frequency of measurement
I. Measurements that should be performed routinely in all patients	• Predialysis or stabilized serum albumin	• Every 4 mo
	• % of usual postdialysis (MHD) or postdrain (CPD) body weight	• Every 6 mo
	• % of standard (NHANES II) body weight	• Every 6 mo
	• SGA	
	• Dietary interview and diary	• Monthly MHD; every 3–4 mo CPD
	• nPNA	
	• Monthly	
	• Monthly	
II. Measures that can be useful to confirm or extend the data obtained from the measures in category	• Predialysis or stabilized serum prealbumin	• As needed
	• Skinfold thickness	• As needed
	• Midarm muscle area, circumference, or diameter	• As needed
	• Dual-energy x-ray absorptiometry	• As needed
III. Clinically useful measures, which, if low, might suggest the need for a more rigorous examination of protein-energy nutritional status	• Predialysis or stabilized serum	
	—Creatinine	• As needed
	—Urea nitrogen	• As needed
	—Cholesterol	• As needed
	• Creatinine index	• As needed

MHD, maintenance hemodialysis; CPD, chronic peritoneal dialysis; NHANES II, Second National Health and Nutrition Evaluation Survey; SGA, subjective global assessment; nPNA, normalized protein equivalent of total nitrogen appearance [determined from the urea nitrogen appearance (183)].
Source: From Am J Kidney Dis, with permission.

measurement is obtained after the patient has stabilized on a given dose of continuous peritoneal dialysis.)

There are other nutritional parameters that, at times, will require monitoring; for example, urine sodium and phosphorus, serum potassium, iron ferritin, transferrin, vitamins, total LDL and HDL cholesterol, triglycerides, and, if relevant, bone radiography (36).

Dietitians are often best qualified to perform anthropometric measurements of nutritional status because of their experience and training, interest in nutritional therapy, and access to the patient. In general, to maintain good dietary compliance and to monitor closely the patient's clinical, fluid and electrolyte, and nutritional status, patients with advanced renal failure should be seen approximately monthly by the physician and the dietitian. It is arguable as to whether patients with slowly progressive mild or moderate renal insufficiency who are clinically stable and adhere well to the diet may see a physician less frequently. However, to maximize compliance to the diet, most patients should continue to see the dietitian more frequently, often monthly. A study by Bergstrom et al. (170) emphasizes the importance of close medical follow-up. These authors observed that frequent clinic visits, apparently independent of dietary prescription, led to a slowing in the rate of progression of renal insufficiency.

In many patients with progressive renal failure, the creatinine clearance decreases more or less linearly with time

(171,172). Transposing the clearance equation, it can be predicted that the log of the serum creatinine level or the 1.0/serum creatinine ratio also should decrease linearly with time. This has been confirmed in several studies (171,172); approximately 60% to 80% of patients with chronic progressive kidney disease lose creatinine clearance in a roughly linear fashion. Thus, for patients with CRF, the creatinine clearance or the 1.0/serum creatinine ratio periodically should be plotted against time. If the rate of progression slows, it may indicate that treatment is beneficial. On the other hand, acceleration of the rate of progression may indicate the development of new causes that are impairing renal function. Such causes include worsening hypertension, drug reactions, urinary tract obstruction, infection, intake of nonsteroidal antiinflammatory drugs, or increased activity of the underlying renal disease. It is well documented that the creatinine clearance is not as precise a measure of the GFR as the clearance of inulin, iothalamate, or several other solutes and may give misleading results (173,174). This is due primarily to variability in the renal tubular secretion of creatinine (175). Indeed, the creatinine clearance has been largely invalidated as a measure of GFR for clinical or laboratory research studies (174,175). However, the creatinine clearance or the mean of the creatinine and urea clearances (176) is often helpful for the clinical management of patients, particularly when serial measurements are taken, and may give a substantially more precise estimate of the actual GFR than the serum creatinine level.

Because the nutritional status may begin to deteriorate in patients with chronic progressive renal disease when the GFR falls to less than 35 to 50 mL per minute per 1.73 m^2 (88), careful attention to nutritional status should begin at this time or earlier. This is particularly important because markers of poor nutritional status at the onset of maintenance dialysis therapy predict increased morbidity and mortality (157). Chronically uremic patients appear to be at greatest risk for malnutrition from the time the GFR falls to less than 10 mL per minute until the patient is established on maintenance dialysis therapy (43). Studies in both children and adults indicate that the nutritional status of patients at the onset of chronic dialysis treatment is a good predictor of their nutritional status 2 to 3 years later (43,177,177a). Hence, particular effort should be given to preventing malnutrition as the patient approaches dialysis therapy and during the first few weeks of maintenance dialysis treatment. These efforts should be directed toward maintaining a good nutritional intake during this period, rapidly instituting therapy for superimposed illnesses, and maintaining good nutritional intake during such illnesses.

Urea Nitrogen Appearance and the Serum Urea Nitrogen : Serum Creatinine Ratio

Because the control of protein intake is central to the nutritional management of patients with acute renal failure (ARF) or CRF, it is important to accurately monitor nitrogen intake. Fortunately, for most patients, this is possible. Patients who are in neutral nitrogen balance should have a total nitrogen output that is equal to nitrogen intake minus about 0.5 g of nitrogen per day from such unmeasured losses as sweat, respiration, flatus, blood drawing, and growth of skin, hair, and nails (178). Thus, nitrogen output should correlate closely with nitrogen intake in patients who are more or less in nitrogen balance. For the clinical management of patients, a slightly positive or negative balance will not substantially alter the use of the nitrogen output measurement to estimate nitrogen intake. In patients who are in very positive or negative nitrogen balance (e.g., from pregnancy or severe infection), nitrogen output may not reflect intake. However, when the patient is in very positive or negative balance, there is usually an accompanying alteration in the patient's clinical status that is readily apparent to the physician.

The measurement of total nitrogen outputs (i.e., the nitrogen losses in urine, fecal, dialysate, or tube or fistula drainage) is too laborious and expensive to be widely applied for clinical uses. However, because urea is the major nitrogenous product of protein and amino acid degradation, the UNA can be used to estimate total nitrogen output and hence nitrogen intake (109,179,180). UNA is the amount of urea nitrogen that appears or accumulates in body fluids and all outputs (e.g., urine, dialysate, fistula drainage). The term UNA is employed

rather than urea production or urea generation because some urea is degraded in the intestinal tract; the ammonia released from urea is largely transported to the liver and converted back to urea (181,182). Thus, the enterohepatic urea cycle leads to an increase in absolute urea synthesis but has little effect on serum urea levels or total nitrogen economy, and this cycle can be ignored without compromising the accuracy of the UNA for estimating total nitrogen output or intake. This offers an important advantage because the recycling of urea cannot be measured without costly and time-consuming isotope studies.

UNA is calculated as follows:

$$
\begin{aligned}
\text{UNA (g/d)} = {} & \text{urinary urea nitrogen (g/d)} \\
& + \text{dialysate urea nitrogen (g/d)} \\
& + \text{change in body urea nitrogen (g/d)} \quad [1]
\end{aligned}
$$

$$
\begin{aligned}
\text{change in body urea nitrogen (g/d)} \\
= {} & (\text{BUN}_f - \text{BUN}_i, \text{g/L/d}) \\
& \times \text{BW}_i \text{ (kg)} \times (0.60 \text{ L/kg}) \\
& + (\text{BW}_f - \text{BW}_i, \text{kg/d}) \\
& \times \text{BUN}_f \text{ (g/L)} (1.0 \text{ L/kg}) \quad [2]
\end{aligned}
$$

where i and f are the initial and final values for the period of measurement; BUN is blood urea nitrogen (grams per liter); BW is body weight (kilograms); 0.60 is an estimate of the fraction of body weight that is water; and 1.0 is the volume of distribution of urea in the weight that is gained or lost.

The estimated proportion of body weight that is water may be increased in patients who are edematous or lean and decreased in individuals who are obese or very young. Changes in body weight during the 1- to 3-day period of measurement of UNA are assumed to be due entirely to changes in body water. In patients undergoing hemodialysis, UNA may be calculated during the interdialytic interval and then normalized to 24 hours. Alternatively, UNA may be calculated by urea kinetic techniques. Two pool models for urea kinetic measurements that take into account delays in equilibration of endogenous urea pools during hemodialysis will give more accurate results for both the UNA method described here and the urea kinetic technique (183). The 24-hour dialysate urea concentration can be readily measured in patients on CAPD or APD. Measurement of total protein as well as urea in peritoneal dialysate may give more accurate measurements of total nitrogen output and, hence, dietary protein intake (184).

In our experience, the relationship between UNA and TNA in chronically uremic patients not undergoing dialysis is as follows (180):

$$
\text{TNA (g/d)} = 1.19 \text{ UNA (g/d)} + 1.27 \quad [3]
$$

If the individual is approximately in neutral nitrogen balance, the UNA also will correlate closely with nitrogen intake. The following equation describes our observed relationship between UNA and dietary nitrogen intake in clinically stable, nondialyzed, patients with CRF.

$$\text{dietary nitrogen intake (g/d)} = 1.20 \text{ UNA (g/d)} + 1.74$$
[4]

When both nitrogen intake and UNA are known, nitrogen balance can be estimated from the difference between nitrogen intake and nitrogen output estimated from the UNA. If the patient is markedly anabolic, such as in pregnancy or in a young person with anorexia nervosa who is being refed, Equation 4 will underestimate nitrogen intake. In patients who have large protein losses (e.g., from the nephrotic syndrome or peritoneal dialysis) or who are acidemic and have sufficient kidney function to excrete large quantities of ammonia, Equations 3 and 4 will underestimate both nitrogen output and nitrogen intake. In most circumstances, however, these conditions are not present, and the UNA provides a powerful tool for monitoring nitrogen output and intake or for estimating balance. Other investigators have described similar approaches to monitoring nitrogen intake and output (185).

The ratio of the BUN : serum creatinine also correlates fairly closely with dietary protein or amino acid intake in nondialyzed patients with CRF (186). This relationship can be used to estimate the recent daily intake of these patients. Although the BUN : serum creatinine ratio is not as precise as the UNA and is influenced by a number of clinical factors (186), it is easy and inexpensive to measure. For clinically stable, nondialyzed, chronically uremic patients, this ratio can also be used to estimate the level at which the BUN will stabilize for any given dietary protein intake and GFR (186).

Protein, Amino Acids, and Keto Acids

Background Information

Low-protein diets have been prescribed for many decades to reduce the accumulation of potentially toxic metabolites of protein metabolism in patients with CRF (187–194). There is considerable evidence that mixtures of essential amino acids can be used more efficiently than protein by uremic patients (195–202). Several investigators reported that in patients with CRF, low-protein diets supplemented with essential amino acids promoted greater nitrogen retention, compared with unsupplemented low-protein diets (e.g., about 0.3 g of protein per kilogram per day) or diets providing very low quantities of essential amino acids (e.g., about 20 g per day) as the sole nitrogen source, and was also effective at improving uremic symptoms (197,199,200). Substitution of α-keto acid or α-hydroxy acid analogs for some essential amino acids may further reduce nitrogen intake while maintaining good nutrition (203–207). α-Keto acids contain a keto group instead of an amino group on the [SC]-carbon; [SC]-hydroxy acids contain a hydroxyl group on this carbon.

Low-protein diets have been reported to slow the rate of progress of CRF (208–212). Some studies suggest that the very-low-protein diets supplemented with keto acids,

hydroxy acids, and essential amino acids may be particularly effective at slowing the rate of loss of renal function (201,202, 213–216). Not all studies confirmed these results (217). The nitrogen-sparing effects of these essential amino acid– or keto acid–supplemented diets are due, in part, to the branched-chain amino acids and keto acids, particularly leucine and its keto acid analog, α-ketoisocaproic acid, which promote protein anabolism (218,219). Recently, there have been primarily three types of low-nitrogen diets that have been used for the treatment of patients with CRF: (a) a low-protein diet providing about 0.55 to 0.60 g of protein per kilogram of body weight per day (165,194,202,208–213); (b) a very-low-protein diet providing approximately 16 to 20 g of protein of miscellaneous quality per day (i.e., about 0.28 g of protein per kilogram per day) supplemented with about 10 to 20 g of the nine L-essential amino acids per day (199,200,217); and (c) a similar diet of 16 to 20 g of protein generally supplemented with four essential amino acids—histidine, lysine, threonine, and tryptophan—and the keto acid or hydroxy acid analogs of the other five essential amino acids sometimes with a few other amino acids added (165,202,204,212,214–216). There is strong evidence that histidine is an essential amino acid for both healthy individuals and patients with CRF (220), and for this reason, histidine is included in all essential amino acid and keto acid preparations. The diet containing 0.55 to 0.60 g of protein per kilogram per day includes primarily high-biologic-value protein (i.e., protein containing a high fraction of the essential amino acids proportioned roughly according to the daily dietary requirements for humans). Because the diets with a very low protein intake (0.28 g per kilogram per day) are supplemented with amino acids or keto acids, it is not important that the protein be of high biologic value.

The largest and most thorough examination of whether dietary control will retard the rate of progression of renal disease was the National Institutes of Health–funded MDRD Study (165). This project investigated, in an intention to treat analysis, the effects of three levels of dietary protein and phosphorus intakes and two blood pressure management goals on the progression of chronic renal disease. Eight hundred forty adults with various types of renal disease, but excluding insulin-dependent diabetes mellitus, were divided into two study groups according to their GFR.

Study A included 585 patients with a GFR, measured by ^{131}I-iothalamate clearances, of 25 to 55 mL per minute per 1.73 m^2. They were randomly assigned to either a usual protein, usual phosphorus diet (1.3 g of protein per kilogram of standard body weight per day and 16 to 20 mg of phosphorus per kilogram per day) or a low-protein, low-phosphorus diet (0.58 g of protein per kilogram per day and 5 to 10 mg of phosphorus per kilogram per day), and to either a moderate or strict blood pressure goal (mean arterial blood pressure 107 mm Hg [113 mm Hg for those 61 years or older] or 92 mm Hg [98 mm Hg for those 61 years or older]). In study B, 255 patients with a baseline GFR of 13 to 24 mL per minute per 1.73 m^2 were randomly assigned to the low-protein and low-phosphorus diet or to a very-low-protein and very-low-phosphorus diet (0.28 g of protein per kilogram per day and 4 to 9 mg of phosphorus per kilogram per day) with a keto acid–amino acid supplement (0.28 g/kg per day). They were also randomly assigned to either the moderate or the strict blood pressure control groups, as in study A. The adherence to the dietary protein prescription in the different diet groups was excellent.

Among participants in study A, those prescribed the low-protein diet had significantly faster declines in GFR during the first 4 months than those on the usual protein diet. Thereafter, the rate of decline of the GFR in the low-protein, low-phosphorus group was significantly slower than in the group fed the usual protein and phosphorus diet. Over the course of the entire treatment period, there was no difference in the overall rate of progression of renal failure in the two diet groups. However, it is likely that the initial greater fall in GFR in the patients prescribed the low-protein diet may reflect a hemodynamic response to the reduction in protein intake, rather than a greater rate of progression of the parenchymal renal disease. This might be beneficial, reflecting a reduction of intrarenal hyperfiltration and intrarenal hypertension. If this explanation is correct—and it is not established that it is correct—the subsequent slower rate of progression of disease after the first 4 months of dietary treatment is consistent with a beneficial effect of this intervention in renal disease. In study B, the very-low-protein group had a marginally slower decline of GFR than the low-protein group; the average rate of decline did not differ significantly between the two groups ($P = 0.066$).

In a secondary analysis of study B in which the decrease in GFR was correlated with the actual quantity of protein ingested, there was no effect of ingesting the low-protein diet versus the very-low-protein diet supplemented with keto acids and amino acids on the progression of renal failure (221). However, if the two diet groups were analyzed together and the protein intake of the latter diet was considered to be the sum of the protein and keto acid–amino acid supplement ingested, a significantly lower rate of decline in GFR was found in the patients who actually ingested lower-protein diets (221). These findings suggest that a lower total protein intake, but not the keto acid–amino acid preparation itself, retarded the rate of progression of renal failure.

In the MDRD Study, the very-low-protein keto acid–amino acid supplemental diet was not compared with the usual protein intake. Also, it is possible that the lack of significant effect of the low-protein diet on the progression of renal failure might reflect the rather short mean duration of treatment in the MDRD Study, 2.2 years. Indeed, if the trend toward slower progression of renal failure in the low-protein-diet groups that was present at the termination of the MDRD Study had persisted during a longer follow-up period, statistically significantly slower progression would have been observed with the 0.60 g/kg-protein diet in study A and the very-low-protein, keto acid–amino acid supplemental diet in study B. This phenomenon is perhaps exemplified with the

Diabetes Control and Complications Trial of intensive versus more conventional serum glucose control. After 2 years of study, there was not even a trend toward less microalbuminuria in the more rigorously controlled glucose group (222). However, when the study was terminated after a mean of 6.5 years, a much lower incidence of microalbuminuria was found in these latter patients. The MDRD Study also included a substantial proportion of patients assigned to each diet who did not show progression of renal failure, and there was a large number of patients with adult polycystic disease enrolled in the study. The presence of both of these subgroups probably reduced the likelihood of showing a slowing effect of low-protein diets on the progression of renal failure.

There was also no significant difference in the rate of decline in the GFR between the moderate and low blood pressure groups in either study A or study B, although the difference in the mean arterial blood pressure during the follow-up period in the two groups was small, 4 mm Hg (165). But in study A, patients assigned to the low blood pressure group who had a baseline urinary protein excretion of more than or equal to 0.25 g per day had a significantly slower rate of decline of GFR than those assigned to the moderate blood pressure level. In study B, patients with baseline urinary protein more than or equal to 1.0 g per day had a slower decline in GFR when assigned to the low blood pressure group (223). Other analyses now confirm that strict blood pressure control (e.g., 130/185 to 125/75 mm Hg or lower) is particularly beneficial for reducing the rate of progression of renal failure in hypertensive patients, particularly in those who have 1 g or more of urinary protein per day or diabetes mellitus (224,225). In general, the dietary and blood pressure treatments were well tolerated, safe, and acceptable to patients. There was a tendency for some patients to develop worsening parameters of protein-energy nutritional status (90). This was particularly evident during the first 4 months of therapy in the patients prescribed the low-protein and very-low-protein diets. It is possible that the lower dietary energy intakes may have contributed to this phenomenon (90), and that it may be more difficult to maintain an adequate energy intake with low-protein diets. No treatment group developed evidence for frank protein-energy malnutrition during the study. Three meta-analyses indicate that low-protein diets are associated with a postponement in the time until chronic dialysis therapy is inaugurated (226,227) or a modest reduction in the rate of decline in GFR in patients with chronic renal disease (228). Thus, taken together with other published research in this field, the results of the MDRD Study are interpreted to indicate that dietary protein and phosphorus restriction will retard the rate of progression of renal failure in patients with progressive renal disease. On average, this effect, although clear-cut, is not dramatic and often requires many months of treatment to become evident. In conjunction with blood pressure control and other medical management, dietary protein and phosphorus restriction appears to offer the patient with chronic renal disease another method for slowing the rate of loss of renal function.

Recommended Protein Intake

GFR of more than 70 mL per minute per 1.73 m^2. There is almost no information concerning the most desirable dietary protein and phosphorus prescription for patients with chronic renal disease and mild impairment in renal function. Indeed, almost all of the studies of the effect of low-protein diets on the rate of progression of renal failure have examined patients with moderately advanced to advanced renal failure (i.e., serum creatinine level of 2.5 mg/dL or more).

It is recommended that protein (and phosphorus) intake be restricted for patients with a GFR of more than 70 mL per minute per 1.73m^2 only if there is evidence that renal function is continuing to decline. In this situation, the patient is treated as indicated in the next paragraph.

GFR of 25 to 70 mL per minute per 1.73 m^2. At present, we discuss with the patient the evidence that low-protein, low-phosphorus diets may retard progression and indicate that the data, although not definitive, are sufficiently convincing to justify prescription of a protein- and phosphorus-restricted diet. If the patient agrees to dietary therapy, he or she is offered a diet providing about 0.60 to 0.75 g of protein per kilogram per day, of which at least 0.35 g is high-biologic-value protein to ensure a sufficient intake of the essential amino acids. This quantity of protein should maintain neutral or positive nitrogen balance and for many patients should not be excessively burdensome. Keto acid preparations are not available in the United States for therapeutic use.

GFR of less than 25 mL per minute per 1.73 m^2. At this level of renal insufficiency, the potential advantages to following a low-protein, low-phosphorus diet become more compelling. First, at this degree of renal failure, potentially toxic products of nitrogen metabolism begin to accumulate in substantial quantities. The low-protein diet will generate less potentially toxic nitrogenous compounds. Second, because the low-protein diet generally contains less phosphorus and potassium, the intake of these minerals can be lowered more readily with this diet (see later sections on recommended phosphorus and potassium intakes). Third, some patients with chronic renal insufficiency eat too little protein, rather than too much. Specific training and encouragement to follow a prescribed diet may increase the likelihood that the patient will not ingest too little protein. Patients should be prescribed 0.60 g of protein per kilogram of body weight per day or, if this is not feasible, up to 0.75 g of protein per kilogram per day (Table 103-5). This diet will generally maintain a neutral or positive nitrogen balance as long as energy intake is not deficient (Table 103-5), should generate a low UNA and reduce the development of uremic symptoms (179,180,194), and may be more effective at retarding the progression of renal failure.

The NKF K/DOQI Clinical Practice Guidelines for Nutrition recommend that "for individuals with CRF (GFR less than 25 mL per minute) who are not undergoing maintenance dialysis, the institution of a planned low-protein diet providing 0.60 g of protein per kilogram per day should be considered. For individuals who will not accept such a diet or who are unable to maintain adequate dietary energy intake with such a diet, an intake of up to 0.75 g of protein per kilogram per day may be prescribed" (229). Allowing the dietary protein intake to increase to 0.75 g of protein per kilogram per day may enable the patient to increase dietary energy intake; this diet also is easier for most people to follow. Dietary protein intakes of more than 0.75 g of protein per kilogram per day may be associated with more rapid rates of progression of renal failure (221). At least 50% of the protein intake with these low-protein diets should be of high biologic value. The protein content of this diet should be increased by 1.0 g per day of high-biologic-value protein for each gram of protein excreted in the urine each day. In the experience of some investigators in this field, roughly 15% of individuals with chronic renal disease are willing and able to adhere to diets providing 0.60 g of protein per kilogram per day or essential amino acid–supplemented very-low-protein diets.

The clinical indications for cessation of low-protein dietary therapy and inauguration of maintenance dialysis therapy or renal transplantation are still somewhat controversial. The NKF K/DOQI Clinical Practice Guidelines for Nutrition recommend a nutritional indicator for inaugurating renal replacement therapy as follows (230): "In patients with CRF (e.g., GFR less than 15 to 20 mL per minute) who are not undergoing maintenance dialysis, if protein-energy malnutrition develops or persists despite vigorous attempts to optimize protein and energy intake and there is no apparent cause for malnutrition other than low nutrient intake, initiation of maintenance dialysis or a renal transplant is recommended." This guideline is based on the rationale that patients who have evidence of protein-energy malnutrition at the onset of MHD therapy have an increased mortality rate, and that inaugurating MHD therapy or performing a renal transplantation will often improve nutritional status in malnourished individuals with advanced CRF (157,231,232).

Maintenance Hemodialysis

There are few studies of dietary protein requirements in patients undergoing MHD. These investigations were all nitrogen balance studies; of the carefully controlled balance studies, most were carried out using dialyzers and schedules of dialysis therapy that are no longer in use (125,233–235). It is apparent that patients on maintenance dialysis have increased dietary protein requirements because of the removal of amino acids and peptides by the dialysis procedure (92–96) and because hemodialysis appears to stimulate protein catabolism, perhaps particularly when it is conducted with less biocompatible dialyzer membranes (125,127,128)

TABLE 103-5. *Recommended dietary nutrient intake for patients with chronic renal failure not undergoing dialysis and for patients undergoing maintenance hemodialysis or chronic peritoneal dialysis*

	Chronic renal failure[a,b,c]	Maintenance hemodialysis (MHD)	Continuous ambulatory or automated peritoneal dialysis (CAPD or APD)
Protein			
Low-protein diet	0.60 g/kg/d; protein may be increased up to 0.75 g/kg/d if necessary to maintain adequate energy intake or if patient will not accept lower protein diets. 50% of protein is of high biologic value.	1.2 gm/kg/day; 50% high biologic value	1.2–1.3 g/kg/d; 50% high biologic value protein
Energy (kj/kg/d)	147 kj/kg/d for individuals younger than 60 years and 142–147 kj/kg/d for patients 60 years or older. Patients with relative body weight of more than 120% or patients who gain or are afraid of gaining unwanted weight may be prescribed lower energy intakes. Energy intake includes energy obtained from diet and, if applicable, from hemodialysate or peritoneal dialysate.		
Fat (percentage of total energy intake)[d,e]	30–40	30–40	30–40
Polyunsaturated: saturated fatty acid ratio[e]	1.0:1.0	1.0:1.0	1.0:1.0
Carbohydrate[e,f]		Rest of nonprotein calories	
Total fiber intake (g/d)[e]	20–25	20–25	20–25
Minerals (range of intake)			
Sodium (mg/d)	1,000 to 3,000	750 to 1,000[g]	1,000 to 2,000[g]
Potassium (mEq/d)	40 to 70	40 to 70	40 to 70
Phosphorus (mg/kg/d)	5 to 10[h]	8 to 17[h]	8 to 17[h]
Calcium (mg/d)	1,400 to 1,600[i]	1,400 to 1,600[i]	800–1,000[i]
Magnesium (mg/d)	200 to 300	200 to 300	200–300
Iron (mg/d)	≥10 to 18[j]	≥10 to 18[j]	10–18[j]
Zinc (mg/d)	15	15	15
Water (ml/d)	Up to 3,000 as tolerated[g]	Usually 750 to 1,500[g]	Usually 1,000 to 1,500[g]
Vitamins	Diets to be supplemented with these quantities		
Thiamin (mg/d)	1.5	1.5	1.5
Riboflavin (mg/d)	1.8	1.8	1.8
Pantothenic acid (mg/d)	5	5	5
Niacin (mg/d)	20	20	20
Pyridoxine HCl (mg/d)	5	10	10
Vitamin B_{12} (μg/d)	3	3	3
Vitamin C (mg/d)	60	60	60
Folic acid (mg/d)	1–15[k]	1–15[k]	1–15[k]
Vitamin A	No addition	No addition	No addition
Vitamin D	See text	See text	See text
Vitamin E (IU/d)	15	15	15
Vitamin K	None[l]	None[l]	None[l]

[a]Glomerular filtration rate of more than 4–5 mL/min/1.73 m² and less than 25 mL/min/1.73 m² (see text for discussion of dietary intake for patients with less severe renal insufficiency).

[b]The protein intake is increased by 1.0 g/d of high biologic value protein for each gram per day of urinary protein loss.

[c]When recommended, intake is expressed per kilogram of body weight; this refers to the adjusted edema-to-body weight (see text).

[d]Refers to percentage of total energy intake (diet plus dialysate); if triglyceride levels are very high, the percentage of fat in the diet may be increased to about 40% of total calories; otherwise, 30% of total calories is preferable.

[e]These dietary recommendations are considered less crucial than the others. They are only emphasized if the patient has a specific disorder that may benefit from this modification or has expressed interest in this dietary prescription and is complying well to more important aspects of the dietary treatment (see text).

[f]Should be primarily complex carbohydrates.

[g]Can be higher in patients on CAPD or in patients on hemodialysis or nondialyzed patients with chronic renal failure who have greater urinary losses.

[h]Phosphate binders (aluminum carbonate, or hydroxide, or calcium carbonate, acetate, or citrate) often are needed to maintain normal serum phosphorus levels.

[i]Dietary intake usually must be supplemented to provide these levels. Higher daily calcium intakes are commonly ingested because of the use of calcium binders of phosphate.

[j]≥10 mg/d for men and nonmenstruating women; ≥18 mg/d for menstruating women. For individuals receiving erythropoietin large iron intakes, usually given intravenously may be necessary (see text).

[k]Folic acid, 1 mg/d, is adequate for patients with chronic renal failure and on maintenance dialysis except with the common occurrence of hyperhomocysteinemia, where folic acid, 5 to 15 mg/d is more effective at maximizing the reduction in plasma homocysteine concentrations (see text).

[l]Vitamin K supplements may be needed for patients who are not eating and who receive antibiotics.

(see previous discussion). Nitrogen balance studies suggest that most patients on MHD require more than 1.0 g of protein per kilogram of body weight per day (125,234,235). The NKF K/DOQI Clinical Practice Guidelines for Nutrition recommend 1.2 g of protein per kilogram of body weight per day for clinically stable patients on MHD (236). To ensure adequate intake of essential amino acids, at least half of the dietary protein should be of high biologic value. This level of protein intake should maintain neutral or positive balance in almost all clinically stable patients on MHD.

Chronic Peritoneal Dialysis

Blumenkrantz et al. (237) studied protein and mineral balances in eight clinically stable men who underwent 13 metabolic balance studies of 14 to 33 days' duration in a clinical research center. Patients were fed diets that provided an average of 0.98 g of protein per kilogram of body weight per day or 1.44 g of protein per kilogram per day. Total energy (caloric) intake (diet plus dialysate) was 173.5 ± 8.0 kJ/kg (41.3 ± 1.9 and 42.1 ± 1.2 kcal/kg) per day with the low- and high-protein diets, respectively. Nitrogen balance, adjusted for changes in BUN but not for unmeasured losses, was +0.35 ± 0.83 g per day with the 1.0 g of protein per kilogram diet and +2.94 ± 0.54 g per day with the higher protein intake (the P value was not significant). Only the latter diet was significantly different from zero, even if nitrogen balances were adjusted by about 1.0 g per day for losses through skin, respiration, flatus, and blood sampling. There was a curvilinear relationship between dietary protein intake and nitrogen balance in the 13 studies (Fig. 103-1). Nitrogen balance rose as protein intake increased until protein intake was 1.09 g of protein per kilogram of body weight per day. At this level, balance was significantly positive. As dietary protein intake increased to more than this level, there was no further increment in nitrogen balance.

These findings are similar to those of Giordano et al. (238), who reported neutral to positive nitrogen balance in seven of eight patients on CAPD who were fed about 1.2 g of protein per kilogram per day. Gahl et al. (239) reported neutral or positive nitrogen balance in five outpatients undergoing CAPD who were ingesting lower protein diets that provided 0.71 to 0.96 g of protein per kilogram per day, but feces were not collected. Lindholm et al. (240) carried out short-term (10- to 14-day) balance studies in ten patients undergoing CAPD who were fed diets containing 0.76 to 1.07 g of protein per kilogram per day. Total energy intake was about 121.8 kJ (29 kcal) per kilogram of body weight per day. Nitrogen balance, adjusted for unmeasured losses, was positive in all patients. However, there was a positive correlation between protein intake and nitrogen balance in these patients.

Based on the foregoing reports, it seems prudent to prescribe 1.2 to 1.3 g of protein per kilogram of body weight per day to patients on CAPD. Indeed, the NKF K/DOQI Clinical Practice Guidelines for Nutrition recommend 1.2 to 1.3 g of

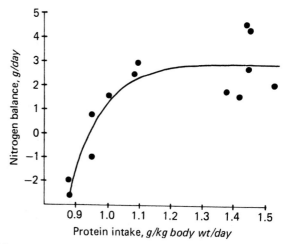

FIG. 103-1. Relationship between dietary protein intake and nitrogen balance measured in 13 studies in eight men undergoing continuous ambulatory peritoneal dialysis. Each circle represents the mean balance data observed in an individual patient fed a constant diet for 14 to 33 days in a clinical research unit. The curved line represents the calculated relationship between nitrogen balance and protein intake. (From Blumenkrantz MJ, Kopple JD, Moran JK, et al. Metabolic balance studies and dietary protein requirements in patients undergoing continuous ambulatory peritoneal dialysis. *Kidney Int* 1982;21:849, with permission.)

protein per kilogram per day for clinically stable patients on CPD (241). As with patients on MHD, at least 50% of the dietary protein should be of high biologic value. It is possible that patients on CAPD who are protein depleted may become more anabolic when they ingest up to 1.5 g of protein per kilogram per day (Fig. 103-1). In most patients on CAPD, BUN levels and uremic toxicity should be adequately controlled with this protein intake, although there may be a need in some patients to increase the number of dialysate exchanges or at least the volume of dialysate outflow.

The author is unaware of any studies concerning dietary protein requirements of patients undergoing APD. Because the protein and amino acid losses with these latter peritoneal dialysis techniques should not be much different than with those with CAPD, the dietary requirements are probably similar to those of the patient receiving CAPD. There have been other nitrogen balance studies in patients on MHD or CPD (242–244). However, nitrogen intake or output was not directly measured in these investigations. Because measurement of nitrogen balances requires rigor and precision to obtain accurate data (245), the results of these latter studies are difficult to interpret.

It has been shown that patients classified as high peritoneal transporters by the peritoneal equilibration test lose more protein and amino acids into peritoneal dialysate than those classified as low transporters (e.g., typical 24-hour losses in high versus low transporters: albumin, 4.9 ± 2 [SD] versus 3.2 ± 1 g per day, P < 0.03; total free amino acids, 15.4 ± 4 versus 10 ± 4 mmol per day, P = 0.002) (193–194a). This trend is shown in all studies of high versus low transporters. The high transporters have also been shown to have lower serum albumin levels (246,247). The difference in protein and amino acid losses with high versus low transporters, however, is not great. Dietary protein intakes of 1.2 to 1.3 g/kg per day should provide sufficient amounts of protein and amino acids to compensate for the increased peritoneal losses if the endogenous synthetic function for serum proteins is normal.

Some nephrologists describe patients on MHD or CPD who have dietary protein intakes of about 0.9 to 1.0 g/kg per day as not appearing protein depleted and leading physically active, rehabilitated lives. These observations have raised questions as to whether the foregoing recommended dietary protein intake may be excessive for patients on MHD. Several comments may be pertinent in this regard. The number of patients on MHD or CPD who have undergone careful nitrogen balance or other studies of their dietary protein requirements is small, and conclusions concerning their dietary protein needs therefore are somewhat imprecise. Moreover, some patients on MHD who appear to be doing well will, on close inspection, turn out to have evidence for protein depletion. On the other hand, the concept of dietary allowances presupposes that to ensure a sufficient nutrient intake for virtually all individuals within a given population, the recommended allowance must be greater than the actual requirement for a large proportion of that population (248). Thus, if the recommended dietary protein allowance is 1.2 to 1.3 g/kg per day, it is to be expected that many patients will tolerate lower protein intakes without developing protein depletion. However, there is no known method that will identify in advance, under the conditions of clinical practice, which patients can safely ingest lower levels of protein. Hence, to be safe, the patients should be prescribed the recommended dietary allowance, an especially relevant consideration given the high incidence of protein malnutrition in patients on MHD and CPD. Finally, subtle forms of malnutrition are particularly difficult to detect. The recommended protein intakes may provide some protection against mild forms of protein malnutrition. In this regard, more recent data suggest that a healthy serum albumin concentration may be about 4.0 to 5.0 g/dL, which is higher than the not uncommonly used standard of 3.5 to 5.0 g/dL (52).

Energy

In nondialyzed patients with CRF and patients undergoing MHD or CAPD, energy expenditure, measured by indirect calorimetry, appears to be normal during resting and sitting, after ingestion of a standard meal, and with defined exercise (235,249–254). In one study of patients on MHD, resting energy expenditure was slightly increased by 7.3% (253). Resting energy expenditure also has been reported to be increased during the hemodialysis procedure in one study (253); but this elevation in energy expenditure may have been due to the specific dynamic action from recently ingested foods. What is most impressive about the foregoing studies is that there is

no report of decreased energy expenditure in patients with CRF, on MHD or CPD.

Nitrogen balance studies in nondialyzed chronically uremic patients ingesting 0.55 to 0.60 g of protein per kilogram per day indicate that the amount of energy intake necessary to ensure neutral or positive nitrogen balance is approximately 147 kJ/kg (35 kcal/kg) per day (235). In clinically stable patients undergoing MHD who ingested 1.13 ± 0.02 (SEM) g of protein per kilogram per day, nitrogen balance study results and anthropometric measurements indicate that close to 159.6 kJ/kg (38 kcal/kg) per day may be necessary to maintain body mass (255). On the other hand, virtually every study of the dietary habits of nondialyzed chronically uremic patients and patients on MHD indicates that their mean energy intakes are lower than this level, usually about 100.8 to 113.4 kJ/kg (24 to 27 kcal/kg) per day (36,42,91,256). Chronically uremic children also have low energy intakes (40,257–259). Indeed, food preferences and eating habits are altered in patients with CRF (256,260). The finding that in nondialyzed patients with advanced CRF or patients undergoing MHD, decreased body fat is one of the more prominent alterations in nutritional status supports the contention that these patients require more energy than they usually ingest (36,38,42).

There are no nitrogen balance studies in patients on CPD in which protein intake has been kept constant while energy intake was varied; although as indicated already, resting energy expenditure in patients on CAPD is not different than that of healthy subjects (252). Many patients undergoing CAPD tend to gain body fat and weight (41), probably due to the glucose uptake from dialysate exchanges. The surges in plasma insulin concentration that accompany the peritoneal instillation of fresh dialysate and enhanced glucose absorption may also contribute to the increase in body fat of patients on CPD. The quantity of glucose absorbed from CAPD is reported to vary between 78 and 316 g per day (102b,261–264). There is a close correlation between the quantity of glucose instilled into the peritoneal cavity each day (x) and the quantity of glucose absorbed (Y) (263); Y (grams per day) $= 0.89x$ (grams per day) -43; R $= 0.91$. In any individual patient, the daily rate of glucose absorption with the same dialysis regimen was very constant.

The NKF K/DOQI Clinical Practice Guidelines for Nutrition recommend that the energy intake for nondialyzed patients with CRF (GFR of less than 25 mL per minute) and for patients on MHD and CPD should be 147 kJ/kg (35 kcal/kg) per day for individuals who are younger than 60 years and 126 to 147 kJ/kg (30 to 35 kcal/kg) per day for those who are 60 or more years of age (Table 103-5) (265,266). This intake includes energy derived from the diet and from any fuels taken up from dialysate in patients on MHD or CPD. Because individuals older than 60 years tend to be more sedentary, their recommended energy intake is somewhat lower. These recommendations are rather similar to those for healthy individuals engaged in light to moderate activity, as put forth in the Recommended Dietary Allowances by the Food and

Nutrition Board, National Academy of Sciences (248). Patients who are obese with an edema-free body weight of more than 120% of desirable body weight may be treated with lower energy intakes. Some patients, particularly those with more mild renal insufficiency and young or middle-aged women, may become obese on this energy intake level or may refuse to ingest the recommended calories out of fear of obesity. These individuals may require a lower energy prescription.

As indicated already, energy (and protein) intake seem to decrease when the GFR falls to about 35 to 50 mL per minute per $1.73m^2$ (see previous discussion) (88). Thus, to prevent malnutrition, it is important to monitor dietary intake and to treat inadequate intakes, even in clinically stable healthy appearing adults, when the GFR decreases to this level. This level of GFR may be associated with a serum creatinine level of as low as 1.4 to 2.5 mg/dL in some adult patients.

There are many commercially available high-calorie foodstuffs that are low in protein, sodium, and potassium. The renal dietitian can recommend these products and other low-protein, high-calorie foods that can be prepared easily at home.

Treatment of Risk Factors for Vascular Disease

Lipids

There are a number of reviews of the causes for the abnormal serum lipids and lipoproteins in these patients (21–23,26). Because these alterations may contribute to the high incidence of atherosclerosis and cardiovascular disease in uremic patients, attention has been directed toward reducing serum triglyceride and LDL cholesterol levels and increasing HDL cholesterol level. Elevated serum triglyceride levels in uremia appear to be caused primarily by impaired catabolism of triglyceride-rich lipoproteins (27,266a,266b). Also, because diets for patients with renal failure are usually restricted in protein, sodium, potassium, and water, it is often difficult to provide sufficient energy without resorting to a large intake of purified sugars that may increase triglyceride production. Activities of plasma and hepatic lipoprotein lipase and lecithin-cholesterol acyltransferase are reduced (21,22,26). CPD, which provides a glucose load, appears to promote a further increase in serum triglyceride and cholesterol levels.

Serum triglyceride levels may be lowered by feeding a diet in which the carbohydrate content is reduced to about 35% of total calories, the fat content is increased to about 55% of total calories, and the polyunsaturated fatty acid : saturated fatty acid ratio is raised to about 1.5 : 1.0 (27,266a). However, the evidence that high cholesterol and fat intakes enhance the risk for arteriosclerotic vascular disease indicates that such a diet is inadvisable, particularly because hypertriglyceridemia is a weak risk factor for arteriosclerotic heart disease. ω-3 Fatty acids (e.g., eicosapentaenoic acid and docosahexaenoic acid, which are found in fish oil) lower serum triglyceride levels and have more variable effects on serum

LDL cholesterol and HDL cholesterol levels (267). Fish oil also decreases platelet aggregation and appears to exert anti-inflammatory effects (268), and ω-3 fatty acids may enhance immune function. Low-fat diets and lipid-lowering medicines retard the rate of progression of renal failure in animal models (269–271). In humans, some research suggests that ω-3 fatty acids may lower the progression of renal failure in patients who have undergone renal transplantation (272). A preponderance of studies suggests that ω-3 fatty acids given as fish oil may retard the rate of progression of immunoglobulin A nephropathy (273–276).

Abnormal carnitine metabolism (see later discussion) has been implicated as a cause of hypertriglyceridemia in CRF. However, the many studies of treatment of hypertriglyceridemia with carnitine in patients with CRF are divided between substantial numbers that show carnitine lowers serum triglyceride levels and substantial numbers that show no change or, rarely, a rise in serum triglyceride levels (278,279). Ingestion of activated charcoal may lower serum cholesterol and triglyceride levels in chronically azotemic rats (280).

Clofibrate also lowers serum triglyceride levels in uremic patients, but because of the altered pharmacokinetics of this drug in patients with renal failure, there is a substantial risk of developing myopathy or other toxicities (281). 3-Hydroxy-3-methylglutaryl coenzyme A (HMG CoA) reductase inhibitors, which block cholesterol synthesis, are the most effective components for lowering serum levels of cholesterol and certain apolipoproteins in patients with the nephrotic syndrome or renal failure (282). The reduction in serum total and LDL cholesterol and in apolipoprotein B-100 concentrations in these individuals averages roughly 30%, and some HMG CoA reductase inhibitors are even more potent at lowering serum total and LDL cholesterol levels (282). These inhibitors may also increase serum HDL cholesterol level by roughly 10% and appear to have antiinflammatory or vascular endothelium.

At present, we recommend a National Cholesterol Education Program (NCEP)–American Heart Association (AHA) Step I diet for nondialyzed patients with CRF and patients on maintenance dialysis (283). This diet provides no more than 30% of total calories from fat, less than 10% of total calories from saturated fat, and 300 mg per day or less of cholesterol. We treat hypertriglyceridemia by dietary modification only when serum triglyceride levels are more than slightly elevated (e.g., at least 50 to 100 mg/dL more than the upper given limit of normal). In this situation, dietary fat intake may be increased, but not more than 40% of total calories. A high proportion of dietary carbohydrates should be complex. These modifications often lower the palatability of the diet; therefore, the patient's total energy intake must be monitored closely to ensure that it does not fall. With high serum triglyceride values that are unresponsive to dietary therapy, clofibrate may be tried cautiously. L-Carnitine, at about 500 to 1,000 mg per day, or for hemodialysis patients, at 10 to 20 mg/kg per day at the end of each dialysis three times weekly, may be tried if hypertriglyceridemia is severe and unresponsive to these treatments. Hypercholesterolemia may be treated with an HMG CoA reductase inhibitor in addition to a Step I or Step II AHA diet (282).

It should be pointed out that there are almost no long-term data on the effects of dietary fat and carbohydrate intake or changing serum lipid levels on the clinical course of patients with specific renal diseases, the nephrotic syndrome, renal failure, or a renal transplant. Paradoxically, in contrast to healthy adults (284,285), patients on MHD in whom the body weight–for-height value is in the upper 50th or higher percentile for individuals undergoing MHD have increased probability of survival (155,156). The recommendations given here are largely based on epidemiologic data or long-term clinical trials in populations without renal disease, on the recognition that patients with renal disease or renal failure have a high incidence of abnormal serum lipid and lipoprotein levels and atherosclerotic vascular disease, as well as on the research indicating that high lipid intakes or elevated lipoprotein levels may accelerate the rate of progression of renal failure in animals with renal disease.

Oxidant and Carbonyl Stress

Evidence suggests that end-stage renal disease is associated with oxidant and carbonyl stress and often with a state of chronic inflammation, and that these factors may promote atherosclerotic and proliferative vascular disease (28–32) (see previous discussion). There are no interventional trials evaluating the effects of reducing these risk factors on morbidity or mortality rate of patients with CRF or on MHD. Nevertheless, the high risk of cardiovascular disease and the evidence for oxidant and carbonyl stress and inflammation in these patients have raised questions as to whether the following treatments may be beneficial for these individuals. Larger flux dialyzers that remove greater amounts of advanced glycation end products, and other reactive carbonyl compounds may be helpful. It is possible to ingest antioxidants or antioxidant precursors, such as Vitamins E or C (see the latter section on vitamins) or selenium. Supplemental selenium must be taken with caution because selenium is primarily excreted in the urine and may accumulate in renal failure (286). Also, it is difficult to measure the body selenium burden because it is protein bound in plasma and the possibility of altered concentrations or binding affinities for the binding protein makes it difficult to identify selenium excess. β-Carotene, one glass per day of an alcoholic drink, perhaps particularly of red wine, HMG CoA reductase inhibitors, and regular exercise may also reduce oxidant stress (287).

Homocysteine

Plasma homocysteine level is increased in nondialyzed patients with CRF as well as in about 85% to 90% of patients on MHD and CPD (288–296). The mechanism for this increase is unclear but may involve impaired remethylation of homocysteine back to methionine (289). Elevated plasma homocysteine level is associated with a high incidence of cardiovascular disease possibly through three biochemical mechanisms (288): homocysteine oxidation generating hydrogen peroxide, decreased methylation reaction due to accumulation of S-adenosylhomocysteine, and acylation of proteins by homocysteine thiolactone. These processes lead to damaged membrane proteins, endothelial injury, inhibition of endothelial cell growth, and other effects. Hyperhomocysteinemia has been shown to be a risk factor for cardiovascular disease in renal failure in some (291–294) but not all (296) epidemiologic studies. In addition to renal failure, low serum folate levels, and possibly protein-energy malnutrition (293), a common mutation in the methylenetetrahydrofolate reductase gene, C677T, is associated with higher plasma homocysteine concentrations (290).

Vitamin B_6 is a cofactor for cystathionine synthetase, which catalyzes the conversion of methionine to cystathionine, and for cystathionase, which converts cystathionine to cysteine. Pyridoxine HCl, a form of Vitamin B_6, generally does not lower plasma homocysteine concentration in patients with CRF or on MHD. The folate metabolite, tetrahydrofolic acid, is necessary for the remethylation of homocysteine to re-form methionine, and folic acid or folinic acid supplements will often decrease plasma homocysteine concentrations in nondialyzed patients with CRF and on maintenance dialysis, although usually not to within the normal range (294–296) (also, see the latter vitamin section). The lowest dose of folic acid associated with the maximum lowering effect on plasma homocysteine level appears to be about 5 to 15 mg per day (294–296).

Carbohydrates

Patients should be encouraged to eat complex rather than purified carbohydrates to reduce triglyceride synthesis and to improve glucose tolerance if it is abnormal.

Carnitine

Carnitine is a naturally occurring compound that is essential for life. It is both synthesized in the body and ingested. Carnitine facilitates the transfer of long-chain (more than 10 carbon) fatty acids into muscle mitochondria (278,279). Because fatty acids are the major fuel source for skeletal and myocardial muscle at rest and during mild to moderate exercise, this activity is considered necessary for normal skeletal and cardiac muscle function. It is also argued that carnitine normally serves a detoxifying function by removing fatty acids from CoA (i.e., from acyl-CoA), thereby forming acylcarnitine and free CoA. Acyl-CoA is toxic or inhibitory for a number of biochemical reactions.

Patients with advanced CRF display low serum free carnitine level and, in some studies, low skeletal muscle free and total carnitine levels (69,278,279,297–300). Also, in CRF, serum and, in some reports, muscle acylcarnitine levels (fatty acid–carnitine compounds) are increased, and serum total carnitine level (i.e., acylcarnitines plus free carnitine) is within the normal range or elevated (69,278,279,299,300). The low serum and skeletal muscle free carnitine levels have led some investigators to postulate that many patients with CRF are carnitine deficient. Such a deficiency could be due to impaired synthesis of carnitine *in vivo,* reduced dietary intake of carnitine, and removal of carnitine by dialysis (278,279). However, the weekly loss of free carnitine by dialysis is approximately equal to the normal weekly urinary excretion of carnitine, and the administration of oral or intravenous carnitine usually does not lead to a sudden change in clinical status of the patient. These findings suggest that a simple deficiency of carnitine is not the sole cause of carnitine disorders in patients with CRF. The theory has been advanced that production of acylcarnitine is enhanced in patients with CRF and those on maintenance dialysis due to alterations in lipid or carnitine metabolism (301). Another theory contends that increased concentrations of acylcarnitines interfere with normal carnitine physiology (279,302).

A number of clinical trials in patients with CRF, particularly those undergoing maintenance dialysis therapy, suggest that L-carnitine may provide clinical benefits. The types of improvement that have been described in randomized, prospective studies include increased physical exercise capacity, reduced interdialytic symptoms of skeletal muscle cramps or hypertension, or improvement in overall global sense of well being (303,304). A decrease in predialysis serum urea level, creatinine level, and phosphorus concentration and an increase in midarm muscle circumference have been reported (303); the mechanisms responsible for these effects are not clear. In this regard, one study suggests that L-carnitine added to peritoneal dialysate may increase nitrogen balance in patients on CAPD who have protein-energy malnutrition (305). Other studies, usually nonrandomized, suggest that carnitine may increase hematocrit level, reduce cardiac arrhythmias, and improve ventricular function in patients on maintenance dialysis (304,306–309).

Many nephrologists remain unconvinced by the published results of carnitine benefits. The reasons are that a number of the studies were not well designed (e.g., not prospective and randomized or not double-blinded), the results were not consistent in all studies, the outcome measures were often soft or difficult to quantify precisely, and it seems that patients may not respond to carnitine treatment for up to several months. Nonetheless, the preponderance of published studies concerning carnitine in patients on maintenance dialysis appears to show benefits. Also, L-carnitine appears to be a safe agent.

The NKF K/DOQI Clinical Practice Guidelines for Nutrition (310) conclude that "there are insufficient data to support the routine use of L-carnitine for maintenance dialysis patients." Although the administration of L-carnitine may improve subjective symptoms such as malaise, muscle weakness, intradialytic cramps and hypotension, and quality of life in selected patients on maintenance dialysis, the totality of evidence is insufficient to recommend its routine provision for any proposed clinical disorder without prior evaluation and attempts at standard therapy. "The most promising of proposed applications is treatment of erythropoietin (EPO)-resistant anemia."

Until more definitive studies are available, it is the author's policy to use L-carnitine for patients on MHD or CPD who satisfy both of the following conditions: (a) disabling or very bothersome skeletal muscle weakness or cardiomyopathy, skeletal muscle cramps or hypotension during hemodialysis treatment, severe malaise, or anemia refractory to EPO therapy for no apparent reason; and (b) the conditions listed do not respond to more standard treatment. The patient is given a 3- to 6-month trial of L-carnitine (up to 9 months for refractory anemia). If there is no measurable improvement in symptoms by the end of the treatment period, carnitine therapy is discontinued. L-Carnitine may be administered orally, intravenously, or into dialysate. Oral L-carnitine is less expensive but has been less well studied than intravenous carnitine for patients on maintenance dialysis. The optimal dose of carnitine is not well defined. Some workers use a carnitine dose of 20 mg/kg at the end of each hemodialysis treatment, three times weekly (300,304).

Sodium

Normally, the renal tubules reabsorb more than 99% of the filtered sodium (311). As renal insufficiency progresses, both the GFR and the fractional reabsorption of sodium fall progressively. Thus, many patients with renal failure are able to maintain sodium balance with a normal sodium intake. In both healthy individuals and patients with CRF, only about 1 to 3 mEq per day of sodium is excreted in the feces, and in the absence of visible sweating, only a few milliequivalents per day of sodium is lost through the skin. Despite the adaptive reduction in the renal tubular reabsorption of sodium, patients with advanced renal failure may be unable to excrete the quantity of sodium ingested, and they may develop edema, hypertension, and congestive heart failure. This syndrome is particularly likely to occur when the GFR is less than 4 to 10 mL per minute. When congestive heart failure, the nephrotic syndrome, or advanced liver disease complicates renal insufficiency, the propensity for sodium retention is increased. In patients with renal failure, hypertension often is more easily controlled when they are sodium restricted, and hypertension may be accentuated by an increased sodium intake, probably because of expanded extracellular fluid volume (312) and possibly due to altered intracellular electrolyte composition within arteriolar smooth muscle cells that increase contractility. With a decreased ability to excrete sodium or an expanded extracellular fluid volume, restriction of sodium and water intake and the use of diuretic medications may be necessary.

Nondialyzed patients with CRF often have an inability to conserve sodium normally (6). A low sodium intake may not be sufficient to replace urinary and extrarenal sodium losses, and the patient may develop sodium depletion, a decrease in extracellular fluid volume, blood volume, and renal blood flow, as well as a further reduction in GFR (i.e., prerenal insufficiency superimposed on CRF). Volume depletion may be difficult to recognize. Unexplained weight loss or reduction in blood pressure may be signs of volume depletion. If the nondialyzed patient with CRF does not show evidence of fluid overload, hypertension, or heart failure, he or she may be cautiously given a greater sodium intake to determine whether the GFR can be improved slightly by extracellular volume expansion.

The antiproteinuric effects of angiotensin-converting enzyme (ACE) inhibitors are substantially abrogated by high-sodium diets; as urinary sodium excretion rises to more than about 100 mEq per day, the antiproteinuric effects abate (313). Treatment with a thiazide diuretic appears to almost completely reestablish the urinary protein lowering effects of the ACE inhibitors in the presence of these higher sodium intakes (313).

Usually, when sodium balance is well controlled, the thirst mechanism will regulate water balance adequately. However, when the GFR falls to less than 2 to 5 mL per minute, the risk of overhydration increases, and water intake should be controlled independently of sodium to prevent overhydration. In patients with diabetes mellitus, hyperglycemia may also increase thirst and enhance positive water balance. For patients with far advanced renal failure whose total body water amount is considered appropriate (as indicated by normal or near-normal blood pressure, absence of edema, and normal serum sodium level), urine volume may be a good guide to water intake; the daily water intake should equal the urine output plus approximately 500 mL to replace insensible losses.

In most nondialyzed patients with advanced renal failure, a daily intake of 1,000 to 3,000 mg (40 to 130 mEq) of sodium and 1,500 to 3,000 mL of fluid will maintain sodium and water balance. The requirement for sodium and water varies markedly, and each patient must be managed individually. Patients undergoing MHD or peritoneal dialysis frequently are oliguric or anuric. For patients on hemodialysis, sodium and total fluid intake generally should be restricted to 1,000 to 1,500 mg per day and 700 to 1,500 mEq per day, respectively. Because sodium and water can be removed easily with CAPD or other forms of CPD, a more liberal salt and water intake is usually allowed. By maintaining a larger dietary sodium and water intake, the patient can increase the quantity of fluid removed, thereby increasing the daily dialysate outflow volume. This may be advantageous, because with CPD, the daily clearance of small- and medium-sized molecules is directly related to the volume of dialysate outflow. Thus, for some patients on CPD, a higher sodium and water intake (e.g., 6 to 8 g of sodium per day and 3 L of water per day) may enable the patient to use more hypertonic glucose exchanges to increase the dialysate outflow volume, thereby increasing dialysate clearances and glucose and energy uptake from dialysate. This treatment may be undesirable for obese or hypertriglyceridemic patients because the greater use of hypertonic glucose exchanges will increase their glucose load. Also, there is the potential disadvantage that some patients may become habituated to high salt and water intakes; if they

change to hemodialysis therapy, they may have difficulty in curtailing their sodium and water intake.

In nondialyzed, chronically uremic patients or patients undergoing maintenance dialysis who are not anuric and who gain excessive sodium or water despite attempts at dietary restriction, a potent diuretic, such as furosemide, may be tried to increase urinary sodium and water excretion.

Potassium

The kidney normally is the major vehicle for potassium excretion. In renal failure, potassium retention may occur and cause fatal hyperkalemia. Three factors may counteract this side effect of renal failure: First, when the urine volume is approximately 1,000 mL per day or more, the tubular secretion of potassium per unit GFR tends to increase, and therefore the renal potassium clearance does not fall as markedly as the GFR. Second, in both nondialyzed patients with CRF and patients on MHD and CPD, the fecal excretion of potassium increases, probably due to enhanced intestinal secretion (194,237). Third, potassium intake tends to fall as a result of anorexia and in response to dietary counseling.

Thus, patients with CRF usually do not become hyperkalemic unless there is (a) excessive intake of potassium; (b) acidemia, oliguria, and hypoaldosteronism (e.g., secondary to decreased renin secretion by the diseased kidney or renal tubular resistance to the actions of aldosterone); (c) catabolic stress; or (d) possibly hypoinsulinism or use of medicines such as potassium-sparing diuretics, nonsteroidal antiinflammatory drugs, ACE inhibitors, and [SC]-receptor blockers (315). Patients with CRF and those undergoing MHD should generally receive no more than 70 mEq of potassium per day.

Magnesium

In nondialyzed patients with CRF and in patients on maintenance dialysis, there is a net absorption of about 40% to 50% of ingested magnesium from the intestinal tract (net absorption is the difference between dietary intake and fecal excretion) (237,316). Because the absorbed magnesium is excreted primarily by the kidney, hypermagnesemia may occur in patients with renal failure (317). Magnesium also commonly accrues in bone in renal failure and may play a causal role in renal osteodystrophy (318). The restricted diets of uremic patients are low in magnesium (usually about 100 to 300 mg per day for a 40-g-protein diet), and the patients' serum magnesium levels are therefore usually within the normal range or only slightly elevated unless the patient takes substances that are high in magnesium content, such as magnesium-containing antacids and laxatives (316,317). Nondialyzed chronically uremic patients require about 200 mg of magnesium per day to maintain neutral magnesium balance (316). The optimal dietary magnesium allowance for the patient on dialysis has not been well defined. Experience suggests that when the magnesium content is about 1.0 mEq/L in hemodialysate or 0.50 to 0.75 mEq/L in peritoneal dialysate, a dietary magnesium intake of 200 to 300 mg per day will maintain the serum magnesium at normal or only slightly elevated levels.

Phosphorus and Phosphate Binders

The rationale for controlling dietary phosphorus and the use of gastrointestinal binders of phosphate is to prevent and treat hyperphosphatemia, a high serum calcium–phosphorus product, calcium phosphate deposition in soft tissue, and hyperparathyroidism. This section considers the prescription of dietary phosphorus intake and phosphate binders. In patients with renal failure, a large dietary phosphorus intake can lead to a high plasma calcium–phosphorus product with increased risk of calcium and phosphate deposition in soft tissues. Also, animal and human studies suggest the possibility that a low phosphorus intake may reduce the rate of progression of renal failure in individuals with chronic renal disease (319–322).

There are few data concerning the optimal level of phosphorus restriction for retarding progressive renal failure or for minimizing or preventing hyperparathyroidism. One approach for nondialyzed patients is to maintain normal renal tubular reabsorption of phosphorus to avoid elevated serum parathyroid hormone levels. This approach requires a very low phosphorus intake, lower than can usually be obtained with the combination of a low-phosphorus diet and phosphate binders unless keto acid– or essential amino acid–supplemented very-low-protein diets are used and the GFR is more than 15 mL per minute. At the very least, in both nondialyzed and dialyzed patients, the morning fasting serum phosphorus concentrations should be always maintained within the normal range. Because there is a rough correlation between the protein and the phosphorus content of the diet, it is much easier to reduce phosphorus intake if a lower protein diet is used.

For patients who have a GFR between 25 and 70 mL per minute per 1.73 m^2 or who have a higher GFR with progressive loss of renal function, 5 to 10 mg of phosphorus per kilogram of body weight per day may be prescribed with the 0.55 to 0.60 g of protein per kilogram per day diet. These individuals generally are not given phosphate binders unless the serum phosphorus concentration increases to more than the upper limit of normal. For nondialyzed patients with a GFR of less than 25 mL per minute per 1.73 m^2 who are prescribed a diet of 0.55 to 0.60 g of protein per kilogram per day, the phosphorus intake generally can be decreased to about 5 to 10 mg/kg per day, although this may increase the burdensomeness of the diet, particularly at the lower end of this range of phosphorus intake. Without phosphate binders, there is a net intestinal phosphate absorption (diet minus fecal phosphorus) of roughly 60% of the phosphorus intake (316). Therefore, this level of dietary phosphorus restriction usually will not maintain normal serum phosphorus concentrations in patients with a GFR of less than about 15 mL per minute, even with a substantial reduction in the renal tubular reabsorption of phosphorus. Hence, phosphate binders are also employed.

The recommended phosphorus intake for patients on MHD or CPD is about 17 mg/kg per day or less. This higher upper limit was chosen because with their greater protein intakes, patients on dialysis cannot readily ingest less phosphorus without making the diet too restrictive. Patients on maintenance dialysis almost always require phosphate binders to prevent hyperphosphatemia.

Traditionally, the two most commonly used phosphate binders have been aluminum carbonate and aluminum hydroxide. Usually, two to four 500-mg capsules taken three to four times per day are needed. Larger dosages may be used if necessary. Evidence that aluminum-induced osteomalacia and other toxicities may be caused by the intake of aluminum phosphate binders has led nephrologists to use calcium salts to bind phosphate (323–326). Calcium carbonate, calcium citrate, and calcium acetate have been used for this purpose (327–330). Of these three compounds, calcium acetate may have the greatest binding affinity to phosphate and may be more effective at lowering serum parathyroid hormone levels (330–332). Intestinal calcium absorption may or may not be lowered with calcium acetate (330–332). However, calcium acetate appears to cause more side effects such as nausea, diarrhea, and constipation (332). This may be the cause of poorer compliance described with calcium acetate tablets (332). Hypercalcemia is reported to be less common with calcium acetate, compared with calcium carbonate (330). Calcium citrate enhances the intestinal absorption of aluminum (329) and should not be given with aluminum salts. Calcium binders should be taken in divided doses with meals and should not be prescribed if the serum phosphorus concentration is very high to avoid precipitation of calcium and phosphate in soft tissues. Thus, hyperphosphatemic patients may be treated with an aluminum binder of phosphate until serum phosphorus concentrations fall to within the normal range or near the normal range. At that time, the regimen may be changed to a calcium binder.

A new calcium-free and aluminum-free phosphate binder polymer, sevelamer hydrochloride, has become available. This is a hydrogel of a cross-linked poly(allylamine), is resistant to digestive degradation, and is not absorbed from the gastrointestinal tract (333–335). Two to four capsules of sevelamer hydrochloride with each meal appears to be roughly as effective as calcium and aluminum binders of phosphate and does not provide a calcium or aluminum load. Sevelamer hydrochloride also has the benefit of lowering serum total cholesterol and LDL cholesterol levels (336). It is generally well tolerated.

Aluminum and probably iron toxicity can cause a syndrome of low bone turnover, which has been referred to as *aplastic bone disease,* and which is characterized by low serum parathyroid hormone levels, decreased bone osteoblasts, and markedly reduced bone turnover (325,326,337). The large intakes of calcium binders, which are used to control serum phosphorus concentrations and in clinical practice may exceed 3 to 5 g per day of elemental calcium, potentially may also cause calcium deposits in soft tissues. It has been suggested that the large calcium intake from dietary calcium supplements or dialysate may also cause this syndrome of low bone turnover (338). Normally, patients should probably not receive more than about 2.0 g per day of elemental calcium to prevent excessive calcium. Because amino acid and keto acid formulations do not contain phosphorus, one advantage of very-low-protein diets supplemented with these preparations is the greater ease with which the phosphorus intake could be reduced, often to as low as 4 to 6 mg/kg per day. There is no well-defined safe lower limit for the serum phosphorus concentration in patients with renal failure. Experience suggests that if the fasting serum phosphorus concentration is maintained higher than the lower limit of normal, patients will not develop phosphate depletion.

Calcium

Nondialyzed patients with CRF and patients undergoing maintenance dialysis therapy have an increased dietary requirement for calcium because they have Vitamin D deficiency and resistance to the actions of Vitamin D. These abnormalities impair the intestinal absorption of calcium. The risk of calcium deficiency in these patients is enhanced because the diets prescribed for uremic patients are almost always low in calcium. Foods high in calcium content are usually high in phosphorus (e.g., dairy products) and are therefore restricted for uremic patients. For example, a 40-g-protein diet generally provides only about 300 to 400 mg of calcium per day, whereas the recommended dietary allowances for healthy, nonpregnant, nonlactating adults is about 800 to 1,200 mg per day (248).

Balance studies indicate that nondialyzed chronically uremic patients usually require about 1,200 to 1,600 mg of calcium per day for neutral or positive calcium balance (316). Total daily calcium intake (diet plus supplement) should therefore be maintained at about 1,400 to 1,600 mg per day (Table 103-5). Thus, the low-protein diets should be supplemented with about 1,000 to 1,400 mg of elemental calcium per day . As indicated already, slightly higher intakes (1,000 to 2,000 mg per day) of elemental calcium may be given as calcium carbonate, acetate, or citrate to bind phosphate in the intestinal tract. To prevent calcium phosphate deposition in soft tissues, the patients should not take the supplemental calcium unless the serum phosphorus concentration is within the normal range or near normal (i.e., 5.5 mg/dL or less). Frequent monitoring of serum calcium concentration also is important because hypercalcemia may develop, particularly if serum phosphorus concentrations fall lower than normal or low levels. Patients undergoing MHD or peritoneal dialysis may need 1.0 g per day of supplemental calcium, even though there is net calcium uptake from dialysis.

In patients on CAPD, the calcium uptake from dialysate is inversely correlated with the serum concentration of total calcium and ionized calcium (237,339,340). Net absorption of calcium from dialysate in patients on CAPD averages about 84 mg per day (237). The calcium balance across dialysate varies according to the serum ionized calcium level and is negative by roughly 80 mg per day in patients on CAPD who have serum ionized calcium values of more than 5 mg/dL and is positive by roughly 40 mg per day in patients with serum ionized calcium levels of less than 4.4 mg/dL (340). Also, the more hypertonic the peritoneal dialysate, the greater the dialysate outflow volume and hence the larger the calcium losses; in one report, a net calcium uptake of roughly 10 mg per exchange occurs with 1.5% dextrose, and a net calcium loss of 21 mg per exchange occurs with 4.25% dextrose (340). In patients on CAPD, calcium balance was usually neutral or positive when dietary calcium intake was 720 mg or more per day (237). Based on these observations, patients on CAPD should probably be given a total dietary calcium intake (diet plus dietary supplement) of about 800 to 1,000 mg per day.

The calcium content is 40% for calcium carbonate, 25% for calcium acetate, 21% for calcium citrate, 18% for calcium lactate, and 9% for calcium gluconate. In general, calcium chloride should not be given to chronically uremic patients because of its acidifying characteristics. Because calcium preparations may contain phosphorus and other ingredients, it is advisable to ascertain the composition of any new calcium preparation before prescribing it to a patient with renal insufficiency. Treatment with 1,25-dihydroxycholecalciferol will decrease the daily calcium requirement by enhancing intestinal calcium absorption (9,341).

Trace Elements

Trace element metabolism in CRF is discussed more extensively in Chapter, and this section covers dietary requirements. A number of factors in patients with renal failure tend to either increase or decrease the body burden of certain trace elements. Many trace elements are excreted primarily in the urine, and with renal failure, they may accumulate. Elements such as iron, zinc, and copper, which are protein bound, may be lost in excessive quantities when there are large urinary protein losses, for example, in the nephrotic syndrome (342). Excessive uptake or losses of trace elements may also occur during dialysis therapy depending on their relative concentrations in plasma and dialysate and the degree of binding to protein or red cells (343–347). Hemodialysis of copper, strontium, zinc, and lead, for example, which are largely bound to plasma proteins or red cells, should be minimal (343,344,348–350). Hemodialysis or hemodiafiltration may remove some trace elements if the dialysate concentrations are sufficiently low (e.g., bromide and zinc [351]). Zinc may be taken up and copper lost from peritoneal dialysis. Because many trace elements are bound avidly to serum proteins, they may be taken up by blood against a concentration gradient when present in even small quantities in dialysate (343,344,349,352). These observations provided part of the justification for purifying dialysate water before use (e.g., the reverse osmosis and ion exchange systems).

Protein-energy malnutrition, by lowering serum concentrations of proteins that bind trace elements, may decrease the serum levels of a number of these elements including zinc, manganese, and nickel (353). Occupational exposure or pica may increase the burden of some trace elements. Therapeutic doses of trace elements may be administered through dialysis, as has been done for zinc (70). The effect of the altered dietary intake of the uremic patient on body pools of trace elements is unknown (353). Oral and possibly intravenous iron supplements are often given to patients who are iron deficient.

Assessment of trace element burden in patients with renal failure is difficult because the binding protein concentrations may be decreased, thereby lowering serum trace element levels, and the binding characteristics of these proteins may be altered in renal failure. Also, red cell concentrations of trace elements may not reflect levels in other tissues. Trace element supplementation should be undertaken with caution because impaired urinary excretion and poor dialysance of trace elements increase the risk of overdosage.

Dietary requirements for trace elements have not been well defined in uremic patients. Iron deficiency is common, particularly in patients on MHD, because intestinal iron absorption is sometimes impaired, there are often substantial blood losses (see previous discussion), iron may bind to the dialyzer membrane, and the EPO-induced rise in hemoglobin levels may deplete the body's iron stores (11,12). Not only do iron requirements increase during the time EPO therapy is initiated and hemoglobin levels rise, but current data indicate that higher serum iron levels and body iron burden are associated with a greater response to EPO (354). Some researchers recommend that in general, patients on MHD or CPD should maintain serum transferrin saturation at 30% to 50% and serum ferritin at about 400 to 800 ng/mL (354–355a).

Although some patients on MHD may maintain these iron values with oral iron supplements, many such individuals will not be able to do so unless they receive parenteral iron therapy (354–355a). Oral ferrous sulfate (300 mg three times per day half an hour after meals) may be tried. Some patients develop anorexia, nausea, constipation, or abdominal pain with ferrous sulfate; these individuals sometimes will tolerate other iron compounds better, such as ferrous fumarate, gluconate, or lactate. Patients who are intolerant to oral iron supplements and the preponderance of patients on MHD or CPD who will not maintain the transferrin saturation level at 30% to 50% and serum ferritin levels of 400 to 800 ng/mL with oral iron may be treated with intramuscular or intravenous iron. Because of pain and risk or staining of skin with intramuscular iron injections, intravenous iron, ferrous gluconate, or iron dextran is generally the preferred method of administration.

Increased body burden of iron or aluminum in patients on hemodialysis or CPD may be reduced by infusion of deferoxamine, which is dialyzable (356). Care must be taken because deferoxamine may promote infection, particularly mucormycosis (357). Injections of EPO with repeated phlebotomy is another method for removing excess body iron (358).

Although the zinc content of most tissues is within the normal range in patients with renal failure (359), usually serum and hair zinc levels are reported to be low and red cell zinc increased (67,70,345,350,360–363). In nondialyzed chronically uremic patients, the fractional urinary excretion of zinc is increased; however, because the GFR is reduced, total urinary excretion of zinc may be decreased (363). Fecal zinc level is increased (350), and a dietary zinc intake of more than the recommended dietary allowance (248) may be necessary to maintain normal body zinc pools. Further studies are needed to confirm this. Some reports indicate that dysgeusia, poor food intake, and impaired sexual function, which are common problems of uremic patients, may be improved by giving patients zinc supplements (70,350,362,364). Other studies, however, have not confirmed this (365). Intestinal absorption of zinc is not affected by administration of 1,25-dihydroxycholecalciferol (366).

The finding that serum selenium level is low in patients on dialysis has raised the question of whether selenium supplements are indicated (367,368). This question is particularly important because selenium participates in the defense against oxidative damage of tissues, which may be increased in renal failure (369). Further research will be necessary to resolve this issue.

Vitamins

Chronically uremic patients have a high incidence of vitamin deficiencies. These are due to several factors. First, in renal failure, 1,25-dihydroxycholecalciferol production is impaired by the diseased kidney (17). Second, vitamin intake is often decreased in uremic patients because of anorexia and reduced food intake. Intercurrent illnesses, which occur frequently in chronically uremic patients (109–111), also impair food intake. Many foods that are high in water-soluble vitamins are often restricted for patients with renal failure because of the elevated protein and potassium content of these foods; the diets prescribed for nondialyzed patients with CRF and patients on maintenance dialysis frequently contain less than the recommended daily allowances for certain water-soluble vitamins (18,370). Third, renal failure appears to alter the absorption, metabolism, or activity of some vitamins. Animal studies indicate that intestinal absorption of riboflavin, folate, and Vitamin D_3 is impaired in renal failure (13–15). The metabolism of folate and pyridoxine appears to be abnormal in CRF (18,371). Fourth, certain medicines interfere with the intestinal absorption, metabolism, or actions of vitamins (18). Fifth, water-soluble vitamins are removed by dialysis (103–106,372).

On the other hand, Vitamin B_{12} deficiency is uncommon in CRF (18,373,377,378) because the daily requirement for this vitamin is small (e.g., 3 μg per day) for healthy nonpregnant, nonlactating adults) (248), the body stores large quantities of this vitamin, and even though Vitamin B_{12} is water soluble, it is protein bound in plasma and hence poorly dialyzed. There is a report of low serum Vitamin B_{12} concentrations in 19 of

60 patients on MHD (105); the serum Vitamin B_{12} concentrations tended to fall progressively over months of dialysis treatment, and serum Vitamin B_{12} levels correlated directly with nerve conduction velocities, which improved with ingestion of large quantities of Vitamin B_{12}. Another study reported low serum Vitamin B_{12} levels in four hemodialysis patients, only one of which demonstrated an intestinal absorption defect for Vitamin B_{12} (378). Their hematocrit level improved after receiving Vitamin B_{12} injections. The explanation for these discrepant reports of low serum Vitamin B_{12} levels in patients on MHD is not known.

Vitamin deficiencies have been observed with particular frequency for 1,25-dihydroxycholecalciferol, folic acid, Vitamin B_6, Vitamin C, and to a lesser extent, other water-soluble vitamins (18,103,104,106,370,373–375,379). Blood folate concentrations were reported to be decreased in patients undergoing MHD who did not take folic acid supplements (373–375). Several investigators found normal serum or red blood cell folate concentrations in patients undergoing MHD (106,373,380). However, although the mean plasma or red cell values may be within the normal range in some patients, a substantial number of patients have deficient levels (106,373,380). In addition, several investigators found hypersegmentation of polymorphonuclear leukocytes in these patients, which decreased after administration of folate supplements (66,375).

Some investigators noted that the reticulocyte count and hematocrit level rose when patients undergoing MHD were given folic acid supplements (66). We have observed normal serum folate concentrations in virtually all patients undergoing MHD who received 1.0 mg of supplemental folic acid per day (*unpublished observations*). Marumo et al. (381) reported higher folate levels in patients on hemodialysis, compared with controls, but the folate intake and type of dialysis were not indicated. Dietary folic acid requirements increase in patients with CRF when they commence EPO therapy and sustain a major rise in their hemoglobin level.

There are substantial losses of Vitamin C into dialysate (103,104,372). Low plasma and leukocyte ascorbic acid concentrations may occur in patients undergoing hemodialysis who were not receiving supplemental Vitamin C (103,372,382). Clinical signs suggestive of mild scurvy have been described in several patients on MHD with very low ascorbic acid concentrations (103). Administration of ascorbic acid orally or into the dialysate prevented negative Vitamin C balance during hemodialysis.

Many workers find evidence for low plasma or red blood cell Vitamin B_6 concentrations in subjects undergoing MHD or CPD who do not take supplemental Vitamin B_6 (66,68, 383–386). Activation coefficients of erythrocyte transaminase enzymes (i.e., the activity of the enzyme divided into the activity of the same enzyme after the Vitamin B_6 cofactor pyridoxal 5-phosphate is added to the assay) are not uncommonly elevated in patients undergoing MHD who do not receive supplemental Vitamin B_6, indicating that these subjects are deficient in Vitamin B_6 (68,383,384). Improve-

ment in the activation coefficient during hemodialysis has been reported, suggesting that there might be an inhibitor of Vitamin B_6 in uremic sera that is removed by dialysis (383). Low stimulation ratios in mixed lymphocyte cultures from these patients have been reported (383). Pyridoxine hydrochloride supplements improve several parameters of immune function in patients on hemodialysis including lymphoblast formation. These observations suggest that Vitamin B_6 deficiency, which is known to cause abnormal immunologic function (383,387), may be one cause of the altered immune response in uremic patients. Interestingly, serum glutamate-oxaloacetate transaminase activity is reduced in renal failure. This effect appears to be related to Vitamin B_6 activity, possibly due to a uremic inhibitor in serum (388–391).

Treatment with pyridoxine hydrochloride has been attempted for the following two metabolic disorders associated with potential adverse clinical consequences in patients with CRF: elevated plasma homocysteine levels and plasma oxalate concentrations. Plasma homocysteine level is increased in nondialyzed patients with CRF and patients on MHD and CPD (see previous discussion) and renal transplant recipients (see later discussion). Elevated plasma homocysteine level is of great concern, because it is a risk factor for occlusive vascular disease (392,393) (see previous discussion). Supplemental pyridoxine hydrochloride or Vitamin B_{12} taken alone has not been shown to reduce plasma homocysteine level in patients on MHD (393). Similarly, it is not evident that adding these vitamins to folic acid therapy lowers plasma homocysteine levels more effectively than equal doses of folic acid alone.

Disorders of folic acid may also contribute to elevated homocysteine levels because the folate metabolite, tetrahydrofolic acid, is necessary for the remethylation of homocysteine to re-form methionine. Folic acid and the combination of folic acid and pyridoxine hydrochloride have decreased plasma homocysteine levels in patients with CRF (392–395). Five to 10 mg of folic acid per day probably maximally lowers plasma homocysteine levels in most cases (296,395); occasionally, 15 mg of folic acid per day may have an additional homocysteine lowering effect (394). However, homocysteine levels, on average, are not reduced to within the normal range with this treatment (295,296,391–396). Folic acid given intravenously, rather than orally, may be more effective at lowering plasma homocysteine levels (393).

It has been suggested that there may be an impairment in conversion of folic acid to 5-methylenetetrahydrofolate (MTHF) and also of the transmembrane transport of MTHF. To circumvent these possible disorders, 37 patients on MHD were given intravenous folinic acid, a precursor of MTHF, 50 mg per week intravenously, and large dosages of pyridoxine hydrochloride, 250 mg three times weekly (396). After a mean of 11.2 months of treatment, mean plasma homocysteine levels decreased significantly to about one-third of pretreatment values, and 78% of the individuals achieved normal plasma homocysteine levels (less than 14.1 μmol). Further research will be helpful to ascertain whether similar beneficial results can be obtained with lower folinic acid and pyridoxine dosages.

Plasma oxalate levels are elevated in renal failure. Increased plasma oxalate level appears to be largely due to impaired urinary excretion, although large doses of Vitamin C (ascorbic acid), a precursor of oxalate, may increase oxalate production (see later discussion). Glyoxylate, a metabolic precursor of oxalate, may also be transaminated to form glycine. Vitamin B_6 is a cofactor for the enzyme that catalyzes this step. Indeed, Vitamin B_6 deficiency increases urinary oxalate excretion in rats with experimental renal insufficiency, as well as in healthy individuals (397). In patients with CRF, some studies indicate that treatment with large doses of pyridoxine hydrochloride decrease plasma oxalate levels, although not to normal values (398,399). Other clinical trials have not been able to confirm these results (400,401).

Five milligrams per day of pyridoxine hydrochloride produced a normal red cell erythrocyte glutamate-pyruvate transaminase activation index in nondialyzed, clinically stable, chronically uremic patients, and 10 mg per day of pyridoxine hydrochloride normalized this index in stable patients on MHD and in nondialyzed patients with CRF with superimposed infections (68).

Despite the water solubility of riboflavin, thiamine, pantothenic acid, and biotin, plasma concentrations of these vitamins are usually not decreased in patients undergoing MHD. It is possible that losses of these vitamins into hemodialysate are offset by the lack of urinary excretion in these patients. Low plasma niacin concentrations have been reported in some patients receiving maintenance dialysis therapy (373). Other investigators did not confirm these findings in patients receiving 7.5 mg of supplemental nicotinic acid per day (66). Low levels of thiamine, and in some patients, thiamine and pyridoxine when they were prescribed low-protein diets, have been described (379).

Serum retinol binding protein and Vitamin A levels are increased in patients with renal failure (402–404). Elevated liver Vitamin A levels were described in two patients with CRF (405), although other investigators could not confirm elevated Vitamin A levels in solid tissues (403). Moreover, even relatively small supplements of Vitamin A, that is, 7,500 to 15,000 IU per day (about 1,500 to 3,000 retinal equivalents per day), appear to cause bone toxicity and hypercalcemia in some patients (406). Normal (407,408), low (369,409), and increased (410) plasma or red cell Vitamin E ([SC]-tocopherol) levels have been described in nondialyzed patients with CRF or on MHD. Vitamin E deficiency may cause oxidative injury to tissues (369). Vitamin K deficiency is uncommon (18). Patients who do not eat (and hence do not ingest foods containing Vitamin K) and who are receiving antibiotics that suppress intestinal bacteria for extended periods of time may require supplemental Vitamin K to prevent deficiency of this vitamin (411).

Blumberg and Sander (370) studied vitamin levels in ten patients on CAPD who were apparently eating an unrestricted protein diet and not receiving vitamin supplements. They reported that plasma Vitamin B_1 (thiamine), Vitamin B_6, folic acid, and Vitamin C levels were frequently reduced. Plasma Vitamin B_2 and B_{12} levels were within the normal range, although Vitamin B_{12} levels tended to decline with time in patients who did not receive supplements of this vitamin. Dietary intake of several vitamins, including Vitamin A, Vitamin B_1, Vitamin B_6, Vitamin B_{12}, and nicotinamide, was often reduced to less than the recommended allowances for healthy adults (370,385). Other investigators have reported low serum folic acid levels in patients on CAPD (412). In patients on CPD not receiving supplements, other investigators have found a high incidence of low (370,404) or normal (413) plasma folate levels, low Vitamin B_1 (370,404), Vitamin B_6 (414), and Vitamin C (404) levels. Reduced plasma Vitamin E levels have been reported in 13% of patients on CPD (404), whereas others found increased plasma Vitamin E levels (414).

Some authors have suggested that many patients on MHD who do not receive vitamin supplementation may subsist for months without developing water-soluble vitamin deficiencies (106,386,415). Based on these observations, these authors have recommended that vitamin supplements should not be prescribed routinely to patients on maintenance dialysis. However, in the studies indicating that patients on maintenance dialysis may maintain normal plasma or blood cell levels of vitamins without supplements, patients were generally followed for less than 1 year; it is possible that with longer periods, the incidence of vitamin deficiency may increase. Moreover, in these studies, some water-soluble vitamins fell to borderline low levels in a number of patients. It is true that many of the studies that indicate a need for routine vitamin supplementation in nondialyzed patients with CRF and patients on maintenance dialysis were carried out in the 1960s and early 1970s when the incidence of poor nutritional intake of these individuals might have been greater than it is today (18). Nonetheless, poor vitamin intake is still common in patients with renal failure (385,415), and many reports continue to show that substantial numbers of patients with renal failure show evidence of vitamin deficiencies (369,379,385,386,414). Because the water-soluble vitamin supplements are generally safe, it would seem wise to use them routinely until these issues are more completely resolved.

The nutritional requirements for most vitamins are not well defined in patients with renal failure, and it is likely that they will be modified. There is evidence that in addition to vitamin intake from foods, the following daily supplements of vitamins will prevent or correct vitamin deficiency (Table 103-5): pyridoxine hydrochloride, 5 mg in nondialyzed patients and 10 mg in patients on MHD or CPD; folic acid, 1.0 to 1.5 mg; and the recommended daily allowance for healthy individuals for the other water-soluble vitamins (248). It is probable that many patients with CRF may need less than 1.0 mg of folic acid per day. Alternatively, for the many nondialyzed patients with CRF and most patients on MHD and CPD who have hyperhomocysteinemia, 5 to 15 mg of folic acid per day may be more appropriate. For these individuals with elevated plasma homocysteine levels, it is probably advisable to start treatment with 5 mg/kg and then increase folic acid doses, if necessary, depending on the response of the plasma homocysteine level. It should be pointed out that no interventional study has been conducted to examine whether lowering plasma homocysteine levels in patients with CRF, in patients on maintenance dialysis, or in renal transplant recipients improves morbidity or mortality rates. Also, there are no studies that have examined the safety of these large folate doses in patients with CRF, in patients on maintenance dialysis, or in transplant recipients, a particularly important consideration because of the reduction in their ability to excrete folate metabolites in the urine.

A supplement of only 60 mg of Vitamin C per day (the recommended daily allowance [248]) is advised because ascorbic acid can be metabolized to oxalate. Large doses of ascorbic acid have been associated with increased plasma oxalate levels in patients with renal failure (416,417). Oxalate is highly insoluble, and there is substantial concern that high plasma oxalate concentrations can lead to precipitation in soft tissues, including the kidney, possibly causing further impairment in renal function in the nondialyzed patient with renal insufficiency.

Supplemental Vitamin A is not recommended because serum levels are increased and there appears to be a high risk of Vitamin A toxicity with supplements (405,406). It is not clear whether Vitamin E supplements are necessary (369). Additional Vitamin K is not needed unless the patient is not eating and receives antibiotics that suppress intestinal bacteria that synthesize Vitamin K. Recommendations for Vitamin D intake are given in Chapter.

Alkalinizing Agents

Nondialyzed patients with advanced renal failure frequently develop metabolic acidosis associated with an increased anion gap, because there is impaired ability of the kidney to excrete acidic metabolites. In the earlier stages of CRF, and occasionally with advanced renal failure, hyperchloremic metabolic acidosis may also be caused by excessive renal losses of bicarbonate. Ingestion of low-protein diets may prevent or decrease the severity of the acidosis because the endogenous generation of acidic products of protein metabolism will be reduced. Metabolic acidemia may engender oxidation of branched-chain amino acids (valine, leucine, and isoleucine) (136) and protein catabolism (135–138), impair albumin synthesis, increase β_2-microglobulin turnover (418), and cause bone loss. Conversely, correction of acidosis has been associated with decreased protein degradation rates (419) and increased plasma branched-chain amino acid levels (420,421), serum albumin level (421), and body weight and midarm circumference (422). Because the exact level of acidemia at which amino acid or protein loss or bone reabsorption is stimulated is not well defined, it would seem prudent to prevent any degree of chronic acidemia. The NKF

K/DOQI Clinical Practice Guidelines recommend that the serum bicarbonate level should be measured once monthly in patients on maintenance dialysis, and that the predialysis or stabilized serum bicarbonate level should be maintained at 22 mmol/L or more in patients on MHD and CPD (423). A similar recommendation concerning the threshold for treating low serum bicarbonate levels would seem appropriate for nondialyzed patients with any level of renal disease. Alkali therapy should be initiated if the arterial pH level is less than 7.35 or regardless of the serum bicarbonate level.

Because in clinically stable patients with CRF, the rate of acid production is usually within the normal range or less than the normal, alkalinizing medicines are usually very effective for preventing or treating the acidemia. Calcium carbonate (5 g per day) may correct mild acidosis, provide needed calcium, and reduce intestinal phosphate absorption. If the acidosis is more severe, sodium bicarbonate or citrate may be administered orally or intravenously. If the nondialyzed, chronically uremic patient is not oliguric and is not particularly likely to develop edema, sodium is usually readily excreted when it is given as sodium bicarbonate or citrate. Oral treatment may be administered with bicarbonate or citrate salts, although the latter may enhance the intestinal absorption of aluminum (329). Before implementing alkali therapy, one must ensure that the low serum bicarbonate level is not a compensatory response to chronic respiratory alkalosis. If acidosis is severe and is not controlled by the foregoing measures, hemodialysis or peritoneal dialysis may be employed.

Fiber

Studies in healthy individuals suggest that a high dietary fiber intake may lower the incidence of constipation, irritable bowel syndrome, diverticulitis, and neoplasia of the colon and possibly improve glucose tolerance (424). In patients with CRF, a high dietary fiber intake also may reduce BUN by decreasing colonic bacterial ammonia generation and enhancing fecal nitrogen excretion (425). Because it seems reasonable that the benefits of a high dietary fiber intake in healthy people would also occur in nondialyzed patients with CRF and in patients on maintenance dialysis, a high dietary fiber intake of 20 to 25 g per day is recommended.

Prioritizing Dietary Goals

The number and magnitude of the changes in the dietary intake for patients with CRF and patients on maintenance dialysis are so great that if they were all presented to the patient at one time, the patient could become demoralized and lose the motivation to comply with the diet. We therefore prioritize goals for dietary treatment. Usually we emphasize the importance of controlling the protein, phosphorus, sodium, energy, potassium, and magnesium intake and the need to take calcium and vitamin supplements. On the other hand, unless the patient has a lipid disorder or other risk factors that indicate odds ration for cardiovascular events, the recommended quantity and types of dietary carbohydrate, fat, and fiber are discussed with the patient, but adherence to these dietary guidelines is not as strongly emphasized. If the patient has complied well with the other, more critical elements of dietary therapy, has a specific lipid disorder that may benefit from dietary therapy, or has expressed an interest in modifying fat, carbohydrate, or fiber intake, then the modification of the dietary intake of these latter nutrients is explored more intensively with the patient.

ADJUSTED EDEMA-FREE BODY WEIGHT

Assessment of nutritional status and assessment and prescription of nutritional intake is often based on body weight. For individuals with renal disease, this represents a special problem because they often not only are obese or underweight but also may be edematous. The NKF Clinical Practice Guidelines for Nutrition address this issue with the following statement (426): "The body weight to be used for assessing or prescribing protein or energy intake is the aBW$_{ef}$ [adjusted edema-free body weight]. For patients on hemodialysis, this should be obtained postdialysis. For patients on peritoneal dialysis, this should be obtained after drainage of dialysate." The aBW$_{ef}$ should be used for individuals with renal disease, including nondialyzed patients with CRF and patients on maintenance dialysis who have an aBW$_{ef}$ that is less than 95% or more than 115% of the median standard weight as determined from the NHANES II data (163). For individuals with an edema-free body weight between 95% and 115% of the median standard weight, the actual edema-free body weight may be used. The guideline goes on to state that "for DXA measurements of total body fat and fat-free mass, the actual edema-free body weight obtained at the time of the DXA measurement should be used. For anthropometric calculations, the postdialysis (for MHD) or postdrain (for CPD) actual edema-free body weight should be used." Clinical judgment and, if desired, body composition measurements can be used to estimate the magnitude of the edema, if any. The aBW$_{ef}$ may be calculated as follows (183,426):

$$aBW_{ef} = BW_{ef} + [(SBW - BW_{ef}) \times 0.25]$$

where *BW$_{ef}$* is the actual edema-free body weight and *SBW* is the standard body weight as determined from the NHANES II data (163).

DIETARY THERAPY FOR PATIENTS WITH THE NEPHROTIC SYNDROME

This syndrome is characterized by albuminuria (more than 3.0 g per day), lipiduria, hypoalbuminemia, hypercholesterolemia, and edema, which can be massive. Serum total protein levels may decrease markedly, from 7 to 8 g/dL to as low as 4 to 5 g/dL, and the resultant fall in plasma oncotic pressure promotes extravascular movement of fluid, sodium retention, and edema formation. Two narrow transverse white bands (Muehrcke's lines) may occur in the fingernails in association with severe hypoproteinemia (427).

Serum triglyceride, phospholipid, and apoproteins B, C-II, C-III, and E levels are increased, whereas apoprotein A-I and A-II levels are within the normal range (428). Plasma Lp(a) level is elevated (429). Both LDL and very-low-density lipoprotein (VLDL) levels may be increased (430). There is increased serum cholesterol ester transport protein (CETP) level and decreased catabolism of LDL apolipoprotein, at least by the more typical receptor pathway. These metabolic changes contribute to the elevated LDL cholesterol level and frequently observed low HDL cholesterol level (428,430–438). Hypercholesterolemia, hypertriglyceridemia, increased LDL cholesterol and VLDL cholesterol levels, increased CETP and Lp(a) levels, and low HDL cholesterol levels all are risk factors for an increased incidence of atherosclerotic cardiovascular disease and cerebrovascular disease in nephrotic patients (428,430,439–441). It has been suggested that the altered serum lipid pattern in the nephrotic syndrome may accelerate the progression of renal failure (442). Altered membrane lipid composition and oxidant injury of the kidney (443) and erythrocytes (444) have been described.

Protein-restricted diets providing less than 30% of calories from fat, less than 200 mg of cholesterol per day, and an abundant amount of polyunsaturated fatty acids, with 10% of calories from linoleic acid, are reported to reduce serum total and LDL cholesterol level and decrease proteinuria in nephrotic patients (445). A vegetarian soy-based low-protein diet may reduce proteinuria and hyperlipidemia in nephrotic patients (446). Reduction in serum lipids by the HMG CoA reductase inhibitor, simvastatin, is reported to cause a partial remission in the nephrotic syndrome in patients (447).

Low serum protein levels are caused by enhanced urinary protein excretion and by degradation of the increased quantity of filtered protein in renal tubular cells (448–450). Also, albumin synthesis may be increased, normal, or decreased, depending at least partly on the adequacy of dietary protein intake. Massive proteinuria may occur (e.g., up to 40 g or more of protein per day) and may be incapacitating or life-threatening (451). Serum levels of many biologically active proteins, including clotting factors and inhibitors, are reduced due to enhanced excretion and renal degradation (452); the clinical importance of these effects are not well defined. However, low plasma concentrations of clotting inhibitors may contribute to the frequency of renal vein thrombosis in the nephrotic syndrome.

The Vitamin D analogs, 25-hydroxycholecalciferol and 1,25-dihydroxycholecalciferol, are bound to an alpha-like globulin (453) and may be lost in urine in the nephrotic syndrome (454,455). In experimental nephrosis, intestinal absorption of Vitamin D appears to be normal (456). Evidence of Vitamin D deficiency with low serum 25-hydroxycholecalciferol and 1,25-dihydroxycholecalciferol levels, decreased ionized and total calcium levels, and bone disease has been found in patients with the nephrotic syndrome (454,457,458). Others have reported normal serum Vitamin D levels and no bone disease (459). There is loss of organic iodide and thyroxine in the urine in the nephrotic syndrome, although hypothyroidism is probably not present (460,461). Also, there may be increased urinary losses of trace elements bound to proteins such as zinc, copper, and iron. These losses may cause nutritional deficiencies (342,462–464).

The severity of nutritional disorders in patients with the nephrotic syndrome varies greatly; in the author's experience, patients with the nephrotic syndrome are not infrequently malnourished and debilitated to a degree that is disproportionate to their renal insufficiency. This is particularly common in patients with more massive proteinuria. The causes of malnutrition and debility include large urinary protein losses, anorexia, the urinary losses of vitamins and trace elements that are protein bound in plasma, glucocorticoid or cytotoxic therapy, and the frequent incidence of infections that result from such treatment.

A high-protein diet providing up to 2.3 g of protein per kilogram of body weight per day has been reported to improve nutritional status, if uremia is not present (465). The findings that low-protein diets may retard progression of renal failure and reduce proteinuria (212,219,227,466) have prompted a reexamination of the use of low-protein diets in this disorder. Kaysen (467) fed isocaloric diets providing 0.8 and 1.6 g of protein per kilogram per day to nine patients with nephrotic syndrome. They reported that with the lower protein intake, urine albumin concentration, renal albumin clearance, and fractional urinary albumin excretion decreased. Serum albumin concentrations and plasma albumin mass were actually greater with the low-protein diet, although total albumin mass did not differ with the two diets. As indicated already, a soy-based protein diet is reported to reduce proteinuria (446).

In rats and humans with proteinuria or the nephrotic syndrome, converting enzyme inhibitors and angiotensin receptor blockers may reduce but not abolish the proteinuria (468–472). The addition of converting enzyme inhibitor medicines seems to allow protein intakes to be increased modestly without increasing urinary protein losses, thereby increasing the likelihood of nutritional repletion. It is likely that angiotensin receptor blockers have similar effects. Reduction of proteinuria is an important goal because large urine protein losses are a risk factor for more rapid progression of renal failure (223). Long-term studies have not shown whether these lower protein intakes will prevent or correct protein malnutrition; this problem is complicated by the difficulty of assessing protein nutrition in nephrotic patients.

It is our policy to prescribe for patients with the nephrotic syndrome diets that provide 0.70 or 0.80 g of protein per kilogram of body weight per day. The higher value would be prescribed for patients with more severe proteinuria. At least 0.35 g of protein per kilogram per day should be of high biologic value. This diet should be supplemented with 1.0 g of high-biologic-value protein for each gram of urine protein excreted each day. Intake of energy and minerals in general is prescribed as described for patients with chronic renal

insufficiency. ACE inhibitors and often angiotensin II receptor blocker antagonists are routinely added to reduce proteinuria. Diuretics and sodium restriction are often used to treat edema and the tendency to retain sodium. When sodium is restricted adequately, thirst will usually regulate water intake to prevent the development of substantial hyponatremia. To maximize the antiproteinuric effects of ACE inhibitors or angiotensin II receptor blockers, the patient must either maintain urinary sodium excretion at or less than 100 mEq per day by dietary sodium restriction or use a diuretic (e.g., a thiazide [see previous discussion]). An NCEP-AHA Step I diet (see previous discussion) may benefit lipid metabolism, although, by itself, it probably will not lower serum lipid levels. Hypercholesterolemia also may be treated with HMG CoA reductase inhibitors. Phosphorus intake may need to be liberalized if the protein intake is much greater than 0.70 g/kg per day. Vitamin supplements should provide the normal daily allowances for the fat-soluble vitamins, including Vitamin D, as well as the water-soluble vitamins.

For patients with moderate or advanced renal insufficiency, 1,25-dihydroxycholecalciferol, 0.25 to 0.50 μg per day, probably should be substituted for Vitamin D_3 or cholecalciferol. The potential benefits of administering trace elements have not been established, although for patients with large amounts of proteinuria, iron, zinc, copper, and probably other trace element supplements should be given. Good blood pressure control is essential (470). More studies are needed to examine these questions and the use of medicines and diet to treat hyperlipidemia and hypercholesterolemia in the nephrotic syndrome.

NUTRITIONAL THERAPY FOR ACUTE RENAL FAILURE

Altered Metabolic and Nutritional Status in Acute Renal Failure

Patients with ARF have widely varying degrees of alterations in metabolic and nutritional status. Some patients maintain nitrogen balance and have normal water balance, plasma electrolyte concentrations, and acid–base status. In general, these patients do not have severely catabolic underlying illnesses. They are usually not oliguric, and the cause of their ARF is typically an isolated, noncatabolic event, such as administration of radiocontrast drugs or aminoglycoside nephrotoxicity. However, most patients with ARF have some degree of net protein breakdown (synthesis minus degradation) and disordered fluid, electrolyte, or acid–base status. There is often excess total body water, azotemia, hyperkalemia, hyperphosphatemia, hypocalcemia, hyperuricemia, and a large anion gap metabolic acidosis.

Net protein degradation in ARF can be massive, with net losses of as high as 200 to 250 g per day (473–475); for comparison, the total noncollagen protein mass of a 70-kg man is about 6 kg (476). Patients are more likely to be catabolic when the ARF is caused by shock, sepsis, or rhabdomyolysis.

In the study of Feinstein et al. (474), mean UNA was $12.0 \pm$ (SD) 7.9 g per day in patients in whom ARF was caused by hypotension, sepsis, or both, and 12.3 ± 7.9 g per day in those with rhabdomyolysis. These UNA rates were significantly greater ($P < 0.001$ and $P < 0.05$, respectively) than in patients with ARF from other causes (3.8 ± 2.4 g per day).

In patients with ARF, marked net protein catabolism may accelerate the rate of rise in plasma concentrations of potassium, phosphorus, nitrogenous metabolites, and non–nitrogen-containing acids. It is therefore not surprising that protein-energy malnutrition is very prevalent in patients with ARF (474,478) and is associated with increased morbidity and mortality rates (478).

There appear to be multiple causes for malnutrition in ARF. Animal studies suggest that acute uremia itself may cause disorders in amino acid and protein metabolism and promote wasting. UNA is increased in rats with ARF compared with sham-operated controls. Livers from acutely uremic rats display increased uptake of several amino acids and enhanced urea production (479). Frohlich et al. (480) studied glucose and urea output in perfused liver from rats with bilateral nephrectomy and reported increased hepatic release of glucose, urea, and the branched-chain amino acids valine, leucine, and isoleucine, which are not well metabolized by the liver. When a mixture of amino acids was added to the perfusate in concentrations that were approximately similar to those found in plasma, the increment in hepatic glucose and urea formation in the acutely uremic rats was significantly greater than that in control rats (480). These observations suggest that in rats, acute uremia per se stimulates both gluconeogenesis and protein degradation in the liver.

Some early studies suggest that protein synthesis may vary independently and according to the organ studied (481,482). However, these investigators did not examine the balance between both synthesis and degradation. Flugel-Link et al. (483) found increased degradation and a trend toward impaired synthesis of protein in the perfused posterior hemicorpus of rats made acutely uremic by bilateral nephrectomy. Clark and Mitch (484) also described reduced protein synthesis and enhanced protein degradation in skeletal muscle from acutely uremic rats. Insulin, added to the incubation media, enhanced protein synthesis and reduced protein degradation in muscle of these animals. The effect of insulin was less marked in the acutely uremic animals compared with the sham-operated controls, indicating that acute uremia causes insulin resistance in muscle. The acidemia that occurs in ARF contributes to the protein catabolism (485). Nonetheless, acute uremia per se seems to engender only a mild increase in catabolism, at least in the commonly studied rat model (483,485). It is when sepsis or hypoxia is superimposed that catabolism increases (473–475,486).

The mechanisms responsible for increased gluconeogenesis and net protein degradation in rats with ARF are not well defined. In the liver of acutely uremic rats, increased activity has been reported for glutamate-oxaloacetate aminotransferase, which catalyzes the transamination of glutamate (487). Elevated activity of two urea cycle enzymes, ornithine transaminase, which catalyzes the conversion of glutamate to ornithine, and arginase, which catalyzes formation of urea and ornithine from arginine, has been observed. Increased activity of serine dehydratase, which oxidizes the gluconeogenic amino acid serine, has been described. In addition, in acutely uremic rats, there is normal hepatic activity of phenylalanine hydroxylase and increased activity of tyrosine aminotransferase, key enzymes in the degradation of phenylalanine and tyrosine (488).

Decreased muscle glycogen has been observed in acutely uremic patients who are catabolic (5) and in rats with bilateral nephrectomy (489). Increased activity of phosphorylase a, which catalyzes glycogenolysis, and decreased activity of glycogen synthetase I, which catalyzes glycogen synthesis, has been observed in muscle of these rats. Supplementing a low-protein diet with serine increased glycogen synthetase I activity in these animals (489).

The catabolic effects of ARF may be induced by several causes. First, the many products of metabolism may be toxic in the high concentrations that occur in uremia. Second, alterations in plasma concentrations of catabolic hormones may promote wasting. Infusion of healthy humans or dogs with cortisone, epinephrine, and glucagon in quantities sufficient to raise plasma concentrations to levels found in acutely catabolic patients causes a sustained increase in glucose production, increased protein turnover and protein degradation, increased energy expenditure, and negative nitrogen balance (490,491). These hormones may be increased in ARF due to associated illnesses (see later discussion). These illnesses are often associated with release of microbial toxins, elevated acute-phase reactants, catabolic cytokines, increase in oxidant levels, and hormonal disorders associated with increased counterregulatory hormones.

A glucocorticoid receptor antagonist blocks the catabolic response in acutely anephric rats (492). Moreover, in patients with CRF, there is evidence for increased sensitivity to the actions of glucagon (144); however, others were unable to demonstrate enhanced sensitivity to glucagon in acutely uremic rats (493). Experience in patients with ARF infused with hypertonic glucose suggests that glucose intolerance is common (474). Parathyroid hormone, which may be increased in ARF (494,495), is another potentially catabolic agent (145,146).

Third, as indicated already, acidemia increases amino acid and protein catabolism (137,485). Fourth, proteolytic activity is increased in the sera of some patients with ARF who are very catabolic (496,497). This suggests that in the sera of hypercatabolic, acutely uremic patients, there may be either increased quantities of proteases, which degrade proteins, a reduction in protease inhibitors, or changes in other factors that lead to enhanced protease activity. In acutely uremic rats that have increased muscle protein degradation, activities of muscle alkaline protease, cathepsin B, and cathepsin D, measured *in vitro*, were found not to be different from those of controls (483).

In addition to the potential catabolic effects of uremia per se, there are clearly other causes of wasting and malnutrition in ARF. These include the following:

1. Many patients are unable to eat adequately because of anorexia or vomiting. These symptoms may be caused by acute uremia, underlying illnesses, or the anorectic effects of dialysis treatment. Other causes of poor food intake are medical or surgical disorders that impair gastrointestinal tract function and the frequent diagnostic studies that require the patient to fast for several hours.
2. The patient's underlying medical disorders often cause a hypercatabolic state. Chief among these catabolic conditions in ARF are infection, hypotension, surgery, trauma, and rhabdomyolysis.
3. Losses of nutrients in draining fistulae and during dialysis therapy may lead to wasting and malnutrition. Moreover, hemodialysis itself may stimulate catabolism (see previous discussion).
4. As indicated previously, blood drawing, gastrointestinal tract bleeding, which may be occult, and blood sequestered in the hemodialyzer are other causes of protein depletion.

Experience with Nutritional Therapy for Acute Renal Failure

Before the mid 1960s, many clinicians recommended severe or total restriction of protein intake for patients with ARF (189,498,499). Small amounts of energy (e.g., 1,680 to 3,360 kJ [400 to 800 kcal] per day) were provided from candy, butterballs, or intravenous infusions of hypertonic glucose to reduce the rate of protein degradation. This therapy was based on Gamble's studies of lifeboat rations for healthy young men. Gamble's observations indicated that administration of 100 g of sugar per day could substantially reduce net protein breakdown in these starving but otherwise healthy volunteers (500).

Anabolic steroids were frequently administered because they could transiently decrease the UNA, the rate of rise of BUN or nonprotein nitrogen, and the development of acidemia (501,502). In the 1960s, the Giordano-Giovannetti diet was developed for patients with CRF (191,195). This diet, which contained about 20 g of protein per day, most of which was usually supplied by two eggs, provided the recommended daily allowances for essential amino acids for young healthy adults. Some clinicians advocated this diet for the acutely uremic patient who was able to eat because they believed that the diet could be used efficiently and would minimize the degree of protein wasting while it reduced the UNA and the accumulation of nitrogenous metabolites (503). In the era before patients could be readily treated with dialysis or hemofiltration, it was thought that anabolic steroids or these low-nitrogen diets might reduce uremic toxicity and maintain life until renal function recovered. Maintaining good nutrition was a secondary aim. When dialysis first became available, it was usually employed only for specific sequelae of renal failure, such as uremic symptoms, congestive heart failure, or hyperkalemia, and great efforts were often made to avoid the need for dialysis therapy. With the development of modern techniques for parenteral and enteral nutrition and the routine use of dialysis, the emphasis on nutritional therapy gradually changed so the maintenance of good nutrition became a primary goal, and dialysis was used as needed to control fluid and electrolyte balance and remove metabolic waste (504).

Lee et al. (505) in 1967 administered solutions containing casein hydrolysate, fructose, ethanol, and soybean oil emulsion (Intralipid) by peripheral vein to several patients with ARF or CRF. Despite the severity of the patients' illnesses, these investigators reported that marked loss of weight did not occur and convalescence was shortened. Wilmore and Dudrick (506) and others (507) treated acutely or chronically uremic patients with intravenous infusions of essential amino acids and hypertonic glucose into the subclavian vein (506,507). They described weight gain, improved wound healing, and stabilization or reduction of BUN levels. Decreased serum potassium and phosphorus concentrations and positive nitrogen balance were often observed. Anephric beagles who received intravenous infusions of essential amino acids and 57% glucose had a lower rise in BUN and a longer survival than similar animals that were given food or infusions of glucose (5% or 57%) alone (508).

A number of authors carried out a series of studies in patients with ARF who were treated with hypertonic glucose and eight essential amino acids, excluding histidine (509–513). Serum potassium, phosphorus, and magnesium concentrations fell, and BUN often stabilized or decreased. These investigators carried out a prospective, double-blind study in 53 patients with ARF who were randomly assigned to receive infusions of either an average of 16 g per day of essential amino acids with hypertonic glucose or hypertonic glucose alone (511). Total energy intake averaged 5,989 to 6,892 kJ (1,426 and 1,641 kcal) per day with the two preparations, respectively. Patients may have eaten some food during the study. There was a higher incidence of survival until renal function recovered in the patients receiving the essential amino acids and glucose. However, overall hospital mortality rate was not significantly less in this group. In patients with more severe renal failure, as indicated by the need for dialysis, and in those with serious complications, such as pneumonia and generalized sepsis, hospital survival rate was significantly greater when essential amino acids and glucose were given than when glucose alone was infused. Sofia and Nicora failed to show improvement in survival from ARF in patients who were treated with essential amino acids and glucose as compared with glucose alone; however, this was a retrospective analysis of patients from a number of centers who may not have been treated with the same protocols (514).

Baek et al. (515) compared results in 63 patients treated with a fibrin hydrolysate and hypertonic glucose with results in 66 subjects who received varying quantities of glucose.

The patients who were given the hydrolysate had lower morbidity and mortality rates. However, it is not clear whether the patients were randomly assigned to the two treatment regimens or whether the two groups of patients were treated concurrently. McMurray et al. (516) and Milligan et al. (517) treated patients with acute tubular necrosis with either hypertonic glucose alone (840 to 1,680 kJ/kg [200 to 400 kcal/kg] per day) or a mixture of essential and nonessential amino acids and hypertonic glucose that provided 12 g of nitrogen per day and more than 8,400 kJ (2,000 kcal) per day. There was no difference in survival rate between the two treatments in the patients with no complications. However, in patients with three or more complications or with peritonitis, those who received 12 g per day of amino acid nitrogen with hypertonic glucose had significantly greater survival, as compared with patients receiving low quantities of glucose alone. The study was carried out retrospectively, and the patients who received amino acids and glucose were treated at a later time than those who received glucose alone. Mocan et al. reported that in 30 patients with ARF, 13.4 g per day of intravenous essential amino acids (517a) with dopamine and 20% glucose reduced the rise in BUN and was associated with higher serum albumin and total protein levels and lower complication and mortality rates as compared with 20 nonrandomized control subjects with ARF receiving dopamine and 20% glucose without amino acids.

Several studies have indicated that nitrogen and energy needs are often high and nitrogen balance is difficult to attain, particularly during the first few days of ARF (473–475,518–522). A few prospective, randomized studies have examined nitrogen balance and requirements in stressed patients with ARF. Leonard et al. (473) randomly assigned patients with ARF to receive infusions of 1.75% essential L-amino acids and 47% dextrose or 47% dextrose alone. Patients who were able to eat or tolerate tube feeding were excluded from the study. Hence, many of the patients studied had severe complicating illnesses. Most patients required dialysis frequently. The rate of rise in BUN was significantly less in the group receiving essential amino acids. However, mean nitrogen balance was approximately 10 g per day negative in both groups, and there was no difference in the rate of survival or recovery of renal function in the two groups.

Feinstein et al. (474) evaluated 30 patients with ARF who were unable to eat adequately. Patients were randomly assigned to receive parenteral nutrition with glucose alone, glucose and 21 g per day of essential amino acids, or glucose and 21 g per day of essential amino acids and 21 g per day of nonessential amino acids (474). Mean energy intake varied from 9,660 to 11,340 kJ (2,300 to 2,700 kcal) per day and did not differ significantly among the groups. Patients were studied in a prospective, double-blind fashion; the duration of the study in the three groups was 9.0 ± (SD) 7.7 days. Many patients were in a markedly catabolic state, as determined from nitrogen balances, UNA, serum protein levels, and plasma amino acid concentrations. Mean nitrogen balance, estimated from the difference between nitrogen

intake and UNA, which underestimates nitrogen losses by about 2 g per day, was −10.4 ± 5.7 g per day with glucose alone, −4.4 ± 7.3 g per day with glucose and essential amino acids, and −8.5 ± 7.9 g per day with glucose and essential and nonessential amino acids. Although nitrogen balance was not different with the three infusates, in a few patients who received essential amino acids or essential and nonessential amino acids, the nitrogen balance was only slightly negative. In one patient receiving essential amino acids, the nitrogen balance was probably neutral or positive. Serum potassium, phosphorus, and urea concentrations often stabilized or decreased in patients from all three treatment groups; these changes in serum levels were probably influenced by dialysis therapy, recovering renal function, or the natural history of the underlying metabolic disorders. There was no difference in the rapidity or incidence of recovery of renal function or in the rate of survival among the three treatment groups, although recovery of renal function and survival tended to be greater in the patients receiving the essential amino acids.

Because these observations suggested that higher nitrogen intakes might be more effective at maintaining nitrogen balance in catabolic patients with ARF, Feinstein et al. (475) carried out another randomized, prospective clinical trial in a small number of patients. Patients received total parenteral nutrition (TPN) providing 21 g per day of essential amino acids or TPN with essential and nonessential amino acids provided in a 1.0 : 1.0 ratio. With the latter treatment, attempts were made to infuse a quantity of nitrogen equal to the UNA. Thirteen patients with ARF were randomly assigned to one of the two treatment groups. The results indicated that although the nitrogen intake was five times greater with the essential and nonessential amino acid regimen, the nitrogen balance, determined from the difference between intake and UNA, was not different. Moreover, the UNA fell significantly only in patients receiving essential amino acids, whereas it tended to rise in patients receiving essential and nonessential amino acids.

These latter two studies, taken together, suggest that high-caloric solutions providing about 21 g per day of essential amino acids may be used more efficiently than isocaloric preparations containing larger quantities of essential and nonessential amino acids (e.g., 40 to 70 g per day provided in an essential to nonessential amino acid ratio of 1.0 : 1.0) (Figs. 103-2 and 103-3) (523). The essential amino acid solutions seem to reduce the UNA and total nitrogen output more than solutions containing both essential and nonessential amino acids. Consequently, nitrogen balance, although negative with both regimens, was no more negative with the low quantities of essential amino acids, but the accumulation of nitrogenous metabolites was less. It would be of interest to examine the response to a TPN regimen that provides larger quantities of essential and nonessential amino acids but that contains a larger proportion of essential amino acids, particularly the branched-chain amino acids (see later discussion).

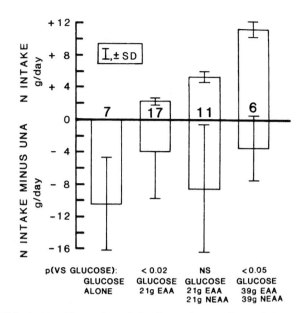

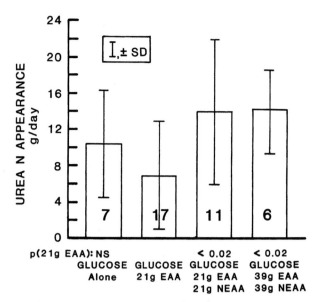

FIG. 103-2. Mean nitrogen intake and approximated nitrogen balance in four groups of patients with acute renal failure who were receiving parenteral nutrition. Individuals were treated with glucose alone, glucose and 21 g of essential amino acids (EAA) per day, glucose and 21 g of EAA and 21 g of nonessential amino acids (NEAA) per day, and glucose and approximately 39 g of EAA and 39 g of NEAA per day. Nitrogen intake was calculated from the measured nitrogen content of the infused parenteral nutrition solutions and is plotted above the horizontal line. The nitrogen balance, estimated as the difference between the nitrogen intake and the nitrogen output, calculated as the urea nitrogen appearance *(UNA)*, is plotted below the horizontal line. Data for patients who received a given parenteral nutrition formulation represent the mean values of the average daily intake and balance data obtained from each of the patients during the parenteral nutrition treatment. The calculated nitrogen intake was not adjusted for the nitrogen received from transfusions of blood or blood products that contain proteins and small amounts of peptides, free amino acids, and other nitrogen-containing compounds. Nitrogen balance was not adjusted for nonurea nitrogen in urine, fecal nitrogen, and other unmeasured nitrogen losses (e.g., from respiration, wound drainage, nasogastric tube or fistula drainage, flatus, sweat, skin desquamation and replacement, and hair and nail growth). The numbers in the vertical bars indicate the sample size of each group. Data from two separate studies (474,475) are combined in this figure. (From Kopple JD. 1995 Jonathan E. Rhoads lecture: the nutrition management of the patient with acute renal failure. *J Parenter Enteral Nutr* 1996;20:3, with permission.)

FIG. 103-3. Urea nitrogen appearance (UNA) in four groups of patients with acute renal failure who were receiving parenteral nutrition (474,475). Data for patients who received a given parenteral nutrition formulation represent the mean values of the daily average UNA for the patients in that treatment group. EAA, essential amino acids; NEAA, nonessential amino acids. (From Kopple JD. 1995 Jonathan E. Rhoads lecture: the nutrition management of the patient with acute renal failure. *J Parenter Enteral Nutr* 1996;20:3, with permission.)

Lopez-Martinez et al. (520) gave parenteral nutrition for 12 days each to 35 septic patients with ARF. The patients were in the polyuric phase, were not very uremic, and had not received dialysis therapy. Patients were given 4.4 g per day of nitrogen from essential amino acids and 8,400 kJ (2,000 kcal) per day (group 1), or 15 g per day of nitrogen from essential and nonessential amino acids and 12,600 kJ (3,000 kcal) per day, provided either by glucose (group 2) or by glucose and fat (group 3). Nitrogen balance, apparently estimated from the difference between nitrogen intake and UNA, was initially negative in all three groups and became more positive with

time, particularly in groups 2 and 3. Over the 12-day period of the study, the mean nitrogen balances were significantly more positive in both group 2 and group 3 than in group 1.

Hasik et al. (524) fed diets varying in protein content to nine patients with ARF when they were polyuric. The authors concluded that these patients, who were probably not severely ill at the time of the study, required 0.97 g of protein per kilogram per day. Mirtallo et al. (525) gave small amounts of essential amino acids or essential and nonessential amino acids to patients with mild ARF. The patients had substantial renal function, and no patient received dialysis in this study. There were no differences in UNA, recovery of renal function, or mortality in the two groups. Because the patients in these last three studies were neither very uremic nor very ill, the results may be more applicable to the patient who is not very catabolic and either has mild ARF or is recovering from ARF.

Effect of CVVH/CVVHD on Nutritional Management of Patients with Acute Renal Failure

Continuous venovenous hemofiltration (CVVH) and continuous venovenous hemodialysis (CVVHD) are commonly used for the management of very ill patients with ARF or other causes of fluid or nitrogen intolerance (e.g., severe liver or congestive heart failure). CVVH and CVVHD offer the following advantages to the patient: (a) Large quantities of water, electrolytes, and metabolites may be removed each day; (b) the rate of removal of water and electrolytes is slow and therefore generally does not cause or worsen hypotension; (c) Because of the high daily clearances of water and small molecules, including metabolic waste products, one may safely administer greater amounts of amino acids and other nutrients to the patient; (d) Because of the high daily clearances of molecules by CVVH or CVVHD, patients receiving CVVH or CVVHD may require hemodialysis therapy less frequently, or in some cases, it may be avoided altogether; and (e) CVVH or CVVHD may be administered by nurses who are not specifically trained in hemodialysis (although special training of nursing personnel is required). Thus, CVVH or CVVHD may be more convenient to use, and the cost for this therapy may be no more or possibly even less expensive than intermittent hemodialysis.

It is not clear that CVVH or CVVHD reduces morbidity or mortality rates more than intermittent hemodialysis in patients with ARF (526). On the other hand, the larger quantities of amino acids that can be given with CVVH or CVVHD have resulted in more positive nitrogen balance than can generally be achieved with thrice-weekly hemodialysis in catabolic patients with ARF. In two recent studies, nutritional support was associated with more positive nitrogen balance when patients with ARF received essential and nonessential amino acids in the amounts of 1.5 to 1.8 g/kg per day as compared with less than 1 g/kg per day (527) or 2.5 g/kg per day as compared with 1.2 g/kg per day (528). These results must be interpreted with some caution because the studies were not randomized, and also with very high protein intakes, the quantity of nitrogen lost through unmeasured routes (e.g., respiration, skin) may increase substantially, making nitrogen balance falsely more positive (245).

Amino acid losses during CVVH or CVVHD are influenced by the permeability characteristics of the filter membrane, the ultrafiltration and dialysis flow rates, and the rate of amino acid infusion, which will influence the plasma amino acid concentrations (529–531). Approximately 4 to 7 g of amino acids per day is removed with CVVH (529). In one study, amino acid losses were about $8.9\% \pm 1.2\%$ (SEM) and $12.1\% \pm 2.2\%$ of the daily quantity of amino acids infused in patients with renal failure undergoing CAVHD with a dialysate flow rate of 1 and 2 L per hour, respectively (530). Thus, the 24-hour amino acid losses with CVVH or CVVHD are similar to the losses during a single hemodialysis treatment (see previous discussion).

Effect of Nutritional Intake on Recovery of Renal Function in Acute Renal Failure

Abel et al. (510) observed that in patients with ARF who were treated with intravenous infusions of essential amino acids and glucose as compared with glucose alone, there was a tendency for the serum creatinine levels to decrease sooner and to lower levels (510). These findings raised the question of whether nutritional therapy may facilitate healing and enhance the rate of recovery of renal function in patients with

ARF. In the proximal tubular cells of rats with acute tubular necrosis caused by injection of mercuric chloride, there is increased synthesis of protein, nucleic acids, and phospholipids and accelerated growth that is apparent as early as the second day after injection (532–534). Toback (535) suggested that this regrowth should increase the requirements for nutrients and that this greater demand for nutrients occurs at a time when food intake is often decreased and uremic toxicity is developing. However, experiments in animals with ARF have given conflicting results as to whether nutritional support will enhance the rate of recovery of ARF (536–539), and no other studies in humans with ARF have shown an effect of nutritional support on recovery of renal function.

Why Benefits of Nutritional Therapy have not been Demonstrated Unequivocally

The foregoing studies, taken together, do not clearly demonstrate that treatment with amino acids and other nutrients will improve the rate or incidence of recovery of renal function, nutritional status, overall clinical condition, or survival. Intuitively, it seems that nutritional therapy should benefit patients with ARF. For patients who have ARF for more than 2 to 3 weeks or who are convalescing from ARF but are still unable to eat, evidence is stronger that oral or parenteral nutritional support should improve nutritional status.

There are probably several reasons why it has been so difficult to demonstrate a beneficial effect of nutritional therapy. These may include the following: (a) The clinical course of patients with ARF is so variable and often so complex that it should be necessary to study large numbers of patients in randomized, prospective studies to show statistically significant advantages to nutritional therapy, if these benefits exist. (b) Many of these studies were retrospective or not randomly controlled. This may have led to unintentional biases in the results. (c) The optimal composition of nutrients in the TPN solutions has not been defined, and the use of suboptimal formulations of nutrients may have made it more difficult to demonstrate the clinical benefits of nutritional therapy. (d) The foregoing studies in patients with ARF did not examine whether parenteral nutrition is beneficial. They compared only the response to different formulations of parenteral nutrition. There has been no prospective controlled comparison between the clinical course of patients with ARF who were receiving nutritional therapy and those who were receiving no special nutritional support. (e) It is probable that catabolic patients or rats with ARF may need both good nutritional intake and metabolic intervention to suppress catabolic processes and promote anabolism in liver and other tissues. Because acutely uremic patients who need nutritional therapy often suffer from underlying catabolic illnesses, they have undergone a metabolic reorganization, so they are more prone to degrade infused amino acids and energy substrates. Thus, the provision of nutrients without altering these metabolic processes may not benefit the nutritional status or clinical outcome. This may be particularly true during the initial days after the onset of ARF.

Effects of Metabolic Interventions to Enhance Recovery of Renal Function

Other types of metabolic intervention have shown varying degrees of promise for preventing or ameliorating the severity of ARF or enhancing recovery of renal failure. These interventions include using calcium channel blockers to inhibit calcium flux into the cell, a preterminal event leading to cell death (540). Other studies addressed maintenance of the cellular energy supply. Siegel et al. (541) infused magnesium chloride with adenosine triphosphate, diphosphate, or monophosphate into rats with ARF secondary to ischemia. The rats that received one of these adenine nucleotides with magnesium chloride had less impairment of inulin clearance, renal blood flow, and osmolar clearance, a lower fractional excretion of sodium, and less histologic evidence of renal injury as compared with rats that either received no infusion or received adenosine triphosphate, adenosine, or magnesium chloride alone. Rats with ARF caused by potassium dichromate injections who received thyroxine showed a greater rise in inulin clearance, a greater fall in fractional excretion of sodium and an increase in urine osmolality, and a more rapid recovery of renal function as compared with control animals (542). However, a study in humans with ARF did not confirm that thyroxine enhanced recovery of renal function (543).

Recently, growth factors have been employed in experimental models of ARF both to accelerate recovery of renal function and to enhance anabolism. Research suggests that epidermal growth factor (544), hepatocyte growth factor (545), IGF-1, and IGF-1 analogs (546–548) may enhance the rate of recovery of renal function in rats with ARF.

Most of the experimental work in this field has been carried out with recombinant human IGF-1 (rhIGF-1). Published studies are virtually uniform in describing that in rats with ARF, rhIGF-1 stimulates mitosis of the proximal tubular cells and possibly elsewhere in the kidney and increases the rate of recovery of both renal blood flow and GFR (546–548). This effect of IGF-1 is observed with ARF caused by ischemic injury (546–548), but not when caused by large doses of radiocontrast media (549). Recovery of renal function is enhanced regardless of whether rhIGF-1 is given concurrently with the renal insult or even several hours afterward (547). Interestingly, rhIGF-1 also stimulates an anabolic response in these rats with ARF (547). Notwithstanding these promising animal studies, one recent prospective, randomized, double-blind clinical trial failed to show that rhIGF-1 enhanced recovery of renal function in patients with established ARF (550). Another randomized, double-blind clinical trial in patients undergoing vascular surgery indicated that there was a slightly lower reduction in creatinine clearance in the individuals randomized to receive preventative treatment with rhIGF-1 (551).

Atrial natriuretic peptide is another potentially valuable agent. In a preliminary study in patients with ARF, atrial natriuretic peptide was reported to increase the creatinine or inulin clearance and reduce the dialysis requirement (552). Large-scale randomized, prospective clinical trials have been carried out to test the potential value of atrial natriuretic peptide for the treatment of patients with ARF. The data suggest that atrial natriuretic peptide has little or no effect on reducing the need for dialysis therapy and no effect on morbidity (553).

Recommended Nutritional Therapy for Acute Renal Failure

General Principles

From the current data, it is not possible to develop definitive protocols for the nutritional therapy for patients with ARF. The following therapeutic approach, summarized in Table 103-6, is based on the author's analysis of the literature and personal experience. In general, the policy is to administer sufficient quantities of nutrients to prevent or minimize the development of malnutrition.

Because the clinical status of patients with ARF is so diverse, the prescribed nutrient intake may vary greatly and should depend on the patient's nutritional status, catabolic rate, residual GFR, and the indications for initiating dialysis therapy or CVVH or CVVHD. A patient who is malnourished or hypercatabolic might receive a surfeit of nutrients and be given dialysis or CVVH or CVVHD as needed. Patients with a high residual GFR also may be given large quantities of nutrients, because there is less risk of developing fluid and electrolyte disorders or accumulating metabolic waste products. For a patient who has little or no urine flow and is not very catabolic or uremic, a reduced intake of water, minerals, and amino acids, often given as the essential amino acids, may decrease the need for dialysis; this may be particularly beneficial if the patient does not tolerate dialysis well because of underlying illnesses.

Similarly, a patient who is beginning to recover from ARF may be given small quantities of water, electrolytes, and amino acids to postpone the need for dialysis until renal function becomes adequate. In these latter patients, high-calorie diets or infusates providing small amounts of essential amino acids with little or no protein may be used for a limited amount of time. As indicated already, such nutritional therapy may maintain near neutral nitrogen balance for short periods. In patients with ARF, fluid and mineral balance should be carefully monitored to avoid overhydration or electrolyte disorders. In general, the intake of water (including the water content from wet foods) should equal the output from urine and all other measured sources (e.g., nasogastric aspirate and fistula drainage) plus about 400 mL per day. This regimen takes into account the contributions of endogenous water production from metabolism and insensible water losses (e.g., from respiration and skin) to water balance. On the other hand, if

TABLE 103-6. *Composition of solutions for total parenteral nutrition in patients with acute renal failure*

Volume	1.0	(L)	**Vitamins**	
			Vitamin A[f]	2,100 IU/day
Essential and nonessential free crystalline amino acids (4.25–5.0%)[b]				
	42.5–50	g/L	Vitamin D	(see text)
			Vitamin K[g]	7.5 mg/week
			Vitamin E[h]	10 IU/d
			Niacin	20 mg/d
Essential amino acids (5%)[b]	12.5–25	g/L	Thiamine HCl (B₁)	2 mg/d
			Riboflavin (B₂)	2 mg/d
Dextrose (D-glucose)[c]	350	g/L	Pantothenic acid (B₃)	10 mg/d
			Pyridoxine HCl	10 mg/d
Energy (approximately)[c]	4800	kj/L	Ascorbic Acid (C)	60 mg/d
			Biotin	200 mg/d
Electrolytes[d]			Folic Acid[g]	1 mg/d
Sodium[e]	40–50	mmol/L	Vitamin B₁₂[g]	3 μg/d
Chloride[e]	25–35	mmol/L		
Potassium	≤35	mmol/day		
Acetate	35–40	mmol/day		
Calcium	5	mmol/day		
Phosphorus	8	mmol/day		
Magnesium	4	mmol/day		
Iron	2	mmol/day		
Other trace elements	(see text)			

CAPD, continuous ambulatory peritoneal dialysis; APD, automated peritoneal dialysis; CVVH, continuous ???venovenous hemofiltration; CVVAD, continuous ???venovenous hemodialysis; TPN, total parenteral nutrition.

[a]The nutrients listed are present in each bottle containing 50 mL of 8.5–10% crystalline amino acids or 250 to 500 mL of 5% essential amino acids and 500 mL of 70% D-glucose. The vitamins and trace elements are an exception because they are added to only one bottle per day. For those doses of nutrients that are expressed as concentrations rather than as quantities per day, the dose refers to the quantity present in each liter of dextrose and amino acids. The patient's fluid status and serum electrolytes and glucose values must be monitored closely. The composition and volume of the infusate may be modified according to the nutritional status of the patient (see text).

[b]For patients who are more catabolic (e.g., UNA ≥5 g/d), who are undergoing regular dialysis treatments (particularly for 2 or more weeks), or who are very wasted, essential and nonessential amino acids may be infused; about 1.0–1.2 g/d for patients on hemodialysis and 1.0–1.3 g/kg/d for patients on intermittent peritoneal dialysis, CAPD, or APD, (see text). 1.5–2.5 g/kg/d of essential and nonessential amino acids may be given to patients undergoing CVVH or CVVHD. For patients who are not very wasted, who are less catabolic, who are not undergoing regular dialysis therapy, and who will not be receiving TPN for more than 2 or 3 weeks, 21–40 g/d of the nine essential amino acids may be infused. See text for discussion of the formulations of amino acids.

[c]70% D-glucose is added as necessary to obtain an energy intake of 126–136 kj/kg/d (see text); lower energy intakes may be used in very obese patients. For the higher levels of energy intake (i.e., 141 kj/kg/d), additional 70% D-glucose may be added to the solutions. Generally lipids are infused each day to provide 20–30% of total calories in order to balance the sources of calories and to prevent essential fatty acid deficiency. For patients who are septic or at high risk for sepsis, about 10–20% of calories may be given as lipids. The lipids probably should be infused over 12 to 24 hours to reduce the hyperlipidemia that occurs with intravenous infusion of lipid emulsions and to avoid impairment of the reticuloendothelial system. The lipids may be infused through a separate line or mixed with the amino acid and dextrose solutions and infused soon after mixing (see text). Usually a 20% lipid emulsions (250–500 mL) is used to reduce the water load. The approximate caloric values are dextrose monohydrate, 3.4 kcal/g; amino acids, 3.5 kcal/g.

[d]When adding electrolytes, the amounts intrinsically present in the amino acid solution should be taken into account.

[e]Refers to the final concentrations of electrolytes after any additional 70% dextrose or other solutions have been added.

[f]See text

[g]Should be given orally or parenterally and not in the TPN solution because of antagonisms.

[h]May need to be increased with use of lipid emulsions.

the patient is catabolic and in negative calorie and nitrogen balance, weight should be allowed to decrease by about 0.2 to 0.5 kg per day to avoid excessive accumulation of fluid. The intake of sodium, potassium, phosphorus, magnesium, calcium, and trace elements should be restricted to prevent accumulation of these minerals. Sodium intake should equal output but should also be coordinated with the water balance to prevent hyponatremia and hypernatremia. Potassium and phosphorus intake should be designed to prevent abnormally high or low blood levels. By controlling the water and electrolyte intake and lowering the rate of accumulation of urea and other nitrogenous metabolites, the patient may be able to reduce the need for dialysis treatments.

Insulin should be used to maintain normal plasma glucose concentrations. Glucose intolerance is very common in patients with ARF. With the large glucose loads frequently administered, hyperglycemia will occur in a large proportion of patients (474). Insulin is also a potent anabolic hormone. Some studies indicate that in nonuremic patients who have catabolic illnesses, insulin can reduce nitrogen output and improve negative nitrogen and protein balance (554,555). Recombinant human growth hormone (rhGH) may also promote nitrogen balance in patients with acute catabolic stress or chronic illness, including CRF (556,557). However, recent studies in acutely ill patients indicate that rhGH may increase mortality (558).

The following discussion of specific nutrient intakes for patients with ARF can be applied to individuals receiving oral, enteral, or intravenous nutrition. TPN has been emphasized because this is frequently the route of choice for nutritional therapy in the sicker, more catabolic patients with ARF, and it is usually the most complicated of the techniques.

Nitrogen Intake

The physician is most likely to maximally benefit the patient's metabolic and clinical status if the nitrogen intake is tailored to the clinical condition of the patient. A low protein or amino acid intake, provided orally, enterally, or intravenously, may be prescribed for patients who have a small UNA (i.e., equal to or less than 4 to 5 g of nitrogen per day), who have no evidence of severe protein malnutrition, and who will probably recover renal function within 1 to 2 weeks. A severely reduced GFR and the desire to avoid or reduce the frequency of dialysis therapy are other indications for low nitrogen intakes. One may give 0.30 to 0.50 g/kg of aBW_{ef} per day (183,426) of essential amino acids with or without arginine. More than 40 g of the nine essential amino acids per day is not prescribed because larger quantities may cause serious amino acid imbalances (see later discussion) (523,559,560). For patients who can eat, diets providing 0.10 to 0.30 g of miscellaneous protein per kilogram per day or 10 to 20 g of essential amino acids per day may be used. These treatment protocols should promote a low rate of accumulation of nitrogenous metabolites, and unless the patient is very catabolic, he or she will usually maintain neutral or only mildly negative nitrogen

balance. Hence, the need for dialysis therapy may be minimized or avoided.

If the patient has substantial residual renal function (i.e., a GFR of 5 to 10 mL per minute), is not very catabolic, and can eat well, he or she may be treated as a nondialyzed patient with CRF, receiving 0.55 to 0.60 g/kg of aBW_{ef} per day (183,426) of primarily high-biologic-value protein or about 0.28 g of protein per kilogram per day supplemented with 6 to 10 g of essential amino acids per day. If such a patient cannot be fed enterally, he or she may be given 0.55 to 0.60 g/kg per day of essential and nonessential amino acids intravenously. For patients who are more catabolic, have a higher UNA (more than 5 g of nitrogen per day), are severely wasted, and either have or are expected to have ARF for more than 2 weeks, a higher protein or amino acid intake is usually prescribed. This prescribed intake is generally 1.0 to 1.2 g/kg per day for patients undergoing regular hemodialysis but is often greater, approximately 1.5 to 2.5 g/kg per day, for individuals receiving CVVH or CVVHD (527,528,561,562). Most patients with ARF receiving TPN will merit one of these latter two dosages.

Compared with small quantities of essential amino acids, these larger nitrogen intakes may improve nitrogen balance, particularly after the first 1 or 2 weeks of dialysis treatments. However, the UNA will almost invariably rise, and the increased azotemia and water load (in patients treated with TPN) may increase the need for dialysis. Patients undergoing CVVH or CVVHD appear to tolerate increased amino acid and water loads more effectively because of the greater weekly clearances. Peak BUN levels tend to be lower with CVVH or CVVHD, and if blood levels of metabolites become excessive, these latter patients can be treated with regular hemodialysis as well.

As indicated already, studies in patients with ARF or CRF suggest that essential amino acids may be used more efficiently than mixtures of essential and nonessential amino adds (198,474,523). On the other hand, large dosages (i.e., more than 40 g per day) of essential amino acids alone may be hazardous. Several reports describe patients with ARF who were infused with relatively large quantities, for their body weight, of essential amino acids (523,559,560). Their plasma amino acid concentrations were bizarre; many plasma amino acid levels were markedly increased. Blood ammonia levels were high, and a metabolic acidosis occurred. Some patients became comatose. The plasma amino acid pattern improved markedly when patients were given an infusion of essential and nonessential amino acids provided in a 1.0 : 1.0 ratio. These considerations suggest that the inclusion of some nonessential amino acids in the mixture may enable the patient to tolerate a larger quantity of essential amino acids. Because solutions with a high ratio of essential : nonessential amino acids may be more anabolic than preparations with a 1.0 : 1.0 ratio (see previous discussion) and may be safer than high dosages (more than 30 to 40 g per day) of essential amino acids alone, the use of such formulations for patients with ARF should be examined (563).

Branched-chain amino acids, particularly leucine, may promote anabolism (218,219). Studies in catabolic patients without renal failure suggest that the intravenous infusion of amino acid solutions containing a large proportion of branched-chain amino acids (e.g., isoleucine, leucine, and valine) may have a modest anabolic effect (566,567); not all reports confirm these findings.

Keto acid analogs of the branched-chain amino acids also enhance anabolism in *in vitro* tissue preparations and in clinical studies carried out in nonuremic individuals who were not hypercatabolic (219,568). In postoperative patients who were receiving TPN, intravenous infusion of the salt complex of α-ketoglutarate and ornithine appears to decrease UNA and improve nitrogen balance (569). Further investigation into the anabolic properties and potential clinical usefulness of these preparations for patients with ARF is necessary.

Energy

The energy expenditure and requirements for patients with ARF are primarily determined by the same factors that affect nonuremic individuals and include weight, age, sex, associated diseases, and physical activity, if any. Whether ARF affects energy expenditure or requirements is not known. In nonuremic individuals, the energy intake necessary to obtain neutral or positive nitrogen balance rises when nitrogen intake is low. Because patients with ARF are often given low quantities of nitrogen, this may indicate a need for greater energy intake. The fact that patients with ARF are often fluid intolerant sometimes influences the quantity of energy that may be given safely. Mault et al. (522) reported that patients with ARF had about a 30% increase in resting energy expenditure as determined by indirect calorimetry; many, if not all, of these patients had associated catabolic illnesses. In a nonrandomized comparison, the authors found that patients who died had a more negative energy balance than those who survived (522). We have also observed that patients with ARF given higher energy intakes had greater survival (474). Although this might reflect a clinical benefit of high energy intakes, it is also possible that the patients with more negative energy balance were sicker and had medical disorders that made them more difficult to nourish (e.g., shock and pulmonary edema).

One standard method for assessing energy needs is based on the Harris-Benedict equations, which estimate basal energy expenditure (BEE) from age, sex, body weight, and height. The Harris-Benedict equations are as follows (570):

For men: BEE − 66.5 + [13.8 × weight(kg)] + [5.0 × height(cm)] − [6.8 × age(yr)]
For women: BEE − 655.1 + [9.6 × weight(kg)] + [1.8 × height(cm)] − [4.7 × age(yr)].

The value calculated from these equations is then multiplied by an adjustment factor for the increase in energy expenditure caused by different clinical conditions. Some of these factors

TABLE 103-7. *Adjustment factors for estimating energy expenditure during illness*

Type of stress	Fraction of normal basal energy expenditure[a]
Malnutrition (chronic, severe)	0.70
Nondialyzed chronic renal failure	1.00
Maintenance hemodialysis	1.00–1.05
Elective surgery	
Early (1–4 d)[b]	1.00
Late (18–21 d)	0.95
Peritonitis	1.15
Soft tissue trauma	1.15
Fractures	1.20–1.25
Infections	
Mild	1.00
Moderate	1.20–1.40
Severe	1.40–1.60
Burns (percentage of body surface)	
0–20%	1.00–1.50
20–40%	1.50–1.85
40–100%	1.85–2.05

[a]The basal energy expenditure values during the normal healthy state may be multiplied by these approximate factors to estimate resting energy expenditure during acute or chronic illness.
[b]Associated with early starvation.
Source: From Wilmore DW. *The metabolic management of the critically ill.* New York: Plenum, 1977:34; and Monteon FJ et al. Energy expenditure in patients with chronic renal failure. *Kidney Int* 1986;30:741.

are shown in Table 103-7. Finally, the energy requirement is increased by 25% to adjust for individual variability, physical activity, and the potentially greater needs associated with a low nitrogen intake and ARF. Thus, the calculation of energy requirements in ARF is as follows:

$$\text{energy requirements} = \text{estimated BEE} \times \text{adjustment for illness} \times 1.25$$

Another method used to estimate energy requirements is to measure energy expenditure by indirect calorimetry and multiply this value by 1.25. In practice, the estimated energy requirements for patients with ARF requiring nutritional support usually fall between 126 to 168 kJ/kg (30 and 40 kcal/kg) of aBW_{ef} per day.

The higher energy intakes (i.e., 168 kJ/kg [40 kcal/kg] per day) generally are prescribed for patients who have a higher UNA, who are severely ill, and who are not very obese. For example, if nitrogen balance, estimated from the difference between the patient's nitrogen intake and the nitrogen output calculated from the UNA (see previous discussion), is negative, despite an appropriate amino acid intake, we try to provide an energy intake close to 168 kJ/kg (40 kcal/kg) per day.

Larger energy intakes are not used because there appears to be little nutritional advantage to administering more than 168 kJ (40 kcal) per day to catabolic patients. Indeed, because high energy intakes generate more carbon dioxide from the infused carbohydrates and fat, they can promote hypercapnia if pulmonary function is impaired (572). Carbon dioxide retention is particularly likely to occur with very high carbohydrate loads, because, in comparison to fat, more carbon atoms are provided with carbohydrate to provide the same quantity of energy. Also, very high energy intakes may cause obesity and fatty liver, and because of the large volume of fluids in the intravenous solutions, they may increase the water load to the patient (573).

Because most patients with ARF do not tolerate large water intakes, glucose is usually administered in a 70% solution. Glucose is added to intravenous solutions as glucose monohydrate, which is 90% anhydrous glucose. The energy available from glucose monohydrate is 14.3 kJ/g (3.4 kcal/g), or from 70% dextrose, about 9.99 kJ/mL (2.38 kcal/mL). Amino acids provide about 14.7 kJ/g (3.5 kcal/g). The glucose and amino acid solutions are mixed so the amino acids and calories are provided simultaneously (Table 103-7).

Patients receiving TPN for more than about 5 days should receive lipid emulsions. The optimal amount of fat for TPN is somewhat controversial, especially because lipid clearance is impaired in ARF (574). Twenty-five grams of lipids per day will prevent essential fatty acid deficiency. Some investigators recommend infusing up to 30% to 40% of calories as lipid emulsions to provide more normal amounts of fatty acids to organs that use lipids for energy and to more closely approximate the normal American dietary intake. Some findings suggest that infusion of lipid emulsions may lower host resistance. Several researchers report that infusions of large amounts of fat emulsions (e.g., 50 g over 8 hours) may impair reticuloendothelial system function (575), presumably by overwhelming the phagocytic capacity of this system. Neonates receiving TPN with lipid emulsions are reported to have a higher incidence of bacteremia than similar infants given TPN without lipids (576).

A prudent approach may be to infuse lipid emulsions over 12 to 24 hours to minimize increases in plasma lipid levels and to avoid overwhelming the reticuloendothelial system. Patients who are not septic may be given up to 20% to 30% of calories as lipid emulsions. Patients who are severely septic probably should not receive intravenous lipid emulsions for several days. Lipids are available as 10% and 20% fat emulsions that provide 4.6 and 8.4 kJ/mL (1.1 and 2.0 kcal/mL), respectively. Traditionally, lipids have been infused separately from the glucose and amino acid mixtures. With careful attention to aseptic techniques, one may mix the lipid emulsions with glucose and amino acids; the mixtures should be infused shortly after preparation (577). Several studies suggest that ω-3 fatty acids may enhance immune function and host resistance (578–580).

Minerals

Minerals can be added to parenteral nutrition solutions for ARF as shown in Table 103-6. Recommended intakes of minerals should be considered tentative and must be modified according to the clinical status of the patient. The patient must be monitored closely because the hormonal and metabolic changes that often occur in ARF may cause serum electrolyte concentrations to rise or fall dramatically. If the serum concentration of an electrolyte is increased, it may be advisable to reduce the quantity infused or to refrain from administering it at the onset of parenteral nutrition. However, parenteral nutrition may rapidly lower certain serum electrolyte concentrations, particularly potassium and phosphorus. On the other hand, a low serum concentration of a mineral may indicate that there is a need for a greater than usual intake of that element. Again, metabolic changes and the impaired GFR can lead to a rapid rise in the serum concentrations of electrolytes or glucose.

With the exception of iron and possibly zinc, trace elements are probably not necessary in parenteral nutrition solutions for ARF, unless this is the sole source of nutritional support for at least 2 to 3 weeks. The nutritional requirements for trace elements have not been established for uremic patients receiving TPN.

Vitamins

The vitamin requirements have not been well defined for patients with ARF, and there is a clear need for more research on this subject. Tentative recommendations for vitamin intake for patients receiving parenteral nutrition are shown in Table 103-6. Much of the recommended intake is based on information obtained from studies in chronically uremic patients, healthy individuals, or nonuremic acutely ill patients. There is a need to provide water-soluble vitamins to patients with ARF because they often eat inadequate quantities, lose vitamins in dialysate, may have increased vitamin needs, and receive medicines that antagonize the actions of many vitamins (see previous discussion). Recently, it has been reported that serum concentrations of the fat-soluble Vitamin A, Vitamin E, 25-hydroxycholecalciferol, and 1,25-dihydroxycholecalciferol are decreased, those of parathyroid hormone and Vitamin K are elevated, and those of retinol binding protein are within the normal range in patients with ARF (581). Another group has reported increased serum Vitamin A levels in patients with ARF (582).

The quantities needed for the prevention or treatment of deficiencies of these vitamins are not known. Caution must be exhibited with Vitamin A therapy because in CRF, serum Vitamin A levels are elevated and rather small supplements of Vitamin A are reported to cause toxicity in chronically uremic patients (402,405,406). Until more data are available that are specifically related to the fat-soluble vitamin requirements for patients with ARF, it is recommended that these individuals should receive Vitamin A, 2,100 IU (i.e., two-thirds of the American Medical Association–Food and Drug Administration [AMA-FDA] adult formula), and Vitamin E, 10 IU. These recommendations are a modification of the 1975 recommendations of the Nutrition Advisory Group of the AMA for intravenous vitamin formulations for adult patients. These AMA recommendations were approved by the FDA in 1979 (583) and have been referred to as the AMA-FDA adult formula (584).

Vitamin K deficiency may occur in patients without renal failure who are not eating and are receiving antibiotics that may suppress Vitamin K, producing intestinal bacteria (411). Vitamin K supplements therefore should be given routinely to patients receiving parenteral nutrition (Table 103-6). Ten milligrams per day of pyridoxine hydrochloride (8.2 mg per day of pyridoxine) is recommended because studies in clinically stable or sick patients undergoing MHD indicate that this quantity may be necessary to prevent or correct Vitamin B_6 deficiency (68). Patients should probably not receive more than 60 to 100 mg per day of ascorbic acid because of the risk of increased serum oxalate concentrations (416,417). Indeed, there is one report of a child with ARF from the hemolytic-uremic syndrome who received parenteral nutrition providing 500 mg per day of ascorbic acid (585). The patient was found to have deposits of calcium oxalate in the kidneys and pancreas.

Although Vitamin D is fat soluble and vitamin stores should not become depleted during the few days to weeks that most patients with ARF receive parenteral nutrition, the turnover of its most active analog, 1,25-dihydroxycholecalciferol, is much faster (586). Hence, there may be a need for this analog in patients with ARF. In patients on MHD, intravenous 1,25-dihydroxycholecalciferol can markedly suppress parathyroid hormone secretion (587). The finding that in ARF, some Vitamin D compounds are decreased and hyperparathyroidism may occur and have adverse effects (494,581) suggests a possible therapeutic role for this Vitamin D analog.

The nutrient intake of patients with ARF must be carefully reevaluated, often each day and sometimes more frequently. This is particularly important because the clinical and metabolic condition of these patients may undergo rapid changes.

Amino Acid and Protein Intake may Predispose to Acute Renal Failure

Several studies in rats suggest that high amino acid or protein intakes may increase the susceptibility to ARF caused by ischemia or nephrotoxicity (588–592). The nutrients seem to increase both the incidence and the severity of ARF induced by these agents. Several individual amino acids, particularly D-serine, DL-ethionine, and L-lysine, appear to be nephrotoxic (590,593). In contrast, glycine and alanine may protect against ischemia- or toxic-induced renal tubular cell damage (592), at least in *in vitro* preparations. The mechanisms responsible for these protective effects are not known. If amino acids or protein predisposes to renal failure in humans, then patients who receive nephrotoxic medicines or who are at high risk for renal ischemia might benefit from low amino acid or protein intakes. On the other hand, if glycine and alanine are protective *in vivo,* it is possible that administration of these amino acids could reduce the likelihood of ARF in high-risk patients. Clearly, more research is needed in this area.

Special Techniques for Managing Catabolic or Malnourished Patients with Acute or Chronic Renal Failure

Agents that may Enhance More Positive Protein Balance

In the last several years, there have been a number of reports indicating the potential value of using growth factors to improve protein balance and of administering specific nutrients to enhance immunoreactivity and host resistance. Experience with these agents in nonuremic individuals or animal models suggests that they may be useful for patients with ARF or CRF and superimposed catabolic stress (556,557). In addition to the use of anabolic steroids or insulin (see previous discussion), several studies suggest that rhIGF-1 and rhGH might enhance protein retention in malnourished patients with CRF who are undergoing MHD or CPD (547,595,596). Many studies have demonstrated that growth hormone stimulates growth in children with CRF (597,598). As indicated already, rhIGF-1 has not been shown to enhance recovery from ARF in humans (550), and rhGH administration has been associated with increased mortality in acutely ill patients (558).

Administration of large quantities of glutamine or arginine to acutely ill humans or animals is reported to improve immune function, reduce risk of infection, and for glutamine, to restore intracellular glutamine pools, which fall early in acute stress, improve intestinal mucosal structure and physiology, and reduce the risk of bacterial translocation (599–605). The benefits of this therapy for critically ill patients have not yet been unequivocally demonstrated (606). There are no data as to whether large supplements of glutamine and arginine are beneficial for physically stressed patients with ARF or CRF. However, in rats with ischemic ARF, administration of L-arginine (300 mg/kg for 60 minutes) is reported to acutely increase GFR, probably by increasing nitric oxide production (607).

Peptides in TPN solutions have been used to provide unstable or poorly soluble amino acids to the patient (e.g., dipeptides of glutamine, cysteine, and tyrosine [600]). Peptides also provide amino acids at a lower osmolality. Experimental evidence derived largely from animal or cell studies also indicates that ω-3 fatty acids and supplemental nucleotides may improve a number of parameters of immunologic function and host resistance (578–580,608). The ω-3 fatty acids appear to modify immune responses by altering the pattern of cytokines elaborated by inflammatory cells (578–580). Clinical trials with anticytokine or anti–cytokine receptor antibodies have not yet been shown to be valuable for acutely ill patients.

Methods of Nutrient Administration in Acute or Chronic Renal Failure

Enteral Versus Parenteral Nutrition

Patients with ARF or CRF and superimposed illness should be given oral nutrition whenever feasible. If the patient will not eat adequately, he or she may be offered liquid-formula diets, elemental diets, or tube or enterostomy feeding. Often enteral tube or gastrostomy feeding is the only possible method of nourishment through the alimentary tract (609) in critically ill patients. For patients who must be fed by an enteric tube or gastrostomy, there are many liquid protein or defined-formula (elemental) diets that may be prescribed. Some are specifically designed for patients with renal failure. Dietitians usually can provide information concerning the composition of these preparations. There are a number of reviews of the techniques and complications associated with the use of the chemically defined diets and tube feeding (609–611). Most of the principles are applicable to the patient with renal failure. Although tube feeding has been used extensively in pediatric patients, particularly infants, with CRF (612,613), there has been a reluctance to employ these techniques for adult patients with renal failure. Many patients with ARF do not have well-functioning gastrointestinal tracts, and parenteral nutrition is the only technique that will provide adequate nutrient intake. This is particularly common in the more catabolic patients with ARF. Parenteral nutrition provides greater fluid loads and is more costly. Techniques for parenteral nutrition and the potential complications of this treatment have been reviewed elsewhere (584).

Peripheral parenteral nutrition has been suggested as an alternative to TPN (614). The solutions are infused into a peripheral vein, and the risks of inserting a central catheter are avoided. A limitation of peripheral parenteral nutrition is that the osmolality of the infusate must be restricted to about 600 mOsmol or lower to prevent thrombophlebitis; even then, the needles or catheters must be changed frequently, usually every 18 to 48 hours. Thus, to receive adequate calories and amino acids, the patient must receive large fluid loads, which are not tolerated by most individuals with ARF who require parenteral nutrition. Moreover, the pharmaceutical costs of peripheral parenteral nutrition are usually similar to those of TPN because with the former technique, larger amounts of expensive lipid emulsions must be given to provide calories with a lower osmotic load.

Peripheral partial parenteral nutrition may be useful for patients with ARF who are able to receive only part of their daily nutritional requirements by oral or enteric feeding. The peripheral infusions may allow these patients to receive adequate nutrition without resorting to TPN through a large flow vein. In these individuals, it is often preferable to infuse an 8.5% to 10% amino acid solution or a 20% lipid emulsion into a peripheral vein and administer as much as possible of the other essential nutrients through the enteral tract, including carbohydrates, which provide most of the osmotic load when given intravenously.

To avoid the risk of central vein catheterization, one can use the peripheral vascular access route that is used for hemodialysis for TPN (615). Because the blood flow through the vascular access route is large, hypertonic solutions can be infused and the water load to the patient can be reduced. However, in our experience, this technique increases the hazard of local infection, and it should not be used in patients who will need a hemodialysis access route for extended periods of time.

Intravenous Nutrition Limited to Hemodialysis

For patients who have marginally adequate intakes and who will not ingest more nutrients through foods or food supplements, supplemental amino acids, glucose, or lipids may be infused intravenously during hemodialysis treatment (e.g., IDPN) (161,162,616). The preparation is infused into the blood leaving the dialyzer; IDPN avoids the need for catheterization of a central or peripheral vein and allows the physician to remove excess water and minerals as these chemicals are infused. Evidence does not clearly show that IDPN is beneficial, or that patients may not receive similar advantages from oral supplements or tube feeding (161,162,616). Regretfully, a large-scale prospective, randomized clinical trial with IDPN has never been performed.

A case-control, retrospective study (162) and a nonrandomized, retrospective report (161) provide suggestive data that IDPN may increase survival in malnourished patients on MHD. In the case-control study, those patients with a serum albumin level of 3.3 g/dL or less who were given IDPN had greater survival than those who were not (162). In the retrospective comparison of nonrandomized patients on MHD, those individuals who received IDPN had a reduced mortality rate (161).

Partly because of substantial evidence for overuse of IDPN, third-party payers have become very restrictive in their indications for reimbursement for IDPN. Recent position papers have attempted to define indications for IDPN (617). One such report emphasizes that IDPN is only indicated for malnourished patients on MHD who ingest inadequate nutrients and for whom counseling, food supplements, and tube feeding are not helpful or are contraindicated (617). IDPN is probably of value only for clinically stable patients who have a slightly suboptimal intake of nutrients. This technique is probably inadequate for physically stressed patients with ARF because their oral or enteral intake level is usually very low, their nutrient needs are high, and the nutritional supplements can be given only intermittently, when the patient undergoes hemodialysis.

However, because most patients who need nutritional supplements have decreased intakes of energy and total nitrogen, we give 40 to 42 g of essential and nonessential amino acids and 200 g of D-glucose (150 g of D-glucose if the dialysate contains glucose) and often 250 mL of a 10% or 20% lipid solution (e.g., 25 to 50 g of fat). The nutrients are administered at a constant rate throughout the dialysis procedure to minimize the fall in amino acid and glucose pools that usually occur with hemodialysis. In our experience, about 85% to 90% of the amino acids and a large proportion of the glucose infused are retained; the amino acid losses in dialysate rise by an average of only 4 to 5 g (94). The nutrients may be used more efficiently because they are given continuously rather than as a bolus. Patients who have low serum concentrations of phosphorus or potassium at the start of the dialysis treatment may need supplements of these minerals during the amino acid and glucose infusions. If the dialysate is glucose-free, the infusion is not stopped until the end of hemodialysis to prevent reactive hypoglycemia. Also, the patient should eat a source of carbohydrates 20 to 30 minutes before the end of the infusion. Otherwise, the infusion must be tapered or a peripheral infusion of glucose must be started to avoid hypoglycemia.

Nutritional Hemodialysis and Nutritional Peritoneal Dialysis

A number of investigators have examined the possibility of adding amino acids to the dialysate of patients undergoing CPD or MHD (96,618–620). With hemodialysis, additional glucose may be added. The nutrients diffuse into the body during dialysis. These techniques have the potential advantages of consolidating nutritional and dialysis treatment into one procedure, reducing the risk of fluid and electrolyte disturbances from intravenous nutrition, and decreasing the considerable costs of intravenous feeding. When the nutrients are added to the hemodialysate, some investigators have reduced the dialysis flow rate to increase the fractional extraction of amino acids and glucose from dialysate (618). This has the benefit of reducing the cost of the nutrients given to the patient, but it also decreases the efficiency of dialysis; hence, these patients may require more hours of dialysis therapy, which raises nursing costs. Also, nutritional hemodialysis would have to be performed daily if it were the only or the main source of nutrition for a patient. This procedure, if it were to have value, would probably be of benefit only for hospitalized patients and it would have to be designed so that it was performed by intensive care unit personnel rather than by hemodialysis nurses to save costs. Under these conditions, it would be a variant of CVVHD.

Chazot et al. (96) added amino acids to the dialysate during standard hemodialysis using a cellulose triacetate hemodialyzer. When about 46 g of a mixture of 20 amino acids was added to the concentrate to provide a final dialysate amino acid concentration similar to fasting plasma levels, the amino acid losses into hemodialysate were prevented. When 139 g of this amino acid mixture was added to the hemodialysate concentrate, there was a net transfer of about 39 g of amino acids from the dialysate to the patient during the hemodialysis.

The possibility of adding amino acids to peritoneal dialysate for malnourished patients undergoing CPD has been investigated (619,620). By using amino acids, one can reduce the glucose load from the dialysate. Also, for malnourished patients who are ingesting low-protein diets, the addition of amino acids appears to increase nitrogen balance, protein synthesis, and several serum protein levels (619,620). In general, a mixture of both essential and nonessential amino acids is provided in about a 1.1% solution of standard peritoneal dialysate, except that it is glucose-free. One or two peritoneal dialysate exchanges of this solution are substituted each day for the patient's usual exchanges. Dwell times should last about 4 to 6 hours to ensure an uptake of about 80% of the total dialysate amino acid content and to prevent excessive reabsorption of other compounds in dialysate by an excessively long dwell time. The caloric load from these solutions is very small. Hence, it is preferable that these exchanges are given during the major meals of the day. Again, dietary counseling and food supplements should be attempted and tube feeding should be considered before turning to these more expensive and incomplete nutritional supplements.

DIETARY THERAPY FOR RENAL TRANSPLANTATION

Patients who undergo renal transplantation often develop normal or even supranormal appetites; the latter is probably a result of glucocorticoid therapy. Gain in body weight and fat is common. However, several nutritional disorders appear to be related to other factors associated with renal transplantation. These include impaired growth in children (621), protein wasting (622–627), altered serum lipid and homocysteine concentrations (628–630), and abnormalities in bone, mineral, and vitamin metabolism (362,631–633).

One of the most important causes of these disorders seems to be the administration of prednisone. Glucocorticoids, particularly in large doses, cause pervasive metabolic effects. These have been well reviewed elsewhere (634,635) and include enhanced gluconeogenesis, degradation of protein and nucleic acids, lipolysis, reduced protein synthesis, and glucose uptake in many tissues. Glucocorticoids can increase serum cholesterol level, inhibit intestinal calcium absorption (636,637), and reduce serum levels of 25-hydroxycholecalciferol and 1,25-dihydroxycholecalciferol (637–640). Glucocorticoids also stimulate catabolism or inhibit anabolic processes in many tissues, including bone and connective tissues, and cause negative calcium balance and osteoporosis (641).

Renal transplant recipients who receive large doses of prednisone for antirejection therapy sustain negative nitrogen balance (622–627). Superimposed catabolic illnesses or the development of the nephrotic syndrome may also cause protein wasting in transplant recipients. In one study, patients with cadaveric renal transplants were given prednisone starting at 120 mg per day and tapering to 70 to 90 mg per day over approximately 10 to 14 days (622). The authors reported that a protein and energy intake of 1.30 ± 0.06 (SEM) g/kg per day and 138.6 ± 12.6 kJ/kg (33 ± 3 kcal/kg) per day, respectively, maintained less negative estimated nitrogen balance (-0.02 ± 0.12 g of nitrogen per kilogram per day) than an intake of 0.73 ± 0.03 g of protein per kilogram per day and 84 ± 16.8 kJ/kg (20 ± 4 kcal/kg) per day (estimated nitrogen balance, -0.72 ± 0.12 g/kg per day). These investigators could not distinguish between the relative contributions of the higher nitrogen and caloric intakes to the more positive nitrogen balance. Nitrogen balance was estimated from the difference between nitrogen intake and nitrogen output, calculated from the UNA. Patients were studied prospectively but were not randomly assigned to the two diets.

Whittier et al. (624) examined the hypothesis that postoperative renal transplant recipients appear to be less cushingoid when they are given a high-protein, low-carbohydrate diet. These investigators randomly assigned 12 nondiabetic renal transplant recipients to a diet providing either 1 ± 0.3 (SD) g of carbohydrate per kilogram per day and 117.6 ± 8.4 kJ/kg (28 ± 2 kcal/kg) per day (experimental diet) or 3 ± 0.4 g of carbohydrate per kilogram per day and 130.2 ± 12.6 kJ/kg (31 ± 3 kcal/kg) per day (control diet) (624). The experimental and control diets provided 2 ± 0.3 and 1 ± 0.2 g of protein per kilogram per day, respectively. The patients underwent balance studies for 28 days. Nitrogen balance was significantly more positive, and there was a tendency for potassium and sodium balance to be more positive in patients receiving the experimental diet. Nitrogen and potassium balance correlated with intake in the 12 patients combined. The regression analysis of the relationship between nitrogen balance and intake indicated that nitrogen balance, uncorrected for unmeasured losses, which were probably about 0.5 g per day (178), was zero at a protein intake of 1.3 g/kg per day. The patients who received the experimental diet were less cushingoid, as judged by three independent observers who examined pretreatment and posttreatment photographs. Chronic low doses of prednisone (10 mg per day or less) do not appear to alter body composition, as determined by anthropometry or dual-energy x-ray absorptiometry, or resting energy expenditure (625).

Renal transplant recipients have increased serum triglyceride, LDL cholesterol, and HDL cholesterol concentrations, and the LDL cholesterol : HDL cholesterol ratio may be increased (628,629). Several patterns of hyperlipoproteinemia may be present, including type IV, type 11B, and type 11A (642). Serum triglyceride levels correlate with the daily dose of prednisone, degree of obesity, and severity of renal insufficiency. These findings are of particular concern because several studies have found a correlation between increased serum lipid levels and the risk of cardiovascular disease, graft failure, and fatality in renal transplant recipients (629,643–645). Causes of increased serum triglyceride and cholesterol levels include excessive fat and energy intake, obesity, glucocorticoids, diuretics, cyclosporine, nephrotic-range proteinuria, and underlying disease (e.g., diabetes mellitus) (646,647). In most studies, dietary counseling of renal transplant recipients can reduce their energy intake, weight gain (648,649), and serum total cholesterol, LDL cholesterol, and triglyceride

levels, but without a change in their serum HDL cholesterol level (628,647–653).

A low-cholesterol, high-fiber diet with a polyunsaturated fatty acid : saturated fatty acid ratio of more than 1.0 and an NCEP-AHA Step 1 diet (see previous discussion) can lower serum total cholesterol and LDL cholesterol levels in renal transplant recipients (628,649,650,652). However, the altered lipoprotein pattern may not be affected. A combination of a similar diet with regular exercise may improve the plasma lipid pattern (654). Pagenkemper reported that a dose of fish oil providing 3 g per day of ω-3 fatty acids for 3 months decreased serum triglyceride and VLDL cholesterol levels in hyperlipidemic renal transplant recipients; however, there was no change in their serum total cholesterol or LDL cholesterol levels (655). Combining dietary therapy with serum HMG CoA reductase inhibitors is even more effective for reducing serum total and LDL cholesterol levels (647,656).

Plasma homocysteine concentrations are also elevated in renal transplant recipients. Some evidence indicates that hyperhomocysteinemia is a risk factor for cardiovascular complications and mortality in this population of patients (630–659). In patients on MHD who have had a successful kidney transplant, their plasma homocysteine level decreases but seems to remain more than that in individuals with similar levels of renal function who have not undergone transplantation (660). The causes of hyperhomocysteinemia include reduced GFR, which appears to be the most important determinant (661), low serum folate levels (662), and possibly cyclosporin A therapy. Reports differ as to whether cyclosporin A contributes to hyperhomocysteinemia (663–665). In one study in healthy individuals, large doses of coffee, (e.g., about 1 L of paper-filtered coffee per day) increased plasma total homocysteine level by 1.5 μmol/L, or 18% (666). Folic acid decreases plasma homocysteine levels in renal transplant recipients, but not to within the normal range (665). It has been suggested that the decrease in plasma homocysteine level is greater when pyridoxine hydrochloride (50 mg per day) and Vitamin B_{12} (0.4 mg per day) are added to folic acid (5 mg per day) (667).

Serum folate levels are reported to be reduced in patients who have received transplants but increased slightly with time after the transplantation (630). However, low serum folate levels were observed as long as 6 years after transplantation. Macrocytosis was observed in 52% of patients; it was only observed in patients with good renal graft function who were treated with azathioprine. The authors suggested that azathioprine rather than folate deficiency caused the macrocytosis. Serum Vitamin B_{12} levels are generally within the normal range in transplant recipients (668). After successful renal transplantation, serum Vitamin A levels often remain elevated for extended periods and may not fall to normal levels in some patients for almost 2 years (669).

Cyclosporin A often reduces the glucocorticoid requirement. However, cyclosporin A itself may increase serum cholesterol (646) level, potassium retention with hyperkalemia

(670), and urinary magnesium wasting with hypomagnesemia (671). Mahajan et al. (362) reported low plasma and hair zinc levels and hyperzincuria in 15 patients who had received a renal transplant within 12 months. These patients also had elevated taste detection and recognition thresholds. On the other hand, patients who had received a renal transplant more than 12 months previously that was still functioning had normal plasma, hair, and urine zinc levels and taste detection and recognition thresholds. Patients more than 12 months posttransplantation who had advanced renal failure had low plasma and hair zinc levels and high taste detection and recognition thresholds.

Patients undergoing renal transplantation often have renal osteodystrophy with reduced bone mass. Bone mass may be further diminished after renal transplantation because of continuing suppression of bone formation, hyperparathyroid- and glucocorticoid-induced bone wasting (641), inhibition of intestinal calcium absorption (636,637), and lowering of serum Vitamin D levels (637–640). Calcium and Vitamin D supplements may suppress serum parathyroid hormone and increase serum 1,25-dihydroxyvitamin D levels (636).

Recommended Nutrient Intake

Because there are still few scientific data concerning the nutritional requirements for renal transplant recipients, the following recommendations should be considered tentative. Immediately after renal transplantation, during periods of catabolic stress or high prednisone dosage (e.g., 30 mg per day or more), patients should probably receive about 1.3 to 1.5 g of protein per kilogram per day. If patients are receiving CVVH or CVVHD or have normal or near-normal renal function, protein intake may be increased to 2.0 g/kg per day if their UNA is very high. When the daily dosage of prednisone is reduced to less than 30 mg per day, protein intake can be decreased.

The long-term management of protein intake should probably be directed toward preventing the progression of renal failure and maintaining good nutritional status. One study suggests that low-protein diets may retard the progression of renal failure in renal transplant recipients (672). For patients with a GFR of less than about 60 mL per minute per 1.73 m^2, who show evidence for progression of renal failure, and who are on low doses of glucocorticoids (e.g., 15 mg or less per day), a protein intake of about 0.60 to 0.75 g/kg per day may be prescribed. If higher chronic glucocorticoid doses are given, a greater protein intake is probably necessary (e.g., 0.60 to 1.0 g/kg per day), depending on the glucocorticoid dose. At least 0.35 g/kg per day of the protein should be of high biologic value. Protein intake may be adjusted upward for acute increases in prednisone dosage or for large urinary protein losses, as seen with nephrotic patients (see previous discussion). Fish oil supplements are also reported to retard the progression of renal failure in renal transplant recipients (272).

The observations of Whittier et al. (624) that a diet low in carbohydrate and modestly restricted in calories may reduce the cushingoid appearance suggest that such individuals may be given a low carbohydrate intake (1 g/kg per day), which is limited to 117.6 to 126.0 kJ/kg (28 to 30 kcal/kg) per day. If such a low carbohydrate, moderately restricted energy intake is employed in renal transplant recipients, it should be limited to short periods when the prednisone dosage is very high (e.g., more than 40 mg per day). This level of energy intake may not minimize the catabolic response during acute illness (see previous discussion) and may lead to further wasting. Also, given the abnormalities in lipid metabolism in renal transplant recipients, it is questionable whether such a high-fat diet should be continued for long periods. In general, renal transplant recipients should be encouraged to ingest an AHA Step 1 diet as described previously for the nondialyzed patient with renal failure and the patient on maintenance dialysis. Patients should be encouraged to exercise regularly and to maintain a normal (163,164) or desirable body weight (673). For transplant recipients with superimposed catabolic illnesses, 126 to 168 kJ/kg (30 to 40 kcal/kg) per day may be prescribed. Other maneuvers to correct abnormal serum lipid levels are similar to those described for the patient with renal failure who has not undergone transplantation (see previous discussion). For renal transplant recipients with serum LDL cholesterol levels of more than about 100 mg/dL, an AHA Step 1 diet should be offered. If dietary therapy does not reduce the serum LDL cholesterol level to less than this value, HMG CoA reductase inhibitors should be considered (647,656).

Calcium intake should probably be maintained at 1,400 to 1,600 mg per day to reduce bone wasting. Because high phosphorus intakes may enhance the rate of progression of renal failure in experimental animals and possibly in humans, dietary phosphorus should be restricted proportionately to the reduction in protein intake, as described previously in this chapter. Hyperphosphatemia should be avoided. The regulation of other macrominerals in the diet is usually unnecessary unless the patient has renal insufficiency, other diseases associated with sodium retention (e.g., congestive heart failure or liver failure), or hypertension. The data of Mahajan et al. (362) suggest that patients with a well-functioning kidney transplant might benefit from a small zinc supplement, possibly 15 mg per day of elemental zinc, for the first 12 months after the transplantation.

Patients should receive a daily vitamin supplement containing the recommended dietary intake of water-soluble vitamins for patients with chronic renal insufficiency (Table 103-5). Hyperhomocysteinemia should be treated with folic acid, probably 5 mg per day. Depending on the response, folic acid may be increased up to 15 mg per day. It is not yet demonstrated whether large doses of pyridoxine hydrochloride and Vitamin B$_{12}$ should be routinely given as well (667). Whether 1,25-dihydroxycholecalciferol or another Vitamin D analog should be routinely given to renal transplant recipients is also not yet established.

REFERENCES

1. Kopple JD. Products of nitrogen metabolism. In: *Massry and Glassock's textbook of nephrology*, 4th ed. Philadephia: Lippincott Williams & Wilkins, 2001.

2. Horton ES, Johnson C, Lebovitz HE. Carbohydrate metabolism in uremia. *Ann Intern Med* 1968;68:63.

3. DeFronzo RA, Andres R, Edgar P, et al. Carbohydrate metabolism in uremia: a review. *Medicine (Baltimore)* 1973;52:469.

4. DeFronzo RA, Alvestrand A, Smith D, et al. Insulin resistance in uremia. *J Clin Invest* 1981;67:563.

5. Bergström J, Hultman E. Glycogen content of skeletal muscle in patients with renal failure. *Acta Med Scand* 1969;186:177.

6. Kahn T, Mohammad G, Stein RM. Alterations in renal tubular sodium and water reabsorption in chronic renal disease in man. *Kidney Int* 1972;2:164.

7. Bricker NS. On the pathogenesis of the uremic state. An exposition of the "trade-off hypothesis. " In Seminars in Medicine of the Beth Israel Hospital, Boston. *N Engl J Med* 1972;286:1093.

8. David DS, Hochgelerent E, Rubin AL, et al. Dietary management in renal failure. *Lancet* 1972;2:34.

9. Coburn JW, Hartenbower DL, Massry SG. Intestinal absorption of calcium and the effect of renal insufficiency. *Kidney Int* 1973;4:96.

10. Coburn JW, Hartenbower DL, Brickman AS, et al. Intestinal absorption of calcium, magnesium and phosphorus in chronic renal insufficiency. In: David DS, ed. *Perspectives in hypertension and nephrology—calcium metabolism in renal disease*. New York: Wiley-Liss, 1977:77.

11. Delano BG, Manis JG, Manis T. Iron absorption in experimental uremia. *Nephron* 1977;19:26.

12. Lawson DH, Boddy K, King PC, et al. Iron metabolism in patients with CRF on regular dialysis treatment. *Clin Sci* 1977;41:345.

13. Vaziri ND, Said HM, Hollander D, et al. Impaired intestinal absorption of riboflavin in experimental uremia. *Nephron* 1985;41:26.

14. Said HM, Vaziri ND, Kariger RK, et al. Intestinal absorption of 5-methyltetrahydrofolate in experimental uremia. *Acta Vitaminol Enzymol* 1984;6(4):339.

15. Vaziri ND, Hollander D, Hung EK, et al. Impaired intestinal absorption of Vitamin D_3 in azotemic rats. *Am J Clin Nutr* 1983;37:403.

16. Sterner G, Lindberg T, Denneberg T. In vivo and in vitro absorption of amino acids and dipeptides in the small intestine of uremic rats. *Nephron* 1982;31:273.

17. Gray RW, Weber HP, Dominguez JH, et al. The metabolism of Vitamin D_3, and 25-hydroxyvitamin D_3 in normal and anephric humans. *J Clin Endocrinol Metab* 1974;39:1045.

18. Chazot C, Kopple, JD. Vitamin metabolism and requirements in renal disease and renal failure. In: Kopple JD, Massry SG, eds. *Nutritional management of renal disease*. Baltimore, MD: Williams & Wilkins, 1997:415.

19. Ott SM, Maloney NA, Coburn JW, et al. The prevalence of bone aluminum deposition in renal osteodystrophy and its relation to the response to calcitriol therapy. *N Engl J Med* 1982;307:709.

20. Friedlander MA, Wu YC, Elgawish A, et al. Early and advanced glycosylation end products: kinetics of formation and clearance in peritoneal dialysis. *J Clin Invest* 1996;97:728.

21. Appel G. Nephrology forum: lipid abnormalities in renal disease. *Kidney Int* 1991;39:169.

21a. Loughrey CM, Young IS, Lightbody JH, et al. Oxidative stress in haemodialysis. *Q J Med* 1997;87:679.

22. Attman PO. Hyperlipoproteinaemia in renal failure: Pathogenesis and perspectives for intervention. *Nephrol Dial Transplantation* 1993;8:294.

23. Król E, Rutkowski B, Wróblewska M, et al. Classification of lipid disorders in chronic hemodialyzed patients. *Miner Electrolyte Metab* 1996;22:13.

24. Cocchi R, Viglino G, Cancarini G, et al. Prevalence of hyperlipidemia in a cohort of CAPD patients. *Miner Electrolyte Metab* 1996;22:22.

25. Wanner C, Bartens W, Nauck M, et al. Lipoprotein(a) in patients with the nephrotic syndrome: Influence of immunosuppression and proteinuria. *Miner Electrolyte Metab* 1996;22:26.

26. Wanner C. Lipid metabolism in renal disease and renal failure. In: Kopple JD, Massry SG, eds. *Nutritional management of renal disease* 1st Edition. Baltimore: Williams & Wilkins, 1996.

27. Sanfelippo ML, Swenson RS, Reaven GM. Reduction of plasma triglycerides by diet in subjects with CRF. *Kidney Int* 1977;11:54.

28. Loughrey CM, Young IS, Lightbody JH, et al. Oxidative stress in haemodialysis. *Q J Med* 1997;87:679.

28a. Galli F, Canestrari F, Bellomo G. Physiopathology of the oxidative stress and its implications in uremia and dialysis. *Contrib Nephrol* 1999;127:1.

29. Nilsson-Thorell CB, Muscalu N, Andren AH, et al. Heat sterilization of fluids for peritoneal dialysis gives rise to aldehydes. *Perit Dial Int* 1993;13:208.

30. Linden T, Forsback G, Deppisch R, et al. 3-Deoxyglucosone, a promoter of advanced glycation end products in fluids for peritoneal dialysis. *Perit Dial Int* 1998;18:290.

31. Lamb EJ, Cattell WR, Dawnay AB. In vitro formation of advanced glycation end products in peritoneal dialysis fluid. *Kidney Int* 1995;47:1768.

32. Miyata T, Horie K, Ueda Y, et al. Advanced glycation and lipoxidation of the peritoneal membrane in peritoneal dialysis: respective roles of serum and peritoneal dialysis fluid reactive carbonyl compounds. *Kidney Int* 2000;58:425.

33. Guarnieri G, Faccini L, Lipartiti T, et al. Simple methods for nutritional assessment in hemodialyzed patients. *Am J Clin Nutr* 1980;33:1598.

34. Attman PO, Ewald J, Isaksson B. Body composition during long-term treatment of uremia with amino acid supplemented low-protein diet. *Am J Clin Nutr* 1980;33:801.

35. Bansal VK, Popli S, Pickering J, et al. Protein-calorie malnutrition and cutaneous anergy in hemodialysis maintained patients. *Am J Clin Nutr* 1980;33:1608.

36. Blumenkrantz MJ, Kopple JD, Gutman RA, et al. Methods for assessing nutritional status of patients with renal failure. *Am J Clin Nutr* 1980;33:1567.

37. Thunberg BJ, Swamy AP, Cestero RV. Cross-sectional and longitudinal nutritional measurements in maintenance hemodialysis patients. *Am J Clin Nutr* 1981;34:2005.

38. Young GA, Swanepoel CR, Croft MR, et al. Anthropometry and plasma valine, amino acids, and proteins in the nutritional assessment of hemodialysis patients. *Kidney Int* 1982;21:492.

39. Schoenfeld PY, Henry RR, Laird NM, et al. Assessment of nutritional status of the national cooperative dialysis study population. *Kidney Int* 1983;23:S80.

40. Salusky IB, Fine RN, Nelson P, et al. Nutritional status of children undergoing continuous ambulatory peritoneal dialysis. *Am J Clin Nutr* 1983;38:599.

41. Heide B, Pierratos A, Khanna R, et al. Nutritional status of patients undergoing continuous ambulatory peritoneal dialysis (CAPD). *Perit Dial Bull* 1983;3:138.

42. Wolfson M, Strong CJ, Minturn D, et al. Nutritional status and lymphocyte function in maintenance hemodialysis patients. *Am J Clin Nutr* 1984;37:547.

43. Kopple JD. Nutrition in renal failure. Causes of catabolism and wasting in acute or CRF. In: Robinson RR, ed. *Nephrology*, vol 2. Proceedings of the IXth International Congress of Nephrology. New York: Springer-Verlag New York, 1984:1498.

44. Carvounis CP, Carvounis G, Hung M-H. Nutritional status of maintenance hemodialysis patients. *Am J Clin Nutr* 1986;43:946.

45. Cano N, Femandez JP, Lacombe P, et al. Statistical selection of nutritional parameters in hemodialysed patients. Proceedings of the Fourth International Congress on Nutrition and Metabolism in Renal Disease. *Kidney Int* 1987;32:S178.

46. Fenton SSA, Johnston N, Delmore T, et al. Nutritional assessment of continuous ambulatory peritoneal dialysis patients. *ASAIO Trans* 1987;33:650.

47. Marckmann P. Nutritional status of patients on hemodialysis and peritoneal dialysis. *Clin Nephrol* 1988;29:75.

48. Bilbrey GI, Cohen TL. Identification and treatment of protein calorie malnutrition in chronic hemodialysis patients. *Dial Transplantation* 1989;18:669.

49. Palop L, Martinez JA. Cross-sectional assessment of nutritional and immune status in renal patients undergoing continuous ambulatory peritoneal dialysis. *Am J Clin Nutr* 1997;66:498S.

50. Young GA, Kopple JD, Lindholm B, el al. Nutritional assessment of continuous ambulatory peritoneal dialysis patients. *Am J Kidney Dis* 1991;17:462.

51. Cianciaruso B, Brunori G, Kopple JD, et al. Cross-sectional comparison of malnutrition in continuous ambulatory peritoneal dialysis and hemodialysis patients. *Am J Kidney Dis* 1995;26:475.

52. Lowrie EG, Lew NL. Death risk in hemodialysis patients: the predictive value of commonly measured variables and an evaluation of death rate differences between facilities. *Am J Kidney Dis* 1990;15:458.

53. Kawaguchi Y, et al. Nutritional assessment of patients on continuous ambulatory peritoneal dialysis. *Jpn J Nephrol* 1993;37:843.

54. Pollock CA, Ibels LS, Ayass W, et al. Total body nitrogen as a prognostic marker in maintenance dialysis. *J Am Soc Nephrol* 1995;6:86.

55. Marcen R, Teruel JL, de la Cal MA, et al. The impact of malnutrition in morbidity and mortality in stable hemodialysis patients. Spanish Cooperative Study of Nutrition in Hemodialysis. *Nephrol Dial Transplantation* 1995;12:2324.

56. Dwyer JT, Cunniff PJ, Maroni BJ, et al, for the HEMO Study Group. The hemodialysis (HEMO) pilot study: nutrition program and participant characteristics at baseline. *J Renal Nutr* 1998;8:11.

57. Williams AJ, McArley A. Body composition, treatment time, and outcome in hemodialysis. *J Renal Nutr* 1999;9:157.

58. Aparicio M, Cano N, Chauveau P, et al. Nutritional status of haemodialysis patients: a French national co-operative study. *Nephrol Dial Transplantation* 1999;14:1679.

59. Laidlaw SA, Berg RL, Kopple JD, et al. Patterns of fasting plasma amino acid levels in chronic renal insufficiency: results from the feasibility phase of the modification of diet in renal disease study. *Am J Kidney Dis* 1994;23:504.

60. Jones MR, Blumenkrantz MJ, Kopple JD. Albumin metabolism in patients with CRF. *Fed Proc* 1980;39:561(abst).

61. Kaysen G, Schoenfeld P. Albumin homeostasis during CAPD. *Kidney Int* 1983;23:153.

62. Bodnar D, Schreiber M, Vidt D. Protein status of patients during the first year on CAPD. *CRN Q* 1984;8(3):11.

63. Williams P, Kay R, Harrison J, et al. Nutritional and anthropometric assessment of patients on CAPD over one year: contrasting changes in total body nitrogen and potassium. *Perit Dial Bull* 1981;1:82.

64. Rubin J, Flynn MA, Nolph KD. Total body potassium—a guide to nutritional health in patients undergoing continuous ambulatory peritoneal dialysis. *Am J Clin Nutr* 1981;34:94.

65. Deleted in proofs.

66. Mackenzie JC, Ford JE, Waters AH, et al. Erythropoiesis in patients undergoing regular dialysis treatment (R.D.T.) without transfusion. *Proc Eur Dial Transplant Assoc* 1968;5:172.

67. Mahajan SK, Prasad AS, Lambujon J, et al. Improvement of uremic hypogeusia by zinc: a double-blind study. *Am J Clin Nutr* 1980;33:1517.

68. Kopple JD, Mercurio K, Blumenkrantz MJ, et al. Daily requirement for pyridoxine supplements in CRF. *Kidney Int* 1981;19:694.

69. Bellinghieri G, Savica V, Mallamace A, et al. Correlation between increased serum and tissue L-carnitine levels and improved muscle symptoms in hemodialyzed patients. *Am J Clin Nutr* 1983;38:523.

70. Sprenger KBG, Bundschu D, Lewis K, et al. Improvement of uremic neuropathy and hypogeusia by dialysate zinc supplementation: a double-blind study. *Kidney Int* 1983;24[Suppl 16]:S315.

71. Kopple JD. Pathophysiology of protein-energy wasting in chronic renal failure. *J Nutr* 1999;129:247S.

72. Heimburger O, Lonnqvist F, Danielsson A, et al. Serum immunoreactive leptin concentration and its relation to the body fat content in chronic renal failure. *J Am Soc Nephrol* 1997;8:1423.

73. Young GA, Woodrow G, Kendall S, et al. Increased plasma leptin/fat ratio in patients with chronic renal failure: a cause for malnutrition? *Nephrol Dial Transplantation* 1997;12:2318.

74. Johansen KL, Mulligan K, Tai V, et al. Leptin, body composition and indices of malnutrition in patients on dialysis. *J Am Soc Nephrol* 1998;9:1080.

75. Campfield LA, Smith FH, Guisez Y, et al. Evidence for a peripheral signal linking adiposity and central neural networks. *Science* 1995;269:546.

76. Pelleymounter MA, Cullen MJ, Baker MB, et al. Effect of the obese gene product on body weight regulation in ob/ob mice. *Science* 1995;269:540.

77. Meyer C, Robson D, Rackovsky N, et al. Role of kidney in human leptin metabolism. *Am J Physiol* 1997;273:E903.

78. Malmstrom R, Taskien M-R, Karonen S-L, et al. Insulin increases plasma leptin concentrations in normal subjects and patients with NIDDM. *Diabetologia* 1996;39:993.

79. Stenvinkel P, Lindholm B, Lonnqvist F, et al. Increases in serum leptin levels during peritoneal dialysis are associated with inflammation and a decrease in lean body mass. *J Am Soc Nephrol* 2000;11:1303.

80. Ikizler TA, Wingard RL, Harvell J, et al. Association of morbidity with markers of nutrition and inflammation in chronic hemodialysis patients: a prospective study. *Kidney Int* 1999;55:1945.

81. Iseki K, Tozawa M, Yoshi S, et al. Serum C-reactive protein (CRP) and risk of death in chronic dialysis patients. *Nephrol Dial Transplantation* 1999;14:1956.

82. Kaysen GA, Dubin JA, Muller HG, et al. The acute-phase response varies with time and predicts serum albumin levels in hemodialysis patients. *Kidney Int* 2000;58:346.

83. Yeun JY, Kaysen GA. Acute phase proteins and peritoneal dialysate albumin loss are the main determinants of serum albumin in peritoneal dialysis patients. *Am J Kidney Dis* 1997;30:923.

84. Descamps-Latscha B, Herbelin A, Nguyen AT, et al. Balance between IL-1 beta, TNF alpha, and their specific inhibitors in chronic renal failure and maintenance dialysis. Relationships with activation markers of T cells, B cells and monocytes. *J Immunol* 1995;154:882.

85. Bologa RM, Levine DM, Parker TS, et al. Interleukin-6 predicts hypoalbuminemia, hypocholesterolemia, and mortality in hemodialysis patients. *Am J Kidney Dis* 1998;32:107.

86. McCarthy DO. Tumor necrosis factor alpha and interleukin-6 have differential effects on food intake and gastric emptying in fasted rats. *Res Nurs Health* 2000;23:222.

87. Laye S, Gheusi G, Cremona S, et al. Endogenous brain IL-1 mediates LPS-induced anorexia and hypothalamic cytokine expression. *Am J Physiol Regul Integr Comp Physiol* 2000;279:R93.

88. Kopple JD, Greene T, Chumlea WC, et al. Relationship between nutritional status and GFR: results from the MDRD Study. *Kidney Int* 2000;57:1688.

89. Kopple JD, Berg R, Houser H, et al. Nutritional status of patients with different levels of chronic renal insufficiency. *Kidney Int* 1989;36[Suppl 27]:S184.

90. Kopple JD, Levey AS, Greene T, et al, for the Modification of Diet in Renal Disease Study Group. Effect of dietary protein restriction on nutritional status in the Modification of Diet in Renal Disease (MDRD) Study. *Kidney Int* 1997;52:778.

91. Dwyer JT, Cunniff PJ, Maroni BJ, et al, for the HEMO Study Group. The hemodialysis (HEMO) pilot study: nutrition program and participant characteristics at baseline. *J Renal Nutr* 1998;8:11.

92. Giordano C, de Pascale C, DeCristofaro D, et al. Protein malnutrition in the treatment of chronic uremia. In: Berlyne GM, ed. *Nutrition in renal disease.* Baltimore: Williams & Wilkins, 1968:23.

93. Kopple JD, Swendseid ME, Shinaberger JH, et al. The free and bound amino acids removed by hemodialysis. *Trans Am Soc Artif Intern Organs* 1973;19:309.

94. Wolfson M, Jones MR, Kopple JD. Amino acid losses during hemodialysis with infusion of amino acids and glucose. *Kidney Int* 1982;21:500.

95. Ikizler TA, Flakoll PJ, Parker RA, et al. Amino acid and albumin losses during hemodialysis. *Kidney Int* 1994;46:830.

96. Chazot C, Shahmir E, Matias B, et al. Dialytic nutrition: provision of amino acids in dialysate during hemodialysis. *Kidney Int* 1997;52:1663.

97. Giordano C, DeSanto NG, Capodicasa G, et al. Amino acid losses during CAPD. *Clin Nephrol* 1980;14:230.

98. Kopple JD, Blumenkrantz MJ, Jones MR, et al. Plasma amino acid levels and amino acid losses during continuous ambulatory peritoneal dialysis. *Am J Clin Nutr* 1982;36:395.

99. Randerson DH, Chapman GV, Farrell PC. Amino acid and dietary status in CAPD patients. In: Atkins RC, Thomson NM, Farrell PC, eds. *Continuous ambulatory peritoneal dialysis.* London: Churchill Livingstone, 1981:179.

100. Wathen RL, Keshaviah P, Hommeyer P, et al. The metabolic effects of hemodialysis with and without glucose in the dialysate. *Am J Clin Nutr* 1978;31:1870.

101. Kaplan AA, Halley SE, Lapkin RA, et al. Dialysate protein losses with bleach processed polysulphone dialyzers. *Kidney Int* 1995;47:573.

102. Blumenkrantz MJ, Gahl GM, Kopple JD, et al. Protein losses during peritoneal dialysis. *Kidney Int* 1981;19:593.

102a. Gahl GM, Becker H, Schurig R, et al. Kontinuierliche ambulante peritonealdialyse (CAPD). *Schweitz Med Wochenschr* 1979;109:1990.

102b. Lindholm B, Ahlberg M, et al. Nutritional aspects of continuous ambulatory peritoneal dialysis. In: Legrain M, ed. *Continuous ambulatory peritoneal dialysis.* Amsterdam: Excerpta Medica, 1979:199.

103. Sullivan JF, Eisenstein AB, Mottola OM, et al. The effect of dialysis on plasma and tissue levels of Vitamin C. *Trans Am Soc Artif Intern Organs* 1972;18:277.

104. Bradley DW, Maynard JE, Webster H. Plasma and whole blood concentrations of ascorbic acid in patients undergoing long-term hemodialysis. *Am J Clin Nutr* 1973;60:145.

105. Rostand SG. Vitamin B_{12} levels and nerve conduction velocities in patients undergoing maintenance hemodialysis. *Am J Clin Nutr* 1976;29:691.

106. Anderson KEH. Folic acid status of patients with CRF maintained by dialysis. *Clin Nephrol* 1977;8:510.

107. Linton AL, Clark WF, Dreidger AA, et al. Correctable factors contributing to the anemia of dialysis patients. *Nephron* 1977;19:95.

108. Rosenblatt SG, Drake S, Faden S, et al. Gastrointestinal blood loss in patients with CRF. *Am J Kidney Dis* 1982;1:232.

109. Grodstein GP, Blumenkrantz MJ, Kopple JD. Nutritional and metabolic response to catabolic stress in chronic uremia. *Am J Clin Nutr* 1980;33:1411.

110. Keane WF, Collins AJ. Influence of co-morbidity on mortality and morbidity in patients treated with hemodialysis. *Am J Kidney Dis* 1994;24:1010.

111. United States Renal Data System. *USRDS 1999 annual data report.* Bethesda, MD: National Institutes of Health and National Institute of Diabetes and Digestive and Kidney Diseases, 1999.

112. Kaysen GA, Stevenson FT, Depner TA. Determinants of albumin concentration in hemodialysis patients. *Am J Kidney Dis* 1997;29:658.

113. Koch M, Kutkuhn B, Trenkwalder E, et al. Apolipoprotein B, fibrinogen, HDL cholesterol, and apolipoprotein(a) phenotypes predict coronary artery disease in hemodialysis patients. *J Am Soc Nephrol* 1997;8:1889.

114. Zimmerman J, Herrlinger S, Pruy A, et al. Inflammation enhances cardiovascular risk and mortality in hemodialysis patients. *Kidney Int* 1999;55:648.

115. Yeun JY, Levine RA, Mantadilok V, et al. C-reactive protein predicts all-cause and cardiovascular mortality in hemodialysis patients. *Am J Kidney Dis* 2000;35:469.

116. Moshage H. Cytokines and the hepatic acute phase response. *J Pathol* 1997;191:257.

117. Steel DM, Whitehead AS. The major acute-phase reactants: C-reactive protein, serum amyloid P component and serum amyloid A protein. *Immunol Today* 1994;15:81.

118. Flores EA, Bistrian BR, Pomposelli J, et al. Infusion of tumor necrosis factor/cachectin promotes muscle catabolism in the rat. A synergistic effect with interleukin 1. *J Clin Invest* 1989;83:1614.

119. Moshage HJ, Janssen JAM, Franssen JH, et al. Study of the molecular mechanisms of decreased liver synthesis of albumin in inflammation. *J Clin Invest* 1987;79:1635.

120. Chung SH, Lindholm B, Lee HB. Influence of initial nutritional status on continuous ambulatory peritoneal dialysis patient survival. *Perit Dial Int* 2000;20:19.

121. Memoli B, Postiglione L, Cianciaruso B, et al. Role of different dialysis membranes in the release of interleukin-6 soluble receptor in uremic patients. *Kidney Int* 2000;58:417.

122. Laude-Sharp M, Caroff M, Simard L, et al. Induction of IL-1 during hemodialysis: transmembrane passage of intact endotoxin (LPS). *Kidney Int* 1990;38:1089.

123. Krautzig S, linnenweber S, Schindler R, et al. New indicators to evaluate bacteriological quality of the dialysis fluid and the associated inflammatory response in ESRD patients. *Nephrol Dial Transplantation* 1996;11:S87.

124. Schindler R, Lonnemann G, Shaldon S, et al. Transcription, not synthesis, of interleukin-1 and tumor necrosis factor by complement. *Kidney Int* 1990;37:85.

125. Borah M, Schoenfeld PY, Gotch FA, et al. Nitrogen balance in intermittent hemodialysis therapy. *Kidney Int* 1978;14:491.

126. Gutierrez A, Alvestrand A, Wahren J, et al. Effect of in vivo contact between blood and dialysis membranes on protein catabolism in humans. *Kidney Int* 1990;38:487.

127. Guttierrez A, Bergström J, Alvestrand A. Protein catabolism in sham hemodialysis: the effect of different membranes. *Clin Nephrol* 1992;38:20.

128. Lindsay RM, Bergström J. Membrane biocompatibility and nutrition in maintenance haemodialysis patients. *Nephrol Dial Transplantation* 1994;9[Suppl 2]:150.

129. Davenport A, Crabtree J, Andeonjna C, et al. Tumor necrosis factor does not increase during routine cuprophan hemodialysis in healthy well-nourished patients. *Nephrol Dial Transplantation* 1991;6:435.

130. Powell AC, Bland L, Oettiger CW, et al. Lack of elevation of plasma interleukin-1beta or tumor necrosis alpha during unfavorable hemodialysis conditions. *J Am Soc Nephrol* 1991;2:1007.

131. Heidland A, Horl WH, Heller N, et al. Proteolytic enzymes and catabolism: enhanced release of granulocyte proteinases in uremic intoxication and during hemodialysis. *Kidney Int* 1983;24[Suppl 16]:S27.

132. Horl W, Jochum M, Heidland A, et al. Release of granulocyte proteinases during hemodialysis. *Am J Nephrol* 1983;3:213.

133. Haag-Weber M, Hable M, Schollmeyer P, et al. Metabolic response of neutrophils to uremia and dialysis. *Kidney Int* 1989;36[Suppl 27]:S293.

134. Bergström J. Uremic toxicity. In: Kopple JD, Massry SG, eds. *Nutritional management of renal disease.* Baltimore: Williams & Wilkins, 1997:97.

135. Massry SG, Glassock RJ. Amino acid and protein metabolism in chronic renal failure. In: *Massry and Glassock's textbook of nephrology,* 4th ed. Philadelphia: Lippincott Williams & Wilkins, 2001.

135a. May RC, Kelly RA, Mitch WE. Mechanisms for defects in muscle protein metabolism in rats with chronic uremia. *J Clin Invest* 1987;79:1099.

136. Reaich D, Channon SM, Scrimgeour CM, et al. Ammonium chloride-induced acidosis increases protein breakdown and amino acid oxidation in humans. *Am J Physiol* 1992;263:E735.

137. Mitch WE, Medina R, Greiber S, et al. Metabolic acidosis stimulates muscle protein degradation by activating the ATP-dependent pathway involving ubiquitin and proteasomes. *J Clin Invest* 1994;93:2127.

138. Garibotto G, Russo R, Sofia A, et al. Skeletal muscle protein synthesis and degradation in patients with CRF. *Kidney Int* 1994;45:1432.

139. De Fronzo RA, Tobin JD, Rowe JW, et al. Glucose intolerance in uremia: quantification of pancreatic beta cell sensitivity to glucose and tissue sensitivity to insulin. *J Clin Invest* 1978;62:425.

140. Ferrannini E, Pilo A, Navalesi R, et al. Insulin kinetics and glucose-induced insulin delivery in chronically dialyzed subjects: acute effects of dialysis. *J Clin Endocrinol Metab* 1979;49:15.

141. Phillips LS, Kopple JD. Circulating somatomedin activity and sulfate levels in adults with normal and impaired kidney function. *Metabolism* 1981;30:1091.

142. Fouque D, Peng SC, Kopple JD. Impaired metabolic response to recombinant insulin-like growth factor 1 in dialysis patients. *Kidney Int* 1995;47:876.

143. Ding H, Gao X-L, Hirschberg R, et al. Effects of insulin-like growth factor 1 on protein synthesis and degradation in skeletal muscle of rats with CRF: evidence for a postreceptor defect. *J Clin Invest* 1996;97:1064.

144. Sherwin RS, Bastl C, Finkelstein FO, et al. Influence of uremia and hemodialysis on the turnover and metabolic effects of glucagon. *J Clin Invest* 1976;57:722.

145. Moxley MA, Bell NH, Wagle SR, et al. Parathyroid hormone stimulation of glucose and urea production in isolated liver cells. *Am J Physiol* 1974;227:1058.

146. Kopple JD, Cianciaruso B, Massry SG. Does parathyroid hormone cause protein wasting? *Contrib Nephrol* 1980;20:138.

147. Birge SJ, Haddad JG. 25-Hydroxycholecalciferol stimulation of muscle metabolism. *J Clin Invest* 1974;56:1100.

148. Kuhlmann MK, Kopple JD. Amino acid metabolism and the kidney. *Semin Nephrol* 1990;10:445.

149. Avram MM, Mittman N, Bonomini L, et al. Markers for survival in dialysis: a seven year prospective study. *Am J Kidney Dis* 1995;26:209.

150. Iseki K, Uehara H, Nishime K, et al. Impact of the initial levels of laboratory variables on survival in chronic dialysis patients. *Am J Kidney Dis* 1996;28:541.

151. Owen WF Jr, Lew NL, Liu Y, et al. The urea reduction ratio and serum albumin concentration as predictors of mortality in patients undergoing hemodialysis. *N Engl J Med* 1993;329:1001.

152. Teehan BP, Schleifer CR, Brown JM, et al. Urea kinetic analysis and clinical outcome on CAPD. A five year longitudinal study. *Adv Perit Dial* 1990;6:181.

153. Churchill DN, Taylor DW, Cook RJ, et al. Canadian hemodialysis morbidity study. *Am J Kidney Dis* 1992;3:214.

154. Blake PG, Sombolos K, Abraham G, et al. Lack of correlation between urea kinetic indices and clinical outcomes in CAPD patients. *Kidney Int* 1991;39:700.

155. Leavey SF, Strawderman RL, Jones CA, et al. Simple nutritional indicators as independent predictors of mortality in hemodialysis patients. *Am J Kidney Dis* 1998;31:997.

156. Kopple JD, Zhu X, Lew N, et al. Body weight-for-height relationships predict mortality in maintenance hemodialysis patients. *Kidney Int* 1999;56:1136.

157. Chung SH, Lindholm B, Lee HB. Influence of initial nutritional status on continuous ambulatory peritoneal dialysis patient survival. *Perit Dial Int* 2000;20:19.

158. Han DS, Lee SW, Kang SW, et al. Factors affecting low serum values of serum albumin in CAPD patients. *Adv Perit Dial* 1996;12:288.

159. Qureshi AR, Alvestrand A, Danielsson A, Divino-Filho JC, Gutierrez A, et al. Factors predicting malnutrition in hemodialysis patients: a cross-sectional study. *Kidney Int* 1998;53:773.

160. Stenvinkel P, Heimburger O, Paultre F, et al. Strong association between malnutrition, inflammation, and atherosclerosis in chronic renal failure. *Kidney Int* 1999;55:1899.

161. Capelli JP, Kushner H, Camiscioli TC, et al. Effect of intradialytic parenteral nutrition on mortality rates in end-stage renal disease care. *Am J Kidney Dis* 1994;23:808.

162. Chertow GM, Ling J, Lew NL, et al. The association of intradialytic parenteral nutrition administration with survival in hemodialysis patients. *Am J Kidney Dis* 1994;24:912.

163. Frisancho AR. New standards of weight and body composition by frame size and height for assessment of nutritional status of adults and the elderly. *Am J Clin Nutr* 1984;40:808.

164. Najjar MF, Rowland M, for the National Center for Health Statistics. Anthropometric reference data and prevalence of overweight, United States, 1976–1980. Hyattsville, MD: National Center for Health Statistics; October 1987. Advance data from Vital and Health Statistics, series 11, no 238. DHHS publication no (PHS)87–1688.

165. Klahr S, Levey AS, Beck GJ, et al. The effects of dietary protein restriction and blood pressure control on the progression of chronic renal disease: the Modification of Diet in Renal Disease Study. *N Engl J Med* 1994;330:877.

166. Russell ML. *Behavioral counseling in medicine: strategies for modifying at-risk behavior.* New York: Oxford University Press, 1986.

167. K/DOQI Nutrition Workgroup. *National Kidney Foundation Kidney Disease Outcomes Quality Initiative clinical practice guidelines for nutrition in chronic renal failure.* 2000;35:S56.

168. K/DOQI Nutrition Workgroup. *National Kidney Foundation Kidney Disease Outcomes Quality Initiative clinical practice guidelines for nutrition in chronic renal failure.* 2000;35:S17.

169. Frisancho AR. New standards of weight and body composition by frame size and height for assessment of nutritional status of adults and the elderly. *Am J Clin Nutr* 1984;40:808.

170. Bergström J, Alvestrand A, Bucht H, et al. Progression of CRF in man is treated with more frequent clinical follow-ups and better blood pressure control. *Clin Nephrol* 1986;25:1.

171. Mitch WE, Walser M, Buffington GA, et al. A simple method of estimating progression of CRF. *Lancet* 1976;2:1326.

172. Rutherford WE, Blondin J, Miller JP, et al. Chronic progressive renal disease: rate of change of serum creatinine concentration. *Kidney Int* 1977;11:62.

173. Perrone RD, Steinman TI, Beck GJ, et al. Utility of radioisotopic filtration markers in chronic renal insufficiency. Simultaneous comparison of ^{124}I-iothalamate, ^{169}Yb-DTPA, ^{99m}Tc-DTPA and insulin. *Am J Kidney Dis* 1990;16:224.

174. Levey AS, Greene T, Schluchter MD, et al. Glomerular filtration rate measurements in clinical trials. *J Am Soc Nephrol* 1993;4:1159.

175. Levey AS, Berg RL, Gassman JJ, et al, for the Modification of Diet in Renal Disease (MDRD) Study Group. Creatinine filtration, secretion and excretion during progressive renal disease. *Kidney Int* 1989;36[Suppl 27]:S73.

176. Lavender S, Hilton PJ, Jones NF. The measurement of glomerular filtration rate in renal disease. *Lancet* 1969;2:1216.

177. Salusky IB, Fine RN, Nelson P, et al. Factors affecting growth and nutritional status in children undergoing CAPD. *Kidney Int* 1984;25:260.

177a. Kopple JD. Nutritional status as a predictor of morbidity and mortality in maintenance dialysis patients. *ASAIO J* 1997;43:246.

178. Calloway DH, Odell ACF, Margen S. Sweat and miscellaneous nitrogen losses in human balance studies. *J Nutr* 1971;101:775.

179. Maroni BJ, Steinman TI, Mitch WE. A method for estimating nitrogen intake of patients with CRF. *Kidney Int* 1985;27:58.

180. Kopple JD, Gao XL, Qing DPY. Dietary protein, urea nitrogen appearance and total nitrogen appearance in chronic renal failure and CAPD patients. *Kidney Int* 1997;52:486.

181. Walser M. Urea metabolism in CRF. *Clin Invest* 1974;53:1385.

182. Varcoe R, Halliday D, Carson ER, et al. Efficiency of utilization of urea nitrogen for albumin synthesis by chronically uremic and normal man. *Clin Sci Mol Med* 1975;48:379.

183. Kopple JD, Jones MR, Keshaviah PR, et al. A proposed glossary for dialysis kinetics. *Am J Kidney Dis* 1995;26:963.

184. Bergström J, Fürst P, Alvestrand A, et al. Protein and energy intake, nitrogen balance and nitrogen losses in patients treated with continuous ambulatory peritoneal dialysis. *Kidney Int* 1993;44:1048.

185. Sargent JA, Gotch FA. Mass balance: a quantitative guide to clinical nutritional therapy. *J Am Diet Assoc* 1979;75:547.

186. Kopple JD, Coburn JW. Evaluation of chronic uremia: Importance of serum urea nitrogen, serum creatinine and their ratio. *JAMA* 1974;227:41.

187. Smith M. Case of chronic nephritis maintained for 6 months on an average daily protein intake of 0.26 gram per kilogram of body weight. *Boston Med Surg J* 1927;196:941.

188. Addis T. *Glomerular nephritis: diagnosis and treatment.* New York: Macmillan, 1948.

189. Borst JGG. Protein metabolism in uraemia; effects of protein-free diet, infections and blood-transfusions. *Lancet* 1948;1:824.

190. Berlyne GM, Shaw AB, Nilwarangkur S. Dietary treatment of CRF. Experiences with a modified Giovannetti diet. *Nephron* 1965;2:129.

191. Giovannetti S, Maggiore Q. A low nitrogen diet with proteins of high biological value for severe chronic uraemia. *Lancet* 1964;1:1000.

192. Kopple JD, Sorensen MK, Coburn JW, et al. Controlled comparison of 20-g and 40-g protein diets in the treatment of chronic uremia. *Am J Clin Nutr* 1968;21:553.

193. Ford J, Phillips ME, Toye FE, et al. Nitrogen balance in patients with CRF on diets containing varying quantities of protein. *Br Med J* 1969;i:735.

194. Kopple JD, Coburn JW. Metabolic studies of low protein diets in uremia. I. Nitrogen and potassium. *Medicine* 1973;52:583.

195. Giordano C. Use of exogenous and endogenous urea for protein synthesis in normal and uremic subjects. *J Lab Clin Med* 1963;62:231.

196. Schloerb PR. Essential L-amino acid administration in uremia. *Am J Med Sci* 1966;252:650.

197. Bergström J, Furst P, Josephson B, et al. Factors affecting the nitrogen balance in chronic uremic patients receiving essential amino acids intravenously or by mouth. *Nutr Metab* 1972;14[Suppl]:162.

198. Kopple JD, Swendseid ME. Nitrogen balance and plasma amino acid levels in uremic patients fed an essential amino acid diet. *Am J Clin Nutr* 1974;27:806.

199. Bergström J, Furst P, Noree L-O. Treatment of chronic uremic patients with protein-poor diet and oral supply of essential amino acids. I. Nitrogen balance studies. *Clin Nephrol* 1975;3:187.

200. Noree LO, Bergström J. Treatment of chronic uremic patients with protein-poor diet and oral supply of essential amino acids. II. Clinical results of long-term treatment. *Clin Nephrol* 1975;3:195.

201. Walser M, Mitch WE, Abras E. Supplements containing amino acids and keto acids in the treatment of chronic uremia. *Kidney Int* 1983;24[Suppl 16]:S285.

202. Kopple JD. Treatment with low protein and amino acid diets in CRF. In: Barcelo R, Bergeron M, Carriere S, et al, eds. *Proceedings VIIth International Congress of Nephrology.* Basel: S. Karger, 1978: 497.

203. Giordano C, Phillips ME, de Pascale C, et al. Utilisation of keto acid analogues of valine and phenylalanine in health and uremia. *Lancet* 1972;1:178.

204. Walser M, Coulter AW, Dighe S, et al. The effect of keto-analogues of essential amino acids in severe chronic uremia. *J Clin Invest* 1973;52:678.

205. Walser M, Lund P, Ruderman NB, et al. Synthesis of essential amino acids from their—keto analogues by perfused rat liver and muscle. *J Clin Invest* 1973;52:2865.

206. Gallina DL, Dominguez JM, Hoschoian JC, et al. Maintenance of nitrogen balance in a young woman by substitution of −ketoisovaleric acid for valine. *J Nutr* 1971;101:1165.

207. Rudman D. Capacity of human subjects to utilize keto analogues of valine and phenylalanine. *J Clin Invest* 1971;50:90.

208. Maschio G, Oldrizzi L, Tessitore N, et al. Effects of dietary protein and phosphorus restriction on the progression of early renal failure. *Kidney Int* 1982;22:371.

209. Rossman JB, Meijer S, Sluiter WJ, et al. Prospective randomised trial of early dietary protein restriction in CRF. *Lancet* 1984;2:1291.

210. Locatelli F, Alberti D, Graziani G, et al. Prospective, randomized, multicentre trial of effect of protein restriction on progression of chronic renal insufficiency. *Lancet* 1991;337:1299.

211. Williams PS, Stevens ME, Fass G, et al. A randomized trial of the effects of protein and phosphate restriction on the progression of CRF. *Nephrol Dial Transplantation* 1987;7:285.

212. Ihle BU, Becker G, Whithworth JA, et al. The effect of protein restriction on the progression of renal insufficiency. *N Engl J Med* 1989;321:1773.

213. D'Amico G, Gentile MG, Fellin G, et al. Effect of dietary protein restriction on the progression of renal failure: a prospective randomized trial. *Nephrol Dial Transplantation* 1994;9:1590.

214. Mitch WE, Walser M, Steinman TI, et al. The effect of a keto acid–amino acid supplement to a restricted diet on the progression of CRF. *N Engl J Med* 1984;311:623.

214a. Walser M, Hill S, Ward L, et al. A crossover comparison of progression of CRF. Ketoacids vs. amino acids. *Kidney Int* 1993;43:933.

215. Teschan PE, Beck GJ, Dwyer JT, et al. Effect of a ketoacid–amino acid–supplemented very low protein diet on the progression of advanced renal disease: a reanalysis of the MDRD feasibility study. *Clin Nephrol* 1998;50:273.

216. Walser M, Hill S. Can renal replacement be deferred by a supplemented very low protein diet? *J Am Soc Nephrol* 1999;10:110.

217. Alvestrand A, Ahlberg M, Bergström J. Retardation of the progression of renal insufficiency in patients treated with low-protein diets. *Kidney Int* 1983;24[Suppl 16]:S268.

218. Buse MG, Reid SS. Leucine. A possible regulator of protein turnover in muscle. *J Clin Invest* 1975;56:1250.

219. Mitch WE, Walser M, Sapir DC. Nitrogen sparing induced by leucine compared with that induced by its keto analogue, [SC]-ketoisocaproate, in fasting obese man. *J Clin Invest* 1981;67:553.

220. Kopple JD, Swendseid ME. Evidence that histidine is an essential amino acid in normal and chronically uremic man. *J Clin Invest* 1975;55:881.

221. Levey AS, Adler S, Caggiula AW, et al. Effects of dietary protein restriction on the progression of advanced renal disease in the Modification of Diet in Renal Disease Study. *Am J Kidney Dis* 1996;27:652.

222. The Diabetes Control and Complications Trial Research Group. The effect of intensive treatment of diabetes on the development and progression of long-term complications in insulin-dependent diabetes mellitus. *N Engl J Med* 1993;329:977.

223. Peterson JC, Adler S, Burkart JM, et al. Blood pressure control, proteinuria, and the progression of renal disease: the Modification of Diet in Renal Disease Study. *Ann Intern Med* 1995;123:754.

224. Lazarus JM, Bourgoignie JJ, Buckalew VM, et al. Achievement and safety of a low BP goal in chronic renal disease. The Modification of Diet in Renal Disease Study Group. *Hypertension* 1997;29:641.

225. Klag MJ, Whelton PK, Randall BL, et al. End-stage renal disease in African-American and white men. 16-year MRFIT findings. *JAMA* 1997;277:1293.

226. Pedrini MT, Levey AS, Lau J, et al. The effect of dietary protein restriction on the progression of diabetic and nondiabetic renal diseases: a meta-analysis. *Ann Intern Med* 1996;124:627.

227. Fouque D, Laville M, Boissel JP, et al. Controlled low protein diets in chronic renal insufficiency: Meta-analysis. *Br Med J* 1992;304:216.

228. Kasiske BL, Lakatua JD, Ma JZ, et al. A meta-analysis of the effects of dietary restriction on the rate of decline in renal function. *Am J Kidney Dis* 1998;31:954.

229. K/DOQI Nutrition Workgroup. *National Kidney Foundation Kidney Disease Outcomes Quality Initiative clinical practice guidelines for nutrition in chronic renal failure.* 2000;35:S58.

230. K/DOQI Nutrition Workgroup. *National Kidney Foundation Kidney Disease Outcomes Quality Initiative clinical practice guidelines for nutrition in chronic renal failure.* 2000;35:S64.

231. Parker TF, Wingard RL, Husni L, et al. Effect of membrane biocompatibility on nutritional parameters in chronic hemodialysis patients. *Kidney Int* 1996;49:551.

232. Goldwasser P, Kaldas AI, Barth RH. Rise in serum albumin and creatinine in the first half-year on hemodialysis. *Kidney Int* 1999;56:2260.

233. Ginn HE, Frost A, Lacy W. Nitrogen balance in hemodialysis patients. *Am J Clin Nutr* 1968;21:385.

234. Kopple JD, Shinaberger JH, Coburn JW, et al. Optimal dietary protein treatment during chronic hemodialysis. *Trans Am Soc Artif Intern Organs* 1969;15:302.

235. Kopple JD, Monteon FJ, Shaib JK. Effect of energy intake on nitrogen metabolism in nondialyzed patients with CRF. *Kidney Int* 1986;29:734.

236. K/DOQI Nutrition Workgroup. *National Kidney Foundation Kidney Disease Outcomes Quality Initiative clinical practice guidelines for nutrition in chronic renal failure.* 2000;35:S40.

237. Blumenkrantz MJ, Kopple JD, Moran JK, et al. Metabolic balance studies and dietary protein requirements in patients undergoing continuous ambulatory peritoneal dialysis. *Kidney Int* 1982;21:849.

238. Giordano C, DeSanto NG, Pluvio M, et al. Protein requirement of patients on CAPD: a study on nitrogen balance. *Int J Artif Organs* 1980;3:11.

239. Gahl GM, Baeyer HU, Averdunk R, et al. Out-patient evaluation of dietary intake and nitrogen removal in continuous ambulatory peritoneal dialysis. *Ann Intern Med* 1981;94:643.

240. Lindholm B, Alvestrand A, Furst P, et al. Metabolic effects of continuous ambulatory peritoneal dialysis. *Proc EDTA* 1980;17:283.

241. K/DOQI Nutrition Workgroup. *National Kidney Foundation Kidney Disease Outcomes Quality Initiative clinical practice guidelines for nutrition in chronic renal failure.* 2000;35:S42.

242. Ikizler TA, Greene JH, Yenicesu M, et al. Nitrogen balance in hospitalized chronic hemodialysis patients. *Kidney Int* 1996;57:S53.

243. Mandolfo S, Zucchi A, Caavalieri D'Oro L, et al. Protein appearance in CAPD patients: what is the best formula? *Nephrol Dial Transplantation* 1996;11:1592.

244. Buchwald R, Pena JC. Evaluation of nutritional status in patients on continuous ambulatory peritoneal dialysis (CAPD). *Perit Dial Int* 1989;9:295.

245. Kopple JD. Uses and limitations of the balance technique. *J Parenter Enteral Nutr* 1987;11:S79.

246. Nolph KD, Moore HL, Prowant B, et al. Continuous ambulatory peritoneal dialysis with a high flux membrane. *ASAIO J* 1993;39:904.

247. Ahmed KR, Scognamillo B, Kopple JD. Relationship of peritoneal transport kinetics and nutritional status in chronic peritoneal dialysis patients. *Perit Dial Int* 1995;15[Suppl 1]:S5(abst).

248. Subcommittee on the Tenth Edition of the RDAs, Food and Nutrition Board, National Research Council. Recommended dietary allowances. Washington: National Academy Press, 1989.

249. Monteon FJ, Laidlaw SA, Shaib JK, et al. Energy expenditure in patients with CRF. *Kidney Int* 1986;30:741.

250. Schneeweiss B, Graninger W, Stockenhuber F, et al. Energy metabolism in acute and CRF. *Am J Clin Nutr* 1990;52:596.

251. Olevitch LR, Bowers BM, DeOreo PB. Measurement of resting energy expenditure via indirect calorimetry during adult hemodialysis treatment. *J Renal Nutr* 1994;4:192.

252. Harty J, Conway L, Keegan M, et al. Energy metabolism during CAPD: a controlled study. *Adv Perit Dial* 1995;11:229.

253. Ikizler TA, Wingard RL, Sun M, et al. Increased energy expenditure in hemodialysis patients. *J Am Soc Nephrol* 1996;7:2646.

254. Tabakian A, Juillard L, Laville M, et al. Effects of recombinant growth factors on energy expenditure in maintenance hemodialysis patients. *Miner Electrolyte Metab* 1998;24:273.

255. Slomowitz LA, Monteon FJ, Grosvenor M, et al. Effect of energy intake on nutritional status in maintenance hemodialysis patients. *Kidney Int* 1989;35:704.

256. Hylander B, Barkeling B, Rössner S. Eating behavior in continuous ambulatory peritoneal dialysis and hemodialysis patients. *Am J Kidney Dis* 1992;6:592.

257. Holliday MA. Calorie deficiency in children with uremia: effect upon growth. *Pediatrics* 1972;50:590.

258. Betts PR, Magrath C. Growth pattern and dietary intake of children with chronic renal insufficiency. *Br Med J* 1974;27:189.

259. Rätsch IM, Catassi C, Verrina E, et al. Energy and nutrient intake of patients with mild-to-moderate CRF compared with healthy children: an Italian multicentre study. *Eur J Pediatr* 1992;151:701.

260. Dobell E, Chan M, Williams P, et al. Food preferences and food habits of patients with CRF undergoing dialysis. *J Am Diet Assoc* 1993;93:1129.

261. DeSanto NG, Capodicasa G, Senatore R, et al. Glucose utilization from dialysate in patients on continuous ambulatory peritoneal dialysis. *Int J Artif Organs* 1979;2:119.

262. Baeyer HV, Gahl GM, Riedinger H, et al. Unexpected alteration of nutritional habits in patients undergoing CAPD. In: Gahl GM, Kessel M, Nolph KD, eds. *Advances in peritoneal dialysis.* Amsterdam: Excerpta Medica, 1981:408.

263. Grodstein GP, Blumenkrantz MJ, Kopple JD, et al. Glucose absorption during continuous ambulatory peritoneal dialysis. *Kidney Int* 1981;19:564.

264. Lindholm B, Bergström J, Karlander S. Glucose metabolism in patients on CAPD. In: Gahl GM, Kessel M, Nolph KD, eds. *Advances in peritoneal dialysis.* Amsterdam: Excerpta Medica, 1981: 413.

265. K/DOQI Nutrition Workgroup. National Kidney Foundation Kidney Disease Outcomes Quality Initiative. Clinical Practice Guidelines for Nutrition in Chronic Renal Failure. 2000;35:S60.

266. K/DOQI Nutrition Workgroup. National Kidney Foundation Kidney Disease Outcomes Quality Initiative. Clinical Practice Guidelines for Nutrition in Chronic Renal Failure. 2000;35:S44.

266a. Chan MK, Varghese Z, Persaud JW. Hyperlipidemia in patients on maintenance hemo- and peritoneal dialysis: the relative pathogenic roles of triglyceride production and triglyceride removal. *Clin Nephrol* 1982;17:183.

266b. Sanfelippo ML, Swenson RS, Reaven GM. Response of plasma triglycerides to dietary change in patients on hemodialysis. *Kidney Int* 1978;14:180.

267. Pagenkemper JJ. In: Gussler JD, Silverman E, eds. *Renal nutrition, report of the Eleventh Ross Round-Table on Medical Issues, 1991.* Columbus: Ross Laboratories, 1991:26.

268. Leaf A, Weber PC. Cardiovascular effects of n-3 fatty acids. *N Engl J Med* 1988;318:549.

269. Alderson LM, Endemann G, Lindsay I, et al. LDL enhances monocyte adhesion to endothelial cell in vitro. *Am J Pathol* 1986;123:334.

270. Kasiske BL, O'Donnel MP, Cleary MP, et al. Treatment of hyperlipidemia reduces glomerular injury in obese zucker rats. *Kidney Int* 1988;33:667.

271. Keane WF, O'Donnell MP, Kasiske BL, et al. Lipids and the progression of renal disease. *J Am Soc Nephrol* 1990;1:S69.

272. Homan van der Heide JJ, Bilo HJG, Tegzess AM, et al. The effects of dietary supplementation with fish oil on renal function in cyclosporine-treated renal transplant recipients. *Transplantation* 1990;49:523.

273. Hamazaki T, Tateno S, Shishido H. Eicosapentaenoic acid and IgA nephropathy [Letter to the Editor]. *Lancet* 1984;1:1017.

274. Bennett WM, Walker RG, Kincaid-Smith P. Treatment of IgA nephropathy with eicosapentanoic acid (EPA): a two-year prospective trial. *Clin Nephrol* 1989;31:128.

275. Donadio JV Jr, Holman RT, Holub BF, et al. Effects of omega (ω)-3 polyunsaturated fatty acids (PUFA) in mesangial IgA nephropathy. *Kidney Int* 1990;37:255(abst).

276. Donadio JV Jr, Bergstralh EJ, Offord KP, et al. A controlled trial of fish oil in IgA nephropathy. *N Engl J Med* 1994;331:1194.

277. Deleted in proofs.

278. Guarnieri G, Toigo G, Crapesi L, et al. Carnitine metabolism in CRF. *Kidney Int* 1987;32[Suppl 22]:S116.

279. Wanner C, Horl WH. Carnitine abnormalities in patients with renal insufficiency. Pathophysiological and therapeutic aspects. *Nephron* 1988;50:89.

280. Manis T, Deutsch J, Feinstein EI, et al. Charcoal sorbent-induced hypolipidemia in uremia and diabetes. *Am J Clin Nutr* 1980;33:1485.

281. Pierides AM, Alvarez-Ude F, Kerr DN. Clofibrate-induced muscle damage in patients with CRF. *Lancet* 1975;2:1279.

282. Thomas ME, Harris KPG, Ramaswamy C, et al. Simvastatin therapy for hypercholesterolemic patients with nephrotic syndrome or significant proteinuria. *Kidney Int* 1993;44:1124.

283. Expert Panel on Detection, Evaluation, and Treatment of High Blood Cholesterol in Adults. Summary of the second report of the National Cholesterol Education Program (NCEP) (Adult Treatment Panel II). *JAMA* 1993;269:3015.

284. Kushner RF. Body weight and mortality. *Nutr Rev* 1993;51:127.

285. Manson JE, Willett WC, Stampfer MJ, et al. Body weight and mortality among women. *N Engl J Med* 1995;333:677.

286. Burk RF, Brown DG, Seely RJ, et al. Influence of dietary and injected selenium on whole-body retention, route of excretion, and tissue retention of $^{75}SeO_3^2-$ in the rat. *J Nutr* 1972;102:1049.

287. Goldberg AP, Geltman EM, Hagberg JM, et al. Therapeutic benefits of exercise training for hemodialysis patients. *Kidney Int* 1983;24[Suppl 16]:S303.

288. Perna AF, Ingrosso D, Castaldo P, et al. Homocysteine, a new crucial element in the pathogenesis of uremic cardiovascular complications. *Miner Electrolyte Metab* 1999;25:95.

289. van Guldener C, Kulik W, Berger R, et al. Homocysteine and methionine metabolism in ESRD: a stable isotope study. *Kidney Int* 1999;56:1064.

290. Kimura H, Gejyo F, Suzuki S, et al. The C677T methylenetetrahydrofolate reductase gene mutation in hemodialysis patients. *J Am Soc Nephrol* 2000;11:885.

291. Klusmann A, Ivens K, Schadewaldt P, et al. Is homocysteine a risk factor for coronary heart disease in patients with terminal renal failure? *Med Klin* 2000;95:189.

292. Oishi K, Nagake Y, Yamasaki H, et al. The significance of serum homocysteine levels in diabetic patients on haemodialysis. *Nephrol Dial Transplantation* 2000;15:851.

293. Suliman ME, Qureshi AR, Barany P, et al. Hyperhomocysteinemia, nutritional status, and cardiovascular disease in hemodialysis patients. *Kidney Int* 2000;57:1727.

294. Blacher J, Demuth K, Guerin AP, et al. Association between plasma homocysteine concentrations and cardiac hypertrophy in end-stage renal disease. *J Nephrol* 1999;12:248.

295. Dierkes J, Domrose U, Ambrosch A, et al. Response of hyperhomocysteinemia to folic acid supplementation in patients with end-stage renal disease. *Clin Nephrol* 1999;51:108.

296. Thambyrajah J, Landray MJ, McGlynn FJ, et al. Does folic acid decrease plasma homocysteine and improve endothelial function in patients with predialysis renal failure? *Circulation* 2000;102: 871.

297. Vacha GM, Corsi M, Giorcelli G, et al. Serum and muscle L-carnitine levels in hemodialyzed patients, during and after long-term L-carnitine treatment. *Curr Ther Res* 1985;37:505.

298. Hiatt WR, Koziol BJ, Shapiro JI, et al. Carnitine metabolism during exercise in patients on chronic hemodialysis. *Kidney Int* 1992; 41:1613.

299. Wanner C, Forstner-Wanner S, Schaeffer G, et al. Serum free carnitine, carnitine esters and lipids in patients on peritoneal dialysis and hemodialysis. *Am J Nephrol* 1986;6:206.

300. Golper TA, Wolfson M, Ahmad S, et al. Multicenter trial Of L-carnitine in maintenance hemodialysis patients. I. Carnitine concentrations and lipid effects. *Kidney Int* 1990;38:904.

301. Brass EP. Carnitine in renal failure: overview of carnitine metabolism. In: Kopple JD, Massry SG, eds. *Nutritional management of renal disease.* Baltimore: Williams & Wilkins, 1997:191.

302. Hoppel CL, Ricanati ES. Carnitine requirements in renal disease. In: Gussler JD, Silverman E, eds. *Renal nutrition, report of the Eleventh Ross Roundtable on medical issues.* Columbia: Ross Laboratories, 1991:68.

303. Ahmad S, Robertson HT, Golper TA, et al. Multicenter trial of L-carnitine in maintenance hemodialysis patients. II. Clinical and biochemical effects. *Kidney Int* 1990;38:912.

304. Golper TA, Ahmad S. L-Carnitine administration to hemodialysis patients: has its time come? *Semin Dial* 1992;5:94.

305. Kopple JD, Qing DP. Effect of L-carnitine on nitrogen balance in CAPD patients. *J Am Soc Nephrol* 1999;10:264A.

306. Fagher B, Cederblad G, Monti M, et al. Carnitine and left ventricular function in hemodialysis patients. *Scand J Clin Lab Invest* 1985;45:193.

307. Kooistra MP, Struyvenberg A, van Es A. The response to recombinant human erythropoietin in patients with the anemia of end-stage renal disease is correlated with serum creatinine levels. *Nephron* 1991;57:127.

308. van Es A, Henry FC, Kooistra MP, et al. Amelioration of cardiac function by L-carnitine administration in patients on hemodialysis. *Contr Nephrol* 1992;98:28.

309. Labonia WD. L-Carnitine effects on anemia in hemodialyzed patients treated with erythropoietin. *Am J Kidney Dis* 1995;26:757.

310. K/DOQI Nutrition Workgroup. *National Kidney Foundation Kidney Disease Outcomes Quality Initiative clinical practice guidelines for nutrition in chronic renal failure.* 2000;35:S54.

311. Pitts RF. *Physiology of the kidney and body fluids.* Chicago: Mosby–Year Book, 1974.

312. Koomans HA, Ross JC, Boer P, et al. Salt sensitivity of blood pressure in CRF. Evidence for renal control of body fluid distribution in man. *Hypertension* 1982;4:190.

313. Buter H, Hemmelder MH, Navis G, et al. The blunting of the antiproteinuric efficacy of ACE inhibition by high sodium intake can be restored by hydrochlorothiazide. *Nephrol Dial Transplantation* 1998;13:1682.

314. Deleted in proofs.

315. DeFronzo RA, Smith JD. Clinical disorders of hyperkalemia. In: Narins RG, ed. *Maxwell & Kleeman's clinical disorders of fluid and electrolyte metabolism*, 5th ed. New York: McGraw-Hill, 1994:697.

316. Kopple JD, Coburn JW. Metabolic studies of low protein diets in uremia. II. Calcium, phosphorus and magnesium. *Medicine* 1973;52:597.

317. Randall RE Jr, Cohen MD, Spray CC Jr, et al. Hypermagnesemia in renal failure: Etiology and toxic manifestations. *Ann Intern Med* 1964;61:73.

318. Wallach S. Effects of magnesium on skeletal metabolism. *Magnesium Trace Elem* 1990;9:1.

319. Tomford RC, Karlinsky ML, Buddington B, et al. Effect of thyroparathyroidectomy and parathyroidectomy on renal function and the nephrotic syndrome in rat nephrotoxic serum nephritis. *J Clin Invest* 1981;68:655.

320. Ibels LS, Alfrey AC, Huffer WE, et al. Calcification in end-stage kidneys. *Am J Med* 1981;71:33.

321. Barsotti G, Giannoni A, Morelli E, et al. The decline of renal function slowed by very low phosphorus intake in chronic renal patients following a long nitrogen diet. *Clin Nephrol* 1984;21:54.

322. Lumlertgul D, Burke TJ, Gillum DM, et al. Phosphate depletion arrests progression of CRF independent of protein intake. *Kidney Int* 1986;29:658.

323. Cannata JB, Briggs JD, Junor BJR. Aluminum hydroxide intake: real risk of aluminum toxicity. *Br Med J* 1983;286:1937.

324. Sedman AB, Miller NL, Warady BA, et al. Aluminum loading in children with CRF. *Kidney Int* 1984;26:201.

325. Kaye M. Oral aluminum toxicity in a non-dialyzed patient with CRF. *Clin Nephrol* 1983;20:208.

326. Norris KC, Crooks PW, Nebeker HG, et al. Clinical and laboratory features of aluminum-related bone disease: difference between sporadic and "epidemic" forms of the syndrome. *Am J Kidney Dis* 1985;6:342.

327. Addison JF, Foulks CJ. Calcium carbonate: an effective phosphorus binder in patients with CRF. *Curr Ther Res* 1985;38:241.

328. Hercz G, Coburn JW. Prevention of phosphate retention and hyperphosphatemia in uremia: a consideration of "newer" phosphate-binding agents. Proceedings of the Fourth International Congress on Nutrition and Metabolism in Renal Disease. *Kidney Int* 1987;32:S215.

329. Nolan CR, Califano JR, Butzin CA. Influence of calcium acetate or calcium citrate on intestinal aluminum absorption. *Kidney Int* 1990;38:937.

330. Schaefer K, Scheer J, Asmus G, et al. The treatment of uraemic hyperphosphataemia with calcium acetate and calcium carbonate: A comparison study. *Nephrol Dial Transplantation* 1991;6:170.

331. Mai ML, Emmett M, Sheikh MS, et al. Calcium acetate, an effective phosphate binder in patients with renal failure. *Kidney Int* 1989;36:690.

332. Pflanz S, Henderson IS, McElduff N, et al. Calcium acetate versus calcium carbonate as phosphate-binding agents in chronic haemodialysis. *Nephrol Dial Transplantation* 1994;9:1121.

333. Slatopolsky EA, Burke SK, Dillon MA. Renagel, a nonabsorbed calcium- and aluminum-free phosphate binder, lowers serum phosphorus and parathyroid hormone. The Renagel Study Group. *Kidney Int* 1999;55:299.

334. Bleyer AJ, Burke SK, Dillon M, et al. A comparison of the calcium-free phosphate binder sevelamer hydrochloride with calcium acetate

in the treatment of hyperphosphatemia in hemodialysis patients. *Am J Kidney Dis* 1999;33:694.

335. Chertow GM, Burke SK, Dillon MA, et al. Long-term effects of sevelamer hydrochloride on the calcium × phosphate product and lipid profile of haemodialysis patients. *Nephrol Dial Transplantation* 1999;14:2907.

336. Wilkes BM, Reiner D, Kern M, et al. Simultaneous lowering of serum phosphate and LDL-cholesterol by sevelamer hydrochloride (Renagel) in dialysis patients. *Clin Nephrol* 1998;50:381.

337. Van de Vyver FL, Visser WJ, D'Haese PC, et al. Iron overload and bone disease in chronic dialysis patients. *Nephrol Dial Transplantation* 1990;5:781.

338. Hercz G, Pei Y, Greenwood C, et al. Aplastic osteodystrophy without aluminum: the role of "suppressed" parathyroid function. *Kidney Int* 1993;44:860.

339. Kurtz SB, McCarthy JT, Kumar R. Hypercalcemia in continuous ambulatory peritoneal dialysis (CAPD) patients. Observations on parameters of calcium metabolism. In: Gahl GM, et al, eds. *Advances in peritoneal dialysis*. Amsterdam: Excerpta Medica, 1981:467.

340. Delmez JA, Slatopolsky E, Martin KJ, et al. Minerals, Vitamin D and parathyroid hormone in continuous ambulatory peritoneal dialysis. *Kidney Int* 1982;21:862.

341. Brickman AS, Coburn JW, Friedman GR, et al. Comparison of effects of 1-hydroxyvitamin D_3, and 1,25-dihydroxyvitamin D_3 in man. *J Clin Invest* 1976;57:1540.

342. Cartwright GE, Gubler CJ, Wintrobe MM. Studies on copper metabolism in the nephrotic syndrome. *J Clin Invest* 1954;33:685.

343. Blomfield J, McPherson J, George CRP. Active uptake of copper and zinc during hemodialysis. *Br Med J* 1969;2:141.

344. Blomfield J. Dialysis and lead absorption. *Lancet* 1973;2:666.

345. Tamura T, Vaughn WH, Waldo FB, et al. Zinc and copper balance in children on continuous ambulatory peritoneal dialysis. *Pediatr Nephrol* 1989;3:309.

346. Navarro JA, Granadillo VA, Rodriguez-Iturbe B, et al. Removal of trace metals by continuous ambulatory peritoneal dialysis after desferrioxamine B chelation therapy. *Clin Nephrol* 1991;35:213.

347. Padovese P, Gallieni M, Brancaccio D, et al. Trace elements in dialysis fluids and assessment of the exposure of patients on regular hemodialysis, hemofiltration and continuous ambulatory peritoneal dialysis. *Nephron* 1992;61:442.

348. Mahler DJ, Walsh JR, Haynie GD. Magnesium, zinc, and copper in dialysis patients. *Am J Clin Pathol* 1971;56:17.

349. Blomfield J, Dixon SR, McCredie DA. Potential hepatotoxicity of copper in recurrent hemodialysis. *Arch Intern Med* 1971;128:555.

350. Mahajan SK, Bowersox EM, Rye DL, et al. Factors underlying abnormal zinc metabolism in uremia. *Kidney Int* 1989;27:S269.

351. Van Renterghem D, Cornelis R, Vanholder R. Behaviour of 12 trace elements in serum of uremic patients on hemodiafiltration. *J Trace Elem Electrolytes Health Dis* 1992;6:169.

352. Manzler AD, Schreiner AW. Copper-induced acute hemolytic anemia. A new complication of hemodialysis. *Ann Intern Med* 1970;73:409.

353. Hosokawa S, Oyamaguchi A, Yoshida O. Trace elements and complications in patients undergoing chronic hemodialysis. *Nephron* 1990;55:375.

354. von Bonsdorff M, Sipila R, and Pitkanen E. Correction of hemodialysis-associated anemia by deteroxamine. *Scand J Urol Nephrol* 1990;131:49.

355. Silva J, Andrade S, Ventura H, et al. Iron supplementation in haemodialysis—practical clinical guidelines. *Nephrol Dial Transplantation* 1998;13:2572.

355a. Macdougall IC. Strategies for iron supplementation: oral versus intravenous. *Kidney Int* 1999;69:S61.

356. von Bonsdorff M, Sipila R, Pitkanen E. Correction of hemodialysis-associated anemia by deferoxamine. *Scand J Urol Nephrol* 1990; 131[Suppl]:49.

357. Boelaert JR, de Locht M, Van Cutsem J, et al. Mucormycosis during deferoxamine therapy as a siderophore-mediated infection—in vitro and in vivo animal studies. *J Clin Invest* 1993;91:1979.

358. Nomura S, Osawa G, Karai M. Treatment of a patient with end-stage renal disease, severe iron overload and ascites by weekly phlebotomy combined with recombinant human erythropoietin. *Nephron* 1990;55:210.

359. Rudolph H, Alfrey AC, Smythe WR. Muscle and serum trace element profile in uremia. *Trans Am Soc Artif Intern Organs* 1973;19:456.

360. Mansouri K, Haisted JA, Gombos EA. Zinc, copper, magnesium, and calcium in dialyzed and non-dialyzed uremic patients. *Arch Intern Med* 1970;125:88.

361. Atkin-Thor E, Goddard BW, O'Nion J, et al. Hypogeusia and zinc depletion in chronic dialysis patients. *Am J Clin Nutr* 1978;31:1948.

362. Mahajan SK, Abraham J, Hessburg T, et al. Zinc metabolism and taste acuity in renal transplant recipients. *Kidney Int* 1983; 24[Suppl 16]:S310.

363. Chen SM. Renal excretion of zinc in patients with chronic uremia. *Taiwan I Hsueh Hui Tsa Chih* 1990;89:220.

364. Antoniou LD, Shalhoub RJ, Sudhakar T, et al. Reversal of uremic impotence by zinc. *Lancet* 1977;2:895.

365. Rodger RS, Sheldon WL, Watson MJ, et al. Zinc deficiency and hyperprolactinemia are not reversible causes of sexual dysfunction in uremia. *Nephrol Dial Transplantation* 1989;4:888.

366. Killerich S, Christiansen C, Christensen MS, et al. Zinc metabolism in patients with CRF during treatment with 1,25-dihydroxycalciferol: a controlled therapeutic trial. *Clin Nephrol* 1981;15:23.

367. Kostakopoulos A, Kotsalos A, Alexopoulos J, et al. Serum selenium levels in healthy adults and its changes in CRF. *Int Urol Nephrol* 1990;22:397.

368. Richard MJ, Arnaud J, Jurkovitz C, et al. Trace elements and lipid peroxidation abnormalities in patients with CRF. *Nephron* 1991;57:10.

369. Taccone-Gallucci M, Lubrano R, Del Principe D, et al. Platelet lipid peroxidation in hemodialysis patients: effects of Vitamin E supplementation. *Nephrol Dial Transplantation* 1989;4:975.

370. Blumberg HA, Sander G. Vitamin nutrition in patients on continuous ambulatory peritoneal dialysis (CAPD). *Clin Nephrol* 1983;20:244.

371. Jennette JC, Goldman ID. Inhibition of the membrane transport of folates by anions retained in uremia. *J Lab Clin Med* 1975;86:834.

372. Sullivan JF, Eisenstein AB. Ascorbic acid depletion during hemodialysis. *JAMA* 1972;220:1697.

373. Lasker N, Harvey A, Baker H. Vitamin levels in hemodialysis and intermittent peritoneal dialysis. *Trans Am Soc Artif Intern Organs* 1963;9:51.

374. Hampers CL, Strieff R, Nathan DG, et al. Megaloblastic hematopoiesis in uremia and in patients on longterm hemodialysis. *N Engl J Med* 1967;276:551.

375. Whitehead VM, Comty CH, Posen GA, et al. Homeostasis of folic acid in patients undergoing maintenance hemodialysis. *N Engl J Med* 1968;279:970.

376. Milman N. Serum Vitamin B$_{12}$ and erythrocyte folate in chronic uraemia and after renal transplantation. *Scand J Haematol* 1980; 25:151.

377. Taniguchi H, Eijiri K, Baba S. Improvement of autonomic neuropathy after mecobalamin treatment in uremic patients on hemodialysis. *Clin Ther* 1987;9:607.

378. Bastow MD, Woods HF, Walls J. Persistent anemia associated with reduced serum Vitamin B$_{12}$ levels in patients undergoing regular hemodialysis therapy. *Clin Nephrol* 1979;11:133.

379. Porrini M, Simonetti P, Ciappellano S, et al. Thiamin, riboflavin and pyridoxine status in chronic renal insufficiency. *Int J Vitam Nutr Res* 1989;59:304.

380. Siddiqui J, Freeburger R, Freeman RM. Folic acid, hypersegmented polymorphonuclear leukocytes and the urermic syndrome. *Am J Clin Nutr* 1970;23:11.

381. Marumo F, Kamata K, Okubo M. Deranged concentrations of water-soluble vitamins in the blood of undialyzed and dialyzed patients with CRF. *Int J Artif Organs* 1986;9:17.

382. Sullivan JF, Eisenstein AB. Ascorbic acid depletion in patients undergoing chronic hemodialysis. *Am J Clin Nutr* 1970;23:1339.

383. Dobbelstein H, Komer WF, Mempel W, et al. Vitamin B$_6$ deficiency in uremia and its implications for the depression of immune responses. *Kidney Int* 1974;5:233.

384. Stone WJ, Warnock LG, Wagner C. Vitamin B$_6$ deficiency in uremia. *Am J Clin Nutr* 1975;28:950.

385. Ross EA, Shah GM, Reynolds RD, et al. Vitamin B$_6$ requirements of patients on chronic peritoneal dialysis. *Kidney Int* 1989;36:702.

386. Descombes E, Hanck AB, Fellay G. Water soluble vitamins in chronic hemodialysis patients and need for supplementation. *Kidney Int* 1993;43:1319.

387. Casciato DA, McAdam LP, Kopple JD, et al. Immunologic abnormalities in hemodialysis patients: improvement after pyridoxine therapy. *Nephron* 1984;38:9.

388. Wolf PL, Williams D, Coplon N, et al. Low aspartate transaminase activity in serum of patients undergoing chronic hemodialysis. *Clin Chem* 1972;18:567.

389. Warnock LG, Stone WJ, Wagner C. Decreased SGOT activity in serum of uremic patients. *Clin Chem* 1974;20:1213.

390. Cohen GA, Goffinet JA, Donabedian RK, et al. Observations on decreased SGOT activity in azotaemic patients. *Ann Intern Med* 1976;84:275.

391. Heaf JG. Liver function tests and pyridoxine levels in uremia. *Nephron* 1982;30:131.

392. Wilcken DEL, Dudman NPB, Tyrrell PA, et al. Folic acid lowers elevated plasma homocysteine in chronic renal insufficiency: possible implications for prevention of vascular disease. *Metabolism* 1988;37:697.

393. Tremblay R, Bonnardeaux A, Geadah D, et al. Hyperhomocystinemia in hemodialysis patients: effects of 12-month supplementation with hydrosoluble vitamins. *Kidney Int* 2000;58:851.

394. Sunder-Plassmann G, Fodinger M, Buchmayer H, et al. Effect of high dose folic acid therapy on hyperhomocysteinemia in hemodialysis patients: results of the Vienna multicenter study. *J Am Soc Nephrol* 2000;11:1106.

395. McGregor D, Shand B, Lynn K. A controlled trial of the effect of folate supplements on homocysteine, lipids and hemorheology in end-stage renal disease. *Nephron* 2000;85:215.

396. Touam M, Zingraff J, Jungers P, et al. Effective correction of hyperhomocysteinemia in hemodialysis patients by intravenous folinic acid and pyridoxine therapy. *Kidney Int* 1999;56:2292.

397. Wolfson M, Kopple JD. The effect of Vitamin B$_6$ deficiency on food intake, growth and renal function in chronically azotemic rats. *J Parenter Enteral Nutr* 1987;11:398.

398. Balcke P, Schmidt P, Zazgornik J, et al. Effect of Vitamin B$_6$ administration on elevated plasma oxalic acid levels in haemodialysed patients. *Eur J Clin Invest* 1982;12:481.

399. Morgan SH, Purkiss P, Watts RWE, et al. Oxalate dynamics in CRF. *Nephron* 1987;46:253.

400. Tomson CRV, Channon SM, Parkinson IS, et al. Effect of pyridoxine supplementation on plasma oxalate concentrations in patients receiving dialysis. *Eur J Clin Invest* 1989;19:201.

401. Costello JF, Sadovnic MJ, Smith M, et al. Effect of Vitamin B$_6$ supplementation on plasma oxalate removal rate in hemodialysis patients. *J Am Soc Nephrol* 1992;3:1018.

402. Smith FR, Goodman DS. The effects of diseases of liver, thyroid, and kidneys on the transport of Vitamin A in human plasma. *J Clin Invest* 1971;50:2426.

403. Stein G, Schöne S, Geinitz D, et al. No tissue level abnormality of Vitamin A concentration despite elevated serum Vitamin A of uremic patients. *Clin Nephrol* 1986;25:87.

404. Boeschoten EW, Schrijver J, Krediet RT, et al. Deficiencies of vitamins in CAPD patients: the effect of supplementation. *Nephrol Dial Transplantation* 1988;2:187.

405. Yatzidis H, Digenis P, Fountas P. Hypervitaminosis A accompanying advanced CRF. *Br Med J* 1975;3:352.

406. Farrington K, Miller P, Varghese Z, et al. Vitamin A toxicity and hypercalcaemia in CRF. *Br Med J* 1981;282:1999.

407. Giardini O, Taccone-Gallucci M, Lubrano R, et al. Effects of alpha-tocopherol administration on red blood cell membrane lipid peroxidation in hemodialysis patients. *Clin Nephrol* 1984;21: 174.

408. Yalcin AS, Yurtkuran M, Dilek K, et al. The effect of Vitamin E therapy on plasma and erythrocyte lipid peroxidation in chronic hemodialysis patients. *Clin Chim Acta* 1989;185:109.

409. Ito T, Niwa T, Matsui E. Vitamin B$_2$ and Vitamin E in long term hemodialysis. *JAMA* 1971;217:699.

410. Stein G, Sperschneider H, Koppe S. Vitamin levels in CRF and need for supplementation. *Blood Purif* 1985;3:52.

411. Udall JA. Human sources and absorption of Vitamin K in relation to anticoagulant stability. *JAMA* 1965;194:127.

412. Papadoyanakis N, Ziroyanis P, Papathanasiou E, et al. The effect of peritoneal dialysis on serum folic acid binding capacity. In: Gahl GM, Kessel M, Nolph KD, eds. *Advances in peritoneal dialysis.* Amsterdam: Excerpta Medica, 1981:70.

413. Salahudeen AK, Varma SR, Karim T, et al. Anaemia, ferritin, and vitamins in continuous ambulatory peritoneal dialysis. *Lancet* 1988;i:1049.

414. Mydlik M, Derzsiova K, Valek A, et al. Vitamins and continuous ambulatory peritoneal dialysis. *Int Urol Nephrol* 1985;17:281.

415. Sharman VL, Cunningham J, Goodwin FJ, et al. Do patients receiving regular haemodialysis need folic acid supplements? *Br Med J* 1982;285:96.

416. Balcke P, Schmidt P, Zazgornic J, et al. Ascorbic acid aggravates secondary hyperoxalemia in patients on chronic hemodialysis. *Ann Intern Med* 1984;3:344.

417. Pru C, Eaton J, Kjellstrand C. Vitamin C intoxication and hyperoxalemia in chronic hemodialysis patients. *Nephron* 1985;39:112.

418. Sonikian M, Gogusev J, Zingraff J, et al. Potential effect of metabolic acidosis on beta 2-microglobulin generation: in vivo and in vitro studies. *J Am Soc Nephrol* 1996;7:350.

419. Williams AJ, Dittmer ID, McArley A, et al. High bicarbonate dialysate in haemodialysis patients: effects on acidosis and nutritional status. *Nephrol Dial Transplantation* 1997;12:2633.

420. Kooman JP, Deutz NE, Zijlmans P, et al. The influence of bicarbonate supplementation on plasma levels of branched-chain amino acids in haemodialysis patients with metabolic acidosis. *Nephrol Dial Transplantation* 1997;12:2397.

421. Lofberg E, Wernerman J, Anderstam B, et al. Correction of acidosis in dialysis patients increases branched-chain and total essential amino acid levels in muscle. *Clin Nephrol* 1997;48:230.

422. Stein A, Moorhouse J, Iles-Smith H, et al. Role of an improvement in acid–base status and nutrition in CAPD patients. *Kidney Int* 1997;52:1089.

423. K/DOQI Nutrition Work Group Membership: National Kidney Foundation K/DOQI clinical practice guidelines for nutrition in renal failure. *Amer J Kidney Dis* 2000;35:538.

424. Symposium on role of dietary fiber in health. *Am J Clin Nutr* 1978;31:S1.

425. Rampton DS, Cohen SL, Crammond VD, et al. Treatment of CRF with dietary fiber. *Clin Nephrol* 1984;21:159.

426. K/DOQI Nutrition Workgroup. *National Kidney Foundation Kidney Disease Outcomes Quality Initiative clinical practice guidelines for nutrition in chronic renal failure.* 2000;35:S36.

427. Muehrcke RC. The finger-nails in chronic hypoalbuminaemia: a new physical sign. *Br Med J* 1956;1:1327.

428. Joven J, Villabona C, Vilella E, et al. Abnormalities of lipoprotein metabolism in patients with the nephrotic syndrome. *N Engl J Med* 1990;323:579.

429. Wanner C, Rader D, Bartens W, et al. Elevated plasma lipoproteins(a) in patients with the nephrotic syndrome. *Ann Intern Med* 1993;119:263.

430. Warwick GL, Caslake MJ, Boulton-Jones JM, et al. Low-density lipoprotein metabolism in the nephrotic syndrome. *Metabolism* 1990;39:187.

431. Marsh JB. Lipoprotein metabolism in experimental nephrosis. *J Lipid Res* 1984;25:1619.

432. Garber DW, Gottlieb BA, Marsh JB, et al. Catabolism of very low density lipo-proteins in experimental nephrosis. *J Clin Invest* 1984;74:1375.

433. Staprans I, Felts JM, Couser WG. Glycosaminoglycans and chylomicron metabolism in control and nephrotic rats. *Metabolism* 1987;36:496.

434. Moulin P, Appel GB, Ginsberg HN, et al. Increased concentration of plasma cholesteryl ester transfer protein in nephrotic syndrome: role in dyslipidemia. *J Lipid Res* 1992;33:1817.

435. Dullaart RP, Gansevoort RT, Dikkeschei BD, et al. Role of elevated lecithin: cholesterol acyltransferase and cholesteryl ester transfer protein activities in abnormal lipoproteins from proteinuric patients. *Kidney Int* 1993;44:91.

436. Kaysen GA, Don B, Schambelan M. Proteinuria, albumin synthesis and hyperlipidemia in the nephrotic syndrome. *Nephrol Dial Transplantation* 1991;6:141.

437. Baxter JH, Goodman HC, Allen JC. Effects of infusions of serum albumin on serum lipids and lipoproteins in nephrosis. *J Clin Invest* 1961;40:490.

438. Bogdonoff MD, Linhart J, Klein RF, et al. The effect of serum albumin infusion upon lipid mobilization in the nephrotic syndrome in man. *J Clin Invest* 1961;40:1024.

439. Berlyne GM, Mallick NP. Ischaemic heart disease as a complication of nephrotic syndrome. *Lancet* 1969;2:399.

440. Gherardi E, Rota E, Calandra S, et al. Relationship among the concentrations of serum lipoproteins and changes in their chemical composition in patients with untreated nephrotic syndrome. *Eur J Clin Invest* 1977;7:563.

441. Mallick NP, Short CD. The nephrotic syndrome and ischaemic heart disease. *Nephron* 1981;27:54.

442. Moorhead JF. Lipids and progressive kidney disease. *Kidney Int* 1991;31:S35.

443. Kaplan R, Aynedjian HS, Bank N, et al. Cholesterol feeding causes renal vasoconstriction via oxidized lipoprotein activation of thromboxane. *Kidney Int* 1990;37:371(abst).

444. Clemens MR, Bursa-Zanetti Z. Lipid abnormalities and peroxidation of erythrocytes in nephrotic syndrome. *Nephron* 1989;53:325.

445. D'Amico G, Remuzzi G, Maschio G, et al. Effect of dietary proteins and lipids in patients with membranous nephropathy and nephrotic syndrome. *Clin Nephrol* 1991;35:237.

446. D'Amico G, Gentile MG, Manna G, et al. Effect of vegetarian soy diet on hyperlipidaemia in nephrotic syndrome. *Lancet* 1992;339:1131.

447. Rabelink AJ, Hene RJ, Erkelens DW, et al. Partial remission of nephrotic syndrome in patients on long-term simvastatin. *Lancet* 1990;335:1045.

448. Jensen H, Rossing N, Andersen SB, et al. Albumin metabolism in the nephrotic syndrome in adults. *Clin Sci* 1967;33:445.

449. Strober W, Waldmann TA. The role of the kidney in the metabolism of plasma proteins. *Nephron* 1974;13:35.

450. Kaysen GA, Gambertoglio J, Jiminez I, et al. Effect of dietary protein intake on albumin homeostatis in nephrotic patients. *Kidney Int* 1986;29:572.

451. Coulthard MG. Management of Finnish congenital nephrotic syndrome by unilateral nephrectomy. *Pediatr Nephrol* 1989;3:451.

452. Kaysen GA, Al-Bander H. Metabolism of albumin and immunoglobulins in the nephrotic syndrome. *Am J Nephrol* 1990;10:36.

453. Haddad JG Jr, Walgate J. 25-Hydroxyvitamin D transport in human plasma: Isolation and partial characterization of calcifediol-binding protein. *J Biol Chem* 1976;251:4803.

454. Lambert PW, De Oreo PB, Fu IY, et al. Urinary and plasma Vitamin D metabolites in the nephrotic syndrome. *Metab Bone Dis Rel Res* 1982;4:715.

455. Sato KA, Gray RW, Lemann J. Urinary excretion of 25-hydroxyvitamin D in health and nephrotic syndrome. *J Lab Clin Med* 1982;69:325.

456. Khamiseh G, Vaziri ND, Oveisi F, et al. Vitamin D absorption, plasma concentration and urinary excretion of 25-hydroxyvitamin D in nephrotic syndrome. *Proc Soc Exp Biol Med* 1991;196:210.

457. Goldstein DA, Haldiman B, Sherman D, et al. Vitamin D metabolites and calcium metabolism in patients with nephrotic syndrome and normal renal function. *J Clin Endocrinol Metab* 1981;52:116.

458. Auwerx J, DeKeyser L, Bouillon R, et al. Decreased free 1,25-dihydroxycholecalciferol index in patients with the nephrotic syndrome. *Nephron* 1986;42:231.

459. Korkor A, Schwartz J, Bergfeld M, et al. Absence of metabolic bone disease in adult patients with the nephrotic syndrome and normal renal function. *J Clin Endocrinol Metab* 1983;56:496.

460. Recant L, Riggs DS. Thyroid function in nephrosis. *J Clin Invest* 1952;31:789.

461. Rasmussen H. Thyroxine metabolism in the nephrotic syndrome. *J Clin Invest* 1956;35:792.

462. Alfrey AC, Hammond WS. Renal iron handling in the nephrotic syndrome. *Kidney Int* 1990;37:1409.

463. Perrone L, Gialanella G, Giordano V, et al. Impaired zinc metabolic status in children affected by idiopathic nephrotic syndrome. *Eur J Pediatr* 1990;149:438.

464. Stec J, Podracka L, Pavkovcekova O, et al. Zinc and copper metabolism in nephrotic syndrome. *Nephron* 1990;56:186.

465. Blainey JD. High protein diets in the treatment of the nephrotic syndrome. *Clin Sci* 1954;13:567.

466. Zeller KR, Raskin P, Rosenstock J, et al. The effect of dietary protein restriction in diabetic nephropathy: reduction in proteinuria. *Kidney Int* 1986;29:209.

467. Kaysen GA, Gambertoglio J, Jimenez I, et al. Effect of dietary protein intake on albumin homeostasis in nephrotic patients. *Kidney Int* 1986;29:572.

468. Taguma Y, Kitamoto Y, Futaki G, et al. Effect of captopril on heavy proteinuria in azotemic diabetics. *N Engl J Med* 1985;313:1617.

469. Anderson S, Meyer TW, Rennke HG, et al. Control of glomerular hypertension limits glomerular injury in rats with reduced renal mass. *J Clin Invest* 1985;76:612.

470. Garini G, Mazzi A, Allegri L, et al. Effectiveness of dietary protein augmentation associated with angiotensin-converting enzyme inhibition in the management of the nephrotic syndrome. *Miner Electrolyte Metab* 1996;22:123.

471. Ravid M, Savin H, Jutrin I, et al. Long-term stabilizing effect of angiotensin-converting enzyme inhibition on plasma creatinine and on proteinuria in normotensive type II diabetic patients. *Ann Intern Med* 1993;118:577.

472. The GISEN Group. Randomised placebo controlled trial of effect of ramipril on decline in glomerular filtration rate and risk of terminal renal failure in proteinuric, non-diabetic nephropathy. *Lancet* 1997;349:1857.

473. Leonard CD, Luke RG, Siegel RR. Parenteral essential amino acids in acute renal failure. *Urology* 1975;6:154.

474. Feinstein EI, Blumenkrantz MJ, Healy H, et al. Clinical and metabolic responses to parenteral nutrition in acute renal failure. A controlled double-blind study. *Medicine* 1981;60:124.

475. Feinstein EI, Kopple JD, Silberman H, et al. Total parenteral nutrition with high or low nitrogen intake in patients with Acute renal failure. *Kidney Int* 1983;26[Suppl 16]:S319.

476. Cahill GF. Starvation in man. *N Engl J Med* 1970;282:668.

477. Ikizler TA, Himmelfarb J. Nutrition in acute renal failure patients. *Adv Renal Repl Ther* 1997;4:S54.

478. Fiaccadori E, Lombardi M, Leonardi S, et al. Prevalence and clinical outcome associated with preexisting malnutrition in acute renal failure: a prospective cohort study. *J Am Soc Nephrol* 1999;10:581.

479. Lacy WW. Effect of acute uremia on amino acid uptake and urea production by perfused rat liver. *Am J Physiol* 1969;216:1300.

480. Frohlich J, Scholmerich J, Hoppe-Seyler G, et al. The effect of acute uremia on gluconeogenesis in isolated perfused rat livers. *Eur J Clin Invest* 1974;4:453.

481. McCormick GJ, Shear L, Barry KG. Alteration of hepatic protein synthesis in acute uremia. *Proc Soc Exp Biol Med* 1966;122:99.

482. Shear L. Internal redistribution of tissue protein synthesis in uremia. *J Clin Invest* 1969;48:1252.

483. Flugel-Link RM, Salusky IB, Jones MR, et al. Enhanced muscle protein degradation and urea nitrogen appearance (UNA) in rats with acute renal failure. *Am J Physiol* 1983;244:E615.

484. Clark AS, Mitch WE. Muscle protein turnover and glucose uptake in acutely uremic rats. Effect of insulin and the duration of renal insufficiency. *J Clin Invest* 1983;72:836.

485. May RC, Kelly RA, Mitch WE. Metabolic acidosis stimulates protein degradation in rat muscle by a glucocorticoid-dependent mechanism. *J Clin Invest* 1986;77:614.

486. Kuhlmann MK, Shahmir E, Massrani E, et al. A new experimental model of acute renal failure and sepsis in rats. *J Parenter Enteral Nutr* 1994;18:477.

487. Shear L, Sapico V, Litwack G. Induction of hepatic enzymes and translocation of cytosol tyrosine amino transaminase (TAT) in uremic rats. *Clin Res* 1973;21:707A.

488. Sapico V, Shear L, Litwack G. Translocation of inducible tyrosine aminotransferase to the mitochondrial fraction. *J Biol Chem* 1974;249:2122.

489. Horl WH, Heidland A. Glycogen metabolism in muscle in uremia. *Am J Clin Nutr* 1980;33:1461.

490. Eigler N, Sacca L, Sherwin RS. Synergistic interactions of physiologic increments of glucagon, epinephrine and cortisol in the dog. A model for stress-induced hyperglycemia. *J Clin Invest* 1979;63:114.

491. Bessey PQ, Watters JM, Aoki TT, et al. Combined hormonal infusion simulates the metabolic response to injury. *Ann Surg* 1984;200:264.

492. Schaefer RM, Riegel W, Stephan E, et al. Normalization of enhanced hepatic gluconeogenesis by the antiglucocorticoid RU 38486 in acutely uraemic rats. *Eur J Clin Invest* 1990;20:35.

493. Mondon CE, Reaven GM. Evaluation of enhanced glucagon sensitivity as the cause of glucose intolerance in acutely uremic rats. *Am J Clin Nutr* 1980;33:1456.

494. Massry SG, Arieff AI, Coburn JW, et al. Divalent ion metabolism in patients with acute renal failure: studies on the mechanism of hypocalcemia. *Kidney Int* 1974;5:437.

495. Pietrek J, Kokot F, Kuska J. Serum 25-hydroxyvitamin D and parathyroid hormone in patients with acute renal failure. *Kidney Int* 1978;13:178.

496. Horl WH, Heidland A. Enhanced proteolytic activity—cause of protein catabolism in acute renal failure. *Am J Clin Nutr* 1980;33:1423.

497. Horl WH, Stepinski J, Schafer RM, et al. Role of proteases in hypercatabolic patients with renal failure. *Kidney Int* 1983;24[Suppl 16]:S37.

498. Bull GM, Joekes AM, Lowe KG. Conservative treatment of anuric uremia. *Lancet* 1949;2:229.

499. Blagg CR, Parsons FM, Young BA. Effects of dietary glucose and protein in acute renal failure. *Lancet* 1962;1:608.

500. Gamble JL. Physiological information from studies on the life-raft ration. *Harvey Lect* 1946–1947;42:247.

501. McCracken BH, Parsons FM. Nilevar (17-ethyl-19-nor-testosterone) to suppress protein catabolism in acute renal failure. *Lancet* 1958;2:885.

502. Gjorup S, Thavsen JH. The effect of anabolic steroid (Durabolin) in the conservative management of acute renal failure. *Acta Med Scand* 1960;167:227.

503. Berlyne GM, Bazzard FJ, Booth EM, et al. The dietary treatment of acute renal failure. *Q J Med* 1967;141:59.

504. Teschan PE, Baxter CR, O'Brien TF, et al. Prophylactic hemodialysis in the treatment of acute renal failure. *Ann Intern Med* 1960;53:992.

505. Lee HA, Sharpstone P, Ames AC. Parenteral nutrition in renal failure. *Postgrad Med J* 1967;43:81.

506. Wilmore DW, Dudrick SJ. Treatment of acute renal failure with intravenous essential L-amino acids. *Arch Surg* 1969;99:669.

507. Dudrick SJ, Steiger E, Long JM. Renal failure in surgical patients-treatment with intravenous essential amino acids and hypertonic glucose. *Surgery* 1970;68:180.

508. Van Buren CT, Dudrick SJ, Dworkin L, et al. Effects of intravenous essential L-amino acids and hypertonic dextrose on anephric beagles. *Surg Forum* 1972;23:83.

509. Abbott WM, Abel RM, Fischer JE. Treatment of acute renal insufficiency after aortoiliac surgery. *Arch Surg* 1971;103:590.

510. Abel RM, Abbott WM, Fischer JE. Intravenous essential L-amino acids and hypertonic dextrose in patients with acute renal failure. *Am J Surg* 1972;123:631.

511. Abel RM, Beck CH Jr, Abbott WM, et al. Improved survival and acute renal failure after treatment with intravenous essential L-amino acids and glucose. *N Engl J Med* 1973;288:695.

512. Abel RM, Abbott WM, Beck CH Jr, et al. Essential L-amino acids for hyperalimentation in patients with disordered nitrogen metabolism. *Am J Surg* 1974;128:317.

513. Abel RM, Shih VE, Abbott WM, et al. Acid metabolism in acute renal failure. *Ann Surg* 1974;180:350.

514. Sofio C, Nicora R. High calorie essential amino acid parenteral therapy in acute renal failure. *Acta Chir Scand* 1976;466[Suppl]:98.

515. Baek SM, Makaboli GG, Bryan-Brown CW, et al. The influence of parenteral nutrition on the course of acute renal failure. *Surg Gynecol Obstet* 1975;141:405.

516. McMurray SD, Luft FC, Maxwell DR, et al. Prevailing patterns and predictor variables in patients with acute tubular necrosis. *Arch Intern Med* 1978;138:950.

517. Milligan SL, Luft FC, McMurray SD, et al. Intra-abdominal infection and acute renal failure. *Arch Surg* 1978;113:467.

517a. Mocan MZ, Mocan H, Gacar MN, et al. Effect of essential amino acid supplementation in acute renal failure. *Int Urol Nephrol* 1996;27:503.

518. Abitbol CL, Holliday MA. Total parenteral nutrition in anuric children. *Clin Nephrol* 1976;3:153.

519. Blackburn GL, Etter G, MacKenzie T. Criteria for choosing amino acid therapy in acute renal failure. *Am J Clin Nutr* 1978;31:1841.

520. Lopez-Martinez J, Caparros T, Perez-Picouto F, et al. Nutrition parenteral en enfermos septicos con fracaso renal agudo en fase poliurica. *Rev Clin Exp* 1980;157:171.

521. Spreiter SC, Myers BD, Swenson RS. Protein-energy requirements in subjects with acute renal failure receiving intermittent hemodialysis. *Am J Clin Nutr* 1980;33:1433.

522. Mault JR, Bartlett RH, Dechert RE, et al. Starvation: a major contribution to mortality in acute renal failure? *Trans Am Soc Artif Intern Organs* 1983;29:390.

523. Kopple JD. 1995 Jonathan E. Rhoads lecture: the nutrition management of the patient with acute renal failure. *J Parenter Enteral Nutr* 1996;20:3.

524. Hasik J, Hryniewiecki L, Baczyk K, et al. An attempt to evaluate minimum requirements for protein in patients with acute renal failure. *Pol Arch Med Wewn* 1979;61:29.

525. Mirtallo JM, Schneider PJ, Mavko K, et al. A comparison of essential and general amino acid infusions in the nutritional support of patients with compromised renal function. *J Parenter Enteral Nutr* 1982;6:109.

526. Mehta RL. Continuous renal replacement therapies in the acute renal failure setting: current concepts. *Adv Renal Repl Ther* 1997;4[Suppl 1]:82.

527. Macias WL, Alaka KJ, Murphy MH, et al. Impact of the nutritional regimen on protein catabolism and nitrogen balance in patients with acute renal failure. *J Parenter Enteral Nutr* 1996;20:56.

528. Bellomo R, Seacombe J, Daskalakis M, et al. A prospective comparative study of moderate versus high protein intake for critically ill patients with acute renal failure. *Renal Fail* 1997;19:111.

529. Davenport A, Roberts NB. Amino acid losses during continuous high-flux hemofiltration in the critically ill patient. *Crit Care Med* 1989;17:1010.

530. Davies SP, Reaveley DA, Brown EA, et al. Amino acid clearances and daily losses in patients with acute renal failure treated by continuous arteriovenous hemodialysis. *Crit Care Med* 1991;19:1510.

531. Mehta RL. Therapeutic alternatives to renal replacement for critically ill patients in acute renal failure. *Semin Nephrol* 1994;14:64.

532. Toback FG, Havener LH, Dodd RC, et al. Phospholipid metabolism during renal regeneration after acute tubular necrosis. *Am J Physiol* 1967;232:E216.

533. Cuppage FE, Chiga M, Tate A. Cell cycle studies in the regenerating rat nephron following injury with mercuric chloride. *Lab Invest* 1972;26:122.

534. Nicholls DM, Ng K. Regeneration of renal proximal tubules after mercuric chloride injury is accompanied by increased binding of aminoacyltransfer ribonucleic acid. *Biochem J* 1976;160:357.

535. Toback FG. Amino acid treatment of acute renal failure. In: Brenner BM, Stein JH, eds. *Acute renal failure.* London: Churchill Livingstone, 1980:202.

536. Toback FG, Dodd RC, Maier ER, et al. Amino acid enhancement of renal protein synthesis during regeneration after acute tubular necrosis. *Clin Res* 1979;27:432A.

537. Toback FG. Amino acid enhancement of renal regeneration after acute tubular necrosis. *Kidney Int* 1977;12:193.

538. Toback FG, Tegarden DE, Havener LJ. Amino acid–mediated stimulation of renal phospholipid biosynthesis after acute tubular necrosis. *Kidney Int* 1979;15:542.

539. Oken DE, Sprinkel FM, Kirschbaum BB, et al. Amino acid therapy in the treatment of experimental acute renal failure in the rat. *Kidney Int* 1980;17:14.

540. Burke TJ, Arnold PE, Gordon JA, et al. Protective effect of intrarenal calcium membrane blockers before or after renal ischemia. *J Clin Invest* 1984;74:1830.

541. Siegel NJ, Glazier WB, Chaudry IH, et al. Enhanced recovery from acute renal failure by the postischemic infusion of adenine nucleotides and magnesium chloride in rats. *Kidney Int* 1980;17:338.

542. Siegel NJ, Gaudio KM, Katz LA, et al. Beneficial effect of thyroxin on recovery from toxic acute renal failure. *Kidney Int* 1984;25:906.

543. Acker CG, Singh AR, Flick RP, et al. A trial of thyroxine in acute renal failure. *Kidney Int* 2000;57:293.

544. Humes HD, Cieslinski DA, Coimbra TM, et al. Epidermal growth factor enhances renal tubule cell regeneration and repair and accelerates the recovery of renal function in postischemic acute renal failure. *J Clin Invest* 1989;84:1757.

545. Miller SB, Martin DR, Kissane J, et al. Hepatocyte growth factor accelerates recovery from acute ischemic renal injury in rats. *Am J Physiol* 1994;266:F129.

546. Miller SB, Martin DR, Kissane J, et al. Insulin-like growth factor-1 accelerates recovery from ischemic acute tubular necrosis in the rat. *Proc Natl Acad Sci USA* 1992;89:11876.

547. Ding H, Kopple JD, Cohen A, et al. Recombinant human insulin-like growth factor-1 accelerates recovery and reduces catabolism in rats with ischemic acute renal failure. *J Clin Invest* 1993;91:2281.

548. Clark R, Mortensen D, Rabkin R. Recovery from acute ischaemic renal failure is accelerated by des (1-3) insulin-like growth factor-1. *Clin Sci* 1994;86:709.

549. Fuchs S, Jaffe R, Beeri R, et al. Failure of insulin-like growth factor 1 (IGF-1) to improve radiocontrast nephropathy. *J Am Soc Nephrol* 1995;6:997(abst).

550. Hirschberg R, Kopple J, Lipsett P, et al. Multicenter clinical trial of recombinant human insulin-like growth factor I in patients with acute renal failure. *Kidney Int* 1999;55:24223.

551. Franklin SC, Moulton M, Sicard GA, et al. Insulin-like growth factor I preserves renal function postoperatively. *Am J Physiol* 1997;272:F257.

552. Rahman SN, Kim GE, Mathew AS, et al. Effects of atrial natriuretic peptide in clinical acute renal failure. *Kidney Int* 1994;45:1731.

553. Lewis J, Salem MM, Chertow GM, et al. Atrial natriuretic factor in oliguric acute renal failure. Anaritide Acute Renal Failure Study Group. *Am J Kidney Dis* 2000;36:767.

554. Hinton P, Allison SP, Littlejohn S, et al. Insulin and glucose to reduced catabolic response to injury in burned patients. *Lancet* 1971;1:767.

555. Woolfson AMJ, Heatley RV, Allison SP. Insulin to inhibit protein catabolism after injury. *N Engl J Med* 1979;300:14.

556. Ponting GA, Teale JD, Halliday D, et al. Postoperative positive nitrogen balance with intravenous hyponutrition and growth hormone. *Lancet* 1988;1:438.

557. Wilmore DW. Catabolic illness. Strategies for enhancing recovery. *N Engl J Med* 1991;325:695.

558. Takala J, Ruokonen E, Webster NR, et al. Increased mortality associated with growth hormone treatment in critically ill adults. *N Engl J Med* 1999;341:785.

559. Motil KJ, Harmon WE, Grupe WE. Complications of essential amino acid hyperalimentation in children with acute renal failure. *J Parenter Enteral Nutr* 1980;4:32.

560. Nakasaki H, Katayama T, Yokoyama S, et al. Complication of parenteral nutrition composed of essential amino acids and histidine in adults with renal failure. *J Parenter Enteral Nutr* 1993;17:86.

561. Chima CS, Meyer L, Hummell AC, et al. Protein catabolic rate in patients with acute renal failure on continuous arteriovenous hemofiltration and total parenteral nutrition. *J Am Soc Nephrol* 1993;3:1516.

562. Bellomo R, Mansfield D, Rumble S, et al. A comparison of conventional dialytic therapy and acute continuous hemodiafiltration in the management of acute renal failure in the critically ill. *Renal Fail* 1993;15(5):595.

563. Kung SP, Lui WY, P'eng FK. A 24-patient experience in hyperalimentation for acute renal insufficiency: emphasis on amino acid determination. *Chung Hua I Hsueh Tsa Chih (Taipei)* 1995;56:252.

564. Deleted in proofs.

565. Deleted in proofs.

566. Cerra FB, Upson D, Angelica R, et al. Branched chains support postoperative protein synthesis. *Surgery* 1982;92:192.

567. Daly M, Mihranian MH, Kehoe JI, et al. Effects of post-operative infusion of branched-chain amino acids on nitrogen balance and forearm muscle substrate flux. *Surgery* 1983;94:151.

568. Tischler ME, Desautels M, Goldberg AL. Does leucine, leucyl-tRNA, or some metabolite of leucine regulate protein synthesis and degradation in skeletal and cardiac muscle? *J Biol Chem* 1982;257:1613.

569. Leander U, Furst P, Vesterberg K, et al. Nitrogen sparing effect of Ornicetil in the immediate postoperative state. Clinical biochemistry and nitrogen balance. *Clin Nutr* 1985;4:43.

570. Harris JA, Benedict FG. *A biometric study of basal metabolism in man.* Washington: Carnegie Institute; 1919. Publication no 279.

571. Wilmore DW. *In the metabolic management of the critically ill.* New York: Plenum Publishing, 1977:34.

572. Askanazi J, Rosenbaum SH, Hyman AL, et al. Respiratory changes induced by the large glucose loads of total parenteral nutrition. *JAMA* 1980;243:1444.

573. Jeejeebhoy KN, Langer B, Tsallas G, et al. Total parenteral nutrition at home: studies in patients surviving 4 months to 5 years. *Gastroenterology* 1976;71:943.

574. Druml W, Laggner A, Widhalm K, et al. Lipid metabolism in acute renal failure. *Kidney Int* 1983;24:S139.

575. Seidner DL, Mascioli EA, Istfan NW, et al. Effects of long chain triglyceride emulsions on reticuloendothelial system functions in humans. *J Parenter Enteral Nutr* 1989;13:614.

576. Freeman J, Goldmann DA, Smith NE, et al. Association of intravenous lipid emulsion and coagulase-negative staphylococcal bacteremia in neonatal intensive care units. *N Engl J Med* 1990;323:301.

577. Driscoll DF, Baptista BJ, Bistrian BR, et al. Practical considerations regarding the use of total nutrient admixtures. *Am J Hosp Pharm* 1986;43:416.

578. Wan JM-F, Teo TC, Babayan VK, et al. Invited comment: lipids and the development of immune dysfunction and infection. *J Parenter Enteral Nutr* 1988;12:43S.

579. Endres S, Ghorbani R, Kelley VE, et al. The effect of dietary supplementation with n-3 polyunsaturated fatty acids on the synthesis of interleukin-1 and tumor necrosis factor by mononuclear cells. *N Engl J Med* 1989;320:265.

580. Kinsella JE, Lokesh B, Broughton S, et al. Dietary polyunsaturated fatty acids and eicosanoids—potential effects on the modulation of inflammatory and immune cells—an overview. *Nutrition* 1990;6:24.

581. Druml W, Schwarzenhofer M, Apsner R, et al. Fat-soluble vitamins in patients with acute renal failure. *Miner Electrolyte Metab* 1998;24:220.

582. Gleghorn EE, Eisenberg LD, Hack S, et al. Observations of Vitamin A toxicity in three patients with renal failure receiving parenteral alimentation. *Am J Clin Nutr* 1986;44:107.

583. Vanamee P, Shils ME, Burke AW, et al. Multivitamin preparations for parenteral use: a statement by the Nutrition Advisory Group. *J Parenter Enteral Nutr* 1979;3:258.

584. Shils ME, Brown RO. Parenteral nutrition. In: Shils ME, Olson JA, Shine M, et al, eds. *Modern nutrition in health disease,* 9th ed. Baltimore: Williams & Wilkins, 1999:1657.

585. Friedman AL, Chesney RW, Gilbert EF, et al. Secondary oxalosis as a complication of parenteral nutrition in acute renal failure. *Am J Nephrol* 1983;3:248.

586. Audran M, Kumar R. The physiology and pathophysiology of Vitamin D. *Mayo Clin Proc* 1985;60:851.

587. Slatopolsky E, Weerts C, Thielan J, et al. Marked suppression of secondary hyperparathyroidism by intravenous administration of 1,25-dihydroxycholecalciferol in uremic patients. *J Clin Invest* 1984;74:2136.

588. Zager RA, Johannes G, Tuttle SE, et al. Acute amino acid nephrotoxicity. *J Lab Clin Med* 1983;101:130.

589. Zager RA, Venkatachalam MA. Potentiation of ischemic renal injury by amino acid infusion. *Kidney Int* 1983;24:620.

590. Malis CD, Racusen C, Solez K, et al. Nephrotoxicity of lysine and of a single dose of aminoglycoside in rats given lysine. *J Lab Clin Med* 1984;103:660.

591. Andrews PM, Bates SB. Dietary protein prior to renal ischemia dramatically affects ischemic kidney function. Proceedings of the Fourth International Congress on Nutrition and Metabolism in Renal Disease. *Kidney Int* 1987;32:S76.

592. Weinberg JM: The effect of amino acids on ischemic and toxic injury to the kidney. *Semin Nephrol* 1990;10:491.

593. Kaltenbach JP, Ganote CE, Carone FA. Renal tubular necrosis induced by compounds structurally related to D-serine. *Exp Mol Pathol* 1979;30:209.

594. Kopple JD. The rationale for the use of growth hormone or insulin-like growth factor-1 in adult patients with renal failure. *Miner Electrolyte Metab* 1991;18:269.

595. Ziegler TR, Lazarus JM, Young LS, et al. Effects of recombinant human growth hormone in adults receiving maintenance hemodialysis. *J Am Soc Nephrol* 1991;2:1130.

596. Schulman G, Wingard RL, Hutchison RL, et al. The effects of recombinant human growth hormone and intradialytic parenteral nutrition in malnourished hemodialysis patients. *Am J Kidney Dis* 1993;21:527.

597. Fine RN, Pyke-Grimm K, Nelson PA, et al. Recombinant human growth hormone treatment of children with CRF: long-term (1- to 3-year) outcome. *Pediatr Nephrol* 1991;5:477.

598. Van Renen MJ, Kogg RJ, Sweeney AL, et al. Accelerated growth in short children with CRF treated with both strict dietary therapy and recombinant growth hormone. *Pediatr Nephrol* 1992;6:451.

599. Hammarqvist F, Wenerman J, Ali R, et al. Addition of glutamine to total parenteral nutrition after elective abdominal surgery spares free glutamine in muscle, counteracts the fall in muscle protein synthesis and improves nitrogen balances. *Ann Surg* 1989;209:455.

600. Stehle P, Mertes N, Puchstein CH, et al. Effect of parenteral glutamine peptide supplements on muscle glutamine loss and nitrogen balance after major surgery. *Lancet* 1989;1:231.

601. Daly JM, Reynolds J, Thom A, et al. Immune and metabolic effects of arginine in the surgical patient. *Ann Surg* 1988;208:512.

602. Barbul A. Arginine: biochemistry, physiology and therapeutic implications. *J Parenter Enteral Nutr* 1986;10:227.

603. Souba WW, Herskowitz K, Augsten TR, et al. Glutamine nutrition: theoretical considerations and therapeutic impact. *J Parenter Enteral Nutr* 1990;14[Suppl]:237S.

604. Ziegler TR, Young LS, Benfell K, et al. Clinical and metabolic efficacy of glutamine-supplemented parenteral nutrition after bone marrow transplantation. A randomized, double-blind, controlled study. *Ann Intern Med* 1992;116:821.

605. Gianotti L, Alexander JW, Pyles T, et al. Arginine-supplemented diets improve survival in gut-derived sepsis and peritonitis by modulating bacterial clearance. *Ann Surg* 1993;217:644.

606. Schloerb PR, Amare M. Total parenteral nutrition with glutamine in bone marrow transplantation and other clinical applications (a randomized, double-blind study). *J Parenter Enteral Nutr* 1993;17:407.

607. Schramm L, Heidbreder E, Schmitt A, et al. Role of L-arginine–derived NO in ischemic acute renal failure in the rat. *Renal Fail* 1994;16:555.

608. Rudolph FB, Kulkarni AD, Fanslow WC, et al. Role of RNA as a dietary source of pyrimidines and purines in immune function. *Nutrition* 1990;6:45.

609. Rombeau JL, Palacio JC. Feeding by tube enterostomy. In: Rombeau JL, Caldwell MD, eds. *Enteral and tube feeding,* 2nd ed, vol 2. Philadelphia: WB Saunders, 1990.

610. DeWitt RC, Kudsk KA. Enteral nutrition. *Gastroenterol Clin North Am* 1998;27:371.

611. Kopple JD. Therapeutic approaches to malnutrition in chronic dialysis patients: the different modalities of nutritional support. *Am J Kidney Dis* 1999;33:180.

612. Warady BA, Weis L, Johnson L. Nasogastric tube feeding in infants on peritoneal dialysis. *Perit Dial Int* 1996;16:S521.

613. Kuizon BD, Nelson PA, Salusky IB. Tube feeding in children with end-stage renal disease. *Miner Electrolyte Metab* 1997;23:306.

614. Freeman JB, Fairfull-Smith RJ. Physiologic approach to peripheral parenteral nutrition. In: Fischer JE, ed. *Surgical nutrition.* Boston: Little, Brown and Company, 1983:703.

615. Shils ME, Wright WL, Turnbull A, et al. A long-term parenteral nutrition through an external arteriovenous shunt. *N Engl J Med* 1970; 283:341.

616. Foulks CJ. An evidence-based evaluation of intradialytic parenteral nutrition. *Am J Kidney Dis* 1999;33:186.

617. Kopple JD, Foulks CJ, Piraino B, et al. Proposed health care financing administration guidelines for reimbursement of enteral and parenteral nutrition. *Am J Kidney Dis* 1995;26:995.

618. Feinstein EI, Collins JF, Blumenkrantz MJ, et al. Nutritional hemodialysis. *Prog Artif Organs* 1984;1:421.

619. Kopple JD, Bernard D, Messana J, et al. Treatment of malnourished CAPD patients with an amino acid based dialysate. *Kidney Int* 1995;47:1148.

620. Brulez HF, van Guldener C, Donker AJ, et al. The impact of an amino acid–based peritoneal dialysis fluid on plasma total homocysteine levels, lipid profile and body fat mass. *Nephrol Dial Transplantation* 1999;14:154.

621. Lewy JE, New MI. Growth in children with renal failure. *Am J Med* 1975;58:65.

622. Cogan MG, Sargent JA, Yarbrough SG, et al. Prevention of prednisone-induced negative nitrogen balance. Effect of dietary modification of urea generation rate in patients on hemodialysis receiving high-dose glucocorticoids. *Ann Intern Med* 1981;95:158.

623. Steinmuller DR, Richards C, Novick A, et al. Protein catabolic rate post transplant. *Dial Transplantation* 1983;7:504.

624. Whittier FC, Evans DH, Dutton S, et al. Nutrition in renal transplantation. *Am J Kidney Dis* 1985;6:405.

625. van den Ham EC, Kooman JP, Christiaans MH, et al. Relation between steroid dose, body composition and physical activity in renal transplant patients. *Transplantation* 2000;69:1591.

626. Seagraves A, Moore EE, Moore FA, et al. Net protein catabolic rate after kidney transplantation: impact of corticosteroid immunosuppression. *J Parenter Enteral Nutr* 1986;10:453.

627. Edelstein CL, van Zyl J, Moosa MR, et al. Protein catabolic rate after renal transplantation. *Transplant Proc* 1992;24:1775.

628. Nelson J, Beauregard H, Gelinas M, et al. Rapid improvement of hyperlipidemia in kidney transplant patients with a multifactorial hypolipidemic diet. *Transplant Proc* 1988;20:1264.

629. Dimëny E, Fellström B, Larsson E, et al. Lipoprotein abnormalities in renal transplant recipients with chronic vascular rejection. *Transplant Proc* 1992;24:366.

630. Socha MW, Polakowska MJ, Socha-Urbanek K, et al. Hyperhomocysteinemia as a risk factor for cardiovascular diseases. The association of hyperhomocysteinemia with diabetes mellitus and renal transplant recipients. *Ann Transplantation* 1999;4:11.

631. Zazgornik J, Druml W, Balcke P, et al. Diminished serum folic acid levels in renal transplant recipients. *Clin Nephrol* 1982;18:306.

632. Bagni B, Gilli P, Cavalini A, et al. Continuing loss of vertebral mineral density in renal transplant recipients. *Eur J Nucl Med* 1994;21:108.

633. Kelleher J, Humphrey CS, Homer D, et al. Vitamin A and its transport proteins in patients with CRF receiving maintenance haemodialysis and after renal transplantation. *Clin Sci* 1983;65:619.

634. Baxter JD, Rousseau GG. In: Baxter JD, Rousseau GG, eds. *Glucocorticoid hormone action.* New York: Springer-Verlag New York, 1979.

635. Reid IR. Steroid osteoporosis. *Calcif Tissue Int* 1989;45:63.

636. Klein RG, Amaud SB, Gallagher JC, et al. Intestinal calcium absorption in exogenous hypercortisolism: role of 25-hydroxyvitamin D and corticosteroid dose. *J Clin Invest* 1977;60:253.

637. Jahn TJ, Halstead LR, Baran DT. Effects of short term glucocorticoid administration on intestinal calcium absorption and circulating Vitamin D metabolite concentrations in man. *J Clin Endocrinol Metab* 1981;52:111.

638. Chesney RW, Hamstra AJ, Mazess RB, et al. Reduction of serum-1,25-dihydroxyvitamin-D$_3$ in children receiving glucocorticoids. *Lancet* 1978;2:1123.

639. Seeman E, Kumar R, Hunder GG, et al. Production, degradation and circulating levels of 1,25-dihydroxyvitamin D in health and in chronic glucocorticoid excess. *J Clin Invest* 1980;66:664.

640. Braun JJ, Juttmann JR, Visser TJ, et al. Short-term effect of prednisone on serum 1,25-dihydroxyvitamin D in normal individuals and in hyper- and hypo-parathyroidism. *Clin Endocrinol* 1982;17:21.

641. LoCascio V, Bonucci E, Imbimbo B, et al. Bone loss after glucocorticoid therapy. *Calcif Tissue Int* 1984;36:435.

642. Ibels LS, Alfrey AC, Weil R III. Hyperlipidemia in adult, pediatric and diabetic renal transplant recipients. *Am J Med* 1978;64:634.

643. Isoniemi H, Nurminen M, Tikkanen M, et al. Risk factors predicting chronic rejection of renal allograft. *Transplantation* 1994;57:68.

644. Roodnat JI, Mulder PG, Zietse R, et al. Cholesterol as an independent predictor of outcome after renal transplantation. *Transplantation* 2000;69:1704.

645. Wissing KM, Abramowicz D, Broeders N, et al. Hypercholesterolemia is associated with increased kidney graft loss caused by chronic rejection in male patients with previous acute rejection. *Transplantation* 2000;70:464.

646. Markell MS, Altura BT, Barbour RL, et al. Ionized and total magnesium levels in cyclosporin-treated renal transplant recipients: relationship with cholesterol and cyclosporin levels. *Clin Sci* 1993;85:315.

647. Foldes K, Maklary E, Vargha P, et al. Effect of diet and fluvastatin treatment on the serum lipid profile of kidney transplant, diabetic recipients: a 1-year follow up. *Transplant Int* 1998;11:S65.

648. Patel MG. The effect of dietary intervention on weight gains after renal transplantation. *J Renal Nutr* 1998;8:137.

649. Lopes IM, Martin M, Errasti P, et al. Benefits of a dietary intervention on weight loss, body composition, and lipid profile after renal transplantation. *Nutrition* 1999;15:7.

650. Moore RA, Callahan MF, Cody M, et al. The effect of the American Heart Association Step One diet on hyperlipidemia following renal transplantation. *Transplantation* 199049:60.

651. Tonstad S. Holdaas H, Gorbitz C, et al. Is dietary intervention effective in post-transplant hyperlipidaemia? *Nephrol Dial Transplantation* 1995;10:82.

652. Barbagallo CM, Cefalu AB, Gallo S, et al. Effects of Mediterranean diet on lipid levels and cardiovascular risk in renal transplant recipients. *Nephron* 1999;82:199.

653. Hines L. Can low-fat/cholesterol nutrition counseling improve food intake habits and hyperlipidemia of renal transplant patients? *J Renal Nutr* 2000;10:30.

654. Triolo G, Segoloni GP, Tetta C, et al. Effect of combined diet and physical exercise on plasma lipids of renal transplant recipients. *Nephrol Dial Transplantation* 1989;4:237.

655. Pagenkemper JJ. Attaining nutritional goals for hyperlipidemic and obese renal patients. In: Gussler JD, Silverman E, eds. *Renal nutrition, report of the Eleventh Ross Roundtable on Medical Issues.* Columbia: Ross Laboratories, 1991:26.

656. Lal SM, Gupta N, Georgiev O, et al. Lipid-lowering effects of fluvastatin in renal transplant patients. A clinical observation. *Int J Artif Organs* 1997;20:18.

657. Duclous D, Motte G, Challier B, et al. Serum total homocysteine and cardiovascular disease occurrence in chronic, stable renal transplant recipients: a prospective study. *J Am Soc Nephrol* 2000;11:134.

658. Dimeny E, Hultberg B, Wahlberg J, et al. Serum total homocysteine concentration does not predict outcome in renal transplant recipients. *Clin Transplantation* 1998;12:563.

659. Massy ZA, Chadefaux-Vekemans B, Chevalier A, et al. Hyperhomocysteinaemia: a significant risk factor for cardiovascular disease in renal transplant recipients. *Nephrol Dial Transplantation* 1994;9:1103.

660. Arnadottir M, Hultberg B, Wahlberg J, et al. Serum total homocysteine concentration before and after renal transplantation. *Kidney Int* 1998;54:1380.

661. Bostom AG, Gohh RY, Beaulieu AJ, et al. Determinants of fasting plasma total homocysteine levels among chronic stable renal transplant recipients. *Transplantation* 1999;68:257.

662. Ducloux D, Ruedin C, Gibey R, et al. Prevalence, determinants, and clinical significance of hyperhomocyst(e)inaemia in renal-transplant recipients. *Nephrol Dial Transplantation* 1998;13:2890.

663. Arnadottir M, Hultberg B, Vladov V, et al. Hyperhomocysteinemia in cyclosporine-treated renal transplant recipients. *Transplantation* 1996;61:509.

664. Ducloux D, Fournier V, Rebibou JM, et al. Hyperhomocyst(e)inemia in renal transplant recipients with and without cyclosporine. *Clin Nephrol* 1998;49:232.

665. Fernandez-Miranda C, Gomez P, Diaz-Rubio P, et al. Plasma homocysteine levels in renal transplanted patients on cyclosporine or tacrolimus therapy: effect of treatment with folic acid. *Clin Transplantation* 2000;14:110.

666. Urgert R, van Vliet T, Zock PL, et al. Heavy coffee consumption and plasma homocysteine: a randomized controlled trial in healthy volunteers. *Am J Clin Nutr* 2000;72:1107.

667. Bostom AG, Gohh RY, Beaulieu AJ, et al. Treatment of hyperhomocysteinemia in renal transplant recipients. A randomized, placebo-controlled trial. *Ann Intern Med* 1997;127:1089.

668. Milman N. Serum Vitamin B$_{12}$ and erythrocyte folate in chronic uraemia and after renal transplantation. *Scand J Haematol* 1980;25:151.

669. Yatzidis H, Digenis P, Koutsicos D. Hypervitaminosis in CRF after transplantation. *Br Med J* 1976;2:1075.

670. Kahan BD. Cyclosporine. *N Engl J Med* 1989;321:1725.

671. Barton CH, Vaziri ND, Martin DC, et al. Hypomagnesemia and renal magnesium wasting in renal transplant recipients receiving cyclosporine. *Am J Med* 1987;83:693.

672. Salahudeen AK, Hostetter TH, Raatz SK, et al. Effects of dietary protein in patients with chronic renal transplant rejection. *Kidney Int* 1992;41:183.

673. Metropolitan height and weight tables. *Stat Bull Metrop Insur Co* 1983:64.

CHAPTER 104

Use of Drugs in Patients with Renal Failure

Suzanne K. Swan and William M. Bennett

The metabolism and excretion of many drugs and their pharmacologically active metabolites depend on normal renal function. Accumulation and toxicity can develop rapidly if dosages are not adjusted in patients with impaired renal function. Likewise, many drugs that are not dependent on the kidneys for elimination may exert untoward effects in the uremic milieu. Since renal patients often have serious comorbid conditions requiring pharmacologic intervention, drug interactions are also very common in this population. In addition, a large part of the difficulty in prescribing drugs for the rapidly growing numbers of older patients is due to age-related declines in renal function. Lastly, the effects of dialysis on drug elimination and the need for supplemental dosing must also be considered in patients receiving renal replacement therapy.

In this chapter, the basic principles of drug prescribing in patients with renal disease are reviewed, the changes in drug pharmacokinetics/pharmacodynamics are highlighted, and practical guidelines for drug dosing in these patients are provided. However, no specific dosing formulas can be given confidently because individual patient factors such as age, diabetes, gender, nutrition, and body fluid volume status as well as many other variables influence pharmacokinetics and pharmacodynamics significantly. To provide safe and effective pharmacotherapy, the clinician must have a working knowledge of altered pharmacologic parameters and the patient's physiologic status to administer drugs to a renal patient population. Comprehensive recent reviews offering an array of approaches to drug dosing in patients with reduced renal function exist (1–9). The present discussion is limited to therapeutic issues that pertain to the care of renal patients for prescribing clinicians.

S. K. Swan: Department of Medicine, University of Minnesota; and Division of Nephrology, Hennepin County Medical Center, Minneapolis, Minnesota

W. M. Bennett: Transplant Services, Legacy Good Samaritan Hospital, Portland, Oregon

PHARMACOKINETIC PRINCIPLES

The term *pharmacokinetics* refers to a mathematic analysis of the time course of a drug in the body that can be used to predict serum concentrations and thus, drug activity. A simplified scheme of drug pharmacokinetics is illustrated in Fig. 104-1. The pharmacologic effect of any drug depends on the concentration of the parent drug or a metabolite at the tissue receptor site of action. The blood and tissue levels of a compound are functions of the amount administered, the degree and rate of its absorption, its volume of distribution, the amount bound to plasma proteins, its rate of metabolism or biotransformation, and its rate of excretion.

Drug Absorption

Drug absorption and bioavailability relate to the amount of drug that reaches the systemic circulation after oral administration. These parameters are often highly specific for a given compound and vary with the physical and chemical properties of the drug, its formulation, the integrity of the absorptive surface, and the presence of other agents and/or food in the gastrointestinal tract. Absorption rates of many therapeutic agents may be slowed by uremia-induced vomiting or sluggish peristalsis secondary to enteropathy. Both calcium- and aluminum-containing phosphate binders may form insoluble complexes with certain drugs such as antibiotics or ferrous sulfate, impeding absorption. Bowel wall edema in patients with hypoalbuminemia may also diminish drug absorption. The first-pass effect, wherein drugs absorbed from the stomach and intestine must first pass through the intestinal mucosa or liver before reaching the systemic circulation, may inactivate various agents, resulting in decreased bioavailability despite normal absorption. Erythromycin, for example, increases the bioavailability of cyclosporine by inhibition of intestinal and hepatic cytochrome P-450 biotransformation to less active drug metabolites (10).

Volume of Distribution

The volume of distribution (Vd) for a specific drug is derived by dividing the fractional absorption of a dose by the

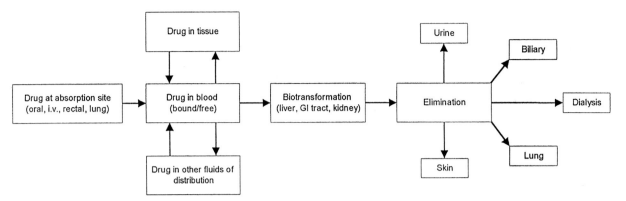

FIG. 104-1. Pharmacokinetic factors involved in drug distribution.

plasma concentration. A drug distributes in the body in a characteristic manner based on its physicochemical properties and individual patient variables. It does not refer to a specific anatomic compartment per se; rather, it is the volume of fluid in which the drug would need to be dissolved to give the observed plasma concentration. It is used mathematically to determine the dose of a drug necessary to achieve a desired plasma concentration. While the Vd is relatively constant for a given drug, many factors such as obesity, extracellular fluid volume status, age, gender, thyroid function, renal function, and cardiac output influence drug distribution. Highly lipid-soluble drugs such as diazepam have a large Vd with little retention of drug in the plasma. Drugs that are highly tissue-bound, such as digoxin, will also have a large Vd. If tissue binding of drugs is decreased by azotemia, a decrease in Vd results. Digoxin is highly bound to cardiac and other tissue $Na^+–K^+–ATPase$ transporters, accounting for its large Vd of 300 to 500 L and very low plasma concentrations. Waste products that accumulate in the azotemic patient serve to displace digoxin from its tissue-binding sites and thus reduce its Vd (11). Further, such waste products cross-react with the antidigoxin antibody used in drug monitoring assays, producing "therapeutic" digoxin levels in patients not even taking the drug. Insulin and methotrexate similarly have diminished Vd in the uremic state. As a general rule, plasma concentrations of a drug correlate inversely with its Vd.

Protein Binding

Plasma protein binding of a drug is a key determinant of its distribution and is often altered in the patient with impaired renal function. Drugs that are highly protein bound are largely confined to the vascular space and thus have a Vd of 0.2 L per kg or less. Protein-bound drugs are pharmacologically inactive, while the unbound or "free" fraction of a drug exerts its biologic effect. Altered physiologic conditions, often associated with renal failure, may increase or decrease protein binding. Specifically, uremic toxins may

decrease the affinity of albumin for a variety of drugs (12–14) (Table 104-1). Organic acids that accumulate in renal failure compete with acidic drugs for protein binding sites. This results in a larger fraction of acidic compounds existing in the unbound or active state. Conversely, basic drugs bind more readily to nonalbumin serum proteins such as α_1-acid glycoprotein and may demonstrate increased protein binding because this acute phase reactant is often elevated in patients with renal impairment (15–17). Malnutrition and proteinuria lower serum protein levels, which may increase the free fraction of a compound as well. Alterations in a drug's protein binding and subsequent effects on drug disposition may be difficult to predict. Generally, the Vd for a given agent increases as its protein binding decreases and diminishes as its protein-bound fraction increases.

Drug Metabolism or Biotransformation

The total body clearance of a drug is equal to the sum of renal clearance plus nonrenal clearance. Obviously, in patients with renal insufficiency, the contribution of renal clearance to total body clearance will be reduced. Nonrenal clearance, however, may be compensatorily increased,

TABLE 104-1. *Clinically relevant drugs with protein binding decreases in renal failure*

Acids	Bases	Tissue binding
Barbiturates	Diazepam	Cardiac glycosides
Clofibrate	Mexiletine	Methotrexate
Diazoxide	Triamterene	
Digitoxin		
Furosemide		
Methotrexate		
Metolazone		
Penicillins		
Phenytoin		
Probenecid		
Salicylates		
Sulfonamides		
Warfarin		

TABLE 104-2. *Pharmacologically active metabolites of common drugs accumulated in renal failure*

Parent drug	Metabolite	Pharmacologic action of metabolite
Acetohexamide	Hydroxyhexamide	Hypoglycemic
Allopurinol	Oxypurinol	Same as parent drug; enhanced desquamative skin eruptions due to xanthine oxidase inhibition
Azathioprine	6-Mercaptopurine	Immunosuppressive
Clofibrate	Chlorophenoxy-isobutyric acid	Increased skeletal muscle damage
Diazepam	Oxazepam	Anxiolytic
Lidocaine	Glycinexlidide	CNS reactions including seizures
Meperidine	Normeperidine	Seizures
Nitroprusside	Thiocyanate	CNS toxicity
Procainamide	N-Acetylprocainamide	Antiarrhythmic
Propranolol	4-Hydroxypropranolol	β-Blocker
Rifampicin	Desacetylrifampin	Antibiotic
Sulfonamides	Acetylated metabolites	Nausea, vomiting, skin reactions

CNS, central nervous system.

unchanged, or reduced in such patients. Specifically, hepatic pathways of drug metabolism or biotransformation including acetylation, oxidation, reduction, and hydrolysis may be slowed or accelerated depending on the drug under consideration. Sulfisoxazole acetylation, propranolol oxidation, hydrocortisone reduction, and cephalosporin hydrolysis are all slowed in uremic patients (18). Most drugs undergo biotransformation to more polar but less pharmacologically active compounds that require intact renal function for elimination from the body. Active or toxic metabolites of parent compounds may accumulate in patients with renal failure. The antiarrhythmic agent procainamide is metabolized to N-acetylprocainamide, which is excreted by the kidney. Thus, the antiarrhythmic properties and toxicity of procainamide and its active metabolite are additive, particularly in patients with renal failure. Meperidine, a commonly used narcotic, is biotransformed to normeperidine, which undergoes renal excretion. Although normeperidine has little narcotic effect, it lowers the seizure threshold as it accumulates in uremic patients. Active metabolites that undergo renal elimination are listed in Table 104-2.

Renal Elimination

Specific processes involved in the renal handling and elimination of drugs include glomerular filtration, tubular secretion and reabsorption, and renal epithelial cell metabolism. Since plasma proteins are too large to pass through a normal glomerulus, only unbound compounds will be freely filtered across this barrier. When proteinuria exists, protein-bound molecules may move into the tubular fluid and be eliminated from the circulation. Binding of furosemide to intraluminal albumin in nephrotic states may contribute to the diuretic resistance characteristic of such conditions (19). When renal disease reduces nephron numbers, the kidney's ability to eliminate drugs declines in proportion to the decline in glomerular filtration rate (GFR). As patients progress toward dialysis dependency, drugs usually filtered and excreted

accumulate, leading to a high prevalence of adverse reactions unless dosage adjustments are instituted.

Drugs that are extensively bound to protein either have a low clearance or enter the filtrate by tubular secretion. Tubular handling of a drug is an energy-requiring, active transport process and involves two separate and distinct pathways in the proximal tubule that are used for the secretion and reabsorption of organic acids and bases. These processes are dependent on renal blood flow but not GFR. Accumulation of organic acids in the setting of renal failure competes with acidic drugs for tubular transport and secretion into the urinary space. This, in turn, may lead to drug accumulation and adverse reactions as serum concentrations of agents such as methotrexate, sulfonylureas, penicillins, and cephalosporins rise. Diuretics gain access to their intraluminal sites of action via organic acid secretory pumps. Competition for these secretory pathways by accumulated uremic wastes results in diuretic resistance and necessitates increased diuretic doses to elicit the desired natriuretic effect.

Drug metabolism occurs in the kidney due to a high parenchymal concentration of cytochrome P-450 enzymes. Endogenous Vitamin D metabolism and insulin catabolism are examples of processes that decline as renal failure progresses (20,21).

First-order pharmacokinetics describe the manner in which most drugs and their metabolites are eliminated from the body. Specifically, the amount of drug eliminated over time is a fixed proportion of the body stores. The half-life ($t_{1/2}$) of a given agent is most commonly used to express its elimination rate from the body and equals the time required for the drug's plasma concentration to fall by 50%. Half-life can be expressed mathematically as follows:

$$t_{1/2} = \frac{0.693}{Kr + Knr}$$

where *Kr* represents the renal elimination rate constant and *Knr* represents the nonrenal elimination rate constant. As renal elimination declines with renal function, $t_{1/2}$ is prolonged.

DOSIMETRY FOR THE PATIENT WITH RENAL FAILURE

The following outline provides a stepwise approach to prescribing drug therapy for patients with renal failure. Again, it must be emphasized that these steps simply provide a framework for dosage adjustments in patients with renal impairment and must be modified on a case-by-case basis.

Initial Assessment

A history and physical examination constitute the first step in assessing dosimetry in any patient but particularly in those with renal impairment. Renal dysfunction should be defined as acute or chronic and the cause ascertained if possible. In addition, a history of previous drug intolerance or toxicity should be determined. The patient's current medication list must be reviewed, including both prescription as well as nonprescription formulations to identify potential drug interactions and nephrotoxins. Calculation of ideal body weight will be based on physical examination findings. For men, the ideal body weight is 50 kg plus 2.3 kg for each 2.5 cm (1 inch) over 152 cm (5 feet). For women, the formula is 45.5 kg plus 2.3 kg per 2.5 cm over 152 cm. An assessment of extracellular fluid volume is also key because significant shifts can affect the Vd of many pharmacologic agents. The presence of hepatic dysfunction may also require additional dosage adjustments.

Calculating Creatinine Clearance

The rate of drug excretion by the kidney is proportional to the GFR. Serum creatinine per se is a crude marker of renal function. Though an overestimate of GFR, creatinine clearance (Ccr) more accurately approximates the GFR and can be estimated conveniently by the Cockcroft and Gault equation (22):

$$Ccr = \frac{(140 - age)(ideal\ body\ weight\ in\ kg)}{72 \times serum\ creatinine\ in\ mg/dL}$$

For women, the calculated value is multiplied by 0.85. The use of this formula implies that the patient is in a steady-state with respect to serum creatinine. There is no accurate method to quantitate GFR when renal function is rapidly changing, and as such it is best to assume a GFR value of less than 10 mL/minute in acute renal failure to avoid drug accumulation and toxicity.

Choosing a Loading Dose

Loading doses are intended to achieve a therapeutic steady-state drug level within a short period of time. As such, the loading dose generally is not reduced in the setting of renal failure. Loading doses can be calculated if the Vd and desired peak level are known, as will be discussed. If extracellular volume depletion exists, the Vd may be reduced for certain pharmacologic agents, and slight reductions in the loading dose would be prudent. Specifically, drugs with narrow therapeutic–toxic profiles such as digoxin and ototoxic aminoglycosides should be administered with a 10% to 25% reduction in their loading dose when volume contraction is present in patients with renal failure.

Choosing a Maintenance Dose

Maintenance doses of a drug ensure steady-state blood concentrations and lessen the likelihood of subtherapeutic regimens or overdosage. In the absence of a loading dose, maintenance doses will achieve 90% of their steady-state level in three to four half-lives. One of two methods can be used to adjust maintenance doses for patients with renal insufficiency. The "dosage reduction" method involves reducing the absolute amount of drug administered at each dosing interval proportional to the patient's degree of renal failure. The dosing interval remains unchanged, and more constant drug concentrations are achieved. The "interval extension" method involves lengthening the time period between individual doses of a drug, reflecting the extent of renal insufficiency. This method is particularly useful for drugs with a wide therapeutic range and long half-life.

Monitoring Drug Levels

Blood, serum, and plasma drug concentrations may not be equivalent. As a result, drug levels can only be interpreted if the dosage schedule is known including the dose administered, timing, and route of administration. A peak level is usually obtained 30 minutes following intravenous administration and 60 to 120 minutes after oral ingestion. It reflects the maximum level achieved after the rapid distribution phase and before significant elimination has occurred. A trough level is obtained just prior to the next dose, reflects total body clearance, and may be a marker of drug toxicity. If the concentration of a drug and its Vd are known, the dose required to achieve a desired therapeutic level can be calculated by the following formula where Vd in liters per kilogram is multiplied by ideal body weight in kilograms (IBW) and the desired plasma concentration in milligrams per liter (Cp):

$$Dose = Vd \times IBW \times Cp$$

The difference between a trough and desired peak concentration can be substituted for Cp.

Drug-level monitoring is a clinically useful tool when used properly. Clinical judgment is paramount because toxicity can occur with "therapeutic" drug levels. For example, digitalis intoxication can occur in the presence of therapeutic serum levels if hypokalemia or metabolic alkalosis coexists. In addition, an increase in the unbound or biologically active fraction of a given drug may not be reflected in therapeutic monitoring because most assays measure total drug concentration (bound plus free fractions).

TABLE 104-3. *Drug and dialysis properties that affect dialytic clearance of pharmacologic agents*

Drug properties that affect dialytic clearance
    Molecular weight
    Protein binding
    Volume of distribution
    Charge
    Water or lipid solubility
    Membrane binding
    Alternative excretory pathway
Dialysis properties that affect drug clearance
    Membrane properties
        Pore size
        Blood flow rate
        Surface area
        Membrane binding
Dialysate properties
    Dialysate flow rate
    Solute concentration
    pH
    Temperature
Convection

DIALYSIS AND DRUG DOSING

Patients undergoing dialytic therapy require special attention in terms of dosimetry because many therapeutic agents are significantly removed by dialysis membranes. An array of modalities including high efficiency, high flux, continuous, and conventional hemodialysis exist and differ from one another based on membrane porosity, surface area, and blood as well as dialysate flow rates. These differences, in turn, affect drug removal. Table 104-3 summarizes drug properties and dialysis parameters that determine dialytic clearance of pharmacologic agents.

Drug Properties Affecting Dialytic Clearance

A drug's molecular weight is a major determinant of its dialyzability (23,24). Specifically, drugs larger than 1,000 daltons are primarily cleared by convection as opposed to diffusion. If too large to pass through a given membrane, the drug will not be cleared from the circulation. An inverse semilogarithmic relationship exists between molecular weight and dialysis clearance (25).

Protein binding represents another major determinant of drug dialyzability. Compounds that are highly protein bound have a smaller fraction of unbound drug available for removal by dialysis. Since heparin stimulates lipoprotein lipase, free fatty acid levels may increase during dialysis (26,27). Free fatty acid levels may displace sulfonamides, salicylates, and phenytoin from their protein binding sites, resulting in increased free fractions of each drug. In contrast, free fatty acids can increase protein binding of certain cephalosporins (28). The free fraction of phenytoin is increased by free fatty acids (29).

As discussed earlier, drugs with a large Vd (greater than 2 L/kg) tend to have low concentrations in the intravascular space and are thus not readily dialyzable. The lower the Vd (less than 1 L/kg), the greater the drug's availability to the circulation and, similarly, to the dialyzer.

Larger molecular-weight compounds do not equilibrate rapidly between the extracellular and intracellular compartments during dialysis; little change is detected in intracellular concentrations while extracellular levels may fall significantly (30,31). As such, postdialysis rebound may occur in which pharmacologic agents move down their concentration gradients into the extracellular space (32). Rebound can be sizable as well as highly unpredictable in its time course, as demonstrated by vancomycin (33). Ultrafiltration raises hematocrit, which can influence the dialytic clearance of drugs that partition into red blood cells. Drugs such as ethambutol, procainamide, and acetaminophen partition into red blood cells and demonstrate decreased dialytic clearance due to hemoconcentration following dialysis ultrafiltration (34,35).

Thus, parent compounds and their metabolites will be eliminated by dialysis to a greater extent if they possess a low molecular weight, limited Vd, and are water-soluble. An increase in drug clearance of 30% or greater by dialytic therapy is considered significant and may warrant supplemental dosing following dialysis (36,37).

Dialytic Factors Affecting Drug Clearance

Dialysis membranes, dialysate flow rates, and the dialytic technique used can significantly alter drug clearance (Table 104-3). A wide variety of membranes have been developed including cellulose, cellulose acetate, polysulfone, polyamide, polyacrylonitrile (PAN; AN69), and polymethylmethacrylate (PMMA) in an effort to improve membrane permeability for larger uremic toxins. Similarly, albumin can cross polysulfone membranes to a limited extent (38). Vancomycin clearance is significantly increased when polysulfone or PAN membranes are used (39–41). Likewise, cuprammonium rayon membranes allow greater aminoglycoside removal compared to cellulose fibers (42). Two endogenous compounds that are poorly dialyzed, phosphate and β_2-microglobulin, undergo enhanced clearance when PAN, PMMA, and polysulfone membranes are used due to the increased surface area of these membranes (43–45). The electrical charge of a dialysis membrane as well as the drug may help or hinder clearance (46,47). Like charges will repel one another, while opposite charges between membrane and drug may lead to drug adsorption to the membrane, ultimately reducing clearance (48–53).

Drug clearance is achieved primarily by two processes, diffusion and convection. Diffusion of a compound increases as its molecular weight decreases and is negligible when standard membranes are used for substances larger than 1,000 daltons (54). Diffusion of a drug is enhanced when the concentration gradient between blood and dialysate is maximized by countercurrent flow and increased blood and dialysate flow rates. Flow rates have less impact on the diffusion of middle-sized and large molecules, but the surface area and hydraulic permeability of the membrane assume greater significance. Diffusion can be hindered, however, when high ultrafiltration rates lead to mixing of dialysate and ultrafiltrate. This results in a decreased concentration gradient between blood and dialysate, reducing diffusive clearance (55–57). Convection refers to the movement of solute by way of ultrafiltration, which affects molecules of all sizes but particularly large molecular-weight substances, which diffuse poorly (58–60). To be removed by dialysis, compounds greater than 1,000 daltons require ultrafiltration when cellulose membranes are used, while those greater than 2,000 daltons demonstrate limited clearance (61). Ultrafiltration, and thus convection, can be reduced by protein binding to membrane surfaces during the dialytic procedure, which ultimately diminishes drug removal (62,63).

Continuous Renal Replacement Therapies and Drug Removal

Critically ill patients may require continuous renal replacement therapies such as hemofiltration or hemodialysis, and an awareness of drug handling by such procedures is crucial to the patient's outcome. Continuous hemofiltration removes solute by convection. The degree to which a solute can convectively cross a membrane can be quantitated by its sieving coefficient (S), the ratio of solute concentration in the ultrafiltrate to solute concentration in the retentate (returning to the patient's circulation). This can be approximated by the formula:

$$S = UF/A$$

where UF = ultrafiltrate and A = arterial concentrations of solute, which will remain relatively constant during hemofiltration because blood flow does not affect sieving (64–68). Clearance of a solute (drug) is determined by multiplying the ultrafiltration rate by the S for that substance. The sieving coefficient for a given molecule can change, however, when comparing different dialysis membranes and is likely due to drug–membrane binding. Sieving can also be reduced by negatively charged solutes (69,70), although exceptions to this exist (71–73). Since inulin can readily cross polysulfone hemofiltration membranes, nearly all therapeutic agents would be expected to permeate such membranes given molecular weights less than that of inulin (74,75). The drug's degree of protein binding will be the major limiting factor to drug removal during hemofiltration (76).

In contrast to hemofiltration, drug removal during continuous hemodialysis occurs primarily via diffusion rather than convection. Protein binding again plays a central role whereby unbound drug diffuses more readily than protein-bound drug and molecular weight correlates inversely with diffusion. It should be noted that during continuous hemodialysis with venovenous access and average blood flow rates of 200 mL/minute, a GFR of 20 to 30 mL/minute can be achieved, which may provide greater drug clearance than

expected. As previously discussed, when supplemental dosing is indicated, the amount of drug required to achieve a desired blood level can be calculated by multiplying the drug's Vd by the patient's ideal body weight and the difference between the desired drug concentration and the trough concentration.

Lastly, peritoneal dialysis generally provides minimal drug removal, as dialysate flow rates are significantly slower than other forms of dialytic therapy (77). Drugs that are dialyzable via peritoneal dialysis must be small in size and have a low Vd. Drugs that are highly protein bound, however, may undergo greater clearance with peritoneal dialysis versus hemodialysis given the large protein losses commonly seen with peritoneal therapy.

SPECIFIC CONSIDERATIONS FOR DRUG PRESCRIBING IN RENAL FAILURE

In this section, the effects of renal insufficiency on drug pharmacokinetics and pharmacodynamics are reviewed and dosimetry guidelines are provided. It is imperative to recognize that the following recommendations provide a framework for dosage adjustments that must be applied to individual patients in a prudent manner. Continual monitoring and modification of drug therapy are mandated by concurrent illnesses, clinical response, and side effects present in the individual patient. Drugs are listed in tabular form (Tables 104-4 through 104-13) by generic name in alphabetical order and are grouped into categories based on therapeutic effect. General comments about each group precede the individual dosing table. For reference, the standard dose given to patients with normal renal function is included. Specific dosing guidelines are provided for each drug based on the patient's level of renal function in terms of GFR. It should be remembered that creatinine clearance always overestimates true GFR.

The maintenance dosage regimen may be modified by either extending the interval between doses, decreasing the individual dose while maintaining normal dosing intervals, or a combination of the two methods. As outlined previously, the variable interval method allows a more convenient and less costly dosing schedule but may result in periods of subtherapeutic drug levels. The variable dose method maintains more constant drug levels because the dosing interval remains unchanged but risks greater toxicity because the difference between peak and trough levels is diminished. When the interval extension method (I) is used, the dosing interval length (in hours) is indicated. When the dosage reduction method (D) is used, the percentage of the standard dose normally used is indicated.

The requirement for supplemental dosing after hemodialysis and special dosing considerations for peritoneal dialysis (77) and continuous renal replacement therapies (78) are also included. For many drugs, specific data are not available on dialytic drug clearance, and the likelihood of dialytic removal is based on molecular weight, Vd, and protein binding.

TABLE 104-4. *Antimicrobial agents*

Drug, toxicity, notes	Dosage for normal renal function	Method	Adjustment failure GFR (mL/min)			Supplement for dialysis
			>50	10–50	<10	
AMINOGLYCOSIDE ANTIBIOTICS						
Ototoxic, nephrotoxic; rare respiratory paralysis; check serum levels to ensure efficacy. Posthemodialysis dose is $\frac{2}{3}$ of normal maintenance dose or $\frac{1}{2}$ of a loading dose. Larger supplement may be required for highly permeable membranes. Volume of distribution larger with obesity, edema, or ascites.						
Amikacin (94–96)	7.5 mg/kg q12h	D, I	70%–100% q8–12h	30%–70% q12h or 100% q24–48h	20%–30% q24–48h or 100% q48–72h	Hemo: $\frac{1}{2}$ loading dose after dialysis CAPD: 30% q24h CRRT: Dose for GFR 10–50
Gentamicin (97–99) Concurrent penicillins may result in subtherapeutic blood levels	1 mg/kg q8h	D, I	70%–100% q8–12h	30%–70% q12h or 100% q24–48h	20%–30% q24–48h or 100% q48–72h	Hemo: $\frac{1}{2}$ loading dose after dialysis CAPD: 30% q24h CRRT: Dose for GFR 10–50
Kanamycin (100)	7.5 mg/kg q12h	D, I	70%–100% q8–12h	30%–70% q12h or 100% of 24–48h	20%–30% q24–48h or 100% q48–72h	Hemo: $\frac{1}{2}$ loading dose after dialysis CAPD: 30% q24h CRRT: Dose for GFR 10–50
Netilmicin (101–103)	5 mg/kg q8h	D, I	70%–100% q8–12h	30%–70% q12h	20%–30% q24–48h	Hemo: $\frac{1}{2}$ loading dose after dialysis CAPD: 30% q24h CRRT: Dose for GFR 10–50
Streptomycin (7,75)	1 g/d	I	q24h	q24–72h	q72–96h	Hemo: $\frac{1}{2}$ normal dose after dialysis CAPD: Dose for GFR 10–50 CRRT: Dose for GFR 10–50
Tobramycin (104,105) Concurrent penicillins may result in subtherapeutic blood levels	1 mg/kg q8h	D, I	70%–100% q8–12h	30%–70% q12h	20%–30% q24–48h	Hemo: $\frac{1}{2}$ loading dose after dialysis CAPD: 30% q24h CRRT: Dose for GFR 10–50
CEPHALOSPORIN ANTIBIOTICS						
Rare allergic interstitial nephritis; absorbed well when administered intraperitoneal, may cause bleeding from impaired prothrombin biosynthesis						
Cefaclor (106,107)	250 mg t.i.d.	D	100%	50%–100%	50%	Hemo: 250 mg after dialysis CAPD: 250 mg q8–12h CRRT: Unknown
Cefadroxil (108)	0.5–1.0 g q12h	I	q12h	q12–24h	q24–48h	Hemo: 0.5–1 g after dialysis CAPD: 0.5 g/d CRRT: Unknown
Cefamandole (109,110)	0.5–1.0 g q4–8h	I	q4–8h	q6–8h	q12h	Hemo: 0.5–1 g after dialysis CAPD: 0.5–1 g q12h CRRT: Dose for GFR 10–50

(Continued)

TABLE 104-4. (*Continued*)

Drug, toxicity, notes	Dosage for normal renal function	Method	Adjustment failure GFR (mL/min) >50	10–50	<10	Supplement for dialysis
Cefazolin (111)	0.5–1.5 g q6h	I	q6–8h	q12h	q24–48h	Hemo: 0.5–1 g after dialysis CAPD: 0.5 g q12h CRRT: Dose for GFR 10–50
Cefepime	250–2000 mg q8h	I	q8–12h	q12–24h	q24–48h	Hemo: 1 g after dialysis CAPD: Dose for GFR <10 CRRT: Not recommended
Cefixime (112)	200 mg q12h	D	100%	75%	50%	Hemo: 300 mg after dialysis CAPD: 200 mg/d CRRT: Not recommended
Cefmenoxime (114,115)	1 g q6h	D, I	1 g q6–8h	750 mg q8–12h	750 mg q12h	Hemo: 750 mg after dialysis CAPD: 750 mg q12 CRRT: Dose for GFR 10–50
Cefmetazole (116,117)	2 g q8h	I	q8–12h	q12–24h	q48h	Hemo: Dose after dialysis CAPD: Dose for GFR <10 CRRT: Dose for GFR 10–50
Cefonicid (118,119)	1 g q24h	D, I	0.5–1.0 g q24h	0.25–0.5 g q24h	0.25 g q48h	Hemo: None CAPD: None CRRT: None
Cefoperazone (120,121) Reduce dose 50% for jaundice	1–2 g q12h	D	100%	100%	100%	Hemo: None CAPD: None CRRT: None
Ceforanide (122,123)	0.5–1.0 g q12h	I	q12h	q12–24h	q24–48h	Hemo: 0.5–1.0 g after dialysis CAPD: None CRRT: 1 g/d
Cefotaxime (124,125)	1 g q6h	I	q6h	q8–12h	q24h	Hemo: 1 g after dialysis CAPD: 1 g/d CRRT: 1 g q12h
Cefotetan (126,127)	1–2 g q12h	D	100%	50%	25%	Hemo: 1 g after dialysis CAPD: 1 g/d CRRT: 150 mg q12h
Cefoxitin (128,129) May raise creatinine by interference with assay	1–2 g q6–8h	I	q6–8h	q8–12h	q24–48h	Hemo: 1 g after dialysis CAPD: 1 g/d CRRT: Dose for GFR 10–50
Cefpodoxime	200 mg q12h	I	q12h	q12–24	q24–48	Hemo: 200 mg after dialysis CAPD: Dose for GFR <10 CRRT: Unknown
Ceftazidime (130–133)	1–2 g q8h	I	q8–12h	q24–48h	q48	Hemo: 1 g after dialysis CAPD: 0.5 g/d CRRT: Dose for GFR 10–50

TABLE 104-4. (*Continued*)

Drug, toxicity, notes	Dosage for normal renal function	Method	Adjustment failure GFR (mL/min)			Supplement for dialysis
			>50	10–50	<10	
Ceftizoxime (134–137)	1–2 g q8–12h	I	q8–12h	12–24h	24h	Hemo: 1 g after dialysis CAPD: 0.5–1 g/d CRRT: Dose for GFR 10–50
Ceftriaxone (138–140)	1–2 g q12h	I	q12h	12–24h	24h	Hemo: Dose after dialysis CAPD: 750 mg q12h CRRT: Dose for GFR 10–50
Cefuroxime (141–143)	0.75–1.5 g q8h (IV) 0.5 g q8h (p.o.)	I	q8h	q8–12h	q24h	Hemo: Dose after dialysis CAPD: Dose for GFR <10 CRRT: Likely to be removed; 1 g q12h
Cephalexin (144)	250–500 mg q6h	I	q8h	q8–12h	q12h	Hemo: 250 mg after dialysis CAPD: Dose for GFR <10 CRRT: Dose for GFR 10–50
Cephalothin (145)	0.5–2.0 q6h	I	q6h	q6–8h	q12h	Hemo: Dose after dialysis CAPD: 1 g q12h CRRT: 1 g q8h
Cephapirin (146)	0.5–2.0 g q6h	I	q6h	q6–8h	q12h	Hemo: Dose after dialysis CAPD: 1 g q12h CRRT: 1 g q8h
Cephradine (147)	0.25–2.0 g q6h	D	100%	50%	25%	Hemo: Dose after dialysis CAPD: Dose for GFR <10 CRRT: Dose for GFR 10–50
Moxalactam (148–150) Sodium 3.8 mEq/g: platelet dysfunction at high doses	1–2 g q8–12h	I	q8–12h	q12–24h	q24–48h	Hemo: Dose after dialysis CAPD: Dose for GFR <10 CRRT: Dose for GFR 10–50
MACROLIDE ANTIBIOTICS						
Azithromycin	250–500 mg q24h	D	100%	100%	100%	Hemo: None CAPD: None CRRT: None
Clarithromycin (151)	250–1000 mg q12h	D	100%	50%–100%	50%	Hemo: Unlikely CAPD: Unlikely CRRT: Unlikely
Erythromycin (152,153) Ototoxicity with high doses in ESRD	250–500 mg q6–12h	D	100%	100%	50%–75%	Hemo: None CAPD: None CRRT: Unlikely
PENICILLINS						
Amoxicillin (7)	500 mg q8h	I	q8h	q8–12h	q24h	Hemo: Dose after dialysis CAPD: 250 mg q12h CRRT: N/A.

(*Continued*)

TABLE 104-4. (*Continued*)

Drug, toxicity, notes	Dosage for normal renal function	Method	Adjustment failure GFR (mL/min)			Supplement for dialysis
			>50	10–50	<10	
Ampicillin	250–2000 mg q6h	I	q6h	q6–12h	q12–24h	Hemo: Dose after dialysis CAPD: 250 mg q12h CRRT: Dose for GFR 10–50
Azlocillin (158,159) Sodium: 2.7 mEq/g	2–3 g q4h	I	q4–6h	q6–8h	q8h	Hemo: Dose after dialysis CAPD: Dose for GFR <10 CRRT: Dose for GFR 10–50 ml/min
Dicloxacillin (7,75)	250–500 mg q6h	D	100%	100%	100%	Hemo: None CAPD: None CRRT: None
Methicillin (7,75)	1–2 g q4h	I	q4–6h	q6–8h	q8–12	Hemo: None CAPD: None CRRT: Dose for GFR 10–50
Mezlocillin (160,161) Sodium: 1.9 mEq/g	1.5–4.0 g q4–6h	I	q4–6h	q6–8h	q8h	Hemo: None CAPD: None CRRT: Dose for GFR 10–50
Nafcillin (7,75) Coagulopathy may develop	1–2 g q4–6h	D	100%	100%	100%	Hemo: None CAPD: None CRRT: Dose for GFR 10–50
Penicillin G (93) Potassium: 1.7 mEq/million U Risk of seizures with high doses in renal insufficiency (6 million U/d upper limit dose in ESRD)	0.5–4.0 million U q6h	D	100%	75%	25%–50%	Hemo: Dose after dialysis CAPD: Dose for GFR <10 CRRT: Dose for GFR 10–50
Piperacillin (162–164) Sodium: 1.9 mEq/g	3–4 g q4h	I	q4–6h	q6–8h	q8h	Hemo: Dose after dialysis CAPD: Dose for GFR <10 CRRT: Dose for GFR 10–50
Ticarcillin (165) Sodium: 5.2 mEq/g	3 g q4h	D, I	1–3 g q4h	1–2 g q8h	2 g q12h	Hemo: 3 g after dialysis CAPD: Dose for GFR <10 CRRT: Dose for GFR 10–50
QUINOLONES						
Ciprofloxacin (83,166,167) Poorly absorbed with antacids	500–750 mg q12h (400 mg i.v.)	I	q12h	q12–24h	q24h	Hemo: 200–400 mg q24h (IV) 500 mg q24h (po) CAPD: 250 mg q12h (po) CRRT: 200 mg IV q12h
Enoxacin (168–170)	200–400 mg q12h	D	100%	50%	50%	Hemo: None CAPD: None CRRT: Unlikely

TABLE 104-4. (*Continued*)

Drug, toxicity, notes	Dosage for normal renal function	Method	Adjustment failure GFR (mL/min)			Supplement for dialysis
			>50	10–50	<10	
Fleroxacin (171)	400 mg q12h	D	100%	50%–100%	50%	Hemo: Dose after dialysis CAPD: 400 mg qd CRRT: None
Levofloxacin	500 mg q24h	D, I	100%	250 mg q24h (500 mg loading dose)	250 mg q48h (500 mg loading dose)	Hemo: Dose for GFR <10 CAPD: Dose for GFR <10 CRRT: Dose for GFR 10–50
Norfloxacin (172)	400 mg q12h	I	q12h	q12–24h	q24h	Hemo: None CAPD: None CRRT: Unlikely
Ofloxacin (173)	200–400 mg/12h	D	100%	200–400 mg q24h	200 mg q24h	Hemo: Dose after dialysis CAPD: Dose for GFR <10 CRRT: Likely to be removed; dose for GFR 10–50
TETRACYCLINE ANTIBIOTICS						
Potentiate acidosis; hyperphosphatemia; increase BUN, antianabolic						
Demeclocycline (82) Nephrotoxicity	300 mg b.i.d.	I	q12h	q24h	q48h	Hemo: None CAPD: Unlikely CRRT: Unlikely
Doxycycline (174) Tetracycline of choice in patients with renal insufficiency; not associated with antianabolic syndrome	100–200 mg/d	D	100%	100%	100%	Hemo: None CAPD: None CRRT: None
Minocycline (174)	100 mg q12h	D	100%	100%	100%	Hemo: None CAPD: None CRRT: None
Oxytetracycline (82)	250–500 mg q.i.d.	I	q8–12h	q24h	q48h	Hemo: Dose after dialysis CAPD: None CRRT: Unlikely
Tetracycline (82)	250–500 q6h	I	q6–8h	q12–24h	Avoid	Hemo: Avoid CAPD: Avoid CRRT: Avoid
MISCELLANEOUS ANTIBACTERIAL ANTIBIOTICS						
Aztreonam (175,176)	1–2 g q8–12h	D	100%	50%–100%	25%	Hemo: 0.5 g after dialysis CAPD: Dose for GFR <10 CRRT: Dose for GFR 10–50
Chloramphenicol (177)	12.5 mg/kg q6h	D	100%	100%	100%	Hemo: None CAPD: None CRRT: None
Cilastatin (178–181) Given with imipenem	See imipenem	D	100%	100%	100%	Hemo: Dose after dialysis CAPD: None CRRT: Dose for GFR 10–50 ml/min

(*Continued*)

TABLE 104-4. (*Continued*)

Drug, toxicity, notes	Dosage for normal renal function	Method	Adjustment failure GFR (mL/min)			Supplement for dialysis
			>50	10–50	<10	
Clindamycin (182)	150–300 mg q6h	D	100%	100%	100%	Hemo: None CAPD: None CRRT: None
Imipenem (178–181) Seizures in ESRD	0.25–1.0 g q6h	D	100%	50%	25%	Hemo: Dose after dialysis CAPD: None CRRT: Dose for GFR 10–50
Lincomycin (7,75)	0.5 g q6h	I	q6h	q6–12h	q12–24h	Hemo: None CAPD: None CRRT: Unlikely
Methenamine mandelate (183) Contributes to uremic gastrointestinal symptoms Not effective for GFR <20 mL/min	1 g q6h	D	100%	Avoid	Avoid	Hemo: Not applicable CAPD: Not applicable CRRT: Not applicable
Metronidazole (184–186) Metabolites accumulate; rare drug-induced lupus	7.5 mg/kg q6h	D	100%	100%	50%	Hemo: Dose after dialysis CAPD: None CRRT: Likely to be removed; dose for GFR 10–50
Nalidixic acid (7,75) Not effective in severe renal insufficiency	1 g q6h	D	100%	Avoid	Avoid	Hemo: Avoid CAPD: Avoid CRRT: Avoid
Nitrofurantoin (7,75) Ineffective at GFR <50 mL/min Polyneuropathy	50–100 mg q6h	D	100%	Avoid	Avoid	Hemo: Avoid CAPD: Avoid CRRT: Avoid
Sulfisoxazole (187) Protein binding decreased in ESRD Use normal dosing for UTI in ESRD	1–2 g q6h	I	q6h	q8–12h	q12–24h	Hemo: 2 g after dialysis CAPD: 3 g/d CRRT: Dose for GFR 10–50
Teicoplanin (188,189)	6 mg/kg/d	I	q24h	q48h	q72h	Hemo: None CAPD: None CRRT: Dose for GFR 10–50
Trimethoprim-sulfamethoxazole (84) Use normal dosing for UTI in ESRD Trimethoprim component interferes with secretion of creatinine	160 mg trimethoprim and 800 mg sulfamethoxazole q12h		q12h	q12–24h	q24h	Hemo: Dose after dialysis CAPD: None CRRT: Likely to be removed; dose for GFR 10–50
Vancomycin (32,38,190,191) Monitor serum levels	1 g q12h	I	q12–24h	q24–96h	4–7 days	Hemo: Dose for GFR <10 CAPD: Dose for GFR <10 CRRT: Dose for GFR 10–50

TABLE 104-4. (*Continued*)

Drug, toxicity, notes	Dosage for normal renal function	Method	Adjustment failure GFR (mL/min)			Supplement for dialysis
			>50	10–50	<10	
ANTIFUNGAL AGENTS						
Amphotericin B (192–196) Nephrotoxicity proportional to total dose: renal tubular acidosis, hypokalemia, hypomagnesemia, nephrogenic diabetes insipidus	0.3–0.5 mg/kg/d	D	100%	100%	100%	Hemo: None CAPD: None CRRT: None
Fluconazole (197–201)	200–400 mg q24h	D	100%	100%	50%	Hemo: Dose after dialysis CAPD: Dose for GFR <10 CRRT: Dose for GFR 10–50
Flucytosine (197,201–203) Hepatic dysfunction Bone marrow suppression more common in azotemic patients Adjust dose to maintain peak serum concentration 40–60 mg/L	150 mg/kg/d in 3–4 divided doses	D, I	25–50 mg/kg q12h	25–50 mg/kg q12–24h	50 mg/kg q24	Hemo: Dose after dialysis CAPD: 0.5–1 g/d CRRT: Dose for GFR 10–50
Griseofulvin (192,193)	125–250 mg q6h	D	100%	100%	100%	Hemo: None CAPD: None CRRT: None
Itraconazole (197,204,205)	100–200 mg q12h	D, I	100%	50–100%	100 mg q12–24h	Hemo: None CAPD: None CRRT: None
Ketoconazole (197,206)	200–400 mg/d	D	100%	100%	100%	Hemo: None CAPD: None CRRT: None
Miconazole (207)	200–1200 mg q8h	D	100%	100%	100%	Hemo: None CAPD: None CRRT: None
ANTIPARASITIC ANTIBIOTICS						
Chloroquine (208,209)	1.5 g over 3 days	D	100%	100%	50%	Hemo: None CAPD: None CRRT: None
Mebendazole (210,211)	100 mg b.i.d. × 3 days Pinworm infection: 100 mg, one dose	D	100%	100%	100%	Hemo: None CAPD: unlikely CRRT: Unlikely
Mefloquine (212)	Nonimmune patients: 1250–1500 mg total in 2–3 doses over 24 h Semi-immune patients: 750–1000 mg total in 2–3 doses over 24 h	D	100%	100%	100%	Hemo: None CAPD: Unknown CRRT: Unknown
Pentamidine (213,214)	4 mg/kg/d	I	q24h	q24–48h	q48h	Hemo: None CAPD: None CRRT: None

(*Continued*)

TABLE 104-4. (*Continued*)

Drug, toxicity, notes	Dosage for normal renal function	Method	Adjustment failure GFR (mL/min)			Supplement for dialysis
			>50	10–50	<10	
Praziquantel (215)	Dose varies	D	100%	100%	100%	Hemo: None CAPD: Unlikely CRRT: Unlikely
Pyrimethamine (208,209)	50–75 mg/d	D	100%	100%	100%	Hemo: None CAPD: None CRRT: None
Quinine (208,209)	10 mg/kg q8h	I	q8h	q8–12h	q24h	Hemo: Dose after dialysis CAPD: None CRRT: Dose for GFR 10–50
Thiabendazole (210)	Dose varies depending on infecting parasite	D	100%	50%–100%	Avoid	Hemo: Unknown CAPD: Unknown CRRT: Unknown
ANTITUBERCULOUS AGENTS						
Capreomycin (216)	1 g qd	I	q24h	q24h	q48h	Hemo: Dose after dialysis only CAPD: None CRRT: Likely to be removed; dose for GFR 10–50
Cycloserine (7,75) CNS toxicity	250 mg q12h	I	q12h	q12–24h	q24h	Hemo: None CAPD: None CRRT: Dose for GFR 10–50
Ethambutol (217) Ocular toxicity Peripheral neuritis	15 mg/kg q24h	I	100%	q24–48h	q48h	Hemo: Dose after dialysis CAPD: Dose for GFR <10 CRRT: Dose for GFR 10–50
Ethionamide (7,75)	250–500 mg q12h	D	100%	100%	50%	Hemo: None CAPD: None CRRT: None
Isoniazid (218) Supplement with 50–100 mg pyridoxine daily to prevent neurotoxicity	300 mg q24h	D	100%	100%	50%	Hemo: Dose after dialysis CAPD: Dose for GFR <10 CRRT: Dose for GFR <10
PAS (*p*-aminosalicylic acid) (7,75) Significant sodium load	50 mg/kg q8h	D	100%	50%–100%	50%	Hemo: Dose after dialysis CAPD: None CRRT: None
Pyrazinamide (219,220) Impairs urate excretion Can precipitate gout	15–30 mg/kg q24h	D	100%	100%	50%	Hemo: Dose after dialysis CAPD: None CRRT: Likely to be removed; dose for GFR 10–50
Rifampin (221) Many drug interactions	600 mg q24h	D	100%	100%	50%–100%	Hemo: None CAPD: None CRRT: None

TABLE 104-4. (*Continued*)

Drug, toxicity, notes	Dosage for normal renal function	Method	Adjustment failure GFR (mL/min) >50	10–50	<10	Supplement for dialysis
ANTIVIRAL AGENTS						
Acyclovir (222–224) Neurotoxic in patients with renal failure; may cause acute renal failure if injected rapidly, intravenously	5 mg/kg q8h	D, I	5 mg/kg q8h	5 mg/kg q12–24h	2.5 mg/kg q24h	Hemo: Dose after dialysis CAPD: Dose for GFR <10 CRRT: 3.5 mg/kg/day
Amantadine (225–227)	100 mg q12h	I	q12–48h	q48–72h	q168h	Hemo: None CAPD: None CRRT: None
Didanosine (228,229)	200 mg q12h	I	q12h	q24h	50% q24h	Hemo: Dose after dialysis CAPD: None CRRT: Likely to be removed; dose for GFR 10–50
Famciclovir	500 mg q8h for herpes zoster 125 mg q12h for genital herpes	D, I	100%	q12–48h	50% q48h	Hemo: Dose after dialysis CAPD: Unknown CRRT: Dose for GFR 10–50
Foscarnet (230) Nephrotoxicity common	60–100 mg/kg q8–12h	D	50%–100%	10%–25%	Avoid	Hemo: Dose after dialysis CAPD: None CRRT: Likely to be removed; dose for GFR 10–50
Ganciclovir (231)	2.5 mg/kg q8h	I	q8–12h	q24h	q48–96h	Hemo: Dose after dialysis CAPD: None CRRT: 2.5 mg/kg q24h
Indinavir Acute renal failure due to crystalluria	800 mg q8h	I	100%	q12h	q12–24h	Hemo: Unknown CAPD: Unknown CRRT: Unknown
Lamivudine	150 mg q12h	D, I	100%	50–150 mg q24h	25–50 mg q24h	Hemo: Dose after dialysis CAPD: Unknown CRRT: Unknown
Ribavirin (232) Loading dose required	200 mg q8h	D	100%	100%	50%	Hemo: None CAPD: Unlikely CRRT: Unlikely
Saquinavir	600 mg q8h	D	100%	100%	100%	Hemo: Unknown CAPD: Unknown CRRT: Unknown
Stavudine	30–40 mg q12h	D, I	100%	50% q12–24h	50% q24h	Hemo: Dose after dialysis CAPD: Unknown CRRT: Unknown
Vidarabine (233)	15 mg/kg infusion q24h	D	100%	100%	50%–100%	Hemo: Infuse after dialysis CAPD: None CRRT: Dose for GFR 10–50
Zidovudine (AZT) (234–237)	200 mg q8h	D	100%	100%	50%	Hemo: Dose after dialysis CAPD: None CRRT: 100 mg q8h

BUN, blood urea nitrogen; *CAPD,* continuous ambulatory peritoneal dialysis; *CNS,* central nervous system; *CRRT,* chronic renal replacement therapy; *D,* dosage reduction method; *ESRD,* end-stage renal disease; *GFR,* glomerular filtration rate; *Hemo,* hemodialysis; *I,* interval extension method; *UTI,* urinary tract infection.

TABLE 104-5. *Analgesics and agents used by anesthesiologists*

Drug, toxicity, notes	Dosage for normal renal function	Method	Adjustment for renal failure GFR (mL/min)		Supplement for dialysis
			10–50	<10	
NARCOTICS AND NARCOTIC ANTAGONISTS					
All agents in this group may cause excessive sedation and respiratory depression.					
Alfentanil (241)	Anesthetic induction	D	100%	100%	Hemo: NA CAPD: NA CRRT: NA
Butorphanol (242)	2 mg q3–4h	D	75%	50%	Hemo: Unlikely CAPD: Unlikely CRRT: Unlikely
Codeine (243)	30–60 mg q4–6h	D	75%	50%	Hemo: Unknown CAPD: Unknown CRRT: Unknown
Fentanyl (244)	Anesthetic induction	D	75%	50%	Hemo: NA CAPD: NA CRRT: NA
Meperidine (239) Normeperidine, an active metabolite, accumulates in ESRD and may cause seizures	50–100 mg q3–4h	D	75%	50%	Hemo: Avoid CAPD: Avoid CRRT: Avoid
Methadone (245)	2.5–10.0 mg q6–8h	D	50–100%	Avoid	Hemo: None CAPD: None CRRT: NA
Morphine (246,247) Metabolites accumulate	20–25 mg PO q4h or 2–10 mg i.v.	D	75%	50%	Hemo: None CAPD: None CRRT: None
Naloxone (238,241)	2 mg	D	100%	100%	Hemo: NA CAPD: NA CRRT: NA
Pentazocine (238,241)	50 mg q4h	D	75%	50%	Hemo: None CAPD: None CRRT: Unlikely
Propoxyphene (248) Active metabolite norpropoxyphene accumulates in ESRD	65 mg PO t.i.d.–q.i.d.	D	50–100%	Avoid	Hemo: Avoid CAPD: Avoid CRRT: Avoid
Sufentanil (238,241)	Anesthetic induction	D	100%	100%	Hemo: NA CAPD: NA CRRT: NA
NON-NARCOTIC ANALGESICS					
Acetaminophen (249,250) Metabolites may accumulate in renal insufficiency Drug is major metabolite of phenacetin	650 mg q4h	I	q6h	q8h	Hemo: None CAPD: None CRRT: None
Methocarbamol (251)	4 g/d in divided doses	D	100%	100%	Hemo: Unknown CAPD: Unknown CRRT: Unknown
Salicylate (252) May decrease GFR when blood flow is prostaglandin-dependent Excretion enhanced in alkaline urine	650 mg q4h	I	q4–6h	Avoid	Hemo: Dose after dialysis CAPD: None CRRT: Likely to be removed

TABLE 104-5. (*Continued*)

Drug, toxicity, notes	Dosage for normal renal function	Method	Adjustment for renal failure GFR (mL/min)		Supplement for dialysis
			10–50	<10	
May add to uremic gastrointestinal symptoms and platelet dysfunction Protein binding reduced					
Salsalate (253)	1500 mg q12h	D	75%–100%	50%	Hemo: 500 mg CAPD: Unknown CRRT: Likely to be removed
NEUROMUSCULAR AGENTS					
Atracurium (254–257)	0.4–0.5 mg/kg load, then 0.08–0.1 mg/kg q15–25 min	D	100%	100%	Hemo: Unknown CAPD: Unknown CRRT: Unknown
Etomidate (255)	0.2–0.6 mg/kg	D	100%	100%	Hemo: Unknown CAPD: Unknown CRRT: Unknown
Gallamine (258) Recurarization may occur up to 24 h after dose; if blockade not responsive to neostigmine, dialysis may be useful	0.5–1.5 mg/kg	D	Avoid	Avoid	Hemo: NA CAPD: NA CRRT: NA
Ketamine (255)	1.0–4.5 mg/kg	D	100%	100%	Hemo: Unknown CAPD: Unknown CRRT: Unknown
Metocurine (259)	0.2–0.4 mg/kg	D	Avoid	Avoid	Hemo: Unknown CAPD: Unknown CRRT: Unknown
Neostigmine (260)	15–375 mg/day	D	50%	25%	Hemo: Unknown CAPD: Unknown CRRT: Unknown
Pancuronium (261) Recurarization may occur up to 24 h after dose	0.04–0.1 mg/kg	D	50%	Avoid	Hemo: Unknown CAPD: Unknown CRRT: Unknown
Propofol (262) High dose may cause rhabdomyolysis and green urine	2.0–2.5 mg/kg load, then 6–12 mg/kg/h	D	100%	100%	Hemo: Unknown CAPD: Unknown RRT: Unknown
Pyridostigmine (263) Renal excretion decreased by basic drugs	60–1500 mg/d	D	35% (GFR >50: 50%)	20%	Hemo: Unknown CAPD: Unknown CRRT: Unknown
Succinylcholine (264) Hyperkalemia in ESRD	0.3–1.1 mg/kg load, then 0.04–0.07 mg/kg prn	D	100%	100%	Hemo: Unknown CAPD: Unknown CRRT: Unknown
Tubocurarine (265) Large or repetitive doses may result in prolonged effect Recurarization may occur	0.1–0.2 mg/kg	D	50% (GFR >50: 75%–100%)	Avoid	Hemo: Unknown CAPD: Unknown CRRT: Unknown
Vecuronium (266)	0.08–0.1 mg/kg load, then 0.01–0.05 mg/kg	D	100%	100%	Hemo: Unknown CAPD: Unknown CRRT: Unknown

CAPD, continuous ambulatory peritoneal dialysis; *CRRT,* chronic renal replacement therapy; *D,* dosage reduction method; *ESRD,* end-stage renal disease; *GFR,* glomerular filtration rate; *Hemo,* hemodialysis; *I,* interval extension method; *NA,* not applicable;

TABLE 104-6. *Antihypertensive and cardiovascular agents*

| Drug, toxicity, notes | Dosage for normal renal function | Method | Adjustment for renal failure GFR (mL/min) | | Supplement for dialysis |
			10–50	<10	
ADRENERGIC MODULATORS					
Clonidine (273,274) Rebound hypertension if drug is suddenly withdrawn; potentiates CNS depressant effects of alcohol, sedatives	0.1–0.6 mg b.i.d.	D	100%	100%	Hemo: None CAPD: None CRRT: None
Doxazosin (275,276)	1–15 mg/d	D	100%	100%	Hemo: None CAPD: None CRRT: None
Guanabenz (277)	8–16 mg b.i.d.	D	100%	100%	Hemo: None CAPD: None CRRT: None
Guanadrel (278,279)	10–50 mg b.i.d.	I	q12–24h	q24–48h	Hemo: Unknown CAPD: Unknown CRRT: Unknown
Guanethidine (7,74)	10–100 mg/d	I	q24h	q48h	Hemo: None CAPD: None CRRT: None
Guanfacine (280,281)	1–2 mg/d	D	100%	100%	Hemo: None CAPD: None CRRT: None
Methyldopa (282) Orthostatic hypotension. Retroperitoneal fibrosis. Elevates serum creatinine by acting as chromogen. Active metabolite with long $t_{1/2}$.	250–500 mg t.i.d.	I	q8–12h	q12–24h	Hemo: 250 mg CAPD: None CRRT: significant removal likely; dose for GFR 10–50
Prazosin (283,284)	1–15 mg b.i.d.	D	100%	100%	Hemo: None CAPD: None CRRT: None
Reserpine (285) Excessive sedation, GI bleeding	0.05–0.25 mg/d	D	100%	Avoid	Hemo: None CAPD: None CRRT: None
Terazosin (286)	1–20 mg/d	D	100%	100%	Hemo: None CAPD: None CRRT: None
ANGIOTENSIN II-RECEPTOR ANTAGONISTS					
Candesartan	4–32 mg qd	D	100%	50%–100%	Hemo: None CAPD: None CRRT: None
Irbesartan	75–300 mg qd	D	100%	50%–100%	Hemo: None CAPD: None CRRT: None
Losartan	50 mg q12h	D	100%	100%	Hemo: None CAPD: None CRRT: None
ANGIOTENSIN-CONVERTING ENZYME INHIBITORS Hypotensive effects exacerbated by diuretics or sodium depletion. May cause hyperkalemia, metabolic acidosis. Acute renal dysfunction with bilateral or transplant renal artery stenosis. Dry cough in 5%–10%.					
Benazepril (287,288)	10–40 mg qd	D	50%–100%	25%–50% (Maximum dose 10 mg/d)	Hemo: None CAPD: None CRRT: None

TABLE 104-6. (*Continued*)

Drug, toxicity, notes	Dosage for normal renal function	Method	Adjustment for renal failure GFR (mL/min)		Supplement for dialysis
			10–50	<10	
Captopril (289–291) Rare nephrotic syndrome, granulocytopenia Increases serum digoxin levels	25–50 mg q8h	D, I	50–100% q12h	50% q24h	Hemo: Dose after dialysis CAPD: None CRRT: Likely to be removed; dose for GFR 10–50 ml/min
Enalapril (292,293)	5–10 mg q12h	D	50%–100%	50%	Hemo: Dose after dialysis CAPD: None CRRT: Likely to be removed; dose for GFR 10–50
Fosinopril (294–296)	10–40 mg qd	D	100%	100%	Hemo: Dose after dialysis CAPD: None CRRT: None
Lisinopril (297,298)	5–40 mg qd	D	50%–100%	25%–50%	Hemo: Dose after dialysis CAPD: None CRRT: None
Ramipril (299,300)	10–20 mg qd	D	50%–100%	25%–50%	Hemo: Dose after dialysis CAPD: None CRRT: Likely to be removed; dose for GFR 10–50

ANTIARRHYTHMIC AGENTS

Blood levels and clinical response best guide to therapy; $t_{1/2}$ may be prolonged in heart failure or with reduced hepatic blood flow.

Amiodarone (301) Thyroid dysfunction; peripheral neuropathy; pulmonary fibrosis	800–1200 mg load 200–600 mg/d	D	100%	100%	Hemo: None CAPD: None CRRT: Unlikely
Bretylium (302,303)	5–30 mg/kg load 5–10 mg i.v. q6h	D	25%–50%	25%	Hemo: None CAPD: None CRRT: Unlikely
Disopyramide (304–306) Urinary retention Variable Vd and extrarenal elimination mandates individualized dosing	100–200 mg q6h	I	q12–24h (GFR >50: q6–8h)	q24–48h	Hemo: None CAPD: None CRRT: None
Encainide (307,308) Active metabolites may accumulate in renal failure	25 mg q8h to 50 mg q6h	D	75%	50%	Hemo: None CAPD: None CRRT: None
Flecainide (309,310) Excretion enhanced in acid urine	100–200 mg q12h	D	100%	50%–75%	Hemo: None CAPD: None CRRT: None
Lidocaine (311) $t_{1/2}$ dependent on hepatic blood flow; active metabolite	Load 1 mg/kg i.v. bolus, then 0.5 mg/kg bolus q8–10 min, up to a total of 3 mg/kg Maintenance: 1–4 mg/min i.v. infusion	D	100%	100%	Hemo: None CAPD: None CRRT: None
Lorcainide (312)	100 mg b.i.d.	D	100%	100%	Hemo: None CAPD: None CRRT: None

(*Continued*)

TABLE 104-6. (*Continued*)

Drug, toxicity, notes	Dosage for normal renal function	Method	Adjustment for renal failure GFR (mL/min)		Supplement for dialysis
			10–50	<10	
Mexiletine (313,314)	100–300 mg q6–8h	D	100%	100%	Hemo: None CAPD: None CRRT: None
Moricizine (315,316)	200–300 mg q8h	D	100%	100%	Hemo: None CAPD: None CRRT: None
N-Acetylprocainamide (317,318)	500 mg q6–8h	D, I	50% q8–12h	25% q12h	Hemo: None CAPD: None CRRT: None
Procainamide (317–319)	350–400 mg q3–4h	I	q6–12h	q12–24h	Hemo: 200 mg CAPD: None CRRT: Replace by blood level
Propafenone (320,321)	150–300 mg q8h	D	100%	100%	Hemo: None CAPD: None CRRT: None
Quinidine (322,323) Active metabolite, increases plasma digoxin and digitoxin; excretion enhanced in acid urine; HD useful in poisoning	200–400 mg q4–6h	D	100%	75%	Hemo: None CAPD: None CRRT: Dose for GFR 10–50
Tocainide (324–326)	200–400 mg q8h	D	100%	50%	Hemo: 200 mg CAPD: None CRRT: Dose for GFR 10–50
β-BLOCKERS					
Acebutolol (327–331) Active metabolites with long $t_{1/2}$	400–600 mg/d or b.i.d.	D	50%	30%–50%	Hemo: Dose after dialysis CAPD: None CRRT: Probably removed; dose for GFR 10–50
Atenolol (332,333) Significant accumulation in ESRD	50–100 mg/d	D, I	50%	25% q48–96h	Hemo: 25–50 mg CAPD: None CRRT: Probably removed; dose for GFR 10–50
Betaxolol (334)	10–20 mg/d	D	100%	50%	Hemo: Dose after dialysis CAPD: None CRRT: Probably removed; dose for GFR 10–50
Carteolol (335,336)	0.5–10 mg/d	D	50%	25%	Hemo: Unknown CAPD: Unknown CRRT: Unknown
Carvedilol	25–50 mg q12–24h	D	100%	100%	Hemo: None CAPD: None CRRT: Dose for GFR 10–50
Dilevalol (337,338)	200–800 mg PO qd	D	100%	100%	Hemo: None CAPD: None CRRT: Unknown
Esmolol (339,340) Active metabolite	50–150 μg/kg/min infusion	D	100%	100%	Hemo: None CAPD: None CRRT: None

TABLE 104-6. (*Continued*)

Drug, toxicity, notes	Dosage for normal renal function	Method	Adjustment for renal failure GFR (mL/min)		Supplement for dialysis
			10–50	<10	
Labetalol (341,342)	200–600 mg b.i.d.	D	100%	100%	Hemo: None CAPD: None CRRT: None
Metoprolol (343)	50–100 mg b.i.d.	D	100%	100%	Hemo: Dose after dialysis CAPD: None CRRT: Likely to be removed; dose for GFR 10–50
Nadolol (344,345)	80–320 mg/d	D	50%	25%	Hemo: 40 mg CAPD: None CRRT: Likely to be removed; dose for GFR 10–50
Penbutolol (346)	10–40 mg/d	D	100%	100%	Hemo: None CAPD: None CRRT: None
Pindolol (347)	10–40 mg b.i.d.	D	100%	100%	Hemo: None CAPD: None CRRT: None
Propranolol (348,349) Metabolites may accumulate & cause increase bilirubin by assay interference hypoglycemia reported in ESRD	80–160 mg b.i.d.	D	100%	100%	Hemo: None CAPD: None CRRT: None
Sotalol (350,351)	160–480 mg/d	D	30%	15%–30%	Hemo: Dose after dialysis CAPD: None CRRT: Likely to be removed; dose for GFR 10–50
Timolol (327,328)	10–20 mg b.i.d.	D	100%	100%	Hemo: None CAPD: None CRRT: None
CALCIUM CHANNEL BLOCKERS					
Amlodipine (352,353)	5 mg qd	D	100%	100%	Hemo: None CAPD: None CRRT: None
Diltiazem (354–356)	30–90 mg q8h	D	100%	100%	Hemo: None CAPD: None CRRT: None
Felodipine (357–359)	10 mg b.i.d.	D	100%	100%	Hemo: None CAPD: None CRRT: None
Isradipine (360–362)	5–10 mg/d	D	100%	100%	Hemo: None CAPD: None CRRT: None
Nicardipine (363)	20–30 mg t.i.d.	D	100%	100%	Hemo: None CAPD: None CRRT: None
Nifedipine (364,365) Nifedipine XL	10–30 mg q8h (XL: 30–120 mg qd)	D	100%	100%	Hemo: None CAPD: None CRRT: None

(*Continued*)

TABLE 104-6. (*Continued*)

Drug, toxicity, notes	Dosage for normal renal function	Method	Adjustment for renal failure GFR (mL/min) 10–50	<10	Supplement for dialysis
Nimodipine (352)	30 mg q8h	D	100%	100%	Hemo: None CAPD: None CRRT: None
Nisoldipine (352)	10 mg b.i.d.	D	100%	100%	Hemo: None CAPD: None CRRT: None
Nitrendipine (366,367)	20 mg b.i.d.	D	100%	100%	Hemo: None CAPD: None CRRT: None
Verapamil (368–370) Verapamil SR	80 mg q8h (SR: 180 mg qd–240 mg q12h)	D	100%	100%	Hemo: None CAPD: None CRRT: None

CARDIAC GLYCOSIDES

Add to uremic gastrointestinal symptoms; serum levels guide therapy; toxicity enhanced by dialysis potassium and magnesium removal.

Drug, toxicity, notes	Dosage for normal renal function	Method	10–50	<10	Supplement for dialysis
Digitoxin (371,372) Protein binding decreased by dialysis; Vd reduced by uremia	0.1–0.2 mg/d	D	100%	100%	Hemo: None CAPD: None CRRT: None
Digoxin (11,373–375) Radioimmunoassay may overestimate serum levels in uremia; clearance reduced by spironolactone, quinidine, verapamil; hypokalemia, hypomagnesemia enhance toxicity	1.0–1.5 mg load 0.25–0.5 mg/d	D, I	25%–75% q24h	10%–25% q48h	Hemo: None CAPD: None CRRT: None
Ouabain (7,75)	0.25 mg load 0.1 mg q12h	I	q24h	q48h	Hemo: None CAPD: None CRRT: None

DIURETICS

Natriuretic drugs may cause volume depletion.

Drug, toxicity, notes	Dosage for normal renal function	Method	10–50	<10	Supplement for dialysis
Acetazolamide (376–378) May potentiate acidemia Ineffective in ESRD	250 mg q6–12h	I	q12h	Avoid	Hemo: Unlikely CAPD: Unlikely CRRT: Unlikely
Amiloride (379) Hyperkalemia Hyperchloremic metabolic acidosis	5–10 mg q24h	D	50%	Avoid	Hemo: NA CAPD: NA CRRT: NA
Bumetanide (380,381) Ototoxicity in combination with aminoglycosides Protein binding reduced in renal failure	1–2 mg q8–12h	D	100%	100%	Hemo: None CAPD: None CRRT: None
Chlorthalidone (382) Ineffective with low GFR	25 mg/d	D	100%	Avoid	Hemo: NA CAPD: NA CRRT: NA
Ethacrynic acid (383) Ototoxicity	50 mg t.i.d.	I	q8–12h	Avoid	Hemo: NA CAPD: NA CRRT: NA

TABLE 104-6. (*Continued*)

Drug, toxicity, notes	Dosage for normal renal function	Method	Adjustment for renal failure GFR (mL/min)		Supplement for dialysis
			10–50	<10	
Furosemide (384–386) Ototoxicity	40–80 mg b.i.d.	D	100%	100%	Hemo: None CAPD: None CRRT: NA
Torsemide Ototoxicity	5–100 mg b.i.d.	D	100%	100%	Hemo: None CAPD: None CRRT: None
Indapamide (387) Hypotensive effect independent of diuretic effect	2.5–5.0 mg/d	D	100%	100%	Hemo: None CAPD: None CRRT: None
Metolazone (376,377)	5–10 mg/d	D	100%	100%	Hemo: None CAPD: None CRRT: None
Piretanide (388,389) Ototoxicity	6–12 mg/d	D	100%	100%	Hemo: None CAPD: None CRRT: None
Spironolactone (390) Hyperkalemia common when GFR <30 mL/min Hyperchloremic acidosis Active metabolites with long $t_{1/2}$	25–50 mg t.i.d.	I	q12–24h	Avoid	Hemo: NA CAPD: NA CRRT: NA
Thiazides (391) Ineffective when GFR <30 mL/min Hyperuricemia	12.5 mg qd 50 mg b.i.d.	D	100%	Avoid	Hemo: NA CAPD: NA CRRT: NA
Triamterene (392) Hyperkalemia common when GFR <30 mL/min Crystalluria in acid urine can cause acute renal failure Active metabolite with long $t_{1/2}$	25–50 mg b.i.d.	D	50%	Avoid	Hemo: NA CAPD: NA CRRT: NA
INOTROPIC AGENTS					
Amrinone (393,394) Nausea in ESRD	5–10 μg/kg min Daily <10 mg/kg	D	100%	50%–75%	Hemo: Unknown CAPD: Unknown CRRT: Unknown
Dobutamine (395,396)	2.5–15.0 μg/kg/min	D	100%	100%	Hemo: None CAPD: None CRRT: None
Milrinone (397,398)	2.5–15.0 mg q6h	D	100%	50%–75%	Hemo: Unknown CAPD: Unknown CRRT: Unknown
NITRATES					
Isosorbide (399–401) Active metabolite	10–20 mg t.i.d.	D	100%	100%	Hemo: Dose after dialysis CAPD: None CRRT: None
Nitroglycerin (399)	Many methods and routes of dosing	D	100%	100%	Hemo: None CAPD: None CRRT: None

(*Continued*)

TABLE 104-6. (*Continued*)

Drug, toxicity, notes	Dosage for normal renal function	Method	Adjustment for renal failure GFR (mL/min)		Supplement for dialysis
			10–50	<10	
VASODILATORS					
Diazoxide (402) Decreased protein binding in renal failure; salt and water retention	150–300 mg bolus	D	75%–100%	50%	Hemo: None CAPD: None CRRT: None
Hydralazine (403) Drug-induced lupus	25–50 mg t.i.d.	I	q8h	q12h	Hemo: None CAPD: None CRRT: None
Minoxidil (404) Fluid retention, pericardial effusion	5–30 mg b.i.d.	D	100%	100%	Hemo: Dose after dialysis CAPD: None CRRT: None
Nitroprusside (405,406) Toxic metabolite thiocyanate accumulates, causing seizures, coma; thiocyanate is hemodialyzable	0.25–8.0 μg/kg/min infusion	D	100%	100%	Hemo: None CAPD: None CRRT: None

CAPD, continuous ambulatory peritoneal dialysis; *CNS,* central nervous system; *CRRT,* continuous renal replacement therapy; *D,* dosage reduction method; *ESRD,* end-stage renal disease; *GFR,* glomerular filtration rate; *Hemo,* hemodialysis; *I,* interval extension method; *NA,* not available; $t_{1/2}$, half-life; *Vd,* volume of distribution.

TABLE 104-7. *Antineoplastic agents*

Drug, toxicity, notes	Dosage for normal renal function	Method	Adjustment for renal failure GFR (mL/min)		Supplement for dialysis
			10–50	<10	
Bleomycin (411) HTN, Dysuria Pulmonary fibrosis	10–20 U/m^2	D	75%	50%	Hemo: None CAPD: None CRRT: Dose for GFR 10–50
Busulfan (412) Hemorrhagic cystitis	4–8 mg/d	D	100%	100%	Hemo: Unknown CAPD: Unknown CRRT: Unknown
Carboplatin (413–415)	400–500 mg/m^2	D	50%–100%	25%	Hemo: 1/2 dose CAPD: Unknown CRRT: Unknown
Chlorambucil (416)	0.1–0.2 mg/kg/d	D	Unknown	Unknown	Hemo: Unknown CAPD: Unknown CRRT: Unknown
Cisplatin (417,418) Nephrotoxic; Mg^{+2} wasting	20–120 mg/m^2	D	75%	50%	Hemo: Unlikely CAPD: None CRRT: Unknown
Cyclophosphamide (419–421) Hemorrhagic cystitis Bladder fibrosis and bladder cancer (SIADH)	1–5 mg/kg/d	D	100%	75%	Hemo: 1/2 Dose after dialysis CAPD: None CRRT: Unknown
Cytarabine (422) Increased risk of neurotoxicity with high-dose therapy (2–3 g/m^2) in patients with renal insufficiency	100–200 mg/m^2	D	100%	100%	Hemo: Unknown CAPD: Unknown CRRT: Unknown
Daunorubicin (423)	30–45 mg/m^2	D	100%	100%	Hemo: Unknown CAPD: Unknown CRRT: Unknown

TABLE 104-7. (*Continued*)

Drug, toxicity, notes	Dosage for normal renal function	Method	Adjustment for renal failure GFR (mL/min)		Supplement for dialysis
			10–50	<10	
Doxorubicin (424)	60–75 mg/m²	D	100%	100%	Hemo: None CAPD: None CRRT: Unlikely
Etoposide (425)	35–100 mg/m²/d	D	50%–100%	50%	Hemo: None CAPD: None CRRT: Unlikely
Fluorouracil (426)	12 mg/kg/d	D	100%	100%	Hemo: 1/2 Dose after dialysis CAPD: Unknown CRRT: Unknown
Formostane (7)	250 mg/m² q2 weeks	D	100%	100%	Hemo: Unknown CAPD: Unknown CRRT: Unknown
Hydroxyurea (7,75)	20–30 mg/kg/d	D	50%	20%	Hemo: Unknown CAPD: Unknown CRRT: Unknown
Idarubicin (427)	12 mg/m²	D	100%	100%	Hemo: Unknown CAPD: Unknown CRRT: Unknown
Ifosfamide Fanconi's syndrome	1.2 g/m²	D	100%	50%–100%	Hemo: Unknown CAPD: Unknown CRRT: Unknown
Melphalan (428,429)	6 mg/day	D	50%–100%	50%	Hemo: Unlikely CAPD: Unlikely CRRT: Unlikely
Methotrexate (409,430,431) Nephrotoxic	Low dose: 15–30 mg/d High dose: 12 g/m² (with leucovorin rescue)	D	50%	Avoid	Hemo: None CAPD: None CRRT: Unlikely
Mitomycin-C (432) Hemolytic-uremic syndrome	20 mg/m² q6–8 weeks	D	100%	75%	Hemo: Unknown CAPD: Unknown CRRT: Unknown
Nitrosureas (433,434)	Varies	D	75%	25%–50%	Hemo: None CAPD: None CRRT: Unlikely
Plicamycin (435)	25–30 μg/kg/d	D	75%	50%	Hemo: Unknown CAPD: Unknown CRRT: Unknown
Streptozocin (436) Nephrotoxic Proteinuria RTA	500 mg/m²/d	D	75%	50%	Hemo: Unknown CAPD: Unknown CRRT: Unknown
Tamoxifen (437) Hot flashes, nausea	10–20 mg b.i.d.	D	100%	100%	Hemo: Unknown CAPD: Unknown CRRT: Unknown
Teniposide (7,75)	50–250 mg/m²	D	100%	100%	Hemo: None CAPD: None CRRT: Unlikely
Vinblastine (438)	3.7 mg/m²	D	100%	100%	Hemo: Unknown CAPD: Unknown CRRT: Unknown
Vincristine (7,75)	1.4 mg/m²	D	100%	100%	Hemo: Unknown CAPD: Unknown CRRT: Unknown

CAPD, continuous ambulatory peritoneal dialysis; *CRRT,* continuous renal replacement therapy; *D,* dosage reduction method; *GFR,* glomerular filtration rate; *Hemo,* hemodialysis; *SIADH,* syndrome of inappropriate antidiuretic hormone.

TABLE 104-8. *Endocrine and metabolic drugs*

Drug, toxicity, notes	Dosage for normal renal function	Method	Adjustment for renal failure GFR (mL/min)		Supplement for dialysis
			10–50	<10	
HYPOGLYCEMIC AGENTS					
Acarbose (449)	50–200 mg t.i.d.	D	25%	Avoid	Hemo: Avoid CAPD: Avoid CRRT: Avoid

Acetohexamide (450)
  Has diuretic effects
  May falsely elevate
    serum creatinine level
  Prolonged
    hypoglycemia in
    azotemic patients
	250–1,500 mg/d	D	Avoid	Avoid	Hemo: None
					CAPD: None
					CRRT: None

Chlorpropamide (450)
  Impairs water excretion
  Prolonged hypoglycemia
    in azotemic patients
	100–500 mg/d	D	Avoid	Avoid	Hemo: Avoid
					CAPD: Avoid
					CRRT: Avoid

Gliclazide (451)	160–320 mg/d	D	50%	Avoid	Hemo: Avoid CAPD: Avoid CRRT: Avoid
Glipizide (452)	2.5–15.0 mg/d	D	100%	50%	Hemo: None CAPD: None CRRT: None
Glyburide (453)	1.25–20.0 mg/d	D	Avoid	Avoid	Hemo: Avoid CAPD: Avoid CRRT: Avoid

Insulin (454)
  Renal metabolism of
    insulin decreases in
    renal insufficiency
  May be given by
    intraperitoneal
    route in CAPD
    patients
	Variable	D	75%	25–50%	Hemo: None
					CAPD: Unlikely
					CRRT: None

Metformin Lactic acidosis	500–850 mg q12h	D	25%	Avoid	Hemo: Avoid CAPD: Avoid CRRT: Avoid
Tolazamide (450)	100–250 mg/d	D	100%	100%	Hemo: Unlikely CAPD: Unlikely CRRT: Unlikely
Tolbutamide (450)	1–2 g/d	D	100%	100%	Hemo: None CAPD: None CRRT: None
HYPOLIPIDEMIC AGENTS					
Monitor creatine kinase levels; rhobdomylosis Atorvastatin	10–40 mg qhs	D	100%	100%	Hemo: None CAPD: None CRRT: None
Bezafibrate (447)	200 mg t.i.d.	D	50%	25%	Hemo: None CAPD: None CRRT: None

Cholestyramine (447)
  Hyperchloremic
    acidosis
  Requires fluids
    for dilution
	4 g q4-6h	D	100%	100% (Use with
				caution)
					Hemo: None
					CAPD: None
					CRRT: None

Clofibrate (455) Impairs H$_2$O excretion	500–1,000 mg b.i.d.	I	q12-24h	Avoid	Hemo: Avoid CAPD: Avoid CRRT: ???

TABLE 104-8. (*Continued*)

| Drug, toxicity, notes | Dosage for normal renal function | Method | Adjustment for renal failure GFR (mL/min) | | Supplement for dialysis |
			10–50	<10	
Colestipol (447) Hyperchloremic acidosis Requires fluids for dilution	13–30 g/d	D	100%	100%	Hemo: None CAPD: None CRRT: None
Fenofibrate (455)	300 mg/d	D	25%–50%	Avoid	Hemo: Avoid CAPD: Avoid CRRT: Avoid
Gemfibrozil (456)	600 mg b.i.d.	D	100%	100%	Hemo: None CAPD: None CRRT: None
Lovastatin (448,457)	20–80 mg/d	D	100%	100%	Hemo: None CAPD: None CRRT: None
Nicotinic acid (458) Aspirin may attenuate flushing	1–2 q t.i.d.	D	50%	25%	Hemo: None CAPD: None CRRT: None
Pravastatin (459)	10–40 mg/d	D	100%	100%	Hemo: None CAPD: None CRRT: None
Probucol (460)	500 mg b.i.d.	D	100%	100%	Hemo: None CAPD: None CRRT: None
Simvastatin (461)	5–40 mg/d	D	100%	100%	Hemo: None CAPD: None CRRT: None
THYROID MEDICATIONS					
L-Thyroxine (71) Adjust dose according to thyroid function tests	100–200 µg/d	D	100%	100%	Hemo: None CAPD: None CRRT: None
Methimazole (462,463)	5–20 mg t.i.d.	D	100%	100%	Hemo: None CAPD: None CRRT: None
Propylthiouracil (462)	5–20 mg t.i.d.	D	100%	100%	Hemo: None CAPD: None CRRT: None

CAPD, continuous ambulatory peritoneal dialysis; *CRRT,* continuous renal replacement therapy; *D,* dosage reduction method; *GFR,* glomerular filtration rate; *Hemo,* hemodialysis; *I,* interval extension method;

Antimicrobial Agents

A primary source of morbidity and mortality for patients with renal failure is infection (79,80). Many antibiotics require dosage adjustment in the setting of renal insufficiency due to alterations in pharmacokinetic parameters. An increased incidence of toxicity is observed in patients with renal insufficiency due, in part, to accumulation of drug and/or active metabolites (81). Specific dosing guidelines for individual antimicrobial agents are provided in Table 104-4. One or more pharmacokinetic parameters may be altered in the patient with renal failure. Decreased absorption may occur for some agents such as tetracycline (82) or ciprofloxacin (83)

if administered concomitantly with antacids or phosphate binders. Although the majority of antibiotics are excreted partially or completely by glomerular filtration, a number of antimicrobials such as trimethoprim–sulfamethoxazole (84) or ciprofloxacin (83) reach the urinary space by tubular secretion. This, in turn, achieves high urinary concentrations of such agents even though the GFR is diminished. This feature is used to therapeutic advantage for treatment of urinary tract infections in patients with renal insufficiency or cyst infections in patients with polycystic kidney disease.

In the majority of cases, the loading dose will be the same as that used in patients with normal renal function because rapid achievement of therapeutic antibiotic levels are critical

TABLE 104-9. *Gastrointestinal drugs*

Drug, toxicity, notes	Dosage for normal renal function	Method	Adjustment for renal failure GFR (mL/min)			Supplement for dialysis
			>50	10–50	<10	
ANTIEMETICS, ANTIDIARRHEALS, MOTILITY AGENTS						
Cisapride (7) Prolonged QT	5–10 mg q.i.d.	D	100%	100%	50%	Hemo: None CAPD: None CRRT: None

Diphenoxylate (7)
   (Each tablet contains
   2.5 mg diphenoxylate
   and 0.025 mg atropine)
	2 tablets q.i.d.	D	100%	50%–100%	Avoid	Hemo: Avoid
						CAPD: Avoid
						CRRT: Avoid

Granisetron (7)	40–160 μg/kg as
	   a 5- to 30-min
	   i.v. infusion
		D	100%	100%	100%	Hemo: Unknown
						CAPD: Unknown
						CRRT: Unknown

Metoclopramide (465,467)
   Extrapyramidal reactions
   increased in ESRD
	10–15 mg q.i.d.	D	100%	50%–100%	50%	Hemo: None
						CAPD: None
						CRRT: None

Ondansetron (468)	0.15 mg/kg as a
	   15-min
	   infusion
		D	100%	100%	100%	Hemo: None
						CAPD: None
						CRRT: None

Prochlorperazine (7)	5–10 mg PO
	   t.i.d.–q.i.d.
	   25 mg PR b.i.d.
		D	100%	100%	100%	Hemo: None
						CAPD: None
						CRRT: None

H$_2$ ANTAGONISTS						

Cimetidine (469–473)
   Increases serum
   creatinine by
   inhibition of tubular
   creatinine secretion
	400 mg b.i.d. or
	   400–800 mg qhs
		D	100%	50%–100%	25%–50%	Hemo: None
						CAPD: None
						CRRT: Dose for
						   GFR 10–50

Famotidine (474–477)	20–40 mg qhs	D	50%–100%	25%–50%	10%	Hemo: None CAPD: None CRRT: None
Nizatidine (478,479)	150–300 mg qhs	D,I	50%–100%	50%	50% q.o.d.	Hemo: None CAPD: None CRRT: None

Ranitidine (480–483)	150–300 mg qhs	D	50%–100%	50%	50%	Hemo: $\frac{1}{2}$ dose
						CAPD: None
						CRRT: Likely to be
						   removed; dose for
						   GFR 10–50

Roxatidine (474)	150 mg qhs	D	50%–100%	50%	25%	Hemo: None CAPD: None CRRT: None

OTHER DRUGS USED FOR PEPTIC DISEASE

Antacids: Calcium, magnesium, and aluminum salts all have absorption of constituent cations, which have reduced elimination in renal failure, producing hypercalcemia, hypermagnesemia, and elevated aluminum levels, respectively. Protracted use may cause nephrolithiasis, metabolic alkalosis, and milk–alkali syndrome. Calcium salts are now the drugs of choice as phosphate binders. For these reasons, other agents are preferred in the treatment of peptic disease in patients with renal failure.

Drug, toxicity, notes	Dosage for normal renal function	Method	>50	10–50	<10	Supplement for dialysis
Enprostil (7)	35 μg b.i.d.	D	100%	100%	100%	Hemo: None CAPD: None CRRT: None
Lansoprazole (484)	30 mg qd	D	100%	100%	100%	Hemo: None CAPD: None CRRT: None
Misoprostol (485)	100–200 μg q.i.d.	D	100%	100%	100%	Hemo: None CAPD: None CRRT: None
Omeprazole (486,487)	20–40 mg/d	D	100%	100%	100%	Hemo: None CAPD: None CRRT: None

Sucralfate (488,489)
   Contains aluminum,
   which may be absorbed
   to produce dementia,
   renal osteodystrophy,
   and anemia; <5% of
   dose absorbed
	1 g q.i.d.	D	50%–100%	Avoid	Avoid	Avoid

CAPD, continuous ambulatory peritoneal dialysis; *CRRT,* continuous renal replacement therapy; *D,* dosage reduction method; *ESRD,* end-stage renal disease; *GFR,* glomerular filtration rate; *Hemo,* hemodialysis; *I,* interval extension method.

TABLE 104-10. *Neurologic agents*

Drug, toxicity, notes	Dosage for normal renal function	Method	Adjustment for renal failure GFR (mL/min)		Supplement for dialysis
			10–50	<10	
ANTICONVULSANTS					
Monitor serum levels					
Carbamazepine (492–494)	200–1,200 mg/d	D	100%	100%	Hemo: None CAPD: None CRRT: None
Ethosuximide (495)	500–1,500 mg/d	D	100%	50%	Hemo: None CAPD: None CRRT: Dose for GFR 10–50
Gabapentin	400 mg t.i.d.	D,I	300 mg q12-24h	300 mg q.o.d.	Hemo: 300 mg after dialysis CAPD: None CRRT: None
Oxcarbazepine (7)	200–400 mg t.i.d.	D	100%	100%	Hemo: None CAPD: None CRRT: None
Phenytoin (491,496) Protein binding decreased and distribution volume increased in renal failure; monitor free dilantin levels	1,000-mg load, then 300–400 mg/d	D	100%	100%	Hemo: None CAPD: None CRRT: None
Primidone (497) Partially converted to phenobarbital and other metabolites with long $t_{1/2}$; excessive sedation; nystagmus	200–500 mg q.i.d.	I	q8-12h	q12-24h	Hemo: $\frac{1}{3}$ dose CAPD: None CRRT: Likely to be removed; dose for GFR 10–50
Trimethadione (7,75)	300–600 mg t.i.d.–q.i.d.	I	q8-12h	q12-24h	Hemo: None CAPD: None CRRT: None
Valproic acid (498,499) Decreased protein binding in uremia Concurrent phenytoin, phenobarbital, and primidone shorten $t_{1/2}$	15–60 mg/kg/d	D	100%	100%	Hemo: None CAPD: None CRRT: None
Vigabatrin (7,75)	2–4 g/d	D	50%	25%	Hemo: None CAPD: None CRRT: Unknown
ANTIPARKINSONIAN AGENTS					
Bromocriptine (500) Orthostatic hypotension	1.25 mg b.i.d.	D	100%	100%	Hemo: None CAPD: None CRRT: None
Carbidopa (501)	1 tablet t.i.d. to 6 tablets daily	D	100%	100%	Hemo: None CAPD: None CRRT: None
Levodopa (501) Active metabolite accumulates in ESRD	250–500 mg b.i.d. to 8 g/d	D	100%	50%	Hemo: None CAPD: None CRRT: None
Trihexyphenidyl (502)	1–2 mg/d to 6–10 mg/d	D	Unknown	Unknown	Hemo: None CAPD: None CRRT: None
AGENTS USED FOR THE TREATMENT OF MIGRAINE HEADACHES					
Ergotamine (7) (Ergotamine, 1 mg; caffeine, 100 mg)	Acute attack: 1 tablet q30 min (maximum 6 tablets)	D	100%	100%	Hemo: None CAPD: None CRRT: None
Dihydroergotamine (7)	Acute attack: 1 mg i.m. or i.v. q1h (maximum 3 mg)	D	100%	100%	Hemo: None CAPD: None CRRT: None

CAPD, continuous ambulatory peritoneal dialysis; *CRRT*, continuous renal replacement therapy; *D*, dosage reduction method; *ESRD*, end-stage renal disease; *GFR*, glomerular filtration rate; *Hemo*, hemodialysis; *I*, interval extension method; $t_{1/2}$, half-life.

TABLE 104-11. *Rheumatologic agents*

Drug, toxicity, notes	Dosage for normal renal function	Method	Adjustment for renal failure GFR (mL/min)		Supplement for dialysis
			10–50	<10	
GOUT AGENTS					
Allopurinol (504,506) Active metabolite; interstitial nephritis; exfoliative dermatitis	300 mg/d	D	50%	33%	Hemo: 100 mg qd CAPD: 100 mg qd CRRT: None
Colchicine (505,507) Increased risk of myopathy and neuropathy in renal failure Monitor creatine kinase values	Acute: 2 mg, then 0.5 mg q6h Chronic: 0.5– 1.0 mg/d	D	50%	25%	Hemo: None CAPD: None CRRT: None
Probenicid (508) Ineffective at decreased GFR	500 mg b.i.d.	D	Avoid	Avoid	Hemo: None CAPD: None CRRT: None
NONSTEROIDAL ANTIINFLAMMATORY DRUGS					
Drugs in this group may be associated with renal dysfunction secondary to prostaglandin inhibition; prostaglandin inhibitors may increase uremic bleeding and gastrointestinal symptoms; nephrotic syndrome; interstitial nephritis, and hyperkalemia reported.					
Diclofenac (509,510)	25–75 mg b.i.d.	D	100%	50%	Hemo: None CAPD: None CRRT: None
Diflunisal (511)	250–500 mg b.i.d.	D	100%	50%	Hemo: None CAPD: None CRRT: None
Etodolac (512)	200–600 mg b.i.d.	D	100%	100%	Hemo: None CAPD: None CRRT: None
Flurbiprofen (513)	100 mg b.i.d.–t.i.d.	D	100%	100%	Hemo: None CAPD: None CRRT: None
Ibuprofen (514)	800 mg t.i.d.	D	100%	100%	Hemo: None CAPD: None CRRT: None
Indomethacin (515)	25–50 mg t.i.d.	D	100%	100%	Hemo: None CAPD: None CRRT: None
Ketoprofen (516)	25–75 mg t.i.d.	D	100%	100%	Hemo: None CAPD: None CRRT: None
Ketorolac (517) Acute hearing loss in ESRD	5–30 mg q.i.d.	D	100%	25–50%	Hemo: None CAPD: None CRRT: None
Meclofenamic acid (509)	50–100 mg t.i.d.–q.i.d.	D	100%	100%	Hemo: None CAPD: None CRRT: None
Mefenamic acid (509)	250 mg q.i.d.	D	100%	100%	Hemo: None CAPD: None CRRT: None
Nabumetone	1–2 g 24 h	D	50%–100%	50%	Hemo: None CAPD: None CRRT: None
Naproxen (518)	500 mg b.i.d.	D	100%	100%	Hemo: None CAPD: None CRRT: None

TABLE 104-11. (*Continued*)

Drug, toxicity, notes	Dosage for normal renal function	Method	Adjustment for renal failure GFR (mL/min)		Supplement for dialysis
			10–50	<10	
Phenylbutazone (509)	100 mg t.i.d.–q.i.d.	D	100%	100%	Hemo: None CAPD: None CRRT: None
Piroxicam (519)	20 mg/d	D	100%	100%	Hemo: None CAPD: None CRRT: None

Sulindac (520)
  Active sulfide
    metabolite
	200 mg b.i.d.	D	100%	100%	Hemo: None
					CAPD: None
					CRRT: None

Tolmetin (509)	400 mg t.i.d.	D	100%	100%	Hemo: None CAPD: None CRRT: None
OTHER AGENTS UTILIZED IN THE TREATMENT OF ARTHRITIS					

Auranofin (521)
  Proteinuria common;
    rarely progresses to
      nephrotic syndrome
	6 mg/d	D	Avoid	Avoid	Hemo: None
					CAPD: None
					CRRT: None

Gold sodium thiomalate (522)
  Nephrotoxic, proteinuria,
    membranous nephritis
	25–50 mg	D	Avoid	Avoid	Hemo: None
					CAPD: None
					CRRT: None

Penicillamine (7,75) Nephrotic syndrome	250–1,000 mg/d	D	Avoid	Avoid	Hemo: None CAPD: None CRRT: None

CAPD, continuous ambulatory peritoneal dialysis; *CRRT,* continuous renal replacement therapy; *D,* dosage reduction method; *ESRD,* end-stage renal disease; *GFR,* glomerular filtration rate; *Hemo,* hemodialysis.

for life-threatening infections. Recently, the postantibiotic effect has been observed with a number of antimicrobials including aminoglycosides, newer macrolides, and the penems (85,86). Clinically, the persistence of antibiotic activity beyond the time point at which blood levels fall below the minimum inhibitory concentration may be used to design extended and more convenient dosing intervals of antimicrobial agents without jeopardizing patient outcomes.

Peritoneal dialysis patients often use the intraperitoneal route of antibiotic administration for treatment of peritonitis (87). Detailed reviews of this therapeutic modality exist elsewhere, and intraperitoneal antibiotic dosing for peritonitis has been reviewed by Keane and colleagues (88).

Patients with renal dysfunction have an increased risk of antimicrobial-induced nephrotoxicity whereby dosage adjustments and close monitoring are required to minimize further renal injury, particularly with aminoglycosides (89). Less predictable, acute interstitial nephritis often complicates courses of antimicrobial therapy, but no known risk factors or preventive measures exist (90). Spurious rises in serum creatinine may result when certain cephalosporins interfere with the creatinine assay or trimethoprim blocks tubular secretion of creatinine (91,92). Lastly, significant potassium and salt loads may accompany the administration of certain antibiotics, particularly penicillins (93).

Analgesics and Agents used by Anesthesiologists

Table 104-5 summarizes dosage recommendations for analgesics and agents used by anesthesiologists. Most analgesics are metabolized by the liver and thus require little dosage adjustment, but renal failure tends to increase the sensitivity to the pharmacologic effects of these drugs (238). Special attention needs to be paid when prescribing meperidine for patients with reduced renal function. Normeperidine, a meperidine metabolite excreted by the kidneys, has central nervous system excitatory properties that can lower the seizure threshold in patients with renal failure (239). Similarly, many of the neuromuscular blocking agents are excreted by the kidney and thus may display prolonged action and recurarization in patients with impaired renal function as the effects of the antagonist dissipate (240).

Antihypertensive and Cardiovascular Agents

Table 104-6 summarizes dosage recommendations for antihypertensive and cardiovascular agents. The most common cause of death in the end-stage renal disease population is cardiovascular disease (267). Hypertension complicates the management of most patients with renal insufficiency and impacts adversely on renal disease progression and increases the risk of cardiovascular events (268,269). Prescribing

TABLE 104-12. *Sedatives, hypnotics, and drugs used in psychiatry*

Drug, toxicity, notes	Dosage for normal renal function	Method	Adjustment for renal failure GFR (mL/min)		Supplement for dialysis
			10–50	<10	
ANTIDEPRESSANTS					
Amoxapine (524)	75–200 mg/d	D	100%	100%	Hemo: None CAPD: None CRRT: None
Bupropion (525)	100 mg q8h	D	100%	100%	Hemo: None CAPD: None CRRT: None
Fluvoxamine	100 mg q24h	D	100%	100%	Hemo: None CAPD: None CRRT: None
Fluoxetine (526,527)	20 mg/d	D	100%	100%	Hemo: None CAPD: None CRRT: None
Maprotiline (7,75)	75–150 mg/d	D	100%	50%	Hemo: None CAPD: None CRRT: None
Paroxetone	20–60 mg q24h	D	50%–100%	50%	Hemo: None CAPD: None CRRT: None
Sertraline	50–200 mg q24h	D	100%	100%	Hemo: None CAPD: None CRRT: None
BARBITURATES					
May cause excessive sedation. Pentobarbital (7,75)	30 mg t.i.d.–q.i.d.	D	100%	100%	Hemo: None CAPD: None CRRT: None
Phenobarbital (7,75) 50% excreted with alkaline diuresis	50–100 mg b.i.d.–t.i.d.	D,I	100% q8-12h	50% q12-24h	Hemo: Dose after dialysis CAPD: 50% q12h CRRT: None
Secobarbital (7,75)	30–50 mg t.i.d.–q.i.d.	D	100%	100%	Hemo: None CAPD: None CRRT: None
Thiopental (528)	Anesthesia induction	D	100%	75%	Hemo: N/A CAPD: N/A CRRT: N/A
BENZODIAZEPINES					
Alprazolam (529,530)	0.25–5.0 mg t.i.d.	D	100%	100%	Hemo: None CAPD: None CRRT: None
Clorazepate (531) Active metabolite	15–60 mg/d	D	100%	100%	Hemo: None CAPD: None CRRT: None
Chlordiazepoxide (532) Active metabolite	15–100 mg/d	D	100%	50%	Hemo: None CAPD: None CRRT: None
Clonazepam (529)	1.5 mg/d	D	100%	100%	Hemo: None CAPD: None CRRT: None
Diazepam (7,75)	5–40 mg/d	D	100%	100%	Hemo: None CAPD: None CRRT: None
Flurazepam (529) Active metabolite	15–30 mg hs	D	100%	100%	Hemo: None CAPD: None CRRT: None

TABLE 104-12. (*Continued*)

Drug, toxicity, notes	Dosage for normal renal function	Method	Adjustment for renal failure GFR (mL/min)		Supplement for dialysis
			10–50	<10	
Lorazepam (533)	1–2 mg b.i.d.–t.i.d.	D	100%	100%	Hemo: None CAPD: None CRRT: None
Midazolam (534)	1.25 mg i.v. initial, titrate to response	D	100%	100%	Hemo: None CAPD: None CRRT: None
Nitrazepam (535)	5–10 mg hs	D	100%	100%	Hemo: None CAPD: None CRRT: None
Oxazepam (536)	30–120 mg/d	D	100%	100%	Hemo: None CAPD: None CRRT: None
Prazepam (529) Active metabolite	20–60 mg hs	D	100%	100%	Hemo: None CAPD: None CRRT: None
Quazepam (537)	15 mg hs	D	100%	100%	Hemo: None CAPD: None CRRT: None
Temazepam (529)	30 mg hs	D	100%	100%	Hemo: None CAPD: None CRRT: None
Triazolam (538,539) Protein binding correlates with α_1-acid glycoprotein concentration	0.125–0.5 mg hs	D	100%	100%	Hemo: None CAPD: None CRRT: None
BENZODIAZEPINE ANTAGONIST					
Flumazenil	0.2 mg IV over 15 sec	D	100%	100%	Hemo: None CAPD: None CRRT: None
PHENOTHIAZINES					
Anticholinergic, urinary retention, orthostatic hypotension, confusion.					
Chlorpromazine (540)	300–800 mg/d	D	100%	100%	Hemo: None CAPD: None CRRT: None
Promethazine (541) Excessive sedation	20–100 mg/d	D	100%	100%	Hemo: None CAPD: None CRRT: None
TRICYCLIC ANTIDEPRESSANTS					
Anticholinergic, urinary retention, orthostatic hypotension, excessive sedation.					
Amitriptyline (542–544)	25 mg t.i.d.	D	100%	100%	Hemo: None CAPD: None CRRT: None
Clomipramine (545)	25–50 mg b.i.d.–t.i.d.	D	100%	100%	Hemo: None CAPD: None CRRT: None
Desipramine (546) Active metabolites	75–150 mg/d	D	100%	100%	Hemo: None CAPD: None CRRT: None
Doxepin (547) Protein binding decrease in ESRD	25 mg t.i.d.	D	100%	100%	Hemo: None CAPD: None CRRT: None

(*Continued*)

TABLE 104-12. (*Continued*)

Drug, toxicity, notes	Dosage for normal renal function	Method	Adjustment for renal failure GFR (mL/min)		Supplement for dialysis
			10–50	<10	
Imipramine (548) Active metabolite	25 mg t.i.d.	D	100%	100%	Hemo: None CAPD: None CRRT: None
Nortriptyline (549)	25 mg t.i.d.–q.i.d.	D	100%	100%	Hemo: None CAPD: None CRRT: None
Protriptyline (550)	15–60 mg/d	D	100%	100%	Hemo: None CAPD: None CRRT: None
MISCELLANEOUS AGENTS					
Buspirone (551) Active metabolite accumulates	5–10 mg t.i.d.	D	100%	50%	Hemo: None CAPD: None CRRT: None
Clozapine (552)	150–200 mg b.i.d.	D	100%	100%	Hemo: None CAPD: None CRRT: None
Chloral hydrate (7,75) Active metabolite Excessive sedation	25 mg t.i.d.	D	Avoid	Avoid	Hemo: Avoid CAPD: Avoid CRRT: Avoid
Ethchlorvynol (7,75) Excessive sedation	500 mg qhs	D	Avoid	Avoid	Hemo: Avoid CAPD: Avoid CRRT: Avoid
Haloperidol (553) Hypotension, excessive sedation	1–2 mg b.i.d.–t.i.d.	D	100%	100%	Hemo: None CAPD: None CRRT: None
Lithium, carbonate (523,524,554) Nephrogenic diabetes insipidus Nephrotoxic; monitor serum levels Toxicity enhanced by volume depletion, diuretics, and NSAIDs	900–1,200 mg total dose/d	D	50%–100%	25%–50%	Hemo: Dose after dialysis CAPD: None CRRT: Dose for GFR 10–50
Meprobamate (7,75) Excessive sedation	300–400 mg q6h	I	q8-12h	q12-24h	Hemo: None CAPD: None CRRT: None
Phenelzine (7,75)	20–30 mg t.i.d.	D	100%	100%	Hemo: None CAPD: None CRRT: None

CAPD, continuous ambulatory peritoneal dialysis; CRRT, continuous renal replacement therapy; D, dosage reduction method; ESRD, end-stage renal disease; GFR, glomerular filtration rate; Hemo, hemodialysis; I, interval extension method; NSAIDs, nonsteroidal anti-inflammatory drugs.

antihypertensive therapy for patients with renal failure is often no different from patients with normal renal functions but exceptions do exist. The angiotensin-converting enzyme (ACE) inhibitors are attractive for use in patients with renal disease, as animal studies and preliminary human studies show benefit in slowing the progression of renal failure (270–272). Hyperkalemia, however, may complicate ACE inhibitor therapy, particularly in patients with type IV renal tubular acidosis as well as insulin-dependent diabetes

mellitus. Since most ACE inhibitors undergo renal excretion, prudent management dictates use of low doses initially and slowly increasing the dose when indicated.

Antineoplastic Agents

Table 104-7 summarizes dosage recommendations for antineoplastic agents. The clinical course of malignancy and its treatment are often complicated by renal failure resulting

TABLE 104-13. *Miscellaneous agents*

Drug, toxicity, notes	Dosage for normal renal function	Method	Adjustment for renal failure GFR (mL/min)		Supplement for dialysis
			10–50	<10	
ANTICOAGULANTS AND ANTIPLATELET AGENTS					
Agents in this group should be carefully titrated to achieve therapeutic effects; may potentiate uremic bleeding.					
Alteplase (tissue-type plasminogen activator [tPA]) (560)	Protocol specific	D	100%	100%	Hemo: None CAPD: None CRRT: None
Clopidogrel	75 mg qd	D	100%	100%	Hemo: None CAPD: None CRRT: None
Dipyridamole (555)	50 mg t.i.d.	D	100%	100%	Hemo: None CAPD: None CRRT: None

Heparin (556)
  $t_{1/2}$ increase with dose
	75 U/kg load,
	  then 0.5 U/kg/min
		D	100%	100%	Hemo: None
					CAPD: None
					CRRT: None

Streptokinase (557)	250,000 U load, then 100,000 U/h	D	100%	100%	Hemo: NA CAPD: NA CRRT: NA
Sulfinpyrazone (558) Acute renal failure	200 mg b.i.d.	D	100%	Avoid	Hemo: Avoid CAPD: Avoid CRRT: Avoid
Ticlopidine (559) Drug-induced TTP	500 mg b.i.d.	D	100%	100%	Hemo: None CAPD: None CRRT: None
Urokinase (7)	4400 U/kg load, then 4,400 U/kg/h	D	100%	100%	Hemo: None CAPD: None CRRT: None

Warfarin (561)
  Follow prothrombin time
	10–15 mg load,
	  then 2–10 mg/d
		D	100%	100%	Hemo: None
					CAPD: None
					CRRT: None

ANTIHISTAMINES					
May cause excessive sedation.					
Astemizole (562,563)	10 mg/d	D	100%	100%	Hemo: None CAPD: None CRRT: None
Brompheniramine (562)	4 mg q4-6h	D	100%	100%	Hemo: None CAPD: None CRRT: None
Cetirizine	5–20 mg q24h	D	50%–100%	25–50%	Hemo: None CAPD: None CRRT: None
Chlorpheniramine (562)	4 mg q4-6h	D	100%	100%	Hemo: None CAPD: None CRRT: None

Diphenhydramine (562)
  Anticholinergic effects
    may cause urine retention
	25 mg t.i.d.–q.i.d.	D	100%	100%	Hemo: None
					CAPD: None
					CRRT: None

Erbastine	10 mg q24h	D	50%–100%	50%	Hemo: None CAPD: None CRRT: None
Flunarizine (7,75)	Unknown	D	100%	100%	Hemo: None CAPD: None CRRT: None

(Continued)

TABLE 104-13. (*Continued*)

| Drug, toxicity, notes | Dosage for normal renal function | Method | Adjustment for renal failure GFR (mL/min) | | Supplement for dialysis |
			10–50	<10	
Hydroxyzine (7,75) Accumulates in ESRD	50–100 mg q.i.d.	D	50%–100%	50%	Hemo: None CAPD: None CRRT: None
Orphenadrine (562)	100 mg b.i.d.	D	100%	100%	Hemo: None CAPD: None CRRT: None
Oxatomide (564)	Unknown	D	100%	100%	Hemo: None CAPD: None CRRT: None
Promethazine (562)	12.5–25.0 mg q.d./q.i.d.	D	100%	100%	Hemo: None CAPD: None CRRT: None
Terfenadine (565) Causes torsades de pointes	60 mg b.i.d.	D	100%	100%	Hemo: None CAPD: None CRRT: None
Tripelennamine (562)	25–50 mg t.i.d.–q.i.d.	D	Unknown	Unknown	Hemo: Unknown CAPD: Unknown CRRT: Unknown
Triprolidine (562)	2.5 mg q4-6h	D	Unknown	Unknown	Hemo: Unknown CAPD: Unknown CRRT: Unknown
BRONCHODILATORS					
Albuterol (566)	2–4 mg t.i.d.–q.i.d. aerosol: 100–200 mg t.i.d.–q.i.d.	D	50%–100%	50%	Hemo: None CAPD: None CRRT: None
Bitolterol (567)	Aerosol: 2 inhalations q8h	D	100%	100%	Hemo: None CAPD: None CRRT: None
Dyphylline (568)	15 mg/kg/d	D	50%	25%	Hemo: $\frac{1}{3}$ dose CAPD: None CRRT: Likely to be removed
Ipratropium (566)	2 inhalations q.i.d.	D	100%	100%	Hemo: None CAPD: None CRRT: None
Terbutaline (566)	2.5–5.0 mg t.i.d.	D	50%	Avoid	Hemo: Avoid CAPD: Avoid CRRT: Avoid
Theophylline (569,570)	200–400 mg q12h	D	100%	100%	Hemo: $\frac{1}{2}$ dose CAPD: Unknown CRRT: Likely to be removed; monitor levels
IMMUNOSUPPRESSIVE DRUGS					
Azathioprine (571,572) Active metabolite	1.5–2.5 mg/kg/d	D	50%–100%	50%	Hemo: Dose after dialysis CAPD: None CRRT: Dose for GFR 10–50
CORTICOSTEROIDS May aggravate azotemia, sodium retention, glucose intolerance, and hypertension.					
Betamethasone (7,75)	0.5–9.0 mg/d	D	100%	100%	Hemo: None CAPD: None CRRT: None

TABLE 104-13. (Continued)

Drug, toxicity, notes	Dosage for normal renal function	Method	Adjustment for renal failure GFR (mL/min)		Supplement for dialysis
			10–50	<10	
Cortisone (7,75)	25–500 mg/d	D	100%	100%	Hemo: None CAPD: None CRRT: None
Dexamethasone (573)	0.75–9.0 mg/d	D	100%	100%	Hemo: None CAPD: None CRRT: None
Hydrocortisone (7,75)	20–500 mg/d	D	100%	100%	Hemo: None CAPD: None CRRT: None
Methylprednisolone (574)	4–48 mg/d	D	100%	100%	Hemo: Yes CAPD: Unknown CRRT: Likely to be removed
Prednisone (575)	5–60 mg/d	D	100%	100%	Hemo: None CAPD: None CRRT: None
Triamcinolone (7,75)	4–48 mg/d	D	100%	100%	Hemo: None CAPD: None CRRT: None

Cyclosporine (576)
  Nephrotoxic
  Hypertension, seizures, tremor
  Inhibitors of hepatic metabolism increase blood levels
	3–10 mg/kg/d	D	100%	100%	Hemo: None
					CAPD: None
					CRRT: None

MISCELLANEOUS					
Acetohydroxamic acid (577) May accumulate in ESRD	10–15 mg/kg/d	D	100%	Avoid	Hemo: Avoid CAPD: Avoid CRRT: Avoid

Deferoxamine (578,579)
  Fungal infections in ESRD
  Use in treatment for iron or aluminum overload
	Chronic iron overload: 0.5–1.0 g/d	D, I	50%–100%	100%	Hemo: Chelation product removed
					CAPD: Chelation product removed
					CRRT: Chelation product removed

Pentoxifylline (580,581)	400 mg q8h	I	q8-12h	q12-24h	Hemo: None CAPD: None CRRT: None

CAPD, continuous ambulatory peritoneal dialysis; CRRT, continuous renal replacement therapy; D, dosage reduction method; ESRD, end-stage renal disease; GFR, glomerular filtration rate; Hemo, hemodialysis; I, interval extension method; $t_{1/2}$, half-life.

from urinary tract obstruction, tumor lysis syndrome, malignancy-associated glomerulonephritis, drug-related nephrotoxicity, or a combination of these (407). Specifically, nephrotoxic renal failure often complicates treatment with cisplatin but may be minimized by hydrating the patient and administering cisplatin in normal or hypertonic saline (408). Tubular damage may be manifested by salt and magnesium wasting, even in the absence of marked azotemia. Likewise, methotrexate-induced renal failure can be minimized by hydration and alkalinization of the urine (409). In addition to

renal failure, mitomycin-C therapy can result in microangiopathic hemolytic anemia and thrombocytopenia (410).

Endocrine and Metabolic Agents

Table 104-8 provides dosage recommendations for endocrine and metabolic agents. Renal failure is associated with peripheral insulin resistance and decreased insulin metabolism by the kidney (439–441). In the presence of renal insufficiency, sulfonylureas that are excreted primarily by the kidney should be avoided, as prolonged hypoglycemia may result from the accumulation of such agents. Peritoneal dialysis allows for intraperitoneal insulin therapy, which has been shown to provide better overall control of plasma glucose when compared to standard subcutaneous injection therapy (442). Hyperlipidemia also complicates renal failure and adds to the increased risk of atherosclerotic complications in this population (443–446). Lipid-lowering agents such as bile acids can add to fluid overload and worsen acidosis in patients with renal failure, while other agents, such as lovastatin and clofibrate, have been associated with rhabdomyolysis (447,448).

Gastrointestinal Drugs

Table 104-9 summarizes dosage recommendations for gastrointestinal drugs. Patients with renal insufficiency experience gastrointestinal disorders more often than the general population, particularly peptic ulcer disease. Prior to the development of H$_2$ blockers, antacid therapy with compounds containing aluminum, calcium, magnesium, or bicarbonate was the mainstay. Excessive intake of calcium carbonate can result in the milk–alkali syndrome, characterized by hypercalcemia, metabolic alkalosis, and renal failure (464). Aluminum toxicity has been well described with chronic ingestion of aluminum-containing antacids in the setting of renal failure.

Neurologic Agents

Table 104-10 provides dosage recommendations for neurologic agents. Unfortunately, seizure disorders complicate renal insufficiency and end-stage renal disease (490). Phenytoin is commonly used as an anticonvulsant, but in patients with renal impairment, its Vd increases while its degree of protein binding decreases (491). As a result, a low total plasma phenytoin level may not reflect subtherapeutic drug levels, as the "free phenytoin" level may be adequate. Following free or unbound phenytoin levels is prudent in patients with markedly reduced renal function.

Rheumatologic Agents

Table 104-11 summarizes dosage recommendations for rheumatologic agents. Although dosage reductions of nonsteroidal antiinflammatory drugs (NSAIDs) are generally not required in renal failure, several precautions must be considered. When renal perfusion is reduced as in congestive heart failure or cirrhotic patients, vasodilatory prostaglandins may be key in maintaining renal blood flow. NSAIDs in such settings may cause reversible abrupt declines in renal function due to prostaglandin inhibition. Impaired potassium, sodium, and water excretion have also been attributed to NSAID use (503).

Patients with gout and renal insufficiency require reductions in allopurinol dosing because accumulation of its metabolite may underlie the complication of exfoliative dermatitis

(504). Similarly, renal failure increases the risk of myopathy and polyneuropathy associated with colchicine use (505).

Sedatives, Hypnotics, and Psychiatric Agents

Table 104-12 provides dosage recommendations for sedatives, hypnotics, and psychiatric agents. The majority of drugs in this category are lipid-soluble, highly protein bound, and excreted primarily by hepatic transformation to inactive metabolites, but increased sensitivity to the sedative side effects occurs in patients with renal impairment. Additionally, though dosage reduction generally is not required, increased sensitivity to the side effects of tricyclic antidepressants mandates a cautious approach in their use. Similarly, renal failure may exacerbate extrapyramidal side effects associated with phenothiazine therapy. In contrast, lithium is water-soluble and undergoes renal elimination. Renal syndromes induced by lithium therapy include nephrogenic diabetes insipidus as well as acute and chronic renal failure (523). Lithium toxicity can be minimized by avoidance of volume depletion and concurrent diuretic therapy.

Miscellaneous Agents

Table 104-13 provides dosage recommendations for a wide variety of miscellaneous agents.

REFERENCES

1. Bennett WM. Geriatric pharmacokinetics and the kidney. *Am J Kidney Dis* 1990;16:283.
2. Swan SK. Adjustment of drug dosage in patients with renal insufficiency. In: Kelley WM, ed. *Textbook of internal medicine.* New York: Lippincott, 1995.
3. Turnheim K. Pitfalls of pharmacokinetic dosage guidelines in renal insufficiency. *Eur J Clin Pharmacol* 1991;40:87.
4. Bennett WM, et al. Drug prescribing in renal failure: dosing guidelines for adults, 3rd ed. Philadelphia: American College of Physicians, 1994.
5. Maderazo E, Sun HE, Jay GT. Simplification of antibiotic dose adjustments in renal insufficiency: the DREM system. *Lancet* 1992;340:767.
6. Maher JF. Principles of dialysis and dialysis of drugs. *Am J Med* 62:475 1977.
7. Seyffart G, ed. *Drug dosage in renal insufficiency.* Dordrecht, The Netherlands: Kluwer Academic Publishers, 1991.
8. Swan SK, Bennett WM. Drug dosing guidelines in patients with renal failure. *West J Med* 1992;156:633.
9. Swan SK, Bennett WM. Use of cardiovascular drugs in chronic renal failure. In: Parfrey PS, Harnett JD, eds. *Cardiac dysfunction in chronic uremia.* Dordrecht: The Netherlands, Kluwer Academic Publishers, 1992:267.
10. Bennett WM. Renal effects of cyclosporine. *J Am Acad Dermatol* 1990;23:1280.
11. Ochs HR, et al. Disease-related alterations in cardiac glycoside disposition. *Clin Pharmacokinet* 1982;7:434.
12. Gulyassy PF, Depner TA. Impaired binding of drugs and endogenous ligands in renal disease. *Am J Kidney Dis* 1983;98:730.
13. McNamara PJ, Lalka D, Gibaldi M. Endogenous accumulation products and serum protein binding in uremia. *J Lab Clin Med* 1981;98:730.
14. Golper TA, Bennett WM. Drug usage in dialysis patients. In: Nissenson A, Fine R, Gentile D, eds. *Clinical dialysis,* 2nd ed. Norwalk, CT: Appleton & Lange, 1988.
15. Lee CC, Marbury TC. Drug therapy in patients undergoing haemodialysis. *Clin Pharmacokinet* 1984;9:42.

16. Vos MC, et al. Drug clearance by continuous hemodiafiltration (CAVHD): II. Results with the AN-69 capillary hemofilter and recommended dose adjustments. *Blood Purif* 1993;11:19.

17. Piafsky KM. Disease-induced changes in the plasma binding of basic drugs. *Clin Pharmacokinet* 1980;5:246.

18. Drayer D. Active drug metabolites and renal failure. *Am J Med* 1977;62:486.

19. Kirchner KA, Voelker JR, Brater DC. Binding inhibitors restore furosemide potency in tubule fluid containing albumin. *Kidney Int* 1991;40:418.

20. DeLuca HF, Krisinger J, Darwish H. The vitamin D system: 1990. *Kidney Int* 1990;29[Suppl]:S2.

21. Rabkin R, et al. Effect of renal disease on renal uptake and excretion of insulin in man. *N Engl J Med* 1970;282:182.

22. Cockcroft DW, Gault MH. Prediction of creatinine clearance from serum creatinine. *Nephron* 1976;16:31.

23. Vincent HH, et al. Drug clearance by continuous haemodiafiltration (CAVHD): analysis of sieving coefficients and mass transfer coefficients of diffusion. *Blood Purif* 1993;11:99.

24. Keller F, et al. Effect of plasma protein binding, volume of distribution, and molecular weight on the fraction of drugs eliminated by hemodialysis. *Clin Nephrol* 1983;19:201.

25. Lasrich M, et al. Correlation of peritoneal transport rates with molecular weight: a method of predicting clearances. *Am Soc Artif Intern Organs J* 1979;2:107.

26. Dromgoole SH. The effect of hemodialysis on the binding capacity of albumin. *Clin Chim Acta* 1973;46:469.

27. Rustein DD, Catelli WP, Nickerson RJ. Heparin and human lipid metabolism. *Lancet* 1969;ii:1003.

28. Suh B, et al. Effect of free fatty acids on protein binding of antimicrobial agents. *J Infect Dis* 1981;143:609.

29. Golper TA, Saad AMA, Morris CD. Gentamicin and phenytoin sieving through hollow-fiber polysulfone hemofilters. *Kidney Int* 1986;30:937.

30. Fabris A, et al. Total solute extraction versus clearance in the evaluation of standard and short hemodialysis. *Trans Am Soc Artif Intern Organs* 1988;34:627.

31. Sprenger KGB, et al. Optimizing of hemodiafiltration with modern membranes? *Contrib Nephrol* 1985;46:43.

32. De Bock V, et al. Pharmacokinetics of vancomycin in patients undergoing hemodialysis and hemofiltration. *Nephrol Dial Transplant* 1989;4:635.

33. Matzke GR, et al. Disposition of vancomycin during hemofiltration. *Clin Pharm Ther* 1986;40:425.

34. Marbury TC, et al. Hemodialysis clearance of ethosuximide in patients with chronic renal disease. *Am J Hosp Pharm* 1981;38:1757.

35. Lee CS, Marbury TC, Benet LZ. Clearance calculations in hemodialysis: application to blood, plasma, and dialysate measurements for ethambutol. *J Pharmacokinet Biopharmacokinet* 1980;8:69.

36. Levy G. Pharmacokinetics in renal disease. *Am J Med* 1977;62:461.

37. Gibson TP. Problems in designing hemodialysis drug studies. *Pharmacotherapy* 1985;5:23.

38. Brunner H, et al. Permeability for middle and higher molecular weight substances. *Contrib Nephrol* 1985;46:33.

39. Lanese DM, Alfrey PS, Molitoris BA. Markedly increased clearance of vancomycin during hemodialysis using polysulfone dialyzers. *Kidney Int* 1989;35:1409.

40. Bastani R, et al. In vivo comparison of three different hemodialysis membranes for vancomycin clearance: cuprophan, cellulose acetate, and polyacrylonitrile. *Dial Transplant* 1988;17:527.

41. Barth RH, et al. Vancomycin pharmacokinetics in high-flux hemodialysis. *ASN Abstract* 1990:348.

42. Agarwal R, Toto RD. Gentamicin clearance during hemodialysis: a comparison of high-efficiency cuprammonium rayon and conventional cellulose ester hemodialyzers. *Am J Kidney Dis* 1993;22:296.

43. Jindal K, McDougall J, Goldstein M. High flux dialyzers: impact of ultrafiltration and surface area on clearance of small and large molecular weight substances. *Natl Kidney Found* 1987;A10(abst).

44. Von Albertini B, et al. Performance characteristics of high flux haemodiafiltration. *Proc Eur Dial Transplant* 1984;21:447.

45. Surian M, et al. Adequacy of haemodiafiltration. *Nephrol Dial Transplant* 1989;4:32.

46. Rumpf KW, et al. Drug elimination by hemofiltration. *J Dial* 1977;1:677.

47. Ernest D, Cutler DJ. Gentamicin clearance during continuous arteriovenous hemodiafiltration. *Crit Care Med* 1992;20:586.

48. Rumpf KW, et al. Binding of antibiotics by dialysis membranes and its clinical relevance. *Proc EDTA* 1978;14:607.

49. Kraft D, Lode H. Elimination of ampicillin and gentamicin by hemofiltration. *Klin Wochenschr* 1979;57:195.

50. Kronfol NO, Lau AH, Barakat MM. Aminoglycoside binding to polyacrylonitrile hemofilter membranes during continuous hemofiltration. *Trans ASAIO* 1987;33:300.

51. Kronfol NO, et al. Effect of CAVH membrane types on drug sieving coefficients and clearances. *Trans ASAIO* 1986;32:85.

52. Lau A, et al. Determinants of drug removal by continuous arteriovenous hemofiltration. *Drug Intell Clin Pharm* 1986;20:467.

53. Kronfol NO, et al. Effect of membrane properties on drug clearances by CAVH. Abstracts from the National Kidney Foundation Annual Meeting 1986;A10.

54. Henderson LW. Hemodialysis: rationale and physical principles. In: Brenner BM, Rector FC, eds. *The kidney* Philadelphia: WB Saunders, 1976:1643.

55. Husted FC, et al. Detrimental effects of ultrafiltration on diffusion in coils. *J Lab Clin Med* 1976;87:435.

56. Nolph KD, New DL. Effects of ultrafiltration on solute clearances in hollow fiber artificial kidneys. *J Lab Clin Med* 1976;88:593.

57. Nolph KD, Hopkins C, Van Stone J. Effects of ultrafiltration on solute clearances in parallel plate dialyzers. *Clin Nephrol* 1977;8:453.

58. Henderson LW, et al. Clinical response to maintenance hemodiafiltration. *Kidney Int Suppl* 1975;2:S58.

59. Hamilton R, et al. Blood cleansing by diafiltration in uremic dog and man. *Trans Am Soc Artif Intern Organs* 1971;17:259.

60. Henderson LW, et al. Uremic blood cleansing by diafiltration using hollow-fiber ultrafilter. *Trans Am Soc Artif Intern Organs* 1970;16:107.

61. Jaffrin MY, Ding L, Laurent JM. Simultaneous convective and diffusive mass transfers in a hemodialyzer. *J Biomech Eng* 1990;112:212.

62. Vincent HH, et al. Solute transport in continuous arteriovenous hemodiafiltration: a new mathematical model applied to clinical data. *Blood Purif* 1990;8:149.

63. Torras J, et al. Pharmacokinetics of vancomycin in patients undergoing hemodialysis with polyacrylonitrile. *Clin Nephrol* 1991;36:35.

64. Colton CK, et al. Kinetics of hemodiafiltration: I. in vitro transport characteristics of a hollow fiber blood ultrafilter. *J Lab Clin Med* 1975;85:355.

65. Golper TA, et al. Drug removal during CAVH: theory and clinical observations. *Intern J Artif Organs* 1985;8:307.

66. Ronco C, et al. Permeability characteristics of polysulfonic membranes in CAVH. In: Sieberth HG, Mann H, eds. *Continuous arteriovenous hemofiltration (CAVH)*. Basel: Karger, 1985:59.

67. Golper TA, Saad AM. Gentamicin and phenytoin in vitro sieving characteristics through polysulfone hemofilters: effect of flow rate, drug concentration and solvent systems. *Kidney Int* 1986;30:937.

68. Frigon RP, et al. Hemofilter solute sieving is not governed by dynamically polarized protein. *Trans ASAIO* 1984;30:486.

69. Lysaght MJ. An experimental model for the ultrafiltration of sodium ion from blood or plasma. *Blood Purif* 1983;1:25.

70. Leypoldt JK, Frigon RP, Henderson LW. Macromolecular charge affects hemofilter solute sieving. *Trans ASAIO* 1986;32:384.

71. Kaplan AA, Longnecker RE, Folkert VW. Continuous arteriovenous hemofiltration—a report of 6 months' experience. *Ann Intern Med* 1984;100:358.

72. Paganini EP, et al. Amino acid balance in patients with oliguric renal failure undergoing slow continuous ultrafiltration (SCUF). *Trans ASAIO* 1982;28:615.

73. Kroh U, et al. Dosisanpassung von pharmaka wahrend kontinuierlicher hamofiltration. *Anaesthesist* 1989;38:225.

74. Leypoldt JK, Frigon RP, Henderson LW. Dextran sieving coefficients of hemofilter membranes. *Trans ASAIO* 1983;29:678.

75. Dodd NJ, et al. Arteriovenous hemofiltration: a recent advance in the management of renal failure. *Br Med J* 1983;287:1008.

76. Bennett WM, et al. *Drug prescribing in renal failure: dosing guidelines for adults*, 2nd ed. Philadelphia: American College of Physicians, 1991.

77. Keller E, Reetze P, Schollmeyer P. Drug therapy in patients undergoing continuous ambulatory peritoneal dialysis. *Clin Pharmacokin* 1990;18(2):104.

78. Reetze-Bonorden P, Böhler J, Keller E. Drug dosage in patients during continuous renal replacement therapy. *Clin Pharmacokin* 1993;24(5):362.

79. Goldman M, Vanherweghem J. Bacterial infections in chronic hemodialysis patients: epidemiologic and pathophysiologic aspects. *Adv Nephrol* 1990;19:315.

80. Mailloux SU, et al. Mortality in dialysis patients: analysis of the causes of death. *Am J Kidney Dis* 1991;18(3):326.

81. Manian FA, Stone WJ, Alford RH. Adverse antibiotic effects associated with renal insufficiency. *Rev Infect Dis* 1990;12(2):236.

82. Siegel D. Tetracyclines: new look at old antibiotic. *NY State J Med* 1978;78:950.

83. Vance-Bryan K, Guay DRP, Rotschafer JC. Clinical pharmacokinetics of ciprofloxacin. *Clin Pharmacokinet* 1990;19(6):434.

84. Paap CM, Nahata MC. Clinical use of trimethoprim/sulfamethoxazole during renal dysfunction. *Ann Pharmacother* 1989;23:646.

85. Gilbert DN. Once-daily aminoglycoside therapy. *Antimicrob Agents Chemother* 1991;35:399.

86. Wood CA, et al. The influence of tobramycin dosage regimens on nephrotoxicity, ototoxicity, and antibacterial efficacy in a rat model of subcutaneous abscess. *J Infect Dis* 1988;158:13.

87. Johnson CA, Zimmerman SW, Rogge M. The pharmacokinetics of antibiotics used to treat peritoneal dialysis-associated peritonitis. *Am J Kidney Dis* 1984;4(1):3.

88. Keane WF, et al. Peritoneal dialysis-related peritonitis treatment recommendations: 1993 update. *Peritoneal Dial Int* 1993;13:14.

89. Humes HD. Aminoglycoside nephrotoxicity. *Kidney Int* 1988;33:900.

90. Cameron JS. Allergic interstitial nephritis: clinical features and pathogenesis. *Q J Med* 1988;66:97.

91. Shouval D, Ligumsky M, Ben-Ishay D. Effect of co-trimoxazole on normal creatinine clearance. *Lancet* 1978;i:244.

92. Ayneck ML, Berardi RR, Johnson RM. Interference of cephalosporins and cefoxitin with serum creatinine determination. Am J Hosp Pharm 1981;38:1348.

93. Baron DN, Hamilton-Miller JMT, Brumfitt W. Sodium content of injectable β-lactam antibiotics. *Lancet* 1984;i:1113.

94. Blaser J, et al. Increase of amikacin half-life during therapy in patients with renal insufficiency. *Antimicrob Agents Chemother* 1983;23:888.

95. Lanao JM, et al. Pharmacokinetics of amikacin (BB-K8) in patients undergoing hemodialysis. *Int J Clin Pharmacol Biopharm* 1979;17:357.

96. Smeltzer BD, Schwartzman MS, Bertino JS. Amikacin pharmacokinetics during continuous ambulatory peritoneal dialysis. *Antimicrob Agents Chemother* 1988;32:236.

97. Goetz DR, et al. Prediction of serum gentamicin concentrations in patients undergoing hemodialysis. *Am J Hosp Pharm* 1980;37:1077.

98. Gyselynck A, Forrey A, Cutler R. Pharmacokinetics of gentamicin: distribution and plasma and renal clearance. *J Infect Dis* 1971;124[Suppl]:S70.

99. Zarowitz BJ, et al. Continuous arteriovenous hemofiltration of aminoglycoside antibiotics in critically ill patients. *J Clin Pharmacol* 1986;26:686.

100. Healy JK, Drum PJ, Elliott AJ. Kanamycin dosage in renal failure. *Aust NZ J Med* 1973;3:474.

101. Campoli-Richards DM, et al. Netilmicin: a review of its antibacterial activity, pharmacokinetic properties and therapeutic use. *Drugs* 1989;38:703.

102. Herrero A, et al. Pharmacokinetics of netilmicin in renal insufficiency and hemodialysis. *Int J Clin Pharmacol Ther* 1988;26:84.

103. Pechere J, Dugal R, Pechere M. Pharmacokinetics of netilmicin in renal insufficiency and haemodialysis. *Clin Pharmacokinet* 1978;3:395.

104. Brogden RN, et al. Tobramycin: a review of its antibacterial and pharmacokinetic properties and therapeutic use. *Drugs* 1976;12:166.

105. Pechère J, Dugal R. Pharmacokinetics of intravenously administered tobramycin in normal volunteers and in renal-impaired and hemodialyzed patients. *J Infect Dis* 1976;134:S118.

106. Wise R. The pharmacokinetics of the oral caphalosporins—a review. *J Antimicrob Chemother* 1990;26[Suppl E]:13.

107. Gartenberg G, et al. Pharmacokinetics of cefaclor in patients with stable renal impairment, and patients undergoing haemodialysis. *J Antimicrob Chemother* 1979;5:465.

108. Leroy A, Humbert G, Godin M. Pharmacokinetics of cefadroxil in patients with impaired renal function. *J Antimicrob Chemother* 1982;10[Suppl B]:39.

109. Bliss M, et al. Disposition kinetics of cefamandole during continuous ambulatory peritoneal dialysis. *Antimicrob Agents Chemother* 1986;29(4):649.

110. Brogard JM, et al. Cefamandole pharmacokinetics and dosage adjustments in relation to renal function. *J Clin Pharmacol* 1979;19(7):366.

111. Bergen T, Brodwall EK, <asO>rjavik <asO>. Pharmacokinetics of cefazolin in patients with normal and impaired renal function. *J Antimicrob Chemother* 1977;3:435.

112. Guay DRP, et al. Pharmacokinetics of cefixime (CL 284635; FK027) in healthy subjects and patients with renal insufficiency. *Antimicrob Agents Chemother* 1986;30(3):485.

113. Campoli-Richards DM, Todd PA. Cefmenoxime: a review of its antibacterial activity, pharmacokinetic properties and therapeutic use. *Drugs* 1987;34:188.

114. Evers J, Borner K, Koeppe P. Elimination of cefmenoxime during continuous haemofiltration. *Eur J Clin Pharmacol* 1993;44[Suppl 1]:S31.

115. Konishi K. Pharmacokinetics of cefmenoxime in patients with impaired renal function and in those undergoing hemodialysis. *Antimicrob Agents Chemother* 1986;30(6):901.

116. Halstenson CE, et al. Disposition of cefmetazole in healthy volunteers and patients with impaired renal function. *Antimicrob Agents Chemother* 1990;34(4):519.

117. Schentag JJ. Cefmetazole sodium: pharmacology, pharmacokinetics, and clinical trials. *Pharmacotherapy* 1991;11(1):2.

118. Blair AD, et al. Cefonicid kinetics in subjects with normal and impaired renal function. *Clin Pharmacol Ther* 1984;35(6):798.

119. Saltiel E, Brogden RN. Cefonicid: a review of its antibacterial activity, pharmacological properties and therapeutic use. *Drugs* 1986;32:222.

120. Greenfield RA, Gerber AU, Craig WA. Pharmacokinetics of cefoperazone in patients with normal and impaired hepatic and renal function. *Rev Infect Dis* 1983;5[Suppl]:S127.

121. Hodler JE, et al. Pharmacokinetics of cefoperazone in patients undergoing chronic ambulatory peritoneal dialysis: clinical and pathophysiological implications. *Eur J Clin Pharmacol* 1984;26:609.

122. Campoli-Richards DM, Lackner TE, Monk JP. Ceforanide: a review of its antibacterial activity, pharmacokinetic properties and clinical efficacy. *Drugs* 1987;34:411.

123. Hess JR, et al. Pharmacokinetics of ceforanide in patients with end stage renal disease on hemodialysis. *Antimicrob Agents Chemother* 1980;17(2):251.

124. Matzke GR, et al. Cefotaxime and desacetyl cefotaxime kinetics in renal impairment. *Clin Pharmacol Ther* 1985;38:31.

125. Todd PA, Brogden RN. Cefotaxime: an update of its pharmacology and therapeutic use. *Drugs* 1990;40(4):608.

126. Ohkawa M, Hirano S, Tokunaga S. Pharmacokinetics of cefotetan in normal subjects and patients with impaired renal function. *Antimicrob Agents Chemother* 1983;23(1):31.

127. Ward A, Richards DM. Cefotetan: a review of its antibacterial activity, pharmacokinetic properties and therapeutic use. *Drugs* 1985;30:382.

128. Greaves WL, et al. Cefoxitin disposition during peritoneal dialysis. *Antimicrob Agents Chemother* 1981;19(2):253.

129. Humbert G, et al. Pharmacokinetics of cefoxitin in normal subjects and in patients with renal insufficiency. *Rev Infect Dis* 1979;1(1):118.

130. Nikolaidis P, Tourkantonis A. Effect of hemodialysis on ceftazidime pharmacokinetics. *Clin Nephrol* 1985;24(3):142.

131. Richards DM, Brogden RN. Ceftazidime: a review of its antibacterial activity, pharmacokinetic properties and therapeutic use. *Drugs* 1985;29:105.

132. Tourkantonis A, Nicolaidis P. Pharmacokinetics of ceftazidime in patients undergoing peritoneal dialysis. *J Antimicrob Chemother* 1983;12[Suppl A]:263.

133. Welage LS, Schultz RW, Schentag JJ. Pharmacokinetics of ceftazidime in patients with renal insufficiency. *Antimicrob Agents Chemother* 1984;25(2):201.

134. Burgess ED, Blair AD. Pharmacokinetics of ceftizoxime in patients undergoing continuous ambulatory peritoneal dialysis. *Antimicrob Agents Chemother* 1983;24(2):237.

135. Gross ML, et al. Ceftizoxime elimination kinetics in continuous ambulatory peritoneal dialysis. *Clin Pharmacol Ther* 1983;34(5):673.

136. Kowalsky SF, et al. Pharmacokinetics of ceftizoxime in subjects with various degrees of renal function. *Antimicrob Agents Chemother* 1983;24(2):151.

137. Richards DM, Heel RC. Ceftizoxime: a review of its antibacterial activity, pharmacokinetic properties and therapeutic use. *Drugs* 1985;29:281.

138. Patel IH, et al. Ceftriaxone pharmacokinetics in patients with various degrees of renal impairment. *Antimicrob Agents Chemother* 1984;25(4):438.

139. Ti T, et al. Kinetic disposition of intravenous ceftriaxone in normal subjects and patients with renal failure on hemodialysis or peritoneal dialysis. *Antimicrob Agents Chemother* 1984;25(1):83.

140. Yuk JH, Nightingale CH, Quintiliani R. Clinical pharmacokinetics of ceftriaxone. *Clin Pharmacokinet* 1989;17(4):223.

141. Höffler D, Koeppe P, Schleith A. Pharmacokinetics of cefuroxime-axetil in patients undergoing haemodialysis therapy. *Acta Therapeutica* 1991;17:107.

142. Konishi K, et al. Pharmacokinetics of cefuroxime axetil in patients with normal and impaired renal function. *J Antimicrob Chemother* 1993;31:413.

143. Weiss LG, et al. Pharmacokinetics of intravenous cefuroxime during intermittent and continuous arteriovenous hemofiltration. *Clin Nephrol* 1988;30(5):282.

144. Bailey RR, Gower PE, Dash CH. The effects of impairment of renal function and haemodialysis on serum and urine levels of cephalexin. *Postgrad Med J* 1970;46[Suppl]:60.

145. Venuto RC, Plaut M. Cephalothin handling in patients undergoing hemodialysis. *Antimicrob Agents Chemother* 1970;10:50.

146. McCloskey RV, et al. Effect of hemodialysis and renal failure on serum and urine concentrations of cephapirin sodium. *Antimicrob Agents Chemother* 1972;1:90.

147. Solomon AE, Briggs JD. The administration of cephradine to patients in renal failure. *Br J Clin Pharmacol* 1975;2:443.

148. Bolton WK, et al. Pharmacokinetics of moxalactam in subjects with various degrees of renal dysfunction. *Antimicrob Agents Chemother* 1980;18(6):933.

149. Carmine AA, et al. Moxalactam: a review of its antibacterial activity, pharmacokinetic properties and therapeutic use. *Drugs* 1983;26:279.

150. Srinivasan S, Neu HC. Pharmacokinetics of moxalactam in patients with renal failure and during hemodialysis. *Antimicrob Agents Chemother* 1981;20(3):398.

151. Peters DH, Clissold SP. Clarithromycin: a review of its antimicrobial activity, pharmacokinetic properties and therapeutic potential. *Drugs* 1992;44(1):117.

152. Disse B, et al. Pharmacokinetics of erythromycin in patients with different degrees of renal impairment. *Int J Clin Pharmacol Ther Toxicol* 1986;24(9):460.

153. Kanfer A, et al. Changes in erythromycin pharmacokinetics induced by renal failure. *Clin Nephrol* 1987;27(3):147.

154. Blum RA, et al. Pharmacokinetics of ampicillin (2.0 grams) and sulbactam (1.0 gram) coadministered to subjects with normal and abnormal renal function and with end-stage renal disease on hemodialysis. *Antimicrob Agents Chemother* 1989;33:1470.

155. Francke EL, Appel GB, Neu HC. Kinetics of intravenous amoxicillin in patients on long-term dialysis. *Clin Pharmacol Ther* 1979;26:31.

156. Humbert G, et al. Pharmacokinetics of amoxicillin: dosage nomogram for patients with impaired renal function. *Antimicrob Agents Chemother* 1979;15:28.

157. Todd PA, Benfield P. Amoxicillin/clavulanic acid: an update of its antibacterial activity, pharmacokinetic properties and therapeutic use. *Drugs* 1990;39:264.

158. Leroy A, et al. Pharmacokinetics of azlocillin in subjects with normal and impaired renal function. *Antimicrob Agents Chemother* 1980;17:344.

159. Whelton A, Stout RL, Delgado FA. Azlocillin kinetics during extracorporeal haemodialysis and peritoneal dialysis. *J Antimicrob Chemother* 1983;11S[Suppl B]:89.

160. Aronoff GR, et al. Mezlocillin pharmacokinetics in renal impairment. *Clin Pharmacol Ther* 1980;28:523.

161. Kampf D, et al. Effects of impaired renal function, hemodialysis, and peritoneal dialysis on the pharmacokinetics of mezlocillin. *Antimicrob Agents Chemother* 1980;18:81.

162. Holmes B, et al. Piperacillin: a review of its antibacterial activity, pharmacokinetic properties and therapeutic use. *Drugs* 1984;28:375.

163. De Schepper PJ, et al. Comparative pharmacokinetics of piperacillin in normals and in patients with renal failure. *J Antimicrob Chemother* 1982;9[Suppl B]:49.

164. Welling PG, et al. Pharmacokinetics of piperacillin in subjects with various degrees of renal function. *Antimicrob Agents Chemother* 1983;23:881.

165. Parry MF, Neu HC. Pharmacokinetics of ticarcillin in patients with abnormal renal function. *J Infect Dis* 1976;133:46.

166. Davies SP, et al. Pharmacokinetics of ciprofloxacin and vancomycin in patients with acute renal failure treated by continuous haemodialysis. *Nephrol Dial Transplant* 1992;7:848.

167. Kowalsky SF, et al. Pharmacokinetics of ciprofloxacin in subjects with varying degrees of renal function and undergoing hemodialysis or CAPD. *Clin Nephrol* 1993;39(1):53.

168. Neuman M. Clinical pharmacokinetics of the newer antibacterial 4-quinolones. *Clin Pharmacokinet* 1988;14:96.

169. Henwood JM, Monk JP. Enoxacin: a review of its antibacterial activity, pharmacokinetic properties and therapeutic use. *Drugs* 1988;36:32.

170. Nix DE, Schultz RW, Frost RW. The effect of renal impairment and haemodialysis on single dose pharmacokinetics of oral enoxacin. *J Antimicrob Chemother* 1988;21[Suppl B]:87.

171. Weidekamm E. Pharmacokinetics of fleroxacin in renal impairment. *Am J Med* 1993;94[Suppl 3A]:70S.

172. Holmes B, Brogden RN, Richards DM. Norfloxacin: a review of its antibacterial activity, pharmacokinetic properties and therapeutic use. *Drugs* 1985;30:482.

173. Lameire N, et al. Ofloxacin pharmacokinetics in chronic renal failure and dialysis. *Clin Pharmacokinet* 1991;21(5):357.

174. Saivin S, Houin G. Clinical pharmacokinetics of doxycycline and minocycline. *Clin Pharmacokinet* 1988;15:355.

175. Fillastre JP, et al. Pharmacokinetics of aztreonam in patients with chronic renal failure. *Clin Pharmacokinet* 1985;10:91.

176. Gerig JS, et al. Effect of hemodialysis and peritoneal dialysis on aztreonam pharmacokinetics. *Kidney Int* 1984;26:308.

177. Ambrose PJ. Clinical pharmacokinetics of chloramphenicol and chloramphenicol succinate. *Clin Pharmacokinet* 1984;9:222.

178. Buckley MM, et al. Imipenem/cilastatin: a reappraisal of its antibacterial activity, pharmacokinetic properties and therapeutic efficacy. *Drugs* 1992;44:408.

179. Gibson TP, Devetriades JL, Bland JA. Imipenem/cilastatin: pharmacokinetic profile in renal insufficiency. *Am J Med* 1985;78[Suppl 6A]:54.

180. Konishi K, et al. Removal of imipenem and cilastatin by hemodialysis in patients with end-stage renal failure. *Antimicrob Agents Chemother* 1991;35(8):1616.

181. Vos MC, Vincent HH, Yzerman EPF. Clearance of imipenem/cilastatin in acute renal failure patients treated by continuous hemodiafiltration (CAVHD). *Intensive Care Med* 1992;18:282.

182. Roberts AP, et al. Serum and plasma concentrations of clindamycin following a single intramuscular injection of clindamycin phosphate in maintenance haemodialysis patients and normal subjects. *Eur J Clin Pharmacol* 1978;14:435.

183. Hamilton-Miller JMT, Brumfitt W. Methenamine and its salts as urinary tract antiseptics: variables affecting the antibacterial activity of formaldehyde, mandelic acid, and hippuric acid in vitro. *Inv Urol* 1977;14(4):287.

184. Guay DR, et al. Pharmacokinetics of metronidazole in patients undergoing continuous ambulatory peritoneal dialysis. *Antimicrob Agents Chemother* 1984;25(3):306.

185. Kreeft JH, Ogilvie RI, Dufresne LR. Metronidazole kinetics in dialysis patients. *Surgery* 1983;93(1):149.

186. Lau AH, et al. Clinical pharmacokinetics of metronidazole and other nitroimidazole anti-infectives. *Clin Pharmacokinet* 1992;23(5):328.

187. Shermantine M, et al. Pharmacokinetics of sulfisoxazole in renal transplant patients. *Antimicrob Agents Chemother* 1985;28(4):535.

188. Bonati M, et al. Teicoplanin pharmacokinetics in patients with chronic renal failure. *Clin Pharmacokinet* 1987;12:292.

189. Campoli-Richards DM, Brogden RN, Faulds D. Teicoplanin: a review of its antibacterial activity, pharmacokinetic properties and therapeutic potential. *Drugs* 1990;40(3):449.

190. Moellering RC, Krogstad DJ, Greenblatt DJ. Vancomycin therapy in patients with impaired renal function: a nomogram for dosage. *Ann Intern Med* 1981;94:343.

191. Nielson HE, Sorenson I, Hansen HE. Peritoneal transport of vancomycin during peritoneal dialysis. *Nephron* 1979;24:274.

192. Daneshmend TK, Warnock DW. Clinical pharmacokinetics of systemic antifungal drugs. *Clin Pharmacokinet* 1983;8:17.

193. Lyman CA, Walsh TJ. Systemically administered antifungal agents: a review of their clinical pharmacology and therapeutic applications. *Drugs* 1992;44:9.

194. Craven PC, et al. Excretion pathways of amphotericin B. *J Infect Dis* 1979;140:329.

195. Morgan DJ, et al. Elimination of amphotericin B in impaired renal function. *Clin Pharmacol Ther* 1983;34:248.

196. Janknegt R, et al. Liposomal and lipid formulations of amphotericin B. *Clin Pharmacokinet* 1992;23:279.

197. Cleary JD, Taylor JW, Chapman SW. Imidazoles and triazoles in antifungal therapy. *Ann Pharmacother* 1990;24:148.

198. Bailey EM, Krakovsky DJ, Rybak MJ. The triazole antifungal agents: a review of itraconazole and fluconazole. *Pharmacotherapy* 1990;10:146.

199. Toon S, et al. An assessment of the effects of impaired renal function and haemodialysis on the pharmacokinetics of fluconazole. *Br J Clin Pharmacol* 1990;29:221.

200. Oono S, et al. The pharmacokinetics of fluconazole during haemodialysis in uraemic patients. *Eur J Clin Pharmacol* 1992;42:667.

201a. Debruyne D, Ryckelynck J. Clinical pharmacokinetics of fluconazole. *Clin Pharmacokinet* 1993;24:10.

201b. Bennett JE. Flucytosine. *Ann Intern Med* 1977;86:319.

202. Cutler RE, Blair AD, Kelly MR. Flucytosine kinetics in subjects with normal and impaired renal function. *Clin Pharmacol Ther* 1978;24:333.

203. Eisenberg ES. Intraperitoneal flucytosine in the management of fungal peritonitis in patients on continuous ambulatory peritoneal dialysis. *Am J Kidney Dis* 1988;11:465.

204. Boelaert J, et al. Itraconazole pharmacokinetics in patients with renal dysfunction. *Antimicrob Agents Chemother* 1988;32:1595.

205. Grant SM, Clissold SP. Itraconazole: a review of its pharmacodynamic and pharmacokinetic properties, and therapeutic use in superficial and systemic mycoses. *Drugs* 1989;37:310.

206. Daneshmen TK, Warnock DW. Clinical pharmacokinetics of ketoconazole. *Clin Pharmacokinet* 1988;14:13.

207. Lewi PJ, et al. Pharmacokinetic profile of intravenous miconazole in man. *Eur J Clin Pharmacol* 1976;10:49.

208. White JW. Clinical pharmacokinetics of antimalarial drugs. *Clin Pharmacokinet* 1985;10:187.

209. White NJ. Antimalarial pharmacokinetics and treatment regimens. *Br J Clin Pharmacol* 1992;34:1.

210. Edwards G, Breckenridge AM Clinical pharmacokinetics of antihelminthic drugs. *Clin Pharmacokinet* 1988;15:67.

211. Keystone JS, Murdoch JK. Mebendazole. *Ann Intern Med* 1979; 91:582.

212. Palmer KJ, Holliday SM, Brogden RN. Mefloquine: a review of its antimalarial activity, pharmacokinetic properties and therapeutic efficacy. *Drugs* 1993;45(3):430.

213. Goa KL, Compoli-Richards DM. Pentamidine isethionate: a review of its antiprotozoal activity, pharmacokinetic properties and therapeutic use in *Pneumocystis carinii* pneumonia. *Drugs* 1987;33:242.

214. Conte JE. Pharmacokinetics of intravenous pentamidine in patients with normal renal function or receiving hemodialysis. *J Infect Dis* 1991;163:169.

215. King CH, Mahmoud AAF. Drugs five years later: praziquantel. *Ann Intern Med* 1989;110:290.

216. Lehmann CR, et al. Capreomycin kinetics in renal impairment and clearance by hemodialysis. *Am Rev Respir Dis* 1988;138:1312.

217. Varughese A, et al. Ethambutol kinetics in patients with impaired renal function. *Am Rev Respir Dis* 1986;134:34.

218. Weber WW, Hein DW. Clinical pharmacokinetics of isoniazid. *Clin Pharmacokinet* 1979;4:401.

219. Lacroix C, et al. Haemodialysis of pyrazinamide in uraemic patients. *Eur J Clin Pharmacol* 1989;37:309.

220. Stamatikis G, et al. Pyrazinamide and pyrazinoic acid pharmacokinetics in patients with chronic renal failure. *Clin Nephrol* 1988;30:230.

221. Acocella G. Clinical pharmacokinetics of rifampicin. *Clin Pharmacokinet* 1978;3:108.

222. Burgess ED, Gill MJ. Intraperitoneal administration of acyclovir in patients receiving continuous ambulatory peritoneal dialysis. *J Clin Pharmacol* 1990;30:997.

223. Laskin OL, et al. Acyclovir kinetics in end-stage renal disease. *Clin Pharmacol Ther* 1982;31:594.

224. O'Brien JJ, Campoli-Richards DM. Acyclovir: an updated review of its antiviral activity, pharmacokinetic properties and therapeutic efficacy. *Drugs* 1989;37:233.

225. Aoki FY, Sitar DS. Clinical pharmacokinetics of amantadine hydrochloride. *Clin Pharmacokinet* 1988;14:35.

226. Horadam VW, et al. Pharmacokinetics of amantadine hydrochloride in subjects with normal and impaired renal function. *Ann Intern Med* 1981;94(1):454.

227. Wu MJ, et al. Amantadine hydrochloride pharmacokinetics in patients with impaired renal function. *Clin Nephrol* 1982;17(1):19.

228. Morse GD, Shelton MJ, O'Donnell AM. Comparative pharmacokinetics of antiviral nucleoside analogues. *Clin Pharmacokinet* 1993;24:101.

229. Faulds D, Brogden RN. Didanosine: a review of its antiviral activity, pharmacokinetic properties and therapeutic potential in human immunodeficiency virus infection. *Drugs* 1992;44(1):94.

230. Chrisp P, Clissold SP. Foscarnet: a review of its antiviral activity, pharmacokinetic properties and therapeutic use in immunocompromised patients with cytomegalovirus retinitis. *Drugs* 1991;41(1):104.

231. Faulds D, Heel RC. Ganciclovir: a review of its antiviral activity, pharmacokinetic properties and therapeutic efficacy in cytomegalovirus infections. *Drugs* 1990;39(4):597.

232. Kramer TH, et al. Hemodialysis clearance of intravenously administered ribavirin. *Antimicrob Agents Chemother* 1990;34(3):489.

233. Aronoff GR, et al. Hypoxanthine-arabinoside pharmacokinetics after adenine arabinoside administration to a patient with renal failure. *Antimicrob Agents Chemother* 1980;18(1):212.

234. Collins JM, Unadkat JD. Clinical pharmacokinetics of zidovudine: an overview of current data. *Clin Pharmacokinet* 1989;17(1):1.

235. Gallicano KD, et al. Pharmacokinetics of single and chronic dose zidovudine in two HIV positive patients undergoing continuous ambulatory peritoneal dialysis (CAPD). *J Acquir Immune Defic Syndr* 1992;5:242.

236. Garraffo R, et al. Influence of hemodialysis on zidovudine (AZT) and its glucuronide (GAZT) pharmacokinetics: two case reports. *Int J Clin Pharmacol Ther Toxicol* 1989;27(11):535.

237. Gleason JR, Brier ME. Zidovudine in renal failure. *Semin Dial* 1990;3(2):101.

238. Chan GLC, Matzke GR. Effects of renal insufficiency on the pharmacokinetics and pharmacodynamics of opioid analgesics. *Drug Intell Clin Pharm* 1987;21:773.

239. Szeto HH, et al. Accumulation of normeperidine active metabolite of meperidine, in patients with renal failure or cancer. *Ann Intern Med* 1977;86:738.

240. Agoston S, Vandenbrom RHG, Wierda JMKH. Clinical pharmacokinetics of neuromuscular blocking drugs. *Clin Pharmacokinet* 1992;22(2):94.

241. Horton MW, Byerly WG. Opioid analgesics. *Semin Dial* 1990; 3(3):187.

242. Heel RC, et al. Butorphanol: a review of its pharmacological properties and therapeutic efficacy. *Drugs* 1978;16:473.

243. Barnes JN, et al. Dihydrocodeine in renal failure: further evidence for an important role of the kidney in the handling of opioid drugs. *Br Med J* 1985;290:740.

244. Mather LE. Clinical pharmacokinetics of fentanyl and its newer derivatives. *Clin Pharmacokinet* 1983;8:422.

245. Kreek MJ, et al. Methadone use in patients with chronic renal disease. *Drug Alcohol Depend* 1980;5:197.

246. Chauvin M, et al. Morphine pharmacokinetics in renal failure. *Anesthesiology* 1987;66(3):327.

247. Säwe J. Odar-Cederlöl I. Kinetics of morphine in patients with renal failure. *Eur J Clin Pharmacol* 1987;32:377.

248. Giacomini KM, Gibson TP, Levy G. Effect of hemodialysis on propoxyphene and norpropoxyphene concentrations in blood of anephric patients. *Clin Pharmacol Ther* 1980;27(4):508.

249. Clissold SP. Paracetamol and phenacetin. *Drugs* 1986;32[Suppl 4]:46.

250. Prescott LF, et al. Paracetamol disposition and metabolite kinetics in patients with chronic renal failure. *Eur J Clin Pharmacol* 1989;36:291.

251. Sica DA, et al. Pharmacokinetics and protein binding of methocarbamol in renal insufficiency and normals. *Eur J Clin Pharmacol* 1990;39:193.

252. Needs CJ, Brooks PM. Clinical pharmacokinetics of the salicylates. *Clin Pharmacokinet* 1985;10:164.

253. Williams ME, Weinblatt M, Rosa RM. Salsalate kinetics in patients with chronic renal failure undergoing hemodialysis. *Clin Pharmacol Ther* 1986;39:420.

254. Davis PJ, Cook DR. Clinical pharmacokinetics of the newer intravenous anaesthetic agents. *Clin Pharmacokinet* 1986;11:18.

255. Pollard BJ. Neuromuscular blocking drugs and renal failure [Editorial]. *Br J Anaesth* 1992;68(6):545.

256. Gramstad L. Atracurium, vecuronium and pancuronium in end-stage renal failure. *Br J Anaesth* 1987;59:995.

257. Mongin-Long D, et al. Atracurium in patients with renal failure: clinical trial of a new neuromuscular blocker. *Br J Anaesth* 1986;58:44S.

258. Ramzan MI, Shanks CA, Triggs EJ. Gallamine disposition in surgical patients with chronic renal failure. *J Clin Pharmacol* 1981;12:141.

259. Brotherton WP, Matteo RS. Pharmacokinetics and pharmacodynamics of metocurine in humans with and without renal failure. *Anesthesiology* 1981;55(3):273.

260. Aquilonius S, Hartvig P. Clinical pharmacokinetics of cholinesterase inhibitors. *Clin Pharmacokinet* 1986;11:236.

261. McLeod K, Watson MJ, Rawlins MD. Pharmacokinetics of pancuronium in patients with normal and impaired renal function. *Br J Anaesth* 1976;48:341.

262. Kirvelä M, et al. Pharmacokinetics of propofol and haemodynamic changes during induction of anaesthesia in uraemic patients. *Br J Anaesth* 1992;68:178.

263. Cronnelly R, et al. Pyridostigmine kinetics with and without renal function. *Clin Pharmacol Ther* 1980;28:78.

264. Bishop M, Hornbein TF. Prolonged effect of succinylcholine after neostigmine and pyridostigmine administration in patients with renal failure. *Anesthesiology* 1983;58:384.

265. Matteo RS, et al. Pharmacokinetics of d-tubocurarine in man: effect of an osmotic diuretic on urinary excretion. *Anesthesiology* 1980;52:335.

266. Lynam DP, et al. The pharmacodynamics and pharmacokinetics of vecuronium in patients anesthetized with isoflurane with normal renal function or with renal failure. *Anesthesiology* 1988;69:227.

267. Agodoa LYC, Held PJ, Port FK. *Causes of death in U.S. Renal Data System, USRDS 1993 Annual Data Report*. Bethesda, MD: National Institutes of Health; National Institute of Diabetes and Digestive and Kidney Diseases, March 1993:49.

268. Parving H, et al. Effective antihypertensive treatment postpones renal insufficiency in diabetic nephropathy. *Am J Kidney Dis* 1993;22:188.

269. Castelli WP. Epidemiology of coronary heart disease: the Framingham Study. *Am J Med* 1984;76:4.

270. Anderson S, Rennke HG, Brenner BM. Therapeutic advantage of converting enzyme inhibitors in arresting progressive renal disease associated with systemic hypertension in the rat. *J Clin Invest* 1986;77:1993.

271. Brunner HR. ACE inhibitors in renal disease. *Kidney Int* 1992;42:463.

272. Lewis EJ, Hunsicker LG, Bain RP. The effect of angiotensin-converting-enzyme inhibition on diabetic nephropathy. *N Engl J Med* 1993;329(20):1456.

273. Hulter HN, et al. Clinical efficacy and pharmacokinetics of clonidine in hemodialysis and renal insufficiency. *J Lab Clin Med* 1979;94:223.

274. Lowenthal DT, Matzek KM, MacGregor TR. Clinical pharmacokinetics of clonidine. *Clin Pharmacokinet* 1988;14:287.

275. Carlson RV, et al. Pharmacokinetics and effect on blood pressure of doxazosin in normal subjects and patients with renal failure. *Clin Pharmacol Ther* 1986;40:561.

276. Young RA, Brogden RN. Doxazosin: a review of its pharmacodynamic and pharmacokinetic properties, and therapeutic efficacy in mild or moderate hypertension. *Drugs* 1988;35:525.

277. Holmes B, et al. Guanabenz: a review of its pharmacodynamic properties and therapeutic efficacy in hypertension. *Drugs* 1983;26:212.

278. Finnerty FA, Brogden RN. Guanadrel: a review of its pharmacodynamic and pharmacokinetic properties and therapeutic use in hypertension. *Drugs* 1985;30:22.

279. Halstenson CE, et al. Disposition of guanadrel in subjects with normal and impaired renal function. *J Clin Pharmacol* 1989;29:128.

280. Carchman SH, et al. Steady-state plasma levels and pharmacokinetics of guanfacine in patients with renal insufficiency. *Nephron* 1989;53:18.

281. Sorkin EM, Heel RC. Guanfacine: a review of its pharmacodynamic and pharmacokinetic properties, and therapeutic efficacy in the treatment of hypertension. *Drugs* 1986;31:301.

282. Myhre E, Rugstad HE, Hansen T. Clinical pharmacokinetics of methyldopa. *Clin Pharmacokinet* 1982;7:221.

283. Lameire N, Gordts J. A pharmacokinetic study of prazosin in patients with varying degrees of chronic renal failure. *Eur J Clin Pharmacol* 1986;31:333.

284. Vincent J, et al. Clinical pharmacokinetics of prazosin—1985. *Clin Pharmacokinet* 1985;10:144.

285. Zsoter TT, et al. Excretion and metabolism of reserpine in renal failure. *Clin Pharmacol Ther* 1973;14:325.

286. Jungers P, et al. Influence of renal insufficiency on the pharmacokinetics and pharmacodynamics of terazosin. *Am J Med* 1986;80[Suppl 5B]:94.

287. Hoyer J, Schulte K, Lenz T. Clinical pharmacokinetics of angiotensin converting enzyme (ACE) inhibitors in renal failure. *Clin Pharmacokinet* 1993;24(3):230.

288. Balfour JA, Goa KL. Benazepril: a review of its pharmacodynamic and pharmacokinetic properties, and therapeutic efficacy in hypertension and congestive heart failure. *Drugs* 1991;42(3):511.

289. Brogden RN, Todd PA, Sorkin EM. Captopril: an update of its pharmacodynamic and pharmacokinetic properties, and therapeutic use in hypertension and congestive heart failure. *Drugs* 1988;36:540.

290. Duchin KL, et al. Elimination kinetics of captopril in patients with renal failure. *Kidney Int* 1984;25:942.

291. Fujimura A, et al. Pharmacokinetics and pharmacodynamics of captopril in patients undergoing continuous ambulatory peritoneal dialysis. *Nephron* 1986;44:324.

292. Fruincillo RJU, et al. Disposition of enalapril and enalaprilat in renal insufficiency. *Kidney Int* 1987;31[Suppl 20]:S117.

293. Todd PA, Goa KL. Enalapril: a reappraisal of its pharmacology and therapeutic use in hypertension. Drugs 1992;43(3):346.

294. Gehr TWB, Sica DA, Grasela DM. Fosinopril pharmacokinetics and pharmacodynamics in chronic ambulatory peritoneal dialysis patients. *Eur J Clin Pharmacol* 1991;41:165.

295. Hui KK, et al. Pharmacokinetics of fosinopril in patients with various degrees of renal function. *Clin Pharmacol Ther* 1991;49:457.

296. Murdoch D, McTavish D. Fosinopril: a review of its pharmacodynamic and pharmacokinetic properties, and therapeutic potential in essential hypertension. *Drugs* 1992;43(1):123.

297. Lancaster SG, Todd PA. Lisinopril: a preliminary review of its pharmacodynamic and pharmacokinetic properties, and therapeutic use in hypertension and congestive heart failure. *Drugs* 1988;35:646.

298. Schaik BAM, et al. Pharmacokinetics of lisinopril in hypertensive patients with normal and impaired renal function. *Eur J Clin Pharmacol* 1988;34:61.

299. Schunkert H, Kindler J, Gassmann M. Pharmacokinetics of ramipril in hypertensive patients with renal insufficiency. *Eur J Clin Pharmacol* 1989;37:249.

300. Todd PA, Benfield P. Ramipril: a review of its pharmacological properties and therapeutic efficacy in cardiovascular disorders. *Drugs* 1990;39(1):110.

301. Gill J, Heel RC, Fitton A. Amiodarone: an overview of its pharmacological properties, and review of its therapeutic use in cardiac arrhythmias. *Drugs* 1992;43(1):69.

302. Josselson J, et al. Bretylium kinetics in renal insufficiency. *Clin Pharmacol Ther* 1983;33:144.

303. Rapeport WG. Clinical pharmacokinetics of bretylium. *Clin Pharmacokinet* 1985;10:248.

304. Brogden RN, Todd PA. Disopyramide: a reappraisal of its pharmacodynamic and pharmacokinetic properties, and therapeutic use in cardiac arrhythmias. *Drugs* 1986;34:151.

305. Burk M, Peters U. Disopyramide kinetics in renal impairment: determinants of interindividual variability. *Clin Pharmacol Ther* 1983;34(3):331.

306. Haughey DB, et al. Protein binding of disopyramide and elevated alpha-1-acid glycoprotein concentrations in serum obtained from dialysis patients and renal transplant recipients. *Am J Nephrol* 1985;5:35.

307. Bergstrand RH, et al. Encainide disposition in patients with renal failure. *Clin Pharmacol Ther* 1986;40(1):64.

308. Brogden RN, Todd PA. Encainide: a review of its pharmacological properties and therapeutic efficacy. *Drugs* 1987;34:519.

309. Forland SC, et al. Oral flecainide pharmacokinetics in patients with impaired renal function. *J Clin Pharmacol* 28:259 1988.

310. Forland SC, et al. Flecainide pharmacokinetics after multiple dosing in patients with impaired renal function. *J Clin Pharmacol* 1988;28:727.

311. Bennett PN, et al. Pharmacokinetics of lidocaine and its deethylated metabolite: dose and time dependency studies in man. *J Pharmacokinet Biopharm* 1982;10(3):265.

312. Eiriksson CE, Brogden RN. Lorcainide: a preliminary review of its pharmacodynamic properties and therapeutic efficacy. *Drugs* 1984;27:279.

313. Monk JP, Brogden RN. Mexiletine: a review of its pharmacodynamic and pharmacokinetic properties, and therapeutic use in the treatment of arrhythmias. *Drugs* 1990;40(3):374.

314. Wang T, et al. Pharmacokinetics and nondialyzability of mexiletine in renal failure. *Clin Pharmacol Ther* 1988;37(6):649.

315. Fitton A, Buckley MM-T. Moricizine: a review of its pharmacological properties, and therapeutic efficacy in cardiac arrhythmias. *Drugs* 1990;40(1):138.

316. Pieniaszek HJ, et al. Moricizine pharmacokinetics in renal insufficiency: reevaluation of elimination half-life. *J Clin Pharmacol* 1992;32:412.

317. Stec GP, et al. N-acetylprocainamide pharmacokinetics in functionally anephric patients before and after perturbation by hemodialysis. *Clin Pharmacol Ther* 1979;26(5):618.

318. Harron DWG, Brogden RN. Acecainide (N-acetylprocainamide): a review of its pharmacodynamic and pharmacokinetic properties, and therapeutic potential in cardiac arrhythmias. *Drugs* 1990;39(5):720.

319. Raehl CL, Moorthy AV, Beirne GJ. Procainamide pharmacokinetics in patients on continuous ambulatory peritoneal dialysis. *Nephron* 1986;44:191.

320. Bryson HM, et al. Propafenone: a reappraisal of its pharmacology, pharmacokinetics and therapeutic use in cardiac arrhythmias. *Drugs* 1993;45(1):85.

321. Burgess E, Duff H, Wilkes P. Propafenone disposition in renal insufficiency and renal failure. *J Clin Pharmacol* 1989;29:112.

322. Crevasse L. Quinidine: an update on therapeutics, pharmacokinetics and serum concentration monitoring. *Am J Cardiol* 1988;62:22.

323. Kessler KM, Perez GO. Decreased quinidine plasma protein binding during hemodialysis. *Clin Pharmacol Ther* 1981;30(1):121.

324. Holmes B, et al. Tocainide: a review of its pharmacological properties and therapeutic efficacy. *Drugs* 1983;26:93.

325. Raehl CL, et al. Tocainide pharmacokinetics during continuous ambulatory peritoneal dialysis. *Am J Cardiol* 1987;60:747.

326. Wiegers U, et al. Pharmacokinetics of tocainide in patients with renal dysfunction and during haemodialysis. *Eur J Clin Pharmacol* 1983;24:503.

327. Borchard U. Pharmacokinetics of beta-adrenoceptor blocking agents: clinical significance of hepatic and/or renal clearance. *Clin Physiol Biochem* 1990;8[Suppl 2]:28.

328. Riddell JG, Harron DWG, Shanks RG. Clinical pharmacokinetics of beta-adrenoceptor antagonists: an update. *Clin Pharmacokinet* 1987;12:305.

329. Kirch W, et al. The influence of renal function on plasma levels and urinary excretion of acebutolol and its main N-acetyl metabolite. *Clin Nephrol* 1982;18(2):88.

330. Roux A, et al. Pharmacokinetics of acebutolol in patients with all grades of renal failure. *Eur J Clin Pharmacol* 1980;17:339.

331. Singh BN, Thoden WR, Ward A. Acebutolol: a review of its pharmacological properties and therapeutic efficacy in hypertension, angina pectoris and arrhythmia. *Drugs* 1985;29:531.

332. Kirch W, et al. Pharmacokinetics of atenolol in relation to renal function. *Eur J Clin Pharmacol* 1981;19:65.

333. Wadworth A, Murdoch D, Brogden RN. Atenolol: a reappraisal of its pharmacological properties, and therapeutic use in cardiovascular disorders. *Drugs* 1991;42(3):468.

334. Beresford R, Heel RC. Betaxolol: a review of its pharmacodynamic and pharmacokinetic properties, and therapeutic efficacy in hypertension. *Drugs* 1986;31:6.

335. Amemiya M, et al. Pharmacokinetics of carteolol in patients with impaired renal function. *Eur J Clin Pharmacol* 1992;43:417.

336. Hasenfub G, et al. Pharmacokinetics of carteolol in relation to renal function. *Eur J Clin Pharmacol* 1985;29:461.

337. Chrisp P, Goa KL. Dilevalol: a review of its pharmacodynamic and pharmacokinetic properties, and therapeutic potential in hypertension. *Drugs* 1990;39:234.

338. Kelly JG, et al. The pharmacokinetics of dilevalol in renal impairment. *J Hum Hypertens* 1990;4[Suppl 2]:59.

339. Benfield P, Sorkin EM. Esmolol: a preliminary review of its pharmacodynamic and pharmacokinetic properties, and therapeutic efficacy. *Drugs* 1987;33:392.

340. Flaherty JF, et al. Pharmacokinetics of esmolol and ASL-8123 in renal failure. *Clin Pharmacol Ther* 1989;45:321.

341. Goa KL, Benfield P, Sorkin EM. Labetalol: a reappraisal of its pharmacology, pharmacokinetics and therapeutic use in hypertension and ischemic heart disease. *Drugs* 1989;37:583.

342. Halstenson CE, et al. The disposition and dynamics of labetalol in patients on dialysis. *Clin Pharmacol Ther* 1986;40:462.

343. Regardh CG, Johnsson G. Clinical pharmacokinetics of metoprolol. *Clin Pharmacokinet* 1980;5:557.

344. Dreyfuss J, et al. Pharmacokinetics of nadolol, a beta-receptor antagonist: administration of therapeutic single- and multiple-dosage regimens to hypertensive patients. *J Clin Pharmacol* 1979;19(11&12):712.

345. Frishman WH. Nadolol: a new beta-adrenoceptor antagonist. *N Engl J Med* 1981;305:678.

346. Bernard N, et al. Pharmacokinetics of penbutolol and its metabolites in renal insufficiency. *Eur J Clin Pharmacol* 1985;29:215.

347. Ohnhaus EE, et al. Metabolism of pindolol in patients with renal failure. *Eur J Clin Pharmacol* 1982;22:423.

348. Stone WJ, Walle T. Massive propranolol metabolite retention during maintenance hemodialysis. *Clin Pharmacol Ther* 1980;28:449.

349. Wood AJ, et al. Propranolol disposition in renal failure. *Br J Clin Pharmacol* 1980;10:561.

350. Blair AD, et al. Sotalol kinetics in renal insufficiency. *Clin Pharmacol Ther* 1981;29(4):457.

351. Singh BN, et al. Sotalol: a review of its pharmacodynamic and pharmacokinetic properties, and therapeutic use. *Drugs* 1987;34a:311.

352. Kelly JG, O'Malley K. Clinical pharmacokinetics of calcium antagonists: an update. *Clin Pharmacokinet* 1992;22(6):416.

353. Laher MS, et al. Pharmacokinetics of amlodipine in renal impairment. *J Cardiovasc Pharmacol* 1988;12[Suppl 7]:S60.

354. Buckley MM, Grant SM, Goa KL. Diltiazem: a reappraisal of its pharmacological properties and therapeutic use. *Drugs* 1990;39(5):757.

355. Grech-Bèlangèr O, Langlois S, LeBoeuf E. Pharmacokinetics of diltiazem in patients undergoing continuous ambulatory peritoneal dialysis. *J Clin Pharmacol* 1988;28:477.

356. Pozet N, et al. Pharmacokinetics of diltiazem in severe renal failure. *Eur J Clin Pharmacol* 1983;24:635.

357. Buur T, et al. Pharmacokinetics of felodipine in chronic hemodialysis patients. *J Clin Pharmacol* 1991;31:709.

358. Edgar B, et al. Pharmacokinetics of felodipine in patients with impaired renal function. *Br J Clin Pharmacol* 1989;27:67.

359. Todd PA, Faulds D. Felodipine: a review of the pharmacology and therapeutic use of the extended release formulation in cardiovascular disorders. *Drugs* 1992;44(2):251.

360. Chandler MHH, et al. The effects of renal function on the disposition of isradipine. *J Clin Pharmacol* 1988;28:1076.

361. Fitton A, Benfield P. Isradipine: a review of its pharmacodynamic and pharmacokinetic properties, and therapeutic use in cardiovascular disease. *Drugs* 1990;40(1):31.

362. Schonholzer K, Marone C. Pharmacokinetics and dialysability of isradipine in chronic haemodialysis patients. *Eur J Clin Pharmacol* 1992;42:231.

363. Sorkin EM, Clissold SP. Nicardipine: a review of its pharmacodynamic and pharmacokinetic properties, and therapeutic efficacy, in the treatment of angina pectoris, hypertension and related cardiovascular disorders. *Drugs* 1987;33:296.

364. Martre H, et al. Haemodialysis does not affect the pharmacokinetics of nifedipine. *Br J Clin Pharmacol* 1985;20:155.

365. Sorkin EM, Clissold SP, Brogden RN. Nifedipine: a review of its pharmacodynamic and pharmacokinetic properties, and therapeutic efficacy, in ischaemic heart disease, hypertension and related cardiovascular disorders. *Drugs* 1985;30:82.

366. Goa KL, Sorkin EM. Nitrendipine: a review of its pharmacodynamic and pharmacokinetic properties, and therapeutic efficacy in the treatment of hypertension. *Drugs* 1987;33:123.

367. Mikus G, et al. Pharmacokinetics, bioavailability, metabolism and acute and chronic antihypertensive effects of nitrendipine in patients with chronic renal failure and moderate to severe hypertension. *Br J Clin Pharmacol* 1991;31:313.

368. Hanyok JJ, et al. An evaluation of the pharmacokinetics, pharmacodynamics, and dialyzability of verapamil in chronic hemodialysis patients. *J Clin Pharmacol* 1988;28:831.

369. McTavish D, Sorkin EM. Verapamil: an updated review of its pharmacodynamic and pharmacokinetic properties, and therapeutic use in hypertension. *Drugs* 1989;38(1):19.

370. Mooy J, et al. Pharmacokinetics of verapamil in patients with renal failure. *Eur J Clin Pharmacol* 1985;28:405.

371. Graves PE, et al. Kinetics of digitoxin and the bis- and monodigitoxosides of digitoxigenin in renal insufficiency. *Clin Pharmacol Ther* 1984;36:607.

372. Vohringer HF, Rietbrock N. Digitalis therapy in renal failure with special regard to digitoxin. *Int J Clin Pharmacol Res* 1981; 19:175.

373. Gibson TP, Nelson HA. The question of cumulation of digoxin metabolites in renal failure. *Clin Pharmacol Ther* 1980;27(2): 219.

374. Keller F, Molzahn M, Ingerowski R. Digoxin dosage in renal insufficiency: impracticality of basing it on the creatinine clearance, body weight and volume of distribution. *Eur J Clin Pharmacol* 1980;18:433.

375. Sonnenblick M, et al. Correlation between manifestations of digoxin toxicity and serum digoxin, calcium, potassium, and magnesium concentrations and arterial pH. *Br Med J* 1983;286:1089.

376. Lant A. Diuretics: clinical pharmacology and therapeutic use (part I). *Drugs* 1985;29:57.

377. Lant A. Diuretics: clinical pharmacology and therapeutic use (part II). *Drugs* 1985;29:162.

378. Chapron DJ, Gomokin IH, Sweeney KR. Acetazolamide blood concentrations are excessive in the elderly: propensity for acidosis and relationship to renal function. *J Clin Pharmacol* 1989;29:348.

379. Spahn H, et al. Pharmacokinetics of amiloride in renal and hepatic disease. *Eur J Clin Pharmacol* 1987;33:493.

380. Pentikäinene PJ, et al. Bumetanide kinetics in renal failure. *Clin Pharmacol Ther* 1985;37:582.

381. Ward A, Heel RC. Bumetanide: a review of its pharmacodynamic and pharmacokinetic properties and therapeutic use. *Drugs* 1984;28:426.

382. Mulley BA, Parr GD, Rye RM. Pharmacokinetics of chlorthalidone. *Eur J Clin Pharmacol* 1980;17:203.

383. Pillary VK, et al. Transient and permanent deafness following treatment of ethacrynic acid in renal failure. *Lancet* 1969;1:77.

384. Brater DC, Anderson SA, Brown-Cartwright D. Response to furosemide in chronic renal insufficiency: rationale for limited doses. *Clin Pharmacol Ther* 1986;40:134.

385. Ponto LLB, Schoenwald RD. Furosemide (frusemide): a pharmacokinetic/pharmacodynamic review (part I). *Clin Pharmacokinet* 1990;18(5):381.

386. Traeger A, et al. Pharmacokinetic and pharmacodynamic effects of furosemide in patients with impaired renal function. *Int J Clin Pharmacol Ther Toxicol* 1984;22(9):481.

387. Acchiardo SR, Skoutakis VA. Clinical efficacy, safety, and pharmacokinetics of indapamide in renal impairment. *Am Heart J* 1983;106:237.

388. Clissold SP, Brogden RN. Piretanide: a preliminary review of its pharmacodynamic and pharmacokinetic properties, and therapeutic efficacy. *Drugs* 1985;29:489.

389. Marone C, et al. Pharmacokinetics of high doses of piretanide in moderate to severe renal failure. *Eur J Clin Pharmacol* 1984;27:589.

390. Skluth HA, Gums JG. Spironolactone: a re-examination. *Ann Pharmacother* 1990;24:52.

391. Niemeyer C, et al. Pharmacokinetics of hydrochlorothiazide in relation to renal function. *Eur J Clin Pharmacol* 1983;24:661.

392. Fairley KF, et al. Triamterene-induced crystalluria and cylinduria: clinical and experimental studies. *Clin Nephrol* 1986;26(4): 169.

393. Bottorff MB, Rutledge DR, Pieper JA. Evaluation of intravenous amrinone: the first of a new class of positive inotropic agents with vasodilator properties. *Pharmacotherapy* 1985;5:227.

394. Ward A, et al. Amrinone: a preliminary review of its pharmacological properties and therapeutic use. *Drugs* 1983;26:468.

395. Majerus TC, et al. Dobutamine: ten years later. *Pharmacotherapy* 1989;9:245.

396. Sonnenblick EH, et al. Dobutamine: a new synthetic cardioactive sympathetic amine. *N Engl J Med* 1979;300:17.

397. Larsson R, et al. Pharmacokinetics and effects on blood pressure of a single oral dose of milrinone in healthy subjects and in patients with renal impairment. *Eur J Clin Pharmacol* 1986;29:549.

398. Young RA, Ward A. Milrinone: a preliminary review of its pharmacological properties and therapeutic use. *Drugs* 1988;36:158.

399. Bogaert MG. Clinical pharmacokinetics of glyceryl trinitrate following the use of systemic and topical preparations. *Clin Pharmacokinet* 1987;12:1.

400. Evers J, et al. Pharmacokinetics of isosorbide-5-nitrate during haemodialysis and peritoneal dialysis. *Eur J Clin Pharmacol* 1987; 32:503.

401. Evers J, et al. Pharmacokinetics of isosorbide-5-nitrate in renal failure. *Eur J Clin Pharmacol* 1986;30:349.

402. Pearson RM. Pharmacokinetics and response to diazoxide in renal failure. *Clin Pharmacokinet* 1977;2:198.

403. Ludden TM, et al. Clinical pharmacokinetics of hydralazine. *Clin Pharmacokinet* 1982;7:185.

404. Halstenson CE, et al. Disposition of minoxidil in patients with various degrees of renal function. *J Clin Pharmacol* 1989;29:798.

405. Rindone JP, Sloane EP. Cyanide toxicity from sodium nitroprusside: risks and management. *Ann Pharmacother* 1992;26:515.

406. Schulz V. Clinical pharmacokinetics of nitroprusside, cyanide, thiosulphate and thiocyanate. *Clin Pharmacokinet* 1984;9:239.

407. Fer MF, et al. Cancer and the kidney: renal complications of neoplasms. *Am J Med* 1981;71:704.

408. Ozols RF, Corden BJ, Jacob J. High-dose cisplatin in hypertonic saline. *Ann Intern Med* 1984;100:19.

409. Sand TE, Jacobsen S. Effect of urine pH and flow on renal clearance of methotrexate. *Eur J Clin Pharmacol* 1981;19:453.

410. Narins RG, et al. The nephrotoxicity of chemotherapeutic agents. *Semin Nephrol* 1990;10(6):556.

411. Crooke ST, et al. Effects of variations in renal function on the clinical pharmacology of bleomycin administered as an IV bolus. *Cancer Treat Rep* 1977;61(9):1631.

412. Ehrsson H, et al. Busulfan kinetics. *Clin Pharmacol Ther* 1983;34:86.

413. Elferink F, et al. Pharmacokinetics of carboplatin after intraperitoneal administration. *Cancer Chemother Pharmacol* 1988;21:57.

414. Motzer RJ, et al. Carboplatin-based chemotherapy with pharmacokinetic analysis for patients with hemodialysis-dependent renal insufficiency. *Cancer Chemother Pharmacol* 1990;27:234.

415. Van der Vijgh WJF. Clinical pharmacokinetics of carboplatin. *Clin Pharmacokinet* 1991;21:242.

416. Newell DR, Calvert AH, Harrap KR. Studies on the pharmacokinetics of chlorambucil and prednimustine in man. *Br J Clin Pharmacol* 1983;15:253.

417. Blachley JD, Hill JB. Renal and electrolyte disturbances associated with cisplatin. *Ann Intern Med* 1981;95:628.

418. Corden BJ, et al. Clinical pharmacology of high-dose cisplatin. *Cancer Chemother Pharmacol* 1985;14:38.

419. Juma FD, Rogers HJ, Trounce JR. Effect of renal insufficiency on the pharmacokinetics of cyclophosphamide and some of its metabolites. *Eur J Clin Pharmacol* 1981;19:443.

420. Moore MJ. Clinical pharmacokinetics of cyclophosphamide. *Clin Pharmacokinet* 1991;20(3):194.

421. Wang LH, et al. Clearance and recovery calculations in hemodialysis: application to plasma, red blood cell, and dialysate measurements for cyclophosphamide. *Clin Pharmacol Ther* 1981;29(3):365.

422. Damon LE, Mass R, Linker CA. The association between high-dose cytarabine neurotoxicity and renal insufficiency. *J Clin Oncol* 1989;7(10):1563.

423. Goto M, et al. Delayed disposition of adriamycin and its active metabolite in haemodialysis patients. *Eur J Clin Pharmacol* 1993;44:301.

424. Speth PA, van Hoesel QG, Haanen C. Clinical pharmacokinetics of doxorubicin. *Clin Pharmacokinet* 1988;15:15.

425. Henwood J. M, Brogden RN. Etoposide: a review of the pharmacodynamic and pharmacokinetic properties, and therapeutic potential in combination chemotherapy of cancer. *Drugs* 1990;39(3):438.

426. Diasio RB, Harris BE. Clinical pharmacology of 5-fluorouracil. *Clin Pharmacokinet* 1989;16:215.

427. Hollingshead LM, Faulds D. Idarubicin: a review of its pharmacodynamic and pharmacokinetic properties, and therapeutic potential in the chemotherapy of cancer. *Drugs* 1991;42(4):690.

428. Alberts DS, et al. Effect of renal dysfunction in dogs on the disposition and marrow toxicity of melphalan. *Br J Cancer* 1981;43:330.

429. Österborg A, et al. Pharmacokinetics of oral melphalan in relation to renal function in multiple myeloma patients. *Eur J Cancer Clin Oncol* 1989;25(5):899.

430. Jolivet J, et al. The pharmacology and clinical use of methotrexate. *N Engl J Med* 1983;309:1094.

431. Shen DD, Azarnoff DL. Clinical pharmacokinetics of methotrexate. *Clin Pharmacokinet* 1978;3:1.

432. Den Hartigh J, et al. Pharmacokinetics of mitomycin C in humans. *Cancer Res* 1983;43:5017.

433. Ellis ME, Weiss RB, Kuperminc M. Nephrotoxicity of lomustine: a case report and literature review. *Cancer Chemother Pharmacol* 1985;15:174.

434. Oliverio VT. Toxicology and pharmacology of the nitrosoureas. *Cancer Chemother Rep* 1985;15:174.

435. Kennedy BJ. Metabolic and toxic effects of mithramycin during tumor therapy. *Am J Med* 1970;49:494.

436. Hall-Craggs M, et al. Acute renal failure and renal tubular squamous metaplasia following treatment with streptozocin. *Hum Pathol* 1982;13:597.

437. Buckley MM, Goa KL. Tamoxifen: a reappraisal of its pharmacodynamic and pharmacokinetic properties, and therapeutic use. *Drugs* 1989;37:451.

438. Owellen RJ, Hartke CA, Hains FO. Pharmacokinetics and metabolism of vinblastine in humans. *Cancer Res* 1977;37:2597.

439. Adroguè HJ. Glucose homeostasis and the kidney. *Kidney Int* 1992;42:1266.

440. Alvestrand A, et al. Glucose intolerance in uremic patients: the relative contributions of impaired beta-cell function and insulin resistance. *Clin Nephrol* 1989;31:175.

441. Hager SR. Insulin resistance of uremia. *Am J Kidney Dis* 1989;4:272.

442. Wideröe T, et al. Intraperitoneal (^{125}I) insulin absorption during intermittent and continuous peritoneal dialysis. *Kidney Int* 1983;23:22.

443. Attman P, Samuelsson O, Alaupovic P. Lipoprotein metabolism and renal failure. *Am J Kidney Dis* 1993;21:573.

444. Cheung AK, et al. Atherogenic lipids and lipoproteins in hemodialysis patients. *Am J Kidney Dis* 1993;22:271.

445. Haffner SM, et al. Increased lipoprotein(a) concentrations in chronic renal failure. *J Am Soc Nephrol* 1992;3:1156.

446. Joven J, et al. Lipoprotein heterogeneity in end-stage renal disease. *Kidney Int* 1993;43:410.

447. Guba EA, Abel SR, Golper TA. Practical guidelines for drug therapy in dialysis: lipid lowering agents. *Semin Dial* 1989;2:186.

448. Corpier CL, et al. Rhabdomyolysis and renal injury with lovastatin use. *JAMA* 1988;260:239.

449. Clissold SP, Edwards C. Acarbose: a preliminary review of its pharmacodynamic and pharmacokinetic properties, and therapeutic potential. *Drugs* 1988;35:214.

450. Ferner RE, Chaplin S. The relationship between the pharmacokinetics and pharmacodynamic effects of oral hypoglycaemic drugs. *Clin Pharmacokinet* 1987;12:379.

451. Palmer KJ, Brogden RN. Gliclazide: an update of its pharmacological properties and therapeutic efficacy in non-insulin-dependent diabetes mellitus. *Drugs* 1993;46:92.

452. Lebovitz HE. Glipizide: a second-generation sulfonylurea hypoglycemic agent. *Pharmacotherapy* 1985;5:63.

453. Feldman J. M. Glyburide: a second-generation sulfonylurea hypoglycemic agent. *Pharmacotherapy* 1985;5:43.

454. Brogden RN, Heel RC. Human insulin: a review of its biological activity, pharmacokinetics and therapeutic use. *Drugs* 1987;34:350.

455. Sherrard DJ, et al. Chronic clofibrate therapy in maintenance hemodialysis patients. *Nephron* 1980;25:219.

456. Manninen V, Malkonin M. Gemfibrozil treatment of dyslipidaemias in renal failure with uraemia or in the nephrotic syndrome. *Res Clin Forums* 1982;4:113.

457. Henwood J. M, Heel RC. Lovastatin: a preliminary review of its pharmacodynamic properties and therapeutic use in hyperlipidaemia. *Drugs* 1988;36:429.

458. Figge HL, et al. Nicotinic acid: a review of its clinical use in the treatment of lipid disorders. *Pharmacotherapy* 1988;8:287.

459. McTavish D, Sorkin EM, Pravastatin: a review of its pharmacological properties and therapeutic potential in hypercholesterolaemia. *Drugs* 1991;42:65.

460. Buckley MM, et al. Probucol: a reappraisal of its pharmacological properties and therapeutic use in hypercholesterolaemia. *Drugs* 1989;37:761.

461. Mauro VF. Clinical pharmacokinetics and practical applications of simvastatin. *Clin Pharmacokinet* 1993;24:195.

462. Kampmann JP, Hansen JM. Clinical pharmacokinetics of antithyroid drugs. *Clin Pharmacokinet* 1981;6:401.

463. Jansson R, Lindstrom B, Dahlberg PA. Pharmacokinetic properties and bioavailability of methimazole. *Clin Pharmacokinet* 1985;10:443.

464. Orwoll ES. The milk-alkali syndrome: current concepts. *Ann Intern Med* 1982;97:242.

465. Lauritsen K, Laursen LS, Rask-Madsen J. Clinical pharmacokinetics of drugs used in the treatment of gastrointestinal diseases (part I). *Clin Pharmacokinet* 1990;19:11.

466. Bateman DN, et al. The pharmacokinetics of single doses of metoclopramide in renal failure. *Eur J Clin Pharmacol* 1981;19:437.

467. Harrington RA, et al. Metoclopramide: an updated review of its pharmacological properties and clinical use. *Drugs* 1983;25:451.

468. Milne RJ, Heel RC. Ondansetron: therapeutic use as an antiemetic. *Drugs* 1991;41:574.

469. Lin JH. Pharmacokinetic and pharmacodynamic properties of histamine H_2-receptor antagonists. *Clin Pharmacokinet* 1991;20:218.

470. Somogyi A, Gugler R. Clinical pharmacokinetic of cimetidine. *Clin Pharmacokinet* 1983;8:463 1983.

471. Larsson R, Bodemar G, Norlander B. Oral absorption of cimetidine and its clearance in patients with renal failure. *Eur J Clin Pharmacol* 1979;15:153.

472. Larsson R, et al. The pharmacokinetics of cimetidine and its sulphoxide metabolite in patients with normal and impaired renal function. *Br J Clin Pharmacol* 1982;13:163.

473. Bjoeldager PA, et al. Pharmacokinetics of cimetidine in patients undergoing hemodialysis. *Nephron* 1983;34:159.

474. Krishna DR, Klotz U. Newer H_2-receptor antagonists: clinical pharmacokinetics and drug interaction potential. *Clin Pharmacokinet* 1988;15:205.

475. Echizen H, Ishizaki T. Clinical pharmacokinetics of famotidine. *Clin Pharmacokinet* 1991;21:178.

476. Gladziwa U, et al. Pharmacokinetics and dynamics of famotidine in patients with renal failure. *Br J Clin Pharmacol* 1988;26:315.

477. Halstenson CE, et al. Disposition of famotidine in renal insufficiency. *J Clin Pharmacol* 1987;27:782.

478. Price AH, Brogden RN. Nizatidine: a preliminary review of its pharmacodynamic and pharmacokinetic properties, and its therapeutic use in peptic ulcer disease. *Drugs* 1988;36:521.

479. Saima S, et al. Hemofiltrability of histamine H_2-receptor antagonist, nizatidine, and its metabolites in patients with renal failure. *J Clin Pharmacol* 1993;33:324.

480. Comstock TJ, et al. Ranitidine bioavailability and disposition kinetics in patients undergoing chronic hemodialysis. *Nephron* 1989;52:15.

481. Grant SM, Langtry HD, Brogden RN. Ranitidine: an updated review of its pharmacodynamic and pharmacokinetic properties, and therapeutic use in peptic ulcer disease and other allied diseases. *Drugs* 1989;37:801.

482. Meffin PJ, et al. Ranitidine disposition in patients with renal impairment. *Br J Clin Pharmacol* 1983;16:731.

483. Zech PY, et al. Ranitidine kinetics in chronic renal impairment. *Clin Pharmacol Ther* 1983;34:667.

484. Barradell LB, Faulds D, McTavish D. Lansoprazole: a review of its pharmacodynamic and pharmacokinetic properties, and its therapeutic efficacy in acid-related disorders. *Drugs* 1992;44(2):225.

485. Jones JB, Bailey RT. Misoprostol: a prostaglandin E_1 analog with antisecretory and cytoprotective properties. *Ann Pharmacother* 1989;23:276.

486. Howden CW. Clinical pharmacology of omeprazole. *Clin Pharmacokinet* 1991;20:38.

487. Naesdal J, et al. Pharmacokinetics of [^{14}C] omeprazole in patients with impaired renal function. *Clin Pharmacol Ther* 1986;40:344.

488. Burgess E, Muruve D, Audette R. Aluminum absorption and excretion following sucralfate therapy in chronic renal insufficiency. *Am J Med* 1992;92:471.

489. Roxe DM, Mistovich M, Barch DH. Phosphate-binding effects of sucralfate in patients with chronic renal failure. *Am J Kidney Dis* 1989;13:194.

490. Fraser CL, Arieff AI. Nervous system complications in uremia. *Ann Intern Med* 1988;109:143.

491. Dasgupta A, Abu-Alfa A. Increased free phenytoin concentrations in predialysis serum compared to postdialysis serum in patients with uremia treated with hemodialysis. *Am J Clin Pathol* 1992;98:19.

492. Eadie MJ. Anticonvulsant drugs: an update. *Drugs* 1984;27:328.

493. Bertilsson L, Tomson T. Clinical pharmacokinetics and pharmacological effects of carbamazepine and carbamazepine-10, 11-epoxide: an update. *Clin Pharmacokinet* 1986;11:177.

494. Lee CS, et al. Hemodialysis clearance and total body elimination of carbamazepine during chronic hemodialysis. *Clin Toxicol* 1980;17:429.

495. Marbury TC, et al. Hemodialysis clearance of ethosuximide in patients with chronic renal disease. *Am J Hosp Pharm* 1981;38:1757.

496. Czajka PA, et al. A pharmacokinetic evaluation of peritoneal dialysis for phenytoin intoxication. *J Clin Pharmacol* 1980;20:565.

497. Lee CS, et al. Pharmacokinetics of primidone elimination by uremic patients. *J Clin Pharmacol* 1982;22:301.

498. Brewster D, Muir NC. Valproate plasma protein binding in the uremic condition. *Clin Pharmacol Ther* 1980;27:76.

499. Zaccara G, Messori A, Moroni F. Clinical pharmacokinetics of valproic acid—1988. *Clin Pharmacokinet* 1988;15:367.

500. Cedarbaum JM. Clinical pharmacokinetics of anti-parkinsonian drugs. *Clin Pharmacokinet* 1987;13:141.

501. Yeh KC, August TF, Bush DF. Pharmacokinetics and bioavailability of sinemet CR: a summary of human studies. *Neurology* 1989;39:25.

502. Burke RE, Fahn S. Pharmacokinetics of trihexyphenidyl after short-term and long-term administration to dystonic patients. *Ann Neurol* 1985;18:35.

503. Clive DM, Stoff FS. Renal syndromes associated with nonsteroidal antiinflammatory drugs. *N Engl J Med* 1984;310:563.

504. Hande K, Noone RM, Stone WJ. Severe allopurinol toxicity: description and guidelines for prevention in patients with renal insufficiency. *Am J Med* 1984;76:47.

505. Wallace SL, et al. Renal function predicts colchicine toxicity: guidelines for the prophylactic use of colchicine in gout. *J Rheumatol* 1991;18:264.

506. Murrel GA, Rapeport WG. Clinical pharmacokinetics of allopurinol. *Clin Pharmacokinet* 1986;11:343.

507. Levy M, Spino M, Read SE. Colchicine: a state of the art review. *Pharmacotherapy* 1991;11:196.

508. Cunningham RF, Israili ZH, Dayton PG. Clinical pharmacokinetics of probenecid. *Clin Pharmacokinet* 1981;6:135.

509. Verbeck RK, Blackburn JL, Loewen GR. Clinical pharmacokinetics of non-steroidal anti-inflammatory drugs. *Clin Pharmacokinet* 1983;8:297.

510. Todd PA, Sorkin EM. Diclofenac sodium: a reappraisal of its pharmacodynamic and pharmacokinetic properties, and therapeutic efficacy. *Drugs* 1988;35:244.

511. Eriksson LO, et al. Influence of renal failure, rheumatoid arthritis and old age on the pharmacokinetics of diflunisal. *Eur J Clin Pharmacol* 1989;36:165.

512. Balfour JA, Buckley MM. Etodolac: a reappraisal of its pharmacology and therapeutic use in rheumatic diseases and pain states. *Drugs* 1991;42:274.

513. Cefali EA, et al. Pharmacokinetic comparison of flurbiprofen in end-stage renal disease subjects and subjects with normal renal function. *J Clin Pharmacol* 1991;31:808.

514. Albert KS, Gernaat CM. Pharmacokinetics of ibuprofen. *Am J Med* 1984;77:40.

515. Skoutakis VA, et al. Dialyzability and pharmacokinetics of indomethacin in adult patients with end-stage renal disease. *Drug Intell Clin Pharm* 1986;20:956.

516. Williams RL, Upton RA. The clinical pharmacology of ketoprofen. *J Clin Pharmacol* 1988;28[Suppl]:S13.

517. Brocks DR, Jamali F. Clinical pharmacokinetics of ketorolac tromethamine. *Clin Pharmacokinet* 1992;23:415.

518. Todd PA, Clissold SP. Naproxen: a reappraisal of its pharmacology, and therapeutic use in rheumatic diseases and pain states. *Drugs* 1990;40:91.

519. Verbeeck RK, Richardson CJ, Blocka KLN. Clinical pharmacokinetics of piroxicam. *J Rheumatol* 1986;13:789.

520. Ravis WR, et al. Pharmacokinetics and dialyzability of sulindac and metabolites in patients with end-stage renal failure. *J Clin Pharmacol* 1993;33:527.

521. Chaffman M, et al. Auranofin: a preliminary review of its pharmacological properties and therapeutic use in rheumatoid arthritis. *Drugs* 1984;27:378.

522. Blocka KL, Paulus HE, Furst DE. Clinical pharmacokinetics of oral and injectable gold compounds. *Clin Pharmacokinet* 1986;11:133.

523. Singer I. Lithium and the kidney. *Kidney Int* 1981;19:374.

524. Levy NB. Psychopharmacology in patients with renal failure. *Int J Psychiatry Med* 1990;20:325.

525. Preskorn SH, Othmer SC. Evaluation of bupropion hydrochloride: the first of a new class of atypical antidepressants. *Pharmacotherapy* 1984;4:20.

526. Aronoff GR, et al. Fluoxetine kinetics and protein binding in normal and impaired renal function. *Clin Pharmacol Ther* 1984;36(1):138.

527. Benfield P, Heel RC, Lewis SP. Fluoxetine: a review of its pharmacodynamic and pharmacokinetic properties, and therapeutic efficacy in depressive illness. *Drugs* 1986;32:481.

528. Christensen JH, Andreasen F, Jansen J. Pharmacokinetics and pharmacodynamics of thiopental in patients undergoing renal transplantation. *Acta Anaesthesiol Scand* 1983;27:513.

529. Garzone PD, Kuoboth PD. Pharmacokinetics of the newer benzodiazepines. *Clin Pharmacokinet* 1989;16:337.

530. Schmith VD, et al. Alprazolam in end-stage renal disease: I. pharmacokinetics. *J Clin Pharmacol* 1991;31:571.

531. Ochs HR, Rauh HW, Greenblatt DJ. Clorazepate dipotassium and diazepam in renal insufficiency: serum concentrations and protein binding of diazepam and desmethyldiazepam. *Nephron* 1984;37:100.

532. Greenblatt DJ, et al. Clinical pharmacokinetics of chlordiazepoxide. *Clin Pharmacokinet* 1978;3:381.

533. Morrison G, et al. Effect of renal impairment and hemodialysis on lorazepam kinetics. *Clin Pharmacol Ther* 1984;35(5):646.

534. Vinik HR, et al. The pharmacokinetics of midazolam in chronic renal failure patients. *Anesthesiology* 1983;59(5):390.

535. Ochs HR, Oberem U, Greenblatt DJ. Nitrazepam clearance unimpaired in patients with renal insufficiency. *J Clin Psychopharmacol* 1992;12(3):183.

536. Greenblatt DJ, et al. Multiple-dose kinetics and dialyzability of oxazepam in renal insufficiency. *Nephron* 1983;34:234.

537. Ankier SI, Goa KL. Quazepam: a preliminary review of its pharmacodynamic and pharmacokinetic properties, and therapeutic efficacy in insomnia. *Drugs* 1988;35:42.

538. Kroboth PD, et al. Triazolam protein binding and correlation with alpha-1 acid glycoprotein concentration. *Clin Pharmacol Ther* 1984;36(3):379.

539. Roth T, Roehrs TA, Zorick FJ. Pharmacology and hypnotic efficacy of triazolam. *Pharmacotherapy* 1983;3:137.

540. Loo JCK, Midha KK, McGilveray IJ. Pharmacokinetics of chlorpromazine in normal volunteers. *Communications Psychopharmacol* 1980;4:121.

541. Taylor G, et al. Pharmacokinetics of promethazine and its sulphoxide metabolite after intravenous and oral administration to man. *Br J Clin Pharmacol* 1983;15:287.

542. Lieberman JA, et al. Tricyclic antidepressant and metabolite levels in chronic renal failure. *Clin Pharmacol Ther* 1985;37:301.

543. Sandoz M, et al. Metabolism of amitriptyline in patients with chronic renal failure. *Eur J Clin Pharmacol* 1984;26:227.

544. Tasset JJ, Singh S, Pesce AJ. Evaluation of amitriptyline pharmacokinetics during peritoneal dialysis. *Ther Drug Monitor* 1985;7:255.

545. McTavish D, Benfield P. Clomipramine: an overview of its pharmacological properties and a review of its therapeutic use in obsessive-compulsive disorder and panic disorder. *Drugs* 1990;39(1):136.

546. DeVane CL, Savett M, Jusko WJ. Desipramine and 2-hydroxy-desipramine pharmacokinetics in normal volunteers. *Eur J Clin Pharmacol* 1981;19:61.

547. Faulkner RD, Senekjian HO, Lee CS. Hemodialysis of doxepin and desmethyldoxepin in uremic patients. *Artif Organs* 1984;8(2):151.

548. Potter WZ, et al. Active metabolites of imipramine and desipramine in man. *Clin Pharmacol Ther* 1982;31(3):393.

549. Dawling S, et al. Nortriptyline metabolism in chronic renal failure: metabolite elimination. *Clin Pharmacol Ther* 1982;32(3):322.

550. Ziegler VE, et al. Protriptyline kinetics. *Clin Pharmacol Ther* 1978;23(5):580.

551. Caccia S, et al. Clinical pharmacokinetics of oral buspirone in patients with impaired renal function. *Clin Pharmacokinet* 1988;14:171.

552. Fitton A, Heel RC. Clozapine: a review of its pharmacological properties, and therapeutic use in schizophrenia. *Drugs* 1990;40(5):722.

553. Froemming JS, et al. Pharmacokinetics of haloperidol. *Clin Pharmacokinet* 1989;17(6):396.

554. Luisier PA, Schultz P, Dick P. The pharmacokinetics of lithium in normal humans: expected and unexpected observations in view of basic kinetic principles. *Pharmacopsychiatry* 1987;20:232.

555. Mahoney G, et al. Dipyridamole kinetics. *Clin Pharmacol Ther* 1982;31:330.

556. Kandrotas RJ. Heparin pharmacokinetics and pharmacodynamics. *Clin Pharmacokinet* 1992;22:359.

557. Grierson DS, Bjornsson TD. Pharmacokinetics of streptokinase in patients based on amidolytic activator complex activity. *Clin Pharmacol Ther* 1987;41:304.

558. Pedersen AK, Jakobsen P, Kampmann JP. Clinical pharmacokinetics and potentially important drug interactions of sulphinpyrazone. *Clin Pharmacokinet* 1982;7:42.

559. McTavish D, Faulds D, Goa KL. Ticlopidine: an updated review of its pharmacology and therapeutic use in platelet-dependent disorders. *Drugs* 1990;40:238.

560. Collen D, et al. Tissue-type plasminogen activator: a review of its pharmacology and therapeutic use as a thrombolytic agent. *Drugs* 1989;38:346.

561. Holford NHG. Clinical pharmacokinetics and pharmacodynamics of warfarin. *Clin Pharmacokinet* 1986;11:483.

562. Paton DP, Webster DR. Clinical pharmacokinetics of H1-freceptor antagonists (the antihistamines). *Clin Pharmacokinet* 1985;10:477.

563. Krstenansky RM, Cluxton RJ. Astemizole: a long-acting, nonsedating antihistamine. *Drug Intell Clin Pharm* 1987;21:947.

564. Richards DM, et al. Oxatomide: a review of its pharmacodynamic properties and therapeutic efficacy. *Drugs* 1984;27:210.

565. Carter CA, et al. Terfenadine, a nonsedating antihistamine. *Drug Intell Clin Pharm* 1985;19:812.

566. Morgan DJ. Clinical pharmacokinetics of beta-agonists. *Clin Pharmacokinet* 1990;18:270.

567. Friedel HA, Brogden RN. Bitolterol: a preliminary review of its pharmacological properties and therapeutic efficacy in reversible obstructive airways disease. *Drugs* 1988;35:22.

568. Lee CC, et al. Pharmacokinetics of dyphylline elimination by uremic patients. *J Pharmacol Exp Ther* 1981;217:340.

569. Bauer LA, Bauer SP, Blouin RA. The effect of acute and chronic renal failure on theophylline clearance. *J Clin Pharmacol* 1982;22:65.

570. Kradjan WA, et al. Effect of hemodialysis on the pharmacokinetics of theophylline in chronic renal failure. *Nephron* 1982;32:40.

571. Chan GLC, Canafax DM, Johnson CA. The therapeutic use of azathioprine in renal transplantation. *Pharmacotherapy* 1987;7(5):165.

572. Salemans J, et al. Pharmacokinetics of azathioprine and 6-mercaptopurine after oral administration of azathioprine. *Clin Transplant* 1987;1:217.

573. Kawai S, Ichikawa Y, Homma M. Differences in metabolic properties among cortisol, prednisolone, and dexamethasone in liver and renal diseases: Accelerated metabolism of dexamethasone in renal failure. *J Clin Endocrinol Metab* 1985;60:848.

574. Sherlock JE, Letteri JM. Effect of hemodialysis on methylprednisolone plasma levels. *Nephron* 1977;18:208.

575. Frey BM, Frey FJ. Clinical pharmacokinetics of prednisone and prednisolone. *Clin Pharmacokinet* 1990;19(2):126.

576. Foliath F, et al. Intravenous cyclosporine kinetics in renal failure. *Clin Pharmacol Ther* 1983;34(5):638.

577. Putcha L, Griffith DP, Feldman S. Pharmacokinetics of acetohydroxamic acid in patients with staghorn renal calculi. *Eur J Clin Pharmacol* 1985;28:439.

578. Boelaert JR, Fenves AZ, Coburn JW. Deferoxamine therapy and mucormycosis in dialysis patients: report of an international registry. *Am J Kidney Dis* 1991;18(6):660.

579. Verpooten GA, et al. Pharmacokinetics of aluminoxamine and ferrioxamine and dose finding of desferrioxamine in haemodialysis patients. *Nephrol Dial Transplant* 1992;7:931.

580. Silver MR, Kroboth PD. Pentoxifylline in end-stage renal disease. *Drug Intell Clin Pharm* 1987;21:976.

581. Ward A, Clissold SP. Pentoxifylline: a review of its pharmacodynamic and pharmacokinetic properties, and its therapeutic efficacy. *Drugs* 1987;34:50.

Subject Index

Beta-blockers. *See* Beta-adrenergic receptor
  blockers
Beta-lipotropin, in uremia, 2842
Betamethasone, 3174*t*
Beta-2-microglobulin, in sickle cell disease,
  2291
Betaxolol, 3158*t*
Bethanechol, for lower urinary tract
  dysfunction, 685
Bezafibrate, 3164*t*
Bicarbonate
  in acute renal failure, 1113, 1113*t*
  deficit, 2675
  excretion, during pregnancy, 2136–2137,
    2137*f*
  plasma levels
    distal potassium secretion and, 184
    potassium excretion and, 179
  reclamation, 204–205, 205*f*
  tubule fluid concentration, distal potassium
    secretion and, 183
  urinary excretion, in chronic renal failure,
    2584–2585
"Big bang" theory, 725
Bile acid sequestrants, for lipid disorders in
  renal failure, 2826
Bilharziasis, 678
Bilirubin, urinary, 320
Biofeedback, for lower urinary tract
  dysfunction, 683
Biologic agents, causing acute renal failure,
  1176*t*, 1181, 1181*f*
Bioluminescence methods, for bacteriuria
  detection, 929
Biopsy guns, 458
Biotransformation enzymes, in cellular injury,
  1074, 1074*f*, 1075*f*, 1075*t*, 1076–1077
Birmingham Reflux Study Group (BRSG),
  734, 744–745
Birth control pills, 1518, 1886, 1970
Bismuth nephrotoxicity, 1266
Bisphosphonates
  for hormone refractory prostate cancer,
    884
  for hypercalcemia, 2643–2644, 2644*t*
  hyperphosphatemia and, 2623
Bitolterol, 3174*t*
Blacks, hypertensive nephrosclerosis and,
  1547–1548
Bladder
  acontractility, 674*f*
  anatomy, 663, 664*f*
  augmentation, 689
  biopsy, 671, 672*f*
  calcifications, plain films of, 371
  catheterization, bacteriuria and, 924
  "Christmas tree," 674*f*, 679
  compliance, 667
  control, development, behavioral aspects
    of, 666–667
  distention, 666
  dysfunction
    AIDS-related, 678–679
    in end-stage renal disease/renal
      transplantation, 681, 684*f*
    inflammatory, 678
    in metabolic disorders, 678
    in neurological disease, 679
    in vesicoureteric reflux, 717
    vesicoureteric reflux and, 728–729

emptying. *See* Micturition
epithelium, 912
filling, 667, 668*f*
function
  "four-phase concept" of, 667, 668*f*, 669*f*
  recovery after micturition, 667, 670*f*
inflammation. *See* Cystitis
neuroanatomic studies, 664–666, 665*f*,
  665*t*
neurogenic
  pyelonephritis and, 949
  surgical treatment of, 688–689, 689*f*
  urinary tract infection in, prevention of,
    963
  with vesicoureteric reflux, 718–720,
    719*f*
  with vesicoureteric reflux, management
    of, 746–747
pressure, 715
spastic, in spinal cord injury, 673, 674*f*
"tower," 679
ultrasonography, 376–377, 377*f*
volume, 667
Bladder cancer
  clinical course, 856–857
  clinical presentation, 854, 865
  deaths from, 851
  diagnosis, 854, 855*f*
  epidemiology, 851
  grading, 857
  incidence, 851
  molecular genetic studies, of pathogenesis,
    852–854, 853*f*
  palliation, 865
  pathogenesis, 852–854, 853*f*, 865
  pathology, 852
  prognosis, 857, 857*t*
  risk factors
    cyclophosphamide, 852
    dietary, 852
    disease-related, 852
    industry-related carcinogens, 851
    phenacetin, 852
    smoking, 851–852
  staging, 854–856, 856*t*
  survival
    improvement of, 862
    by stage, 860*t*
  treatment, 865
    combined-modality approaches,
      862–865, 863*t*
    with comorbid conditions, 862
    of metastatic disease, 861–862, 861*t*
    of muscle-infiltrating disease, 859–861,
      859*t*, 860*t*
    predictive factors for, 857
    of superficial disease, 857–859
Bladder catheterization, for urine collection,
  317–318
Bladder epithelium, as host defense,
  911–912
Bladder neck obstruction, in females, 676
Bladder pressure, vesicoureteric reflux and,
  728–729, 729*f*
Bladder-sparing strategies, for bladder cancer,
  864–865
Bladder washout technique, for
  pyelonephritis diagnosis, 952, 955
Blastomyces dermatitides, 1008
Blastomycosis, 1008–1009

Bleeding complications
  in acute renal failure, management of, 1125
  after renal transplantation, 2907
  postoperative, with hypertension, 1565
Bleeding diathesis, in hemodialysis, 2993
Bleomycin
  dosage, in renal failure, 3162*t*
  for testicular carcinoma, 895–896, 895*t*,
    896*t*
Block Design Learning Test (BDLT), 2772
Blood, in urine, 321
Blood coagulation, in sickle cell disease, 2293
Blood loss, anemia in renal disease and, 2724
Blood pressure
  adult, salt intake reduction and, 1337
  children, salt intake reduction and, 1337,
    1337*f*
  in chronic hemodialysis, 2989–2990
  control
    ESRD in autosomal-dominant polycystic
      kidney disease and, 571–572
    nonsteroidal antiinflammatory drugs
      and, 1200
  coronary heart disease development and,
    1341, 1341*f*
  diastolic, in renovascular hypertension,
    1414
  distribution in population, 1341, 1341*f*
  elevation. *See also* Hypertension
    in malignant hypertension, 1534–1535
    in primary aldosteronism, 1502
    renal mechanisms, 1351–1353
  familial studies, in diabetic nephropathy,
    2090
  increased salt intake
    in normal animals, 1335, 1335*f*, 1336*f*
    in normal humans, 1335–1336
  in malignant hypertension, 1520, 1521*f*
  neonatal, salt intake reduction and,
    1336–1337, 1337*f*
  in preeclampsia, 1468
  preeclampsia development and, 1464
  in pregnancy, 1459, 1463
  reduction
    to glomeruli, 403
    gradual *vs.* rapid for hypertensive crisis
      treatment, 1569–1571, 1570*f*
  regulation, factors in, 1367–1368, 1368*t*
  renal artery. *See* Renal arterial pressure
  salt balance and, 1369–1370, 1370*f*
  salt intake and, 1332–1333
    cross-center analysis, 1334–1335, 1334*f*
    epidemiologic studies, 1333
    migratory studies, 1333–1334
  stroke development and, 1341, 1341*f*
Blood transfusion
  avoidance, use of rHuEPO for, 2727
  iron overload from, 2725–2726
  pre-transplantation, 2881
Blood urea nitrogen (BUN)
  in acute renal failure, 1093, 1108, 1113,
    1113*t*, 1118
  elevation
    as renal biopsy contraindications, 462
    in uric acid nephropathy, 1312
  glomerular filtration rate and, 344–346,
    345*t*
  protein intake and, 346
  as renal function intake, 346
  serum creatinine and, 346